Understanding
Pathophysiology

Understanding Pathophysiology

Sue E. Huether, RN, PhD
Professor, College of Nursing
University of Utah, Salt Lake City, Utah

Kathryn L. McCance, RN, PhD
Professor, College of Nursing
University of Utah, Salt Lake City, Utah

Second Edition
with 1075 illustrations

 Mosby

An Imprint of Elsevier Science

St. Louis   London   Philadelphia   Sydney   Toronto

Vice-President and Nursing Editorial Director: *Sally Schrefer*
Senior Developmental Editor: *Michele D. Hayden*
Project Manager: *John Rogers*
Project Specialist: *Betty Hazelwood*
Designer: *Kathi Gosche*
Cover Art: *William B. Westwood*

Notice
Pharmacology is an ever-changing field. Standard safety precautions must be followed, but as new research and clinical experience broaden our knowledge, changes in treatment and drug therapy may become necessary or appropriate. Readers are advised to check the most current product information provided by the manufacturer of each drug to be administered to verify the recommended dose, the method and duration of administration, and contraindications. It is the responsibility of the licensed health care provider, relying on experience and knowledge of the patient, to determine dosages and the best treatment for each individual patient. Neither the publisher nor the editor assumes any liability for any injury and/or damage to persons or property arising from this publication.

Mosby, Inc.
An Imprint of Elsevier Science
11830 Westline Industrial Drive
St. Louis, MO 63146

Printed in the United States of America

0–323-00791–0

02 03 GW/QWV 9 8 7 6 5 4 3

Contributors

Barbara J. Boss, RN, PhD, CS, CANP
Professor of Nursing, School of Nursing,
University of Mississippi Medical Center,
Jackson, Mississippi

Valentina L. Brashers, MD
Associate Professor of Nursing,
Clinical Assistant Professor of Medicine,
University of Virginia Health Sciences Center,
Charlottesville, Virginia

Jean Anne Connor, RN, MS, CPNP
Pediatric Nurse Practitioner,
Division of Pediatric Cardiology,
University Medical Center;
Clinical Assistant, Maternal Child Health,
School of Nursing,
State University of New York,
Stony Brook, New York

Sheryl S. Davey, RN, MS
Clinical Assistant Professor, College of Nursing,
University of Utah,
Salt Lake City, Utah

Judith A. Farley, RN, MSN, CNRN
Director, Neuroscience Program,
Children's Hospital,
Boston, Massachusetts

Cyrena M. Gilman, RN, MN, CNN
Manager of Clinical Operations,
Pediatric Dialysis,
Riley Hospital for Children,
Clarian Health Partners, Inc.,
Indianapolis, Indiana

Todd C. Grey, MD
Chief Medical Examiner, State of Utah;
Associate Clinical Professor of Pathology,
University of Utah School of Medicine,
Salt Lake City, Utah

Marilyn Hockenberry-Eaton, RN, PhD, CS, PNP, FAAN
Associate Professor, Department of Pediatrics,
Baylor College of Medicine;
Director of Nurse Practitioners,
Texas Children's Hospital,
Houston, Texas

Lynn B. Jorde, PhD
Professor and Associate Chairman,
Department of Human Genetics,
University of Utah School of Medicine,
Salt Lake City, Utah

Nancy E. Kline, RN, PhD, CPNP
Assistant Professor of Pediatrics,
Baylor College of Medicine;
Pediatric Nurse Practitioner,
Texas Children's Cancer Center,
Houston, Texas

Thom J. Mansen, RN, PhD
Associate Professor, College of Nursing,
University of Utah,
Salt Lake City, Utah

Leona A. Mourad, RN, MS, ONC
Associate Professor Emeritus,
Ohio State University, College of Nursing,
Columbus, Ohio;
Nursing Consultant,
Mourad Consultant Associates,
Santa Barbara, California

Stephanie J. Richardson, RN, PhD
Assistant Professor, College of Nursing,
University of Utah,
Salt Lake City, Utah

Lee K. Roberts, PhD
Director of Vaccine Development,
PowderJect Vaccines, Inc.,
Madison, Wisconsin

Kristynia M. Robinson, RN, PhD, FNPc
Associate Professor of Nursing;
Coordinator, Family Nurse Practitioner Program,
Idaho State University,
Pocatello, Idaho

Neal S. Rote, PhD
Professor and Chair,
Microbiology and Immunology;
Professor, Obstetrics and Gynecology,
Wright State University, School of Medicine,
Dayton, Ohio

Jane Shelby, PhD
Associate Professor of Surgery,
University of Utah, Department of Surgery,
Salt Lake City, Utah

Richard A. Sugerman, PhD
Professor of Anatomy,
Western University of Health Sciences,
Pomona, California

Karen M. VanSyckle, RN, MSN, CPNP, CPON
Pediatric Nurse Practitioner,
Texas Children's Hospital;
Instructor, Pediatrics,
Baylor College of Medicine,
Houston, Texas

Reviewers of First and Second Editions

Irene Aguilar, RN, MSN, MEd, CNS
Professor,
Department of Nursing Education,
San Antonio College,
San Antonio, Texas

Paulette M. Archer, RN, MS
Instructor,
St. Francis Medical Center College of Nursing,
Peoria, Illinois

Victor G. Campbell, RN, PhD
Senior Patient Care Director,
Columbus Community Hospital,
Columbus, Ohio

Kathryn Ann Caudell, RN, PhD, AOCN
Assistant Professor,
College of Nursing,
University of New Mexico,
Albuquerque, New Mexico

Joan Parker Frizzell, RN, PhD
Assistant Professor,
School of Nursing,
La Salle University,
Philadelphia, Pennsylvania

Dorothy Hughes, RN, MSc
Associate Professor,
Faculty of Nursing,
University of Calgary,
Calgary, Alberta,
Canada

Lois Kimmel, RN, MSN
School of Nursing,
Pennsylvania State University,
Hershey, Pennsylvania

Carol Ann Barnett Lammon, RN, MSN
Assistant Professor,
Capstone College of Nursing,
University of Alabama,
Tuscaloosa, Alabama

Karen Otterson, RN, MSN
Nursing Instructor,
Chippewa Valley Technical College,
Eau Claire, Wisconsin

Patricia Picketts, RN, BScN, MEd
Instructor,
Grant MacEwen Community College,
Edmonton, Alberta,
Canada

Maria Van Dyke Pringle, RN, MSN
Assistant Professor,
Grandview College,
Des Moines, Iowa

James Rankin, RN, MSc, PhD(c)
Associate Professor,
Faculty of Nursing,
University of Calgary,
Calgary, Alberta,
Canada

Marlene Reimer, RN, MN, PhD(c)
Associate Professor,
Faculty of Nursing,
University of Calgary,
Calgary, Alberta,
Canada

Karen Taylor, RN, MSN
Nursing Instructor,
Chippewa Valley Technical College,
Eau Claire, Wisconsin

Karen Then, RN, MN
Assistant Professor,
Faculty of Nursing,
University of Calgary,
Calgary, Alberta,
Canada

Lorraine Watson, RN, PhD
Associate Professor,
Faculty of Nursing,
University of Calgary,
Calgary, Alberta,
Canada

A. Denyce Watties-Daniels, RN, MSN
Assistant Professor of Nursing,
Helene Fuld School of Nursing,
Coppin State College,
Baltimore, Maryland

Susan B. Zekauskus, RN, MSN, PNP
Assistant Professor of Nursing,
Department of Nursing,
Tulsa Junior College,
Tulsa, Oklahoma

Preface

Welcome to the second edition of *Understanding Pathophysiology*. As in the first edition, the text is written to provide basic and easy-to-comprehend information about pathophysiologic mechanisms and manifestations of disease.

The second edition is dynamite! We undertook the enormous challenge of changing the entire art program, as well as updating and adding new relevant content. Tedious attention was paid to our goal of consolidating and simplifying complex materials for this "elementary" version of pathophysiology. Toward that end the following specific goals were achieved:

- An essential presentation of disease processes across the life span with separate sections on aging and separate chapters on children
- Ceaseless updating of relevant epidemiology, pathophysiology, clinical manifestations, and treatment
- Addition of **full-color** illustrations and high-quality, **full-color** photographs, including pathologic specimens
- Attention to gender differences, especially regarding epidemiology and pathophysiology
- Integration of new, although essential, modern biology for all disease states
- Focus on health promotion/risk reduction by emphasizing Risk Factors in special boxes, nutrition and disease, and addition of new, integrated **Health Alert** boxes

Organization of the Book

The book is organized into two parts: "Basic Concepts of Pathophysiology" (Part One) and "Body Systems and Diseases" (Part Two). Basic principles and processes are introduced in the first part, including descriptions of cellular communication; genes and genetic diseases; forms of cell injury; fluids and electrolytes and acids and bases; immunity; stress, coping, and illness; and tumor biology. Knowledge of these processes is essential to a contemporary understanding of the pathophysiology of common diseases. The application of the principles and concepts in Part One determines the learner's ability to grasp the cellular and tissue responses to the most common diseases presented in Part Two. The content in Part One has been thoroughly updated and revised, and significant revisions include:

- Reorganization and emphasis on types of cell injury, including free radicals and activated oxygen species
- New section on intentional and unintentional injuries
- New summary figures on immunity, strategically placed to help synthesize content
- New separate chapter on cancer in children

Part Two is a presentation of the pathophysiology of the most common alterations according to body system. To guarantee readability and comprehension, we have used a logical and uniform approach for presenting the sequence and content of the units and chapters. Each unit focuses on a specific organ system and begins with anatomy and physiology content to provide students with a basis of comparison for understanding the alterations brought about by disease. A brief summary of normal aging is included at the end of these chapters. The remaining chapters in the unit contain the most common diseases and common alterations in children. The general organization of each disease/disorder entity includes an introductory paragraph of relevant risk factors and epidemiology, pathophysiology, clinical manifestations, and a brief review of treatment. Significant revisions of content in Part Two include:

- New presentation of heart failure and revision of shock and multipe organ dysfunction syndrome
- New sections on silent ischemia and myocardial infarction, and mental stress and heart disease
- More simplified presentation of the integrated cancer sections
- New information on fibromyalgia, ear infection, peptic ulcer disease, and homone receptors
- New presentations on diabetes mellitus and thyroid disorders

Features to Promote Learning

Ease of learning has been enhanced by designing several features that guide and support understanding:

- Beautiful new *full-color design,* with more than 1000 illustrations, the majority in full color, helps simplify complex concepts for students.
- *Chapter Outline* for each chapter, with page numbers, provides quick access to content for review.
- *Quick Checks,* strategically placed throughout the chapters, encourage readers to reflect on what they have just read and to question their understanding and comprehension of the material.
- *Health Alert* boxes cover a broad range of topics and present brief discussions of new biologic research, disease prevention, new diagnostic tests and treatments, or other developments related to health or specific diseases.
- *Risk Factors* for specific diseases are presented in specially designed boxes for easy identification.
- Numerous *algorithms* included throughout the book clearly illustrate all major diseases and disease processes. A list of algorithms with page references is included inside the front cover.
- End of chapter *Did You Understand?* sections summarize the major concepts presented in the chapter.
- *Key Terms* appear in boldface type and are listed at the end of each chapter, with corresponding page numbers for rapid access.

Art Program

The art program is truly outstanding! With the help of several artists and editors, a carefully-crafted, full-color art program was developed. Much care and attention to detail were given to the creation of new drawings, as well as the inclusion of high-quality, full-color photographs of clinical manifestations, pathologic specimens, and clinical imaging techniques. The combination of illustrations, algorithms, photographs, and use of color for tables and boxes helps the student "put it all together."

Life Span Content

Chapter 3 reviews theories and processes of aging and provides a reference for content in Part Two. Content related to normal aging is integrated throughout the book and highlighted with a unique logo ⋈ . The information provides a quick review to help readers differentiate a normal process of change in structure and function from pathophysiologic alterations

Pediatric coverage is in-depth. Selected pediatric ⋀ disorders are presented in Part One as examples of genetic and familial diseases, immune disorders, and cancers. The last chapter in each body system unit discusses pathophysiologic alterations in children. This content is important to include because pathophysiologic processes often are accompanied by different risk factors, pathogenesis, and manifestations in children as compared with adults.

Teaching/Learning Package

For the second edition of this text, an extensive number of ancillary products for instructors and students is offered:

The *CD Companion,* FREE with every text, contains a variety of activities to enhance learning. Included are answers to the text's Quick Check questions, critical thinking questions and answers, algorithm exercises that provide a snapshot progression of the most frequently encountered diseases, key terms with their definitions, and printable chapter summaries for added review.

MERLIN is Mosby's Electronic Resource Links and Information Network, an innovative Web site that provides a wealth of content, resources, and information on pathophysiology, including links to related Web sites. Use the passcode on the sticker in the front of the text to access MERLIN's wide array of information.

The *Study Guide and Workbook* by Clayton Parkinson, PhD, has been revised and updated. Each chapter includes learning objectives and carefully written summaries of key pathophysiologic concepts. Follow-up questions help students test their knowledge and understanding. Numerous case studies help illustrate clinical application of content.

For adopting instructors:

The updated and expanded *Instructor's Resource Manual and Test Bank* is a time-saving resource designed to assist faculty in developing lectures, reinforcing teaching through classroom and clinical activities, and evaluating student comprehension. Content includes learning objectives, lecture outlines, difficult concepts, and critical thinking exercises for each chapter of the text. The *Test Bank* contains approximately 1800 questions and includes page cross-references to the text.

Mosby's Electronic Image Collection CD contains more than 180 full-color illustrations and photos from the text to help instructors develop presentations and explain challenging concepts. All images on the CD can be printed out as acetates for overhead projection.

ACKNOWLEDGMENTS

Once again, we are enormously grateful to our contributors. For your continued commitment to making this textbook current, easy to read, and artistic, we thank you.

We would be lost without the expertise of Sue Meeks. Each time, to our total amazement, Sue not only word processes the entire manuscript but also orchestrates all the individual pieces to "fit and make the whole." Thanks Sue.

Our editor, Sally Schrefer, is key. Noteworthy is her constant and patient skill for directing us into yet another full-color text. She continues to be a steady source of perspective and judgement. Shelly Hayden, our developmental editor, managed the entire process of switching from two-color to four-color art—a mammoth job. We are sincerely grateful for her talents. Betty Hazelwood, as production editor, continues to be the sensitive and thorough critic. Her keen eye and supportive approach always make us feel that "we are in the best of hands." Thank you Betty!

We are constantly astonished by the talent of the artists. Much of the new art for this edition was completed by Barbara Cousins. Seemingly without effort, even with the most complex figures, she transformed our scribbles into sophisticated and aesthetic renditions. Kathi Gosche, our book's designer, did a spectacular job of creating a beautiful, full-color design that is both attractive and helpful in following the flow of the book's content. We are particularly grateful to Bill Westwood for the stunning design of the textbook's cover. Thank you all!

Other people contributed to the art program. Dennis Kunkel, PhD, at the University of Hawaii, provided many color photos of blood cells. Pamela G. Nemzer, MD, who catalogued the photo collection for the Department of Dermatology, School of Medicine, University of Utah, assisted us with the selection of photos. Other contributors of photos included Tony Egan, MB, MRCPI; Kappa P. Meadows, MD; Theresa A. Scholz, MD; Eileen Pazdeida Smith, MD; E. David Wright, MD; Sheryll L. Vanderhooft, MD; Margretta A. O'Reilly, MD; and Tena M. Rallis, MD.

Thank you to our colleagues and friends at the University of Utah College of Nursing. Once again, Deb Bachan was most helpful with tracking and communicating with contributors and mailings. Becky Nielson and Lyn Pearse helped with many details—mailing, scheduling conferences, and just being supportive friends! Thank you Deb, Becky, and Lyn.

Many hard-to-find documents were located and retrieved by the reference librarians at Eccles Medical Library—their help is essential. Thank you!

Special thanks are given to colleagues and students throughout the country, as well as foreign lands. Their critiques and suggestions are imperative, and we thank them all.

Always supportive are our families, especially Mae, John, Anne, Greg, Beth, Mark, and Eric—for they make the work possible!

Sue E. Huether
Kathryn L. McCance

Contents

Detailed Contents

Unit 2: Mechanisms of Self-Defense

Unit 8: The Pulmonary System

CHAPTER

1

Cellular Biology

Kathryn L. McCance

An understanding of cellular biology is increasingly necessary to comprehend disease processes. An overwhelming amount of information reveals how cells behave as a multicellular "social" organism. At the heart of it all is cellular communication (cellular "cross talk")—how messages originate and are transmitted, received, interpreted, and used by the cell. Streamlined conversation between, among, and within cells maintains social acceptance. Cells must demonstrate a "chemical fondness" for other cells to maintain the integrity of the entire organism. When they no longer tolerate this fondness, the conversation breaks down and cells either adapt (sometimes altering function) or become vulnerable to isolation, injury, or disease.

 Check out your CD Companion for chapter-related exercises and answers to the Quick Check questions

PROKARYOTES AND EUKARYOTES

Living cells generally are divided into eukaryotes and prokaryotes. The cells of higher animals and plants are eukaryotes, as are the single-celled organisms fungi, protozoa, and most algae. Prokaryotes include cyanobacteria (blue-green algae), bacteria, and rickettsiae. Prokaryotes traditionally were studied as core subjects of molecular biology. Today emphasis is on the eukaryotic cell; much of its structure and function have no counterpart in bacterial cells.

Eukaryotes (*eu* = good; *karyon* = nucleus) are larger and have more extensive intracellular anatomy and organization than prokaryotes. Eukaryotic cells have a characteristic set of membrane-bound intracellular compartments, called *organelles,* that includes a well-defined nucleus. The **prokaryotes** contain no organelles, and their nuclear material is not encased by a nuclear membrane. Prokaryotic cells are characterized by lack of a distinct nucleus.

Besides having structural differences, prokaryotic and eukaryotic cells differ in chemical composition and biochemical activity. The *nuclei* of prokaryotic cells carry genetic information in a single circular chromosome, and they lack a class of proteins called *histones,* which in eukaryotic cells bind with deoxyribonucleic acid (DNA) and are involved in the supercoiling of DNA. Eukaryotic cells have several or many chromosomes. Protein production, or synthesis, in the two classes of cells also differs because of major structural differences in ribonucleic acid (RNA) protein complexes. Other distinctions include differences in mechanisms of transport across the outer cellular membrane and in enzyme content.

CELLULAR FUNCTIONS

Cells become specialized through the process of differentiation, or maturation, so that some cells eventually perform one kind of function and other cells perform other functions. Cells with a highly developed function, such as movement, often lack some other property, such as hormone production, which is more highly developed in other cells.

The seven chief cellular functions are as follows:
1. *Movement.* Muscle cells can generate forces that produce motion. Muscles that are attached to bones produce limb movements, whereas those that enclose hollow tubes or cavities move or empty contents when they contract, for example, the colon.
2. *Conductivity.* Conduction as a response to a stimulus is manifested by a wave of excitation, an electrical potential, that passes along the surface of the cell to reach its other parts. Conductivity is the chief function of nerve cells.
3. *Metabolic absorption.* All cells can take in and use nutrients and other substances from their surroundings.
4. *Secretion.* Certain cells can synthesize new substances from substances they absorb and secrete the new substances to serve as needed elsewhere.
5. *Excretion.* All cells can rid themselves of waste products

resulting from the metabolic breakdown of nutrients. Membrane-bound sacs (lysosomes) within cells contain enzymes that break down, or digest, large molecules, turning them into waste products that are released from the cell.
6. *Respiration.* Cells absorb oxygen, which is used to transform nutrients into energy in the form of adenosine triphosphate (ATP). Cellular respiration, or oxidation, occurs in organelles called *mitochondria.*
7. *Reproduction.* Tissue growth occurs as cells enlarge and reproduce themselves. Even without growth, tissue maintenance requires that new cells be produced to replace cells that are lost normally through cellular death. Not all cells are capable of continuous division, and some cells, such as nerve cells, cannot reproduce.

STRUCTURE AND FUNCTION OF CELLULAR COMPONENTS

Fig. 1-1 shows a "typical" eukaryotic cell. It consists of three components: an outer membrane called the **plasma membrane,** or **plasmalemma;** a fluid "filling" called **cytoplasm;** and the "organs" of the cell—the membrane-bound intracellular **organelles,** among them the nucleus.

Nucleus

The **nucleus,** which is surrounded by the cytoplasm and generally is located in the center of the cell, is the largest membrane-bound organelle. Two membranes compose the **nuclear envelope** (Fig. 1-2, *A*). The outer membrane is continuous with membranes of the endoplasmic reticulum. The nucleus contains the **nucleolus,** most of the cellular DNA, and the DNA-binding proteins, the histones, that regulate its activity. The DNA in eukaryotic cells is so long that it is easily broken. Therefore the histones that bind to DNA cause DNA to fold into chromosomes (Fig. 1-2, *C*), which decreases the risk of breakage and is essential for cell division in eukaryotes.

The primary functions of the nucleus are cell division and control of genetic information. Other functions include the replication and repair of DNA and the transcription of the information stored in DNA. Genetic information is transcribed into RNA, which can be processed into messenger, transport, and ribosomal RNA and introduced into the cytoplasm, where it directs cellular activities. Most of the processing of RNA occurs in the nucleolus. (The role of DNA and RNA in protein synthesis is discussed in Chapter 2.)

Cytoplasmic Organelles

Cytoplasm is an aqueous solution (cytosol) that fills the **cytoplasmic matrix**—the space between the nuclear envelope and the plasma membrane. The cytosol represents about half the volume of a eukaryotic cell. It contains thousands of enzymes involved in intermediate metabolism and is crowded with ribosomes making proteins. Newly synthe-

Fig. 1-1 *Typical components of a eukaryotic cell.*

sized proteins remain in the cytosol if they lack a signal for transport to a cell organelle.[1] The organelles suspended in the cytoplasm are enclosed in biologic membranes, so they can simultaneously carry out functions requiring different biochemical environments. Many of these functions are directed by coded messages carried from the nucleus by RNA. They include synthesis of proteins and hormones and their transport out of the cell, isolation and elimination of waste products from the cell, metabolic processes, breakdown and disposal of cellular debris and foreign proteins (antigens), and maintenance of cellular structure and motility. Table 1-1 lists the principal cytoplasmic organelles.

✓ QUICK CHECK

Why is the process of differentiation essential to specialization? Give an example.

Why is the cytoplasm necessary for normal cellular function?

Describe the principal cytoplasmic organelles.

Plasma Membranes

Whether they surround the cell or enclose an intracellular organelle, membranes are exceedingly important to normal physiologic function because they control the composition of the space, or compartment, they enclose. Membranes can include or exclude various molecules, and by controlling the movement of substances from one compartment to another, membranes exert a powerful influence on metabolic pathways. The plasma membrane also has an important role in cell-to-cell recognition. Other functions of the plasma membrane include cellular mobility and the maintenance of cellular shape (Table 1-2).

Membrane composition

The major chemical components of all membranes are lipids and proteins, but the percentage of each varies among different membranes. Intracellular membranes have a higher percentage of proteins than plasma membranes have, presumably because most enzymatic activity occurs within organelles. Carbohydrates are associated mainly with plasma membranes, where they combine chemically with lipids, forming glycolipids, and with proteins, forming glycoproteins.

Fig. 1-2 *The nucleus.* The nucleus is composed of a double membrane, called a *nuclear envelope,* that encloses the fluid-filled interior, called *nucleoplasm.* The chromosomes are suspended in the nucleoplasm (here shown much larger than real size to show the tightly packed DNA strands). Swelling at one or more points of the chromosome, shown in **A,** occurs at a nucleolus where genes are being copied into RNA. The nuclear envelope is studded with pores. **B,** The pores are visible as dimples in this freeze etch of a nuclear envelope. **C,** Histone-folding DNA in chromosomes. *(From Raven, P.H. & Johnson, G.B. [1999]. Biology [5th ed.]. New York: McGraw-Hill.)*

Lipids

The basic component of the plasma membrane is a bilayer of lipid molecules—phospholipids, glycolipids, and cholesterol. Lipids are responsible for the structural integrity of the membrane. Each lipid molecule is said to be **amphipathic,** which means that one part is hydrophobic (uncharged, or "water hating") and another part is hydrophilic (charged, or "water loving") (Fig. 1-3).

The membrane spontaneously organizes itself into two layers because of these two incompatible solubilities. The hydrophobic region (hydrophobic tail) of each lipid molecule is protected from water, whereas the hydrophilic region (hydrophilic head) is immersed in it. The bilayer serves as a barrier to the diffusion of water and hydrophilic substances, while allowing lipid-soluble molecules, such as oxygen (O_2) and carbon dioxide (CO_2), to diffuse through it readily.

TABLE 1-1 Principal Cytoplasmic Organelles

Organelle	Characteristics and Description
Ribosomes	RNA-protein complexes synthesized in the nucleolus and secreted into the cytoplasm. Provide sites for cellular protein synthesis.
Endoplasmic reticulum	A network of tubular channels (cisternae) that extend throughout the outer nuclear membrane. Specializes in the synthesis and transport of protein and lipid components of most organelles.
Golgi complex	A network of smooth membranes and vesicles located near the nucleus. Is responsible for processing and packaging proteins into secretory vesicles that break away from the complex and migrate to various intracellular and extracellular destinations, including the plasma membrane.
Lysosomes	Saclike structures that originate from the Golgi complex and contain enzymes for digesting most cellular substances down to their basic form, such as amino acids, fatty acids, and sugars. Cellular injury leads to release of lysosomal enzymes that cause cellular self-destruction.
Peroxisomes	Similar to lysosomes but contain several enzymes that either produce or use hydrogen peroxide; detoxify harmful substances.
Mitochondria	Contain the metabolic machinery needed for cellular energy metabolism. Enzymes of respiratory chain (electron-transport chain), found in inner membrane of mitochondria, generate most of cell's ATP. Has a role in osmotic regulation, pH control, calcium homeostasis and cell signaling.
Cytoskeleton	"Bone and muscle" of cell. Composed of a network of protein filaments, including microtubules and actin filaments (microfilaments); forms cell extensions (microvilli, cilia, flagella).
Caveolae	Newly discovered tiny indentations (caves) can capture extracellular material and shuttle it inside the cell or across the cell.

TABLE 1-2 Plasma Membrane Functions

Cellular Mechanism	Membrane Functions
Structure	Usually thicker than the membranes of intracellular organelles
	Containment of cellular organelles
	Maintenance of relationship with cytoskeleton, endoplasmic reticulum, and other organelles
	Maintenance of fluid and electrolyte balance
	Outer surfaces of plasma membranes in many cells are not smooth but are studded with cilia or even smaller cylindric projections called *microvilli;* both are capable of movement
Protection	Barrier to toxic molecules and macromolecules (proteins, nucleic acid, polysaccharides)
	Barrier to foreign organisms and cells
Activation of cell	Hormones (regulation of cellular activity)
	Mitogens (cellular division, see Chapter 2)
	Antigens (antibody synthesis, see Chapter 7)
	Growth factors (proliferation and differentiation, see Chapter 9)
Transport	Diffusion and exchange diffusion
	Endocytosis (pinocytosis, phagocytosis)
	Exocytosis (secretion)
	Active transport
Cell-to-cell interaction	Communication and attachment at junctional complexes
	Symbiotic nutritive relationships
	Release of enzymes and antibodies to extracellular environment
	Relationships with extracellular matrix

Modified from King, D.W., Fenoglio, C.M., & Lefkowitch, J.H. (1983). General pathology: Principles and dynamics. *Philadelphia: Lea & Febiger.*

Fig. 1-3 *Amphipathic molecule.* In cellular membranes, amphipathic phospholipid molecules are organized in a bimolecular layer. The hydrophilic regions of the molecules are located at the membrane surfaces, and the hydrophobic regions are oriented toward the center of the membrane.

Proteins

Proteins can be classified as integral or peripheral membrane proteins. ***Integral membrane proteins*** are embedded in the lipid bilayer linked to either *phosphatidylinositol,* a minor phospholipid, or a fatty acid chain. The integral proteins can be removed from the membrane only by detergents that solubilize (dissolve) the lipid. ***Peripheral membrane proteins*** are not embedded in the bilayer but reside at one surface or the other, bound to an integral protein.

Proteins exist in densely folded molecular configurations rather than straight chains, so most hydrophilic units are at the surface of the molecule and most hydrophobic units are inside. Although membrane structure is determined by the lipid bilayer, membrane functions are determined largely by proteins. Proteins act as (1) recognition and binding units (receptors) for substances moving into and out of the cell; (2) pores or transport channels for various electrically charged particles called *ions* or *electrolytes,* and specific carriers for amino acids and monosaccharides; (3) specific enzymes that drive active pumps to promote concentration of certain ions, particularly potassium (K^+), within the cell while keeping concentrations of other ions, for example, sodium (Na^+), below concentrations found in the extracellular environment; (4) cell surface markers, such as ***glycoproteins*** (proteins attached to carbohydrates) that identify a cell to its neighbor; (5) cell adhesion proteins allowing cells to hook together and as attachments of the cytoskeleton for maintaining cellular shape; and (6) catalysts of chemical reactions, for example, lactose to glucose (Fig. 1-4).

The interaction of plasma membrane proteins with lipids is complex. The role of proteins in the onset and progression of disease is important because of their enzymatic, transport, and recognition-receptor functions in cellular physiology.

Carbohydrates

The carbohydrate contained within the plasma membrane is generally in the form of glycoprotein. Intercellular recognition, which is required for tissue formation, is an important function of membrane glycoproteins.

Fluid mosaic model

In the 1960s, G.L. Nicholson and S.J. Singer proposed the popular ***fluid mosaic model*** for biologic membranes (Fig. 1-5). The model, which is continually being modified, presents integral proteins as pieces of a mosaic that float singly or as aggregates in the fluid lipid bilayer. The protein molecules (1) transport other molecules into and out of the cell, (2) facilitate (catalyze) membrane reactions, (3) receive messages, thus acting as receptors for extracellular and intracellular signals, and (4) create structural linkages between the external and internal cellular environments.

The fluid mosaic model accounts for the flexibility of cellular membranes, their self-sealing properties, and their impermeability to many substances. The degree of a membrane's fluidity depends on temperature. At lower temperatures the lipids are in a gel crystalline state, and at higher temperatures they become highly fluid. These properties are critical for cellular growth, division, and receptor function. Because *some* proteins are free to move within the plasma membranes (like floating icebergs), certain foreign proteins (antigens) may become buried in the bilayer, emerging at the surface only after injury and then attracting antibodies (proteins produced by the immune system), which attack host cells. Antigens and antibodies, which are integral to the immune response, are discussed in Chapter 5. The burial and reemergence of antigens may cause autoimmune disease, described in Chapter 7.

In the fluid mosaic model, cellular membranes are dy-

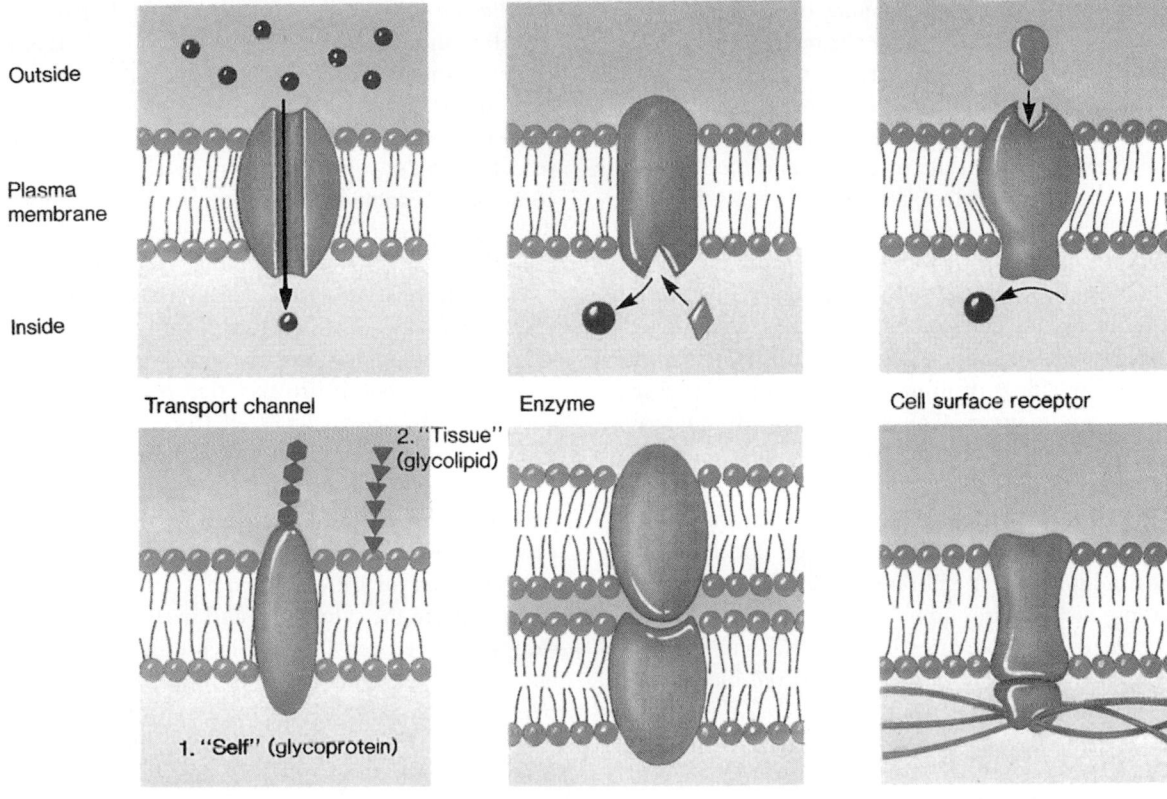

Outside

Plasma membrane

Inside

Transport channel

Enzyme

Cell surface receptor

2. "Tissue" (glycolipid)

1. "Self" (glycoprotein)

Cell surface markers

Cell adhesion

Attachment of cytoskeleton

Fig. 1-4 *Functions of plasma membrane proteins.* The plasma membrane proteins illustrated here show a variety of functions performed by the different types of plasma membranes. *(From Raven, P.H. & Johnson, G.B. [1995]. Understanding biology [3rd ed.]. Dubuque, Iowa: Brown.)*

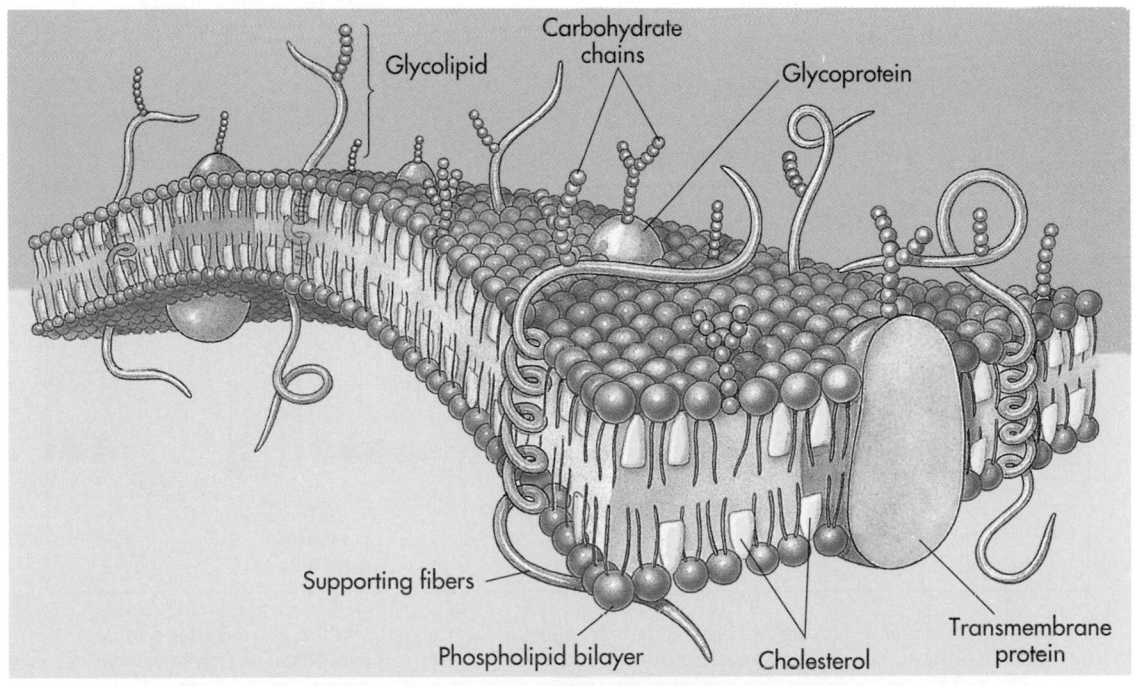

Glycolipid

Carbohydrate chains

Glycoprotein

Supporting fibers

Phospholipid bilayer

Cholesterol

Transmembrane protein

Fig. 1-5 *Fluid mosaic model.* Schematic, three-dimensional view of the fluid mosaic model of membrane structure. The lipid bilayer provides the basic structure and serves as a relatively impermeable barrier to most water-soluble molecules. *(Modified from Thibodeau, G.A. & Patton, K.T. [1997]. Structure and function of the human body [10th ed.]. St. Louis: Mosby.)*

namic. Lipids and proteins move laterally on the membrane, and ions and other molecules move through it. Cells, however, can immobilize specific membrane proteins in a region of the membrane. Confinement may be needed for certain functions to occur. The fluid mosaic model describes the membrane as existing in a state of change and modulation, which allows the cell to protect itself actively against injurious agents. Hormones, bacteria, viruses, drugs, antibodies, chemicals that transmit nerve impulses (neurotransmitters), and other substances attach to the plasma membrane by means of receptor molecules on its outer layer. The number of receptors present may vary at different times, and the cell can modulate the effects of injurious agents by altering receptor number and pattern.[2] This aspect of the fluid mosaic model has drastically modified previously held concepts concerning the onset of disease.

The concentration of cholesterol in the plasma membrane affects membrane fluidity. Increased concentration means less fluidity on the membrane's hydrophilic outer surface and more at its hydrophobic core. Cholesterol content changes are factors in some diseases. In cirrhosis of the liver, for example, the cholesterol content of the red blood cell's plasma membrane increases, causing a decrease in membrane fluidity that seriously affects the cell's ability to transport oxygen.

Cellular Receptors

Cellular receptors are protein molecules on the plasma membrane, in the cytoplasm, or in the nucleus that can recognize and bind with specific smaller molecules called *ligands.* Hormones, for example, are ligands. Recognition and binding depend on the chemical configuration of the receptor and its smaller ligand, which must fit together somewhat like pieces of a jigsaw puzzle (see Chapter 17).

Plasma membrane receptors protrude from or are exposed at the external surface of the membrane, often attached to integral proteins (Fig. 1-6). Some of these recognition units have all the mobile properties related to membrane fluidity. The ligands that bind with membrane receptors include hormones, neurotransmitters, antigens, complement components, lipoproteins, infectious agents, drugs, and metabolites. Many new discoveries concerning the specific interactions of cellular receptors with their respective ligands have provided a basis for understanding disease.

Although the chemical nature of ligands and their receptors differs, receptors are classified based on their location and function (see Cell-to-Cell Communication). Cellular type determines overall cellular function, but plasma membrane receptors determine which ligands a cell will bind with and how the cell will respond to the binding. Specific processes also control intracellular mechanisms.

Receptors for different drugs are found on the plasma membrane, in the cytoplasm, and in the nucleus. Membrane receptors have been found for certain anesthetics, opiates, endorphins, enkephalins, antibiotics, cancer chemotherapeutic agents, digitalis, and other drugs. Membrane receptors for endorphins, which are opiate-like peptides isolated from the pituitary gland, are found in large quantities in pain pathways of the nervous system (see Chapters 12 and 13). With binding, the endorphins (or drugs such as morphine) change the cell's permeability to ions, increase the concentration of molecules that regulate intracellular protein synthesis, and initiate molecular events that modulate pain perception.

Receptors for infectious microorganisms, or antigen receptors, bind bacteria, viruses, and parasites. Antigen receptors on white blood cells (lymphocytes, monocytes,

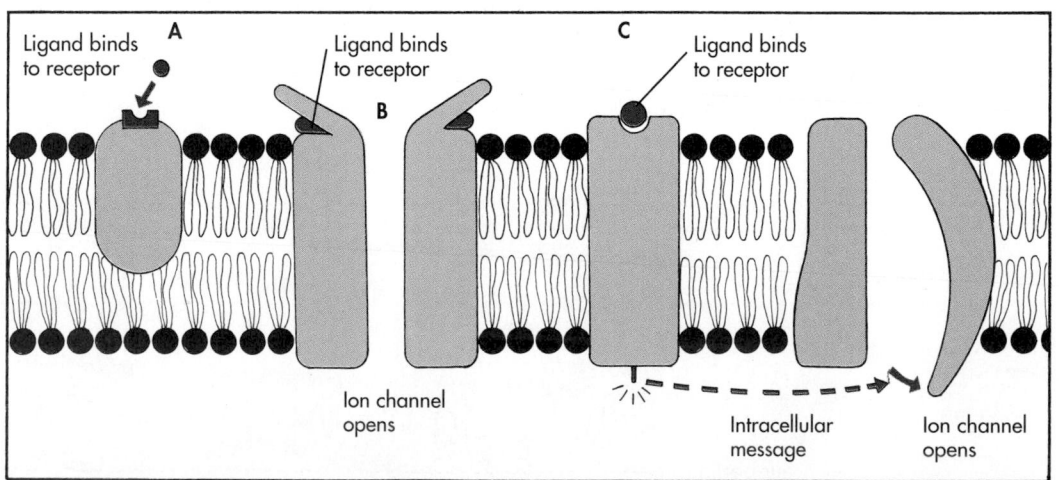

Fig. 1-6 *Cellular receptors.* **A,** Plasma membrane receptor for a ligand (here, a hormone molecule) on the surface of an integral protein. A neurotransmitter can exert its effect on a postsynaptic cell by means of two fundamentally different types of receptor proteins: **B,** channel-linked receptors, and **C,** non-channel-linked receptors. Channel-linked receptors are also known as *ligand-gated channels. (B and C modified from Alberts, B. et al. [1994]. Molecular biology of the cell [3rd ed.]. New York: Garland.)*

macrophages, granulocytes) recognize and bind with antigenic microorganisms and activate the immune and inflammatory responses (see Chapters 5 and 6).

CELL-TO-CELL COMMUNICATION

Cells need to communicate with each other to regulate their growth and division, to oversee their development and organization into tissues, and to coordinate their functions. Cells communicate in three ways: (1) they form protein channels (gap junctions) that directly coordinate the activities of adjacent cells; (2) they display plasma-membrane-bound signaling molecules (receptors) that affect the cell itself and other cells in direct physical contact; and (3) they secrete chemicals that signal to cells some distance away (Fig. 1-7). Alterations in cellular communication affect disease onset and progression. In fact, if a cell cannot perform gap junctional intercellular communication, normal growth control and cell differentiation may not be possible, thereby favoring cancerous tumor development (see Chapter 9). (Communication through gap junctions is discussed on p. 23, and contact signaling by plasma-membrane-bound molecules is discussed on this page and on p. 10.) Secreted chemical signals involve communication locally and at a distance. Four primary modes of chemical signaling are endocrine, paracrine, autocrine, and synaptic (Fig. 1-8).

Endocrine signaling involves specialized endocrine cells that secrete hormone chemicals released by one set of cells that travel through the tissue through the bloodstream to produce a response in other sets of cells (see Chapter 17). In *paracrine signaling,* cells secrete local chemical mediators that are quickly taken up, destroyed, or immobilized. The mediators act only on nearby cells. In *autocrine signaling,* signaling molecules may act back on the cells of origin (i.e., autostimulation). Autocrine circuits function as a component of normal growth—regulatory mechanisms in many adult tissue types. In *synaptic signaling,* cells secrete chemicals, or *neurotransmitters,* at specialized junctions called *chemical synapses;* the neurotransmitter diffuses across the synaptic cleft and acts on the postsynaptic target cell (see

HEALTH ALERT
Intracellular Communication Alterations

Intracellular communication and transmission of messages for many hormones and free radicals occur after the hormones and free radicals bind to their receptors by increasing the activity of guanylase cyclase, the enzyme used in the conversion of guanosine triphosphate to the intracellular messenger cyclic guanosine-3'-5' monophosphate (cyclic GMP). Cyclic GMP promotes growth by increasing DNA, RNA, and protein synthesis. Overactivity of this system is observed in the common disturbance known as traveler's diarrhea. This disturbance can be corrected in vitro by the addition of cyclic GMP.

Data from Vesely, D.L. (1997). Signal transduction: Activation of the guanylate cyclase-cyclic guanosine-3'-5' monophosphate system by hormones and free radicals. American Journal of Medical Science, 314(5), 311-323.

Fig. 1-8). Many of the same signaling molecules are receptors used in endocrine, paracrine, autocrine, and synaptic signaling. Important differences lie in the speed and selectivity with which the signals are delivered to their targets.[1]

Plasma membrane receptors belong to one of three classes that are defined by the signaling (transduction) mechanism used. Table 1-3 summarizes these receptors. Cells respond to external stimuli by activation of a variety of *signal transduction pathways,* or communication pathways. Signals are passed between cells when a particular type of molecule is produced by one cell—the *signaling cell*—and received by another—the *target cell*—by means of a *receptor protein* that recognizes and responds specifically to the signal molecule (Fig. 1-9). In turn, the signaling molecules activate a path of intracellular protein kinases that results in stereotypical responses, such as proliferation, arrest of growth, increase in cellular size (hypertrophy), maturation, or cell death (apoptosis).

Remote signaling by secreted molecules	Contact signaling by plasma membrane–bound molecules	Contact signaling via gap junctions

Fig. 1-7 *Cellular communication.* Three primary ways in which cells communicate with one another. *(Modified from Alberts, B. et al. [1994]. Molecular biology of the cell [3rd ed.]. New York: Garland.)*

Fig. 1-8 *Primary modes of chemical signaling.* Four forms of signaling mediated by secreted molecules. Not all neurotransmitters act in the strictly synaptic mode shown; some act in a paracrine mode as local chemical mediators that influence multiple target cells in the area. *(Modified from Alberts B. et al. [1994]. Molecular biology of the cell [3rd ed.]. New York: Garland.)*

Fig. 1-9 *Schematic of a signal transduction pathway.* Like a telephone receiver that converts an electrical signal into a sound signal, a cell converts an extracellular signal, **A,** into an intracellular signal, **B.** *(Modified from Alberts, B. et al. [1998]. Essential cell biology: An introduction to the molecular biology of the cell. New York: Garland.)*

TABLE 1-3	Classes of Plasma Membrane Receptors
Type of Receptor	**Description**
Channel-linked	Also called ligand-gated channels; involve rapid synaptic signaling between electrically excitable cells. Channels open and close briefly in response to neurotransmitters, changing the ion permeability of the plasma membrane of the postsynaptic cell.
Catalytic	Once activated by ligands, function directly as enzymes.
G-protein-linked	Indirectly activate or inactivate plasma membrane enzyme or ion channel; interaction mediated by *GTP-binding regulatory protein (G-protein).* May also interact with inositol phospholipids, which are significant in cell signaling, and molecules involved in the *inositol-phospholipid transduction pathway.*

CELLULAR METABOLISM

All of the chemical tasks of maintaining essential cellular functions are referred to as *cellular metabolism.* The energy-using process of metabolism is called *anabolism* (*ana* = upward), and the energy-releasing process is known as *catabolism* (*kata* = downward). Metabolism provides the cell with the energy it needs to produce cellular structures.

Dietary proteins, fats, and starches are hydrolyzed in the intestinal tract into amino acids, fatty acids, and glucose.

These constituents are then absorbed, circulated, and taken up by the cell, where they may be used for various vital cellular processes, including the production of ATP. The process by which ATP is produced is one example of a series of reactions called a *metabolic pathway.* A metabolic pathway involves several steps whose end products are not always detectable. A key feature of cellular metabolism involves protein catalysts, or enzymes, most of which respond to a specific enzyme. Each enzyme has a high affinity for a *substrate*—a specific substance converted to a product of the reaction.

Role of Adenosine Triphosphate

For a cell to function, it must be able to extract and use the chemical energy in organic molecules. When 1 mole of glucose is metabolically broken down in the presence of oxygen into carbon dioxide and water, 686 kilocalories (kcal) of chemical energy is released. The chemical energy lost by one molecule is transferred to the chemical structure of another molecule by an energy-carrying or transferring molecule, such as ATP. The energy stored in ATP can be used in various energy-requiring reactions and in the process is generally converted to adenosine diphosphate (ADP) and inorganic phosphate (Pi). The energy available as a result of this reaction is about 7 kcal/mol of ATP. ATP is used by the cell for muscle contraction and active transport of molecules across cellular membranes. ATP not only *stores* energy but also *transfers* it from one molecule to another. Energy stored by carbohydrate, lipid, and protein is catabolized and transferred to ATP.

Food and Production of Cellular Energy

Catabolism of the proteins, lipids, and polysaccharides found in food can be divided into the following three phases (Fig. 1-10):

Phase 1: *digestion.* Large molecules are broken down into smaller subunits—proteins into amino acids, polysac-

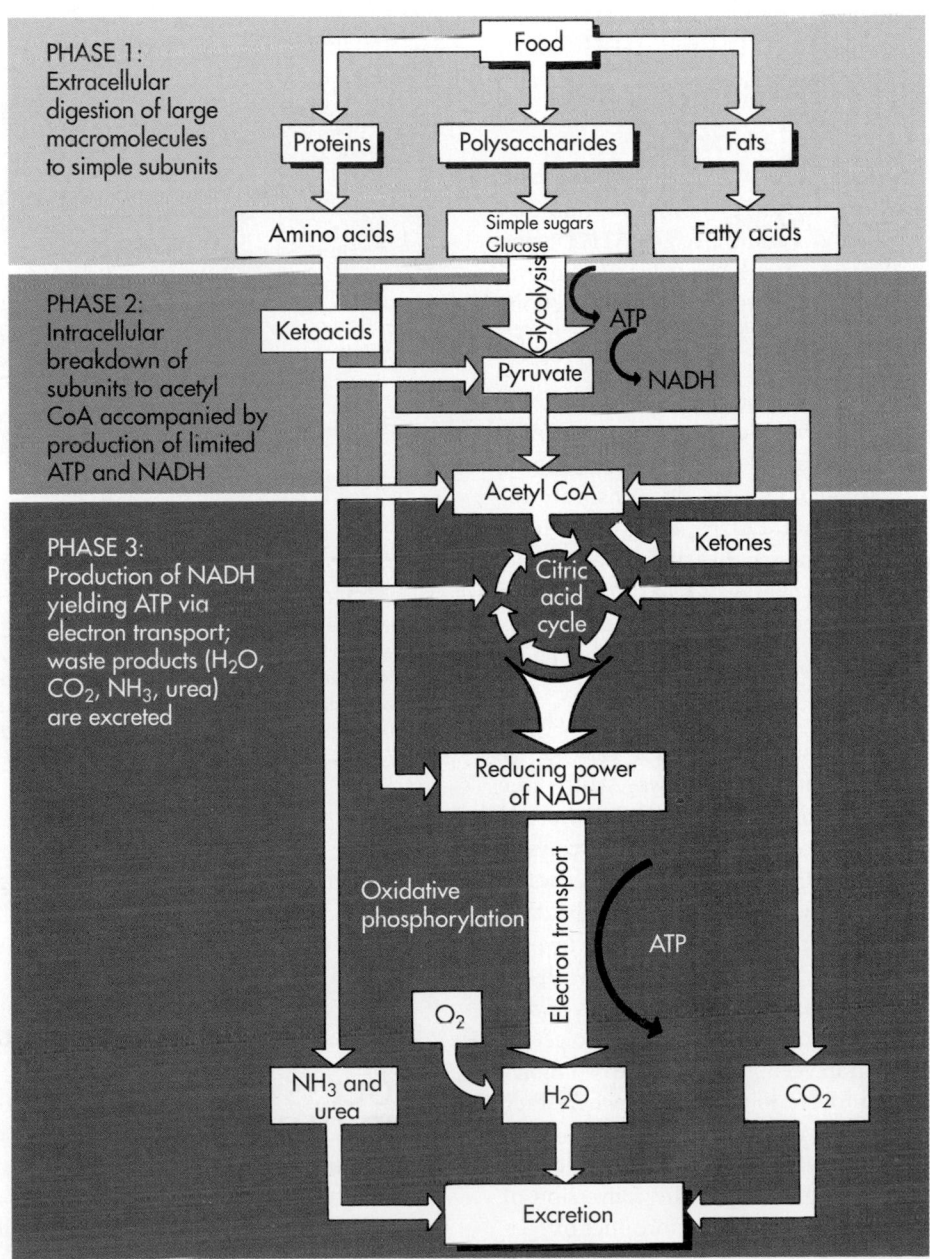

Fig. 1-10 *Three phases of catabolism, which leads from food to waste products.* These reactions produce ATP, which is used to drive other processes in the cell.

charides into simple sugars, and fats into fatty acids and glycerol. These processes occur outside the cell and are activated by secreted enzymes.

Phase 2: *glycolysis* and *oxidation.* The most important part of phase 2 is glycolysis, the splitting of glucose. Glycolysis produces two molecules of ATP per glucose molecule through oxidation, or the removal and transfer of a pair of electrons. The total process is called *oxidative cellular metabolism* and involves nine biochemical reactions (Fig. 1-11).

Phase 3: *citric acid cycle (Krebs cycle, tricarboxylic acid cycle).* Most of the ATP is generated during this final phase. It begins with the citric acid cycle and ends with oxidative phosphorylation. About two thirds of the total oxidation of carbon compounds in most cells is accomplished during this phase. The major end products are CO_2 and two dinucleotides, NADH and $FADH_2$, which transfer their electrons into the electron-transport chain.

Oxidative Phosphorylation

Oxidative phosphorylation occurs in the mitochondria and is the mechanism by which the energy produced from carbohydrates, fats, and proteins is transferred to ATP. During the catabolism of foods, many reactions involve the removal of electrons from various intermediates. These reactions generally require a coenzyme (a nonprotein carrier molecule), such as nicotinamide adenine dinucleotide (NAD), to transfer the electrons and thus are called **transfer reactions.**

Molecules of NAD and flavin adenine nucleotide (FAD) transfer electrons they have gained from the oxidation of substrates to molecular oxygen, O_2. The electrons from reduced NAD and FAD, NADH and $FADH_2$, are transferred to the **electron-transport chain** on the inner surfaces of the mitochondria with the release of hydrogen ions. Some carrier molecules are brightly colored, iron-containing proteins known as *cytochromes* that accept a pair of electrons. These electrons eventually combine with molecular oxygen.

If oxygen is not available to the electron-transport chain, ATP will not be formed by the mitochondria. Instead, an anaerobic (without oxygen) metabolic pathway synthesizes ATP. This process, called **substrate phosphorylation** or **anaerobic glycolysis,** is linked to the breakdown (glycolysis) of carbohydrate (see Fig. 1-11). Because glycolysis occurs in the cytoplasm of the cell, it provides energy for cells that lack mitochondria. The reactions in anaerobic glycolysis involve the conversion of glucose to pyruvic acid (pyruvate) with the simultaneous production of ATP. With the glycolysis of one molecule of glucose, two ATP molecules and two molecules of pyruvate are liberated. If oxygen is present, the two molecules of pyruvate move into the mitochondria, where they enter the citric acid cycle (Fig. 1-12).

If oxygen is absent, pyruvate is converted to lactic acid and released into the extracellular fluid. The conversion of pyruvic acid to lactic acid is reversible; therefore once oxygen is restored, lactic acid is quickly converted back to either pyruvic acid or glucose. The anaerobic generation of ATP from glucose through glycolysis is not as efficient as the aer-

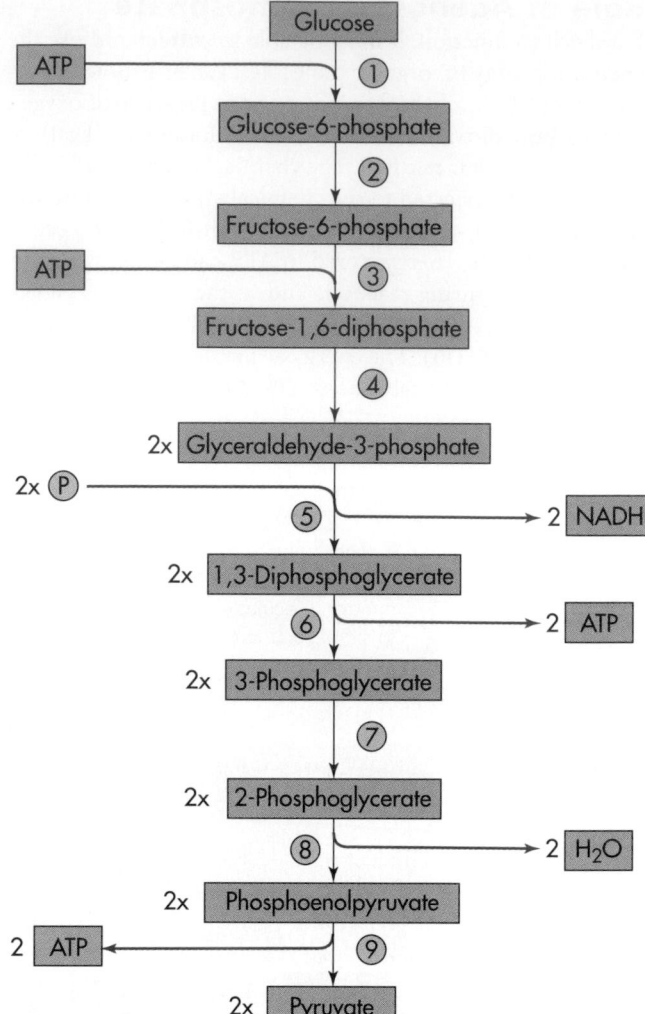

Fig. 1-11 *Glycolysis.* Each of the numbered reactions is catalyzed by a different enzyme. At step 4, a six-carbon sugar is broken down to give two three-carbon sugars, so that the number of molecules at every step after this is doubled. Reactions 5 and 6 are the reactions responsible for the net synthesis of ATP and NADH molecules. *(Modified from Alberts, B. et al. [1994]. Molecular biology of the cell [3rd ed.]. New York: Garland.)*

obic generation process. Adding an oxygen-requiring stage to the catabolic process (phase 3; see Fig. 1-10) provides cells with a much more powerful method for extracting energy from food molecules.

PROCESSES OF CELLULAR INTAKE AND OUTPUT

Cells continually take in nutrients, fluids, and chemical messengers from the extracellular environment and expel metabolites, or the products of metabolism, and end products of lysosomal digestion. The mechanisms involved depend on the characteristics of the substance to be transported. In **passive transport,** water and small, electrically

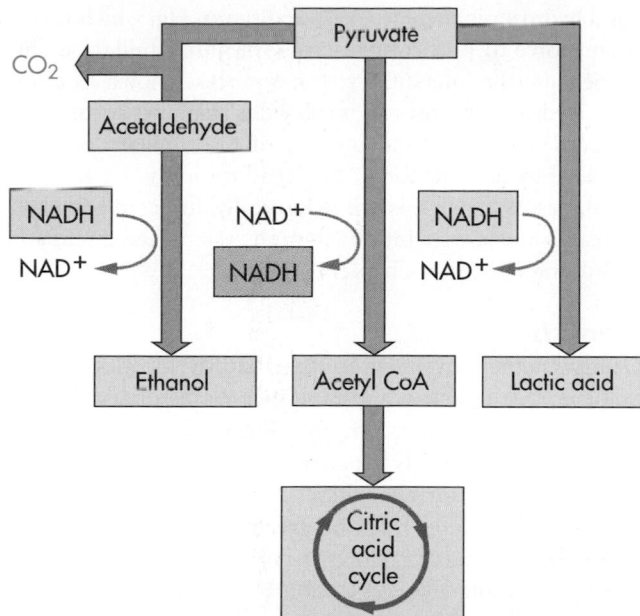

Fig. 1-12 *What happens to pyruvate, the product of glycolysis?* In the presence of oxygen, pyruvate is oxidized to acetyl CoA and enters the citric acid cycle. In the absence of oxygen, pyruvate instead is reduced, accepting the electrons extracted during glycolysis and carried by NADH. When pyruvate is reduced directly, as it is in muscles, the product is lactic acid. When CO_2 is first removed from pyruvate and the remainder is reduced, as it is in yeasts, the product is ethanol.

uncharged molecules move easily through pores in the plasma membrane's lipid bilayer. This process occurs naturally through any semipermeable barrier. It is driven by osmosis, hydrostatic pressure, and diffusion, all of which depend on the laws of physics and do not require life. The process does not require any energy expenditure by the cell.

Other molecules are too large to pass through pores or are ligands bound to receptors on the cell's plasma membrane. Some of these molecules are moved into and out of the cell by *active transport,* which requires life, biologic activity, and the cell's expenditure of metabolic energy. Unlike passive transport, active transport occurs across only living membranes that (1) use energy generated by cellular metabolism and (2) have receptors that can recognize and bind with the substance to be transported. Large molecules (macromolecules), along with fluids, are transported by endocytosis (taking in) and exocytosis (expelling). Water and electrically charged molecules are transported by protein channels embedded in the plasma membrane. Ligands enter the cell by means of receptor-mediated endocytosis.

Movement of Water and Solutes

Cellular membranes are semipermeable and generally allow passage of water and small particles of dissolved substances called *solutes,* depending on their size, solubility, electrical

properties, and concentration on either side of the membrane. Small, lipid-soluble particles, such as oxygen, carbon dioxide, and urea, readily pass through the lipid bilayers of the plasma membrane. Larger, water-soluble particles may pass through pores in the membranes. Although large protein molecules, such as albumin and globulin, pass through membranes by endocytosis, they exert an osmotic effect on the movement of water (see p. 14).

Body fluids are composed of *electrolytes,* which are electrically charged and dissociate into constituent *ions* when placed in solution, and nonelectrolytes, such as glucose, urea, and creatinine, which do not dissociate. Electrolytes account for approximately 95% of the solute molecules in body water. Electrolytes exhibit *polarity* by orienting themselves toward the positive or negative pole. Ions with a positive charge are known as *cations* and migrate toward the negative pole, or cathode, if an electrical current is passed through the electrolyte solution. *Anions* carry a negative charge and migrate toward the positive pole, or anode, in the presence of electrical current. Anions and cations are located in both the intracellular fluid (ICF) and extracellular fluid (ECF) compartments, although their concentration depends on their location. (Fluid and electrolyte balance between body compartments is discussed in Chapter 4.) For example, sodium (Na^+) is the predominant extracellular cation, and potassium (K^+) is the principal intracellular cation. The difference in ICF and ECF concentrations of these ions is important to the transmission of electrical impulses across the plasma membranes of nerve and muscle cells.

Electrolytes are measured in milliequivalents per liter (mEq/L) or milligrams per deciliter (mg/dl). The term *milliequivalent* indicates the chemical-combining activity of an ion, which depends on the electrical charge, or *valence,* of its ions. In abbreviations, valence is indicated by the *number* of plus or minus signs. One milliequivalent of any cation can combine chemically with 1 mEq of any anion: one monovalent anion will combine with one monovalent cation. Divalent ions combine more strongly than monovalent ions. To maintain electrochemical balance, one divalent ion will combine with two monovalent ions (e.g., $Ca^{++} + 2Cl^- = CaCl_2$).

Passive transport
Diffusion

Diffusion is the movement of a solute molecule from an area of greater solute concentration to an area of lesser solute concentration. This difference in concentration is known as a *concentration gradient.* Although particles in a solution move randomly in any direction, if the concentration of particles in one part of the solution is greater than in another part, the particles distribute themselves evenly throughout the solution. The same holds true with respect to permeable membranes. Particles diffuse spontaneously from an area of greater concentration to an area of lesser concentration until equilibrium is reached.

The diffusion rate is influenced by differences of electrical potential across the membrane (see p. 18). Because the

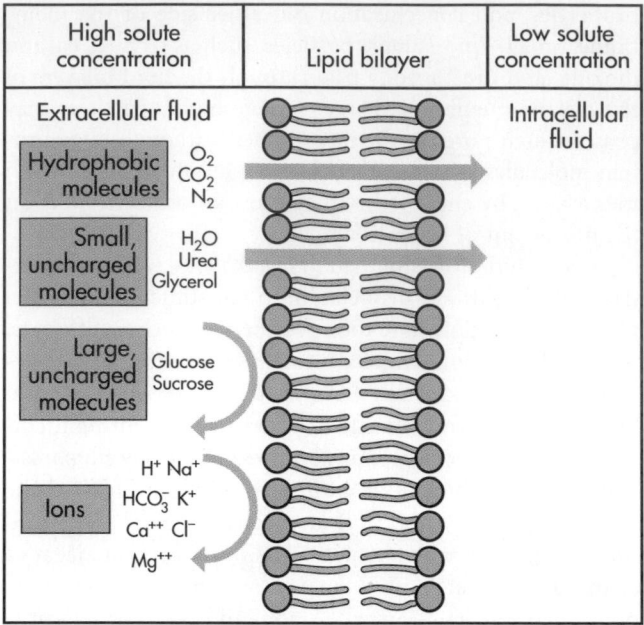

Fig. 1-13 *Passive diffusion of solute molecules across the plasma membrane.* Oxygen, nitrogen, water, urea, glycerol, and carbon dioxide can diffuse readily down the concentration gradient. Macromolecules are too large to diffuse through pores in the plasma membrane. Ions may be repelled if the pores contain substances with identical charges. If the pores are lined with cations, for example, other cations will have difficulty diffusing because the positive charges will repel one another. Diffusion can still occur, but it occurs more slowly.

pores in the lipid bilayer are often lined with Ca^{++}, other cations (e.g., Na^+ and K^+) diffuse slowly because they are repelled by positive charges in the pores.

The rate of diffusion of a substance depends also on its size (diffusion coefficient) and its lipid solubility (Fig. 1-13). Usually, the smaller the molecule and the more soluble it is in oil, the more hydrophobic or nonpolar it is and the more rapidly it will diffuse across the bilayer. Oxygen, carbon dioxide, and steroid hormones are all nonpolar molecules. Water-soluble substances, such as sugars and inorganic ions, diffuse very slowly, whereas uncharged lipophilic ("lipid-loving") molecules, such as fatty acids and steroids, diffuse rapidly. Ions and other polar molecules generally diffuse across cellular membranes more slowly than lipid-soluble substances.

Water readily diffuses through biologic membranes because water molecules are small and uncharged. The dipolar structure of water allows it to cross rapidly the regions of the bilayer containing the lipid head groups. Their groups constitute the two outer regions of the lipid bilayer.

Hydrostatic pressure

Hydrostatic pressure is the mechanical force of water pushing against cellular membranes. In the vascular system, hydrostatic pressure is the blood pressure generated in vessels when the heart contracts. Blood reaching the capillary bed

has a hydrostatic pressure of 25 to 30 mm Hg, which is sufficient force to push water across the thin capillary membranes into the interstitial space, a process known as *filtration*. Hydrostatic pressure is partially balanced by osmotic pressure, with water moving out of the capillary partially balanced by osmotic forces that tend to pull water into the capillaries. Water that is not osmotically attracted back into the capillaries moves into the lymph system (see discussion of Starling's forces in Chapter 4).

Osmosis

Osmosis is the movement of water "down" a concentration gradient, that is, across a semipermeable membrane from a region of higher water concentration to one of lower concentration. For osmosis to occur, (1) the membrane must be more permeable to water than to solutes and (2) the concentration of solutes must be greater so that water moves more easily. Osmosis is directly related to both hydrostatic pressure and solute concentration but *not* to particle size or weight. For example, particles of the plasma protein albumin are small but are more concentrated in body fluids than the larger and heavier particles of globulin. Therefore albumin exerts a greater osmotic force than does globulin.

Osmolality controls the distribution and movement of water between body compartments. The terms *osmolality* and *osmolarity* often are used interchangeably in reference to osmotic activity, but they define different measurements. **Osmolality** measures the number of milliosmoles per kilogram of water, or the concentration of molecules per *weight* of water. **Osmolarity** measures the number of milliosmoles per liter of solution, or the concentration of molecules per *volume* of solution.

In solutions that contain only dissociable substances, such as sodium and chloride, the difference between the two measurements is negligible. In considering all the different solutes in plasma (e.g., proteins, glucose, lipids), however, the difference between osmolality and osmolarity becomes more significant. Less of plasma's weight is water, and the overall concentration of particles is therefore greater. The osmolality will be greater than the osmolarity because of the smaller proportion of water. Osmolality is thus preferred in human clinical assessment.

The normal osmolality of body fluids is 280 to 294 mOsm/kg. The osmolality of intracellular and extracellular fluid tends to equalize and so provides a measure of body fluid concentration and thus the body's hydration status. Hydration is affected also by hydrostatic pressure, since the movement of water by osmosis can be opposed by an equal amount of hydrostatic pressure. The amount of hydrostatic pressure required to oppose the osmotic movement of water is called the **osmotic pressure** of the solution. Factors that determine osmotic pressure are the type and thickness of the plasma membrane, the size of the molecules, the concentration of molecules or the concentration gradient, and the solubility of molecules within the membrane.

Effective osmolality is sustained osmotic activity and depends on the concentration of solutes remaining on one side of a permeable membrane. If the solutes penetrate the membrane and equilibrate with the solution on the other side of the membrane, the osmotic effect will be diminished or lost.

Plasma proteins influence osmolality because they have a negative charge. The principle involved is known as *Gibbs-Donnan equilibrium;* it occurs when fluid in one compartment contains small, diffusible ions, such as Na^+ and Cl^-, together with large, nondiffusible, charged particles, such as plasma proteins. Because the body tends to maintain an electrical equilibrium, the nondiffusible protein molecules cause asymmetry in the distribution of small ions. Anions such as Cl^- are thus driven out of the cell or plasma, and cations such as Na^+ are attracted. The protein-containing compartment maintains a state of electroneutrality, but the osmolality is higher. The overall osmotic effect of colloids, such as plasma proteins, is called the **oncotic pressure,** or *colloid osmotic pressure.*

Tonicity describes the effective osmolality of a solution. (The terms *osmolality* and *tonicity* may be used interchangeably.) Solutions have relative degrees of tonicity. An **isotonic solution** (or isoosmotic solution) has the same osmolality or concentration of particles (285 mOsm) as the ICF or ECF. A **hypotonic solution** has a lower concentration and is thus more dilute than body fluids. A **hypertonic solution** has a concentration more than 285 to 294 mOsm/kg. The concept of tonicity is important when correcting water and solute imbalances by administering different types of replacement solutions (see Chapter 4).

✓QUICK CHECK

Why is glycolysis important?

Why does oxidative phosphorylation require a coenzyme?

Why do water and small, electrically charged molecules move easily through pores in the plasma membrane?

Mediated and active transport
Mediated transport

Mediated transport (passive and active) involves integral or transmembrane proteins with receptors that are highly specific for the substance being transported. Inorganic anions and cations (e.g., Na^+, K^+, Ca^{++}, Cl^-, HCO_3^-) and charged and uncharged organic compounds require specific transport systems to facilitate movement through different cellular membranes. Mediated transport is much faster than simple diffusion.

A **transport protein** *(carrier protein)* is a transmembrane or integral protein that binds with and transfers a specific solute molecule across the lipid bilayer. Each transport protein, or **transporter,** has receptors for a specific solute. When the transporter is saturated—that is, when all receptor sites are occupied by solute molecules—the rate of transport is

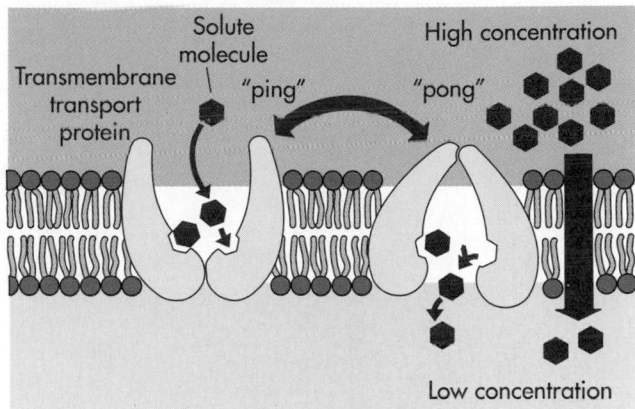

Fig. 1-14 *Conformational-change model of mediated transport (facilitated diffusion).* The transporter protein has two states, "ping" and "pong." In the ping state, sites for molecules of a specific solute are exposed on the outside of the bilayer. In the pong state, the sites are exposed to the inner side of the bilayer.

maximal. Solute binding can be blocked by **competitive inhibitors** that compete for the same receptor site and may or may not be transported by the transport protein. Noncompetitive inhibitors bind elsewhere but can alter the structure of the transporter.

The polypeptide chain of the transport protein crosses the lipid bilayer multiple times. This chain forms a continuous pathway enabling solutes to pass across the membrane without directly contacting the hydrophobic interior of the lipid bilayer (Fig. 1-14).[1]

Another mechanism of mediated transport is the channel protein. The protein transporter creates a water-filled pore or channel across the bilayer through which specific ions can diffuse. These channels are sometimes called *ion channels* or *K^+ leak channels* (Fig. 1-15). The channel is controlled by a gate mechanism that determines which receptor-bound solutes can move into it. Binding stimulates conformational changes in the protein transporter that move the solute through the channel short distances until it reaches the other side of the membrane. Ion channels are responsible for the electrical excitability of nerve and muscle cells and play a critical role in the membrane potential.

Mediated transport systems can move solute molecules singly or two at a time. Two molecules can be moved simultaneously in one direction (a process called **symport**) or in opposite directions (called **antiport**), or a single molecule can be moved in one direction (called **uniport**) (Fig. 1-16).

In **passive mediated transport,** or **facilitated diffusion,** the protein transporter moves solute molecules through cellular membranes without expending metabolic energy. The direction of movement is the same as in simple diffusion—down the concentration gradient. A well-known passive transport system is that for glucose in erythrocytes (red blood cells). Glucose is transported by a uniport mechanism and demonstrates saturation kinetics; that is, the transport system is saturated when all the glucose-specific receptors on

Fig. 1-15 *Channel mode of mediated transport (facilitated diffusion).* A channel protein forms a water-filled pore across the bilayer through which specific ions can diffuse.

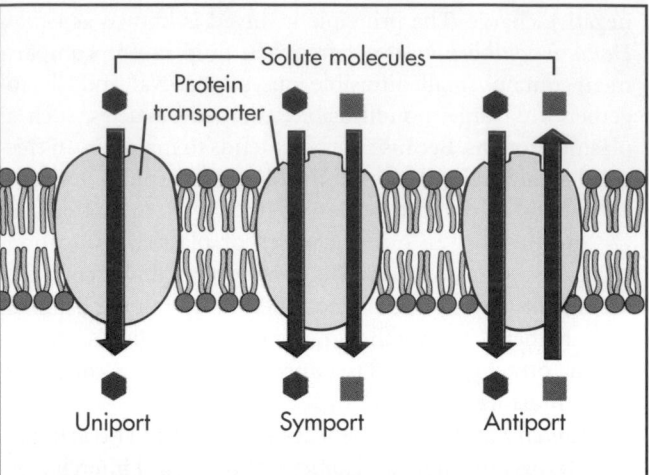

Fig. 1-16 *Mediated transport.* Simultaneous movement of a single solute molecule in one direction (uniport), of two different solute molecules in one direction (symport), and of two different solute molecules in opposite directions (antiport).

Fig. 1-17 *Active mediated transport.* Metabolic energy (ATP; P) controls the active transport of many substances, including Na^+. ATP is necessary for active mediated transport. *(Redrawn from Alberts, B. et al. [1994]. Molecular biology of the cell [3rd ed.]. New York: Garland.)*

the membrane are occupied and operating at their maximal capacity.

In *active mediated transport*, or active transport, the protein transporter moves molecules against, or up, the concentration gradient. Unlike passive mediated transport, active mediated transport requires the expenditure of energy. Many, but not all, active mediated transport systems, or pumps, have ATP as their primary energy source. Some use

the electrochemical gradient of Na^+ across the membrane (Fig. 1-17). Energy in the form of ATP, however, is required for activation of the Na^+ gradient.

A "carrier" mechanism in the plasma membrane mediates the transport of ions and nutrients. The best-known pump is the $Na^+ + K^+$–dependent ATPase pump. It continuously regulates the cells' volume by controlling leaks through pores or protein channels and maintaining the ionic

TABLE 1-4 Major Transport Systems in Mammalian Cells		
Substance Transported	Mechanism of Transport	Tissues
Sugars		
Glucose	Passive: protein channel	Most tissues
	Active: symport with Na^+	Small intestines and renal tubular cells
Fructose	Passive	Intestines and liver
Amino acids	Coupled channels	
Amino acid specific transporters	Active: symport with Na^+	Intestines, kidney, and liver
All amino acids except proline	Active: group translocation	Liver
Specific amino acids	Passive	Small intestine
Other organic molecules		
Cholic acid, deoxycholic acid, and taurocholic acid	Active: symport with Na^+	Intestines
Organic anions, e.g., malate, α-ketoglutarate, glutamate	Antiport with counter-organic anion	Mitochondria of liver cells
ATP-ADP	Antiport transport of nucleotides; can be active	Mitochondria of liver cells
Inorganic ions		
Na^+	Passive	Distal renal tubular cells
Na^+/H^+	Active: antiport, proton pump	Proximal renal tubular cells and small intestines
Na^+/K^+	Active: ATP driven, protein channel	Plasma membrane of most cells
CA^{++}	Active: ATP driven, antiport with Na^+	All cells, antiport in red cells
H^+/K^+	Active	Parietal cells of gastric cells secreting H^+
Cl^-/HCO_3^- (perhaps other anions)	Mediated: antiport	Erythrocytes and many other cells

Data from Alberts, B. et al. (1994). Molecular biology of the cell (3rd ed.). New York: Garland; Devlin, T.M. (Ed.). (1992). Textbook of biochemistry: With clinical correlations (3rd ed.). New York: Wiley; Raven, P.H., & Johnson, G.B. (1995). Understanding biology (ed. 3). Dubuque, Iowa: Brown.
NOTE: *The known transport systems are listed here; others have been proposed. Most transport systems have been studied in only a few tissues, and their sites of activity may be more limited than indicated.*

concentration gradients needed for cellular excitation and membrane conductivity (see p. 18). The maintenance of intracellular K^+ concentrations is required also for enzyme activity, including enzymes involved in protein synthesis.

Active transport of Na+ and K+

The active transport system for Na^+ and K^+ is found in virtually all mammalian cells. The Na^+, K^+ antiport system (i.e., Na^+ moving out of and K^+ moving into the cell) uses the direct energy of ATP to move these cations. The transporter protein is ATPase, which requires Na^+, K^+, and Mg^{++} ions. The concentration of ATPase in plasma membranes is directly related to Na^+, K^+ transport activity. Approximately 60% to 70% of the ATP synthesized by cells, especially muscle and nerve cells, is used to maintain the Na^+, K^+ transport system. Excitable tissues have a high concentration of Na^+, K^+ ATPase, as do other tissues that transport significant amounts of Na^+. For every ATP molecule hydrolyzed, three molecules of Na^+ are transported out of the cell, whereas only two molecules of K^+ move into the cell. The process leads to an electrical potential and is called *electrogenic*, with the inside of the cell more negative than the outside. Although the exact mechanism for this transport is uncertain,

it is possible that ATPase induces the transporter protein to undergo several conformational changes, causing Na^+ and K^+ to move short distances (see Fig. 1-17). The conformational change lowers the affinity for Na^+ and K^+ to the ATPase transporter, resulting in the release of the cations after transport.

Table 1-4 summarizes the major mechanisms of transport through pores and protein transporters in the plasma membranes. Many disease states are caused or manifested by loss of these membrane transport systems.

Transport by Vesicle Formation
Endocytosis and exocytosis

The active transport mechanisms by which the cells move large proteins, polynucleotides, or polysaccharides (macromolecules) across the plasma membrane are very different from those that mediate small solute and ion transport. Transport of macromolecules involves the sequential formation and fusion of membrane-bound vesicles.

In *endocytosis,* a section of the plasma membrane enfolds substances from outside the cell, invaginates (folds inward), and separates from the plasma membrane, forming a

Fig. 1-18 *Endocytosis and exocytosis*. A, Endocytosis and fusion with lysosome and exocytosis. **B,** Electron micrograph of exocytosis. *(B from Raven, P.H. & Johnson, G.B. [1999]. Biology [5th ed.]. New York: McGraw-Hill.)*

vesicle that moves into the cell (Fig. 1-18, *A*). Two types of endocytosis are designated based on the size of the vesicle formed. ***Pinocytosis*** (cell drinking) involves the ingestion of fluids and solute molecules through formation of small vesicles, and ***phagocytosis*** (cell eating) involves the ingestion of large particles, such as bacteria, through formation of large vesicles (vacuoles).

Because most cells continually ingest fluid and solutes by pinocytosis, the terms *pinocytosis* and *endocytosis* often are used interchangeably. In pinocytosis the vesicle containing fluids, solutes, or both fuses with a lysosome, and lysosomal enzymes digest them for use by the cell. In phagocytosis the large molecular substances are engulfed by the plasma membrane and enter the cell so that they can be isolated and destroyed by lysosomal enzymes (see Chapter 6). Substances that are not degraded by lysosomes are isolated in residual bodies and released by exocytosis. Both pinocytosis and phagocytosis require metabolic energy and often involve binding of the substance with plasma membrane receptors before membrane invagination and fusion with lysosomes in the cell.

In eukaryotic cells, secretion of macromolecules almost always occurs by ***exocytosis*** (see Fig. 1-18). Exocytosis has two main functions: (1) replacement of portions of the plasma membrane that have been removed by endocytosis and (2) release of molecules synthesized by the cells into the extracellular matrix.

Receptor-mediated endocytosis

Ligand binding to *some* plasma membrane receptors leads to clustering, aggregation, and immobilization of the receptors in specialized areas of the membrane called ***coated pits*** (Fig. 1-19). The pits, which are coated with bristlelike structures (clathrin), deepen and enfold (invaginate), internalizing ligand-receptor complexes and forming a coated vesicle. The clathrin coat or bristles may be responsible for trapping membrane receptors in coated pits. This internalization process, called ***receptor-mediated endocytosis (ligand internalization),*** is rapid and enables the cell to ingest large amounts of specific ligands without ingesting large volumes of extracellular fluid. The cellular uptake of cholesterol, for example, depends on receptor-mediated endocytosis.

Movement of Electrical Impulses: Membrane Potentials

All body cells are electrically polarized, with the inside of the cell more negatively charged than the outside. The difference in electrical charge, or voltage, is known as the ***resting membrane potential*** and is about -270 to -85 millivolts. The difference in voltage across the plasma membrane results from the differences in ionic composition of ICF and ECF. Sodium ions are more concentrated in the ECF, and potassium ions are in greater concentration in the ICF. The concentration difference is maintained by the active transport of Na^+ and K^+ (the sodium-potassium pump), which trans-

Fig. 1-19 *Ligand internalization by means of receptor-mediated endocytosis.* **A,** The ligand attaches to its surface receptor (through the bristle coat or clathrin coat) and, through receptor-mediated endocytosis, enters the cell. The ingested material fuses with a lysosome and is processed by hydrolytic lysosomal enzymes. Processed molecules can then be transferred to other cellular components. **B,** Electron micrograph of a coated pit showing different sizes of filaments of the cytoskeleton (X82,000). *(B from Erlandsen, S.L. & Magney, J.E. [1992]. Color atlas of histology. St. Louis: Mosby.)*

ports sodium outward and potassium inward (Fig. 1-20). Because the resting plasma membrane is more permeable to K$^+$ than to Na$^+$, K$^+$ diffuses easily from the ICF to the ECF. Because both sodium and potassium are cations, the net result is an excess of anions inside the cell, resulting in the resting membrane potential.

Nerve and muscle cells are excitable and can change their resting membrane potential in response to electrochemical stimuli. Changes in resting membrane potential convey messages from cell to cell. When a nerve or muscle cell receives a stimulus that exceeds the membrane threshold value, a rapid change occurs in the resting membrane potential, known as the *action potential.* The action potential carries signals along the nerve or muscle cell and conveys information from one cell to another. (Nerve impulses are described in Chapter 12.) When a resting cell is stimulated through voltage-regulated channels, the cell membranes become more permeable to sodium, so a net movement of sodium into the cell occurs and the membrane potential decreases, or "moves forward," from a negative value (in millivolts) to zero. This decrease is known as *depolarization.* The depolarized cell is more positively charged, and its polarity is neutralized.

To generate an action potential and the resulting depo-

larization, the *threshold potential* must be reached. Generally this occurs when the cell has depolarized by 15 to 20 millivolts. When the threshold is reached, the cell will continue to depolarize with no further stimulation. The sodium gates open, and sodium rushes into the cell, causing the membrane potential to reduce to zero and then become positive (depolarization). The rapid reversal in polarity results in the action potential.

During *repolarization* the negative polarity of the resting membrane potential is reestablished. As the voltage-gated sodium channels begin to close, voltage-gated potassium channels open. Membrane permeability to sodium decreases, and potassium permeability increases, so potassium ions leave the cell. The sodium gates close, and with the loss of potassium, the membrane potential becomes more negative. The Na$^+$, K$^+$ pump then returns the membrane to the resting potential by pumping potassium back into the cell and sodium out of the cell.

During most of the action potential, the plasma membrane cannot respond to an additional stimulus. This time is known as the *absolute refractory period* and is related to changes in permeability to sodium. During the latter phase of the action potential, when permeability to potassium in-

Fig. 1-20 *Sodium-potassium pump and propagation of an action potential.* **A,** Concentration difference of Na+ and K+ intracellularly and extracellularly. The direction of active transport by the sodium-potassium pump is also shown. **B,** Top diagram represents the polarized state of a neuronal membrane when at rest. The lower diagrams represent changes in sodium and potassium membrane permeabilities with depolarization and repolarization. *(From Thibodeau, G.A. & Patton, K.T. [1999]. Anatomy & physiology [4th ed.]. St. Louis: Mosby.)*

creases, a stronger-than-normal stimulus can evoke an action potential known as the *relative refractory period.*

When the membrane potential is more negative than normal, the cell is in a hyperpolarized (less excitable) state. A stronger-than-normal stimulus is then required to reach the threshold potential and generate an action potential. When the membrane potential is more positive than normal, the cell is in a hypopolarized (more excitable than normal) state and a weaker-than-normal stimulus is required to reach the threshold potential. Changes in the intracellular and extracellular concentration of ions or a change in membrane permeability can cause these alterations in membrane excitability.

✓ QUICK CHECK

Why does sodium's movement into a cell cause depolarization?

Why does potassium diffuse easily from the ICF to the ECF?

Why is it that, during most of the action potential, the plasma membrane cannot respond to an additional stimulus?

CELLULAR REPRODUCTION: THE CELL CYCLE

Cells of the human body are subject to wear and tear, and most do not last for the lifetime of the individual. In most tissues, new cells are created as fast as old cells die. Cellular reproduction is therefore necessary for the maintenance of life. Reproduction of gametes (sperm and egg cells) occurs through a process called *meiosis,* described in Chapter 2. The reproduction, or division, of other body cells (somatic cells) involves two sequential phases: *mitosis,* or nuclear division, and *cytokinesis,* or cytoplasmic division. Before a cell can divide, however, it must double its mass and duplicate all its contents. Separation for division occurs during the growth phase, called *interphase.* The alternation between mitosis and interphase in all tissues with cellular turnover is known as the *cell cycle.*

The four designated phases of the cell cycle (Fig. 1-21) are (1) the *S phase* (S = synthesis), in which DNA is synthesized in the cell nucleus; (2) the *G₂ phase* (G = gap), in which RNA and protein synthesis occurs, namely, the period between the completion of DNA synthesis and the next phase (M); (3) the *M phase* (M = mitosis), which includes both nuclear and cytoplasmic division; and (4) the *G₁ phase,*

Fig. 1-21 *Interphase and the phases of mitosis. (B from Thibodeau, G.A. & Patton K.T. [1999]. Anatomy & physiology [4th ed.]. St. Louis: Mosby.)*

which is the period between the M phase and the start of DNA synthesis.

Phases of Mitosis and Cytokinesis

Interphase (the G_1, S, and G_2 phases) is the longest phase of the cell cycle. During interphase the chromatin consists of very long, slender rods jumbled together in the nucleus. Late in interphase, strands of **chromatin** (the substance that gives the nucleus its granular appearance) begin to coil, causing shortening and thickening.

The M phase of the cell cycle, mitosis and cytokinesis, begins with **prophase,** the first appearance of chromosomes. As the phase proceeds, each chromosome is seen as two identical halves called **chromatids,** which lie together and are attached by a spindle site called a **centromere.** (The two chromatids of each chromosome, which are genetically identical, are sometimes called *sister chromatids.*) The nuclear membrane, which surrounds the nucleus, disappears. **Spindle fibers** are microtubules formed in the cytoplasm. They radiate from two centrioles located at opposite poles of the cell and pull the chromosomes to opposite sides of the cell, beginning **metaphase.** Next, the centromeres become aligned in the middle of the spindle, which is called the **equatorial plate** (or **metaphase plate**) of the cell. In this stage, chromosomes are easiest to observe microscopically, since they are highly condensed and arranged in a relatively organized fashion.

Anaphase begins when the centromeres split and the sister chromatids are pulled apart. The spindle fibers shorten,

causing the sister chromatids to be pulled, centromere first, toward opposite sides of the cell. When the sister chromatids are separated, each is considered to be a chromosome. Thus the cell has 92 chromosomes during this stage. By the end of anaphase, there are 46 chromosomes lying at each side of the cell. Barring mitotic errors, each of the two groups of 46 chromosomes is identical to the original 46 chromosomes present at the start of the cell cycle.

During **telophase,** the final stage, a new nuclear membrane is formed around each group of 46 chromosomes, the spindle fibers disappear, and the chromosomes begin to uncoil. Cytokinesis causes the cytoplasm to divide into roughly equal parts during this phase. At the end of telophase, two identical diploid cells, called **daughter cells,** have been formed from the original cell.

Rates of Cellular Division

Although the complete cell cycle lasts 12 to 24 hours, generally about 1 hour is required for the four stages of mitosis and cytokinesis. All types of cells undergo mitosis during formation of the embryo, but many adult cells, such as nerve cells, lens cells of the eye, and muscle cells, lose their ability to replicate and divide. The cells of other tissues, particularly epithelial cells (e.g., of the intestine, lung, skin), divide continuously and rapidly, completing the entire cell cycle in less than 10 hours.

The difference between cells that divide slowly and cells that divide rapidly is the length of time spent in the G_1 phase of the cell cycle. Once the S phase begins, however, progres-

TABLE 1-5	Examples of Growth Factors and Their Actions
Growth Factor	**Physiologic Actions**
Platelet-derived growth factor (PDGF)	Stimulates proliferation of connective tissue cells and neuroglial cells
Epidermal growth factor (EGF)	Stimulates proliferation of epidermal cells and other cell types
Insulin-like growth factor I (IGF-I)	Collaborates with PDGF and EGF; stimulates proliferation of fat cells and connective tissue cells
Insulin-like growth factor II (IGF-II)	Collaborates with PDGF and EGF; stimulates proliferation of fat cells and connective tissue cells
Transforming growth factor B (TGF-B; multiple subtypes)	Stimulates or inhibits response of most cells to other growth factors; regulates differentiation of some cell types (e.g., cartilage)
Fibroblast growth factor (FGF; multiple subtypes)	Stimulates proliferation of fibroblasts, endothelial cells, myoblasts, and other cell types
Interleukin-2 (IL-2)	Stimulates proliferation of T-lymphocytes
Nerve growth factor (NGF)	Promotes axon growth and survival of sympathetic and some sensory and CNS neurons
Hemopoietic cell growth factors (IL-3, GM-CSF, M-CSF, G-CSF, erythropoietin)	See Chapter 19

sion through mitosis takes a relatively constant amount of time.

The mechanisms that control cell division depend on "social control genes" and protein growth factors. Protein growth factors govern the proliferation of different cell types. Individual cells are members of a complex cellular society in which survival of the entire organism is key—not survival or proliferation of just the individual cells. When a need arises for new cells, as in repair of injured cells, previously nondividing cells must be triggered rapidly to reenter the cell cycle. With continual wear and tear, the cell birth rate and the cell death rate must be kept in balance.

Growth Factors

G*rowth factors,* also called *cytokines,* are peptides (protein fractions) that transmit signals within and between cells. They have a major role in the regulation of tissue growth and development (Table 1-5).[3] Nutrients are not enough for a cell to proliferate; it must also receive stimulatory chemical signals (growth factors) from other cells, usually its neighbors (Fig. 1-22). These signals act to overcome intracellular braking mechanisms that tend to restrain cell growth and block progress through the cell cycle (see Fig. 1-22).

An example of a brake that regulates cell proliferation is the *retinoblastoma (Rb) protein,* first identified through studies of a rare childhood eye tumor called *retinoblastoma,* in which the Rb protein is missing or defective (see p. 440). The Rb protein is abundant in the nucleus of all vertebrate cells. It binds to gene regulatory proteins, preventing them from stimulating the transcription of genes required for cell proliferation (see Fig. 1-22). Extracellular signals, such as growth factors, activate intracellular signaling pathways that inactivate the Rb protein, leading to cell proliferation.

Different types of cells require different growth factors; for example, *platelet-derived growth factor (PDGF)* stimulates the production of connective tissue cells. Table 1-5

summarizes the most significant growth factors. Recent evidence shows that some growth factors also regulate other cell processes, such as cellular differentiation. In addition to growth factors that stimulate cellular processes, there are factors that inhibit these processes; these factors are not well understood. Cells that are starved of growth factors come to a halt after mitosis and enter the *arrested (G_o) state* of the cell cycle (see p. 21 for cell cycle).[1]

TISSUES

Cells of one or more types are organized into tissues, and different types of tissues compose organs. Finally, organs are integrated to perform complex functions as tracts or systems.

All cells are in contact with a network of extracellular macromolecules known as the *extracellular matrix.* This matrix not only holds cells and tissues together but also provides an organized latticework within which cells can migrate and interact with one another.

Tissue Formation

The process by which differentiated cells create tissues and organs is called *pattern formation.*[4] To form tissues, cells must exhibit intercellular recognition and communication, adhesion, and memory. Specialized cells sense their environment through signals, such as growth factors, from other cells. This type of communication ensures that new cells are produced only when and where they are required. Different cell types have different adhesion molecules in their plasma membranes, sticking selectively to other cells of the same type. They can also adhere to extracellular matrix components. Cells have memory because of specialized patterns of gene expression evoked by signals that acted during embryonic development. Memory allows cells to autonomously preserve their distinctive character and pass it on to their progeny.[1]

Fig. 1-22 *How growth factors stimulate cell proliferation.* **A,** Resting cell. With the absence of growth factors, the retinoblastoma (Rb) protein is not phosphorylated; thus it holds the gene regulatory proteins in an inactive state. The gene regulatory proteins are required to stimulate the transcription of genes needed for cell proliferation. **B,** Proliferating cell. Growth factors bind to the cell surface receptors and activate intracellular signaling pathways leading to activation of intracellular proteins. These intracellular proteins phosphorylate and thereby inactivate the Rb protein. The gene regulatory proteins are now free to activate the transcription of genes, leading to cell proliferation. *(Modified from Alberts, B. et al. [1998]. Essential cell biology: An introduction to the molecular biology of the cell. New York: Garland.)*

Intercellular Communication

Cells in direct physical contact with neighboring cells are often linked together at specialized plasma membrane regions called *cell junctions.* Cell junctions have two main functions: (1) to hold cells together and (2) to allow small molecules to pass from cell to cell, allowing coordination of the activities of cells that form tissues.

The three main types of cell junctions are (1) desmosomes (macula adherens), (2) tight junctions (zonula occludens), and (3) gap junctions (Fig. 1-23). Together they form the *junctional complex. Desmosomes* hold cells together by forming either continuous bands or belts of epithelial sheets or buttonlike points of contact. Desmosomes also act as a system of braces to maintain structural stability. *Tight junctions* are barriers to diffusion, prevent the movement of sub-

stances through transport proteins in the plasma membrane, and prevent the leakage of small molecules between the plasma membranes of adjacent cells. *Gap junctions* are clusters of protein channels that allow small ions and molecules to pass directly from the inside of one cell to the inside of another. Cells connected by gap junctions are considered ionically (electrically) and metabolically coupled. Gap junctions coordinate the activities of adjacent cells. They are important, for example, in synchronizing contractions of heart muscle cells through ionic coupling and in permitting action potentials to spread rapidly from cell to cell in neural tissues. Why gap junctions occur in tissues that are not electrically active is unknown. Although most gap junctions are associated with junctional complexes, they sometimes exist as independent structures. Nitric oxide (NO) has recently been

Fig. 1-23 *Junctional complex.* A, Schematic drawing of a belt desmosome between epithelial cells. This junction, also called the *zonula adherens,* encircles each of the interacting cells. The spot desmosomes and hemidesmosomes, like the belt desmosomes, are adhering junctions. This tight junction is an impermeable junction that holds cells together but seals them in such a way that molecules cannot leak between them. The gap junction, as a communicating junction, mediates the passage of small molecules from one interacting cell to the other. **B,** Electron micrograph of desmosomes. *(From Raven, P.H. & Johnson, G.B. [1999]. Biology [5th ed.]. New York: McGraw-Hill.)*

implicated as an important chemical for intracellular communication in the nervous system.[5]

The junctional complex is a highly permeable part of the plasma membrane. Its permeability is controlled by a process called ***gating,*** which depends on concentrations of calcium ions in the cytoplasm. Increased cytoplasmic calcium causes decreased permeability at the junctional complex. Gating enables uninjured cells to seal themselves off from injured neighbors. Calcium is released from injured cells.

Types of Tissues

The four basic types of tissues are nerve, epithelial, connective, and muscle. The structure and function of these four types underlie the structure and function of each organ sys-

tem. Neural tissue is composed of highly specialized cells called *neurons,* which receive and transmit electrical impulses very rapidly across junctions called *synapses* (Fig. 1-24). Different types of neurons have special characteristics that depend on their distribution and function within the nervous system. Epithelial, connective, and muscle tissues are summarized in Boxes 1-1 to 1-3.

✓QUICK CHECK

Why is the cell cycle important?

Do all cells renew themselves through the cell cycle?

Why is the extracellular matrix important for tissue?

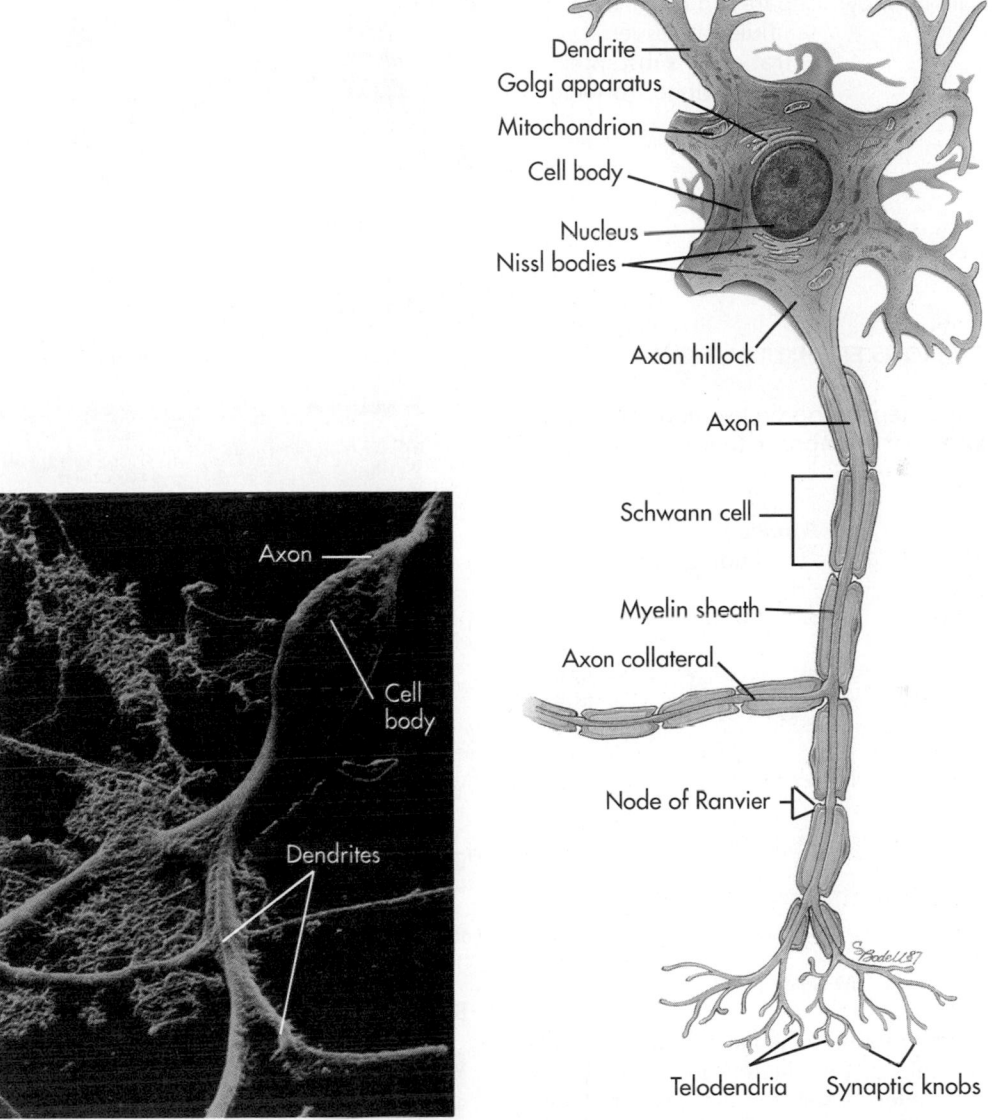

Fig. 1-24 *Typical neuron.* The axon conducts electrical signals away from the cell body. Signals are produced by a flux of ions across the neuron's plasma membrane. At the synapse, the neuron forms a specialized junction with another neuron (or with a muscle cell), across which electrochemical signals (neurotransmitters) pass. The inset is a scanning electron micrograph of a neuron. *(From Thibodeau, G.A. & Patton, K.T. [1999]. Anatomy & physiology [4th ed.]. St. Louis: Mosby.)*

SIMPLE SQUAMOUS EPITHELIUM (FIG. 1-25)

Structure
Single layer of cells

Location
Lining of blood vessels
Lining of pulmonary alve-
   oli (air sacs)
Bowman's capsule (kidney)

Function
Diffusion and filtration
Separation of blood from
   fluids in tissues
Separation of air from
   fluids in tissues
Filtration of substances
   from blood, forming
   urine

Fig. 1-25 *Simple squamous epithelial cell.* Photomicrograph of simple squamous epithelial cell in parietal wall of Bowman's capsule in kidney. *(From Erlandsen, S.L. & Magney, J.E. [1992]. Color atlas of histology. St. Louis: Mosby.)*

STRATIFIED SQUAMOUS EPITHELIUM (FIG. 1-26)

Structure
Two or more layers, depending on location, with cells
   closest to basement membrane tending to be
   cuboidal

Location
Epidermis of skin
Linings of mouth, pharynx,
   esophagus, anus,

Function
Protection and secretion

Cornified layer

Basement membrane   Basal cells   Dermis

Fig. 1-26 *Cornified stratified squamous epithelium.* Diagram of stratified squamous epithelium of the skin. *(From Thibodeau, G.A. & Patton, K.T. [1999]. Anatomy & physiology [4th ed.]. St. Louis: Mosby.)*

TRANSITIONAL EPITHELIUM (FIG. 1-27)

Structure
Vary in shape from cuboidal to squamous depending on
   whether basal cells of the bladder are columnar and
   comprise many layers; when the bladder is full and
   stretched, the cells flatten and stretch like squamous cells

Location
Linings of urinary bladder
   and other hollow structures

Function
Stretching that permits
   expansion of hollow
   organs

Binucleate cell

Stratified transitional
epithelial cells

Basement membrane   Connective tissue

Fig. 1-27 *Stratified squamous transitional epithelium.* Photomicrograph of stratified squamous transitional epithelium of the urinary bladder. *(Copyright Ed Reshke. Used with permission.)*

SIMPLE CUBOIDAL EPITHELIUM (FIG. 1-28)
Structure
Simple cuboidal cells; rarely stratified (layered)

Location	*Function*
Glands (i.e., thyroid, sweat, salivary) Parts of kidney tubule and outer covering of the ovary	Secretion

Fig. 1-28 *Simple cuboidal epithelium.* Photomicrograph of simple cuboidal epithelium of the pancreatic duct. *(From Erlandsen, S.L. & Magney, J.E. [1992]. Color atlas of histology. St. Louis: Mosby.)*

SIMPLE COLUMNAR EPITHELIUM (FIG. 1-29)
Structure
Large amounts of cytoplasm and cellular organelles

Location	*Function*
Lining of digestive tube from stomach to anus Ducts of many glands	Secretion and absorption

CILIATED SIMPLE COLUMNAR EPITHELIUM
Structure
Same as simple columnar epithelium but ciliated

Location	*Function*
Linings of bronchi of the lungs, nasal cavity, and oviducts	Secretion, absorption, and propulsion of fluids and particles

STRATIFIED COLUMNAR EPITHELIUM
Structure
Small and rounded basement membrane (columnar cells do not touch basement membrane)

Location	*Function*
Linings of epiglottis, part of pharynx, anus, and male urethra	Protection

Goblet cells

Columnar epithelial cell

A

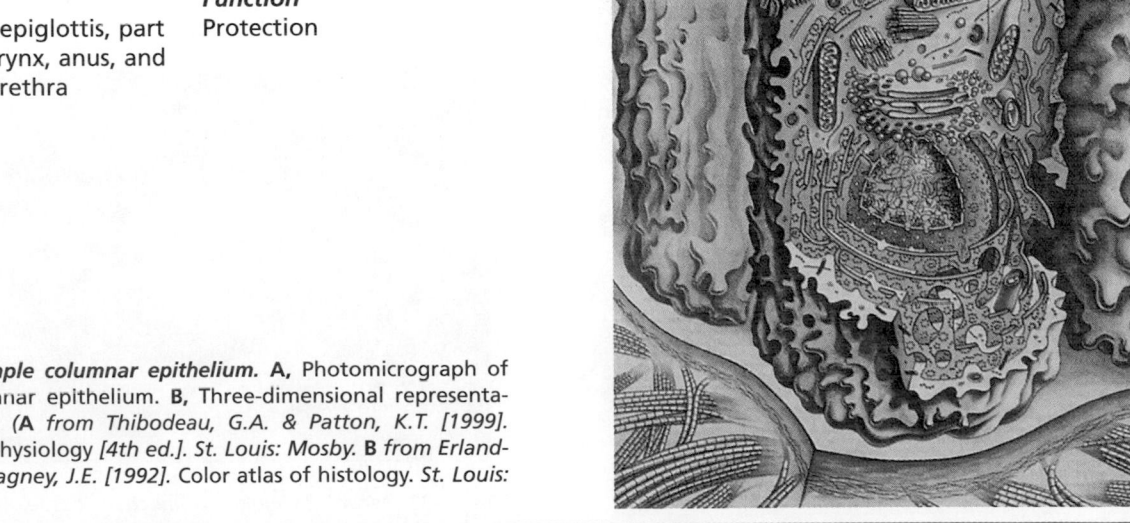

B

Fig. 1-29 *Simple columnar epithelium.* A, Photomicrograph of simple columnar epithelium. **B,** Three-dimensional representation of cells. (**A** from Thibodeau, G.A. & Patton, K.T. [1999]. Anatomy & physiology [4th ed.]. St. Louis: Mosby. **B** from Erlandsen, S.L.,& Magney, J.E. [1992]. Color atlas of histology. St. Louis: Mosby.)

Continued

PSEUDOSTRATIFIED CILIATED COLUMNAR EPITHELIUM (FIG. 1-30)

Structure

All cells in contact with basement membrane
Nuclei found at different levels within the cell, giving stratified appearance
Free surface often ciliated

Location

Linings of large ducts of some glands (parotid, salivary), male urethra, respiratory passages, and eustachian tubes of ears

Function

Transport of substances

Fig. 1-30 *Pseudostratified ciliated columnar epithelium.* Photomicrograph of pseudostratified ciliated columnar epithelium of the trachea. *(Copyright Robert L. Calentine. Used with permission.)*

Connective Tissues

BOX 1-2

LOOSE OR AREOLAR TISSUE (FIG. 1-31)

Structure

Unorganized; spaces between fibers
Most fibers collagenous, some elastic and reticular
Includes many types of cells (fibroblasts and macrophages most common) and large amount of intercellular fluid

Location and Function

Attaches skin to underlying tissue, holds organs in place by filling the spaces between them, supports blood vessels
Intercellular fluid transports nutrients and waste products
Fluid accumulation causes swelling (edema)

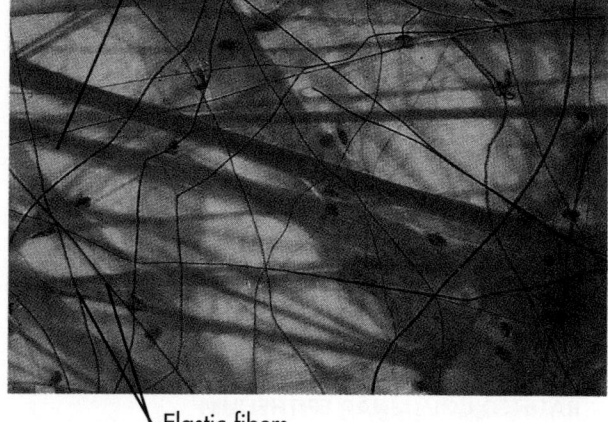

Fig. 1-31 *Loose areolar connective tissue. (From Thibodeau, G.A. & Patton, K.T. [1999]. Anatomy & physiology [4th ed.]. St. Louis: Mosby.)*

DENSE, IRREGULAR TISSUE (FIG. 1-32)

Structure

Dense, compact, and areolar tissue, with fewer cells and more, closely woven collagenous fibers than in loose tissue

Location and Function

Acts as protective barrier; dermis layer of the skin

Fig. 1-32 *Dense, irregular connective tissue. (Copyright Ed Reshke. Used with permission.)*

DENSE, REGULAR (WHITE FIBROUS) TISSUE (FIG. 1-33)
Structure
Collagenous fibers and some elastic fibers, tightly
packed into parallel bundles, with only fibroblast
cells

Location and Function
Forms strong tendons of muscle, ligaments of joints,
some fibrous membranes, and fascia that surrounds
the organs and muscles

Fibroblast   Collagenous fibers

Fig. 1-33 Dense, regular (white fibrous) connective tissue.
(Copyright Phototake. Used with permission.)

ELASTIC TISSUE (FIG. 1-34)
Structure
Elastic fibers, some collagenous fibers, fibroblasts

Location and Function
Lends strength and elasticity to walls of arteries, trachea, vocal chords, and other structures

Fig. 1-34 Elastic connective tissue. *(From Erlandsen, S.L. & Magney, J.E. [1992]. Color atlas of histology. St. Louis: Mosby.)*

ADIPOSE TISSUE (FIG. 1-35)
Structure
Fat cells dispersed in loose tissues; each cell containing
a large droplet of fat flattens nucleus and forces
cytoplasm into a ring around cell's periphery

Location and Function
Stores fat, which provides padding and protection

Storage area for fat   Plasma membrane

A   B

Nucleus of adipose cell

Fig. 1-35 Adipose tissue. A, Fat storage areas—distribution of fat in male and female bodies.
B, Photomicrograph of adipose tissue. (**A** *from Thibodeau, G.A., & Patton, K.T. [1999]. Anatomy
and Physiology [4th ed.] St. Louis: Mosby.* **B** *copyright Ed Reschke. Reprinted with permission.)*

Continued

CARTILAGE (HYALINE, ELASTIC, FIBROUS) (FIG. 1-36)
Structure
Collagenous fibers embedded in a firm matrix (chondrin); no blood supply

Location and Function
Gives form, support, and flexibility to joints, trachea, nose, ear, vertebral disks, embryonic skeleton, and many internal structures

Fig. 1-36 *Cartilage.* **A**, Hyaline cartilage. **B**, Elastic cartilage. **C**, Fibrous cartilage. (*A* and *C* copyright Robert L. Calentine; *B* copyright Ed Reshke. Used with permission.)

BONE (FIG. 1-37)
Structure
Collagenous fibers and inorganic salts called *osteoblasts*
Well supplied by blood vessels (see Chapter 36)

Location and Function
Lends skeleton rigidity and strength

SPECIAL CONNECTIVE TISSUES
• Plasma
Structure
Fluid

Location and Function
Serves as matrix for blood cells

• Macrophages in tissue, reticuloendothelia, or macrophage system
Structure
Scattered macrophages (phagocytes) called Kupffer's cells (in liver), alveolar macrophages (in lungs), microglia (in central nervous system)

Location and Function
Facilitate inflammatory response and carry out phagocytosis in loose connective, lymphatic, digestive, medullary (bone marrow), splenic, adrenal, and pituitary tissues

Fig. 1-37 *Bone.* (Copyright Phototake. Used with permission.)

SKELETAL (STRIATED) MUSCLE (FIG. 1-38)

Structure Characteristics of Cells

Long, cylindric cells that extend throughout length of
muscles

Striated myofibrils (proteins)

Many nuclei on periphery

Location
Attached to bones directly
or by tendons

Function
Voluntary movement of
skeleton; maintenance
of posture

Cross striations of muscle cell

Nuclei of muscle cell

Muscle fiber

Fig. 1-38 *Skeletal (striated) muscle. (From Thibodeau, G.A. &
Patton, K.T. [1999]. Anatomy & physiology [4th ed.] St. Louis:
Mosby.)*

CARDIAC MUSCLE (FIG. 1-39)

Structure Characteristics of Cells

Branching networks throughout muscle tissue

Striated myofibrils

Location
Cells attached end-to-end
at intercalated disks;
tissue forms walls of
heart (myocardium)

Function
Involuntary pumping ac-
tion of heart

Nucleus

Intercalated disks

Fig. 1-39 *Cardiac muscle. (Copyright Ed Reshke. Used with permission.)*

SMOOTH (VISCERAL) MUSCLE (FIG. 1-40)

Structure Characteristics of Cells

Long spindles that taper to a point

Absence of striated myofibrils

Location
Walls of hollow internal
structures, such as di-
gestive tract and blood
vessels (viscera)

Function
Voluntary and involuntary
contractions that move
substances through
hollow structures

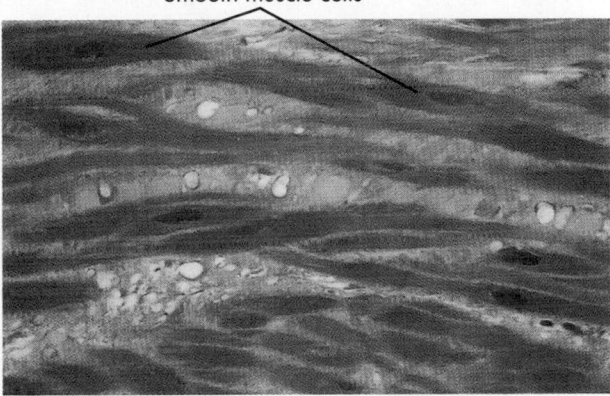

Smooth muscle cells

Fig. 1-40 *Smooth (visceral) muscle. (Copyright Phototake. Used
with permission.)*

Cellular Functions

1. Cells become specialized through the process of differentiation or maturation.

2. The seven specialized cellular functions are movement, conductivity, metabolic absorption, secretion, excretion, respiration, and reproduction.

3. The eukaryotic cell consists of three general components: the plasma membrane, the cytoplasm, and the intracellular organelles.

4. The nucleus is the largest membrane-bound organelle and is found usually in the cell's center. The chief functions of the nucleus are cell division and control of genetic information.

5. Cytoplasm, or the cytoplasmic matrix, is an aqueous solution (cytosol) that fills the space between the nucleus and the plasma membrane.

6. The organelles are suspended in the cytoplasm and are enclosed in biologic membranes.

7. The endoplasmic reticulum is a network of tubular channels (cisternae) that extend throughout the outer nuclear membrane. It specializes in the synthesis and transport of protein and lipid components of most of the organelles.

8. The Golgi complex is a network of smooth membranes and vesicles located near the nucleus. The Golgi complex is responsible for processing and packaging proteins into secretory vesicles that break away from the Golgi complex and migrate to a variety of intracellular and extracellular destinations, including the plasma membrane.

9. Lysosomes are saclike structures that originate from the Golgi complex and contain digestive enzymes. These enzymes are responsible for digesting most cellular substances down to their basic form, such as amino acids, fatty acids, and sugars.

10. Cellular injury leads to a release of the lysosomal enzymes causing cellular self-digestion.

11. Peroxisomes are similar to lysosomes but contain several enzymes that either produce or use hydrogen peroxide.

12. Mitochondria contain the metabolic machinery necessary for cellular energy metabolism. The enzymes of the respiratory chain (electron-transport chain), found in the inner membrane of the mitochondria, generate most of the cell's ATP.

13. The cytoskeleton is the "bone and muscle" of the cell. The internal skeleton is composed of a network of protein filaments, including microtubules and actin filaments (microfilaments).

14. The plasma membrane encloses the cell and, by controlling the movement of substances across it, exerts a powerful influence on metabolic pathways.

15. Protein receptors (recognition units) on the plasma membrane enable the cell to interact with other cells and with extracellular substances.

16. The plasma membrane is a bilayer of lipids (phospholipids, glycolipids) and cholesterol, which gives the membrane its structural integrity.

17. Membrane functions are determined largely by proteins. These functions include recognition by protein receptors and transport of substances into and out of the cell.

18. The fluid mosaic model accounts for the fluidity of the lipid bilayer and the flexibility, self-sealing properties, and selective impermeability of the plasma membrane.

19. Cellular receptors are protein molecules on the plasma membrane, in the cytoplasm, or in the nucleus that are capable of recognizing and binding smaller molecules, called *ligands*.

20. The dynamic nature of the fluid plasma membrane enables it to vary the number of receptors on its surface. The cell is therefore capable of "hiding" from injurious agents by altering receptor number and pattern.

21. The ligand-receptor complex initiates a series of protein interactions, causing adenylate cyclase to catalyze the transformation of cellular ATP to messenger molecules that stimulate specific responses within the cell.

Cell-to-Cell Communication

1. Cells communicate in three ways: (a) they form protein channels (gap junctions); (b) they display receptors that affect intracellular processes or other cells in direct physical contact; and (c) they secrete signals for long-distance communication.

2. Modes of chemical signaling include endocrine, paracrine, autocrine, and synaptic.

Cellular Metabolism

1. The chemical tasks of maintaining essential cellular functions are referred to as *cellular metabolism*. Anabolism is the energy-using process of metabolism, whereas catabolism is the energy-releasing process.

2. Adenosine triphosphate (ATP) functions as an energy-transferring molecule. Energy is stored by molecules of carbohydrate, lipid, and protein, which, when catabolized, transfer energy to ATP.

3. Oxidative phosphorylation occurs in the mitochondria and is the mechanism by which the energy produced from carbohydrates, fats, and proteins is transferred to ATP.

Processes of Cellular Intake and Output

1. Water and small, electrically uncharged molecules move through pores in the plasma membrane's lipid bilayer in the process called *passive transport*.

2. Passive transport does not require the expenditure of energy; rather, it is driven by the physical effects of osmosis, hydrostatic pressure, and diffusion.

3. Larger molecules and molecular complexes (e.g., ligand-receptor complexes) are moved into the cell by active transport, which requires expenditure of energy (by means of ATP) by the cell.

4. The largest molecules (macromolecules) and fluids are transported by the processes of endocytosis (ingestion) and exocytosis (expulsion).

5. Two types of solutes exist in body fluids: electrolytes and nonelectrolytes. Electrolytes are electrically charged and dissociate into constituent ions when placed in solution. Nonelectrolytes do not dissociate when placed in solution.

6. Diffusion is the passive movement of a solute from an area of higher solute concentration to an area of lower solute concentration.

7. Hydrostatic pressure is the mechanical force of water pushing against cellular membranes.

8. Osmosis is the movement of water across a semipermeable membrane from a region of lower solute concentration to a region of higher solute concentration.

9. The amount of hydrostatic pressure required to oppose the osmotic movement of water is called the *osmotic pressure of the solution.*

10. The overall osmotic effect of colloids, such as plasma proteins, is called the *oncotic pressure* or *colloid osmotic pressure.*

11. Mediated transport can be passive or active. Mediated transport includes the movement of two molecules simultaneously in one direction (symport) or in opposite directions (antiport) or the movement of a single molecule in one direction (uniport).

12. Passive mediated transport is also called *facilitated diffusion.* It does not require the expenditure of metabolic energy.

13. Active mediated transport requires metabolic energy (ATP) to move molecules against the concentration gradient.

14. Active transport occurs also by endocytosis, or vesicle formation, in which the substance to be transported is engulfed by a segment of the plasma membrane, forming a vesicle that moves into the cell.

15. Pinocytosis is a type of endocytosis in which fluids and solute molecules are ingested through formation of small vesicles.

16. Phagocytosis is a type of endocytosis in which large particles, such as bacteria, are ingested through formation of large vesicles, called *vacuoles.*

17. In receptor-mediated endocytosis, the plasma membrane receptors are clustered, along with bristlelike structures, in specialized areas called *coated pits.*

18. Endocytosis occurs when coated pits invaginate, internalizing ligand-receptor complexes in coated vesicles.

19. Inside the cell, material ingested by endocytosis is processed and digested by lysosomal enzymes.

20. All body cells are electrically polarized, with the inside of the cell more negatively charged than the outside. The difference in voltage across the plasma membrane is the resting membrane potential.

21. When an excitable (nerve or muscle) cell receives an electrochemical stimulus, cations enter the cell, causing a rapid change in the resting membrane potential known as the *action potential.* The action potential "moves" along the cell's plasma membrane and is transmitted to an adjacent cell. This is how electrochemical signals convey information from cell to cell.

Cellular Reproduction: The Cell Cycle

1. Cellular reproduction in body tissues involves mitosis (nuclear division) and cytokinesis (cytoplasmic division).

2. Only mature cells are capable of division. Maturation occurs during a stage of cellular life called *interphase (growth phase).*

3. The cell cycle is the reproductive process that begins after interphase in all tissues with cellular turnover. There are four phases of the cell cycle: (1) the S phase, during which DNA synthesis takes place in the cell nucleus; (2) the G_2 phase, the period between the completion of DNA synthesis and the next phase (M); (3) the M phase, which involves both nuclear (mitotic) and cytoplasmic (cytokinetic) division; and (4) the G_1 phase (growth phase), after which the cycle begins again.

4. The M phase (mitosis) involves four stages: prophase, metaphase, anaphase, and telophase.

5. The mechanisms that control cell division depend on "social control genes" and protein growth factors.

Tissues

1. Cells of one or more types are organized into tissues, and different types of tissues compose organs. Organs are organized to function as tracts or systems.

2. Three key factors that maintain the cellular organization of tissues are (a) recognition and cell communication, (b) selective cell-cell adhesion, and (c) wmemory.

3. Tissue cells are linked at cell junctions, which are specialized regions on their plasma membranes called *desmosomes, tight junctions,* and *gap junctions.* Cell junctions attach adjacent cells and allow small molecules to pass between them.

4. The four basic types of tissues are epithelial, muscle, nerve, and connective tissues.

5. Neural tissue is composed of highly specialized cells called *neurons* that receive and transmit electrical impulses very rapidly across junctions called *synapses.*

6. Epithelial tissue covers most internal and external surfaces of the body. The functions of epithelial tissue include protection, absorption, secretion, and excretion.

7. Connective tissue binds various tissues and organs together, supporting them in their locations and serving as storage sites for excess nutrients.

8. Muscle tissue is composed of long, thin, highly contractile cells or fibers called *myocytes.* Muscle tissue that is attached to bones enables voluntary movement. Muscle tissue in internal organs enables involuntary movement, such as the heartbeat.

KEY TERMS

Absolute refractory period, 19
Action potential, 19
Active mediated transport, 16
Active transport, 13
Amphipathic, 4
Anabolism, 10
Anaphase, 21
Anion, 13
Antiport, 15
Arrested (G_0) state, 22
Autocrine signaling, 9
Catabolism, 10
Cation, 13
Cell cycle, 20
Cell junction, 23
Cellular metabolism, 10
Cellular receptor, 8
Centromere, 21
Chemical synapse, 9
Chromatid, 21
Chromatin, 21
Citric acid cycle (Krebs cycle, tricarboxylic acid cycle), 12
Coated pit, 18
Competitive inhibitor, 15
Concentration gradient, 13
Cytokinesis, 20
Cytoplasm, 2
Cytoplasmic matrix, 2
Daughter cell, 21
Depolarization, 19
Desmosome, 23
Diffusion, 13
Digestion, 11
Effective osmolality, 14
Electrolyte, 13
Electron-transport chain, 12
Endocrine signaling, 9
Endocytosis, 17
Equatorial plate (metaphase plate), 21
Eukaryote, 2

Exocytosis, 18
Extracellular matrix, 22
Fluid mosaic model, 6
G_1 phase, 20
G_2 phase, 20
Gap junction, 23
Gating, 24
Glycolysis, 12
Glycoprotein, 6
Growth factor, 22
Hydrostatic pressure, 14
Hypertonic solution, 15
Hypotonic solution, 15
Integral membrane protein, 6
Interphase, 20
Ion, 13
Isotonic solution, 15
Junctional complex, 23
Ligand, 8
M phase, 20
Mediated transport, 15
Metabolic pathway, 10
Metaphase, 21
Mitosis, 20
Neurotransmitter, 9
Nuclear envelope, 2
Nucleolus, 2
Nucleus, 2
Oncotic pressure (colloid osmotic pressure), 15
Organelle, 2
Osmolality, 14
Osmolarity, 14
Osmosis, 14
Osmotic pressure, 14
Oxidation, 12
Oxidative phosphorylation, 12
Paracrine signaling, 9
Passive mediated transport (facilitated diffusion), 15
Passive transport, 12

Pattern formation, 22
Peripheral membrane protein, 6
Phagocytosis, 18
Pinocytosis, 18
Plasma membrane (plasmalemma), 2
Plasma membrane receptor, 8
Platelet-derived growth factor (PDGF), 22
Polarity, 13
Prokaryote, 2
Prophase, 21
Receptor protein, 9
Receptor-mediated endocytosis (ligand internalization), 18
Relative refractory period, 20
Repolarization, 19
Resting membrane potential, 18
Retinoblastoma (Rb) protein, 22
S phase, 20
Signal transduction pathway, 9
Signaling cell, 9
Solute, 13
Spindle fiber, 21
Substrate, 10
Substrate phosphorylation (anaerobic glycolysis), 12
Symport, 15
Synaptic signaling, 9
Target cell, 9
Telophase, 21
Threshold potential, 19
Tight junction, 23
Tonicity, 15
Transfer reaction, 12
Transport protein (transporter), 15
Uniport, 15
Valence, 13

REFERENCES

1. Alberts, B. et al. (1998). *Essential cell biology: An introduction to the molecular biology of the cell.* New York: Garland.
2. Catt, K.J. et al. (1979). Hormonal regulation of peptide receptors and target cell responses. *Nature, 280,* 109-116.
3. McGeachie, J. & Tennant, M. (1997). Growth factors and their implications for clinicians: A brief review. *Australian Dental Journal, 42*(6), 375-380.
4. Jorde, L.B. et al. (1999). *Medical genetics.* St. Louis: Mosby.
5. Sawada, M., Ichinose, M., & Stefano, G.B. (1997). Nitric oxide inhibits the dopamine-induced K^+ current via guanylate cyclase in Aplysia neurons. *Journal of Neuroscience Research, 50*(3), 450-456.

Genes and Genetic Diseases

Lynn B. Jorde

In the nineteenth century, microscopic studies of cells led scientists to suspect that the nucleus of the cell contained the important mechanisms of inheritance. Scientists found that chromatin, the substance that gives the nucleus a granular appearance, is observable in nondividing cells. Just before the cell divides, the chromatin condenses to form discrete, dark-staining organelles, which are called **chromosomes.** (Cell division is discussed in Chapter 1.) With the rediscovery of Mendel's important breeding experiments at the turn of the twentieth century, it soon became apparent that the chromosomes contained **genes,** the basic units of inheritance.

The primary constituent of chromatin is **deoxyribonucleic acid (DNA).** Genes are composed of sequences of DNA. By serving as the blueprints of proteins in the body, genes ultimately influence all aspects of body structure and function. Structural genes dictate the makeup of proteins. Estimates suggest that there are approximately 50,000 to 100,000 structural genes. An error in one of these genes often leads to a recognizable genetic disease.

To date, more than 9000 genetic conditions have been identified and cataloged. As infectious diseases come under increasingly effective control, the proportion of beds in pediatric hospitals occupied by children with genetic diseases has risen. In addition, many common diseases that primarily affect adults, such as hypertension, coronary heart disease, diabetes, and cancer, are now known to have important genetic components.

Great progress is being made in the diagnosis of genetic diseases and the understanding of genetic mechanisms underlying them. With the huge strides being made in molecular genetics, "gene therapy"—the insertion of normal genes to correct genetic disease—has begun.

CHAPTER OUTLINE

DNA, RNA, AND PROTEINS: HEREDITY AT THE MOLECULAR LEVEL

Definitions

Composition and structure of DNA

Genes are composed of DNA, which has three basic components: the pentose sugar molecule, deoxyribose; a phosphate molecule; and four types of nitrogenous bases. Two of the bases, *cytosine* and *thymine,* are single carbon-nitrogen rings called *pyrimidines.* The other two bases, *adenine* and *guanine,* are double carbon-nitrogen rings called *purines.* The four bases are commonly represented by their first letters: A, C, T, and G.

Watson and Crick demonstrated how these molecules are physically assembled together as DNA, proposing the *double-helix* model, in which DNA appears like a twisted ladder with chemical bonds as its rungs (Fig. 2-1). The two sides of the ladder are composed of the sugar and phosphate molecules, held together by strong phosphodiester bonds. Projecting from each side of the ladder, at regular intervals, are the nitrogenous bases. The base projecting from one side is bound to the base projecting from the other by a weak hydrogen bond. Therefore the nitrogenous bases form the rungs of the ladder; adenine pairs with thymine, and guanine pairs with cytosine. Each DNA subunit—consisting of one deoxyribose molecule, one phosphate group, and one base—is called a *nucleotide.*

DNA as the genetic code

DNA can direct the synthesis of all the body's proteins. Proteins are composed of one or more *polypeptides,* which are in turn composed of sequences of *amino acids.* The body contains 20 different types of amino acids, with 20 possible amino acids and only four possible bases. To specify 20 different amino acids with only four bases, different combinations of bases, occurring in groups of three, are used. These triplets of bases are known as *codons.*

The genetic code is universal: *all* living organisms use precisely the same DNA codes to specify proteins except mitochondria, cytoplasmic organelles where cellular respiration takes place (see Chapter 1), which have their own extranuclear DNA. Several codons of mitochondrial DNA code for amino acids that differ from those of the same nuclear DNA codons.

Replication of DNA

DNA replication consists of breaking the weak hydrogen bonds between the bases, leaving a single strand with each

Fig. 2-1 *Watson-Crick model of the DNA molecule.* The DNA structure illustrated here is based on that published by James Watson *(photograph, left)* and Francis Crick *(photograph, right)* in 1953. Note that each side of the DNA molecule consists of alternating sugar and phosphate groups. Each sugar group is united to the sugar group opposite it by a pair of nitrogenous bases (adenine-thymine or cytosine-guanine). The sequence of these pairs constitutes a genetic code that determines the structure and function of a cell. *(From Thibodeau, G.A. & Patton, K.T. [1999]. Anatomy & physiology [4th ed.]. St. Louis: Mosby.)*

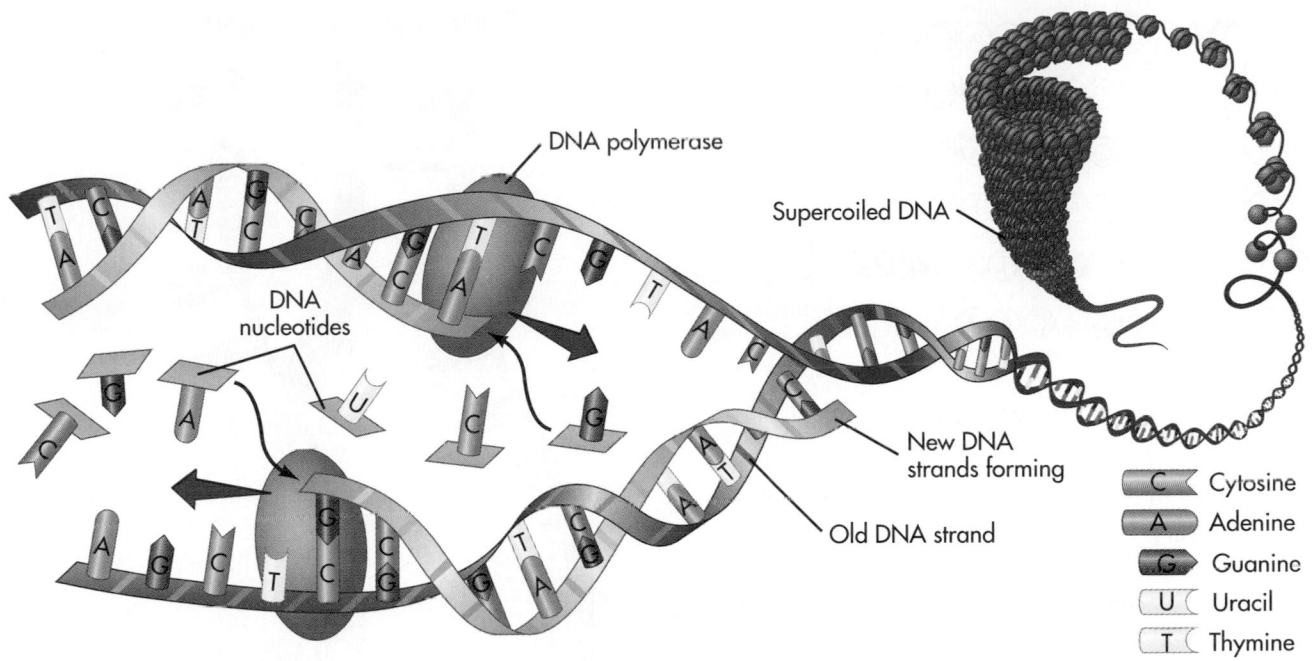

Fig. 2-2 *Replication of DNA.* The two chains of the double helix separate, and each chain serves as the template for a new complementary chain. *(From Thibodeau, G.A. & Patton, K.T. [1999]. Anatomy & physiology [4th ed.]. St. Louis: Mosby.)*

base unpaired. The consistent pairing of adenine with thymine and of guanine with cytosine, known as ***complementary base pairing,*** is the key to accurate replication. The unpaired base attracts a free nucleotide only if the nucleotide has the proper complementary base. When replication is complete, a new double-stranded molecule identical to the original is formed (Fig. 2-2). The single strand is said to be a ***template,*** or molecule on which a complementary molecule is built, and is the basis for synthesizing the new double strand.

Several different proteins are involved in DNA replication. The most important of these proteins is an enzyme known as ***DNA polymerase.*** This enzyme travels along the single DNA strand, adding the correct nucleotides to the free end of the new strand and checking to make sure that its base is actually complementary to the template base. This mechanism of DNA proofreading substantially enhances the accuracy of DNA replication.

Mutation

A ***mutation*** is any inherited alteration of genetic material. Mutations may cause disease or be subtle ***silent substitutions*** that do not change amino acids. One type of mutation is the ***base pair substitution,*** where one base pair is replaced by another.

The ***frameshift mutation*** involves the insertion or deletion of one or more base pairs of the DNA molecule. As Fig. 2-3 shows, these mutations can change the entire "reading frame" of the DNA sequence, greatly altering the amino acid sequence.

Agents known as ***mutagens*** increase the frequency of mutations. Examples include radiation and chemicals such as nitrogen mustard, vinyl chloride, alkylating agents, formaldehyde, and sodium nitrite.

Mutations are rare events. The rate of ***spontaneous mutations*** (those occurring in the absence of exposure to known mutagens) in humans is about 10^{-4} to 10^{-7} per gene per generation. This rate varies from one gene to another. Some chromosome regions have particularly high mutation rates and are known as ***mutational hot spots.***

From Genes to Proteins

DNA is formed and replicated in the cell nucleus, but protein synthesis takes place in the cytoplasm. The DNA code is transported from nucleus to cytoplasm, and subsequent protein is formed through two basic processes: transcription and translation. These processes are mediated by ***ribonucleic acid (RNA),*** which is chemically very similar to DNA except that the sugar molecule is ribose rather than deoxyribose, and uracil rather than thymine is one of the four bases. The other bases of RNA, as in DNA, are adenine, cytosine, and guanine. Uracil is structurally very similar to thymine, so it also can pair with adenine. Whereas DNA usually occurs as a double strand, RNA usually occurs as a single strand.

Transcription

In ***transcription,*** RNA is synthesized from a DNA template, forming ***messenger RNA (mRNA). RNA polymerase*** binds to a ***promoter site,*** a sequence of DNA that specifies the beginning of a gene. RNA polymerase then separates a portion of the DNA, exposing unattached DNA bases. One DNA strand then provides the template for the sequence of mRNA nucleotides.

Fig. 2-3 *Different kinds of mutations.* C, Cytosine; A, adenine; T, thymine; G, guanine.

The sequence of bases in the mRNA is thus complementary to the template strand, and except for the presence of uracil instead of thymine, the mRNA sequence is identical to the other DNA strand. Transcription continues until a *termination sequence* is reached. Then the RNA polymerase detaches from the DNA, and the transcribed mRNA is freed to move out of the nucleus and into the cytoplasm (Fig. 2-4).

Gene splicing

When the mRNA is first transcribed from the DNA template, it reflects exactly the base sequence of the DNA and is called *heterogeneous nuclear RNA (hnRNA).* In eukaryotes, many RNA sequences are removed by nuclear enzymes and the remaining sequences are spliced together to form the functional mRNA that migrates to the cytoplasm. The excised sequences are called *introns,* and the sequences that are left to code for proteins are called *exons.*

Translation

In *translation,* RNA directs the synthesis of a polypeptide (Fig. 2-5), interacting with *transfer RNA (tRNA),* a cloverleaf-shaped strand of about 80 nucleotides. The tRNA molecule has a site where an amino acid attaches. The three-nucleotide sequence at the opposite side of the cloverleaf is called the *anticodon.* It undergoes complementary base pairing with an appropriate codon in the mRNA, which specifies the sequence of amino acids through tRNA.

The site of actual protein synthesis is the *ribosome,* which consists of roughly equal parts of protein and *ribosomal RNA (rRNA).* During translation, the ribosome first binds to an initiation site on the mRNA sequence and then binds to its surface, so that base pairing can occur between tRNA and mRNA. The ribosome then moves along the mRNA sequence, processing each codon and translating an amino acid by the interaction of mRNA and tRNA.

Fig. 2-4 *General scheme of RNA transcription.* (See text for explanation.) *(From Thibodeau, G.A. & Patton, K.T. [1999]. Anatomy & physiology [4th ed.]. St. Louis: Mosby.)*

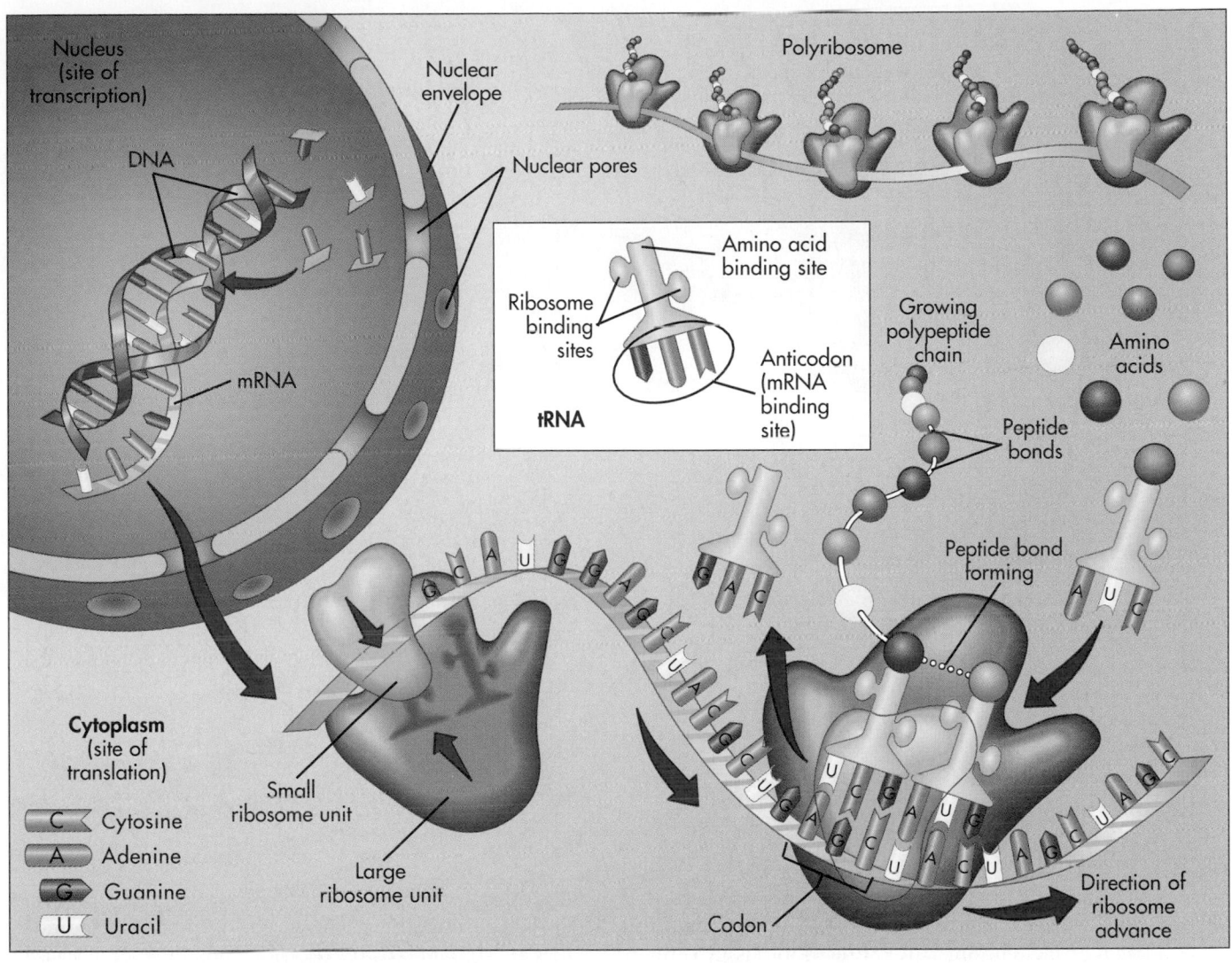

Fig. 2-5 *Protein synthesis.* (*From Thibodeau, G.A. & Patton, K.T. [1999].* Anatomy & physiology *[4th ed.]. St. Louis: Mosby.)*

The ribosome provides an enzyme that catalyzes the formation of covalent peptide bonds between the adjacent amino acids, resulting in a growing polypeptide. When the ribosome arrives at a termination signal on the mRNA sequence, translation and polypeptide formation cease; the mRNA, ribosome, and polypeptide separate from one another; and the polypeptide is released into the cytoplasm to perform its required function.

CHROMOSOMES

Human cells can be categorized into *gametes* (sperm and egg cells) and *somatic cells,* which include all cells other than gametes. Each somatic cell nucleus has 46 chromosomes in 23 pairs (Fig. 2-6). These are *diploid cells,* and the individual's father and mother each donate one chromosome per pair. New somatic cells are formed through *mitosis* and *cytokinesis.* Gametes are *haploid cells:* they have only one member of each chromosome pair, for a total of 23 chromo-

somes. Haploid cells are formed from diploid cells by *meiosis* (Fig. 2-7).

In 22 of the 23 chromosome pairs, the two members of each pair are virtually identical in microscopic appearance; thus they are *homologous.* These 22 chromosome pairs are homologous in both males and females and are termed *autosomes.* The remaining pair of chromosomes, the *sex chromosomes,* consists of two homologous X chromosomes in females and a nonhomologous pair, X and Y, in males.

Fig. 2-8, *A,* illustrates a *metaphase spread,* which is a photograph of the chromosomes as they appear in the nucleus of a somatic cell during metaphase. (Chromosomes are easiest to visualize during this stage of mitosis.) In Fig. 2-8, *B,* the chromosomes are cut out and arranged according to size, with the homologous chromosomes paired together. The 22 autosomes are numbered according to length, with chromosome number 1 the longest and chromosome 22 the shortest. A *karyotype* is an ordered display of chromosomes. Some natural variation in relative chromosome length can

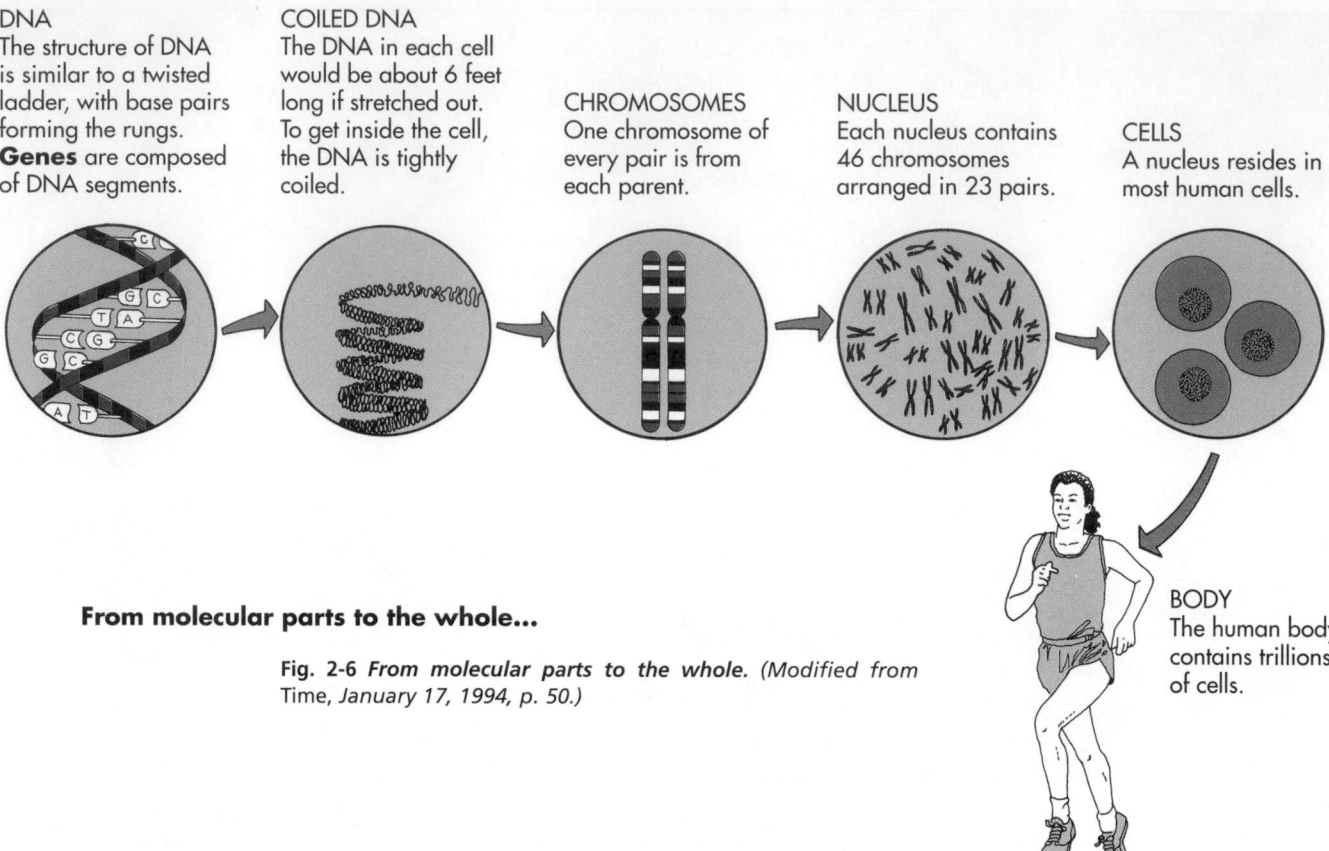

DNA
The structure of DNA is similar to a twisted ladder, with base pairs forming the rungs. **Genes** are composed of DNA segments.

COILED DNA
The DNA in each cell would be about 6 feet long if stretched out. To get inside the cell, the DNA is tightly coiled.

CHROMOSOMES
One chromosome of every pair is from each parent.

NUCLEUS
Each nucleus contains 46 chromosomes arranged in 23 pairs.

CELLS
A nucleus resides in most human cells.

BODY
The human body contains trillions of cells.

From molecular parts to the whole...

Fig. 2-6 *From molecular parts to the whole.* (Modified from Time, *January 17, 1994, p. 50.*)

be expected from person to person, so it is not always possible to distinguish each chromosome by its length. Therefore the position of the centromere also is used to classify chromosomes (Fig. 2-9).

The chromosomes in Fig. 2-8 were stained with Giemsa stain, resulting in distinctive **chromosome bands.** These form various patterns in the different chromosomes so that each chromosome can be distinguished easily. Using banding techniques, researchers can number chromosomes and study individual variations. Missing or duplicated portions of chromosomes, which often result in serious diseases, also are readily identified. More recently, techniques have been devised that permit each chromosome to be visualized with a different color.

Chromosome Aberrations and Associated Diseases

Chromosome abnormalities are the leading known cause of mental retardation and miscarriage. Estimates indicate that a major chromosome aberration occurs in at least 1 in 12 conceptions. Most of these fetuses do not survive to term; about 50% of all recovered first-trimester spontaneous abortuses have major chromosome aberrations.[1] The number of live births affected by these abnormalities is, however, significant; about 1 in 150 has a major diagnosable chromosome abnormality.[1]

Polyploidy

Cells with a multiple of the normal number of chromosomes are **euploid cells** (Greek *eu* = good or true). Because normal gametes are haploid and most normal somatic cells are diploid, they are both euploid forms. When a euploid cell has more than the diploid number of chromosomes, it is said to be a **polyploid cell.** Several types of body tissues, including some liver, bronchial, and epithelial tissues, are normally polyploid. A zygote having three copies of each chromosome, rather than the usual two, has a form of polyploidy called **triploidy. Tetraploidy,** a condition in which euploid cells have 92 chromosomes, has been observed also. Both of these conditions are incompatible with postnatal survival. Nearly all triploid fetuses are spontaneously aborted or stillborn. The prevalence of triploidy among live births is approximately 1:10,000. Tetraploidy has been found primarily in early abortuses, although occasionally, affected infants have been born alive. Like triploid infants, however, they do not survive. Triploidy and tetraploidy are relatively common conditions, accounting for approximately 10% of all known miscarriages.[2]

Aneuploidy

A somatic cell that does not contain a multiple of 23 chromosomes is an **aneuploid cell.** A cell containing three copies of one chromosome is said to be trisomic (a condition

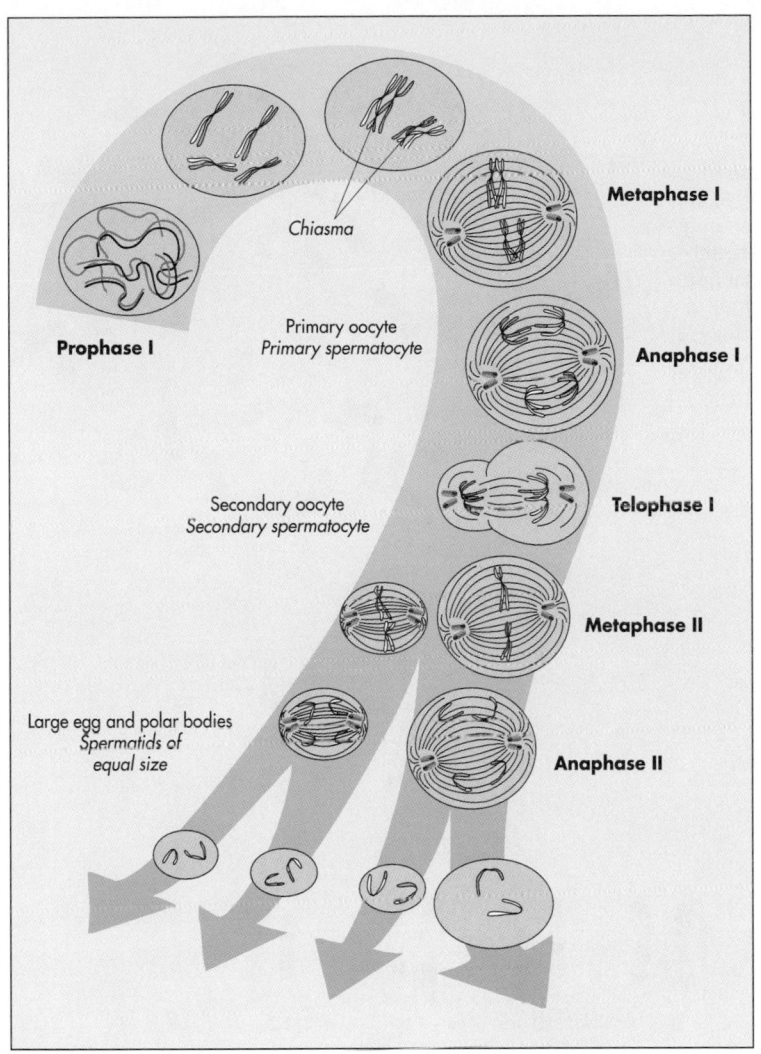

Fig. 2-7 *Phases of meiosis. (From Jorde, L.B. et al. [1999]. Medical genetics [2nd ed.]. St. Louis: Mosby.)*

termed *trisomy*) and is aneuploid. *Monosomy,* the presence of only one copy of a given chromosome in a diploid cell, is the other common form of aneuploidy. Among the autosomes, monosomy of any chromosome is lethal, but newborns with trisomy of some chromosomes can survive. This difference illustrates an important principle: *in general, loss of chromosome material has more serious consequences than duplication of chromosome material.*

Aneuploidy of the sex chromosomes is less serious than that of the autosomes. Very little genetic material seems to be located on the Y chromosome. For the X chromosome, inactivation of extra chromosomes (see p. 53) largely diminishes their effect. A zygote bearing *no* X chromosome, however, will not survive.

Aneuploidy is usually the result of *nondisjunction,* an error in which homologous chromosomes or sister chromatids fail to separate normally during meiosis or mitosis (Fig. 2-10). Nondisjunction during either stage of meiosis produces some gametes that have two copies of a given chromosome and others that have no copies of the chromosome. When such gametes unite with normal haploid gametes, the resulting zygote is monosomic or trisomic for that chromosome. Occasionally, a cell can be monosomic or trisomic for more than one chromosome.

Autosomal aneuploidy

Trisomy can occur for any chromosome, but the only forms seen with an appreciable frequency in live births are trisomies of the thirteenth, eighteenth, or twenty-first chromosomes. Fetuses with most other chromosomal trisomies do not survive to term. Trisomy 16, for example, is the most common trisomy among abortuses, but it is not seen in live births.[3]

Partial trisomy, in which only an extra portion of a chromosome is present in each cell, can occur also. The consequences of partial trisomies are not as severe as those of complete trisomies. Trisomies may occur in only some cells of the body. Individuals thus affected are said to be *chromosomal mosaics,* meaning that the body has two or more different cell lines, each of which has a different karyotype. Mosaics are often formed by early mitotic nondisjunction occurring in one embryo cell but not in others.

Fig. 2-8 *Karyotype of chromosomes.* A, G-banded metaphase of a normal cell showing the bands of all normal chromosomes. **B,** G-banded karyotype of a normal female cell showing the banding patterns of the various chromosomes. Identical patterns character-ize homologous chromosomes. The chromosomes are arranged from largest to smallest in size. *(From Damjanov, I. & Linder, J. [1996]. Anderson's pathology [10th ed., vol. 1]. St. Louis: Mosby.)*

A

B

The best-known example of aneuploidy in an autosome is trisomy of the twenty-first chromosome, which causes **Down syndrome** (named after J. Langdon Down, who first described the disease in 1866). Down syndrome is seen in approximately 1 in 1000 live births[4]; its principal features are shown and outlined in Fig. 2-11 and Table 2-1.

The risk of having a child with Down syndrome in-creases greatly with maternal age. As Fig. 2-12 demonstrates, women younger than 30 years have a risk ranging from about 1 in 1000 births to 1 in 2000 births. The risk begins to rise substantially after 35 years of age, and it reaches 3% to 5% for women older than 45 years. This dramatic increase in risk may be caused by the age of maternal egg cells, which are held in an arrested state of prophase I from the time they are formed in the female embryo until they are shed in ovula-tion. Thus an egg cell formed by a 45-year-old woman is it-self 45 years old. This long suspended state may allow defects to accumulate, leading to nondisjunction. The risk of Down syndrome, as well as other trisomies, does not increase with paternal age.[4]

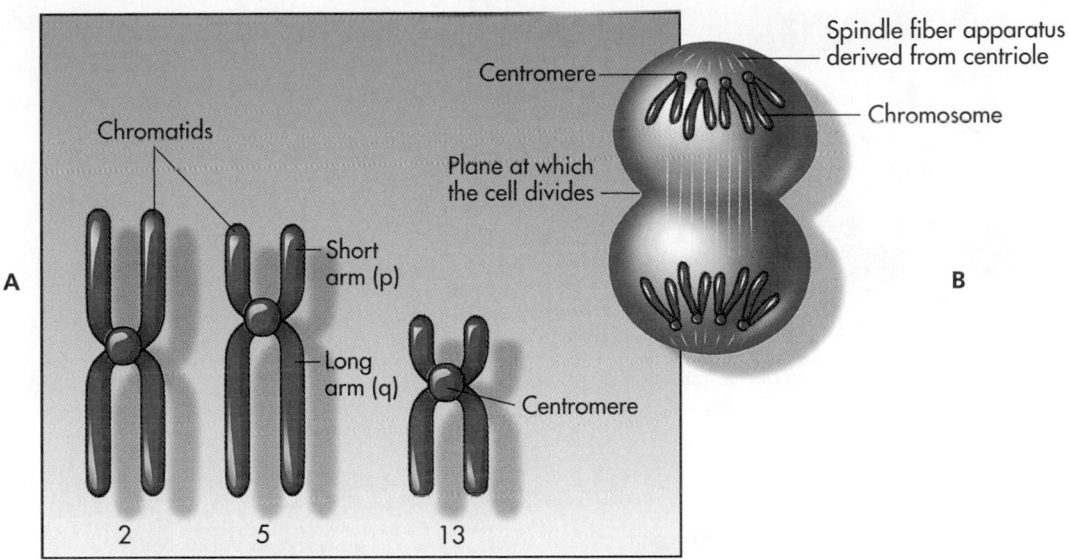

Fig. 2-9 *Structure of chromosomes.* **A,** Human chromosomes 2, 5, and 13. Each is replicated and consists of two chromatids. Chromosome 2 is a metacentric chromosome because the centromere is close to the middle; chromosome 5 is submetacentric because the centromere is set off from the middle; chromosome 13 is acrocentric because the centromere is at or very near the end. **B,** During mitosis the centromere divides and the chromosomes move to opposite poles of the cell. At the time of centromere division, the chromatids are designated as chromosomes.

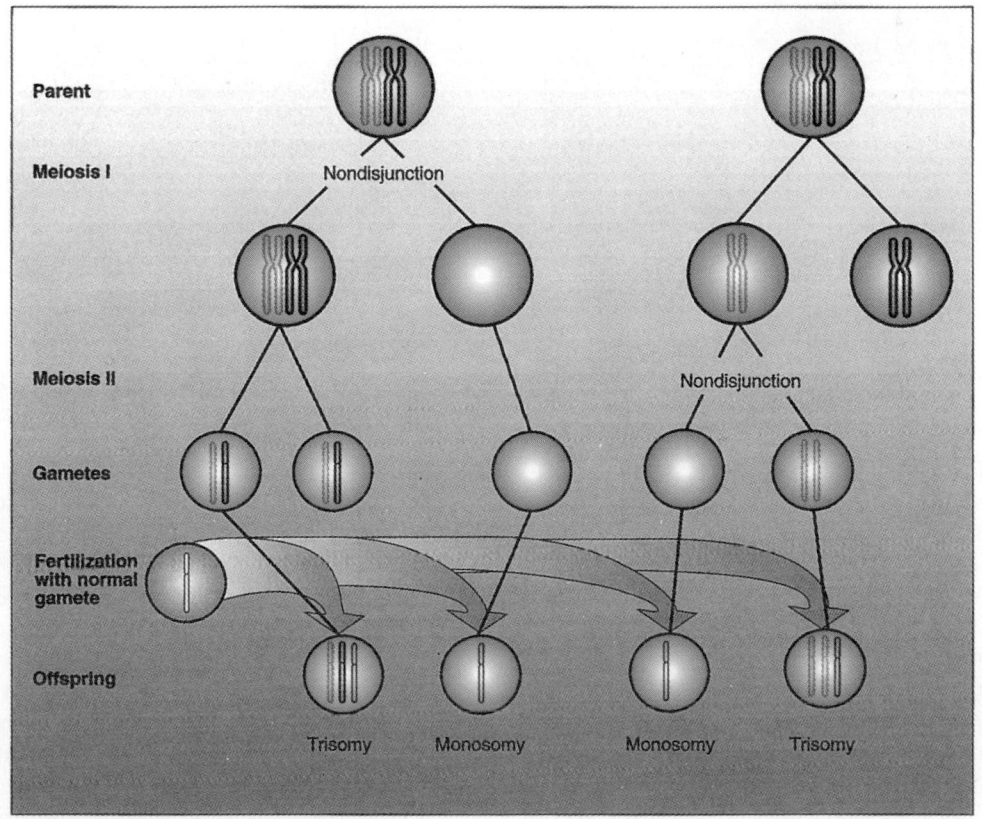

Fig. 2-10 *Nondisjunction.* Causes aneuploidy when chromosomes or sister chromatids fail to divide properly. *(From Jorde, L.B. et al. [1999]. Medical genetics [2nd ed.]. St. Louis: Mosby.)*

Fig. 2-11 *Patient with Down syndrome. (Courtesy Drs. A. Olney and M. MacDonald, University of Nebraska Medical Center, Omaha.)*

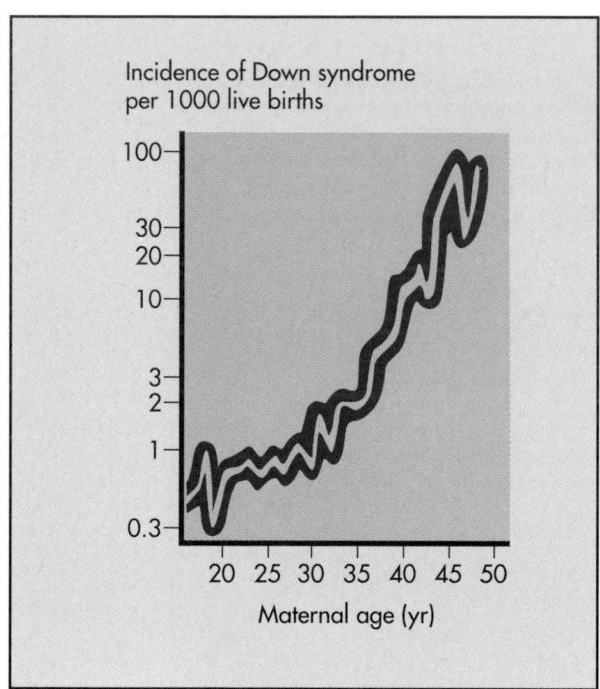

Fig. 2-12 *Down syndrome increases with maternal age.* Rate is per 1000 live births related to maternal age.

Fig. 2-13 *Turner syndrome.* A sex chromosome is missing, and the person's chromosomes are 45,X. Characteristic signs are short stature, female genitalia, webbed neck, shieldlike chest with underdeveloped breasts and widely spaced nipples, and imperfectly developed ovaries. *(From Thibodeau, G.A. & Patton, K.T. [1999].* Anatomy & physiology *[4th ed.]. St. Louis: Mosby.)*

generally have more severe mental retardation and various physical defects.

A condition that leads to somewhat more serious problems is the presence of a single X chromosome and no homologous X or Y chromosome, so that the individual has a total of 45 chromosomes. The karyotype is usually designated 45,X, and it causes a set of symptoms known as *Turner syndrome* (Fig. 2-13; Table 2-1).

Individuals with at least two X chromosomes and one Y chromosome in each cell (47,XXY karyotype) have a disorder known as *Klinefelter syndrome* (Fig. 2-14; Table 2-1).

Abnormalities of chromosome structure

In addition to the loss or gain of whole chromosomes, parts of chromosomes can be lost or duplicated as gametes are formed and the arrangement of genes on chromosomes can be altered. Unlike aneuploidy and polyploidy, these changes sometimes do not have serious consequences for an individual's health. Some of them can even go entirely unnoticed, especially when very small pieces of chromosomes are involved. Nevertheless, abnormalities of chromosome structure can also produce serious disease in individuals or their offspring.

During meiosis and mitosis, chromosomes usually maintain their structural integrity but *chromosome breakage* occasionally occurs. Mechanisms exist to "heal" these breaks and usually repair them perfectly with no damage to

Sex chromosome aneuploidy

The incidence of sex chromosome aneuploidies is fairly high. Among live births, about 1 in 500 males and 1 in 900 females has a form of sex chromosome aneuploidy.[5] Because these conditions are generally less severe than autosomal aneuploidies, all forms except complete absence of an X chromosome allow at least some individuals to survive.

One of the most common sex chromosome aneuploidies, affecting about 1 in 1000 newborn females, is trisomy X. Instead of two X chromosomes, these females have three X chromosomes in each cell. Most of them have no overt physical abnormalities, although sterility, menstrual irregularity, or mental retardation is sometimes seen. Some females have four X chromosomes, and they are more often mentally retarded. Those with five or more X chromosomes

TABLE 2-1	Characteristics of Various Chromosome Disorders	
Disease/Disorder	**Features**	

Down syndrome
Trisomy of chromosome 21

IQ	Usually range from 20-50 (mental retardation)
Male/female findings	Virtually all males are sterile; some females can reproduce
Face	Distinctive: low nasal bridge, epicanthal folds, protruding tongue, low-set ears
Musculoskeletal system	Poor muscle tone (hypotonia), short stature
Systemic disorders	Congenital heart disease (one half to one third of cases), reduced ability to fight respiratory infections, increased susceptibility to leukemia—overall reduced survival rate; by age 40 yr usually develop symptoms similar to those of Alzheimer disease
Mortality	About three fourths of fetuses with Down syndrome abort spontaneously or are stillborn; 20% of infants die before age 10 yr; those who live beyond 10 yr have life expectancy of about 60 yr.
Causative factors	97% caused by nondisjunction during formation of one of parent's gametes or during early embryonic development; 3% result from translocations; in 95% of cases, nondisjunction occurs when mother's egg cell is formed; rest involve paternal nondisjunction; 1% are mosaics—these have a large number of normal cells, and the effects of the trisomic cells are attenuated and symptoms generally less severe

Turner syndrome
(45,X) Monosomy of the X chromosome

IQ	Not considered retarded, although some impairment of spatial and mathematical reasoning ability is found
Male/female findings	Found only in females
Musculoskeletal system	Short stature common, characteristic webbing of the neck, widely spaced nipples, reduced carrying angle at the elbow
Systemic disorders	Coarctation (narrowing) of the aorta, edema of the feet in newborns, usually sterile and have gonadal streaks rather than ovaries; streaks are sometimes susceptible to cancer
Mortality	About 15%-20% of spontaneous abortions with chromosome abnormalities have this karyotype, most common single-chromosome aberration; highly lethal during gestation, only about 0.5% of these conceptions survive to term
Causative factors	Three fourths inherit X chromosome from mother, thus caused by meiotic error in the father; frequency low compared with other sex chromosome aneuploidies (1:5000 newborn females); half have simple monosomy of X chromosome; rest have more complex abnormalities; combinations of 45,X cells with XX, XX, or XY cells common

Klinefelter syndrome
(47,XXY)

IQ	Moderate degree of mental impairment may be present
Male/female findings	Have a male appearance but usually sterile; half develop femalelike breasts (gynecomastia); occurs in 1:1000 male births
Face	Voice somewhat high-pitched
Systemic disorders	Sparse body hair, sterile, testicles small
Causative factors	Half of cases the result of nondisjunction of X chromosomes in mother, frequency rises with increasing maternal age; also involves XXXY and XXXXY karyotypes with degree of physical and mental impairment increasing with each added X chromosome; mosaicism fairly common with most prevalent combination with XXY and XY cells

the daughter cell. However, some breaks remain or heal in a way that alters the chromosome's structure. The extent of chromosome breakage is increased when harmful agents called *clastogens,* such as ionizing radiation, viral infections, or chemicals, are present.

Deletions

Broken chromosomes and lost DNA cause *deletions* (Fig. 2-15). Usually, a gamete with a deletion unites with a normal gamete to form a zygote. The zygote thus has one chromosome with the normal complement of genes and one with some missing genes. Because many genes can be lost in a deletion, serious consequences result even with one normal chromosome. The most often cited example of a disease caused by a chromosomal deletion is the *cri du chat syndrome* (Fig. 2-16). The term literally means "cry of the cat" and describes the characteristic cry of the affected child. Other symptoms include low birth weight, severe mental re-

Fig. 2-14 *Klinefelter syndrome.* This young man exhibits many characteristics of Klinefelter syndrome: small testes, some development of the breasts, sparse body hair, and long limbs. This syndrome results from the presence of two or more X chromosomes with one Y chromosome (genotypes XXY or XXXY, for example). *(From Thibodeau, G.A. & Patton, K.T. [1999].* Anatomy & physiology *[4th ed.]. St. Louis: Mosby.)*

tardation, microcephaly (smaller than normal head size), heart defects, and the typical facial appearance shown in Fig. 2-16. The disease is caused by a deletion of part of the short arm of chromosome 5.

Duplications

A deficiency of genetic material is more harmful than an excess, so **duplications** usually have less serious consequences than deletions. For example, a deletion of a region of chromosome 5 causes cri du chat syndrome but a duplication of the same region causes mental retardation but less serious physical defects.

Inversions

An **inversion** occurs when two breaks take place on a chromosome, followed by the reinsertion of the missing fragment at its original site but in inverted order. Therefore a chromosome symbolized as ABCDEFG might become ABEDCFG after an inversion.

Unlike deletions and duplications, no loss or gain of genetic material occurs, so inversions are "balanced" alterations of chromosome structure and they often have no apparent physical effect. Some genes are influenced by neighboring genes, however, and this **position effect,** a

change in a gene's expression caused by its position, sometimes results in physical defects in these persons.

Inversions can cause serious problems in the offspring of individuals carrying the inversion because the inversion can lead to duplications and deletions in the chromosomes transmitted to the offspring.

Translocations

The interchange of genetic material between nonhomologous chromosomes is called **translocation.** A **reciprocal translocation** occurs when breaks take place in two different chromosomes and the material is exchanged (Fig. 2-17, *A*). As with inversions, the carrier of a reciprocal translocation is usually normal but his or her offspring can have duplications and deletions.

A second, and clinically more important, type of translocation is **robertsonian translocation.** In this disorder, the long arms of two nonhomologous chromosomes fuse at the centromere, forming a single chromosome. Robertsonian translocations are confined to chromosomes 13, 14, 15, 21, and 22 because the short arms of these chromosomes are very small and contain no essential genetic material. The short arms are usually lost during subsequent cell divisions. Because the carriers of robertsonian translocations lose no important genetic material, they are normal, although they have only 45 chromosomes in each cell. Their offspring, however, may have serious monosomies or trisomies. For example, a common robertsonian translocation involves the fusion of the long arms of chromosomes 21 and 14. An offspring who inherits a gamete carrying the fused chromosome can receive an extra copy of the long arm of chromosome 21 and develop Down syndrome. Robertsonian translocations are responsible for approximately 3% to 5% of Down syndrome cases. Parents who carry a robertsonian translocation involving chromosome 21 have an increased risk for producing multiple offspring with Down syndrome.

Fragile sites

A number of areas on chromosomes develop distinctive breaks and gaps (observable microscopically) when the cells are cultured. Most of these **fragile sites** do not appear related to disease. However, one fragile site, located on the long arm of the X chromosome, is associated with *fragile X syndrome.* The most important feature of this syndrome is mental retardation. With a relatively high population prevalence (affecting approximately 1 in 1500 males and 1 in 2500 females), the fragile X syndrome is the second most common genetic cause of mental retardation (after Down syndrome).

In fragile X syndrome, females who inherit the mutation do not necessarily express the disease condition but they can pass it on to descendants who do express it. Ordinarily, a male who inherits a disease gene on the X chromosome expresses the condition, since he has only one X chromosome. Another uncommon feature of this disease is that about one third of carrier females are affected, although less severely than males. Recently, unaffected transmitting males have been shown to have more than about 50 repeated DNA se-

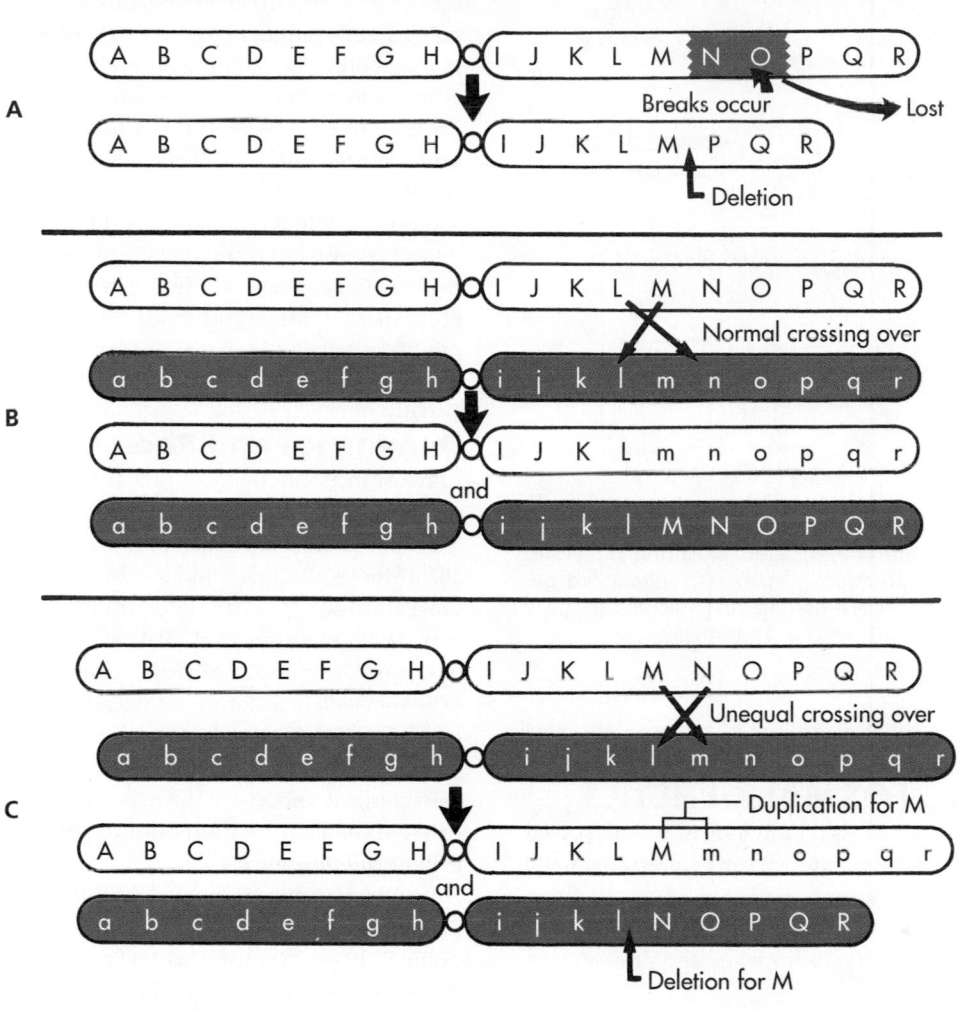

Fig. 2-15 *Abnormalities of chromosome structure.* **A,** Deletion occurs when a chromosome segment is lost. **B,** Normal crossing over. **C,** The generation of duplication and deletion through unequal crossing over.

quences near the beginning of the fragile X gene. These "repeats" consist of CGG sequences duplicated again and again. Affected males have 120 or more.[6] Increased numbers of these repeated sequences in successive generations can lead to expression of the fragile X syndrome. Several other genetic diseases also are caused by this mechanism.[7]

✓QUICK CHECK

Why is mRNA so important in the process of translation?

Define the terms *homologous, autosomes,* and *sex chromosomes.*

Why does an increase in maternal age increase the risk of Down syndrome?

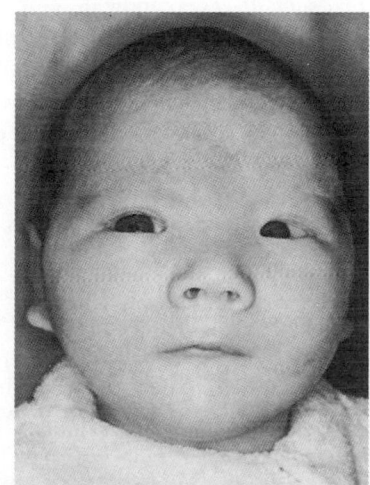

Fig. 2-16 *Infant with cri du chat syndrome.* Caused by deletion of part of the short arm of chromosome 5. *(From Thompson, M.W., McInnes, R.R., & Willard, H.F. [1991]. Genetics in medicine [5th ed.]. Philadelphia: Saunders.)*

Fig. 2-17 *Normal and chromosome translocation.* **A,** Normal chromosomes and reciprocal translocation. **B,** Pairing at meiosis. **C,** Consequences of translocation in gametes; unbalanced gametes result in zygotes that are partially trisomic and partially monosomic and consequently develop abnormally.

ELEMENTS OF FORMAL GENETICS

The mechanisms by which an individual's set of paired chromosomes produces traits are the principles of genetic inheritance. Mendel's work with garden peas first defined these principles. Later geneticists have refined Mendel's work to explain patterns of inheritance for traits and diseases that appear in families.

Analysis of traits that occur with defined, predictable patterns has helped geneticists link the pieces of the human gene map. Current research focuses on assigning genes to specific locations on chromosomes. Eventually, diseases and defects caused by single genes can be traced and therapies to prevent and treat such diseases can be developed.

Traits caused by single genes are called mendelian traits (after Gregor Mendel). Each gene occupies a position along a chromosome known as a *locus.* The genes at a particular locus can take different forms (i.e., they can be composed of different nucleotide sequences), called *alleles.* A locus that has two or more alleles that each occur with an appreciable frequency in a population is said to be *polymorphic* or a *polymorphism.*

Because humans are diploid organisms, each chromosome is represented twice, with one member of the chromosome pair contributed by the father and one by the mother. At a given locus, an individual has one gene whose origin is paternal and one whose origin is maternal. When the two genes are identical, the individual is *homozygous* at that locus. When the genes are not identical, the individual is *heterozygous* at that locus.

Phenotype and Genotype

The composition of genes at a given locus is known as the *genotype.* The outward appearance of an individual, which

is the result of both genotype and environment, is the *phenotype.* For example, an infant who is born with an inability to metabolize the amino acid phenylalanine has the single-gene disorder known as phenylketonuria (PKU) and thus has the PKU genotype. If the condition is left untreated, abnormal metabolites of phenylalanine will begin to accumulate in the infant's brain and irreversible mental retardation will occur. Mental retardation is thus one aspect of the PKU phenotype. By imposing dietary restrictions to exclude food that contains phenylalanine, however, retardation can be prevented. Although the child still has the PKU genotype, a modification of the environment (in this case the child's diet) produces an outwardly normal phenotype.

Dominance and Recessiveness

In many loci, the effects of one allele mask those of another when the two are found together in a *heterozygote.* The allele whose effects are observable is said to be *dominant.* The allele whose effects are hidden is said to be *recessive* (from the Latin root for "hiding"). Traditionally, for loci having two alleles, the dominant allele is denoted by an uppercase letter and the recessive allele is denoted by a lowercase letter. When one allele is dominant over another, the heterozygote genotype *Aa* has the same phenotype as the dominant homozygote *AA.* For the recessive allele to be expressed, it must exist in the *homozygote* form, *aa.* When the heterozygote is distinguishable from both homozygotes, the locus is said to exhibit *codominance.*

A *carrier* is an individual who has a disease gene but is phenotypically normal. Many genes for a recessive disease occur in heterozygotes who carry one copy of the gene but do not express the disease. Because recessive genes can be lethal in the homozygous state, they are eliminated from the population when they occur in homozygotes. By "hiding" in carriers, however, recessive genes for diseases are passed on to the next generation.

TRANSMISSION OF GENETIC DISEASES

The pattern in which a genetic disease is inherited through generations is termed the *mode of inheritance.* Knowing the mode of inheritance can reveal much about the disease gene itself, and reliable genetic counseling can be given to members of families with the disease.

Modes of inheritance were systematically studied by Gregor Mendel, who formulated two basic laws of inheritance. His *principle of segregation* states that homologous genes separate from one another during reproduction and that each reproductive cell carries only one homologous gene. Mendel's second law, the *principle of independent assortment,* states that the hereditary transmission of one gene does not affect the transmission of another. Mendel discovered these laws in the mid−nineteenth century by performing breeding experiments with garden peas, even though he had no knowledge of chromosomes. Early twentieth century geneticists found that chromosomal behavior essentially corresponds to Mendel's laws, which now form the basis for the ***chromosome theory of inheritance.***

The known single-gene diseases can be classified into four major modes of inheritance: autosomal dominant, autosomal recessive, X-linked dominant, and X-linked recessive. The first two types involve genes known to occur on the 22 pairs of autosomes. The last two types occur on the X chromosome; very few disease genes occur on the Y chromosome.

The ***pedigree*** chart summarizes family relationships and shows which members of a family are affected by a genetic disease (Fig. 2-18). Generally, the pedigree begins with one individual in the family, the ***proband,*** also termed the ***propositus*** (male) or ***proposita*** (female). This individual is usually the first person in the family diagnosed or seen in a clinic.

Autosomal Dominant Inheritance
Characteristics of pedigrees

Diseases caused by autosomal dominant genes are rare, with the most common occurring in fewer than 1 in 500 individuals. Therefore it is uncommon for two individuals both affected by the same autosomal dominant disease to produce offspring together. Fig. 2-19, *A,* illustrates this unusual pattern. Affected offspring are usually produced by the union of a normal parent with an affected heterozygous parent. The Punnett square in Fig. 2-19, *B,* illustrates this mating. The affected parent can pass either a disease gene or a normal gene to the next generation. On average, half the children will be heterozygous and will express the disease, and half will be normal.

The pedigree in Fig. 2-20, *A,* shows the transmission of an autosomal dominant gene. Several important characteristics of this pedigree support the conclusion that the trait is caused by an autosomal dominant gene:

1. The two sexes exhibit the trait in approximately equal proportions, and males and females are equally likely to transmit the trait to their offspring.
2. No generations are skipped. If an individual has the trait, one parent must also have it. If neither parent has the trait, none of the children has it (with the exception of new mutations, as discussed later).
3. Affected heterozygous individuals transmit the trait to approximately half their children, and because gamete transmission is subject to chance fluctuations, all or none of the children of an affected parent may have the trait. When large numbers of matings of this type are studied, however, the proportion of affected children closely approaches one half.

Recurrence risks

Parents at risk for producing children with a genetic disease nearly always ask the question, "What is the *chance* that our child will have this disease?" When one child has already been born with a genetic disease, the parents can be given a ***recurrence risk,*** which is the probability that subsequent children will also have the disease. If the parents have not yet

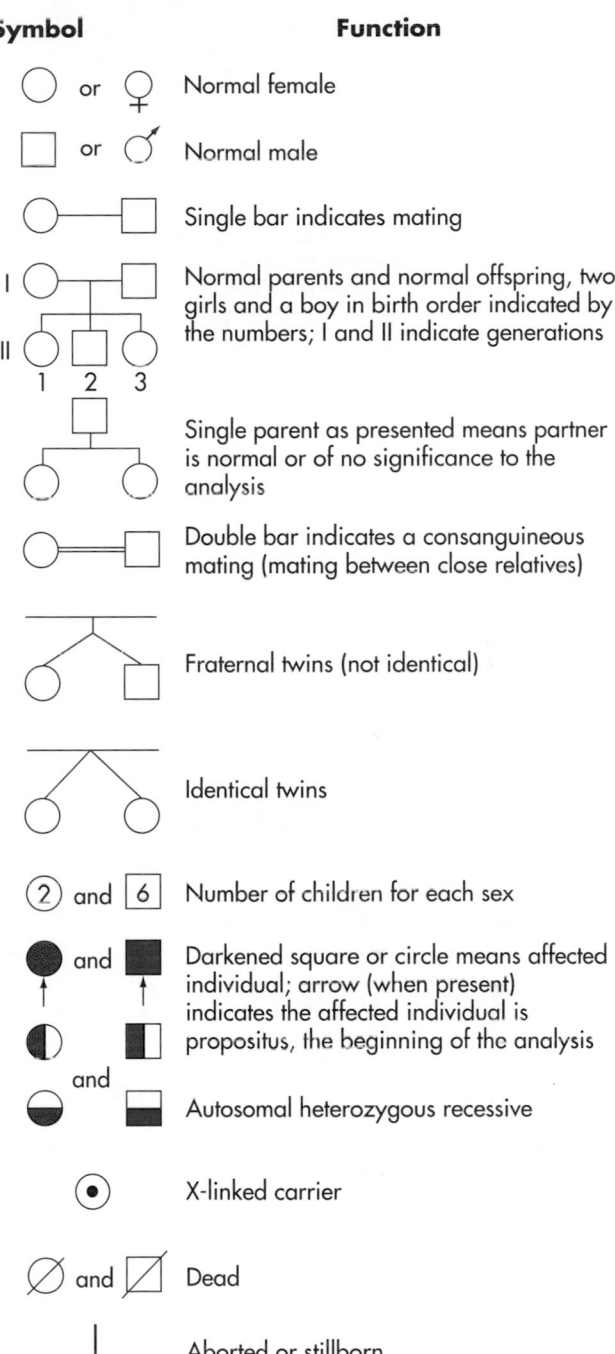

Symbol		Function
○ or ♀		Normal female
□ or ♂		Normal male
○—□		Single bar indicates mating
		Normal parents and normal offspring, two girls and a boy in birth order indicated by the numbers; I and II indicate generations
		Single parent as presented means partner is normal or of no significance to the analysis
○═□		Double bar indicates a consanguineous mating (mating between close relatives)
		Fraternal twins (not identical)
		Identical twins
② and 6		Number of children for each sex
● and ■		Darkened square or circle means affected individual; arrow (when present) indicates the affected individual is propositus, the beginning of the analysis
◐ and ◧	and	Autosomal heterozygous recessive
⊙		X-linked carrier
⊘ and ⊠		Dead
		Aborted or stillborn

Fig. 2-18 *Symbols commonly used in pedigrees.*

had children but are known to be at risk for having children with a genetic disease, an ***occurrence risk*** (the probability that a child will have a specific disease) can be given. When one parent is affected by an autosomal dominant disease (and is a heterozygote) and the other is normal, the occurrence and recurrence risks for each child are one half.

An important principle is that each birth is an independent event, much like a coin toss. Thus even though parents may have already had a child with the disease, their recurrence risk remains one half. Even if they have had several children, all affected (or all unaffected) by the disease, the law of independence dictates that the probability that their

Affected parent

	D	d
D	DD Homozygous affected (usually rare)	Dd Heterozygous affected
d	Dd Heterozygous affected	dd Homozygous normal

Affected parent (left side label) — **A**

Normal parent

	d	d
D	Dd Heterozygous affected	Dd Heterozygous affected
d	dd Homozygous normal	dd Homozygous normal

Affected parent (left side label) — **B**

Fig. 2-19 *Punnett square and autosomal dominant traits.* **A,** Punnett square for the mating of two individuals with an autosomal dominant gene. Here both parents are affected by the trait. **B,** Punnett square for the mating of a normal individual with a carrier for an autosomal dominant gene.

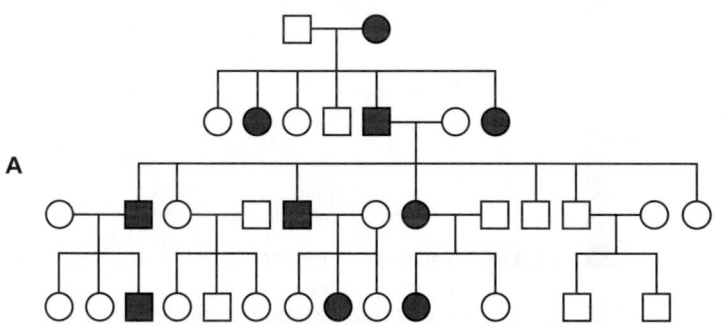

A

Fig. 2-20 *Pedigree for achondroplasia.* **A,** Pedigree showing the transmission of an autosomal dominant disease. **B,** Achondroplasia, an autosomal dominant disorder. *(**B** from McKusick, V.A. [1994]. Mendelian inheritance in man [11th ed.]. Baltimore: Johns Hopkins University Press.)*

B

next child will have the disease is still one half. Parents' misunderstanding of this principle is a common problem encountered in genetic counseling.

If a child is born with an autosomal dominant disease and there is no history of the disease in the family, the child is probably the product of a new mutation. The gene transmitted by one of the parents has thus undergone a mutation from a normal to a disease-causing allele. The genes at this locus in most of the parent's other germ cells are still normal. In this situation the recurrence risk for the parent's subsequent offspring is not greater than that of the general population. The offspring of the affected child, however, will have an occurrence risk of one half. Because these diseases often reduce the potential for reproduction, many autosomal dominant diseases result from new mutations.

Occasionally, two or more offspring have symptoms of an autosomal dominant disease when there is no family history of the disease. Because mutation is a rare event, it is unlikely that this disease would be a result of multiple mutations in the same family. The mechanism most likely responsible is termed **germline mosaicism.** During the embryonic development of one of the parents, a mutation occurred that affected all or part of the germline but few or none of the somatic cells of the embryo. Thus the parent carries the mutation in his or her germline but does not actually express the disease. As a result, the unaffected parent can transmit the mutation to multiple offspring. This phenomenon, although relatively rare, can have significant effects on recurrence risks.[8]

Delayed age of onset

One of the best-known autosomal dominant diseases is Huntington disease, a neurologic disorder whose main features are progressive dementia and increasingly uncontrollable limb movements (chorea; discussed further in Chapter 15). A key feature of this disease is its *delayed age of onset:* symptoms are not seen usually until 40 years of age or later. Thus those who develop the disease often have had children before they are aware that they have the gene. If the disease were present at birth, nearly all affected persons would die before reaching reproductive age and the occurrence of the gene in the population would be much lower. An individual whose parent has the disease has a 50% chance of developing it during middle age. He or she is thus confronted with a torturous question: Should I have children, knowing that there is a 50:50 chance that I may have this disease gene and pass it to half of my children? A DNA test is now used to determine whether an individual has inherited the mutation that causes Huntington disease.

Penetrance and expressivity

The *penetrance* of a trait is the percentage of individuals with a specific genotype who also exhibit the expected phenotype. Incomplete penetrance means that individuals who have the gene for a disease may not exhibit the disease phenotype at all, even though the gene and the associated disease may be transmitted to the next generation. A pedigree illustrating the transmission of an autosomal dominant gene with incomplete penetrance is given in Fig. 2-21. Retinoblastoma, the most common malignant eye tumor affecting children, typically exhibits incomplete penetrance. About 10% of the individuals who are *obligate carriers* of the gene (i.e., those who have an affected parent and affected children and therefore must themselves carry the gene) do not have the disease. The penetrance of the gene is then said to be 90%.

The gene responsible for retinoblastoma has been mapped to the long arm of chromosome 13, and its DNA sequence has been studied extensively. This gene is known as a *tumor-suppressor gene:* the normal function of its protein product is to regulate the cell cycle so that cells do not grow uncontrollably. When the protein is altered, its tumor-suppressing capacity is lost and a tumor can form[15] (see Chapters 9 and 15).

Expressivity is the extent of variation in phenotype associated with a particular genotype. If the expressivity of a disease is variable, penetrance may be complete but the severity of the disease can vary greatly. The best-known example of variable expressivity in an autosomal dominant disease is type 1 neurofibromatosis, or von Recklinghausen disease. The gene that causes neurofibromatosis has been mapped to the long arm of chromosome 17, and studies of its DNA sequence indicate that, like the retinoblastoma gene, it is a tumor-suppressor gene.[9] The expression of this gene varies from a few harmless café-au-lait (light brown) spots on the skin to numerous neurofibromas, scoliosis, seizures, gliomas, neuromas, hypertension, and mental retardation (Fig. 2-22).

A parent with mild expression of the disease can un-

Fig. 2-21 *Pedigree for retinoblastoma showing incomplete penetrance.* Female with marked arrow in line II must be heterozygous, but she does not express the trait.

Fig. 2-22 *Neurofibromatosis.* **A,** Young adult with multiple dermal neurofibromas of the trunk. Note also a café-au-lait spot in the right upper abdomen. **B,** Patient has large plexiform neurofibroma hanging from lower right back, causing considerable inconvenience and discomfort (substantially improved by surgical removal of tumor). *(From Jorde, L.B. et al. [2nd ed.]. St. Louis: Mosby. B courtesy Dr. D. Viskochil, University of Utah Health Sciences Center.)*

Fig. 2-23 *Pedigree for cystic fibrosis.*

	D	d
D	DD Homozygous normal	Dd Heterozygous carrier
d	Dd Heterozygous carrier	dd Homozygous affected

Fig. 2-24 *Punnett square for the mating of heterozygous carriers typical of most cases of recessive disease.*

knowingly transmit the gene to a child, who may exhibit severe expression of the disease. Variable expressivity provides a mechanism by which autosomal dominant genes can be maintained at higher prevalence rates in populations.

Several factors cause variable expressivity. Genes at other loci sometimes modify the expression of a disease gene. Environmental factors can influence expression of a disease gene. Finally, different mutations at a locus can cause variation in severity. For example, a (not defined) mutation that alters only one amino acid usually produces a mild form of hemophilia A, whereas a "stop" codon (premature termination of translation) usually produces a more severe form of this clotting disorder.

Genomic imprinting

Mendel's work with garden peas established that the phenotype is the same whether a given allele is inherited from the mother or the father. Recently, however, this principle has been shown not always to hold. For example, when a deletion on the long arm of chromosome 15 (15q11-q13) is inherited from the father, the offspring manifest a disease known as *Prader-Willi syndrome* (short stature, obesity, hypogonadism). When the deleted chromosome is inherited from the mother, the offspring develop Angelman syndrome (mental retardation, seizures, ataxic gait). Yet the deletions inherited from the father and the mother are usually cytogenetically indistinguishable. This indicates that different genes are active (imprinted) in the maternal and paternal copies of this region of chromosome 15.

Autosomal Recessive Inheritance
Characteristics of pedigrees

Like autosomal dominant diseases, diseases caused by autosomal recessive genes are rare in populations, although there can be numerous carriers. The most common lethal recessive disease in white children, cystic fibrosis, occurs in about 1 in 2000 births. Approximately 1 in 23 whites carries one copy of the gene for cystic fibrosis (see Chapter 27). Carriers are phenotypically normal. Some autosomal recessive diseases are characterized by delayed age of onset, incomplete penetrance, and variable expressivity.

Fig. 2-23 shows a pedigree for cystic fibrosis. The cystic

fibrosis gene, which has been mapped to the long arm of chromosome 7, encodes a chloride ion channel in some epithelial cells. Defective transport of chloride ions leads to a salt imbalance that results in secretions of abnormally thick, dehydrated mucus. Some digestive organs, particularly the pancreas, become obstructed, causing malnutrition, and the lungs become clogged with mucus, making them highly susceptible to bacterial infections. Death from lung disease or heart failure occurs before 30 years of age in about one half of persons with cystic fibrosis.

The important criteria for discerning autosomal recessive inheritance include the following:
1. Males and females are affected in equal proportions.
2. Consanguinity (marriage between related individuals) is sometimes present.
3. The disease is seen in siblings but usually not in their parents.
4. On average, one fourth of the offspring of carrier parents will be affected.

Recurrence risks

In most cases of recessive disease, both of the parents of affected individuals are heterozygous carriers. On average, one fourth of their offspring will be normal homozygotes, one half will be phenotypically normal carrier heterozygotes, and one fourth will be homozygotes with the disease (Fig. 2-24). Thus the recurrence risk for the offspring of carrier parents is 25%. However, in any given family, there are chance fluctuations.

If two parents have a recessive disease, they each must be homozygous for the disease. Therefore all their children also must be affected. This distinguishes recessive from dominant inheritance because two parents both affected by a dominant gene are nearly always both heterozygotes and thus one fourth of their children will be unaffected.

Because carrier parents usually are unaware that they both carry the same recessive gene, they often produce an affected child before knowing of their condition. Increasingly, *carrier detection tests* are used to identify heterozygotes by measuring the reduced amount of a critical enzyme. This enzyme is totally lacking in a homozygous recessive individual, but an essentially normal phenotype is seen in the carrier. Often carriers can also be detected by direct examination of the disease locus for a mutation. Some recessive diseases for which carrier detection tests are now available are PKU, sickle cell disease, cystic fibrosis, Tay-Sachs disease, hemochromatosis, and galactosemia.

Consanguinity

Consanguinity and *inbreeding* are related concepts. *Consanguinity* refers to the mating of two related individuals, and the offspring of such matings are said to be *inbred*. Consanguinity is sometimes an important characteristic of pedigrees for recessive diseases because relatives share a certain proportion of genes received from a common ancestor. The proportion of shared genes depends on the closeness of their biologic relationship. Consanguineous matings produce a significant increase in recessive disorders and are seen most frequently in pedigrees for rare recessive disorders.

X-linked Inheritance

Some genetic conditions are caused by genes located on the sex chromosomes, and that mode of inheritance is termed *sex-linked*. Only a few diseases are known to be inherited as X-linked dominant or Y chromosome traits, so only the much more common X-linked recessive diseases are discussed here.

Because females receive two X chromosomes, one from the father and one from the mother, they can be homozygous for a disease allele at a given locus, homozygous for the normal allele at the locus, or heterozygous. Males, having only one X chromosome, are *hemizygous* for genes on this chromosome. If a male inherits a recessive disease gene on the X chromosome, he will be affected by the disease because the Y chromosome does not carry a normal allele to counteract the effects of the disease gene. Because a single copy of an X-linked recessive gene will cause disease in a male, whereas two copies are required for disease expression in females, males more frequently are affected by X-linked recessive diseases than are females.

X inactivation

In the late 1950s Mary Lyon proposed that one X chromosome in the somatic cells of females is permanently inactivated, a process termed **X inactivation**.[10,11] This proposal, the Lyon hypothesis, explains why most gene products coded by the X chromosome are present in equal amounts in males and females, even though males have only one X chromosome and females have two X chromosomes. This phenomenon is called *dosage compensation*. The inactivated X chromosomes are observable in many interphase cells as highly condensed intranuclear chromatin bodies, termed *Barr bodies* (after Barr and Bertram, who discovered them in the late 1940s). Normal females have one Barr body in each somatic cell, whereas normal males have no Barr bodies.

Inactivation occurs very early in embryonic development—approximately 7 to 14 days after fertilization. In each somatic cell one of the two X chromosomes is inactivated. In some cells the inactivated X chromosome is contributed by the father; in other cells it is contributed by the mother. Once the X chromosome has been inactivated in a

cell, all the descendants of that cell have the same chromosome inactivated. Thus inactivation is said to be *random* but *fixed*.

Some individuals do not have the normal number of X chromosomes in their somatic cells. For example, males with Klinefelter syndrome typically have two X chromosomes and one Y chromosome. These males do have one Barr body in each cell. Females whose cell nuclei have three X chromosomes have two Barr bodies in each cell, and females whose cell nuclei have four X chromosomes have three Barr bodies in each cell. Females with Turner syndrome have only one X chromosome and no Barr bodies. Thus the number of Barr bodies is always one less than the number of X chromosomes in the cell. All but one X chromosome are always inactivated.

Persons with abnormal numbers of X chromosomes, such as those with Turner syndrome or Klinefelter syndrome, are not physically normal. This situation presents a puzzle because they presumably have only one active X chromosome, just as individuals with normal numbers of chromosomes do. This is probably because the distal part of the short arm of the X chromosome, as well as several other regions on the chromosome arm, is not inactivated. Thus X inactivation is also known to be *incomplete*.

Methylation of X chromosome DNA, a process in which DNA is inactivated when cytosine bases are enzymatically converted to 5-methylcytosine, appears to be involved in X inactivation. Inactive X chromosomes can be at least partially reactivated in vitro by administering 5-azacytidine, a demethylating agent.

Sex determination

The process of sexual differentiation, in which the embryonic gonads become either testes or ovaries, begins during the sixth week of gestation. A key principle of sex determination in the human is that one copy of the Y chromosome is sufficient to initiate the process of gonadal differentiation that produces a male fetus. The number of X chromosomes does not alter this process. For example, an individual with two X chromosomes and one Y chromosome in each cell is still phenotypically a male. Thus the Y chromosome must contain a gene that begins the process of male gonadal development.

This gene, termed *SRY* (for "sex-determining region on the Y"), has been located on the short arm of the Y chromosome.[12] The *SRY* gene lies just outside the *pseudoautosomal* region (Fig. 2-25), which pairs with the distal tip of the short arm of the X chromosome during meiosis and exchanges genetic material with it (crossover), just as autosomes do. The DNA sequences of these regions on the X and Y chromosomes are highly similar. The rest of the X and Y chromosomes, however, do not exchange material and are not similar in DNA sequence.

Other genes that contribute to male differentiation are located on other chromosomes. Thus *SRY* appears to trigger the action of genes on other chromosomes. This concept is supported by the fact that the *SRY* protein product is similar to other proteins known to regulate gene expression.

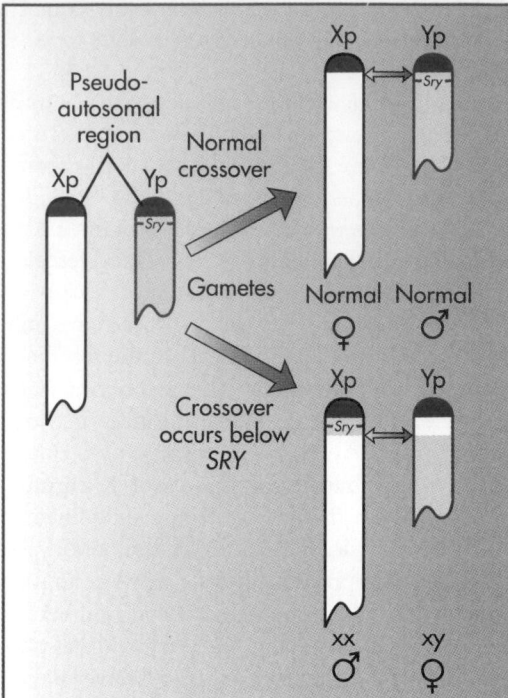

Fig. 2-25 *Distal short arms of the X and Y chromosomes exchange material during meiosis in the male.* The region of the Y chromosome in which this crossover occurs is called the *pseudoautosomal region.* The *SRY* gene, which triggers the process leading to male gonadal differentiation, is located just outside the pseudoautosomal region. Occasionally, the crossover occurs on the centromeric side of the *SRY* gene, causing it to lie on an X chromosome instead of a Y chromosome. An offspring receiving this X chromosome will be an XX male, and an offspring receiving the Y chromosome will be an XY female.

Occasionally, the crossover between X and Y occurs closer to the centromere than it should, placing the *SRY* gene on the X chromosome after crossover. This variation can result in offspring with an apparently normal XX karyotype but a male phenotype. Such XX males are seen in about 1 in 20,000 live births and resemble males with Klinefelter syndrome. Conversely, it is possible to inherit a Y chromosome that has lost the *SRY* gene (the result of either a crossover error or a deletion of the gene). This situation produces an XY female. Such females have gonadal streaks rather than ovaries and have poorly developed secondary sex characteristics.

✓ QUICK CHECK

Why is the influence of environment significant to phenotype?

Why is the recurrence risk for autosomal dominant transmission 50%?

Why are the concepts of variable expressivity, incomplete penetrance, and delayed age of onset so important for genetic diseases?

Why does X inactivation occur only in females, and what are its consequences for disease?

Characteristics of pedigrees

X-linked pedigrees show distinctive modes of inheritance. The most striking characteristic is that females seldom are affected. To express an X-linked recessive trait, a female must be homozygous: either both her parents are affected, or her father is affected and her mother is a carrier. Such matings are rare.

The following are important principles of X-linked recessive inheritance:
1. The trait is seen much more frequently in males than in females.
2. Because a father can give a son only a Y chromosome, the trait is never transmitted from father to son.
3. The gene can be transmitted through a series of carrier females, causing the appearance of a "skipped generation."
4. The gene is passed from an affected father to all his daughters, who, as phenotypically normal carriers, transmit it to approximately half their sons, who are affected.

The most common and severe of all X-linked recessive disorders is Duchenne muscular dystrophy (DMD), which affects approximately 1 in 3500 males. As its name suggests, this disorder is characterized by progressive muscle degeneration. Affected individuals usually are unable to walk by age 10 or 12 years. The disease affects the heart and respiratory muscles, and death caused by respiratory or cardiac failure usually occurs before 20 years of age. Identification of the disease gene (on the short arm of the X chromosome) has greatly increased our understanding of the disorder.[13] The DMD gene is the largest gene ever found in the human, spanning more than 2 million DNA bases. It encodes a previously undiscovered muscle protein, termed **dystrophin.** Extensive study of dystrophin indicates that it plays an essential role in maintaining the structural integrity of muscle cells: it may also help to regulate the activity of membrane proteins. When dystrophin is absent, as in DMD, the cell cannot survive, and muscle deterioration ensues. Most cases of DMD are caused by frameshift deletions of portions of the DMD gene and thus involve alterations of all the amino acids encoded by the DNA following the deletion.

Recurrence risks

The most common mating type involving X-linked recessive genes is the combination of a carrier female and a normal male (Fig. 2-26, *A*). On average, the carrier mother will transmit the disease gene to half her sons (who are affected) and half her daughters (who are carriers).

The other common mating type is an affected father and a normal mother (Fig. 2-26, *B*). In this situation all the sons must be normal because the father can transmit only his Y chromosome to them. Because all the daughters must receive the father's X chromosome, they will all be heterozygous carriers. Because the sons *must* receive the Y chromosome and the daughters *must* receive the X chromosome with the disease gene, these are precise outcomes and not probabilities. None of the children will inherit the disease.

The final mating pattern, less common than the other two, involves an affected father and a carrier mother (Fig. 2-26, *C*). With this pattern, on average, half the daughters

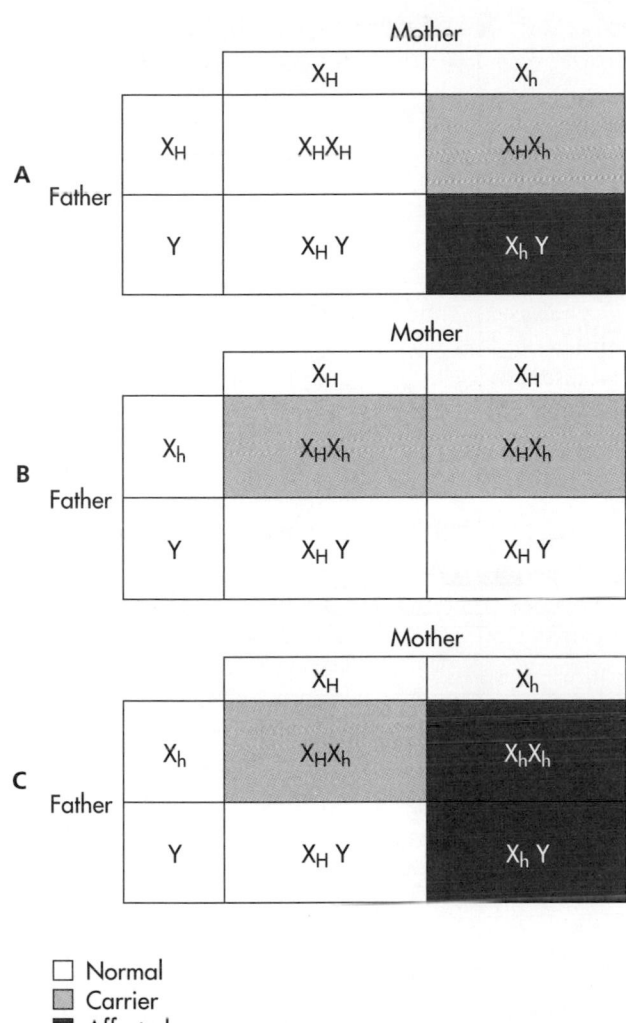

□ Normal
▨ Carrier
■ Affected

Fig. 2-26 *Punnett square and X-linked recessive traits.* **A,** Punnett square for the mating of a normal male ($X_H Y$) and a female carrier of an X-linked recessive gene ($X_H X_h$). **B,** Punnett square for the mating of a normal female ($X_H X_H$) with a male affected by an X-linked recessive disease ($X_h Y$). **C,** Punnett square for the mating of a female who carries an X-linked recessive gene ($X_H X_h$) with a male who is affected with the disease caused by the gene ($X_h Y$).

will be heterozygous carriers, and half will be homozygous for the disease gene and thus affected. Half the sons will be normal, and half will be affected. Some X-linked recessive diseases, such as DMD, are fatal or incapacitating before the affected individual reaches reproductive age, and therefore affected fathers are rare or nonexistent.

Sex-limited and sex-influenced traits

A *sex-limited trait* can occur in only one sex, often because of anatomic differences. Inherited uterine and testicular defects are two obvious examples. A *sex-influenced trait* occurs much more frequently in one sex than the other. For example, male-pattern baldness occurs in both males and females but is much more common in males. In males it is inherited as an autosomal dominant trait, whereas in females it is inherited as an autosomal recessive trait. Because

of their hormonal constitution, females need two copies of the gene to express male-pattern baldness. Autosomal dominant breast cancer, which is now much more commonly expressed in females than males, is another example of a sex-influenced trait.

Evaluation of Pedigrees

With complications such as incomplete penetrance, variable expressivity, delayed age of onset, and sex-influenced traits, it is not always possible simply to look at a disease pedigree and determine the mode of inheritance. A sophisticated statistical methodologic approach has evolved to deal with such complications. Incorporated into computer programs, these statistical techniques assess the probability of observing a certain pedigree if a particular mode of inheritance (e.g., autosomal dominant with incomplete penetrance) is in effect.

LINKAGE ANALYSIS AND GENE MAPPING

Locating genes on chromosomes and on specific areas of chromosomes is one of the most important endeavors in human genetics. The location of a gene can tell much about the function of the gene, its interaction with other genes, and the likelihood that certain individuals will develop a genetic disease.

Classical Pedigree Analysis

Mendel's second law, the principle of independent assortment, states that an individual's genes will be transmitted to the next generation independently of one another. This law is only partly true, however, because genes located close together on the same chromosome *do* tend to be transmitted together to the offspring. Thus Mendel's principle of independent assortment holds true for most pairs of genes but not those that occupy the same region of a chromosome. Such loci demonstrate **linkage** and are said to be linked.

During the first meiotic stage, the arms of homologous chromosome pairs intertwine and sometimes exchange portions of their DNA (Fig. 2-27) in a process known as ***crossing over*** (or ***crossover***). During crossover new combinations of alleles can be formed. For example, two loci on a chromosome have alleles A and a and alleles B and b. Alleles A and B are located together on one member of a chromosome pair, and alleles a and b are located on the other member. The genotype of this individual is denoted as AB/ab.

As Fig. 2-27, *A,* shows, the allele pairs AB and ab would be transmitted together when no crossover occurs. However, when crossover occurs (Fig. 2-27, *B*), all four possible pairs of alleles can be transmitted to the offspring: AB, aB, Ab, and ab. The process of forming such new arrangements of alleles is called **recombination.** Crossover does not necessarily lead to recombination, however, because double crossover between two loci can result in no actual recombination of the alleles at the loci (Fig. 2-27, *C*).

Once a close linkage has been established between a disease locus and a "marker" locus (a DNA sequence that varies

Homologous chromosomes   Meiosis gametes

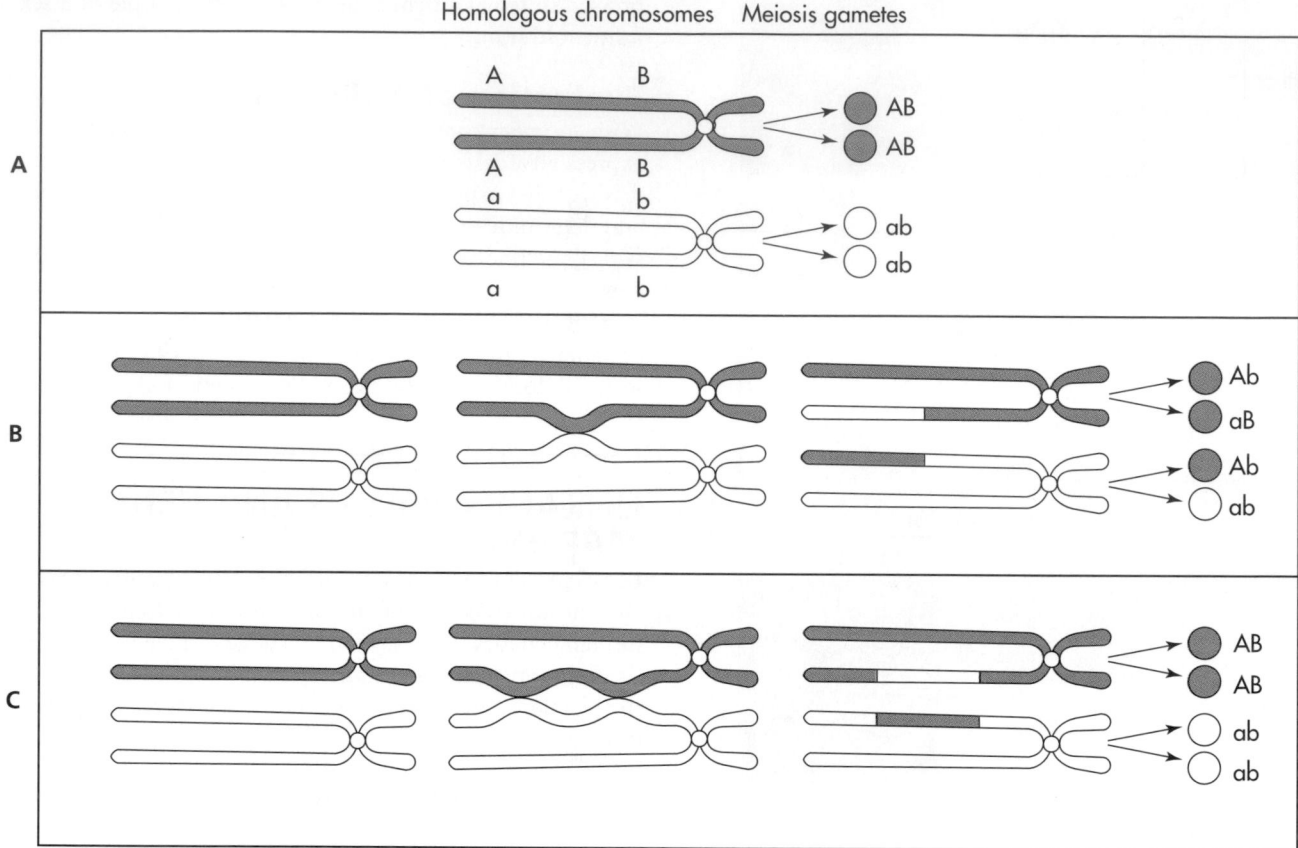

Fig. 2-27 *Genetic results of crossing over.* **A,** No crossing over. **B,** Crossing over with recombination. **C,** Double crossing over, resulting in no recombination.

among individuals) and once the alleles of the two loci that are inherited together within a family have been determined, reliable predictions can be made whether a member of a family will develop the disease. This ability is especially important for diseases with delayed age of onset. Linkage has been established between several DNA polymorphisms and each of the two genes for autosomal dominant breast cancer (about 5% of breast cancer cases are caused by these autosomal dominant genes). Determining this kind of linkage means that it is possible for offspring of an individual with autosomal dominant breast cancer to know whether they also carry the gene and thus could pass it on to their own children. Other diseases for which linked markers have been found include adult polycystic kidney disease, familial Alzheimer disease, Huntington disease, and neurofibromatosis, type 1. In addition, specific mutations that cause these diseases have been identified, enabling direct detection of disease genes.

For some genetic diseases, prophylactic treatment is available if the condition can be diagnosed in time. An example of this is hemochromatosis, a recessive genetic disease in which excess iron is absorbed, causing degeneration of the heart, liver, brain, and other vital organs. The gene for hemochromatosis is closely linked to the human leukocyte antigen (HLA) (see Chapter 5) complex on chromosome 6. Individuals at risk for developing the disease can be determined by testing for a mutation in the hemochromatosis gene, and preventive therapy (periodic phlebotomy) can be initiated to deplete iron stores and ensure a normal life span.

Complete Human Gene Map: Prospects and Benefits

Rapid progress is being made in assigning genes to their chromosomal locations. A number of important genetic diseases have been located on specific areas of individual chromosomes: these include Huntington disease, retinoblastoma, DMD, hemophilia A, cystic fibrosis, PKU, neurofibromatosis, and familial Alzheimer disease (Fig. 2-28).[1,14] Table 2-2 contains a partial list of mapped diseases. The development of thousands of new DNA markers is especially helpful in this effort. Mapping a disease gene is an important step toward isolating and *cloning* the gene (clones are identical

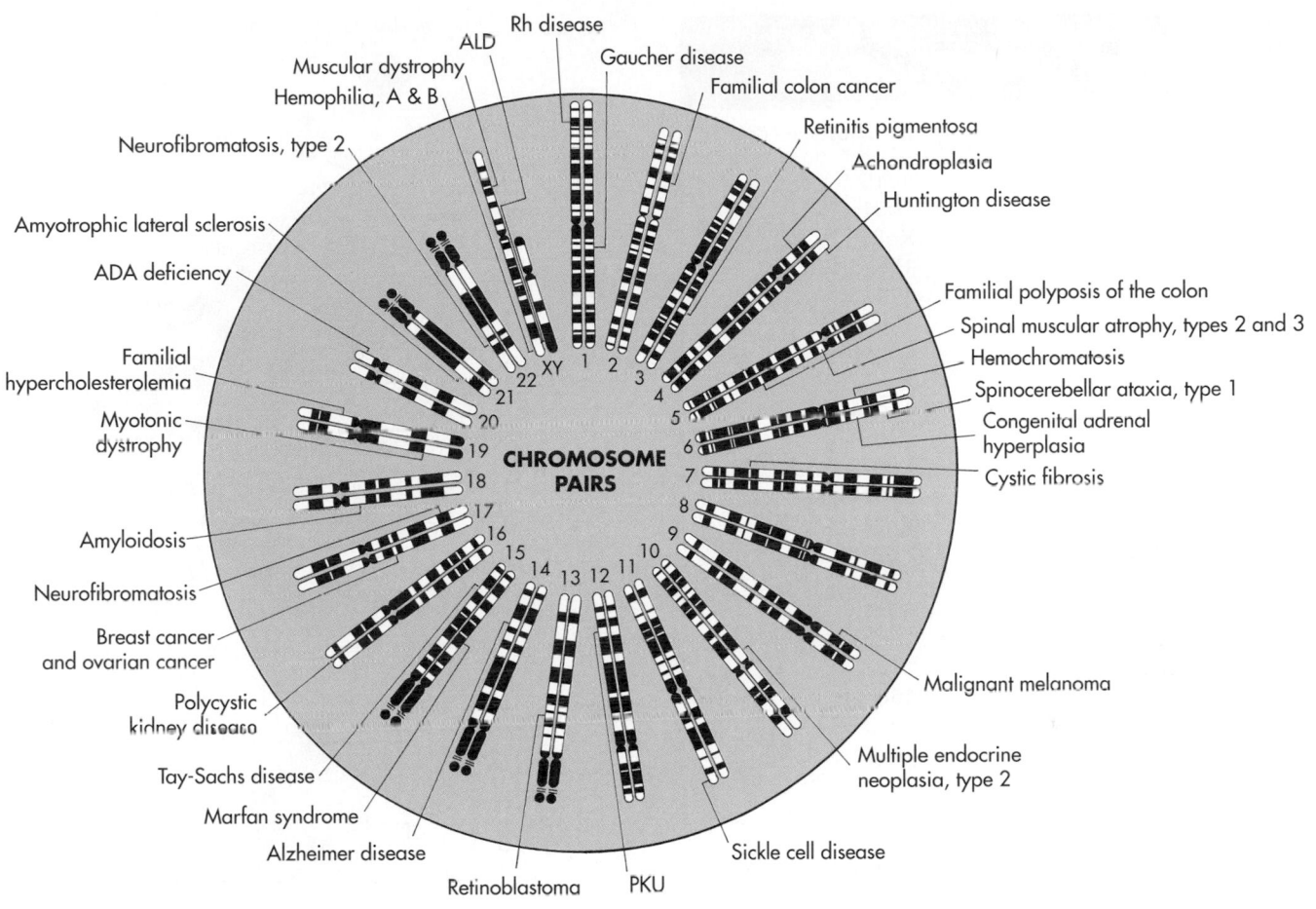

Fig. 2-28 *Example of diseases: a gene map.*

PKU = Phenylketonuria
ALD = Adrenoleukodystrophy
ADA = Adenosine deaminase

copies of genes). Once a gene is cloned, its DNA sequence can be studied to determine the nature and function of the protein encoded by the gene. Cloning the genes that cause diseases such as cystic fibrosis and DMD has contributed immensely to our understanding of the pathophysiology of these disorders. In addition, the ability to clone a gene opens up the possibility of gene therapy for the disorder.

HEALTH ALERT

Gene Therapy

Currently more than 3000 individuals are enrolled in approximately 300 different gene therapy protocols. Most of these protocols involve the genetic alteration of cells to combat various types of cancer. Other protocols involve the treatment of inherited diseases, such as cystic fibrosis and familial hypercholesterolemia.

Data from Anderson, W.F. (1998). Human gene therapy. Nature, *392(Suppl), 25-30; Friedmann, T. (1997). Overcoming the obstacles to gene therapy.* Scientific American, *276, 96-101.*

MULTIFACTORIAL INHERITANCE

Not all traits are produced by single genes; some traits result from several genes acting together. These are called *polygenic traits.* When environmental factors influence the expression of the trait (as is usually the case), the term *multifactorial inheritance* is used. Many multifactorial and polygenic traits tend to follow a normal distribution in populations (the familiar bell-shaped curve). Fig. 2-29 shows how three loci acting together can cause grain color in wheat to vary in a gradual way from white to red, exemplifying multifactorial inheritance. If both the alleles at each of the three loci are white alleles, the color is pure white. If most alleles are white but a few are red, the color is somewhat darker; if all are red, the color is dark red.

Other examples of multifactorial traits include height and IQ. Although both height and IQ are determined in part by genes, they are influenced also by environment. For example, the average height of many human populations has increased by 5 to 10 cm in the past 100 years because of improvements in nutrition and health care. Also, IQ scores can

TABLE 2-2	Some Important Genetic Diseases That Have Been Mapped to Specific Chromosome Locations and Cloned
Disease	**Chromosome Location**
Huntington disease	4p16
Cystic fibrosis	7q31
Hemophilia A	Xq28
Marfan syndrome	15q15-21
Sickle cell anemia	11p15
β-Thalassemia	11p15
α-Thalassemia	16pter-p12
Familial breast cancer	
BRCA1	17q21
BRCA2	13q
Fragile X syndrome	Xq27
Phenylketonuria	12q21-qter
Duchenne muscular dystrophy	Xp21
Becker muscular dystrophy*	Xp21
Retinoblastoma	13q14
Hemochromatosis	6p21
Familial hypercholesterolemia (LDL receptor defect)	19p13
Polycystic kidney disease	16p,4
α₁-Antitrypsin deficiency	14q31-32
Familial Alzheimer disease†	21q11-q21, 14, 19, 1
Tay-Sachs disease	15q22-q25
Neurofibromatosis, type 1 (classical)	17q11
Neurofibromatosis, type 2 (bilateral acoustic form)	22q11-13
Familial polyposis coli	5q21-22

*Becker muscular dystrophy is an allelic form of Duchenne muscular dystrophy.

†Familial Alzheimer disease is a complex, heterogeneous disease. The single genes now located for this disease are associated with only some of the known cases.

Fig. 2-29 *Multifactorial inheritance.* Analysis of mode of inheritance for grain color in wheat. The trait is controlled by three independently assorted gene loci.

be improved by exposing individuals (especially children) to enriched learning environments. Thus both genes and environment contribute to variation in these traits.

A number of diseases do not follow the bell-shaped distribution. Instead they appear to be either present in or absent from an individual. Yet they do not follow the patterns expected of single-gene diseases. Many of these are probably polygenic or multifactorial, but a certain *threshold of liability* must be crossed before the disease is expressed. Below the threshold the individual appears normal; above it the individual is affected by the disease (Fig. 2-30).

One of the best-known examples of such a threshold trait is pyloric stenosis, a disorder characterized by a narrowing or obstruction of the pylorus, the area between the stomach and intestine. Chronic vomiting, constipation, weight loss, and electrolyte imbalance can result from the

condition, but it is easily corrected by surgery. The prevalence of pyloric stenosis is about 3 in 1000 live births in whites. This disorder is much more common in males than females, affecting 1 in 200 males and 1 in 1000 females. The apparent reason for this difference is that the threshold of liability is much lower in males than females, as shown in Fig. 2-30. Thus fewer defective alleles are required to generate the disorder in males. This situation also means that the offspring of affected females are more likely to have pyloric stenosis because affected females necessarily carry more disease-causing alleles than do most affected males.

A number of other common diseases are thought to correspond to a threshold model. They include cleft lip and cleft palate, neural tube defects (anencephaly, spina bifida), clubfoot (talipes), and some forms of congenital heart disease.

Although recurrence risks can be given with confidence

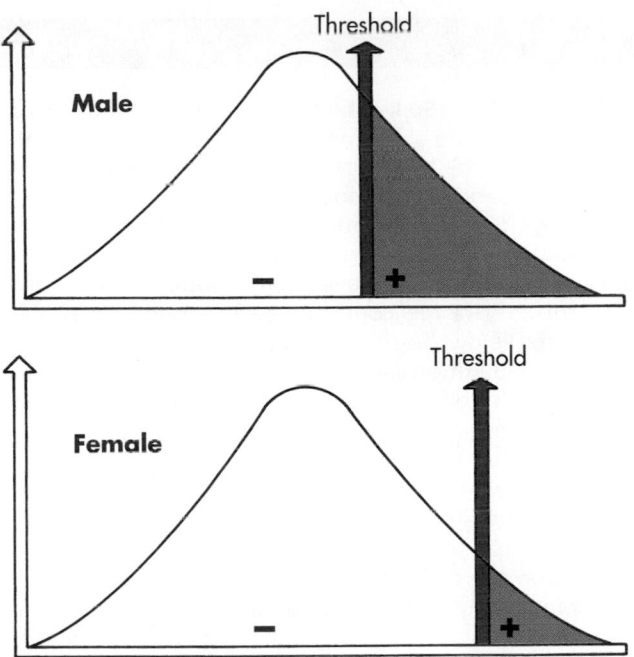

Fig. 2-30 *Threshold of liability for pyloric stenosis in males and females.*

for single-gene diseases (e.g., 50% for autosomal dominants, 25% for autosomal recessives), it is considerably more difficult to do so for multifactorial diseases. The number of genes contributing to the disease is not known, the precise allelic constitution of the parents is not known, and the extent of environmental effects can vary from one population to another. For most multifactorial diseases, *empirical risks* (i.e., those based on direct observation) have been derived. To determine empirical risks, a large sample of families in which one child has developed the disease is examined. Then the siblings of each child are surveyed to calculate what percentage of them also develop the disease.

Another difficulty is distinguishing polygenic or multifactorial diseases from single-gene diseases that have incomplete penetrance or variable expressivity (Box 2-1).

Large data sets and good epidemiologic data often are necessary to make the distinction. Box 2-1 lists criteria that are commonly used to define multifactorial diseases.

The genetics of common disorders such as hypertension, heart disease, and diabetes is complex and often confusing. Nevertheless, the public health impact of these diseases, together with the evidence for hereditary factors in their etiology, demands that genetic studies be pursued. The next decade will undoubtedly witness substantial advancements in our understanding of these disorders.

Criteria Used to Define Multifactorial Diseases   BOX 2-1

1 The recurrence risk becomes higher if more than one family member is affected. For example, the recurrence risk for neural tube defects in a British family increases to 10% if two siblings have been born with the disease. By contrast, the recurrence risk for single-gene diseases remains the same regardless of the number of siblings affected.
2 If the expression of the disease is more severe, the recurrence risk is higher. This is consistent with the liability model; a more severe expression indicates that the individual is at the extreme end of the liability distribution. Relatives of the affected individual are thus at a higher risk for inheriting disease genes. Cleft lip and/or cleft palate is a condition in which this has been shown to be true.
3 Relatives of probands of the less commonly affected are more likely to develop the disease. As with pyloric stenosis, this occurs because an affected individual of the less susceptible sex is usually at a more extreme position on the liability distribution.
4 Generally, if the population frequency of the disease is *f*, the risk for offspring and siblings of probands is approximately *f*. This does not usually hold true for single-gene traits.
5 The recurrence risk for the disease decreases rapidly in more remotely related relatives. Although the recurrence risk for single-gene diseases decreases by 50% with each degree of relationship (e.g., an autosomal dominant disease has a 50% recurrence risk for siblings, 25% for uncle-nephew relationship, 12.5% for first cousins), the risk for multifactorial inheritance decreases much more quickly.

✓ QUICK CHECK

Why is autosomal dominant breast cancer considered a sex-influenced trait?

Define linkage analysis; cite an example.

Why is "threshold of liability" an important consideration in multifactorial inheritance?

Discuss the concept of multifactorial inheritance, and include two examples.

▣ DID YOU UNDERSTAND?

DNA, RNA, and Proteins: Heredity at the Molecular Level

1. Genes, the basic units of inheritance, are composed of deoxyribonucleic acid (DNA) and are located on chromosomes.
2. DNA is composed of deoxyribose, a phosphate molecule, and four types of nitrogenous bases. The physical structure of DNA is a double helix.
3. The DNA bases code for amino acids, which in turn make up proteins. The amino acids are specified by triplet codons of nitrogenous bases.
4. DNA replication is based on complementary base pairing, in which a single strand of DNA serves as the template for attracting bases that form a new strand of DNA.
5. DNA polymerase is the primary enzyme involved in replication. It adds bases to the new DNA strand and performs "proofreading" functions.
6. A mutation is an inherited alteration of genetic material (i.e., DNA).
7. Substances that cause mutations are called *mutagens.*
8. The mutation rate in humans varies from locus to locus and ranges from 10^{-4} to 10^{-7} per gene per generation.
9. Transcription and translation, the two basic processes in which proteins are specified by DNA, both involve ribonucleic acid (RNA). RNA is chemically similar to DNA, but it is single-stranded, has a ribose sugar molecule, and has uracil rather than thymine as one of its four nitrogenous bases.
10. Transcription is the process by which DNA specifies a sequence of messenger RNA (mRNA).
11. Much of the RNA sequence is spliced from the mRNA before the mRNA leaves the nucleus. The excised sequences are called *introns,* and those that remain to code for proteins are called *exons.*
12. Translation is the process by which RNA directs the synthesis of polypeptides. This process takes place in the ribosomes, which consist of proteins and ribosomal RNA (rRNA).
13. During translation mRNA interacts with transfer RNA (tRNA), a molecule that has an attachment site for a specific amino acid.

Chromosomes

1. Human cells consist of diploid somatic cells (body cells) and haploid gametes (sperm and egg cells).
2. Humans have 23 pairs of chromosomes. Twenty-two of these pairs are autosomes. The remaining pair consists of the sex chromosomes. Females have two homologous X chromosomes as their sex chromosomes; males have an X and a Y chromosome.
3. A karyotype is an ordered display of chromosomes arranged according to length and the location of the centromere.
4. Various types of stains can be used to make chromosome bands more visible.

5. About 1 in 150 live births has a major diagnosable chromosome abnormality. Chromosome abnormalities are the leading known cause of mental retardation and miscarriage.
6. Polyploidy is a condition in which a euploid cell has some multiple of the normal number of chromosomes. Humans have been observed to have triploidy (three copies of each chromosome) and tetraploidy (four copies of each chromosome); both conditions are lethal.
7. Somatic cells that do not have a multiple of 23 chromosomes are aneuploid. Aneuploidy is usually the result of nondisjunction.
8. Trisomy is a type of aneuploidy in which one chromosome is present in three copies in somatic cells. A partial trisomy is one in which only part of a chromosome is present in three copies.
9. Monosomy is a type of aneuploidy in which one chromosome is present in only one copy in somatic cells.
10. In general, monosomies cause more severe physical defects than do trisomies, illustrating the principle that the loss of chromosome material has more severe consequences than the duplication of chromosome material.
11. Down syndrome, a trisomy of chromosome 21, is the best-known disease caused by a chromosome aberration. It affects 1 in 800 live births and is much more likely to occur in the offspring of women older than 35 years.
12. Most aneuploidies of the sex chromosomes have less severe consequences than those of the autosomes.
13. The most commonly observed sex chromosome aneuploidies are the 47,XXX karyotype, 45,X karyotype (Turner syndrome), 47,XXY karyotype (Klinefelter syndrome), and 47,XYY karyotype.
14. Abnormalities of chromosome structure include deletions, duplications, inversions, and translocations.

Elements of Formal Genetics

1. Mendelian traits are caused by single genes, each of which occupies a position, or locus, on a chromosome.
2. Alleles are different forms of genes located at the same locus on a chromosome.
3. At any given locus in a somatic cell, an individual has two genes, one from each parent. An individual may be homozygous or heterozygous for a locus.
4. An individual's genotype is his or her genetic makeup, and the phenotype reflects the interaction of genotype and environment.
5. In a heterozygote, a dominant gene's effects mask those of a recessive gene. The recessive gene is expressed only when it is present in two copies.

■ DID YOU UNDERSTAND? —cont'd

Transmission of Genetic Diseases

1. Genetic diseases caused by single genes usually follow autosomal dominant, autosomal recessive, or X-linked recessive modes of inheritance.
2. Pedigree charts are an important tool in the analysis of modes of inheritance.
3. Recurrence risks specify the probability that future offspring will inherit a genetic disease. For single-gene diseases, recurrence risks remain the same for each offspring, regardless of the number of affected or unaffected offspring.
4. The recurrence risk for autosomal dominant diseases is usually 50%.
5. Germline mosaicism can alter recurrence risks for genetic diseases since unaffected parents can produce multiple affected offspring. This situation occurs because the germline of one parent is affected by a mutation but the parent's somatic cells are unaffected.
6. Skipped generations are not seen in classical autosomal dominant pedigrees.
7. Males and females are equally likely to exhibit autosomal dominant diseases and to pass them on to their offspring.
8. Many genetic diseases have a delayed age of onset.
9. A gene that is not always expressed phenotypically is said to have incomplete penetrance.
10. Variable expressivity is a characteristic of many genetic diseases.
11. Genomic imprinting, which may involve methylation, results in differing expressions of a disease gene, depending on which parent transmitted the gene.
12. Most commonly, parents of children with autosomal recessive diseases are both heterozygous carriers of the disease gene.
13. The recurrence risk for autosomal recessive diseases is 25%.
14. Males and females are equally likely to be affected by autosomal recessive diseases.
15. Consanguinity is sometimes present in families with autosomal recessive diseases, and it becomes more prevalent with rarer recessive diseases.
16. Carrier detection tests for an increasing number of autosomal recessive diseases are available.
17. The frequency of genetic diseases approximately doubles in the offspring of first-cousin matings.
18. In each normal female somatic cell, one of the two X chromosomes is inactivated early in embryogenesis.
19. X inactivation is random, fixed, and incomplete (i.e., only part of the chromosome is actually inactivated). It may involve methylation.
20. Gender is determined embryonically by the presence of the *SRY* gene on the Y chromosome. Embryos that have a Y chromosome (and thus the *SRY* gene) become males, whereas those lacking the Y chromosome become females. When the Y chromosome lacks the *SRY* gene, an XY female can be produced. Similarly, an X chromosome that contains the *SRY* gene can produce an XX male.
21. X-linked genes are those that are located on the X chromosome. Nearly all known X-linked diseases are caused by X-linked recessive genes.
22. Males are hemizygous for genes on the X chromosome.
23. X-linked recessive diseases are seen much more frequently in males than in females because males need only one copy of the gene to express the disease.
24. Fathers cannot pass X-linked genes to their sons.
25. Skipped generations often are seen in X-linked recessive disease pedigrees because the gene can be transmitted through carrier females.
26. Recurrence risks for X-linked recessive diseases depend on the carrier and affected status of the mother and father.
27. A sex-limited trait is one that occurs only in one sex (gender).
28. A sex-influenced trait is one that occurs more frequently in one sex than in the other.

Linkage Analysis and Gene Mapping

1. During meiosis I, crossover occurs and can cause recombinations of alleles located on the same chromosome.
2. The frequency of recombinations can be used to infer the map distance between loci on the same chromosome.
3. A marker locus, when closely linked to a disease-gene locus, can be used to predict whether an individual will develop a genetic disease.
4. A more complete gene map will facilitate marker studies, gene cloning, studies of gene function and interaction, and gene therapy.

Multifactorial Inheritance

1. Traits that result from the combined effects of several loci are polygenic. When environmental factors also influence the trait, it is multifactorial.
2. Many multifactorial traits have a threshold of liability. Once the threshold of liability has been crossed, the disease may be expressed.
3. Empiric risks, based on direct observation of large numbers of families, are used to estimate recurrence risks for multifactorial diseases.
4. Recurrence risks for multifactorial diseases become higher if more than one family member is affected or if the expression of the disease in the proband is more severe.
5. Recurrence risks for multifactorial diseases decrease rapidly for more remote relatives.

KEY TERMS

Adenine, 36
Allele, 48
Amino acid, 36
Aneuploid cell, 40
Anticodon, 38
Autosome, 39
Barr body, 53
Base pair substitution, 37
Carrier, 48
Carrier detection test, 52
Chromosomal mosaic, 41
Chromosome band, 40
Chromosome breakage, 44
Chromosome theory of inheritance, 49
Clastogen, 45
Cloning, 56
Codominance, 48
Codon, 36
Complementary base pairing, 37
Consanguinity, 53
Cri du chat syndrome, 45
Crossing over (crossover), 55
Cytokinesis, 39
Cytosine, 36
Delayed age of onset, 51
Deletion, 45
Deoxyribonucleic acid (DNA), 35
Diploid cell, 39
DNA polymerase, 37
Dominant, 48
Dosage compensation, 53
Double helix, 36
Down syndrome, 42
Duplication, 46
Dystrophin, 54
Empirical risk, 59
Euploid cell, 40
Exon, 38
Expressivity, 51
Fragile site, 46
Frameshift mutation, 37
Gamete, 39

Gene, 35
Genotype, 48
Germline mosaicism, 50
Guanine, 36
Haploid cell, 39
Hemizygous, 53
Heterogeneous nuclear RNA (hnRNA), 38
Heterozygote, 48
Heterozygous, 48
Homologous, 39
Homozygote, 48
Homozygous, 48
Inbreeding, 53
Intron, 38
Inversion, 46
Karyotype, 39
Klinefelter syndrome, 44
Linkage, 55
Locus, 48
Meiosis, 39
Messenger RNA (mRNA), 37
Metaphase spread, 39
Methylation, 53
Mitosis, 39
Mode of inheritance, 48
Monosomy, 41
Multifactorial inheritance, 57
Mutagen, 37
Mutation, 37
Mutational hot spot, 37
Nondisjunction, 41
Nucleotide, 36
Obligate carrier, 51
Occurrence risk, 49
Partial trisomy, 41
Pedigree, 49
Penetrance, 51
Phenotype, 48
Polygenic trait, 57
Polymorphic (polymorphism), 48

Polypeptide, 36
Polyploid cell, 40
Position effect, 46
Principle of independent assortment, 48
Principle of segregation, 48
Proband (propositus/proposita), 49
Promoter site, 37
Pseudoautosomal, 53
Purine, 36
Pyrimidine, 36
Recessive, 48
Reciprocal translocation, 46
Recombination, 55
Recurrence risk, 49
Ribonucleic acid (RNA), 37
Ribosomal RNA (rRNA), 38
Ribosome, 38
RNA polymerase, 37
Robertsonian translocation, 46
Sex chromosome, 39
Sex-influenced trait, 55
Sex-limited trait, 55
Sex-linked (inheritance), 53
Silent substitution, 37
Somatic cell, 39
Spontaneous mutation, 37
Template, 37
Termination sequence, 38
Tetraploidy, 40
Threshold of liability, 58
Thymine, 36
Transcription, 37
Transfer RNA (tRNA), 38
Translation, 38
Translocation, 46
Triploidy, 40
Trisomy, 41
Tumor-suppressor gene, 51
Turner syndrome, 44
X-inactivation, 53

REFERENCES

1. Jorde, L.B. et al. (1999). *Medical genetics* (2nd ed.). St. Louis: Mosby.
2. Hassold, T.J. (1986). Chromosome abnormalities in human reproductive wastage. *Trends in Genetics, 2,* 105-110.
3. Hassold, T., Hunt, P.A., & Sherman, S. (1993). Trisomy in humans: Incidence, origin and etiology. *Current Opinions in Genetics and Development, 3,* 398-403.
4. Epstein, C.J. (1995). Down syndrome (trisomy 21). In C.R. Scriver, A.L. Beaudet, W.S. Sly, & D. Valle (Eds.). *The metabolic basis of inherited disease* (vol. 1, pp. 749-794). New York: McGraw-Hill.
5. Robinson, A. & de la Chapelle, A. (1997). Sex chromosome abnormalities. In D.L. Rimoin, J.M. Connor, & R.E. Pyeritz (Eds.). *Emery and Rimoin's principles and practice of medical genetics* (vol. 1, pp. 973-997). New York: Churchill Livingstone.
6. Warren, S.T. (1997). Trinucleotide repetition and fragile X syndrome. *Hospital Practice, 32,* 73-98.
7. Reddy, P.S. & Housman, D.E. (1997). The complex pathology of trinuclcotide repeats. *Current Opinions in Genetic Development, 9,* 364-372.
8. Bernards, A. & Gusella, J.F. (1994). The importance of genetic mosaicism in human disease. *New England Journal of Medicine, 331,* 1447-1449.
9. Shen, M.H., Harper, P.S., & Upadhyaya, M. (1996). Molecular genetics of neurofibromatosis type 1 (NF1). *Journal of Medical Genetics, 33,* 2-17.
10. Lyon, M.F. (1992). Some milestones in the history of X-chromosome inactivation. *Annual Review of Genetics, 26,* 17-28.
11. Lee, J.T. & Jaenisch, R. (1997). The (epi)genetic control of mammalian X-chromosome inactivation. *Current Opinions in Genetic Development, 7,* 274-280.
12. Schafer, A.J. & Goodfellow, P.M. (1996). Sex determination in humans. *BioEssays, 18,* 955-963.
13. Brown, R.J. (1997). Dystrophin-associated proteins and the muscular dystrophies. *Annual Review of Medicine, 48,* 457-446.
14. Collins, F.S. (1997). Sequencing the human genome. *Hospital Practice, 32,* 35-54.
15. Cavanee, W.K. & White, R.L. (1995). The genetic basis of cancer. *Scientific American 272,* 72-79.

CHAPTER

3

Altered Cellular and Tissue Biology

Kathryn L. McCance and Todd C. Grey

Knowledge of the structural and functional reactions of cells and tissues to injurious agents, including genetic defects, is key for the understanding of disease processes. Altered cellular and tissue biology can result from adaptation, injury, neoplasia, aging, or death. (Neoplasia is discussed in Chapters 9 to 11.) Adaptation occurs in response to both normal, or physiologic, conditions and adverse, or pathologic, conditions. For example, the uterus adapts to pregnancy—a normal physiologic state—by enlarging. Enlargement occurs because of an increase in the size and number of uterine cells. In an adverse condition such as high blood pressure, myocardial cells are stimulated to enlarge by the increased work of pumping. Like most of the body's adaptive mechanisms, however, cellular adaptations to adverse conditions are usually only temporarily successful. Severe or long-term stressors overwhelm adaptive processes, and cellular injury or death ensues.

Injury may be reversible (sublethal) or irreversible (lethal) and is classified broadly as chemical, hypoxic (lack of sufficient oxygen), free radical, or infectious. Cellular injuries from various causes have different clinical and pathophysiologic manifestations. Cellular death is confirmed by structural changes seen when cells are stained and examined under a microscope.

Cellular aging causes structural and functional changes that eventually may lead to cellular death or a decreased capacity to recover from injury. Mechanisms explaining how and why cells age are not known, and distinguishing between pathologic changes and physiologic changes that occur with aging is often difficult. Aging clearly causes alterations in cellular structure and function, yet senescence is both inevitable and normal.

CHAPTER OUTLINE

 Check out your CD Companion for chapter-related exercises and answers to the Quick Check questions

CELLULAR ADAPTATION

Cells adapt to their environment to escape and protect themselves from injury. An adapted cell is neither normal nor injured—its condition lies somewhere between these two states. Cellular adaptations, however, are a common and central part of many disease states. In the early stages of a successful adaptive response, cells may have enhanced function; thus it is hard to know whether the response is pathologic or an extreme adaptation to an excessive functional demand.[1] The most significant adaptive changes in cells include atrophy (decrease in cell size), hypertrophy (increase in cell size), hyperplasia (increase in cell number), and metaplasia (reversible replacement of one mature cell type by another, less mature cell type). Dysplasia (deranged cellular growth) is not considered a true cellular adaptation, but rather an *atypical hyperplasia.* These changes are shown in Fig. 3-1.

Atrophy

Atrophy is a decrease or shrinkage in cellular size. If atrophy occurs in a sufficient number of an organ's cells, the entire organ shrinks or becomes atrophic. Atrophy can affect any

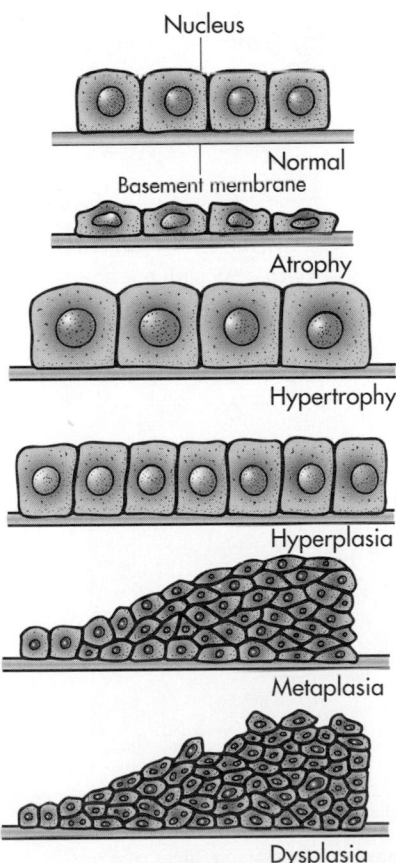

Fig. 3-1 *Adaptive and dysplastic alterations in simple cuboidal epithelial cells. (From Lewis, S.M., Collier, I.C., & Heitkemper, M.M. [1996].* Medical-surgical nursing: Assessment and management of clinical problems *[4th ed.]. St. Louis: Mosby.)*

organ, but it is most common in skeletal muscle, the heart, secondary sex organs, and the brain. The causes of atrophy include decreases in workload, use, blood supply, nutrition, hormonal stimulation, and nervous stimulation. Individuals immobilized in bed for a prolonged time exhibit a type of skeletal muscle atrophy called *disuse atrophy.* Aging causes brain cells to become atrophic (presumably as arteriosclerosis obstructs the brain's blood supply) and endocrine-dependent organs, such as the gonads, to shrink as hormonal stimulation decreases. Whether atrophy is caused by normal physiologic conditions or by pathologic conditions, atrophic cells exhibit the same basic changes.

The atrophic muscle cell contains less endoplasmic reticulum and fewer mitochondria and myofilaments (part of the muscle fiber that controls contraction) than does the normal cell. In muscular atrophy caused by nerve loss, oxygen consumption and amino acid uptake are immediately reduced.

Atrophy resulting from chronic malnutrition is often accompanied by more *autophagic vacuoles,* which are membrane-bound vesicles within the cell that contain cellular debris and hydrolytic enzymes. The level of hydrolytic enzymes rises rapidly in atrophy. The enzymes are isolated in autophagic vacuoles to prevent uncontrolled cellular destruction. Thus the vacuoles form as needed to protect uninjured organelles from the injured organelles and are eventually taken up and destroyed by lysosomes. Certain contents of the autophagic vacuole may resist destruction by lysosomal enzymes and persist in membrane-bound residual bodies. An example of this is granules that contain *lipofuscin,* the yellow-brown age pigment. Lipofuscin accumulates primarily in liver cells, myocardial cells, and atrophic cells.

Hypertrophy

Hypertrophy is an increase in the size of cells and consequently in the size of the affected organ (Fig. 3-2). The cells of the heart and kidneys are particularly prone to enlargement. The increased cellular size is associated with an increased accumulation of protein in the cellular components (plasma membrane, endoplasmic reticulum, myofilaments, mitochondria) and not with an increase in cellular fluid. How hypertrophy develops in various cells remains uncertain. Muscular hypertrophy might involve an increase in the rate of protein synthesis, a decrease in the rate of protein degradation, or both. If protein degradation decreases and protein synthesis is normal or slightly increased, the net effect is an accumulation of cellular protein. Muscular hypertrophy tends to diminish if the excessive workload diminishes.

After removal of one kidney, the other kidney adapts to increased demand for work with an increase in both the size and the number of cells. The major contribution to renal enlargement is hypertrophy. An example of normal or physiologic hypertrophy is the increased growth of the uterus and mammary glands in response to pregnancy.

Hyperplasia

Hyperplasia is an increase in the number of cells resulting from an increased rate of cellular division. Hyperplasia, as a

HEALTH ALERT

Coronary Angioplasty and Cell Injury

Coronary angioplasty has been used clinically for more than a decade (see figure below). Its initial promise as an alternative to coronary bypass surgery has only partially been fulfilled because of the high rate of postoperative restenosis (narrowing). Restenosis is a frequent long-term complication secondary to mechanically induced injury by the balloon. The injury causes an adaptive response of hypertrophy of the smooth muscle cells and an increase in macrophage activity. The rate of reocclusion is thought to accelerate because the macrophages release potent cytokines and growth factors that may recruit new cells into the intima and cause intimal cell proliferation. In addition, reactive oxygen species may be involved in the intimal response to injury.

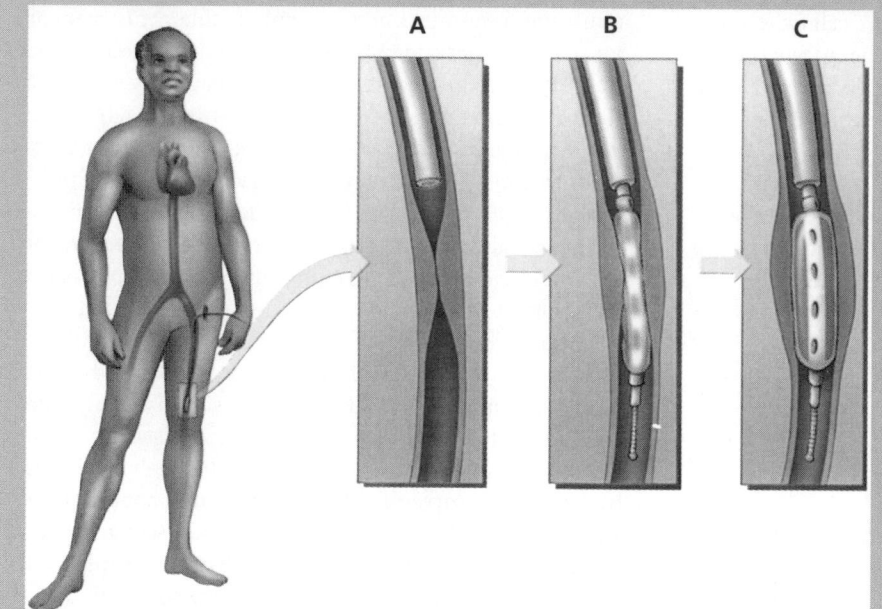

Balloon angioplasty. **A,** A catheter is inserted into the vessel until it reaches the affected region. **B,** A probe with a metal tip is pushed out the end of the catheter into the blocked region of the vessel. **C,** The balloon is inflated, pushing the walls of the vessel outward. Sometimes metal coils or tubes, called *stents*, are inserted to keep the vessel open. *(From Thibodeau, G.A. & Patton, K.T. [1999]. Anatomy & physiology [4th ed.]. St. Louis: Mosby.)*

Data from Ferns, G.A. & Woolaghan, E. (1995). Recent insights into the mechanisms of iatrogenic arteriosclerosis [editorial]. Journal of Pathology, *176(4), 331; Voisard, R. et al. High dose diltiazem prevents migration and proliferation of vascular smooth muscle cells in various in-vitro models of human coronary restenosis.* Coronary Artery Disease, *8(3-4), 189-201.*

Fig. 3-2 *Hypertrophy of cardiac muscle in response to valve disease.* **A,** Transverse slices of a normal heart and a heart with hypertrophy of the left ventricle (*L,* normal thickness of left ventricular wall; *T,* thickened wall from heart in which severe narrowing of aortic valve caused resistance to systolic ventricular emptying). **B,** Histology of cardiac muscle from the normal heart. **C,** Histology of cardiac muscle from a hypertrophied heart. *(From Stevens, A. & Lowe, J. [1995]. Pathology. St. Louis: Mosby.)*

response to injury, occurs when the injury has been severe and prolonged enough to have caused cell death.[1] Loss of epithelial cells and cells of the liver and kidney triggers deoxyribonucleic acid (DNA) synthesis and mitotic division. Increased cell growth is a multistep process involving the production of growth factors, which stimulate the remaining cells to synthesize new cell components and, ultimately, to divide. Hyperplasia and hypertrophy often occur together, and both take place if the cells can synthesize DNA, which enables mitotic division to occur.

Two types of normal, or physiologic, hyperplasia are (1) compensatory and (2) hormonal. *Compensatory hyperplasia* is an adaptive mechanism that enables certain organs to regenerate. For example, removal of part of the liver leads to hyperplasia of the remaining liver cells (hepatocytes) to compensate for the loss. Even with removal of 70% of the liver, regeneration is complete in about 2 weeks. A relatively recently identified new protein, *hepatocyte growth factor* (HGF), is thought to be a mediator of liver regeneration.[2]

Some cells, such as nerve, skeletal muscle, and myocardial cells and the lens cells of the eye, do not regenerate. Additional skeletal muscle cells, however, can be made by the fusion of myoblasts.[3] Significant compensatory hyperplasia occurs in epidermal and intestinal epithelia, hepatocytes, bone marrow cells, and fibroblasts, and some hyperplasia is noted in bone, cartilage, and smooth muscle cells. Another example of compensatory hyperplasia is the callus, or thickening, of the skin as a result of hyperplasia of epidermal cells in response to a mechanical stimulus.

Hormonal hyperplasia occurs chiefly in estrogen-dependent organs, such as the uterus and breast. After ovulation, for example, estrogen stimulates the endometrium to grow and thicken for reception of the fertilized ovum. If pregnancy occurs, hormonal hyperplasia, as well as hypertrophy, enables the uterus to enlarge. (Hormone function is described in Chapters 17 and 31.)

Pathologic hyperplasia is the abnormal proliferation of normal cells, usually in response to excessive hormonal stimulation. The most common example is pathologic hyperplasia of the endometrium (caused by an imbalance between estrogen and progesterone secretion, with oversecretion of estrogen). Pathologic endometrial hyperplasia, which causes excessive menstrual bleeding, is under the influence of regular growth-inhibition controls. If these controls fail, hyperplastic endometrial cells can undergo malignant transformation.

Dysplasia

Dysplasia refers to abnormal changes in the size, shape, and organization of mature cells. Dysplasia is not considered a true adaptive process but is related to hyperplasia and is often called *atypical hyperplasia.* Dysplastic changes frequently are encountered in epithelial tissue of the cervix and respiratory tract, where they are strongly associated with common neoplastic growths and often are found adjacent to cancerous cells. Dysplasia is often classified as mild, moderate, or severe; however, this subjective scheme has prompted recommendations to use either "low grade" or "high grade." Data indicate that atypical hyperplasia is a strong predictor of breast cancer development.[4] Neoplasia is a term associated with malignant tumors. If the inciting stimulus is removed, dysplastic changes often are reversible.

Metaplasia

Metaplasia is the reversible replacement of one mature cell type by another, sometimes less differentiated, cell type. The best example of metaplasia is replacement of normal columnar ciliated epithelial cells of the bronchial (airway) lining by stratified squamous epithelial cells (Fig. 3-3). The newly formed cells do not secrete mucus or have cilia, causing loss of a vital protective mechanism. Bronchial metaplasia can be reversed if the inducing stimulus, usually cigarette smoking,

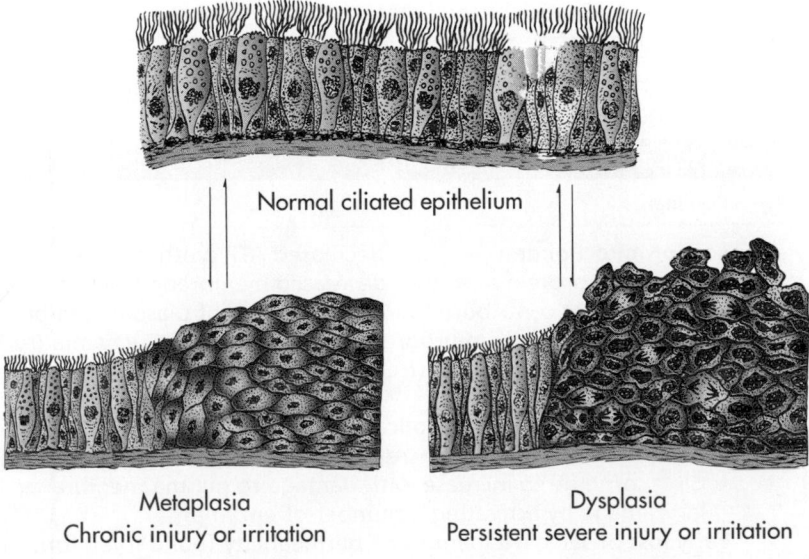

Normal ciliated epithelium

Metaplasia
Chronic injury or irritation

Dysplasia
Persistent severe injury or irritation

Fig. 3-3 *Reversible changes in cells lining the bronchi.*

is removed. With prolonged exposure to the inducing stimulus, however, cancerous transformation can occur.

CELLULAR INJURY

Most diseases begin with cell injury. Cellular injury occurs if the cell is unable to maintain homeostasis—a normal or adaptive steady state—in the face of injurious stimuli. Injured cells may recover (***reversible injury***) or die (***irreversible injury***). Injurious stimuli include chemical agents, lack of sufficient oxygen (hypoxia), free radicals, infectious agents, physical and mechanical factors, immunologic reactions, genetic factors, and nutritional imbalances. Types of injuries and their responses are summarized in Table 3-1 and Fig. 3-4.

The extent of cellular injury depends on the type, state (including level of cell differentiation and increased susceptibility to fully differentiated cells), and adaptive processes of the cell, as well as the type, severity, and duration of the injurious stimulus. Two individuals exposed to an identical stimulus may incur varying degrees of cellular injury. Modifying factors, such as nutritional status, can profoundly influence the extent of injury. The precise "point of no return" that leads to cellular death is a biochemical puzzle, and the exact mechanisms responsible for the transition from reversible to irreversible cellular damage are currently debated.

General Mechanisms of Cell Injury

Four common biochemical themes are important to cell injury and cell death regardless of the injuring agent (Table 3-2). New information exists on cell injury caused by free radicals, including activated oxygen species. Therefore this discussion is expanded to include three common forms of cell injury: (1) hypoxic injury, (2) free radicals and reactive oxygen species injury, and (3) chemical injury.

Hypoxic Injury

Hypoxia, or lack of sufficient oxygen, is the single most common cause of cellular injury (Fig. 3-5). Hypoxia can result from a decreased amount of oxygen in the air, loss of hemoglobin or hemoglobin function, decreased production of red blood cells, diseases of the respiratory and cardiovascu-

TABLE 3-1	Progressive Types of Cell Injury and Responses
Type	**Responses**
Adaptation	Atrophy, hypertrophy, hyperplasia, metaplasia
Active cell injury	Immediate response of "entire" cell
Reversible	Loss of adenosine triphosphate (ATP), cellular swelling, detachment of ribosomes, autophagy of lysosomes
Irreversible	"Point of no return" structurally when severe vacuolization of the mitochondria occurs and Ca^{++} moves into the cell
Necrosis	Common types of cell death with severe cell swelling and breakdown of organelles
Apoptosis, or programmed cell death	Cellular self-destruction for elimination of unwanted cell populations
Chronic cell injury (subcellular alterations)	Persistent stimuli response may involve only specific organelles or cytoskeleton, e.g., phagocytosis of bacteria
Accumulations or infiltrations	Water, pigments, lipids, glycogen, proteins
Pathologic calcification	Dystrophic and metastatic calcification

TABLE 3-2	Common Themes in Cell Injury and Cell Death
Theme	**Comments**
ATP depletion	Loss of mitochondrial ATP and decreased ATP synthesis; results include cellular swelling, decreased protein synthesis, decreased membrane transport, and lipogenesis, all changes that contribute to loss of integrity of plasma membrane
Oxygen and oxygen-derived free radicals	Lack of oxygen is key in progression of cell injury in ischemia (reduced blood supply); activated oxygen species (free radicals, O_2^-, H_2O_2, OH·) cause destruction of cell membranes and cell structure
Intracellular calcium and loss of calcium steady state	Normally intracellular cytosolic calcium concentrations are very low; ischemia and certain chemicals cause an increase in cytosolic Ca^{++} concentrations; sustained levels of Ca^{++} continue to increase with damage to plasma membrane; Ca^{++} causes intracellular damage by activating a number of enzymes
Defects in membrane permeability	Early loss of selective membrane permeability found in all forms of cell injury

ATP, Adenosine triphosphate.

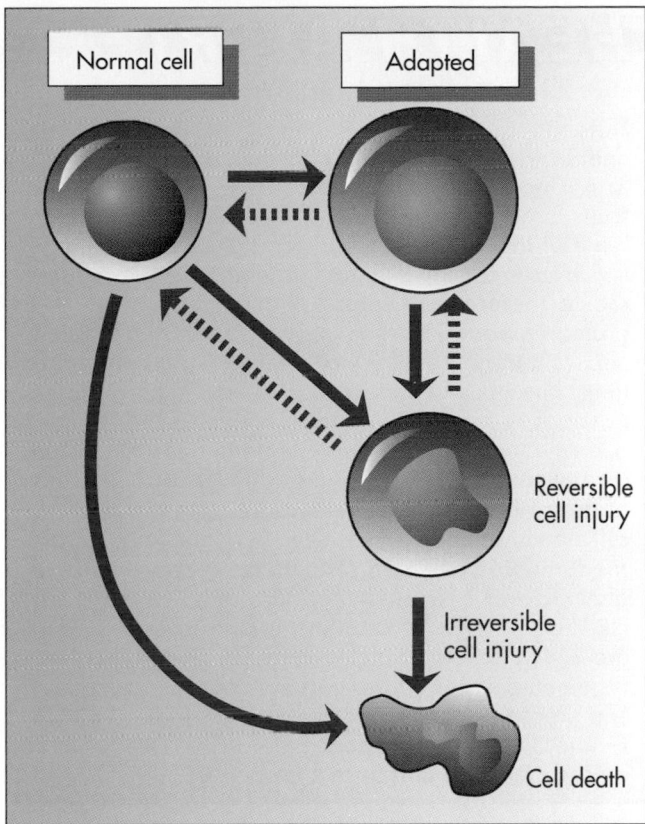

Fig. 3-4 *Cellular injury and responses.* Relationship among normal, adapted (hypertrophied), and reversibly injured cells and cell death of myocardial cells is depicted here.

lar systems, and poisoning of the oxidative enzymes (cytochromes) within the cells. The most common cause of hypoxia is *ischemia* (reduced blood supply).

Ischemic injury often is caused by gradual narrowing of arteries (arteriosclerosis) and complete blockage by blood clots (thrombosis). Progressive hypoxia caused by gradual arterial obstruction is better tolerated than the sudden acute *anoxia* (total lack of oxygen) caused by a sudden obstruction, as with an embolus (a blood clot or other plug in the circulation). An acute obstruction in a coronary artery can cause myocardial cell death (infarction) within minutes if the blood supply is not restored, whereas gradual onset of ischemia usually results in myocardial adaptation. Myocardial infarction and stroke, which are common causes of death in the United States, generally result from atherosclerosis (a type of arteriosclerosis) and consequent ischemic injury. (Vascular obstruction is discussed in Chapter 23.)

Cellular responses to hypoxic injury caused by ischemia have been demonstrated in studies of the heart muscle. Within 1 minute after blood supply to the myocardium is interrupted, the heart becomes pale and has difficulty contracting normally. Within 3 to 5 minutes, the ischemic portion of the myocardium ceases to contract because of a rapid decrease in mitochondrial phosphorylation, causing insufficient adenosine triphosphate (ATP) production. Lack of ATP leads to increased anaerobic metabolism, which generates ATP from glycogen when there is insufficient oxygen. When glycogen stores are depleted, even anaerobic metabolism ceases.

Fig. 3-5 *Hypoxic injury induced by ischemia.*

A reduction in ATP levels causes the plasma membrane's sodium-potassium pump and sodium-calcium exchange to fail, which leads to an intracellular accumulation of sodium and calcium and diffusion of potassium out of the cell. Sodium and water then can enter the cell freely, and cellular swelling, as well as early dilation of the endoplasmic reticulum, results. Dilation causes the ribosomes to detach from the rough endoplasmic reticulum, reducing protein synthesis. With continued hypoxia, the entire cell becomes markedly swollen, with increased concentrations of sodium, water, and chloride and decreased concentrations of potassium. These disruptions are reversible if oxygen is restored. If oxygen is not restored, however, vacuolation (formation of vacuoles) occurs within the cytoplasm, as well as marked mitochondrial swelling resulting from damage to this membrane. Structurally, this stage is associated with irreversible cell injury. With plasma membrane damage, extracellular calcium moves into the cell and accumulates in the mitochondria. Restoration of oxygen, however, can cause additional injury called **reperfusion injury.** Reperfusion injury results from the generation of high reactive oxygen intermediates, including hydroxyl radical ($OH\cdot$), superoxide (O_2^-), and hydrogen peroxide (H_2O_2). These radicals can *all* cause further membrane damage. Antioxidants can decrease the amount of damage, especially superoxide dismutase (SOD) and vitamin E.[5]

All cells in the body are bathed in a fluid rich in calcium ions. In muscle cells, calcium is needed to activate the contractile proteins, actin and myosin. If the plasma membrane's barrier to calcium ions is eliminated or damaged, calcium readily enters and accumulates in the mitochondria, resulting in mitochondrial swelling and rapid death of the cell, caused by calcium accumulation compromising ATP production by the mitochondria.[6,7] In hypoxic injury caused by atherosclerosis, failure of ATP production further deprives the myocardium of the energy needed for contraction.

✓ QUICK CHECK

Why is atypical hyperplasia not considered a true adapted change?

Why do cells become irreversibly injured?

Why do cells become markedly swollen with hypoxic injury?

Free Radicals and Reactive Oxygen Species Injury

An important mechanism of cellular injury is injury induced by free radicals, especially by activated oxygen species. A *free radical* is an electrically uncharged atom or group of atoms having an unpaired electron. Having one unpaired electron makes the molecule unstable; thus to stabilize it gives up an electron to another molecule or steals one. Therefore it is capable of injurious chemical bond formation with proteins, lipids, and carbohydrates—key molecules in membranes and nucleic acids. Free radicals are difficult to control and initiate chain reactions.

Free radicals may be initiated within cells by (1) the absorption of extreme energy sources (e.g., ultraviolet light, radiation); (2) endogenous reactions when oxygen is reduced to water created by systems involved in electron and oxygen transport (redox reactions; all biologic membranes contain redox systems important for cell defense, iron update, growth, and proliferation and signal transduction) (Fig. 3-7); and (3) enzymatic metabolism of exogenous chemicals or drugs (e.g., CCl_3, a product of carbon tetrachloride [CCl_4]). Table 3-3 describes the most significant free radicals.

Free radicals cause several damaging effects by (1) **lipid peroxidation,** which is the destruction of polyunsaturated lipids (the same process by which fats become rancid) leading to membrane damage and increased permeability; (2) attacking critical proteins that affect ion pumps and transport mechanisms; (3) fragmenting DNA, causing decreased protein synthesis; and (4) damaging mitochondria, causing the liberation of calcium into the cytosol (see pp. 69-70). Because of increased understanding of free radicals, a growing number of diseases and disorders have been linked either directly or indirectly to these reactive species (Table 3-4).

It is fortunate that the body can sometimes rid itself of

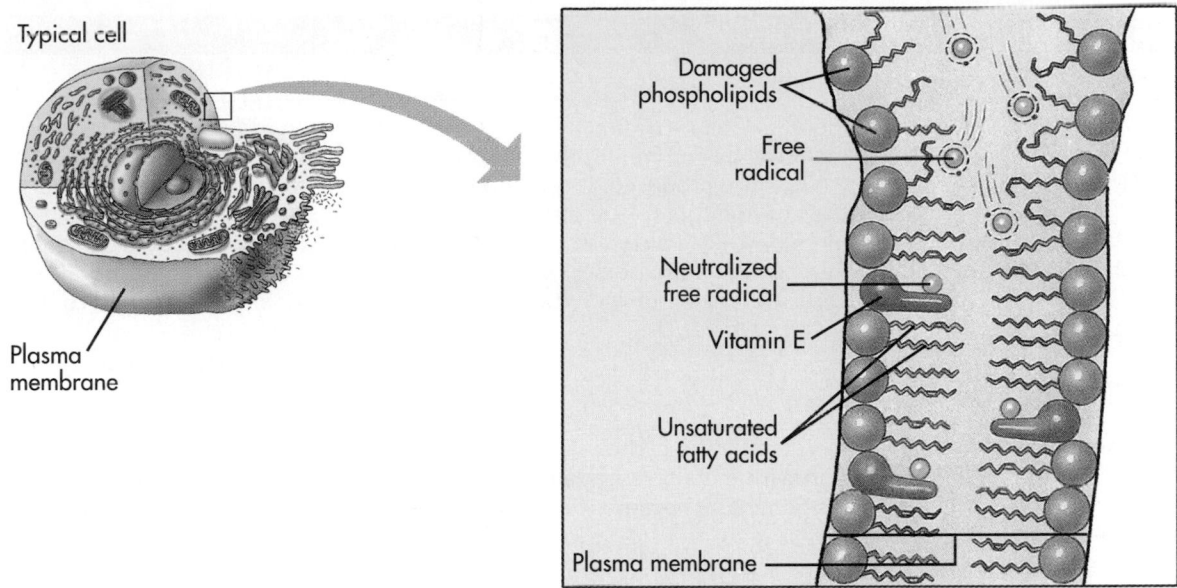

Fig. 3-6 *Role of vitamin E.* Vitamin E can act as an antioxidant, attracting and neutralizing molecules with unpaired electrons. *(From Thibodeau, G.A. & Patton, K.T. [1999].* Anatomy & physiology *[4th ed.]. St. Louis: Mosby.)*

Fig. 3-7 *Generation of reactive oxygen species and antioxidant mechanisms in biologic systems.* O_2 is converted to superoxide (O_2^{-}) by oxidative enzymes in the mitochondria, endoplasmic reticulum (ER), plasma membrane, peroxisomes, and cytosol. O_2 is converted to H_2O_2 by superoxide dismutase (SOD) and further to OH· by the Cu^{++}/Fe^{++} Fenton reaction. Superoxide catalyzes the reduction of Fe^{++} to Fe^{+++}, thus increasing OH· formation by the Fenton reaction. H_2O_2 is also derived from oxidases in peroxisomes. The three reactive oxygen species (O_2^{-}, H_2O_2, OH·) cause free radical damage to lipids (peroxidation of the membrane), proteins (ion pump damage), and DNA (impaired protein synthesis). The major antioxidant enzymes include SOD, catalase, and glutathione peroxidase. *(Modified from Cotran, R.S., Kumar, V., & Robbins, S.L. [1994].* Robbins pathologic basis of disease *[5th ed.]. Philadelphia: Saunders.)*

TABLE 3-3   Biologically Relevant Free Radicals

Free Radical	Comments
Reactive oxygen species (ROS) Superoxide O_2^- $O_2 \xrightarrow{oxidase} O_2^-$	Generated either (1) directly during autooxidation in mitochondria or (2) enzymatically by enzymes in the cytoplasm, such as xanthine oxidase or cytochrome P-450; once produced, it can be inactivated spontaneously or more rapidly by the enzyme superoxide dismutase (SOD): $O_2^- + O_2^- + 2H^- \xrightarrow{SOD} H_2O_2 + O_2$
Hydrogen peroxide (H_2O_2) $O_2^- + O_2^- + 2H \xrightarrow{SOD} H_2O_2 + O_2$ or oxidases present in peroxisomes O_2 peroxisome $O_2^- \xrightarrow{SOD} H_2O_2$	Generated by the enzyme superoxide dismutase (SOD) or directly by oxidases in intracellular peroxisomes; NOTE: SOD is considered an antioxidant because it converts superoxide to H_2O_2; catalase (another antioxidant) can then decompose H_2O_2 to $O_2 + H_2O$
Hydroxyl radicals (OH^-) $H_2O \rightarrow H\cdot + OH\cdot$ or $Fe^{++} + H_2O_2 \rightarrow Fe^{+++} + OH\cdot + OH^-$ or $H_2O_2 + O_2^- \rightarrow OH\cdot + OH^- + O_2$	Generated by the hydrolysis of water caused by ionizing radiation or by interaction with metals—especially ion (Fe) and copper (Cu). Iron is important in toxic oxygen injury because it is required for maximal oxidative cell damage
Nitric oxide (NO) $NO\cdot + O_2^- \rightarrow ONOO^- + H^+$	NO by itself is an important mediator that can act as a free radical; it can be converted to another radical—peroxnitrite anion ($ONOO^-$), as well as NO_2^- and NO_3^-

Data from Cotran RS, Kumar V, Collins, T. (1999). Robbins' pathologic basis of disease (6th ed.). Philadelphia: Saunders.

TABLE 3-4   Diseases and Disorders Linked to Oxygen-Derived Free Radicals

Deterioration noted in aging	Iron overload
Atherosclerosis	Lung disorders
Heart disease	Asbestosis
Stroke	Oxygen toxicity
Brain disorders	Emphysema
Ischemic brain injury	Nutritional deficiencies
Aluminum toxicity	Radiation injury
Alzheimer disease	Reperfusion injury
Neurotoxins	Rheumatoid arthritis
Cancer	Skin disorders
Cardiac myopathy	Solar radiation
Chronic granulomatous disease	Burns
Diabetes mellitus	Contact dermatitis
Eye disorders	Bloom syndrome
Macular degeneration	Toxic states
Cataracts	Xenobiotics (CCl_4, paraquat, cigarette smoke, etc.)
Inflammatory disorders	Metal ions (Ni, Cu, Fe, etc.)

Data from Knight, J.A. (1995). Annals of Clinical Laboratory Science, 25(2), 111.

---

free radicals. Superoxide may spontaneously decay into oxygen and hydrogen peroxide. Table 3-5 summarizes other methods that contribute to inactivation or termination of free radicals. The toxicity of certain drugs and chemicals can be attributed to either conversion of these chemicals to free radicals or the formation of oxygen-derived metabolites (see Mechanisms of Chemical Injury).

Mechanisms of Chemical Injury

Chemical injury begins with a biochemical interaction between a toxic substance and the cell's plasma membrane, which is ultimately damaged, leading to increased permeability. Not all the mechanisms causing chemically induced membrane destruction are known; however, the two general mechanisms include (1) direct toxicity by combining with a

TABLE 3-5	Methods Contributing to Inactivation or Termination of Free Radicals
Method	**Process**
Antioxidants	Endogenous or exogenous; either blocks synthesis or inactivates (e.g., scavenges) free radicals; includes vitamin E, vitamin C, cysteine, glutathione, albumin, ceruloplasmin, transferrin
Enzymes	Superoxide dismutase,* which converts superoxide to H_2O_2; catalase* (in peroxisomes) decomposes H_2O_2; glutathione peroxidase* decomposes $OH\cdot$ and H_2O_2

These enzymes are important in modulating the cellular destructive effects of free radicals, also released in inflammation.

molecular component of the cell membrane or organelles and (2) reactive free radicals and lipid peroxidation.

Because it has been investigated extensively, carbon tetrachloride (CCl_4) injury is a useful example of chemical injury. Carbon tetrachloride, an agent formerly used in dry cleaning, is converted by an enzyme system in the smooth endoplasmic reticulum of liver cells into CCl_3 (chloromethyl), a highly toxic free radical. The newly formed CCl_3 rapidly destroys the endoplasmic reticulum of the liver cell by lipid peroxidation, breaking down the reticulum's lipid component.

The lipid molecules accumulate within the cytoplasm, starting within cisternae of the endoplasmic reticulum (Fig. 3-8). Fatty liver develops because CCl_4 poisoning blocks the synthesis of **lipid-acceptor proteins (apoproteins)** that normally bind with triglycerides to form lipoproteins, which are transported out of the cell. Blockage of triglyceride (lipoprotein) secretion begins 10 to 15 minutes after CCl_4 exposure. Fat droplets that accumulate in cisternae of the endoplasmic reticulum combine to form larger droplets and fill vacuoles that, in turn, fill the entire cytoplasm. Approximately 10 to 12 hours later, the liver appears grossly enlarged and pale because of the accumulation of fat. Fatty change is reversible if the abnormality responsible is removed. At this point, the cellular changes are the same as in hypoxic injury (see p. 68).

Chemical agents

Many chemical agents cause cellular injury. Highly toxic substances are known as poisons. Minute amounts of some, such as arsenic and cyanide, can rapidly destroy enough cells to cause death of the individual. Chronic exposure to air pollutants, insecticides, and herbicides can cause cellular injury. Carbon monoxide, carbon tetrachloride, and social drugs, such as alcohol, can significantly alter cellular function and injure cellular structures. Recreational, over-the-counter, and prescribed drugs also may cause cellular injury, sometimes leading to death. Accidental or suicidal poisonings by chemical agents cause numerous deaths. The injurious effects of some agents—lead, carbon monoxide, ethyl alcohol—are common cellular injuries.

Lead

Heavy metals, such as lead, cause a significant number of childhood poisonings. Lead-based paint has a sweet taste and is often ingested by children. Other sources of lead include dust and soil in inner-city urban and possibly rural areas, debris from household renovations, formula mixed with lead-contaminated tap water, newsprint, lead water pipes, hair dyes, soldered tin cans, pottery glazes, and contamination from leaded gasoline.[8] Recently, rigid vinyl miniblinds were found to contain lead dust.[9] Children are particularly vulnerable to lead toxicity because, compared with adults, they absorb lead more readily through the intestines. If nutrition is compromised, especially if dietary intake of iron, calcium, and vitamin D is insufficient, lead's toxic effects are enhanced.[10]

The organ systems primarily affected by lead include the nervous system, the hematopoietic system (tissues that produce blood cells), and the kidneys. A suggested mechanism by which lead acts on the central nervous system (CNS) is interference with neurotransmitters, which may cause hyperactive behavior and proliferation of capillaries of the white matter and intercerebral arteries.[1] Lead inhibits several enzymes involved in hemoglobin synthesis and causes anemia as a result of lysis of red blood cells (hemolysis). Manifestations of brain involvement include convulsions and delirium and, with peripheral nerve involvement, wrist, finger, and sometimes foot paralysis. Renal lesions can cause tubular dysfunction resulting in glycosuria (glucose in the urine), aminoaciduria (amino acids in the urine), and hyperphosphaturia (excess phosphate in the urine). Gastrointestinal symptoms are less severe and include nausea, loss of appetite, weight loss, and abdominal cramping.

Carbon monoxide

Gaseous substances can be classified according to their ability to asphyxiate (interrupt respiration) or irritate. Toxic asphyxiants, such as carbon monoxide, hydrogen cyanide, and hydrogen sulfide, directly interfere with cellular respiration.

Carbon monoxide is odorless, colorless, and undetectable unless it is mixed with a visible or odorous pollutant. It is produced by the incomplete combustion of fuels such as gasoline. Although carbon monoxide is a chemical agent, the ultimate injury it produces is a hypoxic injury—namely, oxygen deprivation. Normally, oxygen molecules are carried to tissues bound to hemoglobin in red blood cells (see Chapter 25). Because carbon monoxide's affinity for hemoglobin is 300 times greater than that of oxygen, it quickly binds with the hemoglobin, preventing oxygen molecules from doing so. Minute amounts of carbon monoxide can produce significant percentages of carboxyhemoglobin (carbon monoxide bound with hemoglobin).

Symptoms related to carbon monoxide poisoning include headache, giddiness, tinnitus (ringing in the ears), nausea, weakness, and vomiting. At risk for carbon monox-

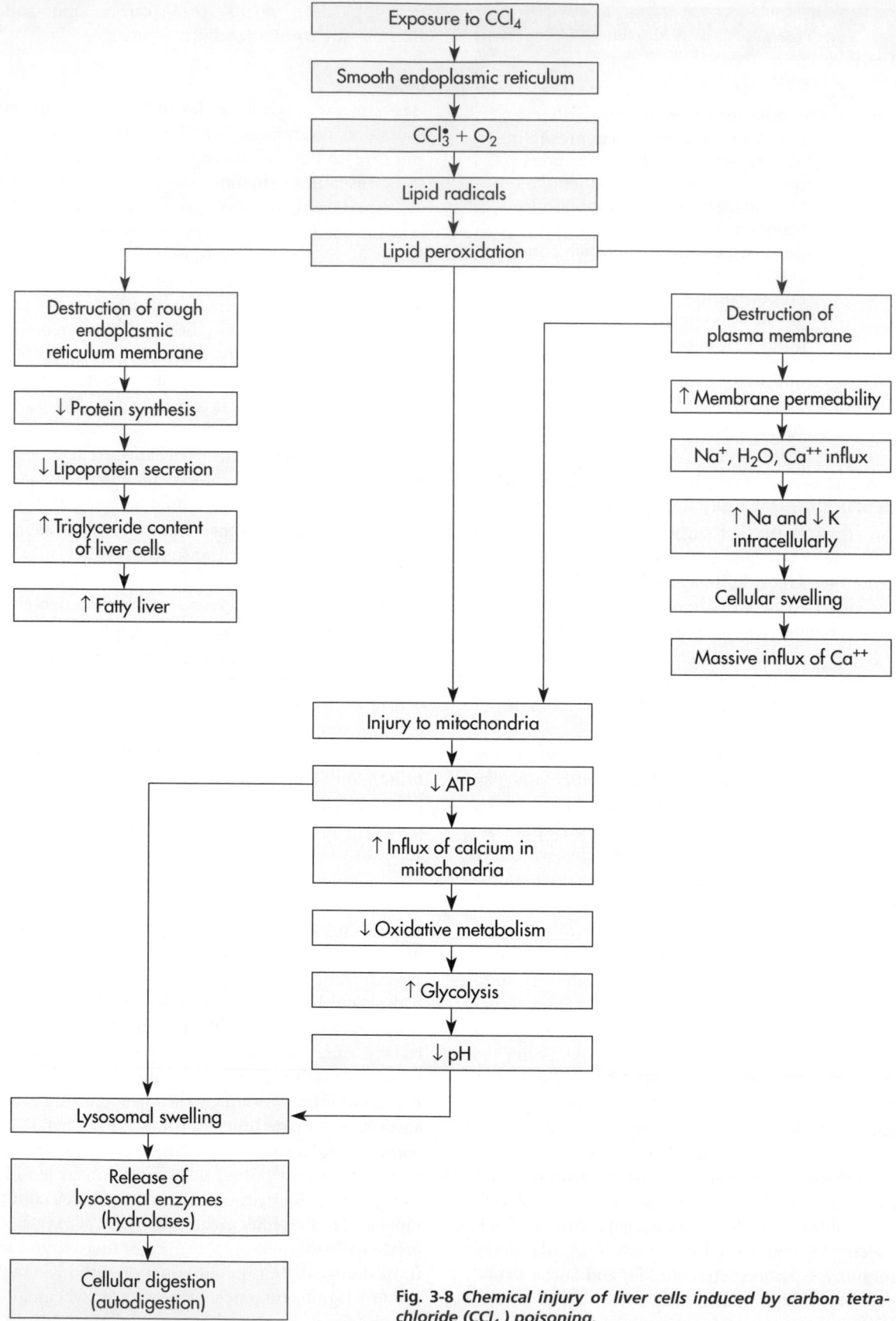

Fig. 3-8 *Chemical injury of liver cells induced by carbon tetra-chloride (CCl$_4$) poisoning.*

ide exposure are those who (1) breathe air polluted by gasoline engines or defective furnaces; (2) work in occupations such as coal mining, fire fighting, or engine repair; and (3) smoke cigarettes, cigars, or pipes. The fetus is especially at risk from the effects of carbon monoxide because fetal carboxyhemoglobin levels are likely to be 10% to 15% more than maternal levels.

Ethanol

Alcohol (ethanol) is the primary choice among mood-altering drugs in the United States. Because alcohol is not only a psychoactive drug but also a food, it is considered part of the basic food supply in many societies. A large intake of alcohol has enormous effects on nutritional status. Liver and nutritional disorders are the most serious consequences of alcohol abuse. New understandings of the mechanisms of ethanol-induced liver injury have emerged through the clarification of a new pathway for ethanol oxidation, the microsomal P-450 oxidase pathway.

The major effects of acute alcoholism involve the CNS. After alcohol is ingested, it is absorbed, unaltered, in the stomach and small intestine. Fatty foods and milk slow absorption. Alcohol then is distributed to all tissues and fluids of the body in direct proportion to the blood concentration.

Most of the alcohol in the blood is metabolized in the liver through one major and two accessory pathways. The major pathway involves hepatic alcohol dehydrogenase (ADH), an enzyme of the cytosol that catalyzes the conversion of ethanol to acetaldehyde (Fig. 3-9).

The microsomal ethanol oxidizing system (MEOS) depends on cytochrome P-450, an enzyme needed for cellular oxidation.[11] Activation of MEOS requires a high ethanol concentration and thus is thought to be important in the accelerated ethanol metabolism (i.e., tolerance) noted in persons with chronic alcoholism.[11]

Individuals differ in their capability to metabolize alcohol. Genetic differences in metabolism of liver alcohol, including aldehyde dehydrogenases, have been identified.[12] Persons with chronic alcoholism develop tolerance because of production of enzymes, leading to an increased rate of metabolism (e.g., P-450).

Acute alcoholism affects mainly the CNS but may induce reversible hepatic and gastric changes.[13-15] The hepatic changes, initiated from acetaldehyde, include deposition of fat, enlargement of the liver, interruption of microtubular transport of proteins and their secretion, increase in intracellular water, depression of fatty acid oxidation in the mitochondria, increased membrane rigidity, and acute liver cell necrosis (see Chapter 34). In the CNS, alcohol is, itself, a depressant, initially affecting subcortical structures (probably the brain stem reticular formation).[13] Consequently, motor and intellectual activity becomes disoriented. At higher blood levels, medullary centers become depressed, affecting respiration. Much investigation is underway on the relationship of alcohol and snoring and obstructive sleep apnea (cessation of breathing).[16]

Chronic alcoholism causes structural alterations in prac-

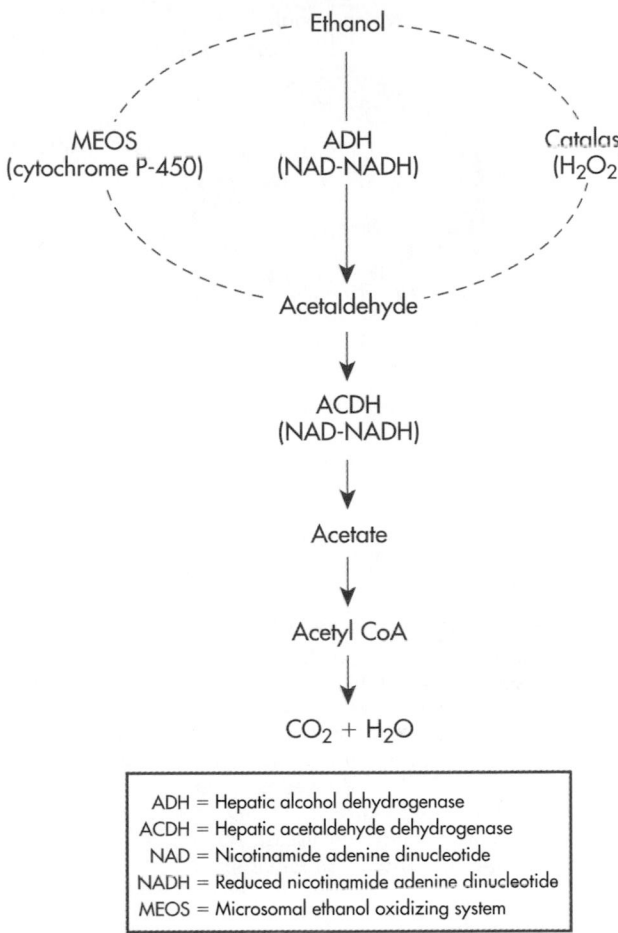

Fig. 3-9 *Major pathway of metabolism of alcohol in the liver through ADH. (Modified from Cotran, R.S., Kumar, V., & Robbins, S.L. [1994].* Robbins pathologic basis of disease *[5th ed.]. Philadelphia: Saunders.)*

tically all organs and tissues in the body, especially the liver and stomach. Acetaldehyde, because of its reactive nature, is proposed as the mediator of the widespread tissue and organ damage.[11] Chronic alcoholism is related to several disorders, including increased tendency to hypertension, a higher incidence of acute and chronic pancreatitis, and regressive changes in skeletal muscle (see Chapter 34).[17]

Ethanol is implicated in the onset of a variety of immune defects, including effects on the production of cytokines involved in inflammatory responses (tumor necrosis factor, interleukin-1, interleukin-6).[18] The deleterious effects of prenatal alcohol exposure (e.g., *fetal alcohol syndrome*), including growth retardation and cerebral malformations, have also been noted (Fig. 3-10). Animal laboratory studies have shown that enthanol at moderate concentrations inhibits epidermal growth factor—dependent replication of hepatocytes. This finding may account for the growth and development impairment associated with fetal alcohol syndrome and decreased liver regeneration in alcoholic liver disease.[19]

Fig. 3-10 *Fetal alcohol syndrome.* When alcohol enters the fetal blood, the potential result can cause tragic congenital abnormalities, such as microcephaly ("small head"), low birth weight, and cardiovascular defects, as well as developmental disabilities, such as physical and mental retardation, and even death. Note the small head, thinned upper lip, small eye openings (palpebral fissures), epicanthal folds, and receded upper jaw (retrognathia) typical of fetal alcohol syndrome. *(From Simon, C. & Janner, M. [1988]. Color atlas of pediatric disease [4th ed.]. Chapman and Hall, ITP International Thompson Publishing.)*

Whatever the cause, persons with chronic alcoholism have a significantly shortened life span related mainly to damage to the liver, stomach, brain, and heart. Alcohol is a well-known cause of hepatic injury, terminating in cirrhosis (Fig. 3-11) (see Chapter 34). Although findings are still controversial, moderate amounts of alcohol may decrease the incidence of coronary heart disease (see Chapter 23).

Social or street drugs

The social or "recreational" use of psychoactive drugs is widespread around the world. Most popular and dangerous are the drugs marijuana, cocaine, and heroin. The real prevalence of marijuana and heroin use is unknown. Although the prevalence of cocaine use in the general population decreased in 1986, morbidity and mortality related to cocaine increased sharply in the 1990s. Drug trafficking is a prevalent risk behavior among adolescents. Table 3-6 summarizes the effects of these drugs.

✓QUICK CHECK

Why is lipid peroxidation so injurious to cells?

What are some of the systemic effects of cocaine, marijuana, and heroin use?

Unintentional and Intentional Injuries

Unintentional and intentional injuries are an important health problem in the United States. In 1995 there were 150,809 deaths, an injury death rate of 57.4/100,000.[20] Death is significantly more common for men than women; the overall rate for men is 83.34/100,000 versus 32.6/100,000 for women. There are also significant racial differences in the death rate, with whites at 54.9/100,000, blacks at 79.9/100,000, and other racial groups at a combined rate of 39.39/100,000. There also is a bimodal age distribution for injury-related deaths, with peaks in the young adult and elderly groups. Unintentional injury is the leading cause of death for people between the ages of 1 and 34 years, with intentional injury (suicide, homicide) ranking between the second and fourth leading cause of death in this age-group. Statistics on nonfatal injuries are harder to document accurately, but they are known to be a significant cause of morbidity and disability and to cost society billions of dollars annually. The more common terms used to describe and classify unintentional and intentional injuries and brief descriptions of important features are discussed here.

Blunt force injuries

Injuries by **blunt force** are the result of the application of mechanical energy to the body resulting in the tearing, shearing, or crushing of tissues. They are the most common type of injuries seen in most health care settings. Blunt force injury may be caused by blows (where a moving object strikes the body), impacts (where the moving body strikes a fixed object), or a combination of both. Motor vehicle accidents and falls are the most common causes, accounting for 43,484 and 11,275 deaths, respectively, in 1995.

Contusion

A **contusion** (bruise) is bleeding into the skin and/or underlying tissues as a consequence of a blow that squeezes or crushes the soft tissues and ruptures blood vessels without breaking the skin. It may take several hours after injury before any change in skin color is seen. A bruise will be red-purple initially, eventually becoming blue-black, and then gradually changing to yellow-brown and/or green before fully disappearing (see Fig. 3-21). These color changes reflect the progression of tissue damage and healing that develops in the area of underlying injury. The length of time depends on factors such as the extent and location of the injury and the degree of vascularization in the area. Small contusions may resolve in a matter of days, whereas larger ones can take weeks to completely heal. Bruising of soft tissues may sometimes be confined to deeper structures; thus no injury is visible externally. Blood in deeper structures may dissect along fascial planes so discoloration of the skin may be seen in areas not directly injured by the initiating blow or impact, such as bruising of the thigh in a hip or pelvis fracture or "black eyes" in orbital plate fractures. Contusions may also be seen in internal organs in cases of severe injury.

A collection of blood in soft tissues or an enclosed space may also be referred to as a **hematoma. A subdural hema-**

TABLE 3-6	Social or Street Drugs
Type of Drug	**Comments**
Marijuana	Active substance: delta 9-tetrahydrocannabinol (THC) found in resin of the cannabis sativa plant; with smoking (e.g., "joints"), about 50% is absorbed through the lungs; when ingested only 10% is absorbed; with heavy use the following adverse effects have been reported: alterations of sensory perceptions, cognitive and psychomotor impairment (e.g., inability to judge time, speed, distance); smoking 3 or 4/day is similar to 20 cigarettes/day with frequency of chronic bronchitis, unknown but may contribute to lung cancer; from animal studies only reproductive changes include reduced fertility, decreased sperm motility, decreased circulatory testosterone; fetal abnormalities include low birth weight and increased frequency of childhood leukemia; increased frequency of infectious illnesses thought to be the result of depressed cell-mediated and humoral immunity.
Cocaine and crack	Extracted from the leaves of the coca plant and sold as a water-soluble powder (cocaine hydrochloride) liberally diluted with talcum powder or other white powders; extraction of pure alkaloid from cocaine hydrochloride is "free-base" called *crack* because it cracks when heated; crack is more potent than cocaine; cocaine is widely used as an anesthetic, usually in procedures of the oral cavity; it is a potent CNS stimulant, blocking reuptake of neurotransmitters norepinephrine, dopamine, and serotonin; also increases synthesis of norepinephrine and dopamine; dopamine induces a sense of euphoria, and norepinephrine causes adrenergic potentiation, including hypertension, tachycardia, and vasoconstriction; cocaine can therefore cause severe coronary artery narrowing and ischemia; not clear is why cocaine increases thrombus formation; other cardiovascular effects include dysrhythmias, sudden death, dilated cardiomyopathy, rupture of descending aorta (i.e., secondary to hypertension); effects to the fetus include premature labor, retarded fetal development, stillbirth, hyperirritability.
Heroin	An opiate closely related to morphine, methadone, and codeine; highly addictive, and withdrawal causes intense fear ("I'll die without it"); sold "cut" with similar-looking white powder; dissolved in water it is often highly contaminated; feeling of tranquility and sedation lasts only a few hours and thus encourages repeated intravenous or subcutaneous injections; acts on the receptors enkaphalins, endorphins, and dynorphins, which are widely distributed throughout the body with high affinity to the CNS; effects can include infectious complications, especially *Staphylococcus aureus,* granulomas of the lung, septic embolism, and pulmonary edema—in addition, viral infections from casual exchange of needles and HIV; sudden death is related to overdosage secondary to respiratory depression, cardiac output, and severe pulmonary edema.

Data from Cotran, R.S., Kumar, V., Collins, T. (1999). Robbins pathologic basis of disease (6th ed.). Philadelphia: Saunders; Nahas, G. & Latour, C. (1992). Medical Journal of Australia 156, 495.

Fig. 3-11 *Alcoholic hepatitis.* Chicken-wire fibrosis in zone 3. (Mallory trichrome stain.) *(From Damjanov, I. & Linder J. [Eds.] [1996]. Anderson's pathology [10th ed.]. St. Louis: Mosby.)*

toma is a collection of blood between the inner surface of the dura mater and the surface of the brain, resulting in the shearing of small veins that bridge the subdural space. Subdural hematoma can result from blows, falls, or sudden acceleration/deceleration of the head, as occurs in *shaken baby syndrome*. An **epidural hematoma** is a collection of blood between the inner surface of the skull and the dura. It is caused by a torn artery and is almost always associated with a skull fracture.

Contusions of the brain may result from (1) a blow or (2) a fall or impact. In blows, when a moving object strikes the stationary head, a cerebral contusion grouped in the portions of the brain underlying the area of scalp and skull injury is known as a *coup* pattern of injury. In falls or impacts, when the moving head strikes a fixed object, a cerebral contusion seen in the area of the brain opposite the external injury is known as a *contrecoup* pattern of injury. Contrecoup injury results when the head accelerates and the brain lags behind and presses into the areas of the skull directly opposite the direction of motion. When the head suddenly stops, the areas of the brain pressing into the skull are injured. For example, a person who falls directly backward, striking the occiput (back of the head), will have cerebral contusions of the frontal and temporal tips (these injuries are discussed further in Chapter 14).

Abrasion

An **abrasion** (scrape) results from removal of the superficial layers of the skin caused by friction between the skin and the injuring object. Abrasions vary in size and severity from fine, thin scratches to large areas of denudation (road rash). In cases where force is applied in a tangential, nonperpendicular direction to the skin surface, tags of tissue may be heaped up at the training or downstream edge of the abrasion. An abrasion will have a pale, moist, yellow-brown appearance at first. The color darkens to brown or even black as the injury dries. The injury may ooze fluid for 1 or 2 days until it is completely covered by a crust, or scab, which eventually flakes off of the underlying regenerated skin.

Abrasions and contusions may have a patterned appearance that mirrors the shape and features of an injuring object (Fig 3-12). Patterning of injuries can be of crucial importance in cases of automobile accidents, assaults, or homicides by documenting the connection between the victim's injuries and a suspect vehicle or weapon. Bite marks (usually a combination of abrasion and contusion) are another example of a patterned injury that can demonstrate a link between an assailant and a victim.

Laceration

A **laceration** is a tear or rip resulting when the tensile strength of the skin or tissue is exceeded. Unlike an incision, where the tissue is cleanly divided by a sharp edge, a laceration is much more jagged and irregular, and the edges will be abraded. The depths of the laceration will be irregular, and there are often tissue "bridges" of small vessels or nerves that have been stretched but not broken, crossing from one side

Fig. 3-12 *Patterned abrasion caused by a piece of rebar.* Note the tissue tags at the inferior margins indicating a downward direction to the blow that caused this injury.

of the wound to the other. If the injuring force is applied perpendicularly to the skin, there will be crushing of the surrounding tissue with associated abrasion and contusion. If force is applied tangentially, there will also be undermining of the wound, with tissues at the trailing edge of the wound lifted away from the underlying structures creating a pocket in the direction opposite from where the blow came. An extreme example is an **avulsion** (Fig. 3-13), in which a wide area of tissue may be pulled away creating a large flap. Usually, the shallower the angle of incidence of the blow, the more extensive the undermining.

Lacerations of internal organs are common in blunt impact injuries. Lacerations of the liver, spleen, kidneys, and bowel may occur in cases of blows to the abdomen, often with no visible injury to the abdominal wall seen externally. The thoracic aorta may be lacerated in sudden deceleration accidents. This results from the fact that the arch of the aorta is freely mobile, whereas the descending portion is attached

Fig. 3-13 *Avulsed laceration In motor vehicle accident victim.* The victim was the driver, and this injury most likely was caused by the brake pedal.

to the spinal column. Rapid deceleration will cause horizontal shearing with either partial or complete transection just below the take-off of the left subclavian artery. Severe blows or impacts to the chest may also cause rupturing of the heart with lacerations of the atria or ventricles.

Fractures

Blunt force blows or impacts can also cause bone to break or shatter. Fractures are extensively covered in Chapter 37 and are not discussed here.

Sharp force injuries

Cutting and piercing injuries accounted for 3367 deaths in 1995. As with all injuries, men have a higher rate (1.92/100,000) than women (0.67/100,000). There are also differences among races, with rates in whites 0.89/100,000, blacks 3.9/100,000, and other racial groups 1.18/100,000.

Incised wounds

An *incised wound* is a cut that is *longer* than it is *deep*. The wound may be straight or jagged, depending on the object used and how the injury occurred, with sharp, distinct edges without abrasion. Because the wound is caused by a sharp edge, the tissues are cleanly divided and there is no tissue bridging or undermining. An incised wound may be thin and narrow or more elliptic and gaping in appearance because of varying lines of tension in the skin, location, and orientation. They tend to produce significant external bleeding with minimal internal hemorrhage. These wounds are often seen in sharp force injury suicides. In most cases, in addition to a deep, lethal cut, there will be multiple superficial incisions grouped in the area known as *hesitation marks* (Fig. 3-14).

Stab wounds

A *stab wound* is a penetrating sharp force injury that is *deeper* than it is *long*. Because a sharp instrument is used, the depths of the wound are clean and distinct with no underlying or associated crushing injury. The edges usually are clean but may be abraded if the object is inserted deeply with enough force so that a wider, blunter portion of the instru-

Fig. 3-14 *Self-inflicted incised wound of the neck with multiple hesitation marks.*

ment (e.g., hilt of a knife) impacts the skin. Fig. 3-15 illustrates this type of wound.

A number of features about the blade used may be determined from careful examination of the stab wound. If a *single-edge* blade was used, one margin of the wound will be sharp and the other blunt; if a *double-edge* blade caused the wound, both margins will have a sharp appearance. Stab wounds produced by a *serrated-edge* blade are often indistinguishable from those made by a *smooth-edge* blade. If there was any hesitation or scraping of the skin edges by the blade, an interrupted pattern of abrasion may be seen but is uncommon. As with incised wounds, skin tension may cause the wound to gap giving it an elliptic appearance. The edges must be brought into opposition so there is no distortion before trying to determine if the margins are sharp or blunt. The length of the stab wound may or may not correlate with the width of the blade, depending on whether there was any cutting or twisting when the blade was inserted or withdrawn. Once the edges are in opposition, the thickness of the blade may be estimated from the width of the wound. Depth of the wound may not correlate with the length of the blade because the blade was not inserted fully, or, as a consequence of compression of tissues from a forceful thrust, the wound may be deeper than the length of the blade.

Depending on size and location of the stab wound, the amount of external bleeding may be surprisingly small. Af-

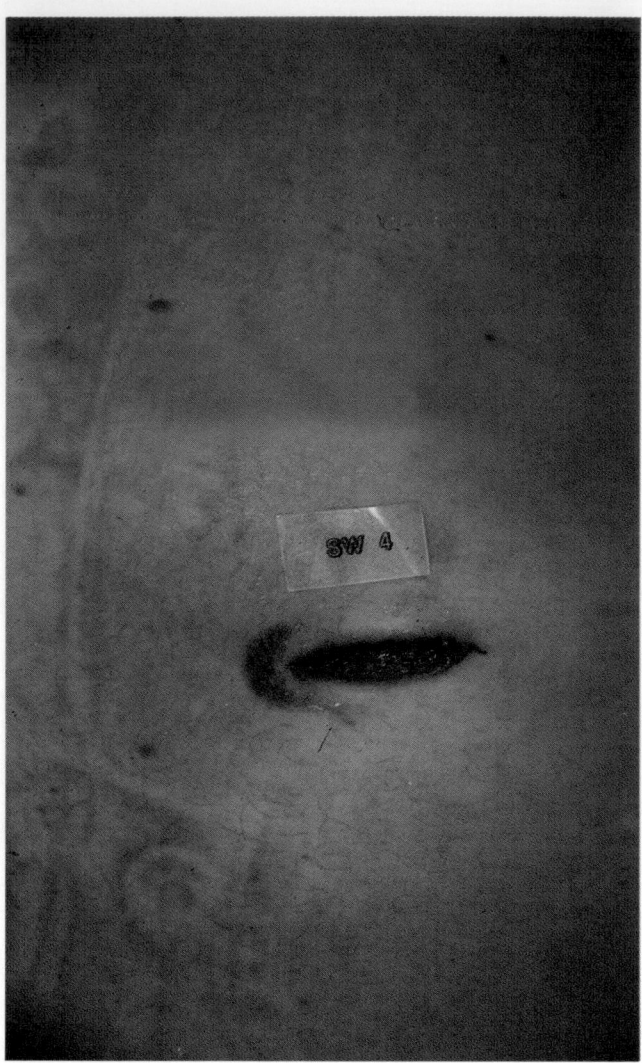

Fig. 3-15 *Stab wound with associated hilt mark.* Note the sharp margin away from the hilt mark with the blunt margin toward it. This wound was caused by a single-edge knife.

ter an initial spurt, even if a major vessel or the heart is struck, the wound track may be almost completely closed by tissue pressure, allowing only a trickle of visible blood despite copious internal bleeding.

Puncture wounds

Instruments or objects with sharp points but without sharp edges may produce penetrating *puncture wounds.* A classic example is a wound of the foot caused by stepping on a nail. These injuries often will have abrasion of the edges of the wound, are prone to infection, and can also be quite deep despite a sometimes innocuous external appearance.

Chopping wounds

Heavy, edged instruments (axes, hatchets, propeller blades) will produce injuries—*chopping wounds*—with a combination of sharp and blunt force characteristics. In addition to cutting, there will usually be associated crushing of the wound edges and underlying tissues.

Gunshot wounds

Injuries caused by gunfire accounted for more than 35,957 deaths in the United States in 1995. Of these, 18,503 were suicides, 15,835 homicides, 1225 accidents, and 394 classified as undetermined. These figures represent a 21.5% increase in the number of deaths from gunfire since 1985. Men are much more likely to die from gunshot injury than women. The male death rate in 1995 was 23.9/100,000, and it was only 3.9/100,000 for women. Black men between the ages of 15 and 24 years have the greatest gunfire injury death rate: 140.2/100,000. To put this statistic into perspective, if this was the rate for the United States as a whole, there would be more than 340,000 gunshot wound deaths per year.

Gunshot wounds may be either penetrating (bullet retained in the body) or perforating (bullet exits). In some cases the bullet may fragment so pieces of the missile are retained even though there is an exit wound. The most important factors determining the appearance of a gunshot injury are whether it is an entrance or an exit wound and the range of fire.

Entrance wounds

Although all **entrance wounds** share some common features, the overall appearance is most affected by the range of fire.

Contact range entrance wounds occur when the gun is held so the muzzle rests on or presses into the skin surface, causing a distinctive type of wound. In addition to the hole made by the bullet, there will be searing of the edges of the wound from the flame, hot gases exiting the barrel, and soot or smoke deposited on the edges of and in the depths of the wound. In hard contact wounds, where the barrel is firmly pressed into the skin, there may be minimal soot and searing on the outside of the wound but deep penetration of smoke, burning gunpowder fragments, and hot gases into the depths of the injury. In hard contact wounds of the head, where there is only a thin layer of skin and muscle overlying bone, the large amount of gas and explosive energy sent into the wound may cause severe tearing and disruption of the tissues, giving the wound a large, gaping, and jagged appearance—a phenomenon known as *blow back.* In areas of the body with thicker layers of soft tissue, the blow back may not cause tearing but will forcefully drive the skin back onto the end of the barrel, producing a patterned abrasion that mirrors the features of the weapon, known as a *muzzle imprint* (Fig. 3-16).

Intermediate range entrance wounds are surrounded by gunpowder tattooing or stippling (Fig. 3-17). *Tattooing* results from fragments of burning or unburned pieces of gunpowder exiting the barrel and striking the skin surface with enough force to be driven into the epidermis or superficial dermis. *Stippling* results when fragments of powder strike with enough force to abrade the skin but not actually penetrate the surface. This phenomenon can be seen when the muzzle-to-target range of most handguns is less than 48 inches. Beyond this distance, pieces of gunpowder disperse and slow down so much that tattooing or stippling cannot

Fig. 3-16 *Contact range gunshot wound of the chest with a muzzle abrasion.*

Fig. 3-17 *Intermediate range gunshot wound with stippling and tattooing.*

occur. The closer the muzzle is to the skin, the tighter the distribution and greater the density of powder fragments will be around the actual entrance hole. Soot may also be deposited.

An *indeterminate (distant) range entrance wound* occurs when flame, soot, or gunpowder does not reach the skin surface and the only thing striking the body is the bullet. The term *indeterminate* is used rather than *distant* because it does not imply that one can actually determine the range of fire from the appearance of the wound. For example, if an individual is shot through multiple layers of clothing, the entrance wound may have no soot, searing, or stippling even though the actual range of fire is only a matter of inches; the wound would look the same as if the shot came from a range of 6 meters (20 feet) or more. Indeterminate wounds are characterized by a hole surrounded by a rim of abrasion. The size of the hole can vary according to a number of factors. It is important to remember that one cannot say what caliber of weapon inflicted the wound based solely on the size of the entrance wound. The collar of abrasion results from the fact that the bullet first causes stretching and scraping of the skin before it actually perforates. If the bullet strikes perpendicular to the skin, the margin of abrasion collar is concentrically disturbed about the defect; if it strikes at an angle, the collar is eccentric, with the wider margin pointing in the direction from which the bullet came (Fig. 3-18). If the bullet has struck an intermediary target before hitting the skin, it can be turning and tumbling, producing an irregular abrasion collar.

Exit wounds

Exit wounds have the same general appearance no matter what the range of fire. Their shape can vary from round to slitlike to completely irregular. As with entrance wounds, the size does not correlate very well with the caliber of the projectile making the wound. The most important factors affecting exit wounds are the speed of the projectile and the degree of deformation. A smaller, highly deformed bullet ex-

Fig. 3-18 *Indeterminate range entrance wound with eccentric collar of abrasion resulting from the bullet striking the skin at an angle.*

iting at high speed can produce a large, irregular wound, whereas a larger, intact, slower-moving bullet may make only a small hole. Size *cannot* be used to determine if the hole is an exit or entrance wound. In most cases, the margins of an exit wound will *not* have an abrasion collar. An exit wound will have clean edges that can often be reproximated to cover the defect. The exception is when something is pressing against the skin surface at the exit site, such as tight clothing or the back of a chair. In this situation, the bullet will push the skin against the supporting surface, causing rubbing and scraping around the exit defect as it comes out, known as a *shored exit wound.*

It is important to remember that because the skin is so elastic and deformable, it is one of the toughest structures for a bullet to go through. It is not uncommon for a bullet to pass entirely through the body and be stopped just beneath the skin. There will often be no visible injury of the overlying skin; however, careful palpation of the area may allow one to locate the bullet.

Wounding potential of firearms

The amount of damage done by a bullet is a function of a number of variables. For the most part, the damage caused is a result of the amount of energy transferred to the tissues impacted. The energy a bullet has is determined by the following formula:

$$KE = \frac{1}{2} MV_2$$

where KE is the energy, M is the mass, and V is the speed.

Clearly, increasing the speed of a bullet has a much greater effect on its potential to cause damage than increasing its size. As the bullet passes through tissue and slows down, its energy is dissipated into the surrounding structures. This energy transfer causes tissue destruction in a zone that can be much larger than the actual size of the bullet; the zone of destruction may be several inches in diameter with very high-powered bullets. This transfer of energy in head wounds may lead to orbital plate fractures and palpebral ecchymosis (black eyes) or blood draining from the ears even though the path of the bullet does not come near the base of the skull. The amount of damage caused may be exacerbated by the generation of secondary missiles of bone fragments when portions of the skeleton are struck. Some bullets are designed to expand or fragment when they strike an object, thereby increasing the cross-sectional area of the projectile, increasing drag, and enhancing the transfer of energy into the tissues. "Hollow-point" ammunition is an example of this kind of bullet.

Obviously the lethality of a gunshot injury depends on what structures are damaged. Depending on the extent of damage, even gunshot wounds of the brain may not be lethal; however, they are usually immediately incapacitating and lead to significant long-term disability. It is important to remember that a victim with a "lethal" injury (wound of the heart or aorta) may not be immediately incapacitated and may engage in varying degrees of physical activity after being injured. Just because the victim is active or even combative when first evaluated does not mean the individual may *not* have experienced a potentially lethal injury.

Asphyxial injuries

Asphyxial injuries are caused by a failure of cells to receive or utilize oxygen. Deprivation of oxygen may be partial (*hypoxia*) or total (*anoxia*). Asphyxial injuries can be grouped into four general categories: suffocation, strangulation, chemical, and drowning.

Suffocation

Suffocation, or oxygen failing to reach the blood, can result from a lack of oxygen in the environment (entrapment in an enclosed space or filling the environment with a suffocating gas) or blockage of the external airways. Classic examples of these types of asphyxial injuries are a child who is trapped in an abandoned refrigerator or a person who commits suicide by putting a plastic bag over his or her head. A reduction in the ambient oxygen level to 16% (normal is 21%) is immediately dangerous. If the level is below 5%, death can ensue within a matter of minutes. The diagnosis of these types of asphyxial injuries depends on the history of what happened because there will be no specific physical findings.

Diagnosis and treatment in *choking asphyxiation* (obstruction of the internal airways) depend on locating and removing the obstructing material. Injury or disease also may cause swelling of the soft tissues of the airway leading to partial or complete obstruction and subsequent asphyxiation. Suffocation also may result from compression of the chest or abdomen (mechanical or compressional asphyxia) preventing normal respiratory movements. Usual signs and symptoms include florid facial congestion and petechiae (pinpoint hemorrhages) of the eyes and face.

Strangulation

Strangulation is caused by compression and closure of the blood vessels and air passages resulting from external pressure on the neck. This causes cerebral hypoxia or anoxia secondary to the alteration or cessation of blood flow to and from the brain. It is important to remember that the amount of force needed to close the jugular veins (2 kg [4.5 lb]) or carotid arteries (5 kg [11 lb]) is significantly less than that required to crush the trachea (15 kg [33 lb]). It is the alteration of cerebral blood flow in most types of strangulation that causes injury or death—not the lack of air flow. With complete blockage of the carotid arteries, unconsciousness can occur within 10 to 15 seconds.

A noose is placed around the neck, and the weight of the body is used to cause constriction of the noose and compression of the neck in *hanging strangulations.* The body does not need to be completely suspended to produce severe injury or death. Depending on the type of ligature used, there will usually be a distinct mark on the neck, an inverted V with the base of the V pointing toward the point of suspension. Internal injuries of the neck are actually quite rare in hangings, and only in judicial hangings, where the body is weighted and dropped, will significant soft tissue or cervical spinal trauma be seen. Petechiae of the eyes or face may be seen, but they are rare.

In *ligature strangulation,* the mark on the neck is horizontal without the inverted V pattern seen in hangings. Petechiae may be more common because intermittent opening and closure of the blood vessels may occur as a result of the victim's struggles. Internal injuries of the neck are rare.

There will be variable amounts of external trauma on the neck with contusions and abrasions in *manual strangulation* caused either by the assailant or the victim clawing at his or her own neck in an attempt to remove the assailant's hands. Internal damage can be quite severe, with bruising of deep structures and even fractures of the hyoid bone, and tracheal and cricoid cartilages. Petechiae are common.

Chemical asphyxiants

Chemical asphyxiants either prevent the delivery of oxygen to the tissues or block its utilization. Carbon monoxide is the most common chemical asphyxiant (see p. 73). *Cyanide* acts as an asphyxiant by combining with the ferric iron atom in cytochrome oxidase, thereby blocking the intracellular utilization of oxygen. A victim of cyanide poisoning will have the same cherry-red appearance as a carbon monoxide intoxication victim because cyanide blocks the utilization of circulating oxyhemoglobin. An odor of bitter almonds may also be detected. (The ability to smell cyanide is a genetic trait that is absent in a significant portion of the general population.) *Hydrogen sulfide* (sewer gas) is a chemical asphyxiant in which victims of hydrogen cyanide poisoning may have brown-tinged blood in addition to the nonspecific signs of asphyxiation.

Drowning

Drowning is an alteration of oxygen delivery to tissues resulting from the breathing in of fluid, usually water. In 1995 there were 5071 drowning deaths in the United States. Although research in the 1940s and 1950s indicated that changes in blood electrolyte levels and volume as a result of absorption of fluid from the lungs may be an important factor in some drownings, the major mechanism of injury is hypoxemia (low blood oxygen levels). Even in freshwater drownings, where large amounts of water can pass through the alveolar-capillary interface, there is no evidence that increases in blood volume cause significant electrolyte disturbances or hemolysis or that the amount of fluid loading is beyond the compensatory capabilities of the kidneys and heart. Airway obstruction is the more important pathologic abnormality, underscored by that fact that in as many as 15% of drownings little or no water enters the lungs because of vagal nerve-mediated laryngospasms. This phenomenon is called *dry-lung drowning.* No matter what mechanism is involved, cerebral hypoxia will lead to unconsciousness in a matter of minutes. Whether this progresses to death depends on a number of factors, including the age and the health of the individual. One of the most important factors is the temperature of the water. Irreversible injury will develop much more rapidly in warm water than it will in cold water. Submersion times of up to 1 hour with subsequent survival have been reported in children, in very cold water. Complete submersion is not necessary for a person to drown. An incapacitated or helpless individual (epileptic, alcoholic, infant) may drown in water that is only a few inches deep.

It is important to remember that no specific or diagnostic findings *prove* that a person recovered from the water is actually a drowning victim. In cases where water has entered the lung, there may be large amounts of foam coming out of the nose and mouth, although this can be seen also in certain types of drug overdoses. A body recovered from water with signs of prolonged immersion could just as easily be a victim of some other type of injury and has been put in the water to obscure the actual cause of death. When working with a living victim recovered from water, it is essential to keep in mind that an underlying condition may have led to the person's becoming incapacitated and submerged—a condition

that may *also* need to be treated or corrected while correcting hypoxemia and dealing with its sequelae.

Infectious Injury

The pathogenicity (virulence) of microorganisms lies in their ability to survive and proliferate in the human body, where they injure cells and tissues. The disease-producing potential of a microorganism depends on its ability to (1) invade and destroy cells, (2) produce toxins, and (3) produce damaging hypersensitivity reactions. (See Chapter 7 for a description of infection and infectious organisms.)

Immunologic and Inflammatory Injury

Cellular membranes are injured by direct contact with cellular and chemical components of the immune and inflammatory responses, such as phagocytic cells (lymphocytes, macrophages) and substances such as histamine, antibodies, lymphokines, complement, and proteases (see Chapter 6). Complement is responsible for many of the membrane alterations that occur during immunologic injury.

Membrane alterations are associated with rapid leakage of K^+ out of the cell and rapid influx of water. Antibodies can interfere with membrane function by binding to and occupying receptor molecules on the plasma membrane. Antibodies also can block or destroy cellular junctions, interfering with intercellular communication. Other mechanisms of cellular injury are genetic factors, nutritional imbalances, and physical agents. These are summarized in Table 3-7.

MANIFESTATIONS OF CELLULAR INJURY

Cellular accumulations, also known as *infiltrations,* not only occur when injury is sublethal and sustained in injured cells, but also can occur in normal cells. Common accumulations consist of substances that are normally present, such as fluids and electrolytes, triglycerides (lipids), glycogen, calcium, uric acid, proteins, melanin, and bilirubin. Abnormal accumulations of these substances can occur in the cytoplasm (frequently in the lysosomes) or in the nucleus if (1) the normal, endogenous substance is produced in excess or

TABLE 3-7 Mechanisms of Cellular Injury

Mechanism	Characteristics	Examples
Genetic factors	Alter cell's nucleus and the plasma membrane's structure, shape, receptors, or transport mechanisms	Sickle cell anemia, Huntington disease, muscular dystrophy, abetalipoproteinemia, familial hypercholesterolemia
Nutritional imbalances	Pathophysiologic cellular effects develop when nutrients are not consumed in diet and transported to the body's cells *or* when excessive amounts of nutrients are consumed and transported	Protein deficiency, protein-calorie malnutrition, glucose deficiency, lipid deficiency (hypolipidemia), hyperlipidemia (increased lipoproteins in the blood causing deposits of fat in the heart, liver, and muscle), vitamin deficiencies
Physical agents		
Temperature extremes	Hypothermic injury results from chilling or freezing of cells, creating high intracellular sodium concentrations; abrupt drops in temperature lead to vasoconstriction and increased viscosity of blood, causing ischemic injury, infarction, and necrosis	Frostbite
	Hyperthermic injury is caused by excessive heat and varies in severity according to the nature, intensity, and extent of the heat	Burns, burn blisters
Atmospheric pressure	Tissue injury caused by compressive waves of air or fluid impinging on the body, followed by a sudden wave of decreased pressure; changes may collapse the thorax, rupture internal solid organs, and cause widespread hemorrhage: carbon dioxide and nitrogen that are normally dissolved in blood come out of solution and form small bubbles (gas emboli), causing hypoxic injury and pain	Blast injury (air or immersion), decompression sickness (caisson disease or "the bends")
Ionizing radiation	Refers to any form of radiation that can remove orbital electrons from atoms; source is usually the environment, and damage is mainly to the DNA molecule, thus causing chromosomal aberrations	X-rays, γ-rays, α- and β-particles cause skin redness, skin damage, chromosomal damage, cancer
Illumination	Fluorescent lighting and halogen lamps create harmful stresses; ultraviolet light has been linked to skin cancer	Eyestrain, obscured vision, cataracts, headaches, melanoma
Mechanical stresses	Injury is caused by physical impact or irritation; they may be overt or cumulative	Faulty occupational biomechanics, leading to overexertion disorders
Noise	Can be caused by acute loud noise or the cumulative effects of various intensities, frequencies, and duration of noise	Hearing impairment or loss; tinnitus, temporary threshold shift (TTS)

at an increased rate; (2) an endogenous substance (normal or abnormal) is not effectively catabolized, usually because of lack of a vital lysosomal enzyme; or (3) harmful exogenous materials, such as heavy metals, mineral dusts, or microorganisms, accumulate because of inhalation, ingestion, or infection.

In all storage diseases, the cells attempt to digest, or catabolize, the "stored" substances. As a result, excessive amounts of metabolites (products of catabolism) accumulate in the cells and are expelled into the extracellular matrix, where they are taken up by phagocytic cells called *macrophages* (see Chapter 6). Some of these scavenger cells circulate throughout the body, whereas others remain fixed in certain tissues, such as the liver or spleen. As more and more macrophages and other phagocytes migrate to tissues that are producing excessive metabolites, the affected tissues begin to swell. This is the mechanism that causes enlargement of the liver (hepatomegaly) or the spleen (splenomegaly) as a clinical manifestation of many storage diseases.

Water

Cellular swelling, the most common degenerative change, is caused by the shift of extracellular water into the cells. In hypoxic injury, movement of fluid and ions into the cell is associated with acute failure of metabolism and loss of ATP production. Normally, the pump that transports sodium

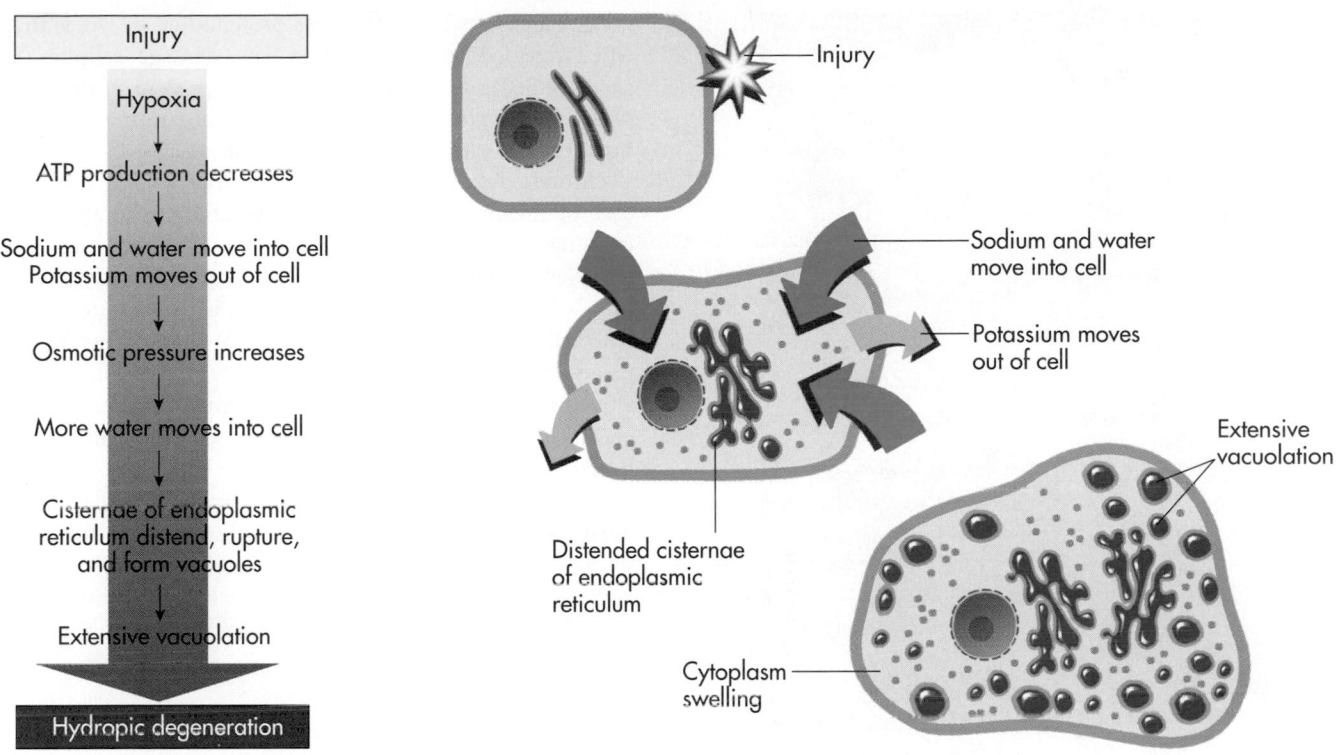

Fig. 3-19 *The process of hydropic degeneration.* *ATP,* Adenosine triphosphate.

ions out of the cell is maintained by the presence of ATP and ATPase, the active-transport enzyme. In metabolic failure caused by hypoxia, reduced ATP and ATPase permit sodium to accumulate in the cell while potassium diffuses outward. The increased intracellular sodium increases osmotic pressure, drawing more water into the cell. The cisternae of the endoplasmic reticulum become distended, rupture, and coalesce to form large vacuoles that isolate the water from the cytoplasm, a process called ***vacuolation.*** Progressive vacuolation results in ***hydropic degeneration*** or swelling (degeneration by water) (Fig. 3-19). If cellular swelling affects all the cells in an organ, the organ increases in weight and becomes distended and pale.

Cellular swelling is reversible and is considered sublethal. It is, in fact, an early manifestation of almost all types of cellular injury, including severe or lethal cell injury. It is also associated with high fever, hypokalemia (abnormally low concentrations of potassium in the blood; see Chapter 4), and certain infections.

Lipids and Carbohydrates

Certain metabolic disorders result in the abnormal intracellular accumulation of carbohydrates and lipids. These substances may accumulate throughout the body but are found primarily in the spleen, liver, and CNS. Accumulations in cells of the CNS can cause neurologic dysfunction and severe mental retardation. Lipids accumulate in Tay-Sachs disease, Niemann-Pick disease, and Gaucher disease, whereas in the

diseases known as mucopolysaccharidoses, carbohydrates are in excess. The mucopolysaccharidoses are progressive disorders that usually involve multiple organs, including liver, spleen, heart, and blood vessels. The accumulated mucopolysaccharides are found in reticuloendothelial cells, endothelial cells, intimal smooth muscle cells, and fibroblasts throughout the body. These carbohydrate accumulations can cause clouding of the cornea, joint stiffness, and mental retardation.[1]

Although lipids sometimes accumulate in heart and kidney cells, the most common site of intracellular lipid accumulation, or ***fatty change,*** is liver cells. Because hepatic metabolism and secretion of lipids are crucial to proper body function, imbalances and deficiencies in these processes lead to major pathologic changes. Lipid accumulation in liver cells causes fatty liver, or fatty change (Fig. 3-20). As lipids fill the cells, vacuolation pushes the nucleus and other organelles aside. Grossly, the liver looks yellowish and greasy.

Lipid accumulation in liver cells occurs after cellular injury sets one or more of the following mechanisms in motion:

1. Increased movement of free fatty acids into the liver (Starvation, for example, increases breakdown of triglycerides in adipose tissue, releasing fatty acids that subsequently enter liver cells.)
2. Failure of the metabolic process that converts fatty acids to phospholipids, resulting in the preferential conversion of the fatty acids to triglycerides

Fig. 3-20 *Fatty liver of an alcoholic.* The liver is enlarged, swollen, greasy, and yellow. *(From Damjanov, I. & Linder, J. [Eds.]. [1996]. Anderson's pathology [10th ed.]. St. Louis: Mosby.)*

3. Increased synthesis of triglycerides from fatty acids (Increases in an enzyme, α-glycerophosphatase, can accelerate triglyceride synthesis.)
4. Decreased synthesis of apoproteins (lipid-acceptor proteins)
5. Failure of lipids to bind with apoproteins and form lipoproteins
6. Failure of mechanisms that transport lipoproteins out of the cell

Glycogen

Intracellular accumulations of glycogen are seen in genetic disorders called *glycogen storage diseases* and in disorders of glucose and glycogen metabolism. Like water and lipid accumulation, glycogen accumulation results in excessive vacuolation of the cytoplasm. The most common cause of glycogen accumulation is the disorder of glucose metabolism, diabetes mellitus (see Chapter 18).

Proteins

Proteins provide cellular structure and constitute most of the cell's dry weight. They are synthesized on ribosomes in the cytoplasm from the essential amino acids lysine, threonine, leucine, isoleucine, methionine, tryptophan, valine, phenylalanine, and histidine. Protein accumulation probably damages cells in two ways. First, metabolites, produced when the cell attempts to digest some proteins, are enzymes that, when released from lysosomes, can damage cellular organelles. Second, excessive amounts of protein in the cytoplasm push against cellular organelles, disrupting organelle function and intracellular communication.

Protein excess accumulates primarily in the epithelial cells of the renal convoluted tubule and in the antibody-forming plasma cells (B lymphocytes) of the immune system. Several types of renal disorders cause excessive excretion of protein molecules in the urine (proteinuria). Normally, little or no protein is present in the urine and its presence in significant amounts indicates cellular injury and altered cellular function. Protein accumulations in the cytoplasm of renal tubular cells do not cause direct cellular dysfunction, but they do signify a pathologic process.

Accumulations of protein in B lymphocytes can occur during active synthesis of antibodies during the immune response. The excess aggregates of protein are called *Russell bodies* (see Chapter 5). Russell bodies have been identified in multiple myeloma (plasma cell tumor) (see Chapters 20 and 37).

Pigments

Pigment accumulations may be normal or abnormal, endogenous (produced within the body) or exogenous (produced outside the body). Endogenous pigments are derived, for example, from amino acids (e.g., tyrosine, tryptophan). They include melanin and the blood proteins—porphyrins, hemoglobin, and hemosiderin. Lipid-rich pigments, such as lipofuscin (the aging pigment), give a yellow-brown color to cells undergoing slow, regressive, and often atrophic changes. Exogenous pigments include mineral dusts containing silica and iron particles, lead, silver salts, and dyes for tattoos.

Melanin

Melanin accumulates in epithelial cells (keratinocytes) of the skin and retina. It is an extremely important pigment because it protects the skin against long exposure to sunlight and is considered an essential factor in the prevention of skin cancer (see Chapters 10 and 39). Ultraviolet light (e.g., sunlight) stimulates the synthesis of melanin, which probably absorbs ultraviolet rays during subsequent exposure. Melanin also may protect the skin by trapping the injurious free radicals produced by the action of ultraviolet light on skin.

Melanin is a brown-black pigment derived from the amino acid *tryptosine.* It is synthesized by epidermal cells called *melanocytes* and is stored in membrane-bound cytoplasmic vesicles called *melanosomes.*

Melanin also can accumulate in melanophores (melanin-containing pigment cells), macrophages, or other phagocytic cells in the dermis. Presumably these cells acquire the melanin from nearby melanocytes or from pigment that has been extruded from dying epidermal cells. This is the mechanism that causes freckles. Melanin also occurs in the benign form of pigmented moles called *nevi* (see Chapter 39). Malignant melanoma is a cancerous skin tumor that contains melanin.

A decrease in melanin production occurs in the inherited disorder of melanin metabolism called *albinism*. Albinism is often diffuse, involving all the skin, the eyes, and the hair. Albinism is also related to phenylalanine metabolism. In classic types, the person with albinism is unable to convert tyrosine to DOPA (3,4-dihydroxyphenylalanine), an intermediate in melanin biosynthesis. Melanin-producing cells are present in normal numbers, but they are unable to make melanin. Individuals with albinism are very sensitive to sunlight and quickly become sunburned. They are also at high risk for skin cancer.

Hemoproteins

Hemoproteins are among the most essential of the normal endogenous pigments. They include hemoglobin and the oxidative enzymes, the *cytochromes*. Central to an understanding of disorders involving these pigments is knowledge of iron uptake, metabolism, excretion, and storage (see Chapter 19). Hemoprotein accumulations in cells are caused by excessive storage of iron, which is transferred to the cells from the bloodstream. Iron enters the blood from three primary sources: (1) tissue stores; (2) the intestinal mucosa; and (3) macrophages that remove and destroy dead or defective red blood cells. The amount of iron in blood plasma depends also on the metabolism of the major iron-transport protein, *transferrin*.

Iron is stored in tissue cells in two forms: as ferritin and, when increased levels of iron are present, as hemosiderin. *Hemosiderin* is a yellow-brown pigment derived from hemoglobin. With pathologic states, excesses of iron cause hemosiderin to accumulate within cells, often in areas of bruising and hemorrhage and in the lungs and spleen after congestion caused by heart failure. With local hemorrhage, the skin first appears red-blue and then lysis of the escaped red blood cells occurs, causing the hemoglobin to be transformed to hemosiderin. The color changes noted in bruising reflect this transformation (Fig. 3-21).

Hemosiderosis is a condition in which excess iron is stored as hemosiderin in the cells of many organs and tissues. This condition is common in individuals who have received repeated blood transfusions or prolonged parenteral administration of iron. Hemosiderosis is associated also with increased absorption of dietary iron, conditions in which iron storage and transport are impaired, and hemolytic anemia. Excessive alcohol (wine) ingestion also can lead to hemosiderosis. Normally, absorption of excessive dietary iron is prevented by an iron-absorption process in the intestines. Failure of this process can lead to total body iron accumulations in the range of 60 to 80 g, compared with normal iron stores of 4.5 to 5 g. Excessive accumulations of iron, such as occur in hemochromatosis (a genetic disorder of iron metabolism and the most severe example of iron overload), are associated with liver and pancreatic cell damage.

It is debatable whether iron accumulation itself causes

Fig. 3-21 *Hemosiderin accumulation is noted as the color changes in a "black eye."*

cellular injury or whether injury is the result of the basic defect that leads to iron storage. The finding that the extent of liver injury (cirrhosis) is related to the extent of iron accumulation[21] suggests that excessive iron accumulation does injure cells.

Bilirubin is a normal, yellow-to-green pigment of bile derived from the porphyrin structure of hemoglobin. Excess bilirubin within cells and tissues causes jaundice (icterus), or yellowing of the skin. Jaundice occurs when the bilirubin level exceeds 1.5 to 2 mg/dl of plasma, compared with the normal values of 0.4 to 1 mg/dl. Hyperbilirubinemia occurs with (1) destruction of red blood cells (erythrocytes), such as in hemolytic jaundice; (2) diseases affecting the metabolism and excretion of bilirubin in the liver; and (3) diseases that cause obstruction of the common bile duct, such as gallstones or pancreatic tumors. Certain drugs (specifically chlorpromazine and other phenothiazine derivatives), estrogenic hormones, and halothane, an anesthetic, can cause the obstruction of normal bile flow through the liver.

Because unconjugated bilirubin is lipid soluble, it can injure the lipid components of the plasma membrane. Albumin, a plasma protein, provides significant protection by binding unconjugated bilirubin in plasma. Unconjugated bilirubin causes two cellular effects: uncoupling of oxidative phosphorylation and a loss of cellular proteins. These two effects could cause structural injury to the various membranes of the cell.

Calcium

Calcium salts accumulate in both injured and dead tissues (Fig. 3-22). An important mechanism of cellular calcification is the influx of extracellular calcium in injured mitochondria (see p. 70). Another mechanism that causes calcium accumulation in alveoli (gas-exchange airways of the lungs), gastric epithelium, and renal tubules is the excretion of acid at these sites, leading to the local production of hydroxyl ions. Hy-

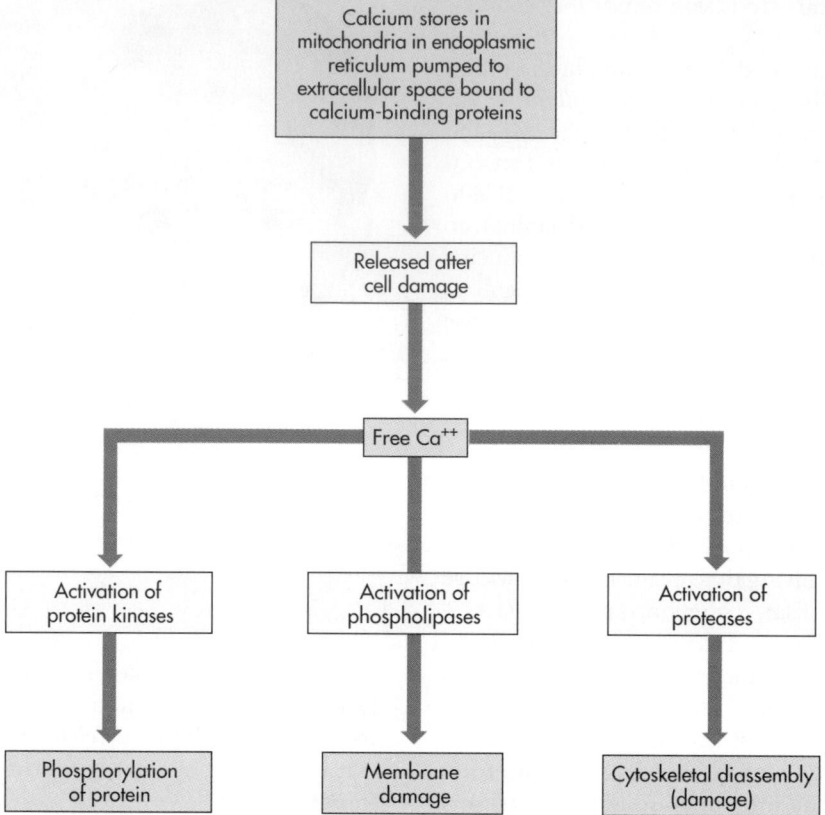

Fig. 3-22 *Free cytosolic calcium: a destructive agent.* Normally, calcium is removed from the cytosol by ATP-dependent calcium pumps. In normal cells, calcium is bound to buffering proteins, such as calbindin or paralbumin, and is contained in the endoplasmic reticulum and the mitochondria. If there is abnormal permeability of calcium-ion channels, direct damage to membranes, or depletion of ATP (i.e., hypoxic injury), calcium increases in the cytosol. If the free calcium cannot be buffered or pumped out of cells, uncontrolled enzyme activation takes place, causing further damage. Uncontrolled entry of calcium into the cytosol is an important final common pathway in many causes of cell death. *(Modified from Stevens, A. & Lowe, J. [1995].* Pathology. *St. Louis: Mosby.)*

droxyl ions result in precipitation of calcium hydroxide ($Ca[OH]^2$) and hydroxyapatite ($3Ca^3[PO^4]^2Ca[OH]^2$), a mixed salt. Damage occurs when calcium salts clump and harden, interfering with normal cellular structure and function.

Pathologic calcification can be dystrophic or metastatic. ***Dystrophic calcification*** occurs in dying and dead tissues, chronic tuberculosis of the lungs and lymph nodes, advanced atherosclerosis (narrowing as a result of plaque accumulation), and heart valve injury (Fig. 3-23). Calcification of the heart valves interferes with their opening and closing, causing heart murmurs (see Chapter 23). Calcification of the coronary arteries predisposes them to severe narrowing and thrombosis, which can lead to myocardial infarction. Another site of dystrophic calcification is the center of tumors. Over time, the center is deprived of its oxygen supply, dies, and becomes calcified. The calcium salts appear as gritty, clumped granules that can become hard as stone. When several layers clump together, they resemble grains of sand and are called ***psammoma bodies.***

Metastatic calcification consists of mineral deposits that occur in undamaged normal tissues as the result of hypercalcemia (excess calcium in the blood; see Chapter 4). Conditions that cause hypercalcemia include hyperparathyroidism, toxic levels of vitamin D, hyperthyroidism, idiopathic hypercalcemia of infancy, Addison disease (adrenocortical insufficiency), systemic sarcoidosis, milk-alkali syndrome, and the increased bone demineralization that results from bone tumors, leukemia, and disseminated cancers. Hypercalcemia also may occur in advanced renal failure with phosphate retention, resulting in hyperparathyroidism.[1]

Urate

In humans, uric acid (***urate***) is the major end product of purine catabolism in the absence of urate oxidase. Serum urate concentration is, in general, stable: approximately 5 mg/dl in postpubertal males and 4.1 mg/dl in postpubertal females. Disturbances in maintaining serum urate levels result in hyperuricemia and the deposition of sodium urate crystals in the tissues, leading to painful disorders collectively called *gout.* These disorders include acute arthritis,

Fig. 3-23 *Aortic valve calcification.* **A,** This aortic valve was unable to close because of calcification caused by rheumatic heart disease. **B,** Algorithm showing the dystrophic mechanism of calcification. *(A from Damjanov, I. & Linder, J. [Eds.]. [1996]. Anderson's pathology [10th ed.]. St. Louis: Mosby.)*

TABLE 3-8	Systemic Manifestations of Cellular Injury
Manifestation	**Cause**
Fever	Release of endogenous pyrogens (interleukin-1, tumor necrosis factor-α, prostaglandins) from bacteria or macrophages; acute inflammatory response
Increased heart rate	Increase in oxidative metabolic processes resulting from fever
Increase in leukocytes (leukocytosis)	Increase in total number of white blood cells because of infection; normal is 5000-9000/mm³ (increase is directly related to the severity of the infection)
Pain	Various mechanisms, such as release of bradykinins, obstruction, pressure
Presence of cellular enzymes in extracellular fluid	Release of enzymes from cells of tissue*
Lactate dehydrogenase (LDH) (LDH isoenzymes)	Release from red blood cells, liver, kidney, skeletal muscle
Creatine kinase (CK) (CK isoenzymes)	Release from skeletal muscle, brain, heart
Aspartate aminotransferase (AST/SGOT)	Release from heart, liver, skeletal muscle, kidney, pancreas
Alanine aminotransferase (ALT/SGPT)	Release from liver, kidney, heart
Alkaline phosphatase (ALP)	Release from liver, bone
Amylase	Release from pancreas
Aldolase	Release from skeletal muscle, heart

The rapidity of enzyme transfer is a function of the weight of the enzyme and the concentration gradient across the cellular membrane. The specific metabolic and excretory rates of the enzymes determine how long levels of enzymes remain elevated.

chronic gouty arthritis, tophi (firm, nodular, subcutaneous deposits of urate crystals surrounded by fibrosis), and nephritis (inflammation of the nephron) (see Chapter 37). Chronic hyperuricemia results in the deposition of urate in tissues, cell injury, and inflammation. Because urate crystals are not degraded by lysosomal enzymes, they persist in dead cells.

Systemic Manifestations

Systemic manifestations of cellular injury include a general sense of fatigue and malaise, a loss of well-being, and altered appetite. Fever frequently is present because of biochemicals produced during the inflammatory response. Table 3-8 summarizes the most significant systemic manifestations of cellular injury.

CELLULAR DEATH
Necrosis

Cellular death eventually leads to cellular dissolution, or **necrosis**. Necrosis is the sum of cellular changes after local cell death and the process of cellular self-digestion known as autodigestion, or **autolysis** (Fig. 3-24). The structural signs that indicate irreversible injury and progression to necrosis are dense clumping and progressive disruption of genetic material and disruption of the plasma and organelle membranes. In later stages of necrosis, most organelles are disrupted, and **karyolysis** (nuclear dissolution from the action of hydrolytic enzymes) is underway. In some cells, the nucleus shrinks and becomes a small, dense mass of genetic material (**pyknosis**). The pyknotic nucleus eventually dissolves (by karyolysis) as a result of the action of hydrolytic lysosomal enzymes on DNA.

Different types of necroses tend to occur in different organs or tissues and sometimes can indicate the mechanism or cause of cellular injury. The four major types of necroses are coagulative, liquefactive, caseous, and fatty. Another type, gangrenous necrosis, is *not* a distinctive type of cell death but refers to larger areas of tissue death. These are summarized as follows:

1. **Coagulative necrosis.** Occurs primarily in the kidneys, heart, and adrenal glands; commonly results from hypoxia caused by severe ischemia or hypoxia caused by chemical injury, especially ingestion of mercuric chloride. Coagulation is caused by protein denaturation, which causes the protein albumin to change from a gelatinous, transparent state to a firm, opaque state (Fig. 3-25).

2. **Liquefactive necrosis.** Commonly results from ischemic injury to neurons and glial cells in the brain (Fig. 3-26). Dead brain tissue is readily affected by liquefactive necrosis because brain cells are rich in the digestive hydrolytic enzymes and lipids and the brain contains little connective tissue. Cells are digested by their own hydrolases so the tissue becomes soft, liquefies, and is walled off from

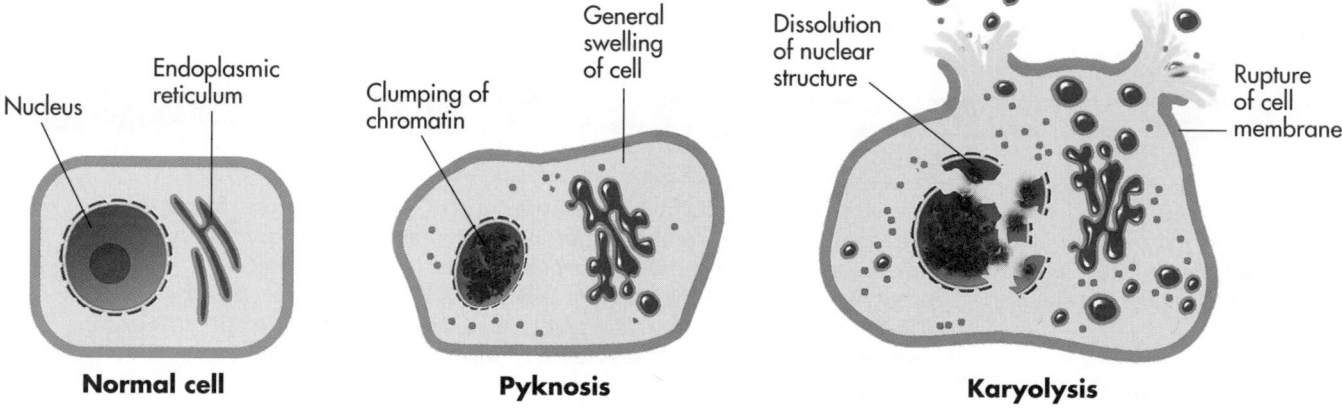

Fig. 3-24 *Stages of necrosis.*

Fig. 3-25 *Coagulative necrosis of myocardium of posterior wall of left ventricle of heart.* A large, anemic *(white)* infarct is readily apparent; note also the necrosis of papillary muscle. *(From Damjanov, I. & Linder, J. [Eds.]. [1996]. Anderson's pathology [10th ed.]. St. Louis: Mosby.)*

Fig. 3-26 *Liquefactive necrosis of the brain developed at a large cerebral infarct caused by ischemia.* *(From Damjanov, I. & Linder, J. [Eds.]. [1996]. Anderson's pathology [10th ed.]. St. Louis: Mosby.)*

Fig. 3-27 *Granuloma with central caseous necrosis typical of pulmonary tuberculosis.* (From Damjanov, I. & Linder, J. [Eds.]. [1996], Anderson's pathology [10th ed.]. St. Louis: Mosby.)

Fig. 3-28 *Fat necrosis of pancreas.* Interlobular adipocytes are necrotic; these are surrounded by acute inflammatory cells. *(From Damjanov, I. & Linder, J. [Eds.]. [1996]. Anderson's pathology [10th ed.]. St. Louis: Mosby.)*

healthy tissue, forming cysts. This can be caused by bacterial infection, especially staphylococci, streptococci, and *Escherichia coli.*

3. *Caseous necrosis.* Usually results from tuberculous pulmonary infection, especially by *Mycobacterium tuberculosis* (Fig. 3-27). It is a combination of coagulative and liquefactive necroses. The dead cells disintegrate, but the debris is not completely digested by the hydrolases. Tissues resemble clumped cheese, soft and granular. A granulomatous inflammatory wall encloses areas of caseous necrosis.

4. *Fat necrosis.* Occurs in the breast, pancreas, and other abdominal structures (Fig. 3-28). This is a specific type of cellular dissolution caused by powerful enzymes called *lipases,* which break down triglycerides, releasing free fatty acids, which then combine with calcium, magnesium, and sodium ions, creating soaps (saponification). The necrotic tissue appears opaque and chalk white.

5. *Gangrenous necrosis.* Refers to death of tissue and results from severe hypoxic injury, commonly occurring because of arteriosclerosis, or blockage, of major arteries, particularly those in the lower leg (Fig. 3-29). With hypoxia and

subsequent bacterial invasion, the tissues can undergo necrosis. *Dry gangrene* is usually the result of coagulative necrosis. The skin becomes very dry and shrinks, resulting in wrinkles, and its color changes to dark brown or black. *Wet gangrene* develops when neutrophils invade the site, causing liquefactive necrosis. This usually occurs in internal organs, causing the site to become cold, swollen, and black. A foul odor is present, and if systemic symptoms become severe, death can ensue.

6. *Gas gangrene.* This special type of gangrene is caused by infection of injured *tissue* by one of many species of *Clostridium.* These anaerobic bacteria produce hydrolytic enzymes and toxins that destroy connective tissue and cellular membranes and cause bubbles of gas to form in muscle cells. This can be fatal if enzymes lyse the membranes of red blood cells, destroying their oxygen-carrying capacity. Death is caused by shock.

Apoptosis

Apoptosis (Greek for "dropping off") is an important, distinct type of cell death that differs from necrosis in several respects. Apoptosis is an active process of cellular self-

Thrombosis or embolism

Strangulated hernia

Volvulus

Intussusception

Gangrene

Fig. 3-29 *Gangrene is a complication of necrosis.* In certain circumstances necrotic tissue will be invaded by putrefactive organisms that are both saccharolytic and proteolytic. Foul-smelling gases are produced, and the tissue becomes green or black as a result of breakdown of hemoglobin. Obstruction of the blood supply to the bowel almost inevitably is followed by gangrene.

destruction implicated in both normal and pathologic tissue changes. Unlike necrosis, *apoptosis* affects scattered, single cells. It is nuclear and cytoplasmic shrinkage of a cell followed by fragmentation into membrane-bound fragments and subsequent phagocytosis by neighboring healthy cells.[13,22] As a controlled process in normal development, apoptosis determines the size, patterning, and function of many tissues.[23,24] It is responsible for local deletion of cells during tissue turnover and normal embryonic development, neurons dying during synaptogenesis (i.e., to match the number of neurons to their synaptic targets),[23] lymphocytes dying during receptor repertoire selection, and so on.[25,26] Recently, apoptosis has been shown to play a major role in endocrine-dependent tissues undergoing atrophic change,[27,28] and in hemopoietic cells it is linked to the production of free radicals.[29] Apoptosis can occur spontaneously in malignant tumors and in normal, rapidly proliferating cells treated with cancer chemotherapeutic agents and ionizing radiation.[30] Apoptotic cell antigens have been identified as targets of autoantibodies in autoimmune diseases, such as systemic lupus erythematosus.[31]

Normal cells that die might kill themselves by activating a "suicide program."[25,28] The survival of many developing vertebrate neurons depends on neurohormonal factors secreted by the target cells they innervate; those that fail to get enough die, apparently by active suicide because their death can be prevented for days by drugs that inhibit ribonucleic acid (RNA) or protein synthesis.[25] Among nonneural tissues, blood cell precursor cells require one or more colony-stimulating factors, T lymphoblasts (immature lymphocytes) require interleukin-2 (a cytokine), and endothelial cells require growth factors, such as fibroblast growth factor. In all these examples, cells deprived of survival signals die by programmed (normal) cell death. It seems reasonable that dependence on specific survival signals provides a simple way to eliminate misplaced cells for regulating cell numbers and, perhaps, to select the fittest cells.[22,25,26,32,33]

> ✓ **QUICK CHECK**
>
> Why does cell injury cause calcification?
>
> List several systemic manifestations of cellular injury.
>
> Why is apoptosis significant?

AGING AND ALTERED CELLULAR AND TISSUE BIOLOGY

Aging usually is defined as a normal physiologic process that is both universal and inevitable. The basic mechanisms of aging depend on the irreversible and universal processes at the cellular and molecular level. To understand aging requires the separation of irreversible processes from potentially reversible mechanisms (i.e., those that result from disease or age-related debilities).

Aging traditionally has not been considered a disease because it is "normal"; disease is usually considered "abnormal." Conceptually, this distinction seems clear until the concept of injury is introduced; disease has been defined by some pathologists as the result of injury. Aging has been defined as the time-dependent loss of structure and function that proceeds very slowly and in such small increments that it appears to be the result of the accumulation of small, imperceptible injuries—a gradual result of "wear and tear."

Injuries may result from unavoidable and universal microinsults caused by continuous bombardment by ultraviolet light, countless mechanical insults, and reactions to metabolites (Fig. 3-30).[33] In this context, the distinction between aging and disease is unclear. For example, some degree of atrophy of the brain is considered normal in old age until it proceeds far enough to cause clinically significant disabil-

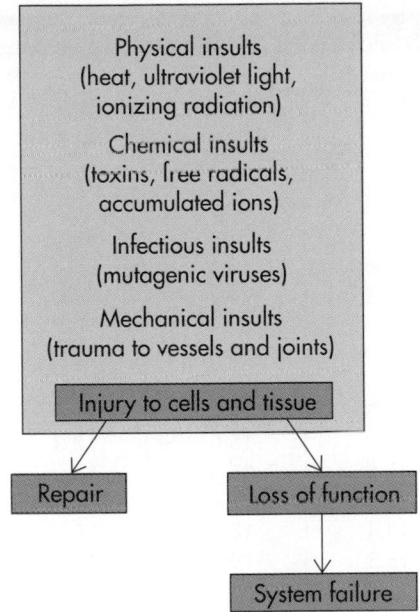

Fig. 3-30 *Microinsults. (Redrawn from Johnson, H.A. [Ed.]. [1985].* Is aging physiological or pathological? Relations between normal aging and disease. *New York: Raven.)*

ity and is called *disease.* Likewise, most human beings have atherosclerosis, and the plaques progress with age, but at what point in this progression is atherosclerosis considered abnormal? These conceptual distinctions have given rise to two general categories of theories of aging. The first category proposes that aging is the result of the accumulation of random injuries and events. The second category proposes that aging is the result of a genetically controlled developmental program, or built-in self-destructive processes.

Normal Life Span

The *maximal life span* of humans is between 80 and 100 years and does not vary significantly among populations. However, in primitive societies few individuals reach the maximal life span; most die in infancy or the early years. In societies with improved sanitation, housing, nutrition, and health care, many persons attain the maximal life span. Although the maximal life span has not changed significantly over time, the average life span, or *life expectancy,* has increased. Recently, the death rate for people 65 years of age and older has declined significantly, largely as a result of decreased cardiovascular disease.[34]

Life Expectancy and Gender Differences

Life expectancy for females exceeds that for males (the *gender gap*) except in Bangladesh, Bhutan, India, Nepal, and Pakistan.[35,36] The female advantage ranges from 4 to 8 years. Swedish data (most reliable recorded data) for 1950 to 1987 show plateau values of around 75 years for males and 80 years for females. In Japan, however, women had a life expectancy of 81.8 years and males 79.5 years; these figures are

still rising.[3,37] Thus the Japanese are the longest-lived population. The average life expectancy in the United States is 9.1 years for 80-year-old white women and 7.0 years for 80-year-old white men.

Race has a key impact on gender mortality differences in the United States. Between 1920 and 1970, the gender gap increased among whites by a factor of 6 and among blacks by a factor of 8 (Table 3-9). Since 1970, however, the gap has narrowed sharply among whites and has begun to narrow among blacks.[38]

Factors responsible for these differences in the gender gap in the United States include (1) more rapid *improvement* in female compared with male death rates and (2) an *increasing* male disadvantage in death rates from the chronic conditions that are the leading causes of death in developed countries.[33] The narrowing of the gender gap between 1970 and 1986 in the United States was the result of two factors: (1) a *decline* in the rate of increase in female life expectancy and (2) a sharp *increase* in life expectancy by males.[36,38]

Causes of the gender gap may be biologic, behavioral, or sociocultural (Table 3-10).

Theories and Mechanisms of Aging

Relatively little indisputable knowledge exists on the subject of aging. Table 3-11 presents the historical development of aging research. Many theories have focused on a single mechanism—the so-called magic bullet approach to arrest aging. It is doubtful that a single theory will explain all the mechanisms of aging.

Evidence exists both for and against any particular theory of aging. Three major mechanisms of aging have retained their appeal or have been extensively tested, however:

TABLE 3-9 Life Expectancy at Birth, at 65 Years, and at 75 Years, by Race and Sex: Selected Years, 1900-02 to 1991

Age and Year	All Races			White		Black	
	Both Sexes	Male	Female	Male	Female	Male	Female
	Remaining Life Expectancy in Years						
At birth							
1900-1902[1,2]	47.3	46.3	48.3	46.6	48.7	32.5[3]	33.5[3]
1950[2]	68.2	65.6	71.1	66.5	72.2	58.9	62.7
1960[2]	69.7	66.6	73.1	67.4	74.1	60.7	65.9
1970	70.8	67.1	74.7	68.0	75.6	60.0	68.3
1980	73.7	70.0	77.4	70.7	78.1	63.8	72.5
1991	75.5	72.0	78.9	72.9	79.6	64.6	73.8
At 65 years							
1900-1902[1,2]	11.9	11.5	12.2	11.5	12.2	10.4	11.4
1950[2]	13.9	12.8	15.0	12.8	15.1	12.9	14.9
1960[2]	14.3	12.8	15.8	12.9	15.9	12.7	15.1
1970	15.2	13.1	17.0	13.1	17.1	12.5	15.7
1980	16.4	14.1	18.3	14.2	18.4	13.0	16.8
1991	17.4	15.3	19.1	15.4	19.2	13.4	17.2
At 75 years							
1980	10.4	8.8	11.5	8.8	11.5	8.3	10.7
1991	11.1	9.5	12.1	9.5	12.1	8.7	11.2

[1]Death registration area only. The death registration area increased from 10 states and the District of Columbia in 1900 to the coterminous United States in 1933.
[2]Includes deaths of nonresidents of the United States.
[3]Figure is for the Black and other races population.
Source: National Center for Health Statistics, Health, United States, 1993, Hyattsville, Md, Public Health Service, 1994, Table 27.

TABLE 3-10 Causes of the Current Longevity and Health Differences Between Men and Women

Biologic Hypotheses	Comments
Genetic	
Female genotype (XX) compared with male genotype (XY)	Little known about Y chromosome compared with X chromosome, especially significance of X chromosome to longevity; however, certain genes on X chromosome involved in vital functions, including blood clotting, muscle function, protection against oxidative damage, DNA synthesis, nucleotide synthesis, and immune response; thus question raised, To what extent are these genes critical to longevity?
Increased male mortality during the prenatal period	Incidence of excess male mortality or early die-off during prenatal period may be attributed to homozygosity of genes of X chromosome (one allele instead of two alleles for each gene)
Characteristics of the Y chromosome	Y chromosome about one third of size of X chromosome; few recognize genes mapped to Y chromosome
Genetic and/or hormonal	
Sex hormones	Levels of balance of cholesterol-carrying lipoproteins by sex hormones major factors in gender gap; sex hormones result in *healthier* pattern of lipoproteins in women than in men; exogenous extrogens raise protective lipoproteins (high-density lipoproteins [HDL]) and lower nonprotective lipoproteins (low-density lipoproteins [LDL]); male androgens have opposite effect (see Chapter 31); pattern in women undergoes disadvantageous change after menopause; however, increased death rate for women from cardiovascular disease lags behind that of men by several years
Neuroendocrine effects, hormones, and the immune system	Sex hormones regulate longevity through their effects on behavior and through immune system; these effects interrelated and the CNS is center of these relationships; behaviorally, sex hormones affect aggressiveness, territoriality, mate selection, and mating behavior; how these behaviors affect longevity incompletely understood; reproductive senescence, although life-threatening, can contribute to increasing "wear and tear" and includes cell depletion, cell death, and organ involution; CNS affects immune system through neuroendocrine mechanisms; sex hormones also affect immune system; important question, How do men and women differ in their perception, handling, and physiologic consequences of stress, and how do these differences relate to the gender gap?

TABLE 3-10	Causes of the Current Longevity and Health Differences Between Men and Women—cont'd
Biologic Hypotheses	**Comments**
Immune function	Immune system in female mice does appear more robust than that in males; not clear whether this is related to antibody genes that map to X chromosome (Smith & Warner, 1990)
Cardiovascular effect	Increased myocyte cell loss and myocyte cellular "reactive" hypertrophy are significant in men and women; thus gender differences may play a large role in the bad effects of aging on the heart; an increase in mean arterial pressure with age persisted in women beyond 62 yr but not in women younger than 62 yr or in men of any age; endogenous and exogenous androgens are known to decrease HDL cholesterol in men (Bagatell & Bremner, 1995)
Social roles	
Multiple roles held by middle-aged women	Differing social roles of men and women often cited as major causes of gender gap; key question, To what extent do the different roles become sources of stress and thus differentially affect longevity?; data from women 45-55 yr old reveal that majority of these women perform multiple roles; although these roles are sources of stress, surprisingly the reported stresses were not translated into negative health outcomes (Barer, 1994; Poehlman et al, 1995); working may play protective role by alleviating stress of nurturing roles and thereby prevent morbidity
Occupations and social class	There continues to be increase in relative mortality disadvantage of manual relative to nonmanual workers (for many causes of death) for both men and women; from 1957 to 1983, age-adjusted incidence of myocardial infarction in both white and blue collar male workers declined; however, decline in white collar workers was double that of blue collar workers (National Center Health Statistics, 1996); no consistent trends in myocardial infarction observed in women
Risky behavior and social class	Social class differences in smoking behavior (most documented risky behavior) do correspond to observed gender and social class mortality relationships; men with lower levels of education substantially more likely to smoke than either better educated men or women (National Center Health Statistics, 1996); however, as prevalence of smoking among men has declined more rapidly than among women, gender differences in smoking within blue collar group, although still present, have become less marked
Health service use and morbidity differences	Although women report greater use of physician services (particularly preventive services) than men, elderly men have higher hospitalization rates than women; with fewer work obligations, women are more likely to curtail activities and get more bed rest when ill; more flexible daily schedule made possible by lower employment rate is key reason women make more physician visits for long-term problems (Verbrugge, 1990); overall, however, women have higher rates of morbidity and therapeutic care than men; women more frequently have short-term illnesses, with higher rates of daily symptoms and higher incidence rates for acute illnesses; thus women have higher prevalence of many nonfatal long-term conditions, such as arthritis, chronic sinusitis, and digestive conditions; by contrast, men have higher prevalence rates of heart disease, atherosclerosis, emphysema, and other fatal conditions
Other social, psychologic, and emotional issues	Women's excess morbidity in contemporary life driven by social factors, risks from less satisfying employment, keenly "felt" stress and unhappiness, stronger feelings of illness vulnerability, fewer formal time constraints, and less physically strenuous leisure activities

Data from Smith, D.W.E. & Warner, H.R. (1990). Overview of biomedical perspectives: Possible relationships between genes on the sex chromosomes and longevity. In M.G. Ory & H.R. Warner (Eds.). Gender, health, and longevity: Multidisciplinary perspectives. New York: Springer; Bagatell, C.J. & Bremner, W.T. (1995). Androgen and progestogen effects on plasma lipids. Progress in Cardiovascular Diseases, 38(3), 255; Barer, B.M. (1994). Men and women aging differently. International Journal of Aging and Human Development, 38(1), 29; Poehlman, E.T. et al. (1995). Physiological predictors of increasing total and central adiposity in aging men and women. Archives of Internal Medicine, 155(22), 2433; National Center for Health Statistics, Health, United States, 1993, Hyattsville, Md, Public Health Service, 1996; Verbrugge, L.M. (1990). The twain meet: Empirical explanations of sex differences in health and mortality. In M.G. Ory & H.R. Warner (Eds.). Gender, health, and longevity: Multidisciplinary perspectives. New York: Springer.

TABLE 3-11	Theories of Aging	
Theory	Year	Proponent
Waste product theory	1923	Carrell & Ebeling
Wear-and-tear theory	1924	Pearl
Rate of living theory*	1928	Pearl
Endocrine theory	1947	Korenchevsky & Jones
Free-radical theory	1955	Harman
Collagen theory†	1957	Verzar
Metabolic theory*	1957; 1961	Carlson et al; Johnson et al.
Somatic mutation theory	1959	Sziliard
Error-catastrophe theory	1963; 1970	Orgel
Cross-linking theory†	1968	Bjorksten
Programmed senescence theory	1969	Hayflick
Immunologic theory	1969	Walform
Evolution theory	1977	Kirkwood

From Schneider, E.L. (1987). Theories of aging: A perspective. In H.R. Warner, et al. (Eds.). Modern biological theories of aging. New York: Raven; Vijg, J.U. & Wei, J.Y. (1995). Journal of the American Geriatrics Society, 43, 426.
*May represent the same theory.
†May represent the same theory.

(1) cellular changes produced by genetic and environmental factors; (2) changes in cellular regulatory, or control, mechanisms, especially in cells of the neuroendocrine, immune, and central nervous systems; and (3) degenerative extracellular and vascular alterations.[39,40]

Genetic and environmental factors

Cellular aging results from wear and tear that causes functional changes and eventual cellular death. Cellular damage may occur during replication as a result of factors within the cell, such as DNA and protein mechanisms, or factors outside the cell, such as ionizing radiation. Cells may already be programmed at birth or injured during life so as to cause errors in mitotic division and in the replication of genetic material, eventually leading to either cellular atrophy or death. Atrophy is common in the thymus, testis, ovary, uterus, and breast of aged individuals, although these organs age differently.

One genetic mechanism of aging is programmed aging. Regardless of damaging environmental factors, some investigators think that each normal cell may have a finite life span during which it can replicate. A classic experiment done by Hayflick[41] demonstrated that fibroblasts are limited to a finite number of generations (40 to 60 doublings). Proponents believe that an intrinsic program within the human genome progressively slows or shuts down certain physiologic mechanisms, including mitosis.

The *somatic mutation hypothesis* proposes that aging is the result of DNA damage, inefficiency of repair, and loss of integrity of DNA synthesis. Most experimental evidence thus far does not support the hypothesis that aging is the result of somatic mutation.

The *catastrophic* or *error-prone theory,* initially proposed by Orgel in 1963, stated that the presence of errors in those enzymes involved in transcription and translation, and thus their own synthesis, leads to an increase in errors and eventually to the death of the cell. Most of the evidence, however, argues against this theory as originally formulated. The accumulation of altered proteins in aging may result from an increased production or a decreased ability of aged cells to degrade their cellular proteins or both.

Alterations of cellular control mechanisms

The overall effects of aging may be caused by changes in certain cell populations that exert regulatory or control functions, such as cells of the CNS, neuroendocrine system, and immune system. The *neuroendocrine theory* of aging purports that a genetic program for aging is encoded in the brain and is controlled and relayed to peripheral tissues through hormonal and neural agents. Possible mechanisms include (1) increased hormonal degradation, (2) decreased rate of hormonal synthesis and secretion, and (3) decreased target-organ sensitivity related to the number of cellular receptors for hormonal ligands, ligand-receptor binding, or ligand internalization.

Proponents of immune theories of aging believe that the immune system is implicated in aging because (1) immune function declines with age; (2) the decline in immune function is related to certain diseases, such as cancer, and to many other secondary effects; and (3) the number of autoantibodies (antibodies that attack body tissues) increases with age.

Degenerative extracellular changes

Extracellular factors that affect the aging process include the binding of collagen; the increase in free radicals' effects on cells; the structural alterations of fascia, tendons, ligaments, bones, and joints; and peripheral vascular disease, particularly arteriosclerosis (see Chapter 23).

Aging affects the extracellular matrix with increased cross-linking (e.g., aging collagen becomes more insoluble, chemically stable but rigid, resulting in decreased cell permeability), decreased synthesis, and increased degradation of collagen. These changes, together with the disappearance of elastin and changes in proteoglycans and plasma proteins, cause disorders of the ground substance that result in dehydration and wrinkling of the skin (see Chapter 39). Other age-related defects in the extracellular matrix include skeletal muscle alterations (e.g., atrophy, decreased tone, loss of contractility), cataracts, diverticula, hernias, and rupture of intervertebral disks.

Free radicals of oxygen that result from oxidative cellular metabolism (e.g., respiratory chain, phagocytosis, prostaglandin synthesis) may damage tissues during the aging process. The oxygen radicals produced include superoxide radical, hydroxyl radical, and hydrogen peroxide (see p. 70). These oxygen products are extremely reactive and can damage nucleic acids, destroy polysaccharides, oxidize proteins, peroxidize unsaturated fatty acids, and kill and lyse cells. Oxidant effects on target cells can give rise to malignant transformation through DNA damage. That progressive and cumulative damage from oxygen radicals may lead to harmful alterations in cellular function is consistent with those alterations of aging. This hypothesis is founded on the wear-and-tear theory of aging, which states that damages accumulate with time, decreasing the organism's ability to maintain a steady state. Because these oxygen-reactive species not only can permanently damage cells but also may lead to cell death, there is new support for their role in the aging process.

Of much interest is the relationship between aging and the disappearance or alteration of extracellular substances important for vessel integrity. With aging, lipid, calcium, and plasma proteins are deposited in the walls of vessels. These depositions cause serious basement membrane thickening and alterations in smooth muscle functioning, resulting in arteriosclerosis (a progressive disease that causes such problems as stroke, myocardial infarction, renal disease, and peripheral vascular disease).

Cellular Aging

Cellular changes characteristic of aging include atrophy, decreased function, and loss of cells, possibly caused by apoptosis. Loss of cellular function from any of these causes initiates the compensatory mechanisms of hypertrophy and hyperplasia of remaining cells, which can lead to metaplasia, dysplasia, and neoplasia. All these changes can alter receptor placement and function, nutrient pathways, secretion of cellular products, and neuroendocrine control mechanisms. In the aged cell, DNA, RNA, cellular proteins, and membranes are most susceptible to injurious stimuli. DNA is particularly vulnerable to such injuries as breaks, deletions, and additions. Lack of DNA repair increases the cell's susceptibility to mutations that may be lethal or may promote the development of neoplasia (see Chapter 9).

Tissue and Systemic Aging

It is probably safe to say that every physiologic process functions less efficiently with increasing age. The most characteristic tissue change with age is a progressive stiffness or rigidity that affects many systems, including the arterial, pulmonary, and musculoskeletal systems. A consequence of blood vessel and organ stiffness is a progressive increase in peripheral resistance to blood flow. The movement of intracellular and extracellular substances also decreases with age, as does the diffusion capacity of the lung. Blood flow through organs also decreases.

Changes in the endocrine and immune systems include thymus atrophy. Although this occurs at puberty, causing a decreased immune response to T-dependent antigens (foreign proteins), increased autoantibodies and immune complexes (antibodies that are bound to antigens) and an overall decrease in the immunologic tolerance for the host's own cells further diminish the effectiveness of the immune sys-

tem later in life. In women, the reproductive system loses ova, and in men, spermatogenesis is decreased. Responsiveness to hormones decreases in the breast and endometrium.

The stomach experiences decreases in the rate of emptying and secretion of hormones and hydrochloric acid. Muscular atrophy diminishes mobility by decreasing motor tone and contractility. *Sarcopenia,* or muscle loss, can occur into old age. The skin of the aged individual is affected by atrophy and wrinkling of the epidermis and alterations in underlying dermis, fat, and muscle.

Total body changes include a decrease in height; a reduction in circumference of the neck, thighs, and arms; widening of the pelvis; and lengthening of the nose and ears. Several of these changes are the result of tissue atrophy and of decreased bone mass caused by osteoporosis and osteoarthritis. Although growth hormone function, reflected in diminished levels of insulin-like growth factor-1, is a current hypothesis for explaining decreased bone and lean body mass, recent research has found advancing age rather than declining levels of these hormones as a major determinant.[42] Body composition changes with age. With middle age, there is an increase in body weight (men gain until 50 years of age and women until 70 years) and fat mass followed by a decrease in stature, weight, *fat-free mass* (FFM; includes all minerals, proteins, and water plus all other constituents except lipids), and body cell mass at older ages. As fat increases, total body water decreases. Increased body fat and centralized fat distribution (abdominal) are associated with non-insulin-dependent diabetes and heart disease. Total body potassium also decreases because of decreased cellular mass. An increased sodium/potassium ratio suggests that the decreased cellular mass is accompanied by an increased extracellular fluid compartment.

Although some of these alterations are probably inherent in aging, others represent consequences of the process. Advanced age increases susceptibility to disease, and death occurs after an injury or insult because of diminished cellular, tissue, and organic function.

SOMATIC DEATH

Somatic death is death of the entire organism. Unlike the changes that follow cellular death in a live body, *postmortem change* is diffuse and does not involve components of the inflammatory response. Within minutes after death, postmortem changes appear, eliminating any difficulty in determining that death has occurred. The most notable manifestations are complete cessation of respiration and circulation. The surface of the skin usually becomes pale and yellowish; however, the lifelike color of the cheeks and lips may persist after death that is caused by carbon monoxide poisoning, drowning, and chloroform poisoning.[43]

Body temperature falls gradually immediately after death and then more rapidly (approximately 1.0° to 1.5° F/hr) until, after 24 hours, body temperature equals that of the environment.[44] After death caused by certain infective diseases, body temperature may continue to rise for a short time. Postmortem reduction of body temperature is called *algor mortis.*

Blood pressure within the retinal vessels decreases, causing muscle tension to decrease and the pupils to dilate. The face, nose, and chin become sharp or peaked-looking as blood and fluids drain away.[38] Gravity causes blood to settle in the most dependent, or lowest, tissues, which develop a purple discoloration called **livor mortis.** Incisions at this time usually fail to cause bleeding. The skin loses its elasticity and transparency.

Within 6 hours after death, acidic compounds accumulate within the muscles because of the breakdown of carbohydrate and depletion of ATP. This interferes with ATP-dependent detachment of myosin from actin (contractile proteins), and muscle stiffening, or **rigor mortis,** sets in. The smaller muscles are usually affected first, particularly the muscles of the jaw. Within 12 to 14 hours, rigor mortis usually affects the entire body.

Signs of putrefaction are generally obvious about 24 to 48 hours after death. Rigor mortis gradually diminishes, and the body becomes flaccid at 36 to 62 hours. Putrefactive changes vary depending on the temperature of the environ-ment. The most visible is greenish discoloration of the skin, particularly on the abdomen. The discoloration is thought to be related to the diffusion of hemolyzed blood into the tissues and the production of sulfhemoglobin.[39] Slippage or loosening of the skin from underlying tissues occurs at the same time. After this, swelling or bloating of the body and liquefactive changes occur, sometimes causing opening of the body cavities. At a microscopic level, putrefactive changes are associated with the release of enzymes and lytic dissolution called **postmortem autolysis.**

✓ QUICK CHECK

Why is the free radical theory of aging gaining support?

Why has the gender gap in life expectancy been decreasing?

What are the body composition changes with aging?

Define postmortem autolysis.

▣ DID YOU UNDERSTAND?

Cellular Adaptation

1. Cellular adaptation is an alteration that enables the cell to maintain a steady state despite adverse conditions.
2. Atrophy is a decrease in cellular size caused by aging, disuse, or lack of blood supply, hormonal stimulation, or neural stimulation. Amounts of endoplasmic reticulum, mitochondria, and microfilaments are decreased.
3. Hypertrophy is an increase in the size of cells caused by increased work demands or hormonal stimulation. Amounts of protein in the plasma membrane, endoplasmic reticulum, microfilaments, and mitochondria are increased.
4. Hyperplasia is an increase in the number of cells caused by an increased rate of cellular division. Normal hyperplasia is stimulated by hormones or the need to replace lost tissues.
5. Dysplasia, or atypical hyperplasia, is an abnormal change in the size, shape, and organization of mature tissue cells.
6. Metaplasia is the reversible replacement of one mature cell type by another, less mature cell type.

Cellular Injury

1. Cellular injury occurs if the cell is unable to maintain homeostasis. Injured cells may recover (reversible injury) or die (irreversible injury). Injury is caused by lack of oxygen (hypoxia), free radicals, caustic or toxic chemicals, infectious agents, in-flammatory and immune responses, genetic factors, insufficient nutrients, or physical trauma from many causes.
2. Four biochemical themes are important to cell injury: (a) ATP depletion, (b) oxygen and oxygen-derived free radicals, (c) intracellular calcium and loss of calcium steady state, and (d) defects in membrane permeability.
3. The sequence of events leading to cell death is commonly decreased ATP production, failure of active-transport mechanisms (the sodium-potassium pump), cellular swelling, detachment of ribosomes from the endoplasmic reticulum, cessation of protein synthesis, mitochondrial swelling as a result of calcium accumulation, vacuolation, leakage of digestive enzymes from lysosomes, autodigestion of intracellular structures, lysis of the plasma membrane, and death.
4. The initial insult in hypoxic injury is usually ischemia (the cessation of blood flow into vessels that supply the cell with oxygen and nutrients).
5. Free radicals cause cellular injury because they have an unpaired electron that makes the molecule unstable. To stabilize itself, the molecule gives up an electron to another molecule or steals one. Therefore it forms injurious chemical bonds with proteins, lipids, and carbohydrates—key molecules in membranes and nucleic acids.
6. The damaging effects of free radicals, especially activated oxygen species (e.g., O_2^-, $OH\cdot$, H_2O_2), in-

clude (a) lipid peroxidation, (b) alteration of ion pumps and transport mechanisms, (c) fragmentation of DNA, and (d) damage to mitochondria-releasing calcium into the cytosol.

7. Restoration of oxygen, however, can cause additional injury called reperfusion injury.

8. The initial insult in chemical injury is damage or destruction of the plasma membrane. Examples of chemical agents that cause cellular injury are carbon tetrachloride, lead, carbon monoxide, and ethyl alcohol.

9. Unintentional and intentional injuries are an important health problem in the United States. Death is more common for men than women and higher among blacks than whites and other racial groups.

10. Injuries by blunt force are the result of the application of mechanical energy to the body, resulting in tearing, shearing, or crushing of tissues. The most common types of blunt force injuries include motor vehicle accidents and falls.

11. A contusion is bleeding into the skin or underlying tissues as a consequence of a blow. A collection of blood in soft tissues or an enclosed space may be referred to as a hematoma.

12. An abrasion (scrape) results from removal of the superficial layers of the skin caused by friction between the skin and injuring object. Abrasions and contusions may have a patterned appearance that mirrors the shape and features of an injuring object.

13. A laceration is a tear or rip resulting when the tensile strength of the skin or tissue is exceeded.

14. An incised wound is a cut that is longer than it is deep. A stab wound is a penetrating sharp force injury that is deeper than it is long.

15. Gunshot wounds may be either penetrating (bullet retained in the body) or perforating (bullet exits). The most important factors determining the appearance of a gunshot injury are whether it is an entrance or an exit wound and the range of fire.

16. Asphyxial injuries are caused by a failure of cells to receive or utilize oxygen. These injuries can be grouped into four general categories: suffocation, strangulation, chemical, and drowning.

17. Activation of inflammation and immunity, which occurs after cellular injury or infection, involves powerful biochemicals and proteins capable of damaging normal (uninjured and uninfected) cells.

18. Genetic disorders injure cells by altering the nucleus and the plasma membrane's structure, shape, receptors, or transport mechanisms.

19. Deprivation of essential nutrients (proteins, carbohydrates, lipids, vitamins) can cause cellular injury by altering cellular structure and function, particularly of transport mechanisms, chromosomes, the nucleus, and DNA.

20. Injurious physical agents include temperature extremes, changes in atmospheric pressure, ionizing radiation, illumination, mechanical stresses (e.g., repetitive body movements), and noise.

Manifestations of Cellular Injury

1. Cellular manifestations of cellular injury include accumulations of water, lipids, carbohydrates, glycogen, proteins, pigments, hemosiderin, bilirubin, calcium, and urate.

2. Accumulations harm cells by "crowding" the organelles and by causing excessive (and sometimes harmful) metabolites to be produced during their catabolism. The metabolites are released into the cytoplasm or expelled into the extracellular matrix.

3. Cellular swelling, the accumulation of excessive water in the cell, is caused by the failure of transport mechanisms and is a sign of many types of cellular injury.

4. Accumulations of organic substances—lipids, carbohydrates, glycogen, proteins, pigments—are caused by disorders in which (a) cellular uptake of the substance exceeds the cell's capacity to catabolize (digest) or use it or (b) cellular anabolism (synthesis) of the substance exceeds the cell's capacity to use or secrete it.

5. Dystrophic calcification (accumulation of calcium salts) is always a sign of pathologic change because it occurs only in injured or dead cells. Metastatic calcification, however, can occur in uninjured cells in individuals with hypercalcemia.

6. Disturbances in urate metabolism can result in hyperuricemia and deposition of sodium urate crystals in tissue—leading to a painful disorder called *gout*.

7. Systemic manifestations of cellular injury include fever, leukocytosis, increased heart rate, pain, and serum elevations of enzymes in the plasma.

Cellular Death

1. Cellular death is manifested as cellular dissolution, or necrosis. Necrosis is the sum of the changes after local cell death and includes the process of autolysis, or cellular self-destruction.

2. There are four major types of necroses: coagulative, liquefactive, caseous, and fat necroses. Different types of necroses occur in different tissues.

3. Structural signs that indicate irreversible injury and progression to necrosis are the dense clumping and disruption of genetic material and the disruption of the plasma and organelle membranes.

4. Apoptosis, a distinct type of cellular death, is a process of selective cellular self-destruction that occurs in both normal and pathologic tissue changes.

5. Gangrenous necrosis, or gangrene, is tissue necrosis caused by hypoxia and subsequent bacterial invasion.

Continued

▣ DID YOU UNDERSTAND?—cont'd

◩ Aging

1. It is difficult to determine the physiologic (normal) from the pathologic changes of aging.
2. Humans have an inherent maximal life span (80 to 100 years) that is dictated by currently unknown intrinsic mechanisms.
3. Although the maximal life span has not changed significantly over time, the average life span, or life expectancy, has increased. Life expectancy for men is about 75 years, and for women it is 80 years.
4. The physiologic mechanisms of aging apparently are associated with (a) cellular changes produced by genetic and environmental factors, (b) changes in cellular regulatory or control mechanisms, and (c) degenerative extracellular and vascular alterations.

Somatic Death

1. Somatic death is death of the entire organism. Postmortem change is diffuse and does not involve the inflammatory response.
2. Manifestations of somatic death include cessation of respiration and circulation, gradual lowering of body temperature, pupil dilation, loss of elasticity and transparency in the skin, muscle stiffening (rigor mortis), and skin discoloration (livor mortis). Signs of putrefaction are obvious about 24 to 48 hours after death.

KEY TERMS

Abrasion, 78
Algor mortis, 98
Anoxia, 68
Apoptosis, 91
Asphyxial injuries, 82
Atrophy, 65
Atypical hyperplasia, 65
Autolysis, 90
Autophagic vacuole, 65
Avulsion, 78
Bilirubin, 87
Blow back, 80
Blunt force, 76
Caseous necrosis, 91
Catastrophic (error-prone) theory, 96
Cellular accumulation (infiltration), 83
Cellular swelling, 84
Chemical asphyxiants, 82
Choking asphyxiation, 82
Chopping wound, 80
Coagulative necrosis, 90
Compensatory hyperplasia, 66
Contact range entrance wound, 80
Contusion, 76
Cyanide, 83
Disuse atrophy, 65
Drowning, 83
Dysplasia (atypical hyperplasia), 66
Dystrophic calcification, 88
Entrance wound, 80
Epidermal hematoma, 78
Exit wound, 81

Fat necrosis, 91
Fat-free mass, 97
Fatty change, 85
Fetal alcohol syndrome, 75
Free radical, 69
Gangrenous necrosis, 91
Gas gangrene, 91
Gender gap, 93
Hanging strangulation, 82
Hematoma, 76
Hemoprotein, 87
Hemosiderin, 87
Hemosiderosis, 87
Hepatocyte growth factor, 66
Hormal hyperplasia, 66
Hydrogen sulfide, 83
Hydropic degeneration, 85
Hyperplasia, 65
Hypertrophy, 65
Hypoxia, 68
Incised wound, 79
Indeterminate (distance) range entrance wound, 81
Intermediate range entrance wound, 80
Irreversible injury, 67
Ischemia, 68
Karyolysis, 90
Laceration, 78
Life expectancy, 93
Ligature strangulation, 82
Lipid peroxidation, 70
Lipid-acceptor protein (apoprotein), 73

Lipofuscin, 65
Liquefactive necrosis, 90
Livor mortis, 98
Manual strangulation, 82
Maximal life span, 93
Melanin, 86
Metaplasia, 66
Metastatic calcification, 88
Muzzle imprint, 80
Necrosis, 90
Neuroendocrine theory, 96
Pathologic hyperplasia, 66
Postmortem autolysis, 98
Postmortem change, 97
Psammoma body, 88
Puncture wound, 80
Pyknosis, 90
Reperfusion injury, 69
Reversible injury, 67
Rigor mortis, 98
Sarcopenia, 97
Shored exit wound, 81
Somatic death, 97
Somatic mutation hypothesis, 96
Stab wound, 79
Stippling, 80
Strangulation, 82
Subdural hematoma, 76
Suffocation, 82
Tattooing, 80
Urate, 88
Vacuolation, 85

REFERENCES

1. Damjanov, I. & Linder, J. (Eds.). (1996). *Anderson's pathology* (10th ed.). St. Louis: Mosby.

2. Bottaro, D.P. et al. (1991). Identification of the hepatocyte growth factor receptor as the c-met proto-oncogene product. *Science, 251*(495), 802-805.

3. Alberts, B. et al. (1998). *Essential cell biology: An introduction to molecular biology of the cell.* New York: Garland.

4. London, S.J. et al. (1992). A prospective study of benign breast disease and the risk of breast cancer. *Journal of the American Medical Association, 267*(7), 941-944.

5. Ferrari, R. (1995). Metabolic disturbances during myocardial ischemia and reperfusion. *American Journal of Cardiology, 76*(6), 178.

6. Farber, J.L. (1981). Minireview: The role of calcium in cell death. *Life Sciences, 29,* 1289.

7. Kristian, T. & Siesjo, B.K. (1998). Calcium in ischemic cell death. *Stroke, 29*(3), 705-718.

8. Holtz M., Kneipmann, K., & Kohn, L. (1998). Occupational therapy in pediatric lead exposure prevention. *American Journal of Occupational Therapy, 52*(1), 53-59.

9. Norman, E.H. et al. (1997). Childhood lead poisoning and vinyl miniblind exposure. *Archives of Pediatric and Adolescent Medicine, 151,* 1033-1037.

10. *Science News.* (1994). Country kids: No let up from lead. *Science News, 146*(5), 65-80.

11. Lieber, C.S. (1991). Hepatic, metabolic, and toxic effects of ethanol: 1991 update. *Alcoholism Clinical and Experimental Research, 15*(4), 574-592.

12. Lieber, C.S. (1991). Metabolic effects of ethanol and its interaction with other drugs, hepatoxic agents, vitamins, and carcinogens: A 1988 update. *Seminars in Liver Disease, 8*(1), 47-68.

13. Cotran, R.S., Kumar, V., & Collins, T. (1999). *Robbins pathologic basis of disease* (6th ed.). Philadelphia: Saunders.

14. Cohen, S.D. & Khairalla, E.A. (1997). Selective protein arylation and acetaminophen-induced hepatotoxicity. *Drug Metabolism Review, 29*(1), 59-77.

15. Kurose, I. et al. (1997). CD188/ICAM-1-dependent nitric oxide production of Kupffer cells as a cause of mitochondrial dysfunction in hepatoma cells: Influence of chronic alcohol feeding. *Free Radical and Biologic Medicine, 22*(1-2), 229-239.

16. Stradling, J.R. & Crosby, J.H. (1991). Predictors and prevalence of obstructive sleep apnea and snoring in 1001 middle-aged men. *Thorax, 46*(2), 85-90.

17. Coca, A. et al. (1992). Chronic alcohol intake induces reversible disturbances on cellular Na metabolism in humans: Its relationship with changes in blood pressure. *Alcoholism Clinical and Experimental Research, 16*(4), 714-720.

18. Martinez, F. et al. (1992). Ethanol and cytokine secretion. *Alcohol, 9*(6), 455-458.

19. Devi, B.G., Henderson, G.I., & Schenker, S. (1993). Effect of ethanol on rat fetal hepatocytes: Studies in cell replication, lipid peroxidation and glutathione. *Hepatology, 18*(3), 648-659.

20. Centers for Disease Control. (1997). Injury Statistics Webside. Washington, DC: The Author.

21. Powell, L.W. & Kerr, J.F.R. (1975). Pathology of the liver in hemochromatosis. *Pathobiological Annual, 5,* 317.

22. al Rubeai, M. (1998). Apoptosis and cell culture technology. *Advanced Biochemical Engineering and Biotechnology, 59,* 225-249.

23. D'Mello, S.R. (1998). Molecular regulation of neuronal apoptosis. *Current Topics in Developmental Biology, 39,* 187-213.

24. Zakeri, Z.F. & Ahuja, H.S. (1997). Cell death/apoptosis: Normal, chemically induced, and teratogenic effect. *Mutation Research, 396*(1-2), 149-161.

25. Raff, M.C. (1992). Social controls on cell survival and cell death. *Nature, 356,* 397-401.

26. Chow, S.C., Kass, C.E., & Orrenius, S. (1997). Purines and their roles in apoptosis. *Neuropharmacology, 36*(9), 1149-1156.

27. Sandford, N.L., Searle, J.W., & Kerr, J.F.R. (1984). Successive waves of apoptosis in the rat prostate after repeated withdrawal of testosterone stimulation. *Pathology, 16*(4), 406-410.

28. Tomei, L.D. & Cope, F.O. (Eds.). (1991). *Apoptosis: The molecular basis of cell death.* New York: Cold Spring Harbor Laboratory Press.

29. Garland, J.M., Sondergaard, K.L., & Jolly, J. (1997). Redux regulation of apoptosis in interleukin-3-dependent haemopoietic cells. *British Journal of Haematology, 99*(4), 756-765.

30. Wyllie, A.H., Kerr, J.F.R., & Currie, A.R. (1980). Cell death: The significance of apoptosis. *International Review of Cytology, 68,* 251-306.

31. Koh, J.S. & Levine, J.S. (1997). Apoptosis and immunity. *Current Opinion in Nephrology and Hypertension, 6*(3), 259-266.

32. Raff, M.C. et al. (1993). Programmed cell death and control of cell survival: Lessons from the nervous system. *Science, 262*(5130-5136), 695-700.

33. Johnson, H.A. (Ed.). (1985). Is aging physiological or pathological? In *Relations between normal aging and disease.* New York: Raven.

34. Cassel, C.K. et al. (1990). *Geriatric medicine* (2nd ed.). New York: Springer-Verlag.

35. Trussel, J. (1995). Women's longevity [letter], *Science, 270*(5237), 719-720.

36. Manton, K.G. (1997). Demographic trends for the aging population. *Journal of the American Medical Association, 52*(3), 99-105.

REFERENCES

37. Simonton, D.K. (1997). Achievement domain and life expectancies in Japanese civilization. *International Journal of Aging and Human Development, 44*(92), 103-114.

38. Nathanson, C.A. (1990). The gender-mortality differential in developed countries: Demographic and sociocultural dimensions. In M.G. Ory & H.R. Warner (Eds.). *Gender, health, and longevity: Multidisciplinary perspectives.* New York: Springer.

39. Riley, M.W. (1990). Foreword: The gender paradox. In M.G. Ory & H.R. Warner (Eds.). *Gender, health, and longevity: Multidisciplinary perspectives.* New York: Springer.

40. Norwood, T.H. (1990). Cellular aging. In C.K. Cassel et al. (Eds.). *Geriatric medicine* (2nd ed.). New York: Springer-Verlag.

41. Hayflick, L. (1965). The limited in vitro lifetime of human diploid cell strains. *Experimental Cell Research, 37,* 614.

42. O'Connor, K.G. et al. (1998). Serum levels of insulin-like growth factor-1 are related to age and not to body composition in healthy women and men. *Journal of Gerontology, 53*(3), M176-M182.

43. Shennan, T. (1935). *Postmortems and morbid anatomy* (3rd ed.). Baltimore: William Wood.

44. Minckler, J., Anstall, H.B., & Minckler, T.M. (1971). *Pathobiology: An introduction.* St. Louis: Mosby.

CHAPTER 4

Fluids and Electrolytes, Acids and Bases

Sue E. Huether

The cells of the body live in a fluid environment that requires an electrolyte concentration and pH value maintained within a narrow range. Changes in electrolyte concentration affect electrical potentials of excitatory cells and cause shifts of fluid from one compartment to another. Alterations in pH disrupt the cellular function of enzyme systems. Fluid fluctuations affect blood volume and cellular function. Disturbances in these functions are common and can be life threatening. Understanding how alterations occur and how the body compensates or corrects the disturbance is important to understanding many pathophysiologic conditions.

CHAPTER OUTLINE

TABLE 4-1	Total Body Water (%) in Relation to Body Weight		
Body Build	Adult Male	Adult Female	Infant
Normal	60	50	70
Lean	70	60	80
Obese	50	42	60

NOTE: Total body water is a percentage of body weight.

TABLE 4-2	Distribution of Body Water	
	Percentage of Body Weight	Volume (L)
Intracellular fluid (ICF)	40	28
Extracellular fluid (ECF)	20	14
Interstitial	(15)	(11)
Intravascular	(5)	(3)
Total body water (TBW)	60	42

TABLE 4-3	Normal Water Gains and Losses (70-Kg Man)		
	Daily Intake (ml)		Daily Output (ml)
Drinking	1400-1800	Urine	1400-1800
Water in food	700-1000	Stool	100
Water of oxidation	300-400	Skin	300-500
		Lungs	600-800
TOTAL	2400-3200	TOTAL	2400-3200

DISTRIBUTION OF BODY FLUIDS

The sum of fluids within all compartments constitutes *total body water (TBW)*—about 60% of body weight (Table 4-1). The volume of TBW is usually expressed as a percentage of body weight in kilograms. One liter of water weighs 2.2 lb (1 kg), and 1 milliliter equals 1/1000 of a liter. The rest of the body weight is made up of fat and fat-free solids, particularly bone.

Body fluids are distributed among functional compartments, or spaces, and provide a transport medium for cellular and tissue function. *Intracellular fluid (ICF)* comprises all the fluid within cells. *Extracellular fluid (ECF)* is all the fluid outside the cells and is divided into smaller compartments. The two main ECF compartments are the *interstitial fluid* (the space between cells and outside the blood vessels) and the *intravascular fluid* (blood plasma) (Table 4-2). Other ECF compartments include lymph and transcellular fluids, such as synovial, intestinal, and cerebrospinal fluid; sweat; urine; and pleural, synovial, peritoneal, pericardial, and intraocular fluids.

Although the amount of fluid within the various compartments is relatively constant, solutes and water are exchanged between compartments to maintain their unique compositions. The percentage of TBW varies with the amount of body fat and age. Because fat is water-repelling (hydrophobic), very little water is contained in adipose cells. Individuals with more body fat have proportionately less TBW and tend to be more susceptible to fluid imbalances that cause dehydration.

Maturation and the Distribution of Body Fluids

The distribution and the amount of TBW change with age (see Pediatric and Aging boxes), and although daily fluid in-

PEDIATRICS & *Distribution of Body Fluids*

NEWBORN INFANTS
At birth, TBW represents about 75% to 80% of body weight and decreases to about 67% during the first year of life. Physiologic loss of body water amounting to 5% of body weight occurs as an infant adjusts to a new environment. Infants are particularly susceptible to significant changes in TBW because of a high metabolic rate and greater body surface area. Renal mechanisms of fluid and electrolyte conservation may not be mature enough to counter losses, allowing dehydration to occur.

CHILDREN AND ADOLESCENTS
TBW slowly decreases to 60% to 65% of body weight. At adolescence, the percentage of TBW approaches adult levels and differences according to gender appear. Males have a greater percentage of body water because of increased muscle mass, and females have more body fat because of the influence of estrogen and thus less water.

AGING & *Distribution of Body Fluids*

The further decline in the percentage of TBW in the elderly is in part the result of an increased amount of fat and decreased muscle, as well as reduced ability to regulate sodium and water balance. Kidneys are less efficient in producing concentrated urine, and sodium-conserving responses are sluggish. With stress, when disease is present, this normal decrease in TBW can become life-threatening.

take may fluctuate widely, the body regulates water volume within a relatively narrow range. The primary sources of body water are drinking, ingestion of water in food, and water derived from oxidative metabolism. Normally, the largest amounts of water are lost through renal excretion, with lesser amounts lost through the stool and through vaporization from the skin and lungs (insensible water loss) (Table 4-3).

A. Normal osmotic equilibrium

280 mOsm/kg 17 L

280 mOsm/kg
25 L
ICF

ECF

Addition of solute to ECF

B. Osmotic disequilibrium with higher milliosmolarity of ECF

300 mOsm/kg 17 L

280 mOsm/kg
25 L
ICF

ECF

Reestablishment of osmotic gradient

C. Reestablishment of osmotic equilibrium

290 mOsm/kg 18 L

290 mOsm/kg
24 L
ICF

ECF

Fig. 4-1 *Model of osmotic equilibrium.*

Water Movement Between ICF and ECF

Water moves between ICF and ECF compartments primarily as a function of osmotic forces (see Chapter 1). Water crosses cell membranes freely, so the osmolality of TBW is normally at equilibrium. Sodium is responsible for the ECF osmotic balance, and potassium maintains the ICF osmotic balance. The osmotic force of ICF proteins and other nondiffusible substances is balanced by the active transport of ions out of the cell. Normally the ICF is not subject to rapid changes in osmolality, but when ECF osmolality changes, water moves from one compartment to another until osmotic equilibrium is reestablished. A model of the maintenance of osmotic equilibrium is illustrated in Fig. 4-1.

Water Movement Between Plasma and Interstitial Fluid

The distribution of water and the movement of nutrients and waste products among the capillary, plasma, and interstitial spaces occur as a result of changes in hydrostatic (blood) pressure (pushes water) and osmotic forces (pull water) at the arterial and venous ends of the capillary. Because water, sodium, and glucose readily move across the capillary membrane, plasma proteins maintain effective osmolality by generating plasma oncotic pressure. Osmotic forces within the capillary are balanced by the hydrostatic pressure, which arises from cardiac contraction. The movement of fluid back and forth across the capillary wall is called ***net filtration*** and is best described by ***Starling's hypothesis:***

$$\text{Net filtration} = \text{Force favoring filtration} - \text{Forces opposing filtration}$$

Filtration is the movement of water out of the capillary and into the interstitial space. Forces favoring filtration include capillary hydrostatic pressure and interstitial oncotic pressure. Opposing forces are plasma oncotic pressure and interstitial hydrostatic pressure. Normally only a small percentage of plasma proteins cross the capillary membrane, so interstitial fluid moves into cells or is drawn back into the plasma.

As the plasma flows from the arterial to the venous end of the capillary, changes in hydrostatic pressure facilitate water's outward movement across the capillary membrane. Oncotic pressure remains fairly constant because plasma proteins normally do not cross the capillary membrane. At the arterial end of the capillary, hydrostatic pressure exceeds capillary oncotic pressure and water filters into the interstitial space. Some water moves back into the capillary, but the net effect is loss of water from the capillary (filtration). At the venous end of the capillary, oncotic pressure exceeds hydrostatic pressure. Fluids are attracted back into the circulation (reabsorption), balancing the movement of fluids between the plasma and the interstitial space (Fig. 4-2). A small amount of fluid is reabsorbed from the interstitial space by the lymph channels.

The integrity of the capillary membrane is an important factor. Changes in membrane permeability may permit plasma proteins to escape into the interstitial space. The osmotic movement of water into the interstitial space causes tissue edema.

ALTERATIONS IN WATER MOVEMENT
Edema

Edema is the accumulation of fluid within the interstitial spaces. It can indicate a fluid excess or sequestered fluids. The forces favoring fluid movement from the capillaries or lymphatic channels into the tissues are increased hydrostatic pressure, lowered plasma oncotic pressure, increased capillary membrane permeability, and lymphatic obstruction (Fig. 4-3).

Pathophysiology

Hydrostatic pressure increases as a result of venous obstruction or salt and water retention. Venous obstruction causes hydrostatic pressure to increase, which pushes fluid from capillaries into the interstitial spaces. Thrombophlebitis, hepatic obstruction, tight clothing around the extremities, and prolonged standing are common causes of venous obstruction. Congestive heart failure and renal failure are associated with salt and water retention, which cause volume overload and edema.

Arterial Capillary Pressures		Venous Capillary Pressures	
Blood hydrostatic pressure	37 mm Hg	Blood hydrostatic pressure	18 mm Hg
Interstitial fluid hydrostatic pressure	2 mm Hg	Interstitial fluid hydrostatic pressure	3 mm Hg
Net pushing pressure	**35 mm Hg**	**Net pushing pressure**	**15 mm Hg**
Blood oncotic pressure	27 mm Hg	Blood oncotic pressure	25 mm Hg
Interstitial fluid oncotic pressure	2 mm Hg	Interstitial fluid oncotic pressure	0 mm Hg
Net pulling pressure	**25 mm Hg**	**Net pulling pressure**	**25 mm Hg**
Net filtration pressure	**+10 mm Hg**	Net filtration pressure	**−10 mm Hg**

Fig. 4-2 *Movement of fluids between the capillary and interstitial space.* A small amount of fluid moves to the lymph vessels, accounting for the net filtration difference between the arterial and venous ends of the capillary.

Lost or diminished plasma albumin production (liver disease or protein malnutrition) contributes to decreased plasma oncotic pressure. Plasma proteins are lost in glomerular diseases of the kidney, serous drainage from open wounds, hemorrhage, burns, and cirrhosis of the liver. The decreased oncotic attraction of fluid within the capillary causes fluid to move into the interstitial space, resulting in edema.

Capillaries become more permeable with inflammation and immune responses, especially trauma such as burns or crushing injuries; neoplastic disease; and allergic reactions. Proteins escape from the vascular bed and produce edema through lost capillary oncotic pressure and interstitial fluid protein accumulation.

The lymphatic system normally absorbs interstitial fluid and a small amount of proteins. When lymphatic channels are blocked or surgically removed, proteins and fluid accumulate in the interstitial space. For example, lymphedema of the arm or leg occurs after surgical removal of axillary and femoral lymph nodes for treatment of carcinoma. Inflam-

mation or tumors may cause lymphatic obstruction, leading to edema.

Clinical Manifestations

Edema may be localized or generalized. Localized edema may be limited to the site of trauma, as in a sprained finger. Another kind of localized edema occurs within particular organ systems and includes cerebral edema, pulmonary edema, pleural effusion, pericardial effusion, and ascites (accumulation of fluid in the peritoneal space). Generalized edema is manifest by a more uniform distribution of fluid in interstitial spaces. Dependent edema, in which fluid accumulates in gravity-dependent areas of the body, might signal more generalized edema. Dependent edema appears in the feet and legs when standing and in the sacral area and buttocks when lying down. It can be identified by pressing on tissues overlying bony prominences. A pit left in the skin indicates edema (hence the term *pitting edema*).

Edema usually is associated with weight gain, swelling and puffiness, tight-fitting clothes and shoes, limited move-

Fig. 4-3 *Mechanisms of edema formation.*

ment of the affected area, and symptoms associated with the underlying pathologic condition. Fluid accumulations increase the distance required for nutrients and waste products to move between capillaries and tissues. Blood flow may be impaired also. Therefore wounds heal more slowly and the risks of infection and pressure sores increase. Edema of specific organs, such as the brain, lung, or larynx, can be life threatening.[1]

Although excess fluid accumulates, it is trapped in a "third space" and unavailable for metabolic processes. Therefore dehydration can develop as a result of the sequestering. Such sequestration occurs with severe burns, where large amounts of vascular fluid are lost to the interstitial spaces, reducing plasma volume and causing shock (see Chapter 39).

SODIUM, CHLORIDE, AND WATER BALANCE

Because water follows the osmotic gradients established by changes in salt concentration, sodium and water balance are intimately related. Water balance is regulated primarily by antidiuretic hormone (ADH; also known as *vasopressin*); sodium is regulated by aldosterone.

Water Balance

Water balance is regulated by the secretion of ADH and the perception of thirst. Thirst stimulates water drinking and is experienced when water loss equals 2% of an individual's body weight or when there is an increase in osmolality. Dry mouth, hyperosmolality, and plasma volume depletion activate *osmoreceptors* (neurons in the hypothalamus), which then cause thirst. Drinking water restores plasma volume and dilutes the ECF osmolality.

ADH is secreted when plasma osmolality increases or circulating blood volume decreases and blood pressure drops. Increased plasma osmolality occurs with water deficit or sodium excess in relation to water. The increased osmolality results in a fall in extracellular and interstitial fluid volume and stimulates hypothalamic osmoreceptors. In addition to causing thirst, these osmoreceptors cause the posterior pituitary gland to release ADH. ADH increases the permeability of renal tubular cells to water, so the water can

Fig. 4-4 *The antidiuretic hormone system. (From Thibodeau G.A. & Patton, K.T. [1999]. Anatomy & physiology [4th ed.]. St. Louis: Mosby.)*

TABLE 4-4	Distribution of Electrolytes in Body Compartments	
	ECF (mEq/L)	**ICF (mEq/L)**
Cations		
Sodium	142	10
Potassium	5	156
Calcium	5	4
Magnesium	2	26
TOTALS	154	196
Anions		
Bicarbonate	24	12
Chloride	104	4
Phosphate	2	40-95
Proteins	16	54
Other anions	8	31-86
TOTALS	154	141(196)-251

ECF, *Extracellular fluid;* ICF, *intracellular fluid.*

be reabsorbed into the plasma from the distal tubules and collecting ducts of the kidney. Urine concentration increases, and the reabsorbed water decreases plasma osmolality, returning it toward normal.

With dehydration from vomiting, diarrhea, or excessive sweating, **volume-sensitive receptors** and **baroreceptors** (nerve endings that are sensitive to changes in volume and pressure) stimulate the release of ADH from the pituitary gland. The volume receptors are located in the right and left atria and thoracic vessels; baroreceptors are found in the aorta, pulmonary arteries, and carotid sinus. ADH secretion also occurs when atrial pressure drops, as occurs with decreased blood volume. The reabsorption of water mediated by ADH then promotes the restoration of plasma volume (Fig. 4-4).

Sodium and Chloride Balance

Sodium accounts for 90% of the ECF cations (positively charged ions) and is the most powerful cation in the ECF. (The distribution of electrolytes in body compartments is summarized in Table 4-4.) Along with its constituent anions (negatively charged ions), chloride and bicarbonate, sodium regulates osmotic forces and therefore regulates water balance. Sodium is important in other functions, including regulation of osmolality (interstitial and intravascular fluid volume), working with potassium and calcium to maintain neuromuscular irritability for conduction of nerve impulses, regulation of acid-base balance (through sodium bicarbonate and sodium phosphate), participation in cellular chemical reactions, and membrane transport.

Chloride is the major anion in the extracellular fluid and provides electroneutrality, particularly in relation to sodium. The transport of chloride is generally passive and follows the active transport of sodium, so that increases or decreases in chloride are proportional to changes in sodium. The concentration of chloride tends to vary inversely with changes in concentration of bicarbonate, the other major anion.

The kidney maintains normal serum sodium concentration within a narrow range (136 to 145 mEq/L) primarily through renal tubular reabsorption. Neural and hormonal mediators also play a role. Hormonal regulation of sodium balance is mediated by **aldosterone,** a mineralocorticoid synthesized and secreted from the adrenal cortex (see Chapter 17). Aldosterone secretion is influenced by both circulating blood volume and plasma concentrations of Na^+ and K^+ (aldosterone is secreted when sodium levels are depressed or potassium levels are increased). Aldosterone increases the reabsorption of sodium and the secretion of potassium by the distal tubule of the kidney. As a result, sodium concentration of the ECF is enhanced, and potassium is excreted with the urine.

When circulating blood volume is reduced, **renin,** an enzyme secreted by the juxtaglomerular cells of the kidney, is released. Renin stimulates the formation of **angiotensin I,** an inactive polypeptide, which is then converted into **angiotensin II,** which stimulates the secretion of aldosterone and causes vasoconstriction. The aldosterone then promotes sodium and water reabsorption, increasing blood volume (Fig. 4-5). Vasoconstriction elevates the systemic blood pressure and restores renal perfusion. This restoration inhibits the further release of renin. This complete mechanism is known as the **renin-angiotensin system** (see Chapter 28).

Natriuretic hormone promotes urinary excretion of sodium. It also decreases renal tubular reabsorption of sodium, thus causing a loss of salt and water. Atrial natriuretic factor is produced by the atrial muscle of the heart

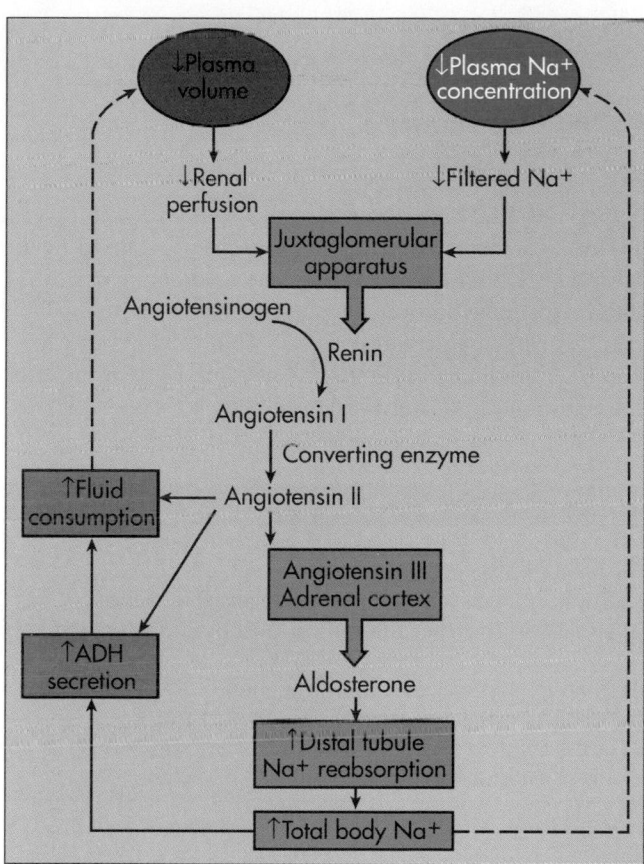

Fig. 4-5 *The renin-angiotensin-aldosterone system.* *(From Thibodeau, G.A. & Patton, K.T. [1999]. Anatomy & physiology [4th ed.]. St. Louis: Mosby.)*

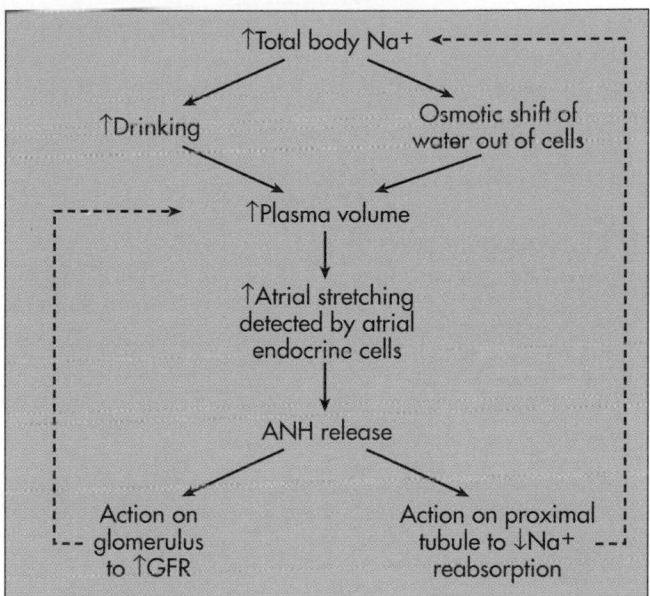

Fig. 4-6 *The atrial natriuretic hormone (ANH) system.* *(From Thibodeau, G.A. & Patton, K.T. [1999]. Anatomy & physiology [4th ed.]. St. Louis: Mosby.)*

and functions in renal elimination of sodium to control sodium and water balance. Natriuretic hormone is sometimes called the *third factor* in sodium regulation, after increased glomerular filtration rate and aldosterone.[2] Its effect is apparent when there is prolonged aldosterone elevation from chronic retention of fluid or excessive secretion from an adrenal tumor. The sodium-retaining action of aldosterone is overcome, and salt is excreted, followed by a water diuresis (Fig. 4-6).

ALTERATIONS IN SODIUM, CHLORIDE, AND WATER BALANCE

Alterations in sodium and water balance are closely related.[3] Water imbalances may develop with gains or losses of salt.

Likewise, sodium imbalances occur with alterations in body water volume. Generally, these alterations can be classified as changes in tonicity—the change in the concentration of solutes with relation to water (see Chapter 1). Alterations can therefore be classified as isotonic, hypertonic, or hypotonic (Table 4-5).

Isotonic Alterations (Fluid Volume Deficits)

Isotonic alterations occur when TBW changes are accompanied by proportional changes in electrolytes. For example, if an individual loses pure plasma or ECF, fluid volume is depleted but the number and type of electrolytes and the osmolality remain in the normal range. Excessive amounts of isotonic body fluids can result from excessive administration of intravenous normal saline or oversecretion of aldosterone with renal retention of both sodium and water. Losses of isotonic body fluids include hemorrhage, severe wound drainage, and excessive diaphoresis.

Isotonic fluid loss (isotonic dehydration) causes contraction of the ECF volume with weight loss, dryness of skin and mucous membranes, decreased urine output, and symptoms of hypovolemia. Indicators of hypovolemia include a rapid heart rate, flattened neck veins, and normal or decreased blood pressure. In severe states, hypovolemic shock can occur (see Chapter 23).

Isotonic fluid excesses are most commonly the result of excessive administration of intravenous fluids, hypersecretion of aldosterone, or the effects of drugs such as cortisone. As plasma volume expands, hypervolemia develops, with weight gain, decreased hematocrit, and fewer plasma proteins because of the diluting effect of excess plasma volume.

The neck veins may distend, and the blood pressure increases. Increased capillary hydrostatic pressure leads to edema formation. Ultimately, pulmonary edema and heart failure may develop.

Hypertonic Alterations

Hypertonic fluid alterations develop when the osmolality of the ECF is elevated above normal. The most common causes are increased concentration of ECF sodium (hypernatremia) or deficit of ECF water. In both instances, ECF hypertonicity attracts water from the intracellular space, causing ICF dehydration. A primary increase in ECF sodium causes an osmotic attraction of water and symptoms of hypervolemia. In contrast, a hypertonic state caused primarily by water loss leads to hypovolemia (Table 4-6).

Hypernatremia

Pathophysiology

Hypernatremia occurs when serum sodium levels exceed 147 mEq/L. Increased serum sodium may be caused by an acute gain in sodium or a loss of water. Sodium gains cause intracellular dehydration; the movement of water to the ECF may cause hypervolemia. With an accompanying water loss, both ICF and ECF dehydration may occur. Hyperosmolality is a common result of hypernatremia.

TABLE 4-5	Water and Solute Imbalances
Tonicity	**Mechanism**
Isotonic (isoosmolar) imbalance	Gain or loss of ECF resulting in a concentration equivalent to a 0.9% sodium chloride (salt) solution (normal saline); no shrinking or swelling of cells
Hypertonic (hyperosmolar) imbalance	Imbalances that result in an ECF concentration more than 0.9% salt solution, i.e., water loss or solute gain; cells shrink in a hypertonic fluid
Hypotonic (hypoosmolar) imbalance	Imbalance that results in an ECF less than 0.9% salt solution, i.e., water gain or solute loss; cells swell in a hypotonic fluid

TABLE 4-6	Causes and Consequences of Hypertonic Imbalances		
Causative Factor	**Mechanism**	**ECF Effects**	**ICF Effects**
Increased sodium (hypernatremia)	**Excessive intake** Intravenous hypertonic sodium Saline-induced abortions Selected infant formulas **Decreased sodium loss** Hyperaldosteronism Cushing syndrome Renal failure Congestive heart failure	**Hypervolemia** Weight gain Bounding pulse Increased blood pressure Edema Venous distintion **Neuromuscular symptoms** Muscle weakness Seizures	**Intracellular dehydration** Thirst Fever Decreased urine output Shrinkage of brain cells Confusion Coma Cerebral hemorrhage
Water deficit	**Water deprivation** Confusion or coma Inability to communicate Loss of thirst Inability to swallow **Water loss** Watery diarrhea Diabetes insipidus ($\downarrow$ ADH) Excessive diuresis Excessive diaphoresis	**Hypovolemia** Weight loss Weak pulses Postural hypotension Tachycardia	**Intracellular dehydration** See above
Other factors	Hyperglycemia	Initial dilutional hyponatremia Polyuria Polydipsia Weight loss Hypovolemia Late hypernatremia	**Intracellular dehydration** See above

High amounts of dietary sodium rarely cause hypernatremia. More commonly, high sodium levels occur with inappropriate administration of hypertonic saline solution (e.g., as sodium bicarbonate for treatment of acidosis during cardiac arrest). High sodium levels can occur also with oversecretion of aldosterone, as in primary hyperaldosteronism or Cushing syndrome caused by excess secretion of adrenocorticotropic hormone (ACTH), which also causes increased secretion of aldosterone.

Increased sodium in relation to water loss is associated with fever or respiratory infections, which increase the respiratory rate and enhance water loss from the lungs. Diabetes insipidus, diabetes mellitus, polyuria, profuse sweating, and diarrhea also cause water loss in relation to sodium. Infants with severe diarrhea are particularly vulnerable. Insufficient water intake can cause hypernatremia, particularly in individuals who are comatose, confused, or immobilized.

Clinical Manifestations

Water is redistributed to the extracellular space, and intracellular dehydration ensues. Convulsions and pulmonary edema are the most serious symptoms. Thirst, fever, dry mucous membranes, and restlessness are associated with hypernatremia as a result of water loss.

Water deficit

Pathophysiology

Dehydration describes water deficit but also is commonly used to indicate both sodium loss and water loss (isotonic or isoosmolar dehydration).[4] Pure *water deficits* (hyperosmolar or hypertonic dehydration) are rare because most people have access to water. Individuals who are comatose or paralyzed continue to have insensible water losses through the skin and lungs with a minimal obligatory formation of urine. Hyperventilation caused by fever also may precipitate water deficit. The most common cause of water loss is increased renal clearance of free water as a result of impaired tubular function or inability to concentrate the urine, as with diabetes insipidus (decreased ADH) (see Chapter 18).

Clinical Manifestations

Marked water deficit is manifested by symptoms of dehydration: thirst, dry skin and mucous membranes, elevated temperature, weight loss, and concentrated urine (with the exception of diabetes insipidus). Skin turgor may be normal or decreased. Symptoms of hypovolemia include tachycardia, weak pulses, and postural hypotension.

TABLE 4-7	Causes and Consequences of Hypotonic Imbalances		
Causative Factor	**Mechanism**	**ECF Effects**	**ICF Effects**
Decreased sodium (hyponatremia)	**Inadequate intake** **Hyperaldosteronism** **Increased loss** Diuresis Profuse sweating Gastrointestinal losses	**Extracellular volume contraction and hypovolemia** (but may not be if there is water excess)	**Increased intracellular water; edema** Brain cell swelling, irritability, depression, confusion Systemic cellular edema, including weakness, anorexia, nausea, and diarrhea
Water excess	**Sodium dilution** Excessive administration of hypotonic intravenous solutions Drinking water to replace isotonic fluid losses Tap water enemas Psychogenic polydipsia Renal water retention Increased antidiuretic hormone	**Extracellular volume expands with hypervolemia** (but may not be if fluid is trapped in intracellular space)	**Edema** (see above)
Other factors	Isotonic dehydration treated with intravenous D_5W; glucose in D_5W solution is metabolized to water, contributing to hyponatremia Nephrotic syndrome Cirrhosis Cardiac failure	**Hypervolemia** or **hypovolemia**	**Edema** (see above)

Hyperchloremia

Hyperchloremia occurs clinically when there is too much sodium or too little bicarbonate. More than normal amounts of chloride can be expected with hypernatremia or metabolic acidosis (see p. 119). Ingestion of excessive chloride infrequently accompanies the use of an ammonium chloride diuretic. No specific symptoms are associated with chloride excess.

Hypotonic Alterations

Hypotonic fluid imbalances occur when the osmolality of the ECF is less than normal. The most common causes are sodium deficit *(hyponatremia)* or water excess. Either leads to intracellular overhydration (edema). When there is a sodium deficit, the osmotic pressure of the ECF decreases and water moves into the cell, where the osmotic pressure is greater. The plasma volume then decreases, leading to symptoms of hypovolemia. With a water excess, increases in both the ICF and ECF volume occur, causing symptoms of hypervolemia (Table 4-7).

Hyponatremia

Pathophysiology

Hyponatremia develops when the serum sodium concentration falls below 135 mEq/L. Sodium deficits usually cause hypoosmolality with movement of water into cells. Among the clinical syndromes causing hyponatremia are sodium loss, inadequate sodium intake, or dilution of the body's sodium level.

Pure sodium deficits usually are caused by extrarenal losses, such as vomiting, diarrhea, gastrointestinal suctioning, or burns. *Inadequate intake* of dietary sodium is rare but possible in individuals on low-sodium diets, particularly when diuretics are taken. *Dilutional hyponatremias* occur when the proportion of TBW to total body sodium is excessive. Replacement of fluid loss with intravenous 5% dextrose in water also can cause a dilutional hyponatremia once the glucose is metabolized, leaving a hypotonic solution with a diluting effect. Excessive sweating may stimulate thirst and intake of large amounts of water, which dilute sodium. Hyponatremia also may be hypoosmolar or hypertonic. During acute oliguric renal failure, severe congestive heart failure, or cirrhosis, renal excretion of water is impaired. Both TBW and sodium levels are increased, but TBW exceeds the increase in sodium, producing a *hypoosmolar hyponatremia.* *Hypertonic hyponatremia* develops with hyperlipidemia, hyperproteinemia, and hyperglycemia. Increases in plasma lipids and proteins displace water volume and decrease sodium concentration. Hyperglycemia increases ECF osmolality and attracts water from the ICF compartment. The osmotic fluid shift to the ECF in turn dilutes the concentration of sodium and other electrolytes.

Clinical Manifestations

Deficits of sodium alter the cell's ability to depolarize and repolarize normally (see Chapter 1). Behavioral and neurologic changes characteristic of hyponatremia include lethargy, confusion, apprehension, seizures, and coma. Pure sodium losses may be accompanied by loss of ECF, causing an isotonic *hypovolemia* with symptoms of hypotension, tachycardia, and decreased urine output. Weight gain, edema, ascites, and jugular vein distention are characteristic of dilutional hyponatremias.

Water excess

≋ *Pathophysiology*

When the body is functioning normally, it is almost impossible to produce an excess of TBW. Some individuals with psychogenic disorders develop water intoxication from *compulsive water drinking.* Acute renal failure, severe congestive heart failure, and cirrhosis can precipitate water excess during intravenous infusion of 5% dextrose in water. *Decreased urine formation* from intrinsic renal disease or decreased renal blood flow contributes to water excess. The overall effect is dilution of the ECF with water moving to the intracellular space by osmosis. Water excess produces a hypotonic or hypoosmolar water imbalance.

The *syndrome of inappropriate secretion of ADH (SIADH)* occurs when factors other than hyperosmolality or hypovolemia stimulate the secretion of ADH. Several clinical conditions that result in SIADH are fear, pain, acute infection, brain trauma, surgery, and drugs such as analgesics and anesthetics. The most common cause is bronchogenic cancer. SIADH is not caused by excess water intake but by decreased renal excretion of water. Therefore SIADH increases the risk of water excess if intravenous fluids are being administered. Serum sodium and osmolality are reduced. The kidney continues to excrete sodium, and urine specific gravity is elevated, but urine volume is decreased.

≋ *Clinical Manifestations*

The symptoms of water excess are related to the rate at which water loading has occurred. Acute excesses cause confusion and convulsions. Weakness, nausea, muscle twitching, headache, and weight gain are common symptoms of long-term water accumulation.

Hypochloremia

Loss of chloride, *hypochloremia,* is usually the result of hyponatremia or elevated bicarbonate concentration, as in metabolic alkalosis (see p. 120). Hypochloremia develops with vomiting and loss of hydrochloric acid. Sodium deficit related to restricted intake or use of diuretics is accompanied by chloride deficiency. Cystic fibrosis, for example, also is characterized by hypochloremia.

✓ QUICK CHECK

What causes isotonic imbalance?

Give two examples of hypertonic alterations, and explain the mechanisms of action for each.

What is a hypotonic imbalance? Give two examples.

ALTERATIONS IN POTASSIUM AND OTHER ELECTROLYTES
Potassium

Potassium is the major intracellular electrolyte and contributes to many important cellular functions. Total body potassium content is about 4000 mEq, with most of it (98%) located in the cells. The ICF concentration of K^+ is 150 to 160 mEq/L; the ECF concentration is 3.5 to 4.5 mEq/L. The difference in concentration is maintained by a sodium-potassium active transport system (Na^+, K^+ ATPase pump).

As the predominant ICF ion, potassium exerts a major influence in regulating ICF osmolality and fluid balance and for intracellular electrical neutrality in relation to H^+ and Na^+. Potassium is required for glycogen and glucose deposition in liver and skeletal muscle cells. It also maintains the resting membrane potential, as reflected in transmission and conduction of nerve impulses, maintenance of normal cardiac rhythms, and skeletal and smooth muscle contraction.

Although potassium is found in most body fluids, the kidney provides the most efficient regulator of potassium balance. Potassium is freely filtered by the renal glomerulus, and 90% is reabsorbed by the proximal tubule and loop of Henle. The distal tubule secretes potassium and determines the amount of K^+ excreted from the body. The transport is passive; unlike sodium, however, the renal mechanism for conserving K^+ is weak, even when total body potassium stores are depleted.[5]

Concentration gradients, changes in pH, changes in electrical potential differences across the distal tubule, and aldosterone levels all aid in renal regulation of potassium.

The potassium concentration in the distal tubular cell is determined primarily by the plasma concentration in the peritubular capillaries. When plasma K^+ concentration increases from increased dietary intake or shifts of K^+ from the ICF occur, potassium is secreted into the urine by the distal tubules. Decreased plasma potassium results in decreased distal tubular secretion, although approximately 5 to 15 mEq/day continues to be lost. Changes in the rate of filtrate flow through the distal tubule also influence the concentration gradient for K^+ secretion. When the flow rate is high, as with the use of diuretics, K^+ concentration in the distal tubular urine is lower, leading to the secretion of potassium.

Changes in pH and thus in hydrogen ion concentration also affect K^+ balance. During acidosis, hydrogen ions accumulate in the ICF and potassium shifts out of the cell to the ECF to maintain a balance of cations across the cell membrane. This decreased ICF K^+ results in decreased secretion of K^+ by the distal tubular cells, contributing to hyperkalemia. In alkalosis, however, intracellular fluid levels of hydrogen diminish and potassium shifts into the cell, so that the distal tubular cells increase their secretion of K^+, contributing to hypokalemia.

Besides conserving sodium, aldosterone also regulates potassium. When potassium concentration increases, aldosterone is released, stimulating the release of potassium into the urine by the distal renal tubules. Aldosterone also increases the secretion of K^+ from the sweat glands.

Insulin helps regulate plasma potassium levels by promoting the movement of potassium into liver and muscle cells. Therefore it can be used to treat hyperkalemia, and dangerously low levels of plasma potassium can result when insulin is given while potassium levels are depressed. Potassium balance is especially significant in the treatment of conditions requiring insulin administration, such as insulin-dependent diabetes.

The body can adapt to increased levels of potassium intake over time. A sudden increase in potassium may be fatal, but if the intake of potassium is slowly increased by amounts more than 120 mEq/day, the kidney can increase the urinary excretion of potassium and maintain potassium balance. This tolerance to increasing amounts of potassium is known as **potassium adaptation.**

HEALTH ALERT
Potassium and Stroke Risk

Potassium intake has been associated with a reduction in blood pressure and other beneficial vascular effects. When potassium was combined with the use of potassium-losing diuretics in men with hypertension, the incidence of stroke was significantly reduced. Although causal relationships cannot be supported, the study supports theories that potassium supplements may have beneficial vascular effects.

Data from Ascherio, A. et al. (1998). Intake of potassium, magnesium, calcium, and fiber and risk of stroke among U.S. men. Circulation, 98(12), 1198-1204.

Hypokalemia

Pathophysiology

Potassium deficiency, or **hypokalemia,** develops when the serum potassium concentration falls below 3.5 mEq/L. Because cellular and total body stores of potassium are difficult to measure, changes in potassium balance are described, although not always accurately, by the plasma concentration. Generally, lowered serum potassium indicates loss of total body potassium. With potassium loss from the ECF, the concentration gradient change favors movement of K^+ from the cell to the ECF. The ICF/ECF concentration ratio is maintained, but total body K^+ is depleted.

Extracellular fluid hypokalemia can develop without losses of total body potassium. For example, potassium shifts into the cell during respiratory or metabolic alkalosis or after administration of insulin. In alkalosis, K^+ shifts into the cell in exchange for H^+ to maintain plasma acid-base balance. Insulin also promotes cellular uptake of K^+, causing an ECF potassium deficit.

Potassium shifts from the ICF to the ECF in conditions such as diabetic ketoacidosis, in which the increased hydrogen ion concentration in the ECF causes H^+ to shift into the

TABLE 4-8   Clinical Manifestations of Potassium Alterations

Organ System	Hypokalemia	Hyperkalemia
Cardiovascular	Dysrhythmias Electrocardiogram changes Cardiac arrest Weak irregular pulse Postural hypotension	Dysrhythmias Bradycardia Heart block Cardiac arrest
Nervous	Lethargy Fatigue Confusion Paresthesias	Anxiety Tingling Numbness

Gastrointestinal	Nausea and vomiting
	Decreased motility
	  Distention
	  Decreased bowel sounds
	  Ileus
		Nausea and vomiting
		Diarrhea
		Colicky pain

Kidney	Water loss Thirst Inability to concentrate urine Kidney damage	Oliguria Kidney damage
Skeletal muscle	Weakness Flaccid paralysis Respiratory arrest	Early: hyperactive muscles Late: weakness and flaccid paralysis

cell in exchange for potassium. A normal level of potassium is maintained in the plasma, but potassium continues to be lost in the urine, causing a deficit in total body potassium. Severe, even fatal, hypokalemia may occur if insulin is administered without also providing potassium supplements. Thus total body potassium depletion becomes evident when insulin treatment and rehydration therapy are initiated. Potassium replacement is instituted cautiously. Potassium loss also occurs through normal body functions without causing hypokalemia.

Factors contributing to the development of hypokalemia include reduced intake of potassium, increased entry of potassium into cells, and increased losses of body potassium. Dietary deficiency of potassium is a rare cause but may occur in elderly individuals with both low protein intake and inadequate intake of fruits and vegetables and in individuals with alcoholism or anorexia nervosa. Generally, reduced potassium intake becomes a problem when combined with other causes of potassium depletion.

Shifts of potassium from the extracellular to intracellular space cause apparent deficits in total body potassium. Alkalosis, particularly respiratory alkalosis, is the most common clinical problem. Extracellular fluid potassium exchanges with ICF hydrogen and corrects alkalosis by increasing the pH of the ECF. Treatment of pernicious anemia with vitamin B_{12} or folate may also precipitate hypokalemia if new red blood cell formation causes enough potassium uptake to cause an extracellular decrease in potassium.

Losses of potassium from body stores are usually caused by gastrointestinal and renal disorders. Diarrhea, intestinal drainage tubes or fistulae, and laxative abuse also result in hypokalemia. Normally, only 5 to 10 mEq of potassium and 100 to 150 ml of water are excreted in the stool each day. With diarrhea, fluid and electrolyte losses can be voluminous, with several liters of fluid and 100 to 200 mEq of potassium lost per day. Vomiting or continuous nasogastric suctioning frequently is associated with potassium depletion, partly because of the potassium lost from the gastric fluid but principally because of renal compensation for volume depletion and the metabolic alkalosis (elevated bicarbonate levels) that occurs from sodium, chloride, and hydrogen ion losses. The loss of fluid and sodium stimulates the secretion of aldosterone, which in turn causes renal losses of potassium. The elevated flow of bicarbonate at the distal tubule contributes to renal excretion of potassium because of increased tubular lumen electronegativity.

Renal potassium losses occur with increased secretion of potassium by the distal tubule. Use of K^+-wasting diuretics, excessive aldosterone secretion, increased distal tubular flow rate, and low plasma magnesium concentration all may contribute to urinary losses of potassium. Many diuretics inhibit the reabsorption of sodium chloride, causing the diuretic effect. The distal tubular flow rate then increases, promoting potassium secretion. If sodium loss is severe, the compensating aldosterone secretion may further deplete potassium stores. Primary hyperaldosteronism with excessive secretion of aldosterone from an adrenal adenoma also causes potassium wasting. Many kidney diseases result in a reduced ability to conserve sodium. The disordered sodium reabsorption produces a diuretic effect, and the increased distal tubule flow rate favors the secretion of potassium. Magnesium deficits stimulate renin release and hyperaldosteronism, causing hypokalemia. Several antibiotics are known to cause hypokalemia.

Clinical Manifestations

A wide range of metabolic dysfunctions may result from potassium deficiency (Table 4-8). Carbohydrate metabolism is affected because hypokalemia depresses insulin secretion and alters hepatic and skeletal muscle glycogen synthesis. Renal function is impaired, with a decreased ability to concentrate urine. Polyuria (increased urine) and polydipsia (increased thirst) are associated with decreased responsiveness to ADH. Long-term potassium deficits lasting more than 1 month may damage renal tissue, with interstitial fibrosis and tubular atrophy.

Neuromuscular and cardiac effects of hypokalemia produce the most common symptoms. Neuromuscular excitability is decreased, causing skeletal muscle weakness, smooth muscle atony, and cardiac dysrhythmias.

Symptoms occur in relation to the rate of potassium depletion. Because the body can accommodate slow losses of potassium, the decrease in ECF concentration may allow potassium to shift from the intracellular space, restoring the potassium concentration gradient toward normal, with less severe neuromuscular changes. With acute losses of potassium, changes in neuromuscular excitability are more profound. Skeletal muscle weakness occurs initially in the larger muscles of the legs and arms and ultimately affects the diaphragm and depresses ventilation. Paralysis and respiratory arrest can occur. Loss of smooth muscle tone is manifested by constipation, intestinal distention, anorexia, nausea, vomiting, and paralytic ileus.

The cardiac effects of hypokalemia are related also to changes in membrane excitability. Because potassium contributes to the repolarization phase of the action potential, hypokalemia delays ventricular repolarization. Various dysrhythmias may occur, including sinus bradycardia, atrioventricular block, and paroxysmal atrial tachycardia. The characteristic changes in the electrocardiogram reflect delayed repolarization. For instance, the amplitude of the T wave is decreased, the amplitude of the U wave is increased, and the ST segment is depressed (Fig. 4-7). In severe states of hypokalemia, P waves peak and the QRS complex is prolonged. Hypokalemia also increases the risk of digitalis toxicity.

Hyperkalemia

Pathophysiology

Elevation of ECF potassium *above 5.5 mEq/L* constitutes **hyperkalemia.** Because of efficient renal excretion, increases in total body potassium are relatively rare. Acute increases in serum potassium are handled quickly through increased cel-

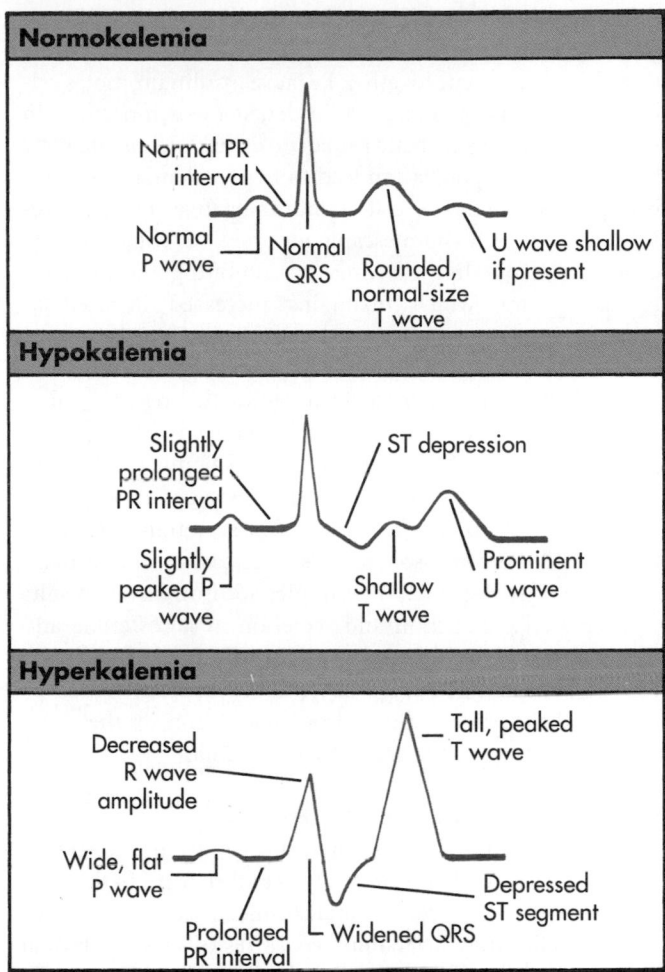

Fig. 4-7 *Electrocardiogram changes with potassium imbalance.*

lular uptake and renal excretion of body potassium excesses. Excretion is partially mediated by the secretion of aldosterone, because it facilitates losses of potassium in the urine.

Potassium excesses may be caused by increased intake, a shift of potassium from cells to the ECF, or decreased renal excretion. If renal function is normal, slow, long-term increases in potassium intake are usually well tolerated through potassium adaptation, although short-term potassium loading can exceed renal excretion rates. Use of stored whole blood and intravenous boluses of penicillin G or replacement potassium can precipitate hyperkalemia, particularly with impaired renal function. Dietary excesses of potassium are uncommon, but accidental ingestion of potassium salt substitutes can cause toxicity.

Potassium moves from the ICF to the ECF with cell trauma or a change in cell membrane permeability, acidosis, insulin deficiency, or cell hypoxia. Burns, massive crushing injuries, and extensive surgeries can cause loss of potassium to the ECF. If renal function is sustained, potassium is excreted. As cell repair begins, hypokalemia develops without an adequate intake of potassium.

In acidosis, hydrogen ions shift into the cells in exchange for ICF potassium and sodium; hyperkalemia and acidosis therefore often occur together. Because insulin promotes cellular entry of potassium, insulin deficits, which occur with such conditions as diabetic ketoacidosis, are accompanied by hyperkalemia. Hypoxia can lead to hyperkalemia by diminishing the efficiency of cell membrane active transport, resulting in the potassium escaping to the ECF. Digitalis overdose may cause hyperkalemia by inhibiting the Na^+, K^+ ATPase pump, which maintains increased intracellular potassium and extracellular sodium (see Chapter 1).

Decreased renal excretion of potassium commonly is associated with hyperkalemia. Renal failure that results in oliguria (urine output 30 ml/hr) is accompanied by elevations of serum potassium. The severity of hyperkalemia is related to the amount of potassium intake, the degree of acidosis, and the rate of cell damage. Decreases in the secretion or renal effects of aldosterone also can cause decreases in the urinary excretion of potassium. For example, Addison disease results in decreased production and secretion of aldosterone and thus contributes to hyperkalemia. Potassium-sparing diuretics (e.g., spironolactone, which inhibits sodium reabsorption) and potassium and hydrogen secretion by the distal tubule also may contribute to hyperkalemia.

🔳 *Clinical Manifestations*

Symptoms of hyperkalemia vary, but common characteristics are muscle weakness or paralysis and changes in the electrocardiogram. During mild attacks, increased neuromuscular irritability may be manifested as restlessness, intestinal cramping, and diarrhea. Severe hyperkalemia causes muscle weakness, loss of muscle tone, and paralysis. In mild states of hyperkalemia, the more rapid repolarization is reflected in the electrocardiogram as narrow and taller T waves with a shortened QT interval. Severe hyperkalemia depresses the ST segment, prolongs the PR interval, and widens the QRS complex (see Fig. 4-7). Bradydysrhythmias are common in hyperkalemia, with alterations in cardiac conduction causing ventricular fibrillation or cardiac arrest.

As with hypokalemia, changes in the ratio of intracellular to extracellular potassium concentration contribute to the symptoms of hyperkalemia (see Table 4-8). The neuromuscular effects of hyperkalemia are related to the increase in rate of repolarization and the presence of other contributing factors, such as acidosis and calcium balance. Long-term increases in ECF potassium concentration result in shifts of potassium into the cell, because the tendency is to maintain a normal ratio of ICF to ECF potassium concentrations. Acute elevations of extracellular potassium affect neuromuscular irritability as this ratio is disrupted.

Increases in extracellular fluid calcium concentration can override the effects of hyperkalemia.

Other Electrolytes

The specifics of balance for the other body electrolytes—calcium, phosphate, magnesium—are summarized in Table 4-9.

✓ QUICK CHECK

What role does potassium play in the body? What metabolic dysfunctions occur in potassium deficiency? In potassium excess?

What other body electrolytes must be in balance for proper functioning? Briefly summarize the effects of excess and deficiency of each.

ACID-BASE BALANCE

Hydrogen ion concentration must be regulated within a narrow range for the body to function normally. Slight changes in amounts of hydrogen can significantly alter biologic processes in cells and tissues. Hydrogen ion is needed to maintain membrane integrity and the speed of enzyme reactions. Most pathologic conditions disturb acid-base balance, producing conditions possibly more harmful than the disease process itself.

Hydrogen Ion and pH

The concentration of hydrogen ion $[H^+]$ in body fluids is very small—approximately 0.0000001 mg/L. This number may be expressed as 10^{-7}, and, for convenience, the concentration of 10^{-7} is indicated as pH 7.0. The symbol pH represents the power of hydrogen. As the pH changes one unit (e.g., 7.0 to 6.0), the $[H^+]$ changes tenfold. The greater the $[H^+]$, the more acidic the solution and the lower the pH. The lower the $[H^+]$, the more basic the solution and the higher the pH. In biologic fluids, a pH of less than 7.4 is defined as acidic and a pH greater than 7.4 is defined as basic or alkaline (Table 4-10).

Body acids are formed as end-products of the metabolism of protein, carbohydrates, and fats. This must be balanced by the amount of basic substances in the body. The lungs, kidneys, and bones are the major organs involved in regulating acid-base balance. The systems work together to regulate short- and long-term changes in acid-base status.

Body acids exist in two forms: *volatile* (can be eliminated as CO_2 gas) and *nonvolatile.* The volatile acid is carbonic acid (H_2CO_3), a weak acid (does not release its hydrogen easily). With carbonic anhydrase, it readily dissociates into carbon dioxide (CO) and water (H_2O). The carbon dioxide is then eliminated by pulmonary ventilation.

Sulfuric, phosphoric, and other organic acids are nonvolatile strong acids (readily give up their hydrogen). Nonvolatile acids are eliminated by the renal tubules in amounts of about 150 mEq of hydrogen per day.

Buffer Systems

Buffering occurs in response to changes in acid-base status. *Buffers* can absorb excessive H^+ (acid) or OH^- (base) and prevent a significant change in pH. The buffer systems are located in both the ICF and ECF compartments, and they function at different rates (Table 4-11). The most important plasma buffer systems are carbonic acid-bicarbonate and he-

TABLE 4-9	Alterations in Other Body Electrolytes		
Parameter	**Calcium**	**Phosphate**	**Magnesium**
Normal values	Serum: (total) 9.0-10.5 mg/dl, (ionized) 4.5-5.6 mg/dl; 99% in bone as hydroxyapatite; the rest in plasma and body cells with 50% bound to plasma proteins, 40% free or ionized; ionized form most important physiologically	Serum: 2.5-4.5 mg/dl, but may be as high as 6.0-7.0 mg/dl in infants and young children; mainly in bone with some in ICF and ECF; exists as phospholipids, phosphate esters, and inorganic phosphate (ionized form)	Serum: 1.8-2.4 mEq/L; 40%-60% stored in muscle and bone, one third bound to plasma proteins
Function	Needed for fundamental metabolic processes; major cation for structure of bone and teeth; enzymatic cofactor for blood clotting; required for hormone secretion and the function of cell receptors; directly related to plasma membrane stability and permeability, as well as transmission of nerve impulses and contraction of muscles	Intracellular and extracellular anion buffer in regulation of acid-base balance; provides energy for muscle contraction (as ATP)	A cofactor in intracellular enzymatic reactions and causes neuromuscular excitability; often interacts with calcium and potassium in reactions at cellular level and has an important role in smooth muscle contraction and relaxation
Excess	Hypercalcemia (serum concentrations >1 mg/dl)	Hyperphosphatemia (serum concentrations >6.0 mg/dl)	Hypermagnesemia (serum concentrations >3.0 mEq/dl)
Causes	Hyperparathyroidism; bone metastases with calcium resorption from breast, prostate, and cervical cancer; sarcoidosis; excess vitamin D; many tumors that produce PTH	Acute or chronic renal failure with significant loss of glomerular filtration; treatment of metastatic tumors with chemotherapy that releases large amounts of phosphate into serum; long-term use of laxatives or enemas containing phosphates; hypoparathyroidism	Usually renal failure; also excessive intake of magnesium-containing antacids, adrenal insufficiency
Effects	Many nonspecific; fatigue, weakness, lethargy, anorexia, nausea, constipation; impaired renal function, kidney stones; dysrhythmias, bradycardia, cardiac arrest; bone pain, osteoporosis	Symptoms primarily related to low serum calcium levels, similar to the results of hypocalcemia; when prolonged, calcification of soft tissues in lungs, kidneys, joints	Skeletal smooth muscle contraction; excess nerve function; loss of deep tendon reflexes; nausea and vomiting; muscle weakness; hypotension; bradycardia; respiratory distress.
Deficit	Hypocalcemia (serum calcium concentration <8.5 mg/dl)	Hypophosphatemia (serum phosphate concentration <2.0 mg/dl)	Hypomagnesemia (serum magnesium concentration <1.5 mEq/L)
Causes	Related to inadequate intestinal absorption, deposition of ionized calcium into bone or soft tissue, blood administration, or decreases in PTH and vitamin D; nutritional deficiencies occur with inadequate sources of dairy products or green leafy vegetables	Most commonly by intestinal malabsorption related to vitamin D deficiency, use of magnesium- and aluminum-containing antacids, long-term alcohol abuse, and malabsorption syndromes; respiratory alkalosis; increased renal excretion of phosphate associated with hyperparathyroidism	Malnutrition, malabsorption syndromes, alcoholism, renal tubular dysfunction, loop diuretics

PTH, *Parathyroid hormone.*

Continued

TABLE 4-9   Alterations in Other Body Electrolytes—cont'd

Parameter	Calcium	Phosphate	Magnesium
Effects	Increased neuromuscular excitability; tingling, muscle spasm; Chvostek sign, Trousseau sign; severe cases show convulsions and tetany; prolonged QT interval, cardiac arrest; intestinal cramping, hyperactive bowel sounds	Conditions related to reduced capacity for oxygen transport by red blood cells and disturbed energy metabolism; leukocyte and platelet dysfunction; deranged nerve and muscle function; in severe cases, irritability, confusion, numbness, coma, convulsions; possibly respiratory failure (because muscle weakness), cardiomyopathies, bone resorption (leading to rickets or osteomalacia)	Behavioral changes, irritability, increased reflexes, muscle cramps, ataxia, nystagmus, tetany, convulsions, tachycardia, hypotension

TABLE 4-10   pH of Body Fluids

Body Fluid	pH	Factors Affecting pH
Gastric juices	1.0-3.0	Hydrochloric acid production
Urine	5.0-6.0	H^+ ion excretion from waste products
Arterial blood	7.38-7.42	pH is slightly higher because there is less carbonic acid (H_2CO_3)
Venous blood	7.37	pH is slightly lower because there is more carbonic acid
Cerebrospinal fluid	7.32	Decreased bicarbonate and higher carbon dioxide content decreases pH
Pancreatic fluid	7.8-8.0	Contains bicarbonate produced by exocrine cells

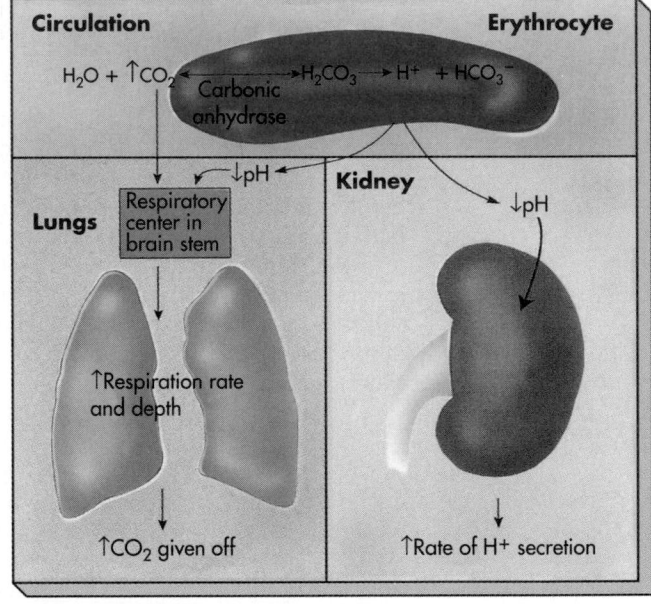

Fig. 4-8 *Integration of pH control mechanisms.* Elevated CO_2 levels result in increased formation of carbonic acid in red blood cells. The resulting increase in hydrogen ions, coupled with elevated CO_2 levels, results in an increase in respiratory rate and secretion of hydrogen ions by the kidneys, thus helping to regulate the pH of body fluids. *(From Thibodeau, G.A. & Patton, K.T. [1999]. Anatomy & physiology [4th ed.]. St. Louis: Mosby.)*

moglobin (Fig. 4-8). Phosphate and protein are the most important intracellular buffers.

Carbonic acid–bicarbonate buffering

The carbonic acid–bicarbonate buffer pair operates in both the lung and the kidney. The lungs can decrease the amount of carbonic acid by blowing off CO_2 and leaving water. The kidneys can reabsorb bicarbonate or regenerate new bicarbonate from CO_2 and water. The relationship between bicarbonate and carbonic acid is usually expressed as a ratio. Normal bicarbonate level is about 24 mEq/L, and normal carbonic acid level is about 1.2 mEq/L, producing a 20:1 ratio and the normal pH of 7.4. These two systems are very effective together because acid concentration can be adjusted rapidly by the lungs and bicarbonate is easily reabsorbed or regenerated by the kidneys.

This type of adjustment in pH is known as *compensation.* The respiratory system compensates for changes in pH by increasing or decreasing ventilation. The renal system compensates by producing more acidic or more alkaline urine. *Correction* occurs when the values for both components of the buffer pair return to normal.

Protein buffering

Both intracellular and extracellular proteins have negative charges and can serve as buffers for H^+, but because most

TABLE 4-11	Buffer Systems		
Buffer Pairs	**Buffer System**	**Reaction**	**Rate**
HCO_3^-/H_2CO_3	Bicarbonate	$H^+ + HCO_3^- \rightleftarrows H_2O + CO_2$	Instantaneous
Hb^-/HHb	Hemoglobin	$HHb \rightleftharpoons H^+ + Hb^-$	Instantaneous
HPO_4^-/H_2PO_4	Phosphate	$H_2PO_4 + H^+ + HPO_4^-$	Instantaneous
Pr^-/HPr	Plasma proteins	$HPr \rightleftharpoons H^+ + Pr^-$	Instantaneous
Organs	**Mechanism**		**Rate**
Lungs	Regulates retention or elimination of CO_2 and therefore H_2CO_3 concentration		Minutes-hours
Ionic shifts	Exchange of intracellular potassium and sodium for hydrogen		2-4 hours
Kidneys	Bicarbonate reabsorption and regneration, ammonia formation, phosphate buffering		Hours-days
Bone	Exchanges of calcium and phosphate and release of carbonate		Hours-days

proteins are inside cells, they are primarily an intracellular blood buffer system. Hemoglobin (Hb) is an excellent intracellular buffer because it can bind with H^+ (forming HHb) and carbon dioxide ($HHbCO_2$). Hemoglobin bound to H^+ becomes a weak acid. Unsaturated hemoglobin (venous blood) is a better buffer than hemoglobin saturated with oxygen (arterial blood). The hemoglobin buffer system is illustrated in Fig. 4-8.

Renal buffering

The distal tubule of the kidney regulates acid-base balance by secreting hydrogen into the urine and reabsorbing bicarbonate. Dibasic phosphate (HPO_4^-) and ammonia (NH_3) are two important renal buffers. The renal buffering of hydrogen ions requires the use of CO_2 and H_2O to form H_2CO_3. The enzyme carbonic anhydrase catalyzes the reaction. The hydrogen is then secreted from the tubular cell and buffered in the lumen by phosphate and ammonia. The bicarbonate is reabsorbed. The end effect is the addition of new bicarbonate, which contributes to the alkalinity of the plasma because the hydrogen ion is excreted from the body.

Acid-Base Imbalances

Pathophysiologic changes in the concentration of hydrogen ion in the blood lead to acid-base imbalances.[7] In *acidemia* the pH of arterial blood is less than 7.4. A systemic increase in hydrogen ion concentration is termed *acidosis*. In *alkalemia* the pH of arterial blood is greater than 7.4. A systemic decrease in hydrogen ion concentration is termed *alkalosis.* These changes may be caused by metabolic or respiratory processes. Fig. 4-9 summarizes the relationship among pH, PCO_2, and bicarbonate during different acid-base states.

Metabolic acidosis

In *metabolic acidosis* noncarbonic acids increase or bicarbonate is lost from extracellular fluid (Table 4-12). This can occur either quickly (e.g., in lactic acidosis caused by poor oxygenation) or over an extended period (e.g., in renal failure or diabetic ketoacidosis).[6]

The buffering systems normally compensate for excess acid and maintain arterial pH within normal range. When

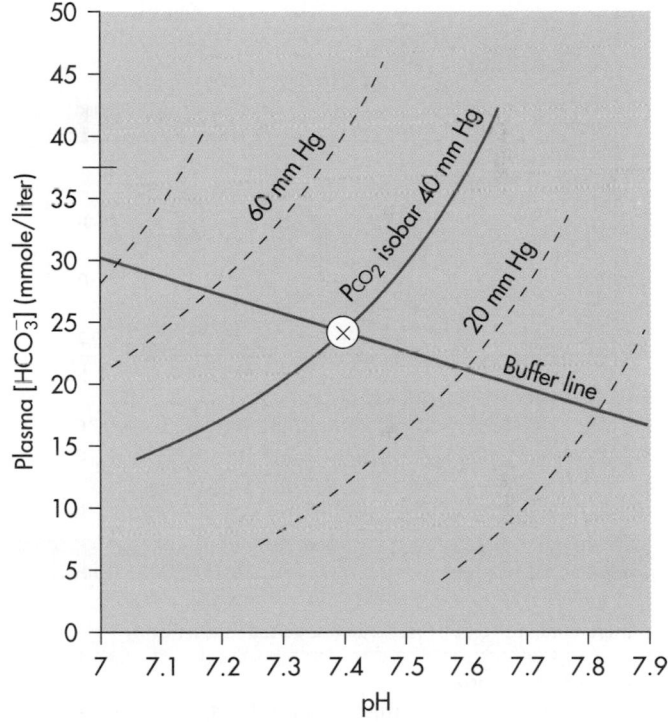

Fig. 4-9 *Davenport diagram: classic working diagram for studying acid-base imbalance. (Redrawn from Groer, M.W. [1981]. Physiology and pathophysiology of body fluids. St. Louis: Mosby.)*

acidosis is severe, buffers cannot compensate and the ratio of bicarbonate to carbonic acid decreases to less than 20:1 (Fig. 4-10). The specific type of acidosis can be determined by examining the anion gap (Box 4-1).

Metabolic acidosis is manifested by changes in the neurologic, respiratory, gastrointestinal, and cardiovascular systems. Early symptoms include headache and lethargy, which progress to coma in severe acidosis. The respiratory system's efforts to compensate result in Kussmaul respirations, which are deep and rapid. This represents the body's attempt to increase pH by blowing off CO_2, which decreases carbonic acid. Other symptoms include anorexia, nausea, vomiting, diarrhea, and abdominal discomfort. Death can result.

Fig. 4-10 *Metabolic acidosis. (Modified from Thibodeau, G.A. & Patton, K.T. [1993]. Anatomy and physiology [2nd ed.]. St. Louis: Mosby.)*

Fig. 4-11 *Metabolic alkalosis. (Modified from Thibodeau, G.A. & Patton, K.T. [1993]. Anatomy and physiology [2nd ed.]. St. Louis: Mosby.)*

TABLE 4-12	Causes of Metabolic Acidosis	
Increased Noncarbonic Acids (Elevated Anion Gap)		**Bicarbonate Loss (Normal Anion Gap)**
Increased H^+ load		Diarrhea
Ketoacidosis (e.g., diabetes mellitus, starvation)		Ureterosigmoidoscopy
Lactic acidosis (e.g., shock)		Renal failure
Ingestion (e.g., ammonium chloride, ethylene glycol, methanol, salicylates, paraldehyde)		Proximal renal tubule acidosis
Decreased H^+ excretion		
Uremia		
Distal renal tubule acidosis		

Metabolic alkalosis

When excessive loss of metabolic acids occurs, bicarbonate increases, causing *metabolic alkalosis.* When acid loss is caused by vomiting, renal compensation is not very effective because loss of chloride in HCl acid stimulates renal retention of bicarbonate. Hyperaldosteronism can also lead to alkalosis as a result of sodium bicarbonate retention and loss of hydrogen and potassium. Diuretics may produce a mild alkalosis because they promote greater excretion of sodium, potassium, and chloride than of bicarbonate (Fig. 4-11).

Some common signs and symptoms are weakness; muscle cramps; hyperactive reflexes; tetany; shallow, slow respirations; confusion; convulsions; and atrial tachycardia. The manifestations vary with the cause of the alkalosis.

Respiratory acidosis

A decrease in alveolar ventilation in relation to the metabolic production of carbon dioxide produces *respiratory acidosis* by an increase in carbonic acid. This occurs with depression of ventilation, resulting in an excess of carbon dioxide (hyper-

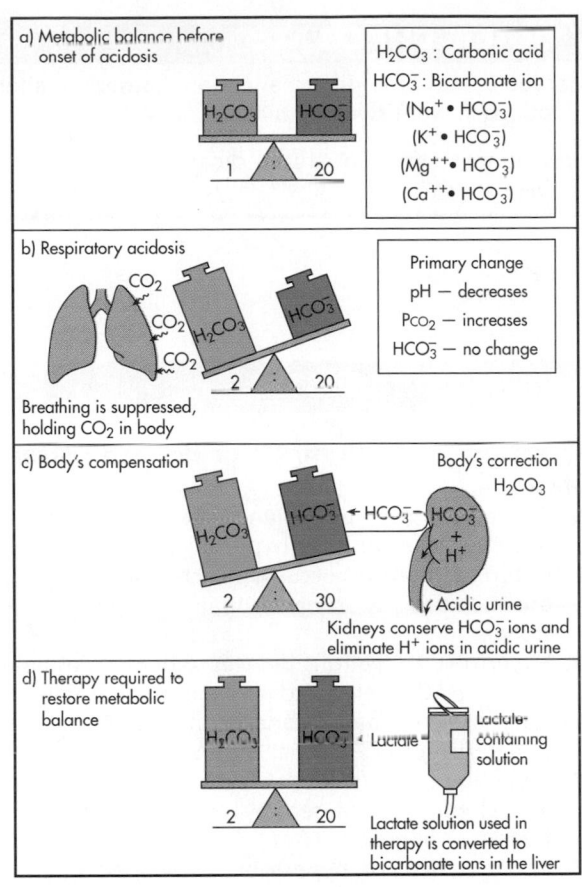

Fig. 4-12 *Respiratory acidosis. (Modified from Thibodeau, G.A. & Patton, K.T. [1993]. Anatomy and physiology [2nd ed.]. St. Louis: Mosby.)*

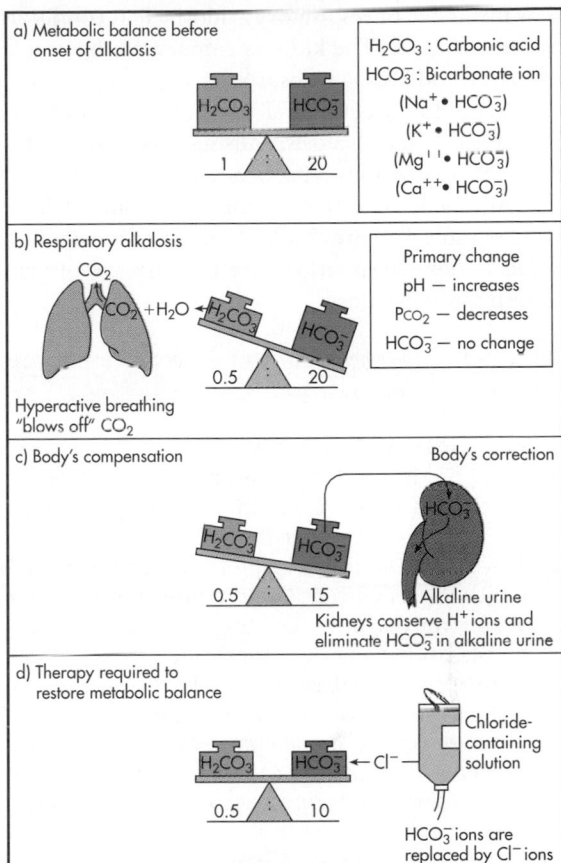

Fig. 4-13 *Respiratory alkalosis. (Modified from Thibodeau, G.A. & Patton, K.T. [1993]. Anatomy and physiology [2nd ed.]. St. Louis: Mosby.)*

capnia). Common causes include depression of the respiratory center, respiratory muscle paralysis, disorders of the chest wall (kyphoscoliosis, pickwickian syndrome, flail chest), and disorders of the lung parenchyma (pneumonia, pulmonary edema, emphysema, asthma, bronchitis). Respiratory acidosis can be acute or chronic. Renal compensation occurs by elimination of H^+ and retention of HCO_3^- (Fig. 4-12).

The signs and symptoms seen include restlessness and apprehension followed by lethargy, muscle twitching, tremors, convulsions, and coma. Respiratory rate is rapid at first and gradually becomes depressed as the respiratory center adapts to increasing levels of CO_2.

Respiratory alkalosis

Respiratory alkalosis occurs when there is alveolar hyperventilation and excessive reduction in carbon dioxide levels (hypocapnia). Hypoxemia (caused by pulmonary disease, congestive heart failure, or high altitudes), hypermetabolic states (fever, anemia, thyrotoxicosis), early salicylate intoxication, hysteria, cirrhosis, and gram-negative sepsis stimulate hyperventilation. Improper use of mechanical ventilators also can cause iatrogenic respiratory alkalosis, and secondary alkalosis may develop as a result of hyperventilation stimu-

Anion Gap   BOX 4-1

The evaluation of the anion gap can be useful for distinguishing different types of metabolic acidosis. Normally the concentrations of cations and anions in the plasma are equivalent. Some anions, such as protein, sulfates, phosphates, and organic acids, however, are not measured in the common laboratory evaluations of the blood. Therefore the normal anion gap represents the difference between the sum of Na^+ and K^+ and the sum of HCO_3 and Cl^-, or about 10 to 12 mEq.

In metabolic acidosis a normal anion gap is characteristic of conditions related to bicarbonate loss with retention of chloride to maintain an ionic balance. This is called *hyperchloremic metabolic acidosis.* An elevated anion gap is characteristic of acidosis associated with accumulation of anions other than chloride (e.g., lactate, ketoacids) (see Table 4-12).

lated by metabolic or respiratory acidosis. This condition can be chronic or acute. The kidneys compensate by decreasing H^+ excretion and HCO_3^- reabsorption (Fig. 4-13).

The central and peripheral nervous systems are stimulated by respiratory alkalosis, causing dizziness, confusion, tingling of extremities (paresthesias), convulsions, and coma. Carpopedal spasm and other symptoms of hypocalcemia (see Table 4-9) are similar to those of metabolic alkalosis. Deep, rapid respirations are primary symptoms that cause respiratory alkalosis.

✓ QUICK CHECK

Metabolic acid-base disturbances are caused by alterations in what two chemicals?

How do alterations in carbon dioxide influence acid-base states?

▣ DID YOU UNDERSTAND?

Distribution of Body Fluids

1. Body fluids are distributed among functional compartments and are classified as intracellular fluid (ICF) and extracellular fluid (ECF).
2. The sum of all fluids is the total body water (TBW), which varies with age and amount of body fat.
3. Water moves between the ICF and ECF compartments principally by osmosis.
4. Water moves between the plasma and interstitial fluid by osmosis and hydrostatic pressure, which occur across the capillary membrane.
5. Movement across the capillary wall is called *net filtration* and is described according to Starling's law.

Alterations in Water Movement

1. Edema is a problem of fluid distribution that results in accumulation of fluid within the interstitial spaces.
2. The pathophysiologic process that leads to edema is related to an increase in forces favoring fluid filtration from the capillaries or lymphatic channels into the tissues.
3. Edema is caused by arterial dilation, venous or lymphatic obstruction, and increased vascular volume.
4. Edema may be localized or generalized and usually is associated with weight gain, swelling and puffiness, tighter-fitting clothes and shoes, and limited movement of the affected area.

Sodium, Chloride, and Water Balance

1. Sodium and water balance are intimately related; chloride levels are generally proportional to change in sodium levels.
2. Water balance is regulated by the sensation of thirst and by antidiuretic hormone, which is initiated by an increase in plasma osmolality or a decrease in circulating blood volume.
3. Sodium balance is regulated by aldosterone, which increases reabsorption of sodium by the distal tubule of the kidney.
4. Renin and angiotensin are enzymes that promote or inhibit secretion of aldosterone and thus regulate sodium and water balance.
5. Atrial natriuretic hormone also is involved in decreasing tubular resorption and promoting urinary excretion of sodium.

Alterations in Sodium, Chloride, and Water Balance

1. Alterations in water balance may be classified as isotonic, hypertonic, or hypotonic.
2. Isotonic alterations occur when changes in TBW are accompanied by proportional changes in electrolytes.
3. Hypertonic alterations develop when the osmolality of the ECF is elevated above normal, usually because of an increased concentration of ECF sodium or a deficit of ECF water.
4. Hypernatremia (sodium levels more than 147 mEq/L) may be caused by an acute increase in sodium or a loss of water.
5. Water deficit, or hypertonic dehydration, is rare but can be caused by lack of access to water, pure water losses, hyperventilation, arid climates, and increased renal clearance.
6. Hyperchloremia is caused by an excess of sodium or a deficit of bicarbonate.
7. Hypotonic alterations occur when the osmolality of the ECF is less than normal.
8. Hyponatremia (serum sodium concentration less than 135 mEq/L) usually causes movement of water into cells.
9. Hyponatremia may be caused by sodium loss, inadequate sodium intake, or dilution of the body's sodium level.
10. Water excess is rare but can be caused by compulsive water drinking, decreased urine formation, or the syndrome of inappropriate secretion of ADH.
11. Hypochloremia usually is the result of hyponatremia or elevated bicarbonate concentrations.

Alterations in Potassium and Other Electrolytes

1. Potassium is the predominant ICF ion; it functions to regulate ICF osmolality, maintain the resting membrane potential, and deposit glycogen in liver and skeletal muscle cells.
2. Potassium balance is regulated by the kidney, by aldosterone and insulin secretion, and by changes in pH.
3. A mechanism known as potassium adaptation allows the body to accommodate slowly to increased levels of potassium intake.

■ DID YOU UNDERSTAND? —cont'd

4. Hypokalemia (serum potassium concentration less than 3.5 mEq/L) indicates loss of total body potassium, although ECF hypokalemia can develop without losses of total body potassium and plasma K^+ levels may be normal or elevated when total body potassium is depleted.

5. Hypokalemia may be caused by reduced potassium intake, increased ICF/ECF potassium concentration, loss of potassium from body stores, increased aldosterone, and increased renal excretion.

6. Hyperkalemia (potassium levels that are more than 5.5 mEq/L) may be caused by increased potassium intake, a shift from ICF to ECF potassium, or decreased renal excretion.

7. Calcium is a necessary ion in the structure of bones and teeth, in blood clotting, in hormone secretion and the function of cell receptors, and in membrane stability.

8. Phosphate acts as a buffer in acid-base regulation and provides energy for muscle contraction.

9. Calcium and phosphate concentrations are rigidly controlled by parathyroid hormone (PTH), vitamin D, and calcitonin.

10. Hypocalcemia (serum calcium concentration less than 8.5 mg/dl) is related to inadequate intestinal absorption, deposition of calcium into bone or soft tissue, blood administration, or decreased PTH and vitamin D levels.

11. Hypercalcemia (serum calcium concentration more than 12 mg/dl) can be caused by a number of diseases, including hyperparathyroidism, bone metastases, sarcoidosis, and excess vitamin D.

12. Hypophosphatemia is usually caused by intestinal malabsorption and increased renal excretion of phosphate.

13. Hyperphosphatemia develops with acute or chronic renal failure with significant loss of glomerular filtration.

14. Magnesium is a major intracellular cation and is regulated principally by PTH.

15. Magnesium functions in enzymatic reactions and often interacts with calcium at the cellular level.

16. Hypomagnesemia (serum magnesium concentrations less than 1.5 mEq/L) may be caused by malabsorption syndromes.

17. Hypermagnesemia (serum magnesium concentrations more than 2.5 mEq/L) is rare and usually is caused by renal failure.

Acid-Base Balance

1. Hydrogen ions, which maintain membrane integrity and the speed of enzymatic reactions, must be concentrated within a narrow range if the body is to function normally.

2. Hydrogen ion concentration is expressed as pH, which represents the negative logarithm of hydrogen ions in solution.

3. Different body fluids have different pH values.

4. The renal and respiratory systems, together with the body's buffer systems, are the principal regulators of acid-base balance.

5. Buffers are substances that can absorb excessive acid or base without a significant change in pH.

6. Buffers exist as acid-base pairs; the principal plasma buffers are carbonic acid–bicarbonate, protein (hemoglobin), and phosphate.

7. The lungs and kidneys act to compensate for changes in pH by increasing or decreasing ventilation and by producing more acidic or more alkaline urine.

8. Correction is a process different from compensation; correction occurs when the values for both components of the buffer pair return to normal.

9. Acid-base imbalances are caused by changes in the concentration of H^+ in the blood; an increase causes acidosis, and a decrease causes alkalosis.

10. An abnormal increase or decrease in bicarbonate concentration causes metabolic acidosis or metabolic alkalosis; changes in the rate of alveolar ventilation of carbon dioxide produce respiratory acidosis or respiratory alkalosis.

11. Metabolic acidosis is caused by an increase in noncarbonic acids or loss of bicarbonate from the extracellular fluid.

12. Metabolic alkalosis occurs with an increase in bicarbonate usually caused by loss of metabolic acids from conditions such as vomiting, gastrointestinal suctioning, excessive bicarbonate intake, hyperaldosteronism, and diuretic therapy.

13. Respiratory acidosis occurs with a decrease of alveolar ventilation and an increase in levels of carbon dioxide, which in turn causes hypercapnia.

14. Respiratory alkalosis occurs with alveolar hyperventilation and excessive reduction of carbon dioxide, or hypocapnia.

KEY TERMS

Acidemia, 119
Acidosis, 119
Aldosterone, 108
Alkalemia, 119
Alkalosis, 119
Angiotensin I and II, 108
Baroreceptor, 108
Buffering, 116
Buffer, 116
Chloride, 108
Compensation, 118
Compulsive water drinking, 112
Correction, 118
Decreased urine formation, 112
Dehydration, 111
Dilutional hyponatremia, 112
Edema, 105
Extracellular fluid (ECF), 104

Hyperchloremia, 112
Hyperkalemia, 115
Hypernatremia, 110
Hypertonic hyponatremia, 112
Hypochloremia, 112
Hypokalemia, 113
Hyponatremia, 112
Hypoosmolar hyponatremia, 112
Hypovolemia, 112
Inadequate intake, 112
Interstitial fluid, 104
Intracellular fluid (ICF), 104
Intravascular fluid, 104
Isotonic fluid excess, 109
Isotonic fluid loss, 109
Metabolic acidosis, 119
Metabolic alkalosis, 120
Natriuretic hormone, 108

Net filtration, 105
Nonvolatile, 116
Osmoreceptor, 107
Potassium adaptation, 113
Pure sodium deficit, 112
Renin, 108
Renin-angiotensin system, 108
Respiratory acidosis, 120
Respiratory alkalosis, 121
Sodium, 108
Starling's hypothesis, 105
Syndrome of inappropriate secretion of ADH (SIADH), 112
Total body water (TBW), 104
Volatile, 116
Volume-sensitive receptor, 108
Water deficit, 111

REFERENCES

1. Rose, D.B. (1994). *Clinical physiology of acid-base and electrolyte disorders.* New York: McGraw-Hill.
2. Schafer, J.A. (1994). 1993 Homer W. Smith Award. Salt and water homeostasis: Is it just a matter of good housekeeping? *Journal of the American Society of Nephrology, 4*(12), 1929-1950.
3. Kumar, S. & Berl, T. (1998). Sodium. *Lancet, 352*(9123), 220-228.
4. Lee, C.A.B., Barrett, C.A., & Ignatavicius, D. (1996). *Fluids and electrolytes: A practical approach* (4th ed.). Philadelphia: Davis.
5. Kokko, P. & Tannen, R.L. (Eds.). (1996). *Fluids and electrolytes.* Philadelphia: Saunders.
6. Preston, R.A. (1997). *Acid-base, fluid, and electrolytes made ridiculously simple.* Miami: MedMaster Inc.
7. Williams, A.J. (1998). ABC of oxygen: Assessing and interpreting arterial blood gases and acid-base balance. *BMJ, 317*(7167), 1213-1216.

CHAPTER

5

Immunity

Neal S. Rote

The body's first lines of defense are anatomic barriers: the skin and mucous membranes lining the respiratory, gastrointestinal, and genitourinary tracts. These surfaces are biochemical barriers as well. Sebaceous glands in the skin secrete antibacterial and antifungal fatty acids and lactic acid. Perspiration, tears, and saliva contain an enzyme (lysozyme) that attacks the cell walls of grampositive bacteria. As a result of these glandular secretions, the surface of the skin is acidic (pH 3 to 5), making it inhospitable to most bacteria.

If an injurious chemical, foreign body, or microorganism penetrates these defenses, the body attempts to eliminate it by mechanical clearance. It may be sloughed off with skin, caught in respiratory mucus and coughed up, vomited from the stomach, or flushed from the urinary tract by urine. Auxiliary defenses are present in the form of the body's normal population of bacteria, or flora, which produce chemicals that inhibit the growth of some invading bacteria. All these defenses are both external and nonspecific; that is, they protect the host as needed against any and all invaders.

Once external barriers have been compromised, permitting harmful chemicals, foreign bodies, or microorganisms to penetrate cells and tissues, the **inflammatory response,** or **inflammation,** occurs. This response, which begins within seconds of injury or invasion, is also nonspecific. It begins with the immediate marshaling of resources by vascular structures at the site of invasion. The affected tissues are soon surrounded by cells and fluids that are equipped to isolate, destroy, and remove the invaders and thereby to promote healing.

The third and last line of defense is the **immune response,** or **immunity.** It occurs much more slowly than the inflammatory response and is specific in that it can confer permanent or long-term protection against specific microorganisms. It can also be induced by vaccination or inoculation. Unlike inflammation, which involves many different plasma systems and cell types,

immunity is effected by one type of serum protein (immunoglobulin, or **antibody**) and one type of blood cell (lymphocyte). The many defenses against microorganisms are summarized in Table 5-1.

CHAPTER OUTLINE

HEALTH ALERT
Nutrition and Immune Function

Nutrition is a critical determinant of immune responses and malnutrition the most common cause of immuno-deficiency worldwide. Protein-energy malnutrition is associated with a significant impairment of cell-mediated immunity, phagocyte function, complement system, secretory immunoglobulin A antibody concentrations, and cytokine production. Deficiency of single nutrients also results in altered immunity—even when the deficiency state is relatively mild. Of the micronutrients, zinc; selenium; iron; copper; vitamins A, C, E, and B-6; and folic acid have significant influences on immune responses. Overnutrition and obesity reduce immunity. Low-birth-weight infants have a prolonged impairment of cell-mediated immunity that can be partly restored by providing extra amounts of dietary zinc. In the elderly, impaired immunity can be increased by modest amounts of a combination of micronutrients.

Data from Chandra, R.K. (1997). Nutrition and the immune system: An introduction. American Journal of Clinical Nutrition, 66(2), 460S-463S.

TABLE 5-1	Defenses Against Infection
Type of Defense	**Specific Mechanism**
Surface defenses	Physical barriers: skin, conjunctivae, mucous membranes
	Mechanical removal: desquamation of skin, tears, mucus, ciliary action, coughing, salivation, swallowing, urination, defecation
	Normal bacterial flora: antibacterial factors
	Chemical inhibitors: gastric acid, lactic acid, fatty acids, spermine, lactoperoxidase, bile salts
	Antimicrobial substances: lysozyme, secretory IgA
Nonspecific resistance factors	Fever, interferons, complement, lysozyme, C-reactive protein (reacts with bacterial surface polysaccharides and activates complement), lactoferrin (binds and removes iron as a bacterial nutrient), α_1-antitrypsin (inhibits bacterial enzymes)
Inflammation	Soluble factors
	Clotting system: Hageman factor (factor XII)
	Complement system: chemotactic factors, anaphylatoxins
	Kinin system: bradykinin
	Phagocytes
	Circulating neutrophils, eosinophils, monocytes, macrophages
	Fixed cells (of mononuclear phagocyte system) in alveoli, spleen, liver, bone marrow
Immune response	Humoral immune response: B cells, plasma cells, immunoglobulins
	Cell-mediated immune response: T cells, lymphokines

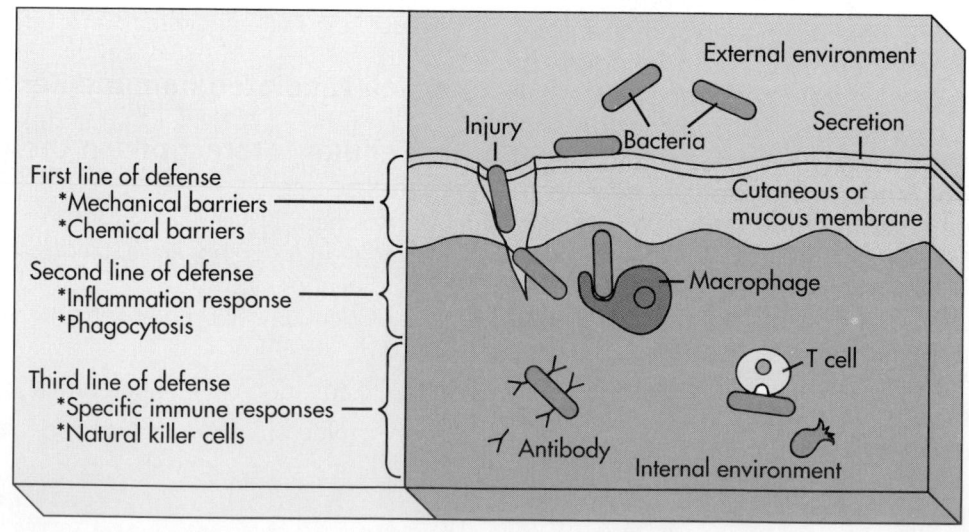

Unn Fig. 5-A *Lines of defense. (From Thibodeau, G.A. & Patton, K.T. [1999]. Anatomy & physiology [4th ed.]. St. Louis: Mosby.)*

Fig. 5-1 *Myeloid and lymphoid pathways of differentiation.*

CHARACTERISTICS OF THE IMMUNE RESPONSE

The immune system of the normal adult continually is challenged by a spectrum of substances that it recognizes as foreign, or "nonself." These substances are called *antigens.* Some antigens are on infectious agents, such as viruses, bacteria, fungi, or parasites; some are on noninfectious substances from the environment, such as pollens, foods, and bee venoms; and others are on drugs, vaccines, transfusions, and transplanted tissues.

Leukocytes are white blood cells (WBCs) that are cells of the inflammatory and immune responses. These cells are the most important cellular components participating in the body's defense. WBCs are divided into three main types: granulocytes, monocytes, and lymphocytes. All three types originate from two lines of differentiation—*lymphoid* lineage and *myeloid* lineage. The lymphoid lineage produces lymphocytes, and the myeloid lineage produces granulocytes and monocytes (Fig. 5-1; also see Fig.19-9). All blood cells are discussed in detail in Chapter 19.

The body's reaction to antigenic challenges is the immune response, in which physiologic and biochemical interactions cause the maturation and activation of two types of *lymphocytes, B lymphocytes (B cells)* and *T lymphocytes (T cells),* which act in different ways to recognize and destroy specific antigens (Fig. 5-2). They differ from the cells involved in inflammation in two ways. First, they are specific, so that each individual B or T cell recognizes only one specific antigen. The B cells produce antibodies, which incapacitate the antigen, and the T cells attack the antigen directly. Second, once B and T cells have been exposed to a particular antigen, some, called *memory cells,* can "remember" the antigen and act even faster if it invades the host again. Thus the

Fig. 5-2 *Scanning electron micrograph shows a mixed population of B and T lymphocytes. Arrows* designate red blood cells; *L* denotes lymphocytes. *(From King, D.W., Fenoglio, C.M., & Lefkowitch, J.H. [1983].* General pathology: Principles and dynamics. *Philadelphia: Lea & Febiger.)*

immune system possesses memory and specificity and creates long-lasting protection against specific antigens. This process is termed **immunity.**

Some exogenous factors, such as trauma, disease, pollutants, radiation, ultraviolet light, and drugs, profoundly affect an individual's immune system. Endogenous factors, such as the individual's age, gender, nutritional status, genetic background, and reproductive status, also modulate the immune response. The quality and intensity of the immune response are therefore a sum of the effects of all these factors: antigenic challenge, exogenous modulators, and endogenous factors.

Sometimes the normal immune response does not function in the best interests of the host and must be suppressed. For example, transplanted organs from donors are in danger of rejection because of the immune response. Lessening the likelihood of rejection involves matching host tissues and donor tissues for antigenic compatibility, or histocompatibility. Pharmacologic suppression of the immune response also may be used.

Another example of a functioning but detrimental immune response is an allergic reaction. Allergies are detrimental immune responses in which the host's immune system overreacts, or is hypersensitive, to the antigenic properties of substances in the environment. (Immune deficiency diseases, autoimmune diseases, and allergic hypersensitivity are the subjects of Chapter 7.)

Natural Versus Acquired Immunity

Natural immunity, also called *native* or *innate resistance,* is not produced by the immune response. One type of natural immunity, present at birth, is species-dependent. Human beings are naturally immune to some infectious agents that cause illness in other species. For example, humans do not contract canine distemper or serious cases of cowpox. The other type of natural immunity is host-dependent and involves the specific individual's characteristics. (Analysis of risk factors, as described in Chapter 2, has identified some of these characteristics.)

Acquired immunity is gained after birth as a result of the immune response. It can be either active or passive, depending on whether the components of the immune response have been produced by the host or by a donor. **Active acquired immunity** is produced by the host after either natural exposure to an antigen or immunization. In **passive acquired immunity,** preformed antibodies or T lymphocytes are transferred to the recipient. This can occur naturally, as in the passage of maternal antibodies to the fetus, or artificially, as in a clinical treatment. Clinically preformed antibodies from a donor (human or animal) are administered in the form of immune serum, which is antibody-containing blood from which the clotting factors and cells have been removed. Passive immunity is temporary and is used in the treatment of clinical emergencies, such as rabies exposure, tetanus, and snake bite.

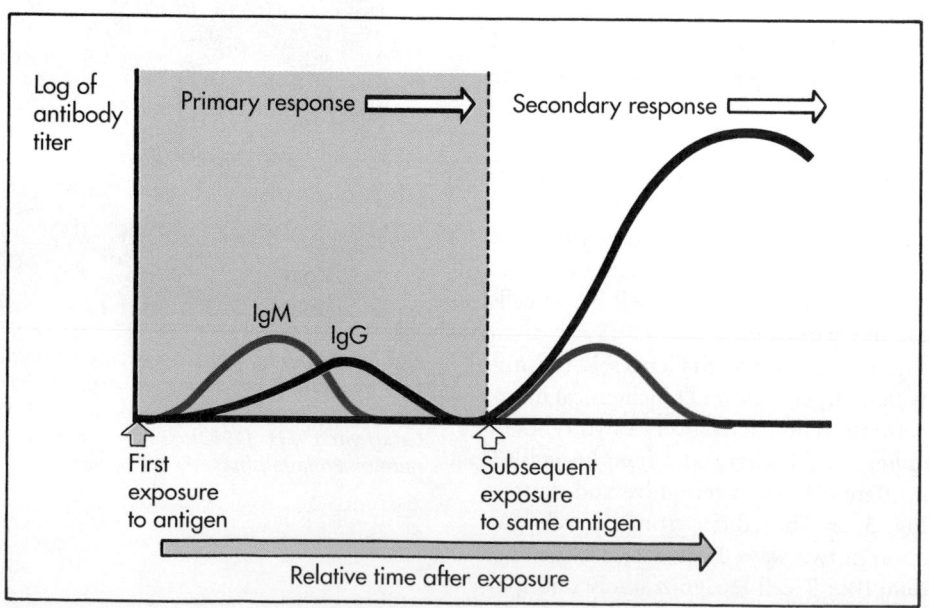

Fig. 5-3 *Primary and secondary immune responses.* The introduction of antigen induces a response dominated by two classes of immunoglobulins, IgM and IgG. IgM predominates in the primary response, with some IgG appearing later. After the host's immune system is primed, another challenge with the same antigen induces the secondary response, in which some IgM and large amounts of IgG are produced.

Primary and Secondary Immune Responses

The immune response to antigenic challenge has classically been divided into two phases—the primary and secondary responses. These phases can be demonstrated by serologic tests that measure plasma concentrations of antibody over time (Fig. 5-3). The initial administration of (or exposure to) most antigens is followed by a latent period during which B cells produce no detectable antibodies (immunoglobulin [Ig]). After approximately 5 days, one class of antibody (IgM) can be detected in the circulation. This marks the beginning of the initial or *primary immune response,* which is usually dominated by IgM, with lesser amounts of IgG (another class of immunoglobulin). With no further exposure to the antigen, the circulating antibody is catabolized (broken down) and measurable quantities fall. The individual's immune system, however, has been primed. A second challenge by the same antigen results in the *secondary* (*anamnestic*) *immune response,* which is characterized by the more rapid production of a larger amount of antibody (titers) than the primary response. The rapidity of the secondary immune response results from the presence of memory cells. IgG is the predominant antibody class of the secondary response and frequently is present in concentrations several times those of IgM.

The primary and secondary immune responses confer active acquired immunity. When an antigen or vaccine, such as that on rubella virus, enters the host for the first time, the primary immune response occurs. After a lag phase, during which the antigen is processed, the initial antibody levels are not high. When the host undergoes a second exposure to the same antigen or vaccine, the secondary response occurs; antibody levels rise immediately and may remain elevated for many years. *Vaccines* do not cause disease because they are killed, made less infectious (*attenuated*), or otherwise altered before administration so that they are capable of eliciting an immune response but are not capable of causing illness in a healthy individual.

Humoral Versus Cell-Mediated Immunity

The primary cell of the immune response is the lymphocyte (Fig. 5-4). The mature *lymphocyte* is a small, round, white blood cell approximately 6 to 10 micrometers (μm) in diameter.

Lymphocytes originate in the liver, spleen, and bone marrow of the fetus and child as lymphocyte precursors or stem cells. They are not capable of implementing the immune response. To become mature immunocompetent cells, they must migrate through lymphoid tissues in various parts of the body (Fig. 5-5, *A* and *B*). While passing through these tissues, they mature and undergo changes that commit them to one of two cellular lineages. The lymphocytes that migrate through bone marrow become B lymphocytes, or B cells. When B cells encounter antigens, they are stimulated into mature plasma cells that secrete antibodies. B cells are ultimately responsible for *humoral immunity.*

Fig. 5-4 *Scanning electron micrograph of lymphocytes and macrophages.* The lymphocytes are small and spherical; the macrophages are larger and more irregular in shape. *(From Raven, P.H. & Johnson, G.B. [1999]. Biology [5th ed.]. New York: McGraw-Hill.)*

The lymphocytes that migrate through the thymus gland become T lymphocytes, or T cells. T cells are capable of becoming sensitized to and recognizing specific antigens, which they attack directly. They are responsible for *cell-mediated immunity.*

The success of the immune response depends on the interaction between the humoral and cell-mediated responses, which share some components and processes. Differentiation (maturation) of T cells and B cells is shown in Fig. 5-6.

✓ QUICK CHECK

Define immunity.

Why are lymphocyte precursor cells unable to cause an immune response?

Why is the antibody titer greater in the secondary immune response?

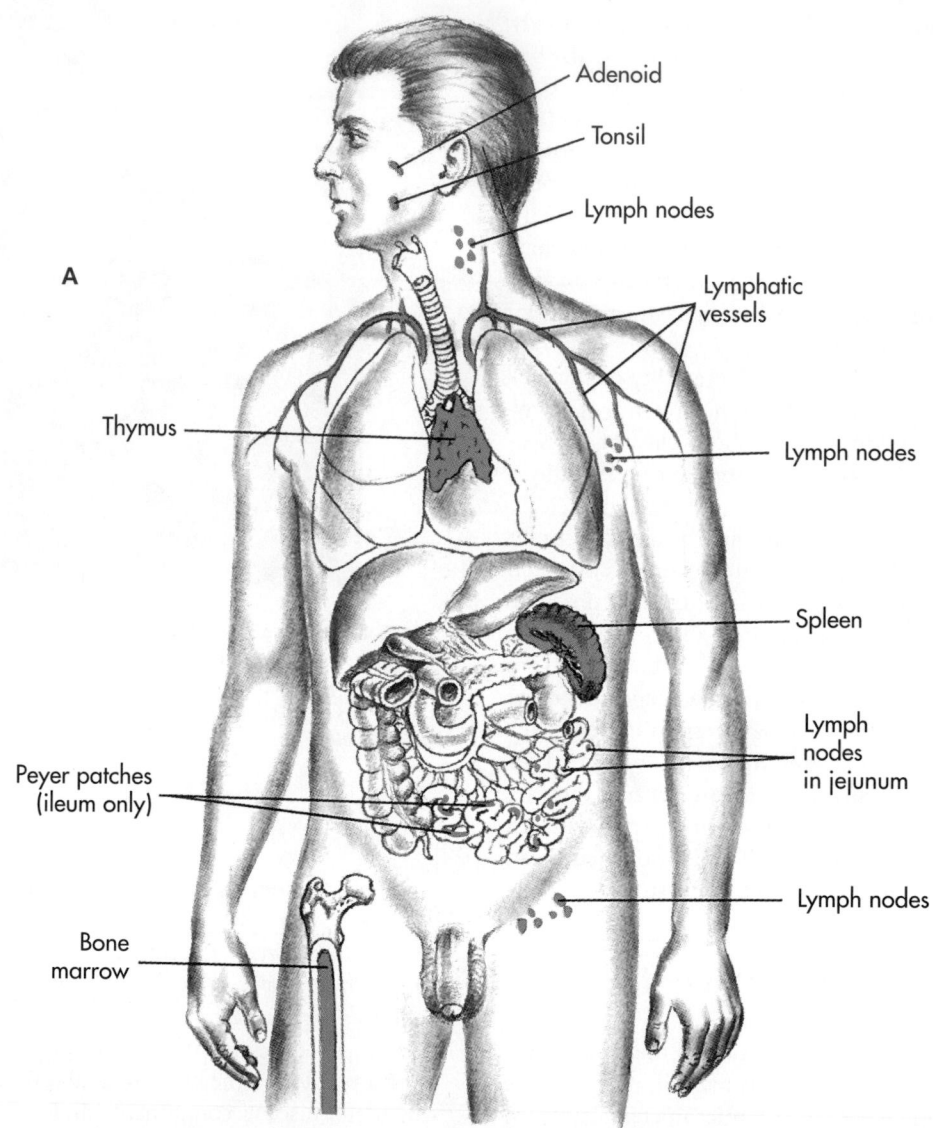

Fig. 5-5 A, *Lymphoid tissues: sites of B cell and T cell differentiation.* Immature lymphocytes migrate through central lymphoid tissues: the bone marrow (probable central lymphoid tissue for B lymphocytes) and the thymus (central lymphoid tissue for T lymphocytes). Mature lymphocytes later reside in the T and B lymphocyte–rich areas of the peripheral lymphoid tissues.

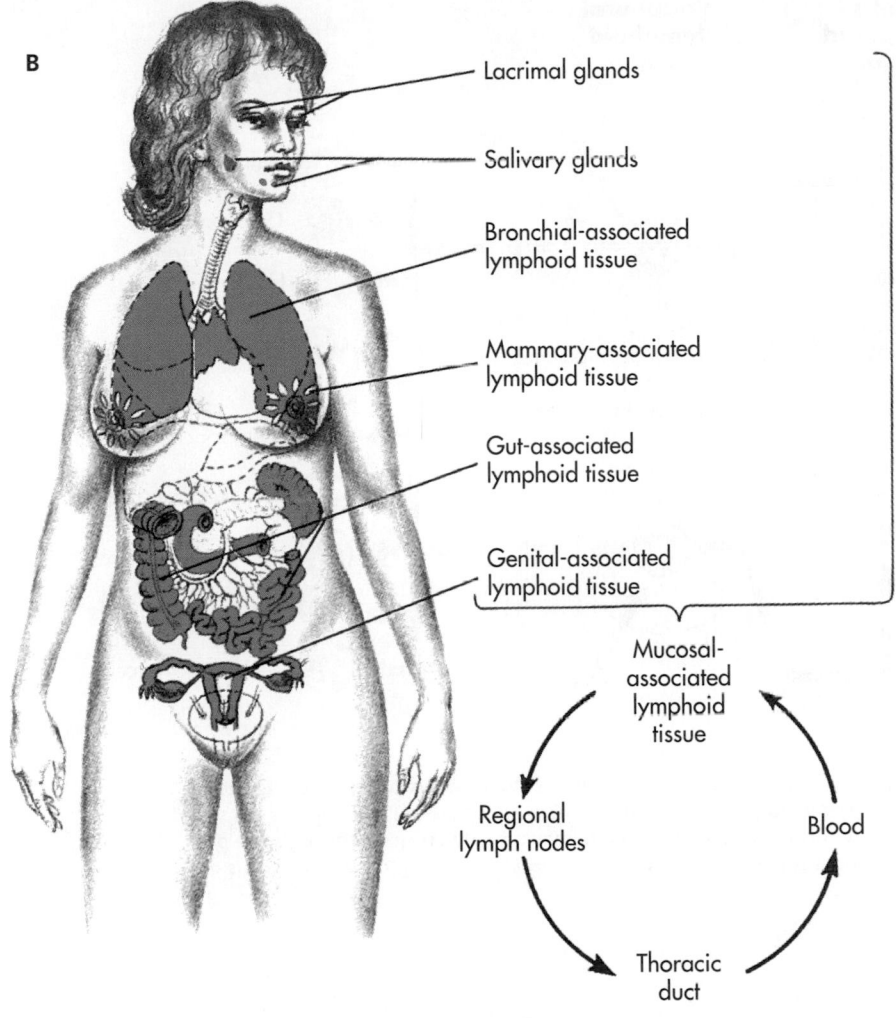

B

Lacrimal glands

Salivary glands

Bronchial-associated lymphoid tissue

Mammary-associated lymphoid tissue

Gut-associated lymphoid tissue

Genital-associated lymphoid tissue

Mucosal-associated lymphoid tissue

Regional lymph nodes

Blood

Thoracic duct

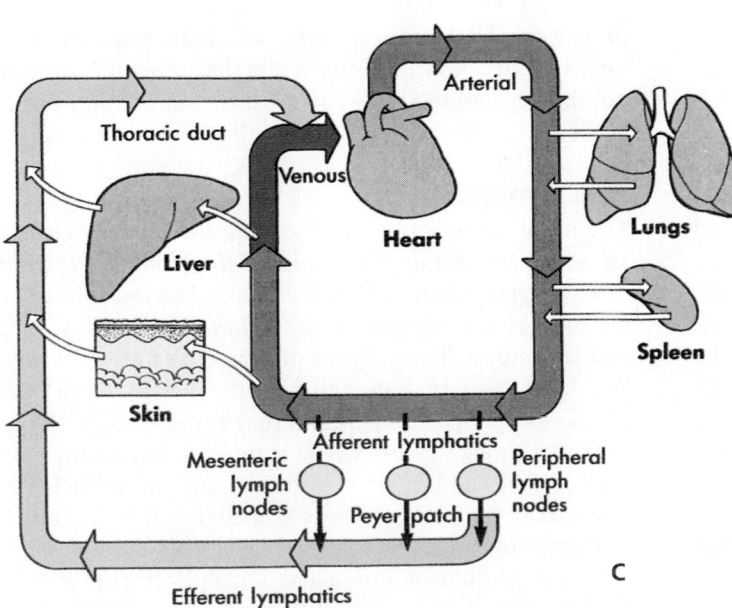

Thoracic duct

Arterial

Venous

Heart

Lungs

Liver

Spleen

Skin

Afferent lymphatics

Mesenteric lymph nodes

Peyer patch

Peripheral lymph nodes

Efferent lymphatics

C

Fig. 5-5, cont'd B, *Mucosal-associated lymphoid tissues of the secretory immune system.* Lymphocytes from the mucosal-associated lymphoid tissues circulate throughout the body in a pattern separate from other lymphocytes. For example, lymphocytes from the gut-associated lymphoid tissue circulate through the regional lymph nodes, the thoracic duct, and the blood and return to other mucosal-associated lymphoid tissues rather than to lymphoid tissue of the systemic immune system. **C,** *Pathways of lymphocyte travel. (C from Mudge-Grout, C. [1992].* Immunologic disorders. *St. Louis: Mosby.)*

Fig. 5-6 *Outcome of T (thymus-derived) and B (bursal-derived) pathways of lymphocyte maturation.* Mature cells of the T cell lineage that have different functions usually develop from separate immature T cells. Mature B cells, on the other hand, may directly progress through the production of different classes of antibody against the same antigen. *Immunoglobulin D (IgD) is not shown because it does not circulate in the blood.*

INDUCTION OF THE IMMUNE RESPONSE
Antigens

An **antigen** is a molecule or molecular complex that reacts with components of the immune system, such as lymphocytes and antibodies. Antigenicity is the molecule's innate capacity *to react with* those components and is determined by the chemical structure of the antigen molecule. The portion of the antigenic molecule that is configured for recognition and binding is called an **antigenic determinant,** or **epitope.** The matching portion of the receptor on the lymphocyte or antibody is sometimes referred to as an *antigen-binding* or *antigen-combining, site.*

The immune system has the exquisite ability to distinguish self (**self-antigens**) from nonself (foreign antigens). Under normal conditions the immune system is in a state of **tolerance** with the host's tissues but is able to reject foreign tissues and destroy infectious agents.

Histocompatibility Antigens

How does the body actually recognize that a substance is foreign? The code that brings about this recognition consists of the major **histocompatibility antigens** (also called **HLA antigens** or **HLA determinants**), which are proteins found on the surface of nearly every cell in the body. HLA antigens not only defend the body against infection but also distinguish each individual's tissue from the tissues of others.

HLA complex

The major group of *genes* producing the HLA antigens is known as the **major histocompatibility complex (MHC).** This complex consists of four closely linked loci located on the short arm of chromosome 6. They are labeled A, B, C, and D complex. The antigens produced by the A, B, and C loci (class I antigens) are found on the surfaces of virtually all cells except erythrocytes, and they are involved in the rejection of foreign tissue. The D complex (class II antigens), on the other hand, consists of other independent loci (DR, DP, DZ/DO, and DQ) and are confined mostly to B lymphocytes, macrophages, and some epithelial cells and transiently to subpopulations of stimulated T lymphocytes (Fig. 5-7). HLA-A, -B, and -C genes and their products are commonly referred to as MHC class I genes or proteins; similarly, HLA-DR, -DP, and -DQ genes and proteins are commonly referred to as MHC class II genes or proteins. Class III proteins

Chromosome 6: Site of genes that encode HLA antigens

Fig. 5-7 *Human leukocyte antigen (HLA).* The major histocompatibility complex (MHC) is located on chromosome 6. *(Modified from Mudge-Grout, C. [1992]. Immunologic disorders. St. Louis: Mosby.)*

(some complement components and cytokines) are located between class I and class II antigens on chromosome 6 of the MHC.

Each HLA locus has many alleles. Therefore many possible allele combinations exist, making it unlikely that two unrelated individuals will have the same HLA composition.

The specific alleles at the six HLA loci on one chromosome are termed the *haplotype.* Each individual has two HLA haplotypes, one for each chromosome. Because the loci are closely linked, the haplotypes usually are not disrupted by recombination and are thus transmitted intact to the offspring from each parent. Each parent passes *one* HLA haplotype to his or her offspring. The offspring then share one haplotype with each parent, and (on the average) they share one haplotype with one half of their siblings, both haplotypes with one fourth of their siblings, and no haplotypes with one fourth of their siblings. Monozygotic twins, of course, have identical HLA haplotypes. This coexpression and polymorphism make the HLA antigen system useful in determining paternity.

The HLA complex is particularly important in determining the success of tissue grafts and organ transplants. The more similar two individuals are in their HLA make-up, the more likely the success of a transplant from one to the other (they also must have the same ABO blood type).

Role of HLA antigens

One normal function of MHC class I and class II antigens appears to be distinguishing self from nonself. Genetic loci within the MHC also control the quality and quantity of an immune response. These are part of a group of genes referred to as *immune response genes,* or *Ir genes.*

Blood Group Antigens

The HLA antigens are not found on the surfaces of erythrocytes, but several other antigens that determine compatibility are found. These are known collectively as the *blood group antigens.* More than 80 different red cell antigens are

grouped into several dozen blood group systems, each determined by a different locus or set of loci. The most important of these, because they provoke the strongest humoral immune response, are the ABO and Rh systems.

Rh system

The *Rh blood group* (named after the rhesus monkey, the animal in which it was first discovered), with its high degree of polymorphism, is a protein antigen system second in complexity only to the HLA system. At least five major antigens and a large number of rare variants have been identified and are expressed only on erythrocytes.[1,2] The Rh system appears to consist of three very tightly linked genetic loci, labeled C, D, and E. Each locus has two alleles labeled C and c, D and d, or E and e. Distinct antigens are expressed by C, c, E, e, and D, whereas no distinct antigen has been observed for d. Therefore d is considered a lack of D. The locus of greatest interest is the D locus, more commonly expressed as $Rh_o(D)$, because it is responsible for Rh maternal-fetal incompatibility and the resulting hemolytic disease of the newborn (see Chapter 21). Persons who have the DD or Dd genotype have the Rh antigen on their erythrocytes and are called Rh-positive. The recessive homozygotes, with genotype dd, are Rh-negative and do not have the Rh antigen. About 85% of North Americans are Rh-positive, and about 15% are Rh-negative.

ABO system

The *ABO blood group* consists of two major carbohydrate antigens, labeled A and B (Fig. 5-8). These are codominant, so individuals can have one of four blood types. Individuals with blood type A carry the A antigen on their erythrocytes; individuals with blood type B carry the B antigen; those with blood type AB carry both A and B; and those with type O carry neither antigen. A person with type A blood also has anti-B antibodies in the blood. If this person receives blood containing B antigens (i.e., blood from a type AB or B individual), a severe antibody reaction occurs. Similarly, a type B individual (whose blood contains anti-A antibodies) cannot receive blood from a type A or AB donor. Type O individuals, who have neither antigen but have both anti-A and anti-B antibodies, cannot accept blood from any of the other three types. These naturally occurring antibodies are immunoglobulins of the IgM class and are called *isohemagglutinins.*

Because individuals with type O blood lack both types of antigens, they can be universal donors and anyone can accept small volumes of their blood. Similarly, type AB individuals are universal recipients, because they lack both anti-A and anti-B antibodies. When large volumes of *whole* blood are transfused, however, the donor's antibodies can bind to antigenic determinants on the recipient's erythrocytes. This reaction causes clumping of erythrocytes in the blood. Clumping (agglutination) and lysis cause harmful transfusion reactions, which can be prevented only by complete and careful ABO matching between donor and recipient.

Fig. 5-8 *Blood types.* The relationship of antigens and antibodies involved in the ABO blood group system.

HUMORAL IMMUNE RESPONSE
B Lymphocytes

In birds, an organ called the *bursa of Fabricius* is responsible for the maturation of B lymphocytes.[3] Humans have no discrete bursa but do have tissues (probably the bone marrow) that make up the so-called *human bursal equivalent* (see Fig. 5-5). Lymphocytes destined to become B cells circulate through the bursal equivalent, where they undergo hormonally directed proliferation that gives them the capacity to react with antigen and generate diverse antibodies that protect the host against infection (see Fig. 5-6). B cell precursors cannot react with antigen, whereas postbursal B cells produce plasma membrane-bound antibodies of the IgM and IgD classes, which can bind antigen.

More than 10^8 different antigenic determinants may be recognized by the B cells. The *clonal selection* theory postulates that a large number of B cells with plasma membrane receptors for all potential antigenic determinants are spontaneously generated during fetal life, independent of the presence of antigen (Fig. 5-9). Each B cell, however, responds to only one specific antigen. When the immunocompetent B cells encounter an antigen for the first time, those with specific membrane antibody receptors complementary to that antigen's determinant sites are stimulated to proliferate. B cells that have undergone this process are called *plasma cells* and can be found in the blood, secondary lymphoid organs (primarily spleen and lymph nodes), and some inflammatory sites.

Thus two proliferative steps take place before antibody production can occur. The first, the generation of clonal diversity, probably takes place in the bursal-equivalent tissues,

is hormonally driven and antigen-independent, and results in the generation of immunocompetent mature B cells with plasma membrane receptors that can recognize virtually any antigenic molecule. The second, clonal selection, occurs in the peripheral lymphoid organs, is antigen-specific and antigen-driven, and results in the proliferation and maturation of antibody-secreting plasma cells. At about the eighth week of gestation in humans, antigen-driven differentiation may begin, although generation of clonal diversity probably continues in the bone marrow throughout most of adult life.

The immune response is initiated when an antigen binds and interacts with antibody receptors on the surface of the mature B cell, triggering it into a sequence of proliferation and differentiation that results in the production of (1) immunoglobulin-secreting plasma cells and (2) a set of long-lived memory cells (see Figs. 5-6 and 5-9).

Immunoglobulins

Antibodies, or immunoglobulins, are serum glycoproteins produced by plasma cells in response to a challenge by an antigen. The term *immunoglobulin* is used to denote all molecules of this type. *Antibodies,* on the other hand, are immunoglobulins known to have specificity for a particular antigen. The five molecular classes of immunoglobulins are IgG, IgA, IgM, IgE, and IgD (Table 5-2). These classes are characterized by antigenic, structural, and functional differences. Within the classes are several distinct subclasses, including four subclasses of IgG and two subclasses of IgA.

Structure of immunoglobulin molecules

Enzymatic analysis of the immunoglobulins revealed three fragments, two of which were identical (Fig. 5-10).[4] The two

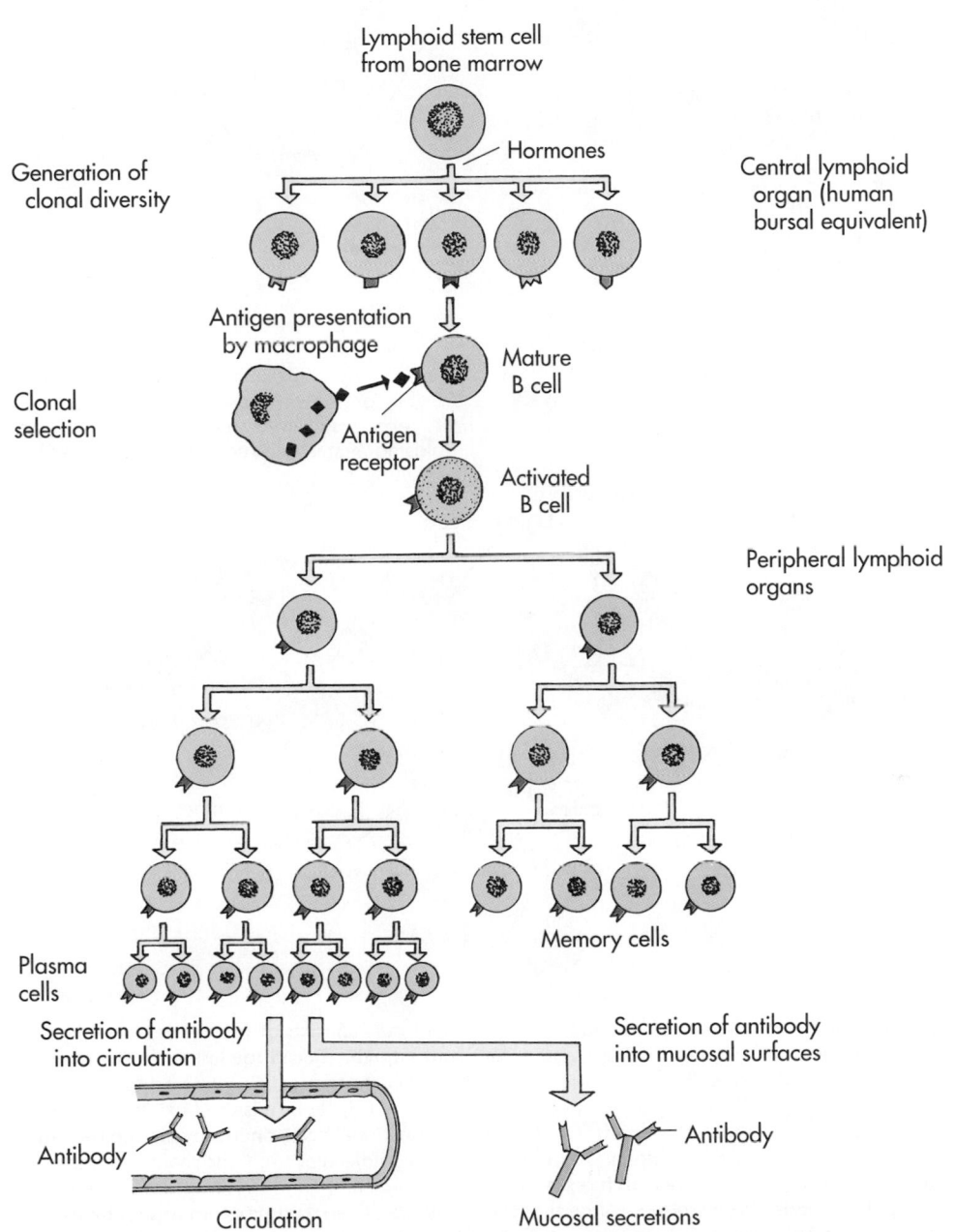

Fig. 5-9 *Antibody production: generation of clones of antigen-specific B lymphocytes (B cells).*
Under the control of hormones and without antigen, B lymphocyte precursors undergo cellular division in the central lymphoid organs (bursal-equivalent tissues, probably bone marrow) and generate receptors against all possible antigens that may be encountered in the host's adult life. Later, primarily in the peripheral lymphoid organs (spleen, lymph nodes), antigen, either directly or presented by macrophages (phagocytic cells of inflammation), reacts with the clones of B cells having appropriate receptors on their surfaces, causing those cells to proliferate and produce antibody.

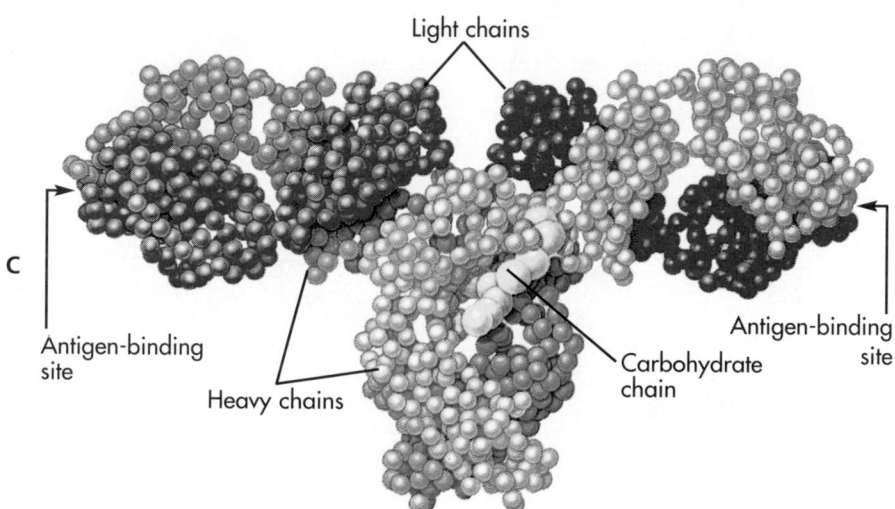

Fig. 5-10 *Molecular structure of an antibody.* **A,** The molecule consists of four chains—two light *(L)* and two heavy *(H)*—held together by intrachain and interchain disulfide linkages. The molecule can be divided into regions with variable *(V)* and relatively constant *(C)* amino acid structures (CH$_1$, CH$_2$, and CH$_3$ on the heavy chain). Between the CH$_1$ and CH$_2$ regions is the flexible hinge region *(Hi).* **B,** Experimental fragmentation of IgG into its functional components by limited papain digestion. **C,** In this molecular model of a typical antibody molecule, the light chains are represented by strands of *red spheres* (each represents an individual amino acid). Heavy chains are represented by strands of *blue spheres.* Note that the heavy chains can complex with a carbohydrate chain. *(C from Thibodeau, G.A. & Patton, K.T. [1999]. Anatomy & physiology [4th ed.]. St. Louis: Mosby.)*

identical fragments were found to retain the antigen-binding activity of the molecule and were termed ***antigen-binding fragments (Fab).*** The third piece crystallized when separated from the Fab portions and was termed the ***crystalline fragment (Fc).***

The Fab portions contain the recognition sites (receptors) for antigenic determinants and confer specificity. The Fc portion is responsible for most of the biologic functions of the molecule, including interactions with various systems of inflammation, such as the complement cascade (see p. 156); for transport of maternal antibody to the fetus; and for binding to the surface of the effector cells of inflammation (polymorphonuclear neutrophils, macrophages, lymphocytes, mast cells, platelets).

The antibody molecule consists of four polypeptide chains—two identical light (L) chains and two identical heavy (H) chains. Both light and heavy chains are divided into variable (V) and constant (C) regions. Among different antibodies the variable region is characterized by a large number of amino acid differences. The light chains of an an-

Fig. 5-11 *Structure of different immunoglobulins.* Secretory IgA, IgD, IgE, IgG, and IgM.

TABLE 5-2	Immunoglobulins and Serum Levels		
Class	Subclass	Heavy Chain	Adult Serum Levels (mg/dl)
IgG	IgG1	γ_1	800-900
	IgG2	γ_2	280-300
	IgG3	γ_3	90-100
	IgG4	γ_4	50
IgM	IgM	μ	120-150
IgA	IgA1	α_1	280-300
	IgA2	α_2	50
	sIgA	α_1, α_2	5
IgD	IgD	δ	3
IgE	IgE	ϵ	0.03

✓ QUICK CHECK

Define antigen.

Why is the MHC important in the immune response?

Why are the blood cell antigens—Rh and ABO systems—important for blood transfusions?

Why are the Fab and Fc regions of the antibody so important?

tibody molecule are of either the kappa or lambda type and also consist of a variable (VL) and a constant (CL) region. Each class of antibody has a unique type of heavy chain: gamma (IgG), mu (IgM), alpha (IgA), epsilon (IgE), or delta (IgD) (Fig. 5-11). The light and heavy chains are held together by two major forces: noncovalent bonds and disulfide linkages.

The interaction of the variable region's amino acid sequences on both the heavy and light chains determines the conformation of the antigen-combining site and therefore the antigenic specificity of the immunoglobulin molecule (Fig. 5-12). In some cases the substitution of a single critical amino acid may significantly affect the shape of the combin-

ing site and the specificity of the antibody molecule. The antigen fits into this binding site like a key into a lock and is held there by noncovalent chemical interactions.

Function of antibodies

The chief functions of antibodies are to protect the host by (1) neutralizing bacterial toxins, (2) neutralizing viruses, (3) opsonizing bacteria (i.e., promoting phagocytosis [see p. 163]), and (4) activating components of the inflammatory response (Fig. 5-13 and Table 5-3).

Normally an antibody circulates in the blood or is suspended in body secretions until it encounters and binds to its appropriate antigen. At that time the antibody may play two roles: (1) it may have a direct effect on the antigen, and (2) it may have an indirect effect on other mechanisms of self-defense. Directly, the antibody may produce *agglutination* (clumping together), *precipitation* (falling out of solu-

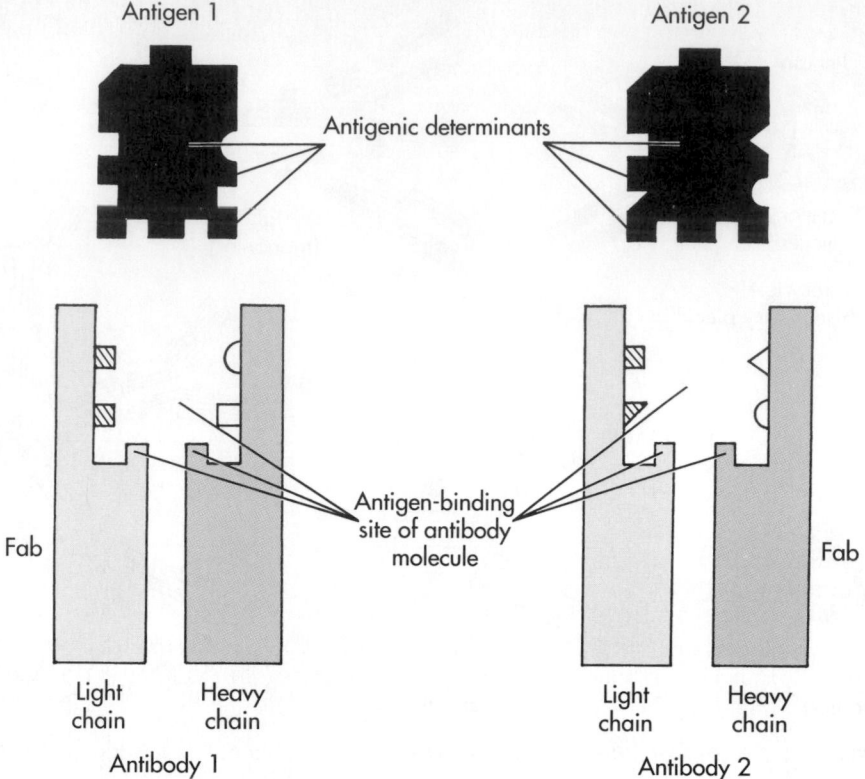

Fig. 5-12 *Antigen-antibody binding.* The specificity required for antibody binding with an antigen is determined by the shape of the combining site on the antibody.

Fig. 5-13 *Functions of antibody.* Protective activities of antibodies include neutralization of bacterial exotoxins, neutralization of viruses and prevention of their interactions with cellular membranes, and opsonization of bacteria. All of these mechanisms are followed by removal of the antigen by phagocytosis, drainage along with body fluid, or both.

TABLE 5-3 | Biologic Properties of Immunoglobulins

| Subclass | Complement Activation | | Binding to Fc Receptors on | | | | Placental Transfer | Presence in Secretions | Induction of Agglutination |
	Classical	Alternate	Macrophages	PMNs	Mast Cells	Platelets			
IgG1	++	−	+	+	−	+	+++	±	+
IgG2	+	−	−	−	−	+	+	±	+
IgG3	+++	−	+	+	−	+	+++	±	+
IgG4	−	−	−	±	+	+	++	±	+
IgM	++++	−	−	−	−	−	−	+	+++
IgA1	−	+	−	±	−	−	−	+	−
IgA2	−	+	−	±	−	−	−	+	−
sIgA	−	−	−	−	−	−	−	++++	−
IgD	−	±	−	−	−	−	−	−	−
IgE	−	±	?	−	+++	−	−	+	−

Fc, *Crystalline fragment;* PMN, *polymorphonuclear neutrophil;* Ig, *immunoglobulin;* −, *lack of activity;* +, *relative degree of activity;* sIgA, *secretory immunoglobulin A. (Complement activation and the function of monocytes, PMNs, mast cells, and platelets are described in the section on inflammation, beginning on p. 162.)*

tion), or **neutralization** (inactivation) of the antigen. Which of these occurs is determined by the class of antibody and the characteristics of the antigen. Antibody function always begins with antigen-antibody binding. The antibody molecule's Fab portions bind with antigenic determinant sites on the antigen. Binding results in **antigen-antibody complexes,** also called **immune complexes.** Antigen-antibody binding may directly affect the antigen by occupying its antigenic determinant sites, rendering them unable to bind with receptors on host cells. For example, viruses that are neutralized in this way cannot infect cells because they cannot bind with receptors on the cell's plasma membrane.

Indirect effects of antibody result as it acts as a bridge that lends specificity to the inflammatory response. One end of the molecule, Fab, specifically binds to antigens, and the other end, Fc, informs the nonspecific amplifiers of the inflammatory response, both molecular and cellular, that an unwanted substance has invaded the body, either from the outside (e.g., infectious agents) or from within (e.g., a malignancy) the body. Antigenic molecules are usually complex, have multiple antigenic determinants, and bind several antibodies so that when an antigen reacts with the Fab regions of the antibody, the Fc portions are held close to other Fc regions. The clustering of Fc regions results in (1) the binding to and activation of the complement cascade and (2) the recognition of and binding to receptors (Fc receptors) on the surfaces of inflammatory cells (e.g., macrophages, neutrophils).

Neutralization of bacterial toxins

Many bacteria produce toxins that enhance their pathogenic effects and harm the host. (The injurious effects of bacterial toxins are described in Chapter 7.) Fortunately for the host, bacterial toxins can initiate the humoral immune response. A principal role of the antibodies subsequently produced is to function as antitoxins that neutralize bacterial toxins.

Neutralization proceeds with the formation of antigen-antibody complexes (in this case, toxin-antitoxin complexes)

(see Figs. 5-12 and 5-13). Simply stated, the antibodies capture the toxin molecules by occupying their antigenic determinant sites. This prevents the toxins from binding to tissue cells and exerting their harmful effects. Once the antigen-antibody complexes are formed, they may be removed from the body by **phagocytosis** (ingestion by phagocytic cells; see p. 163).

Detecting the presence of specific antitoxins can aid in diagnosing diseases. For example, laboratory tests that detect antistreptolysin O or anti-DNase B measure antibodies produced against those toxins and can be useful in diagnosing group A streptococcal infections.

Actively induced immunity against many pathogens can be achieved by immunization (vaccination) with their toxins. To prevent harming the recipient, the toxins are chemically inactivated, resulting in a toxoid that has few toxic properties but remains an antigen. Vaccines against such diseases as diphtheria and tetanus are toxoids.

Neutralization of viruses

Antibodies protect the host against some viral infections by preventing the attachment and entrance of viruses into host cells. The mechanism of viral neutralization is shown schematically in Fig. 5-13. Neutralized viral particles may agglutinate or be ingested and removed by phagocytes.

Many viruses (e.g., measles, herpes) are usually inaccessible to antibody because they do not circulate in the bloodstream. Instead they remain in cells and tend to spread by direct cell-to-cell contact. Antibodies against these viruses are most effective in preventing the initial infection but usually play only a minor role in recovery from a primary (initial) infection or in preventing recurrent infection. Other viruses, such as polio and influenza, spread from cell to cell through the blood and are more susceptible to the effects of circulating antibodies. These viruses can be controlled by antibodies even after the initial infection.

Protection against many viral infections, such as rubella, can be elicited effectively by vaccination with inactivated viruses. Levels of circulating IgG are usually a good indication of the degree of protection. Because antibody protects against reinfection, some vaccines have been designed to induce antibody production at the site of viral entrance into the body. For example, both oral and injected polio vaccines prevent systemic infection in the recipient, but only the oral preparation readily protects against the carrier state by inducing a secretory IgA response at the usual site of viral entry, which is the gastrointestinal tract.

Opsonization of bacteria

An *opsonin* is a substance that renders bacteria susceptible to phagocytosis. Antibodies themselves are opsonins; antibodies also induce opsonization by complement component C3b (see p. 156). *Opsonization,* the process of opsonin-enhanced phagocytosis, is necessary because many bacteria have an outer capsule that resists phagocytosis unless antibody is produced against it.

Classes of immunoglobulins

Fig. 5-11 illustrates the structure of the immunoglobulins. IgG constitutes 80% to 85% of the circulating immunoglobulins. IgG has four subclasses: IgG1, IgG2, IgG3, and IgG4; the most predominant are IgG1 and IgG2. IgG is the major class of immunoglobulin in the immune response and is responsible for most of the antibody functions, such as precipitation, agglutination, and complement activation. As a result of selective transport across the placenta, maternal IgG is also the major antibody found in fetal blood.

IgA has two subclasses, IgA1 and IgA2. The predominant antibody in normal body secretions is secretory IgA, which is predominantly IgA2. IgA in the blood is predominantly IgA1. The secretory piece is attached to IgA dimers in the mucosal cells and may protect the molecule against degradative enzymes in secretions. (The biologic role of IgA is discussed on p. 141.)

IgM is the largest immunoglobulin and has 10 theoretic antigenic binding sites, although only 5 are functional. It is the first antibody produced during the initial, or primary, response to antigen (see Fig. 5-3). IgM is synthesized early in neonatal life, and its synthesis may be increased as a response to infection in utero. The trophoblast cells that cover the surface of the placenta lack Fc receptors for IgM; therefore the molecule does not cross the placenta under normal conditions.

IgD is located on the surfaces of developing B lymphocytes. Information about its role is limited.

IgE is the least concentrated of any of the immunoglobulins in the circulation. It is also the principal antibody in the allergic response (see Chapter 7) and in the prevention of parasitic infections.

Monoclonal antibodies

Most humoral immune responses are polyclonal; that is, a mixture of antibodies is produced from multiple clones of B lymphocytes (see Fig. 5-9). This occurs because most antigenic molecules have multiple antigenic determinants and may stimulate proliferation of a spectrum of B lymphocytes. Each clone secretes antibody that differs slightly from that secreted by other clones, even though all the B cells were stimulated to proliferate by the same antigen. The antibodies are heterogeneous in immunoglobulin class, amino acid sequence, specificity, and function, and some react more strongly with the antigen than others.

Laboratory procedures have been devised to isolate and clone individual B lymphocytes, resulting in the production of a pure monoclonal antibody, in which each molecule is completely identical.

The advantages of monoclonal antibodies over conventional antisera (antibody-containing sera) are that (1) a single antibody of known antigenic specificity is generated rather than a mixture of different antibodies; (2) monoclonal antibodies have a single, constant binding affinity; (3) monoclonal antibodies can be diluted to a constant titer (concentration in fluid) because the actual antibody concentration is known; and (4) the antibody can be easily purified to homogeneity.

The generation of monoclonal antibodies is creating new therapeutic and diagnostic possibilities, particularly in the treatment of cancer and early detection of viral infections. Detection of viral infections thus far has been limited to verification that a particular virus is the cause of disease because diagnosis generally is performed by measuring the specific antibody response against the virus and any antibody that is produced immediately reacts with circulating antigen and therefore cannot be detected by routine serologic tests. Diagnosis is made after viral antigen has been removed from the blood and the patient is recovering. Monoclonal antibody, on the other hand, can be selected against specific antigenic determinants of the virus, produced in large quantities, and used in tests to detect elevations in circulating viral antigen that appears early in disease.

Secretory Immune System

The immune system within the body is called the *systemic immune system.* A distinct set of lymphoid tissues make up another, partially independent, immune system at the external surfaces of the body, the *secretory (mucosal) immune system.*[5] Most humoral immune responses occur when antibodies or B cells encounter antigens in the blood or tissues, but sometimes this encounter occurs in other body fluids. Some antibodies are present in secretions such as tears, sweat, saliva, mucus, and breast milk, where they can protect the body (or the neonate) against antigens that have not yet penetrated the skin or mucous membranes. IgA is the predominant secretory antibody, although IgM and IgG are present in secretions also.

Although antibodies in both blood and secretions are produced by B cells that have matured into plasma cells, antibodies in blood are produced by cells of the systemic immune system, whereas antibodies in secretions are produced by cells of the secretory (mucosal) immune system. The B cells of these two systems follow a different pattern of migration once they leave the bone marrow and enter the lymphatics. Lymphocytes of the systemic immune system travel through the spleen and most lymph nodes (see Fig. 5-5, *A* and *B*). Lymphocytes of the secretory immune system travel through the lacrimal (tear-producing) and salivary glands and lymphoid tissues in the breast, bronchi, intestines, and genitourinary tract (see Fig. 5-5, *C*).

Local protection is necessary to combat antigens (chiefly infectious microorganisms) that are inhaled, swallowed, or otherwise contact external body surfaces. Once they have taken up residence in the external layers of the body, harmful microorganisms can multiply and the host becomes a carrier. These microorganisms may (1) cause local disease (e.g., cholera); (2) penetrate the skin or mucosa and cause systemic disease (e.g., gram-negative bacterial infection of the blood [septicemia] if the integrity of the gut is disturbed); (3) not cause disease in the carrier (because of effective systemic immunity) but be spread to other individuals; or (4) pass out of the body without any ill effects (e.g., in feces).

The primary role of secretory IgA is to prevent the attachment and invasion of pathogens through mucosal membranes, such as those of the gastrointestinal, pulmonary, and genitourinary tracts. To induce protective immunity against some pathogens that enter through these routes, it is preferable to induce local immunity as well as systemic immunity. The Sabin vaccine against polio is administered orally as an attenuated live virus. This route causes a transient, limited infection and induces effective systemic and secretory immunities, preventing both the disease and the establishment of a carrier state. The Salk vaccine, on the other hand, consists of killed viruses that are administered intradermally. It induces adequate systemic protection but does not generally prevent an intestinal carrier state.

The breast-associated lymphoid tissue is in the trafficking pattern of cells of the secretory immune system, so most antigens to which the mother has been exposed gastrointestinally induce sensitized lymphocytes that migrate to the breast and secrete IgA, IgM, and IgG into the milk.[6] Antibodies against infectious disease agents are found in the milk and may provide protection to the newborn against those pathogens, such as polio, that invade through the gut. Colostral antibodies do not cross the newborn's gut after the first 24 hours of life and do not have a role in the newborn's systemic immunity.

The mechanisms of antigen-antibody binding are the same in the secretory and systemic immune systems; that is, binding neutralizes or opsonizes the antigen, preventing it from harming the host. The major differences between the two systems are the following:

1. Their lymphocytes follow different paths of migration and pass through different lymphoid tissues.
2. The secretory immune response is one of the body's first lines of defense, whereas the systemic response is the body's final defense.
3. The secretory response occurs locally and externally (in body secretions), whereas the systemic response occurs systemically and internally (in blood and tissues).

✓ QUICK CHECK

Which antibody is responsible for most of the antibody functions?

Why have monoclonal antibodies created new therapeutic possibilities?

Why is the secretory immune system important?

CELL-MEDIATED IMMUNE RESPONSE

There are five types of mature T cells, each with a different immune function (Box 5-1). *Memory cells* induce the secondary immune response; *lymphokine-producing cells* transfer delayed hypersensitivity (Td) and secrete proteins (lymphokines) that activate other cells, such as macrophages (see Chapter 7); *cytotoxic (Tc) cells* attack antigens directly and destroy cells that bear foreign antigens; and *helper T (Th)* and *suppressor T (Ts) cells* control both cell-mediated and humoral processes. The Td and Ts cell phenotypes are probably subsets of Th cells that produce the appropriate lymphokines for activating macrophages or for suppressing other Th cells' functions but do not provide any other helper function.

The process of T cell proliferation and differentiation shown in Fig. 5-15 is similar to that for B cells. The chief difference is that clonal diversity takes place in the thymus for T cells and in the human bursal equivalent for B cells.

Lymphocytes destined to become T cells journey through the *thymus,* where, under the pressure and guidance of the thymic hormones and without the presence of antigen, they are driven to proliferate and simultaneously become able to recognize the diversity of antigens the host will encounter throughout life.[7] They exit the thymus as antigenically committed (immunocompetent) mature T cells.[8] These T cells produce plasma membrane receptors that are not antibody but are related molecules with similar specificity for antigens. The thymus, which atrophies at puberty and practically disappears in adulthood, consists of a cortex and a medulla interspersed with connective tissue.

During maturation, T cells begin producing new proteins that are differentiation related and inserted into the plasma membrane of the cell. These proteins have been identified using monoclonal antibodies and are classified as "cluster of differentiation" (CD) antigens. Several important CD antigens participate in the development of the immune response, and several are markers for particular cells of the immune system. The most important of these are listed in Table 5-4.

The thymic epithelium produces several hormones involved in the maturation of T cells, including forms of thymosin, thymopoietin, ubiquitin, thymostimulin, and several other hormones. Thymic peptide hormones are involved in T cell differentiation both within the thymus and in the bloodstream, influencing uncommitted lymphocytes in the

Major Effects of the Cell-Mediated Immune Response

BOX 5-1

Cytotoxicity. Cytotoxic T cells mediate the direct cellular killing of target cells, such as virally infected cells, tumors, or foreign grafts. This function requires cellular contact, binding, and release of toxic substances from the Tc cell (Fig. 5-14).

Delayed hypersensitivity. The Td cells are involved in the inflammatory response and produce soluble mediators (lymphokines) that influence other cells, such as macrophages.

Memory. Memory cells are also responsible for the accelerated response to a second antigenic challenge (the secondary immune response).

Control. Helper T cells facilitate and suppressor T cells inhibit both humoral and cell-mediated immune responses.

 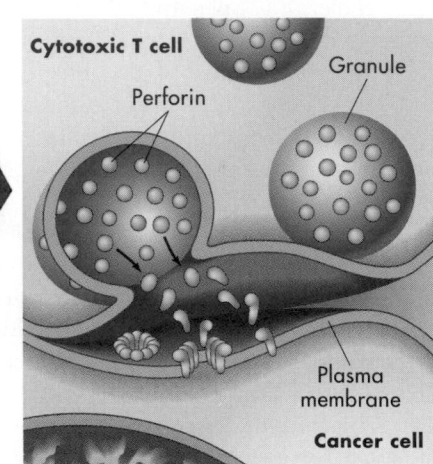

Fig. 5-14 *Cytotoxic T cells.* The *blue spheres* seen in this scanning electron microscope view are cytotoxic T cells attacking a much larger cancer cell. T cells are a significant part of the body's defense against cancer and other abnormal or foreign cells. The *inset* shows how the lymphotoxin *perforin* acts to kill cells by puncturing holes in their plasma membranes. *(From Thibodeau, G.A. & Patton, K.T. [1999]. Anatomy & physiology [4th ed.]. St. Louis: Mosby.)*

TABLE 5-4	CD Antigenic Markers of T Cell Development
CD No.	**Cell Type**
1	Early thymocytes
2	Early thymocytes, receptor for sheep RBCs
3	T cells, interacts with T cell receptor
4	Th cells, adhesion molecule for class II MHC binding
5	T cells
7	Early thymocytes
8	Tc and Ts cells, adhesion molecule for class I MHC binding

bone marrow and peripheral lymphoid tissues to travel to the thymus.

Antigenically committed T cells exit the thymus through the blood vessels and lymphatics. When these T cells encounter an antigen they can bind with, they are stimulated to proliferate. This step differs from the proliferation that occurred in the thymus in that (1) all the cells produced can recognize the same antigen and (2) proliferation is driven by antigen and not dependent on thymic hormones. Therefore the end product of antigen-driven proliferation is a large number of T cells capable of acting against the same antigen.

Another specialized lymphocyte, the ***NK cell,*** appears to have undergone only partial commitment to the T cell lineage. The NK cell expresses only the earliest markers of T cell differentiation such as CD2, does not bind antigen, and is not induced to proliferate by immunization with antigen. The NK cell can, however, recognize yet undefined chemical changes on the surface of virally infected cells or malignant cells, binding to its target and killing the infected or malignant cell by mechanisms similar to the Tc cell. The NK cell also has Fc receptors that can bind to the Fc region of antibody that has coated a target cell. Through these receptors the NK cell can adhere indirectly to and kill an antibody-coated target. This process is called ***antibody-dependent cellular cytotoxicity (ADCC),*** and when the cell performs this function, it has been referred to as a ***K cell.***

CELLULAR INTERACTIONS IN THE IMMUNE RESPONSE

Few antigens can directly induce B lymphocytes to become antibody-producing plasma cells. Antigens with this capacity are likely to have repeating antigenic determinants (multiple identical antigenic determinant sites). Because these antigens can stimulate B cells without the help of T cells, they are called *T-independent antigens* (Fig. 5-16). The repeating antigenic determinants interact with the B cell's membrane receptors at multiple sites, inducing the cross-linking of receptors and the activation of antibody production. Antigens that cannot induce the immune response independently must first interact with several populations of

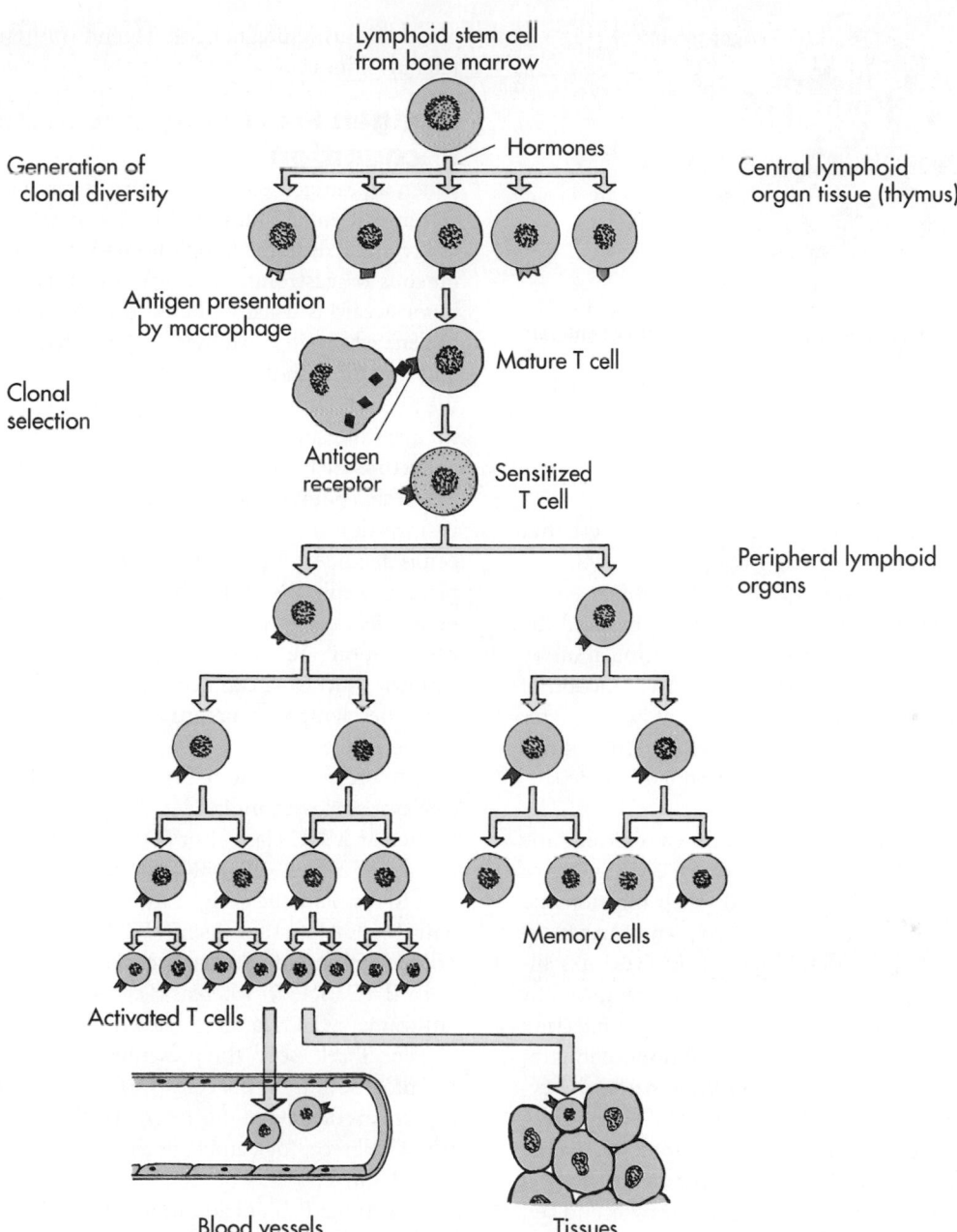

Fig. 5-15 *T cell production: generation of clones of antigen-reactive T lymphocytes.* Under the control of hormones and without antigen, T lymphocyte precursors undergo cellular division in the central lymphoid organ (the thymus) and generate receptors against all possible antigens that may be encountered in the host's adult life. Later, antigen encountered in the peripheral lymphoid organs reacts with the clones of cells expressing appropriate receptors on their surfaces, causing those cells to proliferate and produce functional T lymphocytes.

cells, including T helper (Th) cells and *antigen-presenting cells (APCs).* APCs are usually macrophage or macrophage-like cells in tissue (i.e., Langerhans cells in the skin), B cells, and endothelial cells (see Figs. 5-9 and 5-15). The immune response begins after the antigen interacts with Th cells and APCs.

Cytokines

Cytokines are secreted by cells participating in the immune response and function as messengers, providing communi-

cation among macrophages and various lymphocytes[9] (Table 5-5). During an immune response, one participant may produce a cytokine that is released, binds to a specific receptor on a neighboring cell, and instructs that target cell to respond in a genetically programmed fashion. Cytokines produced by lymphocytes are referred to as *lymphokines,* and those produced by monocytes/macrophages are called *monokines.* Because of their communications role, cytokines have been called the *hormones of the immune response.* Their effects may be on neighboring cells

Antigen receptor

T-independent antigen with repeating antigenic determinants

IgM production

B cell

Fig. 5-16 *Activation of a B cell by a T cell–independent antigen.* Repeating and identical antigenic determinants interact with several receptors on the surface of the B cell and mainly induce the production of IgM.

(paracrine), or they may bind to and affect the same cell that produced them (autocrine).

The *interleukins* (ILs) are biochemical messengers sent from one leukocyte to another. They are produced by macrophages or lymphocytes in response to stimulation by an antigen or by-products of inflammation. The function of these messengers is to enhance the response of lymphocytes and other cells to antigens and other foreign substances. They have effects on many other cells, frequently independent of antigen stimulation.

Interferon is a type of lymphokine known to defend the body against tumor cell growth and viruses. Three types of interferons have been identified, based on their function and cell origin: alpha interferon, beta interferon, and gamma interferon (IFN-α, IFN-β, and IFN-γ). Other cytokines include *tumor necrosis factors* (*TNF*-α, TNF-β) produced by macrophages, T cells, and NK cells in response to infection with gram-negative bacteria and other conditions of inflammation (see Chapter 6). *Colony-stimulating factors* are cytokines known to stimulate differentiation of blood cells. These factors are discussed in detail in Chapter 19. *Transforming growth factors* (α, β) are produced by many types of cells in response to inflammation, tumor growth, and cellular differentiation.

After cytokine stimulation, a target cell may respond in several ways. One common response is increased production of proteins that are inserted in the plasma membrane and function as receptors. Many of these receptors are specific for various cytokines. Some protect against infectious agents, such as receptors for complement component C3b or receptors for the Fc portion of antibody. Most cytokines also cause the target cell to initiate proliferation and differentiation. Because this effect is common among cytokines, different cytokines have similar effects on the same target. Cytokines must participate to develop an adequate immune response.

Cytokines are produced by various cells and guide many cellular activities. Cytokines that are growth factors induce the proliferation and differentiation of cells other than lymphocytes, for example, other hemopoietic blood cells (see Chapter 19). In addition, the development and growth of the placenta during pregnancies depend on both maternal and fetal cytokines.

Antigen Processing, Presentation, and Recognition

When an antigen enters the host, it circulates through the spleen if it enters intraperitoneally or intravenously and to the regional draining lymph nodes if it enters by the subcutaneous or gastrointestinal route. Antigen entering by the bloodstream is usually filtered through the red pulp of the spleen, where it encounters splenic lymphocytes. Antigen entering through the interstitial spaces usually is drained by the afferent lymphatics to the regional lymph nodes, where it enters the sinusoids. These spaces in the lymph node architecture are lined with phagocytic cells that ingest antigen.

At this point *antigen processing* occurs (Fig. 5-17). After its ingestion by a macrophage in the lymph node, the antigen is degraded. A portion is reexposed, or expressed, on the plasma membrane of the phagocyte, which "presents" it to T or B cells (see Figs. 5-9 and 5-15). Antigen processing and presentation are necessary for most immune responses. Antigen processing can occur at various other sites, including other lymphoid organs, the skin, and mucous membranes.

For presentation to occur effectively, the antigen must be in a complex with molecules of the MHC antigens.[10-12] The particular MHC class (I or II) that bears the antigen helps determine which cell will respond to that antigen. For Th cells to respond, the antigen must be presented in a complex with MHC class II antigens (HLA-DR, -DP, and -DQ). Th cell recognition of antigen, therefore, is referred to as "MHC class II restricted," whereas Tc and Ts cell recognition of antigen is "MHC class I restricted."

The T cell "sees" the presented antigen through a set of receptors found on the cell's surface. At least two sets of receptors participate in this interaction; one is antigen specific (the T cell receptor), and the other is independent of the presented antigen (CD4 or CD8). The *T cell receptor (TCR)* is similar to the Fab portion of an antibody, consisting of two protein chains and containing a combining site that specifically recognizes antigen. The TCR is inserted into the membrane in association with a complex referred to as CD3. CD4 (on Th cells) and CD8 (on Tc cells) are on the lymphocyte surface, independent of the TCR, and will not recognize the presented antigen directly.[13] Rather, each binds specifically to regions of the HLA molecule away from where the antigen is being presented. CD4 recognizes a particular amino acid sequence found on MHC class II molecules, and CD8 recognizes a sequence found on MHC class I molecules. Because the TCR/CD3 complex and CD4 or CD8 are holding onto the same MHC/antigen complex, the cytoplasmic portions of CD3 and CD4 or CD8 come into close proximity. The interaction of these two molecules results in communication of a signal to the cell for differentiation to begin. Additional signals are provided by other independent surface molecules that provide adhesion between the APC and Th cell.

The macrophage also produces a hormone, *interleukin-*

TABLE 5-5 Cytokines

Types	Source	Main Functions
Interleukins (IL)		
IL-1 (α and β)	Predominantly macrophages	↑ Immune response; inflammatory mediator; activates T cells; activates phagocytes; ↑
IL-2 (T cell growth factor [TCGF])	Predominantly helper T lymphocytes; NK cells	↑ T lymphocytes and NK cells; ↑ growth and ↑ T cells
IL-3 (multiple colony-stimulating factor [CSF])	T lymphocytes, mast cells, NK cells	Hematopoietic growth factor for immature hematopoietic precursor cells, ↑ NK cells
IL-4 (B cell growth factor [BCGF])	T lymphocytes, mast cells	Growth factor for T cells, activated B cells, and mast cells; macrophage-activating factor, ↑ IgE reactions
IL-5	T lymphocytes, macrophages	↑ Growth and proliferation of activated B cells, ↑ eosinophils, ↑ T cell production
IL-6	Monocytes, T and B lymphocytes, fibroblasts, endothelial cells	B cell stimulatory and differentiation factor; ↑ hematopoiesis, ↑ inflammatory response, fever
IL-7	Bone marrow, thymus	↑ Lymphoid cells
IL-8 (monocyte-derived neutrophil chemotactic factor)	Macrophages, monocytes, endothelial cells	Triggers chemotactic activity of neutrophils and lymphocytes
IL-9	Helper T cells	T cell and mast cell growth factor; maturation of erythroid progenitors
IL-10	Helper T cells	↓ Proliferation of helper T cells; ↑ cytotoxic T cell differentiation; induces MHC antigen expression, ↓ cytokines
IL-11	Fibroblasts	↑ Monocyte and B cell function, ↓ some inflammatory cytokines
IL-12	Macrophages	↑ Helper T cells and production of other lymphocytes and cytokines
IL-13	Activated T cells	↑ Gene expression in nerve and intestinal cells, ↑ osteoclasts, ↑ progenitor cells in bone marrow
IL-14	T cells	B cell growth factor
IL-15	Macrophages	Activity identical to that of IL-2
IL-16	CD8+ T cells	Chemotactic factor and growth factor for CD4+ T cells, chemotactic for eosinophils
IL-17	Helper T cells	↑ IL-6 and IL-8
Interferon (IFN)		
IFN-α	T and B lymphocytes, macrophages	Provides antiviral protection; ↓ B cell proliferation; ↓ IL-8, ↓ tumor growth, ↑ NK cell
IFN-β	Fibroblasts, macrophages, epithelial cells	Provides antiviral protection; ↑ IL-6, ↓ IL-8
IFN-γ	T lymphocytes, NK cells	Activates macrophages; ↑ B cell differentiation and NK cell activity, ↓ tumor growth
Tumor necrosis factor (TNF)		
TNF-α	Macrophages, lymphocytes, fibroblasts, endothelial cells	↑ Cytokines, ↑ inflammatory and immune responses
TNF-β	T cells	Cytotoxic to tumor cells, ↑ phagocytosis by macrophage and neutrophil, ↑ macrophages, ↑ B cell proliferation
Colony-stimulating factors (CSFs)		
G-CSF	Monocytes, fibroblasts	Myeloid growth factor
GM-CSF	T cells, fibroblasts, monocytes, endothelial cells	Myelocytic growth factor
M-CSF	Monocytes, lymphocytes, fibroblasts, endothelial and epithelial cells	Macrophage growth factor
Transforming growth factor (TGF-β)		
	Lymphocytes, macrophages, platelets, bone	Chemotactic for macrophages, ↑ IL-1 production; stimulates fibroblasts for wound healing; inhibits immune response; potentially inhibits mitotic division in other cells

↑, Increased; ↓, decreased; see text for other abbreviations.

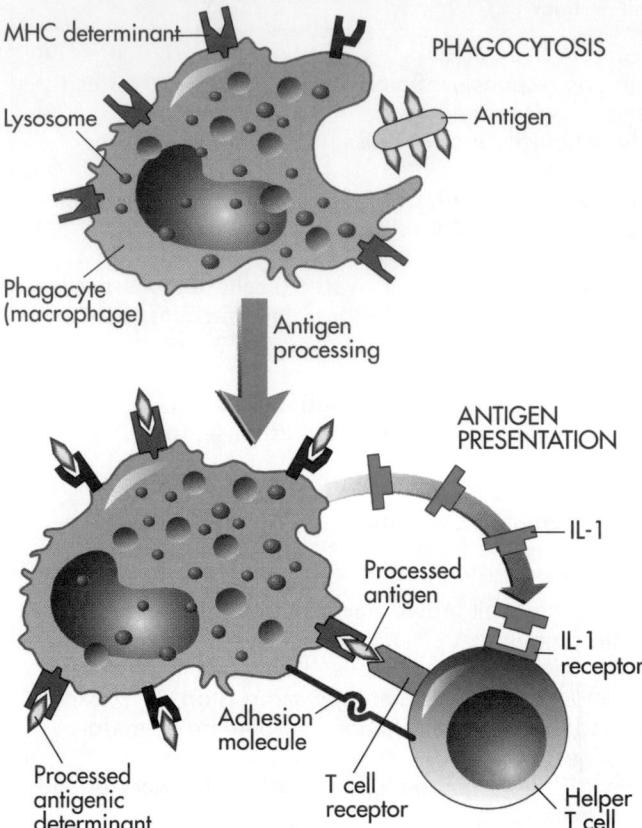

Fig. 5-17 *Antigen processing and presentation.* Circulating antigen is phagocytosed by macrophages. Remnants of the digested antigen are expressed on the membrane of the phagocyte and, in conjunction with MHC molecules, are presented to lymphocytes to initiate the immune response. The macrophage and T cell are also held together by adhesion molecules, and the macrophage produces interleukin-1 (IL-1) that helps the T cell respond to antigen.

1 (IL-1), that helps the T cell respond. During antigen presentation, IL-1 is released by the macrophage and binds to specific receptors on the surface of the Th cell. In response to these multiple signals, the Th cell produces another cytokine, IL-2, without which the Th cell cannot efficiently mature into a functional helper cell. IL-2 has an autocrine effect in that it binds to specific IL-2 receptors on the surface of the same cell that is producing it. The results of the interaction of IL-2 and its receptor are increased production of both IL-2 and IL-2 receptor, further differentiation of the Th cell, proliferation of the Th cell, and the production of other cytokines, such as IL-4 and IL-6. A summary of cellular interactions and the immune response is presented in Fig. 5-18.

A recently recognized group of antigens has the property of binding simultaneously to certain groups of TCRs at sites away from the normal antigen-specific combining site and to class II antigens (Fig. 5-19).[14] Because the antigen is not limited to reacting with only a few T cells that bear the appropriate antigen-specific TCR, many more T cells will be given an activation signal and initiate differentiation and cytokine production. The resultant increase in the immune re-

sponse has led to these antigens being referred to as *super-antigens.* Several bacteria (e.g., bacteria that cause toxic shock syndrome) secrete superantigens that induce excessive production of cytokines that cause most of the clinical symptoms of the disease.

T Cell and B Cell Differentiation
T cell differentiation
Cytotoxic T cells (Tc), which are responsible for the cell-mediated destruction of tumor cells or virally infected cells, develop when foreign antigens are presented in association with MHC class I antigens. Tc cells can see antigen on the surface of antigen-presenting cells or other target cells. The Tc cell binds presented antigen with a TCR identical with that found on Th cells. CD8 interacts with class I molecules and provides another differentiation signal. Additional adhesion molecules also must participate. A cytokine must also interact with the Tc cell to induce complete maturation and development of cytotoxic activity. IL-2 from the Th cell fulfills this role.

B cell differentiation
B lymphocytes also can recognize antigen, either on the surface of antigen-presenting cells or in soluble form. The antibody response of the B lymphocyte is controlled by hormones (IL-4 and other interleukins) secreted by the activated Th cell. Some of these hormones probably mimic the effects of antigens. Interleukins are not antigen-specific, so the Th cell activated by one antigenic determinant can produce a factor that facilitates the production of antibody against another antigenic determinant.

B cell differentiation proceeds through multiple stages, under the control of cytokines. After interacting with antigen, B cells proliferate and differentiate into plasma cells with no further capacity to undergo cell division. IL-4 and IL-5 most likely provide some of the signals to begin differentiation and proliferation. Most cytokines are produced by Th cells, and each binds to its target through specific cell membrane receptors. As a result of this process, individual B cells may change the class of antibody they are producing from IgM to IgG, IgA, or IgE (class switch).

Control of B Cell and T Cell Development
The immune system is activated only during time of need and then completely or partially turned off after the threat to the individual has been repelled. It is normally prevented from recognizing and rejecting its own tissue.

Helper T lymphocytes recently have been divided into two subsets (Th1, Th2). Th1 cells may be important to the development of Tc cells, whereas Th2 cells may play more of a role in B cell development.

Several suppressor cells, including Ts cells and some monocytes and macrophages, may control both the humoral and cell-mediated activities of the immune system. Suppressor cells vary in specificity, with some being antigen-specific

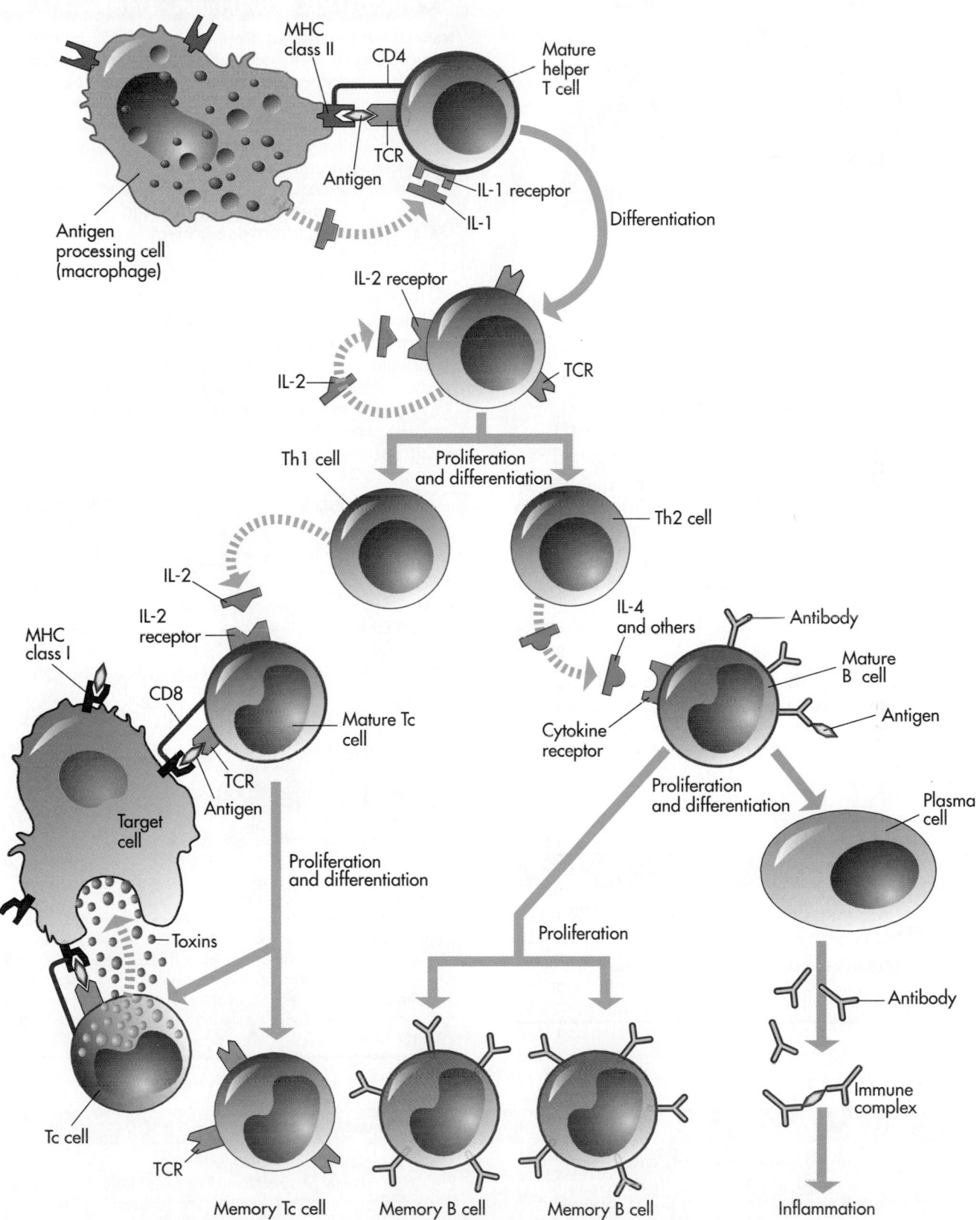

Fig. 5-18 Cellular interactions and the immune response. Schematic showing activation and differentiation of T and B cell immune responses. *Solid arrows* indicate differentiation steps. *Hatched arrows* indicate indirect effects through cytokine.

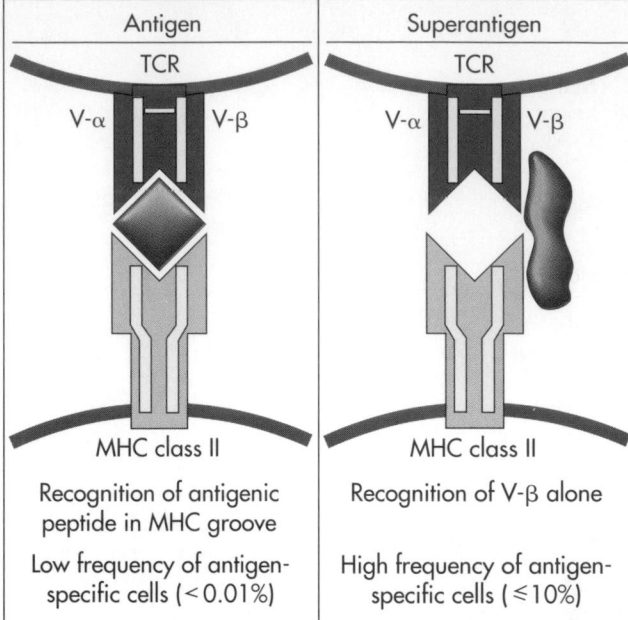

Antigen	Superantigen
TCR	TCR
V-α V-β	V-α V-β
MHC class II	MHC class II
Recognition of antigenic peptide in MHC groove	Recognition of V-β alone
Low frequency of antigen-specific cells (<0.01%)	High frequency of antigen-specific cells (≤10%)

Fig. 5-19 *Superantigens.* The T cell receptor (TCR) and major histocompatibility complex (MHC) class II molecule are normally held together by processed antigen. Superantigens, such as some bacterial exotoxins, bind directly to the variable region of the TCR-β chain and the MHC class II molecule. Each superantigen activates distinct sets of V-β chains independently of the antigen specificity of the TCR.

and others relatively nonspecific. Some suppressor cells affect the recognition of antigen, and others suppress the proliferative steps that follow antigen recognition. Some suppression appears to result from differential functions of Th1 and Th2 cells.

✓ QUICK CHECK

Why is the macrophage important for antigen processing?

Why are cytokines important to the immune response?

How are B and T cells differentiated?

⚠ PEDIATRICS & *Immune Function*

Normal human infants are immunologically immature when born, with deficiencies in antibody production, phagocytic activity, and complement activity.

The fetus in the last trimester can produce a primary immune response (IgM; T-cell independent) to antigenic challenge in utero and to infections (e.g., cytomegalovirus, rubella virus, and *Toxoplasma gondii*) but cannot produce sufficient IgG response, and only limited amounts of IgA can be detected.

Maternal antibodies provide protection within the fetal circulation.

Trophoblasts separate maternal and fetal blood so that immunoglobulins cannot cross; however, trophoblast cells actively **transport** immunoglobulins.

At birth, total IgG levels are near adult levels.

After birth, antibody titers drop as maternal antibody is catabolized, reaching a minimum at 5 to 6 months; transient hypogammoglobulinemia can then occur.

Recurrent respiratory tract infections are common during this period of immune insufficiency.

Unn Fig. 5-B, *Transport of IgG across the trophoblast.* The transport of maternal IgG across the trophoblast and into the fetal circulation is an active process. Maternal IgG binds to Fc receptors on the surface of the trophoblast and is enclosed in vacuoles by the process of endocytosis. Receptors on the trophoblast are specific for the Fc portion of IgG and do not bind other classes of immunoglobulins. The interaction of IgG with the receptors protects the antibody from digestion during transport of the vacuole across the cell. On the fetal side, IgG is released into the fetal circulation by exocytosis (see Chapter 1).

⚠ AGING & *Immune Function*

Immune function decreases with age, with diminished T cell function and antibody responses to antigenic challenge; however, circulating autoantibodies and immune complexes increase.

Spontaneous monoclonal antibody production also increases without B cell malignancies (myeloma).

Thymus reaches maximum size at sexual maturity and then undergoes involution until it is vestigial remnant by middle age; by 45 to 50 years of age thymus is only 15% of maximum size.

Thymic hormone production drops, as does the organ's ability to mediate T cell differentiation.

T cell function deteriorates although the number of T cells does not drop.

Those older than 60 years have decreased delayed hypersensitivity responses, decreased T cell–mediated responses to infections, and decreased T cell activity.

⊞ DID YOU UNDERSTAND?

Characteristics of the Immune Response

1. Immunity is a state of protection, primarily against infectious agents, characterized by memory and specificity.
2. Antigens are substances that react with components of the immune response. Most antigens can also induce an immune response.
3. Self-antigens are antigens on host cells. Self-antigens are normally not recognized as immunogenic by the host's immune system, a condition known as *tolerance*.

Induction of the Immune Response

1. The immune response is characterized by the activation of two types of immunocytes: B lymphocytes (B cells) and T lymphocytes (T cells). The activities of B cells compose the humoral immune response; those of T cells compose the cell-mediated immune response.
2. A B cell develops from a stem cell that matures under hormonal control in bursal-equivalent tissues and develops into a mature plasma cell capable of producing antibody against a specific antigen.
3. Antibodies are plasma glycoproteins that can be classified by chemical structure and biologic activity as IgG, IgM, IgA, IgE, or IgD.
4. Antibodies may protect the host from harmful antigens by recognizing and binding with the antigen's antigenic determinant sites. Occupied antigenic determinants on viruses and bacterial toxins cannot bind with receptors on host cells and therefore cannot have injurious effects.
5. The protective effects of antibodies vary with the identity of the antigen. Antibodies opsonize bacteria, neutralize toxins and viruses, and activate inflammatory processes.
6. Antibodies of the systemic immune system function internally, in the bloodstream and tissues. Antibodies of the secretory, or mucosal, immune system function externally, in the secretions of mucous membranes.
7. A T cell develops from a stem cell that matures under hormonal control in the thymus and develops into a cytotoxic T cell, which can kill target cells directly; a delayed hypersensitivity T cell, which produces lymphokines that affect other cells (especially macrophages); a helper T cell, which induces B cells to produce antibody; or a suppressor T cell, which suppresses immune function.
8. Antibody production is the final stage of a process requiring the interaction of B cells, helper T cells, and antigen-presenting cells.

Cellular Interactions in the Immune Response

1. Antigens that cannot induce the immune response independently must first interact with several populations of cells, including T helper cells and macrophages (as antigen-presenting cells).
2. Cytokines are proteins or glycoproteins secreted by cells participating in the immune response. They function as messengers, enabling communication among macrophages and lymphocytes.
3. When an antigen enters a host, it first equilibrates throughout body fluids. Eventually, antigen encounters macrophages, for example, by circulating through interstitial spaces in the lymph node. At this point, antigen processing occurs.
4. For antigen presentation to lymphocytes to occur, it must be in a complex with molecules of MHC class I antigens or MHC class II antigens. For Th cells to respond, the antigen must be presented in a complex with MHC class II antigens. For Tc cells and Ts cells to respond, the antigen must be presented in a complex with MHC class I antigens. During antigen presentation, interleukin-1 (IL-1) is released by the macrophage and binds to receptors of the Th cell. The Th cell then responds by producing IL-2. IL-4, IL-5, and others most likely provide a signal to begin differentiation and proliferation of B lymphocytes for antibody production.

⩗ PEDIATRICS & IMMUNE FUNCTION

1. Mechanisms of self-defense are naturally somewhat deficient in the fetus, the neonate, and the elderly individual (see below).
2. The T cell−independent immune response is adequate in the fetus and neonate, but the T cell−dependent immune response develops slowly during the first 6 months of life.
3. Maternal IgG antibodies protect the neonate for the first 6 months, after which they are catabolized.

⋀ AGING & IMMUNE FUNCTION

1. T cell function and antibody production in response to specific antigenic challenge are somewhat deficient in elderly persons. Elderly individuals also tend to have increased levels of circulating autoantibodies (antibodies against self-antigens).

KEY TERMS

ABO blood group, 133
Acquired immunity, 128
Active acquired immunity, 128
Agglutination, 137
Antibody, 125, 134
Antibody-dependent cellular
    cytotoxicity (ADCC), 142
Antigen, 127, 132
Antigen-antibody complex, 139
Antigen-binding fragment (Fab), 136
Antigenic determinant (epitope), 132
Antigen processing, 144
Antigen-presenting cell (APC), 143
B lymphocyte (B cell), 127
Blood group antigen, 133
Cell-mediated immunity, 129
Clonal selection, 134
Colony-stimulating factor, 144
Crystalline fragment (Fc), 136
Cytokine, 143
Cytotoxic (Tc) cell, 141
Helper T (Th) cell, 141
Histocompatibility antigen (HLA
    antigen, HLA determinant), 132
Human bursal equivalent, 134

Humoral immunity, 129
Immune complex, 139
Immune response (immunity), 125
Immune response gene (Ir gene), 133
Immunity, 128
Immunoglobulin, 134
Inflammatory response
    (inflammation), 125
Interferon, 144
Interleukin, 144
Interleukin-1 (IL-1), 144
Isohemagglutinin, 133
K cell, 142
Leukocyte, 127
Lymphocyte, 127, 129
Lymphoid, 127
Lymphokine, 143
Lymphokine-producing cell, 141
Major histocompatibility complex
    (MHC), 132
Memory cell, 141
Monokine, 143
Myeloid, 127
Natural immunity, 128
Neutralization, 139

NK cell, 142
Opsonin, 140
Opsonization, 140
Passive acquired immunity, 128
Phagocytosis, 139
Plasma cell, 134
Precipitation, 137
Primary immune response, 129
Rh blood group, 133
Secondary (anamnestic) immune
    response, 129
Secretory (mucosal) immune
    system, 140
Self-antigen, 132
Superantigen, 146
Suppressor T (Ts) cell, 141
Systemic immune system, 140
T cell receptor (TCR), 144
T lymphocyte (T cell), 127
Thymus, 141
Tolerance, 132
Transforming growth factor, 144
Tumor necrosis factor (TNF), 144
Vaccine, 129

REFERENCES

1. Rote, N.S. (1982). Pathophysiology of Rh isoimmunization. *Clinical Obstetrics and Gynecology, 25,* 243-254.

2. Huang, C.H. (1997). Molecular insights into the Rh protein family and associated antigens. *Current Opinion in Hematology, 4,* 94-103.

3. Glick, B., Chang, T.S., & Jaap, R.G. (1956). The bursa of Fabricius and antibody production. *Poultry Science, 35,* 224-225.

4. Porter, R.R. (1959). The hydrolysis of rabbit gamma-globulin and antibodies with crystalline papain. *Biochemistry Journal, 73,* 119.

5. Brown, T.A. (1996). Immunity at mucosal surfaces. *Advances in Dental Research, 10,* 62-65.

6. Orlando, S. (1995). The immunologic significance of breast milk. *Journal of Obstetric, Gynecologic, & Neonatal Nursing, 24,* 678-683.

7. Roitt, I., Brostoff, J., & Male, D. (1998). *Immunology* (5th ed.). St. Louis: Mosby.

8. McCoy, K.L. (1998). Programmed B and T cell development. *Nutrition Reviews, 56,* S19-S26.

9. Bellanti, J.A., Kadlee, J.V., & Escobar-Gutierrez, A. (1994). Cytokines and the immune response. *Pediatric Clinics of North America, 41,* 597-621.

10. Krensky, A.M. (1997). The HLA system, antigen processing and presentation. *Kidney International, 58*(Suppl.), S2-S7.

11. Yewdell, J.W. et al. (1998). TAP-independent delivery of antigenic peptides to the endoplasmic reticulum: Therapeutic potential and insights into TAP-dependent antigen processing. *Journal of Immunotherapy, 21,* 127-131.

12. Fourie, A.M. & Yang, Y. (1998). Molecular requirements for assembly and intracellular transport of class I major histocompatibility complex molecules. *Current Topics in Microbiology and Immunology, 232,* 49-74.

13. Zamoyska, R. (1998). CD4 and CD8: Modulators of T-cell receptor recognition of antigen and of immune responses? *Current Opinion in Immunology, 10,* 82-87.

14. Michie, C.A. & Cohen, J. (1998). The clinical significance of T-cell superantigens. *Trends in Microbiology, 6,* 61-65.

CHAPTER

6

Inflammation

Neal S. Rote

Inflammation is a biochemical and cellular process that occurs in vascularized tissues. Most of the essential components of the inflammatory process are found in the circulation, and most of the early mediators (facilitators) of inflammation increase the movement of plasma and blood cells from the circulation into the tissues surrounding the injury. These substances, known collectively as **exudate**, defend the host against infection and facilitate tissue repair and healing.

The superficial hallmarks of inflammation include redness (rubor), swelling (tumor), heat (calor), pain (dolor), and loss of function (functio laesa). In the nineteenth century, Julius Cohnheim observed three characteristic changes in the microcirculation (arterioles, capillaries, venules) near the site of an injury. He saw that (1) blood vessels were dilated, increasing blood flow to the area; (2) vascular permeability was increased, resulting in the outward leakage of plasma, which formed an inflammatory exudate; and (3) white blood cells adhered to the inner walls of vessels and then emigrated through vessel walls to the site of injury.

Inflammation and repair can be divided into several phases (Fig. 6-1). Early inflammatory responses differ from later responses, and each phase involves different biochemical mediators and cells that function together to (1) destroy injurious agents and remove them from the inflammatory site; (2) wall off and confine these agents so as to limit their effects on the host; (3) stimulate and enhance the immune response; and (4) promote healing.

In contrast to the immune system, which is antigen-specific and has memory, the inflammatory response is nonspecific because it takes place in about the same way no matter what the stimulus and occurs in the same manner even on second exposure to the same stimulus. Unlike chronic inflammation, the acute response is self-limiting; that is, it continues only until the threat to the host is eliminated. This usually takes 8 to 10 days from onset to healing. Inflammation is considered chronic if it persists longer than 2 weeks.

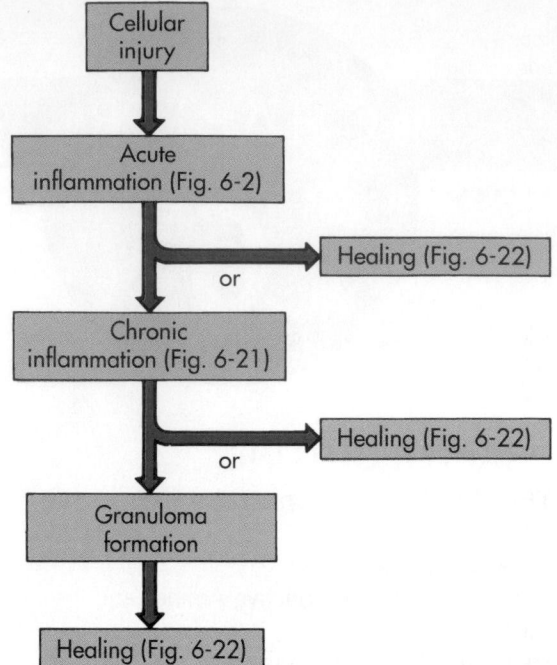

Fig. 6-1 *The inflammatory process.* Cellular injury leads to acute inflammation, which may result either in resolution and healing of the injured site or in progression into chronic inflammation. Chronic inflammation, in turn, may result either in healing or in progression into the development of a granuloma. The final step of the process is usually healing and reconstruction of the damaged tissue. For more detailed information on each portion of the process, see the figures referred to in the illustration.

THE ACUTE INFLAMMATORY RESPONSE

The acute inflammatory response begins after lethal or non-lethal cellular injury (Fig. 6-2) from trauma (mechanical forces), oxygen or nutrient deprivation, genetic or immune defects, chemical agents, microorganisms, temperature extremes, or ionizing radiation. (Mechanisms of cellular injury are described in Chapter 3.) Inflammation also is triggered by the presence of dead cells, which may be host cells, microorganisms, or cells of dead parasites.

Unlike the immune response, which takes days to develop, the vascular effects of inflammation are immediate, occurring in seconds. First, arterioles near the site of injury constrict briefly. Then they dilate, which increases blood flow to the inflamed site, increases pressure in the microcirculation, and increases the exudation of plasma and blood cells into the tissues, leading to edema and swelling. As plasma moves outward, blood remaining in the microcirculation flows more slowly and becomes more viscous (thick and sticky). Leukocytes (white blood cells) migrate to vessel walls and adhere there, while biochemical mediators stimulate the endothelial cells that line capillaries and venules to retract, creating spaces at junctions between the cells. (Inter-

cellular junctions are described in Chapter 1.) The leukocytes, which otherwise could not penetrate vessel walls, are able to squeeze out through the spaces created by endothelial retraction (Fig. 6-3).

This state of vascular permeability continues throughout acute inflammation, permitting blood cells and plasma proteins to move continuously into inflamed tissues. Once in the tissues, these cells and proteins (1) stimulate and control subsequent inflammatory processes and (2) interact with components of the immune response.

Neutrophils are the first phagocytic leukocytes to arrive at the inflamed site. They ingest bacteria, dead cells, and cellular debris and then die and are removed as pus through the epithelium or the lymphatic system. (The lymphatic system is described in Chapter 22.) The next phagocytes on the scene are monocytes and macrophages, which perform many of the same functions as neutrophils but for a longer time and later in the inflammatory response. Other cells found in inflamed tissues are eosinophils, which help to control the inflammatory response or act directly against parasites; basophils, which have a function similar to that of mast cells (described below); and ***platelets,*** which are cytoplasmic fragments that stop bleeding if vascular injury has occurred (see Chapter 19).

The cells and platelets carry out their roles with the assistance of the complement, clotting, and kinin systems and immunoglobulins. All of these cells and protein systems, along with the substances they produce, act at the site of tissue injury to kill microorganisms and remove the debris of "battle," including exudate and dead cells. This prepares the lesion for tissue regeneration or repair, the process known as resolution.

Like inappropriate immune processes, inappropriate or exaggerated inflammatory processes have deleterious effects on the host. Even appropriate inflammation can be painful and harm healthy tissues. Further, because it is complex and nonspecific and can be triggered and maintained by many different stimuli, inflammation is often difficult to control with drugs. (See Chapter 7 for a discussion of exaggerated, deficient, or inappropriate immune and inflammatory processes.)

The acute inflammatory response is a complex system of interactions that frequently begins with degranulation of mast cells and ends with healing.

THE MAST CELL

The mast cell is probably the most important activator of the inflammatory response (Fig. 6-4). *Mast cells* are cellular bags of granules located in the loose connective tissues close to blood vessels.[1] *Basophils* are found in the blood and probably function in the same way as tissue mast cells. Mast cells activate the inflammatory response through (1) *degranulation,* by which they release preformed granular contents into the extracellular matrix, and (2) synthesis of certain mediators in response to a stimulus.

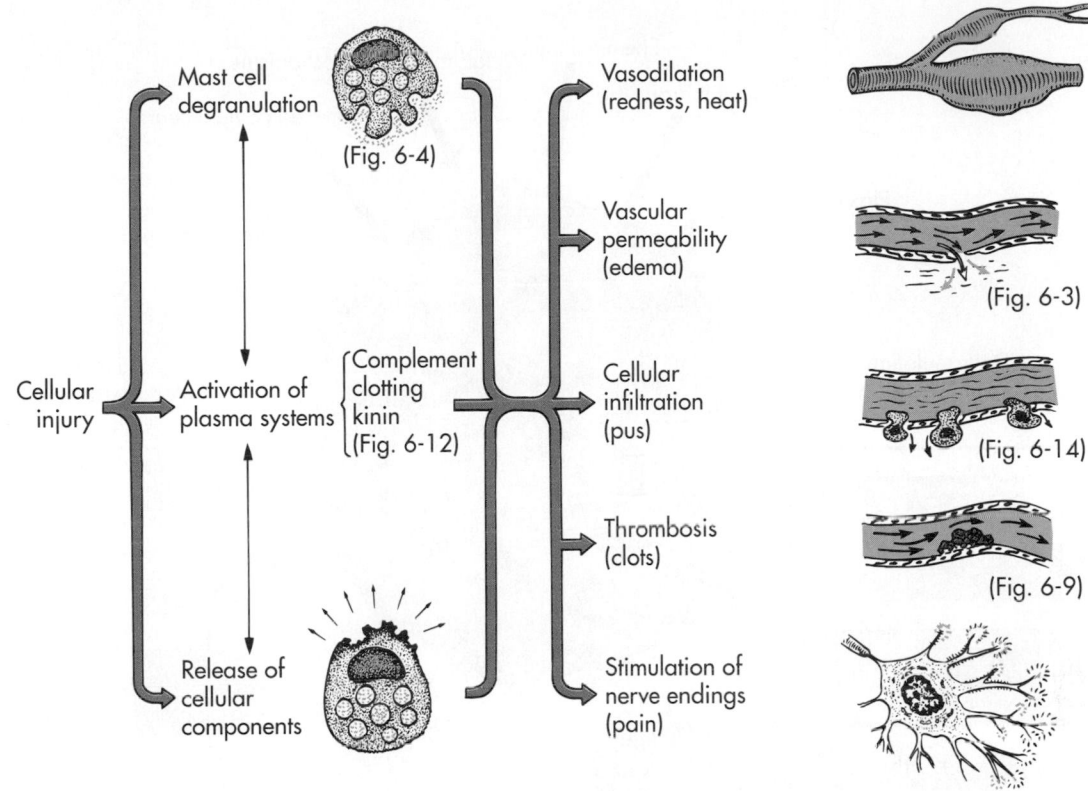

Fig. 6-2 *The acute inflammatory response.* Inflammation is initiated usually by cellular injury. Mast cell degranulation, the activation of three plasma systems, and the release of subcellular components from the damaged cells occur as a consequence of cellular injury. These systems are interdependent, so that induction of one (e.g., mast cell degranulation) can result in the induction of the other two. The end result is the development of microscopic changes in the inflamed site, as well as characteristic clinical manifestations. For more detailed information on each portion of the response, see the figures referred to in the illustration.

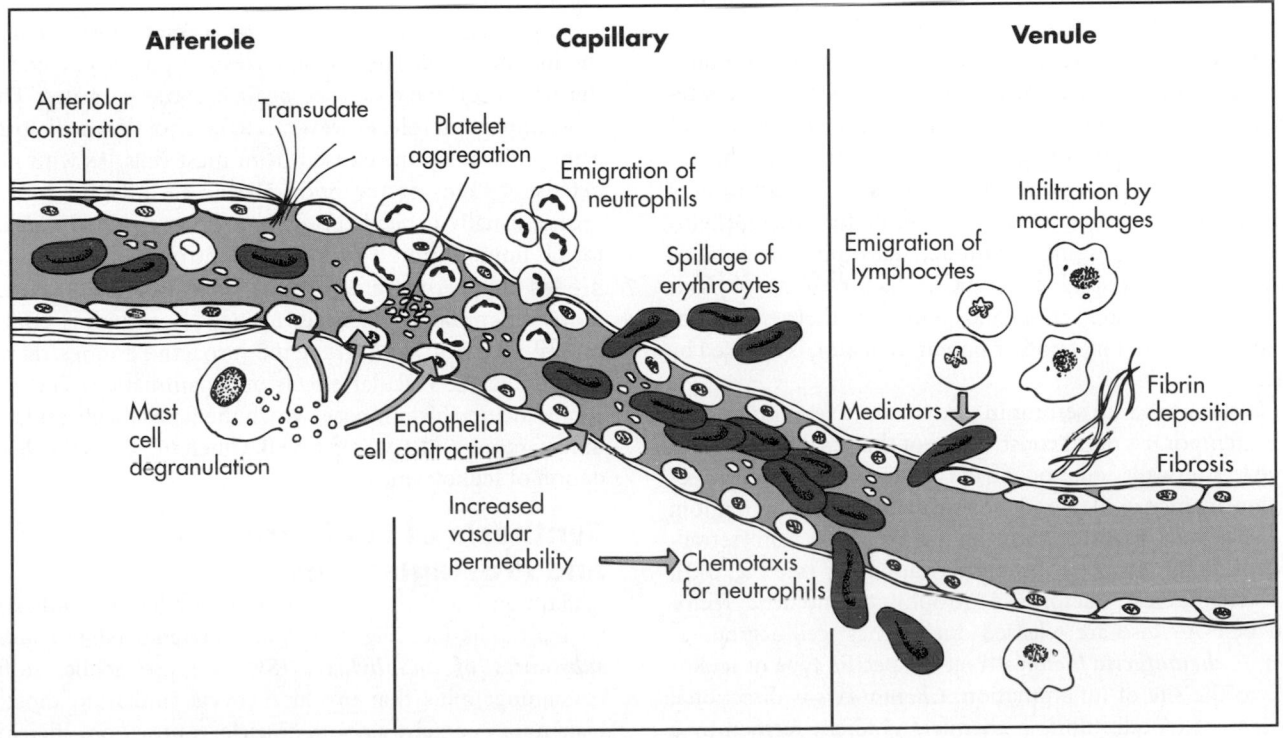

Fig. 6-3 *The sequence of events in the process of inflammation.* See text for details.

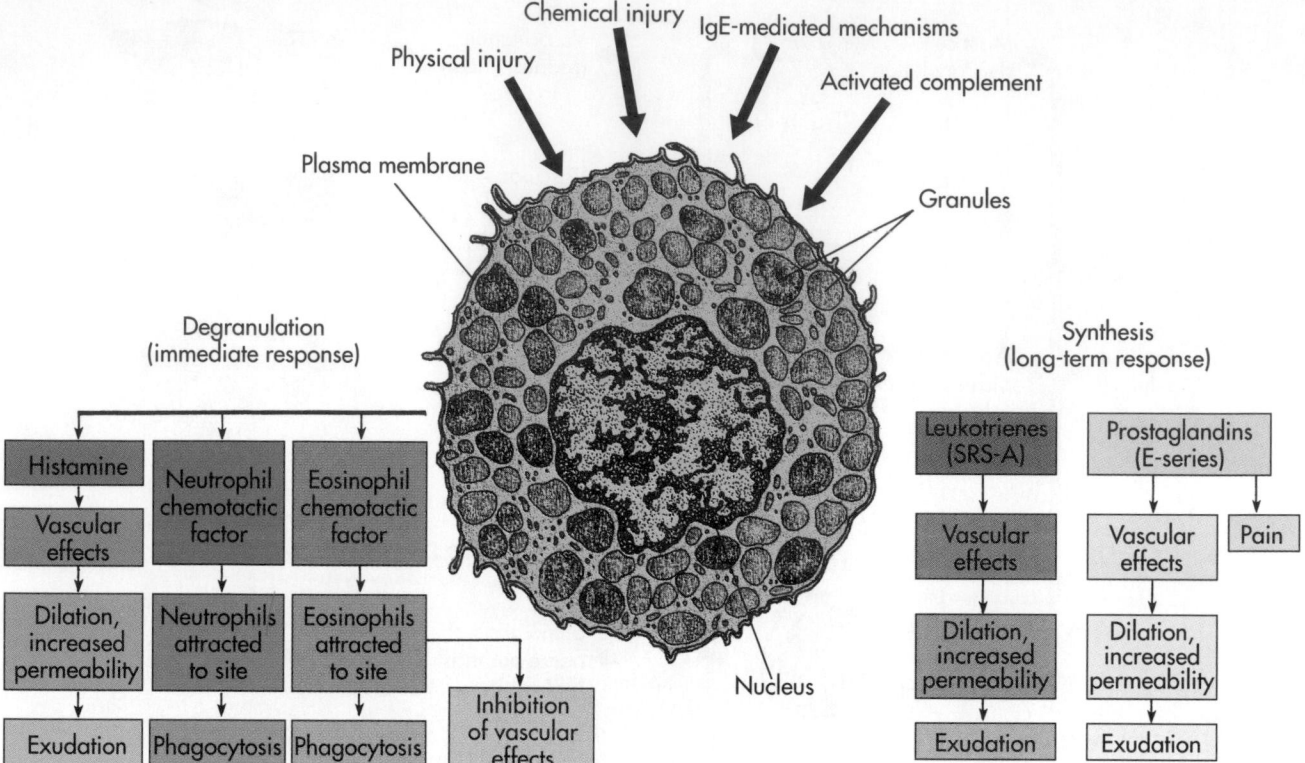

Fig. 6-4 *Effects of degranulation* (left) *and synthesis* (right) *by mast cells.* The electron micrograph of a tissue mast cell shows darkly stained granules in the cytoplasm (x9200). SRS-A, Slow-reacting substances of anaphylaxis.

Degranulation of Vasoactive Amines and Chemotactic Factors

Mast cell degranulation is stimulated by (1) physical injury, such as heat, mechanical trauma, ultraviolet light, or x-rays; (2) chemical agents, such as toxins, snake and bee venoms, tissue proteases (enzymes), dextran, or a cationic protein released from neutrophils; or (3) immunologic means, such as the triggering of immunoglobulin E (IgE)–mediated hypersensitivity reactions, or direct processes, such as activation of complement components (see p. 156). Preformed biochemical mediators, including histamine, neutrophil chemotactic factor, and eosinophil chemotactic factor of anaphylaxis (ECF-A), are released in seconds and exert their effects immediately. Serotonin, another potent mediator, is released by platelets.

Histamine and serotonin are vasoactive amines that cause temporary, rapid constriction of the smooth muscle of large vessel walls; dilation of the postcapillary venules, resulting in increased blood flow into the microcirculation; and increased vascular permeability, resulting from retraction of endothelial cells lining the capillaries (see Fig. 6-3). Two chemotactic factors—neutrophil chemotactic factor and ECF-A—also are released during mast cell degranulation. A *chemotactic factor* attracts a specific type of leukocyte to the site of inflammation. *Chemotaxis* is directional movement of cells along a chemical gradient formed by a chemotactic factor (Fig. 6-5). Neutrophil chemotactic factor

attracts neutrophils to the site of inflammation. Neutrophils are the predominant leukocytes at work during the early phases of acute inflammation.

Eosinophil chemotactic factor attracts eosinophils to the inflamed site. These leukocytes are phagocytic and are the body's primary defense against some parasites. Their most important role, however, is to control the mediators of acute inflammation released from mast cells. As with most defense systems of the body, the acute inflammatory response usually is needed only in a circumscribed area and for a limited time. Therefore control mechanisms are needed to prevent biochemical mediators from evoking more inflammation than is needed. Eosinophils contain several enzymes that degrade the vasoactive amines, thereby controlling the vascular effects of inflammation. These enzymes include histaminase, which mediates the degradation of histamine, and arylsulfatase B, which mediates the degradation of leukotrienes.

Synthesis of Leukotrienes and Prostaglandins

Leukotrienes and prostaglandins are mediators synthesized by mast cells (see Fig. 6-4).[2] *Leukotrienes (slow-reacting substances of anaphylaxis [SRS-A])* are acidic, sulfur-containing lipids that produce effects similar to those of histamine—namely, smooth muscle contraction, increased vascular permeability, and neutrophil and eosinophil

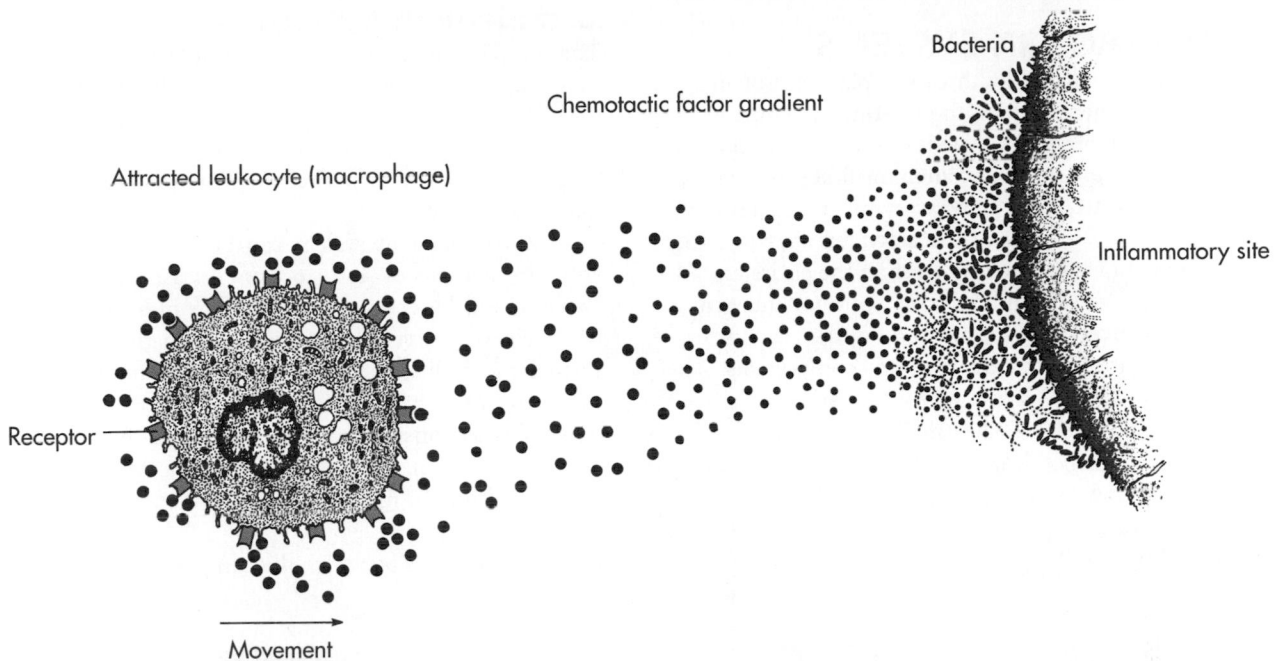

Fig. 6-5 *Chemotaxis.* Multiple receptors on the leukocyte's plasma membrane sense the area of highest concentration of a chemotactic factor *(dots)*, and the leukocyte (usually a phagocyte) moves toward this area.

chemotaxis. Leukotrienes appear to be important in the later stages of the inflammatory response, because they stimulate slower and more prolonged responses than do histamines. Leukotrienes are produced from a lipid, arachidonic acid, released from mast cell membranes.

The mast cell also synthesizes ***prostaglandins,*** which cause increased vascular permeability and neutrophil chemotaxis and induce pain. Prostaglandins are long-chain, unsaturated fatty acids produced from arachidonic acid. They are classified into groups (E, A, F, B) according to their structure. Prostaglandins E_1 and E_2 probably cause increased vascular permeability and smooth muscle contraction; they appear to act directly on postcapillary venules. They can also inhibit some aspects of inflammation by suppressing the release of histamine from mast cells and lysosomal enzymes from neutrophils, and they cause pain. Enhancement or suppression of the inflammatory response may be related to concentrations of prostaglandins. Aspirin and some other nonsteroidal antiinflammatory agents block the synthesis of prostaglandins, thereby inhibiting inflammation.

HEALTH ALERT

New Antiinflammatory Drugs

A new class of nonsteroidal antiinflammatory drugs (NSAIDs) has recently been developed for the control of pain and inflammation. The new agents, known as *cyclooxygenase-2 (COX-2) inhibitors,* are thought to specifically inhibit inflammation. The COX-2 inhibitors do not block the prostaglandin synthesis responsible for gastric mucus production, and thus there are fewer gastric side effects or toxic responses. They may also protect against colon cancer and lessen brain damage associated with Alzheimer disease.

Data from Bolten, W.W. (1998). Scientific rationale for specific inhibition of COX-2. Journal of Rheumatology, 51(Suppl.), 2-7; Cryer, B. & Feldman, M. (1998). Cyclooxygenase-1 and cyclooxygenase-2 selectivity of widely used nonsteroidal anti-inflammatory drugs. American Journal of Medicine, 104(5), 413-421; Vane, J.R. & Botting, R.M. (1998). Mechanism of action of antiinflammatory drugs. International Journal of Tissue Reactions, 20(1), 3-15.

✓ QUICK CHECK

What are cytokines? How do they promote inflammation?

PLASMA PROTEIN SYSTEMS

Inflammation is mediated by three key plasma protein systems: the complement system, the clotting system, and the kinin system. Each of these systems consists of a series of inactive enzymes, or **proenzymes.** When the first proenzyme in the series is converted to an active enzyme, it initiates a cascade in which the substrate of the activated enzyme is the next component of the system. Therefore the entire cascade is activated upon activation of the first component. Activation usually involves the enzyme cleaving the inactive precursor (proenzyme) into two or more components. The larger one is an active enzyme whose substrate is the next component in the system. The smaller component is frequently a potent biochemical mediator of the inflammatory response. Most of these components are short-lived, since they are inactivated rapidly by other naturally occurring plasma proteins.

Complement System

The complement system consists of at least 10 proteins and makes up 10% of the serum proteins in the circulation (Fig. 6-6).[3] This system is perhaps the most important of the plasma protein systems of inflammation because, once activated, its components participate in virtually every inflammatory response.[4]

The complement system can be activated by antigen-antibody complexes, by products released from invading bacteria, and by components of other plasma protein systems (Fig. 6-7). Even when the complement system is activated by a specific mechanism—namely, antigen-antibody complexes (the immune system)—it mediates inflammation, which is nonspecific. Thus proteins of the complement system (sometimes called *complement components*) are among the body's most potent defenders against bacterial infection.

The two routes by which the **complement cascade** is ac-

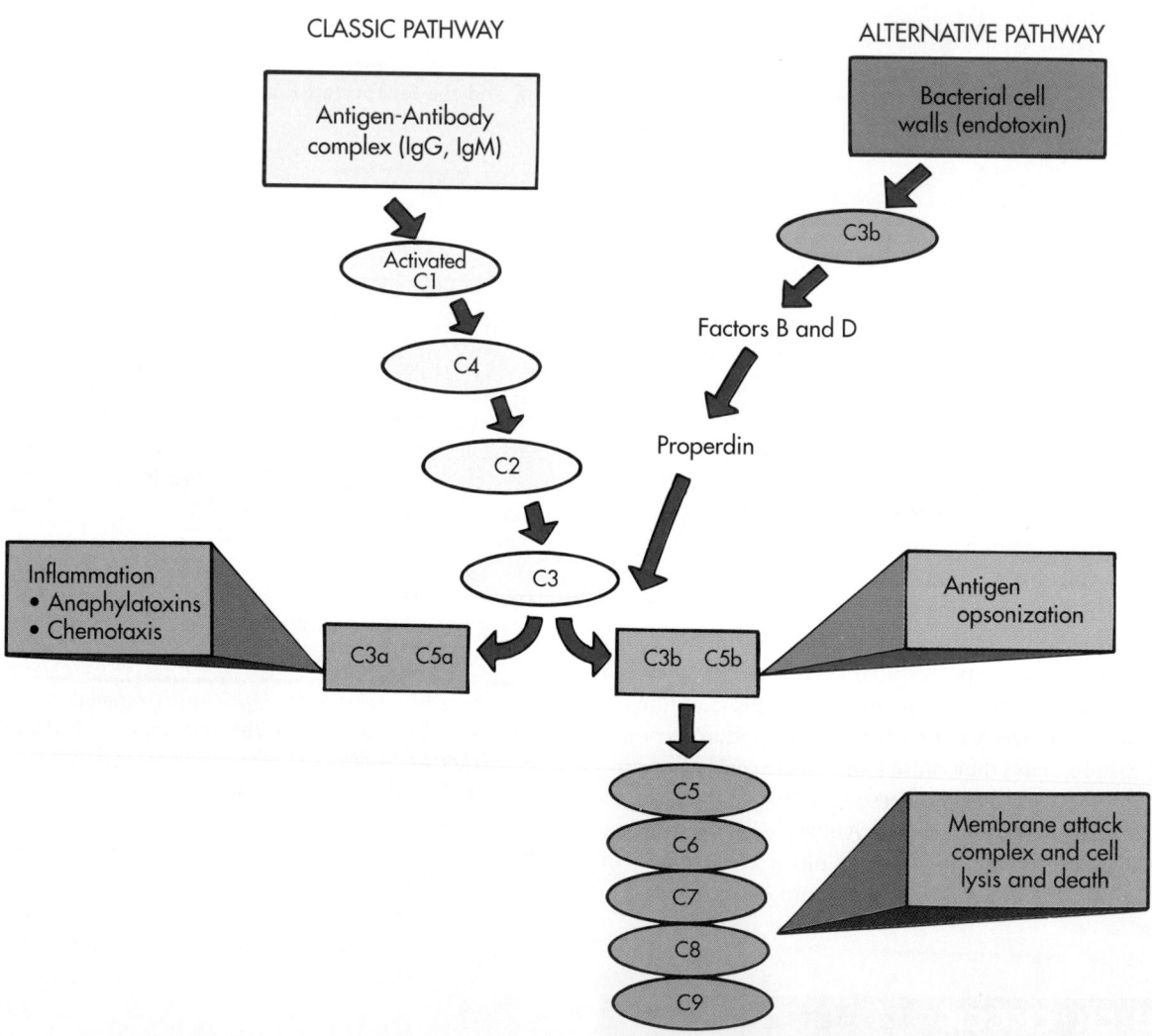

Fig. 6-6 *Pathways of activation of the complement cascade.* Complement components are cleaved into fragments (denoted by *lowercase letters*) during activation. Many of the fragments are biochemical mediators of inflammation. The classic pathway usually is activated by antigen-antibody complexes through component C1, whereas the alternative pathway is activated by many agents, such as bacterial polysaccharides, through component C3b.

Fig. 6-7 *Immunologic mechanisms that activate the inflammatory response.* Immunologic factors may affect inflammation through three mechanisms: (1) IgE can bind to the surface of a mast cell and, after binding antigen, induce the cell's degranulation; (2) antigen and antibody can form immune complexes that activate the complement cascade, releasing small polypeptide fragments, primarily C5a, that have potent biologic activities resulting in mast cell degranulation and neutrophil chemotaxis; and (3) antigen may also react with T lymphocytes, resulting in the production of lymphokines that may contribute to the development of either acute or chronic inflammation.

tivated are shown in Fig. 6-6. The *classic pathway* is activated when an antigen-antibody complex containing IgG or IgM interacts with the first component of the complement cascade, C1. The *alternative pathway* can be activated by several biologic substances, chiefly bacterial and fungal cell wall polysaccharides (especially endotoxin on gram-negative bacteria). (Bacterial endotoxins are described in Chapter 3.)

Activation of components C1 through C5 produces subunits that enhance inflammation by (1) opsonizing bacteria, (2) attracting leukocytes by chemotaxis, and (3) acting as *anaphylatoxins,* that is, inducing degranulation of mast cells. Components C6 through C9 form complexes that can create pores in cell or bacterial membranes. The pores disrupt the cell's rigid outer membrane and permit water and ions to enter, causing the cell to burst or at least preventing its reproduction. (Cellular injury is discussed in Chapter 3.)

Classic pathway

Activation of the classic pathway is preceded by formation of an *antigen-antibody (immune) complex.* Because molecules or cells tend to have more than one antigenic determinant, multiple antibodies are bound in the complex. Complement activation occurs when antibody crystallizable fragment (Fc) regions are held in close proximity. The Fc contains a site that binds C1 so that C1 is "fixed" to adjacent antibody molecules attached to the antigen. The complex formed by antigen-antibody-complement binding is shown in Fig. 6-8.

Activation of C1 results in the sequential enzymatic activation of other components of the cascade. Although the cascade continues through the terminal components C6, C7, C8, and C9, whose activation results in the lysis of cells, the importance of the complement system resides in the activi-

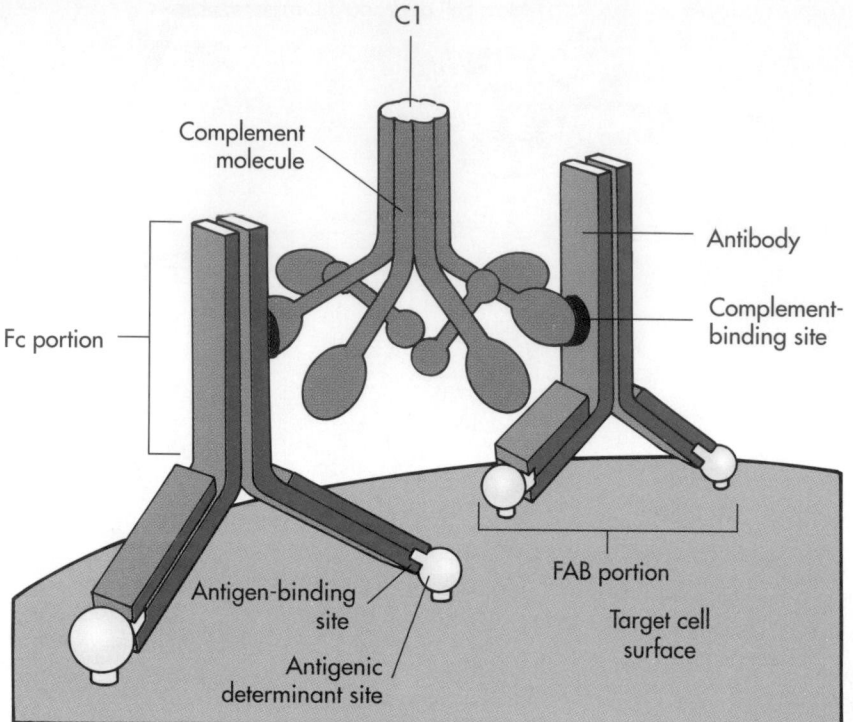

Fig. 6-8 *Activation of the first component of complement (C1).* It takes two IgG molecules to activate one complement component. Activation of complement cannot occur unless (1) antigen-antibody binding has occurred, placing two Fc regions of the antibody molecule into close proximity, and (2) the complement component can span the gap between two adjacent Fc portions.

ties of the small fragments. A fragment, C3b, that adheres to the surface of a target cell (e.g., bacterium) is an efficient opsonin. C3a and C5a, which are soluble, low-molecular-weight fragments, are potent activators of the acute inflammatory response, causing vasodilation and increased vascular permeability. C3a and C5a are anaphylatoxins; that is, they induce the rapid degranulation of mast cells, with release of histamine[5] (see Fig. 6-4).

C3a and C5a are also chemotactic for neutrophils. The dual functions (chemotactic factor and anaphylatoxin) are not needed simultaneously or to the same degree. Anaphylatoxic activity is necessary early in inflammation and close to the inflammatory site to induce local mast cell degranulation and increase the number of soluble mediators available to enhance vascular permeability. Degranulation of mast cells away from the site of injury is contrary to the protective nature of the inflammatory response because the substances released would needlessly affect healthy neighboring tissues. Chemotactic activity, on the other hand, is required for a much longer period and distal to the inflammatory site to attract leukocytes from the circulation. Therefore enzymes in the exudate can destroy the anaphylatoxic activity of C3a and C5a without affecting chemotactic activity.

Alternative pathway

There are several non-antibody-mediated (alternate) avenues of entrance into the complement cascade. (Both pathways are shown in Fig. 6-6.) The components of the alternative pathway include those listed in Fig. 6-6.

Clotting System

The clotting (coagulation) system is a plasma protein system that forms a fibrous exudate, or meshwork, at the inflamed site to trap exudates, microorganisms, and foreign bodies.[6] This (1) prevents the spread of infection and inflammation to adjacent tissues, (2) keeps microorganisms and foreign bodies at the site of greatest phagocytic activity, and (3) forms a clot that stops bleeding and provides a framework for future repair and healing. The main substance in this mesh is an insoluble protein called *fibrin*, which is the end product of the coagulation cascade.

Like the complement cascade, the coagulation cascade can be activated through two different pathways that converge where each pathway produces the same substance (Fig. 6-9). In the complement cascade the classic and alternative pathways converge when each has activated C5 (see Fig. 6-6). In the coagulation cascade the *extrinsic pathway* and the *intrinsic pathway* converge at factor X. (The coagulation cascade is discussed further and illustrated in Chapter 19.)

The clotting system can be activated by many substances released during tissue destruction and infection, including collagen, proteases, kallikrein, plasmin, and bacterial endotoxins. In addition, activation of the clotting cascade produces two low-molecular-weight fibrinopeptides. They are

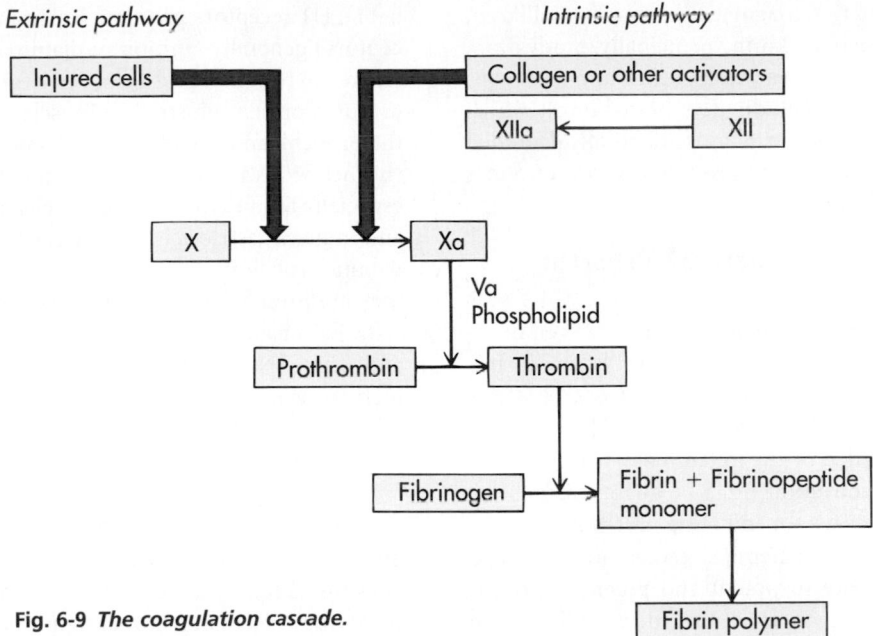

Fig. 6-9 *The coagulation cascade.*

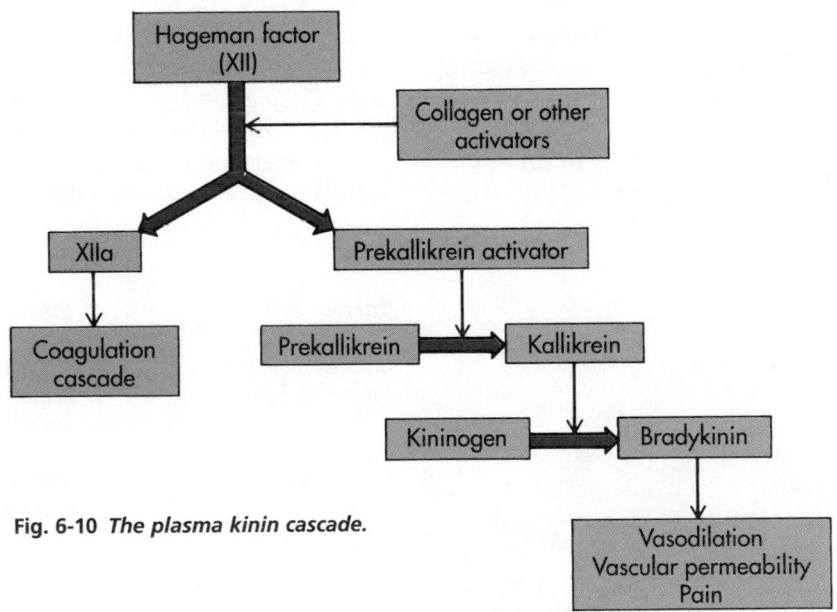

Fig. 6-10 *The plasma kinin cascade.*

released from fibrinogen during fibrin production (especially fibrinopeptide B), are chemotactic for neutrophils, and increase vascular permeability by enhancing the effects of bradykinin (formed from the kinin system).

Kinin System

The primary kinin is *bradykinin,* which, at low doses, causes dilation of vessels, acts with prostaglandins to induce pain, causes extravascular smooth muscle contraction, increases vascular permeability, and may increase leukocyte chemotaxis.[7] Bradykinin induces smooth muscle contraction more slowly than histamine and may be more important during the later phase of inflammation. Along with prostaglandins, it probably causes endothelial cell retraction (see Fig. 6-3) and increased vascular permeability.

The kinin system is activated by stimulation of the *plasma kinin cascade* (Fig. 6-10). Plasma prekallikrein is converted to kallikrein through a subunit, *prekallikrein acti-*

vator, generated from the coagulation cascade. Kallikrein then converts kininogen to kinin, principally bradykinin. Tissue kallikreins in saliva, sweat, tears, urine, and feces convert serum kininogens to kallidin (lys-bradykinin), which may be converted to bradykinin. Kinins are rapidly degraded and therefore controlled by kininases, which are enzymes present in plasma and tissues.

Control and Interaction of Plasma Protein Systems

The activation of the plasma protein systems involved in inflammation produces many potent, biologically active substances that protect the host from infection. Control of this process is essential for two reasons:

1. The protection afforded by the inflammatory process is so important that its activation must be guaranteed; therefore multiple means exist for initiating inflammation.
2. The activities of the biochemical mediators generated during this process are so potent and potentially detrimental to the host that their actions must be limited to injured or infected tissues.

Control is apparent at many levels. Many components of inflammation are destroyed within seconds by plasma enzymes. Two components of the complement cascade, C3a and C5a, are inactivated by *carboxypeptidase,* and histamine and leukotrienes are inactivated by *histaminase* and *arylsulfatase.* Other natural inhibitors include antagonists for histamine, kinins, complement components, kallikrein, and plasmin.

Histamine activity is controlled, in part, by receptors on the host's target cells, particularly H1 and H2 receptors[8] (Fig. 6-11). H1 receptors promote inflammation, whereas H2 receptors generally inhibit inflammation by suppressing leukocyte function and mast cell degranulation. The H1 receptor is present on smooth muscle cells, especially those of the bronchi, and cause bronchial smooth muscle to contract (bronchoconstriction) when stimulated. The H2 receptor is especially abundant on parietal cells of the stomach mucosa and induces gastric acid secretion when stimulated. The distribution of both types of receptors varies, and frequently they are present on the same cells and may act antagonistically. For instance, both receptors are present on neutrophils and when H1 receptors are stimulated, chemotaxis is augmented. When H2 receptors are stimulated, chemotaxis is inhibited (see discussion of allergic reactions in Chapter 7).

Most control processes interact, so that the activation of one plasma system results in a similar effect on the others (Fig. 6-12). Plasmin controls clot formation (by degrading fibrin and fibrinogen), activates the complement cascade (as does thrombin), and activates the plasma kinin cascade by activating Hageman factor and producing prekallikrein activator. The activation of Hageman factor has four effects: (1) activation of the clotting cascade through factor XI; (2) activation of the fibrinolytic systems through conversion of plasminogen proactivator to plasminogen activator, resulting in the generation of plasmin; (3) activation of the kinin system by a Hageman factor fragment, prekallikrein activator; and (4) activation of C1 in the complement cascade. Plasmin itself exists as a proenzyme, plasminogen, which is activated by several factors.

The interaction of control mechanisms is exemplified by the effects of *C1 esterase inhibitor.* Hereditary angioneu-

Target cell	Effect of histamine
Smooth muscle cell	Contraction
Endothelial cell	Contraction (retraction at endothelial junctions)
Neutrophil	Increased chemotaxis
Mast cell	Prostaglandin synthesis
Parietal cell of stomach mucosa	Secretion of gastric acid
Lymphocyte	Decreased activity
Eosinophil	Decreased activity
Neutrophil	Decreased chemotaxis
Mast cell	Decreased degranulation

Fig. 6-11 *Effects of histamine through H1 and H2 receptors.* Effects depend on (1) density and affinity of H1 and/or H2 receptors on the target cell and (2) the identity of the target cell. *GTP,* Guanosine triphosphate; *cGMP,* cyclic guanosine monophosphate; *ATP,* adenosine triphosphate; *cAMP,* cyclic adenosine monophosphate.

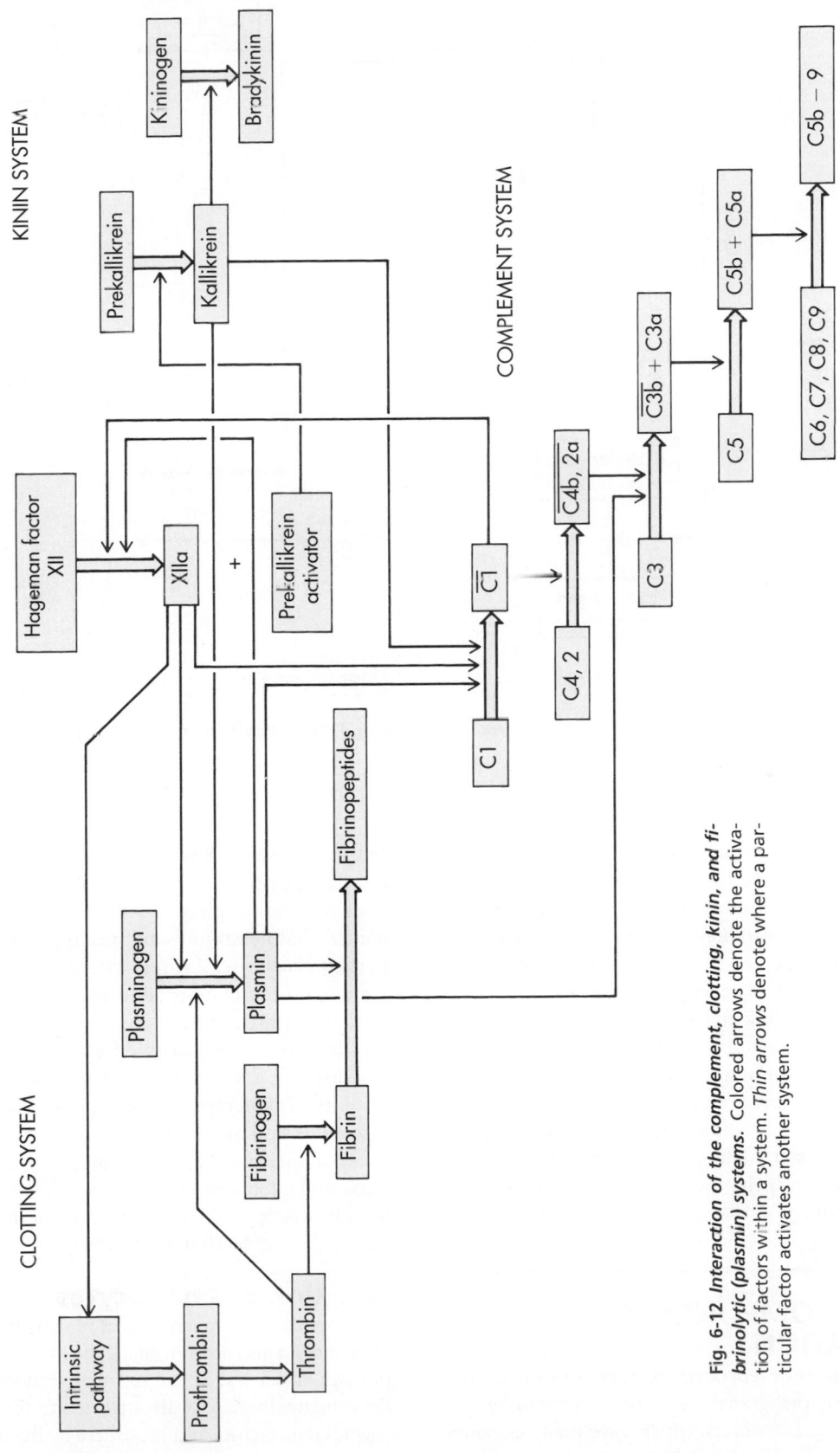

Fig. 6-12 *Interaction of the complement, clotting, kinin, and fibrinolytic (plasmin) systems.* Colored arrows denote the activation of factors within a system. *Thin arrows* denote where a particular factor activates another system.

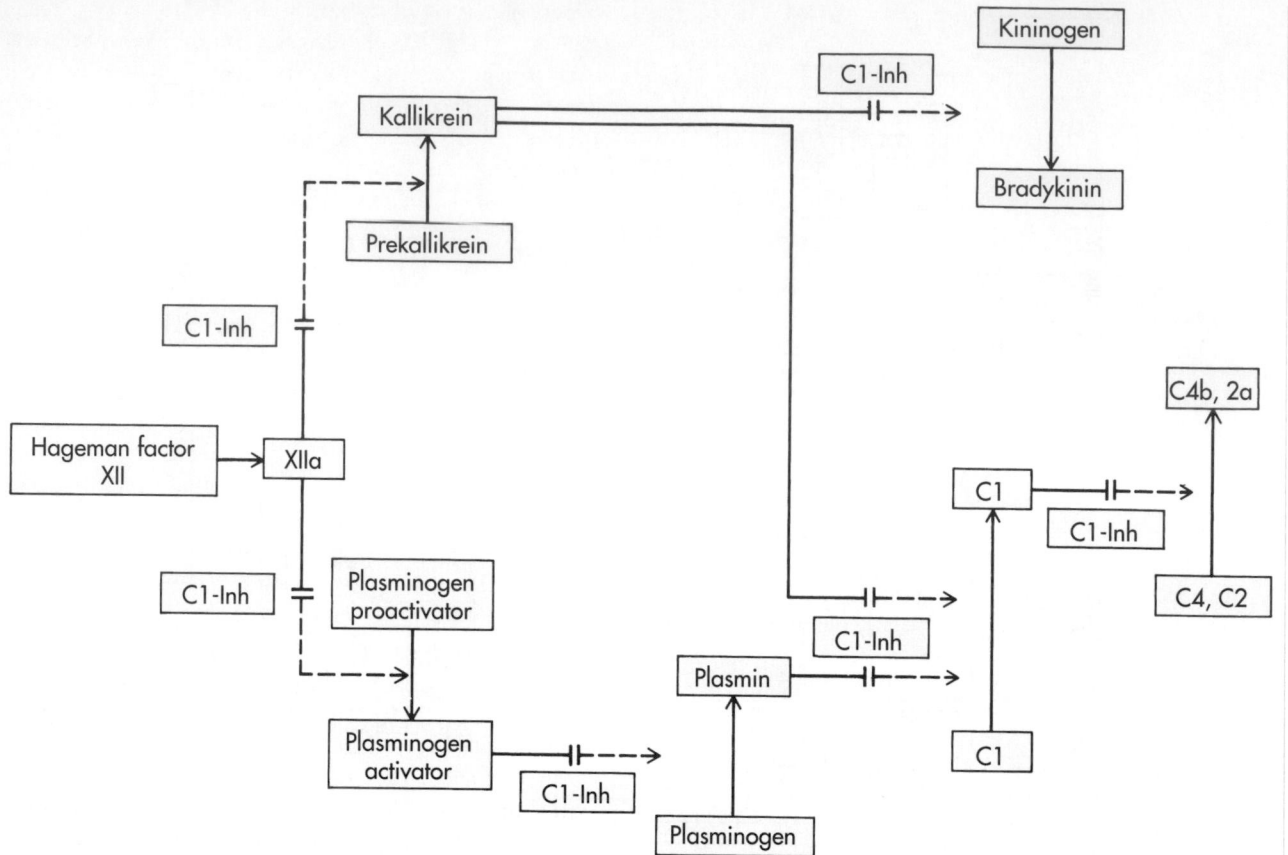

Fig. 6-13 *Common control of the complement, clotting, and kinin systems by C1 esterase inhibitor (C1-Inh).*

rotic edema is an autosomal dominant disease characterized by a deficiency of this inhibitor. In individuals with this disease, emotional stress and other stimuli frequently cause recurrent edema in the gastrointestinal tract, respiratory tract, and skin, with laryngeal swelling sometimes causing death. The mechanism appears to be episodic, uncontrolled activation of plasmin, resulting in Hageman factor activation, bradykinin production, and C1 activation. C1 esterase inhibitor blocks several steps in the activation of all three cascades (Fig. 6-13). Activation of plasmin may be the most important single cause of hereditary angioneurotic edema, as indicated by the fact that attacks are prevented by ε-aminocaproic acid, which prevents the conversion of plasminogen to plasmin.

CELLULAR COMPONENTS OF INFLAMMATION

The two main classes of leukocytes to carry out inflammatory processes are the granulocytes and the monocytes/macrophages. The granulocytes, which have many enzyme-containing lysosomal granules in their cytoplasm, include neutrophils, eosinophils, and basophils. Monocytes (the immature form in the blood) and macrophages (the mature

cell in the tissues) have fewer and larger lysosomes in their cytoplasm than do granulocytes. All of these cells are phagocytes (capable of phagocytosis, the ingestion of particulate matter), but neutrophils and macrophages are the most important phagocytes. Lymphocytes also participate in inflammation, primarily by producing soluble mediators (see the section on immunity).

Platelets are cytoplasmic fragments that circulate in the bloodstream until vascular injury occurs. After injury, platelets (1) interact with components of the coagulation cascade to stop bleeding and (2) degranulate, releasing biochemical mediators such as serotonin, which has vascular effects similar to those of histamine. Their activation is stimulated by many products of inflammation. (Platelet function is described in detail in Chapter 19.)

Function of Phagocytes

Neutrophils and macrophages normally circulate in the bloodstream and are stimulated by inflammation to migrate through vessel walls near an inflammatory lesion.[9] Once in the exudate, these cells are attracted to the lesion by specific chemotactic factors and kept there by the meshwork formed by fibrinous exudate. Once at the site, they phagocytose (ingest) foreign or dead cells until their life span is over. Dead phagocytes then become part of the purulent exudate, or

Phagocytes
in circulation

Basement membrane   Endothelial cell

Intercellular junction

Margination
(pavementing)

Diapedesis

Retracted
intercellular junction

Exudation into
inflamed
tissue

Fig. 6-14 *Diapedesis of a phagocyte.* Phagocytes are capable of ameboid movement, which allows them to squeeze through intercellular junctions and migrate to inflammatory lesions.

pus, which leaves the body through the lymphatic system or through the epithelium. Neutrophils and monocytes/macrophages differ chiefly in (1) the speed with which they arrive at the site, with the neutrophils arriving first; (2) the length of time they remain active, with the macrophages being longer-lived; (3) the chemotactic factors capable of attracting them; (4) the enzymatic content of their lysosomes, or digestive vacuoles; and (5) their participation in the immune response, with the macrophages being involved in antigen processing and responding to lymphokines.

The phagocytes' role begins when the inflammatory response causes them to stick tightly to capillary and venule walls in *margination,* or *pavementing* (Fig. 6-14). Margination is caused by increased stickiness of the phagocytes and increased adsorption by the endothelial cells lining the vessels as a result of adhesion proteins produced on the surface of each cell. This is followed by *diapedesis,* or emigration through the retracting endothelial junctions and the basement membrane and out into the surrounding tissues (see Fig. 6-3).

Once they enter the inflammatory exudate, phagocytes

progress to the inflammatory site by chemotaxis. They can detect, through chemoreceptors at multiple locations on their plasma membrane, where chemotactic factors are most highly concentrated (see Fig. 6-5) and migrate there. The primary chemotactic factors for neutrophils, eosinophils, and monocytes include bacterial products, complement components C5a and C3a, kallikrein and plasminogen activator, fibrinopeptides, products of fibrin degradation, prostaglandins, the activated C567 complex from the complement system, the eosinophil and neutrophil chemotactic factors released from mast cells, and a monocyte chemotactic factor released from the neutrophil. Histamine, although not chemotactic itself, may facilitate chemotaxis.

Phagocytosis begins when the phagocytic cell enters the inflammatory site. There are four steps: (1) recognition of the target and its adherence to the phagocyte, (2) engulfment (ingestion, or endocytosis), (3) fusion with lysosomes within the phagocyte, and (4) destruction of the target by lysosomal enzymes (lysosomes are described in Chapter 1). Throughout the process, both target and digestive enzymes are isolated within membrane-bound vesicles. Isolation protects the phagocyte from the harmful effects of target microorganisms and its own enzymes. Phagocytosis of an opsonized bacterium is illustrated in Fig. 6-15.

Most phagocytes can trap and engulf bacteria that have not been "coated" with an opsonin, but the process is slow and inefficient. Opsonization, usually by antibody or complement component C3b, greatly enhances both recognition and binding (also called *adherence*). Opsonins function as "glue" between the phagocyte and the target cell because receptors on the phagocyte are specific for sites on the opsonin (Fc receptors for antibody, C3b receptors for C3b). Thus the phagocyte can bind opsonized bacteria tightly to its surface.

Engulfment is carried out by small pseudopods that extend from the plasma membrane and surround the adhered microorganism (Fig. 6-16), forming an intracellular phagocytic vacuole, or *phagosome.* The membrane that surrounds the phagosome consists of inverted plasma membrane. After the phagosome is formed, lysosomes converge, fuse with the phagosome, and discharge their contents, creating a *phagolysosome,* where bacteria are destroyed (see Fig. 6-15).

Phagocytosis is accompanied by a burst of metabolic activity in the phagocyte, producing several oxygen-containing molecules that are highly damaging to cells (oxygen-dependent killing mechanism). The principal oxygen-dependent killing mechanism is hydrogen peroxide, especially when combined with myeloperoxidase and halide anions (I^-, Cl^-, Br^-).

The oxygen-independent mechanisms of killing are (1) acid pH (3.5 to 4.0) of the phagolysosome caused by lactic acid production; (2) cationic proteins, which bind to and damage target cell membranes; (3) lysozyme and elastase, which attack mucopeptides in the target cell wall; and (4) lactoferrin, which inhibits bacterial growth by binding iron.

When the phagocyte dies at the inflammatory site, it lyses (breaks open) and its cytoplasmic contents, including the

Fig. 6-15 *Phases of phagocytosis.* **A,** Opsonized microorganisms *(1)* bind to the surface of a phagocyte and *(2)* are ingested into a phagocytic vacuole, or phagosome *(3)*. Lysosomes fuse with the phagosome *(4)*, releasing their digestive enzymes into the vacuole. This results in the formation of a phagolysosome *(5)*, within which the microorganism is killed and digested. **B,** Enlargement showing bacterium opsonization. *IgG,* Immunoglobulin G; *C3b,* complement component.

lysosomal enzymes, are released. Enzymes released from lysosomes can digest the connective tissue matrix, causing much of the tissue destruction associated with inflammation. α_1-Antitrypsin, a plasma protein produced by the liver, inhibits the destructive effects of many enzymes released by dead phagocytes. An inherited deficiency of α_1-antitrypsin often results in long-term lung damage and emphysema as a result of tissue destruction. (The pulmonary effects of α_1-antitrypsin deficiency are described in Chapter 26.)

Released lysosomal products contribute to other aspects of inflammation, including increased vascular permeability, chemotaxis for monocytes, breakdown of connective tissues, and activation of the complement and kinin systems. [10]

Polymorphonuclear Neutrophils

The *neutrophil,* or *polymorphonuclear neutrophil (PMN),* is the predominant phagocytic cell in the early inflammatory response, entering the inflammatory site 6 to 12 hours after the initial injury. Neutrophils are attracted by the immediately generated chemotactic factors, such as complement fragments. Macrophages and lymphocytes enter the site later, usually after 24 hours, and gradually replace the neutrophils.

Because the neutrophil is a mature cell incapable of division and is sensitive to the acidic environment of inflammatory lesions, it is short-lived in the inflammatory site. Its primary roles are removal of debris in sterile lesions, such as burns, and phagocytosis of bacteria in nonsterile lesions.

Monocytes and Macrophages

The *monocyte* is the largest normal blood cell (14 to 20 μm in diameter) and has a single nucleus that is usually indented or horseshoe shaped.[11] It is produced in the bone marrow, enters the circulation, and migrates to the inflammatory site, where it develops into a macrophage. The *macrophage* is generally larger (20 to 40 μm) and is a more active phagocyte than the monocyte (see Fig. 6-16). Monocytes also appear to be the precursors of macrophages that are fixed in tissues (tissue macrophages), including Kupffer cells of the liver and alveolar macrophages of the lungs. (Tissue macrophages are discussed in Chapter 5.)

Macrophage and lymphocyte infiltration is characteristic of chronic rather than acute inflammation. Macrophages may appear at the inflammatory site within 24 hours of injury but usually arrive 3 to 7 days later. They migrate to the site slowly because (1) many of the chemotactic factors that attract them, such as macrophage chemotactic factor, are released by neutrophils and (2) monocytes move somewhat sluggishly.

Macrophages are well suited to long-term defense against infectious agents because they can survive and divide in the acidic inflammatory site. They can also fuse into larger cells capable of phagocytosing larger targets.

Macrophages are responsive to the soluble products (lymphokines) secreted by T cells, participate in activating the immune response by processing antigen for presentation to lymphocytes (see Figs. 5-17 and 5-18), and are a source of a soluble factor (colony-stimulating factor) that stimulates the growth and differentiation of granulocytes and monocytes in the bone marrow. Macrophages also secrete substances that promote the regrowth of tissues during wound healing.

Several bacteria can survive and even thrive inside macrophages. Microorganisms such as *Mycobacterium tuberculosis* (tuberculosis), *Mycobacterium leprae* (leprosy), *Salmonella typhi* (typhoid fever), *Brucella abortus* (brucellosis), and *Listeria monocytogenes* (listeriosis) can remain dormant or multiply inside the phagolysosomes of macrophages. The immune system helps to prevent this (see Fig. 6-7). Macrophages are further activated, or "turned on," by lymphokines secreted by T cells. Lymphokines increase the killing capacity of the macrophage by increasing its phagocytic activity, size, plasma membrane area, glucose metabolism, and number of lysosomes (Fig. 6-17).

Macrophages may not be activated because of defective T cell responses to certain microorganisms. For example, a form of leprosy called *lepromatous leprosy* is characterized by the survival of *M. leprae* organisms that have been phagocytosed by macrophages. In individuals with lepromatous leprosy, T cells fail to secrete the lymphokines needed to trans-

Fig. 6-16 *Steps in phagocytosis.* This scanning electron micrograph shows the progressive steps in phagocytosis. **A,** Red blood cells *(R)* attach to the surface of a macrophage *(M).* **B,** Part of macrophage *(M)* membrane starts to enclose the red cell *(R).* **C,** The red blood cells *(R)* are almost totally engulfed by the macrophage *(M). (From King, D.W., Fenoglio, C.M., & Lefkowitch, J.H. [1983]. General pathology: Principles and dynamics. Philadelphia: Lea & Febiger.)*

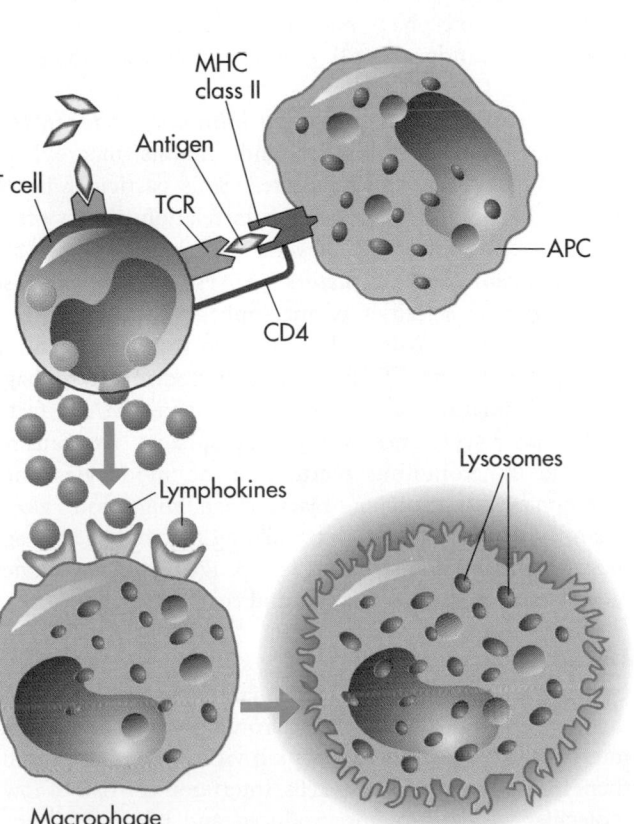

Fig. 6-17 *Activation of a macrophage by a lymphokine (macrophage-activating factor [MAF]).* Lymphokine is produced by T cells that have been stimulated by an antigen. The ruffled plasma membrane indicates macrophage activation. *MHC,* Major histocompatibility complex; *TCR,* T cell receptor; *APC,* antigen-presenting cell.

form the macrophages into cells more highly dedicated to killing.

Eosinophils

Eosinophils are granulocytes with many lysosomes containing (1) biochemical mediators that control the vascular effects of serotonin and histamine (see p. 154) and (2) a caustic protein that can dissolve the surface membranes of parasites.[12] Eosinophils do not phagocytose parasites, many of which are multicellular organisms. Rather, they bind to and degranulate highly caustic cationic proteins onto the parasite's outer membrane. This causes extensive damage to the parasite, and the tight fit between the eosinophil and its target prevents lysosomal contents from damaging neighboring host tissues. This is preceded by the processes shown in Fig. 6-18.

IgE is the chief immunoglobulin involved in allergic hypersensitivity reactions. Although the role of IgE in allergic reactions that are detrimental to the host (see Chapter 7) is most clearly understood, IgE may also mediate normal defenses against some pathogenic organisms (see Fig. 6-7). Multicellular parasites, particularly worms, elicit an IgE-mediated allergic response that benefits the host by destroying the parasite.

✓ QUICK CHECK

Describe the basic steps in acute inflammation.

Describe how acute inflammation differs from chronic inflammation. What characteristics do they share?

List the type of exudate produced in inflammation.

CELLULAR PRODUCTS
Inflammatory Cytokines

Some host cells produce cytokines that contribute to nonspecific mechanisms of defense by affecting other, neighboring host cells. (Cytokines are also discussed in Chapter 5.) Although some cytokines are produced in response to specific antigenic stimulation and govern the development of antigen-specific immunity, all of them also act in a nonspecific manner to enhance the inflammatory response.[13]

Many cells cooperate in producing an effective inflammatory response. Cytokines govern these interactions. Although most effects of cytokines are over short distances (e.g., between cells that are in contact), some effects are mediated over long distances within the body (e.g., the induction of fever by cytokines that are produced at an inflammatory site and act directly on the brain). The binding of cytokines to a particular cell is mediated through specific receptors, which are themselves under the regulation of cytokines. The same cytokine may have a large variety of different biologic activities depending on the target cell to which it binds. Cytokines may be synergistic (so that their combined activity exceeds the sum of their individual activities) or antagonistic (so that they inhibit each other). Mediators associated with stages of inflammation are illustrated in Fig. 6-19.

Tumor necrosis factor (TNF) is produced primarily by macrophages in response to infection with gram-negative bacteria. TNF facilitates inflammation in a variety of ways. It causes vascular endothelial cells to become stickier by increasing expression of surface adhesion molecules. This results in increased adherence of neutrophils and their emigration from the vessels. TNF also increases the phagocytic activity of neutrophils. Systemically, TNF acts directly on the hypothalamus in the brain to induce fever and on cells of the liver to produce some of the plasma proteins that are needed during inflammation and whose levels rise in the acute inflammatory response (acute-phase reactants; see p. 169). Very high doses of TNF can be directly lethal and are probably responsible for fatalities from shock caused by gram-negative bacterial infections. TNF also controls the production of other cytokines, especially IL-1, by other cells.

Interleukin-1 (IL-1) is also produced mostly by macrophages stimulated by substances associated with tissue injury, including bacteria, endotoxins (bacterial pyrogens), interferon, antigen-antibody complexes, and antigen. IL-1 has many properties in common with TNF, such as a direct effect on the hypothalamus and induction of fever, induction of liver cells to produce the same acute-phase reactants as are induced by TNF, and activation of vascular endothelial cells. IL-1 controls the production of several other cytokines, especially IL-6. Like IL-1, IL-6 also induces the production of acute-phase reactants by liver cells, although some of those induced by IL-6 differ from those induced by TNF and IL-1.[14]

One cytokine, called *migration-inhibitory factor (MIF),* is produced by lymphocytes and inhibits macrophage migration from the inflamed site.[15] This particular factor has not been characterized, and its relationship to other cytokines is unknown. Several other cytokines are *macrophage-activating factors (MAFs),* which increase the phagocytic activities of macrophages (see Fig. 6-17). MAF activity is attributable mostly to interferon-gamma (INF-γ), although TNF and granulocyte-macrophage colony-stimulating factor (GM-CSF) also have MAF effects. Many other cytokines affect macrophages by causing chemotaxis, promoting maturation of monocytes into macrophages, enhancing macrophage migration along chemotactic gradients, and stimulating macrophages to aggregate or fuse into giant cells (see p. 170). Some cytokines are chemotactic for neutrophils and eosinophils.

Interferons

One of the body's defenses against viral infection is the production of *interferon.* Interferon-alpha (IFN-α) and interferon-beta (IFN-β) do not kill viruses but can prevent them from infecting healthy cells. Interferon consists of low-molecular-weight proteins produced and released by host cells that have been invaded by a virus. Once released, inter-

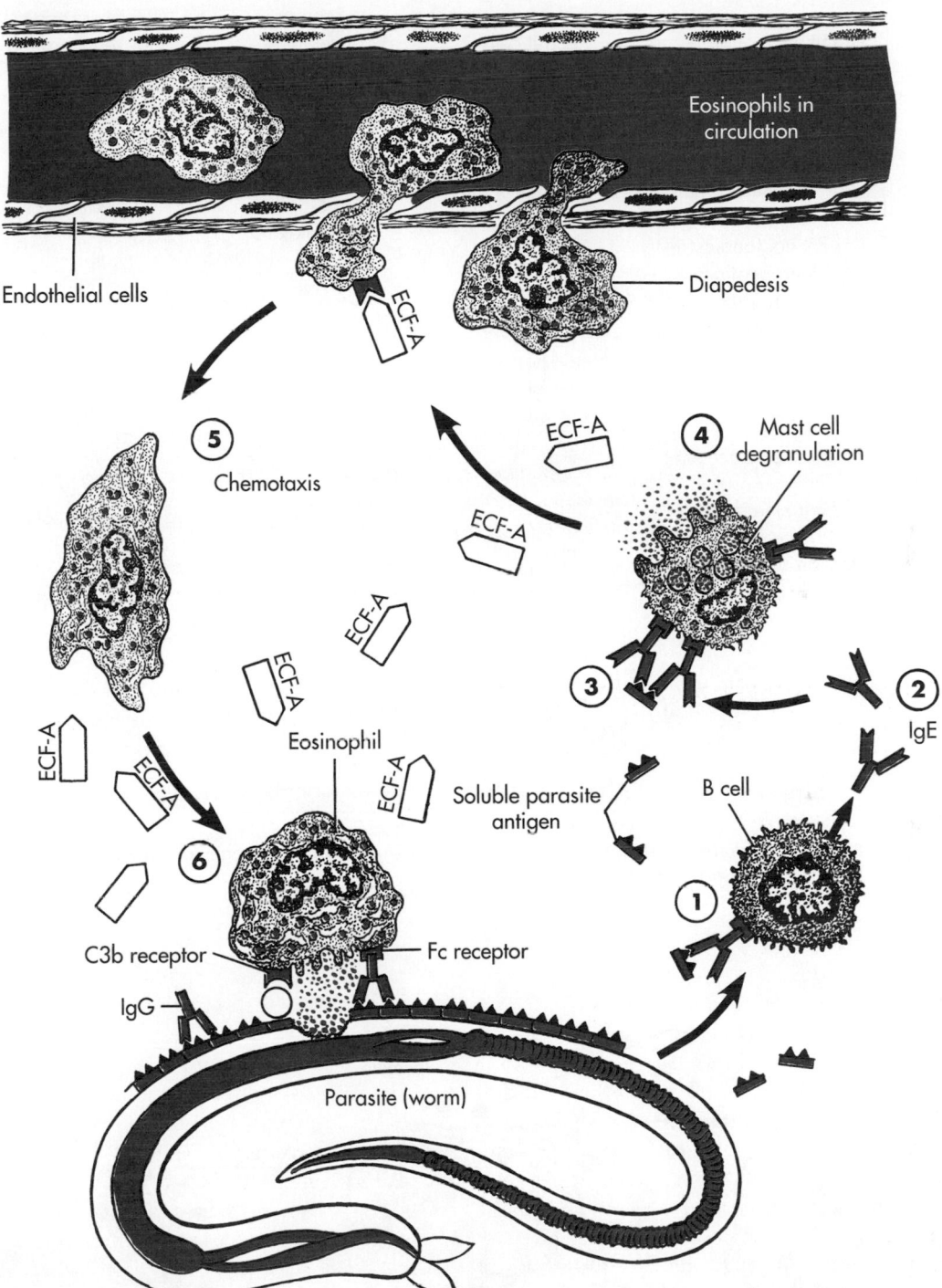

Fig. 6-18 *IgE-mediated destruction of a parasite by an eosinophil.* Soluble antigen from a para-site binds to an IgE-bearing B cell *(1)*, stimulating the B cell to produce IgE *(2)*, which binds to Fc receptors on a mast cell. Soluble antigen also binds to IgE on the mast cell *(3)*, causing the mast cell to degranulate *(4)*. ECF-A released from the mast cell granules attracts eosinophils out of the circulation and toward the site of inflammation *(5)*. IgG and complement component C3b are the opsonins that bind the eosinophil to the parasite. Once bound to the parasite, the eosinophil tries to ingest it and in the process releases its lysosomal enzymes onto the parasite, damaging its outer membrane *(6)*.

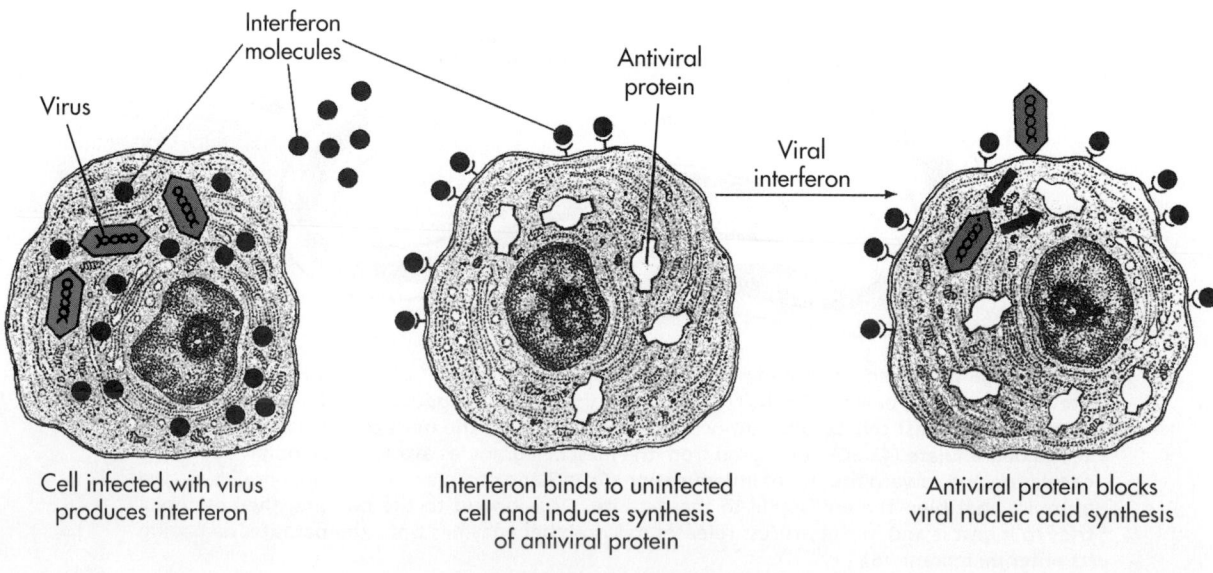

Fig. 6-19 *Mediators associated with stages of inflammation.* The stages of inflammation overlap and can be concurrent.

Fig. 6-20 *The action of interferon.*

TABLE 6-1	Circulating Levels of Acute-Phase Reactants During Inflammation	
Function	**Increased**	**Decreased**
Coagulation components	Fibrinogen	None
	Prothrombin	
	Factor VIII	
	Plasminogen	
Protease inhibitors	α_1-Antitrypsin	Inter-α-antitrypsin
	α_1-Antichymotrypsin	
Transport proteins	Haptoglobin	Transferrin
	Hemopexin	
	Ceruloplasmin	
	Ferritin	
Complement components	C1s, C2, C3, C4, C5, C9, factor B, C1 inhibitor	Properdin
Miscellaneous proteins	α_1-Acid glycoprotein	Albumin
	Fibronectin	Prealbumin
	Serum amyloid A (SAA)	α_1-Lipoprotein
	C-reactive protein (CRP)	β-Lipoprotein

feron molecules attach themselves to receptors on neighboring host cells. If a neighboring cell is uninfected, the interferon stimulates it to produce a number of antiviral proteins (Fig. 6-20). Interferon has no effect on a cell that is already infected by the virus.

SYSTEMIC MANIFESTATIONS OF ACUTE INFLAMMATION

The three primary systemic changes associated with the acute inflammatory response are fever, leukocytosis (a transient increase in circulating leukocytes), and an increase in circulating plasma proteins. Fever appears to be induced primarily by IL-1 released from neutrophils and macrophages.[16] IL-1 acts directly on the hypothalamus, which controls the body's thermostat. Its release occurs after phagocytosis or after exposure of the cell to bacterial endotoxin or to antigen-antibody complexes. (Mechanisms of temperature regulation are discussed in Chapter 13.)

A febrile response can be beneficial to defense because some microorganisms (e.g., those causing syphilis or gono-coccal urethritis) are sensitive to even small increases in body temperature. Fever may also have harmful side effects, enhancing the host's susceptibility to the endotoxins accompanying gram-negative bacterial infections.

During many infections, circulating leukocyte levels, primarily neutrophils, increase with a "left shift" in the ratio of immature to mature neutrophils (more immature neutrophils, such as band cells, metamyelocytes, and, occasionally, myelocytes, in greater-than-normal proportions). (See Chapter 19 for a discussion of the development and maturation of blood cells.) Leukocyte production is stimulated by several products of inflammation. Colony-stimulating factors produced by phagocytes also induce granulopoiesis (formation of granulocytes, namely, neutrophils, eosinophils, and basophils) in the bone marrow (see Chapter 19).

Many plasma proteins, mostly from the liver, are increased during inflammation and are termed ***acute-phase reactants*** (Table 6-1). These antiinflammatory proteins reach maximal circulating levels in 10 to 40 hours.

Acute inflammation can be verified by hematologic tests (see Chapter 19). Increased blood levels of acute-phase reactants, primarily fibrinogen (see Table 6-1), are usually associated with an increased erythrocyte sedimentation rate. Plasma protein alterations probably lead to enhanced erythrocyte rouleaux formation (stacking of erythrocytes, as in a stack of coins) and increased sedimentation rates. Although nonspecific, increased erythrocyte sedimentation is considered a good indicator of an acute inflammatory response.

CHRONIC INFLAMMATION

Superficially, the difference between acute and chronic inflammation is purely one of duration, with chronic cases lasting weeks or longer, regardless of cause. There also may be characteristic histologic and mechanistic differences (Fig.

Fig. 6-21 *The chronic inflammatory response.* Inflammation usually becomes chronic because of the persistence of an infection, an antigen, or a foreign body in the wound. Chronic inflammation is characterized by the persistence of many of the processes of acute inflammation. In addition, large amounts of neutrophil degranulation and death, the activation of lymphocytes, and the concurrent activation of fibroblasts result in the release of mediators that induce the infiltration of more lymphocytes and monocytes/macrophages and the beginning of wound healing and tissue repair. For more detailed information on each portion of the response, see the figures referred to in the illustration.

6-21). Chronic inflammation can be preceded by an unsuccessful acute inflammatory response. For example, if bacterial contamination or foreign objects (e.g., dirt, wood splinter, glass) persist in a traumatic wound, an inflammatory response that is difficult to differentiate from the acute response will continue beyond 2 weeks. Suppuration, pus formation, and incomplete wound healing characterize this chronic inflammation.

Chronic inflammation can occur also without much acute inflammation. Some microorganisms (e.g., mycobacteria) have cell walls with a very high lipid and wax content, making them relatively insensitive to degradation by phagocytes. The persistence of these bacteria continues to stimulate inflammation. Other microorganisms, such as the ones that cause tuberculosis, leprosy, syphilis, and brucellosis, can survive within the macrophage. In addition, some microorganisms produce toxins that stimulate tissue-damaging reactions even after they are killed. Persistent inflammation can also result from prolonged irritation by chemicals, particulate matter, or physical irritants (e.g., inhaled dusts, wood splinters, suture material).

Chronic inflammation is characterized by a dense infiltration of lymphocytes and macrophages. If macrophages cannot protect the host from tissue damage, the body attempts to wall off and isolate the infected site, forming a *granuloma.* Infections caused by some bacteria (listeriosis, brucellosis), fungi (histoplasmosis, coccidioidomycosis), parasites (leishmaniasis, schistosomiasis, toxoplasmosis), and perhaps large antigen-antibody complexes (rheumatoid arthritis) result in granuloma formation.

Granulomas form when some macrophages differentiate into large *epithelioid cells,* which cannot phagocytose but can take up debris and other small particles. Other macrophages fuse into multinucleated *giant cells,* which are active phagocytes and can engulf particles too large to be engulfed by single macrophages. The granuloma itself is usually encapsulated by fibrous deposits of collagen and may be hyalinized or calcified by deposits of calcium. The classic granuloma associated with tuberculosis is characterized by a wall of epithelioid cells surrounding a center of dead and decaying tissue (caseous necrosis; see Chapter 3) and mycobacteria.

Cells decay within the granuloma and release acids and the enzymatic contents of dead phagocytes' lysosomes. In this inhospitable environment, cellular debris is broken down into its basic constituents and a clear fluid (liquefaction necrosis; see Chapter 3) remains in the granuloma. Eventually this fluid diffuses out and leaves a thick-walled structure in the tissue that may remain for the life of the individual.

LOCAL MANIFESTATIONS OF INFLAMMATION

Because inflammation is a nonspecific defense mechanism, it generally proceeds in the same way, no matter what type of injury has occurred. All local manifestations of acute inflammation are caused by vascular changes and exudation. As exudate accumulates, swelling accompanied by pain occurs, caused by pressure from the accumulation and by the presence of soluble biochemical mediators (prostaglandins, bradykinin). Heat and redness result from increased perfusion (increased blood flow through the area).

The vascular changes and exudation deliver leukocytes, plasma proteins, and their biochemical mediators to the site of injury. Exudate and its contents have three functions: (1) to dilute toxins produced by bacteria and toxic products released by dying cells; (2) to carry plasma proteins (including antibody) and leukocytes (both phagocytes and lymphocytes) to the site; and (3) to carry away bacterial toxins, dead cells, debris, and other products of inflammation. This third function occurs via channels through the epithelium (sinuses) or through lymphatic vessels. Antigens in lymphatic fluid pass through the lymph nodes, where they stimulate B lymphocytes to become antibody-producing plasma cells or T lymphocytes to become effector T cells, thus helping the immune response. (The lymphatic system is described in Chapter 22.)

The composition of exudate varies, depending on the stage of the inflammatory response and, to some extent, the injurious stimulus. In early or mild inflammation the exudate is watery (*serous exudate*) with very few plasma proteins or leukocytes, like fluid in a blister. In more severe or advanced inflammation the exudate may be thick and clotted (*fibrinous exudate*), as in the lungs of individuals with lobar pneumonia. If many leukocytes accumulate, as in persistent bacterial infections, the exudate consists of pus and is called a *purulent (suppurative) exudate.* Purulent exudate is characteristic of walled-off lesions (*cysts* or *abscesses*). If bleeding occurs, the exudate is filled with erythrocytes (*hemorrhagic exudate*).

The local manifestations of inflammation can affect all vascularized tissues, but lesions vary, depending on the organ or tissue involved. With widespread cellular death (necrosis), different lesions occur in myocardial (heart muscle), brain, and hepatic (liver) tissue. Cellular death resulting from myocardial infarction (deprivation of oxygen caused by cessation of blood flow) causes a response that proceeds to replacement of the dead tissue with a fibrinous scar. The same injury to brain tissue is more likely to result in the formation of an abscess filled with necrotic tissue (types of necrosis are described in Chapter 3). Destruction of liver tissue stimulates the regrowth, or regeneration, of liver cells.

Local manifestations of inflammation also accompany all types of nonlethal cellular and tissue injury, from fractures or strains of the musculoskeletal system to burn injuries (see Chapter 3). No matter what the cause or where the lesion, inflammation occurs without fail because without it, healing could not occur.

RESOLUTION AND REPAIR

Tissue destruction is followed by a period of healing that begins during acute inflammation and may not be complete for as long as 2 years. The most favorable outcome of healing is complete return to normal structure and function.[17] This is possible if damage is minor, no complications occur, or destroyed tissues *regenerate* (mitotic proliferation of remaining cells; mitosis is described in Chapter 1). Restoration of original structure and physiologic function is called *resolution.*

If extensive damage is present (particularly in tissues incapable of regeneration), if infection results in abscess or granuloma formation, or if fibrin persists in the lesion, resolution is not possible and repair takes place instead. *Repair* is the replacement of destroyed tissue with scar tissue composed of *collagen.* It fills in the lesion and restores tensile strength but cannot carry out the physiologic functions of destroyed tissue.

Both regeneration and repair begin during inflammation, with phagocytosis of particulate matter in the inflammatory exudate. This cleanup of the lesion, which also involves dissolution of fibrin clots (or scabs) by fibrinolytic enzymes, is called *débridement.* After débridement, exudate, toxic products, and particulate matter are drained away and vascular dilation and permeability are reversed, preparing the lesion for either regeneration or repair.

Repair, which ends in the formation of scar tissue, always involves processes that (1) fill in the wound, (2) cover or seal the wound, and (3) shrink the wound. These common denominators of wound healing vary in importance and duration among different types of wounds. A clean incision, such as a paper cut or a sutured surgical wound, heals primarily through the process of collagen synthesis. Because sealing of this type of wound has already been facilitated by minimal tissue loss and joining of the wound edges, very little sealing (epithelialization) and shrinkage (contraction) are required for healing. Wounds that heal under conditions of minimal tissue loss are said to heal by *primary intention* (Fig. 6-22, A to D).

Healing of an open wound, such as a stage IV pressure sore (decubitus ulcer), requires a great deal more tissue replacement than healing of a surgical incision. With an open wound, epithelialization, scar formation, and contraction take longer and healing occurs through *secondary intention*

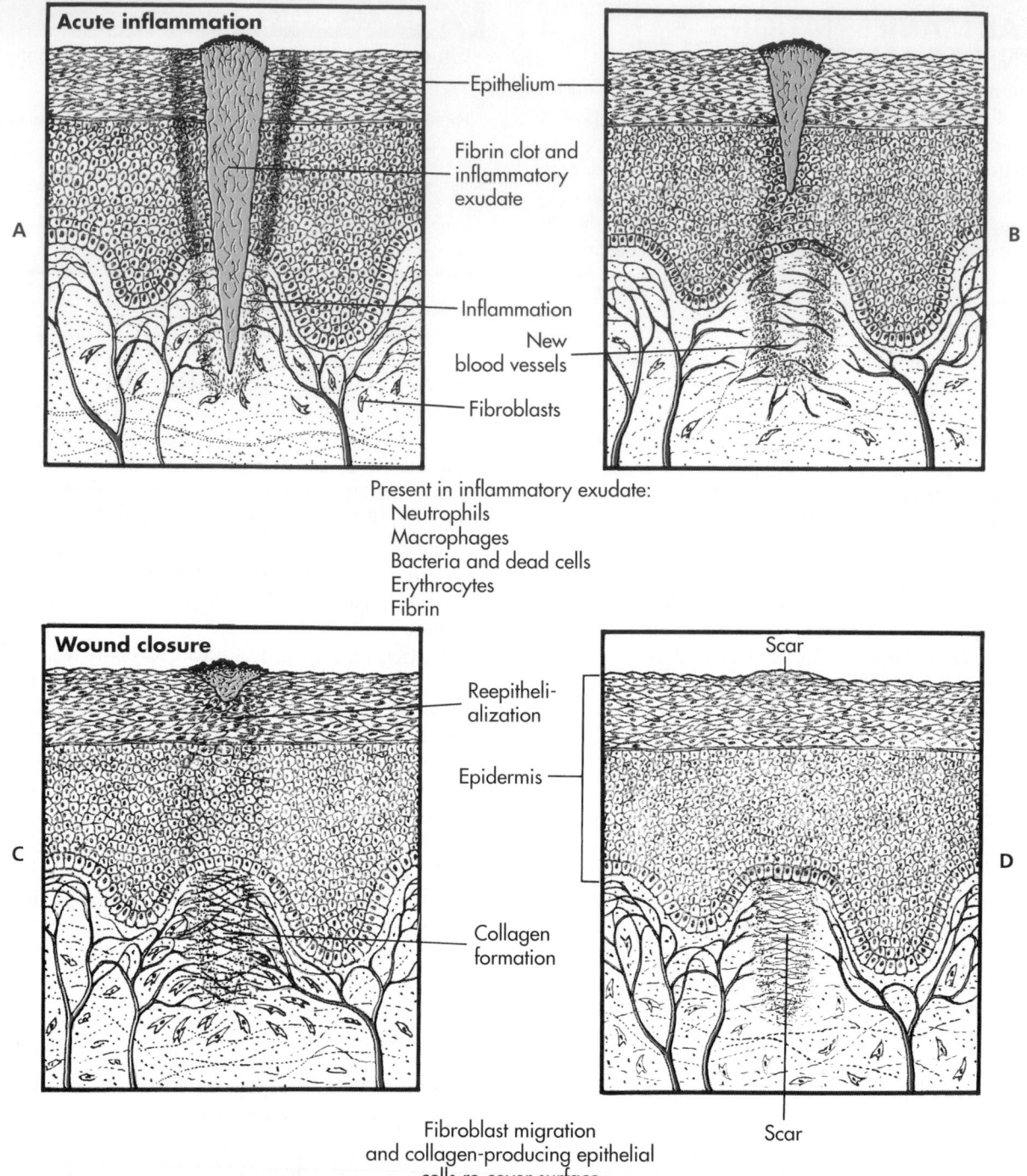

Present in inflammatory exudate:
Neutrophils
Macrophages
Bacteria and dead cells
Erythrocytes
Fibrin

Fibroblast migration
and collagen-producing epithelial
cells re-cover surface

Fig. 6-22 *Wound repair by primary or secondary intention.* **A** to **D,** Healing by primary intention.

(Fig. 6-22, *E* to *I*). Healing by either primary or secondary intention may occur at different rates for different types of tissue and for different types of injury.

Resolution and repair occur in two overlapping phases. The first phase, called the ***reconstructive phase*** (or reconstructive, proliferative, fibroblastic, or connective) begins 3 to 4 days after the initial injury and continues for as long as 2 weeks. During the reconstructive phase the lesion is char-

acterized by fibroblast (connective tissue cell) proliferation, which is followed by collagen synthesis by the fibroblasts, epithelialization, and cellular differentiation.

The second phase, the ***maturation phase*** (or differentiation, remodeling, or plateau), begins several weeks after injury and is normally complete within 2 years. With maturation there is continuing differentiation of cells, contraction of the wound, scar formation, and remodeling of the scar.

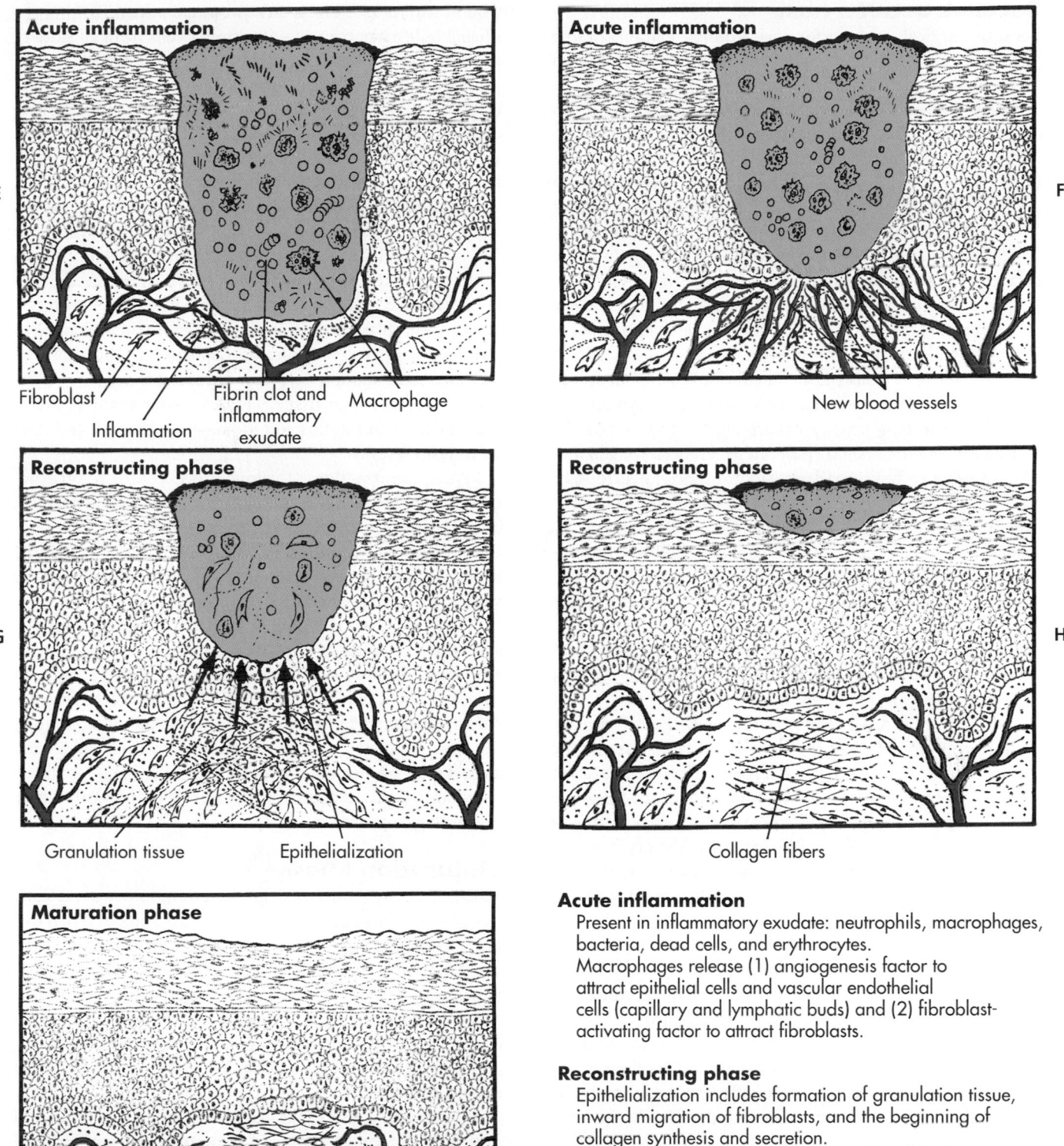

Acute inflammation

E — Fibroblast · Inflammation · Fibrin clot and inflammatory exudate · Macrophage

F — New blood vessels

Reconstructing phase

G — Granulation tissue · Epithelialization

H — Collagen fibers

Maturation phase

I — Scar tissue

Acute inflammation

Present in inflammatory exudate: neutrophils, macrophages, bacteria, dead cells, and erythrocytes.
Macrophages release (1) angiogenesis factor to attract epithelial cells and vascular endothelial cells (capillary and lymphatic buds) and (2) fibroblast-activating factor to attract fibroblasts.

Reconstructing phase

Epithelialization includes formation of granulation tissue, inward migration of fibroblasts, and the beginning of collagen synthesis and secretion.
Granulation tissue becomes scar tissue, contraction begins, and differentiation begins.

Maturation phase

This phase includes completion of contraction, differentiation, and remodeling of scar tissue, and disappearance of capillaries from scar tissue.

Fig. 6-22, cont'd E to I, Healing by secondary intention.

Reconstructive Phase

Because surgical and perforative wounds exhibit all the phases of resolution and repair, they are useful models of both normal and abnormal (dysfunctional) healing. The wound initially is sealed off by a blood clot containing fibrin and trapped cells (erythrocytes, leukocytes). The cross-linked mesh of fibrin is created by activation of the coagulation cascade. The fibrin mesh traps platelets, which further seal damaged vessels by forming a platelet plug (see Chapter 19). Most surgical wounds are completely sealed with fibrin several hours after they have been closed. Sealing creates a barrier to bacterial invasion, although it does not always prevent it, and helps unite the wound edges. Fibrin provides a framework for the collagen molecules or regenerated tissue cells that will ultimately fill the wound.

For healing to proceed, the fibrin clot must be dissolved and replaced by normal tissue or scar tissue. Enzymatic digestion of the clot usually occurs after activation of the plasma fibrinolytic system (plasmin generation; see Chapter 19) or release of lysosomal enzymes from dead neutrophils. Macrophages invade the dissolving clot and clear away debris and dead cells by phagocytosis. Débridement by macrophages and remaining neutrophils is followed by simple resolution with regeneration of destroyed cells or, if regeneration is not possible, by repair and scar formation (see Fig. 6-22).

In repair, *granulation tissue* grows inward from surrounding healthy connective tissue. It is filled with new capillaries that give it a red, granular appearance and is surrounded by fibroblasts and macrophages. First, capillary buds sprout out of vascular endothelial cells around the wound and extend into the débrided areas. Loops form when the young capillaries join *(anastomose)*. The loops are more fragile and permeable than mature vessels, resulting in a leakage of erythrocytes and neutrophils. The erythrocytes are phagocytosed by macrophages, and the neutrophils participate in further débridement of the inflammatory lesion. Many of the new capillaries differentiate into arterioles and venules as repair continues. New lymphatic vessels grow into the granulation tissue by a similar process.

Besides acting as the primary phagocyte of débridement, the macrophage secretes biochemical mediators that promote healing, namely, (1) fibroblast-activating factor, which stimulates fibroblasts to enter the lesion and synthesize and secrete the collagen precursor, procollagen; (2) angiogenesis factor, which stimulates vascular endothelial cells to form capillary buds that grow into the lesion; and (3) a factor that stimulates epithelial cells to grow over and seal the wound's surface. Macrophages also secrete collagenase, which débrides injured collagen fibers in the wound.

As the clot or scab is being dissolved and granulation tissue is being formed, the healing wound must be protected. *Epithelialization* is the process by which epithelial cells grow into the wound from surrounding healthy tissue. Attracted by a factor secreted by macrophages, the epithelial cells migrate under the clot or scab, using proteolytic enzymes to sever the connection between the clot and the wound surface (see Fig. 6-22). Eventually the migrating epithelial cells make contact with similar cells from all sides of the wound and seal the wound, after which migration and proliferation cease. The epithelial cells remain active, however, undergoing differentiation to give rise to the various epidermal layers (see Chapter 39). Epithelialization of a skin wound can be hastened if the wound is kept moist, preventing the fibrin clot from becoming a scab.

Fibroblasts are the most important cells during the reconstructive phase of wound healing because they synthesize and secrete collagen. Collagen is the most abundant protein in the body, present in skin, bones, teeth, blood vessels, tendons, cartilage, and connective tissue. Fibroblasts are stimulated by fibroblast-activating factor (from macrophages) to proliferate and enter the lesion. Collagen is laid down in débrided areas about 6 days after fibroblasts have entered the lesion and forms scar tissue. The scar tissue matures over a period of several months and increases in strength and ability to resist stress.

Wound *contraction* is the final process of the reconstructive phase of healing. It is necessary for closure of all wounds, but especially those wounds that heal by secondary intention. Contraction is noticeable 6 to 12 days after injury. In normal healing, contraction may amount to inward movement of the wound edge by approximately 0.5 mm/day.

The granulation tissue contains *myofibroblasts*—specialized cells that probably cause wound contraction. As the name implies, myofibroblasts have features of both smooth muscle cells and fibroblasts. Wound contraction occurs as structures extending from the plasma membrane of the myofibroblast establish connections with neighboring cells. Once connected, myofibroblasts can exert pull on neighboring cells and anchor themselves to the wound bed, promoting contraction.

Maturation Phase

Collagen deposition, tissue regeneration, and wound contraction all begin during the reconstructive phase. When this phase ends, about 2 weeks after injury, these processes are usually incomplete and continue into the maturation phase, which can last for years. During the maturation phase, scar tissue is remodeled and capillaries disappear, leaving an avascular scar. Within 2 to 3 weeks after maturation has begun, the scar tissue gains about two thirds of its eventual maximum strength.

Epidermal wounds that heal by secondary intention and unsutured internal lesions are seldom completely restored by healing. At best, repaired tissue regains 80% of its original tensile strength. Only epithelial, hepatic (liver), and bone marrow cells perform complete mitotic regeneration (compensatory hyperplasia, described in Chapter 3). In fibrous connective tissue, such as joints and ligaments, normal healing results in the replacement of the original tissue, but the new tissue does not have exactly the same structure as the original. Some damaged tissue heals without replacement. For instance, the damage resulting from myocardial infarction heals with a scar composed of fibrous tissue rather than cardiac muscle. Although the composition of healed tissue may differ, the healing process of soft tissues is the same for all wounds.

Dysfunctional Wound Healing

Dysfunctional healing may occur during any phase of the wound-healing process and may involve insufficient repair, excessive repair, or infection.[18] The cause of dysfunctional healing can be related to a predisposing disorder, such as diabetes mellitus; to an acquired condition, such as hypoxemia (insufficient oxygen in arterial blood); or to numerous drugs and nutrients. Wound repair delays healing by reactivating inflammatory processes.

Dysfunction during the inflammatory response

Healing may be prolonged if bleeding is not stopped during acute inflammation. A clot increases the amount of space that granulation tissue must fill and serves as a mechanical barrier to oxygen diffusion. The accumulation of excess blood cells resulting from hemorrhage prolongs the inflammatory process, since these cells must be cleared before repair. Accumulated blood is an excellent culture medium for bacteria and promotes infection, prolonging inflammation by increasing exudation and pus formation. In addition to slowing healing, sepsis can promote excessive scar formation or prevent healing completely.

Excessive amounts of fibrin also are detrimental to healing. The great amount of fibrin released in response to injury must eventually be reabsorbed so it will not organize into fibrous adhesions. Adhesions are clinically significant when they form in the pleural, pericardial, or abdominal cavities, where they can bind organs together by fibrous bands, the shrinkage of which can distort or strangulate the affected organ.

Hypovolemia—decreased blood volume—also inhibits inflammation. The physiologic response to hypovolemia is vessel constriction rather than the dilation required to deliver inflammatory cells to the site of injury. Antiinflammatory steroids prevent macrophages from migrating to the site of injury and inhibit their release of collagenase and plasminogen activator.[19] Antiinflammatory steroids also inhibit fibroblast migration into the wound during the reconstructive phase.

Optimal nutrition is important during all phases of healing because metabolic needs are increased. The substances most needed for healing are glucose, oxygen, and protein. Because leukocytes need glucose to produce the adenosine triphosphate $5'$(ATP) needed for chemotaxis, phagocytosis, and intercellular killing, the wounds of persons with diabetes who receive insufficient insulin heal poorly, mainly because of infection. Persons with diabetes are at risk for ischemic wounds because they are likely to have both small-vessel diseases that impair the microcirculation and altered (glycosylated) hemoglobin, which has an increased affinity for oxygen and thus does not readily release oxygen in tissues. (Hemoglobin's function as the oxygen-carrying

component of blood is described in Chapter 19.) Oxygen delivery is compromised also by hypoxemic states. Ischemic tissue is susceptible to infection, which prolongs inflammation. Hypoproteinemia also prolongs inflammation because it impairs fibroblast proliferation.

Wound sepsis is treated in several ways. Most important is the removal or débridement of necrotic tissue and foreign bodies. Débridement is accomplished by surgery or use of absorbent dressings. Wound irrigation and antibiotic therapy also combat infection.

Dysfunction during the reconstructive phase
Impaired collagen synthesis
Most of the factors that interfere with the production of collagen in healing tissues are nutritional.[20] Scurvy, for example, is caused by lack of ascorbic acid—one of the cofactors required for collagen formation by fibroblasts. The results of scurvy are poorly formed connective tissue and greatly impaired healing.

Protein and other nutrients are required for collagen synthesis. These include iron, oxygen, α-ketoglutarate, manganese, copper, and calcium. Usually such minute amounts of these substances are required as cofactors that deficiencies are not clinically significant.

Collagen synthesis may be impaired, for example, in individuals with Ehlers-Danlos syndrome (type VII). This disease prevents formation of normal connective tissue, causing the skin to be thin and fragile. All forms of Ehlers-Danlos syndrome are characterized by defects in collagen formation. (The role of collagen in bone formation is described in Chapter 36.)

Dysfunctional collagen synthesis also may involve excessive production of collagen, causing surface overhealing as manifested by a keloid or a hypertrophic scar (Fig. 6-23). Both keloid and hypertrophic scars are caused by increased collagen synthesis with decreased collagen lysis. A *keloid* is a raised scar that extends beyond the original boundaries of the wound. It invades surrounding tissue and is likely to recur after surgical removal. A familial tendency to keloid formation has been observed, with a greater incidence in blacks than whites. A *hypertrophic scar* is raised but remains within the original boundaries of the wound. Hypertrophic scars tend to regress over time.

Impaired epithelialization
Epithelialization is suppressed by antiinflammatory steroids, hypoxemia, ionizing radiation, and zinc deficiencies. Wound care technique may greatly influence epithelial cell migration.

External wounds that are draining or healing by secondary intention often are débrided and protected with dressings. The ideal dressing absorbs some drainage without being incorporated into the clot or granulation tissue. Because epithelial cells must migrate across the wound during healing, dressings that débride healthy epithelial cells along with necrotic tissue prolong epithelialization.

Many solutions that traditionally have been used to clean or irrigate wounds are deleterious to the fragile new cells in

Fig. 6-23 *Keloid (scar) formation.* Scar caused by excessive synthesis of collagen. Keloid from suture marks in a black individual. *(From Habif, T.P. [1990]. Clinical dermatology [2nd ed.]. St. Louis: Mosby.)*

the wound bed. Normal saline is the most innocuous solution that can be used to cleanse or irrigate a wound that is healing primarily by epithelialization. Solutions such as povidone-iodine and hydrogen peroxide are very drying and subsequently inhibit rather than promote epithelial cell migration.

Wound disruption

A potential complication of wounds that are sutured closed is **dehiscence,** in which the wound pulls apart at the suture line. Dehiscence generally occurs 5 to 12 days after suturing, when collagen synthesis is at its peak. Approximately one half of dehiscence occurrences are associated with wound sepsis, but they also may be the result of sutures breaking because of excessive strain. Obesity increases the risk for dehiscence because adipose tissue is difficult to suture. Wound dehiscence usually is heralded by increased serous drainage from the wound and a feeling that "something gave way." Prompt surgical attention is required.

Impaired contraction

Wound contraction, although necessary for healing, may become pathologic when contraction is excessive, resulting in a deformity or **contracture.** Burns are especially susceptible to contracture development. Internal contracture may occur in cirrhosis of the liver. Scar tissue that becomes contracted constricts vascular flow and contributes to the development of portal hypertension and esophageal varices. Other internal contraction deformities include duodenal strictures caused by dysfunctional healing of an ulcer and esophageal strictures caused by lye burns.

Proper positioning and range-of-motion exercises and surgery are among the physical means used to overcome myofibroblast pull and prevent contractures. Biochemical means include control of myofibroblast contraction by the administration of smooth muscle inhibitors (e.g., colchicine) and attempts to inhibit collagen synthesis with drugs that prevent collagen cross-linking or collagenase ac-

tivity. This treatment is based on the knowledge that collagen can "lock" contracted myofibroblasts into position. Clinical use of pharmacologic methods for control of wound contracture is still largely experimental.

PEDIATRICS & *Factors Affecting Mechanisms of Self-Defense*

Immature or depressed immune function in neonates
Transiently depressed inflammatory function
Neutrophils incapable of chemotaxis, lacking fluidity in plasma membrane
Tendency for infections associated with chemotactic defects, e.g., cutaneous abscesses caused by staphylococci and cutaneous candidiasis
Diminished oxidative and bacterial responses in those stressed by in utero infection or respiratory insufficiency
Partial deficiency in complement, especially components of alternative pathways (e.g., factor B)
Tendency to develop severe overwhelming sepsis and meningitis when infected by bacteria against which no maternal antibodies are present

---

AGING & *Factors Affecting Mechanisms of Self-Defense*

At risk for impaired wound healing—often associated with chronic illness, e.g., diabetes mellitus or cardiovascular disease[21]
Taking required medications that may interfere with healing, e.g., antiinflammatory steroids
At risk for sustaining wounds because of impaired sensation or mobility and physiologic changes in skin
Loss of subcutaneous fat, which diminishes layer of protection
Thickened and less elastic collagen fibers, which contributes to less protection
Diminished immune function, which impairs natural ability to fight infection
Atrophied epidermis, including underlying capillaries, which decreases perfusion and increases risk of hypoxia in wound bed

---

✓ QUICK CHECK

How does regeneration of tissue differ from repair of tissue?

What does it mean to heal by primary intention?

What is the role of fibroblasts in wound healing?

Describe various ways wound healing may be dysfunctional.

◻ DID YOU UNDERSTAND?

The Acute Inflammatory Response

1. Inflammation is a rapid and nonspecific protective response to cellular injury from any cause. It can occur only in vascularized tissue.
2. The macroscopic hallmarks of inflammation are redness, swelling, heat, pain, and loss of function of the inflamed tissues.
3. The microscopic hallmark of inflammation is an accumulation of fluid and cells at the inflammatory site.

The Mast Cell

1. The most important activator of the inflammatory response is the mast cell, which initiates inflammation by releasing biochemical mediators (histamine, chemotactic factors) from preformed cytoplasmic granules and synthesizing other mediators (prostaglandins, leukotrienes) in response to a stimulus.
2. Histamine and serotonin are the major vasoactive amines of inflammation. Both cause constriction of vascular smooth muscles, dilation of capillaries, and retraction of endothelial cells lining the capillaries, which increases vascular permeability.

Plasma Protein Systems

1. Inflammation is mediated by three key plasma protein systems: the complement system, the clotting system, and the kinin system. The components of all three systems are a series of inactive proteins (proenzymes) that are activated in cascade fashion.
2. The complement system can be activated by antigen-antibody reactions (through the classic pathway) or by other products, especially bacterial polysaccharides (through the alternative pathway), resulting in the production of biologically active (anaphylatoxic or chemotactic) fragments and target cell lysis.
3. The clotting system stops bleeding, localizes microorganisms, and provides a meshwork for repair and healing.
4. Bradykinin is the most important kinin protein and causes vascular permeability, smooth muscle contraction, and pain.

Cellular Components of Inflammation

1. The cells involved in the inflammatory process include phagocytic leukocytes (neutrophils, macrophages, eosinophils), platelets, and lymphocytes.
2. Phagocytic cells engulf and destroy microorganisms by enclosing them in phagocytic vacuoles (phagolysosomes), within which toxic products (especially metabolites of oxygen) and degradative lysosomal enzymes kill and digest the microorganisms.
3. Opsonins, such as antibody and complement component C3b, coat microorganisms and make them more susceptible to phagocytosis by binding them more tightly to the phagocyte.
4. The polymorphonuclear neutrophil (PMN), the predominant phagocytic cell in the early inflammatory response, exits the circulation by diapedesis through the retracted endothelial cell junctions and moves to the inflammatory site by chemotaxis.
5. The macrophage, the predominant phagocytic cell in the late inflammatory response, is highly phagocytic, responsive to lymphokines, and responsible for antigen processing and presentation to lymphocytes.
6. Eosinophils release products that control the inflammatory response and are induced by IgE-mediated mechanisms of hypersensitivity to kill parasitic organisms directly.

Cellular Products

1. The cells involved in immunity and inflammation stimulate other cells by secreting lymphokines, interferons, or interleukins.
2. Lymphokines are produced by T cells and have their most important effects on macrophages. These effects include chemotaxis, inhibition of migration once the macrophage has entered the inflammatory site, and activation of the macrophage, which makes it a more powerful phagocyte.
3. Interferons are produced by host cells that are already infected by viruses. Once released from infected cells, interferons can stimulate neighboring healthy cells to produce substances that prevent viral penetration.

Systemic Manifestations of Acute Inflammation

1. The systemic effects of inflammation are fever and increases in levels of circulating leukocytes and plasma proteins.

Chronic Inflammation

1. Chronic inflammation lasts 2 weeks or longer. It can occur as a distinct process without much acute inflammation.
2. Chronic inflammation is characterized by a dense infiltration of lymphocytes and macrophages. The body walls off and isolates the host from tissue damage, forming a granuloma.

Local Manifestations of Inflammation

1. Local manifestations of inflammation all involve the same hallmarks of inflammation, but types of exudate and necrosis vary with the injury and the tissue or organ affected.

Continued

▣ DID YOU UNDERSTAND? —cont'd

Resolution and Repair

1. Inflammatory lesions proceed to resolution if little tissue has been lost or injured tissue is capable of regeneration. This is called *healing by primary intention.*

2. Inflammatory lesions that involve extensive damage or tissues incapable of regeneration heal by repair. This process is called *healing by secondary intention.*

⚠ AGING AND FACTORS AFFECTING MECHANISMS OF SELF-DEFENSE

1. Neonates frequently have transiently depressed inflammatory function. Elderly persons are at risk for impaired wound healing.

2. Diminished immune function may interfere with elderly persons' natural ability to ward off infection in a wound.

KEY TERMS

Abscess, 171
Acute-phase reactant, 169
Alternative pathway, 157
Anaphylatoxin, 157
Antigen-antibody (immune) complex, 157
Arylsulfatase, 160
Basophil, 152
Bradykinin, 159
C1 esterase inhibitor, 160
Carboxypeptidase, 160
Chemotactic factor, 154
Chemotaxis, 154
Classic pathway, 157
Collagen, 171
Complement cascade, 156
Contraction, 174
Contracture, 176
Cyst, 171
Débridement, 171
Degranulation, 152
Dehiscence, 176
Diapedesis, 163

Eosinophil, 166
Epithelialization, 174
Epithelioid cell, 170
Extrinsic pathway, 158
Exudate, 151
Fibrinous exudate, 171
Fibroblast, 174
Giant cell, 170
Granulation tissue, 174
Granuloma, 170
Hemorrhagic exudate, 171
Histaminase, 160
Hypertrophic scar, 175
Interferon, 166
Interleukin-1 (IL-1), 166
Intrinsic pathway, 158
Keloid, 175
Leukotriene (slow-reacting substance of anaphylaxis [SRS-A]), 154
Macrophage, 164
Macrophage-activating factor (MAF), 166
Margination (pavementing), 163

Mast cell, 152
Maturation phase, 172
Migration-inhibitory factor (MIF), 166
Monocyte, 164
Myofibroblast, 174
Neutrophil, 164
Phagocytosis, 163
Phagolysosome, 163
Phagosome, 163
Plasma kinin cascade, 159
Platelet, 152
Polymorphonuclear neutrophil (PMN), 164
Primary intention, 171
Proenzyme, 156
Prostaglandin, 155
Purulent (suppurative) exudate, 171
Reconstructive phase, 172
Regenerate, 171
Repair, 171
Resolution, 171
Secondary intention, 171
Serous exudate, 171

REFERENCES

1. Metcalfe, D.D., Baram, D., & Mekori, Y.A. (1997). Mast cells. *Physiological Reviews, 77,* 1033-1079.
2. Sala, A., Zarini, S., & Bolla, M. (1998). Leukotrienes: Lipid bioeffectors of inflammatory reactions. *Biochemistry, 63,* 84-92.
3. Whaley, K. & Schwaeble, W. (1997). Complement and complement deficiencies. *Seminars in Liver Disease, 17,* 297-310.
4. Kirschfink, M. (1997). Controlling the complement system in inflammation. *Immunopharmacology, 38,* 51-62.
5. Erdie, A., Kerekes, K., & Pecht, I. (1997). Role of C3a and C5a in the activation of mast cells. *Experimental and Clinical Immunogenetics, 14,* 16-18.
6. McGilvray, I.D. & Rotstein, O.D. (1998). Role of the coagulation system in the local and systemic inflammatory response. *World Journal of Surgery, 22,* 179-186.
7. Kaplan, A.P. et al. (1997). The intrinsic coagulation/kinin-forming cascade: Assembly in plasma and cell surfaces in inflammation. *Advances in Immunology, 66,* 225-272.
8. Hill, S.J. et al. (1997). Classification of histamine receptors. *Pharmacological Reviews, 49,* 253-278.
9. Imhof, B.A. & Dunon, D. (1997). Basic mechanism of leukocyte migration. *Hormone and Metabolic Research, 29,* 614-621.
10. Dallegi, F. & Ottonello, L. (1997). Tissue injury in neutrophilic inflammation. *Inflammation Research, 46,* 382-391.
11. Vignola, A.M. et al. (1998). Monocytes. *Journal of Allergy and Clinical Immunology, 101,* 149-152.
12. Weller, P.F. (1997). Human eosinophils. *Journal of Allergy and Clinical Immunology, 100,* 283-287.
13. Papanicolaou, D.A. (1997). Role of pro- and anti-inflammatory cytokines during inflammation: Experimental and clinical findings. *Journal of Biological Regulators and Homeostatic Agents, 11,* 91-103.
14. Papanicolaou, D.A. et al. (1998). The pathophysiologic roles of interleukin-6 in human disease. *Annals of Internal Medicine, 128,* 127-137.
15. Metz, C.N. & Bucala, R. (1997). Role of macrophage migration inhibitory factor in the regulation of the immune response. *Advances in Immunology, 66,* 197-223.
16. Rowsey, P.J. (1997). Pathophysiology of fever. I. The role of cytokines. *Dimensions of Critical Care Nursing, 16,* 202-207.
17. Martin, P. (1997). Wound healing—Aiming for perfect skin regeneration. *Science, 276,* 75-81.
18. Thornton, F.J., Schaffer, M.R., & Barbul, A. (1997). Wound healing in sepsis and trauma. *Shock, 8,* 391-401.
19. Mathers, S.J. & Mullenken, B.R. (1995). Wound healing. In J.H. Davis & G.F. Sheldon (Eds.). *Surgery: A problem-solving approach* (2nd ed.). St. Louis: Mosby.
20. Kiy, A.M. Nutrition wound healing: A bio-psychosocial perspective. *Nursing Clinics of North America, 32,* 849-462.
21. Desai, H. (1997). Aging and wounds. II. Healing in old age. *Journal of Wound Care, 6,* 237-239.

CHAPTER

7

Hypersensitivities, Infection, and Immunodeficiencies

*Neal S. Rote, Sue E. Huether, and
Kathryn L. McCance*

The immune system is a finely tuned network that protects the host against foreign antigens, particularly infectious agents. Sometimes this network breaks down, causing the immune system to react inappropriately. Inappropriate immune responses may be (1) exaggerated against environmental antigens (allergy), (2) misdirected against the host's own cells (autoimmunity), or (3) directed against beneficial foreign tissues, such as transfusions or transplants (alloimmunity). All of these can be serious or life threatening. Allergies are the most common and usually the least life threatening.

CHAPTER OUTLINE

Check out your CD Companion for chapter-related exercises and answers to the Quick Check questions

ALTERATIONS IN IMMUNITY AND INFLAMMATION

Hypersensitivity: Allergy, Autoimmunity, and Alloimmunity

The three types of inappropriate responses just listed can be collectively classified as *hypersensitivity,* or an altered immunologic reaction to an antigen that results in a pathologic immune response after reexposure. Allergy, autoimmunity, and alloimmunity (old term is isoimmunity) are differentiated by the source of the antigen against which the hypersensitivity response is directed (Table 7-1). The term *allergy* originally denoted both parts of the immune response: immunity, which is beneficial, and hypersensitivity, which is harmful. Allergy has come to mean the deleterious effects of hypersensitivity to environmental antigens, and immunity refers to the protective responses to antigens expressed by disease-causing agents.

Autoimmunity is a disturbance in the immunologic tolerance of self-antigens. Many clinical disorders are associated with autoimmunity and are referred to as *autoimmune diseases* (Table 7-2). In autoimmune diseases, the immune system reacts against self-antigens and destroys host tissues. Antibodies against self-antigens, termed *autoantibodies,* also are produced by healthy individuals, particularly elderly people, in response to tissue damage without concurrent overt autoimmune disease. In fact, the aging process may, in part, represent a deterioration of tolerance to self-antigens. The presence of small quantities of autoantibodies does not necessarily indicate disease.

Alloimmune diseases occur when the immune system of one individual produces an immunologic reaction against tissues of another individual. Alloimmunity can be observed during immunologic reactions against transfusions, grafted tissue, or the fetus during pregnancy.

Mechanisms of hypersensitivity

Diseases caused by hypersensitivity are characterized by immune mechanisms that initiate inflammation and result in the destruction of healthy tissue (see Table 7-1). These mechanisms are apparent in most hypersensitivity reactions and have been divided into four distinct types: (1) type I (IgE-mediated allergic reactions), (2) type II (tissue-specific reactions), (3) type III (immune-complex-mediated reactions), and (4) type IV (cell-mediated reactions) (Table 7-3).

Hypersensitivity reactions are immediate or delayed, depending on the time required for the reaction to appear after reexposure to the antigen. *Immediate hypersensitivity reactions* occur in minutes to a few hours; *delayed hypersensitivity reactions* may take several hours and are at maximum severity days after reexposure to the antigen.

The most severe immediate hypersensitivity reaction is *anaphylaxis,* which is a rapid and severe response occurring within minutes of reexposure to the antigen.[2-4] It can be either systemic (generalized) or cutaneous (localized).[5] Symptoms of systemic anaphylaxis include itching, erythema, vomiting, abdominal cramps, diarrhea, and breathing difficulties. In severe cases, laryngeal edema and vascular collapse may result in respiratory distress, decreased blood pressure, shock, and death. Cutaneous anaphylaxis causes the less severe symptoms of local inflammation.

IgE-mediated reactions

Type I reactions are characterized by the production of antigen-specific IgE after exposure to an antigen. Most common allergic reactions are mediated by IgE and therefore are type I reactions. In addition, most type I reactions are against en-

TABLE 7-1	Relative Incidences and Examples of Hypersensitivity Reactions*			
	Mechanism			
Target Antigen	**Type I (IgE-Mediated)**	**Type II (Tissue-Specific)**	**Type III (Immune-Complex)**	**Type IV (Cell-Mediated)**
Allergy Environmental antigens	++++ Hay fever	+ Hemolysis in drug allergies	+ Gluten (wheat allergy)	++ Poison ivy allergy
Autoimmunity Self-antigens	± May contribute to some type III reactions	++ Autoimmune thrombocytopenia	+++ Systemic lupus erythematosus	+ Hashimoto thyroiditis
Alloimmunity Other person's antigens	± May contribute to some type III reactions	++ Hemolytic disease of the newborn	+ Anaphylaxis to IgA in IV γ-globulin	++ Graft rejection

The frequency of each reaction is indicated in a range from rare (±) to very common (++++). An example of each reaction is given.

TABLE 7-2   Disorders Associated With Autoimmunity

System Disease	Organ or Tissue	System Disease	Organ or Tissue
Endocrine system		**Eye**	
Hyperthyroidism (Graves disease)	Thyroid gland	Sjögren syndrome	Lacrimal gland
Autoimmune thyroiditis	Thyroid gland	Uveitis	Uveal structures
Primary myxedema	Thyroid gland		
Insulin-dependent diabetes	Pancreas	**Connective tissue**	
Addison disease	Adrenal gland	Ankylosing spondylitis	Joints
Premature gonadal failure	Ovary	Rheumatoid arthritis	Joints
Male infertility	Testis	Systemic lupus erythematosus	Multiple sites
Orchitis	Testis	Mixed connective tissue disease	Multiple sites
Female infertility	Ovary		
Idiopathic hypoparathyroidism	Parathyroid gland	Polyarteritis nodosa (necrotizing vasculitis)	Arterioles (small arteries)
Partial pituitary deficiency	Pituitary gland	Scleroderma (progressive systemic sclerosis)	Multiple organs
		Felty syndrome	Joints
Skin			
Pemphigus vulgaris	Skin	**Renal system**	
Bullous pemphigoid	Skin	Immune-complex glomerulonephritis	Kidney
Dermatitis herpetiformis	Skin	Goodpasture disease	Kidney
Vitiligo	Skin		
		Hematologic system	
Neuromuscular tissue		Idiopathic neutropenia	Neutrophil
Polymyositis (dermatomyositis)	Muscle	Idiopathic lymphopenia	Lymphocytes
Multiple sclerosis	Neural tissue	Autoimmune hemolytic anemia	Erythrocytes
Myasthenia gravis	Neuromuscular junction	Autoimmune thrombo-cytopenic purpura	Platelets
Polyneuritis	Nerve cell		
Rheumatic fever	Heart	**Respiratory system**	
Cardiomyopathy	Heart	Goodpasture disease	Lung
Postvaccinal or post-infectious encephalitis	Central nervous system		
Gastrointestinal system			
Celiac disease	Intestine		
Ulcerative colitis	Colon		
Crohn disease	Ileum		
Pernicious anemia	Stomach		
Atrophic gastritis	Stomach		
Primary biliary cirrhosis	Liver		
Chronic active hepatitis	Liver		

TABLE 7-3   Immunologic Mechanisms of Tissue Destruction

Type	Name	Rate of Development	Class of Antibody Involved	Principal Effector Cells Involved	Complement Participation	Examples of Disorders
I	IgE-mediated reaction	Immediate	IgE	Mast cells	No	Seasonal allergic rhinitis
II	Tissue-specific reaction	Immediate	IgG IgM	Macrophages in tissues	Frequently	Autoimmune thrombocy-topenic purpura, Graves disease, autoimmune he-molytic anemia
III	Immune-complex-mediated reaction	Immediate	IgG IgM	Neutrophils	Yes	Systemic lupus erythematosus
IV	Cell-mediated reaction	Delayed	None	Lymphocytes Macrophages	No	Contact sensitivity to poison ivy and metals

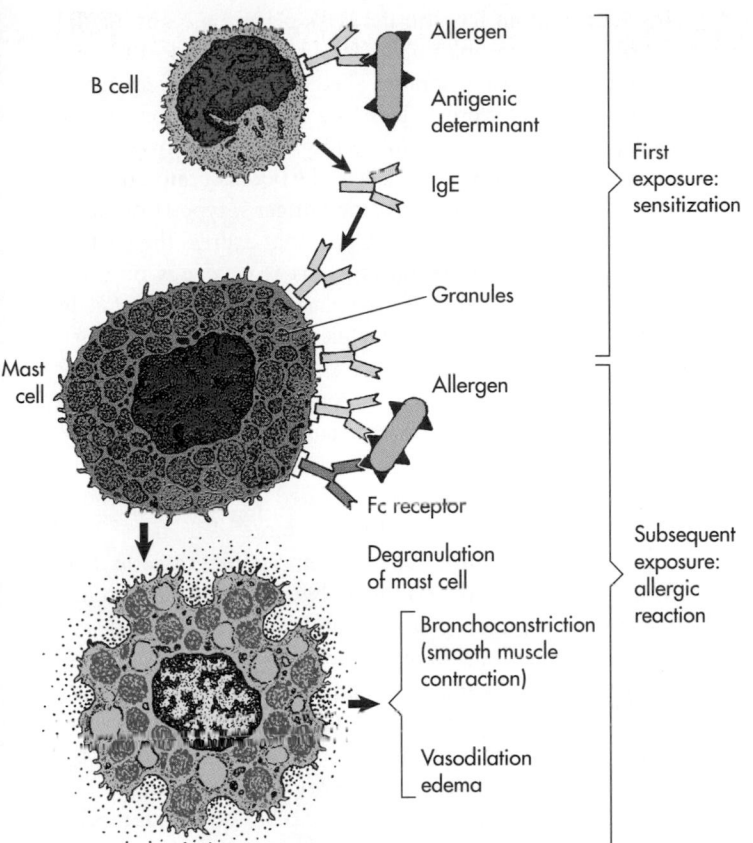

Fig. 7-1 *Mechanism of type I, IgE-mediated reactions.* Initial sensitization to an allergen stimulates B cells to produce IgE. The IgE coats the surface of the mast cell by binding with IgE-specific Fc receptors on the mast cell's plasma membrane. Further exposure to the same allergen cross-links the surface-bound IgE and causes degranulation of the mast cell.

vironmental antigens (*allergens*) and are therefore allergic. Most allergens appear to be proteins that enter the host from the environment.

Role of IgE. Exposure to an allergen can cause IgE production by selected B cells. Repeated exposure to relatively large doses of allergen usually is required to elicit enough IgE so that the person is "sensitized." IgE binds to crystallizable fragment (Fc) receptors on the plasma membranes of mast cells (Fig. 7-1). The Fc receptors on mast cells bind with IgE that has not previously interacted with antigen.

After the individual is sensitized, and with further exposure to the allergen, the allergen's antigenic determinants bind to two molecules of mast-cell-bound IgE (cross-linking two IgE-Fc receptor complexes), initiating degranulation of the mast cell and the release of mast cell products (see Chapter 6). Sometimes the IgE-mediated allergic response is beneficial to the host, as with IgE-mediated destruction of parasites.

Mechanisms of IgE-mediated hypersensitivity. The products of mast cell degranulation can modulate almost all aspects of an acute inflammatory response. The most potent mediator, histamine, affects key target cells. Histamine, acting through H1 receptors, contracts bronchial smooth muscles, causing bronchial constriction; increases vascular

permeability, causing edema; and causes vasodilation, increasing blood flow into the affected area. The interaction of histamine with H2 receptors on target cells results in increased gastric secretion and a decrease of histamine released from mast cells and basophils. The released histamine inhibits release of additional histamine by interacting with histamine receptors on the mast cells.

Although some control of the allergic response is mediated through histamine receptors, the primary mechanism of control is the autonomic nervous system. Its biochemical mediators (e.g., epinephrine, acetylcholine) have profound effects on the behavior of target cells in the host tissue. They bind to appropriate receptors on both mast cells and the target cells of inflammation, thereby controlling (1) release of inflammatory mediators from mast cells and (2) the degree to which target cells respond to inflammatory mediators (see Chapters 5 and 6).

Clinical Manifestations

The clinical manifestations of type I reactions are attributable mostly to the effects of histamine. The target tissues of the type I response contain large numbers of mast cells and are sensitive to the effects of histamine released from them. These tissues are found in the gastrointestinal tract, the skin, and the respiratory tract (Fig. 7-2 and Table 7-4).

Genetic predisposition. Certain individuals appear to be prone to allergies or are *atopic.* Atopic individuals tend to produce higher concentrations of IgE and to have more Fc receptors on their mast cells. The airways and skin of atopic individuals are also more responsive to specific and nonspecific stimuli than the airways and skin of normal individuals. In families in which one parent has an allergy, allergies develop in about 40% of the offspring. If both parents have atopic disease, the incidence in offspring is approximately 80%. Investigators have been accumulating evidence that a gene on chromosome 11 is associated with as many as 60% of atopy cases.[6] Although not totally confirmed, the candidate gene appears to be the gene for the IgE-Fc receptor. In these studies the risk of atopy was higher in children of atopic mothers than in children of unaffected mothers.[6,7]

Tests of IgE-mediated hypersensitivity. Allergic reactions can be life threatening; therefore severely allergic individuals must be made aware of the specific allergen against which they are sensitized and be instructed to avoid contact with that material. Several tests are available to determine the specific allergen, including skin tests with allergens and laboratory tests for allergen-specific IgE.

On injection of an allergen into (intradermal) or onto (epicutaneous or prick test) the skin of a sensitized individual, a local anaphylactic reaction occurs within a few minutes. It consists of a wheal (soft, white center) and flare (reddish skin surrounding the wheal) reaction. The diameter of the flare reaction usually indicates the individual's sensitivity to that allergen. In the most severely allergic individuals, even the extremely small amounts of allergen used for the skin test may evoke systemic anaphylaxis.

Various laboratory tests detect IgE antibodies. *Radioimmunosorbent (RIST) testing* measures circulating levels of

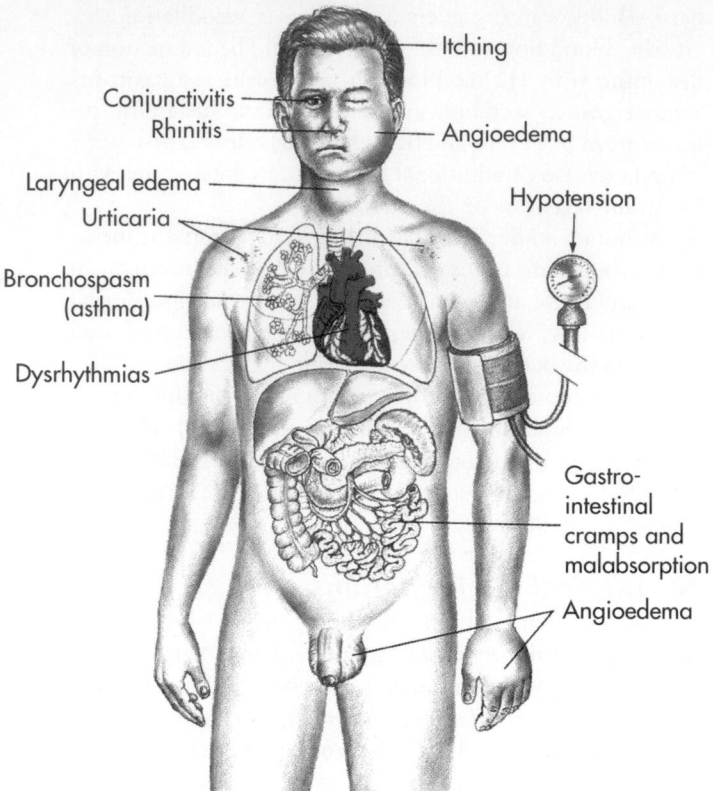

Itching
Conjunctivitis
Rhinitis
Angioedema
Laryngeal edema
Urticaria
Hypotension
Bronchospasm (asthma)
Dysrhythmias
Gastro-intestinal cramps and malabsorption
Angioedema

Fig. 7-2 *Type I hypersensitivity reactions.* Local manifestations of allergic reactions as a result of type I hypersensitivity include itching, angioedema (swelling caused by exudation), edema of the larynx, urticaria (hives), bronchospasm (constriction of airways in the lungs), hypotension (low blood pressure) and dysrhythmias (irregular heartbeat) because of anaphylactic shock, and gastrointestinal cramping caused by inflammation of the gastrointestinal mucosa.

total IgE—with atopic individuals usually having elevated levels. ***Radioallergosorbent (RAST) testing*** measures circulating levels of specific IgE antibodies against many allergens; the amount of IgE has been found to correlate well with the degree of positive skin test and the severity of clinical symptoms.

Desensitization. Clinical desensitization to allergens can be achieved in some individuals. Minute quantities of the allergen are injected in increasing doses over a prolonged period. This procedure may reduce the severity of the allergic reaction in the treated individual. Desensitization may work by inducing the production of large amounts of so-called blocking antibodies. A ***blocking antibody*** presumably competes in the tissues or circulation for binding with antigenic determinants on the allergen. Thus neutralized, the antigen cannot bind with IgE on mast cells. In serum, blocking antibodies are predominantly IgG.

Tissue-specific reactions

Type II hypersensitivity reactions generally are characterized by the destruction of a target cell through the action of anti-

body against an antigen on the cell's plasma membrane. In addition to histocompatibility (HLA) antigens, most tissues have other antigens, generally called ***tissue-specific antigens*** because they are expressed on the plasma membranes of only certain cells. Platelets, for example, have groups of self-antigens found on no other cells of the body. Because of limited distribution of tissue-specific antigens, type II diseases are limited to those tissues or organs that express the particular antigen. Environmental antigens (e.g., drugs or their metabolites) also may bind to the plasma membranes of cells (especially erythrocytes and platelets) and function as targets of type II reactions.

Type II, or tissue-specific, hypersensitivity reactions can destroy or alter cells by four mechanisms (Fig. 7-3). All begin with antibody binding to tissue-specific antigens. The first mechanism, complement-mediated lysis of cells, occurs when antibody that is bound to the target cell "fixes" (attaches) complement, initiating the complement cascade. The second mechanism, phagocytosis by macrophages, occurs when the macrophage recognizes and binds the antibody on the opsonized cell. Antibody-dependent cell-mediated cytotoxicity (ADCC), the third mechanism, involves cell destruction by a subpopulation of cytotoxic cells, which are not antigen-specific. Antibody on the target cell is recognized by and bound to Fc receptors on the cytotoxic cells, which release toxic substances that destroy the cell. The fourth mechanism does not destroy the target cell but, rather, causes it to malfunction. The damage is done by antibody binding alone.

Immune-complex-mediated injury

Mechanisms. Most type III hypersensitivity diseases are caused by antigen-antibody (immune) complexes formed in the circulation and deposited later in vessel walls or extravascular tissues (Fig. 7-4). Type III (immune-complex-mediated) reactions therefore are not organ specific, and symptoms have very little to do with the antigenic target of the antibody.[8] In some instances, immune-complex disease begins with the deposition of antigen in the tissues and is followed by local interactions with antibody and complement. Regardless of whether immune complexes are formed in the circulation or in the tissues, their harmful effects are caused by complement activation, particularly the generation of complement fragments that are chemotactic for neutrophils. The neutrophils attempt to ingest the immune complexes but frequently are unsuccessful because the complexes are bound to the tissues. During the neutrophil's attempts to phagocytose the immune complexes, large quantities of lysosomal enzymes are released into the inflammatory site instead of into phagolysosomes. The attraction of neutrophils and the subsequent release of lysosomal enzymes cause most of the resulting tissue damage.

Immune-complex disease. Immune complexes may change and cause changes in severity of the symptoms. Variations in the ratio of antigen to antibody, the class and subclass of antibody, and the quantity and quality of circulating antigen cause disease activity to be in constant flux.

TABLE 7-4	Causes of Clinical Manifestations of Allergy	
Typical Allergen	Mechanism of Hypersensitivity	Clinical Manifestation
Ingestants		
Foods	Type I	Gastrointestinal allergy
Drugs	Types I, II, III	Urticaria, immediate drug reaction, hemolytic anemia, serum sickness
Inhalants		
Pollens, dust, molds	Type I	Allergic rhinitis, bronchial asthma
Aspergillus fumigatus	Types I, III	Allergic bronchopulmonary aspergillosis
Thermophilic actinomycetes*	Types III, IV	Extrinsic allergic alveolitis
Injectants		
Drugs	Types I, II, III	Immediate drug reaction, hemolytic anemia, serum sickness
Bee venom	Type I	Anaphylaxis
Vaccines	Type III	Localized Arthus reaction
Serum	Types I, III	Anaphylaxis, serum sickness
Contactants		
Poison ivy, metals	Type IV	Contact dermatitis

Modified from Bellanti, J.A. (1985). Immunology III. Philadelphia: Saunders.
An order of fungi that is stimulated by warmth to grow and proliferate.

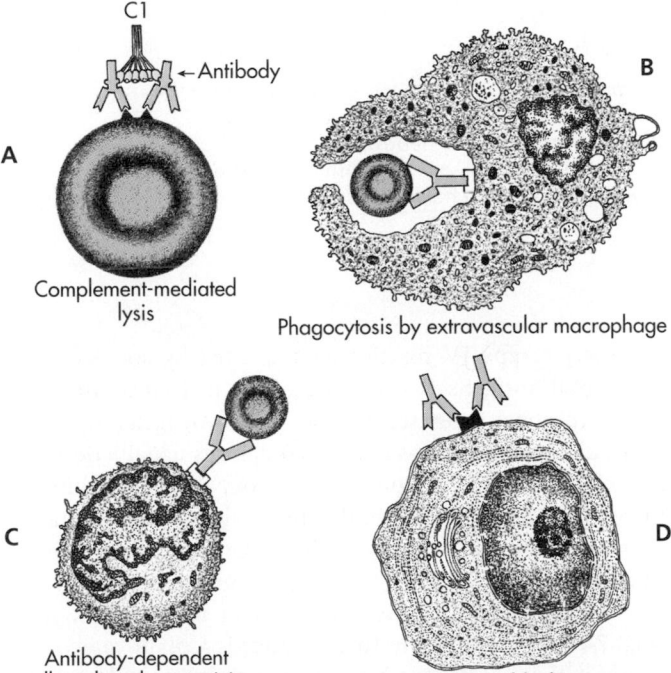

Fig. 7-3 *Mechanisms of type II, tissue-specific reactions.* Antigens on the target cell bind with antibody and are destroyed or prevented from functioning by, **A,** complement-mediated lysis; **B,** clearance by macrophages in tissues; **C,** antibody-dependent, cell-mediated cytotoxicity (ADCC); or **D,** the modulation or blockage of receptors on the target cell.

Because some immune complexes activate complement very effectively and bind some complement components, complement levels in the blood also are in flux. In many conditions in which immune complexes are formed, the individual's blood becomes **hypocomplementemic** (i.e., contains decreased amounts of complement activity). In conditions caused by the other three mechanisms of hypersensitivity (types I, II, and IV) complement levels are unaffected or some components of the complement cascade, such as C3, may even be increased.

Immune-complex formation is dynamic; those immune complexes formed early in a disease may be totally different from those formed later. Several types of immune complexes may be present simultaneously. With the tremendous potential heterogeneity of immune complexes, it is not surprising that these diseases are characterized by various symptoms and periods of remission or exacerbation of symptoms. Table 7-5 describes the two basic forms of immune-complex-mediated disease.

Cell-mediated tissue destruction

Whereas hypersensitivity reactions I, II, and III are mediated by antibody, type IV (cell-mediated) reactions are mediated by specifically sensitized T lymphocytes and do not involve antibody (Fig. 7-5). Type IV mechanisms occur as one of two types involving either cytotoxic T lymphocytes (Tc cells) or lymphokine-producing T cells (Td cells). Tc cells can attack and destroy cellular targets directly. Td cells produce lymphokines that affect various types of cells and can recruit and activate phagocytic cells, especially macrophages, at the inflammatory site. Tissue destruction usually is caused by direct killing by toxins from cytotoxic T cells or the release of

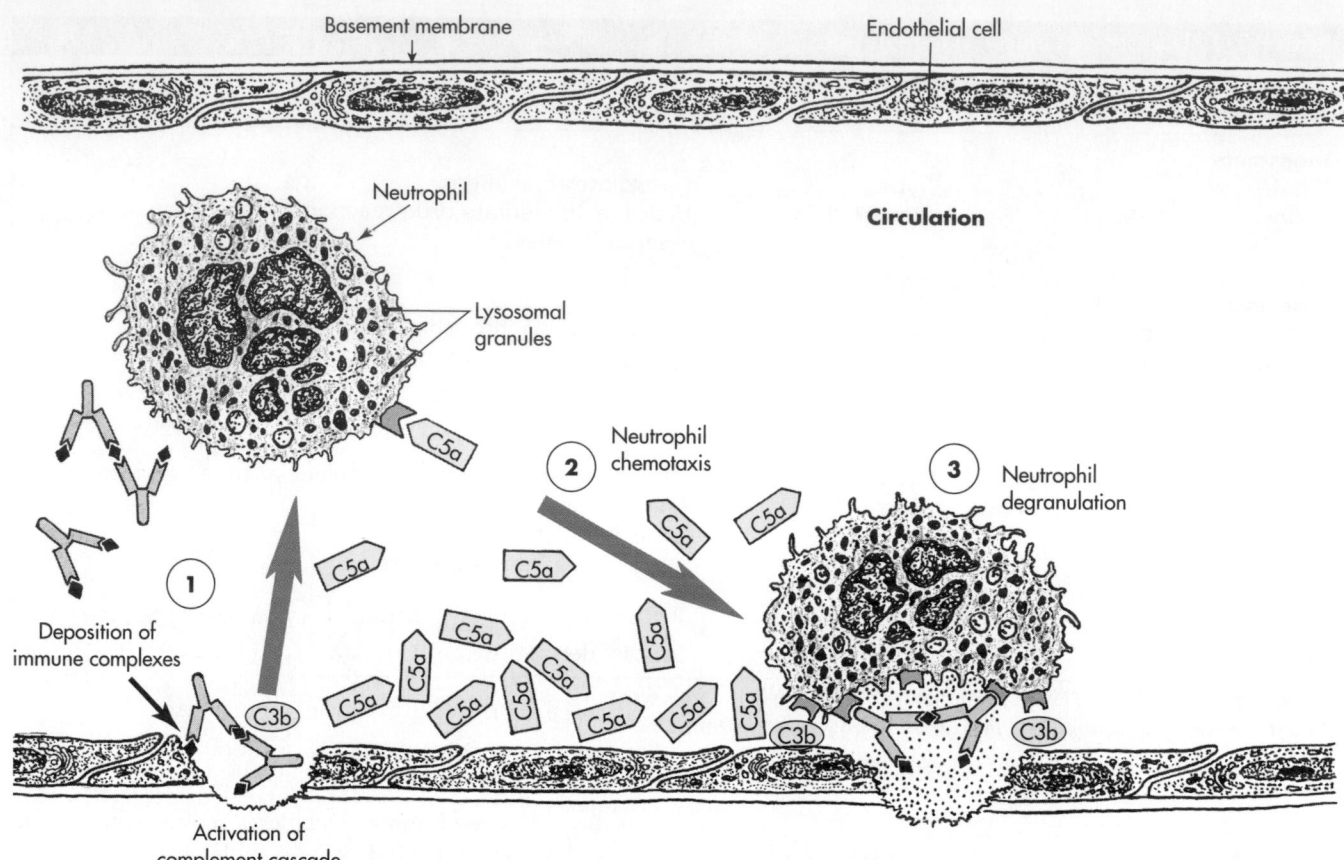

Fig. 7-4 *Mechanism of type III, immune-complex-mediated reactions.* Immune complexes are deposited in the vessels or other healthy tissue, where they activate the complement cascade and generate complement fragments, including C5a *(1)*. C5a is chemotactic for neutrophils, which migrate into the inflamed area *(2)* and attach to the IgG and C3b in the immune complexes. The neutrophils degranulate a variety of degradative enzymes that destroy healthy tissues *(3)*.

soluble factors, such as lysosomal enzymes and toxic oxygen products from macrophages.

Clinical examples of type IV hypersensitivity include graft rejection, tumor rejection, the tuberculin reaction, and allergic reactions resulting from contact with substances such as poison ivy and metals. A type IV component also may be present in autoimmune diseases such as rheumatoid arthritis, in which the self-antigen is apparently type II collagen (a protein present in joint tissues); autoimmune thyroiditis (Hashimoto disease), in which the self-antigen is a protein on thyroid cells; and insulin-dependent diabetes mellitus, in which the self-antigen is a protein on the beta cell of the pancreas (the cell that normally produces insulin).

A type IV hypersensitivity in the skin led to the development of a diagnostic skin test for tuberculosis.[9] The reaction that follows intradermal injection of antigen into a suitably sensitized individual is called a *delayed hypersensitivity skin test* because of its slow onset—24 to 72 hours to reach maximal intensity. It consists of induration (hard, white central area) and erythema (reddish surrounding skin). The reaction site is infiltrated with T lymphocytes and macrophages.

Allergic type IV reactions are elicited by some environmental antigens that are too small to induce an immune response themselves (haptens). Antigens with a molecular weight of less than 1000 daltons usually do not induce an immune response directly but do so after binding with a carrier protein in the host. With allergic contact dermatitis, the carrier protein is in the skin of the host. The best-known example of allergic contact dermatitis is the delayed reaction caused by contact with poison ivy (Fig. 7-6). The antigen in this instance is a plant catechol, *urushiol,* that reacts with normal skin proteins and evokes a cell-mediated immune response. Skin reactions to industrial chemicals, cosmetics, detergents, clothing, food, metals, and topical medicines (e.g., penicillin) are elicited by the same mechanism.

Whether a skin reaction is caused by immediate or delayed hypersensitivity may be determined by the distribution of the lesions. The immediate reaction, termed **atopic dermatitis,** is characterized by widely distributed lesions, whereas **contact dermatitis** (delayed hypersensitivity) consists of lesions only at the site of contact (Fig. 7-7).

TABLE 7-5	Models of Immune-Complex-Mediated Disease	
Name	Causes	Manifestations
Serum sickness, e.g., Raynaud phenomenon	Generalized deposition of immune complexes and inflammation (e.g., from repeated IV administration of certain antigens, such as drugs); Raynaud phenomenon is caused by cold temperature–dependent precipitation of immune complexes in the peripheral circulation	Pain at sites of inflammation: blood vessels, joints, and kidneys are generally affected; fever, enlarged lymph nodes, rash, localized pallor, and numbness followed by cyanosis and gangrene
Arthus reaction	By repeated local exposure to antigen that reacts in the walls of blood vessels with preformed antibody	Begins within 1 hr after exposure and peaks 6-12 hrs later; lesions are characterized by increased vascular permeability, accumulation of neutrophils, edema, hemorrhage, clotting, and tissue damage

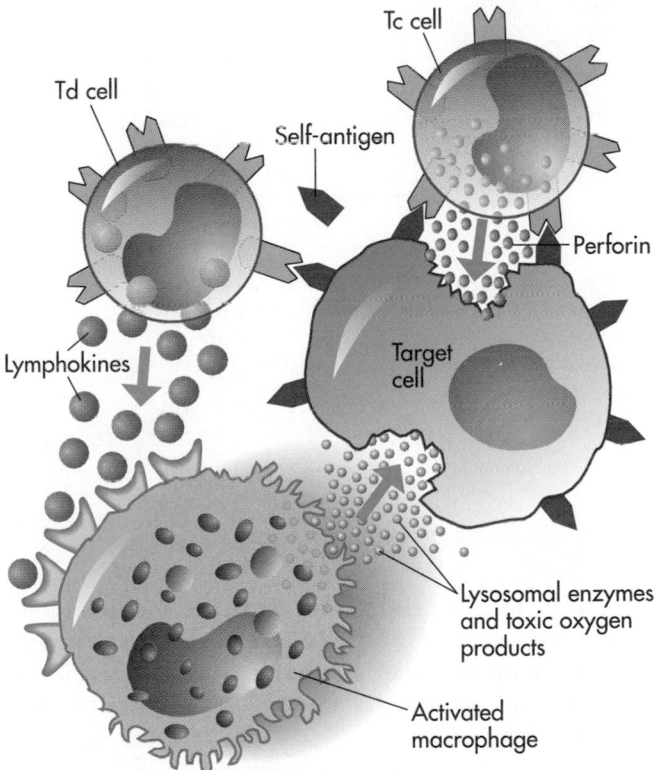

Fig. 7-5 *Mechanism of type IV cell-mediated reactions.* Self-antigens from target cells stimulate T cells to produce cytotoxic T cells *(Tc)*, which have direct cytotoxic activity, and T cells involved in delayed hypersensitivity *(Td)*. Td cells, a form of Th cells, produce lymphokines, some of which attract and activate macrophages. The macrophages and enzymes released by them are responsible for most of the tissue destruction.

✓QUICK CHECK

Distinguish among the four types of hypersensitivity mechanisms.

Why is anaphylaxis a serious problem?

Why does poison ivy cause a delayed hypersensitivity reaction?

Targets of hypersensitivity
Allergy
Allergens are environmental antigens that cause atypically exorbitant immunologic responses in genetically predisposed individuals. Typical allergens include pollens (e.g., ragweed, timothy); molds and fungi (e.g., *Penicillium notatum*); foods (e.g., milk, eggs, fish); animals (e.g., cat dander, dog dander); cigarette smoke; and components of house dust (e.g., fecal pellets of house mites). Frequently, the allergen is contained within a particle that is too large to be phagocytosed or is surrounded by a protective nonallergenic coat. The actual allergen is released after enzymatic breakdown (e.g., by lysozyme in secretions) of the larger particle. Most allergens are either haptens that can react with proteins or small-molecular-weight proteins.

In certain situations an allergen complexes with components of host tissue. The **neoantigen,** or new antigenic determinant, is recognized as foreign, and the tissue is destroyed. This occurs in allergic reactions to drugs (e.g., penicillin, sulfonamides), which are usually haptens and become immunogenic after binding to the host cell's proteins. The immune system attacks the neoantigen on the host cell's membrane and destroys the cell as well. In allergic reactions to penicillin, the immunogenic antigen is a metabolite of penicillin catabolism that binds to the plasma membranes of erythrocytes and induces an antibody response that destroys the cells, causing anemia.

The allergens that induce contact hypersensitivity, a type

Fig. 7-6 *Development of allergic contact dermatitis, a delayed hypersensitivity reaction.* Shown here is the development of allergy to catechols from poison ivy. No dermatitis results from the primary contact because the antigens (catechols) are catabolized before any sensitized T cells are produced. Secondary contact, however, quickly activates a type IV cell-mediated reaction that causes dermatitis.

Fig. 7-7 *Contact dermatitis.* Contact dermatitis caused by a delayed hypersensitivity reaction leading to vesicles and scaling at the sites of contact. *(From Damjanov, I. & Linder, J. [1996]. Anderson's pathology [10th ed.]. St. Louis: Mosby.)*

IV allergic reaction, also are haptens (e.g., metals such as nickel; acetylates and chemicals in rubber; resins in poison ivy and poison oak) that react with normal self-proteins in the skin. When presented in this way, these antigens induce a cell-mediated response.

Autoimmunity

Breakdown of tolerance. Immunologic tolerance develops in humans during the embryonic period, when autoreactive lymphocytes are either eliminated or suppressed. Autoimmunity is a breakdown of tolerance in which the body's immune system begins to recognize self-antigens as foreign.

Original insult. The cause of some immune diseases is quite apparent, as in drug-induced anemia or thrombocytopenia (decreased numbers of circulating platelets) or virus-induced changes, such as rubella infections, in which antigenic alterations result in the destruction of circulating erythrocytes, thrombocytes, or other cells. The causes of other immune diseases, such as rheumatoid arthritis and systemic lupus erythematosus (SLE), are less clear. Most autoimmune diseases are probably sequelae of preexisting infections that leave no traces. The only autoimmune disease, however, that has been associated conclusively with a preceding infection is rheumatic heart disease and a group A streptococcal infection.

Genetic factors. Genetic factors that contribute to autoimmunity are easier to identify than pathogenic agents. It is fairly well established that autoimmune diseases are familial. Affected family members may not all develop the same disease, but several members may have disorders characterized by hypersensitivity.

The association of diseases with specific HLA antigens (see Chapter 5) has been recognized and is a relatively nebulous phenomenon. Individuals with some diseases are more likely than the general population to have a specific HLA allele or alleles. The association of some HLA alleles with inappropriate immune function may directly involve the products of the HLA locus or the histocompatibility-complex-linked immune response (Ir) genes. These genes may determine an individual's susceptibility to specific infectious agents or his or her capacity to mount an immune response against specific antigens.

Alloimmunity

Alloimmunity occurs when an individual's immune system reacts against antigens on the tissues of other members of the same species. There are two clinically relevant examples of this reactivity: (1) transient neonatal diseases (in which the maternal immune system becomes sensitized against antigens expressed by the fetus); and (2) transplant rejection and transfusion reactions (in which the immune system of a recipient of an organ transplant or blood transfusion reacts against antigens on the donor cells).

Because the fetus is a hybrid between the mother and father, it expresses paternal antigens that are not found in the mother. Occasionally, these fetal antigens cross the placenta and elicit an immune response in the mother. Maternal antibody may be transported into the fetal circulation to produce alloimmune disease in the fetus. The mother's immune system produces the antibody, but because her cells do not express the target antigen, she has no manifestations of the disease.

Transient neonatal disease may also be in conjunction with maternal autoimmune diseases. The mother may be producing an IgG autoantibody specific for her self-antigens that are found on fetal cells as well. Therefore symptoms of the same autoimmune disease may affect both mother and child, even though the autoantibody is being produced only by the mother's immune system. This form of disease usually occurs only in association with type II (tissue-specific) reactions. It does not occur in association with type I, type III, or type IV reactions because the immunologic effectors of these reactions (IgE, immune complexes, or T cells) do not readily cross the placenta and enter the fetal circulation in sufficient quantity.

At birth, the source of the antibody in the fetal circulation is removed. Although symptoms of the immune disease may be manifested in utero or immediately after birth and may be fatal to the fetus or neonate, if symptoms are successfully treated at birth, the disease will disappear as the maternal antibody is catabolized.

The child can be affected in the following immunologic diseases:

1. Graves disease, an autoimmune disease in which maternal antibody against the receptor for thyroid-stimulating hormone causes neonatal hyperthyroidism[10]
2. Myasthenia gravis, an autoimmune disease in which maternal antibody binds with receptors for neural transmitters on muscle cells, causing neonatal muscular weakness (see Chapter 15)
3. Immune thrombocytopenic purpura, in which maternal antiplatelet antibody destroys platelets in the fetus and neonate (see Chapter 21)
4. Alloimmune neutropenia, in which maternal antibody against neutrophils destroys neutrophils in the fetus and neonate
5. Systemic lupus erythematosus (SLE), in which diverse maternal autoantibodies induce anomalies (e.g., congenital heart defects) in the fetus
6. Rh and ABO alloimmunization (e.g., erythroblastosis fetalis), in which maternal antibody against erythrocyte antigens induces anemia in the child (see Chapter 21)

Autoimmune and alloimmune diseases

Immunity and alloimmunity are exemplified by two disease states—SLE (an autoimmune disease) and transplant rejection (an alloimmune phenomenon). Most of the classic autoimmune diseases, including disorders of the endocrine system (autoimmune thyroiditis, Graves disease), hematologic system (the hemolytic and pernicious anemias), nervous system (myasthenia gravis), and connective tissue in joints (rheumatoid arthritis) are discussed in Unit II of this book.

Systemic lupus erythematosus

Systemic lupus erythematosus (SLE), which is a chronic, multisystem, inflammatory disease, is one of the most common, complex, and serious of the autoimmune disorders.[11] SLE is characterized by the production of a large variety of autoantibodies against nucleic acids, erythrocytes, coagulation proteins, phospholipids, lymphocytes, platelets, and many other self-components. The most characteristic autoantibodies produced in SLE are against nucleic material: single-stranded deoxyribonucleic acid (DNA), double-stranded DNA, histones, ribonucleoproteins, and others.

Deposition of circulating immune complexes containing antibody against host DNA produces tissue damage in individuals with SLE. DNA and DNA-containing immune complexes may be selectively deposited in the glomerulus. (Kidney structures are described in Chapter 28.) The presence of DNA in the circulation increases from cellular damage in response to trauma, drugs, or infections; it usually is removed in the liver, but removal of circulating DNA is slowed when there are immune complexes, thereby increasing the potential for deposition in the kidney.[12] (The liver's role in removing waste products from the blood is discussed in Chapter 33.) Deposition of immune complexes composed of DNA and antibody also causes inflammatory lesions in the renal tubular basement membranes, brain (choroid plexus), heart, spleen, lung, gastrointestinal tract, skin, and peritoneum.

SLE, as with most autoimmune diseases, is seen more frequently in women, especially in the 20- to 40-year-old age-group. Blacks are affected more frequently than whites. A genetic predisposition for the disease has been implicated on the basis of increased incidence in twins and the existence of autoimmune disease in the families of individuals with SLE.

A transient, lupuslike syndrome that is indistinguishable both clinically and in the laboratory from spontaneously occurring SLE also can develop from the prolonged use of drugs, particularly hydralazine (an antihypertensive agent) and procainamide (an antidysrhythmic drug). In genetically susceptible individuals, certain environmental agents, such as ultraviolet light, and several infectious agents may trigger lupuslike immune reactions.

Clinical manifestations of SLE include arthralgias or arthritis (90% of individuals), vasculitis and rash (70% to 80% of individuals), renal disease (40% to 50% of individuals), hematologic abnormalities (50% of individuals, with anemia being the most common complication), and cardiovascular diseases (30% to 50% of individuals). As with most autoimmune diseases, SLE has frequent remissions and exacerbations. Because the signs and symptoms affect almost every body system and tend to come and go, SLE is extremely difficult to diagnose. This has led to the development of a list of 11 clinical findings. The serial or simultaneous presence of at least four of them indicates that the individual has SLE. The 11 findings are as follows[13]:

1. Facial rash confined to the cheeks (malar rash)
2. Discoid rash (raised patches, scaling)
3. Photosensitivity (skin rash in sunlight)
4. Oral or nasopharyngeal ulcers
5. Nonerosive arthritis of at least two peripheral joints
6. Serositis (pleurisy, pericarditis)
7. Renal disorder (proteinuria of >0.5 g/day or cellular casts)
8. Neurologic disorders (seizures or psychosis)
9. Hematologic disorders (hemolytic anemia, leukopenia, lymphopenia, or thrombocytopenia)
10. Immunologic disorders (positive LE cell preparation, anti-nDNA, anti-Smith [Sm] antigen, or false-positive serologic test for syphilis)
11. Presence of antinuclear antibody (ANA)

Graft rejection

Transplantation of organs commonly is complicated by an immune response against antigens—primarily HLA antigens—on the donated tissue. Based on renal transplant studies, the primary mechanism of the rejection of transplanted organs is a type IV, cell-mediated reaction. Two randomly chosen individuals are almost certainly antigenically different to some degree. Organ transplants between them are rejected in approximately 2 weeks without the extensive use of immunosuppressive drugs. Because HLA antigens are the principal targets of the rejection reaction, HLA matching of donor and recipient greatly enhances the probability of acceptance of the graft. (HLA is discussed in Chapter 5.)

Transplant rejection is classified as hyperacute, acute, or chronic, depending on the amount of time that elapses between transplantation and rejection. Hyperacute rejection is immediate and rare. When the circulation is reestablished to the grafted area, the graft may immediately turn white (the so-called *white graft*) instead of a normal pink color. Hyperacute rejection usually occurs in recipients with preexisting antibody to the antigens in the graft. As circulation to the graft is established, antibody binds to the grafted tissue and activates the inflammatory response, including the coagulation cascade, resulting in stasis of blood flow into the tissue. (Coagulation is described in Chapters 6 and 19.) Biopsies of the graft frequently show deposits of antibody (IgG and IgM), complement, and neutrophils.

Acute rejection is a cell-mediated immune response occurring about 2 weeks after the transplant. This type of rejection occurs when the recipient develops an immune response against unmatched HLA antigens after transplantation. Immunosuppressive drugs may delay or lessen the intensity of acute rejection. A biopsy of the rejected organ shows an infiltration of lymphocytes and macrophages characteristic of a type IV reaction.

Chronic rejection may occur after months or years of normal function. It is characterized by slow, progressive organ failure and may be caused by inflammatory damage to endothelial cells lining blood vessels as a result of a weak immunologic reaction against minor histocompatibility antigens on the grafted tissue.

✓ QUICK CHECK

Why do certain drugs become immunogenic to the host?

Why is SLE considered an autoimmune disease?

Why is transient neonatal disease considered an alloimmune disease?

INFECTION

Modern health care has shown great progress in preventing and treating infectious diseases. In developed countries sanitary living conditions, clean water, uncontaminated food, vaccinations, and antimicrobials make death from infectious disease most common only among those with debilitating diseases or immunosuppression. Infectious disease remains

The Many Relationships Between Humans and Organisms
BOX 7-1

Symbiosis. Benefits only the human; no harm to the organism
Mutualism. Benefits the human and the organism
Commensalism. Benefits only the organism; no harm to the human
Pathogenicity. Benefits the organism; harms the human (*Opportunism* is the situation when benign organisms become pathogenic because of decreased human host resistance.)

TABLE 7-6	Leading Causes of Mortality and Burden of Disease, Estimates for 1998		
	Mortality in all Member States		
	Rank	% of total	(000)
Both sexes			
Ischaemic heart disease	1	13.7	7375
Cerebrovascular disease	2	9.5	5106
Acute lower respiratory infections	3	6.4	3452
HIV/AIDS	4	4.2	2285
Chronic obstructive pulmonary disease	5	4.2	2249
Diarrhoeal diseases	6	4.1	2219
Perinatal conditions	7	4.0	2155
Tuberculosis	8	2.8	1498
Cancer of trachea/ bronchus/lung	9	2.3	1244
Road traffic accidents	10	2.2	1171
Males			
Ischaemic heart disease	1	12.8	3659
Cerebrovascular disease	2	8.2	2340
Acute lower respiratory infections	3	6.1	1753
Chronic obstructive pulmonary disease	4	4.3	1240
HIV/AIDS	5	4.1	1164
Diarrhoeal diseases	6	4.0	1149
Perinatal conditions	7	3.9	1121
Cancer of trachea/ bronchus/lung	8	3.2	911
Tuberculosis	9	3.1	893
Road traffic accidents	10	3.0	855
Females			
Ischaemic heart disease	1	14.6	3717
Cerebrovascular disease	2	10.9	2766
Acute lower respiratory infections	3	6.7	1699
HIV/AIDS	4	4.4	1121
Diarrhoeal diseases	5	4.2	1070
Perinatal conditions	6	4.1	1034
Chronic obstructive pulmonary disease	7	4.0	1010
Tuberculosis	8	2.4	605
Malaria	9	2.1	538
Measles	10	1.7	432

From World Health Report 1999. Geneva: The Organization.

a significant threat to life in many parts of the world, including South America, India, Africa, and Southeast Asia.

Table 7-6 summarizes recent leading causes of mortality as estimated by the World Health Organization. Developing countries with dense populations and poor sanitation are victims of plague, cholera, malaria, tuberculosis, leprosy, and schistosomiasis. Only smallpox has been eradicated by vaccination. Infectious disease other than acquired immunodeficiency syndrome (AIDS) is not the major cause of death in the United States (Table 7-7). Although vaccines and antimicrobials have altered the prevalence of infectious disease, mutant strains of bacteria have emerged for sexually transmitted diseases, tuberculosis, and *Staphylococcus* with resistance to protection previously provided by drug therapy. The emergence of new diseases, such as legionnaires' disease and *Hantavirus*, and the global spread of AIDS are examples of the intense challenge for the prevention and control of infectious disease. Infection is the result of an interaction between an organism and a host; the next section describes how this interaction produces disease.

Microorganisms and Humans: A Dynamic Relationship

Many microorganisms find human bodies to be hospitable sites to grow and flourish, provided with nutrients and appropriate conditions of temperature and humidity. In many cases a mutual relationship exists, in which humans and the microorganisms benefit (Box 7-1). For instance, the human gut is colonized by a large variety of microorganisms that make up normal human flora. The normal flora of different body areas are summarized in Table 7-8. These bacteria are provided with nutrients from ingested food, and in exchange they produce enzymes that facilitate the digestion and utilization of many of the more complex molecules in the human diet, produce antibacterial factors (e.g., bacteriocins, colicins) that prevent colonization by pathogenic organisms, and produce usable metabolites (e.g., vitamin K, B vitamins). This homeostasis normally is maintained through the physical integrity of the skin and mucosal epithelium and other mechanisms that guarantee that the immune and in-

TABLE 7-7 Death Rates and Percent of Total Deaths for the 10 Leading Causes of Death: United States, 1993

Rank Order*	Cause of Death (Ninth Revision, International Classification of Diseases, 1975)	Rate†	Percent of Change, 1992 to 1993
1	Diseases of heart	145.3	0.7
2	Malignant neoplasms, including neoplasms of lymphatic and hematopoietic tissues	132.6	−0.4
3	Cerebrovascular diseases	26.5	1.1
4	Chronic obstructive pulmonary diseases and allied conditions	21.4	7.5
5	Accidents and adverse effects	30.3	3.1
	Motor vehicle accidents	16.0	1.3
	All other accidents and adverse effects	14.4	5.1
6	Pneumonia and influenza	13.5	6.3
7	Diabetes mellitus	12.4	4.2
8	Human immunodeficiency virus infection	13.8	9.5
9	Suicide	11.3	1.8
10	Homicide and legal intervention	10.7	1.9

From (1996). Morbidity and Mortality Weekly Report 45 (8), 161.
Rank based on number of deaths.
†Rates per 100,000 population.

TABLE 7-8 Normal Indigenous Flora of the Human Body

Skin	Predominantly gram-positive cocci and rods. *Staphylococcus epidermidis,* corynebacteria, mycobacteria, and streptococci are primary inhabitants; *S. aureus* in some people; also yeasts (*Candida, Pityrosporum*) in some areas of skin. Numerous transient microorganisms may become temporary residents. In moist areas, gram-negative bacteria. Around sebaceous glands, *Propionibacteria* and brevibacteria. The mite *Demodex folliculorum* lives in hair follicles and sebaceous glands around the face.
Nose	Predominantly gram-positive cocci and rods, especially *S. epidermidis.* Some people are nasal carriers of pathogenic bacteria, including *S. aureus,* β-hemolytic streptococci, and *Corynebacterium diphtheriae.*
Mouth	A complex population of bacteria that includes several species of streptococci, *Actinomyces,* lactobacilli, and *Haemophilus.* Anaerobic bacteria and spirochetes colonize the gingival crevices.
Pharynx	Similar to flora in mouth plus staphylococci, *Neisseria,* and diphtheroids. Some asymptomatic persons also harbor the pathogens pneumococcus, *H. influenzae, N. meningitidis,* and *C. diphtheriae.*
Distal intestine	Enterobacteria, streptococci, lactobacilli, anaerobic bacteria, and *C. albicans.*
Colon	*Bacteroides,* lactobacilli, clostridia, *Salmonella, Shigella, Klebsiella, Proteus, Pseudomonas,* enterococci and other streptococci, bacilli, and *Escherichia coli.*
Distal urethra	Typical bacteria found on the skin, especially *S. epidermidis* and diphtheroids. Also lactobacilli and nonpathogenic streptococci.
Vagina	Birth to 1 mo: similar to adult. 1 mo to puberty: *S. epidermidis,* diphtheroids, *E. coli,* and streptococci. Puberty to menopause: *Lactobacillus acidophilus,* diphtheroids, staphylococci, streptococci, and a variety of anaerobes. Postmenopause: similar to prepubescence.

From Grimes, D.E. (1991). Infectious diseases. Mosby's Clinical Nursing Series. St. Louis: Mosby.

flammatory systems do not attack these symbiotes (see Box 7-1).

Much of the relationship is maintained by the immune and inflammatory systems. If those systems are compromised, many organisms will leave their normal sites and cause infection. Individuals with deficiencies in their immune system become easily infected with opportunistic organisms—those that normally would not cause disease but seize the opportunity provided by the person's decreased immune or inflammatory responses.

True pathogens have devised means to circumvent the normal controls provided by the host's main defensive barriers, the inflammatory system and the immune system. Infection by a pathogen is influenced by several factors:

- *Mechanism of action.* Pathogens directly damage cells, interfere with cellular metabolism, and render the cell dys-

Fig. 7-8 ***The spread of infection.*** *(Redrawn from Mims, C.A. et al. [1993].* Medical microbiology. *St. Louis: Mosby.)*

functional because of the accumulation of pathogenic substances and toxin production (see p. 196)

- *Infectivity.* Ability of the pathogen to invade and multiply in the host; for example, coagulase (an enzyme) that causes coagulation and allows some organisms, such as *Staphylococcus,* to clot and form a sticky layer around themselves, protecting themselves against host defenses
- *Pathogenicity.* Ability of an agent to produce disease depends on its speed of reproduction, extent of tissue damage, and production of toxins (see p. 196)
- *Virulence.* The potency of a pathogen measured in terms of the number of microorganisms or micrograms of toxin required to kill a host—for example, measles is of low virulence; the rabies virus is highly virulent
- *Antigenicity.* Ability of pathogens to induce an immune response, which varies considerably
- *Toxigenicity.* A factor important in determining a pathogen's virulence, such as hemolysin, leukocidin, other exotoxins, and endotoxin. Hemolysin destroys erythrocytes, and leukocidin destroys leukocytes; both are products of streptococci and staphylococci. Not all bacteria produce exotoxins and endotoxins (see p. 196)

The portal of entry for pathogenic organisms may be by direct contact, inhalation, ingestion, or the bite of animals or insects. Spread of infection is facilitated by the ability of

pathogens to attach to cell surfaces, release enzymes that dissolve protective barriers, escape the action of phagocytes, or resist the effect of low pH. After penetrating protective barriers, pathogens then spread through the lymph and blood for invasion of tissues and organs, where they multiply and cause disease. In humans the route of entrance of many pathogenic organisms also becomes the site of shedding, completing a cycle of infection. Fig. 7-8 summarizes the spread of infection in the body.

Classes of Infectious Organisms

Infectious disease can be caused by organisms that range in size from 20 nanometers (poliovirus) to 10 meters (tapeworm). Classes of pathogenic organisms and their characteristics are summarized in Table 7-9.

Innate Host Resistance Mechanisms

The first lines of defense against infectious organisms are external barriers, including the skin and mucous membranes. The digestive, respiratory, and genitourinary tracts form a closed barrier between the internal organs and the environment (Fig. 7-9). The second and third lines of defense are the inflammatory response and the immune system.

Once a microorganism penetrates the first line of defense and invades the tissues, the inflammatory response is

TABLE 7-9   Classes of Human Infectious Organisms

Class	Size	Examples of Disease
Viruses	20-30 nm	Measles
		Hepatitis B
		Pneumonitis
Bacteria	0.8-15 μm	Staphylococcal wound infection
		Cholera
		Streptococcal pneumonia
Chlamydia	200-1000 nm	Trachoma
Rickettsiae	300-1200 nm	Rocky Mountain spotted fever
Mycoplasma	125-350 nm	Mycoplasma pneumonia
Mycobacterium	1-10 μm	Tuberculosis
Fungi	2-200 μm	Tinea pedis (athlete's foot)
		Thrust
		Histoplasmosis
Protozoa	1-50 nm	Giardiasis
		Malaria
Helminths	3 mm to 10 m	Trichinosis
		Filariasis

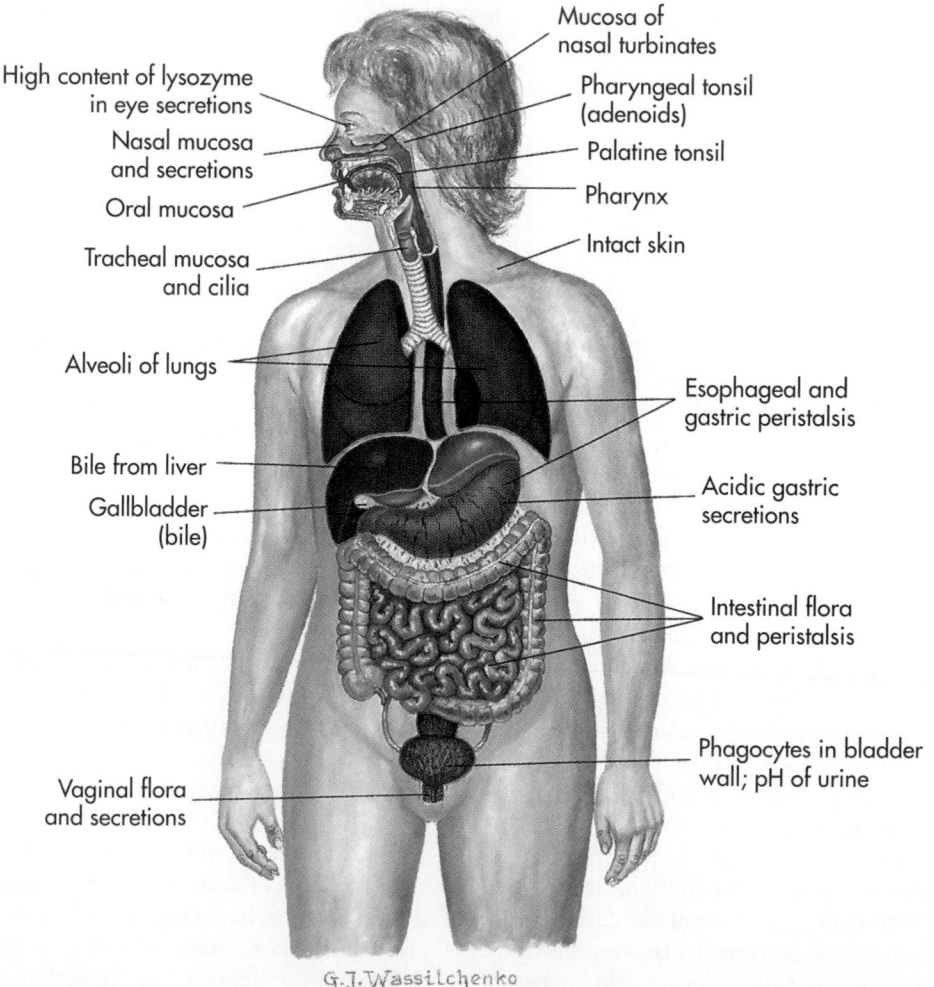

G.J.Wassilchenko

Fig. 7-9 *The closed barrier.* The digestive, respiratory, and genitourinary tracts form closed barriers between the internal organs and the environment. *(From Grimes, D.E. [1991]. Infectious diseases. Mosby's clinical nursing series. St. Louis: Mosby.)*

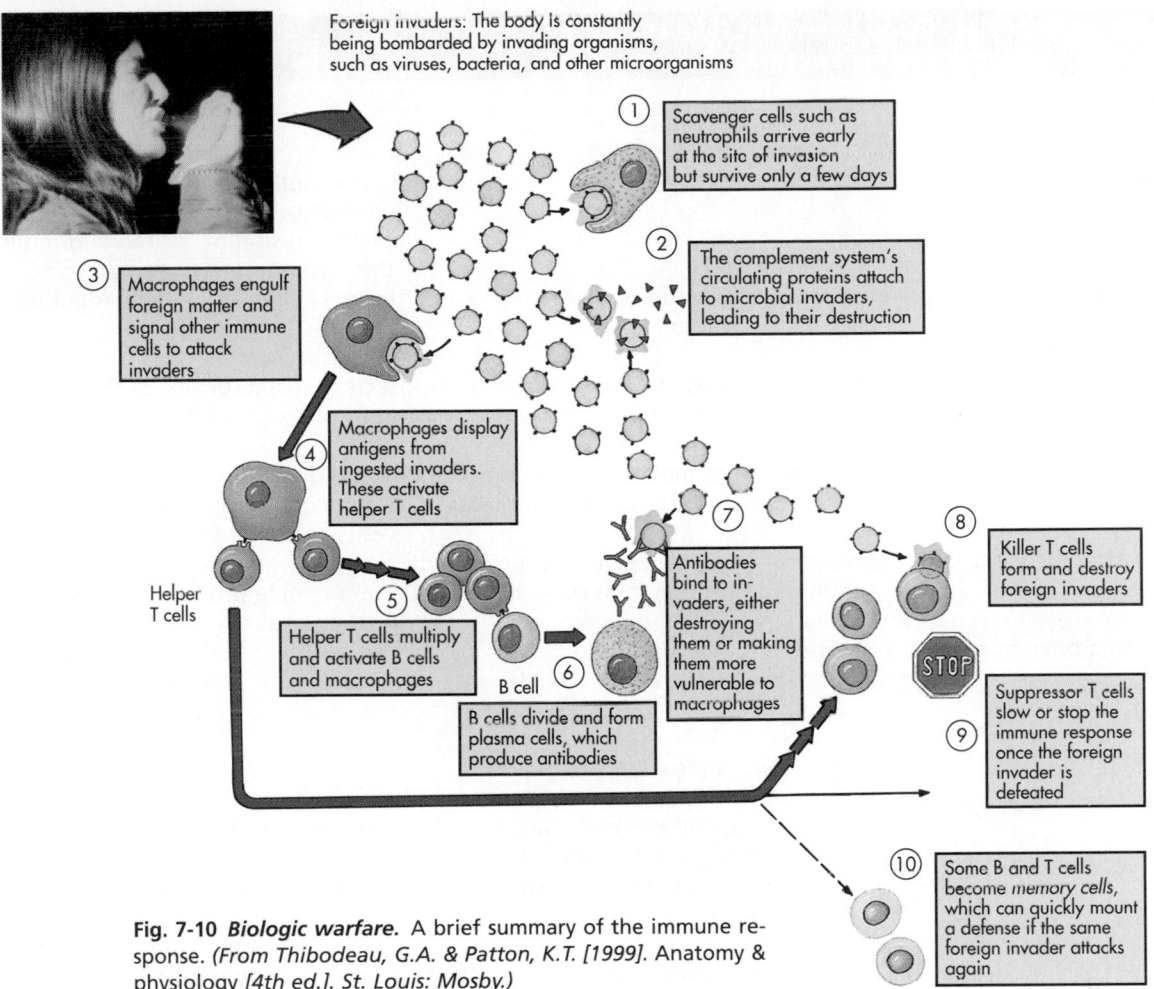

Foreign invaders: The body is constantly being bombarded by invading organisms, such as viruses, bacteria, and other microorganisms

① Scavenger cells such as neutrophils arrive early at the site of invasion but survive only a few days

② The complement system's circulating proteins attach to microbial invaders, leading to their destruction

③ Macrophages engulf foreign matter and signal other immune cells to attack invaders

④ Macrophages display antigens from ingested invaders. These activate helper T cells

Helper T cells

⑤ Helper T cells multiply and activate B cells and macrophages

B cell

⑥ B cells divide and form plasma cells, which produce antibodies

⑦ Antibodies bind to invaders, either destroying them or making them more vulnerable to macrophages

⑧ Killer T cells form and destroy foreign invaders

STOP

⑨ Suppressor T cells slow or stop the immune response once the foreign invader is defeated

⑩ Some B and T cells become *memory cells*, which can quickly mount a defense if the same foreign invader attacks again

Fig. 7-10 *Biologic warfare.* A brief summary of the immune response. *(From Thibodeau, G.A. & Patton, K.T. [1999]. Anatomy & physiology [4th ed.]. St. Louis: Mosby.)*

initiated, especially the phagocytes. The neutrophils actively attack bacteria, engulf them, and destroy the organism (phagocytosis).

The adaptation of the immune system to infection actively neutralizes bacterial defense mechanisms (Fig. 7-10; see Chapter 5 for a complete discussion). The complement system, through the alternative pathway, produces the complement protein C3b, which attaches itself to the surface of bacteria with carbohydrate capsules. C3b functions as a very effective opsonin that allows adherence between the bacterium and C3b receptors on the phagocyte's surface, thus facilitating phagocytosis. B cells also produce antibodies that bind to the surface of bacteria, act as opsonins, and can activate complement. Antibodies also are produced against most of the bacterial toxins, neutralizing their effects.

Pathogenic Defense Mechanisms

Many pathogens have devised ways of preventing destruction by the developing immune system. For example, some bacteria produce thick capsules of carbohydrate or protein that are antiphagocytic, preventing efficient phagocytosis. Others defend themselves by producing toxins that kill neutrophils. Because the primary immune response may take a

week to develop adequately, some pathogens proliferate at rates that surpass the development of a protective response. Some strains of toxin-producing group A streptococci cause destructive skin infections (e.g., flesh-eating bacteria syndrome, or necrotizing fasciitis) and pneumonia that may kill an individual within 2 days.[14] Group B streptococci from the maternal vagina may ascend the birth canal, penetrate fetal membranes, and infect the fluid surrounding the fetus. Table 7-10 contains examples of organisms that fight off the immune system or cause it to attack the host.

Viral pathogens bypass many defense mechanisms by developing intracellularly, thus hiding within tissues and away from normal inflammatory or immune responses. In many cases, however, because viral agents must spread from cell to cell, the developing immune response eventually cures the infection so the disease is self-limiting. (Viruses and viral replication are discussed on p. 198.)

If the immune system is compromised, infections will not be regulated. As a result, a normally limited and clinically mild viral or bacterial infection will become systemic and potentially fatal to the individual. Various immunodeficiency disorders are discussed on p. 204.

TABLE 7-10	Examples of Organisms That Fight Off the Immune System or Cause the Immune System to Attack the Host	
Organism	**Mechanism**	**Comment**
Bacteria		
Staphylococcus *Streptococcus*	Produces toxins	Either kill phagocytes or interfere with chemotaxis
Mycobacterium tuberculosis *Toxoplasma gondii*	Produces toxins	Prevent infusion of lysosomal granules and the formation of phagolysosome
Mycobacteria *Brucella* *Salmonella typhi*	Produces antioxidants (e.g., catalase, superoxide dismutase)	Prevents killing by O_2-dependent mechanisms
Neisseria gonorrhoeae	Produce a protease to digest IgA	Infects mucosal surface of the urethra
Streptococcus pneumoniae *Haemophilus influenzae*	Produce a protease to digest IgA	Causes pneumonia
Staphylococcus Trypanosomes Herpes simplex virus	Produces surface molecules that mimic Fc receptors, which can bind antibody	Protects organism from successful activation of the complement cascade and prevents antibody from functioning as an opsonin
Group A streptococcus	Contains an antiphagocytic capsular antigen, M protein, that resembles human myocardial antigen	Certain people produce antibody against M protein that also reacts with cardiac tissue resulting in rheumatic fever (carditis)
Mycoplasma pneumoniae	Expresses antigens similar to those found on human red blood cells	Antibodies can also react with human red blood cells
Viruses		
Influenza	Antigenic mutations ("drift") of antigen on a yearly basis	The immune response developed against the previous year's strain is no longer protective
	Severe: virus undergoes antigenic "shift" genetic recombination between the human and avian strains of the virus	Because the new virus is now very distinct from those found in previous years, no protective immune function preexists, resulting in serious infection
HIV	Can rapidly mutate its surface antigens (antigenic shift)	Antibodies produced early in the disease will not react with the antigens expressed later
Parasites		
Trypanosoma sp (sleeping sickness) *Borrelia recurrentis* (relapsing fever)	Activates genes that produce different antigens on their surface	Avoids immune rejection because the immune response is unable to identify the parasite

Infection and Injury

Bacterial

Bacteria are prokaryocytes (lacking a discrete nucleus) and are relatively small. They can be aerobic or anaerobic and motile or immotile. Spherical bacteria are called *cocci*, rodlike forms are called *bacilli*, and spiral forms are termed *spirochetes*. Gram stain and acid-fast stain are important for differentiating gram-positive or gram-negative types of bacteria. The different types of gram-positive and gram-negative bacteria are reviewed in Fig. 7-11. The general structure of bacteria is reviewed in Fig. 7-12.

Bacterial survival and growth depend on the effectiveness of the body's defense mechanisms and on the bacterium's ability to resist these defenses. Some bacteria have a coating (capsule) that protects them from ingestion and de-

struction by phagocytes. Such coatings include the thick polysaccharide covering of the pneumococcus, the waxy capsule surrounding the tubercle bacillus, and the M protein cell wall of the streptococcus.

Other bacteria survive and proliferate in the body by producing exotoxins and endotoxins that injure cells and tissues. **Exotoxins** are proteins released during bacterial growth. They are usually enzymes and have highly specific effects on host cells. **Endotoxins** (**lipopolysaccharides**) are contained in the cell walls of gram-negative bacteria and are released during lysis, or destruction, of the bacteria. Endotoxin may be released also from the membrane of the bacteria during bacterial growth or during treatment with antibiotics, which therefore cannot prevent the toxic effects of the endotoxin.[15] Bacteria that produce endotoxins are called *py-*

Gram Positive

- Rods
  - Aerobic
    - Clusters
      - Staphylococcus
    - Chains' pairs
      - Streptococcus
  - Anaerobic
- Spheres (cocci)
  - Aerobic
    - Sporing
      - Bacillus
    - Nonsporing
      - Listeria
  - Anaerobic
    - Sporing
      - Clostridium
    - Nonsporing
      - Propionibacterium

Gram Negative

- Rods
  - Aerobic
    - Simple growth requirements
      - Vibrio
        Escherichia
        Klebsiella
        Salmonella
        Shigella
        Pseudomonas
    - Fastidious growth requirements
      - Legionella
        Haemophilus
        Bordetella
        Brucella
        Campylobacter
  - Anaerobic
    - Bacteroides
- Spheres (cocci)
  - Pairs
    - Neisseria

Fig. 7-11 *Types of gram-positive and gram-negative bacteria.*

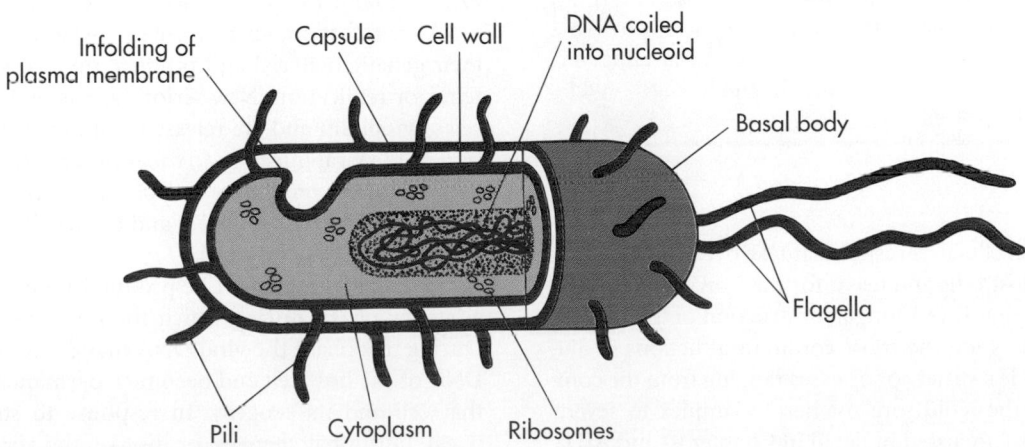

Fig. 7-12 *General structure of bacteria.* (Redrawn from Mims, C.A. et al. [1993]. Medical microbiology. St. Louis: Mosby.)

rogenic bacteria because they activate the inflammatory process and produce fever. The innermost part of the lipopolysaccharide, *lipid A,* is made of polysaccharide and fatty acids and is responsible for the substance's toxic effects.

Inflammation is the body's response to tissue injury or the presence of the bacteria. Vascular permeability is increased, allowing substances involved in bacterial destruction to leave the vessels and access the site of infection. Endotoxins increase vascular permeability further by activating the complement cascade. Vascular permeability may increase sufficiently to permit the escape of large quantities of blood, contributing to hypotension and, in severe cases, cardiovascular shock (see Chapter 23).

Septicemia (bacteremia) is the presence of bacteria in the blood and is caused by a failure of the body's defense mechanisms. The usual cause is proliferation of gram-negative bacteria, although a few gram-positive bacteria and fungi can cause it. (The gram-negative bacteria include *Escherichia coli, Serratia marcescens, Proteus mirabilis, Enterobacter aerogenes, Pseudomonas aeruginosa,* and *Bacteroides* species.) Symptoms of gram-negative septic shock are produced by endotoxins. Once in the blood, endotoxins cause the release of vasoactive peptides that affect blood vessels, producing vasodilation, which reduces blood pressure, causes decreased oxygen delivery, and produces subsequent cardiovascular shock (see Chapter 23). Sepsis is diagnosed from evaluation of blood cultures.

HEALTH ALERT

How to Avoid E. Coli

Shopping: Do not buy unpasteurized milk and milk products. Do not buy unpasteurized fruit juice. Keep raw meat separate from ready-to-eat foods.

Preparing food: Wash your hands and all foods you are going to eat raw. After handling meat, wash hands, cutting boards, and other dishes or utensils with which the meat came into contact. Cook all meat and poultry thoroughly.

Dining out: Avoid eating *rare* meat, especially hamburgers. All food should be well-cooked.

Recreation (swimming): Do not allow toddlers in diapers into swimming pools. Do not take children swimming if they have *had* diarrhea. Avoid swallowing lake water.

Viral

Viruses are intracellular parasites that take over the metabolic machinery of host cells and use it for their own survival and replication, frequently resulting in destruction of the infected cell. Viral diseases are the most common afflictions of humans and include a variety of diseases ranging from the common cold and the "cold sore" of herpes simplex to several types of cancers (discussed in detail in Chapter 9) and AIDS.

Viruses do not produce exotoxins or endotoxins. Although viruses resist phagocytosis because of their extremely small size, they will induce a strong antibody response that usually results in neutralization of the virus (see Chapter 5) and resolution of the disease.

Viral replication

Virions (viral particles) do not possess any of the metabolic organelles found in prokaryotes (e.g., bacteria) or eukaryotes (e.g., human cells). Thus viruses have no metabolism. Unlike bacteria, viruses are incapable of independent reproduction. Their replication depends totally on their ability to infect a **permissive host cell**—a cell that cannot resist viral invasion and replication. The replication cycle of most viruses can be divided into six distinct phases—adsorption, penetration, uncoating, replication, assembly, and release. Infection with a virus begins with a virion binding to a specific receptor on the plasma membrane of a host cell (Fig. 7-13). The specificity of this virus-receptor interaction dictates the range of host cells that a particular virus will infect and therefore the clinical symptoms, which reflect the alteration of the function of the infected cells. For example, the influenza virus binds to a receptor on respiratory epithelial cells, causing symptoms of an upper respiratory tract infection. Once bound, the virion penetrates the plasma membrane by one of several means: by receptor-mediated endocytosis, by viral envelope fusion with the plasma membrane, or by directly crossing the plasma membrane.

Viruses contain their genetic information in either DNA or ribonucleic acid (RNA). The viral genetic material is protected by a protein coat that must be removed in the cytoplasm of the infected host cell (uncoating). The viral genetic material may be processed by one of several paths, depending on the particular virus. Generally, all RNA viruses, except influenza and retroviruses, replicate their genetic material in the cytoplasm of the infected cell, and all DNA viruses, except poxviruses, require the DNA to enter the nucleus and use the cell's DNA polymerases to replicate. Poxviruses provide their own DNA polymerase and replicate their DNA in the cytoplasm of the infected cell. Retroviruses generally convert their RNA genetic information to DNA using an enzyme contained in the virion—reverse transcriptase.

After infection, viruses usually make multiple copies of their genetic material and produce the necessary viral proteins for replication. New virions are assembled in the host cell's cytoplasm and are released from the cell for transmission of the viral infection to other host cells. This cycle is referred to as the *productive* or *lytic cycle* because a large number of progeny are produced, and the result is frequently the destruction of the host cell.

Some viruses will not be productive initially but initiate a latency phase, during which the host cell is *transformed.* During this phase the viral DNA may be integrated into the DNA of the host cell and become a permanent passenger in that cell and its progeny. In response to stimuli, such as stress, hormonal changes, or disease, the virus may exit latency and enter a productive cycle.

Fig. 7-13 *Stages of viral infection of a host cell.* The virion *(1)* becomes attached to the cell's plasma membrane by absorption; *(2)* releases enzymes that weaken the membrane and allow it to penetrate the cell; *(3)* uncoats itself; *(4)* replicates; and *(5)* matures and escapes from the cell by budding from the plasma membrane. The infection then can spread to other host cells.

Cellular effects of viruses

Besides taking over the host cell's metabolic machinery, viral infection can injure cellular structures. In some viral infections, cellular destruction results from large quantities of virus being released from the cell's plasma membrane. Alteration of the plasma membrane by the expression of new antigens as a result of viral infection can incite an immune response with injury of the host's cells (e.g., hepatitis B virus). Once inside the host cell, virions have many harmful effects, including the following:

1. The cessation of protein synthesis
2. Disruption of lysosomal membranes, resulting in release of "digestive" lysosomal enzymes that can kill the cell
3. Fusion of host cells, producing multinucleated giant cells
4. Alteration of the antigenic properties, or "identity" of the host cell, causing the host's immune system to attack the cell as if it were foreign
5. Transformation of host cells into cancerous cells, resulting in uninhibited and unregulated growth
6. Promotion of secondary bacterial infection by cells damaged by virus

Examples of human diseases caused by specific viruses are listed in Table 7-11.

Fungal

Fungi are relatively large organisms with thick walls that grow as either single-celled yeasts (spheres) or multicelled molds (filaments or hyphae) (Fig. 7-14). Some fungi can exist in either form and are called **dimorphic.** The cell walls of fungi are thick and composed of polysaccharides different from the peptidoglycans of bacteria, and they are not motile. The lack of peptidoglycans allows fungi to resist the action of bacterial cell wall inhibitors such as penicillin and cephalosporin. Molds are aerobic, and yeasts are facultative anaerobes. They usually reproduce by simple division or budding.

Diseases caused by fungi are called **mycoses.** Most pathogenic fungi grow as parasites on or near skin or mucous membranes and usually produce mild and superficial disease. Fungi that invade the skin, hair, or nails are known as **dermatophytes.** The diseases they produce are called *tineas* (ringworm), for example, tinea capitis (scalp), tinea pedis (feet), and tinea cruris (groin). Superficial dermatophytes grow in a ringlike, erythematous patch with a raised border. Itching often is intense, and cracking of tissue can occur and lead to secondary bacterial infection. Infections of the scalp are accompanied by scaling and hair loss. (Chapter 39 discusses the various skin disorders caused by fungi.)

Deep infections involving internal organs can be life threatening and are most common in association with other diseases or as an opportunistic infection in immunosuppressed individuals. Fungi causing deep infection enter the body through inhalation or through open wounds. Filamentous forms can multiply extracellularly, but the spherical

TABLE 7-11	Human Diseases Caused by Specific Viruses
Virus	**Pathophysiologic Effects**
Papovaviruses (DNA) (papilloma)	Small viruses that induce tumors and cancers in animals, warts (papilloma) in humans
Adenoviruses (DNA)	Medium-sized viruses that cause various respiratory infections in humans; some cause tumors in animals
Herpesviruses (DNA) (herpes simplex, herpes zoster)	Medium-sized viruses that cause various diseases in humans, such as fever blisters, chickenpox, shingles, and infectious mononucleosis; implicated in a type of human cancer called *Burkitt lymphoma*
Poxvirus (DNA) (variola, cowpox, vaccinia)	Very large, complex, brick-shaped viruses that cause diseases such as smallpox (variola), molluscum contagiosum (wartlike skin lesions), cowpox, and vaccinia; vaccinia virus gives immunity to smallpox
Hepatitis B (DNA)	Widespread throughout the world; blood and blood products are the best-documented routes for transmission
Picornaviruses (RNA) (poliovirus, rhinovirus)	Smallest RNA-containing viruses; at least 70 human picornaviruses are known, including the polioviruses, coxsackieviruses, and echoviruses; more than 100 rhinoviruses exist and are the most common cause of colds
Myxoviruses (RNA) (influenza A, B, C)	Medium-sized viruses with a spiked envelope; have the ability to agglutinate red blood cells; cause influenza
Paramyxoviruses (RNA) (measles, mumps)	Structurally similar to myxoviruses but generally larger; cause parainfluenza, measles, mumps
Coronaviruses (RNA)	Associated with upper respiratory tract infections and the common cold
Retroviruses (RNA)	Tumor-associated viruses; cause leukemia and tumors in animals; some members produce "slow" viral infections; cause of AIDS
Arenaviruses (RNA) (lassa)	Possess RNA-containing granules; some members produce "slow" viral infections in humans
Reoviruses (RNA)	Relation to human disease not clear; may be involved in mild respiratory infections and infantile gastroenteritis
Hepatitis A (RNA)	Isolated from chimpanzees; is known to be transmitted by humans by close person-to-person contact

Modified from Tortora, G.J., Funke, B.R., & Case, C.L. (1989). Microbiology: An Introduction *(3rd ed.). Menlo Park, Calif.: Benjamin Cummings.*

yeasts multiply within cells, including white blood cells. Some fungi are a part of the normal body flora and become pathologic when immunity is compromised, allowing exaggerated growth and translocation. For example, *Candida albicans* is found in the mouth, gastrointestinal tract, and vagina of many healthy individuals. Changes in pH and use of antibiotics that kill bacteria that normally inhibit *Candida* growth permit rapid proliferation, which can lead to superficial or deep infection. Common pathologic fungi are summarized in Table 7-12.

Pathologic fungi release mycotoxins and other enzymes that are damaging to connective tissues, but attachment and invasion by fungi are still not well understood. Phagocytes and T lymphocytes are important in controlling fungi, and low white blood cell counts promote fungal infection.

Fungi are diagnosed by microscopic observation of specimens treated with potassium hydroxide and stained to enhance visualization of spheres and filaments. Specimens also can be cultured. Skin tests are available for species of *Aspergillus*. No vaccines are available to treat fungal disease. Many of the antifungal drugs (e.g., amphotericin B, ketoconazole, fluconazole) used to treat deep or systemic infection are toxic to the host because the fungal cell composition

is similar to the host cell. They also can produce significant drug interactions.

 ## Clinical Manifestations

The progression from infection to infectious disease follows predictable stages (infection, incubation, symptoms, shedding of the organism) as demonstrated by the pathogenesis of measles illustrated in Fig. 7-15. Clinical manifestations of infectious disease vary, depending on the pathogen and the organ system affected. Manifestations can arise directly from the infecting organism or its products; however, the majority of the clinical symptoms result from the host's inflammatory and immune responses. Infectious diseases typically begin with the nonspecific or general symptoms of fatigue, malaise, weakness, and loss of concentration. Generalized aching and loss of appetite are common complaints. However, the hallmark of most infectious diseases is fever.

Fever is not failure of the body to regulate temperature; rather, body temperature is regulated at a higher level than normal. Body temperature is regulated by nervous system feedback to the hypothalamus, which functions as a central thermostat. A large number of agents (pyrogens) can produce fever. In current classification, those pyrogens derived

TABLE 7-12	Common Pathogenic Fungi		
Fungus	**Growth Form**	**Entry**	**Disease**
Superficial dermatophytes			
Microsporum and *Epidermophyton*	Filament	Skin contact	Ringworm, jock itch, athlete's foot
Malassezia furfur	Sphere	Skin contact	Tinea versicolor
Deep			
Pneumocystis carinii	Sphere	Inhalation	Pneumonia
Histoplasma capsulatum	Sphere	Inhalation	Histoplasmosis
Aspergillus fumigatus	Filament	Inhalation	Aspergillosis and pneumonia
Coccidioides immitis	Unusual form	Inhalation	Coccidioidomycosis
Candida albicans	Sphere	Normal flora of skin, mouth, intestine	Thrush, vaginal yeast infections, systemic infections

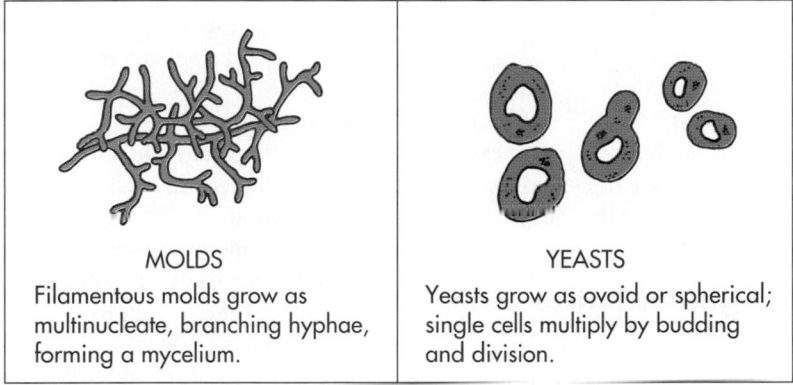

MOLDS
Filamentous molds grow as multinucleate, branching hyphae, forming a mycelium.

YEASTS
Yeasts grow as ovoid or spherical; single cells multiply by budding and division.

Fig. 7-14 *Types of fungi. (Redrawn from Mims, C.A. et al. [1993].* Medical microbiology. *St. Louis: Mosby.)*

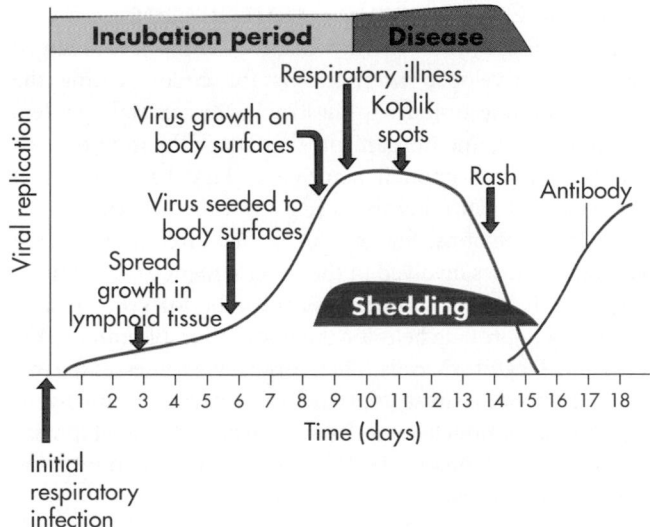

Fig. 7-15 *Pathogenesis of measles.*

from outside the host are known as *exogenous pyrogens* and those produced by the host are known as *endogenous pyrogens*. There is little evidence that exogenous pyrogens cause fever directly. Available data favor an *indirect* effect of such pyrogens on the hypothalamus that is mediated by endogenous pyrogen (EP) released by cells of the host.[16] A number of hormonelike mediators (cytokines) produced during inflammation have been identified as endogenous pyrogens. They are interleukin-1 (IL-1), interleukin-6 (IL-6), interferon, tumor necrosis factor (TNF), and other cytokines.[16] The mechanism by which these cytokines raise the thermoregulatory set point seems to be stimulation of prostaglandin synthesis and turnover in both thermoregulatory (brain) and nonthermoregulatory (peripheral) tissue. (These mechanisms are discussed in detail in Chapter 13.) Although there is a generally accepted belief that fever has a beneficial value in infection, the molecular mechanism behind the beneficial effects has not been established. Many investigators, however, consider fever as an adaptive host-defense response.

Recently recognized is the role played by tumor necrosis factor/cachectin (TNF) in the pathogenesis of endotoxic shock.[15,17,18] TNF is a cytokine (mediator) produced by activated macrophages (e.g., large phagocytic cells) on exposure to endotoxin. It is sometimes called *cachectin* because of its

TABLE 7-13	Recommended Childhood Immunization Schedule
Age	**Vaccine**
Birth	HBV*
2 mo	HBV*†, DTP, OPV, HbCV
4 mo	HBV†, DTP, OPV, HbCV
6 mo	HBV*†, DTP, HbCV
12 mo	HbCV, V
15 mo	DTP, OPV, MMR, HbCV
4-6 yr	DTP, OPV, MMR
14-16 yr	DT

HBV, *Hepatitis B virus*; DTP, *diphtheria, tetanus, pertussis*; OPV, *oral polio vaccine*, HbCV, Haemophilus influenzae *type b*; V, *varicella zoster*; MMR, *measles, mumps, rubella*; DT, *diphtheria toxin (toxoid)*.
*Three injections: one at birth, 1-2 mo, and 6-18 mo.
†At 1-2 mo, 4 mo, and 6-18 mo.

role in promoting cachexia in individuals with cancer. (Cachexia is discussed in Chapter 10; cytokines are discussed in Chapter 5; types of shock are discussed in Chapter 23.)

Countermeasures Against Pathogenic Defenses

Innate

The body's innate and innovative responses against microorganisms are numerous. T lymphocytes increase the phagocytic capacity of macrophages through release of lymphokines. A granulomatous response essentially isolates and excises infection from living tissue and prevents the spread of infection. Interventive therapy also has been developed to prevent the pathogen from initiating disease (vaccines) or to destroy the pathogen once the disease process has started (antimicrobials).

Vaccines

Many vaccines have been developed to protect against pathogens (Table 7-13). Vaccines induce immune responses under conditions that will not result in disease. Most viral vaccines contain live viruses that are weakened or attenuated so they continue to express appropriate antigens but establish only a limited and easily controlled infection. Most bacterial vaccines are killed organisms or extracts of bacterial antigens. Some pathogenic organisms are not invasive, remaining on the mucosal membranes but causing life-threatening disease by the release of powerful toxins that act locally or systemically, including diphtheria, cholera, and tetanus toxins. Vaccination against systemic toxins (e.g., diphtheria, tetanus) has been achieved using toxoids—toxins that have been chemically detoxified without loss of antigenicity. The primary immune response from vaccination is generally short-lived; therefore booster injections are used to push the immune response through multiple secondary responses, resulting in large numbers of memory cells and

long-lasting active immune response with sustained high titers of protective antibody.

Development of successful vaccines frequently is costly and depends on several factors: identification of the protective immune response; appropriate antigen to induce that response; successful development of that antigen into an effective, cost-efficient, stable, and safe vaccine; and compliance of the susceptible population to achieve a protective level of immunization in the total population. Most vaccine development has focused on preventing the most severe and common infections. With the success of other interventions, such as antibiotic therapy, there has been no perceived need for vaccination against many common and non-life-threatening infections. Even with successful development of a vaccine, a certain percent of the population will be genetically unresponsive and unable to produce a protective immune response. Those individuals will be susceptible to the infection and need an effective alternative therapy.

Antimicrobials

During the twentieth century, antimicrobials have had the greatest impact on resisting infection. Antimicrobials are natural products of fungi, bacteria, and related organisms and kill or inhibit the growth of other microorganisms. Numerous chemicals or antimicrobials have been identified that either prevent the growth of microorganisms or directly destroy them (Table 7-14). Antimicrobials act generally by preventing the function of enzymes or cellular structures that are unique to the infecting agent. Because viruses utilize the enzymes of the host's cells, there has been far less success in developing antiviral antimicrobials.

Recent Pathogenic Adaptations

Recently, disease-causing microbial organisms have emerged that have developed mechanisms for circumventing the most modern techniques for destroying or controlling infection, including microorganisms that attack the immune system (human immunodeficiency virus [HIV]) and those that are resistant to antimicrobials (e.g., *M. tuberculosis*).

HIV is one of the few organisms that directly attacks the central processes involved in the development of an immune response. It infects and destroys the T-helper cell, which is necessary to provide help for the maturation of both plasma cells and T-cytotoxic cells. Therefore HIV suppresses the immune response against itself and, secondarily, creates a generalized immunodeficiency by suppressing the development of immune responses against other pathogens and opportunistic organisms.

The development of vaccines against HIV has been frustrating because of the large number of changing antigens expressed on the viral surface. HIV can infect also by intercellular fusion between an infected cell in transmitted body fluids and uninfected cells near the mucosal surface. During this mechanism of infection, the virus may remain sequestered in the cell and be resistant to a vaccine-induced immune response.

Since the development of antimicrobials, some organ-

TABLE 7-14	Chemicals or Antimicrobials Identified That Prevent Growth of or Destroy Microorganisms
Mechanisms of Action	**Agent**
Inhibition of synthesis of cell wall	Penicillins
	Cephalosporins
	Monobactams
	Carbapenems
	Vancomycin
	Bacitracin
	Cycloserine
	Fosfomycin
Damage of cytoplasmic membrane	Polymyxins
	Polyene antifungals
	Imidazoles
Metabolism of nucleic acid	Quinolones
	Rifampin
	Nitrofurans
	Nitroimidazoles
Protein synthesis	Aminoglycosides
	Tetracyclines
	Chloramphenicol
	Macrolides
	Clindamycin
	Spectinomycin
	Mupirocin
Modification of energy metabolism	Sulfonamides
	Trimethoprim
	Dapsone
	Isoniazid

Modified from Ellner, P.D. & Neu, H.C.P. (1992). Understanding infectious disease, St. Louis: Mosby.

isms have mutated and developed resistance to particular antimicrobials. Resistance is developed primarily by inactivation of the drug, alterations of the bacterial membrane so that the antimicrobial is no longer taken up, or alterations of the target molecule. These changes are generally genetic mutations and can be directly transmitted to neighboring organisms. Penicillin resistance, for example, results from the production of an enzyme (β-lactamase) that breaks down the structure of the antimicrobial. Azidothymidine (AZT) is an antimicrobial that suppresses the enzymatic activity of reverse transcriptase, a viral-specific enzyme responsible for the conversion of viral RNA to a DNA strand. HIV frequently will mutate and produce an AZT-resistant reverse transcriptase.

The rapid emergence of multiple-antibiotic-resistant bacteria has been observed during the past decade. These organisms have developed resistance to almost all currently available antimicrobials. For example, *Streptococcus pneumoniae*, which causes pneumonia, meningitis, and acute otitis media (ear infections), was once routinely susceptible to penicillin. Since the 1980s, however, the incidence of penicillin-resistant organisms has risen to 30% in some populations. Many of these are resistant also to multiple antimicrobials. In some areas, almost 20% of tuberculosis cases are

caused by multiple-antimicrobial-resistant *M. tuberculosis.* There also have been dramatic increases in drug-resistant gonorrhea, malaria, salmonellosis, shigellosis, and staphylococcal infections.

Why have multiple-antimicrobial-resistant organisms appeared? Overuse of antimicrobials can lead to the destruction of the normal flora, allowing the selective overgrowth of antimicrobial-resistant strains or pathogens that had previously been kept under control. For example, after treatment with the antimicrobial clindamycin, the normal intestinal flora can become compromised, allowing the overgrowth of *Clostridium difficile* and the development of pseudomembranous colitis. Individuals commonly also do not comply with the instructions of health care providers concerning the necessity of completing the therapeutic regimen with antimicrobials. This practice allows the selective resurgence of organisms that are more relatively resistant to the antimicrobial.

The Future

With the development of multiple-antimicrobial-resistant strains, creativity to address this new challenge must be rekindled. If currently available antimicrobials are no longer effective, alternative forms of therapy must be developed. New antimicrobials may solve a portion of the problem or may exacerbate it further. Other forms of therapy may involve the immune system. If a pathogen is sensitive to destruction by antibody, use of passive immunotherapy, in which preformed antibodies are given to the individual, may be increased. This form of therapy has been used for decades. Horse serum containing antibodies was given to treat diphtheria, pneumococcal pneumonia, tetanus, and other diseases in the early twentieth century. Because of foreign proteins in the serum, many individuals developed an immune reaction against the horse proteins and an immune-complex-mediated serum sickness. Individuals with an immune deficiency of B cells currently are given intravenous immunoglobulin containing various antibodies against most infectious diseases. Several diseases in those with intact immune systems are treated also by the administration of human immunoglobulin preparations, including prophylactic administration to prevent hepatitis A when a traveler will enter a region in which the virus is endemic and therapeutic administration to treat hepatitis B and rabies.

Recurrent administration of the preparations generally confers resistance to most common bacterial and viral infections. More specific therapy with monoclonal antibodies is being evaluated against neonatal infections with the group B *Streptococcus* and against gram-negative bacteria that cause septic shock.

Vaccines induce an active immunotherapy in which the immunized individual produces protective antibodies or T cells. The development and widespread use of vaccines against common antimicrobial-resistant organisms must now be considered. For example, otitis media, a purulent ear infection, is caused primarily by *Streptococcus, Haemophilus,* and *Staphylococcus.* It has been routinely treated successfully with antimicrobials; however, almost half the cases of otitis media in some regions are caused by multiple- antimicrobial-resistant organisms. This may force an evaluation of the use of childhood immunization to prevent this disease. Other vaccines that may be used more widely or may soon be developed include those against cholera, typhoid, malaria, rotavirus, and several others. More novel therapeutic approaches may also require evaluation, such as bacteriophages—viruses that infect bacteria but not humans.

IMMUNODEFICIENCIES

Disorders resulting from immunodeficiency are the clinical results of impaired function of one or more components of the immune or inflammatory response, including B cells, T cells, phagocytic cells, and complement. (Table 7-15 lists defects in phagocytic cells and complement.) An *immunodeficiency* is the failure of these self-defense mechanisms to function at normal capacity. *Congenital (primary) immunodeficiency* is caused by a genetic anomaly,[19,20] whereas *acquired (secondary) immunodeficiency* is caused by another illness, such as cancer or viral infection, or by normal physiologic changes, such as aging. Acquired immunodeficiency is far more common than the congenital form.

Whether congenital or acquired, the chief cause of immunodeficiency is disruption of lymphocyte function. A stem cell defect may prevent normal lymphocyte development and cause total failure of the immune system; a central lymphoid organ dysfunction may prevent maturation of stem cells into B or T cells; or the final stages of B cell maturation may be disrupted, precluding the production of a specific class of immunoglobulin. Other defects may interfere with intercellular cooperation. Sometimes enzyme defects in lymphocytes cause a general accumulation of toxic metabolites. Alterations in the inflammatory response, particularly the chemotactic and phagocytic activities of neutrophils and macrophages or the activity of complement, can also impair host resistance.

The clinical hallmark of immunodeficiency is a tendency to develop unusual or recurrent, severe infections. Preschool and school-age children normally average 6 to 12 infections per year, and adults have 2 to 4. Most are not severe and are limited to viral infections of the upper respiratory tract or recurrent streptococcal pharyngitis. Potential immunodeficiencies are considered if the individual has had severe, documented bouts of pneumonia, otitis media, sinusitis, bronchitis, septicemia, or meningitis or infections with microorganisms that are not normally pathogenic (e.g., *Pneumocystis carinii*). Deficiencies in T cell immune responses are suggested when recurrent infections are caused by certain viruses (e.g., varicella, vaccinia, herpes, cytomegalovirus), fungi and yeasts (e.g., *Candida, Histoplasma*), or certain atypical organisms (e.g., *P. carinii*). B cell deficiencies, however, are suggested if the individual has documented, recurrent infections with microorganisms that require opsonization (e.g., encapsulated bacteria) or viruses against which humoral immunity is normally effective (e.g., rubella).

Many congenital immunodeficiencies also are associated with other defects, some of which appear unrelated to the immune defect yet may be life threatening by themselves. Examples include eczema and thrombocytopenia (in Wiskott-Aldrich syndrome); cardiac anomalies, low levels of calcium in the blood, and structural anomalies of the face (in DiGeorge syndrome); and a severe lack of muscular coordination and dilation of the small blood vessels (in ataxia telangiectasia). The association of these other symptoms sometimes can clarify the pathophysiology of the disease. For instance, in DiGeorge syndrome the defects are the partial or complete absence of a thymus (resulting in depressed T cell immunity), partial or complete absence of the parathyroid gland (resulting in decreased blood calcium levels), and structural defects in the heart. Each of these anatomic structures originates from the same region in the embryo during the twelfth week of gestation; therefore the defect in DiGeorge syndrome can be traced to an abnormal development at a specific time and in a specific region during embryogenesis.

Routine care of individuals with immunodeficiencies must be tempered with the knowledge that the immune system may be totally ineffective. It is unsafe to administer some conventional immunizing agents or blood products to many of these individuals because of the risk that the immunizing agent will cause an uncontrolled infection, which is a particular problem when attenuated vaccines that contain live but weakened microorganisms are used (e.g., rubella virus). Although the virus is attenuated enough to be destroyed by a normal immune system, it can survive, multiply, and cause severe disease in an immunodeficient recipient. Further, even simple procedures, such as penetrating the skin for routine blood tests, may lead to fatal septicemia in the immunodeficient person.

Individuals with immunodeficiencies also are at risk for graft-versus-host (GVH) disease. This occurs if T cells in a graft (e.g., transfused blood or bone marrow) are mature and can destroy tissues in the graft recipient. If the recipient's immune system is normal, the grafted T cells are controlled and no tissue destruction occurs. If, however, the recipient's immune system is deficient, the grafted T cells remain unchecked and can attack the recipient's tissues, leading to death in some cases.

Congenital Immunodeficiencies

Congenital, or primary, immunodeficiency occurs if lymphocyte development is arrested or disrupted in the fetus or embryo (Fig. 7-16). Defects that occur at different stages of stem cell, T cell, or B cell maturation cause different immunodeficiency diseases. Some are caused primarily by a defect in one or the other of the cell lines, although both T and B cell lines may be somewhat deficient. Other congenital immunodeficiency diseases affect stem cells of both cell lines, disrupting both cell-mediated and humoral immune processes. A defect in B cell development results in lower levels of circulating immunoglobulins, or *hypogammaglobulinemia.* The condition in which they are totally or nearly

TABLE 7-15	Congenital Defects of Phagocytosis and Complement Function	
Type of Defect	Characteristic	Clinical Manifestation
Defects of phagocytosis		
Quantitative defects	Neutropenia (decreased granulocyte number)	General increase in bacterial infections
Chemotactic defects	Decreased neutrophil response to chemotactic factors	General increase in bacterial infections
Bacterial killing defects	Decreased bacterial killing because of insufficient H_2O_2 or lysosomal enzymes	Increased bacterial infections—especially with catalase-positive organisms
Complement defects		
Defects in early classic pathway	Decreased activity of C1, C2, or C4	Mild bacterial infections; SLE-like syndrome
Defects in alternative pathway	Decreased activity of alternative pathway components—especially factor B	Increased infections with encapsulated bacteria
Defects in C3	Decreased production of C3b	Severe infections mostly with encapsulated bacteria
Defects in late pathway	Decreased activity of C5, C6, C7, or C8	Recurrent disseminated *Neisseria gonorrhoeae* or *N. meningitidis* infections

Fig. 7-16 *Lymphocyte development defects.* Defects in lymphocyte development that may account for congenital immunodeficiencies: *(1)* reticular dysgenesis; *(2)* severe combined immunodeficiency (SCID); *(3)* DiGeorge syndrome; *(4)* Bruton agammaglobulinemia; *(5)* chronic mucocutaneous candidiasis; and *(6)* selective IgA deficiency. *Ig,* Immunoglobulin.

absent is termed **agammaglobulinemia.** (Normal lymphocyte development is discussed in Chapter 5.)

Although most congenital immunodeficiency diseases are rare, much of our current understanding of how the immune system develops and interacts at the cellular level was developed by studying congenital immunodeficiencies. The

role of bone marrow stem cells in the evolution of the immune system was elucidated by studying children with *severe combined immunodeficiencies (SCID).* The most severe form of SCID is **reticular dysgenesis** (failure of blood cells to develop), in which a common stem cell for all white blood cells is absent; therefore T cells, B cells, and phagocytic cells never develop (see Fig. 7-16). Most children with reticular dysgenesis die in utero or very soon after birth.

The common stem cell normally matures into more developed stem cells for individual populations of white blood cells. Most individuals with SCID are deficient only in a stem cell for lymphocyte development and therefore have normal numbers of all other white cells and few, if any, detectable lymphocytes. T and B lymphocytes are few or totally absent in both the circulation and secondary lymphoid organs (spleen, lymph nodes). The thymus usually is underdeveloped because of the absence of T cells. Immunoglobulin levels, especially IgM and IgA, are absent or greatly reduced, although IgG levels may be almost normal if maternal antibodies are present. Significant impairment of B or T cell functions often presents as viral, bacterial, or fungal infections, including chickenpox, measles, rubella, and infections with *P. carinii.*

Several forms of SCID are caused by autosomal recessive enzymatic defects that result in the accumulation of toxic metabolites to which rapidly dividing cells, such as lymphocytes, are especially sensitive. Deficiencies in adenosine deaminase (*ADA deficiency*) or purine nucleoside phosphorylase (*PNP deficiency*) result in the accumulation of toxic purines.

Stem cells mature in the central or primary lymphoid organs (thymus and bursal equivalence tissue). Children who failed to develop these cells during embryogenesis had either a defective thymus (DiGeorge syndrome) or a defective bursal-equivalent tissue (Bruton agammaglobulinemia). *DiGeorge syndrome* (congenital thymic aplasia or hypoplasia and diminished parathyroid gland development) is caused by the lack, or more commonly partial lack, of the thymus, resulting in lymphopenia with greatly decreased T cell numbers and function (see Fig. 7-16).[21] Lack of the parathyroid gland is accompanied by the inability to regulate calcium. Low blood calcium levels cause the development of tetany or involuntary rigid muscular contraction. Immunodeficiency of T cell function contributes to failure to thrive, oral infections (e.g., candidiasis), chronic diarrhea, pneumonia, and skin rashes. *Bruton agammaglobulinemia* is caused by blocked development of B cell precursors into mature B cells because of the lack of normal B cell development in bursal-equivalent tissue (see Fig. 7-16). There are few or no circulating B cells, although T cell number and function are normal, resulting in repeated infections, such as otitis media, sore throat, and conjunctivitis, and more serious conditions, such as septicemia.

Even if nearly adequate numbers of B and T cells are produced, their cooperation may be defective. The *bare lymphocyte syndrome* is an immunodeficiency characterized by an inability of lymphocytes and macrophages to produce HLA class I or class II antigens. Without HLA antigen expression, antigen presentation and intercellular cooperation cannot occur effectively. Children with this deficiency develop serious, life-threatening infections and usually die before the age of 5 years.

Some immunodeficiencies involve a defect that results in

depressed development of a small portion of the immune system and therefore provide information about the function of that portion. For instance, an individual can be unable to produce a certain class of antibody, as in *Wiskott-Aldrich syndrome* (an X-linked recessive disorder). Here IgM antibody production is greatly depressed, and therefore antibody responses against antigens that elicit primarily an IgM response, such as polysaccharide antigens from bacterial cell walls (e.g., of *P. aeruginosa, S. pneumoniae, Haemophilus influenzae,* and other microorganisms with polysaccharide outer capsules), are deficient. In addition, there are defects in platelets presumably because of the absence of certain glycoproteins. Clinical manifestations include bleeding because of decreases in circulating platelets, eczema, and recurrent infections (e.g., otitis media, pneumonia, herpes simplex, cytomegalovirus).

Another defect in which a particular class of antibody is affected is *selective IgA deficiency,* which occurs in 1 in 700 to 1 in 400 individuals. Individuals with this deficiency produce other classes of immunoglobulins but not IgA. This suggests immature B cells that are committed to IgA production fail to mature into IgA-producing plasma cells (see Fig. 7-16). Many individuals are asymptomatic, although others have a history of severe, recurring sinus, lung, and gastrointestinal infections. Individuals with IgA deficiency frequently have chronic intestinal candidiasis (infection with *C. albicans*). (The secretory, or mucosal, immune system is described in Chapter 5.)

Complications of IgA deficiency include severe atopic disease and autoimmune diseases. Studies of these individuals show that secretory IgA normally may prevent the uptake of allergens from the environment. Therefore IgA deficiency may lead to increased allergen uptake and a more intense challenge to the immune system because of prolonged exposure to environmental antigens.

Other immunodeficiencies are characterized by a defect in the capacity to produce an immune response against a particular antigen. In *chronic mucocutaneous candidiasis,* the T lymphocytes cannot respond to a specific infectious agent, *C. albicans* (see Fig. 7-16). These individuals usually have mild to extremely severe recurrent *Candida* infections involving the mucous membranes and skin.

Acquired Immunodeficiencies

Acquired, or secondary, immunodeficiencies and inflammatory deficiencies develop after birth and are not related to genetic defects. The following physiologic or pathophysiologic conditions are known to be associated with acquired deficiencies:

- Pregnancy
- Infancy
- Infections, such as rubella (congenital), cytomegalovirus (congenital), measles, leprosy, tuberculosis, or coccidioidomycosis
- Down syndrome
- Malignancies, such as Hodgkin disease, acute or chronic leukemia, nonlymphoid malignancy, or myeloma

- Stress caused by surgery or emotional trauma
- Malnutrition caused by insufficient intake of protein, calories, iron, or zinc
- Aging
- Diabetes
- Alcoholic cirrhosis
- Sickle cell anemia
- Immunosuppressive treatment with corticosteroids, cytotoxic drugs, or ionizing radiation
- Anesthesia

Nutritional deficiencies

Nutritional status can profoundly affect immune function, with severe deficits in calorie or protein intake leading to deficiencies in T cell function and numbers. The humoral immune response is less affected by starvation, although complement activity, neutrophil chemotaxis, and bacterial killing within neutrophils frequently are depressed, resulting in infections with organisms that are normally disabled by opsonization and phagocytosis.

Deficient zinc intake can profoundly depress both T and B cell function. Zinc is a cofactor for at least 70 different enzymes, some of which are necessary for lymphocyte function. Secondary zinc deficiencies may be associated with malabsorption syndrome (failure to absorb zinc), chronic renal disease (loss of zinc in the urine), chronic diarrhea (loss of zinc through the gut), or burns or severe psoriasis (loss of zinc through the skin). Deficiencies of other enzyme cofactors, such as vitamins (pyridoxine, pantothenic acid, folic acid, vitamin A, vitamin E), also result in severe depressions of both B and T cell function.

Iatrogenic deficiencies

Iatrogenic disorders are caused by some form of medical treatment. Some drugs (e.g., cancer chemotherapeutic agents) profoundly suppress blood cell formation in the bone marrow, whereas others induce immunologic responses that destroy mature granulocytes. The list of drugs having this effect is growing and includes analgesics, antithyroid medications, anticonvulsants, antihistamines, antimicrobial agents, and tranquilizers.

Many drugs also affect B and T cell function, especially against antigens that require the interaction of T-helper and B cells for antibody production. Depression of B and T cell formation is manifested as a progressive increase in infections with opportunistic microorganisms (especially *P. carinii*, cytomegalovirus, *C. albicans*, and other fungi), the extent and location of which are unusual.

The immunosuppressive effects of chemotherapeutic drugs are exacerbated by concurrent treatment with ionizing radiation (x-rays). Most cytotoxic drugs and x-rays destroy cells that are proliferating or are in susceptible stages in their cell cycles. Therefore these therapies mainly suppress the primary immune response, which involves proliferation of clones of B and T cells.

Surgery and anesthesia also can suppress both T and B cell function. Transient, severe lymphopenia is a common postoperative condition that can last as long as 1 month. Surgery to remove the spleen (splenectomy) results in a depressed humoral response against encapsulated bacteria (especially *S. pneumoniae, H. influenzae, Staphylococcus aureus,* the group A streptococci, and *Neisseria meningitidis*), depressed serum IgM levels, and decreased levels of opsonins.

Deficiencies caused by trauma

Burn victims are susceptible to severe bacterial infections. Thermal burns appear to be associated with decreased neutrophil function (especially chemotaxis), decreased complement levels, decreased cell-mediated immunity, and decreased primary humoral responses, although secondary humoral responses are normal. The mechanism of this immunosuppression may be twofold. Sera from burned individuals contain nonspecific immunosuppressive factors (will suppress all immune responses, regardless of the antigen involved). In addition, burn victims also have increased suppressor cell function, which may increase antigen-specific suppression.

Deficiencies caused by stress

For many decades there have been anecdotal reports of increased incidence of infection and malignancy associated with periods of both intense stress (e.g., the loss of a loved one, divorce) and relatively minor stress (e.g., final examination periods at colleges and universities). In addition, early studies showed that immune function, as demonstrated by delayed hypersensitivity skin test results, could be depressed through posthypnotic suggestion. The mechanisms of this interaction have been investigated. Many lymphoid organs are innervated and can be affected by nerve stimulation. In addition, lymphocytes have receptors for many hormones (i.e., sex hormones, neurotransmitters, neuropeptides) and can respond to changing levels of these chemicals with increased or decreased function. (Further discussion of the effects of stress on susceptibility to disease can be found in Chapter 8.)

Acquired immunodeficiency syndrome (AIDS)

AIDS, or *acquired immunodeficiency syndrome,* is currently the best-known example of an acquired dysfunction of the immune system.[22] It represents a frightening disease because of its extremely high mortality in untreated individuals; the possibility of transmission by asymptomatic individuals who apparently incubate the disease over a period of years; the rapid increase in the number of clinical cases; and the relatively uncontrollable modes of transmission.

This viral disease probably arose in central Africa in the 1950s but is now found throughout the world. Almost every country or territory has reported cases of AIDS. The World Health Organization estimated that about 1.8 million adults died of AIDS worldwide in 1997.[23] More than half of AIDS cases are in Africa, and almost 10% are in Asia. As of the end of June 1998, more than 665,000 cases of AIDS had been reported in the United States alone.[24] In 1995, AIDS became the number one killer of individuals between the ages of 25 and 44 years (Fig. 7-17).[25] The AIDS virus infects and depletes a portion of the immune system, making individuals extremely susceptible to life-threatening infections and malignancies.

Epidemiology

In the United States the groups at highest risk for developing AIDS include homosexual and bisexual men and intravenous drug users (see Health Alert box). The remaining patients consist primarily of female sexual partners of people in AIDS risk groups and children born of mothers at risk. Of all AIDS patients diagnosed in 1977, approximately 22% were women (32% were intravenous drug abusers, and 38% were infected heterosexually).[24] In 1997, 473 new AIDS cases were reported in children younger than 13 years.[24] It is estimated that more than 50% of homosexual men in some urban areas, such as New York City, are infected.[26] In some metropolitan areas, the incidence rates among intravenous drug abusers are beginning to surpass those of the homosexual population.

Although the incidence of apparently heterosexual transmission of AIDS in the United States is rather low (approximately 13% of the total new AIDS cases in 1997, but 38% of cases in women), this route is becoming increasingly more common. It is estimated by the World Health Organization that by the year 2000 approximately 90% of AIDS cases will occur by heterosexual transmission.

Recipients of blood products or of semen for artificial insemination also have developed AIDS, but AIDS tests for screening donors of these products have greatly reduced this risk. Approximately 1% of AIDS patients have been transfusion recipients or received blood products for coagulation disorders. The incidence of HIV seropositivity in hemophiliacs is 70% in individuals with hemophilia A (factor VIII deficiency) and 35% in individuals with hemophilia B (factor IX deficiency), mostly because of pre-1985 exposure.[27]

More than 8000 cases of AIDS have been reported in children, three fourths of which are newborns who contract the virus from their mothers across the placenta during delivery or through the milk during breast-feeding.[24] The remaining pediatric patients are children with hemophilia or transfusion recipients. Symptoms usually develop within 6 months, and the life expectancy is generally less than 3 years. Certain aspects of pediatric AIDS remain enigmatic. Although the fetus is in direct contact with human immunodeficiency virus (HIV) infected maternal blood during the entire pregnancy and HIV can cross the placenta as early as the eighth week of gestation, the incidence of pediatric AIDS is relatively low. Most studies report incidences of infection of approximately 30% or even less.

AIDS appears to be especially prevalent in the black and Hispanic communities.[24] As of January 1998, AIDS cases nationally were distributed as follows: 45% in non-Hispanic whites, 36% in blacks, and 18% in Hispanics. Blacks and Hispanics accounted for 79% of cases in heterosexual men, 76% of heterosexually transmitted cases in

HEALTH ALERT

Risk of HIV Transmission Associated With Sexual Practices

HIGH RISK (IN DESCENDING ORDER OF RISK)
- Receptive anal intercourse with ejaculation (no condom)
- Receptive vaginal intercourse with ejaculation (no condom)
- Insertive anal intercourse (no condom)
- Insertive vaginal intercourse (no condom)
- Receptive anal intercourse with withdrawal before ejaculation
- Insertive anal intercourse with withdrawal before ejaculation
- Receptive vaginal intercourse (with spermicidal foam but no condom)
- Insertive vaginal intercourse (with spermicidal foam but no condom)
- Receptive anal or vaginal intercourse (with a condom)*
- Insertive anal or vaginal intercourse (with a condom)*

SOME RISK (IN DESCENDING ORDER OF RISK)
- Oral sex with men with ejaculation
- Oral sex with women
- Oral sex with men with preejaculate fluid (pre-cum)
- Oral sex with men, no ejaculation or pre-cum
- Oral sex with men (with a condom)

SOME RISK (DEPENDING ON SITUATION, INTACTNESS OF MUCOUS MEMBRANES, ETC.)
- Mutual masturbation with external or internal touching
- Sharing sex toys
- Anal or vaginal fisting

NO RISK
- Masturbating with another person without touching one another
- Hugging/massage/dry kissing
- Frottage (rubbing genitals while remaining clothed)
- Masturbating alone
- Abstinence

UNRESOLVED ISSUES
- The role of pre-cum in transmission
- The protection offered by covering female genitals with a dental dam during oral sex on the woman
- The risk of transmission from wet kissing

Data from Grimes, D.E. & Grimes, R.M. (1994). HIV infection: Progression and management. Mosby's clinical nursing series. St. Louis: Mosby, as modified from Schram, N.R. (1990). Refining safer sex. Focus. 5(7), 3-4.
*Risk lower if no ejaculation and/or if spermicidal foam is used.

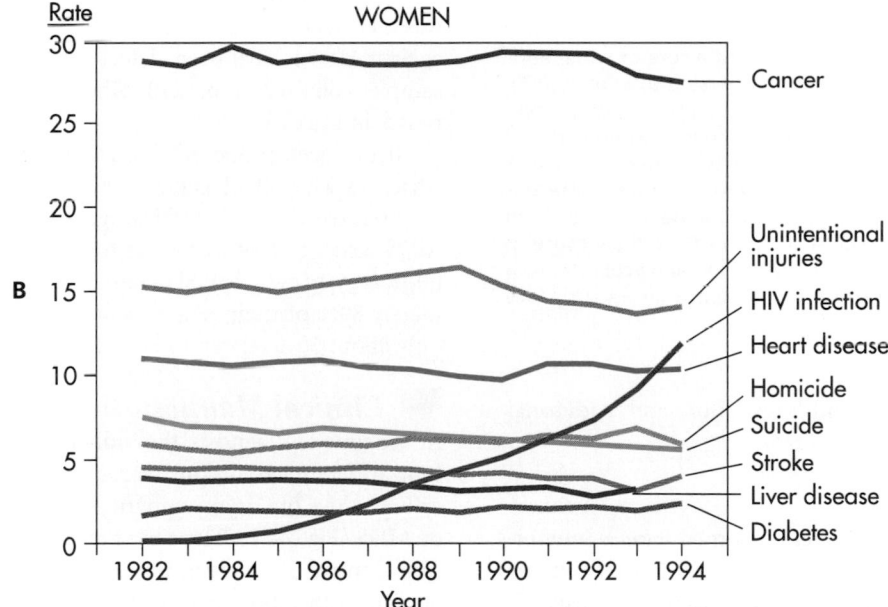

Fig. 7-17 *Death rates (per 100,000 population) from leading causes of death among,* **A,** *men and,* **B,** *women ages 25 to 44 years, by year—United States, 1982-1994.* National vital statistics are based on underlying cause of death using final data for 1982 to 1992 and provisional data for 1993 to 1994. *(Data from Aboulker, J. [1993].* Lancet, 341, *889.)*

women, and 81% of cases in children in the United States. Most were associated with intravenous drug abuse or heterosexual transmission.

The first reported health care provider to become occupationally infected with HIV was an emergency room nurse who became infected in 1986. The route of infection was probably through cuts in her hand that were exposed to contaminated blood through a gauze pad she was holding on a patient's open wound. As of 1998, more than 40,000 health

care workers had become infected with HIV. At least 54 were infected while caring for patients and were health care workers accidentally stuck with needles containing virus-contaminated blood or those who had broken areas of skin exposed to large quantities of contaminated blood.[24] Nurses and clinical laboratory technicians are by far the most commonly exposed health care workers. Because of the potential risk, all health care personnel should routinely follow the guidelines for Universal Precautions published by the Cen-

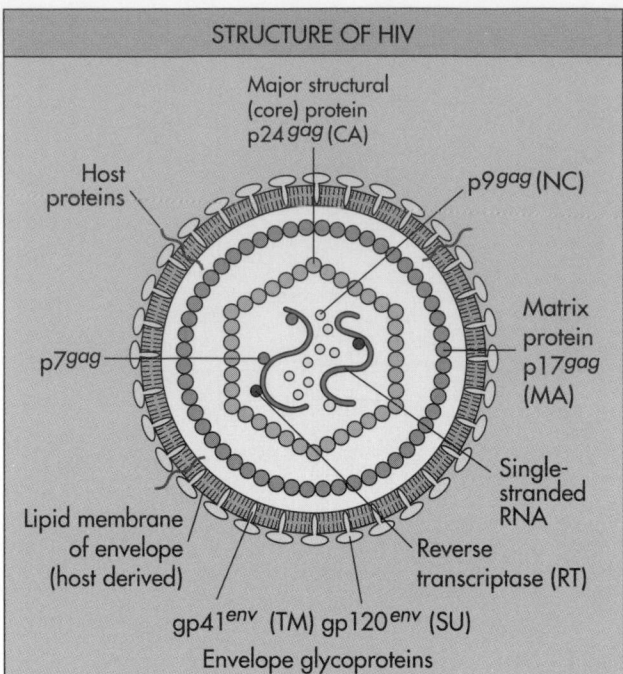

STRUCTURE OF HIV

Major structural
(core) protein
p24 *gag* (CA)

Host
proteins

p9 *gag* (NC)

Matrix
protein
p17 *gag*
(MA)

p7 *gag*

Single-
stranded
RNA

Lipid membrane
of envelope
(host derived)

Reverse
transcriptase (RT)

gp41 *env* (TM) gp120 *env* (SU)

Envelope glycoproteins

Fig. 7-18 *Structure and proteins of human immunodeficiency virus 1 (HIV-1)*. The HIV-1 virion consists of a core of two identical strands of viral RNA, molecules of reverse transcriptase (RT), nucleic acid binding protein (p9, NC), and a proline-rich protein (p7) encoated in a core capsid structure consisting primarily of the structural protein p24 (CA). The core is encased in a matrix consisting primarily of a protein, p17 (MA). The outer surface is an envelope consisting of the plasma membrane of the cell from which the virus budded and containing normal cellular proteins from the infected cell (host cell) and two viral glycoproteins: a transmembrane gp41 (TM) and a noncovalently attached surface protein, gp120 (SU).

ters for Disease Control and Prevention and additional guidelines for infection and control.[28]

Pathogenesis

AIDS is caused by a virus, currently named *human immunodeficiency virus (HIV)*, that has been isolated by researchers at the National Institutes of Health as the human T-lymphotropic virus type III (HTLV-III)[29] and by researchers at the Pasteur Institute as the lymphadenopathy/AIDS virus (LAV) (Fig. 7-18).[30] At least one other AIDS virus (HIV-2) has been identified.[31,32]

HIV is a retrovirus carrying genetic information in RNA rather than DNA (Fig. 7-19). Retroviruses infect cells by binding to the surface of a target cell through a receptor and inserting their RNA into the target cell. Through the use of a viral enzyme, reverse transcriptase, the viral RNA is converted to DNA and inserted into the infected cell's genetic material. If the cell is activated, viral proliferation may occur, resulting in the lysis and death of the infected cell. If, however, the cell remains relatively dormant, the viral genetic material is integrated into the infected cell's DNA, may remain latent for years, and is probably present for the life of the individual.[33]

CD4 is an antigen on the surface of T-helper cells that acts as the primary receptor for the HIV. Several other coreceptors have been identified. The virus infects primarily CD4-positive (CD4+) T-helper lymphocytes but also may infect various other cells of the central nervous system that also express HIV receptors.[34] Once activated, the virus infects other CD4+ cells and kills them, causing a marked decrease in CD4 cells. CD4 cell depletion has a profound effect on the immune system, causing a severely diminished response to a wide array of infectious pathogens and malignant tumors (Fig. 7-20).

A second virus, HIV-2, has been identified in West Africa. The first case of HIV-2 in the United States was diagnosed in December 1987 in a recent visitor from West Africa.[35] HIV-2 is very similar to HIV-1 in route of infection and clinical diagnosis, although it may be less destructive to the immune system and more slowly growing than HIV-1.

Origins of the virus

AIDS may have been around for considerably longer than first suspected. The first unequivocal case in the United States was identified from stored blood samples. The patient was a 15-year-old boy who died in 1969 of AIDS. Antibodies against HIV-1 have been detected also from stored serum samples collected on patients who died of undetermined illnesses in the early 1960s.

It has been proposed that the AIDS virus developed in Africa as a result of genetic mutation from a monkey or chimpanzee virus. The African green monkey does carry an AIDS virus (SIV-agm) similar to HIV-2. Genetic analysis of homology shows that SIV-agm and HIV-2 share approximately 80% of their genetic material. The SIV-agm virus is only about 50% related to HIV-1, however.

Clinical Manifestations

At the time of diagnosis, the individual may manifest one of four different conditions: serologically negative, serologically positive but asymptomatic, early stages of HIV disease, or AIDS (Fig. 7-21). The currently accepted Centers for Disease Control and Prevention (CDC) definition of AIDS relies on both laboratory tests and clinical symptoms. The most common laboratory test is for antibodies against HIV. Without a positive test for antibodies (seropositive), however, individuals can be diagnosed as having AIDS if they have a lymphoma of the brain and are younger than 60 years or if they have lymphoid interstitial pneumonitis and are younger than 13 years. If they are seropositive, the diagnosis of AIDS is made in association with various clinical symptoms, including disseminated coccidioidomycosis or histoplasmosis, extrapulmonary tuberculosis, persistent isosporiasis, recurrent salmonella septicemia, recurrent bacterial infections, HIV encephalopathy, HIV wasting syndrome, lymphoma of the brain at any age, and non-Hodgkin lymphoma. Other clinical symptoms of AIDS include persistent lymphadenopathy, weight loss, recurrent fevers, neurologic abnormalities, recurrent pulmonary infiltrates, and the development of opportunistic infections (e.g., *P. carinii* pneu-

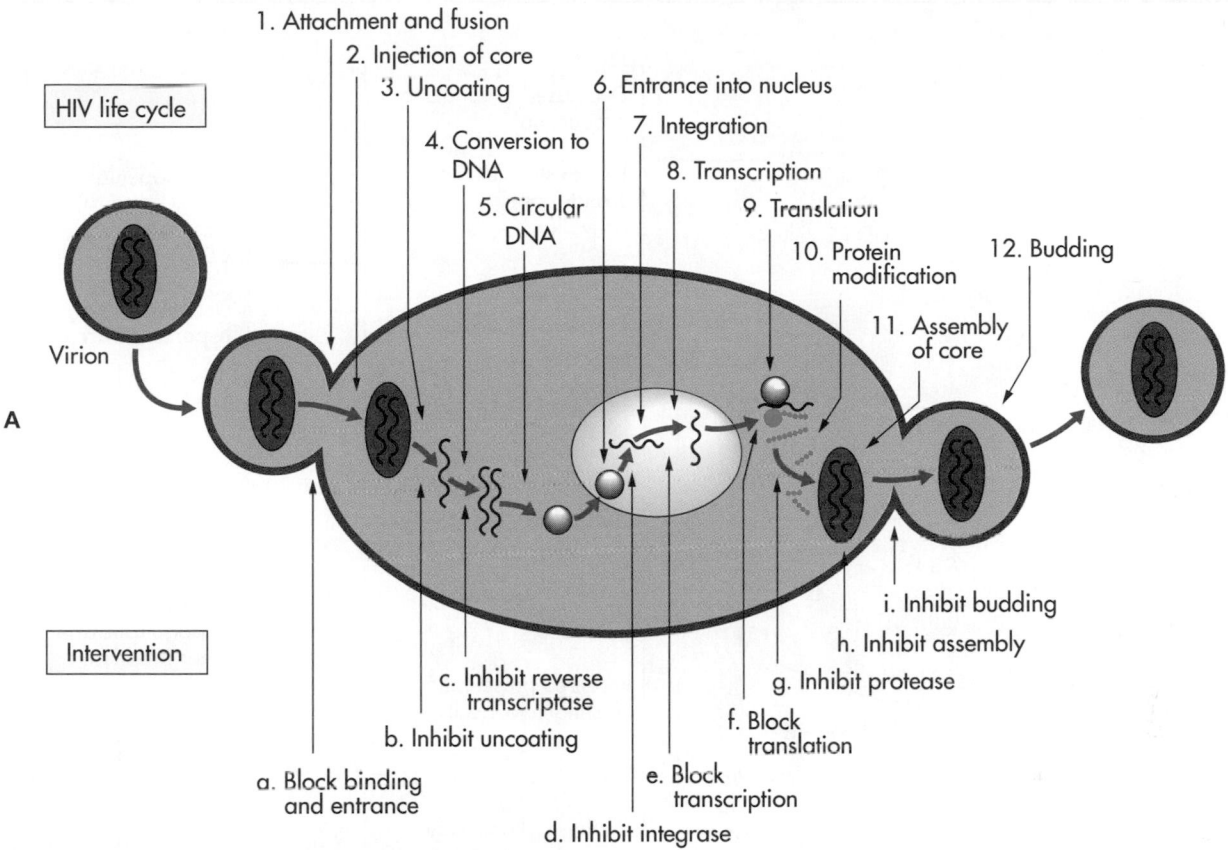

HIV life cycle

1. Attachment and fusion
2. Injection of core
3. Uncoating
4. Conversion to DNA
5. Circular DNA
6. Entrance into nucleus
7. Integration
8. Transcription
9. Translation
10. Protein modification
11. Assembly of core
12. Budding

Virion

A

Intervention

a. Block binding and entrance
b. Inhibit uncoating
c. Inhibit reverse transcriptase
d. Inhibit integrase
e. Block transcription
f. Block translation
g. Inhibit protease
h. Inhibit assembly
i. Inhibit budding

B

Fig. 7-19 *Life cycle and possible sites of therapeutic intervention of human immunodeficiency virus 1 (HIV-1).* **A,** HIV infection begins when a virion, or virus particle, *(1)* binds to specific receptors on the outside of a susceptible cell and the viral envelope and the plasma membrane fuse, and *(2)* the core of the virus is injected into the cytoplasm. Uncoating occurs in the cytoplasm *(3),* during which the core proteins are removed, and the viral ribonucleic acid (RNA) is released into the infected cell's cytoplasm. *(4)* The single-stranded viral RNA is converted to a double-stranded deoxyribonucleic acid copy (cDNA) by the action of reverse transcriptase. The cDNA becomes circular *(5)* and migrates into the nucleus *(6).* The cDNA is integrated as a provirus into the cell's own DNA *(7).* The provirus then either remains latent or *(8)* is transcribed into RNA. Some of the new viral RNA is translated into viral protein precursors at the ribosomes *(9).* The precursor proteins are modified by viral and cellular proteases into smaller proteins *(10).* Additional viral RNA and modified viral proteins are assembled into new virions *(11)* that bud from the cell *(12).* The HIV-1 life cycle is susceptible to blockage at several sites. Some agents (i.e., antibodies against HIV-1 or soluble CD4) could block the binding of the HIV to receptors on the surface of target cells *(a).* Other agents might keep viral RNA and reverse transcriptase from leaving their protein coat *(b).* Drugs such as *azidothymidine (AZT)* and other *dideoxynucleosides* prevent the reverse transcription of viral RNA into DNA *(c).* Drugs may also be able to inhibit the viral integrase and prevent insertion of the viral cDNA into the host's chromosomes *(d). Antisense oligonucleotides* could block the transcription of the provirus *(e)* and translation of mRNA into viral proteins *(f).* New drugs, *protease inhibitors,* specifically inhibit the viral protease and prevent the processing of the pr160, which is the precursor of all *gag* and *pol* proteins *(g).* Certain compounds could interfere with viral assembly by modifying such processes *(h),* and antiviral agents such as *interferon* could keep the virus from assembling itself and budding out of the cell *(i).* **B,** Scanning electromicrograph of HIV-infected CD4 lymphocyte showing virus budding from the plasma membrane. *(B from Morse, S.A., Moreland, A.A., & Holmes, K.K. [Eds.]. [1996]. Atlas of sexually transmitted diseases and AIDS [2nd ed.]. St. Louis: Mosby.)*

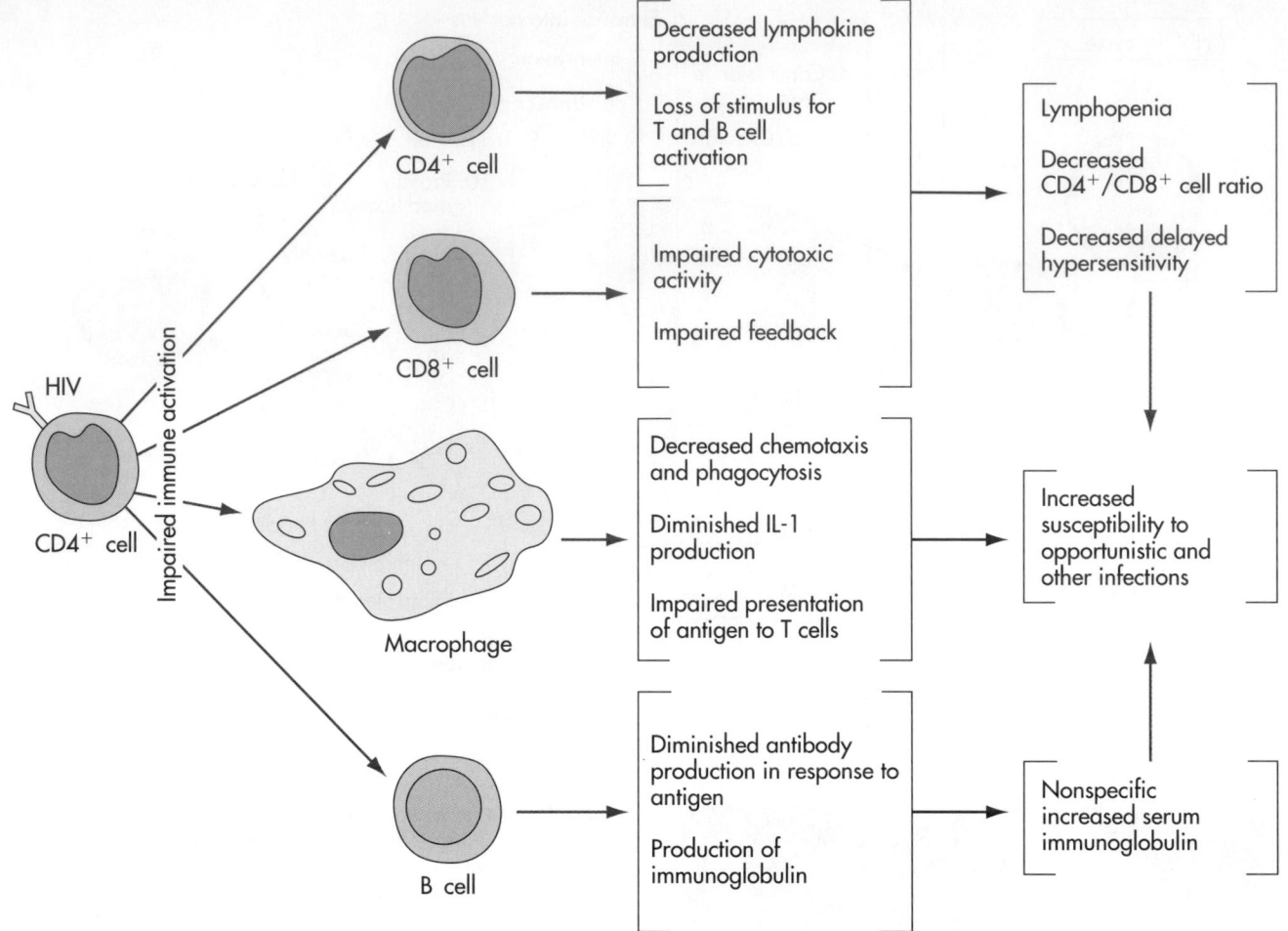

Fig. 7-20 *Summary of human immunodeficiency virus (HIV) infection on the immune system.*
(Redrawn from Morse, S.A., Moreland, A.A., & Holmes, K.K. [Eds.]. [1996]. Atlas of sexually transmitted diseases and AIDS *[2nd ed.]. St. Louis: Mosby.)*

monia) and other atypical malignancies (e.g., Kaposi sarcoma) (Fig. 7-22).

The major immunologic finding in AIDS is the striking decrease in the number of T-helper cells (CD4+ cells). Individuals who are not HIV-infected typically will have 800 to 1000 CD4+ cells per cubic millimeter of blood, with a range from 600/mm³ to 1200/mm³. Numbers of CD8+ cells are usually normal or slightly elevated. This results in a reversal of the normal CD4/CD8 T cell ratio, which is normally about 1.9. Most individuals with AIDS have ratios much lower than 0.9 and frequently near zero. In contrast, B cell numbers are usually normal. In 1993 the CDC added decreased CD4+ T cell numbers (less than 200 CD4+ cells per cubic millimeter of blood) and various other clinical complications, including invasive cervical cancer, pulmonary tuberculosis, and recurrent pneumonia, as indicators of AIDS.[24] These additional criteria have increased the number of reportable AIDS cases dramatically. In 1997 the new cases of AIDS were diagnosed primarily by decreased CD4+ T cell numbers (61% of cases). At diagnosis, 38% had definitive or presumptive pneumocystis pneumonia and 18% had HIV wasting syndrome.

HIV also infects the central nervous system, resulting in AIDS dementia complex in the late stages of the disease.[36] Dementia is present in most individuals because of atrophy of cells of the cerebrum and degeneration of the nerve endings. Symptoms include lack of motor coordination and behavioral changes, including psychosis in the most extreme cases.

An intermediate stage of development formerly was identified as AIDS-related complex (ARC). This description, however, has been dropped from the definition of AIDS, and ARC is now referred to as the early stages of HIV disease. Individuals with early-stage disease present with relatively mild symptoms resembling influenza, such as night sweats, swollen lymph glands, diarrhea, or fatigue. AIDS, however, is characterized by severe symptoms and an increase in infections and malignancies (Fig. 7-23). This stage may last as long as 10 years. Although individuals appear to be in clinical latency, the virus is actively proliferating in lymph nodes.[37]

The presence of circulating antibody against the AIDS virus apparently indicates infection by the virus, although many of these individuals are asymptomatic. Antibody ap-

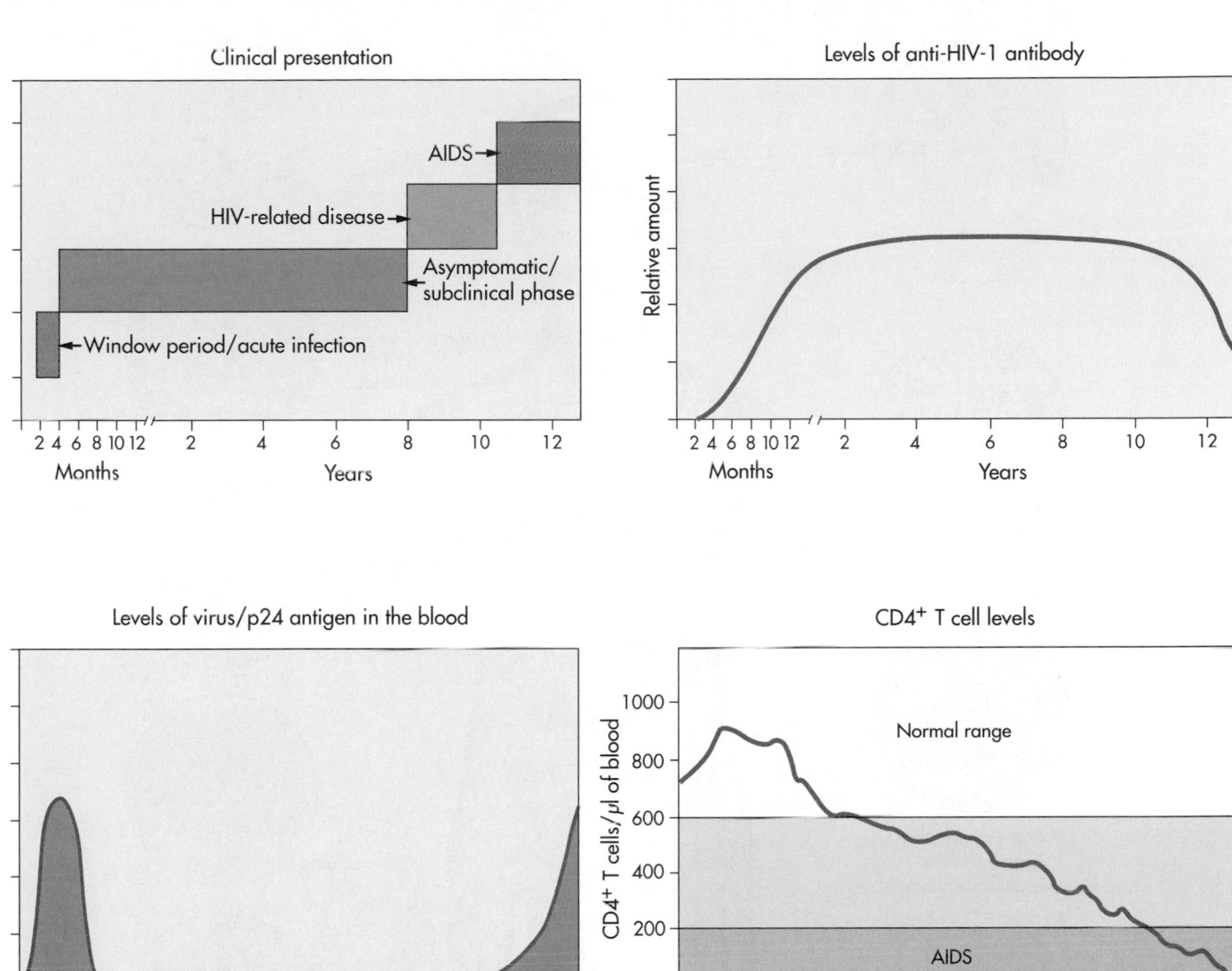

Fig. 7-21 *Changes in laboratory levels during progression from human immunodeficiency virus 1 (HIV-1) infection to acquired immunodeficiency syndrome (AIDS).* The progression from HIV-1 infection to AIDS is divided generally into four stages, the length of which may vary greatly from patient to patient. During the *initial phase* the patient may experience common and unremarkable symptoms of an acute viral infection. Antibodies against HIV-1 are not yet detectable (window period), but viral products, including p24 antigen, viral RNA, and infectious virus, may be detectable in the blood a few weeks after infection. CD4+ T cell levels may increase but will remain within normal ranges. During the *second phase* of infection the patient is generally asymptomatic or has slight chronic lymphadenopathy. The virus is replicating in the lymph nodes and other sites, but viral products are being released into the blood sporadically. The patient is seropositive for multiple antibodies against HIV-1, and CD4+ T cell levels are variable but generally decreasing to below normal ranges. During the *third phase* the patient develops HIV-related disease—a variety of symptoms of acute viral infection without opportunistic infections or malignancies. Viral products remain sporadically detected in the blood, CD4+ T cell levels continue to drop, and antibody levels remain high. During the *fourth,* and last, *phase,* the patient has been diagnosed with AIDS with a CD4+ T cell count of less than 200 or opportunistic infections or malignancies. Viral products are released progressively into the blood. As the immune system becomes severely depressed and excess viral antigen is released into the blood, measurable antibody levels decrease. Disease progression usually ends in the death of the patient.

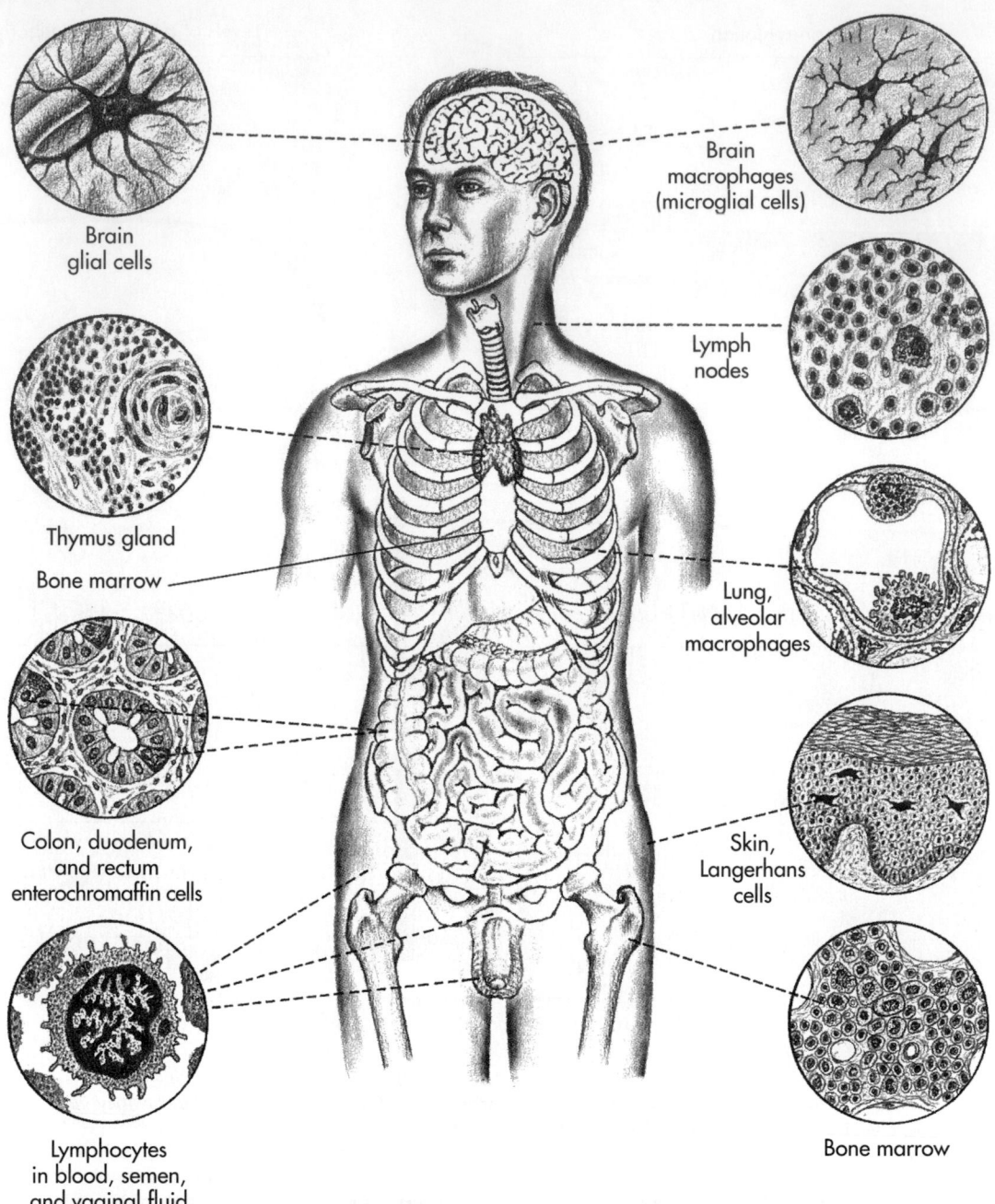

Brain
glial cells

Brain
macrophages
(microglial cells)

Lymph
nodes

Thymus gland

Bone marrow

Lung,
alveolar
macrophages

Colon, duodenum,
and rectum
enterochromaffin cells

Skin,
Langerhans
cells

Lymphocytes
in blood, semen,
and vaginal fluid

Bone marrow

Fig. 7-22 *Distribution of tissues that can be infected by the HIV.* Infection is closely linked to the presence of CD4 receptors on host tissue, with the possible exceptions of glial cells in the brain and chromaffin cells in the colon, duodenum, and rectum. *(Modified from Weber, J.N. & Weiss, R.A. [1989]. HIV infection: The cellular picture. In The science of AIDS: Readings from Scientific American. New York: Freeman.)*

pears rather rapidly after infection through blood products, usually within 4 to 7 weeks. After sexual exposure, however, the individual can be infected yet seronegative for 6 to 14 months, or, in at least one case, for years. In addition, in the late stages of the disease, some individuals become seronegative because of a deficient immune system.

Estimates are that for every diagnosed case of AIDS, approximately 100 others are HIV-infected. It is also estimated that diagnosed cases of AIDS are underestimated by 10% to

15%. The incidence of antibody detected in asymptomatic individuals suggests that more than 2 million people in the United States are infected at the time of this writing, and this will double by the year 2000. Worldwide, approximately 40 million people will become HIV-infected and from 10 to 13 million people will develop AIDS by 2000.

The period between infection and the appearance of antibody is referred to as the *window period* (see Fig. 7-21). Although the patient may not have antibody, he or she may

Fig. 7-23 *Clinical symptoms of acquired immunodeficiency syndrome (AIDS).* **A,** Biopsy-proven Kaposi sarcoma lesions. **B,** Fine, reticulate, white plaques characteristic of oral hairy leukoplakia in a patient with AIDS. **C,** Perianal vesicular and ulcerative lesions of herpes simplex infection. **D,** Magnetic resonance imaging (MRI) scan showing a large lesion, which on biopsy showed lymphoma. *(From Morse S.A., Moreland, A.A., & Holmes, K.K. [Eds.]. [1996]. Atlas of sexually transmitted diseases and AIDS. London: Mosby.)*

have virus growing, be viremic, and be infectious to others within 2 weeks of being infected. The average time from infection to AIDS has been estimated at just over 10 years. Some estimates are that approximately 99% of untreated HIV-infected individuals eventually progress to AIDS.

Treatment and Prevention

Both treatment of ongoing HIV infection and prevention of the initial infection have been very difficult to address. HIV has certain characteristics that frustrate attempts to develop effective treatments and vaccines.

There are two approaches to treatment for AIDS: restoration of immune function and prevention of viral replication. Restoration of immune function has been attempted with bone marrow transplants, transfusions of white blood cells from healthy donors, and the injection of soluble mediators (e.g., interleukin-2, interferons). Attempts

at restoration have met with little or no success because the virus very quickly infects the donor cells.

Several antimicrobials have been tried to prevent viral replication (see Fig. 7-19). Some block reverse transcriptase activity, and some have been successful as antimicrobials against other viruses or parasites (e.g., suramin against trypanosomiasis; ribavirin against cold and flu viruses; acyclovir against herpes simplex virus; azidothymidine [AZT], which suppresses retrovirus-induced leukemia in mice). Although most are effective in preventing AIDS virus replication in vitro, their efficacy in individuals generally has not been good. Initial reports were optimistic but a joint British-French trial (the Concorde trial) showed no improvement in disease prevention or survival when used in asymptomatic individuals.[38] In addition, reverse transcriptase has a very high mutation rate that makes it rapidly become resistant to these antibiotics.

TABLE 7-16 Laboratory Evaluation of Immunodeficiencies

Function Tested	Laboratory Test	Interpretation of Test
Tests of humoral immune function		
Antibody production	Total immunoglobulin levels	Presence of antibody-producing B cells
	Levels of isohemagglutinins	Capacity to produce specific IgM antibodies
	Levels of antibodies against vaccines—especially diphtheria and tetanus toxoids	Capacity to produce specific IgG antibodies
B cell numbers	Numbers of lymphocytes with surface immunoglobulin	Presence of circulating B cells
Tests of cellular immune function		
Delayed hypersensitivity skin test	Skin test reaction against previously encountered antigens—especially *C. albicans* or tetanus toxoid	Presence of antigen-responsive T cells and cellular interactions (e.g., lymphokine activity and macrophage function)
T cell numbers	Numbers of T cells forming rosettes with sheep erythrocytes or expressing membrane CD3 or CD11 antigen	Presence of circulating T cells
T cell proliferation in vitro	Proliferative response to nonspecific mitogens (e.g., phytohemagglutinin)	Capacity of all T cells to divide in response to nonspecific stimulation (mitogens)
	Proliferative response to antigens (e.g., tetanus toxoid)	Capacity of antigen-reactive T cells to respond to antigen

A new battery of therapeutic reagents, protease inhibitors, blocks the viral protease and prevents the production of proteins needed for viral replication. Resistant variants to multiple protease inhibitors have been identified, suggesting resistance to one may result in multiple resistance. Recent trials with protease inhibitors combined with reverse transcriptase inhibitors have yielded highly promising results.[39,40]

Drug therapy for AIDS is difficult because, like most retroviruses, the AIDS virus incorporates into the genetic material of the host and may never be removed by antimicrobial therapy. Therefore drug administration may have to continue for the lifetime of the individual.

The development of an effective AIDS vaccine has been slowed by several major difficulties. *First,* the AIDS virus is genetically and antigenically variable, like the influenza virus, so that a vaccine created against one variant may not provide protection against another variant. As many as 30 to 40 different genetic variants have been isolated from the same individual during the progression of the disease. *Second,* although individuals with AIDS have high levels of circulating antibodies against the virus, these antibodies do not appear to be protective. Therefore even if an antibody response can be induced by vaccine, that response might not be effective. *Third,* the AIDS virus is transmitted from cell to cell and initially may enter the body in an infected cell. Microorganisms that spread by cell-to-cell contact usually are not susceptible to circulating antibody. HIV-infected cells also tend to fuse with other cells, so that infection can spread to uninfected cells without viral particles being produced. It is problematic whether antibodies against HIV prevent intercellular fusion between infected and uninfected cells. *Fourth,* the only good animal model for AIDS experimentation is the chimpanzee, which is a protected species and relatively unavailable for medical research. This means that the efficacy and toxicity of candidate vaccines cannot easily be evaluated.

✓ QUICK CHECK

Why is the development of recurrent or unusual infections the clinical hallmark of immunodeficiency?

Compare and contrast the most common infections in individuals with defects in cell-mediated immune response and those with defects in humoral immune response.

Why has AZT not been as beneficial as initially thought? What type of drugs seems promising?

Clinical Evaluation of Immunity

Individuals with immunodeficiencies first go to the health provider with one common symptom: recurrent infections.

To delineate the pathophysiology of a particular deficiency, certain observations and tests of the immune system are made.[41] Significant information on the specific immunodeficiency can be obtained by noting certain characteristics of the individual, including the presence of any associated anomalies, age, gender, and the types of infections (bacterial, viral, or fungal, and the specific organisms involved). Laboratory evaluation of immunodeficiencies is presented in Table 7-16.

Replacement Therapies for Immunodeficiencies

Individuals with immunodeficiency syndromes usually are treated by replacement therapy. Deficient antibody production is treated by replacement of missing immunoglobulins with commercial gamma (γ)-globulin preparations.[42] Lymphocyte deficiencies are treated with the replacement of host lymphocytes with transplants of bone marrow, fetal liver, or fetal thymus from a donor.

◼ DID YOU UNDERSTAND?

Alterations in Immunity and Inflammation

1. Hypersensitivity is an inappropriate immune response misdirected against the host's own tissues (autoimmunity) or directed against beneficial foreign tissues, such as transfusions or transplants (alloimmunity); or it can be exaggerated responses against environmental antigens (allergy).

2. Mechanisms of hypersensitivity are classified as type I (IgE-mediated) reactions, type II (tissue specific) reactions, type III (immune-complex-mediated) reactions, and type IV (cell-mediated) reactions.

3. Hypersensitivity reactions can be immediate (developing within seconds or hours) or delayed (developing within hours or days).

4. Anaphylaxis, the most rapid immediate hypersensitivity reaction, is an explosive reaction that occurs within minutes of reexposure to the antigen and can lead to cardiovascular shock.

5. Allergens are antigens that cause allergic responses.

6. Type I (IgE-mediated) reactions are mediated through the binding of IgE to Fc receptors on mast cells and cross-linking of IgE by antigens that bind to the Fab portions of IgE. Cross-linking causes mast cell degranulation and the release of histamine and other inflammatory substances.

7. Type II (tissue-specific) reactions are caused by four possible mechanisms: complement-mediated lysis, opsonization and phagocytosis, antibody-dependent cell-mediated cytotoxicity, and modulation of cellular function.

8. Type III (immune-complex-mediated) reactions are caused by the formation of immune complexes that are deposited in target tissues, where they activate the complement cascade, generating chemotactic fragments that attract neutrophils into the inflammatory site.

9. Immune-complex disease can be a systemic reaction, such as serum sickness (Reynaud phenomenon), or localized, such as the Arthus reaction.

10. Type IV (cell-mediated) reactions are caused by specifically sensitized T cells, which either kill target cells directly or release lymphokines that activate other cells, such as macrophages.

11. Allergies can be mediated by any of the four mechanisms of hypersensitivity.

12. Clinical manifestations of allergic reactions are usually confined to the areas of initial intake or contact with the allergen. Ingested allergens induce gastrointestinal symptoms, airborne allergens induce respiratory or skin manifestations, and contact allergens induce allergic responses at the site of contact.

13. Atopic individuals are genetically predisposed to the development of allergies.

14. Alloimmunity is the immune system's reaction against antigens on the tissues of other members of the same species.

15. Alloimmune disorders include transient neonatal disease, in which the maternal immune system becomes sensitized against antigens expressed by the fetus, and transplant rejection and transfusion reactions, in which the immune system of the recipient of an organ transplant or blood transfusion reacts against foreign antigens on the donor's cells.

Infection

1. Bacteria injure cells by producing exotoxins or endotoxins. Exotoxins are enzymes that can damage the plasma membranes of host cells or can inactivate enzymes critical to protein synthesis, and endotoxins activate the inflammatory response and produce fever.

2. Septicemia is the proliferation of bacteria in the blood. Endotoxins released by blood-borne bacteria cause the release of vasoactive enzymes that increase the permeability of blood vessels. Leakage from vessels causes hypotension that can result in septic shock.

3. Viruses enter host cells and use the metabolic processes of host cells to proliferate.

4. Viruses that have invaded host cells may decrease protein synthesis, disrupt lysosomal membranes, form inclusion bodies where synthesis of viral nucleic acids is occurring, fuse with host cells to produce giant cells, alter antigenic properties of the host cell, and transform host cells into cancerous cells.

5. Diseases caused by fungi are called *mycoses,* and

Continued

■ DID YOU UNDERSTAND? —cont'd

Infection—cont'd

they occur in two forms: yeasts (spheres) and molds (filaments or hyphae).

6. Dermatophytes are fungi that infect skin, hair, and nails with diseases such as ringworm and athlete's foot.

7. Fungi release toxins and enzymes that are damaging to tissue.

Immunodeficiencies

1. Immunodeficiency is the failure of mechanisms of self-defense to function in their normal capacity.

2. Immunodeficiencies are either congenital (primary) or acquired (secondary). Congenital immunodeficiencies are caused by genetic defects that disrupt lymphocyte development, whereas acquired immunodeficiencies are secondary to disease or other physiologic alterations.

3. The clinical hallmark of immunodeficiency is a propensity to unusual or recurrent severe infections. The type of infection usually reflects the immune system defect.

4. The most common infections in individuals with defects of cell-mediated immune response are fungal and viral, whereas infections in individuals with defects of the humoral immune response or complement function are primarily bacterial.

5. Severe combined immunodeficiency (SCID) is a total lack of T cell function and a severe (either partial or total) lack of B cell function.

6. DiGeorge syndrome (congenital thymic aplasia or hypoplasia) is characterized by complete or partial lack of the thymus (resulting in depressed T cell immunity), the parathyroid glands (resulting in hypocalcemia), and cardiac anomalies.

7. Defects in B cell function are diverse, ranging from a complete lack of the human bursal equivalent, the lymphoid organs required for B cell maturation (as in Bruton agammaglobulinemia), to deficiencies in a single class of immunoglobulins (e.g., selective IgA deficiency).

8. Acquired immunodeficiencies are caused by superimposed conditions, such as malnutrition, medical therapies, physical or psychologic trauma, or infections.

9. AIDS is an acquired dysfunction of the immune system caused by a retrovirus (HIV) that infects and destroys CD4+ lymphocytes (helper T cells).

10. Immunodeficiency syndromes usually are treated by replacement therapy. Deficient antibody production is treated by replacement of missing immunoglobulins with commercial γ-globulin preparations. Lymphocyte deficiencies are treated with the replacement of host lymphocytes with transplants of bone marrow, fetal liver, or fetal thymus from a donor.

KEY TERMS

Acquired (secondary) immunodeficiency, 204
Acquired immunodeficiency syndrome (AIDS), 207
ADA deficiency (adenosine deaminase deficiency), 206
Agammaglobulinemia, 205
Allergen, 183
Allergy, 181
Alloimmune disease, 181
Alloimmunity, 189
Anaphylaxis, 181
Atopic, 183
Atopic dermatitis, 186
Autoantibody, 181
Autoimmune disease, 181
Autoimmunity, 181
Bare lymphocyte syndrome, 206

Blocking antibody, 184
Bruton agammaglobulinemia, 206
Chronic mucocutaneous candidiasis, 206
Congenital (primary) immunodeficiency, 204
Contact dermatitis, 186
Delayed hypersensitivity reaction, 181
Dermatophyte, 199
DiGeorge syndrome, 206
Dimorphic, 199
Endotoxin (lipopolysaccharide), 196
Exotoxin, 196
Fungi, 199
Hypersensitivity, 181
Hypocomplementemic, 185
Hypogammaglobulinemia, 204
Immediate hypersensitivity reaction, 181
Immunodeficiency, 204

Mycosis (pl., mycoses), 199
Neoantigen, 187
Permissive host cell, 198
PNP deficiency (purine nucleoside phosphorylase deficiency), 206
Radioallergosorbent (RAST) testing, 184
Radioimmunosorbent (RIST) testing, 183
Reticular dysgenesis, 205
Selective IgA deficiency, 206
Septicemia (bacteremia), 198
Severe combined immunodeficiency (SCID), 205
Systemic lupus erythematosus (SLE), 189
Tissue-specific antigen, 184
Virion (viral particle), 198
Window period, 214
Wiskott-Aldrich syndrome, 206

REFERENCES

1. Reference deleted in proofs.
2. Green, T. (1997). The immune system. I. Anaphylaxis. *Nursing Times, 93,* 60-63.
3. Campbell, J. (1997). Anaphylaxis. *Professional Nurse, 12,* 429-432.
4. Sharon, J. (1998). *Basic immunology.* Baltimore: Williams & Wilkins.
5. Portier, P. & Richet, C. (1902). De l'action anaphylactique de certains venins. *Comptes Rendus Societie de Biologie (Paris), 54,* 170-172.
6. Davies, K. (1994). Allergy by mutation. *Nature Genetics, 369,* 506.
7. Sandford, A.J. et al. (1993). Localization of atopy and beta subunit of high affinity FgE receptor (Fc epsilon RI) on chromosome 11q [see Comments]. *Lancet, 341*(8841), 332-334.
8. Rote, N.S. (1985). Immune complex disorders and vasculitis. In N. Gleicher (Ed.). *Principles of medical therapy in pregnancy.* New York: Plenum.
9. Koch, R. (1891). Fortsetzung der mitteilungen über ein hcilmittcl gegen tuberkulose. *Deutsche Medizinische Wochenschrift, 9,* 101-102.
10. McIver, B. & Morris, J.C. (1998). The pathogenesis of Graves's disease. *Endocrinology & Metabolism Clinics of North America, 27,* 73-89.
11. Crispin, J.C. & Alcocer-Varela, J. (1998). Interleukin-2 and systemic lupus erythematosus—Fifteen years later [see Comments]. *Lupus, 7*(4), 214-222.
12. Andreoli, S.P. (1998). Renal manifestations of systemic disease. *Seminars in Nephrology, 18*(3), 270-279.
13. Deftos, M. et al. (1994). Defining the genetic origins of three rheumatoid synovium-derived IgG rheumatoid factors. *Journal of Clinical Investigation, 93*(6), 2545-2553.
14. File, T.M., Jr., Tan, J.S., & DiPersio, J.R. (1998). Group A streptococcal necrotizing fasciitis: Diagnosing and treating the "flesh-eating bacteria syndrome." *Cleveland Clinics Journal of Medicine, 65*(5), 241-249.
15. Calandra, T., Baumgartner, J., & Glauser, M.P. (1991). Anti-lipopolysaccharide and anti-tumor necrosis factor/cachectin antibodies for the treatment of gram-negative bacteremia and septic shock. *Proceedings of Clinical Biological Research, 367,* 141-159.
16. Kozak, W. (1993). Fever: A possible strategy for membrane homeostasis during infection. *Perspectives in Biology and Medicine, 37*(1), 14-34.
17. Cassatella, M.A. et al. (1993). Interleukin 10 (IL-10) inhibits the release of proinflammatory cytokines from human polymorphonuclear leukocytes: Evidence for an autocrine role of tumor necrosis factor and IL-10 beta in mediating the production of IL-8 triggered by lipopolysaccharide. *Journal of Experimental Medicine, 178*(6), 2207-2211.
18. Sherry, B. & Cerami, A. (1988). Cachectin/tumor necrosis factor exerts endocrine, paracrine, and autocrine control of inflammatory responses. *Journal of Cellular Biology, 107,* 1269-1277.
19. Smart, B.A. & Ochs, H.D. (1997). The molecular basis and treatment of primary immunodeficiency disorders. *Current Opinions in Pediatrics, 9,* 570-576.
20. Fischer, A. et al. (1997). Naturally occurring primary deficiencies of the immune system. *Annual Review of Immunology, 15,* 93-124.
21. DiGeorge, A.M. (1968). Congenital absence of the thymus and its immunologic consequences. In D. Bergsma & F.A. McKusick (Eds.). *Immunologic deficiency diseases in man.* Baltimore: National Foundation—March of Dimes Original Article Series, Williams & Wilkins.
22. Stine, G.J. (1995). *AIDS update: 1997.* Englewood Cliffs, N.J.: Prentice-Hall.
23. World Health Organization. (1998). *World health report 1998 executive summary. WHO Web Site: http://www.who.int/whr/1998/exsum98e.htm.* Geneva: The Organization.
24. Centers for Disease Control and Prevention. (1997). *HIV/AIDS surveillance report: U.S. HIV and AIDS cases reported through December 1997.* Atlanta: U.S. Department of Health and Human Services.
25. Update: AIDS among women—United States, 1994. (1995). *Morbidity and Mortality Weekly Report, 44*(5), 81-84.
26. Piot, P. et al. (1988). AIDS: An international perspective. *Science, 239,* 573-579.
27. Human immunodeficiency virus infection in the United States: A review of current knowledge. (1987). *Morbidity and Mortality Weekly Report, 36,* 1-48.
28. Hersey, J.C. & Martin, L.S. (1994). Use of infection control guidelines by workers in health care facilities to prevent occupational transmission of HBV and HIV: Results from a national survey. *Infection Control and Hospital Epidemiology, 15*(4, Pt. 1), 243-252.
29. Gallo, R.C. et al. (1984). Frequent detection and isolation of cytopathic retroviruses (HTLV-III) from patients with AIDS. *Science, 224,* 500-503.
30. Barre-Sinoussi, F. et al. (1983). Isolation of a T-lymphocyte retrovirus from a patient at risk for acquired immune deficiency syndrome (AIDS). *Science, 220,* 868-871.
31. Clavel, F. et al. (1987). Human immunodeficiency virus type 2 infection associated with AIDS in West Africa. *New England Journal of Medicine, 316,* 1180-1185.
32. Ness, P.M., & Ness, C.C. (1994). Blood donor testing for HIV-I/II and HTLV-I/II. *Archives of Pathology and Laboratory Medicine, 118*(4), 337-341.
33. Ho, D.D., Pomerantz, R.J., & Kaplan, J.C. (1987). Pathogenesis of infection with human immunodeficiency virus. *New England Journal of Medicine, 317,* 278-286.

REFERENCES

34. Funke, I. et al. (1987). The cellular receptor (CD4) of the human immunodeficiency virus is expressed on neurons and glial cells in human brain. *Journal of Experimental Medicine, 165,* 1230-1235.

35. Update: Acquired immunodeficiency syndrome (AIDS)—Worldwide. (1988). *Morbidity and Mortality Weekly Report, 37,* 286-295.

36. Price, R.W. (1994). Understanding the AIDS dementia complex (ADC). The challenge of HIV and its effects on the central nervous system. *Research Publications—Association for Research in Nervous and Mental Disease, 72,* 1-45.

37. Pantaleo, G., Graziosi, C., & Fauci, A.S. (1993). The role of lymphoid organs and the pathogenesis of HIV infection. *Seminars in Immunology, 5,* 157-163.

38. Aboulker, J. (1993). Preliminary analysis of the Concorde trial. *Lancet, 341,* 889.

39. Gulick, R.M. et al. (1998). Simultaneous vs sequential initiation of therapy with indinavir, zidovudine, and lamivudine for HIV-1 infection: 100 week follow-up. *Journal of the American Medical Association, 280*(1), 35-41.

40. Carpenter, C.C.J. et al. (1998). Antiretroviral therapy for HIV infection in 1998: Updated recommendations of the International AIDS Society—USA panel. *Journal of the American Medical Association, 280*(1), 78-86.

41. Noroski, L.M. & Shearer, W.T. (1998). Screening for primary immunodeficiencies in the clinical immunology laboratory. *Clinical Immunology and Immunopathology, 86,* 237-245.

42. Lee, M.L., Gale, R.P., & Yap, P.L. (1997). Use of intravenous immunoglobulin to prevent or treat infections in persons with immune deficiency. *Annual Review of Medicine, 48,* 93-102.

CHAPTER 8

Stress and Disease

Jane Shelby and Kathryn L. McCance

Walter B. Cannon used the term stress *in both a physiologic and a psychologic sense as early as 1914.[1] He applied the engineering concept of stress and strain in a physiologic context and believed that emotional stimuli were also capable of causing stress. In 1946 Hans Selye popularized these same findings, viewing stress as a biologic phenomenon.[2] The concept that stress may influence immunity and resistance to disease has been investigated since the 1950s. In the 1970s studies found that life changes or emotions resulting from life changes and occurring over a prolonged time were associated with decreased immune function. More recently we have seen the interactions among social, psychologic, and biologic factors in causing and prolonging or shortening the course of disease. What is emerging from the various disciplines involved—molecular biology, immunology, neurology, endocrinology, and behavioral science—is a more holistic and complex model that involves biochemical relationships of the central nervous system (CNS), autonomic nervous system (ANS), endocrine system, and immune system. A new field—psychoneuroimmunology—has developed.*

CHAPTER OUTLINE

CONCEPTS OF STRESS

The term *stress* has been used persistently and widely in specialties such as biology, health sciences, and social sciences despite numerous disagreements over its definition. Nevertheless, stress has come to be more usefully defined as a *transactional* or *interactional* concept.[3] Transactionally, stress is viewed as the state of affairs arising when a person relates to (i.e., interacts or transacts with) situations in certain ways. People are not disturbed by situations per se but by the ways they appraise and react to situations.[3] In stress, a demand *exceeds* a person's coping abilities, resulting in reactions such as disturbances of cognition, emotion, and behavior that can adversely affect well-being.

General Adaptation Syndrome

Selye[2] originally sought to discover a new sex hormone when he discovered the biologic syndrome of stress. In his attempts to discover the new hormone, Selye injected crude ovarian extracts into rats. Repeatedly he found that the following triad of structural changes occurred: (1) enlargement of the cortex of the adrenal gland, (2) atrophy of the thymus gland and other lymphoid structures, and (3) development of bleeding ulcers of the stomach and duodenal lining. Selye soon discovered that this triad of manifestations was not specific for his ovarian extracts but occurred also after he exposed the rats to other noxious stimuli, such as cold, surgical injury, and restraint. He called these stimuli *stressors.* Selye concluded that this triad or syndrome of manifestations represented a nonspecific response to noxious stimuli. Because many diverse agents caused the same syndrome, Selye suggested that it be called the *general adaptation syndrome (GAS).*

Three successive stages in development of the GAS were identified: (1) the *alarm stage,* in which the CNS is aroused and the body's defenses are mobilized (e.g., "fight or flight") (Fig. 8-1); (2) the *stage of resistance or adaptation,* during which mobilization contributes to "fight or flight"; and (3) the *stage of exhaustion,* in which continuous stress causes the progressive breakdown of compensatory mechanisms (acquired adaptations) and homeostasis. The stage of exhaustion marks the onset of certain diseases *(diseases of adaptation).*

Interactions among the sympathetic branch of the ANS, the pituitary gland, and the adrenal gland produce the nonspecific physiologic responses identified by Selye. The alarm phase begins when a stressor activates the pituitary gland and sympathetic nervous system (Figs. 8-1 and 8-2). The resistance or adaptation phase begins with the actions of the adrenal hormones cortisol, norepinephrine, and epinephrine. Exhaustion occurs if stress continues and adaptation is not successful, ultimately causing impairment of the immune response, heart failure, and kidney failure, leading to death.

Physiologic stress is a chemical or physical disturbance in the cells or tissue fluid produced by a change, either in the external environment or within the body itself, that requires

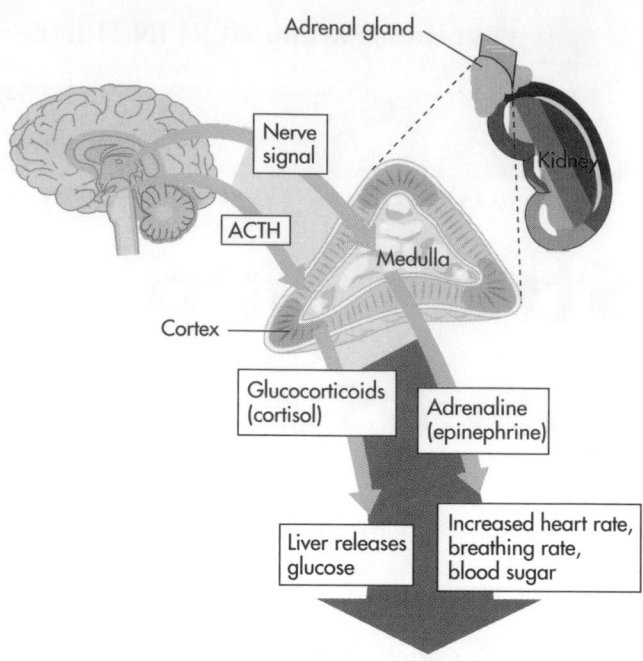

Fig. 8-1 *The alarm reaction.* The alarm reaction includes the hypertrophied adrenal cortex with increased secretion of glucocorticoids (cortisol) and activation of the sympathetic nervous system, including the adrenal medulla gland with increased release of epinephrine. The response from the release of cortisol and sympathetic nerve activation are summarized in Fig. 8-2. ACTH, Adrenocorticotropic hormone. *(From Thibodeau, G.A. & Patton, K.T. [1996].* Anatomy & physiology [3rd ed.]. *St. Louis: Mosby.)*

a response (i.e., begins the GAS) to counteract the disturbance. Selye identified three components of physiologic stress: (1) the exogenous or endogenous stressor initiating the disturbance, (2) the chemical or physical disturbance produced by the stressor, and (3) the body's counteracting (adaptational) response to the disturbance.[2]

Psychologic Mediators and Specificity

Although Selye's identification of the GAS is regarded as tremendously important and the cornerstone of stress research, the idea that stress is a purely physiologic response is oversimplified. Activation of the adrenal cortex occurs in humans in response to psychologic stressors. Several factors, including degrees of discomfort, unpleasantness, or suddenness of the stress, can account for the presence or absence of the physiologic stress response.

Selye believed that stressors cause a general or nonspecific response. However, research done in the past 30 years has shown remarkable sensitivity of the pituitary gland and adrenal cortex to emotional, psychologic, and social influences. Thus it may be the way an individual thinks and feels about a physical stressor or the stressor itself that produces the neuroendocrine responses. In experiments in which psychologic reactions were minimized, physical stressors did not appear to stimulate the pituitary or adrenal cortex in a nonspecific fashion. To support Selye's concept of nonspecificity, hard evidence is needed that increased adrenocortical

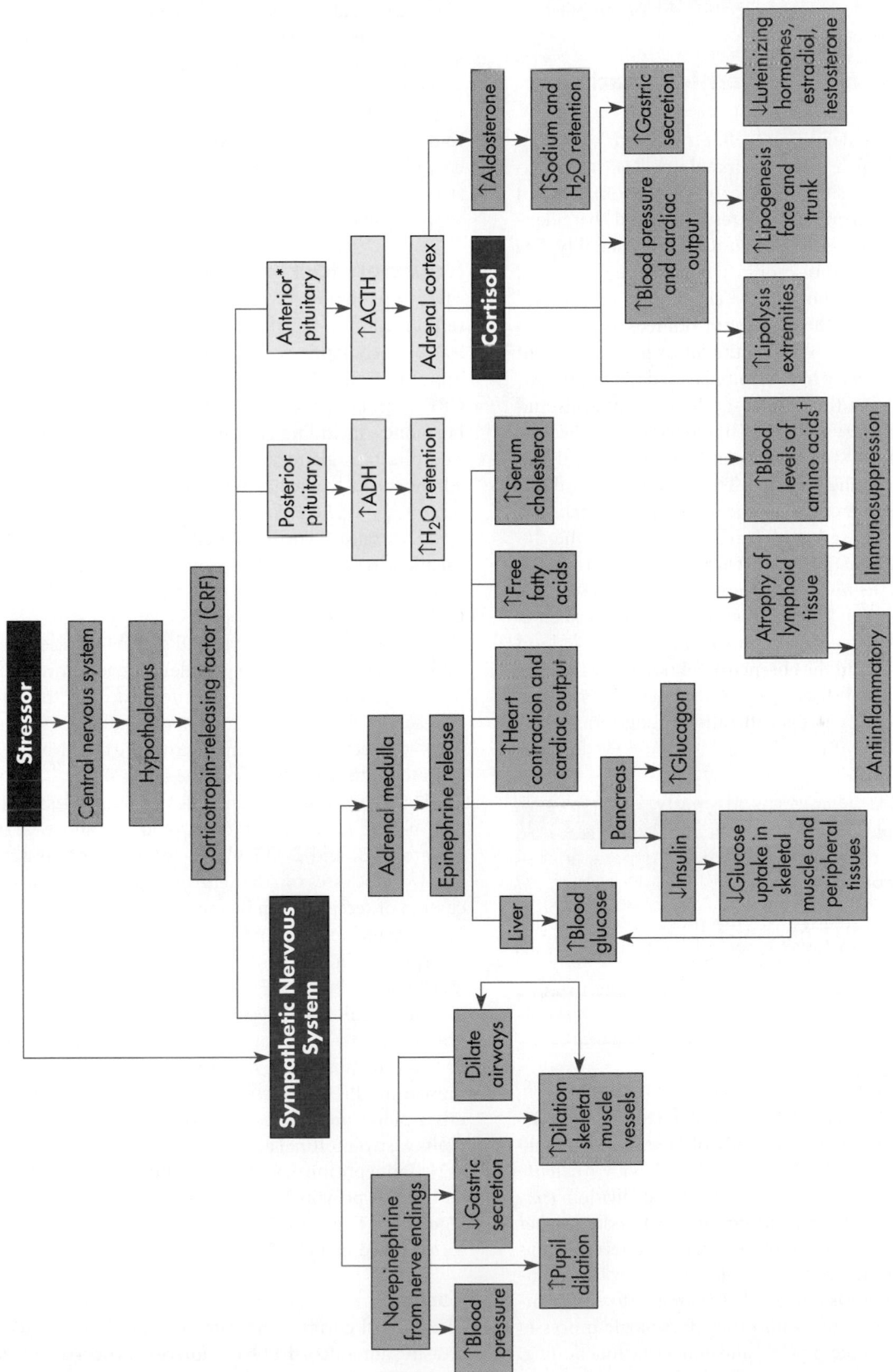

Fig. 8-2 *The stress response.* *Variable changes in β-endorphins, growth hormone, and prolactin (see text). †Caused by protein catabolism in muscle, adipose tissue, skin, bones, lymphoid tissue.

or medullary activity can promote adaptations to both cold and heat. In fact, no single hormone responds to all stressful stimuli in the absolutely nonspecific fashion implied in Selye's definition of the GAS.

Homeostasis as a Dynamic Steady State

Selye used Cannon's definition of *homeostasis* (the sum of the processes by which the body maintains itself at a relatively constant composition) and expanded it to mean that the body's need determines body responses and that adaptive responses are necessary to maintain body stability. Research with various radioisotopes has since demonstrated that homeostasis does not mean "constant composition." Much more accurate is the concept of homeostasis as a *dynamic steady state.* For example, the fat or protein content of the body may not vary much from day to day, but the substances that make up the fat and protein—fatty acids and amino acids—can vary widely.[4] The enzymes in a healthy person are constantly synthesizing fat and proteins and also constantly breaking them down. The process of synthesis and breakdown of all body substances is known as *turnover.*

Stressors cause a series of reactions that alter the dynamic steady state for either short-term or long-term periods. For example, the normal concentration of glucose in the blood is 80 ± 10 mg/dl. It increases with acute stress, such as a burn injury, and then slowly returns to normal. If blood glucose remains high in the absence of a known stressor, it is diagnosed as a sign of disease—probably diabetes mellitus. Prolonged, unrelenting stress can cause a long-term elevation of glucose levels.

✓ QUICK CHECK

Briefly describe the three stages of the general adaptation syndrome.

Why is a dynamic steady state the most accurate definition of homeostasis? How is it related to stressors?

THE STRESS RESPONSE
Psychoneuroimmunologic Regulation

Psychoneuroimmunology is the study of how the consciousness *(psycho),* brain and CNS *(neuro),* and body's defense against external infection and abnormal cell division *(immunology)* interact.[5,6] Psychoneuroimmunology assumes that all immune-mediated disease results from interrelationships among psychosocial, emotional, genetic, neurologic, endocrine, and immune systems and behavioral factors. The immune system is integrated with other physiologic processes and is sensitive to changes in CNS and endocrine functioning, such as those that accompany psychologic states.[6] Stressors can elicit the *stress response* through the action of the nervous and endocrine systems, specifically corticotropin-releasing

factor (CRF) from the hypothalamus, the sympathetic nervous system, the pituitary gland, and the adrenal gland (see Fig. 8-2).[7,8] Adaptive energy is redirected to the CNS and stressed body sites. The sympathetic system stimulates the release of norepinephrine throughout the brain, promoting arousal, increased vigilance, increased anxiety, and other protective emotional responses. Reproduction, growth, and thyroid hormone are suppressed during stress and may conserve energy during stress. The adrenocortical hormones and the sympathetic nervous system may mediate enhancement or suppression of immune functioning.[6-10]

Neuroendocrine Regulation

The sympathetic nervous system is aroused during the stress response and causes the medulla of the adrenal gland to release catecholamines (epinephrine, norepinephrine, dopamine) into the bloodstream. Simultaneously, hypothalamic CRF stimulates the pituitary gland to release a variety of hormones, including antidiuretic hormone from the posterior pituitary gland and prolactin, growth hormone, and adrenocorticotropic hormone (ACTH) from the anterior pituitary gland. ACTH stimulates the cortex of the adrenal gland to release cortisol. (Relationships between the neuroendocrine and immune systems are discussed on p. 227.)

Catecholamines

Epinephrine goes to the liver and skeletal muscle but is then rapidly metabolized. Very little adrenal norepinephrine reaches distal tissue; thus its effects during the stress response are primarily from the sympathetic nervous system.[4,11] Catecholamines cannot cross the blood-brain barrier and are synthesized locally in the brain.[12]

The catecholamines stimulate two major classes of receptors: α-adrenergic receptors (α_1 and α_2) and β-adrenergic receptors (β_1 and β_2). Table 8-1 summarizes the actions of the two subclasses of adrenergic receptors. (A thorough discussion of receptors can be found in Chapters 1, 17, and 22.) Epinephrine binds to and activates both α- and β-receptors. Norepinephrine at physiologic concentrations binds primarily to α-receptors.[12]

The circulating catecholamines essentially mimic direct sympathetic stimulation. Norepinephrine regulates blood pressure because it is the primary constrictor of smooth muscle in all blood vessels. During stress, norepinephrine raises blood pressure by constricting peripheral vessels, inhibits gastrointestinal activity, and dilates the pupils (see Fig. 8-2). Epinephrine has greater influence on cardiac action and is the principal catecholamine involved in metabolic regulation. The physiologic effects of the catecholamines are summarized in Table 8-2.

Cortisol

The adrenal cortex is activated during stress by ACTH, increasing adrenocortical secretion of glucocorticoid (steroid) hormones, primarily cortisol (see Fig. 8-2). (Cortisol is known also as *hydrocortisone.*) Cortisol circulates in the plasma, both protein bound and free. The unbound, or free,

TABLE 8-1	Summary of the Physiologic Actions of α- and β-Receptors*
Receptor	**Physiologic Actions**
α_1	Increased glycogenolysis; smooth muscle contraction (blood vessels, genitourinary tract)
α_2	Smooth muscle relaxation (gastrointestinal tract); smooth muscle contraction (some vascular beds); inhibition of lipolysis, renin release, platelet aggregation, and insulin secretion
β_1	Stimulation of lipolysis; myocardial contraction (increased rate, increased force of contraction)
β_2	Increased hepatic gluconeogenesis; increased hepatic glycogenolysis; increased muscle glycogenolysis; increased release of insulin, glucagon, and renin; smooth muscle relaxation (bronchi, blood vessels, genitourinary tract, gastrointestinal tract)

From Granner, D.K. (1993). Hormones of the adrenal medulla. In R.K. Murray et al. (Eds.). Harper's biochemistry (21st ed.). New York: Lange Medical Books.

Some of these responses require glucocorticoids (e.g., cortisol) for maximal activity (see text for explanation).

TABLE 8-2	Physiologic Effects of the Catecholamines*
Organ	**Process or Result**
Brain	Increased blood flow
	Increased glucose metabolism
Cardiovascular system	Increased rate and force of contraction
	Peripheral vasoconstriction
Pulmonary system	Increased oxygen supply
	Bronchodilation
	Increased ventilation
Muscle	Increased glycogenolysis
	Increased contraction
	Increased dilation of skeletal muscle vasculature
Liver	Increased glucose production
	Increased gluconeogenesis
	Increased glycogenolysis
	Decreased glycogen synthesis
Adipose tissue	Increased lipolysis
	Increased fatty acids and glycerol
Skin	Decreased blood flow
Skeleton	Decreased glucose uptake and utilization (decreases insulin release)
Gastrointestinal and genitourinary tracts	Decreased protein synthesis
Lymphoid tissue	Increased protein breakdown (lymphoid tissue shrinks)

From Granner, D.K. (1993). Hormones of the adrenal medulla. In R.K. Murray et al. (Eds.). Harper's biochemistry (21st ed.). New York: Lange Medical Books.

Some of these responses require glucocorticoids (e.g., cortisol) for maximal activity (see text for explanation).

fraction is approximately 8% of the total plasma cortisol and is the most biologically active fraction of cortisol.[12] Cortisol mobilizes substances needed for cellular metabolism and stimulates gluconeogenesis, or the formation of glycogen from noncarbohydrate sources, such as amino or free fatty acids in the liver. In addition, cortisol enhances the elevation of blood glucose promoted by other hormones, such as epinephrine, glucagon, and somatotropic growth hormone. This action is said to be *permissive* for the actions of other hormones. Cortisol also inhibits the uptake and oxidation of glucose by many body cells. Overall, cortisol's actions on carbohydrate metabolism result in increased blood glucose levels. The physiologic effects of cortisol are summarized in Table 8-3.

Why is cortisol secretion during stress beneficial? Perhaps gluconeogenesis promoted by cortisol ensures an adequate source of glucose (energy) for body tissues, and nerve cells in particular. The pooling of amino acids from catabolized proteins may ensure amino acid availability for protein synthesis in certain cells. The redistribution of protein to sites where replacement is critical, such as muscle or cells of damaged tissue, is beneficial. Short-term, cortisol-induced alterations in immune cell distribution (e.g., traffic) patterns may be adaptive. In addition, decreased immune cell activity may prevent immune-mediated tissue damage by prolonged cell exposure to high levels of certain cytokines. Whether cortisol-induced effects are adaptive or destructive may depend on the intensity, type, and duration of the stressor and the subsequent concentration and length of cortisol exposure that target cells of the individual experience.

TABLE 8-3	Physiologic Effects of Cortisol
Functions Affected	Physiologic Effects
Carbohydrate and lipid metabolism	Diminishes peripheral uptake and utilization of glucose; promotes gluconeogenesis in liver cells; enhances the gluconeogenic response to other hormones; promotes lipolysis in adipose tissue
Protein metabolism	Increases protein synthesis in the liver and decreases protein synthesis (including immunoglobulin synthesis) in muscle, lymphoid tissue, adipose tissue, skin, and bone; increases plasma level of amino acids; stimulates deamination in the liver
Inflammatory effects	Decreases circulating eosinophils, lymphocytes, and monocytes; increases release of polymorphonuclear leukocytes from the bone marrow; decreases accumulation of leukocytes at the site of inflammation; delays healing; permissive for vasoconstrictive action of norepinephrine
Lipid metabolism	Lipolysis in the extremities and lipogenesis in the face and trunk
Immune reserve	Decreases the tissue mass of all lymphoid tissues (e.g., decreases protein synthesis); promotes rapid decrease in circulating lymphocytes, eosinophils, basophils, and macrophages; inhibits the production of interleukin-1 and interleukin-2; consequently, also blocks cell-mediated immunity and the generation of fever
Digestive function	Promotes gastric secretion
Urinary function	Enhances urinary excretion
Connective tissue function	Decreases proliferation of fibroblasts in connective tissue (thus delaying healing)
Muscle function	Maintains normal contractility and maximal work output for skeletal and cardiac muscle
Bone function	Decreases bone formation
Vascular system and myocardial function	Maintains normal blood pressure; permits increased responsiveness of arterioles to the constrictive action of adrenergic stimulation; optimizes myocardial performance
Central nervous system function	Somehow modulates perceptual and emotional functioning, essential for normal arousal and initiation of daytime activity

Other hormones
Endorphins

β-Endorphins (endogenous opiates) are released into the blood as part of the response to stressful stimuli, including traumatic injury and an acute, intense stress situation, such as first-time parachute jumping.[13-16] Stress-induced β-endorphins appear to regulate ACTH secretion and, with ACTH, inhibit hypothalamic CRF secretion, a possible down-regulation pathway of the stress response.[15]

Growth hormone

Growth hormone (somatotropin) is released from the anterior pituitary gland and affects protein, lipid, and carbohydrate metabolism. Growth hormone levels increase in the blood after a variety of stressful stimuli, such as cardiac catheterization, electroshock therapy, gastroscopy, surgery, fever, and physical exercise.[17,18] Immune cells are affected directly by growth hormone. Growth hormone receptors are present on lymphocytes.[19] Prolonged activation of the stress response (long-term stress) leads to suppression of growth hormone and other growth factor effects on target tissues.[20]

Prolactin

Prolactin is released from the anterior pituitary gland and is necessary for lactation and breast development.[21] Prolactin levels in plasma increase from a variety of stressful stimuli, including procedures such as gastroscopy, proctoscopy, pelvic examination, and surgery.[22] Prolactin also rises during parachute jumping, during motion sickness, after examinations,[23] and after various sexual stimuli, for example, stimu-

lation of the nipple or areola in women (plasma only). Like growth hormone, prolactin appears to require more intense stimuli than those leading to increases in catecholamine or cortisol levels. Immune cells also are affected by prolactin—several classes of lymphocytes have receptors for prolactin.[19]

Sex steroids

Testosterone, a hormone secreted by Leydig cells in the testes, regulates male secondary sex characteristics and libido. Levels decrease after stressful stimuli, including anesthesia, surgery, marathon running, and mountain climbing.[24] In addition, psychologic stimuli decrease testosterone levels, and individuals with respiratory failure, burns, and congestive heart failure show a marked reduction in plasma testosterone.[23] Males have a higher risk for morbidity after injury, and testosterone exhibits immunosuppressive activity.[25] Estrogen is thought to mediate the more robust immunologic profiles of females,[26] resulting in enhanced resistance to infection and risk for autoimmune diseases.

✓ QUICK CHECK

Describe psychoneuroimmunology.

Why is it important to understand the relationship among the nervous, endocrine, and immune systems during the stress response?

How does cortisol suppress the inflammatory response?

TABLE 8-4	Examples of Stree-Related Diseases and Conditions		
Target Organ or System	**Disease or Condition**	**Target Organ or System**	**Disease or Condition**
Cardiovascular system	Coronary artery disease	Gastrointestinal system	Ulcer
	Hypertension		Irritable bowel syndrome
	Stroke		Diarrhea
	Disturbances of heart rhythm		Nausea and vomiting
Muscle	Tension headaches		Ulcerative colitis
	Muscle contraction backache	Genitourinary system	Diuresis
Connective tissues	Rheumatoid arthritis (autoimmune disease)		Impotence
			Frigidity
	Related inflammatory diseases of connective tissue	Skin	Eczema
			Neurodermatitis
Pulmonary system	Asthma (hypersensitivity reaction)		Acne
		Endocrine system	Diabetes mellitus
	Hay fever (hypersensitivity reaction)		Amenorrhea
		Central nervous system	Fatigue and lethargy
Immune system	Immunosuppression or deficiency		Type A behavior
			Overeating
	Autoimmune diseases		Depression
			Insomnia

Role of the Immune System

Many immune-related conditions and diseases are associated with stress. The specific stress-induced mechanisms causing these illnesses are not yet clearly defined. Recent research is focused on the regulatory interactions between the immune system and the nervous and endocrine systems, which may represent mechanistic pathways for stress-associated immune-mediated diseases, including infection, some forms of cancer, allergy, and autoimmunity (Table 8-4).

The immune, nervous, and endocrine systems communicate through similar pathways involving hormones, neurotransmitters, neuropeptides, and immune cell products. Various components of immune system responses can be affected by neuroendocrine-produced factors involved in the stress reaction. Conversely, immune cell–derived cytokines and other products affect neurocrine and endocrine cells.[6,7,10] Several pathways regulate communication among these systems (Fig. 8-3).

The stress response directly influences the immune system through hypothalamic and pituitary peptides and through products of the sympathetic branch of the ANS. Immune cells have surface receptors for ACTH, CRF, endorphins, norepinephrine, growth hormone, steroids, and other products of the stress response.[5] There is direct innervation of the thymus, spleen, lymph nodes, and bone marrow.[7] Cholinergic, adrenergic, and peptinergic nerve terminals are present in the lymphoid organs and tissues. Endogenous opiates are released during stress and have concentration-dependent, enhancing, and suppressive effects on various immune cells.[7,13-15,27]

The pineal gland regulates immune response and mediates the apparent effects of circadian rhythm on immunity. When melatonin production is blocked (by continuous light or by pharmacologic means), the immune response is suppressed, whereas administration of melatonin reverses these effects.[28] This immunomodulation pathway may effect immune changes found with sleep disturbance and dysregulated circadian rhythm,[29] which are common among acutely ill and stressed patients.

The hypothalamic-pituitary-adrenal (HPA) axis may produce indirect effects on the CNS that modulate immune responses. The result is profound with prolonged severe stress,[6] including enlargement of the adrenal gland with simultaneous involution of the thymus and lymph nodes. Increased levels of circulating glucocorticosteroids (GCSs) may be an important mechanism in stress-related immune structure alterations and in suppression of the immune response.[6] The GCS level increases are attributable to pituitary ACTH production—a result of increased hypothalamic CRF. A number of stress factors initiate CRF production, including high levels of interleukin-1 (IL-1). Production of IL-1 by activated macrophages and monocytes is inhibited by GCS, suggesting a feedback loop with IL-1, CRF, ACTH, and GCS secretion.[7,30]

Lymphocytes also produce ACTH and endorphins in small amounts, which probably influence immune response in an autocrine (same cell stimulation) or paracrine (cell to cell) manner in ongoing immune responses.[7,31] The T cell growth factor, IL-2, can up-regulate pituitary ACTH. Immune-derived cytokines have significant influence on neuroendocrine function, with evidence for direct and indirect cytokine effects on nervous and adrenal cell functions. Thus the immune system has an adaptive role as a "signal" organ to alert other systems of inner threatening stimuli (e.g., infection, tissue damage, tumor cells) that may upset the dynamic steady state. The release of immune inflammatory mediators (IL-6, tumor necrosis factor–β [TNF-β], interferon) is triggered by bacterial or viral infections, cancer, and tissue injury that in turn initiate a stress response through the HPA pathway. Enhanced systemic production of

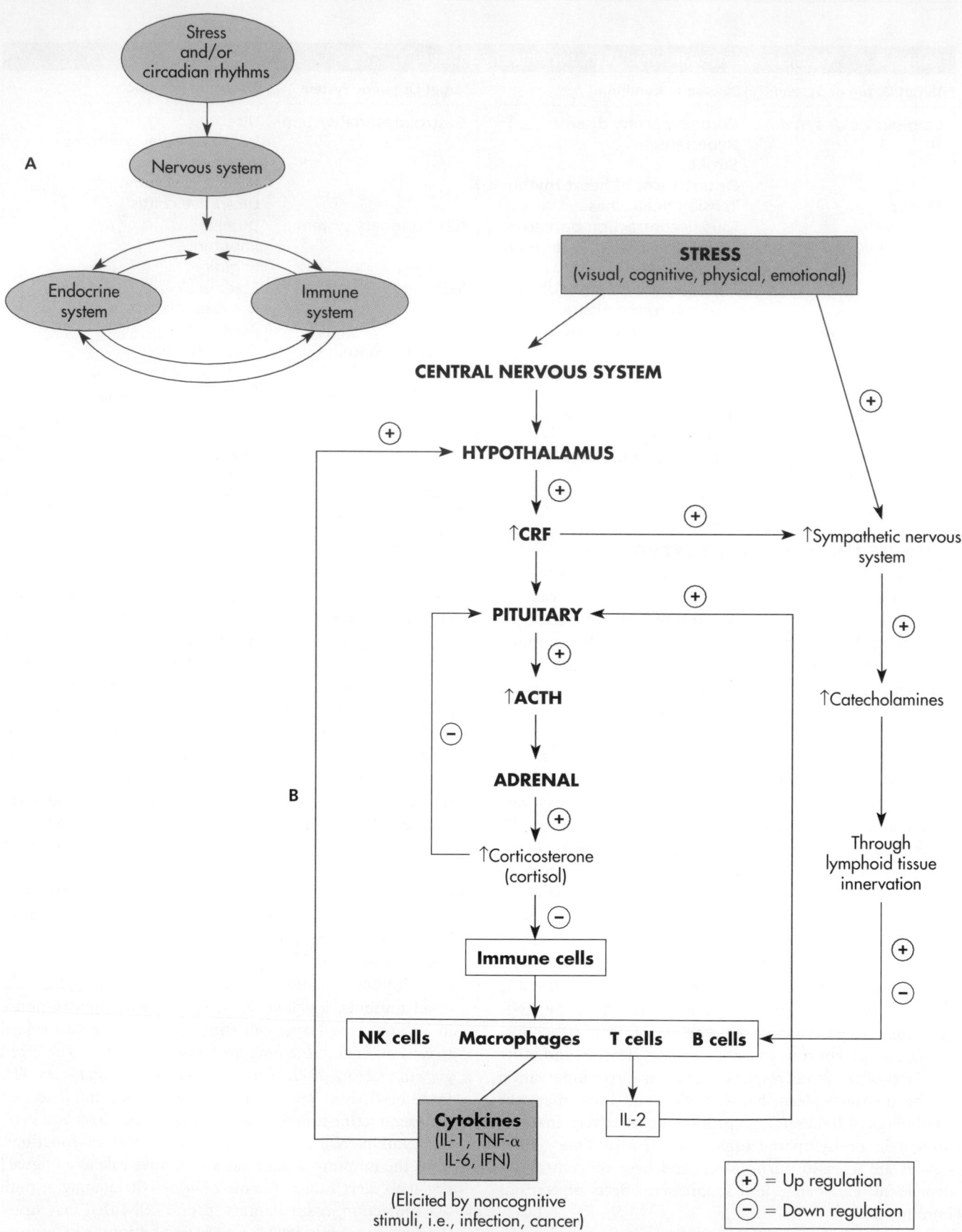

Fig. 8-3 *Nervous system/endocrine system/immune system interactions.* **A,** Interconnections or pathways of communication among the immune, nervous, and endocrine systems. **B,** Communication among these systems specifically involves hormones, neurotransmitters, neuropeptides, and immune cell products. *CRF,* Corticotropin-releasing hormone; *ACTH,* adrenocorticotropic hormone; *NK,* natural killer; *IL,* interleukin; *TNF,* tumor necrosis factor; *IFN,* interferon. (See text for discussion.)

these cytokines also induces other CNS and behavior changes during an acute infectious episode.[32-35]

Neuropeptides and hormones have a significant effect on the immune response. Whether this impact on immune function is suppressive or potentiating depends on the type of factor secreted, with some factors enhancing, some suppressing, and some doing both, depending on the concentration and length of exposure, the target cell, and the specific immune function studies.[32] Neuropeptides and neuroendocrine hormones may directly control biochemical events affecting cell proliferation, differentiation, and function or may indirectly control immune cell behavior by affecting the production or activity of cytokines.[7,10]

In summary, a linkage seems to exist among the nervous, endocrine, and immune systems. The most recent findings are that (1) there are direct effects of CNS and ANS neuropeptides on immune cells; (2) neurologically induced endocrine products influence immune cell and neurologic cell function; and (3) immune cell products (cytokines) affect nervous and endocrine cell function through both direct and indirect pathways.

STRESS, COPING, AND ILLNESS

Extreme physiologic stressors, such as severe burn injury, represent a predictable stimulus for stress responses. A less severe and defined event or situation, however, can be a stressor for one person and not for another. Many stressors, such as fasting or temperature changes, do not necessarily cause a physiologic stress response if psychologic factors are minimized. Stress itself is not an independent entity but a system of interdependent processes moderated by the nature, intensity, and duration of the stressor and the perception, appraisal, and coping efficacy of the affected individual, all of which in turn mediate the psychologic and physiologic response to stress.

Psychosocial distress may be predictive of psychologic, social, and physical health outcomes. In *psychologic distress,* the individual feels a general state of unpleasant arousal after life events. This state is manifested as physiologic, emotional, cognitive, and behavior changes.[36] Periods of depression and emotional upheaval often are associated with adverse life events and place the affected individual at risk for immunologic deficits, increasing the risk of ill health.[6] Examples of triggering circumstances include bereavement, academic pressures, and marital conflict.[37-41] Aging also may increase psychosocial distress and is associated with immune changes[42,43] (see Aging box).

Stressful life events and mood have been reported as important factors preceding the onset or exacerbation of symptoms in AIDS infection, diabetes, and multiple sclerosis.[44-46] In addition, the interaction with health care providers in a clinical setting, the diagnosis of a major illness, and various clinical procedures (e.g., blood sampling, injections, examinations, surgical procedures) may represent significant negative life events to many individuals (Fig. 8-4). These additional stresses may interfere with the efficacy of the medical

⚠ AGING & *Stress: Stress-Age Syndrome*

With aging, sometimes a set of neurohormonal and immune alterations, as well as tissue and cellular changes, develops—these changes recently have been defined as stress-age syndrome. These changes include the following:

- Alterations in the excitability of structures of the limbic system and hypothalamus
- Rise of the blood concentration of catecholamines, ADH, ACTH, and cortisol
- Decrease of testosterone, thyroxine, and others
- Alterations of opioid peptides
- Immunodepression
- Alterations in lipoproteins
- Hypercoagulation of the blood
- Free radical damage of cells

Some of the alterations are adaptational, whereas others are potentially damaging. These stress-related alterations of aging can influence the course of developing stress reactions and lower adaptive reserve and coping.[42]

ADH, *Antidiuretic hormone;* ACTH, *adrenocorticotropic hormone.*

intervention. Identifying and reducing stress in the clinical setting have particular applicability in both disease prevention and illness management.

A beneficial influence during stress has been shown with adaptive coping strategies, especially if they are problem focused and involve social support.[47-52] *Coping* is the process of managing stressful challenges that tax the individual's resources.[47] Adverse consequences of stress may be minimized by effective coping, whereas inadequate coping responses may exacerbate the effects of distress on health, thus augmenting the potential for illness.[47]

Mediating factors that may influence stress susceptibility or resilience include age, socioeconomic status, gender, social support, religious or spiritual factors, personality, self-esteem, genetics, past experiences, and current health status.

HEALTH ALERT

Social Support and Breast Cancer

Social support, including structured psychotherapy, has been shown to enhance adjustment and positively affect survival time in patients with breast cancer. Medical and nursing management of patients with breast cancer ideally would include the availability of psychologic support and treatment to optimize outcome.

Data from Classen, C. et al. (1997). Journal of Psychotherapy Practice and Research, 6(3), 211-218; Classen, C. et al. (1996). Coping styles associated with psychological adjustment to advanced breast cancer. Health Psychology, 15(6), 434-437; Spiegel, D. (1996). Cancer and depression. British Journal of Psychiatry Supplement, (30), 109-116.

Fig. 8-4 *Health outcome determination in stressful life situations is moderated by numerous factors.* Whether a life-challenged individual experiences distress or illness depends on the subject's appraisal of the event and the coping strategies used during the stressful period. Models **A** and **B** reflect possible outcomes in stressed healthy and symptomatic individuals. Model **C** illustrates the dynamic clinical setting in which the diagnosis of a serious illness and subsequent medical interventions may be perceived as stressful challenges and have potentially detrimental influences on physical outcome.

Evidence suggests that effective intervention may result in greater stress resilience and improved psychologic and physiologic outcomes.[54] For example, women with recurrent metastatic breast cancer who were provided weekly group counseling in addition to routine medical treatment lived an average of 19 months longer than control subjects.[52,53]

The importance of social support for seriously ill individuals has focused attention also on the health of caregivers. Significant stress manifested as depression, anxiety, and fatigue has been noted in family caregivers of those with cancer, Alzheimer disease, and burn trauma. Patients and caregivers exhibited suppression of various measures of immune function, with improved function associated with better perceived social support.[48-52]

Interventions to potentially prevent or manage stress-related psychologic or physical problems include both short- and long-term coping strategies. Educational components are specific to the individual's problems. Relaxation techniques may include meditation, imagery, and biofeedback. These approaches may be used on an individual or support group basis. Incorporation of these approaches into clinical training facilitates their use in the clinical arena. Future research should focus on the efficacy of such approaches with various populations.[12]

✓ QUICK CHECK

How do the immune, nervous, and endocrine systems communicate?

Why is psychologic distress an important factor in health?

Why is social support important during stress?

◼ DID YOU UNDERSTAND?

Concepts of Stress

1. Stress recently has been defined as the state of affairs arising when a person relates to (i.e., interacts or transacts with) situations in a certain way. How he or she appraises and reacts to situations is important.
2. Hans Selye identified three structural changes in rats subjected repeatedly to noxious stimuli (stressors): enlargement of the cortex of the adrenal gland, atrophy of the thymus gland and other lymphoid tissues, and gastrointestinal ulceration.
3. Selye believed that the three changes were caused by a nonspecific physiologic response to any long-term stressor. He called this response the general adaptation syndrome (GAS).
4. The GAS occurs in three stages: the alarm stage, the stage of resistance or adaptation, and the stage of exhaustion. Diseases of adaptation develop if the stage of resistance or adaptation does not restore homeostasis.
5. Selye identified three components of physiologic stress: the stressor, the physiologic or chemical disturbance produced by the stressor, and the body's adaptational response to the stressor.
6. Other investigators have shown that the physiologic stress response also occurs in response to psychologic or emotional stress.
7. There is disagreement on the nonspecific nature of the stress response because different processes occur in response to specific stimuli, such as exposure to cold or heat.
8. W.B. Cannon defined homeostasis as the sum of the processes by which the body maintains itself at a relatively constant composition. This definition has since been modified. Homeostasis is now considered to mean the sum of the processes by which the body maintains itself in a dynamic steady state.
9. The function of the physiologic stress response is to maintain the body's dynamic steady state.

The Stress Response

1. The stress response involves the nervous system (sympathetic branch of the autonomic nervous system), the endocrine system (pituitary and adrenal glands), and the immune system.
2. The stress response is initiated when a stressor is present in the body or perceived by the mind.
3. The neuroendocrine response to stress consists of sympathetic stimulation of the adrenal medulla to secrete catecholamines (norepinephrine, epinephrine) and stressor-induced stimulation of the pituitary to secrete ACTH, which in turn stimulates the adrenal cortex to secrete steroid hormones, particularly cortisol.
4. In general, the catecholamines prepare the body to act, and cortisol mobilizes energy (glucose) and other substances needed to fuel the action.
5. Epinephrine exerts its chief effects on the cardiovascular system. Epinephrine increases cardiac output and increases blood flow to the heart, brain, and skeletal muscles by dilating vessels that supply these organs. It also dilates the airways, thereby increasing delivery of oxygen to the bloodstream.
6. Norepinephrine's chief effects complement those of epinephrine. Norepinephrine constricts blood vessels of the viscera and skin; this has the effect of shifting blood flow to the vessels dilated by epinephrine. Norepinephrine also increases mental alertness.
7. Cortisol's chief effects involve metabolic processes. By inhibiting the use of metabolic substances while promoting their formation, cortisol mobilizes glucose, amino acids, lipids, and fatty acids and delivers them to the bloodstream. Cortisol also suppresses immune and inflammatory function.
8. The nervous, endocrine, and immune systems communicate through the common use of signal molecules and their receptors, which in turn regulate the behavior of cells in each system during stress challenge.
9. There are direct and indirect pathways of influence among the nervous, endocrine, and immune systems. Neuropeptides have direct effects on immune cells, as well as indirect influences through neurologically mediated endocrine modulation of immune function. Endocrine products (cortisol) also influence neurologic cell behavior. Immune cell products affect both nervous and endocrine cell function, reflecting an adaptive role for the immune system as a "signal" organ to alert other systems of threatening stimuli.
10. Other hormones are affected by the stress response and include increased circulating levels of β-endorphins, growth hormone, prolactin, and antidiuretic hormone. Testosterone decreases during the stress response.

Stress, Coping, and Illness

1. Stress is a system of interdependent processes that are moderated by the nature, intensity, and duration of the stressor and coping efficacy of the affected individual, all of which in turn mediate the psychologic and physiologic response to stress.
2. Many studies have linked psychologic distress with altered immune function, and there is now evidence that strengthens the association of stress with potential for illness in humans.

KEY TERMS

Alarm stage, 222
Coping, 229
Diseases of adaptation, 222
Dynamic steady state, 224
General adaptation syndrome (GAS), 222
Homeostasis, 224

Permissive, 225
Physiologic stress, 222
Psychologic distress, 229
Psychoneuroimmunology, 224
Psychosocial distress, 229
Stage of exhaustion, 222

Stage of resistance or adaptation, 222
Stress response, 224
Stressor, 222
Turnover, 224

REFERENCES

1. Cannon, W.B., Bringer, C.A.L., & Fritz, R. (1914). Experimental hyperthyroidism. *American Journal of Physiology, 36,* 363.

2. Selye, H. (1946). The general adaptation syndrome and the diseases of adaptation. *Journal of Clinical Endocrinology, 6,* 117-230.

3. Ostell, A. (1991). Coping, problem-solving, and stress: A framework for intervention strategies. *British Journal of Medical Psychology, 64,* 11-24.

4. Dickman, S.R. (1988). *Pathways to wellness.* Champaign, Ill.: Life Enhancement Publishers.

5. Cohen, S. & Herbert, T.B. (1996). Health-psychology: Psychological factors and physical disease from the perspective of human psychoneuroimmunology. *Annual Review of Psychology, 47,* 113-142.

6. Ader, R. & Cohen, N. (1993). Psychoneuroimmunology: Conditioning and stress. *Annual Review of Psychology, 44,* 35-85.

7. Chambers, D.A., Cohen, R.L., & Perlman, R.L. (1993). Commentary neuroimmune modulation: Signal transduction and catecholamines. *Neurochemistry International, 22*(2), 95-110.

8. Cacioppo, J.T. et al. (1998). Autonomic, neuroendocrine, and immune responses to psychological stress: The reactivity hypothesis. *Annals of the New York Academy of Science, 840,* 664-673.

9. Houldin, A.D. et al. (1991). Psychoneuroimmunology: A review of literature. *Holistic Nursing Practice, 5*(4), 10-21.

10. Maier, S.F. & Watkins, L.R. (1998). Cytokines for psychologists: Implications of bidirectional immune-to-brain communication for understanding behavior, mood, and cognition. *Psychological Reviews, 105,* 83-107.

11. Herd, J.A. (1991). Cardiovascular response to stress. *Physiological Reviews, 71*(1), 305-330.

12. Granner, D.K. (1993). Hormones of the adrenal medulla. In R.K. Murray et al. (Eds.). *Harper's biochemistry* (23rd ed.). New York: Lange Medical Books.

13. Guillemin, R. et al. (1977). Beta-endorphin and adrenocorticotropin are secreted concomitantly by the pituitary gland. *Science, 197,* 1367-1369.

14. Schedlowski, M. et al. (1995). Beta-endorphin, but not substance-P, is increased by acute stress in humans. *Psychoneuroendocrinology, 20*(1), 103-110.

15. McCubbin, J.A. (1993). Stress and endogenous opioids: Behavioral and circulatory interactions. *Biological Psychology, 35*(2), 91-122.

16. Hetz, W. et al. (1996). Stress hormones in accident patients studied before admission to hospital. *Journal of Accident and Emergency Medicine, 13*(4), 243-247.

17. Nerlich, M.L. et al. (1994). Neuropepetide levels early after trauma: Immunomodulatory effects? *Journal of Trauma, 37*(5), 759-768.

18. Rose, R.M. (1985). Psychoendocrinology. In J.D. Wilson & D.W. Foster (Eds.). *Williams textbook of endocrinology* (7th ed.). Philadelphia: Saunders.

19. Berne, R.M. & Levy, M.N. (Eds.). (1996). *Principles of physiology* (2nd ed.). St. Louis: Mosby.

20. Schalach, D.S. (1967). The influence of physical stress and exercise on growth hormone and insulin secretion in man. *Journal of Laboratory and Clinical Medicine, 69,* 256-269.

21. Reichlin, S. (1993). Neuroendocrine-immune interactions. *New England Journal of Medicine, 329*(17), 1246-1253.

22. Burguera, B. et al. (1990). Dual and selective actions of glucocorticoid upon basal and stimulated growth hormone release in man. *Neuroendocrinology, 51,* 51-58.

23. Shiu, R.P.C. & Friesen, H.G. (1980). Mechanisms of action of prolactin in the control of mammary gland function. *Annual Review of Physiology, 42,* 83-96.

24. Noel, G.L. et al. (1972). Human prolactin and growth hormone release during surgery and other conditions of stress. *Journal of Clinical Endocrinology and Metabolism, 35,* 840-851.

25. Matsumoto, K. et al. (1970). Plasma testosterone levels following surgical stress in male patients. *Acta Endocrinology, 65,* 11-17.

26. Bone, R.C. (1992). Toward an epidemiology and natural history of SIRS (systemic inflammatory response syndrome). *Journal of the American Medical Association, 268,* 3452-3455.

27. Paavonen, T. (1994). Hormonal regulation of immune responses. *Annals of Medicine, 26*(4), 255-258.

28. Maestroni, G.J.M. & Conti, A. (1991). Anti-stress role of the immuno-opioid network: Evidence for a physiological mechanism involving T cell–derived, immunoreactive X-endorphin and metenkephalin binding to thymic opioid receptors. *International Journal of Neuroscience, 61,* 289-298.

REFERENCES

29. Shelby, J., Ku, W.W., & Nielson, H.C. (1996). Neurohormone and neuropeptide regulation of the posttraumatic immune response. In E. Faist (Ed.). *Host defense alterations of trauma, shock, and sepsis—Multi-organ failure/immunotherapy of sepsis.* Berlin: Pabst.

30. Sundar, S.K. et al. (1990). Brain IL-1–induced immunosuppression occurs through activation of both pituitary-adrenal axis and sympathetic nervous system by corticotropin-releasing factor. *The Journal of Neuroscience, 10,* 3701-3706.

31. Weigent, D.A., Carr, D.J., & Blalock, J.E. (1990). Bidirectional communication between the neuroendocrine and immune systems: Common hormones and hormone receptors. *New York Academy of Science, 579,* 17-27.

32. Aoki, N., Ohno, Y., & Imamura, M. (1990). Physiological interactions between the immune and endocrine systems: Are cytokines hormones? *Medical Science Research, 18,* 195-201.

33. Busbridge, N.J. & Grossman, A.B. (1991). Stress and the single cytokine: Interleukin modulation of the pituitary-adrenal axis. *Molecular and Cellular Endocrinology, 82,* C209-C214.

34. Hori, T. et al. (1991). Immune cytokines and regulation of body temperature, food intake, and cellular immunity. *Brain Research Bulletin, 27,* 309-313.

35. Navarra, P. et al. (1991). Interleukins-1 and -6 stimulate the release of corticotropin-releasing hormone-41 from rat hypothalamus in vitro via the eicosanoid cyclooxygenase pathway. *Endocrinology, 128*(1), 37-44.

36. Thoits, P.A. (1983). Dimensions of life events that influence psychological distress: An evaluation and synthesis of the literature. In H.B. Kaplan (Ed.). *Psychosocial stress: Trends in theory and research.* Orlando: Academic Press.

37. Biondi, M. & Picardi, A. (1996). Clinical and biological aspects of bereavement and loss-induced depression—A reappraisal. *Psychotherapy and Psychosomatics, 65*(5), 229-245.

38. Anderson, J.L. (1996). The immune system and depression. *Advances in Neuroimmunology, 6*(2), 119-129.

39. Kang, D.H., Coe, C.L., & McCarthy, D.O. (1996). Academic examinations significantly impact immune responses, but not lung function, in healthy and well-managed asthmatic adolescents. *Brain, Behavior, and Immunology, 10*(20), 164-181.

40. Kiecolt-Glaser, J.K. et al. (1997). Marital conflict in older adults: Endocrinological and immunological correlates. *Psychosomatic Medicine, 59*(4), 339-349.

41. Kiecolt-Glaser, J.K. et al. (1998). Marital status: Immunologic, neuroendocrine, and autonomic correlates. *Annals of the New York Academy of Science, 840,* 656-663.

42. FrolKis, V.V. (1993). Stress-age syndrome. *Mechanisms of Ageing and Development, 69*(1-2), 93-107.

43. Hirokawa, K. (1997). Reversing and restoring immune functions. *Mechanisms of Ageing and Development, 93*(1-3), 119-124.

44. Solomon, G.F., Kemeny, M.E., & Temoshok, L. (1991). Psychoneuroimmunologic aspects of human immunodeficiency virus infection. In R. Alder, D.L. Felten, & N. Cohen (Eds.). *Psychoneuroimmunology* (2nd ed.). New York: Academic Press.

45. Surwit, R.S. & Schneider, M.S. (1993). Role of stress in the etiology and treatment of diabetes mellitus. *Psychosomatic Medicine, 55*(4), 380-393.

46. Coyle, P.K. (1996). The neuroimmunology of multiple sclerosis. *Advances in Neuroimmunology, 6*(2), 143-154.

47. Folkman, S. & Lazarus, R.S. (1988). The relationship between coping and emotion: Implications for theory and research. *Social Sciences Medicine, 26,* 309-317.

48. Baron, R.S. et al. (1990). Social support and immune function among spouses of cancer patients. *Journal of Personality and Social Psychology, 59,* 344-352.

49. Fawzy, F.I. et al. (1993). Malignant melanoma: Effects of an early structured psychiatric intervention, coping, and affective state on recurrence and survival 6 years later. *Archives of General Psychiatry, 50*(9), 681-689.

50. Kiecolt-Glaser, J. et al. (1987). Chronic stress and immune function in family caregivers of Alzheimers disease victims. *Psychosomatic Medicine, 45*(5), 523-535.

51. Shelby, J. et al. (1992). Severe burn injury: Effects on psychologic and immunologic function in noninjured close relatives. *Journal of Burn Care & Rehabilitation, 13*(1), 58-63.

52. Spiegel, D. et al. (1998). Effects of psychosocial treatment in prolonging cancer survival may be mediated by neuroimmune pathways. *Annals of the New York Academy of Science, 840,* 670-683.

53. Spiegel, D. (1997). Psychosocial aspects of breast cancer treatment. *Seminars in Oncology, 24*(1, Suppl. 1), S1-36-47.

54. Lazar, J.S. (1996). Mind-body medicine in primary care: Implications and applications. *Primary Care, 23*(1), 169-182.

CHAPTER

9

Biology of Cancer

Kathryn L. McCance and Lee K. Roberts

Perhaps no other disease causes more concern, fear, and disability than cancer. The human responses to cancer are vast and profound, progressing from shock and disbelief, to uncertainty and dread of recurrence, to hope, coping, or cure. Cancer is, in reality, a variety of disorders with differing pathophysiologies. Mechanisms of cancer development vary according to the site of the disease and the precipitating cause.

 Check out your CD Companion for chapter-related exercises and answers to the Quick Check questions

CANCER: A DISEASE OF GROWTH, DIVISION, AND CELL DIFFERENTIATION

Cells of multicellular organisms are specialized members of a *cellular society*. The goal of this cellular society is survival of the entire organism and not just the individual cell. Therefore some cells must refrain from dividing even when nutrients are plentiful.[1] Cell division, proliferation, and differentiation (specialization) are strictly regulated under normal conditions. In this way, organ and tissue mass does not change because a balance is maintained between cell birth rate and cell death rate. When a need arises in an organ or tissue for new cells, however, as in the repair of damage, previously nondividing cells (e.g., resting cells) are rapidly triggered to reenter the division cycle (see Cell Cycle, p. 20). Resting cells must be "turned on" to divide and proliferate and "turned off" to stop dividing and undergo differentiation. The cellular control mechanisms that regulate cell birth and cell death are referred to as *social controls* and require social control genes. Abnormal cells that disobey the social control mechanisms of normal cell division, proliferation, and differentiation proliferate to form tumors in the body. Virtually every cell in the body, if mutated, has the potential to form tumors.

Social Control Genes and Cellular Division

Cell division depends on complex social controls. Proliferation of different cell types is regulated by different combinations of protein growth factors (see Chapter 1). A cell that undergoes a mutation or set of mutations presumably disrupts the social control genes that give rise to growth-factor-regulated cell divisions (Fig. 9-1). In other words, the protein growth factors of these genes "turn on" and "turn off" normal cell division and proliferation. Cancer is caused by the malfunction or mutation of the genes that regulate proliferation and differentiation. All cells in the body are programmed to develop, grow, differentiate, and die in response to a complex system of biologic signals. Thus cancer results when any cell is freed from these constraints and its abnormal progeny are allowed to proliferate (see Fig. 9-1, *B*). The identification and characteristics of many of these social control genes have been one of the great triumphs of molecular biology in the past decade.

Three main genetic mechanisms have a role in the development of most human neoplasms. The first is mutation of genes resulting in inappropriate activity (i.e., hyperactivity) of growth-related gene products that under normal circumstances stimulate growth. Such genes are termed **oncogenes** and act in a dominant manner (see p. 245). That is, the phenotype is affected even if only one of the cell's two gene copies has mutated, which abnormally stimulates growth. The second mechanism is loss of activity of gene products that, under normal circumstances, would inhibit growth. These genes are termed **tumor-suppressor genes** or **antioncogenes** (see p. 247). They act in a recessive manner to produce neoplasms, meaning the malignant phenotype develops only if both alleles fail to suppress growth. The third mechanism is expression of genes resulting in overexpression of products that prevent normal cell death (apoptosis), thus allowing continued growth of tumors.

An important question is, "How do activated oncogenes or inactivated tumor suppressor genes drive a tumor cell to

A

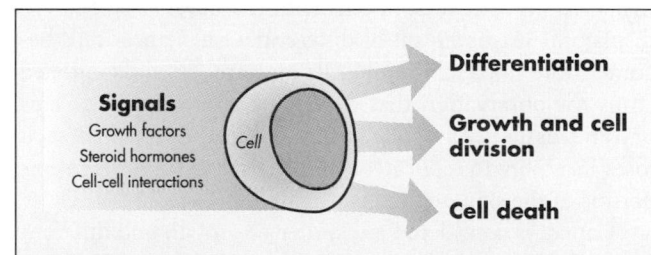

B

Fig. 9-1 *Major features of cellular regulation.* **A,** External growth factors (protein and steroid hormones such as epidermal growth factor) bind to membrane-spanning growth-factor receptors on the cell surface. These activate signal transduction pathways, in which genes such as *ras* participate. Components of the signal transduction pathway in turn interact with nuclear transcription factors, such as *myc* and *fos,* which can bind with other proteins, such as GTPase activating-protein (GAP), to regulatory regions in DNA. **B,** All cells are genetically programmed to develop, grow, differentiate, and die. Occasionally a cell loses its ability to respond to environmental and internal signals. It fails to differentiate, continuing to divide without restraint. The descendants of these cells (progeny) become the founders of neoplasms. *(Modified from Jorde, L.B. et al. [1999]. Medical genetics [2nd ed.]. St. Louis: Mosby.)*

proliferate indefinitely?" Part of the answer involves the enzyme **telomerase.** Telomerase acts on the telomere, the DNA-protein "cap" at the end of each linear chromosome. Normally, the telomere shrinks as the cell divides and differentiates. When the telomere has lost a certain portion of its length, the cell dies. In immortal cancer cells, however, reactivation of telomerase causes the addition of nucleotides back to the telomere; thus with a full-length telomere, cells continue to divide.[2-5]

Cell Differentiation

Cancer cells are defined by two heritable properties: autonomy and anaplasia. **Autonomy** refers to the cancer cell's independence from normal cellular controls. **Anaplasia** is the loss of differentiation, the process of developing specialized functions, and organization, meaning literally "without form." In general, the cancer cell has lost its ability to function normally and to control its growth and division. **Transformation** is the process by which a normal cell becomes a cancer cell (Fig. 9-2). In normal growth and development, cells become irreversibly more specialized or "committed" to a particular line of development, or pathway of differentiation. Thus *differentiation* is the process of acquiring specific new characteristics resulting in observable changes in cellular function. Cells continue to grow and differentiate throughout life.

Genes (proto-oncogenes) normally turned off during differentiation can be mutated or reactivated by carcinogenic agents. Experiments have shown that cells at one level of differentiation can be transformed into less well-differentiated cells by exposing them to carcinogenic agents.[6]

As cells mature, they differentiate to perform the specific functions of the tissue they constitute (Fig 9-3). In the adult, *undifferentiated cells* (not totally committed to a specific function) are known as *pluripotent cells, precursor cells,* or *stem cells.* In comparison, cells within a developing embryo display the least amount of differentiation. Cancer cells become more like embryonic cells and are less differentiated (thus the observation that cancerous tissue resembles embryonic tissue). As a cell becomes more differentiated, it loses its ability to replicate. In some tissues, such as the epidermis of the skin, the cell is destined to die.

Cancer is considered a disorder of growth and differentiation because neoplasms resemble undifferentiated tissue. The less the tumor resembles normal tissue, the more undifferentiated or anaplastic the tumor is said to be. Tumor **grading,** which grades differentiation, is thus a gauge of the tumor's degree of malignancy (Table 9-1). As the malignant cells grow and divide, they often lose their mature characteristics and no longer resemble their tissue of origin.

Cancerous growth often depends on derangements of cell differentiation. Differentiation depends on the functioning of the stem cell. Cell populations are renewed by simple duplication by means of **stem cells** (see Fig. 9-2). The defining properties of a stem cell include the following: (1) it is not at the end of the pathway of differentiation—that is, it is not, itself, **terminally differentiated;** (2) it can divide with-

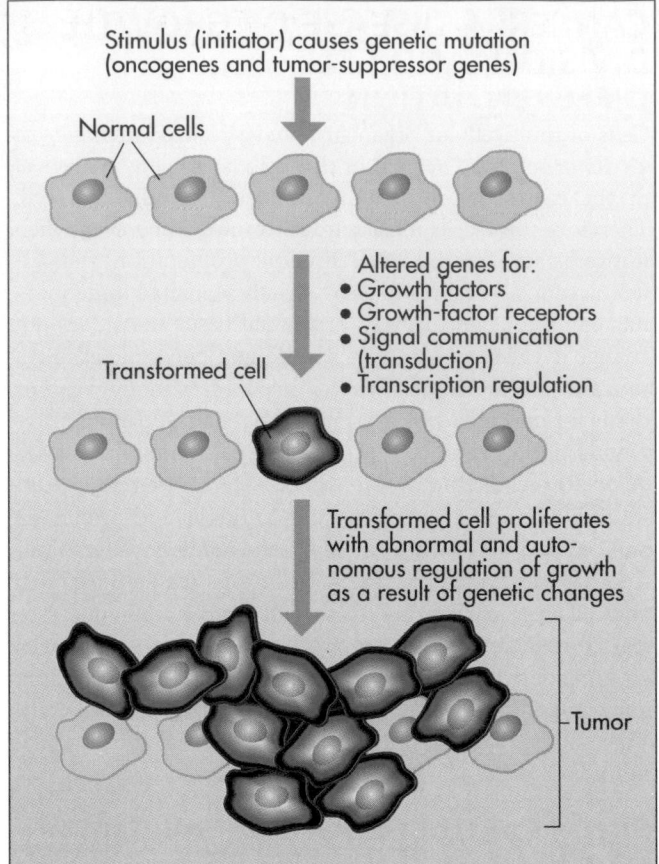

Fig. 9-2 *Transformation by altered genetic changes.*

out limit; and (3) when it divides, each daughter cell has a choice—it can remain a stem cell or it can become irreversibly committed to terminal differentiation (Fig. 9-4). Normally, each stem cell division generates one daughter stem cell and one cell (although it may be pluripotent, giving rise to several types of blood cells, for example) that is committed to terminal differentiation and a cessation of cell division. If the stem cell divides more rapidly, terminally differentiated cells are produced more rapidly. As mentioned, regulation of stem cell proliferation with cell growth and terminal differentiation is required to maintain the balance of new cell production and cell destruction within a tissue. To produce a steadily growing tumor, however, a transformed stem cell must cause an imbalance in cell production and cell destruction. An excessive cell division rate for the stem cells will not by itself have this effect.[1] Two derangements in differentiation, however, could presumably cause an imbalance leading to tumor development (Fig. 9-5).

Tumor Classification and Nomenclature

Tumors are classified on the basis of cell type, tissue of origin, whether benign or malignant, degree of differentiation (well, moderately, or poorly), anatomic site, and function. Table 9-2 shows the differences between benign and malignant tumors. Tumors are named according to the tissues

TABLE 9-1	Tumor Grading: Degrees of Differentiation
Grade	**Tumor Characteristics**
Grade I: well differentiated	Tumor closely resembles tissue of origin and thus retains some specialized functions
Grade II: moderately differentiated	Tumor has less resemblance to tissue of origin; more variation in size and shape of tumor cells; increased mitoses
Grade III: poorly to very poorly differentiated	Tumor does not closely resemble tissue of origin; much variation in size and shape of tumor cells; greatly increased mitoses
Grade IV: very poorly differentiated	Tumor has no resemblance to tissue of origin; great variation in size and shape of tumor cells

Modified from Moosa, A.R., Robson, M.C., & Schimpff, S.C. (Eds.). (1986). Comprehensive textbook of oncology. Baltimore: Williams & Wilkins.

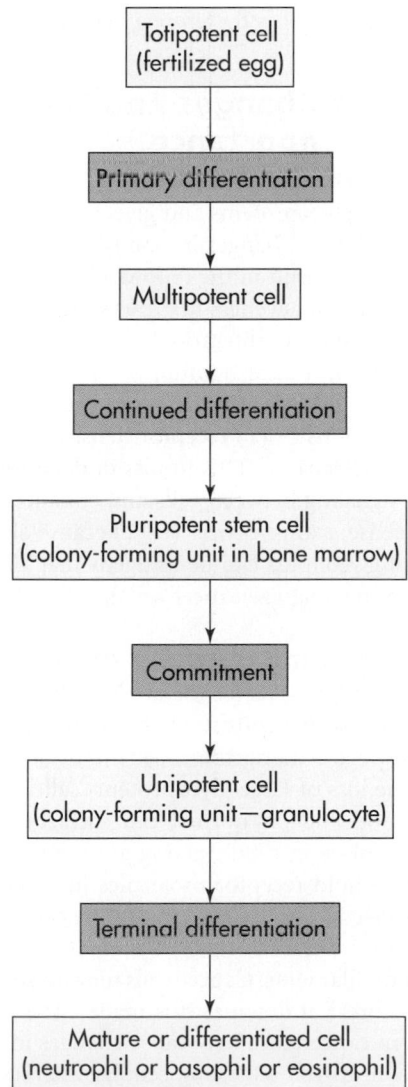

Fig. 9-3 *Example of differentiation.* Differentiation occurs several times in the lifetime of a granulocyte with each step further limiting the cell's potential. Eventually, the cell *terminally* differentiates and can no longer divide, and the mature cell dies.

Fig. 9-4 *Differentiation of a stem cell.* When a stem cell divides, each daughter cell has a choice: it can either remain a stem cell or go on to become terminally differentiated.

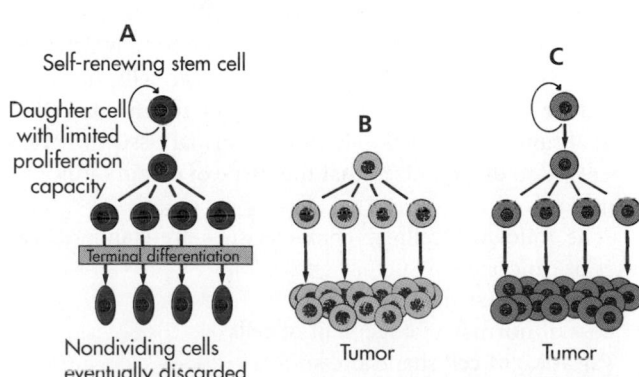

Fig. 9-5 *Differentiated cells and two types of derangements.* **A,** The normal stem cell pathway for producing new differentiated cells. **B,** Stem cell fails to produce one non-stem-cell daughter in each division and thus proliferates to form a tumor. **C,** Daughter cells fail to differentiate normally and thus proliferate to form a tumor.

TABLE 9-2	Important Differences Between Benign and Malignant Tumors	
	Benign	**Malignant**
Differentiation/anaplasia	Well-differentiated; resembles cell of origin	Some lack of differentiation; anaplasia, often atypical
Spread and boundaries	Remains localized; well-demarcated masses that do not invade or infiltrate surrounding normal tissue	Locally invasive, infiltrates surrounding normal tissues; irregular and ill-defined borders, nonencapsulated; rarely cohesive, likely metastases
Rate of growth	Progressive and slow	Erratic; often rapid
Host effects	Produced by pressure on vessels, nerves, organs, etc.; removal will alleviate	Destructive to normal tissue; removal does not necessarily restore function

from which they arise, generally with the suffix "oma." Cancers include those of epithelial tissue *(carcinomas),* connective tissue *(sarcomas),* lymphatic tissue *(lymphomas),* glial cells of the central nervous system *(gliomas),* and blood-forming organs, primarily the bone marrow *(leukemias).* The leukemias usually involve an abnormal growth or proliferation of blood-forming cells that infiltrate and replace normal bone marrow and lymphatic tissue. Table 9-3 presents the nomenclature and classification of tumors.

Carcinoma in situ refers to preinvasive epithelial tumors of glandular or squamous cell origin. These tumors have not broken through basement membranes of the epithelium. Carcinoma in situ occurs in the cervix, skin, oral cavity, esophagus, and bronchus. In glandular epithelium, in situ lesions occur in the stomach, endometrium, breast, and large bowel. These lesions may erroneously be confused with benign tumors, but both the squamous and glandular cell types show disorganization and atypical changes of epithelium. The time that such lesions remain in situ before becoming invasive is unknown. Some carcinomas of the cervix are known to be preinvasive lesions in situ for several years before they progress to invasive carcinoma or metastatic tumors (see Fig. 9-12, *C*).

CHARACTERISTICS OF CANCER CELLS

Cancer cells differ according to the cell type from which they derive. To apply any definition to all cancer cells, however, would be presumptuous. Some tumors retain somewhat normal functions and closely mimic normal tissue, whereas others are so disorganized that the tissue of origin cannot be identified.

The following cellular characteristics are standard features of cancerous tissue:
1. Local increase in cell number
2. Loss of normal arrangement of cells
3. Variation of cell shape and size
4. Increase in nuclear size and density of staining (reflects an increase in total deoxyribonucleic acid [DNA])
5. Increase in mitotic activity
6. Abnormal mitoses and chromosomes

Cancer cells are disordered cells that proliferate rapidly and vary greatly in size and shape. They divide in an uncoordinated fashion, invading and destroying neighboring tissue, a process termed *progression.* Progression is an increase of abnormal biologic properties and not necessarily a progression in tumor size. A cancer is therefore a delinquent cell mass.

Cell Surface Changes and Their Functional Importance
Glycolipids and glycoproteins
The cell surface glycoproteins and glycolipids of cancer cells are lost or modified. Changes in one type of glycolipid, the *glycosphingolipids,* result in the following:
1. Altered cell responsiveness to growth factors
2. Abnormal cellular proliferation[6]
3. Impaired cell-to-cell recognition[7]

Other effects of lost or modified glycoproteins and glycolipids are alterations of (1) receptor density or (2) configuration of the cell surface. This results in decreased communication or signaling between cells and enhancement of the immune defense against cancer (e.g., because altered glycoproteins and glycolipids can be antigens that allow the immune system to recognize cancer cells).[6,8]

Altered membrane transport or permeability
Cancer cells exhibit a greater metabolic demand for certain substrates, so it seems consistent that they would have enhanced transport. Among the most important cell surface changes is the loss of large glycoproteins called *fibronectin,* found in blood and on normal cell surfaces. Fibronectin holds cells in place in tissue, acting as an anchoring molecule, and may hold receptor molecules in certain arrangements. Fibronectin also contributes to the cell's internal organization (e.g., cytoskeleton) by interacting with the spanning actin filaments. Cancer cells may make defective fibronectin or break it down as it is made.[6] The low levels of fibronectin in cancer cells may cause changes in cellular organization, cell-to-cell adhesion, cellular migration, and cytoskeletal structure. It should be noted that plasma fibronectin levels rise in the blood of individuals with cancer.

Protease
Cancer cells secrete plasminogen-activating factor, which activates the inactive protease, plasminogen, into the active

TABLE 9-3   Nomenclature and Classification of Benign and Malignant Tumors*

Cell or Tissue of Origin	Benign Tumor	Malignant Tumor
Tumors of epithelial origin		
Squamous cells	Squamous cell papilloma	Squamous cell carcinoma
Basal cells	—	Basal cell carcinoma
Glandular or ductal epithelium	Adenoma	Adenocarcinoma
	Cystadenoma	Cystadenocarcinoma
Transitional cells	Transitional cell papilloma	Transitional cell carcinoma
Bile duct	Bile duct adenoma	Bile duct carcinoma (cholangiocarcinoma)
Liver cells	Hepatocellular adenoma	Hepatocellular carcinoma
Melanocytes	Nevus	Malignant melanoma
Renal epithelium	Renal tubular adenoma	Renal cell carcinoma
Skin adnexal glands		
Sweat glands	Sweat gland adenoma	Sweat gland carcinoma
Sebaceous glands	Sebaceous gland adenoma	Sebaceous gland carcinoma
Germ cells (testis and ovary)	—	Seminoma (dysgerminoma)
		Embryonal carcinoma, yolk sac carcinoma
Tumors of mesenchymal origin		
Hematopoietic/lymphoid tissue		
Leukocytes		Leukemias
Granular leukocytes and		Granulocytic leukemia
precursors		Myelocytic leukemias
		Myelogenous leukemias
Plasma cells		Multiple myeloma
Lymphoid		
Nongranular leukocytes and		Lymphomas
prelymphocytes		
Proliferating lymphocytes and		Lymphocytic leukemia
monocytes		
Proliferating immature		Lymphoblastic leukemia
precursor monocytes		
Solid tumors of lymph tissue		Lymphoma or lymphosarcoma
(thymus, spleen, lymph nodes)		
Neural and retinal tissue		
Nerve sheath	Neurilemoma, neurofibroma	Malignant peripheral nerve sheath tumor
Nerve cells	Ganglioneuroma	Neuroblastoma
Retinal cells (cones)	—	Retinoblastoma
Connective tissue		
Fibrous tissue	Fibromatosis (desmoid)	Fibrosarcoma
Fat	Lipoma	Liposarcoma
Bone	Osteoma	Osteogenic sarcoma
Cartilage	Chondroma	Chrondrosarcoma
Muscle		
Smooth muscle	Leiomyoma	Leiomyosarcoma
Striated muscle	Rhabdomyoma	Rhabdomyosarcoma
Endothelial and related tissues		
Blood vessels	Hemangioma	Angiosarcoma
		Kaposi sarcoma
Lymph vessels	Lymphangioma	Lymphangiosarcoma
Synovium	—	Synovial sarcoma
Mesathelium	—	Malignant mesothelioma
Meninges	Meningioma	Malignant meningioma
Tumors of uncertain origin		
????	—	Ewing tumor

Modified from Murphy GP et al. (1995). American Cancer Society's textbook of clinical oncology (2nd ed.). New York: American Cancer Society. Reprinted by permission of the American Cancer Society, Inc.
*This list is intended to provide only an introduction to tumor nomenclature.

Fig. 9-6 *Anchoring junctions.* Schematized drawing of anchoring junctions joining cytoskeletal filaments from cell to cell or from cell to extracellular matrix.

form, plasmin. Plasmin can degrade a variety of proteins. Plasminogen activator may play a role in the degradation of the extracellular matrix during tumor cell invasion. Protease secretion or activation may be needed before the expression or phenotype of the malignant cell can be changed.

Altered anchoring junctions and gap junctions

Anchoring junctions connect the cytoskeleton of a cell to its neighbor cell or to the extracellular matrix (a loose meshwork of large, extracellular organic molecules that bind cells together) (Fig. 9-6 and see Fig. 1-23). Normal cells presumably do not divide and proliferate unless they are anchored (see Fig. 9-6). In contrast, cancer cells exhibit **anchorage-independence.** Without anchorage, the transformed cell is allowed to **metastasize,** or grow in new environments. Tumor cells continue to divide when they are missing the necessary requirement for anchorage.

Gap junctions are actually narrow gaps or channels between adjacent cells, allowing inorganic ions and small water-soluble molecules to pass directly from the cytoplasm of one cell to the cytoplasm of the other (see Fig. 1-23). Gap junctions are important in regulating metabolic communication and cooperation among cells, so altered gap-junctional intercellular communication may play an essential role in cancer development.[9] Investigators have found that many tumor promoters, such as chemicals or growth factors, disrupt or block gap junction function.[10-13] Further, the more metastatic a tumor becomes, the greater the loss or decrease in intercellular communication.[14]

Tumor Cell Markers

Tumor cell markers are substances produced by cancer cells that are found on tumor plasma membranes or in the blood, spinal fluid, or urine (Table 9-4). Also called *biologic markers,* tumor cell markers have been associated with cancer for many decades. They include hormones, enzymes, genes, antigens, and antibodies. Tumor cell markers, which vary with the degree of tumor progression, are produced by the cancer cell's genetic material when it is activated during car-

cinogenesis. Tumor cell markers can be used in three ways: (1) to screen and identify individuals at high risk for cancer; (2) to help diagnose the specific type of tumor in individuals with clinical manifestations relating to cancer; and (3) to follow the clinical course of cancer.

A significant problem in diagnosing cancer from tumor marker assays is that many nonmalignant diseases are associated with tumor markers. The presence of a tumor marker may increase the suggestion of cancer, but it is not used alone as a diagnostic test. The need to identify ideal tumor markers remains a high priority because improvement in cancer therapy will depend on earlier detection and tumor identification.

Intracellular Changes in Cancer Cells
Cytoskeleton

The internal structures of the cell constitute the *cytoskeleton.* The cytoskeleton maintains the cell's shape and internal organization, permits the movement of substances within the cell, and permits movement of external projections (cilia or microvilli) from the plasma membrane. The internal skeleton is composed of a network of protein filaments, of which the most important are microtubules and actin filaments (microfilaments). Microfilaments and microtubules are not well organized in cancer cells or in normal cells during division.

In normal cells, bundles of actin filaments pull on the extracellular matrix at sites called *focal contacts,* or *adhesion plaques,* that bind to another cell.[1] In cancer cells, diminished adhesion to extracellular surfaces causes the cell to assume a rounded appearance.

Microtubules control cell shape, cell locomotion, and cellular division. While the cell is not dividing, only a few microtubules are assembled. During division (mitosis) or defense (phagocytosis), microtubules assemble and disassemble rapidly. Antimitotic drugs, such as vinblastine and vincristine, disrupt microtubular function preferentially, killing many rapidly dividing cells.

Cytoplasmic organelles and altered metabolism

The mitochondrial changes and the metabolism of glucose were among the first cellular systems investigated. Cancer cells engage in anaerobic glycolysis and rapid use of glucose even when oxygen is present. The increase in glycolysis most likely results from increased rates of cellular division. Any rapidly growing tissue requires more glucose. Many normal tissues, however, have glycolytic rates greater than those of tumors, and many neoplasms have been found to have normal glycolytic rates.[6]

Other metabolic observations include changes in enzymatic patterns and relationships between enzyme patterns and growth rates in cancer cells and normal cells.[15,16] Currently, however, there is no evidence of any unique metabolic change that accounts for differences between normal cells and cancer cells.

TABLE 9-4	Tumor Cell Markers
Marker	**Tumor**
Cytology	Aspirates, exudates, urine, brushings
Antigens	
Carcinoembryonic antigen	Many solid tumors
α-Fetoprotein	Liver, ovary, testis
Prostate-specific antigen	Prostate
Tumor-specific cell-mediated reactions	
Cytotoxicity tests	Many solid tumors
Delayed hypersensitivity reaction to tumor extracts	Many solid tumors
Ectopic hormones	
Human chorionic gonadotropin	Many tumors
Parathormone	Kidney, lung
Adrenocorticotropic hormone	Lung
Antidiuretic hormone	Lung
Melanin-stimulating hormone	Lung
Thyroid-stimulating hormone	Placenta (choriocarcinoma)
Insulin	Lung
Isoenzymes	
Acid phosphatase	Carcinoma of the prostate; breast cancer
Placental alkaline phosphatase	Choriocarcinoma; carcinomas of ovary, pancreas, colon, breast, uterus, bronchus; testicular cancers; reticulum cell sarcoma; Hodgkin disease; multiple myeloma
Nonplacental alkaline phosphatase	Osteogenic sarcoma; parathyroid carcinoma; cancers metastatic to bone from prostate, breast, multiple myeloma, infiltrative cancers of the liver, leukemia, reticulum cell sarcoma
Galactosyl transferase	Carcinomas of lung, breast, esophagus, stomach, pancreas, colon, gallbladder; chronic lymphocytic leukemia
Aminopeptidases	Carcinomas of pancreas, liver, stomach lining; carcinoma metastatic to liver
γ-Glutamyl transpeptidase	Carcinomas metastatic to liver
Ribonuclease	Carcinoma of pancreas
Sialyltransferase	Carcinoma of breast, colon, lung, prostate; leiomyosarcoma; leukemia; lymphoma; melanoma
Elevated normal substances	
Immunoglobulins	Multiple myeloma
Insulin	Islet cell tumors
Serotonin	Carcinoid tumors
Parathormone	Parathyroid tumors
Prolactin	Pituitary tumors
Gastrin	Islet cell tumors
Human chorionic gonadotropin	Choriocarcinoma
Calcium	Medullary carcinoma (thyroid), parathyroid tumors
Genes*	Various tumors

From King, D.W., Fenoglio, C.M., & Lefkowitch, J.H. (1984). General pathology: Principles and dynamics. Philadelphia: Lea & Febiger.
Additional markers include chromosomes and oncogenes (e.g., DNA-binding proteins c-myc, myb, fos).

Density-dependent inhibition of growth

In the laboratory, when two or more normal cells grown in a single-layer culture come in contact with each other, they tend to stop dividing (proliferating) and form a single layer or sheet of cells called a *confluent monolayer*. This phenomenon is known as **density-dependent inhibition of growth.** Cancer cells, however, usually continue to grow and pile up on top of one another after they have formed a confluent monolayer (Fig. 9-7).

Growth requirements: inducers of differentiation

The proliferation of cells is governed by specific combinations of protein growth factors (see Chapter 1). Growth factors act at very low concentrations, most as local chemical mediators—initiators and inhibitors—to help regulate cell population densities. Cancer may result when these factors become unbalanced or when cells cannot respond to growth-suppressor factors or perhaps are chronically stimu-

Density-dependent inhibition of growth in normal cells

Multilayer of uninhibited cancer cells

Growth   Culture
medium   dish

Fig. 9-7 *Cancer cell uninhibited growth.* Cancer cells, unlike most normal cells, usually continue to grow and pile up on top of one another after they have formed a confluent monolayer.

lated. Investigators suggest that whereas normal cells depend on other cells for growth inducers, either cancer cells need little or no growth inducers or they make their own.[17] Examples of growth factors and their physiologic actions are presented in Table 1-5.

Autocrine stimulation hypothesis

Transformed cells become independent of growth factors by producing their own growth factors by *autocrine secretion.*

(Chemical signaling is discussed in Chapter 1.) Malignant and transformed cells have surface receptors for growth factors and can release growth factors. This discovery led to the hypothesis of ***autostimulation,*** or the ***autocrine stimulatory hypothesis,*** of cancer. Several mechanisms are proposed by which transformed and malignant cells become *autonomous* with respect to growth factors, including (1) manufacture by transformed cells of their own growth factors; (2) reduction in the amount of growth factor necessary for division; (3) defects of the growth factor receptor on the plasma membrane; and (4) alteration of the receptor signal pathway for second messengers.[18] Chapter 1 describes how growth factor binding to membrane receptors initiates a cascade of metabolic events leading to cell division.

All this evidence suggests that the normal processes of cell division and cell differentiation are driven and guided by growth factors and that the cancer cell produces its own. Growth factors are produced by a highly organized sequence of gene activation and gene suppression. Unraveling these complex genetic sequences may lead to enormous breakthroughs in cancer therapy.

Transformed cells commonly exhibit complex abnormalities. These abnormalities and their functional significance are summarized in Tables 9-5 and 9-6.

Changes in the nucleus and cell protein

The nuclei of malignant cells are often *pleomorphic,* that is, enlarged and variably shaped. Chromatin may clump along the periphery of the nucleus. Nuclear membrane alterations include projections, pockets, blebbing, and fewer nuclear pores, which are associated with DNA replication sites. The rate of mitosis frequently is increased in cancerous tissues. Changes in chromosomes include breaks, deletions, ring

TABLE 9-5	Comparison of Normal and Tumor Cells: Cellular Changes Commonly Observed		
Growth Characteristics		**Normal Cells**	**Neoplastic Cells**
Density-dependent inhibition of growth		Present	Absent
Growth-factor requirements		High	Low
Anchorage dependence		Present	Absent
Proliferative life span		Finite	Indefinite
Adhesiveness		High	Low
Morphology		Flat	Rounded; various shapes; abnormal change
Fibronectin		Present	Reduced
Plasminogen activator		Present	Increased

TABLE 9-6	Functional Significance of Cellular Changes in Tumor Cells	
Change		**Functional Significance**
Decreased adhesion		Decreased cell-to-cell adherence, therefore maintenance of a
Disorganized actin filaments (cytoskeleton)		rounded morphology; increased plasminogen activation, therefore increased extracellular proteolysis
Reduced fibronectin		
Increased production of plasminogen activator		
Indefinite proliferative life span		Abnormalities of growth and mitotic division; increased potential
Lowered requirement for growth factors		for invasion and metastasis
Less anchorage dependence		
Density-dependent inhibition of growth		

forms, and abnormal chromosome karyotypes. For example, frequent changes are reported in chromosomes 1 and 17 in a number of hematologic cancers. A change in chromosome 22 (the Philadelphia chromosome), whereby the long arm is translocated to chromosome 9, is well known in chronic myelocytic leukemia (see Chapter 20).

Other genetic changes are phenotypic, or "translated and transcribed" into protein. Transfer ribonucleic acid (RNA), for example, may have too few or too many methyl groups (CH_3) attached. Proteins that regulate genes and enzymes involved in nucleic acid synthesis may exhibit phenotypic changes, all of which are potential expressions of the malignant state. Pathologists rely on phenotypic changes, along with functional and growth-requirement changes, to identify the transformed state and diagnose cancer. The evidence is strong that phenotypic and other changes result from a defect in the genetic information of the cell.

✓ QUICK CHECK

Why do mutations in social control genes cause cancer?

Why is the concept of differentiation important to cancer?

Why do autonomy and anaplasia increase the chances of cancer development?

Why are tumor cell markers important?

CAUSES OF CANCER
Genetics and Cancer Families

Genetic events are the primary basis of carcinogenesis. Most of the genetic alterations that cause cancer occur during the lifetime of the individual, in their somatic tissues. The frequency of these events can be altered by exposure to **mutagens,** that is, agents causing mutations. Thus mutagens establish the link to environmental carcinogens. Because these genetic events occur in somatic cells as opposed to germ cells, they *are not* transmitted to future generations. Even

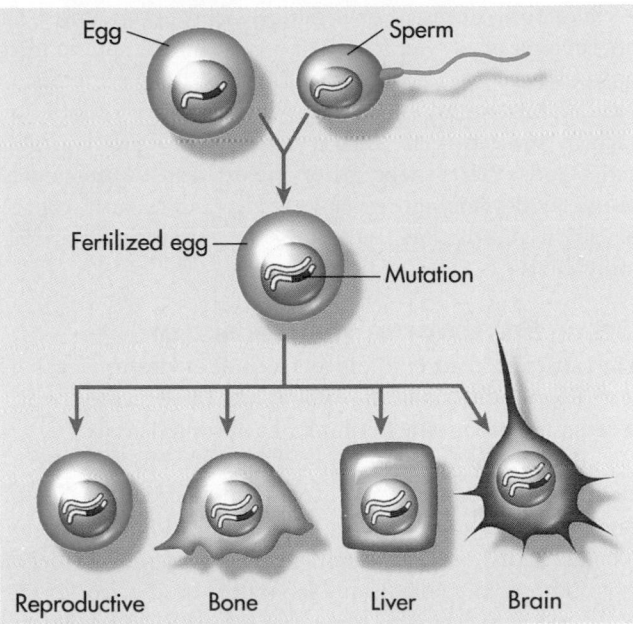

Fig. 9-8 *Germline mutation.* Inherited mutations are carried in the DNA of reproductive cells. When reproductive cells containing mutations combine to produce offspring, the mutation will be present in *all* the offspring's body cells. *(Modified from Lea, D.H., Jenkins, J.F., & Francomano, C.A. (1998).* Genetics in clinical practice. *Boston: Bartlett.)*

though they are *genetic* events, they are not *inherited!* It is possible, however, for cancer-predisposing mutations to occur in germline cells (cells that produce gametes) (Fig. 9-8).[19] Mutations in germline cells result in the vertical transmission of cancer-causing genes from one generation to the next, producing families with a high incidence of specific cancers.

Although rare, such "cancer families" demonstrate that inheritance of a mutated gene can cause cancer (Fig. 9-9). In these families, inheritance of one mutant allele seems sufficient to cause a specific form of cancer: almost all individuals who inherit the germline mutant allele will develop the tumor.[19] Examples of inherited human cancers are retinoblastoma, a childhood cancer of the eye; Wilms tumor,

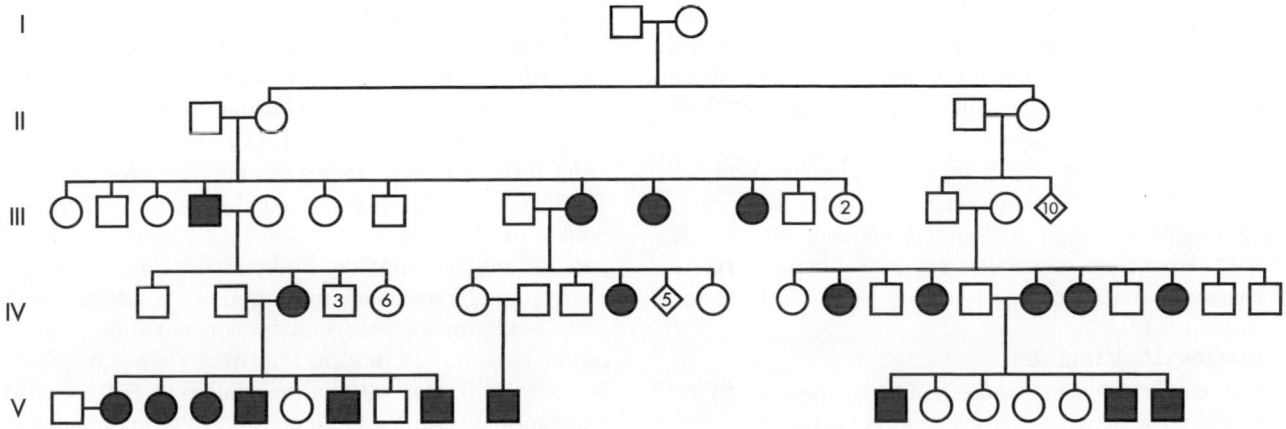

Fig. 9-9 *A familial colon cancer pedigree.* Darkened symbols represent individuals diagnosed with cancer. *(From Jorde, L.B. et al. [1999].* Medical genetics *[2nd ed.]. St. Louis: Mosby.)*

a childhood cancer of the kidney; neurofibromatosis; fibrosarcoma of nerves; inherited breast cancer; and familial polyposis coli, or adenomas of the colon. A specific oncogene and/or tumor suppressor gene has been isolated for each of these cancers. Characterization of cancer-causing genes and other genetic factors helps identify individuals prone to developing cancer (see Fig. 2-28). Early cancer detection and therapy result in better prognosis for at-risk individuals.

Gene-Environment Interaction

The causes of "common" cancers include environmental factors. Reportedly, environmental agents cause cancer by increasing the frequency of mutations in somatic cells.[20,21]

Two lines of evidence support the idea that exposure to environmental agents can increase an individual's risk of cancer. The first is based on the identification of environmental agents that have carcinogenic properties.[20] Evidence from both epidemiologic and laboratory studies, for example, shows that cigarette smoke causes lung cancer. Environmental agents, such as chemical carcinogens, x-rays, and ultraviolet radiation, can cause certain types of cancer.

The second line of evidence is based on comparisons of populations of different life-styles. Breast cancer, for example, is prevalent among northern Europeans and Americans, but it is relatively rare among women in developing countries. The difficulty lies in determining whether these differences between populations are attributable to life-style factors, to genetics, or to both. The influence of environmental agents was demonstrated in studies of Japanese who immigrated to Hawaii and the U.S. mainland. Researchers studied the changes in incidence of colon and stomach cancer after emigration. In Japan, colon cancer is a rare form of cancer. Among the first Japanese immigrants (first generation) in Hawaii, colon cancer incidence rose several-fold but not as high as overall incidence on the U.S. mainland. Among second-generation Japanese on the U.S. mainland, colon cancer rates rose to the U.S. average. Conversely, stomach cancer is common in Japan but relatively rare in the United States. Japanese on the U.S. mainland have the same low incidence of stomach cancer as the U.S. average. Although these observations implicate environment and life-style in the cause of colon and stomach cancer, they do not rule out genetic factors. The difference in incidence rates could be the result of predisposing genes. One could argue that these genes are less penetrating for colon cancer in Japan because of environmental differences.[19-21]

Environmental factors play important roles in cancer development. Because some individuals within the same environment develop cancer and others do not, cancer risk seems to depend on interaction between inherited factors and environmental agents.

Oncogenic Viruses

Viruses were first isolated from certain types of tumors in the early 1900s. These viruses caused cancers when transferred into normal healthy animals. A number of *oncogenic viruses* (cancer-causing viruses) have been isolated, including several that cause human cancers. These oncogenic viruses are true pathogenic agents because they cause a specific type of malignant or benign tumor in susceptible individuals. From a genetic standpoint, these viruses represent an exogenous source of oncogenes. Cells infected by these viruses are transformed when the viral oncogene is activated.

Classification of oncogenic viruses

Oncogenic viruses are divided into two major groups, according to the nucleic acid content (DNA or RNA) of the viral particle (Table 9-7). The three main types of oncogenic DNA viruses are papovaviruses, adenoviruses, and herpesviruses. DNA viruses penetrate host cells by the action of their coat proteins. Inside the cell the viral DNA is uncoated and enters the cell's nucleus, where it is inserted (integrated) into the host's DNA. The integrated viral DNA then is transcribed to mRNA (see Chapter 7).

Oncogenic DNA viruses cause tumors in various tissues of different animals. Hepatitis B virus, Epstein-Barr virus, and human papillomavirus (HPV) are associated with about 15% of all human cancers worldwide.[22] Cancer of the cervix and hepatocellular carcinoma account for about 80% of virus-linked cancer. Hepatitis B virus infection is considered a high-risk factor for hepatocellular carcinoma. In immune-suppressed individuals, Epstein-Barr virus is the causative agent of Burkitt lymphoma, nasopharyngeal cancer, and B cell lymphoma. Sixty different substrains of HPV have been isolated from benign and malignant human tumors. Certain strains of HPV cause warts, or benign tumors of the skin, anus, and genitalia. Other strains of HPV cause anogenital carcinoma, oral carcinoma, laryngeal carcinoma, nasal and paranasal carcinomas, and conjunctival carcinoma. Except in individuals with the rare disease epidermodysplasia verruciformis, evidence is lacking that HPVs play a role in the induction of either squamous cell carcinoma or melanoma of the skin.[23]

Oncogenic RNA viruses are termed *retroviruses* because they contain a certain unique enzyme, *reverse transcriptase*. This enzyme is required for successful infection by the virus. Before viral replication can occur in the host cell, the viral genome must be transcribed from viral RNA to viral DNA by the reverse transcriptase enzyme (Fig. 9-10). Once the viral genome has been transcribed to viral DNA, it can be integrated into the host's DNA, where it is transcribed and replicated by the host's genetic machinery. Human T cell leukemia-lymphoma virus (HTLV) is an oncogenic retrovirus. It is critical for development and progression of adult T cell leukemia-lymphoma (ATLL). HTLV is transmitted both vertically, that is, inherited by children from infected parents, and horizontally, by breast-feeding, sexual intercourse, blood transfusions, and exposure to infected needles.

Infection by an oncogenic virus is not enough to cause cancer. For example, in some industrialized regions, Epstein-Barr virus can infect 90% of the adolescent and young adult population, yet only a small percentage of these individuals develop cancer. Long latency periods, often lasting decades,

1 Oncogenic retrovirus

2 Absorption—virus binds to cell surface

3 Penetration—virus enters cytoplasm

4 Eclipse—viral RNA freed from core (uncoat)

5 Reverse transcriptase—viral RNA to viral DNA

6 Viral DNA incorporated into host DNA

7 Transcription of host DNA—virus replication
   a. Transcribed *v-onc* causes transformation
   b. Viral mRNA released to cytoplasm: core protein translated on free polysomes and coat proteins processed on rough endoplasmic reticulum and Golgi apparatus

8 Maturation—core and capsid are assembled in cytoplasm

9 Coat proteins are inserted into plasma membrane

10 Release—virus cores bind to coat proteins and "bud" from cell surface

11 Infectious virus particles

Fig. 9-10 *Stages of oncogenic RNA viral infection.* *ER,* Endoplasmic reticulum; *mRNA,* messenger ribonucleic acid; *DNA,* deoxyribonucleic acid.

the low number of infected individuals that eventually develop cancer, monoclonality of the tumors, and in some cases exposure to other carcinogenic or promoting agents before the appearance of cancer suggest that additional modifications are required to cause a virally infected cell to develop a malignant phenotype.

Oncogenes

In addition to the genes required by the virus to maintain its integrity as an infectious agent (i.e., virus core proteins, envelope glycoproteins, or reverse transcriptase), the oncogenic virus also possesses specific oncogenes, termed **v-onc** (identifying them as viral oncogenes). Cellular oncogenes, **c-onc,** are incorporated into the genomes of various organisms, including humans. Because normal, nontransformed cells carry *c-onc,* conclusions have been drawn concerning the origin

and function of these genes. The term *proto-oncogene* sometimes is used to refer collectively to the various *c-onc.*

First, the existence of *c-onc* throughout evolution in various unrelated animal species suggests they play an important role in the normal function of the cell. This terminology also indicates *c-onc* and *v-onc* genes are likely derived from a common prototype gene. Proto-oncogenes encode for growth factors, growth-factor receptors, signal transducers, nuclear proteins, and tumor suppressor proteins. Therefore **proto-oncogenes** both are normal genetic components of the cell and encode for viral products or activities required for cell growth and differentiation. Many viral oncogenes may originate from normal cellular DNA sequences.

Second, some viruses, especially the retroviruses, can incorporate infected host cell genes into their viral genome during their replication process. This explains how onco-

TABLE 9-7	Classification and Examples of Oncogenic Viruses	
Viral Class	**Virus**	**Species of Isolation**
Oncogenic DNA viruses		
Papovaviruses	Papilloma	Rabbit, human, others
	Polyoma	Mouse
	SV 40	Monkey
Adenoviruses*	Adenovirus 12	Human
Herpesviruses	Epstein-Barr	Human
	Frog herpesvirus	Frog
	Marek disease	Chicken
Oncogenic RNA viruses†		
Acute-acting type	Rous sarcoma	Chicken
	Maloney sarcoma	Mouse
	Harvey/Kirsten sarcoma	Rat
Subacute type	Avian leukosis	Chicken
	Mouse mammary tumor	Mouse
	Bovine leukemia	Cow
	Human T leukemia/lymphoma virus	Human

Modified from Ruddon, R. (1981). Cancer biology. New York: Oxford University Press.
There are 31 types of adenoviruses that have been isolated from humans; three of these (types 12, 18, and 31) are highly oncogenic when inoculated into newborn rodents.
†*The oncogenic RNA viruses are divided into two classes: the acute-acting types transform cells in vitro, induce rapid disease in vivo, and carry oncogenes in their genome; the subacute types do not cause cell transformation in vitro, have long latency periods for disease induction in vivo, do not possess oncogenes, and appear to be horizontally transmitted.*

genic viruses obtain their proto-oncogenes. Although this suggests the origin of *v-onc,* it does not explain how these viruses transform cells into cancers.

A tremendous amount of research has been directed toward understanding the mechanism or mechanisms by which oncogenic viruses are able to cause cell transformation. This has led to the development of the oncogene hypothesis. This hypothesis states that virtually all cells possess oncogenes. Because these *c-onc* are similar to the v-*onc* carried by oncogenic viruses, their activation during viral infections leads to transformation of the cell, which can result in neoplastic cells that are able to form benign or malignant tumors. How oncogenes are activated in normal cells and their role in maintaining the transformed cell phenotype are unknown.

Mechanisms of viral carcinogenesis

Several mechanisms for viral carcinogenesis are proposed. It should be appreciated, however, that cancer is a complex disease process that can involve many factors. As with other diseases, the pathogenic agents may have either (1) a direct effect, in which the tumor cells are or were at some stage infected with the oncogenic virus; or (2) an indirect effect, in which the neoplastic cells were not altered by the virus but were stimulated to grow because of the viral infection.

Direct mechanisms

During the infection process, the virus may cause mutations in surviving cells that could lead to neoplastic changes. This process may not cause cellular transformation, although viral genes may persist within the noninfected tumor cells. Interestingly, viral genes appear to be incorporated into the host genome randomly, suggesting that the viral genes do not cause transformation directly.

Most oncogenic viruses seem to cause transformation by **insertional mutagenesis.** In this process, the viral genes are incorporated into the host's genome at specific sites. Insertion of the *v-onc* within the host genome can lead to activation of the *v-onc* or *c-onc* genes associated with cell transformation. These inserted genes become an inherited trait of all the cancer cells derived from the original transformed cell.

Indirect mechanisms

Because viral infections lead to tissue damage, there is a burst of cell proliferation in the damaged tissue after the infection subsides that is associated with the normal repair and healing processes. Actively dividing cells are known to be at higher risk of mutation than resting cells. As a result, these cells are more susceptible to both spontaneous mutagenesis and transformation by a physical or chemical carcinogen. Alternatively, during some viral infections, the host's immune system can become compromised. This reduced immunologic protection can allow neoplastic cells to emerge that normally would be rejected by the host. The role of the immune system in cancer is discussed in more detail on p. 259. In conclusion, viral infections may affect carcinogenesis by increasing the individual's risk for neoplasia induced by other means.

Tumor suppressor genes

By definition, oncogenes encode for proteins that cause cancer. Because most of the oncogene-derived proteins are cell growth and differentiation factors, it is thought that their unregulated overexpression plays a role in cell transformation. Thus an imbalance in positive growth signals received by the cell causes it to assume the transformed phenotype. Proliferation of normal cells may be regulated by growth-promoting oncogenes counterbalanced by growth-constraining tumor suppressor genes.[24]

Tumor suppressor genes encode for proteins that act as negative transducers of growth-factor stimulation. The negative growth signals produced by tumor suppressor gene proteins block specific phases of the cell cycle, induce end-stage differentiation, and stimulate cell senescence or death. Carcinogenesis involves *inactivation* of tumor suppressor genes and activation of oncogenes. Examples of suppressor genes are the deleted in colon cancer *(DCC)* gene, the neurofibromatosis *(NF1)* gene, the retinoblastoma *(rb)* gene, the *p53* gene, the Wilms tumor *(WT1)* gene, *BRCA1* in breast cancer, and the multiple tumor suppressor 1 *(MTS1)* gene.[25] Future therapeutic strategies based on genetic alterations in cancer include reintroduction of tumor suppressor function to cells lacking the gene. For example, the *p53* gene is normally a molecular "police officer" that prevents proliferation of genetically damaged cells. The *p53* gene binds to DNA and causes cells to arrest in the G_1 phase of the cell cycle (see Chapter 1). With loss of this guardian, cells exposed to mutagenic agents replicate the damaged DNA, possibly leading to malignant transformation.

Several tumor suppressor genes are involved in inherited human cancers, for example, *rb* in retinoblastoma, *NF1* in neurofibromatosis, and *WT1* in Wilms tumor. These inherited genes are mutant forms of normal cell growth-regulating genes. These mutated genes encode for defective regulatory proteins that allow cell transformation. Thus individuals inheriting these genes are prone to develop cancer, having lost normal cell growth and differentiation controls.

CARCINOGENESIS

Our understanding of the process of tumor development, *carcinogenesis,* is very limited. Within the past 2½ decades, several theories have greatly influenced our view of the carcinogenic process. These theories or proposed mechanisms of carcinogenesis suggest that the formation of a cancerous tumor is not a "one-hit" event. Instead, *all* evidence supports, overwhelmingly, that there is an evolution of phenotypic and, hence, presumably genotoxic (DNA toxic) changes from the normal cell to the invasive, metastasizing cell.

The multistep process of cancer seems to involve the loss of the ability for the cell to terminally differentiate (see p. 236) and to control growth. In addition, the process includes traveling to distant tissues and invading and colonizing these tissues. The tumor, once formed, appears to be derived from a single "outlaw" stem cell.

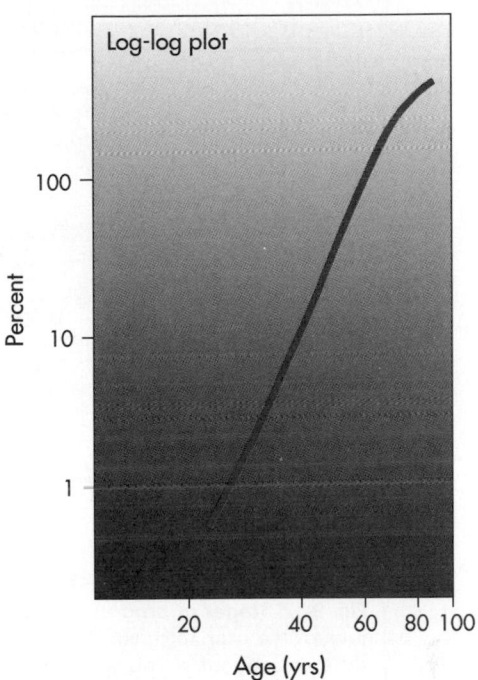

Fig. 9-11 *Incidence of cancer rises steeply as a function of age.* A cell must accumulate the abnormal effects of several independent accidents before it will give rise to a tumor. *(Modified from Alberts, B. et al. [1994]. Molecular biology of the cell [3rd ed.]. New York: Garland.)*

Monoclonal Origin

Where evidence is available, it usually confirms that the cancer arose from a single "outlaw" cell (monoclonal origin). For example, the leukemic white blood cells of individuals with chronic myelogenous leukemia are distinguished from normal cells by a specific chromosomal abnormality (Philadelphia chromosome) (see p. 549). It is doubtful that the genetic mistake responsible for this abnormality would have occurred in several cells at once in the same individual. It is more likely that all the leukemic cells are descendants of the same mutant cell.

Cell Accidents: A Requisite for Cancer Development

Many lines of evidence indicate that tumor development requires several *independent* rare accidents to occur together in one cell. The evidence involves the relationship of tumor development to age. If a single mutation were responsible, the chance of developing cancer in any given year would be independent of age. For most types of cancer, however, the chance increases with age at a rapid rate (Fig. 9-11). Theoretically, several independent random events are required to alter a normal cell into a cancer cell; the smaller numbers of random events apply to leukemias, the larger to carcinomas.[1]

The Slow Stages of Cancer Development

Tumor development almost always involves a long delay between the initial causal event and the onset of the disease; for

A   **B**   **C**   **D**

Mitosis   Basal lamina

Normal epithelium   Dysplasia   Preinvasive carcinoma (carcinoma in situ)   Invasive malignant carcinoma

Fig. 9-12 *Stages of progression.* Stages of progression of development of cancer of the epithelium of the uterine cervix. **A,** Normal. **B,** In dysplasia, the most superficial cells still show signs of differentiation, but this is incomplete and proliferating cells are seen far above the basal layer. **C,** In carcinoma in situ, the cells in all the layers are proliferating and apparently undifferentiated. **D,** Malignancy begins when the cells cross the basal lamina and begin to invade the underlying connective tissue. Several years may elapse from the first signs of dysplasia to the onset of full-blown malignant cancer. *(Modified from Alberts, B. et al. [1994]. Molecular biology of the cell [3rd ed.]. New York: Garland.)*

example, the incidence of lung cancer rises steeply after 10 to 20 years of heavy smoking. During this latent period, the cancer cells undergo multiple and successive changes. It appears for most cancers as though cells of the initial mutant clone undergo further mutation that enables them to divide more rapidly before they terminally differentiate, that is, come to the end of a pathway of specialization (see Figs. 9-3 and 9-4). Because of the rapid division and therefore proliferation of cells, cancer cells begin to outnumber normal cells, as well as those with the primary mutation.

Cancers of the uterine cavity provide a clear example of the early steps in the development of a tumor. These cancers originate from the multilayered cervical epithelium, which is similar to the epidermis of the skin. Normally, proliferation occurs only in the basal and parabasal layers, and the differentiating cells travel outward from their site of origin. It seems logical that among these basal cells is at least one cell whose line of descendants will not die out in one lifetime—an *immortal stem cell.* Cells moving out toward the surface differentiate into flattened, keratin-rich, nondividing cells as they go and, finally, are sloughed off from the surface (Fig. 9-12, *A*). Examination of Papanicolaou (Pap) specimens from different women shows patches of *dysplasia,* where dividing cells are no longer confined to the basal layer and there is disorder in the process of differentiation (Fig. 9-12, *B*). These cells, obtained by a Pap smear, can be viewed under the microscope. If these cells are allowed to progress over a period of years, they give rise to *carcinoma in situ* (Fig. 9-12, *C*). In carcinoma in situ, the cells in all the layers are proliferating and apparently undifferentiated. However, the ab-

normal cells are still confined to the epithelial side of the basal lamina and are highly variable in size and karyotype. Without treatment, the carcinoma in situ cells may remain harmless or over a period of several years give rise to a malignant clinical carcinoma whose cells cross the basal lamina (see Fig. 9-12, *C*) and begin to invade the underlying connective tissue (Fig. 9-12, *D*).

Oncogenes and Tumor Suppressor Genes

Proto-oncogenes are known to represent an array of cell growth and differentiation regulatory genes. Oncogenes generally are considered to encode for factors that stimulate cell growth. In contrast, tumor- suppressor genes encode for proteins that counteract cell growth signals. Mutations or gene activation of growth-promoting oncogenes and inactivation of tumor suppressor genes can lead to transformation. Because transformation involves complex processes, it is not surprising that cancers express multiple oncogenes and tumor suppressor genes. Further, synergy between specific oncogenes is required for tumor induction.[26] All this suggests that as transformed cells grow and metastasize, different growth and regulatory pathways are activated, as represented by oncogenes and tumor suppressor genes.

Other genetic abnormalities occur in many cancers, including deletions, translocations, and inversions of genes, as well as terminal deletions, monosomy, and trisomy of specific chromosomes. Because these chromosome abnormalities are consistent for certain types of cancer, it is believed they are involved in the carcinogenesis process.[27]

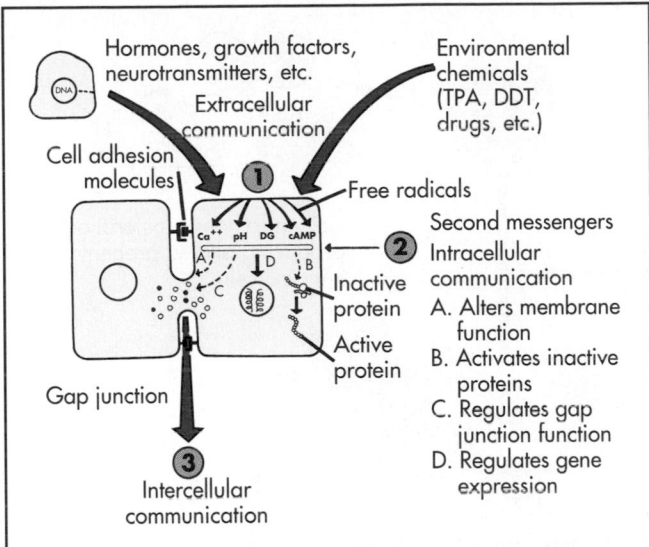

Fig. 9-13 *Cellular communication.* Proposed link between extracellular and intracellular communication. Schema shows the proposed link between extracellular communication and intercellular communication through various intracellular signaling mechanisms (e.g., transmembrane). It provides a holistic view (mind/body connection) of how the neuroendocrine immune system and other coordinations could occur. Although not shown here, activation or altered expression of various oncogenes and tumor suppressor genes could contribute to the regulation of gap junction function. *DNA,* Deoxyribonucleic acid; *TPA,* tissue plasminogen activator; *DDT,* dichlorodiphenyl trichlorethane; *DG,* diocyl glyceride; *cAMP,* cyclic adenosine monophosphate.

Stem Cell or Blocked Differentiation

The concept of cancer as a stem cell disease or a disease of differentiation was derived from several observations: (1) the stem cell and the cancer cell both proliferate extensively; (2) cancer cells and stem cells both appear to self-renew or self-generate (see Fig. 9-4); (3) both types of cells act similarly with radiation therapy; and (4) terminal differentiation can be experimentally (in vitro) induced for both types of cells with natural differentiation factors (see p. 236).

Differentiation depends on the natural functioning of the stem cell progeny (see Fig. 9-4). A transformed stem cell causes cell production and cell destruction to be unbalanced in a normal tissue (see Fig. 9-5). Cancer as a disease of abnormal differentiation is discussed on p. 236.

Intercellular Communication

All cells that are part of a multicellular organism are able to "talk to" or influence each other (see Chapter 1). Delicate integration of three major types of communication is required: *extracellular, intracellular,* and *intercellular* (Fig. 9-13). Extracellular communication involves signals from different molecules or ligands, such as neurotransmitters, chemicals, and hormones. These signals are received by specific cell receptors or directly taken into the cell through coated pits and carrier proteins. Intracellular communication occurs when second messengers are activated inside the cell membrane. Intercellular communication involves ions

and other small molecules that communicate directly with neighboring cells through gap junctions (see Chapter 1, Fig. 1-23, and Fig. 9-14). Normal tissue growth and differentiation depend on cellular feedback mechanisms that take place through intercellular communication. These three types of cell communication are closely related and are capable of controlling cellular function.

Investigators propose that gap junction intercellular communication is either blocked or down-regulated in transforming cancer cells and therefore communication between the transformed cells and normal surrounding cells is lost.[28,29] Investigators have reported that gap junctions can be down-regulated or blocked by many tumor promoters, such as chemicals or growth hormones.

Oncogenes produce abnormal proteins that can take the place of normal hormones, chemicals, or receptors.[9] These oncogene proteins can block normal up- and down-regulation of intercellular communication and gap junction function and therefore stimulate tumor cell growth.[9]

Further research is needed on the relationship between intercellular communication and carcinogenesis. Studies show that intercellular communication between transformed cells and normal cells is decreased or blocked and that transformed cells communicate with each other. The exact mechanisms are still unclear, however, and are being investigated.

Initiation-Promotion-Progression Theory of Carcinogenesis

In 1941 Rous and Kidd hypothesized a two-stage mechanism for the development of cancer, involving first an initiation stage (transformation) induced by a mutagen followed by a promotion stage mediated by another agent.[30] The third stage, progression, was added later (see p. 250) (Fig. 9-14). In the late 1940s, Berenblum and Shubik devised a series of experiments that demonstrated the two-stage mechanism for skin cancer (Fig. 9-15). The initiating agent was methylcholanthrene, and the promoting agent was croton oil. Neither agent alone would cause carcinogenesis (i.e., the cancer-causing process required both agents). When two such agents are required to initiate and promote carcinogenesis, they are called **cocarcinogens.**

Initiation or DNA damage (mutation) is the irreversible developmental stage of the cancer precursor cell after exposure to the carcinogen. The initiated cell may not be considered cancerous, however, until a promoting agent acts to produce an altered, autonomous phenotype. **Promotion** appears to involve cell proliferation and tumor development, thus accelerating the process by which the initiated cells become cancerous. Initiation and promotion mechanisms have not been shown to apply to all cancers, but the process has been applied to chemical agents, such as benzo[*a*]pyrene found in coal tar or cigarette smoke. Other carcinogens are part of the physical environment (e.g., ionizing and nonionizing radiation) or are biologic agents (e.g., viruses or hormones).

Initiators cause alterations in the DNA. These changes can include one or more complete interruptions of the DNA chain, errors in DNA repair, or an elimination of a base pair

Fig. 9-14 *Multistage theory.* Tumor development according to the multistage theory: initiation, promotion, progression. *DNA,* Deoxyribonucleic acid.

(pyrimidine or purine) or sugar. Promoters may affect cell proliferation by altering cell-to-cell communication or by producing oxygen radicals.[9,31] Promoters include hormones, drugs, chemicals, plant products, and other environmental factors. These factors induce initiated cells to divide within a tissue. Several agents induce cell division, but only promoters induce tumor development. Promoting agents may interfere with differentiation, usually after division has occurred. In the early stages of epidermal carcinogenesis, the biologic effects of promotion are reversible and are modified by diet, hormones, and related factors. Table 9-8 compares initiation and promotion substances.

Boutwell suggested that tumor *progression* may be a late phase of promotion.[32] The biologic difference between promotion and progression is unknown, but progression may depend on structural changes in the chromosome and promotion may not cause chromosome abnormalities. Thus progression is considered a stage of biological worsening.

Environmental risk factors

The past 2 decades have led to a greater understanding of the genetic basis of neoplastic development. At the level of the cell, cancer is genetic. The frequency and consequences of these mutations can be altered by a large number of environmental factors. In experimental animals, many agents cause cancer; thus they are called ***carcinogens.*** Neither genetics nor environment is the sole determinant of carcinogenesis—they both play key roles.

Table 9-9 summarizes the estimated new cases and deaths caused by cancer, by gender, for specified sites. Although population trends in incidence rates of cancer are the focus of epidemiologists, laboratory scientists use experimental approaches to determine the effect and nature of environmental factors as initiators or promoters of carcinogenesis. To identify an agent as an initiator, laboratory scientists must demonstrate that altered DNA changes occur in response to variable doses of that agent—a difficult task at best. Thus the relationship between life-style and carcinogenesis of a given human population can be explored and evaluated from two divergent but equally important approaches: epidemiologic and experimental. Each approach has strengths and weaknesses and requires cautious interpretations. These two perspectives, however, do indicate some agreement about particular agents or conditions that either *cause* cancer (i.e., genetic disposition) or are *associated* with increased cancer incidence rates.

Fig. 9-15 *Initiation and promotion.* Procedure demonstrating initiation and promotion of tumors.

TABLE 9-8	Initiation and Promotion Substances
Initiators	**Promoters**
Single exposure to alter cell	Contact after initiator and requires prolonged exposure
Irreversible process	Reversible during early stage
Metabolically converted to reactants that bind covalently to DNA	Neither metabolic conversion nor covalent binding necessary
High doses carcinogenic	Only weakly carcinogenic without prior treatment of initiator

Personal behaviors

Tobacco use. Both epidemiologic and experimental data support the conclusion that cigarette smoke is carcinogenic and remains the most important cause of cancer. In the United States, smoking kills more than 430,000 people each year and is estimated to contribute to 30.5% of all cancer-related deaths.[33] In developed countries as a whole, tobacco is responsible for 24% of all male deaths and 7% of female deaths; these figures rise to more than 40% in men in some countries of central and eastern Europe and to 17% in women in the United States.[34] Worldwide, smoking is killing 3 million people each year and the figure is increasing. It is estimated that by the time the young smokers of today reach middle or old age, there will be about 10 million deaths/yr from tobacco.[34]

The prevalence of cigarette smoking is higher among blacks than among whites. Blacks have higher rates of lung cancer than whites. A preference for mentholated cigarettes by blacks is well documented and is being investigated as an explanation for the black-white differences in rates of cancers of the lung and upper respiratory and digestive tracts.[35]

By late middle age, cancer of the lung is more than 10 times greater in cigarette smokers than in lifelong nonsmokers. In addition, cigarette smoking increases the incidence of cancer of the bladder, pancreas, kidney, larynx, oral cavity, esophagus,[36,37] and certain blood cells (especially acute myeloid leukemia).[34] Cigarette smoking is a direct cause of ischemic heart disease, respiratory heart disease, aortic aneurysm, chronic obstructive lung disease, stroke, pneumonia, cirrhosis, and cancer of the liver.[34] These correlations are not surprising, considering the chemical composition of cigarette smoke. These chemicals possess mutagenic capabilities, are absorbed from the lungs into the blood, through their distribution by the circulation gain access to distant organs, and are present in increased concentration in the urine of smokers.

The harmful effects of cigarette smoke are worse than those of pipe or cigar smoke. This difference may be attributable to the increased alkalinity of pipe and cigar smoke, which may decrease nicotine absorption rates in the blood. Alkaline smoke is also more irritating than cigarette smoke and is therefore less readily inhaled into the lungs. The greatest risk among the numerous causes of cancer of the lung is related to the inhalation of tobacco smoke. Low-tar cigarettes do not reduce the risk of lung cancer.

There are hazards for nonsmokers who breathe the smoke of others' cigarettes (passive smoking or environmental tobacco smoke [ETS]). Passive smoking is associated with a modestly increased risk of lung cancers and possibly other cancers.[37,38]

The use of forms of smokeless tobacco (plug, leaf, snuff) has increased. "Dipping snuff" (in which a coarse, moist powder is placed between the cheek and gum and nicotine and other carcinogens are directly absorbed through the oral tissue) has caused the greatest concern. Oral cancer occurs more frequently among snuff dippers (as well as pipe and cigar smokers) compared with persons who are not tobacco users.[37]

Diet. Perhaps no other area of cancer investigation has proven more difficult than identifying the carcinogenic nature of dietary practices. Reliable information is increasing,

TABLE 9-9   Estimated New Cancer Cases and Deaths by Gender for Specified Sites, 1999

Types of Cancer	Estimated New Cases			Estimated Deaths		
	Total	Male	Female	Total	Male	Female
Oral cavity and pharynx	29,800	20,000	9,800	8,100	5,400	2,700
Esophagus	12,500	9,400	3,100	12,200	9,400	2,800
Stomach	21,900	13,700	8,200	13,500	7,900	5,600
Pancreas	28,600	14,000	14,600	28,600	13,900	14,700
Colon (large intestine)	94,700	43,000	51,700	47,900	23,000	24,900
Rectum	34,700	19,400	15,300	8,700	4,800	3,900
Lung and bronchus	171,600	94,000	77,600	158,900	90,900	68,000
Bones and joints	2,600	1,400	1,200	1,400	800	600
Skin (melanoma)	44,200	25,800	18,400	7,300	4,600	2,700
Breast	176,300	1,300	175,000	43,700	400	43,300
Cervix	12,800	—	12,800	4,800	—	4,800
Corpus, endometrium	37,400	—	37,400	6,400	—	6,400
Ovary	25,200	—	25,200	14,500	—	14,500
Prostate	179,300	179,300	—	37,000	37,000	—
Testis	7,400	7,400	—	300	300	—
Bladder	54,200	39,100	15,100	12,100	8,100	4,000
Brain and central nervous system	16,800	9,500	7,300	13,100	7,200	5,900
Thyroid	18,100	4,600	13,500	1,200	500	700
Leukemias	30,200	16,800	13,400	22,100	12,400	9,700
Hodgkin disease	7,200	3,800	3,400	1,300	700	600
TOTAL	1,005,500	502,500	503,000	443,100	227,300	215,800

From American Cancer Society. (1999). Cancer facts and figures—1999 (p. 4). Atlanta, GA: Author.

particularly about the cancer-causing effects of substances occurring naturally in food or produced during the processes of food storage, cooking, and digestion.

Diet seems also to function over time to place an individual at risk for cancer. In women, who have a much higher incidence of hormone-dependent cancer than men, diet has been suggested as the main single determinant in causing these cancers.[36,37,39,40] Studies find a consistent relationship between increasing weight in women and the risk of cancer, although this is not true for men. Obesity is a consistent risk factor for endometrial cancer, possibly because "overnutrition" causes excessive exposure to estrogen. After menopause, the only natural estrogens produced are those from the adrenal glands and adipose tissue, so more adipose tissue causes more estrogen exposure. High consumption of dietary fat is also linked to endometrial, breast, prostatic, ovarian, and rectal cancer.[37,39-42] Experiments on animals indicate that polyunsaturated vegetable oils, especially those with high polyunsaturated ω-6 fatty acids found in vegetable oils and margarines, promote cancer (e.g., increase free radical formation) more effectively than do saturated fats, whereas in humans total dietary fat correlates more significantly with cancer incidence and mortality in the epidemiologic data (see pp. 253-254).[41]

Much controversy concerns the need to limit the amount of preservatives added to foods. Food preservation is needed because food is grown in one part of the world and eaten in another, sometimes months or even years later. Advocates argue that preservatives allow people more dietary freedom

and actually may encourage better diets. However, consumers may ingest chemicals unknowingly, unnecessarily, and without judicious knowledge for making responsible choices. Most noteworthy among the preservatives and artificial additives under study are saccharin and nitrites. Studies in humans have failed to show a relationship between cancer and saccharin intake.

Nitrites are used as preservatives in fish and meat and may concentrate in the soil and water of some regions. The reaction of nitrites to other nitrosable compounds causes cancer of the glandular stomach in animals. Potentially harmful nitrite reactions can occur when foods are cooked. For example, nitrite-cured bacon, when cooked, yields nitrous acid, which reacts with amines (derivatives of ammonia present in many foods) in the meat to form dimethylnitrosamine (DMN). This reaction is favored at an acidic pH and therefore occurs when nitrites and secondary amines are ingested and encounter the acidic gastric juice. Dietary salts also seem to enhance this reaction. By decreasing the formation of carcinogenic nitrosamines, vitamins C and E (in lettuce and salad greens) exert a protective effect when ingested at the same time as salt and nitrites.[37] The inhabitants of countries with high rates of gastric cancer (e.g., China) ingest large quantities of salted fish and similarly preserved foods.

Three primary mechanisms whereby dietary factors may affect cancer production are suggested.[36] These are (1) direct-acting carcinogens or their precursors, (2) indirect-acting carcinogens (those that affect the formation of body carcino-

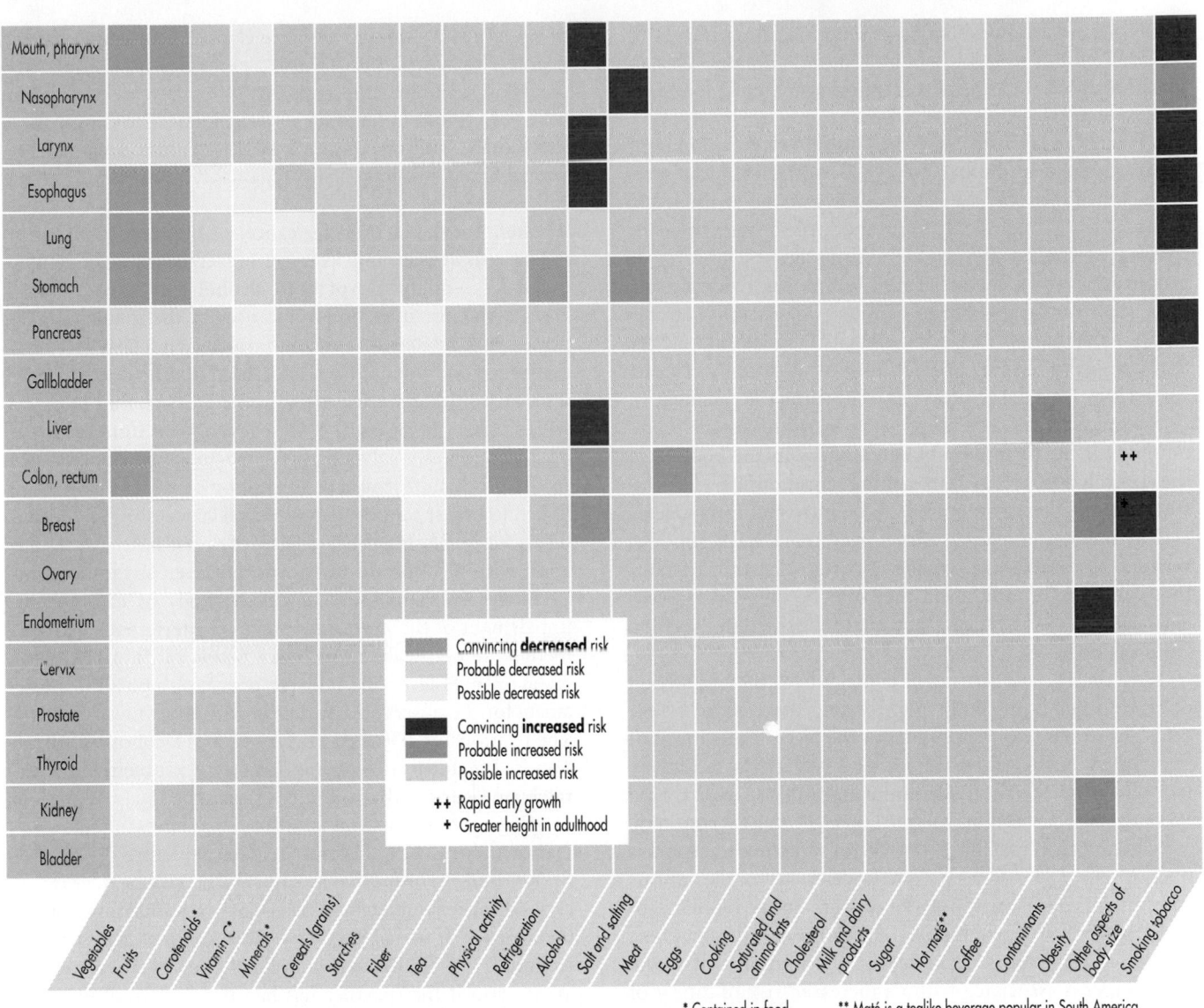

Fig. 9-16 *Diet and cancer. (Redrawn from* Nutrition Action Healthletter *[Dec. 1998].)*

gens), and (3) dietary factors that affect transport, activation, and deactivation of carcinogens.

Direct-acting carcinogens include dietary substances in natural foodstuffs, carcinogens produced by cooking, and carcinogens produced by microorganisms in stored foods. The thorough search for naturally occurring carcinogenic food substances is incomplete, especially for humans. Compounds such as hydrazines found in some mushrooms and aflatoxin produced by some food-related fungi are known to cause cancer in experimental animals. Aflatoxin is likely to be carcinogenic also for humans because human liver cells contain the enzymes needed to activate the agent metabolically. High intakes of aflatoxin by people in the tropics are associated with a high rate of liver cancer, at least among those chronically affected with the hepatitis B virus.[43] Afla-

HEALTH ALERT

Diet and Cancer Prevention

Some foods increase the risk for cancer (Fig. 9-16). Observing the following dietary guidelines might reduce the risk for cancer:

- Low-fat (especially avoidance of omega-6 fatty acids), high-fiber diet
- Increased intake of fruits and vegetables
- Vitamins A, C, and E
- Epigallocatechin gallate (found in green tea)
- Phytoestrogens (soy products)
- Decreased use of foods with high amounts of preservatives
- Decreased use of grilled, blackened foods
- Decreased alcohol intake

toxin is found in contaminated peanuts and other staple carbohydrate foods stored in hot and humid climates. This association raises the possibility that other toxins in food may be carcinogenic.

Some carcinogens may be produced by cooking.[44] Benzo[*a*]pyrene and other polycyclic hydrocarbons are produced when meat or fish is excessively smoked or broiled or when fat is used repeatedly to fry food. Food must be nearly charred or cooked at very high temperatures, however, to produce these potentially harmful substances. Evidence suggests that airborne cancer-causing heterocyclic amines (HCAs) are emitted after grilling meats.[45] These data suggest that those who fry a large amount of meat (e.g., short-order cooks) may have the greatest risk of inhaling the carcinogens.

Indirect-acting carcinogens provide necessary compounds for the formation of carcinogens in the body (e.g., the production of *N*-nitrosamine compounds). Animal studies show these compounds to be powerful carcinogenic agents; their carcinogenic effects in humans have not been verified. Nitrosable compounds can occur naturally in many foods such as fish and meat; they may be ingested as pesticide residues or drugs; and they may be formed in the colon from amino acids.

Certain ingested fats might contribute to the production of carcinogens in the body by increasing the amount of bile acids and cholesterol metabolites in the feces. These metabolites, which include deoxycholic and lithocholic acids, are found in greater quantities in populations that ingest a typical Western fatty diet and in whom colorectal cancer is common.

The most significant dietary factor affecting transport is fiber. Much work has been done to characterize the various components of dietary fiber. (Fiber refers to the remnants of the plant cell wall not hydrolyzed by human digestive enzymes.) Considerable data support the finding that a diet low in fiber is associated with an increased risk of cancer of the colon.[37] High fiber intake is associated with low levels of sex hormones in plasma (e.g., sex hormone−binding globulin, free estradiol, free testosterone), causing a reduction in the bioavailability of the hormones that, possibly, would reduce the risk of hormone-dependent cancers. It has been suggested recently that because fat intake is related to decreased excretion of biologically active sex hormones and fiber is also related to their levels in plasma, a ratio of fat to total fiber may be a better index of risk than either factor alone.[39]

For many carcinogens, intermediate steps must take place before cellular damage occurs. Some carcinogens must be oxidized, yielding metabolically activated intermediates. These activated metabolites are generated through oxidation and peroxidation and include the short-lived intermediates, the oxidative free radicals (free radical OH^- and the superoxide radical O_2^-) (see Chapter 3). In animals, polyunsaturated fatty acids are readily oxidized to yield free radicals and peroxidates that are toxic to cells and related to tumor development.[46] ω-3 Fatty acids (e.g., fatty fish), a class of polyunsaturated fats, however, decrease the number and size

of tumors and increase the time elapsed before tumors appear.[47] The destruction of toxic peroxides or radicals depends on selenium-containing enzymes. Levels of selenium have been found to be lower in individuals with cancer than individuals without cancer.[48] High-selenium areas in the United States (western plains regions) have the lowest colon cancer rates.[49]

Alcohol. Incidence rates for cancer of the mouth, pharynx, larynx, esophagus, and liver are higher in individuals who ingest large quantities of both alcohol and smoke.[37,50] Increased risk for men only for cancer of the major salivary glands was related to current smoking and heavy alcohol consumption.[51] Wine, beer, and "hard liquor" seem to produce an equivalent effect on cancer risk.[37] Alcohol interacts with smoke, increasing the risk of malignant tumors, possibly by acting as a solvent for the carcinogenic chemicals in smoke products. Alcohol consumption consistently has been linked to breast cancer and colorectal cancer.[37,42,52-54] Mechanisms for increasing the incidence of breast cancer in association with alcohol are unknown; however, suggestions include the liver's inability to rid the body of carcinogens, impairment of the immune system, or interference with cell membrane permeability in breast tissue. Alcohol stimulates rectal cell proliferation in the rat, providing a possible mechanism for the observed association with large bowel cancer.[37] The relationship between cancer risk and alcohol consumption is difficult to determine because of problems in accurately measuring the amount of alcohol ingested and in defining other behavioral habits, such as smoking, that further complicate or confound the clinical picture.

Sexual and reproductive behavior. The risk of developing cervical cancer is related to the age of first sexual intercourse, the number of sexual partners, and sexually transmitted infections.[50,55,56] Women who have had one sexual partner are at risk also if that partner has had previous multiple partners. The possible mechanism may be a virus transmitted between partners. New studies reveal that certain types of human papillomavirus (HPV) are causally involved in the development of cancer of the cervix.[57] Condyloma acuminatum (genital warts) is caused by HPV. The seriousness of genital infection seems to be related to the type of HPV causing the infection. There are about 70 serotypes: types 6 and 11 are identified as benign condyloma; types 16 (50%), 18 (20%), 31, and 33 are associated with genital dysplasia. About 95% of invasive cervical cancers contain these types.[58] The most common cause of abnormal Pap smears is the HPV virus, followed by cervical dysplasia.[59] In recent studies, an increased risk of HPV infection was significantly associated with younger age, Hispanic ethnicity, black race, an increased number of vaginal sex partners, high frequencies of vaginal sex and alcohol consumption, anal sex, and partner characteristics (regular partners having an increased number of lifetime partners and not being in school).[59] The risk of an abnormal Pap smear increased with *persistent* HPV infection, particularly with high-risk individuals. The short duration of most HPV infections (median 8 months) suggests that the cervical dysplasia should be managed conservatively.[59] Multiple other types of HPV are associated with cancers of the cervix, vulva, penis, and anus.[22] Although HPV may be a prime determinant worldwide, the importance of cofactors could vary by geographic area. Recently, a report by local inhabitants of a town in Utah implicated nearby toxic waste as causing a substantial increase in the incidence of cervical cancer by 150%.[60] Cancer of the cervix is one of the most prevalent virus-linked cancers.[22]

Herpes simplex virus 2 (HSV-2) has not been shown to be a causative agent, but antibodies to the virus increase with the severity of cervical dysplasia, and invasive carcinoma is associated with higher antibody titers. Studies have failed to provide strong evidence of HSVs in human cancers.[22,57]

The incidence of invasive cervical cancer is two and one-half times greater in black women than in white women in the United States.[50] Cervical malignancy also is found more often in women from lower socioeconomic groups.[61]

Air pollution

A person inhales about 20,000 L of air in 1 day; thus even modest contamination of the atmosphere can result in inhalation of appreciable doses of pollutants. Concerns recently have focused on industrial emissions, including arsenicals, benzene, chloroform, formaldehyde, sulfuric acid, mustard gas, vinyl chloride, and acrylonitrile.[62] Living close to certain industries is a recognized cancer risk factor although it is difficult to determine cancer risk from outdoor pollution because investigators must accurately control for smoking and radon. One team of investigators estimates that one must breathe Los Angeles smog for 1 year to inhale the same amount of burnt material that a two-pack/day smoker inhales in 1 day.[43] Other studies that controlled or stratified for smoking demonstrate associations between excess lung cancer rates and heavy metal and aromatic hydrocarbon emissions in polluted air.[63]

Indoor pollution generally is considered worse than outdoor pollution, partly because of cigarette smoke.[31] Environmental tobacco smoke (ETS; passive smoking) is also an important contaminant. ETS causes the formation of reactive oxygen free radicals and thus DNA damage.[64,65] Another significant indoor air pollutant may be radon gas. Radon is a natural radioactive gas that is present in soil, is trapped in houses, and gives rise to radioactive decay products known to be carcinogenic to humans.[66-69] About 10% of lung cancer cases are attributed to radon pollution in houses.[31] A large Swedish study found the risk for all histologic types of lung cancer, particularly small cell carcinoma, increased progressively with increased radon exposure.[67] The most hazardous houses can be identified and modified to prevent radon contamination. Radon increases the risk of lung cancer in underground miners whether or not they smoke.[70]

Occupation

One way to provide useful information about occupational practices and exposures to subsequent cancer risk is to iden-

tify cancers associated with occupational hazards. Table 9-10 identifies occupational hazards causally associated with cancers in humans.

A substantial percentage of cancers of the upper respiratory passages, lung, bladder, and peritoneum are attributed to occupational factors. Metalworking fluids (MWFs) commonly are used in a number of industrial machining and grinding operations. Recent findings have found an increased risk of cancer at several sites (larynx, rectum, pancreas, skin, scrotum, bladder) with some MWFs used before the 1970s.[71] One notable occupational factor is asbestos, which may cause as many as 5% of all lung cancers.[36,72] Carcinoma of the bladder has been linked with the manufacture of dyes, rubber, paint, and aromatic amines, especially β-naphthylamine and benzidine. Benzol inhalation is linked to leukemia in shoemakers and in workers in the rubber cement, explosives, and dyeing industries.

Ultraviolet radiation

Ultraviolet (UV) sunlight or solar radiation *causes* basal cell carcinoma and squamous cell carcinoma, two common skin cancers found in white individuals. UV radiation is now known to cause specific gene mutations in tumor suppressor gene *p53* associated with skin cancers.[73] In addition, UV light induces the release of tumor necrosis factor-α (TNF-α) in the epidermis, which may reduce immune surveillance against skin cancer.[74]

Basal cell carcinoma commonly occurs on the head and neck. Individuals with these tumors generally have light complexions, light eyes, and fair hair. They tend to sunburn rather than tan and live in areas of high sunlight exposure. Usually these cancers arise on areas of the body that receive the greatest sun exposure, although they are not necessarily restricted to these skin sites. Squamous cell carcinoma is found more commonly in men who work outdoors. These tumors are distributed over the head, neck, and exposed areas of the upper extremities (see Chapter 39).

The incidence of melanoma, a malignant pigmented mole, *correlates* with the amount of exposure to UV light.[75] Although the nonmelanoma skin cancers are related to cumulative exposure to UV radiation, melanoma is related to episodes of severe, blistering sunburn at a young age.[37,76] The relatively recent worldwide increase in melanoma among white-skinned people is attributed largely to changes in clothing that promote greater exposure. The body areas receiving greater sun exposure vary between the sexes because of clothing differences. Malignant melanomas occur on the upper back and the dorsum of the hands of both genders and the legs of females. There has been an alarming increase in the incidence of melanoma over the past 4 decades. It has been suggested that changing habits of sun exposure and the use of sunscreen lotions may reverse this trend by 2020.[77] Recent controversy about sunscreen use and sunscreens' prevention of actinic damage and neoplasia has stimulated a reexamination of their use.[78]

Xeroderma pigmentosum is a rare autosomal disease

TABLE 9-10	Occupational Exposures Related to Cancer		
Cancer Site and Causal Agent	**Related Occupation**	**Cancer Site and Causal Agent**	**Related Occupation**
Lung		**Skin**	
Bischloro-methyl-ether	Ion exchange resin producers	UV light	Outdoor workers, fishermen
		Liver	
Chromium	Ore and pigment manufacturers	Vinyl chloride	Vinyl chloride workers
Mustard gas	Poison gas producers	Alcohol	Brewery workers
Mixed solvents	Painters		
		Bladder	
Lung, pleura		Aromatic amines	Dye and rubber workers
Asbestos	Miners, insulation installers, ship-yard workers		
		Leukemia	
		Benzene	Workers using glue and varnish
Lung and skin			
Arsenic	Smelter and pesticide workers	**Nasal**	
		Isopropyl alcohol	Isopropyl alcohol manufacturers
Lung and nasal		Wood dusts	Furniture makers
Nickel	Nickel refiners		
		Cervical	Service and apparel manufacturing, toxic waste
Lung and skin			
Polycyclic hydro-carbons	Workers using mineral oil and tar	**Multiple sites**	
		Ionizing radiation	Radium dial painters, uranium miners

Modified from American Cancer Society (ACS). (1994). Cancer facts and figures, 1994. New York: The Author; Monson, R.R. & Christiani, D.C. (1997). Summary of the evidence: Occupation and environment and cancer. Cancer Causes and Control, 8(3), 529-531; Lynge, E., Antilla, A., & Hemminki, K. (1997). Organic solvents and cancer. Cancer Causes and Control, 8(3), 406-497; Alterman, T. et al. (1997). Occupation and cervical cancer: An opportunity for prevention. Journal of Women's Health, 6(6), 649-657.

characterized by pigmentation abnormalities and malignancies. Persons with this disease demonstrate excessive skin damage caused by sun exposure at very young ages. People with xeroderma pigmentosum lack enzymes that repair sun-damaged DNA.

Ionizing radiation

Much of the knowledge of the effects of ionizing radiation on human cancer has stemmed from observations of the Hiroshima and Nagasaki atomic bomb exposures. These unfortunate exposures caused acute leukemias in adults and children and increased frequencies of thyroid and breast carcinomas. Lung, stomach, colon, esophageal, and urinary tract cancers and multiple myeloma have lately been added to the list. At Nagasaki and Hiroshima, leukemia incidence in individuals 15 years or younger reached its peak 6 to 7 years after the explosions and has steadily declined since 1952. Middle-aged people, 45 years and older at the time of exposure, had a latent period of 20 years before developing acute leukemia. Children conceived after the exposure of their parents to the atomic bombs surprisingly have shown no increase in any cancer thus far. Human exposure to ionizing radiation includes emissions from x-rays, radioisotopes, and other radioactive sources.

Carcinogenesis. An important effect of ionizing radiation is thought to be inhibition of cell division. Cells of lym-

phoid tissue, bone marrow, and intestinal epithelium are normally short-lived, rapidly dividing cells. Symptoms and causes of death from exposure to large doses of whole-body radiation are related to the inability of these cells to divide. For example, the suppression of stem cell division in the bone marrow can cause the disappearance of granulocytes and repopulation of tissues with the remaining stem cells. Depending on how many cells are lost, repopulation may require days, weeks, or more, which may be too late to reverse the effects.

At low doses of radiation, few dividing cells may be damaged and in some tissues may lead to no detectable change in function. Smaller doses, however, can alter the developing fetus.[79] Organ development occurs early and extremely rapidly during pregnancy; exposure of the fetus to radiation can greatly alter cellular integrity and normal development. These effects depend on the number of stem cells available and the stage of fetal development.

Carcinogenesis can occur from mutation or cell transformation caused by radiation (see Chapter 3). Radiation can cause dominant and recessive mutations in the DNA and chromosome aberrations (Fig. 9-17). To produce a carcinogenic effect, these DNA alterations must survive in cells capable of cell division. Radiation can directly damage macromolecules or carbohydrates, proteins, lipids, and nucleic acids. Indirectly, radiation interacts with substances (gener-

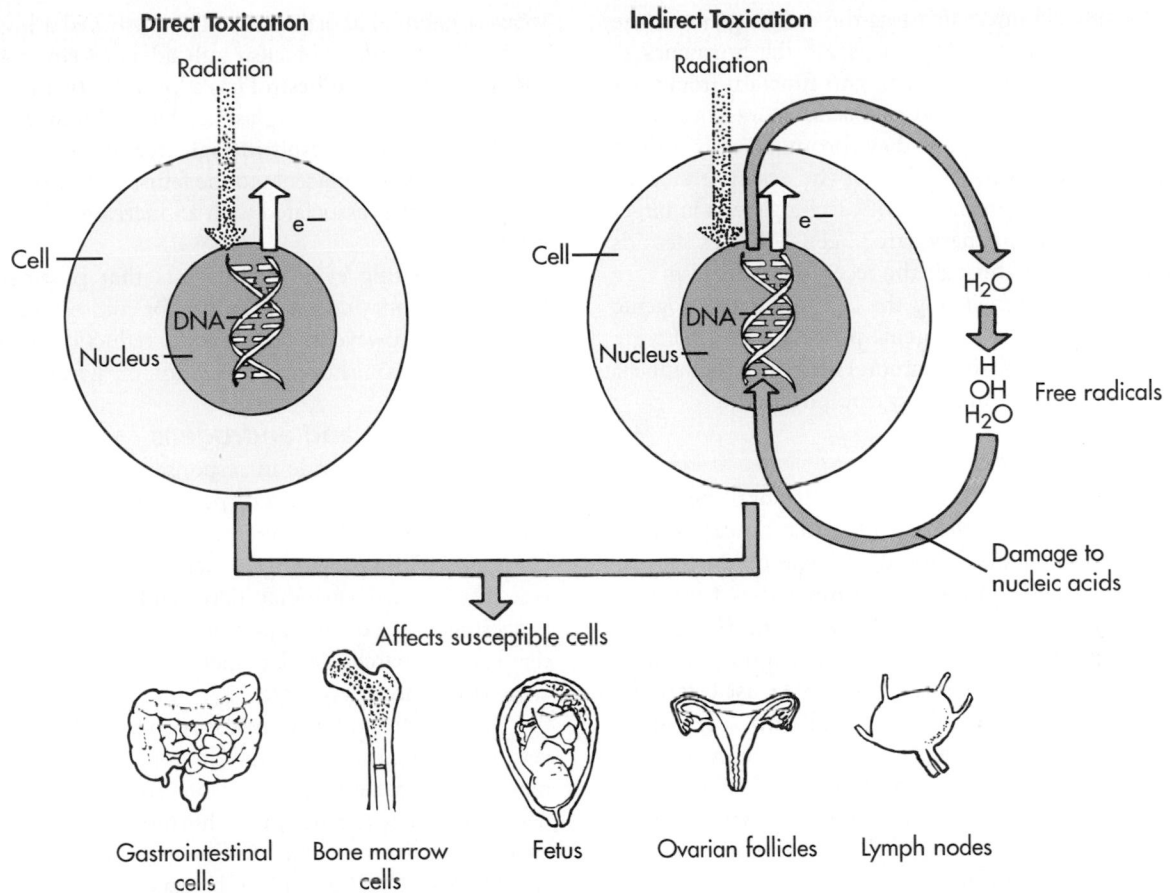

Direct Toxication

Indirect Toxication

Fig. 9-17 *Cellular damage caused by ionizing radiation.* Radiation can damage macromolecules in two ways: (1) directly, where the micromolecules are ionized; and (2) indirectly, where water is ionized and produces free radicals that in turn damage macromolecules. Cells that are particularly susceptible to damage are those of the gastrointestinal tract, bone marrow, lymph nodes, fetus, and ovarian follicles.

ally water) within the cell, producing reactive-free radicals that then interact and damage DNA.

Carcinogenesis also can result from gene-environment interactions. Host factors can influence the carcinogenic effects of radiation. For example, although cells can repair some lesions in DNA, some genetic abnormalities alter the repair mechanism, making the individual sensitive to ionizing radiation. Disturbances in the DNA repair mechanism affect the risk of radiation-induced genetic effects and the risk of cancer.

Many other biologic variables affect responses to radiation, including the part and percentage of the body exposed, the individual's age or developmental stage at time of exposure, hormonal balance (e.g., sex hormones regulate cellular growth), genetic integrity, drugs, and other disease processes. Certain drugs can inhibit the immune response by affecting the surveillance role of the lymphoid cells. In the presence of infections, viral nucleoproteins may be introduced into the DNA, rendering the cell susceptible to transformation. Ionizing radiation can cause leukemias and many solid tumors (e.g., thyroid, breast, salivary gland). Compelling data indicate that diagnostic x-rays to the trunk are related to risk of chronic myelogenous leukemia and that the risk increases with increasing x-ray dose to active bone mar-

row.[80] Solid tumors seldom appear before 10 years after radiation exposure and continue to appear for 30 years or more after exposure. Leukemia is an exception, appearing within a few years after radiation exposure.

Because women constitute nearly half the workforce and most are in their reproductive years, they may be exposed to sources of radiation. Women employed in occupations with exposures to ionizing radiation need evaluation of possible reproductive risk.[81]

Hormones

The relationship between hormones and human cancer has been studied extensively. Interest began in 1919 when Laek reported that removal of the ovaries in female mice prevented the development of breast cancer. Four notable types of human cancer—carcinoma of the breast, endometrium, ovary, and prostate—occur in target or hormone-responsive tissues. (These cancers are discussed in Chapter 32.)

Much of the current research on hormones and cancer focuses on the direct actions of the sex steroids (estrogens, testosterone, progesterone). Prolactin, a major pituitary hormone, has a direct role in rat mammary cancer growth but is not believed to be of primary importance in human breast cancer.

The difficulty in understanding the carcinogenic nature of hormones has been how to separate the hormones as modulators of target tissue growth and function from their potential causative carcinogenic effects. More simply, do hormones cause cancer, do they promote only tumor growth, or do they do both? Most of the evidence thus far supports their role as promoters of carcinogenesis in target tissues rather than as primary carcinogens. The sex steroids produce their actions through the receptor mechanism (see Chapters 1 and 31), sensitizing the cell to the carcinogenic insult, promoting the carcinogenic process, and modifying the growth of the established tumor. Hormones thus appear as promoters rather than primary carcinogens.

Oral contraceptives

Many epidemiologic studies have found that oral contraceptive use has no effect on the risk of breast cancer in most women regardless of dose, brand, or type of estrogen or progestin.[82] Although controversial, some studies have identified subgroups of *current* oral contraceptive users who have an increased risk of breast cancer. Such subgroups include women with many years of oral contraceptive use before the age of 25 years or before the first full-term pregnancy; women who use oral contraceptives at age 45 years or older; women with a history of biopsy-confirmed benign breast disorders; nulliparous, premenopausal women with an early menarche; women with only one child; and women with a family history of breast cancer.[83]

Ovarian cancer seems to develop from the epithelial cells on the surface of the ovary. The main stimulus for division of these cells is ovulation. After each ovulation, epithelial cells replicate to cover the exposed surface of the ovary. Those factors that prevent ovulation help protect against the development of ovarian cancer. Complete and incomplete pregnancies and oral contraceptive use all reduce the risk of ovarian cancer.[84]

Estrogens

Estrogen replacement therapy (ERT) has been prescribed for women to relieve perimenopausal symptoms (e.g., hot flashes), to prevent osteoporosis, and to reduce cardiovascular disease risk. Long-term use of estrogens by these women has been linked to endometrial cancer.[37,50] Current use of postmenopausal ERT is associated with a 30% increase in breast cancer risk.[84] Adding progestin to the estrogen further increases risk by 40%.[84] Furthermore, hormone replacement therapy, especially continuously combined (estradiol-progestin regimens), may increase mammographic density, causing a decrease in clarity and problems with interpretation.[85] Breast cells proliferate in response to estrogens. Accumulating data strongly suggest that breast cancer risk in postmenopausal women is associated with relatively high concentrations of *endogenous* estradiol.[86] The extent to which risk is further increased by exogenous estrogens is unknown.

The synthetic estrogen diethylstilbestrol (DES) also has been linked to cancer. Daughters of women treated with DES

to avert habitual abortion have demonstrated a higher than expected percentage of clear cell adenocarcinomas of the vagina.[42,87] Diethylstilbestrol has a low affinity for binding to its transporter protein, plasma steroid-binding globulin, which may in turn result in high free levels of circulating DES that cross the placenta to the fetus. The use of DES during pregnancy is associated with an increased risk for breast cancer.[42]

Accumulating evidence suggests that postmenopausal hormone use may decrease the risk for colorectal cancer. Recent studies, however, report that the reduction in colorectal cancer risk diminishes upon cessation of therapy.[88]

Progestogens and androgens

Endometrial cells divide in response to estrogen; however, the simultaneous presence of progestogens can decrease or even eliminate such mitotic activity. Estrogen stimulation "unopposed" by progestogen increases endometrial cancer risk. The best evidence that increased levels of estrogen and progestogens, in combination, increase breast cancer risk is that early menarche and late menopause with associated increased hormone levels are such significant risk factors for this disease. Breast cancer risk is reduced 10% to 20% each year menarche is delayed. In addition, for any given age at menarche, rapid establishment of regular menstrual cycles with the associated increased hormone levels further increases risk. Women who stop menstruating before age 45 years have one half the risk of breast cancer of women who continue to menstruate to age 55 years or older. Breast cancer is related to cumulative exposure to estrogens, an effect possibly increased by progesterone.

In men, an increase in risk of breast cancer has been associated with testicular dysfunction and pathologic findings, and a decrease in risk has been related to high fertility, a history of prostate cancer, and exogenous androgens. These observations suggest that risk may be increased by low levels and decreased by high levels of androgens.[89]

Male sex hormones, testosterone and its derivative 5-dihydrotestosterone (DHT), stimulate the growth of target tissues, such as the prostate. Men who take exogenous androgens, however, do not seem to have a higher risk of prostate cancer, whereas women who take estrogens without progestogens after menopause seem to have a higher risk for developing endometrial cancer.

✓ QUICK CHECK

Define *v-onc, c-onc*, proto-oncogene, and tumor suppressor gene. Describe how each contributes to cancer development.

Why is gap junction intercellular communication a significant factor in tumor growth?

Why is initiation, promotion, and progression considered to be linked processes in carcinogenesis? Provide examples of how these processes function to cause cancer.

IMMUNOBIOLOGY OF CANCER
Tumor Immune Surveillance Theory

One conclusion that can be drawn from the viral theory of carcinogenesis is that the induction of altered or abnormal cell products is not necessarily required for cancer cells to develop. The only difference between normal and transformed cells may be the amount, rather than the type, of cellular components (e.g., enzymes, cell surface receptors, plasma membrane-bound proteins) that each possesses. In this regard, the overall structural composition of the plasma membranes of normal and transformed cells may be quite similar, if not identical. Thus any differences between normal and cancer cells may be both subtle and possibly imperceptible by the organism.

The immune system of higher organisms, such as humans, has evolved to recognize antigens that are considered to be "foreign," or "nonself," structures (see Chapter 5). Therefore if the immune system can recognize and reject tumors, cancer cells must express "nonself" antigens. The *tumor immune surveillance theory* is based on this assumption.

For some time, investigators have been intrigued with the idea that the body could defend itself against the development of cancer. In 1908 a biologist, Dr. Paul Ehrlich, proposed that the transformation process was a common event and that, as a result, cancer cells were constantly arising in normal animals. He proposed that most cancer cells express "foreign" antigens that make them susceptible to rejection by their host's immune system.

Since that time, a number of studies have supported Ehrlich's general concept. Based on this work, Sir Macfarlin Burnet formally proposed the tumor immune surveillance theory in 1970. In short, Burnet proposed that cell-mediated cytotoxicity (i.e., tumor cell killing by immunologic cells such as lymphocytes) evolved because the immune system needed to detect cancer cells. Certain experimental and clinical observations support Burnet's theory, including the identification of tumor antigens, increased risk of certain types of cancers in immune-suppressed individuals, tumor-reactive antibodies in the serum of some individuals with cancer, and tumor-specific T cell—mediated cellular immunity (mechanisms of cellular immunity are described in Chapter 5).

Tumor antigens

Human cancer cells express numerous "foreign" molecules on their surface. These can be recognized by the immune system as either *tumor-associated antigens (TAAs)* or *tumor-specific antigens (TSAs)*. Several types of molecules have been identified as TAAs and TSAs. By the strictest definition, TAAs and TSAs are expressed by tumor cells but not by normal cells. In reality, many TAAs expressed by human cancer cells also are expressed by normal cells. This is consistent with the preceding description of cancer. Because cancer is a disease of unregulated cell growth and differentiation, the differences between the molecules expressed on the surfaces of normal and cancer cells are subtle. Thus the recognition of a molecule as a TAA or TSA results from a complex interaction between the tumor and its host's immune system.

Most of our knowledge of human TAAs and TSAs has come from the study of tumor-reactive antibodies that are obtained from individuals' sera or experimental generation of monoclonal antibodies. Serologically defined human TAAs and TSAs include viral antigens, oncofetal antigens, oncogene products, and "mutant" proteins and carbohydrates (Table 9-11).

Immunologic defense against tumors

When a tumor expresses cell surface TSA, the immune system of an immunologically competent host can reject the tumor. A number of clinical observations strongly support the concept of immunologic involvement in the tumor surveillance process. In the 1700s it was noted that individuals with draining, abscessed tumors lived longer than those whose tumors did not appear to be inflamed. Berg, in 1959, reported that women with breast cancer tumors that were infiltrated with lymphocytes had a better prognosis than women whose tumors were free of lymphocytes. For certain types of neoplasia there is an increased risk (2% to 20% increase over the normal population) of developing cancer in individuals who are immunologically suppressed. Such individuals (Table 9-12) include (1) children with immunodeficiency diseases, (2) organ transplant recipients whose immune systems are suppressed with drugs (e.g., cyclosporin A to block graft rejection), (3) individuals with cancer for whom cancer therapy results in the suppression of immune responsiveness (many of the current radiation therapies and chemotherapies that are used to treat various forms of cancer depress the immune system, and these individuals have a high risk of developing secondary tumors), and (4) individuals with acquired immunodeficiency syndrome (AIDS). Immunologic suppression also enhances the growth and recurrence of tumors in individuals with preexisting cancers.[90] These clinical observations strongly support immune surveillance mechanisms and their role in the development of certain types of cancer.

Immune mechanisms for defense against cancer

As with other antigens, TSAs can elicit both protective and suppressive immune responses. Certain immune responses are more beneficial than others for protecting the individual against cancer. The cancer defense mechanisms are summarized in Fig. 9-18. (See Chapters 5 and 7 for discussion on types of immune mechanisms.)

Immune surveillance escape mechanisms

Although the immune system can reject tumors, individuals with normal immunologic function develop cancers. The host-tumor relationship during tumor emergence and progression is thus a complex process. Changes in host immunologic potential (i.e., range of antigenic responses) and characteristics of growing cancer cells (e.g., TAA and TSA expression, growth rate, and metabolism) constantly occur. By taking advantage of these changes, many cancers can by-

TABLE 9-11	Examples of Tumor-Specific Antigens	
Type of Antigens	**Expressed By**	**Comments**
Viral antigens	Virally transformed cells	Examples of tumors caused by viruses appear to include Burkitt lymphoma (Epstein-Barr virus), T cell leukemias (human T cell leukemia virus), cervical carcinomas (human papillomavirus)
Oncofetal-related antigens	Cells during stages of embryogenesis that are usually absent on normal adult cells	Alpha-fetoprotein (α-fetoprotein) is found in individuals with hepatic, pancreatic, and embryonic carcinomas; carcinoembryonic antigen (CEA) has been found in the serum of some individuals with colon, pancreas, and breast cancer; because these antigens are found also in a large number of normal individuals, use as a sole diagnostic marker for cancer screening is not always reliable; one of the best recognized tumor-specific antigens (TSAs) expressed by hematopoietic cancers is the common acute lymphoblastic leukemia-associated antigen (CALLA)
Oncogene-related antigens	Individual tumors suggesting that complex activation of certain oncogenes is required to transform normal cells	Several are expressed by lung cancer, including *ras, myc, neu*; retinoblastoma *(rb)* gene, *p53* gene, Wilms tumor gene, and deleted colon cancer *(DCC)* gene products are expressed as tumor antigens; a cell growth regulatory protein is the *MDR1* gene; multidrug resistance *(MDR1)* increases the excretion of cancer drugs; tumors that express *MDR1* usually are more resistant to drugs used for chemotherapy than those that do not express *MDR1*
Carbohydrate tumor antigens	Alterations in normal glycosylation of proteins or lipids	Examples include the lacto-series of Lewis blood group antigens, Le^a and le^b; these antigens have been detected on gastrointestinal cancers, GM3, GM2, and 9-o-acetyl-GD3 expressed by melanoma and other neuroectodermal cancers; Le^x and G1 have been found on colorectal and lung cancers; expression of the blood group A antigen on lung cancers is associated with a worse prognosis
Protein tumor antigens	These types of TSA are abnormally expressed proteins with normal function: normally function in proliferation, enzymatic processes, as receptors, as cellular structures	HLA-DR is not usually expressed by normal epithelial cells; however, HLA-DR can be expressed by melanomas, carcinomas of the GI tract, larynx, lung, colon, rectum, and breast; TAG-72 is expressed by individuals with breast, colon, ovary, pancreas, stomach, endometrium, and non-small-cell lung carcinoma; prostate-specific antigen (PSA) is expressed by individuals with prostate cancer; CO17-1A is expressed by colorectal cancers; stress-induced or heat shock proteins are

TABLE 9-12	Correlation Between Immunodeficiency and Cancer Risk		
Types of Cancer	**Increased Risk Over Normal Population**	**Types of Cancer**	**Increased Risk Over Normal Population**
Lymphomas	14 times greater	Uterine cervix	13 times greater
Leukemias	6 times greater	Stomach	11 times greater
Carcinomas		Urinary bladder	2 times greater
Skin (low-sun geographic areas)	4-7 times greater		
(high-sun geographic areas)	21 times greater		

Modified from Penn, I. (1981). Depressed immunity and the development of cancer. Clinical and Experimental Immunology, 46, 459-474; Penn, I. (1994). Malignancy. Surgical Clinics of North America, 74(5), 1247-1257.

NOTE: *There is an increased risk for developing specific types of cancer in individuals with various immunodeficiencies versus that of the normal population. The values presented are generalized to include the various immunodeficient conditions. There is no increased risk in immunodeficient individuals for specific cancers not listed.*

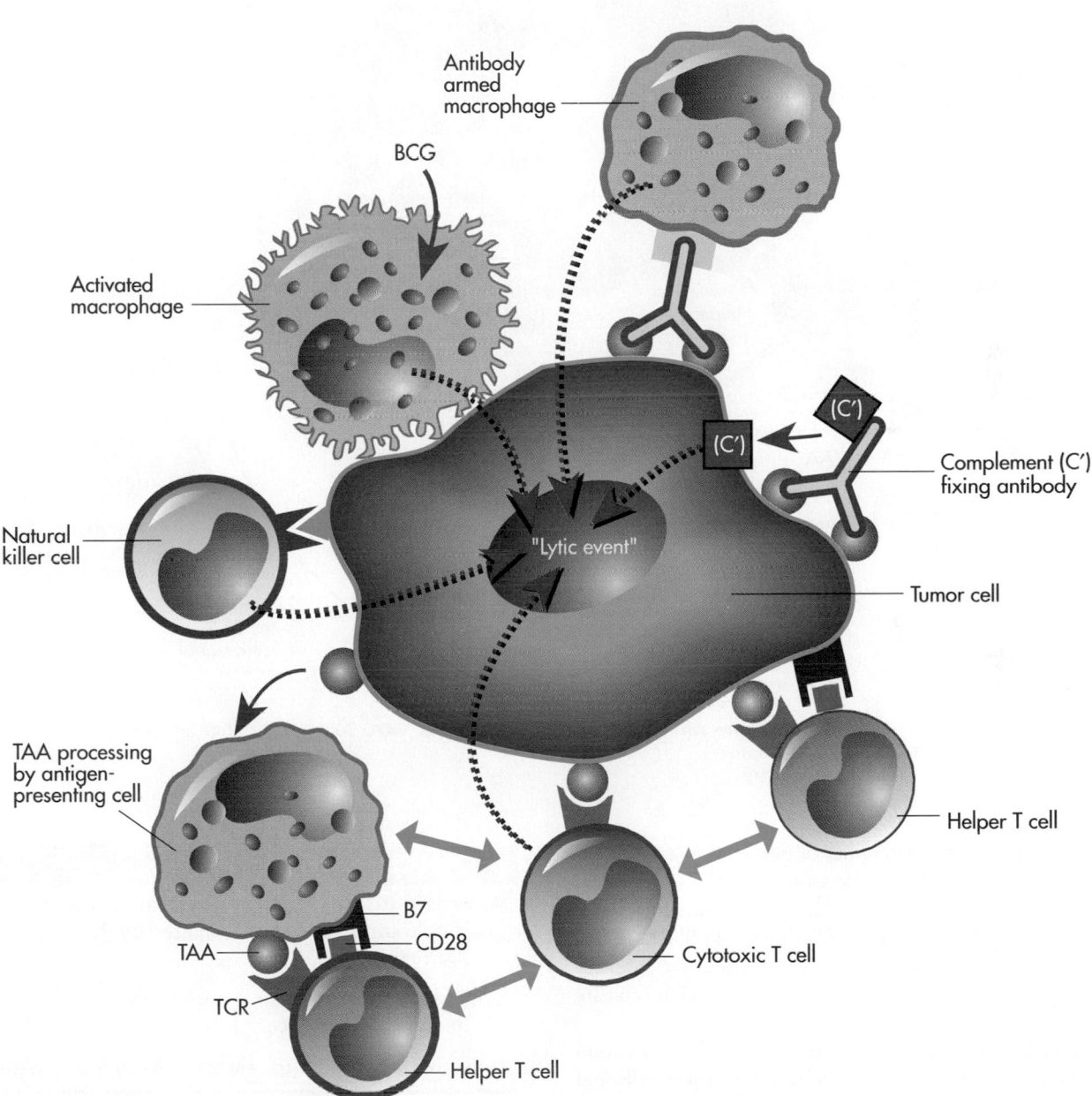

Fig. 9-18 *Tumor immune surveillance mechanisms.* *BCG,* Bacille Calmette-Guerin; *TAA,* tumor-associated antigen; *TCR* , T cell antigen receptor.

Fig. 9-19 *Potential immune surveillance escape mechanisms.* *TAA,* Tumor-associated antigen; *TCR,* T cell antigen receptor.

pass the host's immune surveillance potential. Ways that tumors escape immunologic rejection include (1) antigenic modulation, (2) secretion of immunosuppressive substances, (3) escape and sneaking through, (4) blocking factor, (5) immunostimulation, and (6) TSA-reactive suppressor T lymphocytes (Ts cells). These escape mechanisms are summarized in Fig. 9-19.

In conclusion, it appears that tumor growth or rejection depends on complex interactions between cancer cells and the immune system of their host. A range of immunologic protective mechanisms have been identified that cause tumor lysis. Transformation processes, however, can select for cancer cells that escape the host's tumor surveillance system. Further, many carcinogenic agents can cause immune suppression, making individuals more susceptible to the growth of neoplasia.

✓ QUICK CHECK

According to the tumor surveillance theory, why should cancer cells be eliminated by their host's immune system?

Why are tumor antigens a significant part of tumor immune surveillance?

Why are tumors able to "escape" the immune system?

▢ DID YOU UNDERSTAND?

Cancer: A Disease of Growth, Division, and Cell Differentiation

1. Abnormal cells that disobey the social control mechanisms of normal cell division proliferate to form tumors in the body.
2. Cell division is regulated by different combinations of protein growth factors presumably made by several "social control genes."
3. Three main genetic mechanisms have a role in human carcinogenesis: (a) mutation of genes resulting in hyperactivity of growth-related gene products; such genes are called *oncogenes;* (b) mutation of genes resulting in loss or inactivity of gene products that normally would inhibit growth; such genes are called *tumor suppressor genes;* and (c) mutation of genes resulting in overexpression of products that prevent normal cell death, or *apoptosis,* thus allowing continued growth of tumors.
4. Cancer cells are characterized by anaplasia, or loss of differentiation, and autonomy, or independence from normal cellular controls.
5. In the adult, undifferentiated cells (not totally committed to a specific function) are known as pluripotent cells, precursor cells, or stem cells. Cancer cells become more like embryonic cells and are less differentiated. Cancerous growth depends on derangements of cell differentiation.

Characteristics of Cancer Cells

1. The degree of disorganization varies among tumors, but disordered nuclear and structural components of cells are common.
2. Decreased communication or signaling between cells is the result of alterations in the plasma membranes. Because glycolipid and glycoprotein content is reduced on the cell's surface, cellular communication is thought to be reduced.
3. Loss of fibronectin contributes to the overall loss in shape, cell-to-cell adhesion, and cellular migration.
4. Cancer cells exhibit anchorage independence with decreased cell-cell and cell-extracellular matrix attachments. Without anchorage, cancerous cells are allowed to metastasize.
5. Tumor metastasis has been related to changes in intercellular communication. Gap junctions are important in regulating communication and are thought to be disrupted or blocked in cancer cells.
6. Tumor cell markers are substances, such as hormones, enzymes, genes, antigens, and antibodies, that denote specific tumors.
7. Several intercellular changes occur in cancer cells, including alterations in the cytoskeleton, density-dependent inhibition of growth, growth requirements, and changes in the nucleus and cell protein.

Causes of Cancer

1. Genetic events are the primary basis of carcinogenesis. Most of the genetic alterations that cause cancer during the lifetime of the individual occur in somatic tissues. Because the events occur in somatic cells, as opposed to germ cells, they are *not* transmitted to future generations. Mutations in germ-line cells (gametes) result in inherited cancer-causing genes from one generation to the next.
2. In rare families, cancer is inherited in an autosomal dominant fashion.
3. The mechanism by which environmental agents cause cancer reportedly is through increasing the frequency of mutation in somatic cells. Most human cancers, however, appear to arise without any known prior exposure to a carcinogenic agent.
4. Cancer-causing genes, or oncogenes, can be introduced into an individual (e.g., by oncogenic viruses) or inherited within some families.
5. The three main types of oncogenic DNA viruses are papovaviruses, adenoviruses, and herpesviruses. An example of an oncogenic RNA virus is human T cell leukemia-lymphoma virus.
6. Oncogenic viruses possess specific oncogenes called *v-onc.*
7. It is now known that cellular oncogenes, or *c-onc,* are incorporated into the genomes of a variety of different organisms, including humans.
8. The term *proto-oncogene* is used to refer collectively to the various *c-onc.* The term *proto-oncogene* indicates that *c-onc* and *v-onc* genes were probably derived from a common prototype gene.
9. Proto-oncogenes encode for growth factors, growth-factor receptors, signal transducers, nuclear proteins, and tumor suppressor proteins.
10. Viruses may cause mutations in surviving (e.g., infected) cells that could lead to neoplastic changes. Most oncogenic viruses cause transformation by a mechanism called *insertional mutagenesis.* Here the viral genes are incorporated into the host's genome at specific sites. The inserted genes are associated with cell transformation.
11. During some viral infections, the host's immune system can become compromised, allowing neoplastic cells to emerge that would otherwise be rejected.
12. Tumor suppressor genes encode for proteins that act as inhibitors of growth-factor stimulation. Tumor suppressor gene proteins block specific phases of the cell cycle, induce end-stage (e.g., terminal) differentiation, and stimulate cell senescence or death. Carcinogenesis involves inactivation of tumor suppressor genes and activation of oncogenes.

Carcinogenesis

1. Carcinogenesis is the process of tumor development.
2. Most evidence confirms that cancer has a monoclonal origin.
3. Because of the complexity of transformation processes, it is not surprising that cancers express multiple oncogenes and tumor suppressor genes.

Continued

◼ DID YOU UNDERSTAND? —cont'd

Carcinogenesis—cont'd

4. Researchers propose that gap junction intercellular communication is either blocked or down-regulated in transforming cancer cells, and therefore communication between the transformed cancer cells and normal surrounding cells is lost.

5. One theory of carcinogenesis suggests that cancer development occurs in stages: (a) an *initiation* stage that causes irreversible changes in DNA after exposure to a carcinogen; (b) a *promotion* stage in which the initiated cells become cancerous; and (c) a *progression* stage in which the cells become more biologically defective.

6. Initiators and promoters include hormones, drugs, environmental agents, and a variety of personal behaviors. Although the precise biochemical cause of cancer is unknown, these are actually risk factors associated with increased incidence of cancer.

7. Personal behaviors associated with increased cancer risk include smoking and chewing smokeless tobacco, as well as sexual and reproductive behavior.

8. Smoking is associated with cancers of the lung, bladder, larynx, oral cavity, esophagus, kidney, and certain blood cells; lung cancer is related to inhalation of tobacco smoke, which contains known carcinogenic compounds.

9. Passive smoking, namely by nonsmokers who breathe the smoke of others' cigarettes (environmental tobacco smoke [ETS]) may be related to a slightly increased risk of lung cancer.

10. Oral cancer is associated with "dipping snuff."

11. Dietary factors can act as cancer-promoting or cancer-inhibiting agents.

12. Obesity is associated with endometrial cancer, and high-fat diets, especially those with high polyunsaturated ω-6 fatty acids (found in vegetable oils and margarines), are associated with endometrial, breast, and colon cancer. Obesity and the Western diet likely stimulate insulin resistance, leading to increased levels of bioavailable estrogen.

13. Artificial additives and preservatives in food may include some compounds that are carcinogenic; particularly controversial is the use of nitrites, which react to form direct- or indirect-acting carcinogens when food is cooked.

14. Three primary mechanisms by which dietary factors affect cancer production are direct-acting carcinogens or their precursors; indirect-acting carcinogens; and dietary factors that affect transport, activation, and deactivation of carcinogens.

15. Direct-acting carcinogens may occur in natural foodstuffs, may be produced by cooking, or may be produced by microorganisms in stored foods.

16. Indirect-acting carcinogens provide compounds that act to form carcinogens in the body. Compounds currently being studied include nitrites, fats, and cholesterol.

17. Dietary factors that affect transport, activation, or deactivation of carcinogens include dietary fiber, which probably promotes rapid passage of food through the digestive tract, and selenium, which appears to destroy cytotoxic radicals when reacting at low levels.

18. Age at first sexual intercourse and number of sexual partners are related to development of cervical cancer.

19. Human papillomavirus appears to be the causal agent of warts and cervical cancer.

20. Pregnancy and childbearing seem to be protective factors against cancer of the endometrium, ovary, and breast; other reproductive factors related to decreased risk for breast cancer include late onset of menstruation and early menopause.

21. Air pollution is a concern for causing cancer because of inhalation of emissions, including arsenicals, benzene, chloroform, vinyl chloride, and acrylonitrite. Indoor pollution is considered worse than outdoor pollution because of cigarette smoke and possibly radon gas.

22. Cancers of the upper respiratory tract, lung, bladder, and peritoneum often are attributed to occupational exposures, including asbestos, fossil fuels, dyes, rubber, and paint.

23. Ultraviolet sunlight causes basal cell and squamous cell carcinomas, is associated with malignant melanoma, and also is implicated in increasing the severity of xeroderma pigmentosum.

24. Ultraviolet light damages DNA, inhibits cell division, and can lead to cell death. Damaged DNA can cause cancer by misrepairing itself and creating mutagenic cells that are susceptible to tumor development.

25. Exposure to ionizing radiation is caused by emissions from x-rays, radioisotopes, and other radioactive sources, some of which are industry- or occupation-related exposures.

26. Ionizing radiation inhibits cell division, especially in lymphoid tissue, bone marrow, and intestinal epithelium, which contain normally short-lived, rapidly dividing cells.

27. Carcinogenesis can occur from radiation-induced mutations or cell transformations; mutations may be dominant or recessive and also may cause chromosome aberrations.

28. Genetic factors can alter the repair mechanisms for DNA, so that an individual is particularly sensitive to the carcinogenic effects of ionizing radiation.

29. Biologic variables that affect responses to radiation include the part and percentage of the body exposed, the individual's age or stage of development at the time of exposure, genetic integrity, drugs, and other disease processes.

30. Radiation exposure in the neonate, infant, or child also can cause growth retardation; the younger the child, the more vulnerable the child is to the effects of radiation.

31. For cancers that occur in hormone-responsive target tissues, hormones probably act as promoters of carcinogenesis rather than as primary carcinogens.

▣ DID YOU UNDERSTAND? —cont'd

Immunobiology of Cancer

1. Cancer cells express tumor-associated antigens, which are not found on normal, nontransformed cells.
2. Tumor-associated antigens (TAAs) and tumor-specific antigens (TSAs) may be caused by synthesis of new molecules, by unmasking of potential TAAs, by loss of plasma membrane components, by biochemical modification, or by release of intracellular components.
3. Tumor antigens include viral antigens, oncofetal antigens (e.g., α-fetoprotein, carcinoembryonic antigen), oncogene-related antigens, carbohydrate, and protein tumor antigens.
4. When a developing tumor expresses a TAA or a TSA, an immunologically competent host can recognize these antigens and produce a range of immune responses to reject the tumor.
5. In spite of the immune system's ability to reject cancer cells, some cancer cells apparently are capable of bypassing the host's immune surveillance and by "escaping" can cause cancer.
6. Proposed immune surveillance escape mechanisms include antigenic modulation, secretion of immunosuppressive substances, escape and sneaking through , selective stimulation of suppressor cells, production of blocking antibodies, and immunostimulation.

KEY TERMS

Anaplasia, 236
Anchorage-independence, 240
Anchoring junction, 240
Anti-oncogene, 235
Autocrine stimulatory hypothesis, 242
Autonomy, 236
Autostimulation, 242
Carcinogen, 250
Carcinogenesis, 247
Carcinoma, 238
Carcinoma in situ, 238
Cocarcinogen, 249
c-onc, 245
Density-dependent inhibition of growth, 241

Fibronectin, 238
Gap junction, 240
Glioma, 238
Grading, 236
Immortal stem cell, 248
Initiation, 249
Insertional mutagenesis, 246
Leukemia, 238
Lymphoma, 238
Metastasize, 240
Mutagen, 243
Oncogene, 235
Oncogenic virus, 244
Progression, 238, 250
Promotion, 249

Proto-oncogene, 245
Retrovirus, 244
Reverse transcriptase, 244
Sarcoma, 238
Stem cell, 236
Telomerase, 236
Terminally differentiated, 236
Transformation, 236
Tumor-associated antigen (TAA), 259
Tumor cell marker, 240
Tumor immune surveillance theory, 259
Tumor-specific antigen (TSA), 259
Tumor suppressor gene, 235
v-onc, 245

REFERENCES

1. Alberts, B. et al. (1998). *Essential cell biology.* New York: Garland.
2. Chong, E.Y. et al. (1998). Telomerase expression in gliomas including the nonastrocytic tumors. *Human Pathology, 29*(6), 599-603.
3. Fossel, M. (1998). Telomerase and the aging cell: Implications for human health. *Journal of the American Medical Association, 279*(21), 1732-1735.
4. Kolquist, K.A. et al. (1998). Expression of TERT in early premalignant lesions and a subset of cells in normal tissue [see Comments]. *Nature Genetics, 19*(2), 301-304.
5. Sano, T. et al. (1998). Telomerase activity in 144 brain tumors. *British Journal of Cancer, 77*(10), 1633-1637.
6. LeMarbre, P.J. & Groenwald, S.L. (1997). Biology of cancer. In S.L. Groenwald, M.H. Frogge, & M. Goodman (Eds.). *Cancer nursing: Principles and practice* (4th ed.). Boston: Jones & Bartlett.
7. Hakomori, S. (1996). Tumor malignancy defined by aberrant glycosylation and sphingo (glyco) lipid metabolism. *Cancer Research, 5b,* 5309-5318.
8. Sames, D., Chen, X.T., & Danishefsky, S.J. (1997). Convergent total synthesis of a tumor-associated mucin motif. *Nature, 389*(6651), 587-591.
9. Templeton, D.J. & Weinberg, R.A. (1995). Principles of cancer biology. In G.P. Murphy, W. Lawrence, Jr., & R.E. Lenhard (Eds.). *ACS textbook of clinical oncology* (2nd ed.). Atlanta: American Cancer Society.
10. Albright, C.D. & Kaufman, D.G. (1995). Transforming growth factor-beta 1 mediates communication between human endometrial carcinoma cells and stromal cells. *Pathobiology, 63,* 314-319.
11. Konishi, N., Donovan, P.J., & Waro, J.M. (1990). Differential effects of renal carcinogenesis tumor promoter on growth promotion and inhibition of gap junctional communication. *Carcinogenesis, 11*(6), 903-908.

REFERENCES

12. Krutovskikh, V.A. et al. (1995). Inhibition of rat liver gap junction intercellular communication by tumor-promoting agents in vivo: Association with aberrant localization of connexin in proteins. *Laboratory Investigation, 72*(5), 571-577.

13. Miki, H. et al. (1990). Effect of TPA on intercellular communication in various clones of mouse epidermal cells. *Cancer Research, 50,* 1324-1329.

14. Hamada, J. et al. (1991). Junctional communication of highly and weakly metastatic variant clones from a rat mammary carcinoma in primary and metastatic sites. *Invasion and Metastasis, 11,* 149-157.

15. Douglas, R.G. & Shaw, J.H.F. (1990). Metabolic effects of cancer. *British Journal of Surgery, 77,* 246-254.

16. Weber, G. (1977). Enzymology of cancer cells. I. *New England Journal of Medicine, 296,* 486-492.

17. Sachs, L. (1987). The molecular control of blood cell development. *Science, 238,* 1374-1379.

18. Kahn, P. & Graf, T. (Eds.). (1986). Malignant transformation as a multistep process. In *Oncogenes and growth control.* New York: Springer-Verlag.

19. Jorde, L.B. et al. (1999). *Medical genetics* (2nd ed). St. Louis: Mosby.

20. Jorde, L.B. et al. (1995). *Medical genetics.* St. Louis: Mosby.

21. Cavanee, W.K. & White, R.L. (1995). The genetic basis of cancer. *Scientific American, 272,* 72-79.

22. Hausen, H.Z. (1991). Viruses in human cancers. *Science, 254,* 1167-1173.

23. Quan, M.B., & Moy, R.L. (1991). The role of human papillomavirus in carcinoma. *Journal of the American Academy of Dermatology, 25,* 698-702.

24. Weinberg, R.A. (1995). The molecular basis of carcinogenesis: Understanding the cell cycle clock. *Cytokines Molecular Therapy, 2*(2), 105-110.

25. Kamb, A. et al. (1994). A cell cycle regulator potentially involved in genesis of many tumor types. *Science, 264,* 436-437.

26. Alberts, J.M. & Cory, S. (1991). Transgenic models of tumor development. *Science, 254,* 1161-1167.

27. Solomon, E., Borrow, J., & Goddard, A.D. (1991). Chromosome aberrations and cancer. *Science, 254,* 1153-1160.

28. Hasler, C.M., Bennick, M.R., & Trosko, J.E. (1991). Inhibition of gap junction–mediated intercellular communication by alpha-linolenate. *Journal of Physiology, 261*(1, Pt. 1), 161-168.

29. Trosko, J.E. & Chang, C.C. (1989). Stem cell theory of carcinogenesis. *Toxicology Letters, 4*(2-3), 283-295.

30. Rous, P. & Kidd, J.G. (1941). Conditional neoplasms and subthreshold neoplastic states. *Journal of Experimental Medicine, 73,* 365.

31. Ames, B.N., Magaw, R., & Gold, L.S. (1987). Ranking possible carcinogenic hazards. *Science, 236,* 271-280.

32. Boutwell, R.K. (1964). Some biological aspects of skin carcinogenesis. *Progress in Experimental Tumor Research, 4,* 207-250.

33. Cinciripnin, P.M. & McClure, J.B. (1998). Smoking cessation: Recent developments in behavioral and pharmacologic interventions. *Oncology - Huntington, 12*(2), 249-256, 259, 260, 265.

34. Boyle, P. (1997). Cancer. Cigarette smoking and premature death in Europe: A review including the recommendations of European Cancer Experts Consensus Meeting, Helsinki, October 1996. *Lung Cancer, 71*(1), 1-60.

35. Richardson, T.L. (1997). African-American smokers and cancers of the lung and of the upper respiratory and digestive tracts. Is menthol part of the puzzle? *Western Journal of Medicine, 166*(3), 189-194.

36. Doll, R. & Peto, R. (1981). *The causes of cancer.* New York: Oxford University Press.

37. Henderson, B.E., Ross, R.K., & Pike, M.C. (1991). Toward the primary prevention of cancer. *Cancer Science, 254,* 1131-1137.

38. Tredaniel, J. et al. (1993). Environmental tobacco smoke and the risk of cancer in adults. *European Journal of Cancer, 29A*(14), 2058-2068.

39. Adlercreutz, H. (1990). Western diet and Western diseases: Some hormonal and biochemical mechanisms and associations. *Scandinavian Journal of Clinical Laboratory Investigation, 50*(Suppl. 201), 3-23.

40. Rose, D.P. (1997). Dietary fatty acids and prevention of hormone-responsible cancer. *Proceedings of the Society for Experimental Biology and Medicine, 216*(2), 224-233.

41. Carroll, K.K. (1991). Dietary fats and cancer. *American Journal of Clinical Nutrition, 53*(4), 10654-10675.

42. Kelsey, J. & Gammon, M.D. (1991). The epidemiology of breast cancer. *CA: A Cancer Journal for Clinicians, 41*(3), 146-165.

43. Ames, B.N. (1983). Dietary carcinogens and anticarcinogens. *Science, 221,* 1256.

44. Spingarn, N.E., Slocum, L.A., & Weisburger, J.H. (1980). Formation of mutagens in cooked foods. II. Foods with high starch content. *Cancer Letters, 9,* 7-12.

45. Raloff, J. (1994). Meaty carcinogens: A risk to the cook? *Science News, 146*(7), 97-112.

46. Odeleye, O.E. et al. (1990). Dietary polyunsaturated fatty acid promoter peroxidation and its role in the promotion of cancer. *Advances in Experimental Medical Biology, 283,* 789-791.

47. Simopoulos, A.P. (1991). Omega-3 fatty acids in health and disease and in growth and development. *American Journal of Clinical Nutrition, 54*(3), 438-463.

48. Shamberger, R.J., Tytko, S.A., & Willis, C.E. (1976). Antioxidants and cancer. VI. Selenium and age adjusted human cancer mortality. *Archives of Environmental Health, 31,* 231-235.

REFERENCES

49. Blott, W.J. & Fraumeni, J.F., Jr. (1982). Geographic epidemiology of cancer in the United States. In D. Schottenfield & J.F. Fraumeni, Jr. (Eds.). *Cancer epidemiology and prevention.* Philadelphia: Saunders.

50. American Cancer Society (ACS). (1997). Cancer statistics 1997. *CA: A Cancer Journal for Clinicians, 47*(1), 54-27.

51. Horn-Ross, P.L., Ljung, B.M., & Morrow, M. (1997). Environmental factors and the risk of salivary gland cancer. *Epidemiology, 8*(4), 414-419.

52. Rohan, T.E. & McMichael, A.J. (1988). Alcohol consumption and risk of breast cancer. *International Journal of Cancer, 41*, 695-699.

53. Willett, W.C. et al. (1987). Fat and the risk of breast cancer. *New England Journal of Medicine, 316*(1), 22-28.

54. Young, T.B. (1989). A case-control study of breast cancer and alcohol consumption habits. *Cancer, 64*, 552-558.

55. Kjaer, S.K. et al. (1996). Human papillomavirus—The most significant risk determinant of cervical intraepithelial neoplasia. *International Journal of Cancer, 65*, 601-606.

56. Fontaine, P. (1998). Endometrial cancer, cervical cancer, and the adnexal mass. *Primary Care, 25*(2), 435-457.

57. Southern, S.A. & Herrington, C.S. (1998). Molecular events in uterine cervical cancer. *Sexually Transmitted Infections, 74*(2), 101-109.

58. Cuzick, J. et al. (1994). Type-specific human papillomavirus DNA in abnormal smears as a predictor of high-grade cervical intraepithelial neoplasia. *British Journal of Cancer, 69*(1), 167-171.

59. Ho, G.Y. et al. (1998). Natural history of cervicovaginal papillomavirus infection in young women. *New England Journal of Medicine, 338*(7), 423-428.

60. Rutter, D.O. (1996). Healing their wounds. *Catalyst, 15*(4), 12.

61. Devesa, S.S. & Diamond, E.L. (1980). Association of breast cancer and cervical cancer incidences with income and education among whites and blacks. *National Cancer Institute, 65*, 515-528.

62. Blair, A. & Kazerowni, N. (1998). Reactive chemicals and cancer. *Cancer Causes and Control, 8*(3), 473-490.

63. Epstein, S.S. & Swartz, J.B. (1981). Fallacies of lifestyle cancer theories. *Nature, 289*, 127.

64. Howard, D.J. et al. (1998). Environmental tobacco smoke in the workplace induces oxidative stress in employees, including increased production of 8-hydroxy-2^1-deoxyguanosine. *Cancer Epidemiology, Biomarkers and Prevention, 7*(2), 141-146.

65. Law, M.R., Morris, J.K., & Wald, N.J. (1997). Environmental tobacco smoke exposure and ischemic heart disease: An evaluation of the evidence. *British Medical Journal, 315*, 973-980.

66. Jenks, S. (1992). Researchers open a molecular window on radon damage in lung cancer. *Journal of the National Cancer Institute, 84*(7), 473-474.

67. Pershagen, G. et al. (1994). Residential radon exposure and lung cancer in Sweden. *New England Journal of Medicine, 330*(3), 159-164.

68. Polpong, E. & Borornkitti, S. (1998). Indoor radon. *Journal of the Medical Association of Thailand, 81*(1), 47-57.

69. Neuberger, T. & Allen, A. (1997). Lung cancer risk from residential radon: Meta-analysis of eight epidemiologic studies. *Journal of the National Cancer Institute, 89*(9), 663-664, discussion 664-665.

70. Vahakangas, K.H. et al. (1992). Mutations of p53 and ras genes in radon-associated lung cancer from uranium miners. *Lancet, 339*(8793), 576-580.

71. Calvert, G.M. et al. (1998). Cancer risks among workers exposed to metalworking fluids: A systematic review. *American Journal of Industrial Medicine, 33*(3), 282-292.

72. Demers, R. (1991). Overview of radon, lead, and asbestos exposure. *American Family Physician, 44*(Suppl. 5), 51S-52S, 55S-61S.

73. McNutt, N.S. et al. (1994). Abnormalities of p53 protein expression in cutaneous disorders [Editorial]. *Archives of Dermatology, 130*(2), 225-232.

74. Streilein, J.W. et al. (1994). Immune surveillance and sunlight-induced skin cancer. *Immunology Today, 15*(4), 174-179.

75. Kricker, A., Armstrong, B.K., & Parkin, D.M. (1993). Measurement of skin cancer incidence. *Health Reports, 5*(1), 63-66.

76. Scotto, J., Fears, T.R., & Gori, G.B. (1976). *Measurements of ultraviolet radiation in the United States and comparisons with skin cancer data* (DHEW Publication No. NIH 76-1029, pp. 3.1-3.10). Washington, D.C.: U.S. Government Printing Office.

77. Thompson, S.C., Jolley, D., & Marks, R. (1993). Reduction of solar keratoses by regular sunscreen use. *New England Journal of Medicine, 329*(16), 1147-1151.

78. Naylor, M.F. & Farmer, K.C. (1997). The case for sunscreens: A review of their use in preventing actinic damage and neoplasia. *Archives of Dermatology, 133*(9), 1146-1154.

79. Doll, R. & Wakeford, R. (1997). Risk of childhood cancer from fetal irradiation [see Comment]. *British Journal of Radiology, 70*, 130-139.

80. Repacholi, M.H. (1998). Low-level exposure to radiofrequency electromagnetic fields: Health effects and research needs. *Bioelectromagnetics, 19*(1), 1-19.

81. Feinberg, J.S. & Kelley, C.R. (1998). Pregnant workers: A physician's guide to assessing safe employment. *Western Journal of Medicine, 168*(2), 86-92.

82. Paul, C., Skegg, D.C.G., & Spears, G.F.S. (1995). Oral contraceptive use and risk of breast cancer in older women. *Cancer Causes and Control, 6*, 485-491.

REFERENCES

83. Gadducci, A. & Genazzani, A. R. (1997). Steroid hormones in endometrial and breast cancer. *European Journal of Gynaecology and Oncology, 18*(5), 371-378.

84. Hulka, B.S. (1997). Epidemiologic analysis of breast and gynecologic cancers. *Progress in Clinical Biology Research, 396,* 17-29.

85. Persson, I., Thurfjell, E., & Holmberg, L. (1997). Effect of estrogen and estrogen-progestin replacement regimens on mammographic breast parenchymal density. *Journal of Clinical Oncology, 15*(10), 3201-3207.

86. Thomas, H.V., Reeves, G.K., & Key, T.J. (1997). Endogenous estrogen and postmenopausal breast cancer: A quantitative review. *Cancer Causes and Control, 8*(6), 922-928.

87. Herbst, A.L., Ultelder, H., & Poskanzer, D.C. (1971). Adenocarcinomas of the vagina: Association of maternal stilbestrol therapy with tumor appearance in young females. *New England Journal of Medicine, 284,* 878-881.

88. Grodstein, F. et al. (1997). Postmenopausal hormone use and risk for colorectal cancer and adenoma. *Annals of Internal Medicine, 128*(9), 705-712.

89. Thomas, D.B. (1993). Breast cancer in men. *Epidemiological Review, 15*(1), 220-231.

90. Penn, I. (1994). De novo malignancy in pediatric organ transplant recipients. *Journal of Pediatric Surgery, 29*(2), 221-226; discussion 227-228.

CHAPTER

10

Tumor Spread and Treatment

Kathryn L. McCance and Lee K. Roberts

Metastasis is the major cause of illness and death from most human malignant diseases. Approximately 40% to 50% of malignant tumors are cured by current therapies.[1] However, most cancer patients experience multiple metastases, too small to be detected, at the time the primary tumor is treated. Consequently, an important goal is to develop new therapies or analytic approaches that can be used to accurately predict the metastatic potential of a tumor. New therapies will likely come from cell-molecular research into the mechanism of invasion and metastases. Basic research in this important field has lagged behind the attention given to other cancer problems, such as carcinogenesis and cancer genetics. Because of the complexities of the metastatic process, investigators only recently have attempted to study the biochemical mechanisms of cancer invasion.

 Check out your CD Companion for chapter-related exercises and answers to the Quick Check questions

TUMOR SPREAD

Tumor spread throughout the body can take several forms: (1) local spread by direct invasion of contiguous organs, (2) metastasis to distant organs by lymphatics and veins, and (3) metastasis by implantation. Spreading of a tumor depends on its rate of growth, its degree of differentiation, the presence or absence of anatomic barriers, and various biologic factors.

Local Spread

Invasion, or local spread, is a prerequisite for metastasis and the first step in the metastatic process. In its earliest stages, local invasion may occur as a function of direct tumor extension.[2] Eventually, however, cells or clumps of cells detach from the primary tumor and invade the surrounding interstitial spaces. Mechanisms thought to be important in local invasion include (1) cellular multiplication, (2) mechanical pressure, (3) release of lytic enzymes, (4) decreased cell-to-cell adhesion (making cancer cells slippery), and (5) increased motility of individual tumor cells.[1-4] These mechanisms are not mutually exclusive, and successful tumor invasion is likely caused by the combined effects of these five mechanisms.

Cellular multiplication

Invasion depends on the rate of cellular multiplication, which is a function of the cell generation time (through the cell cycle), the number of cells that are dividing (growth fraction), and the cell loss from the tumor. Cells from malignant lesions thus can divide rapidly, but the tumor may not grow because cells are dying rapidly. (The cell cycle is discussed in Chapters 1 and 9.)

Mechanical invasion

Invasion related to mechanical pressure is analogous to the way plants force their roots through the soil (i.e., by building up pressure that forces shoots, or fingerlike projections, along the lines of least mechanical resistance). Pressure from the growing mass blocks local blood vessels, leading to local tissue death and a reduced mechanical resistance that further aids the spread.

Lytic enzymes

Normal tissue adjacent to areas of tumor invasion shows considerable lytic damage. Many animal and human tumors secrete lytic enzymes (e.g., proteases and collagenases, plasminogen activators, lysosomal enzymes) that destroy normal tissue. Tumor cells can either release collagenase (e.g., digest collagen) or secrete collagenolytic substances in latent forms that are converted to active forms by lysosomal proteases such as plasmin.[3] Collagenases break down collagens, or the major structural element of the extracellular matrices where invasion begins (see Three-Step Theory of Invasion).

Several proteases, including heparinases and serine proteases such as plasminogen activator, that are attached to or released from the cell surface appear to increase tumor inva-

sion. Plasminogen activator is increased in tumor cells.[2] It converts the serum proenzyme plasminogen into the protease plasmin, which can degrade a variety of proteins. Plasminogen activator may play an important role in the degradation of the extracellular matrix during tumor cell invasion.

Decreased cell adhesion

Cancer cells do not adhere to one another as well as normal cells. This slippery trait has been related to fibronectin, which regulates cell attachment, spreading, phagocytosis, and cell structure effects. Fibronectin also stimulates cell movement and generally acts as an anchoring molecule. Cancer cells may make a defective type of fibronectin, or they may break down fibronectin as they make it.[5,6] Low levels or loss of this fibronectin may help cancer cells slip between normal cells in the process of invasion.

Increased motility

Cell movement is key for tumor cells to invade. The invasion process includes the detachment and subsequent infiltration of cells from the primary tumor into adjacent tissue, the migration of cells through the vascular wall into the circulation (intravasation), and movement out of the vascular wall (extravasation) into a secondary site (Fig. 10-1). Data suggest that tumor cells move under their own power by means of chemotactic factors referred to as *autocrine motility factors.* The *autocrine motility factor hypothesis* specifies that the tumor cell secretes a factor that binds to a specific receptor on the cell surface and stimulates motility (Fig. 10-2). In this way the tumor cell acquires independent and continuous stimulation of its motile behavior, which is necessary for invasion.[1] Investigators have identified motility factors from metastatic melanoma (skin cancer) cells.[7]

The Three-Step Theory of Invasion

A three-step theory has been proposed to describe the sequence of biochemical events during tumor cell invasion of the extracellular matrix (Fig. 10-3). The three steps include tumor cell attachment to the matrix, degradation or dissolution of the matrix, and locomotion into the matrix. The first step, attachment, is mediated by specific attachment factors such as laminin, a complex glycoprotein that is a major constituent of all basement membranes. Membrane vesicles on the cell surface of tumor cells are rich in laminin receptors that allow them to attach to basement membrane.[8] Laminin forms a bridge between the cell-surface *laminin receptor* and type IV collagen (see Fig. 10-3). In step two, the anchored tumor cells either secrete proteolytic enzymes or induce host cells to produce them. These proteolytic enzymes may degrade both the attachment proteins and the structural collagenous proteins of the matrix. *Type IV collagenase,* a powerful proteolytic enzyme, may outnumber the natural protease inhibitors present in the matrix. The third step is tumor cell locomotion into the degraded region of the matrix. Fingerlike projections called *pseudopodia,* which extend from the tumor cell (Fig. 10-4), facilitate movement by

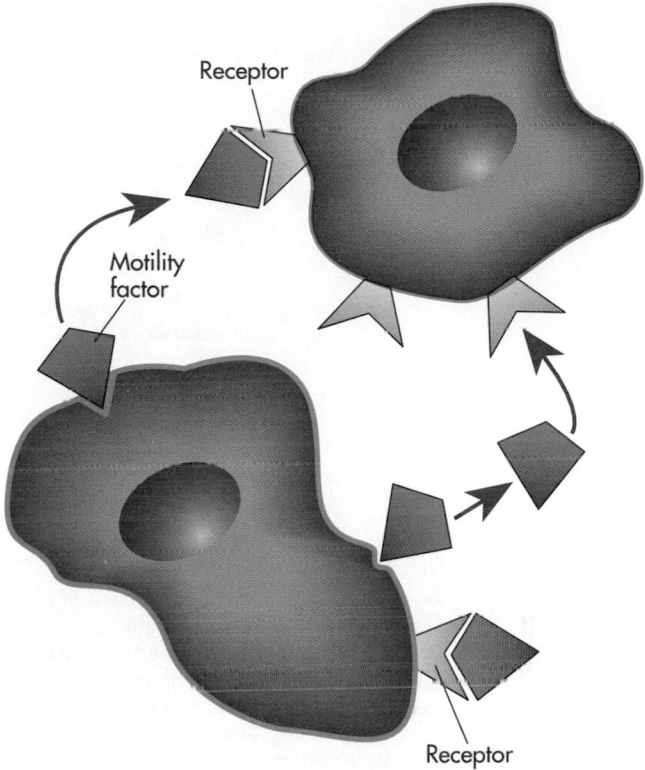

Fig. 10-2 *The autocrine motility factor hypothesis.* Certain tumor cells make and secrete a motility factor that can then activate itself or other tumor cells, presumably through a cell-surface receptor.

Fig. 10-1 *Pathogenesis of metastasis.* Initial neoplastic transformation of susceptible cells gives rise to a small population of tumor cells. Vascularization of this initial neoplastic lesion allows further proliferation of tumor cells and enlargement of the primary tumor. Malignant cells within the primary tumor next begin to invade the surrounding host tissue or tissues. Entry of invading tumor cells into lymphatics or blood vessels serves to transport them to distant sites in the body, where they lodge and become arrested in the capillary beds of various organs. For illustrative purposes, this figure shows arrest of malignant cells in the lung capillary bed. The arrested cells then exit from capillaries into the surrounding lung parenchyma where, subject to provision of a suitable environment, they proliferate to form metastases. *(From Poste, G. & Fidler, I.J. [1980]. The pathogenesis of cancer metastasis.* Nature, 20, *139-145.)*

attaching to blood vessel walls that cross the basement membrane. The tumor cells then extravasate from the vasculature into the interstitial stroma. Theoretically, invasion occurs by cyclic repetition of these steps. The direction of locomotion may be influenced by chemotactic factors (see discussion of autocrine motility factors, p. 270).

Patterns of Spread: Metastasis

Metastasis, the spread of tumor cells from a primary site of origin to a distant site, is the life-threatening characteristic of cancer. Therapies can successfully eradicate *primary tumors* (original sites of tumor origin), but the real challenge for reducing cancer mortality is controlling metastasis, because removal of the primary tumor does not affect tumor growth at other sites. Often the primary tumor is not even diagnosed before secondary spread occurs. Metastasis involves a series of sequential steps: (1) direct or continuous extension of local invasion of tumor cells into surrounding tissue; (2) penetration into lymphatics, blood vessels, or body cavities; (3) release into lymph or blood; (4) transport to secondary sites; and (5) entry and growth in secondary sites (see Fig. 10-1). These steps are not mutually exclusive. Tumor cell spread or dissemination through one pathway often facilitates metastasis through other pathways because tumor cells can access many microscopic anatomic connections.

Steps 1 and 2
Attachment and dissolution

Step 3
Anchoring and locomotion

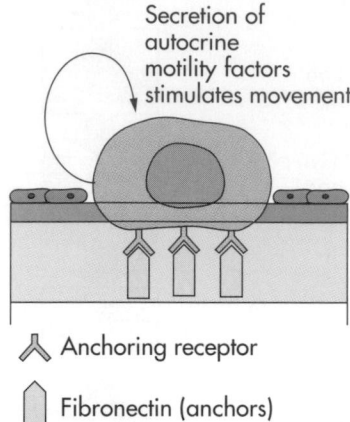

Fig. 10-3 *The three-step hypothesis of tumor invasion: attachment, dissolution, and locomotion.*
Step 1 is tumor cell attachment to the extracellular matrix. Surface receptors on the tumor cell (laminin receptors) bind to parts of the basement membrane (laminin) in the extracellular matrix. Step 2 is degradation of the matrix by tumor cell proteases (type IV collagenase). The anchored tumor cell either secretes proteolytic enzymes or causes the host cell to secrete the proteolytic enzymes that degrade the matrix in a region very close to the tumor cell surface. Step 3 is the migration (locomotion) of the tumor cell through the degraded basement membrane. During this phase, pseudopodia (fingerlike projections) of the tumor cell cross the basement membrane, enabling the cell to extravasate from the blood vessel into the interstitial tissue (see Fig. 10-4).

Fig. 10-4 *Pseudopodia.* Electron micrograph of a breast cancer cell with fingerlike projections called *pseudopodia. (From National Library of Medicine.)*

Direct or continuous extension

The earliest result of invasion could be called *continuous extension.*[5] Cancerous tumors may extend into surrounding tissues as they grow without breaking away from the parent (primary) tumor mass. Direct tumor extension, once thought to result from simple growth pressure only, now is

believed to be initiated by the complex sequence of events discussed earlier. They are initiated by loss of intracellular adhesion that enables cells to slip past one another. Movement of cells through tissue barriers is further influenced by proteases and (autocrine) motility factors (see section on local invasion, p. 270).

Metastasis by lymphatics and bloodstream

Tumor cells spread to distant sites by first penetrating blood vessels or lymphatics. Lymphatics and thin-walled venules offer relatively little mechanical resistance to penetration by tumor cells. Blood vessels within tumors offer malignant cells direct access into the circulation. Clusters, single cells, and fragments of tumor cells become separated from the primary tumor site and disseminate by these routes. Clumps of cells have a better chance of successful metastasis than do single cells. Conversely, cancers close to a serous surface can invade through that surface, implant, and become distant metastases, also known as *seeding.* Cancer seeding occurs in the pleural space surrounding the lung and in the peritoneal space surrounding the abdominal cavity.

The most common route for distant metastases is through the lymphatics. Tumors generally lack a well-formed lymphatic network.[2,4] Lymphatic channels occur at the periphery of the tumor and not within the tumor mass. Tumor cells entering the lymphatic vessels are carried to regional lymph nodes. For many types of cancer, the first evidence of distant spread is a mass in the regional lymph node. For example, an enlarged axillary lymph node may signal breast cancer. Initially, regional lymph nodes may exert a barrier effect, preventing the further spread of tumor cells into the lymphatic system. Host defenses, such as macrophages and natural killer (NK) cells, play an important role in the elimination of circulating metastatic tumor cells.[2] Several events can occur when a cancer cell becomes lodged in a lymph node, including (1) death as a result of a local inflammatory reaction or an incompatible local environment, (2) growth into a discernible lump, (3) sustained dormancy for unknown reasons, or (4) detachment from the node and entrance into the efferent lymphatics.

When small lymphatic vessels are penetrated, tumor cell emboli are released into these lymphatic vessels and are responsible for lymphatic metastasis. Shedding of emboli is influenced by changes in vessel pressure, by turbulent alterations in lymphatic flow, and by movements or manipulation of the tumor during diagnostic tests or surgery. Tumor cells eventually move into the regional or systemic venous drainage because of numerous venolymphatic communications.

Cancer metastasis through the bloodstream is a complex process. Vascularized tumors shed malignant cells constantly as they grow, often releasing millions of cells without producing metastases.[3,9] To establish metastasis, tumor cells must escape host defenses, survive mechanical trauma in the bloodstream, and lodge in the vascular bed of the target organ.[7] About 80% of the tumor cells circulate as single cells and attach directly to the endothelial surface or to preexisting regions of exposed subendothelial basement membrane.[1] Emboli or tumor cells that contain leukocytes, fibrin, or platelets can cause direct embolization in the precapillary venules by mechanical action. The formation of a fibrin-platelet complex may protect tumor cells within the emboli from host defenses and assist in successful attachment to the vascular epithelium.[2] Once arrested in a blood vessel, tumor cells can actively invade the vascular wall, interstitial stroma, and parenchyma of the target organ. Growth in target organ parenchyma requires that a vascular network develop (angiogenesis) and host defenses be ineffective.

Angiogenesis and angiogenesis factors

Growth of cancerous colonies depends on an adequate blood supply. Tumor implants cannot grow more than a few millimeters in diameter without developing new blood vessels to feed them, a process called **angiogenesis**.[10] Several factors can trigger blood vessel formation in a tumor, including vascular endothelial growth factor (VEGF), platelet-derived growth factor (PDGF), transforming growth factor−alpha (TGF-α), and basic fibroblast growth factor (FGF).[11,12] For example, a sudden drop in the cancer cell's production of **thrombospondin**—a protein that inhibits the growth of new blood vessels—can trigger angiogenesis. Normal tissues control the development of new blood vessels by regulating thrombospondin levels.[13] Blood vessels also develop in response to diffusible substances secreted by the tumor, such as **tumor-angiogenesis factor (TAF)** (see Fig. 10-1).

The rate of spread, as well as the growth of the tumor, is correlated with tumor vascularity in clinical situations. For example, small cell carcinoma of the lung arises in highly vascularized capillary beds and spreads easily and widely to other vascular organs, such as the brain.

Growth of metastases and metastatic potential

A metastasis grows and develops when a vascular network is developed, host defenses are evaded, and a compatible environment is available ("the soil"). The metastatic potential of many common carcinomas was thought to be related to the size of the primary tumor.[14] Newer data, however, suggest the "stresses" endured by cancer cells, even in small tumors, promote the emergence of stronger, more aggressive tumors.[15-17] More aggressive malignant cells may evolve into larger tumors that overwhelm their host's immune defense systems.

Distribution and common sites of distant metastases

Distant metastasis in many types of cancer appears to take place in the first capillary bed encountered by the circulating cells.[14,18] Table 10-1 summarizes frequent sites of metastases in various cancers. Patterns of metastasis for certain other tumors, however, are not related to patterns of blood flow or the location of capillary beds.[19] Instead, they show preferential growth in certain organs, called *organ tropism*. Ocular melanoma, for example, frequently metastasizes to the liver, and clear cell kidney carcinomas often spread to bone and the thyroid. Organ tropism may be the result of local growth factors or hormones present in the target organ, preferential adherence to the surface of certain target organs, or the presence of chemotactic factors that diffuse from the target organ and cause circulating tumor cells to leave the vessel and gather in the target organ.[2] Organ tropism is determined genetically. Tumor cells contain organ-specific receptors that can discriminate between various vascular beds and preferentially locate to certain organs.[2,20]

Staging

Tumor staging involves the size of the tumor, the degree to which it has locally invaded, and the extent to which it has spread (metastasized). One common scheme for standardizing staging is the **TNM system;** T is for tumor spread, N is for node involvement, and M is the presence of distant metastasis (Fig. 10-5).

✓ QUICK CHECK

Explain how tumors metastasize, defining each of the steps involved.

List four examples of the frequent sites of metastases of various cancers, and explain why these are targets of metastases.

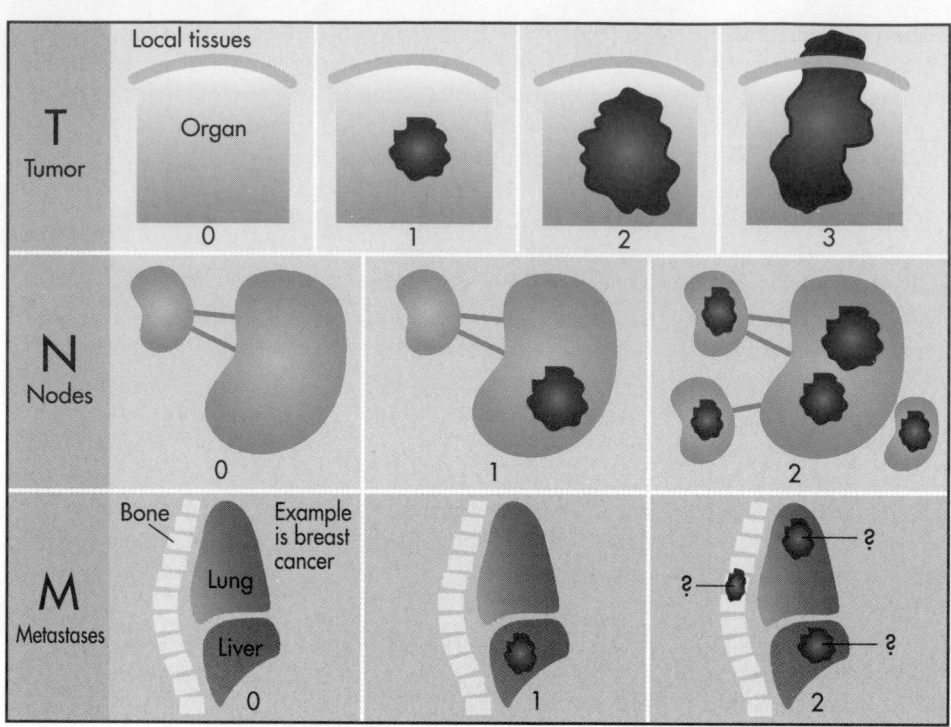

T= Primary tumor; the number equals size of tumor and its local extent. The number can vary according to site.

T0= Breast free of tumor
T1= Lesion < 2 cm in size
T2= Lesion 2-5 cm
T3= Skin and/or chest wall involved by invasion

N= Lymph node involvement; a higher number means more nodes are involved.

N0= No axillary nodes involved
N1= Mobile nodes involved
N2= Fixed nodes involved

M= Extent of distant metastases.

M0= No metastases
M1= Demonstrable metastases
M2= Suspected metastases

Fig. 10-5 *Tumor staging by the TNM system.* (See figure for abbreviations.)

CLINICAL MANIFESTATIONS OF CANCER
Pain

Usually little or no pain is associated with the early stages of malignant disease, but pain occurs in 60% to 80% of those patients who are terminally ill with cancer. Pain is strongly influenced by fear, anxiety, sleep loss, fatigue, and overall physical deterioration. It occurs through an interaction among psychogenic, cultural, and physiologic components.[21,22] (The neurophysiology of pain is discussed in Chapter 13.)

General mechanisms that cause pain associated with cancer include pressure, obstruction, invasion of a sensitive structure, stretching of visceral surfaces, tissue destruction, and inflammation. The pain may be directly related to the malignancy or can result from other problems, such as infection. Bone metastasis causes pain that may be referred away from the involved bone and manifest, for example, as back pain. Bone pain can be caused by periosteal irritation, medullary pressure, and pathologic fractures.

Abdominal pain often is caused by severe stretching from the tumor invasion of the hollow viscus. Tumors that obstruct and distend the bowel cause pain. Small bowel obstructions in persons with known malignant disease commonly result from recurrent cancer, surgical adhesions, or new primary tumors. Surgery often is needed to obtain relief. Hepatic malignancies stretch the liver, resulting in a dull pain or a feeling of fullness over the right upper abdominal quadrant.

Tumors compressing nerve endings create pain. Brain tumors, in particular, have very little space to grow without compressing blood vessels and nerve endings between the tumor and the cranial vault. Infection and necrosis can destroy tissue and cause pain. The oral area, which frequently has ulcerative lesions, often is infected and painful.

The adequacy of pain control should be evaluated regularly. The way that pain is perceived and treated is influenced by one's ethnocultural background.[23] The first priority of treatment is to control pain rapidly and completely as judged by the patient.[22] The second priority is to prevent recurrence of pain.

Fatigue

Fatigue is the most frequently reported symptom of cancer and cancer treatment. The exact mechanisms that produce fatigue are poorly understood. Suggested causes include sleep disturbances, various biochemical changes secondary to disease and treatment, numerous psychosocial factors, level of activity, nutritional status, and other environmental and physical factors.[24]

The physiologic understanding of fatigue probably includes mechanisms for decreased muscle contractility. Overall, studies of muscle function suggest that some individuals with cancer may lose portions of muscle function needed to perform normal physical activities.[24] Other areas of research include muscle function consequences from metabolic products of cancer treatment and associated muscle loss from circulating cytokines (e.g., tumor necrosis factor [TNF] and interleukin-1 [IL-1]).

TABLE 10-1	Frequent Sites of Distant Metastasis in Some Types of Cancer	
Primary Tumor	**Major Anatomic Pathways**	**Common Site of Distant Metastasis**
Lung	Pulmonary vein, left ventricle	Multiple organs, including brain
Colorectal	Mesenteric lymphatics, portal venous system	Liver
	Inferior vena cava, right ventricle, pulmonary artery	Lungs
Testicular	Lymphatics to the periaortic area to the subclavian veins to the right ventricle	Lungs, Liver
Prostate	Batson plexus of paravertebral veins, ilium, lumbar spine	Bones, lungs, liver, endocrine glands, central nervous system
Breast	Batson plexus of paravertebral veins, lymph nodes, superior vena cava	Bony skeleton, lungs
Head and Neck	Direct extension, Batson plexus	Lymphatics, liver, bones
Ovarian	Direct extension	Peritoneal surfaces, diaphragm
	Omentum and mesenteric veins	Omentum, liver
Sarcoma (extremity)	Inferior vena cava, right ventricle, pulmonary artery	Lungs

From Brown, J.M. & Giaccia, A.J. (1998). The unique physiology of solid tumors: Opportunities (and problems) for cancer therapy. Cancer Research 58(7), 1408-1416.

Fig. 10-6 *Cachexia.* Sunken appearance of the eyes, cheeks, and temporal areas; sharp nose; dry, rough skin. *(From Seidel, H.M. et al. [1999]. Mosby's guide to physical examination [4th ed.]. St. Louis: Mosby.)*

Similar to pain, fatigue is a subjective clinical manifestation. Fatigue is described by individuals with cancer as tiredness, weakness, lack of energy, exhaustion, lethargy, inability to concentrate, depression, sleepiness, boredom, lack of motivation, and decreased mental status.[24]

Cachexia

The syndrome of *cachexia* includes anorexia, early satiety (filling), weight loss, anemia, asthenia (marked weakness), taste alterations, and altered protein, lipid, and carbohydrate metabolism (Fig. 10-6). Cachexia is the most severe form of malnutrition associated with cancer and results in wasting, emaciation, and decreased quality of life. Anorexia, or loss of appetite, frequently can be attributed to pain, depression, chemotherapy, or radiotherapy. Alterations in taste also can account for the anorexia in cancer patients by making foods seem bland or distasteful.

Anorexia leads to a protein-energy malnutrition (PEM) of three types: (1) similar to kwashiorkor, (2) similar to marasmus, and (3) a combination of the two. Kwashiorkor is a form of malnutrition that evolves from a protein-deficient diet, in which calories come primarily from carbohydrates. Marasmus is a form of malnutrition resulting from a decreased intake of calories and proteins. There is also an associated prolonged and gradual wasting of muscle mass. A combination of kwashiorkor and marasmus results in hypoalbuminemia, edema, diminished immunologic competence (which depends on normal protein stores), and an overall physical deterioration. (Malnutrition is discussed in detail in Chapter 34.)

Progressive weight loss in the person with cancer occurs despite normal or increased food intake. Starvation usually lowers the basal metabolic rate (BMR), but in cancer patients, BMRs are high. How increased BMR and weight loss relate to a breakdown of protein and nitrogen loss or negative nitrogen balance is unclear. This increase may be a result of accelerated metabolic activity of the tumor itself. Malignant cells replicate more rapidly than normal cells and require more food for their growth at the expense of normal tissue. The normal tissue, over time, is sacrificed, and waste begins to occur. Alterations in protein, lipid, and carbohydrate metabolism undoubtedly play a role.

Altered carbohydrate metabolism causes a syndrome resembling diabetes mellitus. Individuals show hyperinsulinemia, insulin resistance, hyperglycemia, and abnormal glucose tolerance test results. These disturbances cause increased gluconeogenesis, which produces glucose from amino acids. In starvation, protein usually is spared to protect vital structures, but in cancer, protein and fatty acids are used to meet energy needs.

An unusual and frustrating component of cancer care is the person's early satiety, or a sense of being full after only a few mouthfuls of food. Tumor metabolites may be responsible for the cachectic state. Several factors have been identified, including serotonin, bombesin, and lipolytic factors;

TABLE 10-2	Factors Predisposing Individuals With Cancer to Infection
Factor	**Basis**
Age	Many common malignancies occur mostly in older age.
	Immunologic functions decline with age.
	General debility reduces immunocompetence.
	Immobility predisposes to infection.
	Far-advanced cancer often results in immobility and general debility that worsens with age.
	Elderly persons are predisposed to nutritional inadequacies.
	Malnutrition impairs immunocompetence.
Tumor	Nutritional derangements can be caused.
	Sites and circumstances favorable to growth of microorganisms (obstruction, serous or blood effusion, ulceration) can be created.
	Far-advanced disease predisposes patients to debility and immobility.
	Humoral or cellular immune defects may be caused.
	Metastasis to bone marrow may cause leukopenia or other defects in immunity.
Leukemias	Inadequate granulocyte production (impaired phagocytosis) results.
	Thrombocytopenia (bleeding, breaks in skin integrity) can occur.
	Late effect: Chronic lung disease from *Pneumocystis carnii* pneumonia can develop during therapy.
Lymphomas and other reticuloendothelial malignancies	Humoral and cellular immune defects (anergy, altered immunoglobin production) result.
	Late effect: Splenectomy in children can cause increased susceptibility to infection.
Treatment surgery	Invasive procedure interrupts first lines of defense.
	Radical nature of surgery (removal of large blocks of tissue in lengthy procedures) causes hemorrhage, decreased tissue perfusion, creation of dead spaces, devitalization of tissues.
	Procedure may be "dirty" surgery (bowel, infected or contaminated areas).
	Surgery patients are often older and at poor risk.
	Long preoperative hospitalization often precedes surgery.
	Patients may have had previous adrenocorticosteroid therapy.
	Patients may have infections at sites remote from operative area.
	Nutritional derangements (especially important in head and neck surgery) may result.
	Lymph node dissection may predispose patient to local infection and impair containment to area.
	Gynecologic surgery may result in fistulas.
	Lung surgery may cause bronchopleural fistulas.
	Debility and immobility may be caused.

From Donovan, M.I. & Girton, S.F. (1984). Cancer care nursing (2nd ed.). New York: Appleton-Century-Crofts; Murphy, G.P., Lawrence, W., & Lenhard, R.E. (1994). Clinical oncology (2nd ed.). New York: American Cancer Society.

however, they have been measured only in a small number of cancers. What seems to be more important in inducing cancer cachexia is a group of cytokines (e.g., tissue hormones) produced by the body in response to cancer. One of the most significant cytokines is the activated macrophage-produced tumor necrosis factor (TNF), also called *cachectin* because of its role in the cachexia syndrome. TNF plays an important role in the defense against viral, bacterial, and parasitic infections; in autoimmune responses; and in the selective destruction of malignant cells.[25] Its overproduction, however, may be detrimental to the host. Other implicated cytokines include IL-1, IL-6, interferon-γ, leukemia inhibitory factor (LIF), and ciliary neurotrophic factor (CNTF).[26] A cancer cachectic factor (a proteoglycan) that causes cachexia in mice and humans has recently been characterized.[27,27a] (Cytokines are discussed in detail in Chapter 6.)

Anemia

Anemia is commonly associated with malignancy, with 20% of patients having hemoglobin concentrations below 9 g/dl (normal value = 15 g/dl). Mechanisms that cause anemia in persons with cancer include chronic bleeding resulting in iron deficiency, severe malnutrition, medical therapies, or malignancy in blood-forming organs. Chronic bleeding and iron deficiency can accompany colorectal or genitourinary malignancy. Iron also is malabsorbed in persons with gastric, pancreatic, or upper intestinal cancer. Often there is a defect in the reutilization of iron because of lack of transfer of iron from the storage pool to blood cell precursors. This defect may be caused by increased secretion of cytokines, such as IL-1, or alterations in nitric oxide regulation. Defects in erythropoietin production and shortened red cell survival have also been documented. In addition, anorexia can cause iron deficiency, although folate deficiency is more common with anorexia.

Anemia normally does not result from chemotherapy, but normochromic (normal hemoglobin concentration) and normocytic (average red cell size) anemias can occur after prolonged administration of alkylating agents or nitrosoureas, which are chemotherapeutic agents. Megaloblastic (large red cell) anemias may develop after methotrexate treatment.

Malignancy of the blood-forming organs is associated with several hemolytic anemias. An autoimmune hemolytic anemia occasionally develops in persons with chronic lymphocytic leukemia. (Anemia associated with leukemia is discussed in Chapter 20.)

Administration of erythropoietin, which stimulates production of erythrocytes, has been effective in correcting anemia in persons with cancer[28,29]; fewer red blood cell transfusions were required in most of the studied subjects. In addition, anemias occurring after chemotherapy or radiotherapy have been treated successfully with erythropoietin.

Leukopenia and Thrombocytopenia

Direct tumor invasion of the bone marrow causes both leukopenia (a decreased leukocyte count) and thrombocytopenia (a decreased number of platelets). Chemotherapeutic drugs are toxic to the bone marrow, often causing granulocytopenia and thrombocytopenia. Leukopenia can result from chemotherapy or radiotherapy of areas of the bone marrow. Thrombocytopenia is a major cause of hemorrhage in persons with cancer. It usually results from chemotherapy or bone marrow involvement by the malignancy. Thrombocytopenia is an accompanying disorder of disseminated intravascular coagulation that occurs in persons with acute promyelocytic leukemia (see Chapter 20) and prostate cancer (see Chapter 32).

Infection

Infection is the most significant cause of complications and death in persons with malignant disease. When the absolute granulocyte or lymphocyte count falls, the risk of infection increases and persons with cancer have reduced immunologic functions, debility with advanced disease, and immunosuppression from radiotherapy and chemotherapy. (Factors that predispose persons with cancer to infection are summarized in Table 10-2.) Surgery also can lower resistance to infection because removal of large quantities of tissue, together with hemorrhage, dead spaces, and poor tissue perfusion, creates favorable sites for infection. Hospital-related (nosocomial) infections increase because of indwelling medical devices, inadequate wound care, and the introduction of microorganisms from visitors and other patients.

Leukopenia resulting from bone marrow radiation dramatically increases the risk of infection. Mucous membranes and other rapidly dividing cells in the radiation field are prone to irritation and ulceration. Radiation, particularly of the cervix, bladder, and intestinal tract, also can lead to fis-

tula formation or abnormal passages between tissue cavities. Surgery often is required to repair the fistula and eliminate continuous infectious cross contaminations.

CANCER TREATMENT

Cancer currently is treated with chemotherapy, radiotherapy, surgery, immunotherapy, and combinations of these modalities (Table 10-3).

Chemotherapy

Several classes of chemotherapeutic agents are used concurrently to treat different types of cancer tumors (Table 10-4). The mechanism by which each drug acts to eradicate tumor cells depends largely on its effect on the cell cycle (described in Chapter 1). Table 10-5 summarizes the mechanisms of action of certain common chemotherapeutic drugs. To be curative, chemotherapy must eradicate enough tumor cells so that the body's own defenses can eradicate the remaining cells.

HEALTH ALERT

New, Less Toxic Drugs

New, more selective compounds and powerful but less toxic versions of older drugs are now used. Oral and water formulations of injectable drugs have made the delivery of chemotherapy more convenient for patients. In the past 4 years, the U.S. Food and Drug Administration (FDA) approved more than 24 new chemotherapy agents. Companies are racing to develop new antioncogenic factors—to inhibit growth-promoting activity of certain genes; antiangiogenic factors—to block the process of developing new blood vessels; and antimetastatic factors—drugs to keep cancer cells confined to one spot.

Radiation

The goals of ionizing radiation are (1) to eradicate cancer without producing excessive toxicity during treatment and (2) to avoid damage to normal structures. Ionizing radiation damages important macromolecules, especially deoxyribonucleic acid (DNA). The damage may be (1) lethal, in which the cell is killed by radiation; (2) potentially lethal, in which the cell is so severely affected by radiation that modifications in its environment will cause it to die; or (3) sublethal, in which the cell can subsequently repair itself. Cellular compartments with rapidly renewing cells are, in general, more radiosensitive. (Cellular effects of ionizing radiation are discussed in Chapter 3.)

Surgery

Surgical therapy is used when the tumor has not yet spread beyond the limits of surgical excision. Surgeons generally agree that if there is any chance of regional lymph node involvement and there is no evidence of distant disease, the lymph nodes should be removed also.

HEALTH ALERT

Lymphatic Mapping

Surgeons are using a widely available new technique, *lymphatic mapping*, in which dyes and radioactive tracers help them to be more selective in removing lymph nodes.

TABLE 10-3 Examples of Treatment of Site-Specific Cancers

Usual Treatment	Site
Surgery	Colon
	Breast
	Ovary
	Lung
	Thyroid
	Skin
	Uterus
Chemotherapy	Lymphoma
	Leukemia
	Choriocarcinoma
	Ovary
	Breast
Radiation	Breast (all have been combined with surgery)
	Uterus or cervix
	Lymphomas
	Lung
	Combined with surgery in many sites
Hormones	Breast
	Prostate
	Endometrium

Modified from Murphy, G.P., Lawrence, W., & Lenhard, R.E. (1995). Clinical oncology *(2nd ed.). New York: American Cancer Society.*

Curative resections are performed if distant metastasis is not evident. The goals of palliative surgery (alleviation without cure) are (1) prevention of symptoms that would have occurred if the individual were not treated and (2) relief of symptoms that are present. Surgery is indicated also for benign tumors that could progress into malignant tumors.

Immunotherapy

Immunotherapy is a specific method of treatment to eliminate cancer cells without damaging normal tissues. The immune system recognizes antigens and is highly regulated; thus antitumor immune rejection responses (described in Chapter 9) can selectively eliminate cancer cells while sparing normal tissues. Immune memory cells are long-lived and can provide extended protection against the emergence of recurrent primary tumor cells and foci of metastatic cancer cells. Numerous immunologic mechanisms cause rejection of various types of cancer. Current research efforts in anticancer immunotherapies focus on characterizing the immunogenic properties of various tumor-specific antigens and developing methods to selectively enhance tumor rejection immune responses, including the development of new vaccines and monoclonal antibodies.

Immunotherapies for the treatment of cancer generally are referred to as *biologic response modifiers (BRMs)*.[30] BRMs are mammalian gene products, agents, and clinical protocols that modify biologic responses in host-tumor interactions. BRMs have the following actions: (1) a direct cytotoxic effect on cancer cells; (2) the initiation or augmentation of the host's tumor-immune rejection response; and (3) the modification of cancer cell susceptibility to the lytic or tumor-static effects of the immune system. BRMs include immunomodulating agents, interferons and interferon inducers, thymosins, antigens (e.g., vaccines), effector cells (e.g., macrophages, NK cells, cytotoxic T cells), lymphokines, cytokines, and monoclonal antibodies.

✓ QUICK CHECK

Why do patients with cancer experience anorexia?

Why do individuals with cancer frequently develop leukopenia and thrombocytopenia?

How do biologic response modifiers affect tumor growth, and why are they important for cancer treatment?

TABLE 10-4 Examples of Chemotherapeutic Drugs

Drug	Major Toxicity
Alkylating agents Mechlorethamine Chlorambucil Melphalan Thiotepa Busulfan Cyclophosphamide Ifosfamide	Therapeutic doses: moderate depression of peripheral blood cell count; excessive doses: severe bone marrow depression, leukopenia, thrombocytopenia, and bleeding; maximum toxicity may occur 2-3 wk after last dose; alopecia; nausea and vomiting
Antimetabolites Methotrexate 6-Mercaptopurine 6-Thioguanine 5-Fluorouracil 5-Fluorodeoxyuridine Cytarabine Fludarabine 2-Chlorodeoxyadenosine 2′-Deoxycoformycin Gemcitabine	Oral and digestive tract ulcerations; bone marrow depression with leukopenia, thrombocytopenia, and bleeding; toxicity enhanced by impaired kidney function; alopecia
Antibiotics Doxorubicin Bleomycin Dactinomycin Daunorubicin Plicamycin Mitomycin-C Mitoxantrone	Stomatitis, gastrointestinal injury; bone marrow depression; alopecia; cardiac toxicity at cumulative doses over 500 mg/m^2 (doxorubicin, daunorubicin); pneumonitis and pulmonary fibrosis at cumulative doses over 400 U (bleomycin); hypocalcemia; hepatic toxicity (plicamycin); nausea and vomiting.

Steroids and hormonally active agents
Androgen
 Fluoxymesterone
Antiandrogen
 Flutamide
Estrogen
 Ethinyl estradiol
 Diethylstilbestrol
Antiestrogen
 Tamoxifen
Progestin
 Megestrol acetate
Luteinizing hormone-releasing
  hormone agonist
  Leuprolide
Aromatase inhibitor
 Aminoglutethimide
Adrenocortical compound
 Dexamethasone
	Fluid retention; masculinization/feminization; hot flashes (sex hormones); hypertension; diabetes; adrenal insufficiency

Miscellaneous drugs Asparaginase	Anorexia, weight loss, somnolence, lethargy, confusion; hypoproteinemia (including albumin and fibrinogen); hyperlipidemia, abnormal liver function tests, fatty metamorphosis of liver; pancreatitis (rare); azotemia; granulocytopenia, lymphopenia, and thrombocytopenia (usually mild and transient)

From Krakoff, IH. (1996). CA: A Cancer Journal for Clinicians 46, 134.

Continued

TABLE 10-4	Examples of Chemotherapeutic Drugs—cont'd
Drug	**Major Toxicity**
Miscellaneous drugs—cont'd	
Altretamine	Bone marrow depression; peripheral neuropathy
m-AMSA	Bone marrow depression; stomatitis; hepatic dysfunction; nausea and vomiting
Carmustine	Bone marrow depression; thrombocytopenia; nausea and vomiting
Lomustine	Bone marrow depression; thrombocytopenia; nausea and vomiting
Streptozocin	Hypoglycemia; nausea and vomiting
Mitotane	Skin eruptions; diarrhea; mental depression; muscle tremors; adrenal insufficiency; nausea and vomiting
Dacarbazine	Bone marrow depression; nausea and vomiting
Hydroxyurea	Bone marrow depression; nausea and vomiting
Etoposide	Alopecia; nausea and vomiting
Cisplatin	Bone marrow depression; renal tubular damage; deafness; nausea and vomiting
Carboplatin	Bone marrow depression; nausea and vomiting
Procarbazine	Bone marrow depression with leukopenia and thrombocytopenia; mental depression; nausea and vomiting
Vinblastine	Alopecia; areflexia; bone marrow depression
Vincristine	Areflexia; muscular weakness; peripheral neuritis; paralytic ileus; mild bone marrow depression
Levamisole	None
Cis-retinoic acid	Cheilitis; stomatitis; conjunctivitis
Paclitaxel	Leukopenia; peripheral neuropathy
Docetaxel	Leukopenia; peripheral neuropathy

TABLE 10-5	Mechanisms of Action of Common Chemotherapeutic Drugs		
Drug	**Mechanism**	**Drug**	**Mechanism**
Actinomycin D	Prevents transcription; inhibits tRNA, mRNA synthesis	Doxorubicin	Binds to DNA
	Inhibits protein synthesis		Uncoils DNA helix
Bleomycin	Breaks and fragments single strands of DNA		Inhibits DNA-directed RNA polymerase
	Damages nonproliferating as well as proliferating cells	Mitomycin	Produces cross-linking of DNA strands
Cytosine arabinoside	Decreases production of DNA replicating units		
	Inhibits transcription		
	Prematurely terminates nucleic acid chains		

▣ DID YOU UNDERSTAND?

Tumor Spread

1. Tumor spread takes several forms: (a) direct invasion, (b) metastasis to distant organs by lymphatics and veins, and (c) metastasis by implantation.
2. Invasion is the first step in the metastatic process. Mechanisms of local invasion include (a) cellular multiplication, (b) mechanical pressure, (c) release of lytic enzymes, (d) decreased adhesion (slipperiness), and (e) increased motility.
3. The three-step theory of invasion includes (a) tumor cell attachment to the matrix, (b) degradation or dissolution of the matrix, and (c) tumor cell locomotion.
4. Metastasis is the life-threatening characteristic of malignancy. The three mechanisms of metastasis are (a) direct or continuous extension, (b) lymphatic spread, and (c) bloodstream dissemination. These mechanisms are not mutually exclusive.
5. Tumor growth is supported by the development of new blood vessels, a process called *angiogenesis.* Two angiogenic factors thought to be secreted by the tumor include a heparin-binding endothelial growth factor and angiogenin.

■ DID YOU UNDERSTAND? —cont'd

Clinical Manifestations of Cancer

1. Clinical manifestations of cancer include pain, fatigue, cachexia, anemia, leukopenia, thrombocytopenia, and infection.

2. Pain generally is associated with the late stages of cancer. It can be caused by pressure, obstruction, invasion of a structure sensitive to pain, stretching, tissue destruction, and inflammation.

3. Fatigue is the most frequently reported symptom of cancer and cancer treatment.

4. Cachexia (loss of appetite, weakness, inability to maintain weight, taste alterations, altered metabolism) leads to protein-calorie malnutrition and progressive wasting.

5. Anemia associated with cancer usually occurs because of malnutrition, long-term bleeding and resultant iron deficiency, chemotherapy, and malignancies in the blood-forming organs.

6. Leukopenia is usually a result of chemotherapy, which is toxic to bone marrow, or radiation, which kills circulating leukocytes.

7. Thrombocytopenia is usually the result of chemotherapy or malignancy in the bone marrow.

8. Infection may be caused by leukopenia, immunosuppression, or debility associated with advanced disease.

Cancer Treatment

1. Cancer is treated with surgery, radiotherapy, chemotherapy, immunotherapy, and combinations of these modalities.

2. The theoretic basis of chemotherapy is the vulnerability of tumor cells in various stages of the cell cycle. The goal of chemotherapy is to eradicate enough tumor cells so that the body's natural defenses can eradicate remaining cells.

3. Ionizing radiation causes cell damage, so the goal of radiotherapy is to damage the tumor without causing excessive toxicity or damage to undiseased structures.

4. Surgical therapy is used for nonmetastatic disease, for which cure is possible by removing the tumor, and as a palliative measure to alleviate symptoms.

5. Immunotherapy is appropriate for cancers that cannot be managed effectively by chemotherapy or radiation, usually because enough tumor cells are inactive and invulnerable to these modalities.

6. Forms of immunotherapy known as biologic response modifiers include immunomodulating agents, interferons, antigens, effector cells, lymphokines, and monoclonal antibodies.

KEY TERMS

Angiogenesis, 273
Autocrine motility factor hypothesis, 270
Biologic response modifier (BRM), 278
Cachexia, 275
Fatigue, 274

Invasion, 270
Laminin receptor, 270
Metastasis, 271
Primary tumor, 271
Seeding, 272

Thrombospondin, 273
TNM system, 273
Tumor-angiogenesis factor (TAF), 273
Type IV collagenase, 270

REFERENCES

1. Woodhouse, E.C., Chuaqui, R.F., & Liotta, L.A. (1997). General mechanisms of metastasis. *Cancer, 80,* 1529-1537.

2. McCorkle, R. et al. (1996). *Cancer nursing: A comprehensive textbook* (2nd ed.). Philadelphia: Saunders.

3. Fidler, I.J. (1995). Critical factors in the biology of human cancer metastasis. *American Surgery, 61,* 1065-1066.

4. Levin, M.D., Liotta, L.A., & Stracke, M.L. (1995). Stimulation and regulation of tumor cell motility in invasion and metastasis. *EXS, 74,* 157-179.

5. Kupchella, C.E. (1997). Cellular biology of cancer. In S.L. Groenwald, M.H. Frogge, & M. Goodman (Eds.). *Cancer nursing: Principles and practice* (4th ed.). Boston: Jones & Bartlett.

6. Groenwald, S.L. (1997). Differences between normal and cancer cells. In S.L. Groenwald, M.H. Frogge, & M. Goodman (Eds.). *Cancer nursing: Principles and practice* (4th ed.). Boston: Jones & Bartlett.

7. Stracke, M.L., Clair, T., & Liotta, L.A. (1997). Autotaxin, tumor mortality-stimulating exophosphodiesterase. *Advances in Enzyme Regulation, 37,* 135-144.

8. Stetler-Stevenson, W.G., Aznavoorian, S., & Liotta, L.A. (1993). Tumor cell interactions with the extracellular matrix during invasion and metastasis. *Annual Review of Cellular Biology, 9,* 541-573.

9. Liotta, L.A., Kleinerman, J., & Saidel, G.M. (1974). Quantitative relationships of intravascular tumor cells, tumor vessels, and pulmonary metastases following tumor implantation. *Cancer Research, 34,* 997-1004.

10. Winlaw, D.S. (1997). Angiogenesis in the pathobiology and treatment of vascular and malignant diseases. *Annals of Thoracic Surgery, 64,* 1204-1211.

REFERENCES

11. Anan, K. et al. (1996). Vascular endothelial growth factor and platelet-derived growth factor are potential angiogenic and metastatic factors in human breast cancer. *Surgery, 119,* 333-339.

12. Brown, J.M. & Giaccia, A.J. (1998). The unique physiology of solid tumors: Opportunities (and problems) for cancer therapy. *Cancer Research, 58*(7), 1408-1416.

13. Lahav, J. (1993). The functions of thrombospondin and its involvement in physiology and pathophysiology. *Biochemical and Biophysical Acta, 1182*(1), 1-14.

14. Sugarbaker, E.V. (1981). Patterns of metastasis in human malignancies. *Cancer Biology, 2,* 235-245.

15. Graeber, T.G. (1996). Hypoxia-mediated selection of cells with diminished apoptotic potential in solid tumors. *Nature, 379,* 99.

16. Seachrist, L. (1996). Only the strong survive: The evaluation of a tumor favors the meanest, most aggressive cells. *Science News, 149,* 216.

17. Price, J.T., Bonovich, M.T., & Kohn, E.C. (1997). The biochemistry of cancer dissemination. *Critical Review of Biochemistry and Molecular Biology, 322*(3), 175-253.

18. Schirrmacher, V. (1985). Cancer metastasis: Experimental approaches, theoretical concepts, and impacts for treatment strategies. *Advanced Cancer Research, 43,* 1-71.

19. Dudjak, L.A. (1992). Cancer metastasis. *Seminars in Oncology Nursing, 8*(1), 40-50.

20. Borowitz, M.J. (1993). Abnormalities of circulating T-cell subpopulations in patients with cutaneous T-cell lymphoma: Cutaneous lymphocyte-associated antigen expression of T-cells correlates with extent of disease. *Leukemia, 7,* 859.

21. U.S. Department of Health and Human Services, Public Health Service. (1994). Clinical practice guideline. In *Management of cancer pain* (9th vol.). Washington, D.C.: The Author.

22. The Steering Committee on Clinical Practice Guidelines for the Care and Treatment of Breast Cancer. (1998). The management of chronic pain with breast cancer. *Canadian Medical Association Journal, 158*(Suppl. 3), S71-S81.

23. Gordon, C. (1997). The effect of cancer pain on quality of life in different ethnic groups: A literature review. *Nurse Practitioner Forum, 8*(1), 5-13.

24. Winningham, M. et al. (1994). Fatigue and the cancer experience: The state of the knowledge. *Oncology Nursing Forum, 21*(1), 23-36.

25. Fiers, W. (1991). Review: Tumor necrosis factor: Characterization of the molecular, cellular, and in vivo level. *FEBS Letters, 285*(2), 199-212.

26. Matthys, P. & Billian, A. (1997). Cytokines and cachexia. *Nutrition, 13*(9), 763-770.

27. Todorov, P. et al. (1996). Characterization of a cancer cachectic factor. *Nature, 379,* 739.

27a. Todorov, P. et al. (1998). Purification and characterization of a tumor lipid-mobilizing factor. *Cancer Research, 58*(11), 2353-2358.

28. Lange, W. et al. (1991). The role of cytokines in oncology. *International Journal of Cell Cloning, 9,* 252-273.

29. Fisher, J.W. (1997). Erythropoietin: Physiologic and pharmacologic aspects. *Proceedings of the Society for Experimental Biology and Medicine, 216*(3), 358-369.

30. Talmadge, J.E. (1992). Development of immunotherapeutic strategies for the treatment of malignant neoplasms. *Biotherapy, 4,* 215-236.

CHAPTER

11

Cancer in Children

Marilyn Hockenberry-Eaton and
Karen M. VanSyckle

C ancer in children is rare, but because so many
diseases of childhood have been conquered,
cancer is the second leading cause of death in children who survive their first year.[1] (Accidents remain
the leading killer of children and adolescents.) The
unique feature of childhood cancer is the short
latency time—a sharp contrast to adult tumors,
which usually involve a long latent period. Table
11-1 summarizes the differences between childhood and adult cancers.

Kathleen Hardin Mooney, RN, PhD, contributed to this chapter in the
previous edition.

CHAPTER OUTLINE

TABLE 11-1	Comparison of Usual Childhood and Adult Cancers	
Factor	**Childhood Cancers**	**Adult Cancers**
Incidence	Rare, <1% of all cancers	Common, >99% of all cancers
Sites	Involves tissue (e.g., mononuclear phagocyte system, CNS, muscle, bone)	Involves organs (e.g., lung, breast, colon, prostate)
Histology	Most common type—nonepithelial: sarcomas, embryonal, leukemia, lymphoma	Most common type—epithelial: carcinomas
Latency (from initiation to diagnosis)	Relatively short period	Long period; can be well over 20 yr
Influence of environmental factors in causation	Some environmental factors known, few lifestyle factors; overall not strong influence shown; more likely an interaction of genetic alterations and environmental factors, called *ecogenetics*	Strong relationship to environmental exposures and life-style factors
Prevention	Minimal strategies known to date	80% estimated to be preventable
Early detection	Generally accidental; small percentage known to be genetically at high risk can be monitored more closely	Possible with adherence to early detection and screening recommendations
State at diagnosis	80% have metastasized	Local or regional
Response to treatment	Very responsive to chemotherapy; tolerate higher doses	Less responsive to chemotherapy
Treatment side effects	Less difficulty with acute toxicity but more significant long-term consequences	More difficulty with acute toxicity but fewer long-term consequences
Prognosis	>60% cure	<60% cure

Modified from Fernbach, D.J. & Vichi, T. (1991). General aspects of childhood cancer. In D.J. Fernbach & T. Vichi (Eds). Clinical pediatric oncology (4th ed.). St. Louis: Mosby.

INCIDENCE AND TYPES OF CHILDHOOD CANCER

Both incidence rates and types of cancer that develop vary between children and adults. For example, approximately 9000 children up to the age of 15 years are diagnosed with cancer each year, whereas approximately 1,100,000 adults were diagnosed with cancer during the same year.[2] The incidence of cancer in children between birth and the age of 15 years is estimated to be 133 children per million per year (Table 11-2).[3,4] Projections reveal that 1 in every 900 persons between the ages of 16 and 44 years will be a survivor of childhood cancer by the year 2000.[3]

Most childhood cancers originate from the **mesodermal germ layer** that gives rise to connective tissue, bone, cartilage, muscle, blood, blood vessels, gonads, kidney, and the lymphatic system. Thus the more common childhood cancers are leukemias, sarcomas, and embryonic tumors. Embryonic tumors originate during intrauterine life and contain abnormal cells that appear to be immature embryonic tissue unable to mature or differentiate into fully developed functional cells. **Embryonic tumors** are diagnosed early in life (usually by 5 years of age) and therefore are very rare in adults.

Sarcomas and lymphoreticular cancers seen in childhood occur also in adults, but most adult cancers involve epithelial tissue (and are therefore carcinomas). Carcinomas almost never occur in children because these cancers most commonly result from environmental carcinogens and require a long period from exposure to the appearance of the carcinoma. However, epithelial tumors begin to increase between the ages of 15 and 19 years, becoming the most common cancer tissue type after adolescence.

By far the most common malignancy in children is leukemia, which accounts for more than one third of childhood cancers. The second most common group of cancers is tumors of the nervous system, primarily brain tumors. All other pediatric malignancies occur much less frequently. Neuroblastoma is a tumor of the sympathetic nervous system. Wilms tumor is a malignancy of the kidney (named after Max Wilms, who identified the tumor); the histologic name is *nephroblastoma*. Rhabdomyosarcoma is a soft tissue sarcoma of striated muscle. Two major bone tumors also occur in children. These are osteosarcoma and Ewing sarcoma.

Childhood cancers usually are diagnosed during peak times of physical growth and maturation. In general, they are extremely fast-growing cancers. Many childhood cancers have a peak incidence before the child is 5 years of age. Among these are the leukemias, neuroblastoma, Wilms tumor, and retinoblastoma. Central nervous system tumors are more common from ages 5 to 10 years, and bone tumors, soft tissue sarcomas, and lymphomas are more likely to occur from 10 to 15 years of age.[4]

Cancer is 10% to 25% more common in white than in

TABLE 11-2 Annual U.S. Cancer Incidence Rates* Among Children Younger Than 15 Years of Age

Histology	Total†			Males		Females		Male:Female	Whites		Blacks		White:Black
	No.	Rate	(%)	No.	Rate	No.	Rate		No.	Rate	No.	Rate	
All histologic types	10,555	133.3	(100.0)	5711	140.9	4844	125.1	1.13	8756	139.5	1064	108.3	1.29
Acute lymphoid leukemia	2484	30.9	(23.2)	1383	33.7	1101	28.0	1.20	2092	32.9	169	16.9	1.95
All central nervous system (CNS)	2205	27.6	(20.7)	1195	29.3	1010	26.0	1.13	1847	29.3	239	23.8	1.23
Astrocytomas and gliomas	1329	16.8	(12.6)	692	17.1	637	16.2	1.06	1130	17.9	144	14.3	1.25
Primitive neuroectodermal	532	6.6	(5.0)	311	7.7	221	5.6	1.38	433	6.8	58	5.9	1.15
Other CNS	344	4.3	(3.2)	192	4.6	152	3.9	1.18	284	4.6	37	3.6	1.28
Neuroblastoma	754	9.7	(7.3)	389	9.8	365	9.6	1.02	632	10.2	78	7.8	1.31
Non-Hodgkin lymphoma	666	8.4	(6.3)	484	12.0	182	4.6	2.61	578	9.1	53	5.4	1.69
Wilms tumor	638	8.1	(6.1)	287	6.9	351	8.9	0.78	520	8.3	94	9.4	0.88
Hodgkin disease	511	6.6	(5.0)	295	7.4	216	5.6	1.32	451	7.3	46	4.7	1.55
Acute myeloid leukemia	454	5.6	(4.2)	224	5.5	230	6.0	0.92	358	5.8	47	4.8	1.21
Rhabdomyosarcoma	354	4.5	(3.4)	211	5.2	143	3.6	1.44	294	4.7	40	4.1	1.15
Retinoblastoma	306	3.9	(2.9)	144	3.6	162	4.2	0.86	234	3.9	44	4.5	0.87
Osteosarcoma	262	3.4	(2.6)	130	3.3	132	3.4	0.97	197	3.4	38	3.9	0.87
Ewing sarcoma	208	2.8	(2.1)	109	2.8	99	2.6	1.08	194	3.3	3	0.3	11.00
All other histologic types	1713	21.8	(16.4)	860	21.4	853	22.6	0.95	1359	21.3	213	22.7	0.94

From Gurney, J.G. et al. (1995). Incidence of cancer in children in the U.S.: Sex-, race-, and 1-year age-specific rates by histologic type, Cancer, 75(8), 2188.

*Rates are standardized to the 1980 SEER population and reported per million children per year.

†Includes all races and both genders.

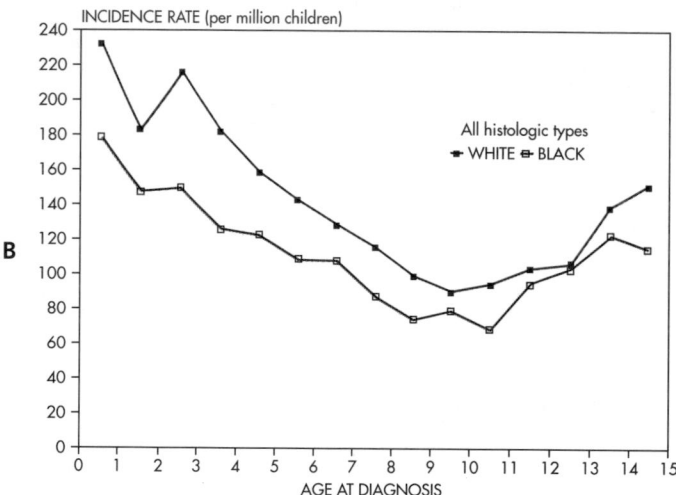

Fig. 11-1 *Incidence rate and gender at diagnosis among U.S. children younger than 15 years of age.* **A,** Age- and gender-specific incidence rates of all histologic types combined among U.S. children younger than 15 years of age. **B,** Age-specific incidence rates of all histologic types combined among U.S. white and black children younger than 15 years. *(Reprinted with permission from Gurney, J.G. et al. [1995]. Incidence of cancer in children in the United States: Sex-, race-, and 1-year age-specific rates by histologic type. Cancer, 75[8], 2187.)*

black children (see Table 11-2 and Fig. 11-1). This is primarily the result of the lower incidence of acute lymphocytic leukemia, lymphomas, and Ewing sarcoma in black children.[2,4] Some geographic differences also are found. These include increases in Burkitt lymphoma in Nigeria, intestinal lymphomas in Israel, Hodgkin disease in Colombia, and retinoblastoma in India.[3] In the United States, childhood cancer also is slightly more common in boys than in girls. The male/female ratio for childhood cancers is 1.2:1.0.[4]

ETIOLOGY

As in adult cancer, the causes of cancer in childhood are largely unknown. Some environmental and host factors are known to predispose a child to cancer, but causal factors have not been established for most childhood cancers. Table 11-3 lists host factors, many of which are genetic risk factors or congenital conditions, implicated in the development of childhood cancer. Childhood cancer most likely can be attributed to the complex interaction of both genetic and environmental factors, now an important area of study called *ecogenetics.*

Most childhood cancers, however, do not lend themselves to early cancer warning signs. Certainly the American Cancer Society's seven warning signs of cancer do not apply because they describe adult, environmentally caused carcinomas. Although host factors are important in identifying populations of children at risk for cancer, most children who are diagnosed with cancer do not demonstrate any predisposing environmental or host factors.

Genetic Factors

Genetic factors may involve chromosome aberrations or single-gene defects or chromosome abnormalities including aneuploidy, deletions, translocations, and fragility. Some congenital malformations herald the onset of pediatric malignancies (see Table 11-3). For example, certain syndromes involve easily diagnosed abnormalities and the children then can be carefully followed and screened for tumor development. One of the more recognized syndromes is the association of trisomy 21 (Down syndrome) with an increased susceptibility to acute leukemia (see Critical Thinking Question). For children with Down syndrome, the risk of developing leukemia is 10 to 18 times greater during the first 10 years of life than the risk in healthy children.[5-8]

Wilms tumor is particularly recognized for its association with a number of malformations, including genitourinary anomalies—for example, horseshoe kidney, cryptorchidism (undescended testicles), and collecting system malformation; aniridia (congenital absence of the iris of the eye); and hemihypertrophy (muscular overgrowth of one half of the body or face).[9] Approximately 15% of children diagnosed with Wilms tumor demonstrate one of these congenital abnormalities. A Wilms tumor gene, named the *WT1* gene, has been found at chromosome 11p13 (Table 11-4).[10,11] Retinoblastoma, a malignant embryonic tumor of the eye, occurs as an inherited defect or as an acquired mutation (see p. 440). The retinoblastoma gene (*RB* gene) remains the most widely studied cause of inherited susceptibility to childhood cancer (see Table 11-4).[12]

More than 150 single-gene defects have been associated with the subsequent development of both childhood and adult cancers. For instance, two autosomal recessive diseases involving increased chromosome fragility, Fanconi anemia and Bloom syndrome, are risk factors that predispose the child to acute nonlymphocytic leukemia.[13-15]

TABLE 11-3	**Host Factors Associated With Childhood Cancer**
Syndrome	**Associated Risk Factors**
Chromosome alterations	
Down syndrome	Acute leukemia
13q syndrome	Retinoblastoma
Chromosome instability	
Ataxia-telangiectasia	Lymphoma
Bloom syndrome	Acute leukemia
Fanconi anemia	Nonlymphocytic leukemia
Hereditary syndromes	
Beckwith-Wiedmann syndrome	Wilms tumor, sarcoma, brain tumors
Neurofibromatosis	Brain tumor, sarcomas, neuroblastomas, Wilms tumor, nonlymphocytic leukemia
Tuberous sclerosis	Brain tumors
Immunodeficiency disorders	
Congenital	
Agammaglobulinemia	Lymphoma, leukemia, brain tumors
Immunoglobulin A (IgA) deficiency	Lymphoma, leukemia, brain tumors
Wiskott-Aldrich syndrome	Leukemia, lymphoma
Acquired	
Aplastic anemia	Leukemia
Organ transplantation	Leukemia, lymphoma
Congenital malformation syndromes	
Aniridia, hemihypertrophy, hamartoma, genitourinary anomalies	Wilms tumor
Cryptorchidism	Testicular tumor
Gonadal dysgenesis	Gonadoblastoma
Family susceptibility	
Twin or sibling with leukemia	Leukemia

The relative ineffectiveness of the immune surveillance system during intrauterine life may explain the occurrence of embryonic tumors. (The immune surveillance system is discussed in Chapter 9.) Because this period requires rapid proliferation and differentiation of cells in the developing fetus, cell mutation theoretically could result in embryonic tumors.

Children with immunodeficiencies experience a striking risk of subsequent cancer over healthy children.[16] These conditions may be either congenital, generally involving X-linked recessive inheritance, or acquired, generally caused by therapeutic immunosuppression after organ transplantation or treatment for aplastic anemia.

Although not determined to be genetically transmitted, a few malignancies seem to demonstrate a familial tendency, suggested by the clustering of specific cancers in a particular family. A child who has a sibling with leukemia has a risk for the development of leukemia that is two to four times greater than for a child with healthy siblings.[17] A strong association for subsequent leukemia also is apparent in children with monozygous twins who have leukemia. The de-gree of risk appears to be age related. If the twin with leukemia was diagnosed when younger than 1 year, the probability is nearly 100%; if diagnosed between the ages of 1 and 4 years, the risk drops to 15%; after 7 years of age the risk is equal to that of the general population.[17]

Environmental Factors

Although many adult cancers are associated with environmental agents, few childhood tumors share a strong association. Because of the lengthy latency period required between exposure and development of cancer, early exposure to carcinogens does not result in a tumor until the child is an adult.

Prenatal exposure

Prenatal exposure to some drugs and to ionizing radiation has been linked to subsequent cancers. Perhaps the most well-known such drug is diethylstilbestrol (DES), a drug taken to avert early abortion. In 1971, DES was identified as a transplacental chemical carcinogen. Adenocarcinoma of the vagina has developed in a small percentage of the daugh-

TABLE 11-4   Selected Oncogenes and Tumor-Suppressor Genes Associated With Childhood Cancer

Gene	Associated Pediatric Tumor
Oncogenes	
abl	Acute lymphoblastoma leukemia
N-*myc*	Neuroblastoma
c-*myb*	Neural tumors, leukemia, lymphomas, rhabdomyosarcoma, Wilms tumor, neuroblastoma
erb B	Glioblastoma
N-*ras*	Neuroblastoma, leukemia
H/K-*ras*	Neuroblastoma, rhabdomyosarcoma, leukemia
Tumor suppressor genes	
rb1 gene	Retinoblastoma
WT1 gene (on chromosome 11)	Wilms tumor
WT2 gene (also on chromosome 11)	Wilms tumor
WT3 gene (familial Wilms tumor gene)	Wilms tumor

Data from Vats, T.S. & Emami, A. (1993). Indian Journal of Pediatrics, 60, 192.

ters of mothers who had taken DES while pregnant. Most of these cancers appeared when the daughters were between 14 and 23 years of age. Increased maternal age has been associated with an increased risk for childhood leukemia.[18]

An area of recent intense study is the role of parental occupational exposures in subsequent childhood cancers in children. The exposure could lead to genetic changes of the egg or sperm or to transplacental transfer of the carcinogen. Several associations have been found consistently in more than one study, including parental occupations with hydrocarbon exposure, petroleum and chemical exposure, and paint exposure. In a recent Canadian study, researchers found a relationship between testicular cancer in sons and paternal employment before conception. Jobs were related to metal, food, and beverage products.[19] Further study is needed because this is a difficult area to study and conflicting results are common.

Intrauterine exposure to radiation during pregnancy may cause an increased risk for all types of childhood cancers.[20,21] Earlier research findings have led to changes in medical practice to prevent exposure to radiation during pregnancy.

Childhood exposure

Childhood exposures to drugs, ionizing radiation, and viruses have been implicated as risk factors that increase susceptibility to specific cancers. In addition to those drug and environmental agents that are known to cause cancer in adults and therefore also are risks for exposure during childhood, a few drugs may particularly increase cancer risk dur-

ing childhood. These drugs include (1) anabolic androgenic steroids, which are used in the treatment of aplastic anemia or used illegally by teenage athletes for body development and have been associated with subsequent hepatocellular carcinoma; (2) cytotoxic agents used in the treatment of pediatric cancers, which may predispose the child to leukemia in later years; and (3) immunosuppressive agents, particularly those used for transplant surgeries, which have been shown to increase the risk of lymphoma. Children infected with hepatitis C are at risk for developing liver cancer as adults (see Health Alert box).

HEALTH ALERT
Hepatitis C Infection

Hepatitis C infection in children may cause only mild symptoms, but once infected, the child is at great risk of liver cancer as an adult. Survivors of childhood cancer who received blood transfusions before the routine screening of all blood products in 1990 are at great risk for hepatitis C infection. One study in Europe showed a prevalence of 43%. HCV-RNA (hepatitis C virus–RNA) detected in serum and liver biopsy samples confirms the diagnosis. Interferon-alpha (IFN-α) is the treatment of choice for infected adults and is being studied for its effectiveness in the pediatric population.

Data from Arico, M. et al. (1994). Hepatitis C virus infection in children treated for acute lymphoblastic leukemia. Blood, 84(9), 2919; Bortolotti, F. et al. (1995). Recombinant interferon alpha therapy in children with chronic hepatitis C. Hepatology, 22, 1623; Tong, M.J. et al. (1995). Clinical outcomes after transfusion associated with hepatitis C. New England Journal of Medicine, 332, 1463; Zellos, A. & Schwartz, K. (1998). What's the latest on hepatitic C? Contemporary Pediatrics, 15(4), 39-58.

Current areas of study focus on the role of childhood environmental exposures to radon gas in the home and electromagnetic fields from residential power lines and the operation of small household appliances. Thus far, results are conflicting and further study is needed to determine the significance of any associations.[22-26] The observation of increased rates of childhood cancer in specific communities has led to investigation of the role of chemical pollution in childhood cancer. Once again, further investigation is needed, but one cluster of childhood cancer in 1979 in the community of Woburn, Massachusetts, was linked to factory-caused water pollution.[27] Parents pressed their case and finally won a legal battle in 1988 linking the contamination to their children's cancer. In addition, a strong association exists between childhood exposure to ultraviolet (UV) radiation and melanoma risk (see Chapter 9).

Although viruses have been implicated in childhood cancers, research has not yet proved a strong association. (The viral theory of carcinogenesis is discussed in Chapter 9.) In children, the strongest carcinogenic relationship has been shown between the Epstein-Barr virus (EBV) and Burkitt lymphoma. Most African children with Burkitt lymphoma have high titers of antibodies against EBV. It is not clear, however, whether EBV infection predisposes the child to African Burkitt lymphoma or if the EBV infection is an essential component of pathogenesis.[28] As many as 50% of American children with Burkitt lymphoma, however, do not have elevated EBV titers. Therefore although EBV can induce lymphocyte transformation in laboratory studies, evidence has not yet shown whether the relationship is causal. Investigators are examining the role of viruses in the development of neuroblastomas, Wilms tumor, and osteosarcoma.

HEALTH ALERT

Parental Smoking Contributes to Childhood Cancer

Statistically significant (P<0.001) associations have been shown between the father's cigarette smoking (with nonsmoking mothers) and the child's risk for cancer.* Parental cigarette smoking accounts for 14% to 15% of all childhood cancers. Cancer risks are increased 3.8-fold for acute leukemia, 4.5-fold for lymphoma, 2.7-fold for brain tumors, and 1.7-fold for all types of cancers among children whose fathers smoke.

Data from Ji, P.T. et al. (1997). Paternal cigarette smoking and the risk of childhood cancer among offspring of nonsmoking mothers. Journal of the National Cancer Institute, 89, 238-244; Sorahan, T. et al. (1997). Childhood cancer and parental use of tobacco: Deaths from 1953 to 1955. British Journal of Cancer, 75, 134-138; Sorahan, T. et al. (1997). Childhood cancer and parental use of tobacco: Deaths from 1971 to 1976. British Journal of Cancer, 76, 1525-1531.
*Only fathers were tested in this study.

PROGNOSIS

Today, childhood cancer should not be considered an inevitably fatal illness. Significant progress has been made in the past 10 years so that more than 60% of children diagnosed with cancer can now be expected to survive. Estimates indicate that 1 of every 900 individuals between 16 and 44 years of age will be a survivor of childhood cancer by the year 2000.[2] These individuals are at increased risk for a second cancer because of their previous exposure to carcinogenic therapy and, possibly, their genetic constitution. The risk of a secondary cancer 20 years after childhood cancer is approximately 8% to 9%.[3] Overall, children have a more favorable prognosis than do adults.[2] Children appear to be both more responsive to available treatments and better able to tolerate the immediate side effects of therapies.

Because childhood cancer should be viewed as a chronic disease instead of a fatal illness, the focus of treatment is on the quality of life. Even those cancers that cannot be cured generally can be treated, resulting in a significant period of quality time. With increasing survival periods, the long-term effects of treatment are under careful investigation. More effective yet less toxic chemotherapy and radiation treatments must be found. Cured children still face residual and late ef-

fects of treatment. These late effects are more significant in children than in adults because childhood treatment occurs in a physically immature, growing individual. Potential effects that need further attention include physical impairments, reproductive dysfunction, soft tissue and bone atrophy, learning disabilities, secondary cancers, and psychologic sequelae. More must be learned about the genetic factors associated with childhood malignancies and about the genetic consequences of treatment. Genetic counseling is appropriate for children cured of cancers known to be transmitted genetically (e.g., retinoblastoma).

✓ QUICK CHECK

What are the most common childhood cancers?

Why are children less likely to get carcinomas?

How are different etiologic factors associated with the development of childhood cancer?

▣ DID YOU UNDERSTAND?

Incidence and Types of Childhood Cancers
1. Childhood cancer is a rare disease, but it remains the second leading cause of death in children.
2. The most common type of childhood cancer is leukemia, and the second most common group of cancers is tumors of the nervous system.

Etiology
1. Because most carcinomas are caused by environmental exposure, these cancers are extremely rare in children because they have not lived long enough to be exposed to carcinogens.
2. Children with immunodeficiencies are at increased risk for developing cancer because of an ineffective immune system.
3. Children with Down syndrome are at increased risk for developing leukemia.
4. Environmental factors associated with childhood cancer include prenatal exposure to some drugs and irradiation and postnatal exposure to certain drugs (i.e., anabolic steroids, cytotoxic and immunosuppressive agents), to radiation, and possibly to certain viruses.

Prognosis
1. Survivors of childhood cancer are at increased risk for developing a second cancer during their lifetime, compared with the general population.
2. Improved survival for children with cancer has led to investigations for less toxic treatments that minimize residual effects and for more research into the genetic factors associated with cancer in childhood.

KEY TERMS

Ecogenetics, 286   Embryonic tumors, 284   Mesodermal germ layer, 284

REFERENCES

1. Woodhouse, E.C., Chuaqui R.F., & Liotta L.A. (1997). General mechanisms of metastasis, *Cancer, 80,* 1529-1537.

2. Landis, S.H. et al. (1998). Cancer statistics 1998. *CA: A Cancer Journal for Clinicians, 48,* 6-29.

3. Robinson, L.L. (1997). General principles of the epidemiology of childhood cancer. In P.A. Pizzo & D.G. Poplack (Eds.). *Principles and practice of pediatric oncology* (3rd ed.). Philadelphia: Lippincott-Raven.

4. Gurney, J.G. et al. (1995). Incidence of cancer in children in the United States: Sex-, race-, and 1-year age-specific rates by histologic type. *Cancer, 75*(8), 2186.

5. Cnattingius, S. et al. (1995). Prenatal and neonatal risk factors for childhood lymphatic leukemia. *Journal of the National Cancer Institute, 87*(12), 908-914.

6. Kempski, H.M., Chessels, J.M., & Reeves, B.R. (1997). Deletions of chromosome 21 restricted to the leukemic cells of children with Down syndrome and leukemia. *Leukemia, 11*(11), 1973-1977.

7. Litz, C.E. et al. (1995). Acute leukemia and the transient myeloproliferative disorder associated with Down syndrome: Morphologic, immunophenotypic, and cytogenic manifestations. *Leukemia, 9*(9), 1432-1439.

8. Shen, J.J. et al. (1995). Cytogenic and molecular studies of Down syndrome individuals with leukemia. *American Journal of Human Genetics, 56*(4), 915-925.

9. Green, D.M. et al. (1996). Wilms tumor. *CA: A Cancer Journal for Clinicians, 460*(1), 46-63.

10. Zhuang, Z. et al. (1997). Identical genetic changes in different histologic components of Wilms' tumors. *Journal of the National Cancer Institute, 89*(15), 1148-1152.

11. Rahman, N. et al. (1996). Evidence for a familial Wilms' tumor gene (FWT1) on chromosome 17q12-q21. *Nature Genetics, 13*(4), 461-463.

12. Weinberg, R.A. (1994). Oncogenes and tumor suppressor genes. *CA: A Cancer Journal for Clinicians, 44*(3), 160-170.

13. Fundia, A., Gorla, N., & Larripa, I. (1995). Non-random distribution of spontaneous chromosome aberrations in two Bloom syndrome patients. *Hereditas, 122*(3), 239-243.

14. Alter, B.P. (1996). Fanconi's anemia and malignancies. *American Journal of Hematology, 53*(2), 99-110.

15. Butturinim, A. et al. (1994). Hematologic abnormalities in Fanconi anemia: An International Fanconi Anemia Registry study. *Blood, 84*(5), 1650-1655.

16. Sondel, P.M. (1997). Tumor immunology and pediatric cancer. In P.A. Pizzo & D.G. Poplack (Eds.). *Principles and practice of pediatric oncology* (3rd ed.). Philadelphia: Lippincott-Raven.

17. Margolin, J.F. & Poplack, D.G. (1997). Acute lymphoblastic leukemia. In P.A. Pizzo & D.G. Poplack (Eds.). *Principles and practice of pediatric oncology* (3rd ed.). Philadelphia: Lippincott-Raven.

18. Wakeford, R. (1995). The risk of childhood cancer from intrauterine and preconceptual exposure to ionizing radiation. *Environmental Health Perspectives, 103*(11), 1018-1025.

19. Knight, J.A. & Marrett, L.D. (1997). Parental occupational exposure and the risk of testicular cancer in Ontario. *Journal of Occupational and Environmental Medicine, 39*(4), 333-338.

20. Doll, R. & Wakeford, R. (1997). Risk of childhood cancer from fetal irradiation. *British Journal of Radiology, 70,* 130-139.

21. Streffer, C. (1997). Health impacts of large releases of radionuclides: Biological effects of prenatal irradiation. *Ciba Foundation Symposium, 203,* 155-164.

22. Feychting, M. et al. (1995). Magnetic fields and childhood cancer—A pooled analysis of two Scandinavian studies. *European Journal of Cancer, 31A*(12), 2035-2039.

23. London, S.J. et al. (1991). Exposure to residential electric and magnetic fields with risk of childhood leukemia. *American Journal of Epidemiology, 134*(9), 923-937.

24. Toren, A., Rechavi, G., & Ramot, B. (1996). Pediatric cancer: Environmental and genetic aspects. *Pediatric Hematology and Oncology, 13*(4), 319-331.

25. Heath, C.W., Jr. (1996). Electromagnetic field exposure and cancer: A review of epidemiologic evidence. *CA: A Cancer Journal for Clinicians, 46*(1), 29-44.

26. Gurney, J.G. et al. (1996). Childhood brain tumor occurrence in relation to residential power line configurations, electric heating sources, and electric appliance use. *American Journal of Epidemiology, 143*(2), 120-128.

27. Lagakos, S.W., Wessen, B.J., & Zelen, M. (1986). An analysis of contaminated well water and health effects in Woburn, MA. *Journal of the American Statistical Association, 81,* 583-596.

28. Shad, A. & Magrath, I. (1997). Malignant non-Hodgkins lymphomas in children. In P.A. Pizzo & D.G. Poplack (Eds.). *Principles and practice of pediatric oncology* (3rd ed.). Philadelphia: Lippincott-Raven.

CHAPTER

12

Structure and Function of the Neurologic System

Richard A. Sugerman

The human nervous system is a remarkable structure responsible for the body's ability to interact with the environment and for the regulation of activities involving internal organs. The nervous system literally drives the other systems of the body. It is a network composed of complex structures that transmit signals—both electrically and chemically—between the body's many organs and tissues and the brain.

Check out your CD Companion for chapter-related exercises and answers to the Quick Check questions

OVERVIEW AND ORGANIZATION OF THE NERVOUS SYSTEM

Although the nervous system functions as a unified whole, structures and functions have been divided to facilitate understanding. Structurally, the nervous system is divided into the central nervous system and the peripheral nervous system. The *central nervous system (CNS)* consists of the brain and spinal cord, enclosed within the protective cranial vault and vertebrae, respectively. The *peripheral nervous system (PNS)* is composed of the *cranial nerves* and the *spinal nerves.* Peripheral nerve pathways are differentiated into *afferent pathways (ascending pathways),* which carry sensory impulses toward the CNS, and *efferent pathways (descending pathways),* which innervate skeletal muscle or effector organs by transmitting motor impulses away from the CNS.

Functionally, the PNS can be divided into the somatic nervous system and the autonomic nervous system. The *somatic nervous system* consists of pathways that regulate voluntary motor control (e.g., skeletal muscle). The *autonomic nervous system (ANS)* is involved with regulation of the body's internal environment (viscera) through involuntary control of organ systems. The ANS is further divided into sympathetic and parasympathetic divisions. Organs innervated by specific components of the nervous system are called *effector organs.*

CELLS OF THE NERVOUS SYSTEM

Two basic types of cells constitute nervous tissue—neurons and supporting cells. The *neuron* is the primary cell of the nervous system, whereas cells such as *neuroglial cells* (CNS) and *Schwann cells* (PNS) provide structural support and nutrition for the neurons.

The Neuron

Working alone or in units, neurons detect environmental changes and initiate body responses to maintain a dynamic steady state. Neuronal structure varies markedly, so that each neuron is adapted to perform specialized functions.

The fuel source for the neuron is predominantly glucose; insulin, however, is not required for cellular glucose uptake in the CNS. Among the cellular constituents of neurons are *microtubules, neurofibrils, microfilaments* (believed to be involved in transport of cellular products), and *Nissl substances* (involved in protein synthesis). Because they lack centrosomes, entire neurons cannot regenerate. Therefore cell division stops at the time of birth, and further replication ceases.

A neuron (Fig. 12-1) has three components: a cell body (soma) and the thin processes of the cell, the dendrites, and the axons. Most cell bodies are located within the CNS; those in the PNS usually are found in groups called *ganglia.* The *dendrites* are extensions that carry nerve impulses toward the cell body. The *dendritic zone* receives a stimulus and continues further conduction. *Axons* are long, conductive projections from the cell body that carry nerve impulses

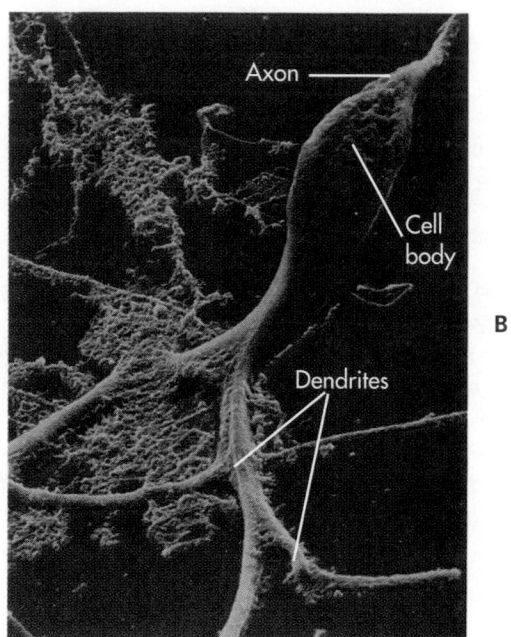

Fig. 12-1 *Neuron with composite parts.* **A,** Multipolar neuron: neuron with multiple extensions from the cell body. **B,** Scanning electron micrograph. *(From Thibodeau, G.A. & Patton, K.T. [1999]. Anatomy & physiology [4th ed.]. St. Louis: Mosby.)*

away from the cell body. The *axon hillock* is the cone-shaped process where the axon leaves the cell body. The first part of the axon hillock has the lowest threshold for stimulation, so action potentials begin here. A typical neuron has only one axon, which may be covered with a segmented layer of lipid material called *myelin,* an insulating substance. This entire membrane is referred to as the *myelin sheath,* and the thin membrane between the myelin sheath and the *endoneurium* (see Fig. 12-22) is the *neurilemma (Schwann sheath).* The neurilemma and the myelin sheath are interrupted at regular intervals by the *nodes of Ranvier.* Axons branch extensively at the nodes of Ranvier.

The principle of *divergence* refers to the ability of axonal branches to influence many different neurons. *Convergence* applies when branches of various numbers of neurons "converge" on and influence a single neuron. Nutrient exchange

Fig. 12-2 *Neuronal transmission and synaptic cleft.* Electrical impulse travels along axon of first neuron to synapse. Chemical transmitter is secreted into synaptic space to depolarize membrane (dendrite or cell body) of next neuron in pathway. *Cell A* represents unipolar cell; *cell B* represents multipolar cell.

is not possible through the myelin sheath, although it can occur at the nodes of Ranvier. Where there is myelin, the velocity of nerve impulses increases. Myelin acts as an insulator that allows ions to flow between segments rather than along the entire length of the membrane, yielding the increased velocity. This mechanism is referred to as *saltatory conduction.* Disorders of the myelin sheath (demyelinating diseases), such as multiple sclerosis and Guillain-Barré syndrome, demonstrate the important role myelin plays in nerve function (see Chapter 15). Conduction velocities depend not only on the myelin coating but also on the diameter of the axon. Larger axons transmit impulses at a faster rate.

Neurons are structurally classified on the basis of the number of processes (projections) extending from the cell body. There are four basic types of cell configuration: (1) unipolar, (2) pseudounipolar, (3) bipolar, and (4) multipolar. *Unipolar neurons* have one process that branches shortly after leaving the cell body. One example is found in

the retina. *Pseudounipolar neurons* (some authors call them *unipolar*) have one process with its dendritic portion extending away from the CNS and its axon portion projecting into the CNS (Fig. 12-2). The configuration is typical of sensory neurons in both cranial and spinal nerves. *Bipolar neurons* have two distinct processes arising from the cell body. This type of neuron connects the rod and cone cells of the retina. *Multipolar neurons* are the most common and have multiple processes capable of extensive branching. A motor neuron is typically multipolar (Fig. 12-2).

Functionally, there are three types of neurons (with their direction of transmission and typical configuration noted in parentheses): (1) sensory (afferent, mostly pseudounipolar), (2) associational (interneurons, multipolar), and (3) motor (efferent, multipolar). *Sensory neurons* carry impulses from peripheral sensory receptors to the CNS. *Associational neurons (interneurons)* transmit impulses from neuron to neuron, that is, sensory to motor neurons. They are located solely within the CNS. *Motor neurons* transmit impulses

TABLE 12-1	Support Cells of the Nervous System
Cell Type	**Primary Functions**
Astrocytes	Form specialized contacts between neuronal surfaces and blood vessels
	Provide rapid transport for nutrients and metabolites
	Believed to form an essential component of the blood-brain barrier
	Appear to be the scar-forming cells of CNS, which may be the foci for seizures
	May play a role in segregating postsynaptic receptor surfaces from other regions
Oligodendroglia (oligodendrocytes)	Formation of myelin sheath and neurilemma in CNS
Schwann cells (neurolemmocytes)	Formation of myelin sheath and neurilemma in PNS
Microglia	Responsible for clearing cellular debris (phagocytic properties)
Ependymal cells	Serve as a lining for ventricles and choroid plexuses involved in production of cerebrospinal fluid

CNS, *Central nervous system;* PNS, *peripheral nervous system.*

away from the CNS to an effector (i.e., skeletal muscle or organ). In skeletal muscle the end processes form a ***neuromuscular (myoneural) junction.***

Neuroglia and Schwann Cells

Neuroglia ("nerve glue") are the general classification of cells that support the neurons of the CNS. They comprise approximately half of the total brain and spinal cord volume and are five to ten times more numerous than neurons. Different types of neuroglia serve different functions. *Astrocytes,* for example, fill the spaces between neurons and surround blood vessels in the CNS; *oligodendroglia (oligondendrocytes)* function to deposit myelin within the CNS. Oligondendroglia are the CNS counterpart of the Schwann cells. Ependymal cells line the cerebrospinal fluid (CSF)-filled cavities of the CNS. *Microglia* remove debris (phagocytosis) in the CNS. (Characteristics of neuroglia and Schwann cells are summarized in Fig. 12-3 and Table 12-1.)

Nerve Injury and Regeneration

Mature nerve cells do not divide, and injury can cause permanent loss of function. When an axon is severed, wallerian degeneration occurs in the distal axon: (1) a characteristic swelling appears within the portion of the axon distal to the cut; (2) the neurofilaments hypertrophy; (3) the myelin sheath shrinks and disintegrates; and (4) the axon degenerates and disappears. The myelin sheaths re-form into Schwann cells that line up in a column between the cut and the effector organ.

At the proximal end of the injured axon, similar changes occur but only back to the next node of Ranvier. The cell body responds to trauma by swelling and the Nissl substance dispersing (chromatolysis). During the repair process the cell increases its metabolic activity, protein synthesis, and mitochondrial activity. Approximately 7 to 14 days after the injury, new terminal sprouts project from the proximal segment and may enter the remaining Schwann cell pathway. (Fig. 12-4 contains a more detailed representation of these

Fig. 12-3 *Types of neuroglial cells.* **A,** Fibrous astrocyte; **B,** oligodendrocytes; **C,** microglia cells; **D,** ependymal cells. *(Modified from Chipps, E., Clanin, N., & Campbell, V. [1992]. Neurologic disorders. St. Louis: Mosby.)*

events.) This process, however, is limited to myelinated fibers and generally occurs only in the PNS. The regeneration of axonal constituents in the CNS is limited by an increased incidence of scar formation and the different nature of myelin formed by the oligodendrocyte.

✓ QUICK CHECK

How do the functions of the somatic and autonomic nervous systems differ?

What are the three components of a neuron?

How does myelin affect nerve impulses?

Name the process through which injured axons are repaired, and describe the process.

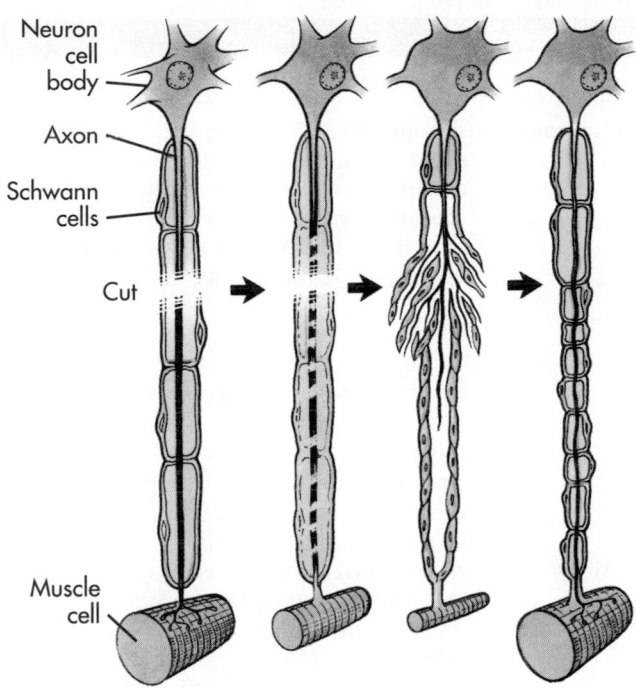

Neuron cell body

Axon

Schwann cells

Cut

Muscle cell

Fig. 12-4 *Repair of a peripheral nerve fiber.* When cut, a damaged motor axon can regrow to its distal connection only if the neurilemma remains intact (to form a guiding tunnel) and if scar tissue does not block its way.

Nerve regeneration depends on many factors, such as location of the injury, type of injury, the inflammatory responses, and the process of scarring. The closer to the cell body of the nerve, the greater the chances that the nerve cell will die and not regenerate. A crushing injury allows recovery more fully than does a cut injury. Crushed nerves sometimes recover fully, whereas cut nerves form connective tissue scars that block or slow regenerating axonal branches.

THE NERVE IMPULSE

Neurons generate and conduct electrical and chemical impulses by selectively changing the electrical potential of the plasma membrane and influencing other nearby neurons by releasing chemicals (neurotransmitters). An unexcited neuron maintains a resting membrane potential (see Chapter 1). When the membrane potential is raised, an action potential is generated and the nerve impulse then flows to all parts of the neuron. The action potential response occurs only when the stimulus is strong enough; if it is too weak, the membrane remains unexcited. This property is termed the *all-or-none response* (see Chapter 1 for a discussion of electrical impulse conduction).

Synapses

Neurons are not physically continuous with one another. The region between adjacent neurons is called a *synapse* (see

Fig. 12-2). Impulses are transmitted across the synapse by chemical and electrical conduction (see Fig. 12-2); only chemical conduction is discussed here. The neurons that conduct a nerve impulse are named according to whether they relay impulses toward (*presynaptic neurons*) or away from (*postsynaptic neurons*) the synapse.

Impulses are transmitted across the synapse by chemical conduction. When an impulse originates in a presynaptic neuron, the impulse reaches the vesicles, where chemicals (*neurotransmitters*) are stored in the **synaptic bouton.** Once released from the vesicles, the neurotransmitters diffuse across the **synaptic cleft** (the space between the neurons) and bind to receptor sites on the plasma membrane of the postsynaptic neuron[1] (see Fig. 12-2).

Neurotransmitters

More than 30 substances are thought to be neurotransmitters, including norepinephrine, acetylcholine, dopamine, histamine, and serotonin. Many of these transmitters have more than one function.[2] For example, norepinephrine in the brain probably helps regulate mood, functions in dreaming sleep, and maintains arousal. Some neurotransmitters are amino acids, including γ-aminobutyric acid (GABA), glutamic acid, and aspartic acid. Small chains of amino acids, such as enkephalins and endorphins, also function as neurotransmitters. Neurotransmitter and neuromodulator substances are listed in Table 12-2.

Because the neurotransmitter is stored on one side of the synaptic cleft and the receptor sites are on the other side, chemical synapses operate in only one direction. Therefore action potentials are transmitted along a multineuronal pathway in only one direction. The binding of the neurotransmitter at the receptor site changes the permeability of the postsynaptic neuron and consequently its membrane potential. Two possible scenarios can then follow: (1) the postsynaptic neuron may be excited (depolarized; *excitatory postsynaptic potentials [EPSPs]*) or (2) the postsynaptic neuron's plasma membrane may be inhibited (hyperpolarized; *inhibitory postsynaptic potentials [IPSPs]*). (Chapter 1 reviews electrical impulses and membrane potentials.)

Usually a single EPSP cannot induce a neuron's action potential and the propagation of the nerve impulse. Whether this occurs depends on the number and frequency of potentials the postsynaptic neuron receives—a concept known as *summation. Temporal summation* (time relationship) refers to the effects of successive impulses received at the same synapse. *Spatial summation* (spacing effect) is the combined effects of impulses a single neuron transmits to different synapses at the same time. *Facilitation* refers to the effect of EPSP on the plasma membrane potential. The plasma membrane is facilitated when summation brings the membrane closer to the threshold potential and decreases the stimulus required to induce an action potential. The effect that a chemical neurotransmitter has on the plasma membrane potential depends on the balance of these effects.

TABLE 12-2 Substances That Are Neurotransmitters and/or Neuromodulators

Substance	Location	Effect	Clinical Example
Acetylcholine	Many parts of the brain, spinal cord, neuromuscular junction of skeletal muscle, and many ANS synapses	Excitatory or inhibitory	Alzheimer disease (a type of senile dementia) is associated with a decrease in acetylcholine-secreting neurons. Myasthenia gravis (weakness of skeletal muscles) results from a reduction in acetylcholine receptors.
Monoamines			
Norepinephrine	Many areas of the brain and spinal cord; also in some ANS synapses	Excitatory or inhibitory	Cocaine and amphetamines,* resulting in overstimulation of postsynaptic neurons.
Serotinin	Many areas of the brain and spinal cord	Generally inhibitory	Involved with mood, anxiety, and sleep induction. Levels of serotonin are elevated in schizophrenia (delusions, hallucinations, withdrawal).
Dopamine	Some areas of the brain and ANS synapses	Generally excitatory	Parkinson disease (depression of voluntary motor control) results from destruction of dopamine-secreting neurons. Drugs used to increase dopamine production induce vomiting and schizophrenia.
Histamine		Generally inhibitory	No clear indication of histamine-associated pathologic conditions. Histamine apparently is involved with arousal, pituitary hormone secretion, control of cerebral circulation, and thermoregulation.
Amino acids			
γ-Aminobutyric acid (GABA)	Most neurons of the CNS have GABA receptors	Majority of postsynaptic inhibition in the brain	Drugs that increase GABA function have been used to treat epilepsy (excessive discharge of neurons).
Glycine	Spinal cord	Most postsynaptic inhibition in the spinal cord	Glycine receptors are inhibited by strychnine.
Glutamate and aspartate	Widespread in the brain and spinal cord	Excitatory	Drugs that block glutamate or aspartate such as riluzole, used to treat amyotrophic lateral sclerosis.[3] These drugs might prevent seizures and neural degeneration from overexcitation.
Neuropeptides			
Endorphins and enkephalins	Widely distributed in the CNS and PNS	Generally inhibitory	The opiates morphine and heroin bind to endorphin and enkephalin receptors on presynaptic neurons and reduce pain by blocking the release of neurotansmitter.
Substance P	Spinal cord, brain, and sensory neurons associated with pain, GI tract	Generally excitatory	Substance P is a neurotransmitter in pain transmission pathways. Blocking the release of substance P by morphine reduces pain.

From Seeley, R., Stephens, T.D., & Tate, P. (1992). Anatomy and physiology (3rd ed.). St. Louis: Mosby.
ANS, *Autonomic nervous system;* CNS, *central nervous system;* PNS, *peripheral nervous system;* GI, *gastrointestinal.*
*Increase the release and block the reuptake of norepinephrine.

TABLE 12-3	Division of the Central Nervous System	
Primary Vesicles	**Secondary Vesicles**	**Associated Structures**
Forebrain (prosencephalon)	Telencephalon	Cerebral hemispheres
		Cerebral cortex
		Rhinencephalon
		Basal ganglia
	Diencephalon	Epithalamus
		Thalamus
		Hypothalamus
		Subthalamus
Midbrain (mesencephalon)	Mesencephalon	Corpora quadrigemina
		Tegmentum
		Cerebral peduncles
Hindbrain (rhombencephalon)	Metencephalon	Cerebellum
		Pons
	Myelencephalon	Medulla oblongata
Spinal cord	Spinal cord	Spinal cord

✓ **QUICK CHECK**

Explain the process of chemical conduction of impulses.

What are neurotransmitters? Give several examples.

Compare *summation* and *facilitation*.

THE CENTRAL NERVOUS SYSTEM
The Brain

The human brain enables us to reason, function intellectually, express personality and mood, and interact with the environment. This pinkish gray organ weighs approximately 3 pounds and receives 15% to 20% of the total cardiac output. The three major divisions of the brain are (1) the forebrain, formed by the two cerebral hemispheres; (2) the midbrain, which includes the corpora quadrigemina, tegmentum, and cerebral peduncles; and (3) the hindbrain, which includes the cerebellum, pons, and medulla (Table 12-3). The midbrain, medulla, and pons make up the ***brain stem,*** which connects the hemispheres of the brain, cerebellum, and spinal cord. A collection of nerve cell bodies (nuclei) within the brain stem makes up the ***reticular formation*** (Fig. 12-5). The reticular formation is a large network of connected tissue that contains portions of vital reflexes, such as those controlling cardiovascular function and respiration. It is essential for maintaining wakefulness and therefore is referred to as the ***reticular activating system*** (see Fig. 12-5). Some nuclei within the reticular formation cause specific motor movements.[4]

Divisions of the brain are associated with different functions, but attributing specific functions to definite regions of the brain is not entirely accurate. Understanding functional destinations is very useful, however, especially in trying to determine or localize the effects of pathologic conditions in

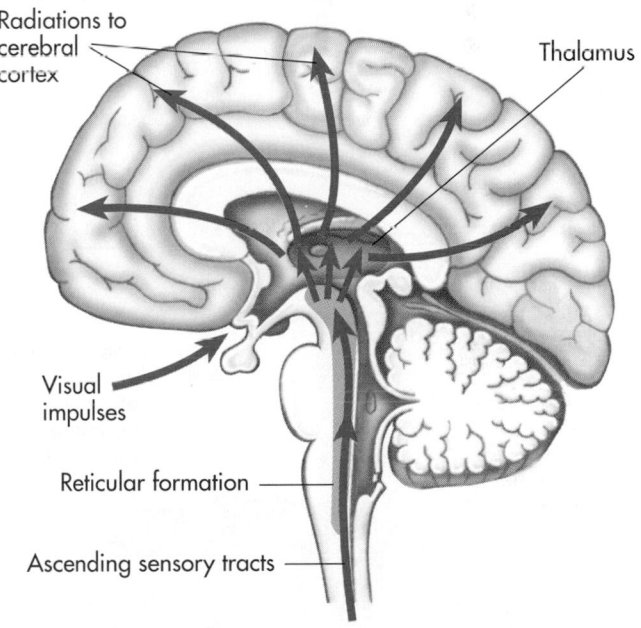

Fig. 12-5 *Reticular activating system.* System consists of nuclei in the brainstem reticular formation plus fibers that conduct to the nuclei from below and fibers that conduct from the nuclei to widespread areas of the cerebral cortex. Functioning of the reticular activating system is essential for consciousness.

various nervous system regions. A neuropsychiatrist (Brodmann) is credited with postulating various activities to many regions of the cerebral cortex. (Fig. 12-6 illustrates these regions and describes some of the areas.)

Forebrain
Telencephalon

The ***telencephalon*** consists of the ***cerebrum*** (the largest portion of the brain), the limbic system, and ***basal ganglia*** composed of several "nuclei." The surface of the cerebrum (cerebral cortex) is covered with convolutions called *gyri* (Fig.

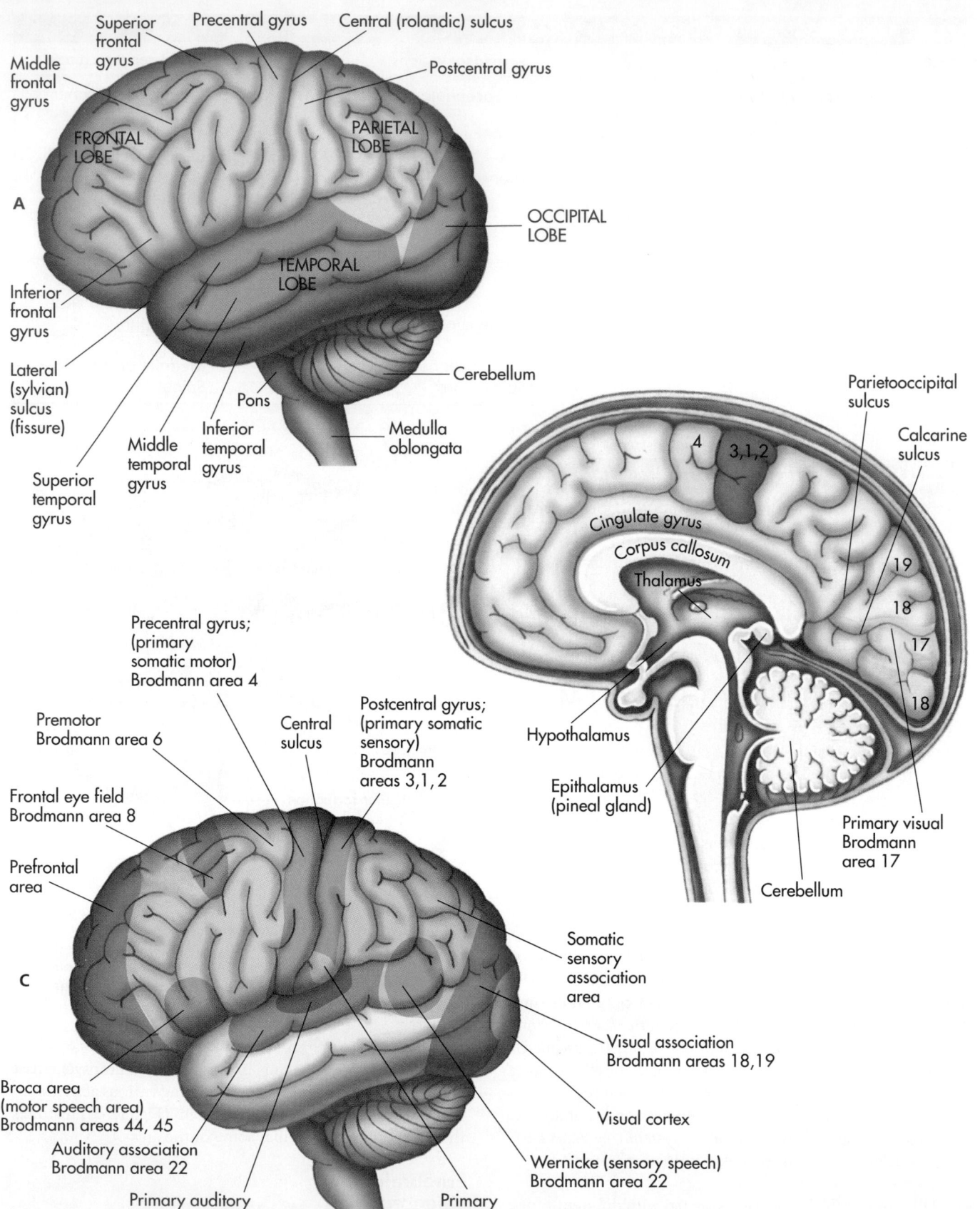

Fig. 12-6 *The cerebral hemispheres.* **A,** Left hemisphere of cerebrum, lateral view. **B,** Functional areas of the cerebral cortex, midsagittal view. **C,** Functional areas of the cerebral cortex, lateral view.

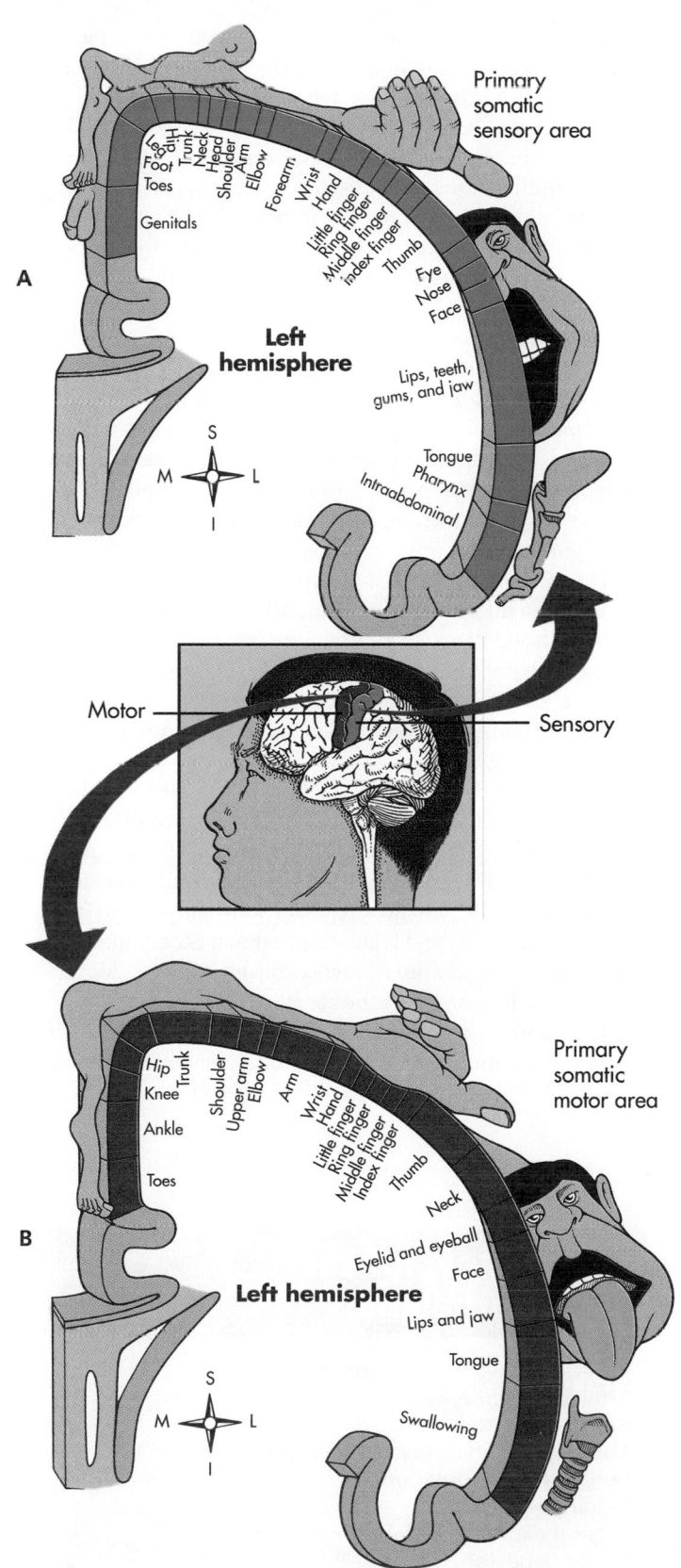

Fig. 12-7 *Primary somatic sensory (A) and motor (B) areas of the cortex.* (From Thibodeau, G.A. & Patton, K.T. [1999]. Anatomy & physiology *[4th ed.]. St. Louis: Mosby.)*

12-7), which increase the surface area where nerve cell bodies can lie, thereby maximizing their function. Grooves between adjacent gyri are termed *sulci;* deeper grooves are *fissures.* The *cerebral cortex* contains the cell bodies of neurons (*gray matter*). *White matter* lies beneath the cerebral cortex and is composed of myelinated nerve fibers.

The two cerebral hemispheres are separated by the longitudinal fissure. The surface of each hemisphere is divided into lobes named after the region of the skull under which each lies. The *frontal lobe's* posterior margin is on the *central sulcus (fissure of Rolando),* and it borders inferiorly on the *lateral sulcus (sylvian fissure, lateral fissure)* (see Fig. 12-6). The *prefrontal area* is responsible for goal-oriented behavior (e.g., ability to concentrate), short-term or recall memory, the elaboration of thought, and inhibition on the limbic areas of the CNS. The *premotor area (Brodmann area 6)* contains motor programs for fine repetitive motor movements and the cell bodies that form part of the *basal ganglia system (extrapyramidal system*—efferent pathways outside the pyramidal pathway that connect the cerebral cortex with spinal nerve pathways). The term *pyramidal* originates from a pyramid shaped structure in the medulla where these pathways converge. The pyramids are also where motor pathways cross over (decussation). Cerebral impulses control function in the opposite side of the body (*contralateral control*) (see Fig. 12-8).

The *primary motor area* is located along the *precentral gyrus* (Fig. 12-7) and forms the *primary voluntary motor pathway.* The axons traveling from the cell bodies in this region are projection fibers that form the *pyramidal system* that descends into the spinal cord. At the inferior edge of the precentral gyrus (usually in the left hemisphere) is *Broca's speech area,* which is responsible for the motor aspects of speech. Damage to this area resulting from a stroke causes speech difficulty or even inability to form words (expressive aphasia or dysphasia) (see Chapter 15).

The *parietal lobe* lies within the borders of the central, parietooccipital, and lateral sulci. It contains the major area for somatic sensory input, located primarily along the *postcentral gyrus* (Fig. 12-7), which is adjacent to the primary motor area. Communication between the motor and sensory areas (and among other regions in the cortex) is provided by *association fibers.* The remainder of this region is involved in sensory association (storage, analysis, and interpretation of sensory stimuli) (see Fig. 12-6, *C*).

The *occipital lobe* lies behind the parietooccipital sulcus and above the cerebellum. The primary visual cortex (visual receptive area) is located in this region. The rest of this lobe is involved primarily in visual association. The *temporal lobe* lies below the lateral fissure. Primary auditory and secondary associational areas account for the primary functional aspects of this region. *Wernicke's area* lies in the superoposterior portion of this region. This area is responsible for reception and interpretation of speech, and dysfunction may cause receptive aphasia or dysphasia. The temporal lobe also is involved in long-term memory and secondary functions such as balance, taste, and smell.

Another lobe, the *insula,* lies hidden from view in the lateral sulci (see Fig. 12-6). Lying directly beneath the longitudinal fissure is a mass of white matter pathways called the **corpus callosum (transverse or commissural fibers).** This structure connects the two cerebral hemispheres and is essential in coordinating activities between hemispheres, especially specific tasks present in only one hemisphere (see Fig. 12-6).

Inside the cerebrum are numerous tracts (white matter) and nuclei (gray matter). The major **cerebral nuclei** are called *basal ganglia* and include the **corpus striatum** and **amygdala.** The corpus striatum consists of the **lentiform nucleus** (lens shaped), the putamen and globus pallidus, and the ram's horn-shaped **caudate nucleus.** The **internal capsule** is a thick white matter region in which afferent and efferent pathways, to and from the cerebral cortex, pass through the center of the cerebral hemispheres. The **corpus striatum** appears striped because of the rostral connections between its gray matter and the white matter of the internal capsule.

The basal ganglia include, in addition to the corpus striatum, the subthalamic nucleus of the diencephalon and the substantia nigra of the mesencephalon. The basal ganglia plus their interconnections with the thalamus, premotor cortex, red nucleus, reticular formation, and spinal cord are part of the basal ganglia system (extrapyramidal system). The basal ganglia system is believed to exert a fine-tuning effect on motor movements. Parkinson disease and Huntington disease are conditions associated with defects of the basal ganglia (see Health Alert: Surgery for Parkinson Disease box). They are characterized by various involuntary or exaggerated motor movements (see Chapter 15).

The **limbic system** is a group of structures surrounding the corpus callosum that mediate emotion through connections in the prefrontal cortex. It is composed of the **Papez circuit** (amygdala, parahippocampal gyrus, **hippocampus,** fornix, mamillary body of the hypothalamus, thalamus, and cingulate gyrus), septal area, habenula, other portions of the hypothalamus, and related autonomic nuclei. It is an extension or modification of the olfactory system. Its principal effects are believed to be involved in primitive behavioral responses, visceral reaction to emotion, feeding behaviors, biologic rhythms, and the sense of smell.

Diencephalon

The **diencephalon,** surrounded by the cerebrum, has four divisions: **epithalamus, thalamus, hypothalamus,** and **subthalamus** (see Table 12-3 and Fig. 12-6). The epithalamus forms the roof of the third ventricle (a brain cavity) and composes the most superior portion of the diencephalon. Its connections and functions are closely associated with those of the limbic system.

The thalamus borders and surrounds the third ventricle. It is a major integrating center for afferent impulses to the cerebral cortex. Various sensations are perceived at this level, but cortical processing is required for interpretation. The thalamus serves also as a relay center for information from the basal ganglia and cerebellum to the appropriate motor area.

The hypothalamus forms the base of the diencephalon. Hypothalamic function may be (1) maintenance of a constant internal environment or (2) implementation of behavioral patterns. Integrative centers control autonomic nervous system (ANS) function, regulate body temperature and endocrine function, and regulate emotional expression. The hypothalamus exerts its influence through the endocrine system, as well as neural pathways (Box 12-1).

The subthalamus flanks the hypothalamus laterally. It serves as an important extrapyramidal center for motor activities.

HEALTH ALERT

Surgery for Parkinson Disease

Surgery to reduce parkinsonian motor symptoms has been an effective treatment procedure for more than 40 years. Precise lesions are made in the subthalamic nucleus, globus pallidus, and thalamus, resulting in rapid reduction of symptoms in a high number of individuals with Parkinson disease. The use of concise imaging techniques allows precision in placement of lesions. Advances in new technologies, including gamma knife radiosurgery and deep brain stimulation from implanted electrodes, provide relief for individuals with advanced disease. Gene therapy to promote dopaminergic neurons is also being explored.

Data from Kumar, R., Lozano, A.M., Kim, Y.J., Hutchison, W.D., Sime, E., Halket, E., & Lange, A.E. (1998). Double-blind evaluation of subthalamic nucleus deep brain stimulation in advanced Parkinson's disease. Neurology, 51*(3), 850-855; Lange, A.E. & Lozano, A.M. (1998). Parkinson's disease.* New England Journal of Medicine, *339(16), 1130-1143.*

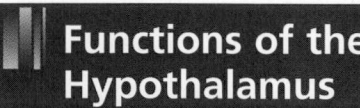

Functions of the Hypothalamus   BOX 12-1

Visceral and somatic responses
Affectual responses
Hormone synthesis
Autonomic nervous system activity
Temperature regulation
Feeding responses
Physical expression of emotions
Sexual behavior
Pleasure-punishment centers
Level of arousal or wakefulness

Midbrain

The *midbrain (mesencephalon)* is composed of three structures: the *corpora quadrigemina (tectum)* (composed of the superior and inferior colliculi), the *tegmentum* (containing the red nucleus and substantia nigra), and the basis pedunculi.*

The *superior colliculi* are involved with voluntary and involuntary visual motor movements (e.g., the ability of the eyes to *track* moving objects in the visual field). The *inferior colliculi* accomplish similar motor activities but involve movements affecting the auditory system (e.g., positioning the head to improve hearing). The *red nucleus* is a major motor output for the basal ganglia system and cerebellum. The last portion of the basal ganglia is the *substantia nigra,* which synthesizes *dopamine,* a neurotransmitter and precursor of norepinephrine. Its dysfunction is associated with Parkinson disease. The *basis pedunculi* are made up of efferent fibers of the corticospinal, corticobulbar, and corticopontocerebellar tracts.

Other notable structures of this region are the nuclei of the third and fourth cranial nerves. The *cerebral aqueduct (aqueduct of Sylvius),* which carries CSF, also traverses this structure. Plugging of this aqueduct is often the cause of hydrocephalus.

Hindbrain

Metencephalon

The major structures of the *metencephalon* are the cerebellum and the pons. The *cerebellum* (see Fig. 12-6) is composed of gray and white matter, and its cortical surface is convoluted like the surface of the cerebrum. It also is divided by a central fissure into two lobes connected by the *vermis.*

The cerebellum is responsible for reflexive, involuntary fine-tuning of motor control and for maintaining balance and posture through extensive neural connections with the medulla through the inferior cerebellar peduncle and with the midbrain through the superior cerebellar peduncle. The two hemispheres are connected to the pons by the middle cerebellar peduncle. These connections allow extensive sampling of visual, vestibular, and proprioceptive data from other regions of the CNS and periphery.

The *pons* (bridge) is easily recognized by its bulging appearance below the midbrain and above the medulla. Primarily it transmits information from the cerebellum to the brain stem and between the two cerebellar hemispheres. The pons is an important center for controlling respiration (i.e., rate and relationship of inspiration to expiration). The nuclei of the fifth through eighth cranial nerves are located in this structure.

Myelencephalon

The *myelencephalon* usually is called the *medulla oblongata* and forms the lowest portion of the brain stem. Reflex

---

** The tegmentum and basis pedunculi are called collectively the **cerebral peduncles.***

activities, such as heart rate, respiration, blood pressure, coughing, sneezing, swallowing, and vomiting, are controlled in this area. The nuclei of cranial nerves IX through XII also are located in this region.

A major portion of the descending motor pathways (i.e., corticospinal tracts) cross to the other side, or decussate, at the medulla (Fig. 12-8). These pathways, together with other areas of decussation in the CNS, are the basis for the phenomenon of contralateral control. Sleep-wake rhythms also are processed by neural influences from lower brain centers and are associated with a complex group of diffuse structures and functions (see Chapter 13), including the reticular activating system (cells that receive collateral signals from the afferent sensory pathways and project the signals to the higher brain centers, thus controlling CNS activity).

✓ QUICK CHECK

Name the three major divisions of the brain and their component parts.

Describe the limbic system's functions.

What are the two major functions of the hypothalamus?

The Spinal Cord

The *spinal cord* lies within the vertebral canal and is surrounded and protected by the *vertebral column.* The spinal cord essentially functions as a large nerve cable connecting the brain and body. It extends from the medulla and ends at the level of the first or second lumbar vertebra in adults (Fig. 12-9). The end of the spinal cord (the *conus medullaris*) is cone-shaped. Spinal nerves continue from the conus medullaris and form the *cauda equina.*

A cross section of the spinal cord (Fig. 12-10) is characterized by a butterfly-shaped inner core of gray matter (containing nerve cell bodies). The *central canal* lies in the center of this region and extends through the spinal cord from its origin in the fourth ventricle. The gray matter of the spinal cord is divided into three regions and displays specific functional characteristics. These regions include the *posterior horn,* or *dorsal horn* (primarily interneurons and axons from sensory neurons whose cell bodies lie in the *dorsal root ganglion*). At the tip of the posterior horn is the *substantia gelatinosa,* a structure involved in pain transmission (see Chapter 13). The *lateral horn* contains cell bodies involved with the ANS, as well as interneurons to connect the dorsal horn cells to the ventral horn. The *anterior horn,* or *ventral horn,* contains the nerve cell bodies for efferent pathways that leave the spinal cord by way of spinal nerves.

Surrounding the gray matter is white matter that forms ascending and descending pathways called *spinal tracts.* Spinal tracts are named to denote their beginning and ending points. For example, the *spinothalamic tract* carries

A

Somatic motor area of cerebral cortex

Internal capsule

Thalamus

Lentiform nucleus

Red nucleus

Midbrain

Cerebral peduncle

Substantia nigra

Upper motor neuron

Pons

Reticular formation

Pyramid

Medulla

Pyramidal decussation

Rubrospinal tract

Lateral corticospinal tract

Reticulospinal tract

Interneuron

Spinal cord

Spinal cord

Motor end plate

Lower (anterior horn) motor neuron

Fig. 12-8 *Examples of somatic motor and sensory pathways.* **A**, Motor: The pyramidal pathway through the lateral corticospinal tract and the extrapyramidal pathways through the rubrospinal and reticulospinal tracts. **B**, Sensory: Pathways of the medial lemniscal system that conducts information about discriminating touch and kinesthesis and the spinothalamic pathway that conducts information about pain and temperature. *(From Thibodeau, G.A. & Patton, K.T. [1999]. Anatomy & physiology [4th ed.]. St. Louis: Mosby.)*

Somatic sensory area of cerebral cortex

Tertiary sensory neuron

Thalamus

Cerebrum

Tertiary sensory neuron

Medial lemniscus

Midbrain

Medial lemniscus

Secondary sensory neuron

B

Nucleus gracilis

Secondary sensory neuron

Pons

Decussation of medial lemniscus

Medial lemniscus

Dorsal root ganglion

Collateral fibers to reticular formation

Dorsal root ganglion

Medulla

Medulla

Primary sensory neuron

Fasciculus gracilis

Lateral spinothalamic tract

Primary sensory neuron

Spinal cord

Receptor

Spinal cord

A

Cervical plexus
Brachial plexus

Cerebellum
Cervical enlargement

Lumbar plexus
Femoral nerve
Sacral plexus
Sciatic nerve
Pudendal nerve

Lumbar enlargement
Filum terminale

Posterior cutaneous nerve of thigh

B

Thalamus

C1
C2
C3
C4
C5
C6
C7
C8
T1
T2
T3
T4
T5
T6
T7
T8
T9
T10
T11
T12
L1
L2
L3
L4
L5
S1
S2
S3
S4
S5

Coccyx

C

T12
L1 — Conus medullaris
L2
L3
Cauda equina
L4
L5
S1
S2
S3
S4
S5
Coccyx

Filum terminale

Fig. 12-9 *Spinal cord within vertebral canal and exiting spinal nerves.* **A,** Posterior view of brain stem and spinal cord in situ with spinal nerves and plexus. **B,** Anterior view of brain stem and spinal cord. **C,** Enlargement of caudal area showing termination of spinal cord (conus medullaris) and group of nerve fibers constituting the cauda equina. *(From Rudy, E.B. [Ed.]. [1984]. Advanced neurological and neurosurgical nursing. St. Louis: Mosby.)*

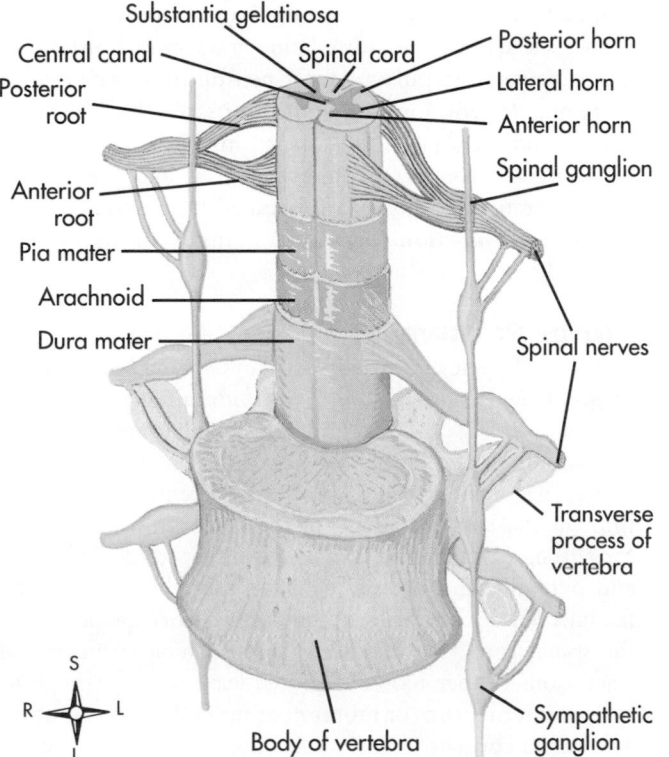

Substantia gelatinosa
Central canal
Spinal cord
Posterior horn
Posterior root
Lateral horn
Anterior horn
Spinal ganglion
Anterior root
Pia mater
Arachnoid
Dura mater
Spinal nerves
Transverse process of vertebra
Body of vertebra
Sympathetic ganglion

S
R — L
I

Fig. 12-10 *Coverings of the spinal cord.* The dura mater is shown in natural color. Note how it extends to cover the spinal nerve roots and nerves. The arachnoid is highlighted in blue and the pia mater in pink. *(Modified from Thibodeau, G.A. & Patton, K.T. [1999]. Anatomy & physiology [4th ed.]. St. Louis: Mosby.)*

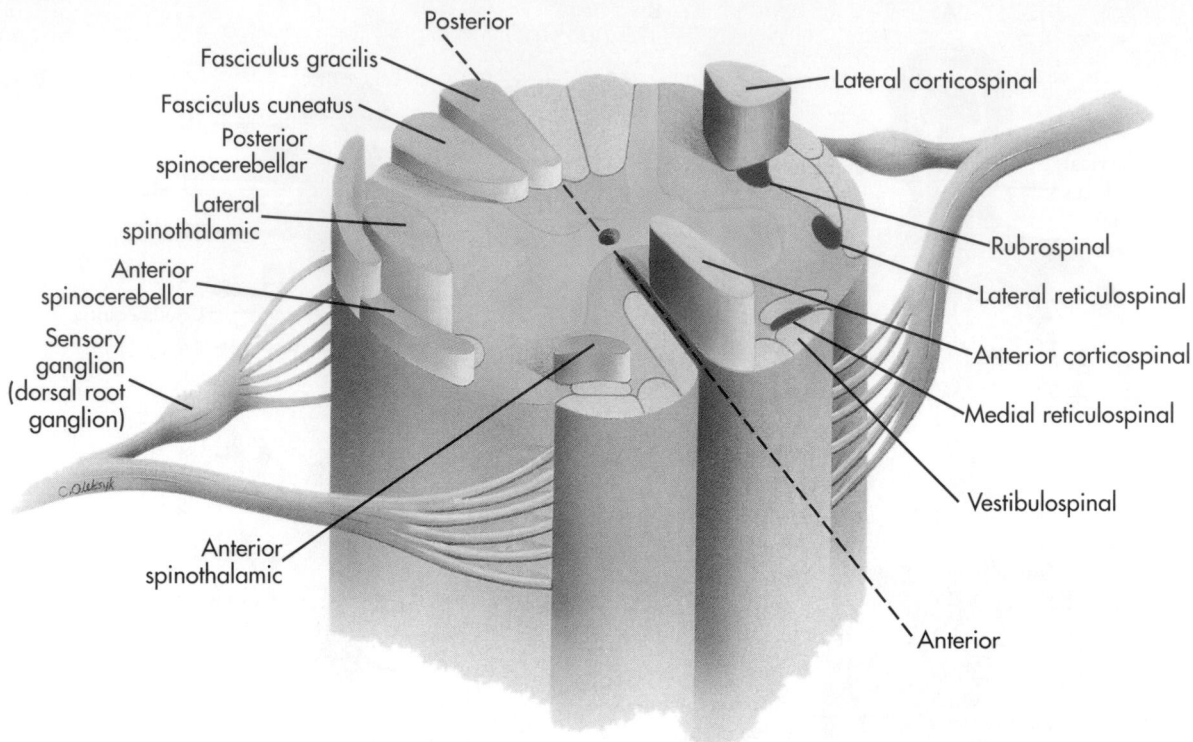

Fig. 12-11 *Major tracts of the spinal cord.* The major ascending (sensory) tracts, shown only on the left here, are highlighted in blue. The major descending (motor) tracts, shown only on the right, are highlighted in red. The broken line indicates the anterior/posterior orientation angle. *(From Thibodeau, G.A. & Patton, K.T. [1999].* Anatomy & physiology *[4th ed.]. St. Louis: Mosby.)*

nerve impulses from the spinal cord to the thalamus in the diencephalon. Numerous spinal tracts are grouped into columns according to their location within the white matter. These include the *anterior columns, lateral columns,* and *posterior (dorsal) columns* (Fig. 12-11).

Neural circuits in the spinal cord, when activated, display specific sets of motor responses. *Reflex arcs* form basic units that respond to stimuli and provide protective circuitry for motor output. Structures needed for a reflex arc are a receptor, an *afferent (sensory) neuron,* an *efferent (motor) neuron,* and an effector muscle or gland. A simple reflex arc may contain only two neurons (Fig. 12-12).

Much internal environmental regulation is mediated by reflex activity involving the ANS. The motor effects of reflex arcs generally occur before the event is perceived in the brain's higher centers.

Afferent pathways transmit information from peripheral receptors and eventually terminate in the cerebral or cerebellar cortex or both. Efferent pathways primarily relay information from the cerebrum to the brain stem or spinal cord. *Upper motor neurons* are completely contained within the CNS. Their primary role is influencing and modifying spinal reflex arcs and circuits. Generally, upper motor neurons form synapses with interneurons, which then form synapses with lower motor neurons before projecting into the periphery. *Lower motor neurons* directly influence muscles. Their cell bodies lie in the gray matter of the spinal cord, but their processes extend out of the CNS and into the

PNS. Destruction of upper motor neurons usually results in initial paralysis followed within days or weeks by partial recovery, whereas destruction of the lower motor neurons often leads to permanent paralysis. Peripheral nerve damage may be followed by nerve regeneration and recovery.

Muscle activity (i.e., stimulation and contraction) is regulated by nerve impulses. Motor neurons innervate one or more muscle cells, forming *motor units,* which consist of a neuron and the skeletal muscles it stimulates. The junction between the axon of the motor neuron and the plasma membrane of the muscle cell is called the *neuromuscular (myoneural) junction* (Fig. 12-13). (Injury to motor neurons is discussed in Chapter 14.)

Motor Pathways

The clinically relevant motor pathways are the *lateral corticospinal, basal ganglia,* and *vestibulospinal.*[5] The corticospinal (see Fig. 12-8, *A*) and corticobulbar are essentially the same tract and consist of a two-neuron chain. The cell bodies originate in and around the precentral gyrus, pass through the corona radiata of the cerebrum, the internal capsule, middle three fifths of the cerebral pedunculus, pons, and pyramid, and decussate (cross contralaterally) in the medulla oblongata and form the lateral corticospinal tract of the spinal cord (see Fig. 12-11). The lateral corticospinal tract axons (upper motor neurons) leave the tract to go to specific interneurons or motor neurons in the anterior horn. The lateral corticospinal tract has the same somatropic or-

Fig. 12-12 *Cross section of spinal cord showing simple reflex arc.* (From Thibodeau, G.A. & Patton, K.T. [1999]. Anatomy & physiology [4th ed.]. St. Louis: Mosby.)

Fig. 12-13 *Neuromuscular junction.* This figure shows how the distal end of a motor neuron fiber forms a synapse, or "chemical junction," with an adjacent muscle fiber. Neurotransmitters (specifically, acetylcholine) are released from the neuron's synaptic vesicles and diffuse across the synaptic cleft. There they stimulate receptors in the motor end-plate region of the sarcolemma. (From Thibodeau, G.A. & Patton, K.T. [1999]. Anatomy & physiology [4th ed.]. St. Louis: Mosby.)

ganization as the body (see Fig. 12-7). These motor neurons project to specific motor units and are lower motor neurons. This tract is involved in precise motor movements. The basal ganglia are part of a system that drives the reticular and rubrospinal descending tracts (see Fig. 12-11). These tracts modulate motor movement by inhibiting and exciting spinal activity. The vestibulospinal tract arises from a vestibular nucleus in the pons and causes the extensor muscles of the body to rapidly contract, most dramatically witnessed when a person starts to fall backward.

Sensory Pathways

The three clinically important spinal afferent pathways are the ***posterior (dorsal) column, anterior spinothalamic,*** and ***lateral spinothalamic*** (Figs. 12-7 and 12-8, *B*). The posterior column (fasciculus gracilis and cuneatus) carries body fine touch, two-point discrimination, and proprioceptive information (i.e., ***epicritic*** information). The posterior column is formed by a three-neuron chain. The primary afferent neuron is the sensory neuron (of the reflex arc), but it sends its axon ipsilaterally up the spinal cord to a specific part of the posterior funiculus and synapses in the posterior column nuclei in the hindbrain. A basketball center has primary afferent neurons that could be more than 6 feet long, running from the great toe up to the pons. The second-order neuron crosses contralaterally and ascends to a specific nucleus of the thalamus and synapses. The third-order neuron, originating in the thalamus, continues the tract into the internal capsule, corona radiata, and postcentral gyrus (Brodmann areas 3, 1, 2) (see Figs. 12-6, *C*, and 12-7). The anterior and

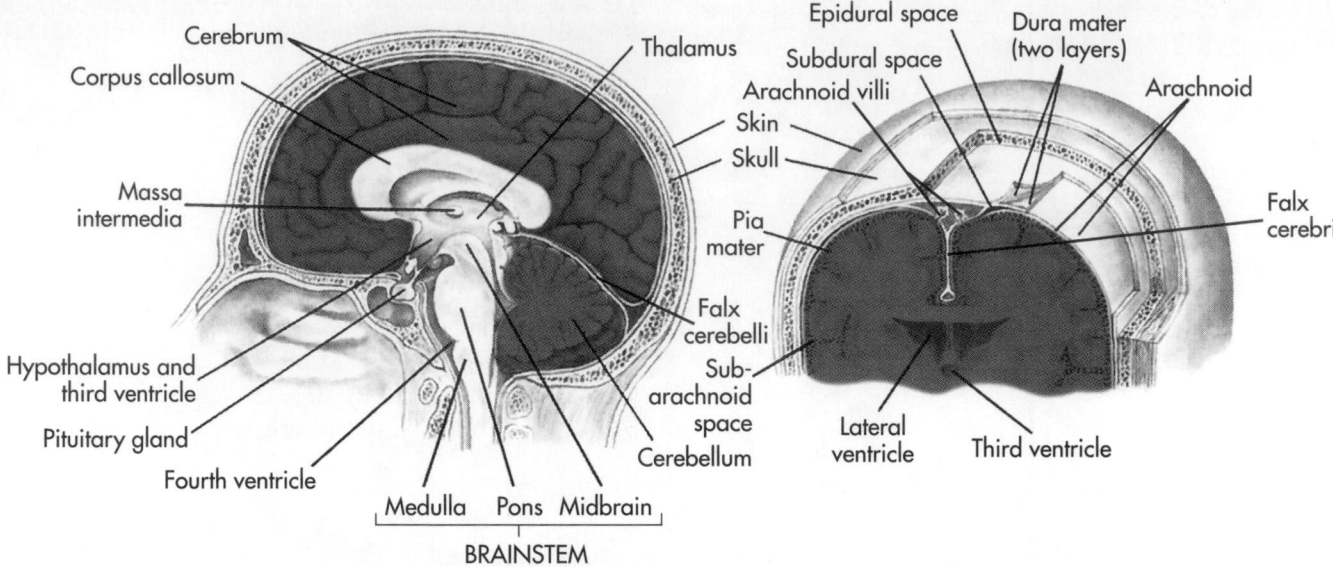

Fig. 12-14 *Meninges of the brain. (From Thompson, J.M. et al. [1997].* Mosby's clinical nursing *[4th ed.]. St. Louis: Mosby.)*

lateral spinothalamic tracts are responsible for vague touch and pain and temperature, respectively (see Fig. 12-8, *B*). These modalities are referred to as *protopathic.* These tracts also form a three-neuron chain. However, the primary afferent neurons synapse in the posterior horn of the spinal cord, not just at the level they enter the intervertebral foramen but in a number of spinal segments above and below their point of entry. This is an example of divergence. The second-order neurons in the posterior horn cross to the contralateral side in the spinal cord and ascend to the same thalamic nucleus as the posterior column pathway and continue on with the posterior column pathway to the postcentral gyrus.

Protective Structures of the Central Nervous System
Cranium

The cranium is composed of eight bones. The cranial vault encloses and protects the brain and its associated structures.

The *galea aponeurotica,* which is a thick, fibrous band of tissue overlying the cranium between the frontal and occipital muscles, affords added protection to the skull. The subgaleal space has venous connections with the dural sinuses and, with increased intracranial pressure, blood can be shunted to the space, thus reducing pressure in the intracranial cavity. The subgaleal space is also a common site for wound drains after intracranial surgery.

The floor of the cranial vault is irregular and contains many foramina (openings) for cranial nerves, blood vessels, and the spinal cord to exit. The cranial floor is divided into three fossae (depressions). The frontal lobes lie in the *anterior fossa,* the temporal lobes and base of the diencephalon lie in the *middle fossa (temporal fossa),* and the cerebellum lies in the *posterior fossa.* These terms are commonly used

anatomic landmarks to describe the location of intracranial lesions.

Meninges

Surrounding the brain and spinal cord are three protective membranes: the dura mater, the arachnoid membrane, and the pia mater. Collectively they are called the *meninges* (Fig. 12-14). The *dura mater* (meaning literally "hard mother") is composed of two layers, with the venous sinuses formed between them. The outermost layer forms the *periosteum (endosteal layer)* of the skull. The *inner dura (meningeal layer)* is responsible for forming rigid plates that support and separate various brain structures.

One of these membranous plates, the *falx cerebri,* dips between the two cerebral hemispheres along the longitudinal fissure. The falx cerebri is anchored anteriorly to the base of the brain at the crista galli of the ethmoid bone. The *tentorium cerebelli,* a common landmark, is a membrane that separates the cerebellum below from the cerebral structures above. Below the dura mater lies the *arachnoid membrane,* a spongy, weblike structure that loosely follows the contours of the cerebral structures.

The *subdural space* lies between the dura and arachnoid membrane. Many small bridging veins that have little support traverse the subdural space. Their disruption results in a subdural hematoma (see Chapter 15). The *subarachnoid space* lies between the arachnoid membrane and the pia mater and contains cerebrospinal fluid (CSF) (see Fig. 12-14).

Unlike the dura mater and arachnoid membrane, the delicate pia mater follows the contours of the brain and spinal cord very closely. It provides support for blood vessels serving brain tissue. The *choroid plexuses,* structures that produce CSF, arise from the pial membrane (see Fig. 12-14).

The spinal cord is anchored to the vertebrae by extension of the meninges. The meninges continue beyond the end of the spinal cord to the lower portion of the sacrum. CSF contained within the subarachnoid space also circulates down to about the second sacral vertebra.

The meninges form potential and real spaces important to understanding functional and pathologic mechanisms. For example, between the dura mater and skull lies a potential space termed the *epidural space* (see Fig. 12-14). The arterial supply to the meninges consists of blood vessels that lie within grooves in the skull.

Cerebrospinal fluid and the ventricular system

Cerebrospinal fluid (CSF) is a clear, colorless fluid similar to blood plasma and interstitial fluid. The intracranial and spinal cord structures float in CSF and are protected from jolts and blows. The buoyant properties of the CSF also prevent the brain from tugging on meninges, nerve roots, and blood vessels. (Constituents of CSF are listed in Table 12-4.) Between 125 and 150 ml of CSF is circulating within the **ventricles** (small cavities) and subarachnoid space at any given time. Approximately 600 ml of CSF is produced daily.

The choroid plexuses in the lateral, third, and fourth ventricles produce the major portion of CSF. (Ventricles are illustrated in Fig. 12-14.) These plexuses are characterized by a rich network of blood vessels, supplied by the pia mater, that lie close to the ependymal cells of the ventricles.

TABLE 12-4	Composition of Cerebrospinal Fluid
Constituent	**Normal Value**
Na^+	148 mM
K^+	2.9 mM
Cl^-	125 mM
HCO_3^-	22.9 mM
Glucose (fasting)	50-75 mg/dl (60% of serum glucose)
pH	7.3
Protein	15-45 mg/dl
Albumin	80%
Globulin	6%-10%
Cells	
White (lymphocytes)	0-6/mm³
Red	

The CSF exerts pressure within the brain and spinal cord. With a person lying down, CSF pressure is about 120 to 180 mm of water pressure, or approximately 9 to 14 mm Hg pressure. CSF flow results from the pressure gradient between the arterial system and the CSF-filled cavities. Beginning in the lateral ventricles, the CSF flows through the *interventricular foramen (foramen of Monro)* into the third ventricle and then passes through the cerebral aqueduct (aqueduct of Sylvius) into the fourth ventricle. From the fourth ventricle the CSF may pass through either the paired *lateral apertures (foramen of Luschka)* or the *median aper-*

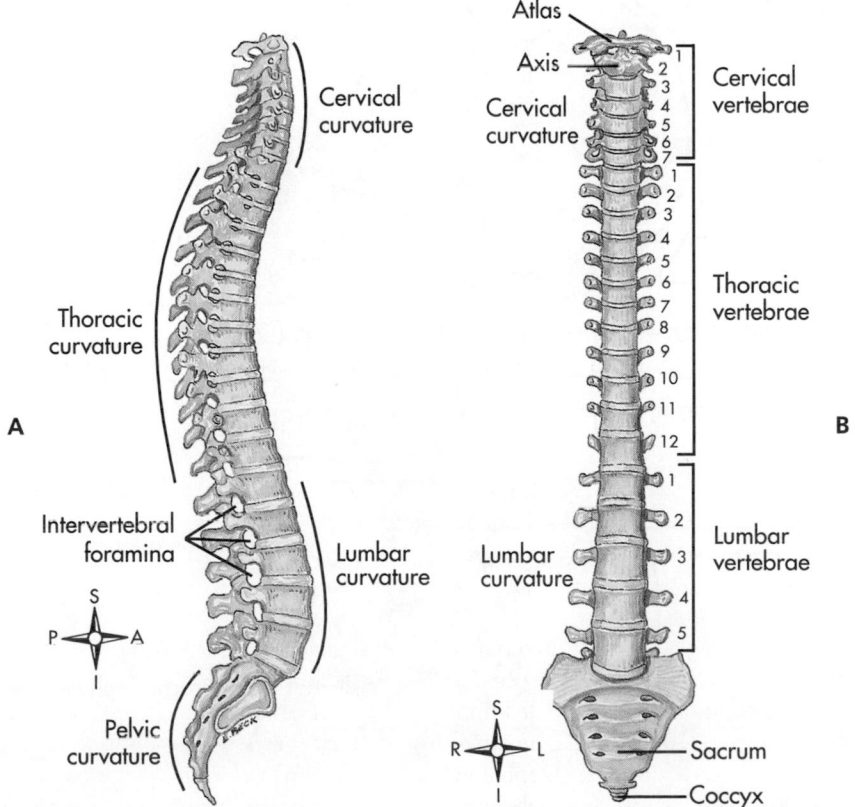

Fig. 12-15 *Vertebral column.* **A,** Right lateral view. **B,** Anterior view. *(From Thibodeau, G.A. & Patton, K.T. [1999]. Anatomy & physiology [4th ed.]. St. Louis: Mosby.)*

Fig. 12-16 *Vertebra and intervertebral disk.* (From Rudy, E.B. [Ed.]. [1984]. Advanced neurological and neurosurgical nursing. St. Louis: Mosby.)

ture (foramen of Magendie) before communicating with the subarachnoid spaces of the brain and spinal cord. The CSF does not, however, accumulate. Instead, it is reabsorbed into the venous circulation through the arachnoid villi. The *arachnoid villi* protrude from the arachnoid space, through the dura mater, and lie within the blood flow of the venous sinuses. CSF is reabsorbed through a pressure gradient between the arachnoid villi and the cerebral venous sinuses. The villi function as one-way valves directing CSF outflow into the blood but preventing blood flow into the subarach-

noid space. Thus CSF is formed from the blood, and after circulating throughout the CNS, it returns to the blood.

Vertebral column

The vertebral column (Fig. 12-15) is composed of 33 vertebrae: 7 cervical, 12 thoracic, 5 lumbar, 5 fused sacral, and 4 fused coccygeal. Between each interspace (except the fused sacral and coccygeal vertebrae) is an *intervertebral disk* (Fig. 12-16). At the center of the intervertebral disk is the *nucleus pulposus,* a pulpy mass of elastic fibers. The intervertebral disk absorbs shocks, preventing damage to the vertebrae. The intervertebral disk is also a common source of back problems. If too much stress is applied to the vertebral column, the disk contents may rupture and protrude into the spinal canal, causing compression of the spinal cord or nerve roots.

✓QUICK CHECK

What information is conveyed in the ascending and descending spinal tracts?

Contrast the functions of upper and lower motor neurons.

Name the protective structures of the central nervous system, and briefly describe each one.

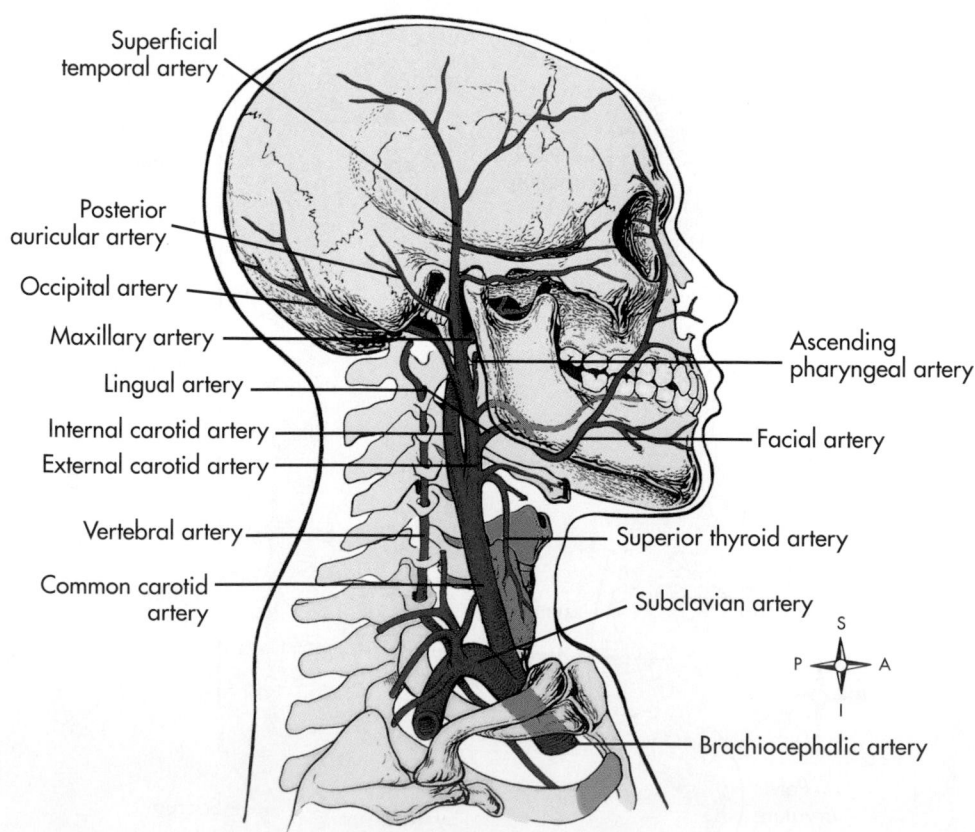

Fig. 12-17 *Major arteries of the head and neck.* (From Thibodeau, G.A., & Patton, K.T. [1999]. Anatomy & physiology [4th ed.]. St. Louis: Mosby.)

Blood Supply of the Central Nervous System

Blood supply to the brain

The brain receives approximately 20% of the cardiac output, or 800 to 1000 ml of blood flow per minute. Carbon dioxide is a primary regulator for blood flow within the CNS. It is a potent vasodilator, and its effects ensure an adequate blood supply.

The brain derives its arterial supply from two systems: the *internal carotid arteries* and the *vertebral arteries* (Fig. 12-17). The internal carotid arteries supply a proportionately greater amount of blood flow. They take their origin from the common carotid arteries, enter the cranium through the base of the skull, and pass through the *cav-ernous sinus.* Just beyond some small branches, these arteries divide into the anterior and middle cerebral arteries. The vertebral arteries originate at the subclavian arteries and pass through the transverse foramina of the cervical vertebrae, entering the cranium through the foramen magnum. They join at the junction of the pons and medulla to form the *basilar artery.* The basilar artery divides at the level of the midbrain to form paired posterior cerebral arteries. The large arteries on the surface of the brain and their branches are called *superficial arteries (conducting arteries).* The small branches that project into the brain are termed *projecting arteries (nutrient arteries).*

The *circle of Willis* (Fig. 12-18) provides an alternative route for blood flow when one of the contributing arteries is

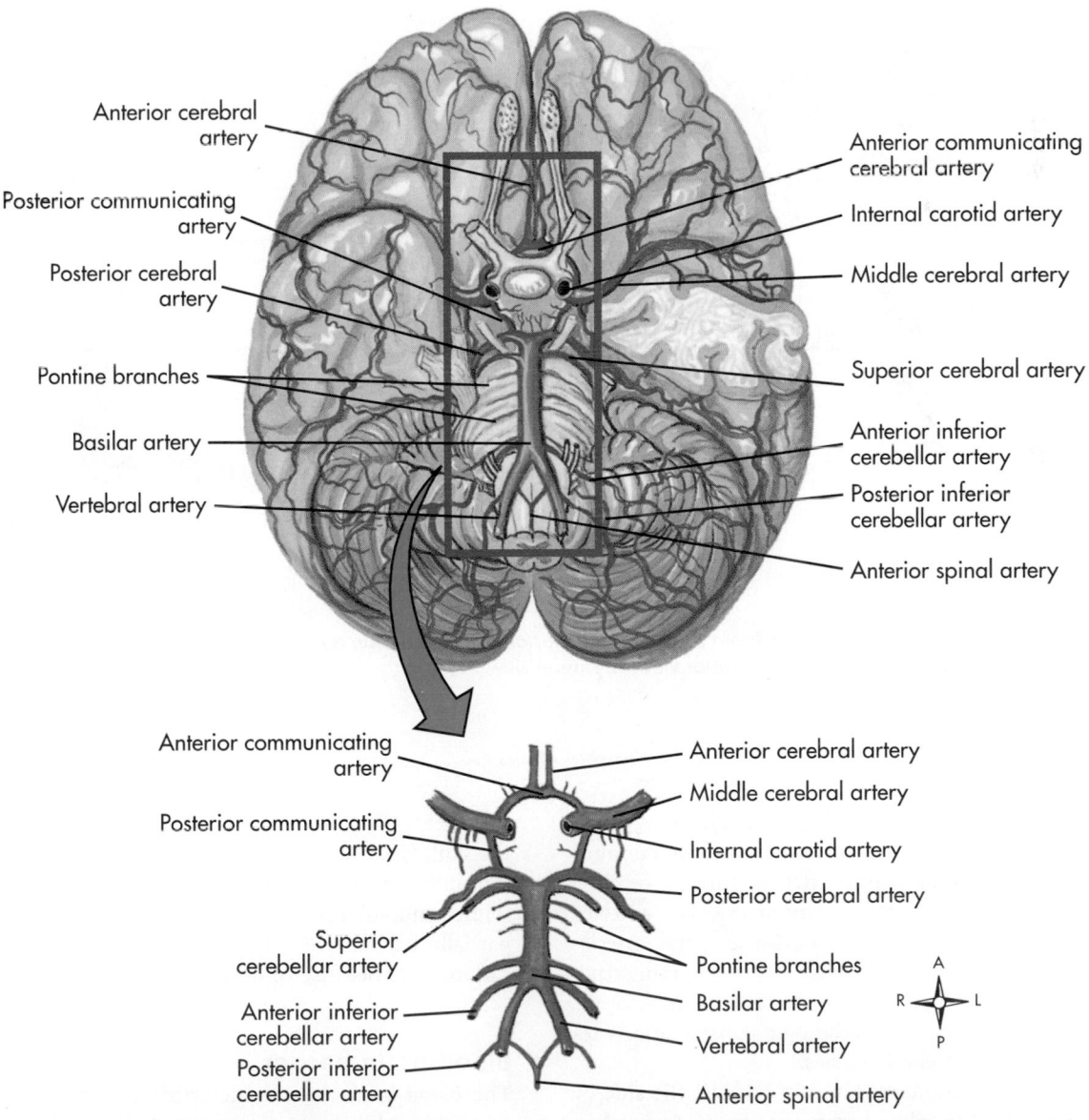

Fig. 12-18 *Arteries at the base of the brain.* The arteries that compose the circle of Willis are the two anterior cerebral arteries, joined to each other by the anterior communicating two short segments of the internal carotids, off of which the posterior communicating arteries connect to the posterior cerebral arteries. *(From Thibodeau, G.A. & Patton, K.T. [1999]. Anatomy & physiology [4th ed.]. St. Louis: Mosby.)*

TABLE 12-5	Arterial Systems Supplying the Brain	
Arterial Origin	**Structures Served**	**Conditions Caused by Occlusion**
Anterior cerebral artery	Basal ganglia; corpus callosum; medial surface of cerebral hemispheres; superior surface of frontal and parietal lobes	Hemiplegia on the contralateral side of the body, greater in the lower than in the upper extremities
Middle cerebral artery	Frontal lobe; parietal lobe; temporal lobe (primarily the cortical surfaces)	Aphasia in dominant hemisphere and contralateral hemiplegia (see Chapter 15)
Posterior cerebral artery	Part of the diencephalon and temporal lobe; occipital lobe	Visual loss; sensory loss; contralateral hemipligia if cerebral peduncle affected

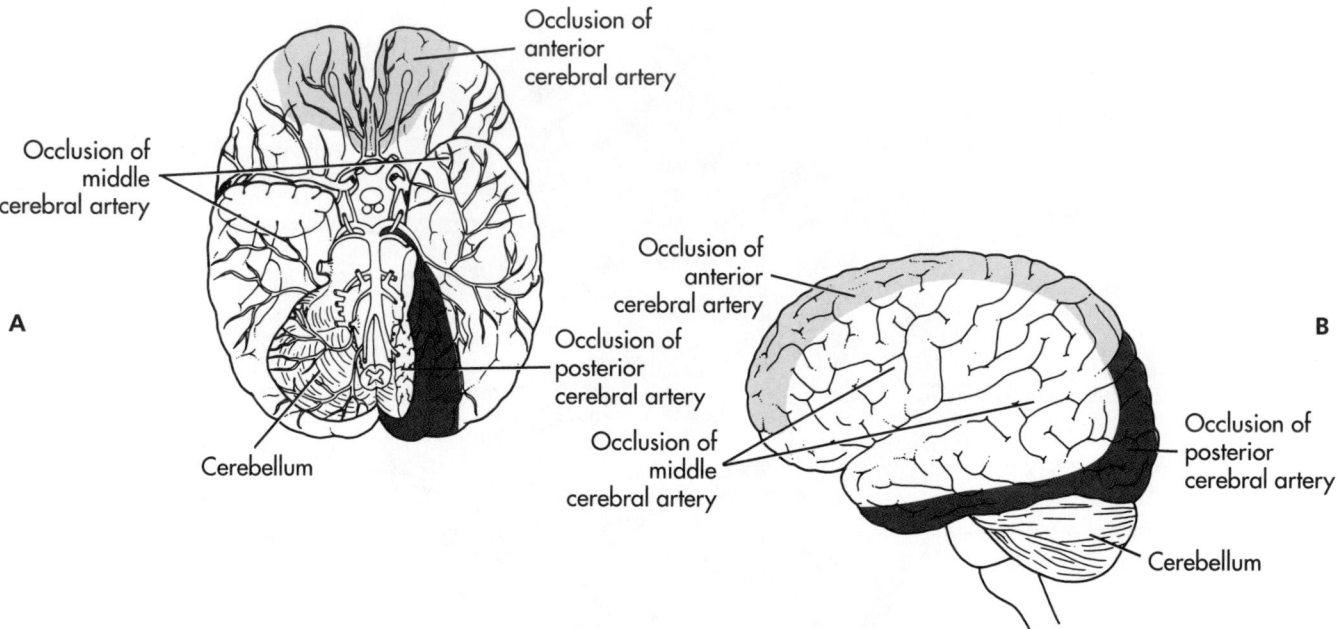

Fig. 12-19 *Areas of the brain affected by occlusion of the anterior, middle, and posterior cerebral artery branches.* **A,** Inferior view. **B,** Lateral view.

obstructed (collateral blood flow). The circle of Willis is formed by the posterior cerebral arteries, posterior communicating arteries, internal carotid arteries, anterior cerebral arteries, and anterior communicating artery. The anterior cerebral, middle cerebral, and posterior cerebral arteries leave the circle of Willis and extend to various brain structures. (Table 12-5 and Fig. 12-19 illustrate structures served, functional relationships, and pathologic considerations related to occlusion of cerebral arteries.)

Cerebral venous drainage does not parallel (lie side by side with) its arterial supply, whereas the venous drainage of the brain stem and cerebellum does parallel the arterial supply of these structures. The cerebral veins are classified as superficial and deep veins. The veins drain into venous plexuses and dural sinuses (formed between the dural layers)

and eventually join the internal jugular veins at the base of the skull (Fig. 12-20). Adequacy of venous outflow can significantly affect intracranial pressure. For example, head-injured individuals who turn or let the head fall to the side partially occlude venous return and intracranial pressure can increase because of decreased flow through the jugular veins.

Blood-brain barrier

The *blood-brain barrier* describes cellular structures that selectively inhibit certain potentially harmful substances in the blood from entering the interstitial spaces of the brain or CSF. Supporting cells (neuroglia), particularly the astrocytes, and tight junctions between endothelial cells of brain cell capillaries (see Chapter 1) are likely involved in forming this

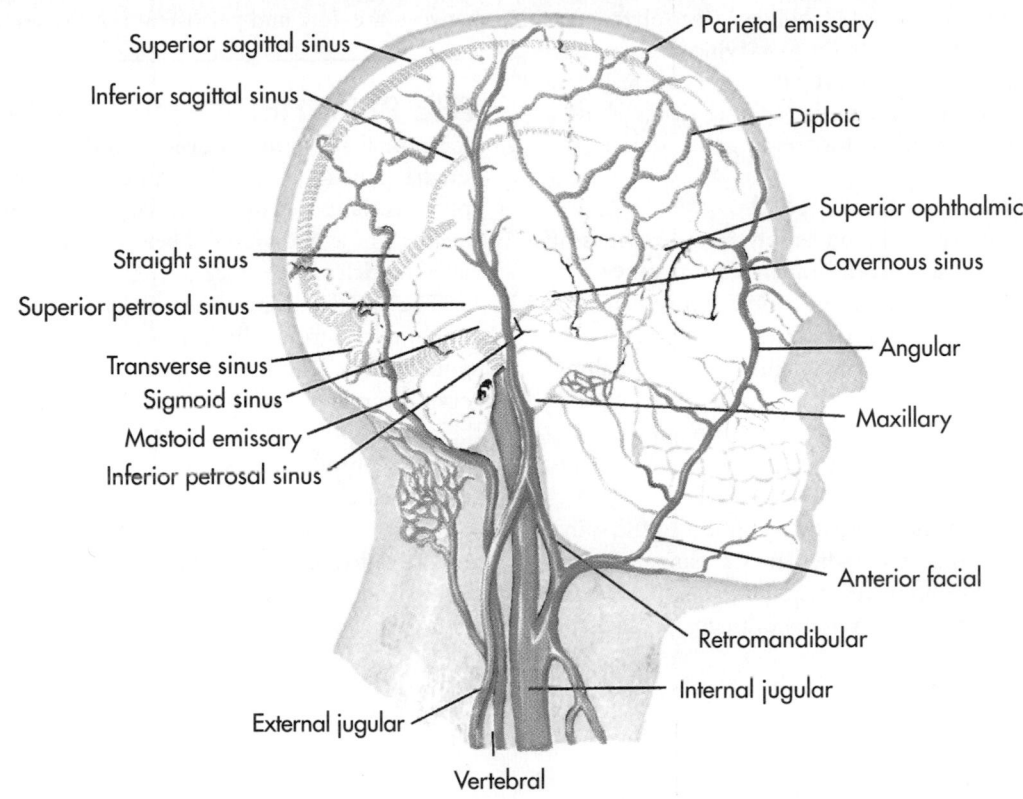

Parietal emissary

Superior sagittal sinus

Inferior sagittal sinus

Diploic

Superior ophthalmic

Cavernous sinus

Straight sinus

Superior petrosal sinus

Angular

Transverse sinus

Sigmoid sinus

Maxillary

Mastoid emissary

Inferior petrosal sinus

Anterior facial

Retromandibular

Internal jugular

External jugular

Vertebral

Fig. 12-20 *Large veins of the head.* Deep veins and dural sinuses are projected on the skull. Note connections (emissary veins) between the superficial and deep veins. *(From Rudy, E.B. [Ed.]. [1984]. Advanced neurological and neurosurgical nursing. St. Louis: Mosby.)*

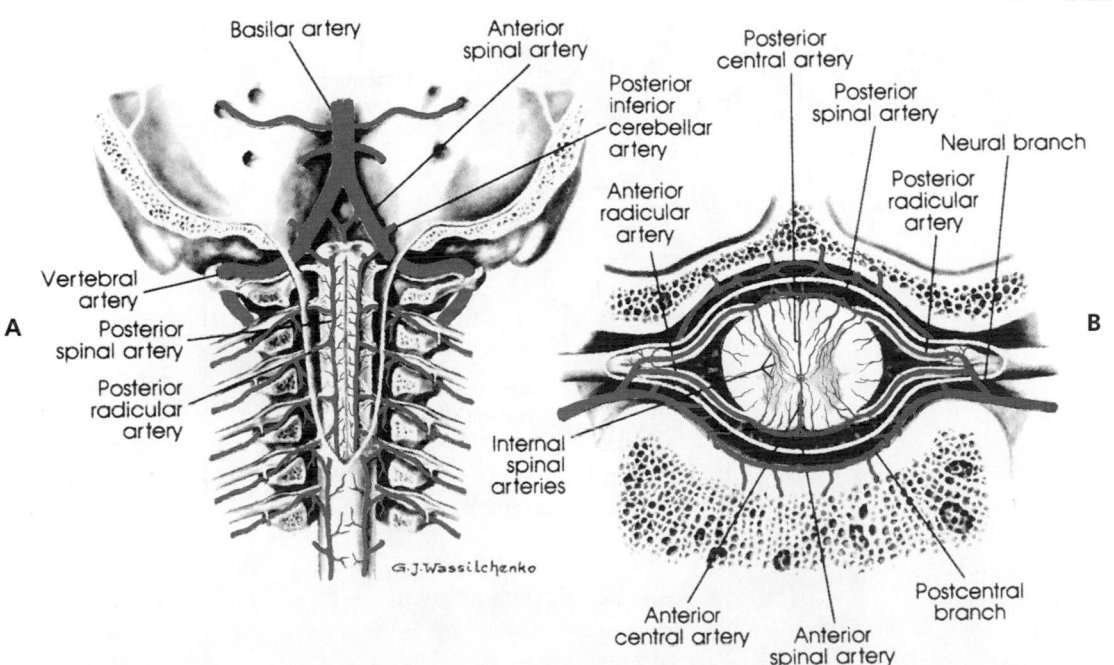

Basilar artery

Anterior spinal artery

Posterior central artery

Posterior inferior cerebellar artery

Posterior spinal artery

Neural branch

Anterior radicular artery

Posterior radicular artery

Vertebral artery

Posterior spinal artery

Posterior radicular artery

A

B

Internal spinal arteries

G.J.Wassilchenko

Anterior central artery

Anterior spinal artery

Postcentral branch

Fig. 12-21 *Arteries of the spinal cord.* **A,** Arteries of cervical cord exposed from the rear. **B,** Arteries of spinal cord diagrammatically shown in horizontal section. *(From Rudy, E.B. [Ed.]. [1984]. Advanced neurological and neurosurgical nursing. St. Louis: Mosby.)*

barrier. The exact nature of this mechanism is controversial, but it appears that certain metabolites, electrolytes, and chemicals can cross into the brain to varying degrees. This has substantial implications for drug therapy because certain types of antibiotics and chemotherapeutic drugs show a greater propensity than others for crossing this barrier.

Blood supply to the spinal cord
The spinal cord derives its blood supply from branches off the vertebral arteries and from branches from various regions of the aorta (Fig. 12-21). The *anterior spinal arteries* and the paired *posterior spinal arteries* branch off the vertebral artery at the base of the cranium and descend alongside the spinal cord. Arterial branches from vessels exterior to the spinal cord follow the spinal nerve through the intervertebral foramina, pass through the dura, and divide into the anterior and posterior radicular arteries.

The radicular arteries eventually reconnect to the spinal arteries. Branches from the radicular and spinal arteries form plexuses whose branches penetrate the spinal cord, supplying the deeper tissues. Venous drainage parallels the

arterial supply closely and drains into venous sinuses located between the dura and periosteum of the vertebrae.

THE PERIPHERAL NERVOUS SYSTEM
The cranial and spinal nerves, including their branches and ganglia, constitute the PNS. A peripheral nerve (cranial or spinal) is composed of individual axons wrapped in a myelin sheath. These individual fibers are arranged in bundles called *fascicles* (Fig. 12-22).

The 31 pairs of spinal nerves derive their names from the vertebral level from which they exit. There are eight cervical spinal nerves. The first cervical nerve exits above the first cervical vertebra, and the rest of the spinal nerves exit below their corresponding vertebrae. From the thoracic region (and interiorly), nerves correspond to the vertebral level above their exit.

Spinal nerves contain both sensory and motor neurons and are called *mixed nerves.* They arise as rootlets from the ventral and dorsal horn cells of the spinal cord. These two spinal nerve roots converge in the region of the interverte-

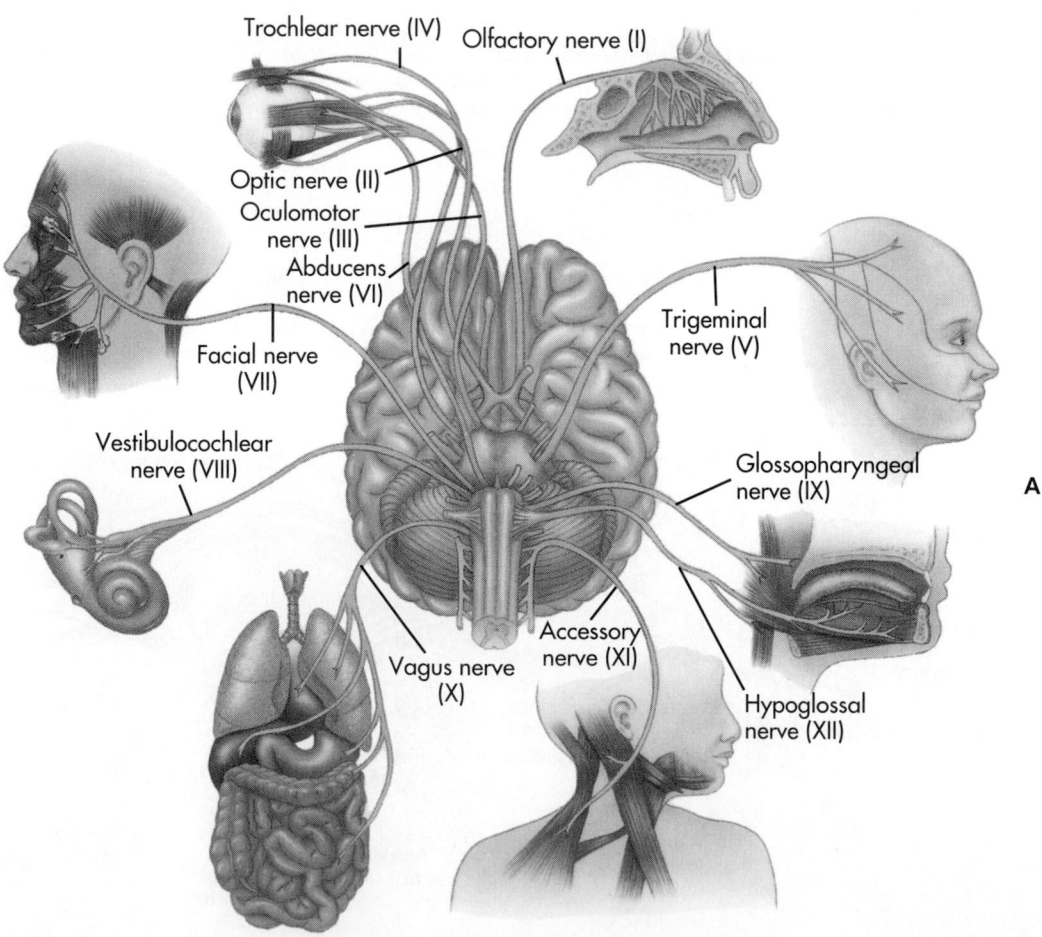

Fig. 12-22 *Cranial and peripheral nerves.* **A,** Ventral surface of the brain showing attachment of the cranial nerves.

bral foramen to form the spinal nerve trunk. Shortly after converging, the spinal nerve divides into anterior and posterior rami (branches). The anterior rami (except the thoracic) initially form **plexuses** (networks of nerve fibers), which then branch into the peripheral nerves. Instead of forming plexuses, the thoracic nerves pass through the intercostal spaces and innervate regions of the thorax.

The main spinal nerve plexuses innervate the skin and the underlying muscles of the limbs. The **brachial plexus,** for example, is formed by the last four cervical nerves (C5 to C8) and the first thoracic nerve (T1). The brachial plexus innervates the nerves of the arm, wrist, and hand. The **lumbar plexus** (L2 to L4) and **sacral plexus** (L5 to S5) contain nerves that innervate the anterior and posterior portions of the lower body, respectively.

The posterior rami of each spinal nerve, with their many processes, are distributed to a specific area in the body. Sensory signals thus arise from specific sites associated with a specific spinal cord segment. Specific areas of cutaneous innervation at these spinal cord segments are called **dermatomes.**

Like spinal nerves, **cranial nerves** are categorized as peripheral nerves. Most of these are mixed nerves (like the spinal nerves), although some are purely sensory or purely motor. Cranial nerves arise from nuclei in the brain and brainstem. (Fig. 12-22 illustrates their structure, and Table 12-6 describes structural and functional characteristics.)

✓ QUICK CHECK

Describe the circle of Willis and its role in supplying blood to the brain.

Where does the spinal cord's blood supply come from?

What are the plexuses? Give two examples in the PNS.

What are the cranial nerves? Give three examples.

Describe the anatomy and function of the PNS.

THE AUTONOMIC NERVOUS SYSTEM

Components of the autonomic nervous system (ANS) are located in both the CNS and the PNS; however, the ANS is considered part of the efferent division of the PNS, even though visceral afferent neurons are certainly an important part of this system. Many neurons of the ANS travel in the spinal nerves and certain cranial nerves. The widespread activity of this system indicates that its components are distributed all over the body. The peripheral autonomic nerves carry mainly efferent fibers. The motor component of the ANS is a two-neuron system consisting of **preganglionic neurons** (myelinated) and **postganglionic neurons** (unmyelinated) (Fig 12-23). This arrangement contrasts with

Fig. 12-22, cont'd B, Peripheral nerve trunk and coverings. **C,** Scanning electron micrograph of a freeze-fractured preparation of peripheral nerve. (*A and C from Thibodeau, G.A. & Patton, K.T. [1999]. Anatomy & physiology [4th ed.]. St. Louis, Mosby.*)

Fig. 12-23 *Locations of neurotransmitters and receptors of the autonomic nervous system.* In all pathways, preganglionic fibers are cholinergic, secreting acetylcholine *(Ach)*, which stimulates nicotinic receptors in the postganglionic neuron. Most sympathetic postganglionic fibers are adrenergic, **A,** secreting norepinephrine *(NE),* thus stimulating α- or β-adrenergic receptors. A few sympathetic postganglionic fibers are cholinergic, stimulating muscarinic receptors in effector cells, **B.** All parasympathetic postganglionic fibers are cholinergic, **C,** stimulating muscarinic receptors in effector cells. *(From Thibodeau, G.A. & Patton, K.T. [1999]. Anatomy & physiology [4th ed.]. St. Louis: Mosby.)*

TABLE 12-6	The Cranial Nerves		
Number and Name	**Origin and Course**	**Function**	**How Tested**
I. Olfactory	Fibers arise from nasal olfactory epithelium and form synapses with olfactory bulbs, which transmit impulses to temporal lobe	Purely sensory; carries impulses for sense of smell	Person is asked to sniff aromatic substances, such as oil of cloves and vanilla, and to identify them
II. Optic	Fibers arise from retina of eye to form optic nerve, which passes through sphenoid bone; two optic nerves then form optic chiasma (with partial crossover of fibers) and eventually end in occipital cortex	Purely sensory; carries impulses for vision	Vision and visual field tested with an eye chart and by testing point at which person first sees an object (finger) moving into visual field; inside of eye is viewed with ophthalmoscope to observe blood vessels of eye interior

TABLE 12-6   The Cranial Nerves—cont'd

Number and Name	Origin and Course	Function	How Tested
III. Oculomotor	Fibers emerge from midbrain and exit from skull to run to eye	Contains motor fibers to inferior oblique, superior, Inferior, and medial rectus extraocular muscles that direct eyeball; levator muscles of eyelid; smooth muscles of iris and ciliary body; and proprioception (sensory) to brain from extraocular muscles	Pupils examined for size, shape, and equality; pupillary reflex tested with a pen light (pupils should constrict when illuminated); ability to follow moving objects
IV. Trochlear	Fibers emerge from posterior midbrain and exit from skull to run to eye	Proprioceptor and motor fibers for superior oblique muscle of eye (extraocular muscle)	Tested in common with cranial nerve III relative to ability to follow moving objects
V. Trigeminal	Fibers emerge from pons and form three divisions that exit from skull and run to face and cranial dura mater	Both motor and sensory for face; conducts sensory impulses from mouth, nose, surface of eye, and dura mater; also contains motor fibers that stimulate chewing muscles	Sensations of pain, touch, and temperature tested with safety pin and hot and cold objects; corneal reflex tested with a wisp of cotton; motor branch tested by asking subject to clench teeth, open mouth against resistance, and move jaw from side to side
VI. Abducens	Fibers leave inferior pons and exit from skull to run to eye	Contains motor fibers to lateral rectus muscle and proprioceptor fibers from same muscle to brain	Tested in common with cranial nerve III relative to ability to move each eye laterally
VII. Facial	Fibers leave pons and travel through temporal bone to reach face	Mixed: (1) supplies motor fibers to muscles of facial expression and to lacrimal and salivary glands and (2) carries sensory fibers from taste buds of anterior part of tongue	Anterior two thirds of tongue tested for ability to taste sweet (sugar), salty, sour (vinegar), and bitter (quinine) substances; symmetry of face checked; subject asked to close eyes, smile, whistle, and so on; tearing tested with ammonia fumes
VIII. Vestibulocochlear (acoustic)	Fibers run from inner ear (hearing and equilibrium receptors in temporal bone) to enter brain stem just below pons	Purely sensory; vestibular branch transmits impulses for sense of equilibrium; cochlear branch transmits impulses for sense of hearing	Hearing checked by air and bone conduction by use of a tuning fork; vestibular tests: Bárány and caloric tests
IX. Glossopharyngeal	Fibers emerge from midbrain and leave skull to run to throat	Mixed: (1) motor fibers serve pharynx (throat) and salivary glands, and (2) sensory fibers carry impulses from pharynx, posterior tongue (taste buds), and pressure receptors of carotid artery	Gag and swallowing reflexes checked; subject asked to speak and cough; posterior one third of tongue may be tested for taste
X. Vagus	Fibers emerge from medulla, pass through skull, and descend through neck region into thorax and abdominal region	Fibers carry sensory and motor impulses for pharynx; a large part of this nerve is parasympathetic motor fibers, which supply smooth muscles of abdominal organs; transmits sensory impulses from viscera	Same as for cranial nerve IX (IX and X are tested in common) because they both serve muscles of throat

Continued

TABLE 12-6   The Cranial Nerves—cont'd

Number and Name	Origin and Course	Function	How Tested
XI. Spinal accessory	Fibers arise from medulla and superior spinal cord and travel to muscles of neck and back	Provides sensory and motor fibers for sternocleidomastoid and trapezius muscles and muscles of soft palate, pharynx, and larynx	Sternocleidomastoid and trapezius muscles checked for strength by asking subject to rotate head and shrug shoulders against resistance
XII. Hypoglossal	Fibers arise from medulla and exit from skull to travel to tongue	Carries motor fibers to muscles of tongue and sensory impulses from tongue to brain	Subject asked to stick out tongue, and any position abnormalities are noted

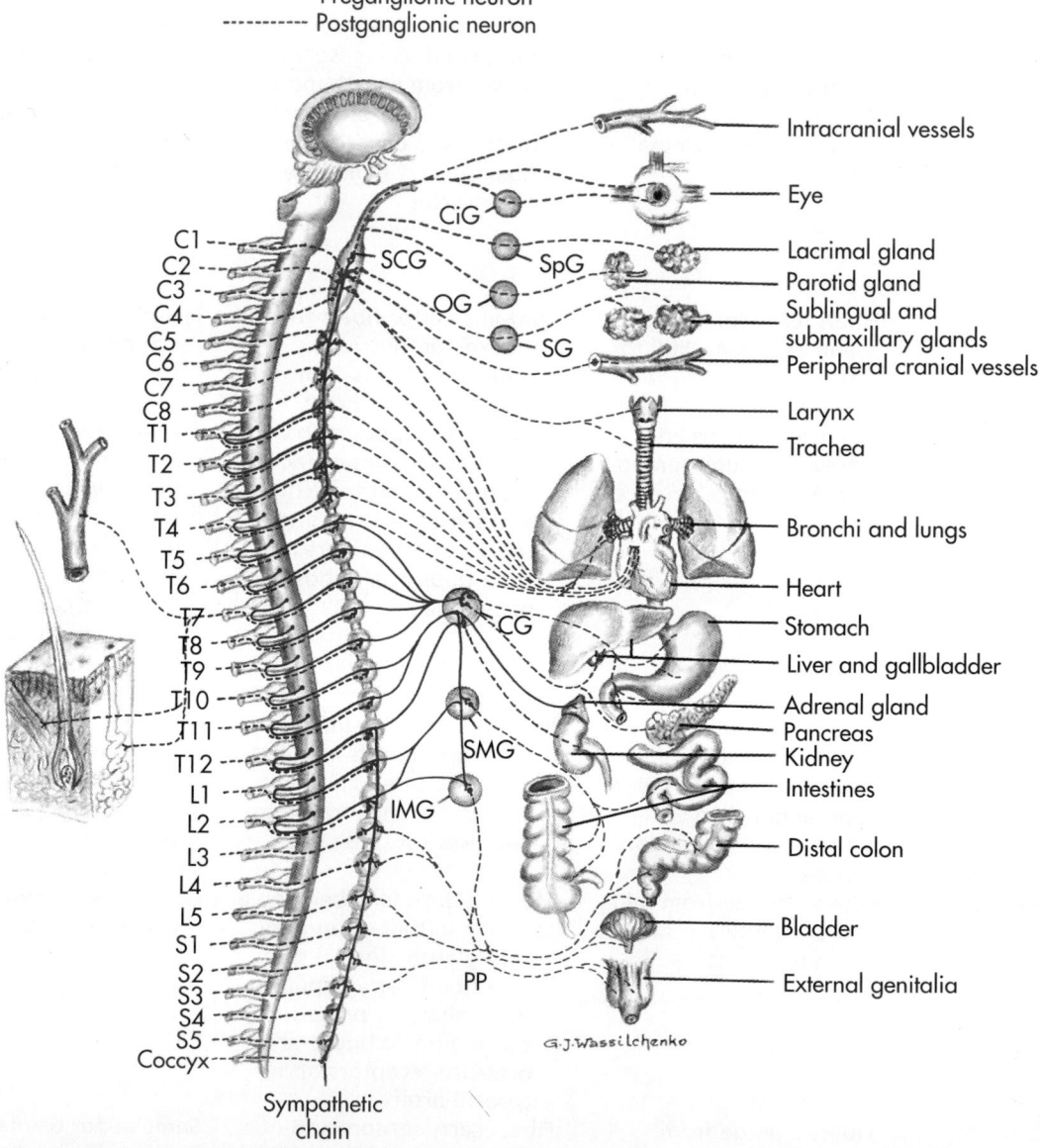

——— Preganglionic neuron
- - - - - Postganglionic neuron

Fig. 12-24 Sympathetic division of the autonomic nervous system. *CiG,* Ciliary ganglion; *SpG,* sphenopalatine ganglion; *SCG,* superior cervical ganglion; *OG,* otic ganglion; *SG,* submandibular ganglion; *CG,* celiac ganglion; *SMG,* superior mesenteric ganglion; *IMG,* inferior mesenteric ganglion; *PP,* pelvic plexus. *(From Rudy, E.B. [Ed.]. [1984]. Advanced neurological and neurosurgical nursing. St. Louis: Mosby.)*

Fig. 12-25 *Parasympathetic division of the autonomic nervous system. CiG,* Ciliary ganglion; *SpG,* sphenopalatine ganglion; *OG,* otic ganglion; *SG,* submandibular ganglion; *VN,* vagus nerve; *PP,* pelvic plexus; *PN,* pelvic nerve. *(From Rudy, E.B. [Ed.]. [1984].* Advanced neurological and neurosurgical nursing. *St. Louis: Mosby.)*

the somatic nervous system, where a single motor neuron travels from the CNS to the innervated structure. Visceral afferent neurons have their cell bodies in some sensory and cranial ganglia and their fiber processes traveling in peripheral nerves. The CNS has autonomic areas in the intermediolateral horns of the spinal cord, cardiovascular and respiratory centers in the reticular formation, and both sympathetic and parasympathetic areas in the hypothalamus. CNS pathways interconnect all these areas.

The ANS coordinates and maintains a steady state among visceral (internal) organs, such as regulation of cardiac muscle, smooth muscle, and the glands of the body. This system is considered an involuntary system because one *generally* cannot "will" these functions to happen. The ANS is separated both structurally and functionally into two divisions: (1) the *sympathetic nervous system* (Fig. 12-24) and (2) the *parasympathetic nervous system* (Fig. 12-25).

Anatomy of the Sympathetic Nervous System

The sympathetic nervous system mobilizes energy stores in times of need (e.g., in the "fight or flight response"). (See Fig. 8-1; see also Chapter 8.) The sympathetic division is innervated by cell bodies located from the first thoracic (T1) through the second lumbar (L2) regions of the spinal cord and therefore is called the *thoracolumbar division.* The preganglionic axons of the sympathetic division form synapses shortly after leaving the cord in the *sympathetic (paravertebral) ganglia.* At this point the impulse may travel several ways: (1) directly across the same ganglion level to form a synapse with the cell bodies of the postganglionic neuron, (2) up or down the sympathetic chain before forming synapses with a higher or lower postganglionic neuron, or (3) through the chain ganglion without synapsing (see Fig 12-24). Some preganglionic axons form pathways called

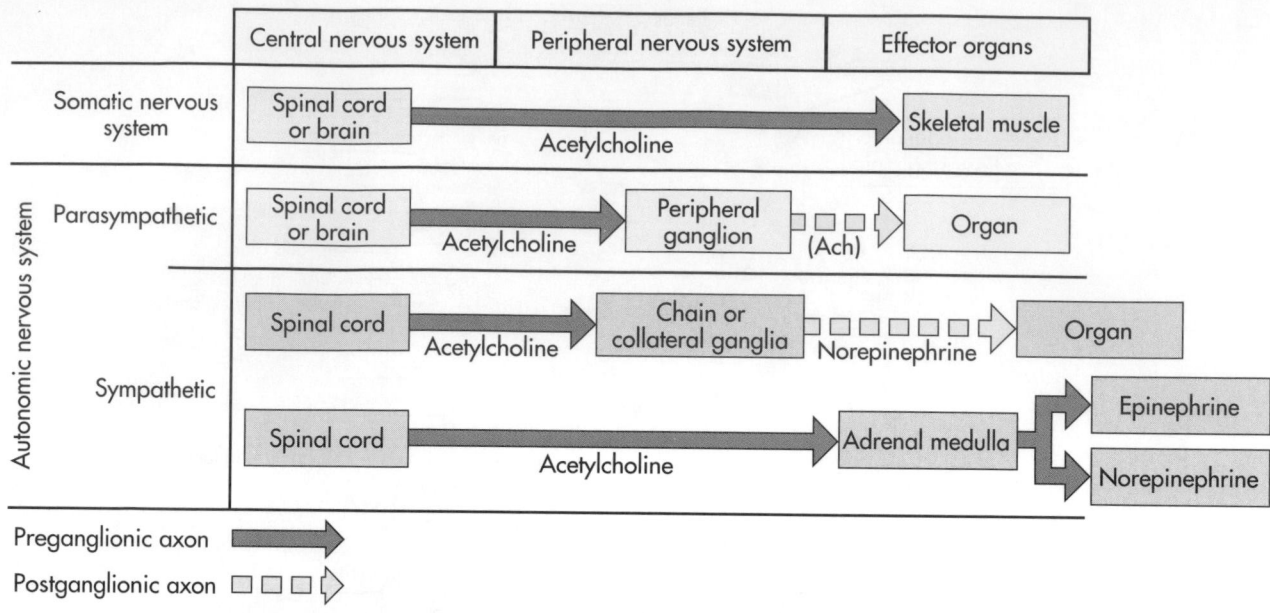

Fig. 12-26 *The autonomic nervous system and the type of neurotransmitters secreted by preganglionic and postganglionic fibers.* Note that all preganglionic fibers are cholinergic *(Ach).* A somatic nerve is used for comparison.

splanchnic nerves, which lead to *collateral ganglia* on the front of the aorta. The collateral ganglia are named according to the branches of the aorta nearest them, namely, the *celiac, superior mesenteric,* and *inferior mesenteric.* The preganglionic neurons synapse with postganglionic neurons within the collateral ganglia. These postganglionic neurons leave the collateral ganglia and innervate the viscera below the diaphragm.

Preganglionic sympathetic neurons that innervate the adrenal medulla also travel in the splanchnic nerves and *do not* synapse before reaching the gland. The secretory cells in the adrenal medulla are considered modified postganglionic neurons. Because preganglionic sympathetic fibers are all myelinated, travel to the adrenal medulla is quick, and innervation causes the rapid release of epinephrine and norepinephrine. Epinephrine and norepinephrine are mediators of the fight or flight response (see Chapter 8).

Anatomy of the Parasympathetic Nervous System

The parasympathetic nervous system conserves and restores energy. The nerve cell bodies of this division are located in the cranial nerve nuclei and in the sacral region of the spinal cord and therefore constitute the *craniosacral division.* Unlike the sympathetic branch, the preganglionic fibers in the parasympathetic division travel close to the organs they innervate before forming synapses with the relatively short postganglionic neurons (see Fig. 12-25). Parasympathetic nerves arising from nuclei in the brain stem travel to the viscera of the head, thorax, and abdomen within cranial nerves—including the oculomotor (III), facial (VII), glossopharyngeal (IX), and vagus (X) nerves.

Preganglionic parasympathetic nerves that originate from the sacral region of the spinal cord run either separately or together with some spinal nerves. The preganglionic axons join together to form the *pelvic nerve,* which innervates the viscera of the pelvic cavity. These preganglionic axons synapse with postganglionic neurons in terminal ganglia located close to the organs they innervate.

Neurotransmitters and Neuroreceptors

Sympathetic preganglionic fibers and parasympathetic preganglionic and postganglionic fibers release *acetylcholine*—the same neurotransmitter released by somatic efferent neurons (Figs. 12-23 and 12-26). These fibers are characterized by *cholinergic transmission.* Most postganglionic sympathetic fibers release *norepinephrine* (adrenaline) and thus are considered to function by *adrenergic transmission.* A few postganglionic sympathetic fibers, such as those that innervate the sweat glands, release acetylcholine.

The action of catecholamines varies with the type of neuroreceptor stimulated. It should be remembered that catecholamines also are released by the adrenal medulla gland that physiologically and biochemically resembles the sympathetic nervous system. Two types of adrenergic receptors exist, α and β. Cells of the effector organs may have only one or both types of adrenergic receptors. The *α-adrenergic receptors* have been further subdivided according to the action produced. α_1-Adrenergic activity is associated mostly with excitation or stimulation; α_2-adrenergic activity is associated with relaxation or inhibition. Most of the α-adrenergic receptors on effector organs belong to the α_1 class. The *β-adrenergic receptors* are classified as β_1-adrenergic recep-

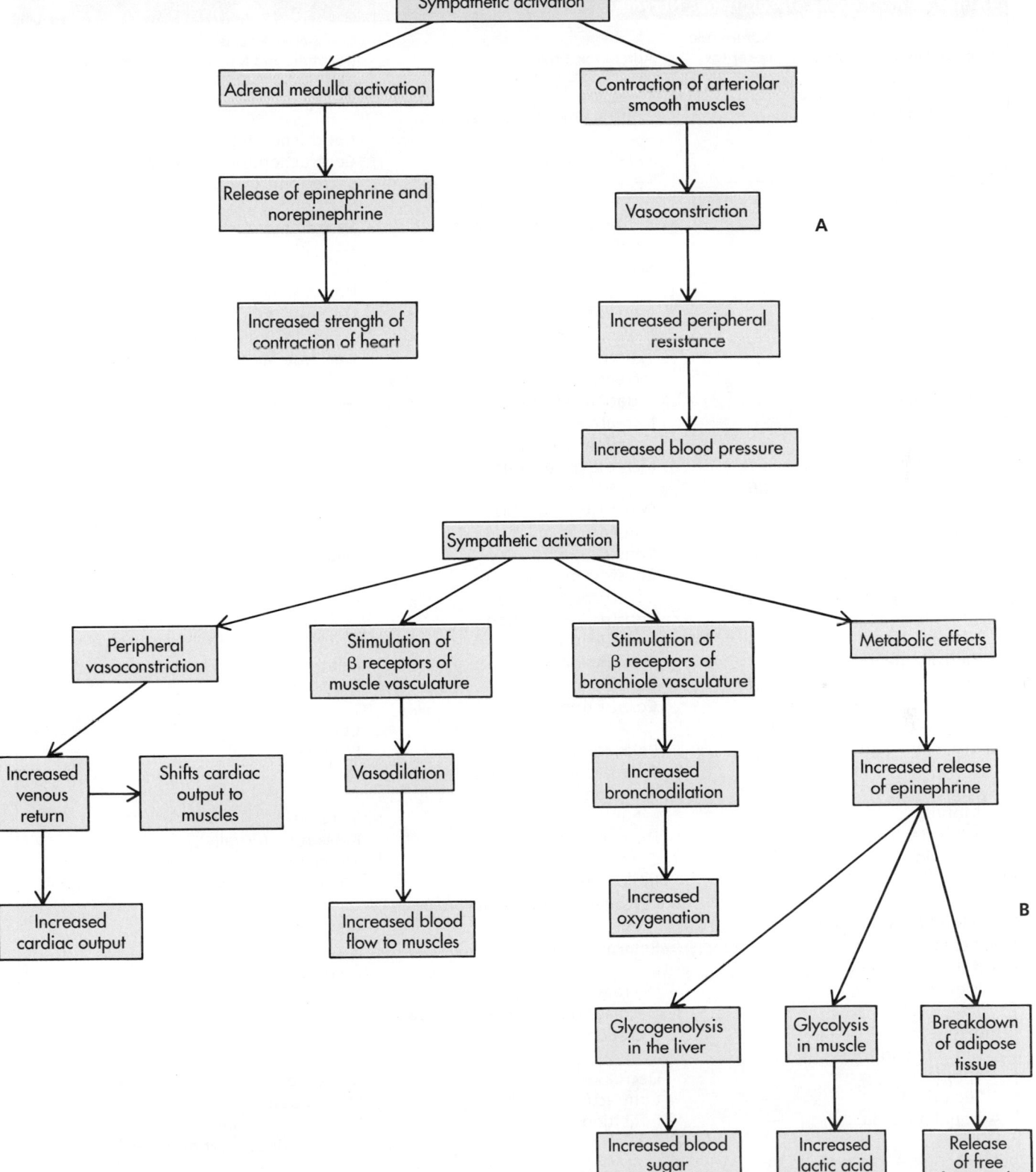

Fig. 12-27 *Some important functions of the sympathetic nervous system.* **A,** Regulation of vasomotor tone. **B,** Regulation of strenuous muscular exercise (fight or flight response). (See also Chapter 8 and Fig. 8-1 for more detail on the stress response.)

TABLE 12-7 Actions of Autonomic Nervous System Neuroreceptors

Effector Organ or Tissue	Adrenergic Receptor $\longrightarrow$	Adrenergic Effects	Cholinergic Effects (Nicotinic and Muscaninic Receptors)
Eye, iris			
Radial muscle	α_1	Contraction (mydriasis)	—
Sphincter muscle		—	Contraction (miosis)
Eye, ciliary muscle	β	Relaxation for far vision	Contraction for near vision
Lacrimal glands	—	—	Secretion
Nasopharyngeal glands	—	—	Secretion
Salivary glands	α_1	Secretion of potassium and water	Secretion of potassium and water
	β	Secretion of amylase	—
Heart			
SA node	β_1		Decrease heart rate; vagus arrest
Atrial	β_1	Increase heart rate	Decrease contractility; shorten action potential duration
		Increase contractility and conduction velocity	
AV junction	β_1	Increase automaticity and propagation velocity	Decrease automaticity and propagation velocity
Purkinje system	β_1	Increase automaticity and propagation velocity	—
Ventricles	β_1	Increase contractility	—
Arterioles			
Coronary	α,β_2		Dilation
Skin	α_2	Constriction, dilation	Dilation
Mucosa	α	Constriction, dilation	Dilation
Skeletal muscle	α,β_2	Constriction	Dilation
Cerebral	α	Constriction, dilation	—
Pulmonary	α,β_2	Constriction (slight)	—
Mesenteric	α	Constriction, dilation	—
Renal	$\alpha,\beta_1,\beta_2,$D	Constriction	—
Salivary glands	α	Constriction, dilation	Dilation
Veins, systemic	α_1,β_2	Constriction	—
Lung		Constriction, dilation	
Bronchial muscle	β_2		Contraction
Bronchial glands	$\alpha_1\beta_2$	Relaxation	Stimulation
		Decrease secretion; increase secretion	
Stomach			
Motility	α_1,β_2		Increase
Sphincters	α	Decrease (usually)	Relaxation (usually)
Secretion	—	Contraction (usually)	Stimulation
Liver	α,β_2	Inhibition (?)	Glyocgen synthesis
		Glycogenolysis and gluconeogenesis	
Gallbladder and ducts	—		Contraction
Pancreas		Relaxation	
Acini	α		Secretion
Islet cells	α_2,β_2	Decrease secretion	—
		Decrease secretion, increase secretion	
Intestine			
Motility and tone	$\alpha_1,\beta_1\beta_2$		Increase
Sphincters	α	Decrease	Relaxation (usually)
Secretion	—	Contraction (usually)	Stimulation
Adrenal medulla	—	Inhibition (?)	Secretion of epinephrine and norepinehrine (nicotinic effect)
		—	

Modified from Vick, R.L. (1984). Contemporary medical physiology, Menlo Park, CA: Addison-Wesley.
D, *Dopaminergic.*

TABLE 12-7   Actions of Autonomic Nervous System Neuroreceptors—cont'd

Effector Organ or Tissue	Adrenergic Receptor $\longrightarrow$ Adrenergic Effects		Cholinergic Effects (Nicotinic and Muscaninic Receptors)
Kidney	β_1		—
Ureter			
Motility and tone	α	Secretion of renin	Increase
Urinary bladder			
Detrusor	β	Increase	Contraction
Trigone and sphincter	α	Relaxation (usually)	Relaxation
Sex organs, male	α	Ejaculation	Erection
Skin			
Pilomotor muscles	α	Contraction	—
Sweat glands	α	Localized secretion	Generalized secretion
Fat cells	α, β_1	Lipolysis	—
Pineal gland	β	Melatonin synthesis	—

tors (which facilitate increased heart rate and contractility and cause the release of renin from the kidney) and β_2-adrenergic receptors (which facilitate all remaining effects attributed to β receptors).[1] Norepinephrine stimulates all α_1 and β_1 receptors and only certain β_2 receptors. The primary response from norepinephrine, however, is stimulation of the α_1-adrenergic receptors that cause vasoconstriction. Epinephrine strongly stimulates all four types of receptors and induces general vasodilation because of the predominance of β receptors in muscle vasculatures. (Table 12-7 summarizes the effects of neuroreceptors on their effector organs.)

Functions of the Autonomic Nervous System

Many body organs are innervated by both the sympathetic and parasympathetic nervous systems. The two divisions frequently cause opposite responses; for example, sympathetic stimulation of the stomach causes decreased peristalsis, whereas parasympathetic stimulation of the intestine increases peristalsis. In general, sympathetic stimulation promotes responses for the protection of the individual. For example, sympathetic activity increases blood sugar levels and temperature and raises the blood pressure. In emergency situations, a generalized and widespread discharge of the sympathetic system occurs. This is accomplished by an increased firing frequency of sympathetic fibers and by activation of sympathetic fibers normally silent and at rest (fibers to the sweat glands, pilomotor muscles, and the adrenal medulla, as well as vasodilator fibers to muscle). Regulation of vasomotor tone is considered the single most important function of the sympathetic nervous system. (Fig. 12-27 illustrates some of the most important functions of the sympathetic nervous system.)

Increased parasympathetic activity promotes rest and tranquility and is characterized by reduced heart rate and enhanced visceral functions concerned with digestion. Stimulation of the vagus nerve (cranial nerve X) in the gastrointestinal tract increases peristalsis and secretion, as well as the relaxation of sphincters. Activation of parasympathetic fibers in the head, provided by cranial nerves III, VII, and IX, causes constriction of the pupil, tear secretion, and increased salivary secretion. Stimulation of the sacral division of the parasympathetic system contracts the urinary bladder and facilitates the process of genital erection.

The parasympathetic system lacks the generalized and widespread response of the sympathetic system. Specific parasympathetic fibers are activated to regulate particular functions. Although the actions of the parasympathetic and sympathetic systems are usually antagonistic, there are exceptions. Peripheral vascular resistance, for example, is increased dramatically by sympathetic activation but is not altered appreciably by activity of the parasympathetic system. Most blood vessels involved in the control of blood pressure are innervated by sympathetic nerves. To decrease blood pressure, therefore, it is more important to block or paralyze the continuous (tonic) discharge of the sympathetic system than to promote parasympathetic activity.

✓ QUICK CHECK

What are the structural and functional divisions of the ANS?

Compare cholinergic and adrenergic transmission.

What does the ANS do?

AGING & *The Nervous System*[6-8]

STRUCTURAL CHANGES WITH AGING
Decreased brain weight and size, particularly frontal regions
Fibrosis and thickening of the meninges
Narrowing of gyri and widening of sulci
Increase in size of ventricles

CELLULAR CHANGES WITH AGING
Decrease in the number of neurons not consistently related to changes in mental function
Decreased myelin
Lipofuscin deposition (a pigment resulting from cellular autodigestion)
Decreased number of dendritic processes and synaptic connections
Intracellular neurofibrillary tangles; significant accumulation in cortex associated with Alzheimer dementia

Imbalance in the amount and distribution of neurotransmitters

CEREBROVASCULAR CHANGES WITH AGING
Arterial athersclerosis (may cause infarcts and scars)
Increased permeability of the blood-brain barrier

FUNCTIONAL CHANGES WITH AGING
Decreased tendon reflexes
Progressive deficit in taste and smell
Decreased vibratory sense
Decrease in accommodation and color vision
Decrease in neuromuscular control with change in gait and posture
Sleep disturbances
Memory impairments
Cognitive alterations associated with chronic disease

DID YOU UNDERSTAND?

Overview and Organization of the Nervous System

1. The divisions of the nervous system have been categorized as either structural (central nervous system [CNS] and peripheral nervous system [PNS]) or functional (somatic nervous system and autonomic nervous system [ANS]).
2. The CNS is contained within the brain and spinal cord.
3. The PNS is composed of cranial and spinal nerves, which carry impulses toward the CNS (afferent) and away from the CNS (efferent) to target organs or skeletal muscle.

Cells of the Nervous System

1. The neuron and neuroglial cells comprise nervous tissue. The neuron is specialized to transmit and receive electrical and chemical impulses, whereas the neuroglial cell provides supportive functions. The neuron is further divided into unipolar, pseudounipolar, bipolar, and multipolar categories, according to its structure and particular mechanics of impulse transmission.
2. The neuron is composed of a cell body, dendrite(s), and an axon. A myelin sheath around selected axons forms an insulation that allows quicker nerve impulse conduction.

The Nerve Impulse

1. The region between the neurons is the synapse, and the region between the neuron and muscle is the myoneural junction. Neurotransmitters are responsible for chemical conduction across the synapse, and myoneural junction nerve impulse is regulated predominantly by a balance of inhibitory postsynaptic potentials (IPSPs) and excitatory postsynaptic potentials (EPSPs), temporal and spatial summation, and convergence and divergence.

The Central Nervous System

1. The brain is contained within the cranial vault and is divided into three distinct regions: (1) forebrain, (2) hindbrain, and (3) midbrain.
2. The forebrain comprises the two cerebral hemispheres and allows conscious perception of internal and external stimuli, thought and memory processes, and voluntary control of skeletal muscles. The deep portion of the forebrain is termed the *diencephalon* and processes incoming sensory data. The center for voluntary control of skeletal muscle movements is located along the precentral gyrus in the frontal lobe, whereas the center for perception is along the postcentral gyrus in the parietal lobe. Broca's area (inferior edge of the postcentral gyrus) and Wernicke's area (superoposterior temporal lobe) are major speech centers.
3. The hindbrain allows sampling and comparison of sensory data, which are received from the periphery and motor impulses of the cerebral hemispheres, for the purpose of coordination and refinement of skeletal muscle movement.
4. The midbrain is primarily a relay center for motor and sensory tracts, as well as a center for auditory and visual reflexes.
5. The spinal cord contains most of the nerve fibers that connect the brain with the periphery. Reflex arcs are completed in the spinal cord and influenced by the higher centers in the brain.
6. The CNS is protected by the scalp, bony cranium, meninges, vertebral column, and cerebrospinal fluid (CSF). CSF is formed from blood components in the choroid plexuses of the ventricles and is reabsorbed in the arachnoid villi (located in the dural venous sinuses) after circulating through the brain and spinal cord.
7. The paired carotid and vertebral arteries supply blood to the brain and connect to form the circle of

▣ DID YOU UNDERSTAND? —cont'd

Willis. The major branches projecting from the circle of Willis are the anterior, middle, and posterior cerebral arteries. Drainage of blood from the brain is accomplished through the venous sinuses and jugular veins.

8. The blood-brain barrier is provided by tight junctions between the cells of brain capillaries and surrounding supporting cells.

9. Blood supply to the spinal cord originates from the vertebral arteries and branches arising from the aorta.

The Peripheral Nervous System

1. The PNS functions to relay information from the CNS to muscle and effector organs through cranial and spinal nerve tracts arranged in fascicles (multiple fascicles bound together form the peripheral nerve).

The Autonomic Nervous System

1. The ANS is responsible for the maintenance of a steady state in the internal environment. Two opposing systems make up the ANS: (1) the sympathetic nervous system responds to stress by mobilizing energy stores and prepares the body to defend itself, and (2) the parasympathetic nervous system conserves energy and the body's resources.

⚠ AGING AND THE NERVOUS SYSTEM

1. Major structural changes with aging include a decrease in number of neurons and a decrease in brain weight and size.

2. Deposition of lipofuscin and the presence of multiple neurofibrillary tangles are common cellular changes with aging.

3. A progressive slowing of neurologic function occurs with advancing age.

KEY TERMS

Acetylcholine, 318
α-Adrenergic receptor, 318
β-Adrenergic receptor, 318
Adrenergic transmission, 318
Afferent pathway (ascending pathway), 292
Afferent (sensory) neuron, 304
Amygdala, 300
Anterior column, 304
Anterior fossa, 306
Anterior horn (ventral horn), 301
Anterior spinal artery, 312
Anterior spinothalamic pathway, 305
Arachnoid membrane, 306
Arachnoid villi, 307
Association fiber, 299
Associational neuron (interneuron), 293
Astrocyte, 294
Autonomic nervous system (ANS), 292
Axon, 292
Axon hillock, 292
Basal ganglia, 297
Basal ganglia pathway, 304
Basal ganglia system (extrapyramidal system), 299
Basilar artery, 308
Basis pedunculi, 301
Bipolar neuron, 293
Blood-brain barrier, 308
Brachial plexus, 313
Brain stem, 297
Broca's speech area, 299
Cauda equina, 301
Caudate nucleus, 300

Cavernous sinus, 307
Celiac, 318
Central canal, 301
Central nervous system (CNS), 292
Central sulcus (fissure of Rolando), 299
Cerebellum, 301
Cerebral aqueduct (aqueduct of Sylvius), 301
Cerebral cortex, 299
Cerebral nuclei, 300
Cerebral peduncle, 301
Cerebrospinal fluid (CSF), 307
Cerebrum, 297
Cholinergic transmission, 318
Choroid plexus, 306
Circle of Willis, 308
Collateral ganglia, 318
Contralateral control, 299
Conus medullaris, 301
Corpora quadrigemina (tectum), 301
Corpus callosum (transverse fibers or commissural fibers), 300
Corpus striatum, 300
Cranial nerve, 292, 313
Craniosacral division, 318
Dendrite, 292
Dendritic zone, 292
Dermatome, 313
Diencephalon, 300
Dopamine, 301
Dorsal root ganglion, 301
Dura mater, 306
Effector organ, 292
Efferent (motor) neuron, 304

Efferent pathway (descending pathway), 292
Endoneurium, 292
Epicritic, 305
Epidural space, 307
Epithalamus, 300
Excitatory postsynaptic potential (EPSP), 295
Facilitation, 295
Falx cerebri, 306
Fascicle, 312
Fissure, 299
Frontal lobe, 299
Galea aponeurotica, 306
Ganglia, 292
Gray matter, 299
Hippocampus, 300
Hypothalamus, 300
Inferior colliculi, 301
Inferior mesenteric, 318
Inhibitory postsynaptic potential (IPSP), 295
Inner dura (meningeal layer), 306
Insula, 300
Internal capsule, 300
Internal carotid artery, 307
Interventricular foramen (foramen of Monro), 307
Intervertebral disk, 307
Lateral aperture (foramen of Luschka), 307
Lateral column, 304
Lateral corticospinal pathway, 304
Lateral horn, 301

KEY TERMS

Lateral spinothalamic pathway, 305
Lateral sulcus (sylvian fissure, lateral fissure), 299
Lentiform nucleus, 300
Limbic system, 300
Lower motor neuron, 304
Lumbar plexus, 313
Median aperture (foramen of Magendie), 307
Meninges, 306
Metencephalon, 301
Microfilament, 292
Microglia, 294
Microtubule, 292
Midbrain (mesencephalon), 301
Middle fossa (temporal fossa), 306
Mixed nerve, 312
Motor neuron, 293
Motor unit, 304
Multipolar neuron, 293
Myelencephalon (medulla oblongata), 301
Myelin, 292
Myelin sheath, 292
Neurilemma (Schwann sheath), 292
Neurofibril, 292
Neuroglia, 294
Neuroglial cell, 292
Neuromuscular (myoneural) junction, 294, 304
Neuron, 292
Neurotransmitter, 295
Nissl substance, 292
Node of Ranvier, 292
Norepinephrine, 318
Nucleus pulposus, 307
Occipital lobe, 299
Oligodendrocyte, 294

Oligodendroglia, 294
Papez circuit, 300
Parasympathetic nervous system, 317
Parietal lobe, 299
Pelvic nerve, 318
Periosteum (endosteal layer), 306
Peripheral nervous system (PNS), 292
Plexus, 313
Pons, 301
Postcentral gyrus, 299
Posterior (dorsal) column, 304, 305
Posterior fossa, 306
Posterior horn (dorsal horn), 301
Posterior spinal artery, 312
Postganglionic neuron, 313
Postsynaptic neuron, 295
Precentral gyrus, 299
Prefrontal area, 299
Preganglionic neuron, 313
Premotor area (Brodmann area 6), 299
Presynaptic neuron, 295
Primary motor area, 299
Primary voluntary motor pathway, 299
Projecting artery (nutrient artery), 308
Protopathic, 306
Pseudounipolar neuron, 293
Pyramidal system, 299
Red nucleus, 301
Reflex arc, 304
Reticular activating system, 297
Reticular formation, 297
Sacral plexus, 313
Saltatory conduction, 293
Schwann cell, 292
Sensory neuron, 293
Somatic nervous system, 292
Spatial summation, 295
Spinal cord, 301

Spinal nerve, 292
Spinal tract, 301
Spinothalamic tract, 301
Splanchnic nerve, 318
Subarachnoid space, 306
Subdural space, 306
Substantia gelatinosa, 301
Substantia nigra, 301
Subthalamus, 300
Sulci, 299
Summation, 295
Superficial artery (conducting artery), 308
Superior colliculi, 301
Superior mesenteric, 318
Sympathetic (paravertebral) ganglia, 317
Sympathetic nervous system, 317
Synapse, 295
Synaptic bouton, 295
Synaptic cleft, 295
Tegmentum, 301
Telencephalon, 297
Temporal lobe, 299
Temporal summation, 295
Tentorium cerebelli, 306
Thalamus, 300
Thoracolumbar division, 317
Unipolar neuron, 293
Upper motor neuron, 304
Ventricle, 307
Vermis, 301
Vertebral artery, 307
Vertebral column, 301
Vestibulospinal pathway, 304
Wernicke's area, 299
White matter, 299

REFERENCES

1. Seigel G.J. et al. (Eds). (1999). *Basic neurochemistry: Molecular, cellular, and medical aspects.* (6th ed.). Philadelphia: Lippincott-Raven.
2. Nolte, J. (1999). *The human brain: An introduction to its functional anatomy.* (4th ed.). St. Louis: Mosby.
3. Kaira, S. et al. (1998). Recovery of N-acetylaspartate in corticomoter neurons of patients with ALS after riluzole therapy. *Neuroreport, 9*(8), 1757-1761.
4. Kiernan, J.A. (1998). *The human nervous system: An anatomical viewpoint.* (7th ed.). Philadelphia: Lippincott-Raven.
5. Cohen, H. (1999). *Neuroscience for rehabilitation.* (2nd ed.) Philadelphia: Lippincott Williams & Wilkins.
6. Albert, M.L. & Knoefel, J.E. (1994). *Clinical neurology of aging.* New York: Oxford University Press.
7. Morrison J.H. & Hof, P.R. (1997). Life and death of neurons in the aging brain. *Science, 278*(5337), 412-419.
8. Perry, E & Kay, D.W. (1997). Some developments in brain ageing and dementia. *British Journal of Biomedical Science, 54*(3), 201-215.

CHAPTER

13

Pain, Temperature, Sleep, and Sensory Function

Sue E. Huether

Alterations in sensory function may involve dysfunctions of the general or the special senses. Dysfunctions of the general senses include chronic pain, abnormal temperature regulation, tactile dysfunction, and proprioceptive dysfunction. Dysfunctions of the special senses include visual, auditory, vestibular, olfactory, and gustatory (taste) dysfunction.

The special senses of vision, hearing, touch, smell, and taste are the means by which individuals perceive stimuli that are essential in interacting with the environment.

All definitions of pain suggest that it is a complex phenomenon composed of sensory experiences that include time, space, intensity, emotion, cognition, and motivation. Pain is an unpleasant phenomenon that is uniquely experienced by each individual; it cannot be adequately defined, identified, or measured by an observer. McCaffery[1] defines pain as "whatever the experiencing person says it is, existing whenever he says it does."

Temperature regulation is measured by clearly defined normal limits. Like pain, however, variations in temperature can signal disease. Fever is a common manifestation of dysfunction and is often the first symptom observed in an infectious or inflammatory condition.

Sleep is a normal cyclic process that restores the body's energy and maintains normal functioning. Sleep is so essential to both physiologic and psychologic function that sleep deprivation causes a wide range of clinical manifestations.

Check out your CD Companion for chapter-related exercises and answers to the Quick Check questions

PAIN
The Experience of Pain
Three systems interact to produce pain.[2] The *sensory/discriminative system* processes information about the strength, intensity, and temporal and spatial aspects of pain. These sensations are mediated through afferent nerve fibers, the spinal cord, the brain stem, and the higher brain centers, and they result in prompt withdrawal from the painful stimulus.

The *motivational/affective system* determines the individual's conditioned or learned approach/avoidance behaviors. These behaviors are mediated through the interaction of the reticular formation, limbic system, and brain stem.

The *cognitive/evaluative system* overlies the individual's learned behavior concerning the experience of pain. The individual's interpretation of appropriate pain behavior is learned through cultural preferences, male and female roles, and experience, among other ways. The influence of the cognitive/evaluative system may block, modulate, or enhance the perception of pain.

Somatogenic versus psychogenic pain
Somatogenic pain, such as the pain of a crushed finger or the pain of a heart attack, is pain with a cause. In contrast, *psychogenic pain* is pain for which there is no known physical cause. Psychogenic pain, however, is *not* imaginary pain and may be just as intense and just as distressing as somatogenic pain. Pain is only *primarily* somatogenic or psychogenic; it is rarely, if ever, purely one type or the other.

Acute versus chronic pain
Acute pain is a protective mechanism that alerts the individual to a condition or experience that is immediately harmful to the body. Acute pain begins suddenly, and the pain is relieved after the chemical mediators that stimulate pain receptors are removed. Acute anxiety is always associated with acute pain and is associated with the threat inherent in the painful experience, including its cause, its treatment, and the prognosis. Hope of recovery also is associated with acute pain. Acute pain mobilizes the individual to take prompt action to relieve it.[3]

Chronic pain is persistent—usually defined as lasting at least 6 months. Its cause often is unknown, and the pain frequently does not respond to usual therapy when the cause is known. The onset may be sudden, but chronic pain often develops insidiously. Individual behavior is adaptive and directed toward modifying the pain. Chronic pain is frequently associated with a sense of hopelessness and helplessness when no cure seems possible and more time elapses. The pain is perceived as meaningless; depression often results. Table 13-1 compares acute and chronic pain.[6]

Pain threshold and pain tolerance
The *pain threshold* is the lowest intensity at which a stimulus is perceived as pain. The threshold does not vary significantly among people or in the same person over time. However, intense pain at one location may increase the threshold in another location. For example, a person with severe pain in one knee is less likely to experience chronic back pain that is less intense (called *perceptual dominance*). Because of perceptual dominance, an individual with many painful sites may report only the most painful one. Then when the dominant pain is diminished, the individual identifies other painful areas.

Pain tolerance is the time or intensity of pain that an individual will endure before initiating overt pain responses. Pain tolerance is influenced by the person's cultural perceptions, expectations, role behaviors, and physical and mental health. It generally decreases with repeated exposure to pain, fatigue, anger, boredom, apprehension, and sleep deprivation. Tolerance increases with alcohol consumption, medication, hypnosis, warmth, distracting activities, and strong beliefs or faith.

Pain tolerance varies greatly among people and in the same person over time because of the body's ability to respond differently to noxious stimuli (Table 13-2). No direct relationship exists between the intensity of painful stimuli and an individual's perception of pain or response to pain.[8]

Neuroanatomy of Pain
The portions of the nervous system responsible for the sensation and perception of pain may be divided into the following three areas:

1. *The afferent pathways.* The afferent pathways are composed of *nociceptors* (pain receptors) in the tissues. Afferent pathways terminate in the dorsal horn of the spinal cord. Some areas have only nociceptor-specific function. Both incoming and descending stimuli modulate pain patterns in the dorsal horn cells.
2. *The central nervous system (CNS).* The portions of the CNS involved in interpreting pain signals are the limbic system, reticular formation, thalamus, hypothalamus, medulla, and cortex. The limbic and reticular tracts probably are involved in alerting, arousal, and motivational behaviors. Parts of the thalamus help in discrimination and localization of pain. The medulla and hypothalamus activate coping responses, such as "fight or flight," the release of corticosteroids, and cardiovascular responses. The regions of the brain that modulate spinal pain transmission are complex and integrated.
3. *The efferent pathways.* The efferent pathways, composed of the fibers connecting the reticular formation, midbrain, and substantia gelatinosa, are responsible for modulating pain sensation.

Role of the afferent and efferent pathways
The nociceptors are at the ends of the small unmyelinated and lightly myelinated afferent neurons and respond to chemical, mechanical, and thermal stimuli (Table 13-3). A gentle touch or warmth may produce a positive, pleasurable sensation. Deep pressure or extreme temperature generally produces pain.

TABLE 13-1	Comparison of Acute and Chronic Pain	
Characteristic	**Acute Pain**	**Chronic Pain**
Experience	An event	State of existence
Source	External agent or internal disease	Unknown or treatment unsuccessful
Onset	Usually sudden	Sudden or develops insidiously
Duration	Transient (up to 6 mo)	Prolonged (months to years)
Pain identification	Painful and nonpainful areas generally well identified	Painful and nonpainful areas less easily differentiated; change in sensations becomes more difficult to evaluate
Clinical signs	Typical response pattern with more visible signs	Response patterns vary; fewer overt signs (adaptation)
Significance	Significant (informs person something is wrong)	Person looks for significance
Pattern	Self-limiting or readily corrected	Continuous or intermittent; intensity may vary or remain constant
Course	Suffering usually decreases over time	Suffering usually increases over time
Actions	Leads to actions to relieve pain	Leads to actions to modify pain experience
Prognosis	Likelihood of eventual complete relief	Complete relief usually not possible

Modified from Black, R.G. (1975). The chronic pain syndrome. Surgical Clinics of North America, 55(4), 999-1011.

TABLE 13-2	Pain Perception in Infants, Children, and Elderly Persons		
	Infants	**Children**	**Elderly Persons**
Pain threshold	Lower than adults	Lower than adults	Increased from middle age or no change
Physiologic symptoms	Increased heart rate, blood pressure, and respiratory rate; flushing or pallor, sweating, and decreased oxygen saturation	Same as infants; nausea and vomiting	Same as infants and children; nausea and vomiting
Behavioral responses	Changes in facial expression, crying and body movements, with lowered brows drawn together; vertical bulge and furrows in the forehead between the brows; broadened nasal root; tightly closed eyes; angular, squarish mouth; chin quiver; withdrawal of affected limbs, rigidity, flailing[4]	Individual responses vary[5]	Individual responses vary[7]

TABLE 13-3	Stimuli That Activate Nociceptors (Pain Receptors)
Location of Receptor	**Provoking Stimuli**
Skin	Pricking, cutting, crushing, burning, freezing
Gastrointestinal tract	Engorged or inflamed mucosa, distention or spasm of smooth muscle, traction on mesenteric attachment
Skeletal muscle	Ischemia, injuries of the connective tissue sheaths, necrosis, hemorrhage, prolonged contraction, injection of irritating solutions
Joints	Synovial membrane inflammation
Arteries	Piercing, inflammation
Head	Traction, inflammation, or displacement of arteries, meningeal structures, and sinuses; prolonged muscle contraction
Heart	Ischemia and inflammation

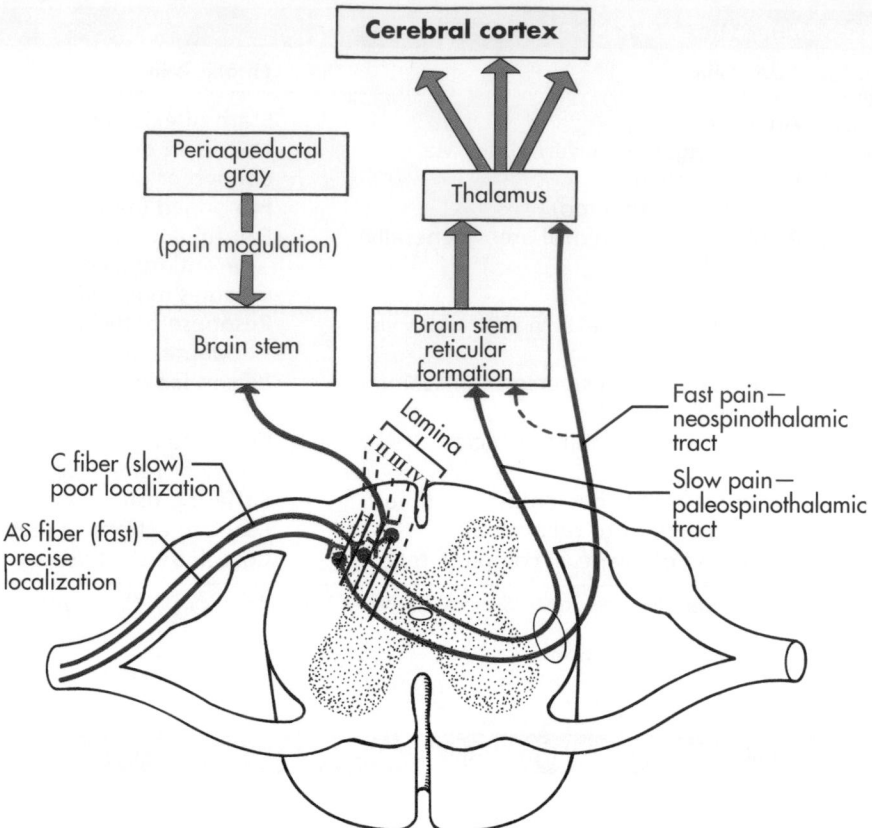

Fig. 13-1 *Aδ fibers transmit acute localized pain sensations.* The fibers synapse in laminae I and V, cross over, and synapse in the midbrain via the neospinothalamic tract. Neurons in lamina I are excited by thermal and mechanical stimuli and are unaffected by touch or movement of hairs. The small C fibers transmit "slow" or chronic burning sensations. The fibers synapse in laminae II and III, cross over, and synapse in the reticular formations and midbrain via the paleospinothalamic tract.

Nociceptors are found under the epidermis (as *Meissner corpuscles*) and within the deep tissues, muscles, tendons, and subcutaneous tissue (as nerve endings termed *pacinian corpuscles*). They also appear as bare endings in the skin. They are not evenly distributed in the body so the relative sensitivity to pain differs according to the area of the body.

As Fig. 13-1 illustrates, stimulated nociceptors produce impulses that are transmitted through small, myelinated A fibers and C fibers to the spinal cord, where they form synapses with neurons in the dorsal horn. From there they are transmitted to the rest of the CNS.

The small unmyelinated C neurons are responsible for the transmission of diffuse burning or aching sensations. C fibers are small and lack a myelin sheath, so transmission is relatively slow (slow pain). Transmission through the slightly larger, myelinated A fibers occurs more quickly. A fibers carry well-localized, sharp pain sensations. The reflex arc to and from the spinal cord is much faster than the transmission of sharp pain sensations by the A fibers, so the injured body part may retract before pain is perceived.

The two divisions of the spinothalamic tract that carry pain information to the brain are (1) the neospinothalamic tract (acute pain) and (2) the paleospinothalamic tract (dull and burning pain). The neospinothalamic tract carries information to the midbrain, postcentral gyrus (where pain is perceived), and cortex. The paleospinothalamic tract carries information to the reticular formation, pons, limbic system, and midbrain.

Afferent stimulation of the *periaqueductal gray (PAG)* (gray matter surrounding the cerebral aqueduct) in the midbrain stimulates the efferent pathway, which modulates or inhibits afferent pain signals.

Neurophysiology of Pain

Melzack and Wall proposed the *gate control theory* in 1965 (Fig. 13-2). According to this theory, pain impulses are transmitted from specialized skin receptors to the spinal cord through large A and small C fibers (see Fig. 13-2). These fibers terminate in the substantia gelatinosa, in the dorsal horn of the spinal cord. Cells in the substantia gelatinosa function as a gate, regulating transmission of impulses to the CNS. Stimulation of larger fibers causes the cells in the substantia gelatinosa to "close the gate," which diminishes pain perception. Small fiber input inhibits cells in the substantia gelatinosa and opens the gate, enhancing pain perception. The CNS, through efferent pathways, may close, partially

Fig. 13-2 *Schematic diagram of the gate control theory of pain mechanism.*

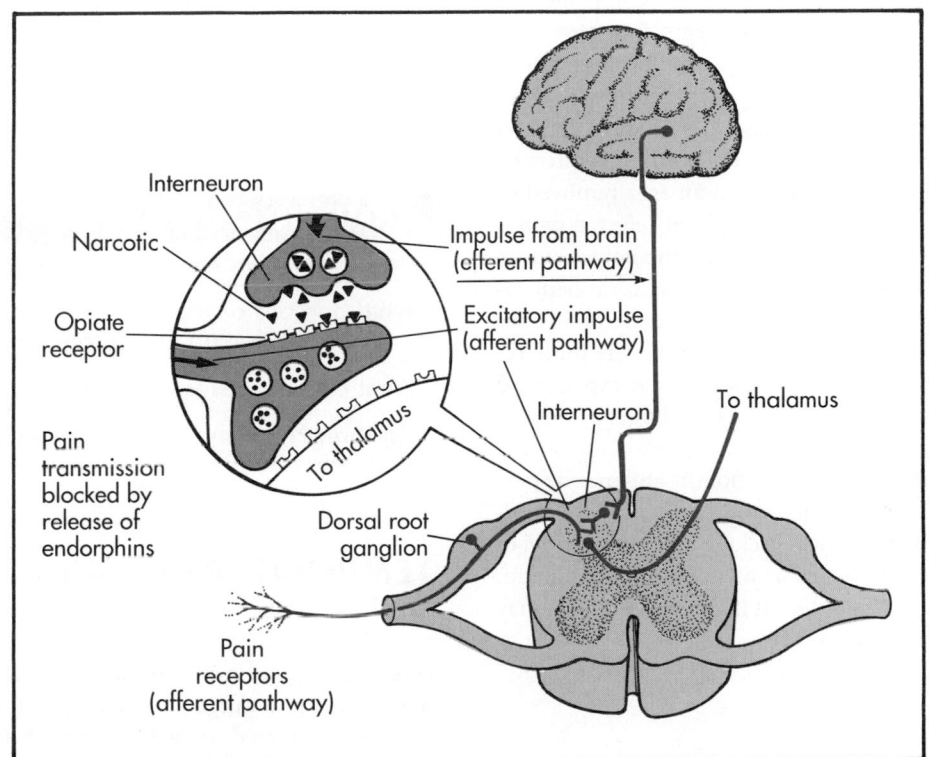

Fig. 13-3 *Descending pathway and endorphin response.* The biologic receptors of the enkephalins and endorphins are located close to known pain receptors in the periphery and ascending and descending pain pathways.

close, or open the gate. The gate control theory is inadequate to explain some chronic pain problems, such as phantom limb pain.[9]

Neuromodulation

Neuromodulators of pain are found in the pathways that mediate information about painful stimuli.[10] Some of the triggering mechanisms to release neuromodulators are tissue injury (prostaglandins, bradykinin) and chronic inflammatory lesions (lymphokines). Neuromodulators include such substances as substance P, norepinephrine, 5-hydroxytryptamine, and calcitonin-gene-related peptide.

Endorphins (endogenous morphines) are a family of neuropeptides that inhibit transmission of pain impulses in the spinal cord and brain. *β-Lipotrophin* (β-, γ-, and α-endorphin) is a potent endorphin located in the hypothalamus and the pituitary gland. It may be responsible for general sensations of well-being. *Enkephalin,* found in the neurons of the brain and spinal cord, is a weaker analgesic than other endorphins but is more potent and longer lasting than morphine. *Dynorphin* is 50 times more potent than β-endorphin and reportedly originates in the neural lobe of the pituitary.[11] Midbrain stimulation in the area of the periaqueductal gray alleviates pain such as that associated with emergency situations.[12]

All endorphins attach to *opiate receptors* on the plasma membrane of the afferent neuron (Fig. 13-3), and the combination inhibits the release of excitatory neurotransmitters.

Opiates relieve pain by attaching to the opiate receptors and enhancing the natural endorphin response.

Stress, excessive physical exertion, acupuncture, intercourse, and other factors increase the levels of circulating endorphins, serotonin, norepinephrine, and other neurotransmitters, raising the pain threshold. Some evidence suggests that high levels of circulating endorphins may play a role in "painless myocardial ischemia and infarction."[13]

Clinical Manifestations of Pain

Acute pain may be (1) somatic, (2) visceral, or (3) referred. *Somatic pain* is superficial (coming from the skin or close to the surface of the body) and is either sharp and well localized or dull, aching, and poorly localized and accompanied by nausea and vomiting. *Visceral pain* is pain in internal organs, the abdomen, or skeleton. It is poorly localized and is associated with nausea and vomiting, hypotension, restlessness, and, in some cases, shock. Visceral pain often radiates (spreads away from the actual site of the pain) or is referred. *Referred pain* is pain that is present in an area removed or distant from its point of origin. The area of referred pain is supplied by the same spinal segment as the actual site of pain. Impulses from many cutaneous and visceral neurons converge on the same ascending neuron, and the brain cannot distinguish between the two. Because there are more receptors in the skin, the painful sensation is experienced there.[14] (Common areas of referred pain and their associated sites of origin appear in Fig. 13-4.)

Chronic pain lasts longer than 6 months and may be persistent (e.g., low back pain) or intermittent (e.g., migraines). Causes or aggravating influences include a decreased level of endorphins or a predominance of a C neuron stimulation. Changes in nerve terminals, afferent fibers, and the CNS may contribute to chronicity of pain.[15]

In contrast, the physiologic responses to chronic pain depend on the persistent or intermittent nature of the pain. Intermittent pain produces responses similar to those of acute pain, whereas persistent pain allows for physiologic adaptation, producing normal heart and respiratory rates and normal blood pressure. However, even though the physiologic responses are normal, the pain is not relieved.

The behavioral and psychologic changes of chronic pain include depression, difficulty sleeping and eating, and preoccupation with the pain.[16] Living with chronic pain requires constant attention to its earliest signs so that the pain-provoking stimuli can be identified and avoided. Persons with chronic pain generally try to keep pain-related behavior to a minimum so that they appear as normal as possible. The desire to relieve pain and the need to hide it are usually conflicting drives for those with chronic pain, who fear being labeled complainers. Several common chronic pain conditions are listed in Table 13-4.

✓ QUICK CHECK

Define the major categories of pain.

What portions of the nervous system are responsible for the sensation and perception of pain?

What physiologic responses are seen in acute pain?

List three common chronic pain conditions.

TEMPERATURE REGULATION

In all homeothermic animals, temperature regulation is achieved through precise balancing of heat production, heat conservation, and heat loss. In humans, body temperature is maintained in a range around 37° C (98.6° F). The normal range is considered to be 36.2° to 37.7° C (96.2° to 99.4° F), but body parts vary in temperature. The extremities are generally cooler than the trunk, and the temperature at the core of the body (as measured by rectal temperature) is generally 0.5° C higher than at the surface (as measured by oral temperature). Internal temperature varies in response to activity, environmental temperature, and daily fluctuation (*circadian rhythm*). Oral temperatures fluctuate within 0.2° to 0.5° C during a 24-hour period. Women tend to have wider fluctuations that follow the menstrual cycle, with a sharp rise in temperature just before ovulation. In both genders the daily fluctuating temperature peaks around 6 PM and is at its lowest during sleep. Maintenance of body temperature within the normal range is necessary for life.

Hypothalamic Control of Temperature

Temperature regulation is mediated primarily by the hypothalamus. Peripheral thermoreceptors in the skin and central thermoreceptors in the hypothalamus, spinal cord, abdominal organs, and other central locations provide the hypothalamus with information about skin and core tempera-

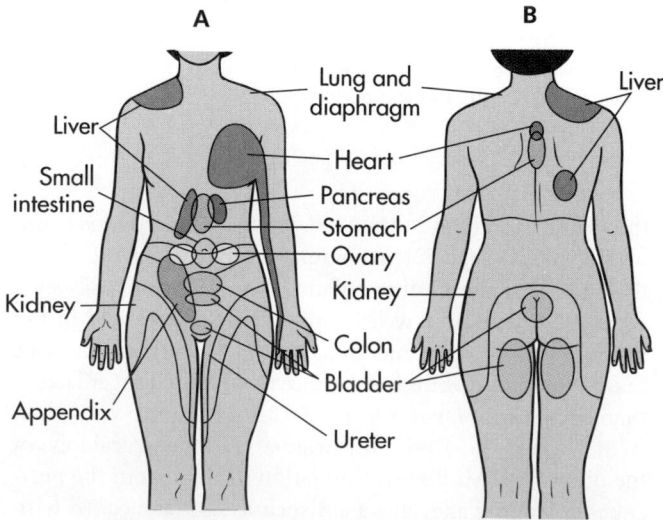

Fig. 13-4 *Sites of referred pain.* **A**, Front. **B**, Back. *(Redrawn from Phipps, W.J., Long, B.C., & Woods, W.F. [1995]. Medical-surgical nursing: Concepts and clinical practice [5th ed.]. St. Louis: Mosby.)*

TABLE 13-4	Common Chronic Pain Conditions
Condition	**Description**
Persistent low back pain	Most common chronic pain condition
	Results from poor muscle tone, inactivity, muscle strain, or sudden, vigorous exercise
Neuralgias	Painful condition resulting from damage to a peripheral nerve
	Common types include causalgia (severe burning pain triggered by various stimuli, such as cold, light touch, or sound) and reflex sympathetic dystrophies (occur after peripheral nerve injury and are characterized by continuous, severe, burning pain associated with vasomotor changes and muscle wasting)
Hyperesthesias	Increased sensitivity and decreased pain threshold to tactile and painful stimuli
	Pain is diffuse, modified by fatigue and emotion and mixed with other sensations
	May result from chronic irritation of CNS areas
Myofacial pain syndromes	Second most common chronic pain condition
	Pain results from muscle spasm, tenderness, and stiffness
	Examples include myositis, fibrositis, myofibrositis, myalgia, and muscle strain—conditions that involve injury to the muscle and fascia
	As disorder progresses, pain becomes increasingly generalized
Hemiagnosia	Loss of ability to identify source of pain on one side of the body
	Painful stimuli on that side produce discomfort, anxiety, moaning, agitation, and distress but no attempt to withdraw from the stimulus
	Associated with stroke
Phantom limb pain	Pain in amputated limb after stump has completely healed; may be immediate or occur months later
	Influenced by emotions/sympathetic stimulation
	Trigger points—small hypersensitive regions in muscle or connective tissues that, when stimulated, produce pain in a specific area
Cancer pain	Can be pain attributed to advance of disease, associated with treatment, or attributed to coexisting disease entities

tures. If these temperatures are low, the hypothalamus triggers heat production and heat conservation mechanisms. The endocrine system also operates in increased heat production. The heat-producing mechanism begins with thyrotropin-stimulating, hormone-releasing hormone (TSH-RH), which stimulates the anterior pituitary to release thyroid-stimulating hormone (TSH), which acts on the thyroid gland, stimulating release of thyroxine. This hormone then acts on the adrenal medulla, causing the release of epinephrine into the bloodstream. Epinephrine causes vasoconstriction, stimulates glycolysis, and increases metabolic rates, thus increasing heat production.

The hypothalamus also triggers heat conservation by stimulating the sympathetic nervous system, which stimulates the adrenal cortex, increasing skeletal muscle tone, initiating the shivering response, and producing vasoconstriction. The hypothalamus also relays information to the cerebral cortex about cold, and voluntary responses result, such as increased body movement. The hypothalamus responds to warmer core and peripheral temperatures by reversing the same mechanisms.

Mechanisms of heat production and loss

Body heat is produced by the chemical reactions of metabolism, skeletal muscle tone and contraction, and chemical thermogenesis. Heat loss is achieved through (1) radiation, (2) conduction, (3) convection, (4) vasodilation, (5) de-

creased muscle tone, (6) evaporation, (7) increased respiration, (8) voluntary measures, and (9) adaptation to warmer climates. For further explanation, see Table 13-5.

Mechanisms of heat conservation

The body conserves heat and protects core temperature through two important mechanisms: (1) involuntary vasoconstriction and (2) voluntary mechanisms. By constricting peripheral blood vessels, centrally warmed blood is shunted away from the periphery to the core of the body, where heat can be retained. This involuntary mechanism takes advantage of the insulating layers of the skin and subcutaneous fat to protect core temperature.

In response to lower body temperatures, individuals typically "bundle up," "keep moving," or "curl up in a ball." These types of voluntary physical activity provide insulation, increase skeletal muscle activity, and decrease the amount of skin surface available for heat loss through radiation, convection, and conduction.[17]

Temperature Regulation in Infants and Elderly Persons

Infants and elderly persons require special attention to maintenance of body temperature. Infants produce sufficient body heat but cannot conserve heat produced because of their small body size and greater ratio of body surface to body weight. Infants also have little subcutaneous fat and

TABLE 13-5	Mechanisms of Heat Production and Loss
Condition	**Description**
Heat production	
Chemical reactions of metabolism	Occur during ingestion and metabolism of food and while maintaining the body at rest (basal metabolism); occur in body core (liver)
Skeletal muscle contraction	Gradual increase in muscle tone or rapid muscle oscillations (shivering)
Chemical thermogenesis	Epinephrine is released and produces rapid, transient increase in heat production by raising basal metabolic rate; quick, brief effect that counters heat lost through conduction and convection; involves brown adipose tissue, which decreases markedly in older adults
Heat loss	
Radiation	Heat loss through electromagnetic waves emanating from surfaces with temperature higher than the surrounding air
Conduction	Heat loss by direct molecule-to-molecule transfer from one surface to another, so that warmer surface loses heat to cooler surface
Convection	Transfer of heat through currents of gases or liquids; exchanges warmer air at body's surface with cooler air in surrounding space
Vasodilation	Diverts core-warmed blood to surface of body, with heat transferred by conduction to skin surface and from there to the surrounding environment; occurs in response to autonomic stimulation under control of hypothalamus
Decreased muscle tone	"Washed out" feeling caused by moderately reduced muscle tone and curtailed voluntary muscle activity
Evaporation	Body water evaporates from surface of skin and linings of mucous membranes; major source of heat reduction connected with increased sweating in warmer surroundings
Increased respiration	Air is exchanged with environment through normal process; minimal effect
Voluntary mechanisms	"Stretching out" and "slowing down" in response to high body temperatures, increasing the body surface area available for heat loss; dressing in light-colored, loose-fitting garments
Adaptation to warmer climates	Gradual process beginning with lassitude, weakness, and faintness, proceeding through increased sweating, lowered sodium content, decreased heart rate, increased stroke volume and extracellular fluid volume, and terminating in improved warm weather functioning and decreased symptoms of heat intolerance (work output, endurance, and coordination increase, and subjective feelings of discomfort decrease)

thus are not as well insulated as adults.[18] Elderly persons respond poorly to environmental temperature extremes because of their slowed blood circulation, structural and functional skin changes, and overall decreased heat-producing activities. In addition, they have a decreased shivering response (delayed onset and decreased effectiveness), slowed metabolic rate, decreased vasoconstrictor response, diminished or absent sweating, decreased peripheral sensation, desynchronized circadian rhythm, decreased perception of heat and cold, undernutrition, and decreased brown adipose tissue.[19]

Pathogenesis of Fever

Fever is "resetting of the hypothalamic thermostat" to a higher level in response to endogenous or exogenous pyrogens. The thermoregulatory mechanisms adjust heat production, conservation, and loss to maintain body core temperature at a normal level. During fever this level is raised so that the thermoregulatory center now adjusts heat production, conservation, and loss to maintain the core temperature at the new, higher temperature, which functions as a new set point.[20]

Exogenous pyrogens, or endotoxins (Fig. 13-5), stimulate the release of substances such as tumor necrosis factor (TNFα), interleukin-1 (IL-1), interleukin-6 (IL-6), and interferon (IF), which raise the set point. In response, the hypothalamus signals an increase in heat production and conservation to raise body temperature to the new level. The individual feels colder, dresses more warmly, decreases body surface area by curling up, and may go to bed in an effort to get warm. Body temperature is maintained at the new level until the fever "breaks," when the set point begins to return to normal. This response is mediated in part by cytokines associated with the inflammatory response.[21] There are decreased heat production and increased heat reduction mechanisms. The individual feels very warm, dons cooler clothes, throws off the covers, and stretches out. Once the body has returned to a normal temperature, the individual feels more comfortable and the hypothalamus adjusts thermoregulatory mechanisms to maintain the new temperature.

Fig. 13-5 *Pathophysiology of fever.* (See text for explanation.)

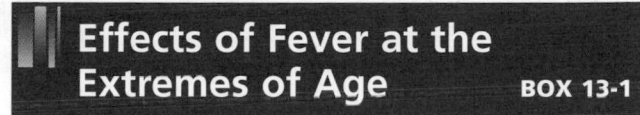

Effects of Fever at the Extremes of Age   BOX 13-1

ELDERLY PERSONS

Decreased or no fever response to infection so benefits decreased

High morbidity and mortality result from lack of beneficial aspects

CHILDREN

Develop higher temperatures than adults for relatively minor infections

Febrile seizures before age 5 years are not uncommon

Benefits of Fever

Fever helps the body respond to infectious processes through several mechanisms[22,23]:

1. Simple raising of body temperature kills many microorganisms and adversely affects their growth and replication.
2. Higher body temperatures decrease serum levels of iron, zinc, and copper—minerals needed for bacterial replication.
3. Increased temperature causes lysosomal breakdown and autodestruction of cells, preventing viral replication in infected cells.
4. Heat increases lymphocytic transformation and motility of polymorphonuclear neutrophils, facilitating the immune response.
5. Phagocytosis is enhanced, and production of antiviral interferon is augmented.[24]

Suppression of fever by treatment with antipyrogenic medications should be used only if a fever produces or is high enough to produce serious side effects, such as nerve damage or convulsion.[25]

Infection and fever responses in elderly persons and children may vary from those in normal adults. Box 13-1 lists the principal features associated with fever at these extremes of age.[26]

Disorders of Temperature Regulation
Hyperthermia

Hyperthermia (marked warming of core temperature) can produce nerve damage, coagulation of cell proteins, and death. At 41° C (105.8° F), nerve damage produces convulsions in the adult. At 43° C (109.4° F), death results. Hyperthermia is not mediated by pyrogens, and the hypothalamic set point is not reset. Hyperthermia may be therapeutic, ac-

cidental, or associated with stroke or head trauma. Prevention of hyperthermia in stroke and head trauma assists in limiting brain injury.[27] Therapeutic hyperthermia, a controversial therapy, is a form of local or general body-induced hyperthermia used to destroy pathologic microorganisms or tumor cells by facilitating the host's natural immune process. The four forms of accidental hyperthermia are summarized as follows:

1. *Heat cramps*—severe, spasmodic cramps in the abdomen and extremities that follow prolonged sweating and associated sodium loss. Usually occur in those not accustomed to heat or those performing strenuous work in very warm climates. Symptoms include fever, rapid pulse, and increased blood pressure.
2. *Heat exhaustion*—results from prolonged high core or environmental temperatures, which cause profound vasodilation and profuse sweating, leading to dehydration, decreased plasma volumes, hypotension, decreased cardiac output, and tachycardia. Symptoms include weakness, dizziness, nausea, and fainting.
3. *Heat stroke*—potentially lethal result of overstressed thermoregulatory center. With very high core temperatures, the regulatory center ceases to function and the body's heat loss mechanisms fail. Symptoms include cerebral edema, degeneration of the CNS, swollen dendrites, renal tubular necrosis, and eventually death if treatment is not undertaken.
4. *Malignant hyperthermia*—potentially lethal complication of a rare inherited muscle disorder that may be triggered by drugs used in anesthesia. The syndrome involves altered calcium function in muscle cells with hypermetabolism, uncoordinated muscle contractions, increased muscle work, increased oxygen consumption, and a raised level of lactic acid production. Acidosis develops, and body temperature rises, with resulting tachycardia and cardiac dysrhythmias, hypotension, decreased cardiac output, and cardiac arrest. Symptoms resemble those of coma—unconsciousness, absent reflexes, fixed pupils, apnea, and a flat electroencephalogram (sometimes). Oliguria and anuria are common. It is most common in children and adolescents.

Defining Characteristics of Hypothermia   BOX 13-2

ACCIDENTAL HYPOTHERMIA
- Results from sudden immersion in cold water or prolonged exposure to cold environments
- Especially common among young and elderly persons, who have altered thermoregulatory mechanisms
- Factors that increase risk
  1. Hypothyroidism
  2. Hypopituitarism
  3. Malnutrition
  4. Parkinson disease
  5. Rheumatoid arthritis
  6. Chronic increased vasodilation
  7. Decreased thermoregulatory control resulting from cerebral injury, ketoacidosis, uremia, and drug overdose
- Mechanisms
  1. Peripheral vasoconstriction—shunts blood away from cooler skin to core to decrease heat loss and produces peripheral tissue ischemia
  2. Intermittent reperfusion of extremities (Lewis phenomenon) helps preserve peripheral oxygenation until core temperature drops dramatically
  3. Hypothalamic center induces shivering; thinking becomes sluggish, and coordination is depressed

  4. Stupor; heart rate and respiratory rate decline; cardiac output diminishes; metabolic rate falls; acidosis; eventual ventricular fibrillation and asystole
- Treatment
  1. Passive rewarming for mild cases
  2. Core temperature greater than 30° C (86° F)—active rewarming (external)
  3. Core temperature less than 30° C (86° F) or with severe cardiovascular problems—active core rewarming (internal)

THERAPEUTIC HYPOTHERMIA
- Used to slow metabolism and preserve ischemic tissue during surgery or limb reimplantation
- Effects and cautions
  1. Stresses the heart, leading to ventricular fibrillation and cardiac arrest (may be desired outcome in open heart surgery when heart must be stopped)
  2. Exhausts liver glycogen stores by prolonged shivering
  3. Surface cooling may cause burns, frostbite, and fat necrosis

Hypothermia

Hypothermia (marked cooling of core temperature) produces vasoconstriction, alterations in microcirculation, coagulation, and ischemic tissue damage. Most tissues can tolerate low temperatures in controlled situations, such as surgery. However, in severe hypothermia, ice crystals form on the inside of the cell, causing cells to rupture and die. Tissue hypothermia slows cell metabolism, increases the blood viscosity, slows microcirculatory blood flow, facilitates blood coagulation, and stimulates profound vasoconstriction. Hypothermia may be accidental or therapeutic (Box 13-2).

Trauma

Major body trauma can affect temperature regulation through various mechanisms. Damage to the CNS, inflammation, increased intracranial pressures, or intracranial bleeding typically produce a fever of greater than 39° C (102.2° F). This sustained temperature, often referred to as a "central fever," appears with or without bradycardia. A central fever does not induce sweating and is very resistant to antipyretic therapy.

Other traumatic mechanisms that produce temperature alterations include accidental injuries, hemorrhagic shock, major surgery, and thermal burns. The severity and type of alteration (hyperthermia or hypothermia) vary with the severity of the cause and the body system affected.

✓ **QUICK CHECK**

Why is temperature regulation important?

What are the principal heat production methods? Heat loss methods?

How does the hypothalamus alter set point to change body temperature?

Compare and contrast hyperthermia and hypothermia and their effects on the body.

SLEEP

Sleep is an active multiphase process. Normal sleep has two phases that can be documented by electrencephalogram (EEG): REM (rapid eye movement) sleep and non-REM, or slow wave, sleep. *Non-REM (slow wave) sleep* is initiated when neurotransmitters withdraw from the reticular formation and arousal mechanisms are blocked. The basal metabolic rate falls by 10% to 15%; temperature decreases 0.5° to 1.0° C (0.9° to 1.8° F); heart rate, respiration, blood pressure, and muscle tone decrease; and knee jerk reflexes are absent. Pupils are constricted. During the various stages, cerebral blood flow to the brain decreases and growth hormone is released, with corticosteroid and catecholamine levels depressed.

Sleep Characteristics of Infants and Elderly Persons
BOX 13-3

INFANTS	ELDERLY PERSONS
Sleep 16 to 17 hours per day; one half in REM sleep, one fourth in non-REM sleep, and one fourth in an indeterminate phase	Total sleep time is decreased with a longer time to fall asleep
Infant sleep cycles are 50 to 60 minutes in length; 20 minutes non-REM and 10 to 45 minutes of REM sleep	Total time in slow wave and final phase of non-REM sleep decreases by 15% to 30%
At 1 year, total sleep time decreases with about equal time in REM and non-REM sleep	Alterations in sleep patterns occur about 10 years later in women than men
	Older adults are less able to tolerate sleep deprivation than younger adults

From Anders, T.F. & Keener, M. (1985). Developmental course of nighttime sleep-wake patterns in full-term and premature infants during the first year of life. Sleep, 8(3), 173-192; Fernsilver, S.H. & Hertz, G. (1994). Sleep in the elderly patient. Clinics in Chest Medicine, 14(3), 405-411.

REM (rapid eye movement) sleep is characterized by desynchronized fast activity that occurs about every 90 minutes beginning 1 to 2 hours after non-REM sleep begins. This sleep is known as *paradoxical sleep* because the EEG pattern is similar to the normal awake pattern. REM and non-REM sleep alternate throughout the night, with lengthening intervals of REM sleep and fewer intervals of deeper stages of non-REM sleep toward morning. The changes associated with REM sleep include rapid eye movement; loss of tone in antigravity muscles; loss of temperature regulation; altered heart rate, blood pressure, and respiration; penile erection in men and clitoral engorgement in women; release of steroids; and many memorable dreams. Respiratory control appears largely independent of metabolic requirements and oxygen variation. Loss of normal voluntary muscle control in the tongue and upper pharynx may produce some respiratory obstruction. Cerebral blood flow increases. About 20% to 25% of sleep time is represented by REM sleep in the adult. Box 13-3 summarizes sleep characteristics in infants and elderly persons.

Many neurotransmitters are associated with excitatory and inhibitory sleep mechanisms, including catecholamines, acetylcholine, serotonin, histamine, L-tryptophan, melatonin, and adenosine.[30] Their mechanism of action is complex and not clearly understood. The reticular formation is primarily responsible for generating REM sleep, and projections from the reticular formation and other areas of the mesencephalon and brain stem produce non-REM sleep.[31]

Sleep Disorders
Sleep disorders are classified by their signs and symptoms rather than by their cause. The four major classifications of sleep disorders are (1) disorders of initiating sleep, (2) disorders of excessive somnolence, (3) disorders of the sleep-wake schedule, and (4) dysfunctions of sleep, sleep stages, or partial arousals.

Disorders of initiating sleep: insomnia
Insomnia is the inability to fall or stay asleep. It may be transient, lasting a few days, and related to travel across time zones, or it may be caused by acute stress. Long-term insomnia is associated with drug or alcohol abuse, chronic pain disorders, chronic depression, or the use of certain drugs.

Disorders of excessive somnolence
Two disorders of excessive sleepiness are **obstructive sleep apnea syndrome** and **hypersomnia sleep apnea (HSA) syndrome.** Substantially more men than women are affected by these syndromes. Both syndromes are associated with periodic breathing and episodes of apnea. The periodic breathing eventually produces arousal, which interrupts the sleep cycle, reducing total sleep time and producing sleep and REM deprivation.[32]

In obstructive sleep apnea syndrome, apneic periods last 10 seconds or longer and generally result from obesity, decreased sensitivity to carbon dioxide and oxygen tensions, or upper airway obstruction. HSA syndrome is associated with upper airway obstruction recurring during sleep with excessive snoring and multiple apneic episodes. Sleep apnea produces low oxygen saturation and eventually leads to polycythemia, pulmonary hypertension, right-sided congestive heart failure, liver congestion, cyanosis, and peripheral edema.[33] Cardiac dysrhythmias during sleep are common. Daytime sleepiness also occurs, and individuals may fall asleep while driving a car, while working, or even while conversing.[34]

Disorders of the sleep-wake schedule
Common disorders of the sleep-wake schedule include rapid time-zone change (or jet-lag syndrome), changing sleep schedule involving 3 hours or more in sleep time, or changing total sleep time from day to day. These changes desynchronize circadian rhythm, which can depress the degree of vigilance, performance of psychomotor tasks, and arousal.

Dysfunctions of sleep, sleep stages, or partial arousals
Three dysfunctions of sleep are common in children. **Somnambulism** (sleepwalking) is a disorder primarily of childhood and appears to resolve within a few years. Sleepwalking is therefore not associated with dreaming, and the child has no memory of the event on awakening.

Night terrors are characterized by sudden apparent arousals in which the child expresses intense fear or emotion. However, the child is not awake and can be difficult to arouse. Once awakened, the child has no memory of the night terror event. Night terrors are not associated with dreams. Although this problem occurs most often in children, adults also may experience it with corresponding daytime anxiety.

Enuresis is possibly the most disturbing childhood sleep dysfunction, and it may be related to a hereditary delay in maturity; organic disorders, including urinary tract infection, small bladder capacity, or reduced nocturnal secretion of antidiuretic hormone; or psychologic distress related to abuse.[35] Most children eventually outgrow the enuretic episodes. Treatment, including alarms and drugs, is effective. Nocturnal enuresis in adults is rare but treatable.[36]

> **✓ QUICK CHECK**
>
> Describe REM and non-REM sleep.
>
> What four types of sleep disorders are seen?
>
> How do medications and alcohol affect sleep?

THE SPECIAL SENSES
Vision

The eyes are complex sense organs responsible for vision. Within a protective casing, each eye has receptors, a lens system for focusing light on the receptors, and a system of nerves for conducting impulses from the receptors to the brain.[37] Visual dysfunction may be caused by abnormal ocular movements or alterations in visual acuity, refraction, color vision, or accommodation. Visual dysfunction also may be the secondary effect of another neurologic disorder.

The eye and its external structures

The wall of the eye is formed of three layers: (1) sclera, (2) choroid, and (3) retina (Fig. 13-6). The *sclera* is the thick, white, outermost layer. It becomes transparent at the *cornea*—the portion of the sclera in the central anterior region that allows light to enter the eye. The choroid is the deeply pigmented middle layer that prevents light from scattering inside the eye. The *iris,* part of the choroid, has a round opening, the *pupil,* through which light passes. Smooth muscle fibers control the size of the pupil so that it adjusts to bright light or dim light and close or distant vision.

The innermost layer of the eye, the *retina,* contains millions of rods and cones—special photoreceptors that convert light energy into nerve impulses. *Rods* mediate peripheral and dim light vision and are densest at the periphery. *Cones,* densest in the center of the retina, are color and detail receptors. There are no photoreceptors where the optic nerve leaves the eyeball, creating the *optic disc,* or blind spot. Lateral to each optic disc is the *fovea centralis*—a tiny area that contains only cones and provides the greatest visual acuity (see Fig. 13-6).

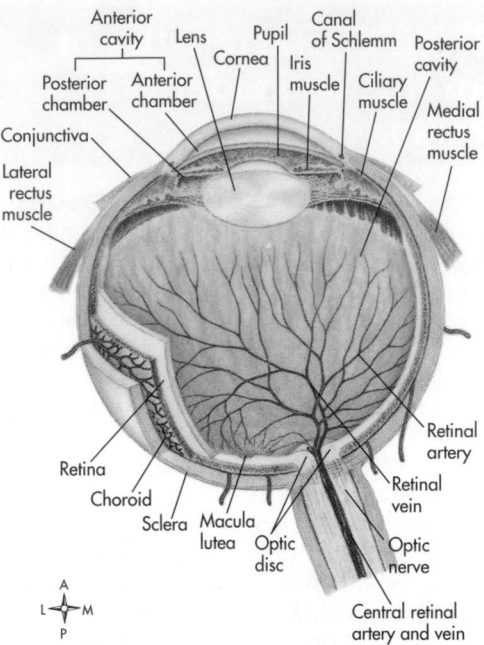

Fig. 13-6 *Internal anatomy of the eye. (From Seidel, H.M. et al. [1999]. Mosby's guide to physical examination [4th ed.]. St. Louis: Mosby.)*

As shown in Fig. 13-10, nerve impulses pass through the optic nerves to the optic chiasm. There nerves from the inner (nasal) halves of the retinas cross to the opposite side and join fibers from the outer (temporal) halves of the retinas to form the optic tracts. The fibers of the optic tracts synapse in the dorsal lateral geniculate nucleus and pass by way of the optic radiation (or geniculocalcarine tract) to the primary visual cortex in the occipital lobe of the brain.[38] Light entering the eye is focused on the retina by the *lens*— a flexible, biconvex, crystal-like structure. With age the lens becomes increasingly hard and opaque. The lens divides the anterior chamber into (1) the aqueous chamber and (2) the vitreous chamber. *Aqueous humor* fills the aqueous chamber and helps maintain pressure inside the eye, as well as provide nutrients to the lens and cornea. Aqueous humor is secreted by the ciliary processes and reabsorbed into the canal of Schlemm. If drainage is blocked, intraocular pressure increases (glaucoma). The vitreous chamber is filled with a gel-like substance called *vitreous humor.* Vitreous humor helps to prevent the eyeball from collapsing inward.

The central retinal artery provides blood to the inner retinal surface, and the choroid supplies nutrients to the outer surface of the retina. Six extrinsic eye muscles allow gross eye movements and permit eyes to follow a moving object (Fig. 13-7).

The external structures protecting the eye include the eyelids (palpebrae), conjunctiva, and lacrimal apparatus (Fig. 13-8). The eyelids are used to control the amount of light reaching the eyes, and the conjunctiva lines the eyelids. Tears released from the lacrimal apparatus bathe the surface of the eye and prevent friction, maintain hydration, and wash out foreign bodies and other irritants.

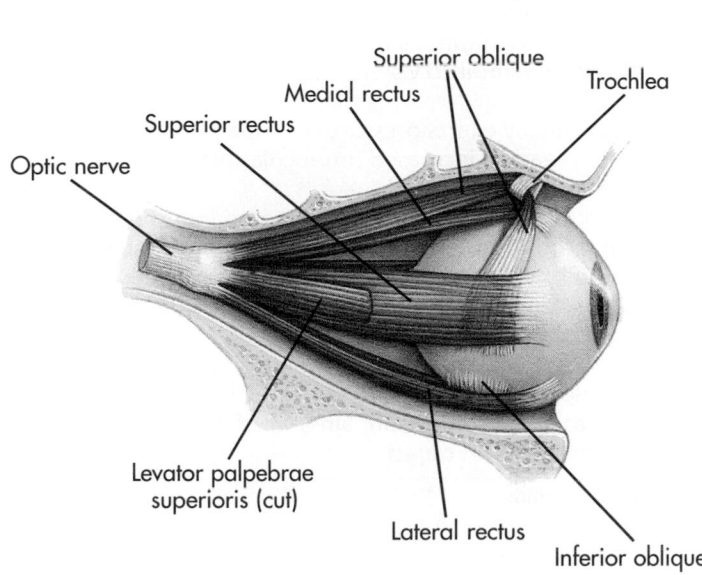

Fig. 13-7 *Extrinsic muscles of the right eye.* *(From Thibodeau, G.A. & Patton, K.T. [1999]. Anatomy and physiology [4th ed.]. St. Louis: Mosby.)*

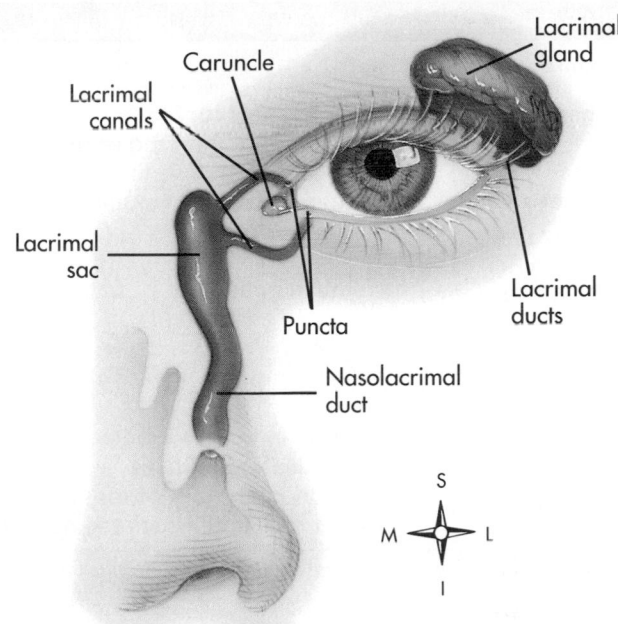

Fig. 13-8 *Lacrimal apparatus.* Fluid produced by lacrimal glands (tears) streams across the eye surface, enters the canals, and then passes through the nasolacrimal duct to enter the nose. *(From Thibodeau, G.A. & Patton, K.T. [1999]. Anatomy and physiology [4th ed.]. St. Louis: Mosby.)*

Visual dysfunction

Alterations in ocular movements

Abnormal ocular movements result from oculomotor, trochlear, or abducens cranial nerve dysfunction (see Table 12-6). The three types of eye movement disorders are (1) strabismus, (2) nystagmus, and (3) paralysis of individual extraocular muscles.

In *strabismus,* one eye deviates from the other when the person is looking at an object. This is caused by a weak or hypertonic muscle in one eye. The deviation may be upward, downward, inward, or outward. Strabismus in children requires early intervention to prevent *amblyopia* (reduced vision in the affected eye caused by cerebral blockage of the visual stimuli). The primary symptom of strabismus is *diplopia* (double vision). Causes of strabismus include neuromuscular disorder of the eye muscle, diseases involving the cerebral hemispheres, or thyroid disease.

Nystagmus is an involuntary unilateral or bilateral rhythmic movement of the eyes. It may be present at rest or when the eye moves. *Pendular nystagmus* is characterized by a regular to-and-fro movement of the eyes. In *jerk nystagmus,* one phase of the eye movement is faster than the other. Nystagmus may be caused by an imbalanced reflex activity of the inner ear, *vestibular nuclei* cerebellum, medial longitudinal fascicle, or nuclei of the oculomotor, trochlear, and abducens cranial nerves (see Table 12-6). Drugs, retinal disease, and diseases involving the cervical cord also may produce nystagmus.

Paralysis of specific extraocular muscles may cause lim-ited abduction, abnormal closure of the eyelid, ptosis (drooping of the eyelid), or diplopia (double vision) as a result of unopposed muscle activity. Trauma or pressure in the area of the cranial nerves or diseases such as diabetes mellitus and myasthenia gravis also paralyze specific extraocular muscles.

Alterations in visual acuity

Visual acuity is the ability to see objects in sharp detail. With advancing age, the lens of the eye becomes less flexible and adjusts slowly. In addition, the sclera changes shape, so that light falls on the macula. Thus visual acuity declines with age. See Table 13-6 for a summary of changes in the eye caused by aging. Specific causes of visual acuity changes are (1) amblyopia, (2) scotoma, (3) cataracts, (4) papilledema, (5) *dark adaptation,* and (6) glaucoma (Table 13-7). There are three types of glaucoma (increased intraocular pressure)[39]:

1. *Open angle.* Outflow obstruction of aqueous humor at trabecular meshwork or canal of Schlemm although there is adequate space for drainage. Often is an inherited disease and a leading cause of blindness with few preliminary symptoms.

2. *Angle closure.* Displacement of the iris toward the cornea with obstruction of the trabecular meshwork and obstruction of outflow of aqueous humor from the anterior chamber. May occur acutely with a sudden rise in intraocular pressure causing pain and visual disturbances.

3. *Congenital closure.* Associated with congenital malformations and other anomalies.

TABLE 13-6   Changes in the Eye Caused by Aging

Structure	Change	Consequence
Cornea	Thicker and less curved	Increase in astigmatism
	Formation of a gray ring at the edge of the cornea (arcus senilis)	Not detrimental to vision
Anterior chamber	Decrease in size and volume caused by thickening of lens	Occasionally exerts pressure on Schlemm canal and may lead to increased intraocular pressure and glaucoma
Lens	Increase in opacity	Decrease in refraction with increased light scattering (blurring) and decreased color vision (green and blue); can lead to cataracts
	Increased firmness, loss of elasticity	Decrease in accommodation for near vision; presbyopia develops by age 50-55 yr
Ciliary muscles	Reduction in pupil diameter, atrophy of radial dilation muscles	Persistent constriction (senile miosis); decrease in critical flicker frequency*
Retina	Reduction in number of rods at periphery, loss of rods and associated nerve cells	Increase in the minimum amount of light necessary to see an object

*The rate at which consecutive visual stimuli can be presented and still be perceived as separate.

TABLE 13-7   Causes of Visual Acuity Changes

Disorder	Description
Amblyopia	Reduced or dimmed vision, cause unknown
	Accompanies such diseases as diabetes mellitus, renal failure, and malaria and the use of drugs such as alcohol and tobacco
Scotoma	Circumscribed defect of central field of vision
	Often associated with retrobulbar neuritis and multiple sclerosis, compression of optic nerve by tumor, inflammation of optic nerve, pernicious anemia, methyl alcohol poisoning, and use of tobacco
Cataract	Cloudy or opaque area in ocular lens
	Incidence increases with age because most commonly a result of degeneration; other causes are congenital
Papilledema	Edema and inflammation of optic nerve where it enters eyeball
	Caused by obstruction of venous return from retina from one of three main sources; increased intracranial pressure, retrobulbar neuritis, or changes in retinal blood vessels
Dark adaptation	With age, the eye does not adapt as readily to dark
	Also, changes in the quantity and quality of rhodopsin are causative; vitamin A deficiencies can produce this at any age
Glaucoma	Increased intraocular pressures (above 12 to 20 mm Hg)
	Loss of acuity results from pressure on the optic nerve, which blocks the flow of nutrients to optic nerve fibers, leading to their death; sixth leading cause of blindness

Alterations in accommodation

Accommodation refers to changes in the thickness of the lens. Accommodation is needed for clear vision and is mediated through the oculomotor nerve. Pressure, inflammation, age, and disease of the oculomotor nerve may alter accommodation, causing diplopia, blurred vision, and headache.[40]

Loss of accommodation with advancing age is termed *presbyopia,* a condition in which the ocular lens becomes larger, firmer, and less elastic. The major symptom is reduced near vision, causing the individual to hold reading material at arm's length.

Alterations in refraction

Alterations in refraction are the most common visual problem. Causes include irregularities of the corneal curvature, the focusing power of the lens, and the length of the eye. The major symptoms of refraction alterations are blurred vision and headache. Three types of refraction are as follows (Fig. 13-9):

Myopia—nearsightedness. Light rays are focused in front of the retina when the person is looking at a distant object.

Hyperopia—farsightedness. Light rays are focused behind the retina when a person is looking at a near object.

Astigmatism—unequal curvature of the cornea. Light rays are bent unevenly and do not come to a single focus on the retina. Astigmatism may coexist with myopia, hyperopia, or presbyopia.

Alterations in color vision

Normal sensitivity to color diminishes with age because of the progressive yellowing of the lens that occurs with aging. All colors become less intense, although color discrimination for blue and green is greatly affected. Color vision deteriorates more rapidly for individuals with diabetes mellitus than for the general population.

Abnormal color vision also may be caused by *color blindness,* an inherited trait. Color blindness affects 8% of the male population and 0.5% of the female population. Although many forms of color blindness exist, most commonly the affected individual cannot distinguish red from green.[41]

Neurologic disorders causing visual dysfunction

Vision may be disrupted at many points along the visual pathway, causing various defects in the visual field. Visual changes may cause defects or blindness in the entire visual field or half a visual field (hemianopia). (Fig. 13-10 illustrates the many areas along the visual pathway that may be damaged and the associated visual changes.)

Injury to the optic nerve causes same-side blindness. In-

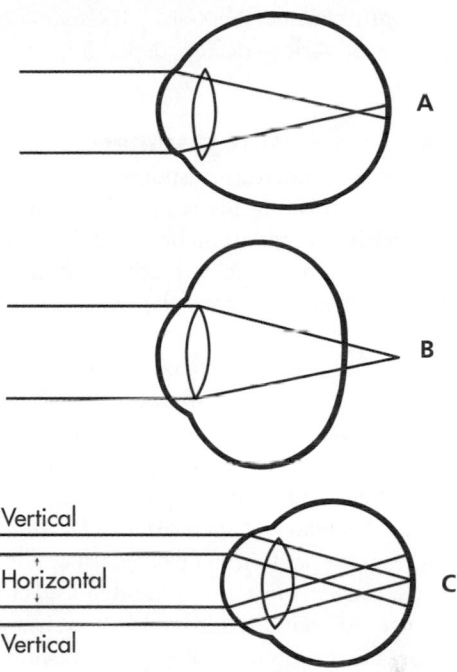

Fig. 13-9 *Alterations in refraction.* **A,** Myopic eye. Parallel rays of light are brought to a focus in front of the retina. **B,** Hyperopic eye. Parallel rays of light come to a focus behind the retina in the unaccommodative eye. **C,** Simple myopic astigmatism. The vertical bundle of rays is focused on the retina; the horizontal rays are focused in front of the retina. *(From Stein, H.A., Slatt, B.J., & Stein, R.M. [1988]. The ophthalmic assistant: Fundamentals and clinical practice [5th ed.]. St. Louis: Mosby.)*

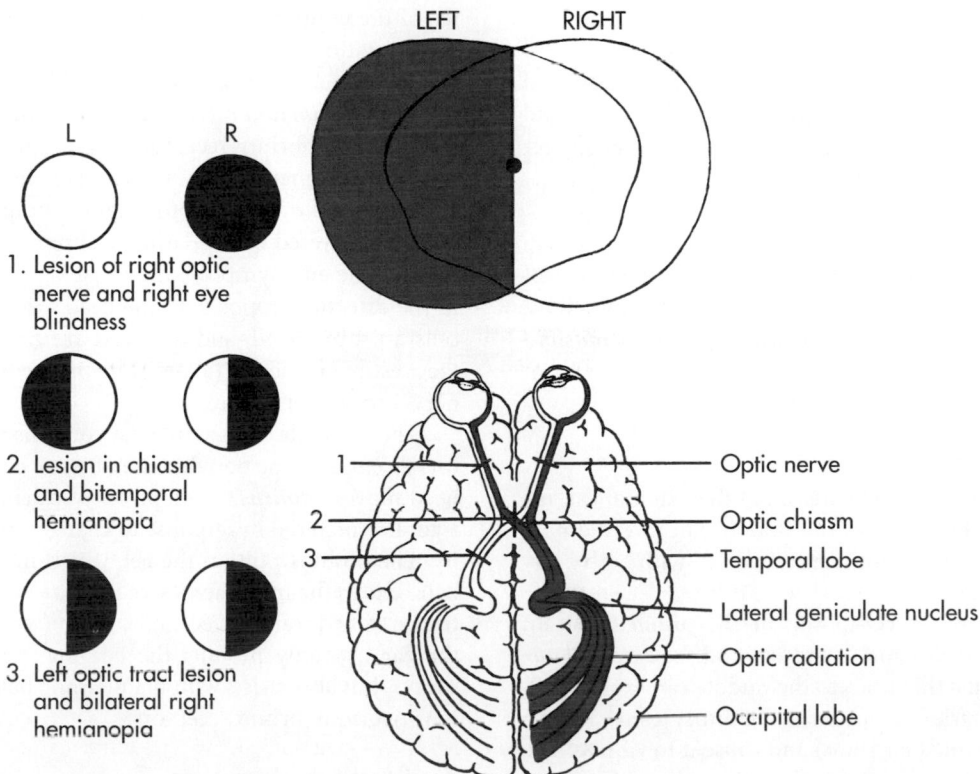

Fig. 13-10 *Visual pathways and defects. (Modified from Thompson, J.M. et al. [1998]. Mosby's clinical nursing [4th ed.]. St. Louis: Mosby.)*

jury to the *optic chiasm* (the X-shaped crossing of the optic nerves) can cause various defects, depending on the location of the injury.

External eye structure disorders

Infection and inflammatory responses are the most common conditions affecting the supporting structures of the eyes. *Blepharitis* is an inflammation of the eyelids caused by *Staphylococcus* or seborrheic dermatitis. A *hordeolum (stye)* is an infection of the sebaceous glands of the eyelids, and a *chalazion* is an infection of the meibomian (oil-secreting) gland. These conditions are treated symptomatically.

Conjunctivitis is an inflammation of the conjunctiva caused by bacteria, viruses, allergies, or chemical irritants.[42] *Acute bacterial conjunctivitis (pinkeye)* is highly contagious and often caused by *Staphylococcus, Haemophilus, Streptococcus pneumoniae,* and *Moraxella catarrhalis,* although other bacteria may be involved. In children younger than 6 years, *Haemophilus* infection often leads to otitis media (conjunctivitis-otitis syndrome).[43] Preventing spread of the microorganism with meticulous handwashing and use of separate towels is important. The disease also is treated with antibiotics.

Viral conjunctivitis is caused by an adenovirus. Again, it is contagious, with watering, redness, and photophobia. *Allergic conjunctivitis* is associated with a variety of antigens, including pollens. *Chronic conjunctivitis* results from any persistent conjunctivitis. *Trachoma* (chlamydial conjunctivitis) is caused by *Chlamydia trachomatis* and often is associated with poor hygiene. It is the leading cause of preventable blindness in the world.

Keratitis is an infection of the cornea caused by bacteria or viruses. Bacterial infections cause corneal ulceration, and type I herpes simplex virus can involve both the cornea and the conjunctiva. Severe ulcerations with residual scarring require corneal transplantation.

Hearing

The external auditory canal is surrounded by the bones of the cranium. The opening (meatus) of the canal is just above the *mastoid process.* The air-filled sinuses, called *mastoid air cells,* of the mastoid process promote conductivity of sound between the external and the middle ear.

The normal ear

The ear is divided into three areas: (1) the external ear, involved only with hearing; (2) the middle ear, involved only with hearing; and (3) the inner ear, involved with both hearing and equilibrium.

The external ear is composed of the *pinna* (auricle), which is the visible portion of the ear, and the *external auditory canal,* a tube that leads to the middle ear (Fig. 13-11). Sound waves entering the external auditory canal hit the *tympanic membrane* (eardrum) and cause it to vibrate. The tympanic membrane separates the external ear from the middle ear.

The middle ear is composed of the *tympanic cavity,* a small chamber in the temporal bone. Three ossicles (small bones known as the *malleus [hammer], incus [anvil],* and *stapes [stirrup]*) transmit the vibration of the tympanic membrane to the inner ear. When the tympanic membrane moves, the malleus moves with it and transfers the vibration to the incus, which passes it on to the stapes. The stapes presses against the oval window, a small membrane of the inner ear. The movement of the *oval window* sets the fluids of the inner ear in motion (Fig. 13-12).

The *eustachian (pharyngeotympanic) tube* connects the middle ear with the thorax. Normally flat and closed, the eustachian tube opens briefly when a person swallows or yawns, and it equalizes the pressure in the middle ear with atmospheric pressure. Equalized pressure permits the tympanic membrane to vibrate freely. Through the eustachian tube the mucosa of the middle ear is continuous with the mucosal lining of the throat.

The inner ear is a system of osseous labyrinths (bony, mazelike chambers) filled with *perilymph.* The bony labyrinth is divided into the *cochlea,* the *vestibule,* and the *semicircular canals* (see Fig. 13-11). Suspended in the perilymph is the endolymph-filled membranous labyrinth that basically follows the shape of the bony labyrinth.

Within the cochlea is the *organ of Corti,* which contains *hair cells* (hearing receptors). Sound waves that reach the cochlea through vibrations of the tympanic membrane, ossicles, and oval window set the cochlear fluids into motion. Receptor cells on the basilar membrane are stimulated when their hairs are bent or pulled by the movement. Once stimulated, hair cells transmit impulses along the cochlear nerve (a division of the vestibulocochlear nerve) to the auditory cortex of the temporal lobe in the brain (see Fig. 13-12). There interpretation of the sound occurs.

The semicircular canals and vestibule of the inner ear contain *equilibrium receptors.* In the semicircular canals the dynamic equilibrium receptors respond to changes in direction of movement. Within each semicircular canal is the *crista ampullaris,* a receptor region composed of a tuft of hair cells covered by a gelatinous cupula. When the head is rotated, the endolymph in the canal lags behind and moves in the direction opposite to the head's movement. The hair cells are stimulated, and impulses are transmitted through the vestibular nerve (a division of the vestibulocochlear nerve) to the cerebellum.

The vestibule in the inner ear contains *maculae*—receptors essential to the body's sense of static equilibrium. As the head moves, *otoliths* (small pieces of calcium salts) move in a gel-like material in response to changes in the pull of gravity. The otoliths pull on the gel, which in turn pulls on the hair cells in the maculae. Nerve impulses in the hair cells are triggered and transmitted to the brain (see Fig. 13-12). Thus the ear not only permits the hearing of a large range of sounds but also assists with maintaining balance through the sensitive equilibrium receptors.

Auditory dysfunction

Between 5% and 10% of the general population have impaired hearing. The major categories of auditory dysfunction are conductive hearing loss, sensorineural hearing loss, mixed

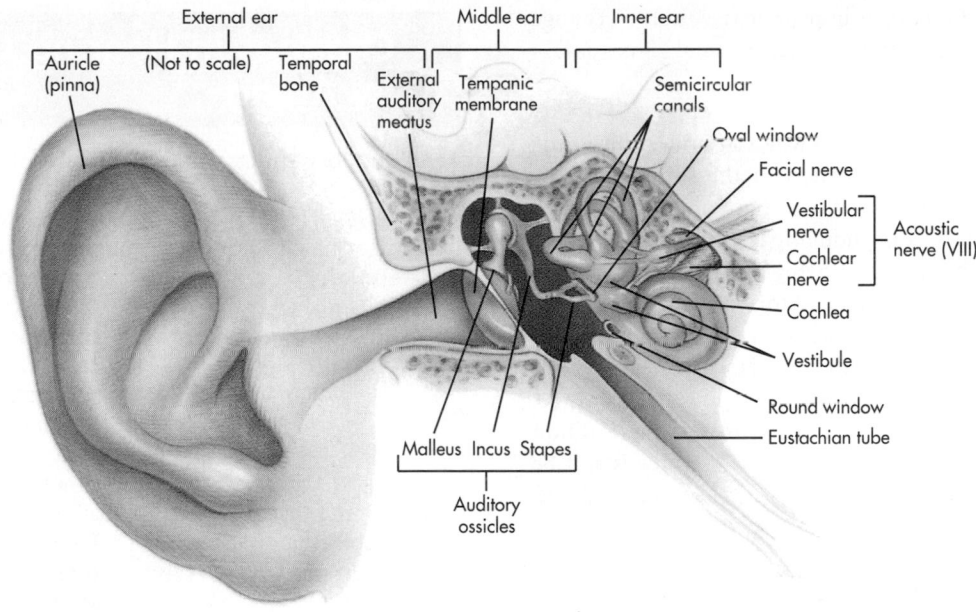

Fig. 13-11 *The ear.* External, middle, and inner ears. (Anatomic structures are not drawn to scale.) *(From Thibodeau, G.A. & Patton, K.T. [1999]. Anatomy and physiology [4th ed.]. St. Louis: Mosby.)*

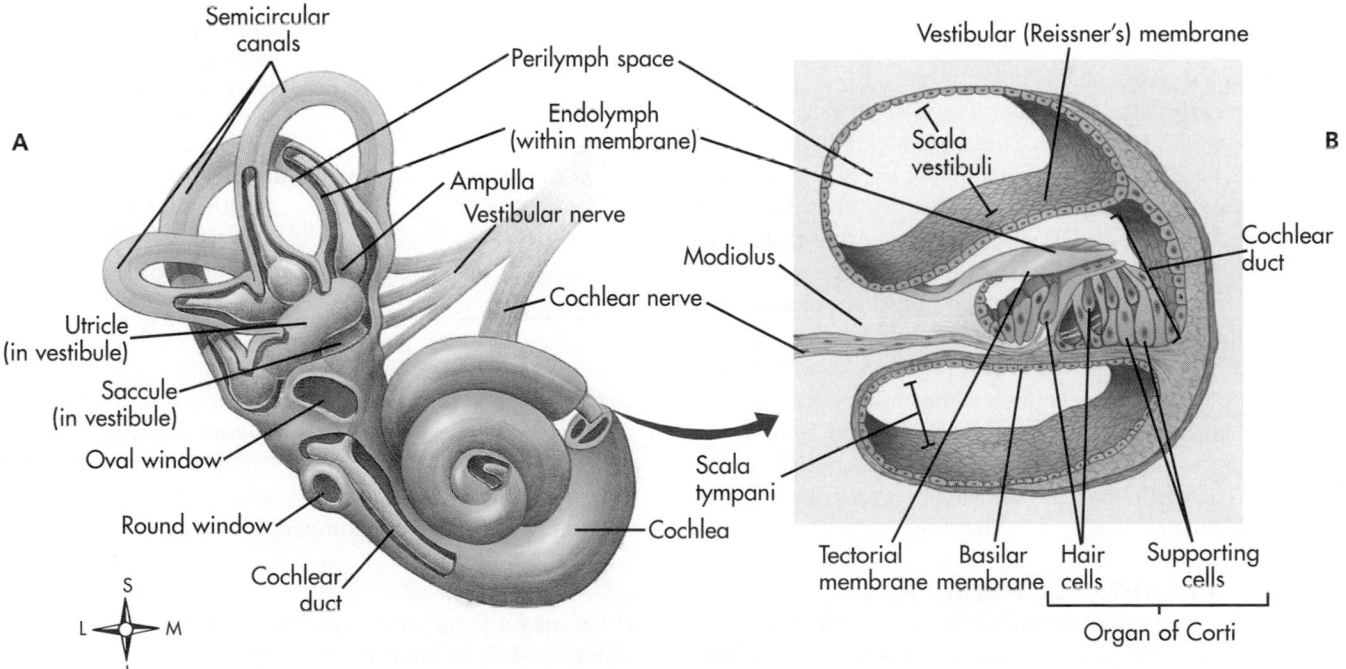

Fig. 13-12 *The inner ear.* **A,** The bony labyrinth *(orange)* is the hard outer wall of the entire inner ear and includes semicircular canals, vestibule, and cochlea. Within the bony labyrinth is the membranous labyrinth *(purple),* which is surrounded by perilymph and filled with endolymph. Each ampulla in the vestibule contains a crista ampullaris that detects changes in head position and sends sensory impulses through the vestibular nerve to the brain. **B,** The inset shows a section of the membranous cochlea. Hair cells in the organ of Corti detect sound and send the information through the cochlear nerve. The vestibular and cochlear nerves join to form the eighth cranial nerve. *(From Thibodeau, G.A. & Patton, K.T. [1999]. Anatomy and physiology [4th ed.]. St. Louis: Mosby.)*

hearing loss, and functional hearing loss. Auditory changes caused by aging are common and incremental (Box 13-4).

Conductive hearing loss

A *conductive hearing loss* occurs when a change in the outer or middle ear impairs conduction of the sound from the outer to the inner ear. Conditions that commonly cause a conductive hearing loss include impacted cerumen, foreign bodies lodged in the ear canal, benign tumors of the middle ear, carcinoma of the external auditory canal or middle ear, eustachian tube dysfunction, otitis media, acute viral otitis media, chronic suppurative otitis media, cholesteatoma, and otosclerosis.

Symptoms of conductive hearing loss include diminished hearing and soft speaking voice. The voice is soft because often the individual hears his or her voice, conducted by bone, as loud.

Sensorineural hearing loss

A *sensorineural hearing loss* is caused by impairment of the organ of Corti or its central connections. The loss may occur gradually or suddenly. Conditions causing sensorineural loss include congenital and hereditary factors, noise exposure, aging, *Ménière disease,* ototoxicity, and systemic disease (syphilis, Paget disease, collagen diseases, diabetes mellitus). Congenital and neonatal sensorineural hearing loss may be caused by maternal rubella, ototoxic drugs, prematurity, traumatic delivery, erythroblastosis fetalis, and congenital hereditary malfunction. Diagnosis often is made when delayed speech development is noted.

Presbycusis is the most common form of sensorineural hearing loss and is especially common in elderly people. Its cause may be atrophy of the basal end of the organ of Corti, loss of auditory receptors, vascular changes, or stiffening of the basilar membranes. Drug ototoxicities (drugs that cause destruction of auditory function) have been observed after exposure to various chemicals; for example, antibiotics such as streptomycin, neomycin, gentamicin, and vancomycin; diuretics such as ethacrynic acid and furosemide; and chemicals such as salicylate, quinine, carbon monoxide, nitrogen mustard, arsenic, mercury, gold, tobacco, and alcohol. In most instances the drugs and chemicals listed initially cause *tinnitus* (ringing in the ear), followed by a progressive high-tone sensorineural hearing loss that is permanent.

Mixed and functional hearing loss

A *mixed hearing loss* is caused by a combination of conductive and sensorineural losses. With *functional hearing loss,* which is rare, the individual does not respond to voice and appears not to hear. It is thought to be caused by emotional or psychologic factors.

Ear infections
Otitis externa

Otitis externa is the most common infection of the outer ear.[44] The most frequently found microorganisms are *Pseudomonas, Escherichia coli,* and *Staphylococcus aureus.* In-

---

Changes in Hearing Caused by Aging   BOX 13-4

Hearing loss affects about one third of older people.

CHANGES IN STRUCTURE	CHANGES IN FUNCTION
Cochlear hair cell degeneration	Inability to hear high-frequency sounds (presbycusis, sensorineural loss); interferes with understanding speech; hearing may be lost in both ears at different times
Loss of auditory neurons in spiral ganglia of organ of Corti	Inability to hear high-frequency sounds (presbycusis, sensorineural loss); interferes with understanding speech; hearing may be lost in both ears at different times
Degeneration of basilar (cochlear) conductive membrane of cochlea	Inability to hear at all frequencies but more pronounced at higher frequencies (cochlear conductive loss)
Decreased vascularity of cochlea	Equal loss of hearing at all frequencies (strial loss); inability to disseminate localization of sound
Loss of cortical auditory neurons	Equal loss of hearing at all frequencies (strial loss); inability to disseminate localization of sound

---

fection usually follows prolonged exposure to moisture (swimmer's ear). The earliest symptoms are inflammation with swelling and clear drainage progressing to purulent drainage with obstruction of the canal. Tenderness and pain with earlobe retraction accompany inflammation.

Otitis media

Otitis media is the most common infection of infants and children. Most children have one episode by 3 years of age. The most common pathogens are *Streptococcus pneumoniae, Haemophilus influenzae,* and *Moraxella catarrhalis.* Predisposing factors include allergy, sinusitis, submucous cleft palate, adenoidal hypertrophy, and immune deficiency. Breast-feeding is a protective factor.

Acute otitis media (AOM) is associated with ear pain, fever, irritability, inflamed tympanic membrane, and fluid in the middle ear. The tympanic membrane progresses from erythema to opaqueness with bulging as fluid accumulates.

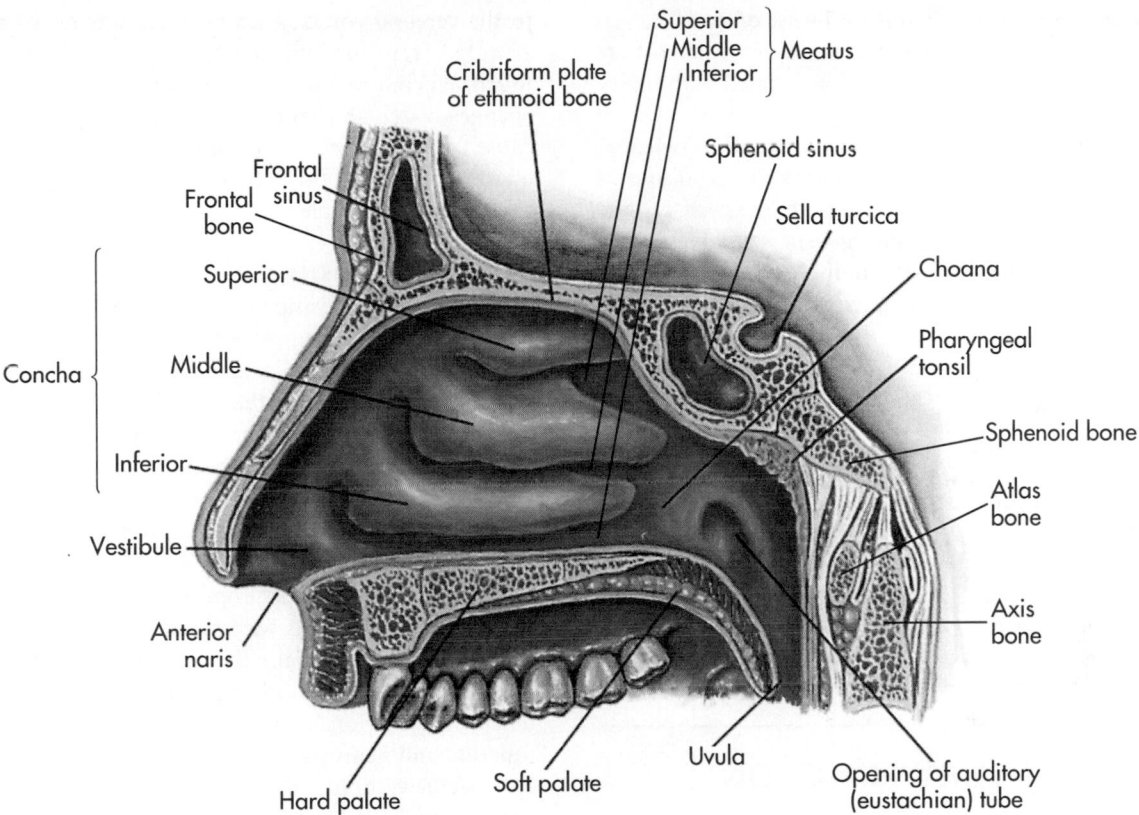

Fig. 13-13 *Olfaction.* Location of olfactory epithelium, olfactory bulb, and neuronal pathways involved in olfaction. *(Modified from Seidel, H.M. et al. [1995].* Mosby's guide to physical examination *[3rd ed.].St. Louis: Mosby.)*

There is an increasing prevalence of AOM caused by penicillin-resistant microorganisms. ***Otitis media with effusion (OME)*** is the presence of fluid in the middle ear without symptoms of acute infection.

Treatment includes antimicrobial therapy for AOM and placement of tympanotomy tubes when there is bilateral effusion persistent for 3 months and significant hearing loss.[45] Complications include mastoiditis, brain abscess, meningitis, and chronic otitis media with hearing loss. Speech, language, and cognitive abilities may be affected by persistent middle ear effusions.

Olfaction and Taste

Olfaction (smell) and taste (gustation) dysfunctions may occur separately or jointly. The strong relationship between smell and taste creates the sensation of flavor. If either sensation is impaired, the perception of flavor is altered. (Olfactory structures are illustrated in Fig. 13-13.)

Olfactory cells, located in the olfactory epithelium, are the receptor cells for smell. Seven different primary classes of olfactory stimulants have been identified: (1) camphoraceous, (2) musky, (3) floral, (4) peppermint, (5) ethereal, (6) pungent, and (7) putrid. The primary sensations of taste are (1) sour, (2) salty, (3) sweet, and (4) bitter. Taste buds sensitive to each of the primary sensations are located in specific areas of the tongue.[46]

Changes in Olfaction and Taste With Aging   BOX 13-5

Decline in sensitivity to odors, usually after 80 years
Loss of olfaction may diminish appetite, taste, and food selection and may affect nutrition
Inability to smell toxic fumes or gases can pose a safety hazard
Decline in taste sensitivity more gradual than smell
Higher concentration of flavors required to stimulate taste
Taste may be influenced by decreased salivary secretion

Sensitivity to odors declines steadily with aging. See Box 13-5 for a summary of changes in olfaction and taste with aging.

Olfactory and taste dysfunctions

Olfactory dysfunctions include the following:
1. ***Hyposmia***—impaired sense of smell
2. ***Anosmia***—complete loss of smell
3. ***Olfactory hallucinations***—smelling odors that are not really present

4. *Parosmia*—abnormal or perverted sense of smell

The sense of taste can be impaired by injury. Altered taste may be attributed to impaired smell associated with injury near the hippocampus.

Hypogeusia is a decrease in taste sensation, whereas *ageusia* is an absence of the sense of taste. These disorders result from cranial nerve injuries and can be specific to the area of the tongue innervated. *Parageusia* is a perversion of taste in which substances possess an unpleasant flavor. Alterations in taste may compromise adequate nutrition or cause anorexia.[47]

✓ QUICK CHECK

List the major structures of the eye.

Visual disorders fall into several categories; name them.

How does fluid accumulate in the middle ear during otitis media?

What factors are involved in the sensation of flavor?

SOMATOSENSORY FUNCTION
Touch

The sensation of touch involves the fusion of several qualities, including modality, intensity, location, and duration of the sensory stimulus. Receptors sensitive to touch are present in the skin, mainly in the fingers and lips. Meissner and pacinian corpuscles are rapidly adapting receptors, whereas Merkel disks and Ruffini endings are slowly adapting touch receptors. Four afferent fiber types mediate tactile sensation.[48] Specific sensory input is carried to the higher levels of the CNS by the dorsal column of the spinal cord and the anterior spinothalamic tract.

The cutaneous senses develop before birth, but structural growth continues into early adulthood. Then a gradual decline occurs, with loss in tactile sensitivity with advancing age.[49]

Abnormal tactile perception may be caused by alterations at any level of the nervous system, from the receptor to the cerebral cortex. Factors that interrupt or impair reception, transmission, perception, or interpretation of touch, including trauma, tumor, infection, metabolic changes, vascular changes, and degenerative diseases, may cause tactile dysfunction. In addition, most tactile sensations evoke affective responses that determine whether the sensation is unpleasant, pleasant, or neutral.

Proprioception

Awareness of the position of the body and its parts depends on impulses from the inner ear and from receptors in joints and ligaments. Sensory data are transmitted to higher centers, primarily through the dorsal columns and the spinocerebellar tracts, with some data passing through the medial lemnisci and thalamic radiations to the cortex. These stimuli are necessary for the coordination of movements, the grading of muscular contraction, and the maintenance of equilibrium.

A progressive loss of proprioception has been reported in elderly persons.[50] As with tactile dysfunction, any factor that interrupts or impairs the reception, transmission, perception, or interpretation of proprioceptive stimuli also alters proprioception. Two common causes are vestibular dysfunction and neuropathy.

Specific vestibular dysfunctions are vestibular nystagmus and vertigo. *Vestibular nystagmus* is the constant, involuntary movement of the eyeball caused by ear disturbances. This condition occurs when the semicircular canal system is overstimulated. *Vertigo* is the sensation of spinning that occurs with inflammation of the semicircular canals in the ear. The individual may feel either that he or she is moving in space or that the world is revolving. Vertigo often causes loss of balance, and nystagmus may occur. Ménière disease can cause loss of proprioception during an acute attack, so that standing or walking is impossible.

Peripheral neuropathies also can cause proprioceptive dysfunction. They may be caused by several conditions and commonly are associated with renal disease and diabetes mellitus. Although the exact sequence of events is unknown, neuropathies cause a diminished or absent sense of body position or position of body parts. Gait changes often occur. (Neuropathies are discussed further in Chapter 14.)

■ DID YOU UNDERSTAND?

Pain

1. Pain is a complex phenomenon composed of sensory experiences (time, space, intensity) and emotion, cognition, and motivation.
2. Categories of pain include somatogenic pain (with a known physiologic cause), psychogenic pain (without a physiologic cause), acute pain (signal to the person of a harmful stimulus), and chronic pain (persistence of pain of unknown cause or unusual response to therapy).
3. Pain threshold is the point at which pain is perceived. Pain threshold does not vary significantly among people or within the same person over time.
4. Pain tolerance is the duration of time or the intensity of pain that an individual will endure before initiating overt pain response. Tolerance varies widely among individuals and in the same individual over time.
5. Newborns and young children have anatomic and

■ DID YOU UNDERSTAND? —cont'd

functional ability to perceive pain. Older individuals tend to have a slightly higher pain threshold, probably because of changes in the thickness of the skin and peripheral neuropathies. In all age-groups, women appear to be more sensitive to pain than are men.

6. The portions of the nervous system responsible for the sensation and perception of pain may be divided into three areas: (a) the afferent fibers, (b) the central nervous system, and (c) the efferent pathways.

7. The afferent system is composed of nociceptors, A and C fibers, the dorsal horn of the spinal column, and afferent neurons in the spinothalamic tract.

8. Efferent pathways from the periaqueductal gray are responsible for modulation or inhibition of afferent pain signals.

9. The thalamus, cortex, and postcentral gyrus perceive, describe, and localize pain. The reticular formation and limbic system control the emotional and affective response to pain.

10. According to the gate control theory, there are specialized cells within the substantia gelatinosa that act as a gate, opening and closing the afferent pathways to transmission of painful stimuli.

11. Endorphins inhibit transmission of the pain impulse. They are present in varying concentrations in the neurons in the brain, spinal cord, and gastrointestinal tract.

12. Acute pain may be (a) somatic (superficial), (b) visceral (internal), or (c) referred (present in an area distant from its origin). The area of referred pain is supplied by the same spinal segment as the actual site of pain.

13. Physiologic responses to acute pain include increased heart rate, respiratory rate, and blood pressure; pallor or flushing; dilated pupils; diaphoresis; and nausea and vomiting. Blood sugar is elevated; gastric secretion and motility are decreased; and blood flow to the viscera and skin is decreased.

14. Psychologic, behavioral, and physiologic responses to chronic pain include depression, difficulty in sleeping, preoccupation with pain, life-style changes, and physiologic adaptation.

15. Chronic pain may be a result of decreased levels of endorphins, predominance of C neuron stimulation, or leukokinin.

16. Chronic pain conditions include lower back pain, neuralgias, reflex sympathetic dystrophies, hyperesthesias, myofascial pain syndrome, pain hemiagnosia, phantom limb pain, migraine, and chronic pain associated with cancer.

Temperature Regulation

1. Temperature regulation is achieved through precise balancing of heat production, heat conservation, and heat loss. Body temperature is maintained in a range around 37° C (98.6° F).

2. Temperature regulation is mediated by the hypothalamus. Peripheral thermoreceptors in the skin and central thermoreceptors in the hypothalamus, spinal cord, and abdominal organs provide the hypothalamus with information about skin and core temperatures.

3. Heat is produced through chemical reactions of metabolism, skeletal muscle contraction, and chemical thermogenesis.

4. Heat is lost through radiation, conduction, convection, vasodilation, decreased muscle tone, evaporation of sweat, increased respiration, and voluntary mechanisms.

5. Heat conservation is accomplished through vasoconstriction and voluntary mechanisms.

6. Infants and elderly people require special attention to maintenance of body temperature. Because of their greater body surface/mass ratio and decreased subcutaneous fat, infants do not conserve heat well. Elderly persons have poor responses to environmental temperature extremes as a result of slowed blood circulation, structural and functional changes in skin, and overall decrease in heat-producing activities.

7. Fever is triggered by the release of pyrogens from leukocytes, bacteria, and other cells involved in the immune response. Fever is both a symptom of a disease and a normal immunologic mechanism.

8. Fever involves the "resetting of the hypothalamic thermostat" to a higher level. When the fever breaks, the set point returns to normal.

9. Fever production aids responses to infectious processes. Higher temperatures kill many microorganisms and decrease serum levels of iron, zinc, and copper that are needed for bacterial replication.

10. Hyperthermia (marked warming of core temperature) can produce nerve damage, coagulation of cell proteins, and death. Forms of accidental hyperthermia include heat cramps, heat exhaustion, heat stroke, and malignant hyperthermia. Heat stroke and malignant hyperthermia are potentially lethal developments.

11. Hypothermia (marked cooling of core temperature) slows the rate of chemical reaction (tissue metabolism), increases the viscosity of the blood, slows blood flow through the microcirculation, facilitates blood coagulation, and stimulates profound vasoconstriction. Hypothermia may be accidental or therapeutic.

Sleep

1. Sleep may be divided into REM and non-REM stages, each of which has its own series of stages. While asleep, an individual progresses through

Continued

☐ DID YOU UNDERSTAND? —cont'd

Sleep—cont'd

REM and non-REM (slow wave) sleep in a predictable cycle.

2. Sleep is initiated by the withdrawal of neurotransmitters from the afferent formation and by the inhibition of arousal mechanisms in the cerebral cortex. REM sleep is controlled by mechanisms in the pontine reticular formation.

3. The sleep patterns of the newborn and young child vary from those of the adult in total sleep time, cycle length, and percentage of time spent in each sleep cycle. Elderly persons experience a total decrease in sleep time.

4. During sleep the body is actively engaged in restoring and repairing itself. Sleep deprivation can cause profound changes in personality and functioning.

5. The restorative, reparative, and growth processes occur during slow wave sleep.

6. Sleep disorders include (a) disorders of initiating sleep (insomnia), (b) disorders of excessive somnolence (obstructive sleep apnea syndrome, hypersomnia sleep apnea syndrome), (c) disorders of the sleep-wake schedule (jet lag, shift work), and (d) dysfunctions of sleep, sleep stages, or partial arousals (somnambulism, night terrors, enuresis).

7. Ingestion of alcohol and some medications can alter or suppress sleep stages, producing sleep disorders.

The Special Senses

1. The eyelids, conjunctiva, and lacrimal apparatus protect the eye. Infections are the most common disorders; they include blepharitis, conjunctivitis, chalazion, and hordeolum.

2. Conjunctivitis can be acute or chronic, bacterial, viral, or allergic. Redness, edema, pain, and lacrimation are common symptoms. Chlamydial conjunctivitis is the leading cause of blindness in the world and is associated with poor sanitary conditions.

3. Keratitis is a bacterial or viral infection of the cornea that can lead to corneal ulceration. Photophobia, pain, and tearing are common symptoms.

4. The wall of the eye has three layers: sclera, choroid, and retina. The retina contains millions of baroreceptors known as rods and cones that receive light through the lens and then convey signals to the optic nerve and subsequently to the visual cortex of the brain.

5. The eye is filled with vitreous and aqueous humor, which prevent it from collapsing.

6. Structural eye changes caused by aging result in decreased visual acuity.

7. The major alterations in ocular movement include strabismus, nystagmus, and paralysis of the extraocular muscles.

8. Alterations in visual acuity can be caused by amblyopia, scotoma, cataracts, papilledema, macular degeneration, and glaucoma.

9. Alterations in accommodation develop with increased intraocular pressure, inflammation, and disease of the oculomotor nerve. Presbyopia is loss of accommodation caused by loss of elasticity of the lens with aging.

10. Alterations in refraction, including myopia, hyperopia, and astigmatism, are the most common visual disorders.

11. Trauma or disease of the optic nerve pathways, or optic radiations, can cause blindness in the visual fields. Homonymous hemianopsia is caused by damage of one optic tract.

12. The ear is composed of external, middle, and inner structures. The external structures are the pinna, auditory canal, and tympanic membrane. The tympanic cavity (containing three bones: the malleus, the incus, and the stapes), oval window, eustachian tube, and fluid compose the middle ear and transmit sound vibrations to the inner ear.

13. The inner ear includes the bony and membranous labyrinths that transmit sound waves through the cochlea to the division of the eighth cranial nerve. The semicircular canals and vestibule help maintain balance through the equilibrium receptors.

14. Approximately one third of all people older than 65 years have hearing loss.

15. Hearing loss can be classified as conductive, sensorineural, mixed, or functional.

16. Conductive hearing loss occurs when sound waves cannot be conducted through the middle ear.

17. Sensorineural hearing loss develops with impairment of the organ of Corti or its central connections.

18. A combination of conductive and sensorineural loss is a mixed hearing loss.

19. Loss of hearing with no known organic cause is a functional hearing loss.

20. Otitis externa is an infection of the outer ear associated with prolonged exposure to moisture.

21. Otitis media is an infection of the middle ear that is common in children. Accumulation of fluid (effusion) behind the tympanic membrane is a common finding.

22. The perception of flavor is altered if olfaction or taste dysfunctions occur. Sensitivity to odor and taste decreases with aging.

23. Hyposmia is a decrease in the sense of smell, and anosmia is the complete loss of the sense of smell. Inflammation of the nasal mucosa and trauma or tumors of the olfactory nerve lead to diminished sense of smell.

24. Hypogeusia is a decrease in taste sensation, and ageusia is the absence of the sense of taste. Loss of taste buds or trauma to the facial or glossopharyngeal nerves decreases taste sensation.

◼ DID YOU UNDERSTAND? —cont'd

Somatosensory Function

1. Tactile sensation is a function of receptors present in the skin (pacinian corpuscles), and the sensory response is conducted to the brain through the dorsal column and anterior spinothalamic tract.

2. Alterations in touch can result from disruption of skin receptors, sensory transmission, or central nervous system perception.

3. Proprioception is the position and location of the body and its parts. Proprioceptors are located in the inner ear, joints, and ligaments. Proprioceptive stimuli are necessary for balance, coordinated movement, and grading of muscular contraction.

4. Disorders of proprioception can occur at any level of the nervous system with impaired balance and lack of coordinated movement.

KEY TERMS

Acute bacterial conjunctivitis (pinkeye), 340
Acute otitis media (AOM), 342
Acute pain, 326
Ageusia, 344
Allergic conjunctivitis, 340
Amblyopia, 337
Anosmia, 343
Aqueous humor, 336
Astigmatism, 339
Blepharitis, 340
Chalazion, 340
Chronic conjunctivitis, 340
Chronic pain, 326
Circadian rhythm, 330
Cochlea, 340
Cognitive/evaluative system, 326
Color blindness, 339
Conductive hearing loss, 342
Cone, 336
Conjunctivitis, 340
Cornea, 336
Crista ampullaris, 340
Dark adaptation, 337
Diplopia, 337
Dynorphin, 329
Enkephalin, 329
Enuresis, 336
Equilibrium receptor, 340
Eustachian (pharyngeotympanic) tube, 340
Exogenous pyrogen, 332
External auditory canal, 340
Fovea centralis, 336
Functional hearing loss, 342
Gate control theory, 328
Hair cell, 340
Heat cramp, 333
Heat exhaustion, 333
Heat stroke, 333

Hordeolum (stye), 340
Hyperopia, 338
Hypersomnia sleep apnea (HSA) syndrome, 335
Hyperthermia, 333
Hypogeusia, 344
Hyposmia, 343
Hypothermia, 334
Incus (anvil), 340
Insomnia, 335
Iris, 336
Jerk nystagmus, 337
Keratitis, 340
Lens, 336
β-Lipotrophin, 329
Macula, 340
Malignant hyperthermia, 333
Malleus (hammer), 340
Mastoid air cell, 340
Mastoid process, 340
Meissner corpuscle, 328
Ménière disease, 342
Mixed hearing loss, 342
Motivational/affective system, 326
Myopia, 338
Night terrors, 335
Nociceptor, 326
Non-REM (slow wave) sleep, 334
Nystagmus, 337
Obstructive sleep apnea syndrome, 335
Olfactory hallucination, 343
Opiate receptor, 329
Optic chiasm, 340
Optic disc, 336
Organ of Corti, 340
Otitis externa, 342
Otitis media, 342
Otitis media with effusion (OME), 342
Otolith, 340
Oval window, 340

Pacinian corpuscle, 328
Pain threshold, 326
Pain tolerance, 326
Parageusia, 344
Parosmia, 344
Pendular nystagmus, 337
Perceptual dominance, 326
Periaqueductal gray (PAG), 328
Perilymph, 340
Pinna, 340
Presbycusis, 342
Presbyopia, 338
Psychogenic pain, 326
Pupil, 336
Referred pain, 330
REM (rapid eye movement) sleep, 335
Retina, 336
Rod, 336
Sclera, 336
Semicircular canal, 340
Sensorineural hearing loss, 342
Sensory/discriminative system, 326
Somatic pain, 330
Somatogenic pain, 326
Somnambulism, 335
Stapes (stirrup), 340
Strabismus, 337
Tinnitus, 342
Trachoma, 340
Tympanic cavity, 340
Tympanic membrane, 340
Vertigo, 344
Vestibular nuclei, 337
Vestibular nystagmus, 344
Vestibule, 340
Viral conjunctivitis, 340
Visceral pain, 330
Vitreous humor, 336

REFERENCES

1. McCaffery, M. (September 1980). Understanding your patient's pain. *Nursing 80,* 26-31.
2. Sanders, S.H. (1979). Behavioral assessment and treatment of clinical pain: Appraisal of current status. *Progress in Behavior Modification, 8,* 249-285.
3. Wall, P.D. & Melzack, R. (1994). *Textbook of pain.* Edinburgh: Churchill Livingstone.
4. Buchholz, M. et al. (1998). Pain scores in infants: A modified infant pain scale versus visual analogue. *Journal of Pain Symptom Management, 15*(2), 117-124.
5. Hain, R.D. (1997). Pain scales in children: A review. *Palliative Medicine, 11*(5), 341-340.
6. Fishbain, D.A. et al. (1997). Chronic pain-associated depression: Antecedent or consequence of chronic pain? A review. *Clinical Journal of Pain, 13*(2), 116-137.
7. Gagliese, L. & Melzack, R. (1997). Chronic pain in elderly people. *Pain, 70*(1), 3-14.
8. Zeltzer, L., Bursch, B., & Walco, G. (1997). Pain responsiveness and chronic pain: A psychobiological perspective. *Journal of Development and Behavioral Pediatrics, 18*(6), 413-422.
9. Melzack, R. (1993). Pain: Past, present, and future. *Canadian Journal of Experimental Psychology, 47*(4), 615-629.
10. Aimone, L.D. (1992). Neurochemistry and modulation of pain. In R.S. Sinatra et al. (Eds.). *Acute pain: Mechanisms and management.* St. Louis: Mosby.
11. Henry, J.L. (1986). Role of circulating opioids in the modulation of pain. *Annals of the New York Academy of Sciences, 467,* 169-181.
12. Willis, W.D. & Westlund, K.N. (1997). Neuroanatomy of the pain system and of the pathways that modulate pain. *Journal of Clinical Neurophysiology, 14*(1), 2-31.
13. Sheps, D.S. et al. (1987). Endorphins are related to pain perception in coronary artery disease. *American Journal of Cardiology, 59,* 523-527.
14. Seeley, R.R., Stephens, T.D., & Tate, P. (1992). *Anatomy and physiology* (2nd ed.). St. Louis: Mosby.
15. Russo, C.M. & Brose, W.C. (1998). Chronic pain. *Annual Review of Medicine, 49,* 123-133.
16. Kanner, R. (1997). *Pain management secrets.* Philadelphia: Hanley & Belfus.
17. Rothwell, N.S. (1994). CNS regulation of thermogenesis. *Critical Reviews in Neurobiology, 8*(1-2), 1.
18. Hammarlund, K., Stromberg, B., & Sedin, G. (1986). Heat loss from the skin of preterm and full-term newborn infants during the first weeks after birth. *Biology of the Neonate, 50*(1), 1-10.
19. Florez-Duquet, M. & McDonald, R.B. (1998). Cold-induced thermoregulation and biological aging. *Physiology Review, 78*(2), 339-358.
20. Dinarello, C.A. & Bunn, P.P., Jr. (1997). Fever. *Seminars in Oncology, 24*(3), 288-298.
21. Mackowiak, P.A. (1998). Concepts of fever. *Archives of Internal Medicine, 158*(17), 1870-1882.
22. Hanson, D.F. (1997). Fever, temperature, and the immune response. *Annals of the New York Academy of Science, 15*(813), 453-464.
23. Rowsey, P.J. (1997). Pathophysiology of fever. II. Relooking at cooling interventions. *Dimensions of Critical Care Nursing, 16*(5), 251-256.
24. Saper, C.B. & Breder, C.D. (1994). The neurologic basis of fever. *New England Journal of Medicine, 330*(26), 1880-1886.
25. Bruce, J.L. & Grove, S.K. (1992). Fever: Pathology and treatment. *Critical Care Nurse, 12*(1), 40-49.
26. Kenney, W.L. (1997). Thermoregulation at rest and during exercise in healthy older adults. *Exercise & Sports Science Review, 25,* 41-76.
27. Ginsberg, M.D. & Busto, R. (1998). Combating hyperthermia in acute stroke: A significant clinical concern. *Stroke, 29*(2), 529-534.
28. Anders, T.F. & Keener, M. (1985). Developmental course of nighttime sleep-wake patterns in full-term and premature infants during the first year of life. *Sleep, 8*(3), 173-192.
29. Fernsilver, S.H. & Hertz, G. (1994). Sleep in the elderly patient. *Clinics in Chest Medicine, 14*(3), 405-411.
30. Brzezinski, A. (1997). Melatonin in humans. *New England Journal of Medicine, 336*(3), 186-195.
31. Steiger, A. & Holsboer, F. (1997). Neuropeptides and human sleep. *Sleep, 20*(11), 1038-1052.
32. Wiegand, L. & Zwillich, C.W. (1994). Obstructive sleep apnea. *Disease-a-Month, 40*(4), 197-252.
33. Khalil, M.M. & Rifaie, O.A. (1998). Electrocardiographic changes in obstructive sleep apnea syndrome. *Respiratory Medicine, 92*(1), 25-27.
34. El-Ad, B. & Korczyn, A.D. (1998). Disorders of excessive daytime sleepiness—An update. *Journal of Neurological Science, 153*(2), 192-202.
35. Wan, J. & Greenfield, S. (1997). Enuresis and common voiding abnormalities. *Pediatric Clinics of North America, 44*(5), 1117-1131.
36. Gimpel, G.A. et al. (1998). Clinical perspectives in primary nocturnal enuresis. *Clinical Pediatrics (Philadelphi), 37*(1), 23-29.
37. Thibodeau, G.A. & Patton, K.T. (1999). *Anatomy & Physiology* (4th ed.). St. Louis: Mosby.
38. Nolte, J. (1999). *The Human Brain* (4th ed.). St. Louis: Mosby.
39. Apple, D.J. & Robb, M.F. (1998). *Ocular pathology: Clinical application and self-assessment* (5th ed.). St. Louis: Mosby.
40. Palay, D.A. & Krachmer, J.H. (1997). *Ophthalmology for the primary care physician.* St. Louis: Mosby.
41. Gordon, B. (1998). Colour blindness. *Public Health, 112*(2), 81-84.

REFERENCES

42. Morrow, G.L. & Abbott, R.L. (1998). Conjunctivitis. *American Family Physician, 57*(4), 735-746.

43. Wald, E.R. (1997). Conjunctivitis in infants and children. *Pediatric Infectious Diseases Journal, 16*(2, Suppl), S17-S20.

44. Schlossberg, D. (1996). *Current therapy of infectious disease.* St. Louis: Mosby.

45. Eowell, S.F. et al. (1998). Otitis media—Principles of judicious use of antimicrobial agents. *Pediatrics, 101,* 165-167.

46. Jones, N. & Rog, D. (1998). Olfaction: A review. *Journal of Laryngology and Otology, 112*(91), 11-24.

47. Nelson, G.M. (1998). Biology of taste buds and the clinical problem of taste loss. *Anatomical Record, 253*(3), 70-78.

48. Bolanowski, S.J. et al. (1988). Four channels mediate the mechanical aspects of touch. *Journal of Acoustical Society of America, 85*(5), 1680-1694.

49. Stevens, J.C. (1992). Age and spatial acuity of touch. *Journal of Gerontology, 47*(1), 35-40.

50. Hay, L. et al. (1996). Availability of visual and proprioceptive afferent messages and postural control in elderly adults. *Experimental Brain Research, 108*(1), 129-139.

CHAPTER

14

Concepts of Neurologic Dysfunction

Barbara J. Boss

A *person achieves functional adequacy (competence) through complex integrated processes. Three major neural networks account for this functional adequacy: cognitive networks, sensory networks, and motor networks. Alterations in any or all of these affect functional adequacy. Alterations in cognitive and motor networks are discussed in this chapter.*

The neural networks that are basic (core) to cognitive function are (1) attentional networks that provide arousal and maintenance of attention over time, (2) memory and language networks by which information is communicated, and (3) affective or emotive systems that mediate feeling tone. These core networks are fundamental to the processes of abstract thinking and reasoning. The products of abstraction and reasoning are organized and made operational through the executive attentional network. The normal functioning of these networks manifests through the motor network in a behavioral array viewed by others as appropriate to human activity and successful living.

Check out your CD Companion for chapter-related exercises and answers to the Quick Check questions

ALTERATIONS IN COGNITIVE NETWORKS

Full consciousness is a state of awareness of oneself and the environment and a set of responses to that environment. The fully conscious individual responds to external stimuli with a wide array of responses. Any decrease in this state of awareness and varied responses is a decrease in consciousness.

Consciousness involves arousal and content of thought. *Arousal* is the state of awakeness of an individual. It is mediated by the reticular activating system. When cerebral function is lost, the reticular activating system and brain stem can maintain a crude waking state known as a **vegetative state.** Cognitive cerebral functions, however, cannot occur without a functioning reticular activating system. **Content of thought** encompasses all cognitive functions, including awareness of self, environment, and affective states (i.e., moods). Content of thought is mediated by all of the core networks under the guidance of executive attention networks.

Alterations in Arousal

An altered level of arousal (awareness) with acute onset may be caused by various factors (i.e., **structural arousal alteration, metabolic arousal alteration, psychogenic arousal alteration**). Structural causes are divided according to whether the original location of the pathologic condition is above or below the tentorial plate. Pathologic processes include infectious, vascular, neoplastic, traumatic, congenital (developmental), degenerative, polygenic, and metabolic causes. Metabolic causes are further divided into hypoxia, electrolyte disturbances, hypoglycemia, drugs, and toxins (both endogenous and exogenous). All the systemic diseases that eventually produce nervous system dysfunction are part of this metabolic category. Alterations in arousal range from slight drowsiness to coma.

⬛ *Pathophysiology*

Processes above the tentorial plate (supratentorial) produce changes in arousal by either diffuse or localized dysfunction. Disease processes may produce diffuse dysfunction (e.g., encephalitis) and may affect the cerebral cortex or the underlying subcortical white matter. Localized dysfunction generally is caused by masses that directly impinge on deep diencephalic structures or that secondarily compress these structures in the process of herniation. Such localized destructive processes directly impair function of the thalamic or hypothalamic activating systems.

Disorders outside the brain but within the cranial vault can produce diffuse dysfunction. Examples include neoplasms, closed-head trauma with subsequent subdural bleeding, and accumulation of pus in the subdural space. Disorders within the brain substance—bleeding, infarcts and emboli, tumors—function primarily as masses.

Arousal is reduced by direct destruction of the reticular activating system and its pathways or the entire brain stem either by direct invasion or by indirect impairment of its blood supply. In addition, decreased awareness may result from compression of the reticular activating system by a disease process. This compression may result from direct pressure or compression as structures either expand or herniate. Causes include accumulations of blood or pus, neoplasms, and demyelinating disorders.

Psychogenic unresponsiveness, although uncommon, may signal general psychiatric disorders. Despite apparent unconsciousness, the person actually is physiologically awake.

⬛ *Clinical Manifestations and Evaluation*

The cause of an altered level of arousal may be organic or functional. Further distinction is then made between metabolic and structural factors (Table 14-1).

Patterns of clinical manifestations help in determining the extent of brain dysfunction and serve as indexes for identifying increasing or decreasing central nervous system (CNS) function. The types of manifestations suggest the cause of the altered arousal state (Table 14-2). Five categories of neurologic function are critical to the evaluation process: (1) level of consciousness, (2) pattern of breathing, (3) size and reactivity of pupils, (4) eye position and reflexive responses, and (5) skeletal muscle motor responses.

Level of consciousness

Level of consciousness is the most critical clinical index of nervous system function, with alterations indicating either improvement or deterioration of the individual's condition. A person who is alert and oriented to self, others, place, and time is considered to be functioning at the highest level of consciousness, which implies full use of all the person's cognitive capacities. From this normal alert state, levels of consciousness diminish in stages, each of which is clinically defined (Table 14-3).

Pattern of breathing

Characteristic respiratory patterns help evaluate the level of brain dysfunction and coma (Fig. 14-1). Rate, rhythm, and pattern should be evaluated. Breathing patterns can be categorized as hemispheric or brain stem patterns (Table 14-4).

With normal breathing, a neural center in the forebrain (cerebrum) produces a rhythmic pattern. When consciousness decreases, lower brain stem centers regulate the breathing pattern, responding only to changes in $PaCO_2$ levels. The result is the irregular breathing associated with posthyperventilation apnea (PHVA).

Cheyne-Stokes respirations result from an increased ventilatory response to carbon dioxide stimulation, causing hypercapnia and diminished ventilatory stimulus. Changes in $PaCO_2$ produce irregular breathing, contributing to overbreathing with carbon dioxide stimulation. The $PaCO_2$ level then decreases to below normal, and breathing stops until the carbon dioxide reaccumulates to bring the $PaCO_2$ level to normal. With opiate or sedative drug overdose, the respiratory center is depressed so the rate of breathing gradually decreases until respiratory failure occurs.

TABLE 14-1	Clinical Manifestations of Metabolic and Structural Causes of Comas	
Manifestations	**Metabolically Induced Coma**	**Structurally Induced Coma**
Blink to threat (cranial nerves II, VII)	Equal	Asymmetric
Discs (cranial nerve II)	Flat, good pulsation	Papilledema
Extraocular movement (cranial nerves III, IV, VI)	Roving eye movements; normal doll's eyes and calorics	Gaze paresis, nerve III palsy
Pupils (cranial nerves II, III)	Equal and reactive, may be large (e.g., atropine), pinpoint (e.g., opiates), or midposition and fixed (e.g., glutethimide [Doriden])	Asymmetric and/or nonreactive; may be midposition (midbrain injury), pinpoint (pons injury), large (tectal injury)
Corneal reflex (cranial nerves V, VII)	Symmetric response	Asymmetric response
Grimace to pain (cranial nerve VII)	Symmetric response	Asymmetric response
Motor function movement	Symmetric	Asymmetric
Tone	Symmetric	Paratonic, spastic, flaccid, especially if asymmetric
Posture	Symmetric	Decorticate, especially if symmetric; decerebrate, especially if asymmetric
Deep tendon reflexes	Symmetric	Asymmetric
Babinski sign	Absent or symmetric response	Present
Sensation	Symmetric	Asymmetric

Modified from Heilman, D.M., Watson, R.T., & Greer, M. (1977). Handbook for differential diagnosis of neurologic signs and symptoms. *New York: Appleton-Century-Crofts.*

TABLE 14-2	Differential Characteristics of States Causing Coma
Mechanism	**Manifestations**
Supratentorial mass lesions compressing or displacing the diencephalon or brain stem	Initiating signs usually of focal cerebral dysfunction
	Signs of dysfunction progress rostral to caudal
	Neurologic signs at any given time point to one anatomic area (e.g., diencephalon, mesencephalon, medulla)
	Motor signs often asymmetric
Infratentorial mass of destruction causing coma	History of preceding brain stem dysfunction or sudden onset of coma
	Localizing brain stem signs precede or accompany onset of coma and always include oculovestibular abnormality
	Cranial nerve palsies usually manifest "bizarre" respiratory patterns that appear at onset
Metabolic coma	Confusion and stupor commonly precede motor signs
	Motor signs usually are symmetric
	Pupillary reactions usually are preserved
	Asterixis, myoclonus, tremor, and seizures are common
	Acid-base imbalance with hyperventilation or hypoventilation is common
Psychiatric unresponsiveness	Lids close actively
	Pupils reactive or dilated (cycloplegics)
	Oculocephalic reflexes are unpredictable; oculovestibular reflexes are physiologic (nystagmus is present)
	Motor tone is inconsistent or normal
	Eupnea or hyperventilation is usual
	No pathologic reflexes are present
	Electroencephalogram (EEG) is normal

Modified from Plum, F. & Posner, J.B. (1980). The diagnosis of stupor and coma. *Philadelphia: F.A. Davis.*

TABLE 14-3	Levels of Altered Consciousness
State	**Definition**
Confusion	Loss of ability to think rapidly and clearly; impaired judgment and decision making
Disorientation	Beginning loss of consciousness; disorientation to time followed by disorientation to place and impaired memory; lost last is recognition of self
Lethargy	Limited spontaneous movement or speech; easy arousal with normal speech or touch; may or may not be oriented to time, place, or person
Obtundation	Mild to moderate reduction in arousal (awakeness) with limited response to the environment; falls asleep unless stimulated verbally or tactilely; answers questions with minimum response
Stupor	A condition of deep sleep or unresponsiveness from which the person may be aroused or caused to open eyes only by vigorous and repeated stimulation; response is often withdrawal or grabbing at stimulus
Coma	No verbal response to the external environment or to any stimuli, noxious stimuli such as deep pain or suctioning do not yield motor movement
Light coma	Associated with purposeful movement on stimulation
Coma	Associated with nonpurposeful movement only on stimulation
Deep coma	Associated with unresponsiveness or no response to any stimulus

TABLE 14-4	Patterns of Breathing	
Breathing Pattern	**Description**	**Location of Injury**
Hemispheric breathing patterns		
Normal	After a period of hyperventilation that lowers the arterial carbon dioxide pressure ($Paco_2$), the individual continues to breathe regularly but with a reduced depth.	Response of the nervous system to an external stressor—not associated with injury to the CNS
Posthyperventilation apnea	Respirations stop after hyperventilation has lowered the Pco_2 level below normal. Rhythmic breathing returns when the Pco_2 level returns to normal.	Associated with diffuse bilateral metabolic or structural disease of the cerebrum
Cheyne-Stokes respirations	The breathing pattern has a smooth increase (crescendo) in the rate and depth of breathing (hyperpnea), which peaks and is followed by a gradual smooth decrease (decrescendo) in the rate and depth of breathing to the point of apnea, when the cycle repeats itself. The hyperpneic phase lasts longer than the apneic phase.	Bilateral dysfunction of the deep cerebral and/or diencephalic structures, seen with supratentorial injury and metabolically induced coma states
Brain stem breathing patterns		
Central neurogenic hyperventilation	A sustained deep, rapid, but regular pattern (hyperpnea) occurs, with a decreased $Paco_2$ and a corresponding increase in pH and Po_2.	May result from CNS damage or disease that involves the midbrain and upper pons; seen after increased intracranial pressure and blunt head trauma
Apneusis	A prolonged inspiratory cramp (a pause at full inspiration) occurs. A common variant of this is a brief end-inspiratory pause of 2 or 3 sec often alternating with an end-expiratory pause.	Indicates damage to the respiratory control mechanism located at the pontine level; most commonly associated with pontine infarction but documented with hypoglycemia, anoxia, and meningitis
Cluster breathing	A cluster of breaths has a disordered sequence with irregular pauses between breaths.	Dysfunction in the lower pontine and high medullary areas
Ataxic breathing	Completely irregular breathing occurs, with random shallow and deep breaths and irregular pauses. Often the rate is slow.	Originates from a primary dysfunction of the medullary neurons controlling breathing
Gasping breathing pattern (agonal gasps)	A pattern of deep "all-or-none" breaths is accompanied by a slow respiratory rate.	Indicative of a failing medullary respiratory center

Fig. 14-1 *Abnormal respiratory patterns with corresponding level of central nervous system activity.* (From Thelan, L.A., Davie, J.K., Urden, L.D., & Lough, M.E. [1998]. Critical care nursing: Diagnosis and management [3rd ed.]. St. Louis: Mosby.)

Fig. 14-2 *Pupils at different levels of consciousness.*

Vomiting

Yawning, vomiting, and hiccups are complex reflexlike motor responses that are integrated by neural mechanisms in the lower brain stem. These responses may be produced by compression or diseases involving tissues of the medulla oblongata (e.g., infection, neoplasm, infarct) but also occur relative to other more benign stimuli to the vagal nerve.

Most CNS disorders produce nausea and vomiting. Vomiting without nausea indicates direct involvement of the central neural mechanism (or pyloric obstruction; see Chapter 34). Vomiting frequently accompanies CNS injuries that (1) involve the vestibular nuclei or its immediate projections, particularly when double vision (diplopia) also is present; (2) impinge directly on the floor of the fourth ventricle; or (3) produce brain stem compression secondary to increased intracranial pressure.

Pupillary changes

Anatomically, brain stem areas that control arousal are adjacent to areas that control the pupils. Pupillary changes thus indicate the presence and level of brain stem dysfunction (Fig. 14-2). For example, severe ischemia and hypoxia usually produce dilated, fixed pupils. Hypothermia also may cause fixed pupils.

Some drugs affect pupils and must be considered in evaluating individuals in comatose states. Large concentrations of atropine and scopolamine fully dilate and fix pupils. Glutethimide doses sufficient to produce a coma cause the pupils to become midposition or moderately dilated, unequal, and frequently fixed to light. Opiates cause pinpoint pupils. Severe barbiturate intoxication may produce fixed pupils.

Oculomotor responses

Resting, spontaneous, and reflexive eye movements change at various levels of brain dysfunction. Persons with metabolically induced coma, except with barbiturate-hypnotic and phenytoin poisoning, generally retain ocular reflexes even when other signs of brain stem damage are present. If brisk oculocephalic reflexes and roving eye movements are present without nystagmus when cold or warm water is instilled into the external ear canal, decreased consciousness but an intact brain stem may be seen (Figs. 14-3 and 14-4). Destructive or compressive injury to the brain stem causes specific abnormalities of the oculocephalic and oculovestibular reflexes. Those that involve an oculomotor nucleus or nerve cause the involved eye to deviate outward, producing a resting dysconjugate lateral position of the eye.

Motor responses

Motor responses help evaluate the level of brain dysfunction and determine the most severely damaged side of the brain. The pattern of response noted may be (1) purposeful; (2) inappropriate, generalized motor movement; or (3) not present. Motor signs indicating loss of cortical inhibition that are commonly associated with decreased consciousness include reflex grasping, reflex sucking, snout reflex, palmomental re-

flex, and rigidity (paratonia) (Fig. 14-5). Abnormal flexor and extensor responses in the upper and lower extremities are defined in Table 14-5 and illustrated in Fig. 14-6.

✓**QUICK CHECK**

Why are structural as well as metabolic factors capable of producing coma?

Why is level of consciousness the most critical index of central nervous system function?

Why do Cheyne-Stokes respirations appear in coma?

Why are oculomotor changes associated with levels of coma?

Outcomes

Two forms of neurologic death—cerebral death and brain death—result from severe pathologic conditions and are associated with coma. Irreversible coma, or ***cerebral death,*** is death of the cerebral hemispheres exclusive of the brain stem and cerebellum. Brain damage is permanent, and the individual is forever unable to respond behaviorally in any significant way to the environment. The brain may continue to maintain internal homeostasis.

Brain death occurs when the brain is damaged so completely that it can never recover and cannot maintain the body's internal homeostasis. State laws define brain death as irreversible cessation of function of the entire brain.[1] Destruction includes the brain stem and cerebellum. On postmortem examination the brain is autolyzing (self-digesting) or already autolyzed.

Brain death has occurred when there is no evidence of function in the cerebral hemispheres or brain stem for an extended period. The abnormality of brain function must result from structural or known metabolic disease and *not* be caused by a depressant drug, alcohol poisoning, or hypothermia. An isoelectric, or flat, electroencephalogram (EEG) (electrocerebral silence) for 6 to 12 hours in a person who is not hypothermic and has not ingested depressant drugs indicates brain death.[1] The clinical criteria used to determine brain death are noted in Box 14-1.

Vegetative states

The vegetative state is a clinical condition of complete unawareness of the self or surrounding environment. Sleep-wake cycles are present, but cerebral function is lost. The person's eyes open spontaneously, and blood pressure and breathing are maintained without support. Brain stem reflexes (pupillary, oculocephalic, chewing, swallowing) are intact. There is bowel and bladder incontinence. The individual does not speak any comprehensible words or follow commands. Recovery is unlikely if the state persists for 12 months.[2]

A ***locked-in syndrome*** differs in that both the content of thought and level of arousal are intact but the efferent path-

G.J.Wassilchenko

Fig. 14-3 *Test for oculocephalic reflex response (doll's eyes phenomenon).* **A,** Normal response—eyes turn together to side opposite from turn of head. **B,** Abnormal response—eyes do not turn in conjugate manner. **C,** Absent response—eyes do not turn as head position changes. *(From Rudy, E.B. [1984]. Advanced neurological and neurosurgical nursing. St. Louis: Mosby.)*

ways are disrupted. Thus the individual cannot communicate through speech or body movement but is fully conscious, with intact cognitive function. The person retains vertical eye movement and blinking as a means of communication.

Seizures

A *seizure* results from a sudden, explosive, disorderly discharge of cerebral neurons and is characterized by a sudden, transient alteration in brain function, usually involving motor, sensory, autonomic, or psychic clinical manifestations and altered level of arousal. Seizure disorders represent a syndrome, however, and not a specific disease entity. The alteration in level of arousal is temporary.

Convulsion, a term sometimes applied to seizures, refers to the jerky, contract-relax (tonic-clonic) movement associated with some seizures. *Epilepsy* is a condition of recurrent seizures that are unprovoked by any immediate identified cause.[3]

Fig. 14-4 *Test for oculovestibular reflex (caloric ice water test).* **A,** Normal response—conjugate eye movements. **B,** Abnormal response—dysconjugate or asymmetric eye movements. **C,** Absent response—no eye movements.

Fig. 14-5 *Pathologic reflexes.* **A,** Grasp reflex. **B,** Snout reflex. **C,** Palmomental reflex. **D,** Suck reflex.

TABLE 14-5 Abnormal Motor Responses With Decreased Responsiveness

Motor Response	Description	Location of Injury
Abnormal motor responses, upper extremity flexion with or without extensor responses in the leg (decorticate rigidity)	Slowly developing flexion of the arm, wrist, and fingers with adduction in the upper extremity and extension, internal rotation, and plantar flexion of the lower extremity	Suggest hemispheric damage above midbrain
Extensor responses in the upper and lower extremities (decerebrate posturing, decerebrate rigidity)	Opisthotonos (hyperextension of the vertebral column) with clenching of the teeth; extension, abduction, and hyperpronation of the arms; and extension of the lower extremities	Associated with severe damage involving caudal diencephalon or midbrain
	In acute brain injury, shivering and hyperpnea may accompany unelicited recurrent decerebrate spasms	Acute injury frequently causes limb extension regardless of location
Extensor responses in the upper extremities accompanied by flexion in the lower extremities		Indicates pontine level dysfunction
Flaccid state with little or no motor response to stimuli		Damage to lower pons and upper myelencephalon

Fig. 14-6 *Decorticate and decerebrate responses.* **A,** Decorticate response. Flexion of arms, wrists, and fingers with adduction in upper extremities. Extension, internal rotation, and plantar flexion in lower extremities. **B,** Decerebrate response. All four extremities in rigid extension, with hyperpronation of forearms and plantar extension of feet. **C,** Decorticate response on right side of body and decerebrate response on left side of body. *(From Rudy, E.B. [1984]. Advanced neurological and neurosurgical nursing. St. Louis: Mosby.)*

Criteria for Brain Death
BOX 14-1

1. Completion of all appropriate and therapeutic procedures
2. Unresponsive coma (no motor or reflex movements)
3. No spontaneous respiration
4. No ocular responses to head turning or caloric stimulation; dilated, fixed pupils
5. Isoelectric (flat) EEG (electrocerebral silence)
6. Persistence of these signs for 30 minutes to 1 hour and for 6 hours after onset of coma and apnea
7. Confirming test indicating absence of cerebral circulation (optional)

Modified from Plum, F. & Posner, J.B. (1980). The diagnosis of stupor and coma. Philadelphia: F.A. Davis; Walker, A.E. (1985). Cerebral death (3rd ed.). Baltimore: Urban & Schwarzenberg.

Conditions associated with seizure disorders

Any disorder that alters the neuronal environment may cause seizure activity, so, theoretically, anyone may experience a seizure. The seizure threshold of some persons, however, apparently is genetically lower.

A seizure disorder can be produced by diseases or other processes that involve the nervous system. The onset may indicate the presence of an ongoing primary neurologic disease. Etiologic factors in seizures generally include (1) cerebral lesions, (2) biochemical disorders, (3) cerebral trauma, and (4) epilepsy, which can result from the following conditions:

Metabolic defects	Infection
Congenital malformation	Brain tumor
Genetic predisposition	Vascular disease
Perinatal injury	Fever
Postnatal trauma	Drug or alcohol abuse
Myoclonic syndromes	

Causes of recurrent seizures are age related (Table 14-6). Seizures may be precipitated by hypoglycemia, fatigue or lack of sleep, emotional or physical stress, febrile illness, large amounts of water ingestion, constipation, use of stimulant drugs, withdrawal from depressant drugs (including alcohol), hyperventilation (respiratory alkalosis), and some environmental stimuli, such as blinking lights, a poorly adjusted television screen, loud noises, certain music, certain odors, or merely being startled. Women may have increased seizure activity immediately before or during menses.

Types of seizure disorders

Seizures are classified in different ways—by clinical manifestations, site of origin, EEG correlates, or response to therapy. A simplified version of the international classification of epileptic seizures is presented in Table 14-7. Terms used to describe seizure activity are defined in Table 14-8.

Pathophysiology

A group of neurons may exhibit a proxysmal depolarization shift and function as an *epileptogenic focus.* These neurons are hypersensitive and are more easily activated by hyperthermia, hypoxia, hypoglycemia, hyponatremia, repeated sensory stimulation, and certain sleep phases.

Epileptogenic neurons fire more and more often and with greater amplitude. When the intensity reaches a threshold point, cortical excitation spreads. Excitation of the subcortical, thalamic, and brain stem areas corresponds to the *tonic phase* (muscle contraction with increased muscle tone) and is associated with loss of consciousness.

The *clonic phase* (alternating contraction and relaxation of muscles) begins when inhibitory neurons in the cortex, anterior thalamus, and basal ganglia react to the cortical excitation. The seizure discharge is interrupted, producing intermittent muscle contractions that gradually decrease and finally cease. The epileptogenic neurons are exhausted.

During seizure activity, oxygen is consumed at a high rate—about 60% over normal. Although cerebral blood flow also increases, O_2 is rapidly depleted, along with glucose, and lactate accumulates in brain tissue. Continued, severe seizure activity holds the potential for progressive brain injury and irreversible damage. In addition, if a seizure focus is active for a prolonged period, a *mirror focus* may develop in normal tissue.

Clinical Manifestations

The clinical manifestations associated with seizure depend on its type (see Table 14-7). Two types of symptoms signal a generalized tonic-clonic seizure: an *aura,* a partial seizure that immediately precedes the onset of a generalized tonic-clonic seizure; and a *prodroma,* an early manifestation occurring hours to days before a seizure. Both may become familiar to the person experiencing recurrent generalized seizures and may enable the person to prevent injuries during the seizure.

HEALTH ALERT

Recurrent Seizures

The 5-year risk for a second seizure after a single unprovoked seizure in adults has been found to be 33%, and the majority of these second seizures occurred within 12 months after the initial seizure. Those persons with recurrence are likely to have additional seizures.

Data from Hauser, W.A., Rich, S.S., Lee, J.R., Annegers, J.F., & Anderson, V.E. (1998). Risk of recurrent seizures after two unprovoked seizures. New England Journal of Medicine, 338, 429-434.

Evaluation and Treatment

The health history, physical examination, and laboratory tests of blood and urine (blood glucose, serum calcium, blood urea nitrogen, urine sodium, creatinine clearance) can identify systemic diseases known to promote seizures. Radiographic studies and cerebrospinal fluid (CSF) examination help identify neurologic diseases associated with seizures. The EEG is used to assess the type of seizure and determine its focus.

Treatment involves correcting or controlling the cause and, if none is identified, administering antiseizure medications to suppress seizure activity. Counseling also may be of value.

✓ QUICK CHECK

Why is irreversible coma different from brain death?

Why is a seizure different from epilepsy?

Why can so many conditions precipitate seizures?

Why is continued seizing dangerous? How does an epileptogenic focus differ from a mirror focus?

TABLE 14-6	Causes of Recurrent Seizures in Different Age-Groups
Age of Onset	**Probable Cause**
Neonatal	Congenital maldevelopment, birth injury, metabolic disorders (hypocalcemia, hypoglycemia), vitamin B deficiency, phenylketonuria
Infancy (1-6 mo)	As above, infantile spasms
Early childhood (6 mo to 3 yr)	Infantile spasms, febrile convulsions, birth injury and anoxia, infections, trauma
Childhood (3-10 yr)	Perinatal anoxia, injury at birth or later, infections, thrombosis of cerebral arteries or veins, indeterminant cause (idiopathic epilepsy)
Adolescence (10-18 yr)	Idiopathic epilepsy, including genetically transmitted types, trauma
Early adulthood (18-35 yr)	Trauma, neoplasm, idiopathic epilepsy, withdrawal from alcohol or other sedative-hypnotic drugs
	Neoplasm, trauma, vascular disease, alcohol or other drug withdrawal
Middle age (35-60 yr)	Vascular disease, tumor, degenerative disease, trauma

From Adams, R.D. (1985). The convulsive state and idiopathic epilepsy. In G.W. Thorn et al. (Eds.). Harrison's principles of internal medicine. New York: McGraw-Hill.

TABLE 14-7	International Classification of Epileptic Seizures
Traditional Terminology	**New Nomenclature**
Focal motor; jacksonian seizures (occasionally become secondarily generalized)	**I. Partial seizures** (seizures beginning locally) 　A. Simple (without impairment of consciousness) 　　1. With motor signs 　　2. With special sensory or somatosensory symptoms 　　3. With autonomic symptoms or signs 　　4. With psychic symptoms
Temporal lobe or psychomotor seizures	B. Complex (with impairment of consciousness) 　　1. Simple partial onset followed by impaired consciousness—with or without automatisms 　　2. Impaired consciousness at onset—with or without automatisms 　C. Secondarily generalized (partial onset evolving to generalized tonic-clonic seizures)
	II. Generalized seizures (bilaterally symmetric and without local onset)
Petit mal	A. Absences
Minor motor	B. Myoclonic seizure
Limited grand mal	C. Clonic seizure
	D. Tonic seizure
Grand mal	E. Tonic-clonic seizure
Drop attacks	F. Atonic seizure
	G. Infantile spasms
	III. Unclassified seizures (because of incomplete data)
	IV. Status epilepticus (prolonged partial or generalized recovery between attacks)

TABLE 14-8	Terminology Applied to a Seizure Disorder
Term	**Definition**
Aura	A partial seizure experienced as a peculiar sensation preceding the onset of generalized seizure that may take the form of gustatory, visual, or auditory experience or a feeling of dizziness, numbness, or just "a funny feeling"
Prodroma	Early clinical manifestations, such as malaise, headache, or a sense of depression, that may occur hours to a few days before the onset of a seizure
Tonic phase	A state of muscle contraction in which there is excessive muscle tone
Clonic phase	A state of alternating contraction and relaxation of muscles
Postictal state	The time period immediately following the cessation of seizure activity

TABLE 14-9	Clinical Manifestations of Cognitive Network Deficits	
Deficit	**Clinical Signs**	**Symptoms**
Attention		
Selective attention (orienting)	Inability to focus attention; decreased eye, head, and body movements associated with focusing on the stimuli; decreased search and scanning; faulty orientation to stimuli, causing safety problems	Person reports inability to focus attention, failure to perceive objects and other stimuli (history of injuries, falls, safety problems)
Memory		
Recent (anterograde memory)	*Left hemisphere:* disorientation to time, situation, place, name, person (verbal identification); impaired language memory (e.g., names of objects); impaired semantic memory *Right hemisphere:* disorientation to self, person (visual), place (visual); impaired episodic memory (personal history); impaired emotional memory Either or both hemispheres: confusion; behavioral change	Person reports disorientation, confusion, "not listening," "not remembering"; reports by others of person being disoriented, not able to remember, not able to learn new information
Pattern recognition (remote)	*Left hemisphere:* inability to retrieve personal history, past medical history; unaware of recent current events *Right hemisphere:* inability to recognize persons, places, objects, music, etc., from past	Person reports remote memory problems; others report that person cannot recall formerly known information
Image and semantic processing	Inability to categorize (identify similarities and differences), sort; inability to form concepts; inability to analyze relationships; misinterpretations; inability to interpret proverbs	Reports by others of frequent misinterpretation of data, failure to conceptualize or generalize information
	Inability to perform deductive reasoning (convergent reasoning); inability to perform inductive reasoning (divergent reasoning); inability to abstract; concrete reasoning demonstrated; delusions	Reports by others of predominantly concrete thinking; lack of understanding of everyday situations, health care regimens, and such; delusional thinking
Executive attentional networks		
Vigilance	Failure to stay alert and orient to stimuli	Person reports decreased alertness or ability to orient
Detection	Lack of initiative (anergy); lack of ambition; lack of motivation; flat affect; no awareness of feelings; appears depressed, apathetic, and emotionless; fails to appreciate deficit; disinterested in appearance; lacks concern about childish or crude behavior	Reports by others of laziness or apathy, flat affect or lack of emotional expression, failing to exhibit or be aware of feelings
Mild	Responds to immediate environment but no new ideas; grooming and social graces are lacking	Reports by others of lack of ambition, motivation, or initiative, failure to carry out adult tasks, lack of social graces and new ideas
Severe	Motionless, lack of responding to even internal cues, does not respond to physical needs, does not interact with surroundings	Reports by others of failure to groom or toilet self, unawareness of surroundings and own physical needs
	Inability to use feedback regarding behavior; failure to recognize omissions and errors in self-care, speech, writing, and arithmetic; impaired cue utilization; overestimation of performance	Reports by others of not changing behavior when requested; unawareness of limitations; does not recognize and correct errors in dressing, grooming, toileting, eating, and such; fails to recognize speech and arithmetic errors; careless speech
	Failure to shift response set; failure to change behavior when conditions change; cue utilization may be impaired	Reports by others of failure to use feedback; inability to incorporate feedback (does not correct when feedback is given)

Continued

TABLE 14-9   Clinical Manifestations of Cognitive Network Deficits—cont'd

Deficit	Clinical Signs	Symptoms
Executive attentional networks—cont'd		
Working memory	Inability to set goals or form goals; indecisiveness	Reports by others of failure to set goals, indecisiveness
	Failure to make plans; inability to produce a complete line of reasoning; inability to make up a story; appears impulsive	Reports by others of failure to plan, impulsiveness, "does not think things through"
	Failure to initiate behavior; failure to maintain behavior; failure to discontinue behavior; slowness to alternate response for the next step; motor perseveration	Reports by others of not knowing where to begin, inability to carry out sequential acts (maintain a behavior), inability to cease a behavior

Cognitive Disorders

Selective attention (orienting) refers to the ability to select from available environmental and internal stimuli specific information to be processed.[4] Certain midbrain and thalamic structures contribute to selective attention, so the etiologic factors for coma potentially can alter selective attention. Selective attention also is mediated by the right parietal lobe.[4] An isolated (pure) *selective attention deficit* rarely occurs clinically. Causes of temporary, permanent, or progressive deficits include seizure activity, parietal lobe contusions, subdural hematomas, stroke, gliomas or metastatic tumor, and late Alzheimer and Pick diseases (see Chapter 15). Table 14-9 summarizes cognitive networks deficits.

Pathophysiology

Very generally, the primary pathophysiologic mechanisms that operate in cognitive networks disorders are (1) direct destruction caused by direct ischemia and hypoxia or indirect destruction resulting from compression and (2) the effects of toxins and chemicals. Disorders of selective attention, at least as they relate to visual orienting behavior, are produced by disease that involves portions of the midbrain. Disease affecting the superior colliculi manifests as a slowness in orienting attention. Parietal lobe disease may produce disengagement from a stimulus or unilateral neglect syndrome. *Sensory inattentiveness* is a form of neglect. The person is able to recognize individual sensory input from the dysfunctional side when called on to do so but ignores the sensory input from the dysfunctional side when stimulated from both sides *(extinction)*. The entire complex of denial of dysfunction, loss of recognition of one's own body parts, and extinction sometimes is referred to as the *neglect syndrome.* A disorder in vigilance may be produced by disease in the prefrontal areas. Right dysfunction in the anterior cingulate gyrus and basal ganglia may cause detection problems, whereas problems with working memory may be produced with left frontal axis injury.

Clinical Manifestations

Clinical manifestations of selective attention deficits, pattern recognition deficits, and executive attention function deficits are presented in Table 14-9.

Evaluation and Ttreatment

Immediate medical management is directed at diagnosing the cause and treating reversible factors. Rehabilitative measures generally focus on compensatory or restorative activities and recently have been greatly facilitated by computer technology and other electronic-assisted devices.

Attention deficits masquerade as other cognitive deficits. Differential diagnosis is blocked and learning potential is largely obscured when an attention deficit is present. Therefore the diagnosis and treatment of attention deficits are fundamental.

Data Processing Deficits
Agnosia

Agnosia is a defect of pattern recognition—a failure to recognize the form and nature of objects. Agnosia can be tactile, visual, or auditory, but generally only one sense is affected. For example, an individual may be unable to identify a safety pin by touching it with a hand but is able to name it when looking at it. Agnosia may be as minimal as a finger agnosia (failure to identify by name the fingers of one's hand) or more extensive, such as a color agnosia.

Although agnosia is associated most commonly with cerebrovascular accidents, it may arise from any pathologic process that injures specific areas of the brain.[5]

Dysphasia

Dysphasia is impairment of comprehension or production of language (semantic processing). Comprehension or use of symbols, in either written or verbal language, is disturbed or lost. *Aphasia* is loss of the comprehension or production of language.

Dysphasias usually are associated with cerebrovascular accident involving the middle cerebral artery or one of its many branches. Language disorders, however, may arise from a variety of injuries and diseases—vascular, neoplastic, traumatic, degenerative, metabolic, or infectious causes. Dysphasia results from dysfunction in the left cerebral hemisphere, usually the frontotemporal region (Fig. 14-7; see also Fig. 12-6). Most language disorders result from acute processes or a chronic residual deficit of the acute process.

Fig. 14-7 *Development of dysphasia.* Portion of the left cerebral hemisphere considered most important in the development of dysphasia.

Some progressive language disorders are the result of degenerative disorders. One or more genes located on chromosome 7 recently have been linked to language and speech.[6]

Dysphasias have been classified both anatomically and functionally. Other classifications describe fluency, volume, or quantity of speech, although pure forms of any language dysfunction are rare. *Expressive dysphasias* involve primarily expression deficits, but verbal comprehension deficit also may be present. Receptive dysphasias may have expressive deficits. (Table 14-10 compares types of dysphasias; Table 14-11 illustrates some of the language disturbances.)

Some dysphasias are referred to as *transcortical dysphasias* and involve the ability to repeat *(echolalia)* and to recite. Speech is fluent but with striking paraphrases. The individual cannot read or write and has impaired comprehension. These dysphasias are caused by hypoxia or other mechanisms that destroy the border zone between the cerebral arteries (see Fig. 12-19). The sensory and motor speech areas are functional, but connections with other sensory or motor areas are impaired. Information cannot be transmitted to Wernicke area and transformed into language.

Acute confusional states

Acute confusional states result from cerebral dysfunction secondary to drug intoxication, metabolic disorder, or nervous system disease. Withdrawal from alcohol, barbiturate, or other sedative drug ingestion is a common cause. Acute confusional states may begin either suddenly or gradually, depending on the amount of exposure to the toxin. These states often occur with febrile illnesses, systemic diseases (e.g., heart failure), head injury, or anesthesia.[7]

Pathophysiology

Three pathophysiologic mechanisms probably underlie the development of acute confusional states: (1) injury to nervous tissue, (2) action of toxin or chemical agent on neuronal cells, and (3) disinhibition and overactivity of a previously depressed brain center.

Clinical Manifestations

The predominant feature of an acute confusional state is impaired or lost detection. The person is highly distractible and unable to concentrate on incoming sensory information or on any one particular mental or motor task.

The onset of an acute confusional state usually is abrupt. The first clinical manifestations are difficulty in concentration, restlessness, irritability, tremulousness, insomnia, and poor appetite. Later there are misperceptions, illusions, hallucinations, and delirium. Obsessions, compulsive behavior, and rituals may be evident.

In acute confusional states with associated underactivity, the individual exhibits decreases in mental function, specifically alertness, attention span, accurate perception, interpretation of the environment, and reaction to the environment. Forgetfulness is prominent, and the individual dozes frequently.

Delirium, an acute confusional state associated with overactivity, typically develops over 2 to 3 days and is seen initially as difficulty in concentrating, restlessness, irritability, insomnia, tremulousness, and poor appetite. Some persons experience seizures. Unpleasant, even terrifying, dreams may occur.

In a fully developed delirium state, the individual is com-

TABLE 14-10 Major Types of Dysphasia

Type	Expression	Verbal Comprehension	Repetition
Expressive			
Broca dysphasia, motor	Nonfluent; cannot find words, difficulty writing	Relatively intact	Impaired
Receptive			
Wernicke dysphasia, sensory	Fluent; can produce verbal language but it is meaningless, with inappropriate words, with similar sounds or meaning substituted for correct words, and neologisms that may be so extensive that speech is incomprehensible; unable to monitor language for correctness, so errors are not recognized. Intonation, accent, cadence, rhythm, and articulation normal	Impaired (disturbance in understanding all language)	Impaired
Word deafness or auditory verbal agnosia, sensory	Fluent; self-initiated speech is normal	Impaired; hears noise rather than language; language has no meaning and is perceived as foreign	Impaired, unable to repeat what is said
Others			
Global, conductive, anomia, transcortical motor, or transcortical sensory	Ranges from nonfluent and producing little speech to fluent with paraphrasia or impaired ability for naming	Can be relatively intact, impaired, or completely lost	Can be intact or impaired with an inability to repeat

Modified from Mancall, E.L. (1981). Alper's and Mancall's essentials of the neurologic examination. Philadelphia: F.A. Davis.

TABLE 14-11 Examples of Language Disturbances

Disorder		Example
Verbal paraphrasia	Question:	What did the car do?
	Patient:	The car would spit sweetly down the road. (The car sped swiftly down the road.)
Literal paraphrasia	Request:	Say "persistence is essential to success."
	Patient:	Mesastence is instans to success.
Neologism	Question:	What do you call this? (Pointing to a plant.)
	Patient:	It's a logper.
Circumlocution	Question:	What do you call this? (Pointing to a plant.)
	Patient:	Something that grows.
Anomia	Question:	What do you call this? (Pointing to a plant.)
	Patient:	It's . . .
		or
	Question:	What did you do this morning?
	Patient:	Reading.
	Question:	Were you reading a book or a newspaper?
	Patient:	One of those.
Telegraphic style	Question:	Where is your daughter?
	Patient:	New Orleans . . . home . . . Monday.

From Boss, B.J. (1984). Dysphasia, dyspraxia, and dysarthria: Distinguishing features (Part I). Journal of Neurosurgical Nursing, *16(3), 151-160.*

Reading Comprehension	Writing	Location of Lesion	Cause of Lesion
Variable	Impaired	Posteroinferior frontal lobe (Broca area)	Occlusion of a branch of the left middle cerebral artery supplying the inferior frontal gyrus
Impaired	Impaired	Posterosuperior temporal lobe (Wernicke area)	Occlusion of inferior division of left middle cerebral artery
Intact; able to read	Intact; able to write	Pathways connecting the primary auditory cortex and the auditory association areas in the middle third of the left superior temporal gyrus	Small, superficial injury typically associated with occlusion of a branch of the middle cerebral artery
Variable; may be impaired or completely lost	Variable or impaired	Various areas including frontotemporal lobe; arcuate fasciculus, supramarginal gyrus, bundle of fibers from the temporal lobe that project anteriorly to the premotor area; angular gyrus; and anterior or posterior presylvian fissures	Occlusion of the left middle cerebral artery of the left internal carotid artery, tumors, other mass lesions, hemorrhage, embolic occlusion of the ascending parietal or posterior temporal branch of the middle cerebral artery

pletely inattentive and perceptions are grossly altered, with extensive misperception and misinterpretation. Hallucinations may be present. The person appears distressed and often perplexed; conversation is incoherent. Frank tremor and high levels of restless movement are common. Violent behavior may be present. The individual cannot sleep, is flushed, and has dilated pupils, a rapid pulse (tachycardia), temperature elevation, and profuse sweating (diaphoresis). Delirium typically abates suddenly or gradually in 2 to 3 days, although occasionally delirium states persist for weeks.

➤ *Evaluation and Treatment*

The initial goal is to establish (1) that the individual is confused and (2) the cause (organic or functional) (Table 14-12). Next, is the confusion a delirium, an acute confusional state with associated underactivity, or an underlying dementia? A complete history and physical examination as well as laboratory tests (electrocardiogram and blood, urine, cerebrospinal fluid, and radiologic studies) are needed. Once the cause is established, treatment is directed at controlling the primary disorder, with supportive measures used as appropriate.

Dementia

The dementias are characterized by the loss of more than one cognitive (intellectual) function. The result may be a decrease in orienting, recent memory, remote memory, and language and executive attentional networks. Because of declining intellectual ability, the individual exhibits alterations in behavior. Dementias may be primary (without a well-defined cause) or secondary (with well-defined etiologies often with associated systemic illness).

➤ *Pathophysiology*

Mechanisms leading to dementia include degeneration, compression, atherosclerosis, and trauma. For example, aging and genetic predisposition are associated with the degenerative diseases of Alzheimer and Huntington disease. CNS infections, including the human immunodeficiency virus (HIV) and slow-growing viruses associated with Creutzfeldt-Jakob disease, are associated with dementia in addition to changes in motor function (see Chapter 15). Progressive dementias produce nerve cell degeneration and brain atrophy.

TABLE 14-12   Differences Between Organic and Functional Confusion

Factor	Organic Confusion	Functional Confusion
Memory impairment	Recent, more impaired than remote	No consistent difference between recent and remote
Disorientation		
Time	Within own lifetime or reasonably near future	May not be related to patient's lifetime
Place	Familiar place or one where patient might easily be	Bizarre or unfamiliar places
Person	Sense of identity usually preserved	Sense of identity diminished
	Misidentification of others as familiar	Misidentification of others based on delusion system
Hallucinations	Visual, vivid	Auditory more frequent
	Animals and insects common	Bizarre and symbolic
Illusions	Common	Not prominent
Delusions	Concern everyday occurrences and people	Bizarre and symbolic
Confused	Spotty confusion	More consistent
	Clear intervals mixed with confused episodes	No tendency to become worse at night
	Worse at night	

From Morris, M. & Rhodes, M. (1972). Guidelines for the care of confused patients. American Journal of Nursing, *72(9), 1632.*

TABLE 14-13   Clinical Manifestations of Dementia

Type	Manifestation
Cortical dementia	Agnosias
	Apraxia
	Difficulty with naming
	Decreased language comprehension
	Loss of recent memory
	Loss of remote memory
	Decreased mathematic skill
	Altered visuospatial relationships
Subcortical dementia	Forgetfullness
	Apathy
	Depression
	Slowed thought processes
	Accident prone
	Personality changes and inappropriate affect
	Loss of motor function: wide shuffling gait with small steps, muscle rigidity, flexion posturing, tendency to fall, abnormal reflexes, bowel and bladder incontinence, immobility

Clinical Manifestations

Symptoms of dementia may be categorized as cortical, subcortical, or both (Table 14-13).

Evaluation and Treatment

Establishing the cause for dementia may be complicated, but individuals with clinical manifestations of dementia should be evaluated with laboratory and neuropsychologic testing to identify underlying conditions that may be treatable. Unfortunately, no specific treatment or cure exists for most progressive dementias. Therapy is directed at maintaining and maximizing use of the remaining capacities, restoring functions if possible, and accommodating to lost abilities. Assisting the family to understand the process and to learn ways to assist the individual is essential.

✓ QUICK CHECK

Why are there so many cognitive disorders?

Why can so many disorders cause dysphasia?

Why is impaired detection the most common feature of acute confusional states (ACS)?

How is an ACS different from dementia?

ALTERATIONS IN CEREBRAL HOMEOSTASIS

Increased Intracranial Pressure

Intracranial pressure (ICP) normally is 5 to 15 mm Hg, or 60 to 180 cm H_2O. *Increased intracranial pressure (IICP)* may result from an increase in intracranial content (as occurs with tumor growth), edema, excess CSF, or hemorrhage. It necessitates an equal reduction in volume of the other cranial contents. The most readily displaced content is CSF. If intracranial pressure remains high after CSF displacement out of the cranial vault, cerebral blood volume is altered.

In *stage 1* of intracranial hypertension, vasoconstriction and external compression of the venous system occur in an attempt to further decrease the intracranial pressure. Thus during the first stage of intracranial hypertension, intracranial pressure may not change because of the effective com-

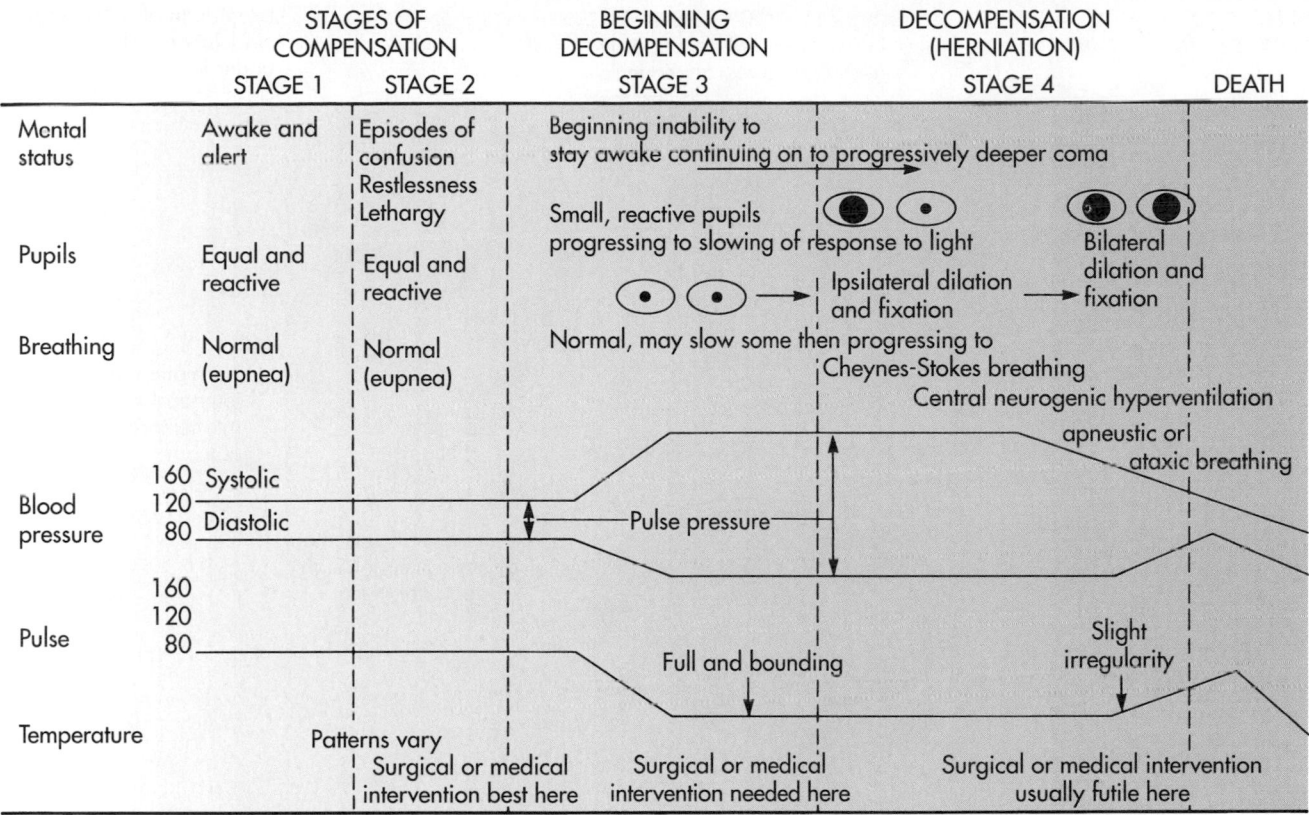

	STAGES OF COMPENSATION		BEGINNING DECOMPENSATION	DECOMPENSATION (HERNIATION)	
	STAGE 1	STAGE 2	STAGE 3	STAGE 4	DEATH
Mental status	Awake and alert	Episodes of confusion Restlessness Lethargy	Beginning inability to stay awake continuing on to progressively deeper coma		
Pupils	Equal and reactive	Equal and reactive	Small, reactive pupils progressing to slowing of response to light → Ipsilateral dilation and fixation	Bilateral dilation and fixation	
Breathing	Normal (eupnea)	Normal (eupnea)	Normal, may slow some then progressing to Cheynes-Stokes breathing	Central neurogenic hyperventilation apneustic or ataxic breathing	
Blood pressure	160 Systolic 120 80 Diastolic		Pulse pressure		
Pulse	160 120 80		Full and bounding	Slight irregularity	
Temperature	Patterns vary Surgical or medical intervention best here		Surgical or medical intervention needed here	Surgical or medical intervention usually futile here	

Fig. 14-8 *Clinical correlates of compensated and uncompensated phases of intracranial hypertension. (From Beare, P.G. & Myers, J.L. [1998].* Principles and practice of adult health nursing *[3rd ed.]. St. Louis: Mosby.)*

pensatory mechanisms and there may be few symptoms (Fig. 14-8). Small increases in volume, however, cause an increase in pressure, and the pressure may take longer to return to baseline. This can be detected with intracranial pressure monitoring.[8]

With continued expansion of the intracranial content, the resulting increase in intracranial pressure may exceed the brain's compensatory capacity to adjust. The pressure begins to compromise neuronal oxygenation, and systemic arterial vasoconstriction occurs in an attempt to elevate the systemic blood pressure sufficiently to overcome the increased intracranial pressure (*stage 2* of intracranial hypertension). Clinical manifestations at this stage usually are subtle and transient, including episodes of confusion, restlessness, drowsiness, and slight pupillary and breathing changes (see Fig. 14-8).

As intracranial pressure begins to approach arterial pressure, the brain tissues begin to experience hypoxia and hypercapnia and the individual's condition rapidly deteriorates. Clinical manifestations include decreasing levels of arousal and/or central neurogenic hyperventilation, widened pulse pressure, bradycardia, and pupils that become small and sluggish (*stage 3* of intracranial hypertension) (see Fig. 14-8).

Dramatic sustained rises in intracranial pressure are not seen until all compensatory mechanisms have been ex-

hausted. Then dramatic rises in intracranial pressure occur over a very short period. *Autoregulation,* the compensatory alteration in the diameter of the intracranial blood vessels designed to maintain a constant blood flow during changes in cerebral perfusion pressure, is lost with progressively increased intracranial pressure. Accumulating carbon dioxide may still cause vasodilation locally, but without autoregulation this vasodilation causes the hydrostatic (blood) pressure in the vessels to drop and blood volume to increase. The brain volume is thus further enhanced, and intracranial pressure continues to rise. Small increases in volume cause dramatic increases in intracranial pressure, and the pressure takes much longer to return to baseline. As the intracranial pressure begins to approach systemic blood pressure, cerebral perfusion pressure falls and cerebral perfusion slows dramatically. The brain tissues experience severe hypoxia and acidosis.

Increased intracranial pressure in one compartment of the cranial vault is not evenly distributed throughout the other vault compartments. In *stage 4* of intracranial hypertension, brain tissue shifts (herniates) from the compartment of greater pressure to a compartment of lesser pressure (see Figs. 14-8 and 14-9). With this shift in brain tissue, the herniating brain tissue's blood supply is compromised, causing further ischemia and hypoxia in the herniating tissues. The volume of content within the lower pressure compart-

Compression
of the opposite
cerebral peduncle
against the
unyielding
tentorium

Herniation of
cingulate gyrus
under falx
cerebri

Herniation of
temporal lobe
into tentorial
notch

Downward displacement
of brain stem through
tentorial notch

Fig. 14-9 *Herniation.* **A,** Normal relationship of intracranial structures. **B,** Shift of intracranial structures. **C,** Downward herniation of the cerebellar tonsils into the foramen magnum.

ment is increased, exerting pressure on the brain tissue that normally occupies that compartment and impairing its blood supply. Small hemorrhages frequently develop in the involved brain tissue. Obstructive hydrocephalus may develop. The herniation process markedly and rapidly increases intracranial pressure. Mean systolic arterial pressure soon equals intracranial pressure, and cerebral blood flow ceases at this point.

The types of herniation syndromes are outlined in Box 14-2.

Cerebral Edema

Cerebral edema is an increase in the fluid content of brain tissue (Fig. 14-10). The result is increased extracellular or intracellular tissue volume. It occurs after brain insult from trauma, infection, hemorrhage, tumor, ischemia, infarct, or hypoxia.[9] The harmful effects of cerebral edema are caused by distortion of blood vessels, displacement of brain tissues, and eventual herniation of brain tissue from one brain compartment to another.

Four types of cerebral edema are (1) vasogenic edema, (2) cytotoxic (metabolic) edema, (3) ischemic edema, and (4) interstitial edema. *Vasogenic edema* is clinically the most important type and is caused by the increased permeability of the capillary endothelium of the brain after injury to the

vascular structure. The blood-brain barrier is disrupted, and plasma proteins leak into the extracellular spaces, drawing water to them and increasing the water content of the brain parenchyma. Vasogenic edema starts in the area of injury and spreads, with fluid accumulating in the white matter of the ipsilateral side because the parallel myelinated fibers separate more easily. Edema promotes more edema because of ischemia from the increasing pressure.

Clinical manifestations of vasogenic edema include focal neurologic deficits, disturbances of consciousness, and a severe increase in intracranial pressure. Vasogenic edema resolves by slow diffusion.

In *cytotoxic (metabolic) edema,* toxic factors directly affect the cellular elements of the brain parenchyma (neuronal, glial, and endothelial cells), causing failure of the active transport systems. The cells lose their potassium and gain larger amounts of sodium. Water follows by osmosis into the cells, so that the cells swell. Cytotoxic edema occurs principally in the gray matter and may increase vasogenic edema.

Ischemic edema follows cerebral infarction. The ischemia has components of both vasogenic and cytotoxic edema. The initial edema is confined to the intracellular compartment, but over several days, brain cells begin to undergo necrosis and die, releasing lysosomes. In this autodi-

Herniation Syndrome

BOX 14-2

SUPRATENTORIAL HERNIATION

1. **Uncal herniation.** Occurs when the uncus or hippocampal gyrus or both shift from the middle fossa through the tentorial notch into the posterior fossa, compressing the ipsilateral third cranial nerve, the contralateral third cranial nerve, and the mesencephalon. Uncal herniation generally is caused by an expanding mass in the lateral region of the middle fossa. The classic manifestations of uncal herniation are a decreasing level of consciousness, pupils that become sluggish before fixing and dilating (first the ipsilateral, then the contralateral pupil), Cheyne-Stokes respirations (which later shift to central neurogenic hyperventilation), and the appearance of decorticate and then decerebrate posturing.

2. **Central herniation.** The straight downward shift of the diencephalon through the tentorial notch. It may be caused by injuries or masses located around the outer perimeter of the frontal, parietal, or occipital lobes, extracerebral injuries around the central apex (top) of the cranium, bilaterally positioned injuries or masses, and unilateral cingulate gyrus herniation. The individual rapidly becomes unconscious; moves from Cheyne-Stokes respirations to apnea; develops small, reactive pupils and then dilated, fixed pupils; and passes from decortication to decerebration.

3. **Cingulate gyrus herniation.** Occurs when the cingulate gyrus shifts under the falx cerebri. Little is known about its clinical manifestations.

INFRATENTORIAL HERNIATION

In the most common syndrome the cerebellar tonsil shifts through the foramen magnum because of increased pressure within the posterior fossa. The clinical manifestations are an arched stiff neck, paresthesias in the shoulder area, decreased consciousness, respiratory abnormalities, and pulse rate variations. Occasionally the force produces an upward transtentorial herniation of a cerebellar tonsil or the lower brain stem. No specific set of clinical manifestations are associated with infratentorial herniation.

Fig. 14-10 *Brain edema.* Intercellular lakes of high protein content fluid. (Hematoxylin-eosin stain; X90.) *(From Kissane, J.M. [Ed.]. [1996]. Anderson's pathology [10th ed.]. St. Louis: Mosby.)*

gestive process, the blood-brain barrier's permeability is increased.

Interstitial edema is seen most often with noncommunicating hydrocephalus (see Chapter 15). The edema is caused by transependymal movement of CSF from the ventricles into the extracellular spaces of the brain tissues. The brain fluid volume increases predominantly around the ventricles, with increased hydrostatic pressure within the white matter. The size of the white matter is reduced because of the rapid disappearance of myelin lipids.

Hydrocephalus

The term *hydrocephalus* refers to various conditions characterized by excess fluid in the cranial vault, subarachnoid space, or both. Hydrocephalus occurs because of interference with CSF flow caused by increased fluid production, obstruction within the ventricular system, or defective reabsorption of the fluid. A tumor of the choroid plexus may, in rare instances, cause overproduction of CSF. The types of hydrocephalus are reviewed in Table 14-14.

Hydrocephalus may develop from infancy through adulthood. Congenital hydrocephalus (i.e., ventricular enlargement before birth) is rare. *Noncommunicating hydrocephalus (internal hydrocephalus, intraventricular hydrocephalus)*—obstruction within the ventricular system—is seen more frequently in children, and *communicating hydrocephalus*—defective resorption of CSF from the cerebral subarachnoid space—is found more frequently in adults.

Most cases of hydrocephalus develop gradually and insidiously over time. *Acute hydrocephalus,* however, may develop in a couple of hours in persons who have sustained head injuries. Acute hydrocephalus contributes significantly to increased intracranial pressure.

Pathophysiology

The obstruction of CSF flow associated with hydrocephalus produces dilation of the ventricles proximal to the obstruction. Obstructed CSF is under pressure, causing atrophy of the cerebral cortex and degeneration of the white matter tracts. There is selective preservation of gray matter. When excess CSF fills a defect caused by atrophy, a degenerative

TABLE 14-14	Types of Hydrocephalus	
Type	**Mechanism**	**Cause**
Noncommunicating	Obstruction of CSF flow between ventricles	Congenital abnormality Aqueduct stenosis Arnold-Chiari malformation (brain extension through foramen magnum) Compression by tumor
Communicating	Impaired absorption of CSF within subarachnoid space	Infection with inflammatory adhesions Compression of subarachnoid space by a tumor High venous pressure in sagittal sinus Head injury Congenital malformation
	Increased CSF secretion by choroid plexus	Secreting tumor

disorder, or a surgical excision, this fluid is not under pressure; therefore atrophy and degenerative changes are not induced.

 ### *Clinical Manifestations*

Acute hydrocephalus presents with signs of rapidly developing increased intracranial pressure. The person quickly deteriorates into a deep coma if not promptly treated. ***Normal-pressure hydrocephalus*** (dilation of the ventricles without increased pressure) develops slowly, with the individual or family noting declining memory and cognitive function. An unsteady, broad-based gait with a history of falling is common. Additional clinical manifestations are apathy, inattentiveness, and indifference to self, family, and the environment. Urinary incontinence is present. In infancy, head enlargement is predominant before closure of the cranial sutures (see Chapter 16).

 ### *Evaluation and Treatment*

The diagnosis is based on physical examination, computed tomography (CT) scan, and magnetic resonance imaging (MRI). A radioisotopic cisternogram may be performed to diagnose normal-pressure hydrocephalus. Hydrocephalus can be treated by surgery to resect cysts, neoplasms, or hematomas or by ventricular bypass into the normal intracranial channel or into an extracranial compartment using a shunting procedure, one of the three most common neurosurgical procedures.[10] Excision or coagulation of the choroid plexus occasionally is needed when a papilloma is present. In normal-pressure hydrocephalus, reduction in CSF through a diuresis regimen often is used.

✓ QUICK CHECK

What are the four stages of intracranial hypertension?

How does supratentorial herniation differ from infratentorial herniation?

What are the different types of edema?

How is communicating hydrocephalus different from noncommunicating hydrocephalus?

ALTERATIONS IN MOTOR FUNCTION

Movements are complex patterns of activity controlled by the CNS. They are influenced by the cerebral cortex, the pyramidal system, the extrapyramidal system, and the motor units. Dysfunction in any of these areas can cause motor dysfunction. General motor dysfunctions may produce changes in muscle tone, movement, and complex motor performance.

Alterations in Muscle Tone

Normal muscle tone involves a slight resistance to passive movement. Throughout the range of motion, the resistance is smooth, constant, and even. The abnormalities of muscle tone are presented in Table 14-15.

Hypotonia

In *hypotonia* (decreased muscle tone) passive movement of a muscle occurs with little or no resistance. Causes include pure pyramidal tract damage (a rare occurrence) and cerebellar damage. A pure pyramidal tract injury produces hypotonia and weakness. The hypotonia contributes to the ataxia and intention tremor in cerebellar damage and manifests with minimal weakness and normal or slightly exaggerated reflexes. Hypotonia or flaccidity (a state in which the muscle may be moved rapidly without resistance) occurs when the nerve impulses needed for muscle tone are lost, such as in spinal cord injury or cerebrovascular accident.

Individuals with hypotonia tire easily (asthenia) or are weak. They may have difficulty rising from a sitting position, sitting down without using arm support, and walking up and down stairs, as well as an inability to stand on their toes. Because of their weakness, accidents during locomotion and self-care activities are common. The joints become hyperflexible, so persons with hypotonia may be able to assume positions that require extreme joint mobility. The joints may appear loose, and the knee jerks are pendulous.

The muscle mass atrophies because of decreased input entering the motor unit, and muscles appear flabby and flat. Muscle cells are gradually replaced by connective tissue and fat. Fasciculations may be present in some cases.

TABLE 14-15	Alterations In Muscle Tone	
Alterations	**Characteristics**	**Cause**
Hypotonia	Passive movement of a muscle mass with little or no resistance	Thought to be caused by decreased muscle spindle activity as a result of decreased excitability of neurons
Flaccidity	Muscles may be moved rapidly without resistance Associated with limp, atrophied muscles and paralysis	Occurs typically when nerve impulses necessary for muscle tone are lost
Hypertonia	Increased muscle resistance to passive movement May be associated with paralysis May be accompanied by muscle hypertrophy	Results when the lower motor unit reflex arc continues to function but is not mediated or regulated by higher centers
Spasticity	A gradual increase in tone causing increased resistance until tone suddenly is reduced, which results in clasp-knife phenomenon	Exact mechanism unclear; appears to arise from an increased excitability of the alpha motor neurons to any input because of absence of the descending inhibition of the pyramidal systems
Gegenhalten (paratonia)	Resistance to passive movement, which varies in direct proportion to force applied	Exact mechanism unclear: associated with frontal lobe injury
Dystonia	Sustained involuntary twisting movement	Produced by slow muscular contraction
Rigidity	Muscle resistance to passive movement of a rigid limb that is uniform in both flexion and extension throughout the motion	Occurs as a result of constant, involuntary contraction of muscle
Plastic, or lead-pipe	Increased muscular tone relatively independent of degree of force used in passive movement; does not vary throughout the passive movement	Associated with basal ganglion damage
Cogwheel	The uniform resistance may be interrupted by a series of brief jerks resulting in movements much like a rachet, "cogwheel" phenomenon	Associated with basal ganglion damage
Gamma and Alpha	Characterized by extensor posturing (decerebrate rigidity)	Loss of excitation of extensor inhibitory areas by the cerebral cortex decreasing the inhibition of alpha and gamma motor neurons Loss of cerebellum input to lateral vestibular nuclei

Hypertonia

In *hypertonia* (increased muscle tone), passive movement of a muscle occurs with resistance. Four types of hypertonia are described: spasticity, gegenhalten (paratonia), dystonia, and rigidity.

Spasticity results from hyperexcitability of the stretch reflexes and is associated with damage to the motor, premotor, and supplementary motor areas, as well as lateral corticospinal tract damage. Increased deep tendon reflexes (hyperflexia) and the spread of reflexes (*clonus*) accompany it.

Gegenhalten (paratonia) manifests as resistance to passive movement that varies in direct proportion to the force applied and is associated with frontal lobe injury. *Dystonia* manifests as sustained, involuntary twisting movements caused by slow muscle contraction and may be caused by lack of appropriate reciprocal inhibition of the muscles. Injury to the putamen or its outflow tracts is associated with hemidystonia.

Rigidity produced by tonic reflex activity mediated by gamma motor neurons may be continuous or intermittent. The involved muscles are firm and tense; the increase in muscle movement is even and uniform throughout the range of passive movement. Four types of rigidity are described: plastic or lead-pipe rigidity, cogwheel rigidity, gamma rigidity, and alpha rigidity (see Table 14-15).

Individuals with hypertonia tire easily (asthenia) or are weak. Passive and active movement is affected equally, except in paratonia, in which more active than passive movement is possible. As a result of hypertonia and weakness, accidents occur during locomotion and self-care activities.

The muscles may atrophy because of decreased use. However, hypertrophy occasionally occurs as a result of overstimulation of muscle fibers. Overstimulation occurs when the motor unit reflex arc remains intact and functioning but is not inhibited by higher centers. This causes continual muscle contraction, resulting in enlargement of the muscle mass and firm muscles.

Alterations in Movement

Movement requires a change in the contractile state of muscles. Abnormal movements occur when CNS dysfunctions alter muscle innervation. Currently, neuropharmacology

TABLE 14-16	Types of Hyperkinesia	
Type	**Characteristics**	**Causes**
Chorea*	Nonrepetitive muscular contractions, usually of the extremities of face; random pattern of irregular, involuntary rapid contractions of groups of muscles; disappears with sleep, decreases with resting; increases with emotional stress and attempted voluntary movement	Associated with excess concentration of or a supersensitivity to dopamine within basal ganglia
Athetosis*	Disorder of distal-muscle postural fixation; slow, sinuous, irregular movements most obvious in the distal extremities, more rhythmic than choreiform movements and always much slower; movements accompany characteristic hand posture; slowly fluctuating grimaces	Occurs most commonly as a result of injury to the putamen of the basal ganglion; exact pathophysiologic mechanism is not known
Ballism	Disorder of proximal-muscle postural fixation with wild flinging movement of the limbs; movement is severe and stereotyped, usually lateral; does not lessen with sleep; ballism is most common on one side of the body, a condition termed *hemiballism*	Results from injury to subthalamus nucleus (one of the nuclei that comprise the basal ganglia); thought to be caused by reduced inhibitory influence in the nucleus, a release phenomenon; hemiballism results from injury to the contralateral subthalamic nucleus
Hyperactivity	State of prolonged, generalized, increased activity that is largely involuntary but may be subject to some voluntary control; not highly stereotyped but rather manifests as continuous changes in total body posture or in excessive performance of some simple activity, such as pacing under inappropriate circumstances	May be caused by frontal and reticular activating system injury
Wandering	Tendency to wander without regard for environment	"Release" phenomenon; associated with bilateral injury to globus pallidus or putamen
Akathisia	Special type of hyperactivity; mild compulsion to move (usually more localized to legs); severe frenzied motion possible; movements are partly voluntary and may be transiently suppressed; carrying out the movement brings a sense of relief; a frequent complication of antipsychotic drugs	Dopaminergic transmission may be involved
Tremor at rest	Rhythmic, oscillating movement affecting one or more body parts	Caused by regular contraction of opposing groups of muscles
Parkinsonian tremor	Regular, rhythmic, slower flexion-extension contraction; involves principally the metacarpophalangeal and wrist joints; alternating movements between thumb and index finger described as "pill rolling"; disappears during voluntary movement	Loss of inhibitory influence of dopamine in the basal ganglia, causing instability of basal ganglial feedback circuit within the cerebral cortex
Postural tremor		
Asterixis (tremor of hepatic encephalopathy)	Irregular flapping movement of the hands accentuated by outstretching arms	Exact mechanisms responsible unknown; thought to be related to accumulation of products normally detoxified by the liver
Metabolic	Rapid, rhythmic tremor affecting fingers, lips, and tongue; accentuated by extending the body part; enhanced physiologic tremor	Occurs in conditions associated with disturbed metabolism or toxicity, as in thyrotoxicosis (hyperthyroidism), alcoholism, and chronic use of barbiturates; amphetamine, lithium, amitriptyline [Elavil]; exact mechanism responsible unknown
Essential (familial)	Tremor of fingers, hands, and feet; absent at rest but accentuated by extension of body part, prolonged muscular activity, and stress	Not associated with any other neurologic abnormalities; cause unknown

*Choreoathetosis involves both chorea and athetosis; precise pathophysiology unknown.

TABLE 14-16	Types of Hyperkinesia—cont'd	
Type	Characteristics	Causes
Intention tremor		
Cerebellar	Tremor initated by movement, maximal toward end of movement	Occurs in disease of the dentate nucleus (one of the deep cerebellar nuclei responsible for efferent output) and the superior cerebellar peduncle (a stalk-like structure connected to the pons); caused by errors in feedback from the periphery and errors in preprogramming goal-directed movement
Rubral	Rhythmic tremor of limbs that originates proximally by movement	Results from lesions involving the dentatorubrothalamic tract (a spinothalamic tract connecting the red nucleus in the reticular formation and the dentate nucleus in the cerebellum)
Myoclonus	Series of shocklike nonpatterned contractions of portion of a muscle, entire muscle, or group of muscles that cause throwing movements of a limb; usually appear at random but frequently triggered by sudden startle; do not disappear during sleep	Associated with an irritable nervous system and spontaneous discharge of neurons; structures associated with myoclonus include the cerebral cortex, cerebellum, reticular formation, and spinal cord

and experimental therapeutic researchers have found that dopamine apparently functions in several movement disorders. Some (e.g., the akinesias) result from too little dopaminergic activity, whereas others (e.g., chorea, ballism, tardive dyskinesia) result from too much. Still others are not primarily related to dopamine function. Movement disorders are not necessarily associated with mass, strength, or tone but are neurologic dysfunctions with either too little or too much movement.

Muscle strength is quantitatively evaluated on a scale of 0 to 4+ or 5+, in which 4+ or 5+ is normal and 0 indicates an inability to move against gravity. Degrees of abnormal muscle strength range from paresis (weakness) to paralysis (inability of a muscle group to overcome gravity). *Hemiparesis* refers to weakness on one side of the body; *hemiplegia* indicates paralysis on one side of the body. These conditions result from dysfunction, such as a tumor or cerebrovascular accident, in the brain or brain stem.

Paraplegia refers to paralysis of the lower extremities, whereas *quadriplegia* refers to paralysis of all four extremities. Both paraplegia and quadriplegia may be caused by dysfunction of the spinal cord. Upper cord damage results in quadriplegia, and lower cord damage preserves upper extremity function and causes paraplegia. (Spinal cord injury is discussed in Chapter 15.)

Hyperkinesia

Hyperkinesia (excessive movements) represents the second broad category of abnormal movements. Within this category are a number of specific dysfunctions (Table 14-16). Also included under the general category of hyperkinesias are dyskinesias, that is, abnormal involuntary movements.

Paroxysmal dyskinesias are abnormal, involuntary movements that occur as spasms. The type of dyskinesia varies depending on the specific disorder.

Tardive dyskinesia is the involuntary movement of the face, trunk, and extremities. Although the condition occurs occasionally in individuals with Parkinson disease, it usually occurs as a side effect of prolonged phenothiazine drug therapy. The most common symptom of tardive dyskinesia is rapid, repetitive, stereotypic movements. Most characteristic is continual chewing with intermittent protrusions of the tongue, lip smacking, and facial grimacing.

Other movement disorders in this category are (1) complex repetitive movements, including automatism, stereotype, complex tics, compulsions, perseverations, and mannerisms; (2) positivism (excessive reactions to certain stimuli); and (3) paroxysmal excessive activity, including cataplexy and excessive startle reaction.

Hypokinesia

Hypokinesia (decreased movement) is loss of voluntary movement despite preserved consciousness and normal peripheral nerve and muscle function. Types of hypokinesia include paresis/paralysis, akinesia, bradykinesia, and loss of associated movement.

Paresis/paralysis

Paresis (weakness) is partial paralysis with incomplete loss of muscle power. *Paralysis* is loss of motor function so that a muscle group is unable to overcome gravity. Two subtypes of paresis/paralysis are described: upper motor neuron paresis/paralysis and lower motor neuron paresis/paralysis (Table 14-17).[11]

TABLE 14-17	Upper and Lower Motor Neuron Syndromes	
Factor	**Upper Motor Neuron Syndromes***	**Lower Motor Neuron Syndromes†**
Distribution of affected muscles	Muscle groups are affected; when movement is possible, the proper relationship among agonists, antagonists, synergists, and fixators is preserved	Individual muscles may be affected
	Synkinesias (residual movements) are present; attempts to move paralyzed part cause a variety of associated movements; movements of normal limb may cause imitative or mirror movements in the paralyzed limb	Individual muscles may be affected
	Hypertonia, specifically spasticity	Hypotonia, flaccidity
Muscle tone	Hyperreflexia with extensor plantar reflex present	Hyporeflexia, no abnormal reflexes present
Tendon reflexes	Slight, caused by disuse	Pronounced atrophy
Atrophy	Absent	May be present

*Pyramidal motor syndromes.
†All are motor unit syndromes.

Upper motor neuron syndromes. Upper motor neuron paresis/paralysis is known also as spastic paresis/paralysis, and many different terms are used to describe the specific disorder. ***Hemiparesis/hemiplegia*** is paresis/paralysis of the upper and lower extremities on one side. ***Diplegia*** is paralysis of both upper or both lower extremities as a result of cerebral hemisphere injuries. ***Paraparesis/paraplegia*** refers to weakness/paralysis of the lower extremities. ***Quadriparesis/quadriplegia*** refers to paresis/paralysis of all four extremities. Both paraparesis/paraplegia and quadriparesis/quadriplegia may be caused by dysfunction of the spinal cord. Upper cord damage results in quadriparesis/quadriplegia, and lower cord damage preserves upper extremity function and causes paraparesis/paraplegia. (Spinal cord injury is discussed in Chapter 15.)

Upper motor neuron paresis/paralysis is associated with a ***pyramidal motor syndrome,*** which involves a series of motor dysfunctions resulting from interruption of the pyramidal system (Figs. 14-11 and 14-12). The injury may be in the cerebral cortex, the subcortical white matter, the internal capsule, the brain stem, or the spinal cord. The clinical manifestations of a pure pyramidal injury are not known, but bilateral interruption of the pyramidal system in monkeys causes temporary hypotonic paralysis. In humans, however, injury generally involves more than interrupting the pyramidal system, so that an upper motor neuron paralysis occurs, indicating involvement of several motor pathways. Excessive movements such as clonus and spasms occur regularly as a result of loss of higher motor center control. There is great variation depending on the suddenness of onset and the age of the individual.

Spinal shock is the complete cessation of spinal cord functions below the lesion (below the level of the pons). It is characterized by complete flaccid paralysis, absence of reflexes, and marked disturbances of bowel and bladder function. A major factor in spinal shock is the sudden destruction of the efferent pathways. If destruction occurs more slowly, spinal shock may not develop (see Chapter 15).

If the pyramidal system is interrupted above the level of the pons, the hand and arm muscles are greatly affected. Paralysis rarely involves all the muscles on one side of the body, even when the hemiplegia results from complete damage to the internal capsule. Bilateral movements, such as those of the eye, jaw, and larynx, as well as those of the trunk, are affected only slightly if at all. Predominantly the limbs are influenced.

Paralysis associated with a pyramidal motor syndrome rarely remains flaccid for a prolonged time. After a few days or weeks, a gradual return of spinal reflexes marks the end of spinal shock. Reflexes then become hyperactive, and muscle tone is significantly increased, particularly in antigravity muscles. Spasticity is common, although rigidity occasionally occurs. Most often, passive range-of-motion movements cause the "clasp-knife" phenomenon, probably by activating the stretch receptors in the muscle spindles and the Golgi tendon organ. (Muscle function is discussed in Chapter 36.) With pyramidal motor syndrome, predominantly the flexors of the arms and extensors of the legs are affected.

Lower motor neuron syndromes. Lower (primary, alpha) motor neurons are the large motor neurons in the anterior (or ventral) horn of the spinal cord, the motor nuclei of the brain stem, and the axons that originate from these nerve cell bodies (to course in the anterior spinal roots or in the cranial nerves to reach skeletal muscles) (Fig. 14-13). Dysfunction in this motor system impairs both voluntary and involuntary movement. The degree of paralysis or paresis is proportional to the number of lower motor neurons affected. If only a portion of the motor units that supply a muscle are affected, only partial paralysis (or paresis) results. If all motor units are affected, a complete paralysis results. Other clinical manifestations also are proportional to the degree of dysfunction, but the precise manifestations depend

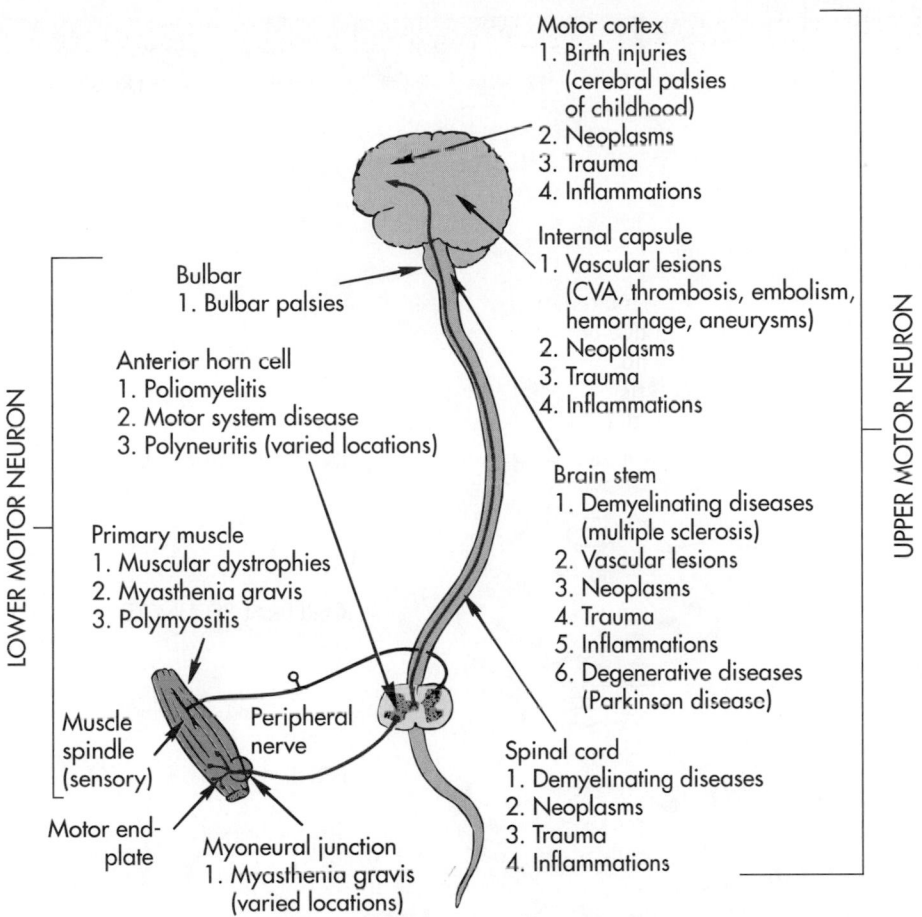

Fig. 14-11 *Disturbances in motor function.* Disturbances in motor function are classified pathologically along upper and lower motor neuron structures. It should be noted that the same pathologic condition occurs at more than one site in an upper motor neuron, *above right.* A few pathologic conditions involve both upper and lower motor neuron structures, as in amyotrophic lateral sclerosis, for example. Other lesion sites include myoneural junction and primary muscle, making it possible to classify conditions as neuromuscular and muscular, respectively. *CVA,* Cerebrovascular accident.

on the location of the dysfunction in the motor unit and in the CNS.

Small motor (gamma) neurons, which maintain muscle tone and protect the muscle from injury, are needed for normal motor movement. They depend on input from the muscle spindle (arriving through an afferent limb rising to the cord). Dysfunction in this motor system impairs tone and reduces the tendon reflexes, causing hyporeflexia. The muscles become susceptible to damage from hyperextensibility.

Generally, the large and small motor neuron systems are equally affected. Therefore the muscle has reduced or absent tone and is accompanied by hyporeflexia or *areflexia* (loss of tendon reflexes) and *flaccid paresis/paralysis.*

Denervated muscles (i.e., muscles that have lost their nervous system input) atrophy over weeks to months, mostly from disuse, and demonstrate fasciculations (muscle rippling or quivering under the skin). Occasionally, denervated muscles cramp. *Fibrillation* (isolated contraction of a single muscle fiber) also may occur, although it is not visible clinically.

Amyotrophies. Lower motor neuron syndromes originating in the anterior horn cells or the motor nuclei of the cranial nerves are called **amyotrophies.** Paralytic poliomyelitis is the prototype of these disorders. It involves a severe inflammatory reaction in motor neurons, some of which do not survive, leaving a permanent lower motor neuron syndrome.

A virally induced or postinfectious/postvaccination inflammatory process may injure or destroy anterior horn cells or cranial nerve cell bodies. Most of these inflammatory processes are mild and are followed by rapid cellular recovery.

In the amyotrophies, muscle strength, muscle tone, and muscle bulk are affected in the muscles innervated by the involved motor neurons. The paresis and paralysis associated with anterior horn cell injury are segmental, but because each muscle is supplied by two or more roots, the segmental character may be difficult to see. When cranial nerve motor nuclei are affected (these lack nerve roots and have only small rootlets near the point of exit from the brain stem), the distribution of the motor weakness follows that of the pe-

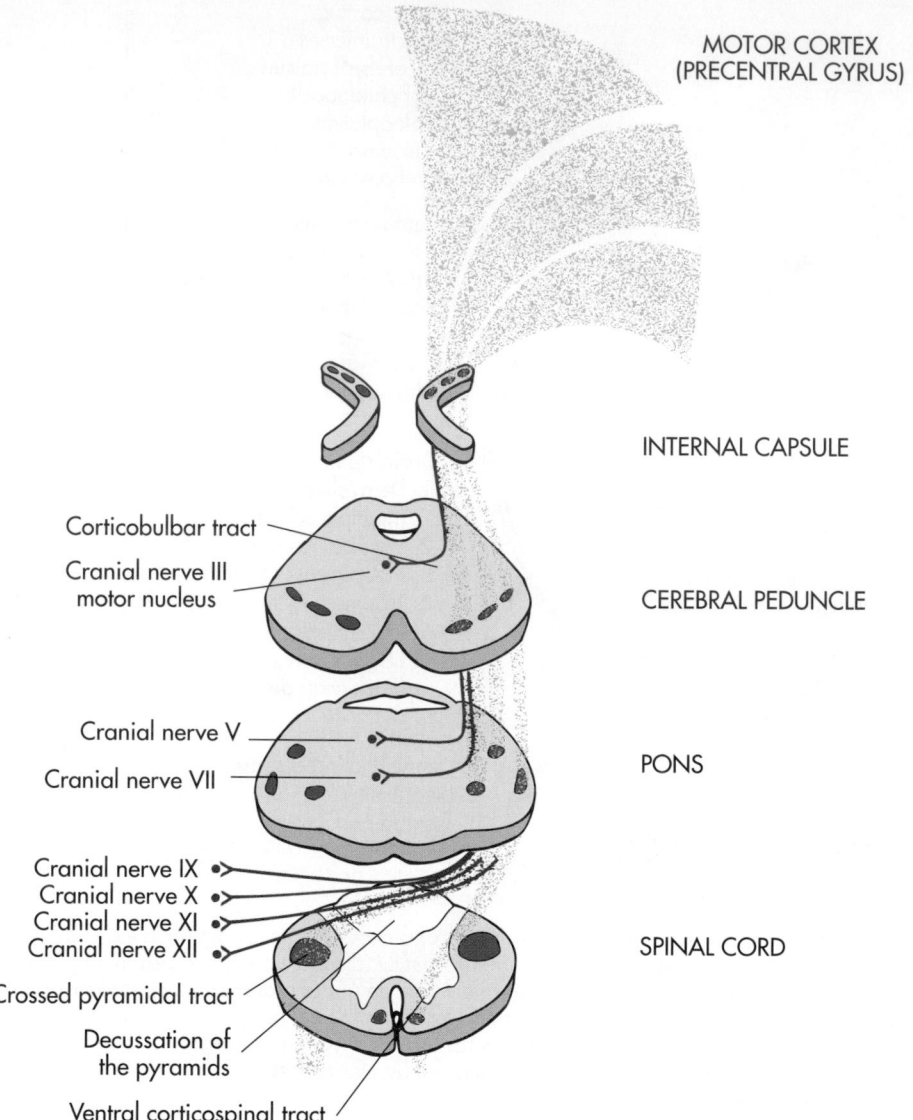

MOTOR CORTEX
(PRECENTRAL GYRUS)

INTERNAL CAPSULE

Corticobulbar tract

Cranial nerve III
motor nucleus

CEREBRAL PEDUNCLE

Cranial nerve V

Cranial nerve VII

PONS

Cranial nerve IX
Cranial nerve X
Cranial nerve XI
Cranial nerve XII

Crossed pyramidal tract

Decussation of
the pyramids

Ventral corticospinal tract

SPINAL CORD

Fig. 14-12 *Structures making up upper motor neuron, or pyramidal, system.* Pyramidal system fibers are shown to originate primarily in cells in precentral gyrus of motor cortex; to converge at internal capsule; to descend to form central third of cerebral peduncle; to descend further through pons, where small fibers are given off to cranial nerve motor nuclei along the way; to form pyramids at medulla, where most of the fibers decussate; and then to continue to descend in lateral column of white matter of spinal cord. A few fibers descend without crossing at medulla level.

ripheral nerve. The weakness may involve distal muscles, proximal muscles, or the muscles of midline structures. Hypotonia and hyporeflexia/areflexia are present.

The atrophy associated with amyotrophy is segmental when the anterior horn cells of the spinal cord are involved and follows the distribution of the peripheral nerve when the motor nuclei of the cranial nerves are affected. It may be in distal, proximal, or midline muscles. Fasciculations are associated particularly with primary motor neuron injury, and muscle cramps and mild fatigue are common. If the pathologic process is limited to the primary motor neuron, no sensory changes are evident.

Several brain stem syndromes, called *nuclear palsies,* in-

volve damage to one or more of the cranial nerve nuclei. Causes include vascular occlusion, tumor, aneurysm, tuberculosis, and hemorrhage.

The anterior horn cells and the motor nuclei of the cranial nerves may be secondarily affected in many severe pathologic processes involving primarily the peripheral nerves. The condition may extend proximally to affect the nerve roots or rootlets and the motor neurons themselves, a process commonly seen, for example, in Guillain-Barré syndrome. If enough motor neurons are destroyed, permanent loss of motor function results because regeneration of the damaged axons requires a living neuronal cell body.

In *progressive spinal muscular atrophy,* the anterior

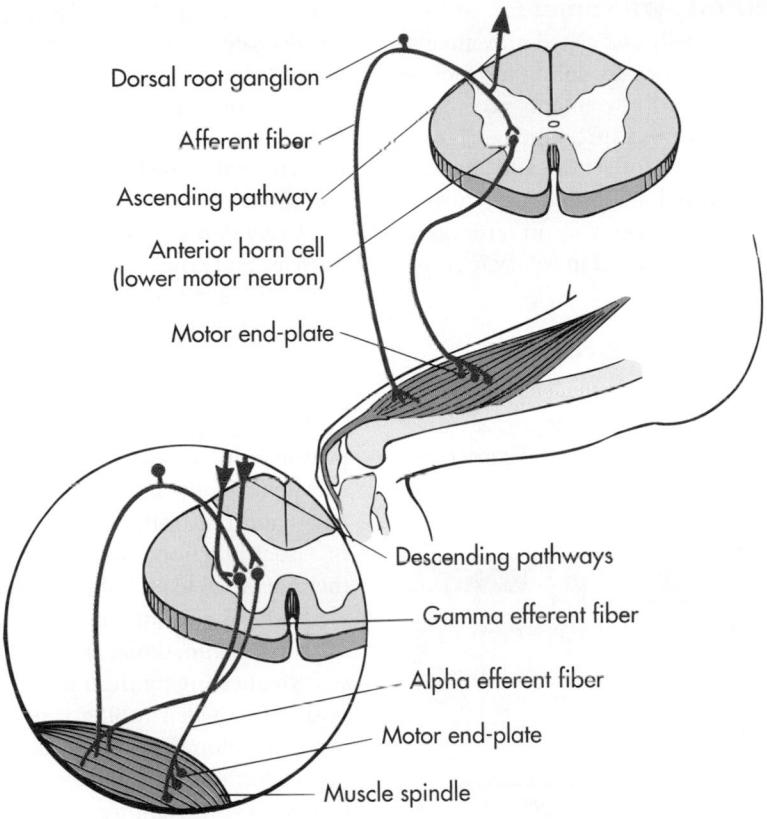

Fig. 14-13 *Structures making up lower motor neuron, including motor (efferent) and sensory (afferent) elements. Top,* Anterior horn cell (in anterior gray column of spinal cord and its axon), terminating in motor end plate as it innervates extrafusal muscle fibers in quadriceps muscle. *Detailed enlargement,* Sensory and motor elements of gamma loop system. Gamma efferent fibers shown innervating polar, or end, region of muscle spindle (sensory receptor of skeletal muscle). Contraction of muscle spindle fibers stretches central portion of spindle and causes afferent spindle fiber to transmit impulse centrally to cord. Muscle spindle afferent fibers in turn synapse on anterior horn cell and are transmitted by way of gamma efferent fibers to skeletal (extrafusal) muscle, causing it to contract. Muscle spindle discharge is interrupted by active contraction of extrafusal muscle fibers.

horn cells of the spinal cord are affected. This disorder occurs in adults and closely resembles the familial progressive muscular atrophies that occur in infants and children and are considered inherited metabolic disorders (see Chapter 38). If the motor nuclei of the cranial nerves are affected instead of the anterior horn cells, the disorder is *progressive bulbar palsy,* so named because the myelencephalon originally was called the *bulb* and a degenerative process causes a progressively more serious condition. When any lower motor neuron syndrome involves the cranial nerves that arise from the bulb (i.e., cranial nerves IX, X, XII), the dysfunction is called a *bulbar palsy.*

The clinical manifestations of bulbar palsy include paresis or paralysis of the jaw, face, pharynx, and tongue musculature. Articulation is affected, especially articulation of the lingual *(r, n, l),* labial *(b, m, p, f),* dental *(d, t),* and palatal *(k, g)* consonants. Modulation is impaired, making the voice rasping or nasal. Pharyngeal reflexes are diminished or lost, palate and vocal cord movement during phonation is im-

paired, and chewing and swallowing are affected. The facial muscles are weak, and the face appears to droop, with decreased jaw jerk. Atrophy and fasciculations eventually become apparent. All these manifestations become progressively worse, leading to aspiration, malnutrition, possible dehydration, and an inability to communicate verbally.

Akinesia and bradykinesia

Akinesia is a decrease in associated and voluntary movements. It is related to dysfunction of the extrapyramidal system and caused by either a deficiency of dopamine or a defect of the postsynaptic dopamine receptors, which occurs in parkinsonism (see Chapter 15). *Bradykinesia* is slowness of voluntary movements. All voluntary movements become slow, labored, and deliberate, with difficulty in (1) initiating movements, (2) continuing movements smoothly, and (3) performing synchronous (at the same time) and consecutive tasks. Both akinesia and bradykinesia involve a disturbance in the time it takes to perform a movement.

Loss of associated neuron syndromes

In hypokinesia the normal, habitually associated movements that provide skill, grace, and balance to voluntary movements are lost. Decreased associated movements accompanying emotional expression cause an expressionless face, a statuelike posture, absence of speech inflection, and absence of spontaneous gestures. Decreased associated movements accompanying locomotion cause reduction in arm and shoulder movements, in hip swinging, and in rotary motion of the cervical spine.

Alterations in Complex Motor Performance

The alterations in complex motor performance include disorders of posture (stance), disorders of gait, and disorders of expression.

HEALTH ALERT

Instability of Gait and Posture in Elderly Persons

Gait and balance abnormalities in elderly persons are associated with patchy white matter changes seen as hypodense areas on computed tomography (CT) or magnetic resonance imagery (MRI) scans.

Briley, D.P., Wasay, M., Sergent, S., & Thomas, S. (1997). Cerebral white matter changes (leukoaraiosis), stroke, and gait disturbance. Journal of American Geriatric Society, 45, 1434-1438; *Tell, G.S., Lefkowitz, S., Diehr, P., & Elster, A.D. (1998). Relationship between balance and abnormalities in cerebral magnetic resonance imaging in older adults.* Archives of Neurology, 55, 73-70.

Disorders of posture (stance)

When the tone in various muscle groups becomes unbalanced because of a loss of normal postural reflexes, posturing of limbs results. Equilibrium and balance are disrupted. Many reflex systems govern tone and posture, but the most important factor in posture control is the stretch reflex, in which extensor (antigravity) muscle stretching causes increased extensor tone and inhibited flexor tone. Four types of disorders of postures are (1) dystonic posture, (2) decerebrate posture, (3) basal ganglion posture, and (4) senile posture.

Dystonia is the maintenance of an abnormal posture through muscular contractions. When muscular contractions are sustained for several seconds, they are called *dystonic movements;* when contractions last for longer periods, they are called *dystonic postures.* Dystonic postures may last for weeks, causing permanent, fixed contractures. Dystonia has been associated with basal ganglia abnormality, but the exact pathophysiologic mechanisms are unknown. One dystonic posture already discussed in this chapter is decorticate (striatal posture or upper motor neuron dysfunction posture), which may be unilateral or bilateral. *Decorticate posture* (also referred to as *antigravity posture* or *hemiplegic posture*) is characterized by upper extremities flexed at the elbows and held close to the body and by lower extremities

that are externally rotated and extended (see Fig. 14-6). Decorticate posture is believed to occur when the brain stem is not inhibited by cerebral cortex motor function. Upper motor neuron posture is more commonly described as the arm flexed at the elbow with a wrist drop, the leg inadequately bent at the knee, the hip excessively circumabducted, and footdrop.

Decerebrate posture refers to increased tone in extensor muscles and trunk muscles, with active tonic neck reflexes. When the head is in a neutral position, all four limbs are rigidly extended. The decerebrate posture is caused by severe injury to the brain and brain stem, resulting in overstimulation of the postural righting and vestibular reflexes.

Basal ganglion posture refers to a stooped, hyperflexed posture with a narrow-based, short-stepped gait. This posture abnormality results from the loss of normal postural reflexes and not from defects in proprioceptive, labyrinthine, or visual function. Dysfunctional equilibrium results when the individual loses stability and cannot make the appropriate postural adjustment to tilting or loss of balance, falling instead. Dysfunctional righting is the inability to right oneself when changing from a lying or crouching to a standing position or when rolling from the supine to the lateral or prone position. Dysfunctional postural fixation is the involuntary flexion of the head and neck, causing the person difficulty in maintaining an upright trunk position while standing or walking. Basal ganglion dysfunction accounts for this posture.

Senile posture is characterized by an increasingly flexed posture similar to that caused by basal ganglion dysfunction. The posture is associated with frontal lobe dysfunction, but the primary pathophysiology is not known.

Disorders of gait

Four predominant types of gait are (1) upper motor neuron dysfunction gait, (2) cerebellar (ataxic) gait, (3) basal ganglion gait, and (4) senile gait (pseudoparkinsonian gait). As with posture, equilibrium and balance are affected with gait disturbances.

Several upper motor neuron gaits exist. With mild forms, the individual may have footdrop with fatigue and hip and leg pain. A *spastic gait,* which is associated with unilateral injury, manifests by a shuffling gait with the leg extended and held stiff, causing a scraping over the floor surface. The leg swings improperly around the body rather than being appropriately lifted and placed. The foot may drag on the ground, and the person tends to fall to the affected side. A *scissors gait* is associated with bilateral injury and spasticity. The legs are abducted so they touch each other. As the person walks, the legs are swung around the body but then cross in front of each other because of adduction. Injury to the pyramidal system accounts for these gaits.

A *cerebellar gait* is wide-based with the feet apart and often turned outward or inward for greater stability. The pelvis is held stiff, and the individual staggers when walking. Cerebellar dysfunction accounts for this particular gait.

A *basal ganglion gait* and a *senile gait* are both broad-based gaits in which the person walks with small steps and a decreased arm swing. The head and body are flexed and the arms semiflexed and abducted while the legs are flexed and rigid in more advanced states. Basal ganglion and frontal lobe dysfunction, respectively, account for these two gaits.

Disorders of expression

Disorders of expression involve the motor aspects of communication and include (1) hypermimesis, (2) hypomimesis, and (3) dyspraxias/apraxias. Hypermimesis commonly manifests as pathologic laughter or crying. Pathologic laughter is associated with right hemisphere injury, and pathologic crying is associated with left hemisphere injury. The exact pathophysiology is not known. Hypomimesis manifests as aprosody—the loss of emotional language. Receptive aprosody involves an inability to understand emotion in speech and facial expression, whereas expressive aprosody involves the inability to express emotion in speech and facial expression. Aprosody is associated with right hemisphere damage.

Dyspraxia/apraxia is the inability to perform purposeful or skilled motor acts in the absence of paralysis, sensory loss, abnormal posture and tone, abnormal involuntary movement, incoordination, or inattentiveness. It is associated with vascular disorders, trauma, tumors, degenerative disorders, infections, and metabolic disorders. Because the performance of any activity is composed of three parts—(1) the development of the idea, (2) the formulation of the plan of execution, and (3) the motor performance of the activity—three types of dyspraxia have been described. Dyspraxia may also be related to specific types of motor activity (Table 14-18).

True dyspraxias occur when the connecting pathways between the left and right cortical areas are interrupted (Fig. 14-14). Dyspraxias may result from any pathologic process that disrupts the cortical areas necessary for the conceptualization and execution of a complex motor act or the communication pathways within the left hemisphere or between the hemispheres.

> ### ✓ QUICK CHECK
>
> Why are there so many causes of hypertonia?
>
> How is chorea different from athetosis?
>
> Why is paresis/paralysis a type of hypokinesia?
>
> What structures are involved in alterations of complex motor performance?

Extrapyramidal Motor Syndromes

Because the extrapyramidal system encompasses all the motor pathways except the pyramidal system, two types of motor dysfunction make up the *extrapyramidal motor syndromes:* (1) the basal ganglia motor syndromes and (2) the cerebellar motor syndromes.[9] Unlike pyramidal motor syn-

Fig. 14-14 *Pathways disrupted in dyspraxias.* Formulation of the idea of the motor act is believed to originate in the region of the supramarginal gyrus in the inferior left parietal lobe. This area is connected via associational pathways to the left premotor cortex. The left premotor cortex is connected through the corpus callosum to the right premotor and motor areas. An injury that interrupts the pathways between the left supramarginal gyrus and the premotor region produces a dyspraxia that involves the entire body. An injury that disrupts the callosal pathways produces a dyspraxia of the left side of the body only.

dromes, both extrapyramidal motor syndromes result in movement or posture disturbance without significant paralysis, along with other distinctive symptoms (Table 14-19).

Basal ganglia motor syndromes

Basal ganglia motor syndromes involve either a paucity or an excess of movements. Stress and nervous tension typically worsen the symptoms, whereas relaxation improves motor performance. Akinesia may occur despite normal strength. Involuntary movements, such as tremor, chorea, ballism, athetosis, and dystonia, also may occur and probably are caused by loss of the normal modulating effects of the basal ganglia.

Basal ganglia motor syndromes also are characterized by alterations in muscle tone and posture. Rigidity and the cogwheel phenomenon are present in all muscle groups but most prominent in those that maintain flexed position. Postural abnormalities result from the loss of normal postural reflexes. Dysfunctional equilibrium results from the loss of postural stability.

Basal ganglia motor syndromes are caused by an imbalance of dopaminergic and cholinergic activity in the corpus striatum. A relative excess of cholinergic activity produces akinesia and hypertonia. A relative excess of dopaminergic activity produces hyperkinesia and hypotonia.

Cerebellar motor syndromes

Cerebellar motor syndromes involve the cerebellum and may result in (1) loss of muscle tone, (2) difficulty with coordination of voluntary movements, (3) minor degrees of muscle

TABLE 14-18   The Dyspraxias

Types	Description	Location
Dyspraxias describing the components of a motor act		
Ideational	Impaired ability to comprehend, grasp an idea, or retain the idea of the described act	Diffuse cortical injury, general suppression of cortex
Ideomotor (ideokinetic)	Impaired ability to formulate an organized idea of action (but habitual motor acts may be performed spontaneously or repetitiously)	Left hemisphere dysfunction in the posterosuperior area of temporal lobe and in the inferior areas of parietal and frontal lobes
Motor (limb, kinetic)	Impaired use of kinesthetic memory patterns (engrams) necessary to perform a motor act; automatic tone and position changes necessary for action do not occur	Premotor area dysfunction, usually limited to contralateral extremity
Dyspraxias related to specific types of motor activity		
Constructional	Impaired ability to draw or use shapes and designs accurately	Visual association area dysfunction and with posterior parietal lobe injury; more severe when right posterior hemisphere is involved rather than left hemisphere because right parietooccipital area controls visuospatial orientation
Dressing	Impaired ability to clothe oneself correctly; agnosia and neglect syndrome contribute to dressing dyspraxia and may be entirely responsible for its occurrence	Right parietal injury
Speech	An articulation disorder resulting from impaired capacity to program positioning of speech muscles and sequencing of muscle movements for volitional production of speech sounds (phonemes); a motor dyspraxia	Dysfunction in Broca area in left hemisphere
	When involvement is more extensive than just the muscles used in speech articulation, the dysfunction is called *facial dyspraxia*	Dysfunction in Broca area and premotor areas controlling the facial muscles
Gait (frontal lobe ataxia, frontal lobe gait)	Impaired ability to use extremities effectively and in coordinated manner during ambulation, producing a low, shuffling gait with small, hesitant steps	Loss of integration between cortex and basal ganglion related to stance and locomotion; not a true dyspraxia because dysfunction is not purely cortical
Callosal	An ideomotor dyspraxia in which right arm and leg use is normal but with impaired ability to perform the same movements with left arm and leg	Anterior corpus callosum injury

TABLE 14-19   Pyramidal Versus Extrapyramidal Motor Syndrome

Manifestations	Pyramidal Motor Syndrome	Extrapyramidal Motor Syndrome
Unilateral movement	Paralysis of voluntary movement	Little or no paralysis of voluntary movement
Tendon reflexes	Increased tendon reflexes	Normal or slightly increased tendon reflexes
Babinski sign	Present	Absent
Involuntary movements	Absence of involuntary movements	Presence of tremor, chorea, athetosis, or dystonia
Muscle tone	Spasticity in muscles (e.g., clasp-knife phenomenon)	Plastic (equal throughout movement) rigidity or intermittent (generalized but predominantly in flexors of limbs and trunk) rigidity (cogwheel rigidity)
	Hypertonia present in flexors of arms and extensors of legs	Hypotonia in cerebellar disease

weakness, tendency toward fatigue, and impairment of associated movements, and (4) disorders of equilibrium and gait. Cerebellar effects primarily influence the same side of the body, so that damage to the right cerebellum generally causes symptoms on the right side of the body. Predominant symptoms depend on the area of damage within the cerebellum.

It should be noted that the nervous system often can operate well despite destruction of parts of the cerebellum, although the mechanisms responsible for this retained function are not fully understood.

◻ DID YOU UNDERSTAND?

Alterations in Cognitive Networks

1. Full consciousness is an awareness of oneself and the environment with an ability to respond to external stimuli with a wide variety of responses.
2. Consciousness has two components: arousal and content of thought.
3. Decreased level of arousal occurs by diffuse bilateral cortical dysfunction, bilateral subcortical (reticular formation, brain stem) dysfunction, and localized hemispheric dysfunction.
4. An alteration in breathing pattern and level of coma reflect the level of brain dysfunction.
5. Pupillary changes reflect changes in level of brain stem function, drug action, and response to hypoxia and ischemia.
6. Abnormal eye movements, including nystagmus and divergent gaze, reflect alterations in brain stem function.
7. Level of brain function manifests by changes in generalized motor responses or no responses.
8. Loss of cortical inhibition associated with decreased consciousness includes abnormal flexor and extensor movements.
9. Cerebral death or irreversible coma represents permanent brain damage, with an ability to maintain cardiac, respiratory, and other vital functions.
10. Brain death results from irreversible brain damage, with an inability to maintain internal homeostasis.
11. Arousal returns in vegetative states, but content of thought is absent.
12. Seizures represent a sudden, chaotic discharge of cerebral neurons, with transient alterations in brain function. Seizures may be generalized or focal and can result from cerebral lesions, biochemical disorders, trauma, or epilepsy.
13. With a deficit in selective attention, mediated by midbrain, thalamus, and parietal lobe structures, the individual cannot focus on selective stimuli and thus neglects those stimuli.
14. In dysmnesia and amnesia, some past memories are lost and new memories cannot be stored.
15. Frontal areas mediate vigilance, detection, and working memory.
16. With vigilance deficits, the person cannot maintain alertness.
17. With detection deficits, the person is unmotivated and unable to set goals and plan.
18. Some specific disorders of content of thought (cognition) are agnosias, dysphasias, acute confusional states, and dementias.

19. Agnosias are a defect of recognition and may be tactile, visual, or auditory. They are caused by dysfunction in the primary sensory area or the interpretive areas of the cerebral cortex.
20. Dysphasia is an impairment of comprehension or production of language. Dysphasia may be expressive or sensory.
21. Aphasia is loss of language comprehension or production.
22. Wernicke dysphasia is a disturbance in understanding all language, both verbal and reading comprehension.
23. Conductive dysphasias result from disruption of temporal lobe fibers, with a failure to repeat words but an ability to initiate speech, writing, and reading aloud.
24. Anomic dysphasia is an inability to name objects, persons, or qualities.
25. Transcortical dysphasias involve an inability to repeat and recite.
26. Broca aphasia is an expressive dysphasia of speech and writing but with retention of comprehension.
27. Global aphasia involves both anterior and posterior speech areas, with both expressive and receptive aphasia.
28. Acute confusional states are characterized chiefly by a loss of detection and, in the case of delirium, an intense autonomic nervous system hyperactivity.

Alterations in Cerebral Homeostasis

1. Increased intracranial pressure may result from edema, excess cerebrospinal fluid, hemorrhage, or tumor growth. When intracranial pressure approaches arterial pressure, hypoxia and hypercapnia produce brain damage.
2. Cerebral edema is an increase in the fluid content of the brain resulting from infection, hemorrhage, tumor, ischemia, infarct, or hypoxia.
3. The shifting or herniation of brain tissue from one compartment to another disrupts the blood flow of both compartments and damages brain tissue.
4. Supratentorial herniation involves temporal lobe and hippocampal gyrus shifting from the middle fossa to posterior fossa; transtentorial herniation with a downward shift of the diencephalon through the tentorial notch; and shifting of the cingulate gyrus herniation under the falx.
5. The most common infratentorial herniation is a shift of the cerebellar tonsils through the foramen magnum.

Continued

▣ DID YOU UNDERSTAND? —cont'd

Alterations in Cerebral Homeostasis—cont'd

6. Hydrocephalus comprises a variety of disorders characterized by an excess of fluid within the cranial vault, subarachnoid space, or both. Hydrocephalus occurs because of interference with cerebrospinal fluid flow caused by increased fluid production or obstruction within the ventricular system or by defective reabsorption of the fluid.

Alterations in Motor Function

1. Motor dysfunction may be characterized as alterations of motor tone, movement, and complex motor performance.
2. Hypotonia and hypertonia are the main categories of altered tone.
3. The four types of hypertonia are spasticity, gegenhalten, dystonia, and rigidity.
4. Hyperkinesia and hypokinesia are the main categories of altered movement.
5. Included in the category of hyperkinesia are chorea, athetosis, ballism, akathisia, tremor, and myoclonus.
6. Types of hypokinesia include paresis/paralysis, akinesia, bradykinesia, and loss of associated movements.
7. Two subtypes of paresis/paralysis are described: upper motor neuron paresis/paralysis and lower motor neuron paresis/paralysis.
8. An upper motor neuron syndrome is characterized by paresis/paralysis, hypertonia, and hyperreflexia.
9. Interruption of the pyramidal tract below the pons results in spinal shock.
10. Lower motor neuron syndromes manifest by impaired voluntary and involuntary movements and flaccid paralysis.
11. Partial paralysis occurs with only partial loss of alpha motor neurons, and total paralysis is complete loss of alpha motor neurons. Loss of gamma motor neurons impairs muscle tone and decreases tendon reflexes.
12. Amyotrophy (e.g., poliomyelitis) is a lower motor neuron syndrome involving the anterior horn cells, with loss of muscle tone and strength resulting in segmental paresis and hyporeflexia.
13. Nuclear palsies involve damage to the cranial nerve nuclei.
14. Bulbar palsies involve cranial nerves IX, X, and XII.
15. Alterations in complex motor performance include disorders of posture (stance), disorders of gait, and disorders of expression.
16. Disorders of posture include dystonic posture, decerebrate posture, basal ganglion posture, and senile posture.
17. Disorders of gait include upper motor neuron gaits, cerebellar gait, basal ganglion gait, and senile gait.
18. Disorders of expression include hypermimesis, hypomimesis, and dyspraxia/apraxia.
19. Dyspraxia is an impairment of the conceptualization or execution of a complex motor act.
20. Extrapyramidal motor syndromes include basal ganglia and cerebellar motor syndromes.
21. Basal ganglia disorders manifest by alterations in muscle tone and posture, including rigidity, involuntary movements, and loss of postural reflexes.
22. Cerebellar motor syndromes result in loss of muscle tone, difficulty with coordination, and disorders of equilibrium and gait.

KEY TERMS

Acute confusional state, 363
Acute hydrocephalus, 369
Agnosia, 362
Akinesia, 377
Amyotrophy, 375
Antigravity posture, 378
Aphasia, 362
Apraxia, 379
Areflexia, 375
Arousal, 351
Aura, 359
Autoregulation, 367
Basal ganglia motor syndrome, 379
Basal ganglion gait, 378
Basal ganglion posture, 378
Bradykinesia, 377

Brain death, 355
Bulbar palsy, 377
Cerebellar gait, 378
Cerebellar motor syndrome, 379
Cerebral death, 355
Cerebral edema, 368
Clonic phase, 359
Clonus, 371
Communicating hydrocephalus, 369
Content of thought, 351
Cytotoxic (metabolic) edema, 368
Decerebrate posture, 378
Decorticate posture (antigravity posture, hemiplegic posture), 378
Diplegia, 374
Dysphasia, 362

Dyspraxia, 379
Dystonia, 371, 378
Dystonic movement, 378
Dystonic posture, 378
Echolalia, 363
Epilepsy, 356
Epileptogenic focus, 359
Expressive dysphasia, 363
Extinction, 362
Extrapyramidal motor syndrome, 379
Fibrillation, 375
Flaccid paresis/paralysis, 375
Gegenhalten (paratonia), 371
Hemiparesis, 373, 374
Hemiplegia, 373, 374
Hemiplegic posture, 378

KEY TERMS

Hydrocephalus, 369
Hyperkinesia, 373
Hypertonia, 371
Hypotonia, 370
Increased intracranial pressure
    (IICP), 366
Interstitial edema, 369
Intracranial pressure (ICP), 366
Ischemic edema, 368
Locked-in syndrome, 355
Metabolic arousal alteration, 351
Mirror focus, 359
Neglect syndrome, 362
Noncommunicating hydrocephalus
    (internal hydrocephalus,
    intraventricular hydrocephalus), 369
Normal-pressure hydrocephalus, 370

Nuclear palsy, 376
Paralysis, 373
Paraparesis, 374
Paraplegia, 373, 374
Paresis, 373
Paroxysmal dyskinesia, 373
Prodroma, 359
Progressive bulbar palsy, 377
Progressive spinal muscular atrophy,
    376
Psychogenic arousal alteration, 351
Pyramidal motor syndrome (upper
    motor neuron syndrome), 374
Quadriparesis, 374
Quadriplegia, 373, 374
Rigidity, 371
Scissors gait, 378

Seizure, 356
Selective attention deficit, 362
Senile gait, 378
Senile posture, 378
Sensory inattentiveness, 362
Spastic gait, 378
Spasticity, 371
Spinal shock, 374
Structural arousal alteration, 351
Tardive dyskinesia, 373
Tonic phase, 359
Transcortical dysphasia, 363
Upper motor neuron paresis/paralysis,
    374
Vasogenic edema, 368
Vegetative state, 351

REFERENCES

1. Taylor, R.M. (1997). Reexamining the definition and criteria of death. *Seminars in Neurology, 17*(3), 265-270.
2. The Multi-Society Task Force on Persistent Vegetative State. (1994). Medical aspects of the persistent vegetative state. *New England Journal of Medicine, 330*(21), 1499-1508.
3. American Association of Neuroscience Nurses. (1997). *Seizure assessment.* Chicago: The Author.
4. Posner, M. II & Raichle, M.E. (1994). *Images of mind.* New York: Scientific American Library.
5. Vaina, I.M. (1994). Functional segregation of color and motion processing in the human visual cortex. *Cerebral Cortex, 4*(5), 555-572.
6. Bower, B. (1998). Family gives genetic clue to language. *Scientific News, 153*(4), 71.
7. Feske, S.K. (1998). Coma and confusional states: Emergency diagnosis and management. *Neurology Clinics, 16*(2), 237-256.
8. American Association of Neuroscience Nurses. (1997). *Intracranial pressure monitoring.* Chicago: The Author.
9. Hariri, R.J. (1994). Cerebral edema. *Neurosurgery Clinics of North America, 5*(4), 687-706.
10. Del Bigio, M.R. (1997). Biological reactions to cerebrospinal fluid shunt devices: A review of the cellular pathology. *Neurosurgery, 42*(2), 319-326.
11. Goetz, C.G., Pappert, E.J. (1999). *Textbook of clinical neurology.* Philadelphia: Saunders.

CHAPTER

15

Alterations of Neurologic Function

Barbara J. Boss and Judith A. Farley

Alterations in central nervous system (CNS) function are caused by traumatic injury, vascular disorders, tumor growth, infectious and inflammatory processes, metabolic derangements (including those arising from nutritional deficiencies and drugs or chemicals), and degenerative processes. Alterations in peripheral nervous system function involve the nerve roots (radiculopathies), a nerve plexus, or the nerves themselves (neuropathies). Disorders of the neuromuscular junction occur also.

CHAPTER OUTLINE

 Check out your CD Companion for chapter-related exercises and answers to the Quick Check questions

CENTRAL NERVOUS SYSTEM DISORDERS
Trauma
Head trauma

Major head injury is defined by the National Head Injury Foundation as a traumatic insult to the brain capable of producing physical, intellectual, emotional, social, and vocational changes. Persons at highest risk for traumatic brain injury (TBI) are young persons 15 to 30 years of age, infants 6 months to 2 years, young school-age children, and elderly persons. The male/female ratio for such injury is 3:1. Traumatic brain injury is highest among blacks and in lower−median income families. Persons living in areas with high crime rates are at greater risk.

Head injuries are broadly categorized into *closed (blunt) trauma* and *open (penetrating) trauma.* Blunt trauma is more common and involves the head striking a hard surface or a rapidly moving object striking the head. The dura remains intact, and brain tissues are not exposed to the environment. Blunt trauma may result in both focal brain injuries and diffuse axonal injuries (Table 15-1). When a break in (penetration of) the dura results in exposure of the cranial contents to the environment, open trauma has occurred, which results in focal brain injuries.

The most common types of traumatic brain injury (75% to 90%) are mild concussion and classical cerebral concussion (see p. 389). Focal brain injury and diffuse axonal injury (DAI) each account for half of all injuries. Focal brain injury accounts for more than two thirds of head injury deaths; DAI for fewer than one third. However, more severely disabled survivors, including those in an unresponsive state (Table 15-2), have DAI.

In recent years, the surviving traumatic head injury population has changed, mostly because of focus on reducing severity of injury (e.g., passive seat restraints, air bags), reduced transport time, and improved on-the-scene medical management. Improved management of secondary and tertiary injury also influences the situation; acute care health professionals focus more on morbidity than mortality. As a result, persons with more severe traumatic brain injuries are being admitted to rehabilitation programs.

Cause

Most traumatic brain injuries are caused by transportation-related events, falls, sports-related events, and violence. The causative mechanisms are summarized in Table 15-3.

Pathophysiology

Three mechanisms produce damage: primary, secondary, and tertiary injury. Primary injury is caused by the impact and involves neural injury, primary glial injury, and vascular response. Two types of primary injury may occur—focal and diffuse brain injury.

Focal brain injury. *Focal brain injuries* are specific, grossly observable brain lesions—cortical contusions, epidural

hemorrhage, subdural hematoma, and intracerebral hematoma. The force of impact typically produces *contusions* from direct contact (as well as injury to the vault, vessels, and supporting structures) that, in turn, produces epidural hemorrhage and subdural and intracerebral hematomas. The mechanisms of injury are depicted in Fig. 15-1. Damage results from compression of the skull at the point of impact and rebound effect. Contusion and bleeding occur from small tears in blood vessels caused by these forces. The severity of contusion varies with the amount of energy transmitted by the skull to underlying brain tissue. In addition, the smaller the area of impact, the greater the severity of injury because the force is concentrated into a smaller area. The focal injury may be coup or contrecoup. Brain edema forms around and in damaged neural tissues, contributing to the increasing intracranial pressure. Within the contused areas, infarction, necrosis, multiple hemorrhages, and edema occur. The tissue has a pulpy quality. The maximum effects of these injuries peak 18 to 36 hours after severe head injury.

Contusions are found most commonly in the frontal lobes, particularly at the poles and along the inferior orbital surfaces; in the temporal lobes, especially in the anterior poles and along the inferior surface; and at the frontotemporal junction. They result in changes in attention, memory, executive attention functions (see Chapter 14), affect, emotion, and behavior. Less commonly, contusions occur in the parietal and occipital lobes. Focal cerebral contusions are superficial, involving just the gyri. Hemorrhagic contusions may coalesce into a large confluent intracranial hematoma.

Extradural hematomas (epidural hematomas, epidural hemorrhages) represent 1% to 2% of major head injuries and occur in all age-groups, but most commonly in 20- to 40-year-olds. An artery is the source of bleeding in 85% of extradural hematomas; 15% result from injury to the meningeal vein or dural sinus. The temporal fossa is the most common site of extradural hematoma caused by injury to the middle meningeal artery or vein. The temporal lobe shifts medially, precipitating uncal and hippocampal gyrus herniation through the tentorial notch. Extradural hemorrhages are found occasionally in the subfrontal area, especially in the young and elderly populations, caused by injury to the anterior meningeal artery or a venous sinus, and in the occipital-suboccipital area, resulting in herniation of the posterior fossa contents through the foramen magnum.

Subdural hematomas arise in 10% to 20% of persons with traumatic brain injury. Acute subdural hematomas develop rapidly, commonly within hours, and usually are located at the top of the skull (the cerebral convexities). Bilateral hematomas occur in 15% to 20% of persons. Subacute subdural hematomas develop more slowly, often over 48 hours to 2 weeks. Chronic subdural hematomas (commonly found in elderly persons and persons who abuse alcohol who have some degree of brain atrophy with a subsequent increase in extradural space) develop over weeks to months. Bridging veins tear, causing both rapidly and subacutely de-

TABLE 15-1 Severity of Trauma Related to Trauma Injury, Onset of Clinical Manifestations, and Persistence of Clinical Manifestations

Severity of Trauma	Trauma State Induced		Onset of Clinical Manifestations	Persistence of DAI Clinical Manifestations
	Focal Injury	DAI		
Mild blunt trauma Moderate blunt trauma		Mild concussion	Immediate	Hours to days
		Classic cerebral concussion	Immediate	Up to 6 mo or longer
	Paraplegia (associated with injury to top of head)		Immediate	
	Blindness (associated with occipital injury)		Immediate	
	Delayed development of unresponsiveness (vaso-motor or vasovagal syn-copal episode)		Delayed	
Severe blunt trauma		Mild DAI	Immediate	Permanent Residual
		Moderate DAI	Immediate	
		Severe DAI	Immediate	
	Acute epidural hemorrhage		Immediate to delayed (2-3 hr)	
	Acute contusional swelling		Delayed onset (few hours after injury)	
	Acute subdural hematoma		Delayed onset (few hours to 1 wk after injury)	
	Subacute subdural hema-toma*		Delayed onset (1 to few weeks)	
	Subdural hygroma (fluid accumulation)		Delayed onset	
	Traumatic cerebral hemor-rhage*		Delayed onset (as late as 1 wk after injury)	

May be seen after moderate head injury, especially in elderly people.

TABLE 15-2 Prognosis Related to DAI

	1 Month	3 Months
Mild DAI		78% good recovery or moderate disability
		3% severe disability
		15% die, usually of secondary infection complications or associated extracranial injuries
		4% unaccounted for
Moderate DAI	26% good or moderate disability	38% good recovery
		20% moderate disability
	50% severe disability	18% severe disability
	24% die of complications	
Severe DAI		15% good recovery
		27% moderate to severe disability

veloping subdural hematomas, although torn cortical veins or venous sinuses and contused tissue also may be the source. These subdural hematomas act like expanding masses, increasing intracranial pressure that eventually compresses the bleeding vessels (Fig. 15-2). Herniation syndrome can result.

With a chronic subdural hematoma the existing subdural space gradually fills with blood. A vascular membrane forms around the hematoma in approximately 2 weeks. Further enlargement may take place.

Intracerebral hematomas occur in 2% to 3% of persons with head injuries, may be single or multiple, and are associated with contusions. Although most commonly located in the frontal and temporal lobes, they may occur in the hemispheric deep white matter. Small blood vessels are traumatized by penetrating injury or shearing forces. The intracere-

TABLE 15-3	Causes of Brain Injuries
Type of Injury	**Mechanism**
Coup and contrecoup	Object strikes the front (coup) or rear (coup + contrecoup) of the head; object strikes side of head (coup or contrecoup); head strikes immovable object with little velocity
Extradural hematoma	Vehicular accidents, minor falls, sporting accidents
Subdural hematoma	Vehicular accidents or falls, especially in elderly persons or persons with chronic alcohol abuse
Intracerebral hemorrhage	Contusions caused by forceful impact, usually vehicular accidents or falls from a distance
Compound fracture	Objects strike head with great force or head strikes object forcefully; temporal blows, occipital blows, upward impact of cervical vertebrae (basilar skull fracture)
Penetrating injury	Missiles (bullets) or sharp projectiles (knives, ice picks, axes, screwdrivers)
Diffuse axonal injury	Moving head strikes hard, unyielding surface or moving object strikes stationary head; vehicular accidents (occupant or pedestrian); torsional head motion

Fig. 15-1 *Coup and contrecoup head injury after blunt trauma.* *1,* Coup injury: impact against object; *a,* site of impact and direct trauma to brain; *b,* shearing of subdural veins; *c,* trauma to base of brain. *2,* Contrecoup injury: impact within skull; *a,* site of impact from brain hitting opposite side of skull; and *b,* shearing forces through brain. These injuries occur in one continuous motion—the head strikes the wall (coup) and then rebounds (contrecoup). *(Modified from Rudy, E.B. [1984]. Advanced neurological and neurosurgical nursing.* St. Louis: Mosby.)

Fig. 15-2 *Acute subdural hematoma (dura removed).* Leptomeninges are intact. *(From Damjanov, I. & Linder, J. [1996]. Anderson's pathology [10th ed.]. St. Louis: Mosby.)*

bral hematoma then acts as an expanding mass, increasing intracranial pressure, compressing brain tissues, and causing edema (Fig. 15-3). Delayed intracerebral hematomas may appear 3 to 10 days after the head injury.

Open trauma produces discrete (focal) injuries and includes compound fractures and missile injuries. A compound fracture opens a communication between the cranial contents and the environment and should be investigated whenever lacerations of the scalp, tympanic membrane, sinuses, eye, or mucous membranes are present. Such fractures may involve the cranial vault or the base of the skull (basilar skull fracture). Bone fragments cause tangential injury (injury caused by direct contact) and, occasionally, pen-

Fig. 15-3 *Hematomas.* Recent hematomas, resulting from trauma, in frontal lobes. *(From Kissane, J.M. [Ed.]. [1990]. Anderson's pathology [9th ed.]. St. Louis: Mosby.)*

TABLE 15-4	Categories of Diffuse Brain Injury
Type of Injury	**Mechanism**
Mild concussion	Temporary axonal disturbance affecting attentional and memory systems; consciousness not lost
Grade I	Confusion and disorientation with amnesia (momentary)
Grade II	Momentary confusion and retrograde amnesia after 5-10 min
Grade III	Confusion and retrograde amnesia from impact; also anterograde amnesia
Classic cerebral concussion	Same as grade IV mild concussion—diffuse cerebral disconnection from brain stem reticular activating system; physiologic neurologic dysfunction without substantial anatomic disruption; immediate loss of consciousness lasting less than 6 hr; retrograde and anterograde amnesia (posttraumatic); may be uncomplicated or complicated
Diffuse axonal injury (DAI)	Prolonged traumatic coma (longer than 6 hr)
Mild	Posttraumatic coma lasts 6-24 hr; death uncommon; persistent residual cognitive, psychologic, and sensorimotor deficits; rare—only 8% of severe head injuries
Moderate	Widespread physiologic impairment throughout the cerebral cortex and diencephalon; actual tearing of axons in both hemispheres; prolonged coma (longer than 24 hr); incomplete recovery among survivors; common—20% of severe head injuries
Severe	Formerly called primary brain stem injury or brain stem contusion; severe mechanical disruption of axons in both hemispheres, diencephalon, and brain stem; 15% of severe head injuries

etrating injuries. Cranial nerves may be damaged with a basilar skull fracture.

Missiles include bullets, rocks, shell fragments, knives, and blunt instruments. They cause tangential injury to the coverings and the brain (scalp and brain lacerations), skull fractures, laceration of the meninges, and cerebral lacerations. Projectiles and debris from scalp and skull injury, when driven into the brain substance, produce a penetrating brain injury. Occasionally, projectiles are so forceful that they pass completely through the cranial vault.

Diffuse brain injury. **Diffuse brain injury** (diffuse axonal injury [DAI]) results from a shaking effect (inertial effects of mechanical input to the head associated with high levels of acceleration and deceleration, effects of head motion). Rotational acceleration (twisting movement) is the primary mechanism of injury, producing strains and distortions within the brain (see Fig. 15-1). The freely moving head is attached to the neck, allowing rotational forces to set up shearing forces on brain tissues. The most severe axonal injuries are located more peripheral to the brain stem, causing extensive cognitive and affective impairments, as seen in survivors of traumatic brain injury from vehicular crashes. Damage reduces the speed of informational processing and responding and disrupts attention.

Pathophysiologically, axonal damage can be seen only with an electron microscope and involves numerous axons, either alone or in conjunction with actual tissue tears. Areas where axons and small blood vessels are torn appear as small hemorrhages, particularly in the corpus callosum and dorsolateral quadrant of the rostral brain stem at the superior cerebellar peduncle. More and more damaged axons are visible 12 hours to several days after the injury. Severity of the diffuse injury correlates with how much shearing force was

applied to the brain stem. DAI is not associated with intracranial hypertension immediately after injury, but acute brain swelling caused by increased intravascular blood within the brain, vasodilation, and increased cerebral blood volume is seen frequently.

Several categories of diffuse brain injury exist: mild concussion, classic concussion, mild DAI, moderate DAI, and severe DAI. An organic component is present within each category. These are summarized in Table 15-4.

Clinical Manifestations, Evaluation, and Treatment

Focal brain injury. A contusion may be evidenced by immediate loss of consciousness (generally accepted to last no longer than 5 minutes), loss of reflexes (individual falls to the ground), transient cessation of respiration, brief period of bradycardia, and decreased blood pressure (lasting 30 seconds to a few minutes). Increased cerebrospinal fluid (CSF) pressure and electrocardiogram (ECG) and electroencephalogram (EEG) changes occur on impact. Vital signs may stabilize to normal values in a few seconds, and then reflexes return and the person regains consciousness over minutes to days. Residual deficits may persist, and in some persons, full level of consciousness never really returns.

Evaluation includes a complete history and physical examination. Skull and spinal x-ray films frequently are taken, and a computed tomography (CT) scan or magnetic resonance imaging (MRI) may be done. Large contusions and lacerations with hemorrhage may be surgically excised. Otherwise, treatment is directed at controlling intracranial pressure and managing symptoms.

Individuals with classic temporal extradural hematomas lose consciousness at injury, and then one third become lucid for a few minutes to a few days (if a vein is bleeding). As the hematoma accumulates, a headache of increasing severity, vomiting, drowsiness, confusion, seizure, and hemiparesis may develop. As temporal lobe herniation occurs, level of consciousness is rapidly lost, with ipsilateral pupillary dilation and contralateral hemiparesis.

A CT scan or MRI usually is needed to diagnose extradural hematoma. The prognosis is good if intervention is initiated before bilateral dilation of the pupils. Extradural hematomas are almost always medical emergencies, requiring surgical ligation of bleeding vessels.

In acute, rapidly developing subdural hematomas, the expanding clots directly compress the brain. As intracranial pressure rises, bleeding veins are compressed. Thus bleeding is self-limiting, although cerebral compression and displacement of brain tissue can cause temporal lobe herniation.

An acute subdural hematoma classically begins with headache, drowsiness, restlessness or agitation, slowed cognition, and confusion. These symptoms worsen over time and progress to loss of consciousness, respiratory pattern changes, and pupillary dilation (i.e., the symptoms of temporal lobe herniation). Homonymous hemianopia (defective vision in either the right or the left field), dysconjugate gaze, and gaze palsies also may occur.

Of persons affected by chronic subdural hematomas, 80% have chronic headaches and tenderness over the hematoma on percussion. Most persons appear to have a progressive dementia with generalized rigidity (paratonia). Chronic subdural hematomas require a craniotomy to evacuate the gelatinous blood. Percutaneous drainage for chronic subdural hematomas has proved successful. However, reaccumulation often occurs unless the surrounding membrane is removed.

Intracerebral hematomas cause a decreasing level of consciousness. Coma or a confusional state from other injuries, however, can make the cause of this increasing unresponsiveness difficult to detect. Contralateral hemiplegia also may occur, and as intracranial pressure rises, temporal lobe herniation may appear. In delayed intracerebral hematoma, the presentation is similar to that of a hypertensive brain hemorrhage: sudden, rapidly progressive decreased level of consciousness with pupillary dilation, breathing pattern changes, hemiplegia, and bilateral positive Babinski reflexes.

History and physical examination help to establish the diagnosis, and CT scan, MRI, and cerebral angiography confirm it. Evacuation of a singular intracerebral hematoma has only occasionally been helpful, mostly for subcortical white matter hematomas. Otherwise, treatment is directed at reducing the intracranial pressure and allowing the hematoma to reabsorb slowly.

With open-head injury, most persons lose consciousness. The depth and duration of the coma are related to the location of injury, extent of damage, and amount of bleeding.

Open-head injury often requires débridement of the traumatized tissues to prevent infection and to remove blood clots, thereby reducing intracranial pressure. Intracranial pressure is managed also with steroids, dehydrating agents, osmotic diuretics, or a combination of these drugs. Broad-spectrum antibiotics are administered.

A compound fracture may be diagnosed through physical examination, skull x-ray films, or both. Basilar skull fracture is determined based on clinical findings. Skull x-rays often do not demonstrate the fracture, although intracranial air or air in the sinuses on x-ray film, CT scan, or MRI is indirect evidence of a basilar skull fracture.

Bed rest and close observation for meningitis and other complications are prescribed for a basilar skull fracture. Prophylactic antibiotics may or may not be given.

Diffuse brain injury. Diffuse axonal injury results in the following:

1. *Physical consequences:* spastic paralysis, peripheral nerve injury, swallowing disorders, dysarthria, visual and hearing impairments, taste and smell deficits
2. *Cognitive deficits:* disorientation and confusion, short attention span, memory deficits, learning difficulties, dysphasia, poor judgment, perceptual deficits
3. *Behavioral manifestations:* agitation, impulsiveness, blunted affect, social withdrawal, depression

Mild concussion is characterized by immediate but transitory clinical manifestations. CSF pressure rises, and ECG and EEG changes occur without loss of consciousness. The initial confusional state lasts for one to several minutes, possibly with amnesia for events preceding the trauma (retrograde amnesia). Anterograde amnesia may also exist transiently. Persons may experience head pain and complain of nervousness and "not being themselves" for up to a few days.

In ***classic cerebral concussion,*** consciousness is lost for up to 6 hours and reflexes fail, causing falls. Reflexes are regained as responsiveness returns. Transiently, breathing stops, bradycardia occurs, and blood pressure falls. Vital signs quickly stabilize to within normal limits. Retrograde and anterograde amnesia exist, with a confusional state for hours to days. Head pain, nausea, fatigue, attentional and memory system impairments (inability to concentrate and forgetfulness), and mood and affect changes (nervousness, anxiety reactions, depression, irritability, fatigability, insomnia) occur. A ***postconcussive syndrome,*** including headache, nervousness or anxiety, irritability, insomnia, depression, inability to concentrate, forgetfulness, and fatigability, may exist. Treatment entails reassurance and symptomatic relief in addition to 24 hours of close observation.

In mild DAI, 30% of persons display decerebrate or decorticate posturing; and they may experience prolonged periods of stupor or restlessness (see Fig. 14-6).

In moderate DAI, the score on the Glasgow Coma Scale (GCS) is 4 to 8 initially and 6 to 8 by 24 hours. Thirty-five percent of victims have transitory decerebration or decortication, with unconsciousness lasting days or weeks. On awakening, the person is confused and suffers a long period of posttraumatic anterograde and retrograde amnesia. There is often permanent deficit in memory, attention, abstraction, reasoning, problem-solving, executive functions, vision or perception, and language. Mood and affect changes range from mild to severe.

In severe DAI, the person experiences immediate autonomic dysfunction that disappears in a few weeks. Increased intracranial pressure appears 4 to 6 days after injury. Pulmonary complications occur frequently. Profound sensorimotor and cognitive system deficits are present. Severely compromised coordinated movements and verbal and written communication, inability to learn and reason, and inability to modulate behavior are found also.

High-resolution CT scan and MRI assist in the diagnosis of focal and diffuse injuries. Medical management must address endocrine and metabolic derangement. Early and late seizures must be prevented and controlled.

✓ QUICK CHECK

How is a concussion different from a contusion?

Why do extradural, subdural, and intracerebral hematomas act like expanding masses?

Why is head motion the principal causative mechanism of diffuse brain injury?

Spinal cord trauma

Each year 10,000 to 12,000 persons experience serious spinal cord injury. Most are men between the ages of 16 and 30 years who sustain injuries from car and motorcycle crashes (55%), sports activities (18%), and penetrating injuries (gunshot or stab wounds) (15%). Elderly people, because of preexisting degenerative vertebral disorders, are particularly at risk for minor trauma that results in serious spinal cord injury; 21% of injuries are attributable to falls in the elderly population.

☰ Pathophysiology

Spinal cord injuries most commonly occur because of vertebral injuries that result from acceleration, deceleration, or deformation forces usually applied at a distance. These forces compress the tissues, pull or exert traction (tension) on the tissues, or shear tissues so that they slide into one another (Figs. 15-4 to 15-7). The bones, ligaments, and joints of the vertebral column may be damaged through fracture and compression of one or more elements, dislocation of elements, or both fracture and dislocation. Vertebral injuries can be classified as (1) simple fracture—a single break usually affecting transverse or spinous processes; (2) compressed (wedged) vertebral fracture—vertebral body compressed anteriorly; (3) comminuted (burst) fracture—vertebral body shattered into several fragments; and (4) dislocation.

The vertebrae fracture readily with both direct and indirect trauma. When the supporting ligaments are torn, the vertebrae move out of alignment and dislocations occur. A horizontal force moves the vertebrae straight forward; if the individual is in a flexed position at the time of injury, the vertebrae are then angulated. Flexion and extension injuries may result in dislocations. (Bone, ligament, and joint injuries are presented in Table 15-5.)

Vertebral injuries occur most frequently at vertebrae C1 to C2 (cervical), C4 to C7, and T10 (thoracic) to L2 (lumbar) (see Fig. 12-9), the most mobile portions of the vertebral column. The cord occupies most of the vertebral canal in the cervical and lumbar regions, so it is easily injured. (Injuries to the cord are summarized in Table 15-6.)

With injury, microscopic hemorrhages appear in the central gray matter and pia-arachnoid, increasing in size until the entire gray matter is hemorrhagic and necrotic. Edema in the white matter occurs, impairing the microcir-

Osteophytes

Disruption of intervertebral disks

Compression of spinal cord

Compressed interspinous ligament

G.J.Wassilchenko

Fig. 15-4 *Hyperextension injuries of the spine.* Hyperextension injuries of the spine can result in fracture or nonfracture injuries with spinal cord damage. *(From Rudy, E.B. [1984]. Advanced neurological and neurosurgical nursing. St. Louis: Mosby.)*

Wedge fracture

Stretched interspinous ligaments

Compressed injury to spinal cord

Disruption of disk with forward dislocation

Rupture of interspinous ligament

Rupture of disk with forward dislocation

Fractured pedicle and disruption of interspinous ligament

Fig. 15-5 *Flexion injury of the spine.* Hyperflexion produces translation (subluxation) of verte-brae that compromises the central canal and compresses spinal cord parenchyma or vascular structures. *(From Rudy, E.B. [1984]. Advanced neurological and neurosurgical nursing. St. Louis: Mosby.)*

Crushed vertebral body with cord compression

Compression fracture without cord compression

G. J. Wassilchenko

Fig. 15-6 *Axial compression injuries of the spine.* In axial compression injuries of the spine, the spinal cord is contused directly by retropulsion of bone or disk material into the spinal canal. *(From Rudy, E.B. [1984]. Advanced neurological and neurosurgical nursing. St. Louis: Mosby.)*

Flexion-rotation dislocation or fracture dislocation

Fig. 15-7 *Flexion-rotation injuries of the spine. (From Rudy, E.B. [1984].* Advanced neurological and neurosurgical nursing. *St. Louis: Mosby.)*

culation of the cord. Localized hemorrhaging and edema are followed by reduced vascular perfusion and development of ischemic areas. Oxygen tension in the tissue at the injury site is decreased. The microscopic hemorrhages and edema are maximal at the level of injury and two cord segments above and below it.

Cellular and subcellular alterations and tissue necrosis occur. Cord swelling increases the individual's degree of dysfunction, so that it is hard to distinguish functions permanently lost from those temporarily impaired. In the cervical region, cord swelling may be life threatening because it may cause impairment of the diaphragm function (phrenic nerves exit at C3 to C5) and vegetative functions (mediated by the medulla oblongata).

Circulation in the white matter tracts of the spinal cord returns to normal in about 24 hours, but gray matter circulation remains altered. Phagocytes appear 36 to 48 hours after injury, and microglia proliferate with altered astrocytes. Red cells then begin to disintegrate, and resorption of hemorrhages begins. Degenerating axons are engulfed by macrophages in the first 10 days after injury. The traumatized cord is replaced by acellular collagenous tissue, usually in 3 to 4 weeks. Meninges thicken as part of the scarring process.

Clinical Manifestations

Normal activity of the spinal cord cells at and below the level of injury ceases because of loss of the continuous tonic discharge from the brain or brain stem and inhibition of suprasegmental impulses immediately after cord injury, thus causing spinal shock. In *spinal shock,* reflex function is completely lost in all segments below the lesion. This condition involves all skeletal muscles; bladder, bowel, and sexual function; and autonomic control. Severe impairment below the level of the lesion is obvious; it includes paralysis and flaccidity in muscles, absence of sensation, loss of bladder and rectal control, transient drop in blood pressure, and poor venous circulation. The condition also results in disturbed thermal control because the sympathetic nervous system is damaged. The hypothalamus cannot regulate body heat through vasoconstriction and increased metabolism; therefore the individual assumes the temperature of the air.

Spinal shock generally lasts 7 to 20 days, with a range of a few days to 3 months. It terminates with the reappearance of reflex activity, hyperreflexia, spasticity, and reflex emptying of the bladder.

Loss of motor and sensory function depends on the level of injury. All motor, sensory, reflex, and autonomic functions cease below any transected area and also may cease below concussive, contused, compressed, or ischemic areas. Table 15-7 summarizes the clinical manifestations of spinal cord injury.

Autonomic hyperreflexia (dysreflexia) may occur after spinal shock resolves. The syndrome is associated with a massive, uncompensated cardiovascular response to stimulation of the sympathetic nervous system (Fig. 15-8). The condition is life threatening and requires immediate treatment. Individuals most likely to be affected have lesions at the T6 level or above. Characteristics include paroxysmal hypertension (up to 300 mm Hg, systolic), a pounding headache, blurred vision, sweating above the level of the lesion with flushing of the skin, nasal congestion, nausea, piloerection caused by pilomotor spasm, and bradycardia (30 to 40 beats/min). The symptoms may develop singly or in combination (syndrome) and often are associated with a distended bladder or rectum.

In hyperreflexia, sensory receptors below the level of the cord lesion are stimulated. The intact autonomic nervous system reflexively responds with an arteriolar spasm that increases blood pressure. Baroreceptors in the cerebral vessels, the carotid sinus, and the aorta sense the hypertension and stimulate the parasympathetic system. The heart rate decreases, but the visceral and peripheral vessels do not dilate because efferent impulses cannot pass through the cord.

The most common cause is a distended bladder or rectum, but any sensory stimulation can elicit autonomic hyperreflexia. Stimulation of the skin or pain receptors may cause autonomic hyperreflexia. Bladder or bowel emptying usually relieves the syndrome, and this may be facilitated by drugs such as phenoxybenzamine.

TABLE 15-5   Mechanisms of Vertebral Injury

Mechanisms of Injury	Vertebral Injury	Forces of Injury	Location of Injury
Hyperextension	Fracture and dislocation of posterior elements, such as spinous processes, transverse processes, laminae, pedicles, or posterior ligaments	Results from forces of acceleration-deceleration and the sudden reduction in the anteroposterior diameter of the spinal cord	Cervical area
Hyperflexion	Fracture or dislocation of the vertebral bodies, disks, or ligaments	Results from sudden and excessive force that propels the neck forward or causes an exaggerated lateral movement of the neck to one side	Cervical area
Vertical compression (axonal loading)	Shattering fractures	Results from a force applied along an axis from the top of the cranium through the vertebral bodies	T12 to L2
Rotational forces (flexion-rotation)	Rupture support ligaments in addition to producing fractures	Adds shearing force to acceleration—acceleration forces	Cervical area

TABLE 15-6   Spinal Cord Injuries

Injury	Description
Cord concussion	Results in a temporary disruption of cord-mediated functions
Cord contusion	Bruising of the neural tissue causing swelling and temporary loss of cord-mediated functions
Cord compression	Pressure on the cord causing ischemia to tissues; must be relieved (decompressed) to prevent permanent damage to the spinal cord
Laceration	Tearing of the neural tissues of the spinal cord; may be reversible if only slight damage sustained by the neural tissues; may result in permanent loss of cord-mediated functions if spinal tracts are disrupted
Transection	Severing of the spinal cord, causing permanent loss of function
Complete	All tracts in the spinal cord completely disrupted; all cord-mediated functions below the transection are completely and permanently lost
Incomplete	Some tracts in the spinal cord remain intact, together with functions mediated by these tracts; has the potential for recovery although function is temporarily lost
Preserved sensation only	Some demonstrable sensation below the level of injury
Preserved motor nonfunctional	Preserved motor function without useful purpose; sensory function may or may not be preserved
Preserved motor functional	Preserved voluntary motor function that is functionally useful
Hemorrhage	Bleeding into the neural tissue as a result of blood vessel damage; usually no major loss of function
Damage or obstruction of spinal blood supply	Causes local ischemia

Evaluation and Treatment

Diagnosis of spinal cord injury is based on physical examination, radiologic examination, CT scan, MRI, and myelography. For a suspected or confirmed vertebral fracture or dislocation, regardless of the presence or absence of spinal cord injury, the immediate intervention is immobilization of the spine to prevent further injury. Decompression and surgical fixation may be necessary. Corticosteroids are given at the time of injury to decrease secondary cord injury from in-flammation and thereafter for several days. Nutrition, lung function, skin integrity, and bladder and bowel management must be addressed. Plans for rehabilitation need early consideration.

In cases of autonomic hyperreflexia, intervention must be prompt because cerebrovascular accident is possible. The head of the bed should be elevated, and the stimulus should be found and removed. Antihypertensive medications may be used if blood pressure remains elevated.

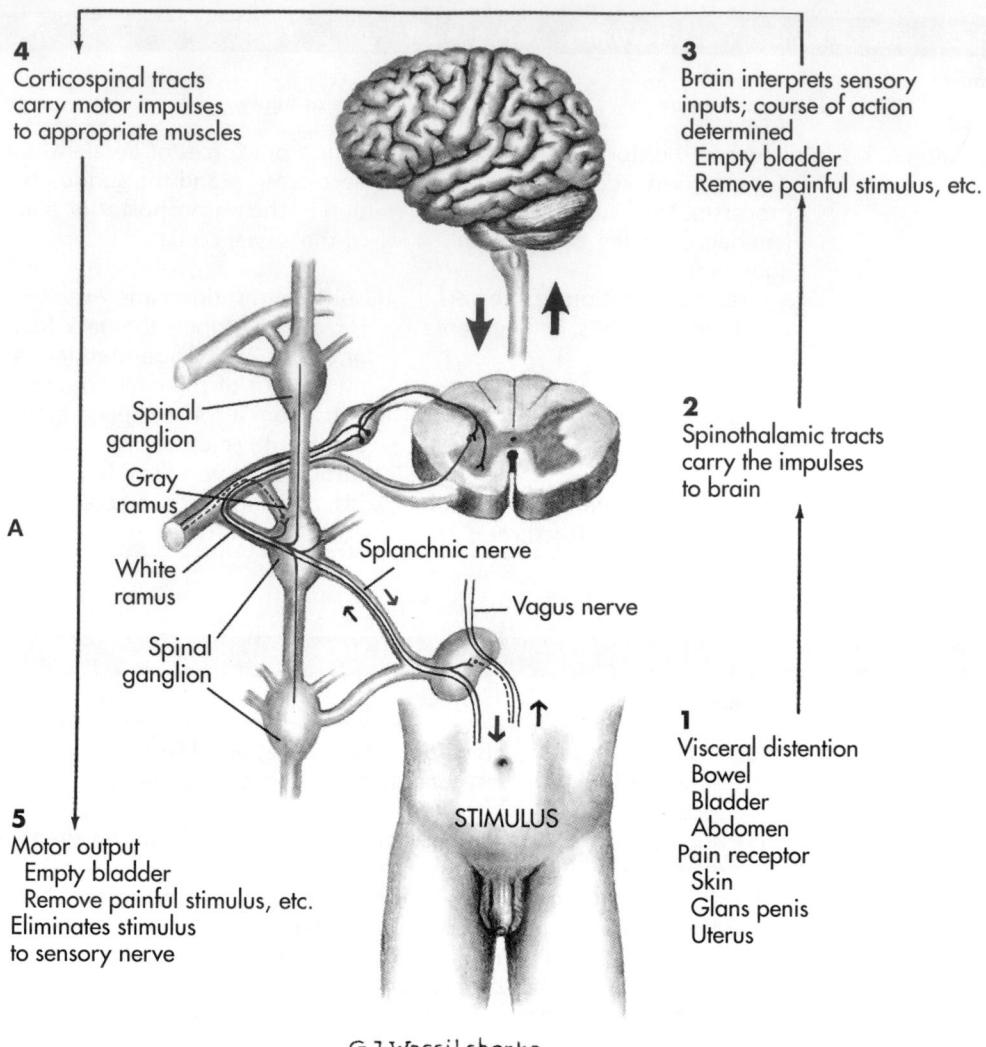

4
Corticospinal tracts
carry motor impulses
to appropriate muscles

3
Brain interprets sensory
inputs; course of action
determined
    Empty bladder
    Remove painful stimulus, etc.

A

Spinal
ganglion

Gray
ramus

White
ramus

Spinal
ganglion

Splanchnic nerve

Vagus nerve

2
Spinothalamic tracts
carry the impulses
to brain

5
Motor output
    Empty bladder
    Remove painful stimulus, etc.
Eliminates stimulus
to sensory nerve

STIMULUS

1
Visceral distention
    Bowel
    Bladder
    Abdomen
Pain receptor
    Skin
    Glans penis
    Uterus

G.J. Wassilchenko

Fig. 15-8 *Autonomic hyperreflexia.* **A,** Normal response pathway.

Low back pain

Low back pain affects the area between the lower rib cage and gluteal muscles and often radiates into the thighs. About 1% of individuals with acute low back pain have sciatica, pain along the distribution of a lumbar nerve root.[1] Sciatica often is accompanied by neurosensory and motor deficits, such as weakness. The percentage of the population affected with low back pain at some point in their lives is 75% to 90%,[1] and the annual prevalence is 16%.[1] Men and women are equally affected; however, women report low back symptoms more often after 60 years of age.

Pathogenesis

Most cases of low back pain are idiopathic, and no precise diagnosis is possible. The local processes involved in low back pain range from tension caused by tumors or disk prolapse, bursitis, synovitis, rising venous and tissue pressure (found in degenerative joint disease), abnormal bone pressures, problems with spinal mobility, inflammation caused by infection (as in osteomyelitis), bony fractures, or liga-

mentous sprains to pain referred from viscera or the posterior peritoneum. General processes resulting in low back pain include bone diseases, such as osteoporosis or osteomalacia, and hyperparathyroidism.

Risk factors include occupations that require repetitious lifting in the forward bent-and-twisted position; exposure to vibrations caused by vehicles or industrial machinery; obesity; and cigarette smoking. Osteoporosis increases the risk of spinal compression fractures and may be why elderly women report more symptoms than men. Genetic predispositions for low back pain include isthmic spondylolisthesis (vertebra slides forward or slips in relation to a vertebra below), spinal osteochondrosis, and spinal stenosis associated with achondroplasia.

The most commonly encountered causes of low back pain include lumbar disk herniation, degenerative disk disease, spondylolysis, spondylolisthesis, and spinal stenosis. Anatomically, low back pain must come from innervated structures, but deep pain is widely referred and varies. The nucleus pulposus has no intrinsic innervation, but when ex-

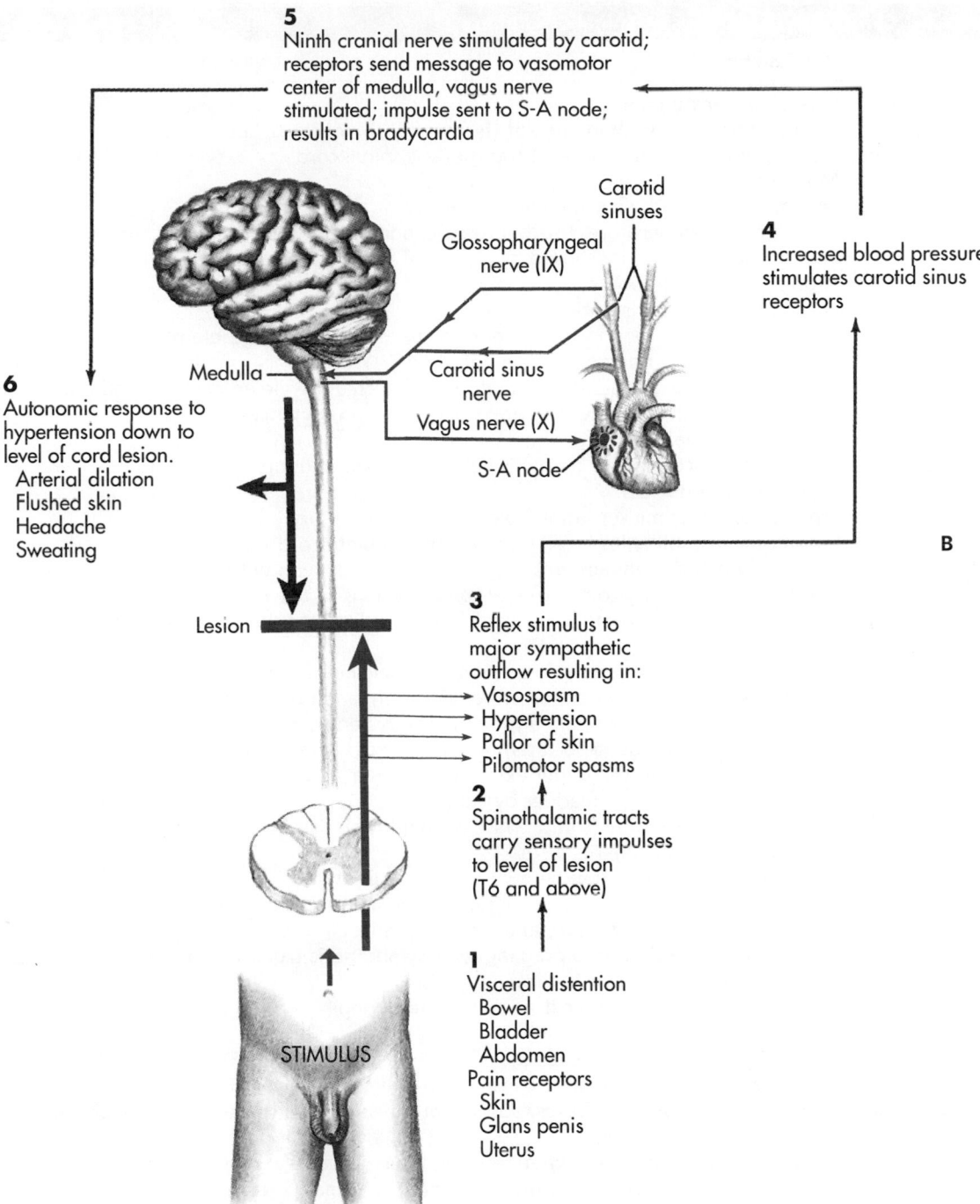

5
Ninth cranial nerve stimulated by carotid; receptors send message to vasomotor center of medulla, vagus nerve stimulated; impulse sent to S-A node; results in bradycardia

Carotid sinuses

Glossopharyngeal nerve (IX)

4
Increased blood pressure stimulates carotid sinus receptors

Medulla

Carotid sinus nerve

Vagus nerve (X)

S-A node

B

6
Autonomic response to hypertension down to level of cord lesion.
  Arterial dilation
  Flushed skin
  Headache
  Sweating

Lesion

3
Reflex stimulus to major sympathetic outflow resulting in:
  Vasospasm
  Hypertension
  Pallor of skin
  Pilomotor spasms

2
Spinothalamic tracts carry sensory impulses to level of lesion (T6 and above)

1
Visceral distention
  Bowel
  Bladder
  Abdomen
Pain receptors
  Skin
  Glans penis
  Uterus

STIMULUS

Fig. 15-8, cont'd B, Autonomic dysreflexia pathway. *S-A,* Sinoatrial. *(From Rudy, E.B. [1984].* Advanced neurological and neurosurgical nursing. *St. Louis: Mosby.)*

truded or herniated through a prolapsed disk, it irritates the dural membranes and causes pain referred to the segmental area (Fig. 15-9). The interspinous bursae can be a source of pain between L3, L4, L5, and S1 but also may affect L1, L2, and L3 spinous processes. The anterior and posterior longitudinal ligaments of the spine and the interspinous and supraspinous ligaments are abundantly supplied with pain receptors, as is the ligamentum flavum. All of these ligaments are vulnerable to traumatic tears (sprains) and frac-

ture. Muscle injury may contribute to low back pain, with sprains and strains the most common diagnoses.

Degenerative disk disease. Degenerative disk disease is common in individuals 30 to 60 years of age and older; however, only a small percentage of people with degenerative disk disease have any functional incapacity because of pain.[2] Causes include biochemical and biomechanical alterations of the intervertebral disk tissue. Fibrocartilage replaces the gelatinous mucoid material of the nucleus pulposus as the

TABLE 15-7	Clinical Manifestations of Spinal Cord Injury
Stage	**Manifestations**
Spinal shock stage Complete spinal cord transection	Loss of motor function a. Quadriplegia with injuries of the cervical spinal cord b. Paraplegia with injuries of the thoracic spinal cord Muscle flaccidity Loss of all reflexes below the level of injury Loss of pain, temperature, touch, pressure, and proprioception below the level of injury Pain at the site of injury caused by a zone of hyperesthesia above the injury Atonic bladder and bowel Paralytic ileus with distention Loss of vasomotor tone in the lower body parts; low and unstable blood pressure Loss of perspiration below the level of injury Loss or extreme depression of genital reflexes such as penile erection and bulbocavernous reflex Dry and pale skin; possible ulceration over bony prominences Respiratory impairment
Partial spinal cord transection	Asymmetric flaccid motor paralysis below the level of injury Asymmetric reflex loss Preservation of some sensation below the level of injury Vasomotor instability less severe than with complete cord transection Bowel and bladder impairment less severe than that seen with complete cord transection Preservation of ability to perspire in some portions of the body below the level of injury **Brown-Séquard syndrome** (associated with penetrating injuries, arises from a relative hemisection of the cord) a. Ipsilateral paralysis or paresis below the level of injury b. Ipsilateral loss of touch, pressure, vibration, and position sense below the level of injury c. Contralateral loss of pain and temperature sensations below the level of injury **Central cord syndrome** (associated with hyperextension or interruption of blood supply) a. Motor deficit in the upper extremities denser than in the lower extremities b. Varying degrees of bladder dysfunction **Anterior cord syndrome** (compromise of the anterior spinal artery by occlusion or the pressure effect of bone fragments or disk) a. Loss of motor function below the level of injury b. Loss of pain and temperature sensations below the level of injury c. Touch, pressure, position, and vibration senses intact **Horner syndrome** (injury to preganglionic sympathetic trunk or postganglionic sympathetic neurons of the superior cervical ganglion) a. Ipsilateral pupil smaller than contralateral pupil b. Sunken ipsilateral eyeball c. Ptosis of the affected eyeball d. Lack of perspiration on the ipsilateral side of the face
Heightened reflex activity stage	Emergence of Babinski reflexes, possibly progressing to a triple reflex; possible development of still later flexor spasms Reappearance of ankle and knee reflexes, which become hyperactive Contraction of reflex detrusor muscle leading to urinary incontinence Appearance of reflex defecation Mass reflex with flexion spasms, profuse sweating, piloerection, and bladder and occasional bowel emptying may be evoked by an autonomic stimulation of skin or from a full bladder Episodes of hypertension Defective heat-induced sweating Eventual development of extensor reflexes, first in muscles of hip and thigh, later in leg Possible paresthesias below the level of transection: dull, burning pain in the lower back, abdomen, buttocks, and perineum

Modified from Boss, B.J. (1984). The nervous system. In Howe, J. et al. (Eds.). The handbook of nursing. New York: John Wiley & Sons.

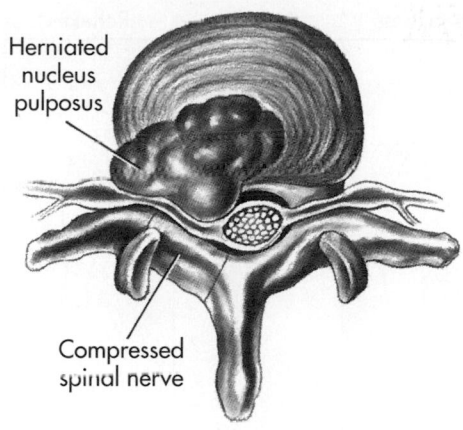

Fig. 15-9 *Herniated nucleus pulposus. (From Thompson, J.M. et al. [1997]. Mosby's clinical nursing [4th ed.]. St. Louis: Mosby.)*

disk ages and variable segmental instability results. The process seems to stabilize then, and the incidence of back pain often decreases.

Spondylolysis. Spondylolysis is a structural defect of the spine involving the lamina or neural arch of the vertebra. The lumbar spine is affected most often, particularly the portion of the lamina between the superior and inferior articular facets (pars interarticularis). Mechanical pressure may cause a forward displacement of the deficient vertebra (spondylolisthesis).

Heredity plays a significant role, and spondylolysis is associated with an increased incidence of other congenital spinal defects. The torsional and rotational "stress" causes "microfractures" at the affected site and eventually the dissolution of the pars interarticularis.

Spondylolisthesis. Spondylolisthesis occurs when a vertebra slides forward in relation to the vertebra below, commonly occurring at L5-S1. Spondylolisthesis is graded from 1 to 4 based on the percentage of slip that occurs. Individuals with grade 3 or 4 usually require operative decompression, stabilization, or both. Grades 1 and 2 usually are managed symptomatically and nonsurgically.

Spinal stenosis. Spinal stenosis may represent several conditions ranging from entrapment of a single nerve root in the lateral recess to diffuse central stenosis involving many roots. It is classified as acquired (more common) or developmental. Surgical decompression is recommended for those with chronic symptoms and those who do not respond to medical management.

Evaluation and Treatment

Diagnosis of low back injury is based on physical examination, electromyelography, CT with or without myelography, MRI, nerve conduction studies, diskography, and epidurography. Most individuals with acute low back pain benefit from a nonspecific short-term treatment regimen of bed rest, analgesic medications, exercises, physical therapy, and education. Surgical treatments, specifically diskectomy and spinal fusions, are used for individuals not responding to

medical management. Individuals with chronic low back pain also are prescribed antiinflammatory and muscle relaxant medications and are instructed to follow exercise programs. Aerobic exercises are a popular treatment and seem to be more effective than traction or low back exercises. Spinal surgery has a limited role in curing chronic low back pain.

Herniated intervertebral disk

Herniation of an intervertebral disk is a protrusion of part of the nucleus pulposus through a tear in the posterior rim of the annulus fibrosus (the fibrous capsule enclosing the gelatinous center of the disk) (see Fig. 15-5). Rupture of an intervertebral disk usually is caused by trauma, degenerative disk disease, or both. Lifting with the trunk flexed and sudden straining when the back is in an unstable position are the most common causes. Men are affected more often than women, with the highest incidence in the 30- to 60-year age-group. Most commonly affected are the lumbosacral disks, that is, L5-S1 and L4-L5. Disk herniation occasionally occurs in the cervical area, usually at C5-C6 and C6-C7. Herniations at the thoracic level are extremely rare. The injury may occur immediately, within a few hours, or months to years after injury.

Pathophysiology

In a herniated disk, the ligament and posterior capsule of the disk are usually torn, allowing the gelatinous material (the nucleus pulposus) to extrude and compress the nerve root. Occasionally the injury tears the entire disk loose, and it protrudes onto the nerve root or compresses the spinal cord. Multiple nerve root compression may be found at the L5-S1 level, where the cauda equina may be compressed. Large amounts of extruded nucleus pulposus or complete disk herniation (i.e., of both the capsule and the nucleus pulposus) may compress the spinal cord.

Clinical Manifestations

The location and size of the herniation into the spinal canal, together with the amount of space in the canal, determine the clinical manifestations associated with the injury (Fig. 15-10). A herniated disk in the lumbosacral area is associated with pain that radiates along the sciatic nerve course over the buttock and into the calf or ankle. The pain occurs with straining, including coughing and sneezing, and usually on straight leg raising. Other clinical manifestations include limited range of motion of the lumbar spine; tenderness on palpation in the sciatic notch and along the sciatic nerve; impaired pain, temperature, and touch sensation in the L5-S1 or L4-L5 dermatomes of the leg and foot; decreased or absent ankle jerk; and mild weakness of the foot.

With the herniation of a lower cervical disk, paresthesias and pain are present in the upper arm, forearm, and hand along the affected nerve root distribution. Neck and nerve root pain may be increased by neck motion and straining, including coughing and sneezing. Neck range of motion is diminished. Slight weakness and atrophy of biceps or triceps

Fig. 15-10 *Clinical features of a herniated lumbar nucleus pulposus.*

may occur; the biceps or triceps reflex may decrease. Occasionally, signs of corticospinal and sensory tract impairments appear, including motor weakness of the lower extremities, sensory disturbances in the lower extremities, and presence of a Babinski reflex.

≣ *Evaluation and Treatment*

Diagnosis of a herniated intervertebral disk is made through the history and physical examination, spinal x-ray films, electromyelography, CT scan, MRI, myelography, diskography, and nerve conduction studies. Multiple avenues of therapy are available. The conservative approach comprises traction, bed rest, heat and ice to the affected areas, and an effective antinflammatory analgesic regimen. The surgical approach is indicated if there is evidence of severe compression (weakness, decreased deep tendon, bladder, or bowel reflexes) or if the conservative approach is unsuccessful.

✓ QUICK CHECK

Why are most spinal cord injuries caused by vertebral injuries?

Why are young men most at risk for spinal cord injury?

Why does spinal shock occur following spinal cord injury?

How is a herniated intervertebral disk different from spondylolisthesis?

Cerebrovascular Disorders

Cerebrovascular disease is the most frequently occurring neurologic disorder, accounting for more than 50% of the persons admitted to general hospitals with neurologic problems. Any abnormality of the brain caused by a pathologic process in the blood vessels is referred to as a *cerebrovascular disease.* Included in this category are lesions of the vessel wall, occlusion of the vessel lumen by thrombus or embolus, rupture of the vessel, and alteration in blood quality such as increased blood viscosity.

The brain abnormalities induced by cerebrovascular disease are either (1) ischemia with or without infarction (death of brain tissues) or (2) hemorrhage. The common clinical manifestation of cerebrovascular disease is a ***cerebrovascular accident (CVA, stroke):*** a sudden, nonconvulsive focal neurologic deficit.

Cerebrovascular accidents (stroke syndromes)

Cerebrovascular accidents are the third leading cause of death in the United States. Stroke occurs mainly among those older than 65 years, but it does occur in individuals younger than 65 years. Stroke tends to run in families and is more common in women. The incidence is greater in blacks than whites, presumably because of the greater incidence of hypertension in blacks. In its mildest form, a cerebrovascu-

lar accident is so minimal as to be almost unnoticed. In its most severe state, hemiplegia, coma, and death result.

Cerebrovascular accidents (stroke syndromes) are classified according to pathophysiology and thus are global hypoperfusion (as in shock), thrombotic, embolic, or hemorrhagic.

HEALTH ALERT

Hypertension

Weight gain and being overweight increased the risk for hypertension in women. Weight loss reduced the risk of hypertension. Since hypertension is a risk factor for stroke, weight loss is an appropriate intervention to decrease stroke risk in women as well.

Data from Huang, A. et al. (1998). Body weight, weight change and risk for hypertension in women. Annals of Internal Medicine, 128, 81-88.

Thrombotic stroke

Thrombotic strokes (cerebral thromboses) occur when arteries supplying the brain or the intracranial vessels are occluded by thrombi that arise from arterial occlusions. The risk factors for cerebrovascular occlusive disease are the following:

- Atherosclerosis, which includes the following risk factors: hypertension, cigarette smoking, elevated blood cholesterol or triglyceride levels, abnormal lipoprotein ratio, diabetes mellitus, sedentary life-style
- Valvular heart disease
- Atrial tachydysrhythmias
- Hypothyroidism
- Use of oral contraceptives
- Sickle cell disease
- Coagulation disorders
- Polycythemia vera
- Arteritis
- Subclavian steal syndrome
- Chronic hypoxia
- Dehydration, especially when combined with any of the preceding conditions

Cerebral thrombosis develops most frequently with atherosclerosis and inflammatory disease processes (arteritis) that damage arterial walls. Increased coagulation can lead to thrombus formation. Conditions causing inadequate cerebral perfusion (e.g., dehydration, hypotension, prolonged vasoconstriction from malignant hypertension) increase the risk of thrombosis. Over 20 to 30 years, atheromatous plaques (stenotic lesion) form at branchings and curves in the cerebral circulation. The smooth stenotic area can degenerate, forming an ulcerated area of the vessel wall. Platelets and fibrin adhere to the damaged wall, and a clot forms, gradually occluding the artery. The clot may enlarge both distally and proximally. Thrombotic strokes occur when parts of the clot break off and travel upstream.

Thrombotic strokes may be further subdivided into transient ischemic attacks, strokes-in-evolution, and completed strokes. *Transient ischemic attacks (TIAs)* probably represent platelet clumps causing an intermittent blockage of circulation or spasm. In a true TIA all the neurologic deficits must be completely clear within 24 hours, leaving no residual dysfunction. Without definitive treatment, 80% of persons have a recurrence of symptoms.

The symptoms of thrombotic strokes occasionally have an abrupt onset but tend to be slowly progressive, evolving in a step-by-step fashion over minutes to hours. The typical development of thrombotic stroke causes the clinical syndrome known as a *stroke-in-evolution (progressive stroke).* An intermittent progression of a neurologic deficit over hours to days is characteristic of thrombotic stroke or slow hemorrhage. The *completed stroke* is a cerebrovascular accident that has reached its maximum destructiveness in producing neurologic deficits, although cerebral edema may not have reached its maximum.

Embolic stroke

An *embolic stroke* involves fragments that break from a thrombus formed outside the brain, in the heart, aorta, or common carotid. Emboli infrequently arise from the ascending aorta or common carotid artery. The embolus usually involves small brain vessels and obstructs at a bifurcation or other point of narrowing, thus causing ischemia. An embolus may plug the lumen entirely and remain in place or break into fragments and move up the vessel. Risk factors for an embolic stroke include atrial fibrillation, myocardial infarction, endocarditis, rheumatic heart disease, valvular prostheses, atrial-septal defects, and disorders of the aorta, carotids, or vertebral-basilar circulation. Less common contributors to embolic stroke are air, fat, and tumors. Fat emboli sometimes develop with fractures of long bones. Air emboli also can develop after certain types of surgery. In persons who experience an embolic stroke, usually a second stroke follows because the source of emboli continues to exist. Embolization is usually in the distribution of the middle cerebral artery.

Hemorrhagic stroke

Hemorrhagic stroke (intracranial hemorrhage) is the third most frequent cause of cerebrovascular accident. Hypertension, ruptured aneurysms or arteriovenous malformation, bleeding into a tumor, and hemorrhage associated with bleeding disorders are common causes.

A hypertensive hemorrhage is associated with significantly increased systolic-diastolic pressure over several years and usually occurs in the brain tissue. A mass of blood is formed and grows, displacing and compressing adjacent brain tissue. Rupture or seepage into the ventricular system occurs in many cases. Hemorrhages are described as massive, small, slit, or petechial. Massive hemorrhages are several centimeters in diameter; small hemorrhages are 1 to 2 cm in diameter; a slit hemorrhage lies in the subcortical area; and a petechial hemorrhage is the size of a pinhead bleed. The most common sites for hypertensive hemorrhages are in the putamen of the basal ganglia (a portion of the lentiform nucleus) (55%), the thalamus (10%), the cortex and subcortex (15%), the pons (10%), and the cerebellar hemispheres (10%).

Lacunar stroke

Lacunar strokes (lacunar infarcts) are smaller than 1 cm in diameter and involve the small perforating arteries, predominantly in the basal ganglia, internal capsules, and pons. They are associated with hypertension and diabetes mellitus. Because of the subcortical location and small area of infarction, these strokes may have pure motor and sensory deficits.

Pathophysiology

Cerebral infarction. Cerebral infarction results when an area of the brain loses its blood supply because of vascular occlusion. Causes include (1) abrupt vascular occlusion (e.g., embolus), (2) gradual vessel occlusion (e.g., atheroma), and (3) vessels that are stenosed but not completely occluded. Cerebral thrombi and cerebral emboli most commonly produce occlusion, but atherosclerosis and hypotension are the dominant underlying processes.

Cerebral infarctions are ischemic or hemorrhagic. In ischemic infarcts, the affected area becomes slightly discolored and softens 6 to 12 hours after the occlusion. Necrosis, swelling around the insult, and mushy disintegration appear by 48 to 72 hours after infarction.

In hemorrhagic infarcts, bleeding occurs into the infarcted area when blood flow is restored. The embolic fragments may be moved or lyzed, or compressive forces may lessen, allowing blood flow to be reestablished.

Cerebral hemorrhage. The primary cause of cerebral hemorrhage is hypertension. Hypertension involves primarily smaller arteries and arterioles, resulting in thickening of the vessel walls, and increased cellularity of the vessels and hyalinization. Necrosis may be present. Microaneurysms in these smaller vessels or arteriolar necrosis may precipitate the bleeding.

A mass of blood is formed as bleeding continues into the brain tissue. Adjacent brain tissue is displaced and compressed, producing ischemia, edema, and increased intracranial pressure. Rupture or seepage of blood into the ventricular system often occurs.

The cerebral hemorrhage resolves through reabsorption. Macrophages and astrocytes appear to clear away the blood. A cavity forms, surrounded by a dense gliosis after removal of the blood.

Clinical Manifestations

Because neurons surrounding the ischemic or infarcted areas undergo changes that disrupt plasma membranes, cellular edema results, causing further compression of capillaries. Cerebral edema reaches its maximum in about 72 hours and takes about 2 weeks to subside. Most persons survive an initial hemispheric ischemic stroke unless there is massive cerebral edema, which is nearly always fatal.

Clinical manifestations of thrombotic stroke vary, depending on the artery obstructed. Different sites of obstruction create different occlusion syndromes.

With hemorrhagic stroke, clinical manifestations vary, depending on the location and size of the bleed. Once a deep unresponsive state occurs, the person rarely survives. The immediate prognosis is grave. If the person survives, however, recovery of function frequently is possible.

Individuals experiencing intracranial hemorrhage from a ruptured or leaking aneurysm have one of three sets of symptoms: (1) onset of an excruciating generalized headache with an almost immediate lapse into an unresponsive state, (2) headache but with consciousness maintained, and (3) sudden lapse into unconsciousness. If the hemorrhage is confined to the subarachnoid space, there may be no local signs. If bleeding spreads into the brain tissue, hemiparesis/paralysis, dysphasia, or homonymous hemianopia may be present. Warning signs of an impending aneurysm rupture include headache, transient unilateral weakness, transient numbness and tingling, and transient speech disturbance. However, such warning signs often are absent.

Evaluation and Treatment

In thrombotic strokes, treatment is directed at prevention of ischemic injury and supportive management to control cerebral edema and increased intracranial pressure. Arresting the disease process by control of risk factors is critical. In embolic strokes, treatment is directed at preventing further embolization by instituting anticoagulation therapy and correcting the primary problem. Rehabilitation is indicated in both thrombotic and embolic strokes. Treatment of an intracranial bleed, regardless of cause, is focused on stopping or reducing the bleeding, controlling the increased intracranial pressure, preventing a rebleed, and preventing vasospasm. Occasionally an attempt is made to evacuate or aspirate the blood.

Intracranial aneurysm. Intracranial aneurysms may result from hemodynamic factors, genetic predisposition, arteriosclerosis, structural abnormality, trauma, inflammation, infection, neoplasm, or radiation.[3] The size may vary from 2 mm to 2 or 3 cm. Most aneurysms are located at bifurcations in or near the circle of Willis, in the vertebrobasilar arteries, or within the carotid system (see Fig. 12-17). Aneurysms may be single, but in 20% to 25% of the cases, more than one is present. In these instances, the aneurysms may be unilateral or bilateral. Peak incidence is 35 to 60 years of age, and women are slightly more susceptible than men.

Pathophysiology

No single pathologic mechanism exists. Aneurysms may be classified on the basis of shape and form. ***Saccular aneurysms (berry aneurysms)*** occur frequently (in approximately 2% of the population) and probably result from congenital abnormalities in the media of the arterial wall. The sac gradually grows over time. A saccular aneurysm may be (1) round with a narrow stalk connecting it to the parent artery, (2) broad-based without a stalk, or (3) cylindric (Fig.

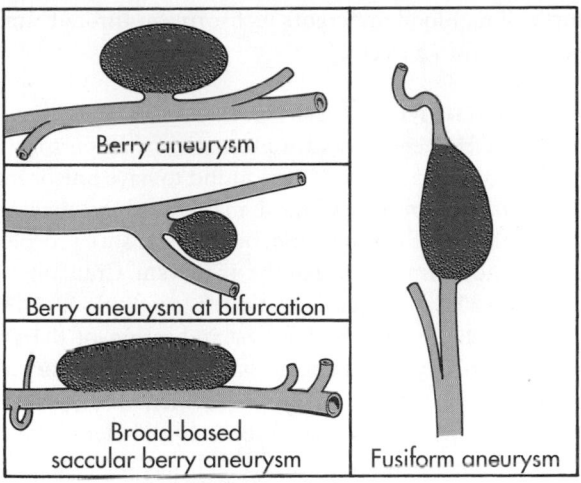

Fig. 15-11 *Types of aneurysms.*

Fig. 15-12 *Ruptured berry aneurysms.* Larger aneurysm is at terminal portion of basilar artery. Smaller aneurysm is in bifurcation angle of middle cerebral artery on right. *(From Kissane, J.M. [Ed.]. [1990]. Anderson's pathology [9th ed.]. St. Louis: Mosby.)*

15-11). Saccular aneurysms are rare in childhood; their highest incidence of rupturing or bleeding is among persons 20 to 50 years of age (Fig. 15-12).

Fusiform aneurysms (giant aneurysms) occur as a result of diffuse arteriosclerotic changes and are found most commonly in the basilar arteries or terminal portions of the internal carotid arteries (see Fig. 15-11). They act as space-occupying lesions.

Aneurysms rupture through thin areas, causing hemorrhage into the subarachnoid space and spreading rapidly, producing localized changes in the cerebral cortex and focal irritation of nerves and arteries (see discussion of the Laplace law in Chapter 22). Bleeding ceases when a fibrin-platelet plug forms at the point of rupture and because of compression. Blood undergoes reabsorption through arachnoid villi within 3 weeks.

 ### Clinical Manifestations

Aneurysms frequently are asymptomatic. Of all persons undergoing routine autopsy, 2% are found to have one or more intracranial aneurysms. Clinical manifestations may arise from cranial nerve compression, but the signs vary, depending on the location and size of the aneurysm. Cranial nerves III, IV, V, and VI are affected most often (see Table 12-6). Unfortunately the most common first indication of the presence of an aneurysm is an acute subarachnoid hemorrhage, intracerebral hemorrhage, or combined subarachnoid-intracerebral hemorrhage (see Subarachnoid Hemorrhage).

 ### Evaluation and Treatment

Diagnosis before a bleeding episode is made through arteriography. After a subarachnoid or intracerebral hemorrhage, a tentative diagnosis of an aneurysm is based on clinical manifestations, history, CT scan, and MRI. The treatment of choice for an aneurysm is surgical management. The location and size of the aneurysm and the person's clinical status determine whether invasive therapy is feasible.

Arteriovenous malformation

An *arteriovenous malformation (AVM)* is a tangled mass of dilated blood vessels creating abnormal channels between the arterial and venous systems (arteriovenous fistula). AVMs may occur in any part of the brain and vary in size from a few millimeters to large malformations extending from the cortex to the ventricle. AVMs occur equally in males and females and occasionally occur in families. Although AVMs are usually present at birth, symptoms exhibit a delayed age of onset and commonly occur between 10 and 20 years of age.

 ### Pathophysiology

AVMs do not have a normal blood vessel structure and are abnormally thin. One or several arteries may feed the AVM and become tortuous and dilated over time. With moderate to large AVMs, sufficient blood is shunted into the malformation to deprive surrounding tissue of adequate blood perfusion.

 ### Clinical Manifestations

Twenty percent of persons with an AVM have a characteristic chronic, nondescript headache, although some experience migraine. Thirty percent of persons experience seizures caused by compression. The other 50% experience an intracerebral, subarachnoid, or subdural hemorrhage. Bleeding from an AVM into the subarachnoid space causes symptoms identical to those associated with a ruptured aneurysm. If bleeding is into the brain tissue, focal signs that develop resemble a stroke-in-evolution. Ten percent of persons experience hemiparesis or other focal signs. At times, noncommunicating hydrocephalus (see Chapter 16) develops with a large AVM that extends into the ventricular lining.

 ### Evaluation and Treatment

A systolic bruit over the carotid artery in the neck, the mastoid process, or the eyeball in a young person is almost diagnostic of an AVM. Confirming diagnosis is made by arteriogram. Treatment of choice is surgical or radiosurgery management or both through dissection or through obliteration by ligation of feeders if dissection is not possible. Embolization may be used.

Subarachnoid hemorrhage

With a *subarachnoid hemorrhage,* blood escapes from a defective or injured vessel into the subarachnoid space. Individuals at risk for a subarachnoid hemorrhage are those with intracranial aneurysm, intracranial arteriovenous malformation, or hypertension and those who have sustained head injuries. Subarachnoid hemorrhages often recur, especially from a ruptured intracranial aneurysm.

 ### Pathophysiology

When a vessel is leaking, blood oozes into the subarachnoid space. When a vessel tears, blood under pressure is pumped into the subarachnoid space. The blood is extremely irritating to the neural tissues and produces an inflammatory reaction. In addition, the blood coats nerve roots, clogs arachnoid granulations (impairing CSF reabsorption), and clogs foramina within the ventricular system (impairing CSF circulation). Intracranial pressure immediately increases to almost diastolic levels but returns to near baseline in about 10 minutes. Cerebral blood flow and cerebral perfusion pressure decrease. The expanding hematoma acts like a space-occupying lesion, compressing and displacing brain tissue. Granulation tissue is formed, and meningeal scarring with impairment of CSF reabsorption and secondary hydrocephalus often results. Mortality in subarachnoid hemorrhage is 50% at 1 month.

 ### Clinical Manifestations

Early manifestations associated with leaking vessels are episodic and include headache, changes in mental status or level of consciousness, nausea and/or vomiting, and focal neurologic defects. A ruptured vessel causes a sudden, throbbing, "explosive" headache, accompanied by nausea and vomiting, visual disturbances, motor deficits, and loss of consciousness related to a dramatic rise in intracranial pressure (ICP). Meningeal irritation and inflammation often occur, causing neck stiffness (nuchal rigidity), photophobia, blurred vision, irritability, restlessness, and low-grade fever. A positive *Kernig sign* (straightening the knee with the hip and knee in a flexed position produces pain in the back and neck regions) and *Brudzinski sign* (passive flexion of the neck produces neck pain and increased rigidity) may appear. No localizing signs are present if the bleed is confined completely to the subarachnoid space.

The Hunt and Hess subarachnoid hemorrhage (SAH) grading system is based on description of the clinical manifestations (Table 15-8). Rebleeding is a significant risk with a high mortality (up to 70%). The period of greatest risk is the first 3 weeks, with the peak incidence of rebleeding during

TABLE 15-8	Subarachnoid Hemorrhage Classification Scale
Category	**Description**
Grade I	Neurologic status intact; mild headache, slight nuchal rigidity
Grade II	Neurologic deficit evidenced by cranial nerve involvement; moderate to severe headache with more pronounced meningeal signs (e.g., photophobia, nuchal rigidity)
Grade III	Drowsiness and confusion with or without focal neurologic deficits; pronounced meningeal signs
Grade IV	Stuporous with pronounced neurologic deficits (e.g., hemiparesis, dysphasia); nuchal rigidity
Grade V	Deep coma state with decerebrate posturing and other brain stem functioning

From Cook, H.S. (1991). Aneurysmal subarachnoid hemorrhage: Neuroscience frontiers and nursing challenges. In C. Winkelman (Ed.), AACN clinical issues in critical care nursing. *Philadelphia: Lippincott.*

the first 24 hours after the initial bleed. Rebleeding is manifested by a sudden increase in blood pressure and ICP, along with a deteriorating neurologic status.

Delayed cerebral ischemia, a syndrome of progressive neurologic deterioration, is associated with cerebral artery vasospasm. From 40% to 60% of persons with a subarachnoid hemorrhage experience vasospasms in adjacent and sometimes in nonadjacent vessels. Vasospasm may occur because of the effects of vasoactive substances (e.g., calcium, prostaglandins, serotonin, catecholamines) on the arteries of the subarachnoid space. Edema, medial necrosis, and proliferation of the intima have been found. Vasospasm causes decreased cerebral blood flow, ischemia, and possibly infarct. The peak time of onset is 3 to 5 days with maximal narrowing at 5 to 14 days after the initial bleed, but it may persist for several weeks.

Seizures occur in 25% of persons with an SAH, and hydrocephalus after a bleed occurs in 20% of cases. Hypothalamic dysfunction, manifested by salt wasting, hyponatremia, and ECG changes, is common.

Evaluation and Treatment

The diagnosis of a subarachnoid hemorrhage is based on the clinical presentation, a noncontrast CT scan, and a lumbar puncture. Arteriography is the definitive diagnostic measure for identifying an aneurysm or arteriovenous malformation. Treatment is directed at controlling intracranial pressure, preventing ischemia and hypoxia of neural tissues, and preventing rebleeding episodes. Antioxidants are being studied for their effectiveness in preventing ischemic brain injury after subarachnoid hemorrhage.[4] The primary problem must be diagnosed and corrected as well.

✓ QUICK CHECK

Why is atherosclerosis a risk factor for thrombotic stroke?

Why do a TIA's signs and symptoms resolve completely?

Why do lacunar strokes involve small infarcts?

How is an AVM different from an aneurysm?

Infection and Inflammation of the Central Nervous System

Bacteria, viruses, fungi, protozoans, and rickettsiae can produce pyogenic, or pus-producing, infections of the CNS. The meninges, neural tissues, and vasculature also may be involved in the inflammatory process.

Meningitis

The causes of *meningitis* (infection of the meninges) include bacteria, viruses, fungi, parasites, or toxins. The infection may be acute, subacute, or chronic, with the pathophysiology, clinical manifestations, and treatment differing for each type of organism.

Bacterial meningitis is primarily an infection of the pia mater and arachnoid, the subarachnoid space, the ventricular system, and the CSF. A systemic or bloodstream infection or a direct extension from an infected area is the access route to the subarachnoid space. Meningococcus (*Neisseria meningitidis*), pneumococcus (*Streptococcus pneumoniae*), and *Haemophilus influenzae* are the most common causes.

Meningococcus has been identified worldwide. Meningococcal meningitis occurs predominantly in men and boys and in the fall, winter, and spring of the year. Epidemics of meningococcal meningitis occur in approximately 10-year cycles, predominantly affecting children and adolescents. With pneumococcal meningitis, young persons and those over 40 years of age are mostly affected. *Haemophilus influenzae* occurs almost exclusively in children 2 months to 7 years of age. Immunization of infants is decreasing its occurrence. Less common causes are staphylococcus, streptococcus, gonococcus, and gram-negative bacteria.

Aseptic meningitis (viral meningitis, nonpurulent meningitis) is believed to be limited to the meninges. It produces various symptoms and is caused by several infectious agents, usually viruses. Enteroviral viruses (echovirus, coxsackievirus, nonparalytic poliomyelitis), mumps, herpes simplex (type 1), adenoviruses, and California virus are the most common agents. Bacterial infections not adequately treated also cause aseptic meningitis.

Fungal meningitis is a chronic, much less common condition than bacterial or viral meningitis. The most common fungal infections of the nervous system are cryptococcosis, coccidioidomycosis, mucormycosis, candidiasis, and aspergillosis. The infection occurs most frequently in persons with impaired immune responses or alterations in normal body flora. It develops insidiously, usually over days or weeks.

 Pathophysiology

The bacteria that usually cause bacterial meningitis are common inhabitants of the nasopharynx, but a predisposing factor such as a prior upper respiratory infection must be present before the bacteria become blood borne. The method of CNS entry is still unclear. The bacteria or their toxins do, however, function as irritants and induce an inflammatory reaction by the meninges (pia and arachnoid), the CSF, and the ventricles. The meningeal vessels become hyperemic and increasingly permeable. Blood cells (neutrophils) migrate into the subarachnoid space, producing an exudate that thickens the CSF and interferes with normal CSF flow around the brain and spinal cord. The exudate can obstruct arachnoid villi and produce hydrocephalus. Further, inflammation occurs as the purulent exudate increases rapidly, especially around the base of the brain, and extends into the sheaths of the cranial and spinal nerves and into the perivascular spaces of the cortex. Meningeal cells become edematous, and the combined exudate and edematous cells increase intracranial pressure. Small and medium-size subarachnoid arteries, veins, and choroid plexuses become engorged, disrupting blood flow and potentially producing thrombosis. Secondary infection of the brain may occur.

Fungi in the nervous system usually produce a granulomatous reaction, forming granulomas or gelatinous masses in the meninges at the base of the brain. Fungi also may extend along the perivascular sites in the subarachnoid space and into the brain tissue, producing arteritis with thrombosis, infarction, and communicating hydrocephalus. Meningeal fibrosis develops later in the inflammatory process. Cranial nerve dysfunction, caused by compression, often results from the granulomas and fibrosis.

 Clinical Manifestations

The clinical manifestations accompanying bacterial meningitis arise from the meningeal inflammation and include generalized, throbbing, severe headache; forceful flexion of the neck onto the chest, causing Brudzinski sign (flexion of the legs and thighs); and Kernig sign (inability to extend the leg with the hip flexed at a right angle). The irritation and damage affect the cranial nerves, the cervical spinal nerves, the vomiting center, and the cortex. Fever is usually present. With meningococcal meningitis, a petechial or purpuric rash covers the skin and mucous membranes. As intracranial pressure increases, papilledema develops and delirium may progress to unconsciousness.

The clinical manifestations of aseptic meningitis are mild compared with those associated with bacterial meningitis. Mild, generalized throbbing headache, mild photophobia, mild neck pain, stiffness, fever, and malaise accompany aseptic meningitis.

Fungal meningitis develops slowly and insidiously. The first manifestations are often those of dementia (see Chapter 14) or communicating hydrocephalus (see p. 370). The individual is characteristically afebrile.

 Evaluation and Treatment

Diagnosis of bacterial meningitis is based on physical examination and cultures of blood and CSF. Bacterial meningitis and fungal meningitis are treated with appropriate antibiotic therapy and other supportive measures. Aseptic meningitis is sometimes managed pharmacologically with antibiotics, antiviral drugs, and steroids.

Abscess

Abscesses are localized collections of pus within the parenchyma of the brain and spinal cord. They occur in about 1 of every 100,000 hospital admissions. Men experience abscesses twice as frequently as women. The median age for abscess formation is 30 to 40 years. They occur (1) after open trauma and during neurosurgery; (2) in association with a contiguous focus of infection, such as the middle ear, mastoid cells, nasal cavity, and nasal sinuses; (3) through metastatic or hematogenous spread from distant foci, such as the heart, lungs, pelvic organs, skin, tonsils, abscessed teeth, osteomyelitis in other than cranial bones, and dirty needles (especially in compromised hosts); and (4) cryptogenically, arising without other associated areas of infection. Streptococci, staphylococci, and *Bacteroides,* often combined with anaerobes, are the most common bacteria that cause abscesses; however, yeast and fungi have been found also. *Toxoplasma gondii* is producing an ever-increasing number of CNS abscesses in persons with acquired immunodeficiency syndrome (AIDS). Eighty percent of CNS abscesses are located in the cerebrum, and 20% are cerebellar, with the frontal and temporal lobes the most common sites. The abscesses are in more than one site in 5% to 20% of cases. Immunosuppressed persons are particularly at risk.

Brain abscesses are classified as extradural or intracerebral. *Extradural brain abscesses* are associated with osteomyelitis in a cranial bone. Unlike *intracerebral brain abscesses,* they rarely arise from a vascular source. *Spinal cord abscesses* are classified as epidural or intramedullary. Individuals with diabetes mellitus show an increased incidence of *spinal epidural abscesses* (which form in the epidural space), whereas debilitated individuals with sepsis more frequently develop *intramedullary spinal cord abscesses* (those within the spinal cord). Epidural spinal abscesses usually originate as osteomyelitis in a vertebra; the infection then spreads into the epidural space. (Osteomyelitis is discussed in Chapter 38.)

 Pathophysiology

Organisms gain entrance to the CNS by direct extension or spread along the wall of a vein. Infective emboli carry organisms from distant sites. Initially, a localized inflammatory process (focal cerebritis) develops, leading to edema, hyperemia, softening, petechial hemorrhage, exudate formation, septic thrombosis of vessels, and aggregates of degenerating leukocytes. The surrounding tissues are edematous (Fig.

Fig. 15-13 *Brain abscess.* Early brain abscess appearing as a poorly demarcated area *(arrow)* of cerebritis at the gray-white junction. *(From Damjanov, I. & Linder, J. [Eds.]. [1996]. Anderson's pathology [10th ed.]. St. Louis: Mosby.)*

15-13), and the veins are filled with fibrin and polymorphonuclear leukocytes (white blood cells [WBCs]). After a few days the intense reaction abates, and fibroblasts from capillaries next to the focal cerebritis deposit collagen fibers to contain and encapsulate the purulent focus. Existing abscesses tend to spread and form daughter abscesses. Nerve damage is associated with compression from edema and the expanding mass of pus.

Clinical Manifestations

Clinical manifestations of brain abscesses are associated with (1) an intracranial infection or (2) an expanding intracranial mass. Early manifestations include low-grade fever, headache (most common symptom), neck pain and stiffness with mild nuchal rigidity, confusion, drowsiness, sensory deficits, and communication deficits. Later clinical manifestations include inattentiveness (distractibility), memory deficits, decreased visual acuity and narrowed visual fields, papilledema, ocular palsy, ataxia, and dementia. The development of symptoms may be very insidious, often making an abscess difficult to diagnose.

Extradural brain abscesses are associated with localized pain, purulent drainage from the nasal passages or auditory canal, fever, localized tenderness, and neck stiffness. Occasionally the individual experiences a focal seizure.

Clinical manifestations of spinal cord abscesses have four stages: (1) spinal aching; (2) severe root pain, accompanied by spasms of the back muscles and limited vertebral movement; (3) weakness caused by progressive cord compression; and (4) paralysis.

Evaluation and Treatment

The diagnosis is suggested by clinical features and confirmed by CT scan. MRI is helpful when the CT scan does not show

a strongly suggested abscess. Aspiration through a burr hole or excision through craniotomy accompanied by antibiotic therapy is the recommended but somewhat controversial treatment for brain abscesses. In addition, intracranial pressure may have to be managed.

Because decompression is necessary, spinal cord abscesses are treated with surgical excision or aspiration. Antibiotic therapy and support therapy also are instituted.

Encephalitis

Encephalitis is an acute febrile illness, usually of viral origin, with nervous system involvement. The most common forms are caused by arthropod-borne (mosquito-borne) viruses and herpes simplex type 1. Referred to as infectious viral encephalitides, encephalitis may occur also as a complication of systemic viral diseases such as poliomyelitis, rabies, or mononucleosis, or it may arise after recovery from viral infections such as rubella or rubeola. Encephalitis also may follow vaccination with a live attenuated virus vaccine if the vaccine has an encephalitis component, for example, measles, mumps, and rubella. Typhus, trichinosis, malaria, and schistosomiasis also are associated with encephalitis. Toxoplasmosis may acutely reactivate in immunosuppressed persons when the once-dormant parasite in cyst form disseminates in brain tissues.

With the exception of the California viral encephalitis, which is endemic, the arthropod-borne (mosquito-borne) encephalitides occur in epidemics, varying in geographic and seasonal incidence (Table 15-9). Eastern equine encephalitis is the most serious but least common of the encephalitides.

Pathophysiology

Meningeal involvement is present in all encephalitides. The various encephalitides may cause widespread nerve cell degeneration related to areas of edema, necrosis with or without hemorrhage, increased intracranial pressure that may progress to herniation, large degenerative injuries, and microscopic areas of injury and degeneration. Infectious encephalitis may result from a postinfectious autoimmune response to the virus or from direct invasion of the CNS.

Clinical Manifestations

Encephalitis ranges from a mild infectious disease to a life-threatening disorder. Dramatic clinical manifestations include fever, delirium, or confusion progressing to unconsciousness, seizure activity, cranial nerve palsies, paresis and paralysis, involuntary movement, and abnormal reflexes. Signs of marked intracranial pressure may be present.

Evaluation and Treatment

Diagnosis is made by history and clinical presentation aided by CSF examination and culture, serology, WBC count, CT scan, or MRI. Most cases of viral meningitis are self-limiting, and until recently no definitive treatment was available. However, herpes encephalitis in immunocompromised

TABLE 15-9	Classification and Characteristics of Viruses Causing Encephalitis			
Viruses	Incubation Period (days)	Location	Season	Affected Population
Eastern equine encephalitis	5-15	Atlantic, Gulf Coast, and Great Lakes regions	Midsummer to early fall	Infants, children, and adults >50 yr
Western equine encephalitis	5-10	All parts of United States, especially western two thirds of country	Summer to early fall	Infants and young children
Venezuelan encephalitis	2-5	Texas, Florida, Mexico; Central and South America	Year round	Infants and young children
St. Louis encephalitis	4-21	United States and Canada, especially Mississippi River, Pacific Coast, Texas, and Florida	Summer and fall	Adults >40 yr; elderly more often affected than younger ages
California encephalitis	5-15	Midwestern United States, eastern seaboard, and Canada	Late summer and early fall	Children <15 yr

Modified from Barker, E. (1994). Neuroscience nursing. *St. Louis: Mosby.*

persons is now being treated with antiviral agents, such as acyclovir. Measures to control intracranial pressure are paramount.

Neurologic complications of AIDS

From 40% to 60% of all persons with AIDS have neurologic complications. On postmortem examination, 75% of AIDS victims have nervous system pathologic findings that result from (1) the primary human immunodeficiency virus (HIV) infection, (2) opportunistic infections, (3) neoplasms, and (4) systemic illness. Complications from the therapeutic drugs used to treat AIDS also may involve the CNS.

The most common neurologic disorder is HIV encephalopathy. Others are peripheral neuropathies, vacuolar (spongy softening) myelopathy, opportunistic infections of the CNS, and neoplasms.

Although HIV has been isolated in the CSF and brain and spinal cord tissues, the mechanism by which HIV infects the CNS is not known. The virus can be isolated in the CSF at approximately the time of seroconversion.

Pathologically, there may be (1) diffuse CNS involvement that produces a variety of clinical manifestations, (2) focal lesions that act as space-occupying lesions, and (3) obstructive hydrocephalus.

HIV encephalopathy

HIV encephalopathy (subacute encephalitis, HIV-associated dementia complex, HIV cognitive motor complex, AIDS encephalopathy, AIDS dementia complex, AIDS-related dementia) may affect adults or children and is characterized by progressive cognitive dysfunction with motor and behavioral alterations. The syndrome typically develops later in the disease but may be an early or singular manifestation in some persons.

It is believed that HIV encephalopathy results from direct brain tissue infection by the virus. HIV is found mostly in white matter subcortical areas causing a demyelinating process, but some viral replication occurs in glial cells and, occasionally, neurons. Multiple small nodules containing inflammatory cells are found scattered throughout the white matter and in subcortical gray matter, such as the basal ganglia and thalami. Multinucleated giant cells and perivascular inflammation are present, with focal and diffuse demyelination of white matter and spongy changes of the spinal cord. Toxins, lymphokines, or other substances also are factors in this process.

HIV encephalopathy is insidious in onset and unpredictable in its course. Most persons experience a steady progression with abrupt accelerations of signs over several months to more than 1 year, although some individuals experience an abrupt onset or an accelerated course. Early clinical manifestations may be vague. Impaired concentration and memory deficits are common, and apathy, lack of motivation, social withdrawal, irritability, and emotional lability appear. Later difficulties with language, spatial or temporal disorientation, and visual construction are present. Some persons manifest an organic psychosis with agitation, inappropriate behavior, and hallucinosis.

Generalized cognitive system deficits occur later in the course of HIV encephalopathy, often accompanied by psychomotor slowing and decreased speech spontaneity and fluency. Progressive loss of balance, gait ataxia, spastic paraparesis or paralysis, and generalized hyperreflexia are common motor signs, sometimes accompanied by decreased writing ability, tremor, myoclonus, and seizure.

Diagnosis is difficult, especially in early stages. History with physical examination findings and supporting CSF and CT scan and MRI data help establish the diagnosis. Treatment is antiviral agents and supportive measures.

Vacuolar myelopathy

Myelopathy involving diffuse degeneration of the spinal cord may occur in persons with AIDS. The most common myelopathy is *vacuolar myelopathy* affecting the lateral and posterior columns of the spinal cord; it is associated with HIV encephalopathy in 60% of individuals. Researchers believe that the pathologic condition is a direct consequence of HIV, although other agents may be involved. Vacuolation in the lumbar cord develops.

Progressive spastic paraparesis with ataxia is the predominant clinical manifestation. Leg weakness, upper motor neuron signs, incontinence, and posterior column sensory loss may be present.

Diagnosis is made on the basis of history, physical findings, and supporting data from diagnostic procedures. Treatment is supportive.

Peripheral neuropathy

The peripheral nervous system may sustain injury in AIDS, manifesting as a peripheral neuropathy, usually of the sensory type and occurring later in the disease. It is unresponsive to treatment.

HIV has been isolated from peripheral nerves, so the virus may directly infect nerves. Persons experience painful, burning dysesthesias and paresthesias, typically in the extremities. Weakness and decreased or absent distal reflexes may be present.

Diagnosis is established through history, physical findings, laboratory data, nerve conduction, and an electromyogram (EMG).

Aseptic viral meningitis

Some persons develop acute aseptic meningitis at approximately the time of seroconversion. This may represent the initial infection of the nervous system by the virus. Symptoms include headache, fever, and meningismus. Cranial nerve involvement, especially V and VII, may appear, but the disease is self-limiting and requires only symptomatic treatment.

Opportunistic viral and nonviral infections

Opportunistic viral infections can produce nervous system disease, with cytomegalovirus encephalitis, in particular, increasing among persons with AIDS. Those with this disease may experience altered cognitive functions, tremor, focal neurologic deficits, and sensory deficits. Herpes encephalitis and herpes varicella zoster radiculitis may develop. Polyomavirus (especially JC virus) in the immunocompromised person with AIDS may produce a demyelinating disorder called progressive multifocal leukoencephalopathy (PML). This virus is found in 90% of healthy persons but is dormant. It reactivates to cause PML in the person with AIDS.

Opportunistic nonviral infections also may cause nervous system disease. *Toxoplasmosis* (a protozoal infection) is the most common CNS disorder associated with AIDS and accounts for almost 50% of CNS disease in some studies. CNS toxoplasmosis typically manifests as a focal encephalitis that is difficult to diagnose but treatable. Persons with AIDS may develop meningitis, encephalitis, or brain abscesses of fungal, mycobacterial, and bacterial origin.

CNS neoplasms

CNS neoplasms associated with AIDS include CNS lymphoma, systemic non-Hodgkin lymphoma, and metastatic Kaposi sarcoma. Primary CNS lymphoma is a large-cell tumor that presents as rapidly developing and expanding multicentric intracranial mass lesions. The meninges and, possibly, the cranial nerves and spinal cord are invaded in systemic non-Hodgkin lymphoma. Metastasis of a Kaposi sarcoma to the CNS is uncommon.

Other CNS complications

Persons with AIDS may develop multifocal ischemic infarctions, hemorrhagic infarctions, hemorrhage into tumors, subdural hematomas, and epidural hemorrhage. Reported neurologic symptoms produced by AIDS therapeutics include extrapyramidal movements, myoclonus, dysphasia, delirium, and acute myelopathy.

✓ QUICK CHECK

Why is bacterial meningitis usually more serious than viral meningitis?

Why can an encephalitis be life threatening?

Why are neurologic complications of AIDS so common?

Degenerative Diseases
Alzheimer disease

Alzheimer disease (AD) (senile disease complex) has been demonstrated to be one of the most common causes of severe cognitive dysfunction in older persons. Its more prevalent forms are early-onset familial Alzheimer disease (FAD), late-onset FAD, and sporadic late-onset AD (75% of cases).[5]

Pathophysiology

The exact cause of Alzheimer disease is unknown, but current theories include loss of neurotransmitter stimulation by choline acetyltransferase; mutation for encoding amyloid precursor protein; alteration in apolipoprotein E, which binds beta amyloid; and mitochondrial defect causing a cell energy failure.[5-7] Early-onset FAD has been linked to mutations on chromosomes 1, 14, and 21, whereas late-onset FAD and sporadic AD are associated with chromosome 19 involved with apolipoprotein E (apo E).[5,8] Accumulation of amyloid occurs with these disorders. Alzheimer disease has also been linked to abnormalities in a lysosomal pathway that yields a neurotoxic substance. A link between the pathologic findings of Alzheimer disease and aluminum has not been established,[5] nor has a viral cause been proved, but submicroscopic proteinaceous infectious particles (prions) have been isolated.[9] An autoimmune cause also is being investi-

Fig. 15-14 *Common pathologic findings in Alzheimer disease. (From Beare, P.G. & Myers, J.L. [1998].* Principles and practice of adult health nursing *[3rd ed.]. St. Louis: Mosby.)*

gated, as are the effects of aging and injury. Apo *E-IV* predisposes to familial late-onset as well as sporadic late-onset cases.[5]

Microscopically, the protein in the neurons becomes distorted and twisted, forming a ***neurofibrillary tangle*** (Figs. 15-14 and 15-15). Tangles are composed of a microtubule-binding protein called *tau protein*.[5] Groups of nerve cells, especially terminal axons, degenerate and coalesce around an amyloid core. Microscopic examination of these areas of degeneration reveals plaquelike material known as **senile plaques,** which disrupt nerve-impulse transmission. Senile plaques and neurofibrillary tangles are more concentrated in the cerebral cortex and hippocampus. Greater numbers of senile plaques and neurofibrillary tangles are associated with AD.

Clinical Manifestations

Initial clinical manifestations are insidious and often attributed to forgetfulness, emotional upset, or other illness. The individual becomes progressively more forgetful over time, particularly in relation to recent events. Memory loss increases as the disorder advances, and the person becomes disoriented and confused and loses the ability to concentrate. Abstraction, problem solving, and judgment gradually deteriorate, with failure in mathematic calculation ability, language, and visuospatial orientation. Dyspraxia may appear. The mental status changes induce behavioral changes, including irritability, agitation, and restlessness. Mood changes also result from the deterioration in cognition. The

person may become anxious, depressed, hostile, emotionally labile, and prone to mood swings. Motor changes may occur if the posterior frontal lobes are involved, causing rigidity (paratonia, gegenhalten), with flexion posturing, propulsion, and retropulsion. Great variability in age of onset, intensity and sequence of symptoms, and location and extent of brain abnormalities is common.

Evaluation and Treatment

The diagnosis of Alzheimer disease is made by ruling out other causes. The history, including a mental status examination and the course of the illness, which may span 5 years or more, is used for diagnosis. Specific diagnosis can be made only by biopsy or at autopsy.

Treatment is directed at using devices to compensate for the impaired cognitive function, such as memory aids; maintaining unimpaired cognitive functions; and maintaining or improving the general state of hygiene, nutrition, and health.

HEALTH ALERT

Alzheimer Disease

An immune gene *(HLA-A2)*, which triggers immune activity and inflammatory reactions mediated by the immune system, is linked to nerve cell damage in Alzheimer disease.

Data from Pennisi, E. (1997). Immune gene tied to Alzheimer's. Science, 277, 1441.

Fig. 15-15 *Pathologic changes in Alzheimer disease.* **A,** Neuritic (senile) plaques and neurofibrillary tangles in Alzheimer disease. (Hortega silver carbonate stain; X135.) **B,** Neurofibrillary change in cell of locus ceruleus in individual with parkinsonism. (Hematoxylin-eosin stain; X600.) *(A from Kissane, J.M. [Ed.]. [1990]. Anderson's pathology [9th ed.]. St. Louis: Mosby; B from Kissane, J.M. [Ed.]. [1985]. Anderson's pathology [8th ed.]. St. Louis: Mosby.)*

Pick disease

Pick disease is a rare, severe degenerative disease of the frontal and anterior frontal lobes that produces death of tissue and dementia. It is difficult to distinguish clinically and pathologically from Alzheimer disease.[10]

Parkinson disease

Parkinson disease is a commonly occurring degenerative disorder of the basal ganglia (corpus striatum) involving failure of the dopaminergic (dopamine-secreting) nigrostriatal pathway. Nigrostriatal disorders produce a syndrome of abnormal movement called *parkinsonism (Parkinson syndrome, parkinsonian syndrome, paralysis agitans)* (Fig. 15-16).

Either primary Parkinson disease or secondary parkinsonism may occur. Secondary parkinsonism is parkinsonism caused by disorders other than Parkinson disease (i.e., trauma, infection, neoplasm, atherosclerosis, toxins, drug intoxication). Drug-induced parkinsonism, caused by neuroleptics, antiemetics, and antihypertensives, is the most common secondary form and usually is reversible.

Parkinson disease begins after the age of 40 years, with peak age of onset between 58 and 62 years.[11] It is slightly more prevalent in males. This disease is one of the most prevalent of the primary CNS disorders and a leading cause of neurologic disability in individuals older than 60 years. The prevalence rate is 130 to 150 per 100,000 persons, with 40,000 new cases in the United States each year.[10]

Pathophysiology

The pathogenesis of Parkinson disease is unknown, but it does not follow a hereditary pattern or familial tendency. Epidemiologic data suggest genetic, viral, and environmental toxins as possible causes.

Nigral and basal ganglial loss of neurons with depletion of dopamine, an inhibitory neurotransmitter, is the principal biochemical alteration in Parkinson disease (Fig. 15-16, *B*). Symptoms in basal ganglial disorders result from an imbalance of dopaminergic (inhibitory) and cholinergic (excitatory) activity in the caudate and putamen of the basal ganglia. In Parkinson disease, degeneration of the dopaminergic nigrostriatal pathway causes dopamine depletion in the basal ganglia and relative excess cholinergic activity in the feedback circuit. This is manifested by hypertonia (tremor and rigidity) and akinesia. Involvement of other neurocenters may contribute to dementia associated with Parkinson disease.[12]

Clinical Manifestations

The classic manifestations of Parkinson disease are tremor at rest (resting tremor), rigidity (muscle stiffness), bradykinesia/akinesia (poverty of movement), postural disturbance, dysarthria, and dysphagia. They may develop alone or in combination, but as the disease progresses, all are usually present. There is no true paralysis. The symptoms are always bilateral but usually involve one side early in the illness. Because the onset is insidious, the beginning of symptoms is difficult to document. Early in the disease, reflex status, sensory status, and mental status usually are normal. Postural abnormalities (flexed, forward leaning), difficulty walking, and weakness develop. Speech may be slurred. Autonomic-neuroendocrine symptoms include inappropriate diaphoresis, orthostatic hypotension, drooling, gastric retention, constipation, and urinary retention. In some cases (up to 40%), dementia may occur.[13] Depression is also prevalent.

Disorders of equilibrium result from loss of postural stability. The person with Parkinson disease cannot make the

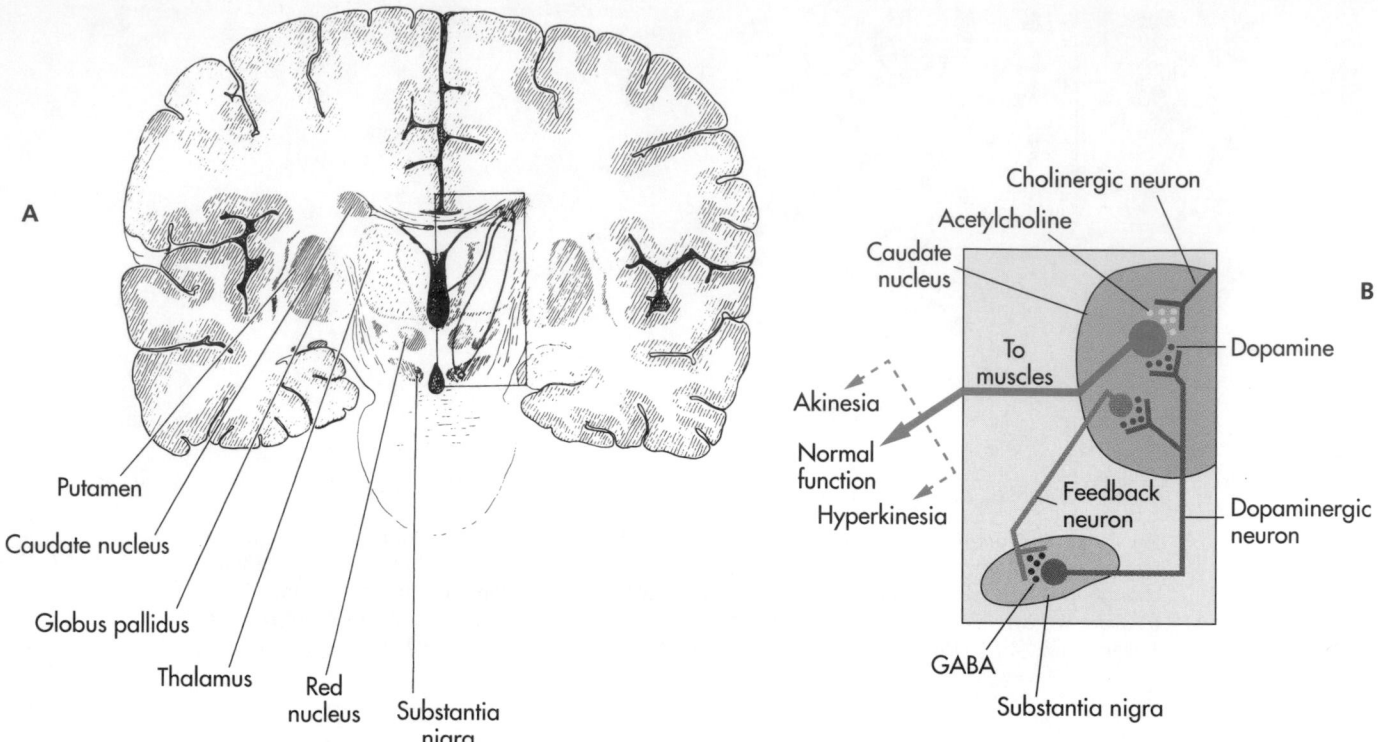

A

Putamen

Caudate nucleus

Globus pallidus

Thalamus   Red
nucleus   Substantia
nigra

B

Cholinergic neuron

Acetylcholine

Caudate
nucleus

To
muscles

Dopamine

Akinesia

Normal
function

Hyperkinesia

Feedback
neuron

Dopaminergic
neuron

GABA

Substantia nigra

Fig. 15-16 *Nigrostriatal disorders produce the Parkinson syndrome.* Coronal section of the brain shows the basal ganglia. Pathways controlling normal and abnormal motor function are depicted in a portion of the basal ganglia (*caudate nucleus*), **A;** they are shown enlarged in **B.** Dopaminergic synaptic activity is mediated by dopamine. Cholinergic synaptic activity is mediated by acetylcholine. A balance between the two kinds of activity produces normal motor function. A relative excess of cholinergic activity produces akinesia and rigidity. A relative excess of dopaminergic activity produces involuntary movements. Neurons in the caudate nucleus contain gamma-aminobutyric acid (GABA) and possibly control dopaminergic neurons in the substantia nigra through a feedback pathway. *(A from Cutler, W.P. [1983].* Degenerative and hereditary diseases *[7th ed.]. Washington, D.C.: Scientific American Medicine.)*

appropriate postural adjustment to tilting or falling and falls like a post when starting to tilt. The festinating gait (short, accelerating steps) of the individual with Parkinson disease is an attempt to maintain an upright position while walking (Fig. 15-17). Individuals are also unable to right themselves when changing from a reclining or crouching position to a standing position and when rolling over from a supine to a lateral or prone position.

Progressive dementia may be associated with the disease and is more common in persons older than 70 years. The person's mental status may be further compromised by the side effects of the medication taken to control symptoms.

Evaluation and Treatment

The diagnosis of Parkinson disease is based on the history and physical examination. Causes of secondary parkinsonism are first excluded. No specific diagnostic tests are available. Treatment of Parkinson disease is symptomatic, involving drug therapy. The drugs used are to decrease akinesia. Because of troublesome side effects and loss of effectiveness, however, drug therapy may not be started until the symp-

toms become incapacitating. Surgical interventions, predominantly pallidotomy, are reemerging.[14] Parkinson disease progresses slowly for 15 to 20 years before producing severe immobility and dependence. Nutrition and exercise are important for maintaining energy and strength.

Huntington disease

Huntington disease (HD), which is also known as *chorea,* is a relatively rare, hereditary, degenerative disorder diffusely involving the basal ganglia and cerebral cortex. The onset of Huntington disease is usually between 30 and 50 years of age, when the trait may already have been passed to the victim's children. The disorder has a prevalence rate of approximately 5 per 100,000 persons and occurs in all races.

Pathophysiology

Huntington disease is inherited as an autosomal dominant trait with high penetrance. The gene has been isolated and cloned on chromosome 4. (Mechanisms of genetic inheritance are discussed in Chapter 2.) The principal pathologic feature of Huntington disease is severe degeneration of the

Fig. 15-17 *Characteristic shuffling gait of individual with Parkinson disease. (Modified from Rudy, E.B. [1984].* Advanced neurological and neurosurgical nursing. *St. Louis: Mosby.)*

basal ganglia, particularly the caudate and putamen nuclei. Early in the disease there is loss of the gamma-aminobutyric acid (GABA) pathway to the globus pallidus. Basal ganglia and nigral depletion of GABA, an inhibitory neurotransmitter, is the principal biochemical alteration in Huntington disease. It alters the integration of motor and mental function. Degeneration of the pallidus pathway to the substantia nigra causes GABA depletion in the substantia nigra with decreased inhibitory GABA activity on dopaminergic neurons in the substantia nigra and relative excess of dopaminergic activity in the basal ganglial feedback circuit with the cerebral cortex. Frontal cerebral atrophy occurs late in the disease.[15] Symptoms progress slowly and include hypotonia and involuntary, fragmentary movements, such as chorea.

Clinical Manifestations

The classic manifestations of Huntington disease are abnormal movement and progressive dysfunction of intellectual and thought processes (dementia). Any one of these features may mark the onset of the disease. Chorea, the most common type of abnormal movement affecting these individuals, begins in the face and arms, eventually affecting the entire body. Cognitive deficits include loss of working memory and reduced capacity to plan, organize, and sequence. Thinking is slow, and apathy is present. Restlessness, disinhibition, and irritability are common. Euphoria or depression may be present.

Evaluation and Treatment

The diagnosis of Huntington disease is based on family history and clinical presentation of the disorder. No known treatment is effective in halting the degeneration or progression of symptoms. Recombinant genetic techniques may someday prevent or control the disorder. Depression or psychosis is treated with drug therapy. Phenothiazines, which are antidopaminergic, may relieve some symptoms of chorea.

Multiple sclerosis

Multiple sclerosis (MS) is a relatively common disorder involving destruction of CNS myelin, sparing the peripheral nervous system. Demyelinating disorders are acquired conditions and are characterized by degeneration of previously normal myelin with relative preservation of axons. CNS demyelinating disorders are subclassified as *primary* and *secondary*, with multiple sclerosis and its variants in the primary category. In secondary disorders, demyelination is caused by disorders other than multiple sclerosis.

The onset of MS is usually between 20 and 50 years of age.[15] Male/female ratio is about 1:2.[16] MS is the most prevalent CNS demyelinating disorder and a leading cause of neurologic disability in early adulthood. The disease is most prevalent in areas far from the equator. In the United States and Canada, the prevalence rate ranges from 30 to 80 per 100,000 persons.[15] MS occurs in all races but is more common in whites. Although the disorder does not exhibit a defined inheritance pattern, 15% of persons with MS have an affected relative.

Pathophysiology

The pathogenesis of MS is unknown. Most theories suggest an immunogenetic-viral cause, and the disease is associated with a possible genetic predisposition and interaction with environmental risk factors (see Chapter 2). The central component of the pathogenic model is the demyelinating process. Pathologic features of this process are (1) interaction between the systemic immune system and the CNS and (2) demyelinating lesions (plaques and diffuse lesions) in the white matter (Fig. 15-18). (The systemic immune system is discussed in Chapter 5.)

The interaction between the immune system and the CNS is complex. An immune response, possibly to a slow viral infection, may cause initial and recurring inflammatory reactions. An autoimmune response may occur during which the body produces antibodies to myelin basic protein, or there may be an autosensitization to an antigen present.

As the inflammation resolves, plaques and diffuse lesions become the pathologic feature of the demyelinating process. Plaques characteristically involve the CNS white matter but occasionally extend into the adjacent gray matter. They often coalesce into larger plaques. In established disease the multifocal, multistaged feature of plaques produces symptoms that are multiple and variable.

The acute (early) stage of plaque formation is characterized by perivenular demyelination with inflammatory

Fig. 15-18 *Chronic multiple sclerosis.* Demyelination plaque at gray-white junction and adjacent partially remyelinated shadow plaque *(arrows). (From Damjanov, I. & Linder, J. [1996]. Anderson's pathology [10th ed.]. St. Louis: Mosby.)*

edema in and around the plaque and partial demyelination. Symptoms usually remit, partially or completely, weeks after the onset of an early episode.

The chronic stage of demyelination and plaque formation is characterized by *gliosis* (glial scarring with late degeneration of axons). Progressive loss of function leads to permanent disability, usually over 20 years or more.

Although plaques are considered diagnostic of MS, diffuse lesions are common pathologic findings in actively progressive cases. Diffuse lesions are small, widespread areas of perivenular demyelination that do not progress through gliosis. These lesions are sometimes accompanied by edema of surrounding normal brain tissue. The relationship of plaques to diffuse lesions is unknown.

Clinical Manifestations

Various events occur immediately before the onset or exacerbation of symptoms and are regarded as precipitating factors. Infection, trauma, and pregnancy are the least debated. Most of the pregnancy-related exacerbations occur 3 months postpartum, suggesting a relation to the stresses of labor and the increased fatigue during the postpartum period rather than to the pregnancy itself.

In 1996 a new classification of types of MS was adopted—benign MS, relapsing-remitting (RR) MS, primary-progressive (PP) MS, secondary-progressive (SP) MS, and

malignant MS.[17] Initially 90% of persons present with a remitting-relapsing course.

The major manifestations of MS are initial syndromes followed by remissions and established syndromes with no remissions. Usually persons with late MS predominantly have one of the following established syndromes—mixed (generalized), spinal, or cerebellar (pontobulbar cerebellar). The syndrome depends on the portion of the CNS most involved. Early cognitive changes are now being found on testing of asymptomatic persons.[18] After years, 50% of individuals appear to have established syndromes of mixed involvement.

Short-lived attacks of neurologic deficits are the temporary appearance or worsening of symptoms. The mechanism of these attacks is complete, reversible conduction block in partially demyelinated axons. Conditions that cause short-lived attacks include (1) minor increases in body temperature or serum Ca^{++} concentration and (2) functional demands exceeding conduction capacity. An increase in body temperature or serum Ca^{++} level increases current leakage through demyelinated neurons. Persons with MS may become dramatically worse when body temperature is raised. Other triggering events include hypercalcemia and physical and emotional stress.

Paroxysmal attacks are sensory or motor symptoms of abrupt onset and short duration (few seconds or minutes) and include paresthesias, dysarthria and ataxia, and tonic head turning. The mechanism of paroxysmal attacks is nonsynaptic transmission, in which nerve impulses are directly transmitted between adjacent demyelinated axons. A common paroxysmal symptom, called Lhermitte sign, is the momentary paresthesia (shocklike or tingling sensation) that shoots down the trunk or limbs during active or passive flexion of the neck. Bending the neck evokes nonsynaptic impulses in demyelinated axons of the dorsal column in the spinal cord. A person with MS may have many paroxysmal attacks each day. Inciting events include sensory stimulation, voluntary movement, hyperventilation, and emotional stress. Paroxysmal attacks tend to persist for weeks or months and may be followed by progressive symptoms of MS.

Evaluation and Treatment

The diagnosis of MS (definite, probable, or possible) is based on the history and physical examination supported by findings from MRI.[19] Persistently elevated CSF immunoglobulin G (IgG) is found in about two thirds of individuals with MS,[15] and oligoclonal (IgG) bands on electrophoresis are found in more than 90%.[19] Evoked response studies aid diagnosis by detecting decreased conduction velocity in visual, auditory, and somatosensory pathways. MRI may be the most sensitive available method of detecting the disease as compared with oligoclonal banding, evoked-response (ER) studies, or CT scanning.

MS is treated from two perspectives[20]: (1) treat exacerbations and (2) treat progression. Drugs with antiinflammatory properties are used to treat exacerbations. Agents that affect the immune system by immunosuppression and immune modulation are used to slow or stop progression.[21] Symptom management is also part of treatment plans.[20] Special problems requiring preventive and symptomatic management are fatigue[22]; weakness; spasticity; bladder, bowel, and sexual dysfunction; pain; tremor and ataxia; depression; and heat intolerance. Supportive and rehabilitative management is directed toward relieving specific symptoms and preventing the complications of immobility—especially pressure sores and infections of the pulmonary and genitourinary systems.

Amyotrophic lateral sclerosis

Amyotrophic lateral sclerosis (ALS, sporadic motor neuron disease, sporadic motor system disease) is a worldwide degenerative disorder diffusely involving lower and upper motor neurons. The term *amyotrophic* (without muscle nutrition or progressive muscle wasting) refers to the predominant lower motor neuron component of the syndrome. Lateral sclerosis, scarring of the corticospinal tract in the lateral column of the spinal cord, refers to the upper motor neuron component of the syndrome.

Classic ALS (Lou Gehrig disease) may begin at any time from the fourth decade of life; its peak occurrence is in the early 50s. Male/female ratio is 3:2, equalizing after menopause. The disorder occurs in approximately 1 of every 100,000 persons. Subtypes of ALS include primary lateral sclerosis, progressive bulbar palsy, and progressive muscular atrophy.

➤ *Pathophysiology*

Current data suggest a genetic factor is involved. Half of persons with familial ALS have a genetic defect on chromosome 21 in the gene that codes for an enzyme that helps destroy free radicals. Glutamate metabolism is altered, and glutamate toxicity is now believed to cause or contribute to major neuron degeneration.[23]

The principal pathologic feature of ALS is lower and upper motor neuron degeneration, although without inflammation. There are fewer large motor neurons in the spinal cord, brain stem, and cerebral cortex (premotor and motor areas), with ongoing degeneration in the remaining motor neurons. Death of the motor neuron results in axonal degeneration and secondary demyelination with glial proliferation and sclerosis (scarring).

Lower motor neuron degeneration denervates motor units. Adjacent, still-viable lower motor neurons attempt to compensate by distal intramuscular sprouting, reinnervation, and enlargement of motor units. The initial symptoms of the disease may be related to lower or upper motor neuron dysfunction or to both.

➤ *Clinical Manifestations*

Weakness may begin in any or all muscles of the body. Both flaccid paralysis and spastic paralysis occur with progressive muscle atrophy. No associated mental, sensory, or autonomic symptoms are present. Normal intellectual and sensory functions are sustained until death.

➤ *Evaluation and Treatment*

The diagnosis of the syndrome is based predominantly on the history and physical examination. Electromyography and muscle biopsy verify lower motor neuron degeneration and denervation. Little treatment is available to alter the overall course of the ALS syndrome. Riluzole (Rilutek) has recently extended time not requiring ventilatory assistance.[24] Supportive management and rehabilitative management are directed toward preventing complications of immobility. Psychologic support of the affected individual and the family is extremely important in this disorder.

The average duration of life is approximately 4 to 5 years from the appearance of symptoms, but the course of the disease may run from a few months to 15 years. Twenty percent of persons survive 5 to 20 years.[8]

✓ QUICK CHECK

Why is Alzheimer disease currently viewed as having a genetic susceptibility?

Why is Parkinson disease classified as a neurotransmitter disease?

Why is multiple sclerosis an autoimmune disease?

Why is amyotrophic lateral sclerosis a motor neuron disease?

PERIPHERAL NERVOUS SYSTEM AND NEUROMUSCULAR JUNCTION DISORDERS

Peripheral Nervous System Disorders

The axons traveling to and from the brain stem and spinal cord neuronal cell bodies may be injured by disease processes. The injury may affect a distinct anatomic area on the axon, or the spinal nerves may be injured at the roots, at the plexus before peripheral nerve formation, or at the nerves themselves. The cranial nerves do not have roots or plexuses and are affected only within themselves. Autonomic nerve fibers may be injured as they travel in certain cranial nerves and emerge through the ventral root and plexuses to travel in the peripheral nerves of the body. The injuries produced are summarized in Table 15-10.

Neuromuscular Junction Disorders

Transmission of the nerve impulse at the neuromuscular junction requires the release of adequate amounts of neurotransmitter from the presynaptic terminals of the axon and effective binding of the released transmitter to the receptors on the membranes of muscle cells (see Fig. 12-13). Nutritional deficits, certain drugs (e.g., reserpine, methyldopa [Aldomet]), and certain disorders that interfere with the synthesis or packaging of the neurotransmitter or its release into the synaptic cleft may result in weakness. Likewise, any

TABLE 15-10	Peripheral Nervous System Disorders	
Disorder	Pathology	Clinical Manifestations
Radiculopathies	Injury to spinal roots as they exit or enter the vertebral canal; caused by compression, inflammation, direct trauma	Affects strength, tone, and bulk of muscles innervated by involved roots; pattern similar to that seen in amyotrophies, with tone and deep-tendon reflexes decreased, rarely absent; fasciculations; mild fatigue; sensory alterations, pain
Plexus injuries	Involve nerve plexus distal to spinal roots but proximal to formation of peripheral nerves; caused by trauma, compression, infiltration, or iatrogenic (positioning or intramuscular injection)	Motor weakness, muscle atrophy, sensory loss in affected areas; paralysis common
Neuropathies	Called sensorimotor if sensory, motor, and reflex effects; pure sensory caused by leprosy, industrial solvents, chloramphenicol, and hereditary mechanisms; motor caused by Guillain-Barré syndrome, infectious mononucleosis, viral hepatitis, acute porphyria, lead, mercury, and triorthocresylphosphates (TCP)	Affects muscle strength, tone, and bulk; whole muscles or groups may be paretic or paralyzed; muscles of feet and legs first, then hands and arms; tone and deep tendon reflexes generally decreased with atrophy and fasciculation; mild fatigue; some specific symptoms of paresthesia and dysesthesia; altered reflexes; autonomic disturbances; deformities; metabolic changes
Guillain-Barré syndrome	Acute onset of motor paralysis (ascending); occurs throughout the world and in both genders and all age-groups, at all seasons; mild respiratory or gastrointestinal viral infection 3 weeks or longer before symptoms appear is common	Paresis of legs to complete quadriplegia, respiratory insufficiency, autonomic nervous system instability; may progress to respiratory arrest or cardiovascular collapse

pathologic process or drug that interferes with the binding of the neurotransmitter to the receptor may cause weakness.

Myasthenia gravis

Myasthenia gravis is a chronic autoimmune disease that affects the neuromuscular junction and is characterized by muscle weakness and fatigability. In 10% to 25% of persons with myasthenia gravis, thymic tumors are found, and in 70% to 80% there are pathologic changes in the thymus.[15] Tumors are more common in males than in females. Myasthenia gravis is an autoimmune disease associated with an increased incidence of other autoimmune diseases, including systemic lupus erythematosus, rheumatoid arthritis, polymyositis, and thyrotoxicosis. (Autoimmune mechanisms are discussed in Chapter 7.) Transitory signs of myasthenia gravis are present in 10% to 15% of infants born to mothers with myasthenia gravis.

The three types of myasthenia gravis are ocular, generalized, and bulbar myasthenia. *Ocular myasthenia,* which is more common in males, involves muscle weakness that is confined to the eye muscles. *Generalized myasthenia* involves the proximal musculature throughout the body and can have periodic remissions, a slowly progressive course, a rapidly progressive course, or a fulminating course. *Bulbar myasthenia* involves the muscles innervated by cranial nerves IX, X, XI, and XII and tends to be rapidly progressive or fulminating.

 Pathophysiology

Myasthenia gravis results from a defect in nerve impulse transmission at the neuromuscular junction. The postsynaptic acetylcholine receptors on the muscle cell's plasma membrane are no longer recognized as "self" and elicit the generation of autoantibodies. IgG antibody is produced against the acetylcholine receptors and fixes onto the receptor sites, blocking the binding of acetylcholine. Eventually the antibody action destroys receptor sites. This causes diminished transmission of the nerve impulse across the neuromuscular junction and lack of muscle depolarization. Why this autosensitization occurs is not known.

 Clinical Manifestations

Myasthenia gravis typically has an insidious onset. Clinical manifestations may first appear during pregnancy, during the postpartum period, or in conjunction with the administration of certain anesthetic agents. The person often complains of fatigue after exercise and has a recent history of recurring upper respiratory tract infections. The muscles of the eyes, face, mouth, throat, and neck usually are affected first. The extraocular (eye) muscles and the levator muscles are most affected. Manifestations include diplopia, ptosis, and ocular palsies.

The muscles of facial expression, mastication, swallowing, and speech are the next most involved. The results are facial droop and an expressionless face; difficulty chewing and swallowing associated with dietary changes and weight loss; drooling and episodes of choking and aspiration; and a nasal, low-volume, but high-pitched monotonous speech pattern.

The muscles of the neck, shoulder girdle, and hip flexors are less frequently affected. When these muscles do become involved, however, the person experiences fatigue requiring periods of rest, weakness of the arms and legs that improves with rest, and difficulty in maintaining head position. The respiratory muscles of the diaphragm and chest wall become weak, and ventilation is impaired. Deep breathing and coughing difficulties predispose the individual to atelectasis and congestion. In the advanced stage of the disease all muscles are weak.

Myasthenic crisis occurs when severe muscle weakness causes extreme quadriparesis or quadriplegia, respiratory insufficiency with shortness of breath, and extreme difficulty in swallowing. The individual in myasthenic crisis is in danger of respiratory arrest.

Cholinergic crisis may arise from anticholinesterase drug toxicity. The clinical picture is like that of myasthenic crisis, but other symptoms are present also. Intestinal motility increases, with episodes of diarrhea and complaints of cramping; fasciculation, bradycardia, pupillary constriction, increased salivation, and increased sweating. These are caused by the smooth muscle hyperactivity secondary to excessive accumulation of acetylcholine at the neuromuscular junctions and excessive parasympathetic-like activity. As in myasthenic crisis, the individual is in danger of respiratory arrest.

⚛ *Evaluation and Treatment*

The diagnosis of myasthenia gravis is made on the basis of a response to edrophonium chloride (Tensilon), an electromyogram (EMG), and antiacetylcholine receptor (anti-AChR) antibody titers. With the intravenous administration of the drug, immediate demonstrable improvement in muscle strength usually persists for several minutes. On EMG, the amplitude of the action potentials of stimulated muscles rapidly declines. Mediastinal tomography and MRI help determine whether a thymoma is present. The progression of myasthenia gravis varies, appearing first as a mild case that spontaneously remits, with a series of relapses and symptom-free intervals ranging from weeks to months. Over time the disease can progress, leading to death. Ocular myasthenia has a very good prognosis.

Anticholinesterase drugs, steroids, and immunosuppressant drugs are used to treat myasthenia gravis and myasthenic crisis. Plasmapheresis may be lifesaving during myasthenic crisis, before and after thymectomy, and at the start of immunosuppressant therapy. For individuals with cholinergic crisis, anticholinergic drugs are withheld until blood levels fall out of the toxic range, while ventilatory support is provided and respiratory complications are prevented. Thymectomy is the treatment of choice in individuals with a thymoma.

Myopathies

Myopathy is the term applied to a primary muscle disorder. Many pathologic processes affect muscles and cause loss of functional muscle cells. In the presence of myopathies, muscle strength, tone, and bulk are affected.

Primary muscle disease invariably is associated with weakness—usually marked. The distribution of the weakness in myopathy is usually symmetric and proximal, although occasionally it is predominantly distal, as in myotonic dystrophy. Mild fatigue is noted. Tone is decreased, as are the tendon reflexes, and atrophy may be present. Some myopathies are associated with muscle hypertrophy (cretinism and the familial progressive muscular dystrophies of childhood), in which muscles are rubbery and weak. Fasciculations are not present with myopathy because no denervation is present. No sensory changes are found. (Specific myopathies are discussed in Chapter 14.)

✓ QUICK CHECK

Why do antibodies contribute to the development of myasthenia gravis?

Why is weakness the primary symptom of a myopathy?

TUMORS OF THE CENTRAL NERVOUS SYSTEM

No proven causative agents for CNS tumors have been established. Carcinogenesis is discussed in Chapter 9.

Cranial Tumors

Tumors within the cranium can be either primary or metastatic as follows:

- *Primary.* Intracerebral tumors originate from brain substance, including neuroglia, neurons, cells of blood vessels, and connective tissue. Extracerebral tumors originate outside substances of brain and include meningiomas, acoustic nerve tumors, and tumors of pituitary and pineal glands.
- *Metastatic.* Found inside or outside brain substance.

CNS tumors include both brain and spinal cord tumors. Primary brain tumors have an incidence rate of 5 per 100,000 in the United States.[24] The incidence of CNS tumors increases to age 70 years and then decreases. CNS tumors are the second most common group of tumors occurring in children.[11,25] Approximately 70% of all intracranial tumors in children are located infratentorially, and in adults 70% are located supratentorially. Peripheral nerve tumors are rare in children and common in adults.

Local effects of cranial tumors are caused by the destructive action of the tumor itself on a particular site in the brain and by compression causing decreased cerebral blood flow. Effects include seizures, visual disturbances, unstable gait, and cranial nerve dysfunction. Generalized effects result

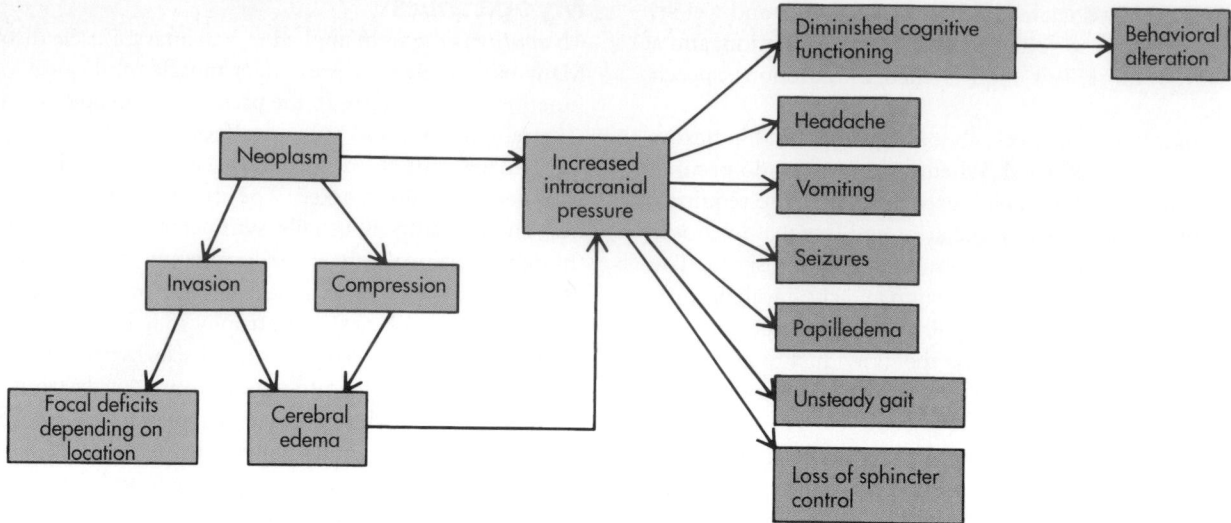

Fig. 15-19 *Origin of clinical manifestations associated with an intracranial neoplasm.*

from increased intracranial pressure (Fig. 15-19) caused by obstruction of the ventricular system, hemorrhages in and around the tumor, or cerebral edema.

Intracranial brain tumors do not metastasize as readily as tumors in other organs because there are no lymphatic channels within the brain substance. If metastasis does occur, it is usually through seeding of cerebral blood or CSF during cranial surgery or through artificial shunts.[25]

Primary intracerebral tumors

Primary intracerebral tumors (*gliomas*) comprise both encapsulated and nonencapsulated or invasive tumors (Table 15-11) and represent 40% to 67% of primary brain tumors.[24] Typically, invasive tumors invade and destroy adjacent normal CNS tissue, and more distal neural and vascular tissues are displaced and compressed, causing ischemia, edema, and increased intracranial pressure. Encapsulated tumors displace and compress adjacent and distal CNS tissues and vasculature. As with invasive tumors, encapsulated tumors produce ischemia, edema, and increased pressure. Both types impair the normal function of the neurons.

Surgical or radiosurgical excision, surgical decompression, chemotherapy, and radiotherapy are used for these tumors. Supportive treatment is directed at reducing edema. (Cancer treatment is discussed in Chapters 9 and 10.)

Astrocytoma

Astrocytomas are the most common primary CNS tumors (30% of all gliomas) and are graded by two classification systems (Table 15-12). Developed from astrocytes, astrocytomas expand and infiltrate into the normal surrounding brain tissues. These tumor cells are believed to have lost normal growth restraint and thus proliferate uncontrollably.

One third of astrocytomas are classified at diagnosis as grade I or grade II astrocytoma. These slow-growing but infiltrative gliomas tend to form cavities (pseudocysts); however, some are firm, noncavitating, avascular, gray-white

masses that are difficult to distinguish from normal white matter. Although these tumors may occur anywhere in the brain or spinal cord, they generally are located in the cerebellum, temporal lobes, frontal lobes, and parietal lobes. Low-grade astrocytomas in adults tend to be located laterally or supratentorially and in a midline or near midline position in children.

Headache and seizures may be early signs. Onset of a focal seizure disorder between the second and sixth decade of life suggests an astrocytoma. Other general or focal neurologic manifestations develop gradually, with increased intracranial pressure occurring late in the tumor's course.

Conventional surgery or radiosurgery is the treatment of choice, often followed by radiotherapy. Survival time from diagnosis is often 6 to 10 years. Grade I and II astrocytomas commonly progress to a higher-grade tumor.

Grade III and IV astrocytomas are found predominantly in the temporal lobes, frontal lobe, and basal ganglia, although they may occur in the brain stem, cerebellum, and spinal cord. Men are twice as likely to have them as women, and those 45 to 55 years old have the highest incidence.

Grade IV astrocytomas, glioblastoma multiforme, are highly vascular and extensively infiltrative. They may become large enough to extend from the meningeal surface through the ventricular wall. Fifty percent of glioblastomas are bilateral or at least occupy more than one lobe at the time of death.

The typical clinical presentation for a glioblastoma multiforme is that of diffuse, nonspecific clinical signs, such as headache, irritability, and "personality changes" that progress to more clear-cut manifestations of increased intracranial pressure, such as headache on position change, papilledema, or vomiting. From 30% to 40% of persons experience seizure activity. Symptoms may progress to include definite focal signs, such as hemiparesis, dysphasia, dyspraxia, cranial nerve palsies, and visual field deficits.

Diagnosis of high-grade astrocytomas most commonly

TABLE 15-11 Brain and Spinal Cord Tumors

Neoplasm	Location	Characteristics	Cell of Origin
Gliomas			
Astrocytoma	Anywhere in brain or spinal cord	Slow-growing, invasive	Astrocytes
Glioblastoma multiforme	Predominantly in cerebral hemispheres	Highly invasive and malignant	Thought to arise from mature astrocytes
Oligodendrocytoma	Most commonly in frontal lobes deep in white matter; may arise in brain stem, cerebellum, and spinal cord	Relatively avascular, tends to be encapsulated; more malignant form called an *oligodendroblastoma*	Oligodendrites
Ependymoma	Intramedullary: well of the ventricles, may arise in caudal tail of the spinal cord	More common in children, variable growth rates; more malignant, invasive form is called *ependymoblastoma;* may extend into the ventricle or invade brain tissue	Ependymal cells
Neuronal cell			
Medulloblastoma	Posterior cerebellar vermis, roof of fourth ventricle	Well-demarcated, rapid-growing, fills fourth ventricle	Embryonic cells
Mesodermal tissue			
Meningioma	Intradural, extramedullary: sylvian fissure region, superior parasagittal surface of frontal and parietal lobes, olfactory groove, wing of sphenoid bone, superior surface of cerebellum, cerebellopontine angle, spinal cord	Slow-growing, circumscribed, encapsulated, sharply demarcated from normal tissues, compressive in nature	Arachnoid cells, may be from fibroblast
Choroid plexus			
Papillomas	Choroid plexus of the ventricular system, lateral ventricle in children, fourth ventricle in adults	Usually benign, slow expansion inducing hemorrhage and hydrocephalus; malignant tumor is rare	Epithelial cells
Cranial nerves and spinal nerve roots			
Neurilemmoma	Cranial nerves (most commonly vestibular division of cranial nerve VIII)	Slow-growing	Schwann cells
Neurofibroma	Extramedullary—spinal cord	Slow-growing	Neurilemma, Schwann cells
Pituitary tumors	Pituitary gland; may extend to or invade floor of the third ventricle	Age-linked, several types, slow-growing, macroadenomas and microadenomas	Pituitary cells, pituitary chromophobes, basophils, eosinophils
Pineal region	Pineal region; pineal parenchyma	Several types (germinoma, pineocytoma, teratoma)	Several types with different cell origins
Blood vessel tumors			
Angioma	Predominantly in posterior cerebral hemispheres	Slow-growing	Arising from congenitally malformed arteriovenous connections
Hemangioblastomas	Predominantly in cerebellum	Slow-growing	Embryonic vascular tissue

TABLE 15-12	Classification Systems for Astrocytomas	
	Kernohen et al. System	Rigertz System
Astrocytoma		Well-differentiated astrocytoma
Grade I	Well-differentiated astrocytoma	
Grade II	More cellular and anaplastic astrocytoma	
Glioblastoma		Malignant anaplastic astrocytoma
Grade III	Poorly differentiated astrocytoma	
Grade IV	Poorly differentiated astrocytoma (glioblastoma multiforme)	Glioblastoma multiforme

takes 3 to 6 months from onset of the first clinical manifestations because the person does not recognize the need to consult a health care provider. The treatment of choice is conventional surgical or radiosurgical resection, which is commonly followed by radiotherapy and then chemotherapy. Fewer than one fifth of persons survive 12 to 18 months beyond the onset of clinical manifestations with a grade IV tumor; fewer than 10% live beyond 2 years. Adding radiotherapy or chemotherapy has extended mean survival time.

Oligodendroglioma

Oligodendrogliomas constitute perhaps 5% to 7% of all intracranial gliomas. They are typically slow-growing tumors, and most oligodendrogliomas are macroscopically indistinguishable from other gliomas. From 40% to 70% develop in the frontal lobes, often in the deep white matter, but they are found also in other parts of the cerebrum, third ventricle, brain stem, cerebellum, and spinal cord. Many are found in young adults with a history of temporal lobe epilepsy. Approximately one half of tumors classified as oligodendrogliomas are actually a mixed type of oligodendroglioma and astrocytoma. Malignant degeneration occurs in approximately one third of persons with oligodendrogliomas, and the tumors are then referred to as *oligodendroblastomas.* If there is extension to the pia mater or ependymal wall (see Fig. 12-14), oligodendrogliomas may metastasize to distant CNS sites through the ventriculoarachnoid spaces.

More than 50% of individuals experience a focal or generalized seizure as the first clinical manifestation. Only one half of those with an oligodendroglioma have increased intracranial pressure at the time of diagnosis and surgery, and only one third develop focal manifestations. The time from first clinical manifestation to surgical intervention ranges from 2 to 6 years, with a mean survival time after operation of 5 years. Recurrences after surgery are common.

Ependymoma

Ependymomas are gliomas that arise from ependymal cells in the walls of the ventricles and grow either into the ventricle or into adjacent brain tissue; they are not encapsulated (Fig. 15-20). They comprise about 5% of all intracranial gliomas in adults and 20% in children and adolescents. About 70% occur in the fourth ventricle, with others found in the third ventricle, lateral ventricles, and caudal portion of the spinal cord. Approximately 40% of infratentorial

ependymomas occur in children younger than 10 years. Cerebral (supratentorial) ependymomas occur at all ages.

Ependymomas in the cerebrum resemble other gliomas clinically. Approximately one third of persons suffer seizures. In fourth ventricle ependymomas, two thirds of persons have increased intracranial pressure. Other clinical manifestations include vomiting, vertigo, difficulty swallowing, head tilt, and paresthesias of the extremities.

The course of ependymomas may be short or long. The interval between first manifestations and surgery may be as short as 4 weeks or as long as 8 years.

Surgery is the treatment of choice. Ependymomas are not very radiosensitive. Some persons benefit from a shunting procedure when the ependymoma has caused a noncommunicating hydrocephalus.

Primary extracerebral tumors
Meningioma

Meningiomas constitute 15% of all intracranial tumors. They are considered benign because they are encapsulated and usually do not invade the surrounding brain. These tumors usually originate from the dura mater or arachnoid membranes and rarely from arachnoid cells of the choroid plexus of the ventricles. Meningiomas are located most commonly in the olfactory grooves, on the wings of the sphenoid bone (at the base of the skull), in the tuberculum sellae (a structure next to the sella turcica), on the superior surface of the cerebellum, and in the cerebellopontine angle and spinal cord.

Small meningiomas (less than 2 cm in diameter) often are found on postmortem examination in middle-age and elderly individuals who experienced no clinical manifestations and died of totally unrelated causes. The cause of meningiomas is unknown.

A meningioma is sharply circumscribed and adapts to the shape it occupies. It may extend to the dural surface and erode the cranial bones or produce an osteoblastic reaction. A few meningiomas exhibit malignant, invasive qualities.

When meningiomas reach a certain size and begin to indent the brain parenchyma, clinical manifestations occur. Focal seizures are frequently the first manifestation. Because of the extremely slow-growing nature of these tumors, increased intracranial pressure is less common than with gliomas.

Surgical excision results in a cure if all the tumor and its

Fig. 15-20 *Large septal ependymoma.* This tumor represents the severity of tissue compression that occurs with a large brain tumor. The area in the upper-right part of the picture represents a secondary hydrocephalus that has further compressed brain tissue. *(Courtesy Dr. J.E. Olivera-Rabiela, Mexico City, Mexico. From Rosai, J. [1989]. Ackerman's surgical pathology [7th ed.]. St. Louis: Mosby.)*

meningeal stem are accessible. If only partial resection is possible, the tumor recurs. Radiation therapies also are used to slow growth.

Neurilemmoma

Neurilemmomas (also called neuromas, schwannomas) arise from the sheath of Schwann cells surrounding the axons of the cranial nerves. These tumors usually affect persons older than 50 years, and women are affected more often than men. The vestibular division of cranial nerve VIII is most commonly affected, although neurilemmomas of the acoustic division of cranial nerve VIII, cranial nerve V, and cranial nerve IX are found.

The tumor generally originates just distal to the junction between the nerve root and the brain stem. As it grows, it extends into the posterior fossa to occupy the cerebellopontine angle and compress adjacent nerves. Eventually the brain stem is displaced, and the CSF flow is obstructed.

Initial clinical manifestations include headache, tinnitus, hearing loss, impaired balance, unsteady gait, facial pain, and loss of facial sensations. Later, vertigo with nausea and vomiting, a sense of pressure in the ear, and moderate to severe unsteadiness with rapid position changes may appear.

CT scan or MRI can establish the diagnosis. Posterior fossa dye studies may be required. Treatment is by surgical excision of the neurilemmoma.

Pituitary tumors are discussed in Chapter 18, and cerebral tumors in children are discussed in Chapter 16.

Metastatic carcinoma

An estimated 25% of persons with cancer develop metastasis to the brain. One third of metastatic brain tumors arise from the lung, approximately one sixth from the breast, and a lesser number from the gastrointestinal tract and kidney. Melanoma and carcinoma of the gallbladder, liver, thyroid, testes, uterus, ovary, and pancreas also may metastasize to the brain. Other tumors that metastasize only occasionally are rhabdomyosarcoma, Ewing tumor, chorioepithelioma, lymphoma, and carcinoma.

Carcinomas are disseminated to the brain through the circulation. In more than three fourths of persons, the metastases are multiple and found scattered through the cerebrum and cerebellum. Metastatic tumors often are located in the meninges and near the brain surface in the gray matter and subcortical white matter. These tumors produce little glial cell reaction in the brain tissue but do cause vasogenic edema in surrounding brain tissue.

Metastatic brain tumors produce signs resembling those of glioblastomas, although several unusual syndromes do exist. Carcinomatous encephalopathy causes headache, nervousness, depressed mood, trembling, confusion, and forgetfulness. In carcinomatosis of the cerebellum, headache, dizziness, and ataxia are found. Carcinomatosis of the craniospinal meninges (carcinomatous meningitis) manifests with headache, confusion, and manifestations of cranial or spinal nerve root dysfunction.

Metastatic brain tumors carry a poor prognosis. If a solitary tumor is found, surgery or radiation therapy is used, but if multiple tumors exist, symptomatic relief only is pursued.

Spinal Cord Tumors

Spinal cord tumors are named to reflect their cell type, growth rate, and structure of origin. They may be *intramedullary tumors* (originating within the neural tissues) or *extramedullary tumors* (originating from tissues outside the spinal cord). Extramedullary tumors arise from the meninges or roots (forming *intradural tumors*) or from epidural tissue or vertebral structure (forming *extradural tumors*). About 5% of spinal cord tumors seen in general hospital settings are intramedullary; 40% are intradural-extramedullary; and 55% are extradural.

Metastatic spinal cord tumors are usually carcinomas, lymphomas, or myelomas. Their location is often extradural, with 50% metastatic, having spread to the spine through direct extension from tumors of the vertebral structures or from extraspinal sources extending through the interventricular foramen or bloodstream.

The most common primary extramedullary spinal cord tumors are neurofibromas and meningiomas. These tumors are intradural more often than extradural. Neurofibromas generally are found in the thoracic and lumbar region, whereas meningiomas are more evenly distributed through the spine. Other extramedullary tumors in order of frequency of occurrence are sarcomas, vascular tumors, chordomas, and epidermoid and similar tumors. Of intradural-extramedullary tumors, 70% are meningiomas, neurofibromas, or sarcomas.

Intramedullary tumors have the same cellular origins as brain tumors. Ependymomas account for 40% of intramedullary spinal cord tumors. Astrocytomas, glioblastomas, oligodendrogliomas, ganglioneuromas, medulloblastomas, hemangiomas, and hemangioblastomas are more or less equally distributed in frequency of occurrence.

Pathophysiology

Extramedullary spinal cord tumors produce dysfunction by compressing adjacent tissue, not by direct invasion. Compression destroys the white matter tracts, and the spinal canal around the cord becomes filled by tumor.

Intramedullary spinal cord tumors produce dysfunction by both invasion and compression. The cord enlarges as the tumor grows inside the cord. Adjacent white matter tracts are then distorted. Metastases from spinal cord tumors occur from seeding through the CSF; medulloblastomas and ependymomas establish distant implants in this way.

Clinical Manifestations

The acute onset of clinical manifestations suggests a vascular insult caused by thrombosis of vessels supplying the spinal cord. Clinical manifestations that are gradual and progressive suggest compression. Three major categories of clinical manifestations are seen: (1) a compressive syndrome, (2) an irritative syndrome, and (3) rarely, a syringomyelic syndrome.

The *compressive syndrome (sensorimotor syndrome)* occurs with compression or, less frequently, invasion and destruction of the spinal cord tracts. Symptoms are usually gradual and progressive, and initial manifestations may be asymmetric. Both motor function and sensory function are affected as the tumor grows and involves both the anterior and posterior spinal tracts.

The *irritative syndrome (radicular syndrome)* combines the clinical manifestations of a cord compression with radicular pain (occurs in the sensory root distribution and indicates root irritation). The segmental manifestations include segmental sensory changes, that is, paresthesias and impaired pain and touch perception; motor disturbances, including cramps, atrophy, fasciculations, and decreased or absent deep tendon reflexes; and ache in the spine.

Evaluation and Treatment

The diagnosis of a spinal cord tumor is made through spinal roentgenograms, CSF studies, CT scan, MRI, myelogram, and spinal angiography. Involvement of specific cord segments is established. Any metastases also are identified. Treatment varies, depending on the nature of the tumor and the person's clinical status.

✓ QUICK CHECK

How is an encapsulated CNS tumor different from a nonencapsulated CNS tumor?

What are three types of spinal cord tumors?

What are some common signs and symptoms of compressive and irritative spinal cord tumor syndromes?

▣ DID YOU UNDERSTAND?

Central Nervous System Disorders

1. Motor vehicle crashes are the major cause of traumatic CNS injury. Traumatic injuries to the head are classified as closed-head trauma (blunt) or open-head trauma (penetrating). Closed-head trauma is the more common type of trauma.

2. Different types of focal brain injury include contusion (bruising of the brain), laceration (tearing of brain tissue), extradural hematoma (accumulation of blood above the dura mater), subdural hematoma (blood between the dura mater and arachnoid membrane), intracerebral hematoma (bleeding into the brain), and open-head trauma.

3. Open-head trauma involves a skull fracture with exposure of the cranial vault to the environment. The types of open-head trauma (compound fracture, perforated fracture) are linear, comminuted, compound, and basilar skull fracture (in the cranial vault or at the base of the skull).

4. Diffuse brain injury (diffuse axonal injury [DAI]) results from the effects of head rotation. The brain experiences shearing stresses resulting in axonal damage ranging from concussion to a severe DAI state.

5. Spinal cord injury involves damage to vertebral or neural tissues by compressing tissue, pulling or exerting tension on tissue, or shearing tissues so that they slide into one another.

6. Spinal cord injury may cause spinal shock with cessation of all motor, sensory, reflex, and autonomic functions below any transected area. Loss of motor and sensory function depends on the level of injury.

7. Paralysis of the lower half of the body with both legs involved is called *paraplegia*. Paralysis involving all four extremities is called *quadriplegia*.

8. Return of spinal neuron excitability occurs slowly. Reflex activity can return in 1 to 2 weeks in most persons with acute spinal cord injury. A pattern of flexion reflexes emerges, involving first the toes, then the feet and the legs. Eventually, reflex voiding and bowel elimination appear and mass reflex (flexor spasms accompanied by profuse sweating, piloerection, and automatic bladder emptying) may develop.

9. Low back pain is pain between the lower rib cage and gluteal muscles and often radiates into the thigh.

■ DID YOU UNDERSTAND? —cont'd

10. Most causes of low back pain are unknown; however, some secondary causes are disk prolapse, tumors, bursitis, synovitis, degenerative joint disease, osteoporosis, fracture, inflammation, and sprain.

11. Herniation of an intervertebral disk is a protrusion of part of the nucleus pulposus. Herniation most commonly affects the lumbosacral disks (L5-S1 and L4-5). The extruded pulposus compresses the nerve root, causing pain that radiates along the sciatic nerve course.

12. Cerebrovascular disease is the most frequently occurring neurologic disorder. Any abnormality of the blood vessels of the brain is referred to as a cerebrovascular disease.

13. Cerebrovascular disease is associated with two types of brain abnormalities: (a) ischemia with or without infarction and (b) hemorrhage.

14. Cerebrovascular accidents are classified according to pathophysiology and include global hypoperfusion, thrombotic (arterial occlusions caused by thrombi), embolic (fragments that break from a thrombus outside the brain), hemorrhagic (intracranial hemorrhage), and lacunar strokes.

15. Intracranial aneurysms result from defects in the vascular wall and are classified on the basis of form and shape. They are frequently asymptomatic, but the signs vary, depending on the location and size of the aneurysm.

16. An arteriovenous malformation (AVM) is a tangled mass of dilated blood vessels. Although sometimes present at birth, AVM exhibits a delayed age of onset.

17. A subarachnoid hemorrhage occurs when blood escapes from defective or injured vasculature into the subarachnoid space. When a vessel tears, blood under pressure is pumped into the subarachnoid space. The blood produces an inflammatory reaction in these tissues.

18. Infection and inflammation of the CNS can occur by bacteria, viruses, fungi, protozoans, and rickettsiae. The resulting infection of bacterial infections is pus producing, or pyogenic.

19. Meningitis (infection of the meninges) is classified as bacterial, aseptic (nonpurulent), or fungal. Bacterial meningitis primarily is an infection of the pia mater and arachnoid and of the fluid of the subarachnoid space. Aseptic meningitis is believed to be limited to the meninges. Fungal meningitis is a chronic, less common type of meningitis.

20. The meningeal vessels become hyperemic, and neutrophils migrate into the subarachnoid space with bacterial meningitis. An inflammatory reaction occurs, and exudate is formed and increases rapidly.

21. Brain abscesses often originate from infections outside the CNS. Organisms gain access to the CNS from adjacent sites or spread along the wall of a vein. A localized inflammatory process develops

with exudate formation, thrombosis of vessels, and degenerating leukocytes. After a few days the infection becomes delimited with a center of pus and a wall of granular tissue.

22. Clinical manifestations of brain abscesses include headache, nuchal rigidity, confusion, drowsiness, and sensory and communication deficits. Treatment includes antibiotic therapy and surgical excision or aspiration.

23. Encephalitis is an acute, febrile illness of viral origin with nervous system involvement. The most common encephalitides are caused by arthropod-borne (mosquito-borne) viruses and herpes simplex. Meningeal involvement appears in all encephalitides.

24. Clinical manifestations of encephalitis include fever, delirium, confusion, seizures, abnormal and involuntary movement, and increased intracranial pressure.

25. Herpes encephalitis is treated with antiviral agents. No definitive treatment exists for the other encephalitides.

26. The common neurologic complications of AIDS are HIV encephalopathy, peripheral neuropathies, vacuolar myelopathy, opportunistic infections of the CNS, and neoplasms. Pathologically, there may be diffuse CNS involvement, focal pathology, and obstructive hydrocephalus.

27. Alzheimer disease is a chronic irreversible dementia that may be related to beta-amyloid metabolism.

28. Pick disease is a rare degenerative disease similar to Alzheimer disease.

29. Parkinson disease is a commonly occurring degenerative disorder of the basal ganglia (corpus striatum) involving degeneration of the dopamine-secreting nigrostriatal pathway. The pathogenesis of Parkinson disease is unknown, but researchers suggest genetic, viral, and environmental toxins as possible causes.

30. Degeneration of the dopaminergic nigrostriatal pathway causes dopamine depletion in the basal ganglia and excess of cholinergic activity in the cortex, basal ganglia, and thalamus. Tremor and rigidity are caused by the excess cholinergic activity. Progressive dementia may be associated with an advanced stage of the disease.

31. Huntington disease (chorea) is a rare hereditary disease involving the basal ganglia and cerebral cortex. It is inherited as an autosomal dominant trait and commonly manifests between 30 and 50 years of age.

32. The major pathologic feature of Huntington disease is severe degeneration of the basal ganglia and the frontal cerebral cortex. The basal ganglia and the substantia nigra exhibit a depletion of gamma-aminobutyric acid (an inhibitory neurotransmitter) secreting neurons. This depletion leads to an excess of dopaminergic activity that causes involuntary, fragmentary movements.

Continued

DID YOU UNDERSTAND? —cont'd

Central Nervous System Disorders—cont'd

33. Multiple sclerosis (MS) is a relatively common degenerative disorder involving CNS myelin. Although the pathogenesis is unknown, the demyelination is thought to result from an immunogenetic-viral cause. Viruses or other antigens may directly attack the myelin or provoke a hypersensitivity reaction.

34. Amyotrophic lateral sclerosis (ALS) is a degenerative disorder diffusely involving lower and upper motor neurons. The pathogenesis of ALS is not fully known; however, there is lower and upper motor neuron degeneration.

Peripheral Nervous System and Neuromuscular Joint Disorders

1. Radiculopathies are disorders of the roots of spinal cord nerves. The roots may be compressed, inflamed, or torn. Clinical manifestations include local pain or paresthesias in the sensory root distribution. Treatment may involve surgery, antibiotics, steroids, radiation therapy, and chemotherapy.

2. Plexus injuries involve the plexus distal to the spinal roots. Paralysis can occur with complete plexus involvement.

3. Neuropathies are the resulting syndrome when the peripheral nerves are affected. Axon and myelin degeneration may be present. Neuropathies are classified as sensorimotor, sensory, or motor. The neuropathies are characterized by varying degrees of sensory disturbance, paresis, and paralysis. Secondary atrophy may be present.

4. Guillain-Barré syndrome is a demyelinating disorder caused by a humoral and cell-mediated immunologic reaction directed at the peripheral nerves. The clinical manifestations may vary from paresis of the legs to complete quadriplegia, respiratory insufficiency, and autonomic nervous system instability. Plasmapheresis is used during the acute phase and followed by aggressive rehabilitation.

5. Myasthenia gravis is a disorder of voluntary muscles characterized by muscle weakness and fatigability. It is considered an autoimmune disease and is associated with an increased incidence of other autoimmune diseases.

6. Myasthenia gravis results from a defect in nerve impulse transmission at the neuromuscular junction. IgG antibody is secreted against the "self" acetylcholine receptors and blocks the binding of acetylcholine. The antibody action destroys the receptor sites, causing decreased transmission of the nerve impulse across the neuromuscular junction.

7. Primary disorders of muscles with weakness and atrophy are known as myopathies.

Tumors of the Nervous System

1. Two main types of tumors occur within the cranium: primary and metastatic. Primary tumors are classified as intracerebral tumors or extracerebral tumors. Metastatic tumors can be found inside or outside the brain substance.

2. CNS tumors cause local and generalized manifestations. The effects are varied, and local manifestations include seizures, visual disturbances, loss of equilibrium, and cranial nerve dysfunction.

3. Spinal cord tumors are classified as intramedullary tumors (within the neural tissues) or extramedullary tumors (outside the spinal cord). Metastatic spinal cord tumors are usually carcinomas, lymphomas, or myelomas.

4. Extramedullary spinal cord tumors produce dysfunction by compression of adjacent tissue, not by direct invasion. Intramedullary spinal cord tumors produce dysfunction by both invasion and compression.

5. The onset of clinical manifestations of spinal cord tumors is gradual and progressive, suggesting compression. Specific manifestations depend on the location of the tumor; for example, there may be paresis and spasticity of one leg with thoracic tumors, followed by involvement of the opposite leg.

KEY TERMS

Alzheimer disease (AD) (senile disease complex), 407
Amyotrophic lateral sclerosis (ALS, sporadic motor neuron disease, sporadic motor system disease), 413
Arteriovenous malformation (AVM), 402
Aseptic meningitis (viral meningitis, nonpurulent meningitis), 403
Autonomic hyperreflexia (dysreflexia), 392

Bacterial meningitis, 403
Brain abscess, 404
Brudzinski sign, 402
Bulbar myasthenia, 414
Cerebrovascular accident (CVA, stroke), 399
Cholinergic crisis, 415
Classic ALS (Lou Gehrig disease), 413
Classic cerebral concussion, 389
Closed (blunt) trauma, 385
Completed stroke, 400

Compressive syndrome (sensorimotor syndrome), 420
Contusion, 385
Degenerative disk disease, 395
Diffuse brain injury, 388
Embolic stroke, 400
Encephalitis, 405
Ependymoma, 418
Extradural brain abscess, 404
Extradural hematoma, 385
Extradural tumor, 419

KEY TERMS

Extramedullary tumor, 419
Focal brain injury, 385
Fungal meningitis, 403
Fusiform aneurysm (giant
    aneurysm), 401
Generalized myasthenia, 414
Glioma, 416
Gliosis, 412
Hemorrhagic stroke (intracranial
    hemorrhage), 400
HIV encephalopathy (subacute
    encephalitis, HIV-associated
    dementia complex, HIV cognitive
    motor complex, AIDS
    encephalopathy, AIDS dementia
    complex, AIDS-related
    dementia), 406
Huntington disease (HD), 410
Intracerebral brain abscess, 404
Intracerebral hematoma, 386
Intradural tumor, 419

Intramedullary spinal cord abscess, 404
Intramedullary tumor, 419
Irritative syndrome (radicular
    syndrome), 420
Kernig sign, 402
Lacunar stroke (lacunar infarct), 400
Meningioma, 418
Meningitis, 403
Multiple sclerosis (MS), 411
Myasthenia gravis, 414
Myasthenic crisis, 415
Myopathy, 415
Neurilemmoma, 419
Neurofibrillary tangle, 408
Ocular myasthenia, 414
Oligodendroblastoma, 418
Oligodendroglioma, 418
Open (penetrating) trauma, 385
Parkinson disease, 409
Parkinsonism (Parkinson syndrome,
    parkinsonian syndrome, paralysis
    agitans), 409

Pick disease, 409
Postconcussive syndrome, 389
Saccular aneurysm (berry
    aneurysm), 401
Senile plaque, 408
Spinal cord abscess, 404
Spinal epidural abscess, 404
Spinal shock, 392
Spinal stenosis, 397
Spondylolisthesis, 397
Spondylolysis, 397
Stroke-in-evolution (progressive
    stroke), 400
Subarachnoid hemorrhage, 402
Subdural hematoma, 385
Thrombotic stroke (cerebral
    thrombosis), 399
Toxoplasmosis, 407
Transient ischemic attack (TIA), 400
Vacuolar myelopathy, 407

REFERENCES

1. Wilkins, R.H. & Rengachary, S.S. (1996). *Neurosurgery* (vol. 3, 2nd ed.). New York: McGraw-Hill.
2. Bovenstein, D.G., Weisel, S.W., & Boden, S.D. (1995). *Low back pain, medical diagnosis, and comprehensive management* (2nd ed.). Philadelphia: Saunders.
3. Wilkins, R.H. & Rengachar, S.S. (1996). *Neurosurgery* (vol. 2, 2nd ed.). New York: McGraw-Hill.
4. Saito, I. et al. (1998). Neuroprotective effect of an antioxidant, Eseben, in patients with delayed neurological deficits after aneurysmal subarachnoid hemorrhage. *Neurosurgery, 42*(2), 269-278.
5. Cummings, J.L. et al. (1998). Alzheimer's disease: Etiologies, pathophysiology, cognitive reserve, and treatment opportunities. *Neurology, 51* (1 Suppl 1), S2-S17, discussion S65-S67.
6. Meier, R.W., Iwangoff, P., & Bertoni-Feddari, C. (1994). What is primary and what is secondary for amyloid deposition in Alzheimer disease. *Annals of the New York Academy of Science, 719,* 230-237.
7. Beal, M.F. (1994). Energy, oxidative damage and Alzheimer's disease: Clues to the underlying puzzle. *Neurobiology of Aging, 15*(Suppl. 2), S171-S174.
8. Strittmatter, W.J. et al. (1993). Apolipoprotein E: High affinity binding to b-amyloid and increased frequency of type 4 allele in familial Alzheimer's. *Proceedings of the National Academy of Science, 90*(5), 1977-1981.
9. Gambetti, P. & Perry, G. (1994). Alzheimer's disease and prion proteins: A meeting made in muscle. *American Journal of Pathology, 145*(6), 1261-1264.
10. Hazzard, W.R. et al. (1994). *Principles of geriatric medicine and gerontology* (3rd ed.). New York: McGraw-Hill.
11. Barker, E. (1994). *Neuroscience nursing.* St. Louis: Mosby.
12. Lang, A.E. & Lozano, A.M. (1998). Parkinson's disease. I. *New England Journal of Medicine, 339*(15), 1044-1053.
13. Albert, C.A. & Knoefel, J.E. (1994). *Clinical neurology of aging* (2nd ed.). New York: Oxford University Press.
14. Guridi, J. & Lozano, A.M. (1997). A brief history of pallidotomy. *Neurosurgery, 41,* 1169-1183.
15. Aylward, E.H. et al. (1998). Frontal lobe volume in patients with Huntington's disease. *Neurology, 50,* 252-258.
16. Adams, R.D., Victor, M., & Ropper, A.H. (1997). *Principles of neurology.* New York: McGraw-Hill.
17. Lublin, F.D. & Reingold, S.C. (1996). Defining the clinical course of multiple sclerosis: Results of an international survey. *Neurology, 46,* 907-911.
18. Amato, M.P. et al. (1995). Cognitive impairment in early onset multiple sclerosis: Patterns, predictors, and impact on everyday life in a 4-year study. *Archives of Neurology, 52*(2), 168-172.
19. Truyen, L. (1994). Magnetic resonance imaging in multiple sclerosis: A review. *Acta Neurologica Belgium, 94*(2), 98-102.
20. Wells, S. (1997). *Multiple sclerosis. The process and medical treatments* (2nd ed.). Cherry Hill, N.J.: MS Association of America.

REFERENCES

21. Miller, A. (1997). Current and investigational therapies used to alter the course of disease in multiple sclerosis. *Southern Medical Journal, 90,* 367-375.
22. Stuifbergen, A.K. & Rogers, S. (1997). The experience of fatigue and strategies of self-care among persons with multiple sclerosis. *Applied Nursing Research, 10,* 2-10.
23. Rothstein, J.D. (1995). Excitotoxic mechanisms in the pathogenesis of amyotrophic lateral sclerosis. In G. Serratrice & T. Munsat, Pathogenesis and therapy of amyotrophic lateral sclerosis. *Advances in Neurology, 68,* 7-20.
24. Miller, R.G. & Sufit, R. (1997). New approaches to the treatment of ALS. *Neurology, 47*(Suppl. 4), S28-S32.
25. Black, P.M. & Loeffler, S.S. (1997). *Cancer of the nervous system.* Cambridge, Mass.: Blackwell Science, Inc.

CHAPTER 16

Alterations of Neurologic Function in Children

Judith A. Farley and Barbara J. Boss

Central nervous system (CNS) malformations are responsible for 75% of fetal deaths and 40% of deaths during the first year of life. During the perinatal period, CNS malformations account for one third of all apparent congenital malformations, and 90% of CNS malformations are defects of neural tube closure. Although embryology is a highly complex and often difficult science, the process of embryonic development explains many of the malformations that occur in children.

Environmental influences also play a significant role in nervous system development. Nutrition, hormones, oxygen levels, and external stimulation all affect normal growth. The proper proportions of essential nutrients are necessary for proliferation of the nervous system tissue. Maternal life-style, nutrition, and state of health also have a crucial impact on nervous system development at certain critical periods of maturation.

Kathleen Hardin Mooney, RN, PhD, contributed to this chapter in the previous edition.

CHAPTER OUTLINE

NORMAL GROWTH AND DEVELOPMENT OF THE NERVOUS SYSTEM

Human neurologic functioning is primarily at a subcortical level at birth (impulses are handled by the brain stem and spinal cord). Many reflex patterns mediated by brain stem and spinal cord mechanisms are present at birth and disappear at predictable times during infancy. Table 16-1 summarizes the age at which reflexes appear and disappear.

Absence of expected reflex responses at the appropriate age indicates general depression of central or peripheral motor functions. Asymmetric responses may indicate lesions in the motor cortex or may occur with fractures of bones after traumatic delivery or postnatal injury. As the infant matures, the neonatal reflexes disappear in a predictable order as voluntary motor functions supersede them. Abnormal persistence of these reflexes is seen in infants with developmental delays or with central motor lesions.

Several differences between adults and children help one to understand the pathophysiology of the nervous system in children. First, the head of a normal infant accounts for approximately one fourth of the total height, whereas an adult's head is one eighth of the total body height. Second, the bones of the infant's skull are separated at the suture lines, thus forming two **fontanelles** or "soft spots": one diamond-shaped anterior fontanelle and one triangular-shaped posterior fontanelle. The posterior fontanelle may be open until 2 to 3 months of age, whereas the anterior fontanelle normally closes by 18 months (Fig. 16-1). Al-

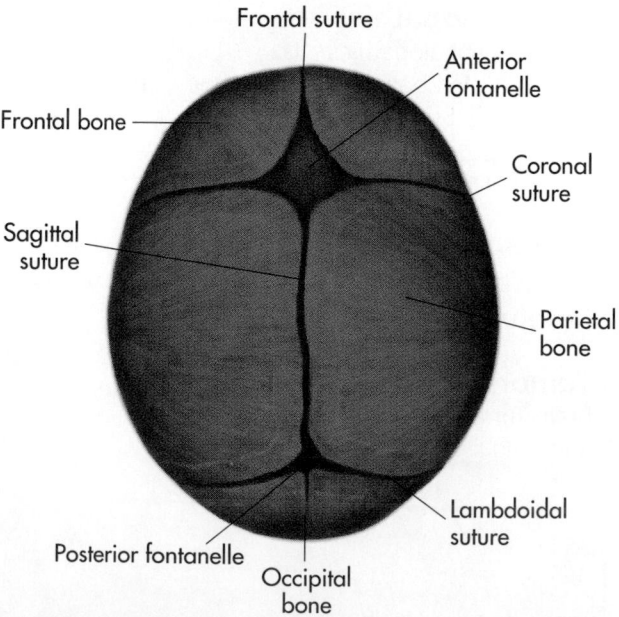

Fig. 16-1 *Cranial sutures and fontanelles in infancy.* Fibrous union of suture lines and interlocking of serrated edges (occurs by 6 months; solid union requires approximately 12 years). *(From Wong, D.L. [1999].* Whaley and Wong's nursing care of infants and children *[6th ed.]. St. Louis: Mosby.)*

Figure labels: Frontal suture; Anterior fontanelle; Frontal bone; Coronal suture; Sagittal suture; Parietal bone; Posterior fontanelle; Occipital bone; Lambdoidal suture

---

Gestation time (days)

Dorsal (posterior) induction (3-4 weeks) | **Ventral (anterior) induction (3-6 weeks)**

Timeline: 0-18 days — 18 — 26 — 28 — 32 — 42

- 0-18 days: Development of three germ layers and formation of early neural plate
- Development of neural plate and groove
- Closure of anterior neurospace
- Closure of posterior neurospace
- Beginning of vascular circulation (near 32)
- Development of five cerebral vesicles, choroid plexus, dorsal root ganglion (near 42)

Disorders

- No effect or death (0-18 days)
- Anterior midline defects (fasciotelencephalopathies): Cyclopia, Holoprosencephaly, cleft lip and/or palate
- Anencephaly
- Posterior midline defects: Myelomeningocele, Encephalocele, Cranium bifidum, Spina bifida occulta
- Microcephaly (primary) (30-175 days)

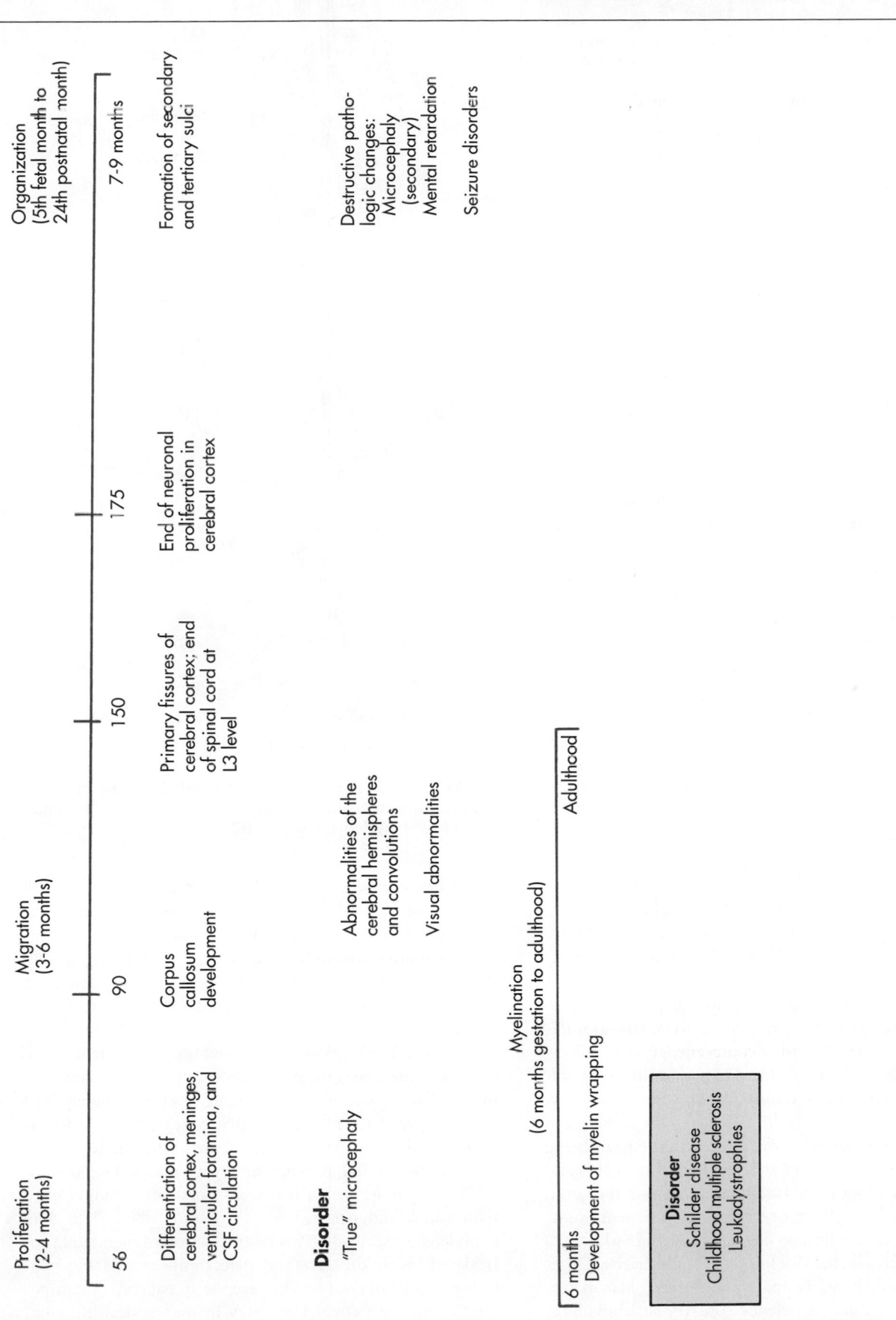

Fig. 16-2 *Disorders associated with specific stages of embryonic development.*

TABLE 16-1	**Reflexes of Infancy**	
Reflex	Age of Appearance of Reflex	Age at Which Reflex Should No Longer Be Obtainable
Moro	Birth	3 mo
Stepping	Birth	6 wk
Sucking	Birth	4 mo awake 7 mo asleep
Rooting	Birth	4 mo awake 7 mo asleep
Palmar grasp	Birth	6 mo
Plantar grasp	Birth	10 mo
Tonic neck	2 mo	5 mo
Neck righting	4-6 mo	24 mo
Landau	3 mo	24 mo
Parachute reaction	9 mo	Persists for

though the adult's cranium is a closed cavity with sutures firmly holding the cranial bones together, the infant's cranium has room for expansion through the fontanelles. An adult's head size will not expand, regardless of intracranial events such as trauma or increased production of cerebrospinal fluid (CSF). The infant's head circumference, on the other hand, increases in size as a result of normal growth up to age 5 years. The head is the fastest growing body part during infancy. Abnormal intracranial conditions, such as those characterized by increased intracranial pressure, also may result in an increased head circumference in excess of that expected with normal growth. Health care providers carefully monitor head growth during the first 5 years of life by measuring head circumference and comparing the results with a standardized growth chart.

STRUCTURAL MALFORMATIONS
Defects of Neural Tube Closure

Neural tube defects occur in 0.7 to 1.0 of every 1000 live births in the United States each year.[1-3] Fetal death often occurs, reducing the actual prevalence of neural defects at birth.[4] These defects are divided into two categories: (1) posterior defects and (2) anterior midline defects. Posterior defects are more common and include anencephaly (*an* = without; *enkephalos* = brain) and a group of disorders collectively referred to as the **myelodysplasias** (*dys* = bad; *plassein* = to form). Anterior midline defects may cause brain and skull abnormalities, with the most extreme form being **cyclopia,** in which the child has a single midline orbit and eye with a protruding noselike appendage above the orbit. Disorders associated with embryonic development are summarized in Fig. 16-2. Folic acid deficiency during early stages of pregnancy increases the risk for neural tube defects. Other risk factors include heredity, maternal obesity, older maternal age, maternal zinc deficiency, use of anticonvulsant drugs, and lower socioeconomic class.[5]

Fig. 16-3 *Normal spine, meningocele, and myelomeningocele.* Diagram showing section through normal spine **(A)**, meningocele **(B)**, and myelomeningocele **(C)**.

In **anencephaly,** the soft, bony component of the skull and part of the brain are missing. This is a relatively common disorder, with an incidence of approximately 0.36 per 1000 total live births in the United States each year.[6] At birth the infant's head, viewed face-on, has a froglike appearance. These infants are stillborn or die within a few days after birth.

Encephalocele refers to a herniation or protrusion of brain and meninges through a defect in the skull, resulting in a saclike structure. The incidence is approximately 0.14 per 1000 live births in the United States each year.[6] Most encephaloceles occur in the occipital area, with the remainder found in the frontal, parietal, or nasopharyngeal regions.

Meningocele, which is a saclike cyst of meninges filled with spinal fluid, occurs when the neural tube fails to close completely (Fig. 16-3). This cystic dilation of meninges protrudes through the vertebral defect and around the malformed tube but does not involve the spinal cord. Meningoceles occur with equal frequency in the cervical, thoracic, and lumbar spine areas.

TABLE 16-2	Functional Alterations in Myelodysplasia Related to Level of Lesion
Level of Lesion	**Functional Implications**
Thoracic	Flaccid paralysis of lower extremities; variable weakness in abdominal trunk musculature; high thoracic level may mean respiratory compromise; absence of bowel and bladder control
High lumbar	Voluntary hip flexion and adduction; flaccid paralysis of knees, ankles, and feet; may walk with extensive braces and crutches; absence of bowel and bladder control
Midlumbar	Strong hip flexion and adduction; fair knee extension; flaccid paralysis of ankles and feet; absence of bowel and bladder control
Low lumbar	Strong hip flexion, extension, and adduction and knee extension; weak ankle and toe mobility; may have limited bowel and bladder function
Sacral	Normal function of lower extremities; normal bowel and bladder function

Modified from Farley, J.A. & Dunleavy, M.J. (1996). Myelodysplasia. In P.L. Jackson & J.A. Vessey (Eds.). Primary care of the child with a chronic condition (2nd ed.). St. Louis: Mosby.

Myelomeningocele (meningomyelocele; spina bifida cystica) is a hernial protrusion of a saclike cyst (containing meninges, spinal fluid, and a portion of the spinal cord with its nerves) through a defect in the posterior arch of a vertebra. Eighty percent of myelomeningoceles are located in the lumbar and lumbosacral regions, the last regions of the neural tube to close. Myelomeningocele is one of the most common developmental anomalies of the nervous system, with an incidence rate ranging from 0.2 to 0.4 per 1000 live births.[2,7]

Clinical Manifestations

A myelomeningocele is the failure of the neural tube to close, resulting in a cystic dilation of meninges and protuberance of the spinal cord through the vertebral defect. A myelomeningocele is evident at birth as a pronounced skin defect on the infant's back (see Fig. 16-3). The bony prominences of the unfused neural arches can be palpated at the lateral border of the defect. The defect usually is covered by a transparent membrane that may have neural tissue attached to its inner surface. This membrane may be intact at birth or may leak CSF, thereby increasing the risks of infection and neuronal damage. Until the defect is surgically closed, CSF may accumulate, resulting in further dilation and enlargement of the sac that may risk further damage to neuronal function.

The actual involvement of the spinal cord has greater implications for the overall function of the infant throughout childhood (Table 16-2). An absence of neurologic function may occur in some infants with myelomeningocele. Function may be attained if underlying fluid or pus accumulation is prevented from stretching and applying pressure to the neural tissue or if the biochemical alterations do not cause neural tissue to die. Residual neural tissue also may be temporarily or permanently lost at birth because of trauma to the tissue during delivery.

One serious, potentially life-threatening problem associated with myelodysplasia is the **Arnold-Chiari II malformation.** This deformity involves the downward displacement of the cerebellum, cerebellar tonsils, brain stem, and fourth ventricle (Fig. 16-4).

Hydrocephalus occurs in 85% of infants with myelo-

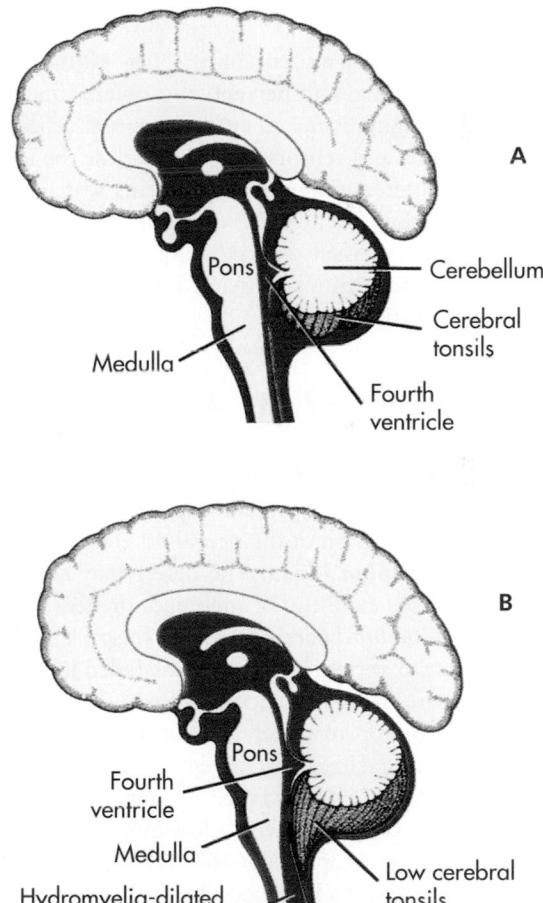

Fig. 16-4 *Normal brain and Arnold-Chiari II malformation.* Diagram showing normal brain, **A,** and brain with Arnold-Chiari II malformation, **B.** *(Modified from Farley, J.A. & Dunleavy, M.J. [1996]. Myelodysplasia. In P.L. Jackson & J.A. Vessey [Eds.]. Primary care of the child with a chronic condition (2nd ed.). St. Louis: Mosby.)*

TABLE 16-3	Causes of Microcephaly	
Defects in Brain Development	**Intrauterine Infections**	**Perinatal and Postnatal Disorders**
Hereditary (recessive) microcephaly	Congenital rubella	Intrauterine or neonatal anoxia
Down syndrome and other trisomy syndromes	Cytomegalovirus infection	Severe malnutrition in early infancy
Fetal ionizing radiation exposure	Congenital toxoplasmosis	Neonatal herpesvirus infection
Maternal phenylketonuria	Congenital syphilis	
Seckel syndrome		
Cornelia de Lange syndrome		
Rubinstein-Taybi syndrome		
Smith-Lemli-Opitz syndrome		
Fetal alcohol syndrome		

Modified from Behrman, R.E., Kliegman, R.M., & Arvin, A.M. (1996). Nelson textbook of pediatrics (15th ed.). Philadelphia: Saunders.

meningocele.[8] Seizures also occur in 30% of those with myelodysplasia.[9] Visual and perceptual problems, including ocular palsies, astigmatism, and visuoperceptual deficits, are common.[10] Motor and sensory functions below the level of the lesions are altered. Often these problems worsen as the child grows and the cord ascends within the vertebral canal, pulling primary scar tissue and tethering the cord.[11] Several musculoskeletal deformities are related to this diagnosis, as are spinal deformities.

Malformations of the Axial Skeleton
Spina bifida occulta
When defects of neural tube closure occur, such as meningocele and myelomeningocele, an accompanying vertebral defect allows the protrusion of the neural tube contents. Such a defect is called *spina bifida.* The defect may also occur without any visible exposure of meninges or neural tissue, and the term *spina bifida occulta* is used. In spina bifida occulta, the posterior vertebral laminae have failed to fuse. Extremely common, the defect occurs to some degree in 10% to 25% of infants. Approximately 80% of these vertebral defects are located in the lumbosacral regions, most commonly in the fifth lumbar vertebra and the first sacral vertebra; they may be detected prenatally with ultrasonic scanning and amniotic fluid alpha-fetoprotein (AFP) testing. About 3% of normal adults have spina bifida occulta of the atlas (cervical vertebra 1).

Certain cutaneous or subcutaneous abnormalities suggest underlying spina bifida, including the following:
1. Abnormal growth of hair along the spine, which often is either very coarse or very silky
2. A midline dimple with or without a sinus tract
3. A cutaneous angioma, usually of the "port wine" variety
4. A subcutaneous mass, usually representing a lipoma or dermoid cyst

Spina bifida occulta usually causes no serious neurologic dysfunctions. When dysfunctions occur, the common lumbosacral defects cause gait abnormalities, positional deformities of the feet as a result of muscle weakness, or sphincter disturbances of the bladder and bowel. These dysfunctions become evident during periods of rapid growth.

Cranial deformities
Skull malformations range from minor, insignificant defects to major defects that are incompatible with life. In *acrania,* the cranial vault is almost completely absent and an extensive defect of the vertebral column often is present. Acrania associated with anencephaly (absence of brain and spinal column) occurs in approximately 1 per 1000 live births and is incompatible with life.

Craniosynostosis (craniostenosis) is the premature closure of one or more of the cranial sutures during the first 18 to 20 months of the infant's life. The incidence of craniosynostosis is 5 per 10,000 live births. Males are affected twice as often as females. Craniosynostosis prevents normal skull expansion and causes asymmetric skull growth. Brain growth may be restricted, and compression may cause neurologic dysfunction from brain damage after age 6 months (Fig. 16-5).

Microcephaly is a defect in brain growth as a whole (see Fig. 16-5). The word microcephaly is derived from the Greek (*mikro* = small; *kephale* = head). Cranial size is significantly below average for the infant's age, gender, race, and gestation. The condition is not treatable.

True (primary) microcephaly can be caused by an autosomal recessive disorder, by a chromosomal abnormality, or by toxin exposure during the period of induction and major cell migration (Table 16-3). Secondary microcephaly is associated with various causes. Infection, trauma, metabolic disorders, and anoxia experienced during the third trimester of pregnancy, the perinatal period, or early infancy may be responsible.

Congenital hydrocephalus is characterized by an increased volume of cerebrospinal fluid (CSF). It may be caused by blockage within the ventricular system where the CSF flows, an imbalance in the production of CSF, or a reduced reabsorption of CSF. The pressure within the ventricular system pushes and compresses the brain tissue against the skull cavity. When hydrocephalus develops before fusion

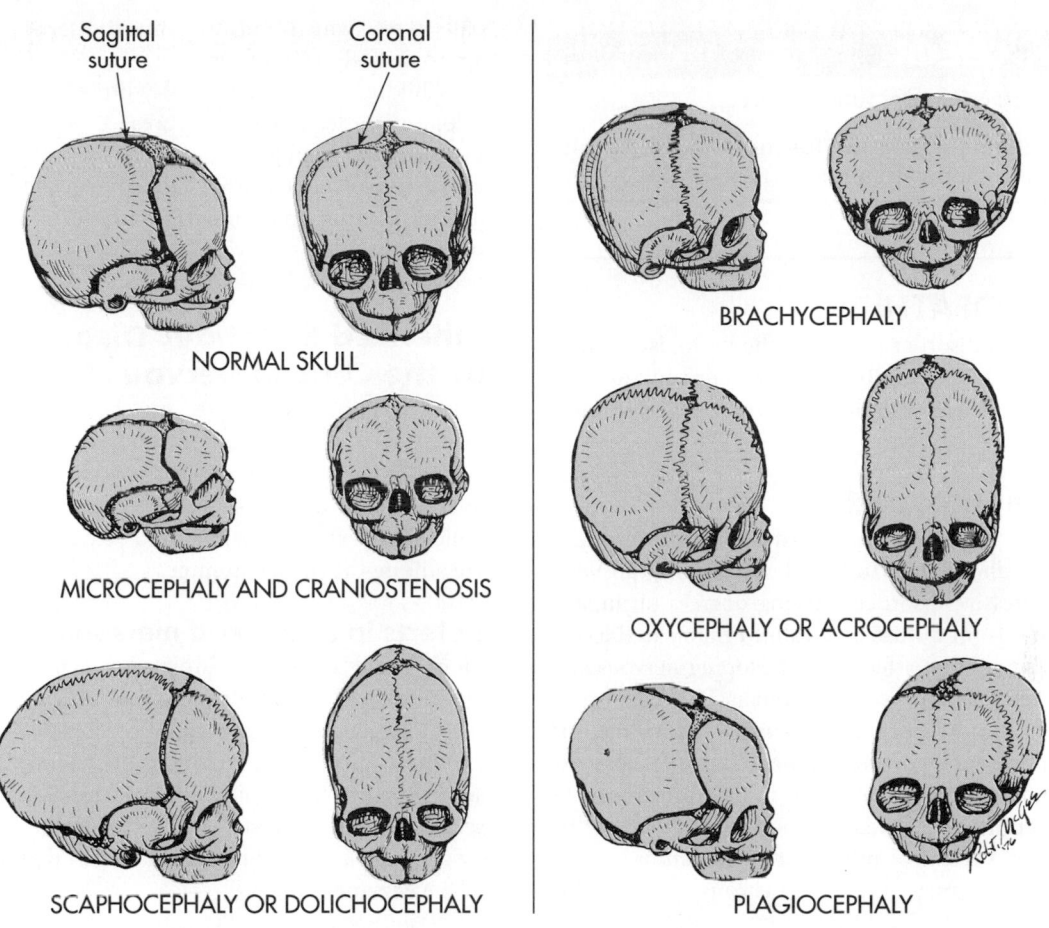

Sagittal suture   Coronal suture

NORMAL SKULL

MICROCEPHALY AND CRANIOSTENOSIS

SCAPHOCEPHALY OR DOLICHOCEPHALY

BRACHYCEPHALY

OXYCEPHALY OR ACROCEPHALY

PLAGIOCEPHALY

Fig. 16-5 *Craniosynostosis.* Abnormal head configuration resulting from premature closing of cranial sutures. *Normal skull,* Bones separated by membranous seams until sutures gradually close. *Microcephaly and craniostenosis,* Microcephaly is head circumference more than 2 standard deviations below the mean for age, gender, race, and gestation and reflects a small brain; craniosynostosis is premature closure of sutures. *Scaphocephaly or dolichocephaly* (frequency 56%), Premature closure of sagittal suture, resulting in restricted lateral growth. *Brachycephaly,* Premature closure of coronal suture, resulting in excessive lateral growth. *Oxycephaly or acrocephaly* (frequency 5.8%-12%), Premature closure of all coronal and sagittal sutures, resulting in accelerated upward growth and small head circumference. *Plagiocephaly* (frequency 13%), Unilateral premature closure of coronal suture, resulting in asymmetric growth. *(From Wong, D.L. [1999].* Whaley and Wong's nursing care of infants and children *[6th ed.]. St. Louis: Mosby.)*

of the cranial sutures, the skull can accommodate this additional space-occupying volume and preserve neuronal function. The overall incidence of hydrocephalus is approximately 2 per 1000 live births. The incidence of hydrocephalus, excluding the hydrocephalus associated with myelomeningocele, is approximately 0.5 to 1 per 1000 live births.[6,12] (Types of hydrocephalus are discussed in Chapter 14.)

Dandy-Walker deformity is a congenital defect of midline cerebellar structures in which hydrocephalus is caused by cystic dilation of the fourth ventricle and aqueductal compression. Other causes of obstructions within the ventricular system that can result in hydrocephalus include brain tumors, cysts, trauma, arteriovenous malformations, blood clots, and infections.

Congenital hydrocephalus may cause fetal death in utero, or the increased head circumference may require cesarean delivery of the infant. Symptoms depend directly on the cause and rate of hydrocephalus development. When there is separation of the cranial sutures, a resonant note sounds when the skull is tapped, a manifestation termed ***Macewen sign*** or ***"cracked pot" sign.*** The eyes may assume a staring expression, with sclera visible above the cornea, called *sunsetting.*

Correlation between the degree of hydrocephalus and impaired cognitive function often is a result of additional complications, such as severe congenital malformations, acute or chronic infections, or progressive brain tumors. Approximately two thirds of children with uncomplicated congenital hydrocephalus treated successfully with shunting may have normal to borderline normal intelligence.[13]

ENCEPHALOPATHIES

Encephalopathy, a disorder involving the brain, is a general category that includes a number of syndromes and diseases (see Chapter 14). These disorders may be acute or chronic, as well as static or progressive.

Static Encephalopathies

Brain injury may occur during gestation or birth or at any time during childhood growth and development, causing a static, nonprogressive disorder. Varying degrees of impairment may result from diffuse or localized injury to the cortex. Prenatal factors that affect the developing nervous system may be endogenous or exogenous. The developing nervous system is most susceptible to injury during the first trimester of pregnancy. Anoxia, trauma, and infections are the most common factors that cause injury to the nervous system in the perinatal period. Infections, metabolic disturbances (acute or a result of inborn errors), trauma, toxins, and vascular disease may injure the nervous system in the postnatal period.

Cerebral palsy is the term given to a diverse group of nonprogressive syndromes that affect the brain and cause motor dysfunction beginning in early infancy. It can be classified on the basis of neurologic signs and symptoms, with the major types involving spasticity, ataxia, dyskinesia, and a mix of one or more of the three. Cerebral palsy is one of the most common crippling disorders of childhood, affecting nearly 400,000 children in the United States alone. Although the exact incidence is unknown, studies suggest that the incidence is 1.5 to 5 cases of cerebral palsy per 1000 live births.[14]

Spastic cerebral palsy is associated with increased muscle tone, prolonged primitive reflexes, exaggerated deep tendon reflexes, clonus, rigidity of the extremities, scoliosis, and contractures. This accounts for approximately 65% to 75% of cerebral palsy cases. *Dyskinetic cerebral palsy* is associated with extreme difficulty in fine motor coordination and purposeful movements. Movements are jerky, uncontrolled, and abrupt, resulting from injury to the basal ganglia or extrapyramidal tracts. This form of cerebral palsy accounts for approximately 20% to 25% of cases. *Ataxic cerebral palsy* manifests with gait disturbances and instability. The infant with this form of cerebral palsy may have hypotonia at birth, but stiffness of the trunk muscles develops by late infancy. Persistence of this increased tone in truncal muscles affects the child's gait and ability to maintain equilibrium. This form of cerebral palsy accounts for approximately 5% of cases. A child may have symptoms of each of these cerebral palsy types, which leads to a mixed disorder accounting for approximately 13% of cases.

Children with cerebral palsy often have associated neurologic disorders, such as seizures (35% to 50%), intellectual impairment ranging from mild to severe (50% to 75%), and visual impairment (50%). Other associated complications include hearing impairment, communication disorders, respiratory problems, bowel and bladder problems, and orthopedic disabilities.[15]

Inherited Metabolic Disorders of the Central Nervous System

A large number of inherited metabolic disorders have been identified. Typically these metabolic disorders damage the entire CNS so extensively that these children do not survive to adulthood. Table 16-4 lists some of these inherited metabolic disorders. Defects in amino acid and lipid metabolism are among the most common.

Defects in amino acid metabolism

Biochemical defects in amino acid metabolism include (1) those in which the transport of amino acid is impaired, (2) those involving an enzyme or cofactor deficiency, and (3) those grouped around certain chemical components, such as sulfur-containing amino acids. Most disorders described to date suggest that the absence of enzymatic activity generally is caused by the genetically determined absence of the enzyme protein.[15]

Phenylketonuria

Phenylketonuria (PKU) is an inborn error of metabolism characterized by the inability of the body to convert the essential amino acid phenylalanine to tyrosine (Fig. 16-6). PKU is caused by phenylalanine hydroxylase deficiency and has an incidence of 1:10,000 worldwide.[16,17] Most natural food proteins contain about 15% phenylalanine, an essential amino acid. Phenylalanine hydroxylase controls the conversion of this essential amino acid to tyrosine in the liver. The body uses tyrosine in the biosynthesis of protein, melanin, thyroxine, and the catecholamines in the brain and adrenal medulla. Phenylalanine hydroxylase deficiency causes an accumulation of phenylalanine in the serum. Abnormalities occur, such as anomalous development of the CNS, defective myelination, cystic degeneration of the gray and white matter, and disturbances in cortical layers. Unfortunately, brain damage occurs before the metabolites can be detected in the urine, and damage continues as long as phenylalanine levels remain high. Nonselective newborn screening is used to detect PKU in the United States and in more than 30 other countries. Most children develop normally on a regular diet.

Defects in lipid metabolism

Disorders of lipid metabolism are termed *lysosomal storage diseases* because each disorder in this group can be traced to a missing lysosomal enzyme. This causes an excessive accumulation of a particular cell product, occurring in the brain,

TABLE 16-4	Inherited Metabolic Disorders of the Central Nervous System
Age of Onset	**Disorder**
Neonatal period	Pyridoxine dependency, galactosemia, maple syrup urine disease and its variant, phenylketonuria (PKU)
Early infancy	Tay-Sachs disease and its variants, infantile Gaucher disease, infantile Niemann-Pick disease, Krabbe disease (leukodystrophy), Farber lipogranulomatosis, Pelizaeus-Merzbacher disease and other sudanophilic leukodystrophies, spongy degeneration, Alexander disease, Alpers disease, Leigh disease (subacute necrotizing encephalomyelopathy), congenital lactic acidosis, Zellweger encephalopathy, Lowe disease (oculocerebrorenal disease)
Late infancy and early childhood	Disorders of amino acid metabolism, metachromatic leukodystrophy, late infantile GM₁ gangliosidosis, late infantile Gaucher and Niemann-Pick diseases, neuroaxonal dystrophy, mucopolysaccharidosis, mucolipidosis, fucosidosis, mannosidosis, aspartylglycosaminuria, amaurotic idiocy (Jansky-Bielschowsky disease, Batten disease, Vogt-Spielmeyer disease, neuronal ceroid lipofuscinosis), Cockayne syndrome
Later childhood and adolescence	Progressive cerebellar ataxias of childhood and adolescence, hepatolenticular degeneration (Wilson disease), Hallervorden-Spatz disease, Lesch-Nyhan syndrome and other uremic states, familial calcification of vessels in basal ganglia and cerebellum, familial polymyoclonus, chronic familial leukodystrophy, homocystinuria, Fabry disease

Fig. 16-6 *Metabolic error and consequences in phenylketonuria.* *(From Wong, D.L. [1999].
Whaley & Wong's nursing care of infants and children [6th ed.]. St. Louis: Mosby.)*

liver, spleen, bone, and lung and thus involving several organ systems. Therapy has been unsuccessful to date.

Perhaps the best known of the lysosomal storage disorders is ***Tay-Sachs disease,*** an autosomal recessive disorder. Approximately 80% of individuals diagnosed are of Jewish ancestry, although sporadic cases appear in the non-Jewish population.[18] In Tay-Sachs disease, the pathologic changes predominate in the CNS, but neurons throughout the body contain characteristic changes in the cytoplasm. Onset of this disease usually occurs when the infant is 3 to 6 months old. Seizures, muscular rigidity, and blindness become prominent after the first year of life, and head size may increase. Death usually occurs by 2 to 5 years of age.

✓ QUICK CHECK

List three types of cerebral palsy.

Why does failure to metabolize phenylaline produce such widespread and devastating consequences?

Seizure Disorders
Epilepsy

Seizures are the abnormal discharge of electrical activity within the brain. Repeated recurrence of seizure activity is known as *epilepsy*. Seizures may result from an underlying disorder of the CNS or a disorder that directly or indirectly affects normal CNS function. Certain types of seizures may have a genetic component or familial predisposition, or they can result from maternal diseases or congenital structural anomalies of the CNS. From the newborn period through childhood, asphyxia, intracranial hemorrhage, CNS infections, injury, electrolyte imbalances, and inborn errors of metabolism may cause seizures. Often the cause of seizures is unknown.

The incidence of epilepsy varies greatly with age. The incidence is highest in infants younger than 1 year, averaging roughly 1 per 1000 in the United States. It decreases with age; 75% to 80% of epilepsy cases initially occur before 20 years of age, with 25% of the cases initially occurring within the first 5 years of life. Approximately 125,000 persons in the United States are newly affected each year.[19-21] Table 16-5 summarizes the major types of seizures.

HEALTH ALERT

Antiepileptic Drug Effectiveness

Several antiepileptic drugs have altered therapeutic effects when combined with common drugs in pediatric care. Caution should be taken when recommending or prescribing antihistamines, antidepressants, aspirin, oral contraceptives, and erythromycin to individuals taking antiepileptic medications.

Data from Farley, J.A. (1996). Epilepsy. In P.L. Jackson & J.A. Vessey (Eds.). Primary care of the child with a chronic condition (2nd ed.). St. Louis: Mosby.

Acute Encephalopathies
Reye syndrome

Reye syndrome is characterized by encephalopathy and fatty changes in various organs, especially the liver. The incidence of Reye syndrome has declined sharply over the past 20 years, coinciding with increased public awareness of the association between ingestion of aspirin during illness and subsequent development of Reye syndrome.[22]

An overview of Reye syndrome is important for the fol-

lowing reasons: (1) it may be considered a prototype for acute hepatic encephalopathies, (2) the potential for recurrence is a factor, and (3) the use of acetaminophen rather than aspirin should be considered important and discussed with the parents when obtaining a history.

Typically, Reye syndrome develops in a previously healthy child who is recovering from varicella, influenza B, upper respiratory infection, or gastroenteritis. The manifestations of the various clinical states are as follows:

- *Stage I:* vomiting, lethargy, drowsiness
- *Stage II:* disorientation, delirium, aggressiveness and combativeness, central neurologic hyperventilation, shallow breathing, hyperactive reflexes, stupor
- *Stage III:* obtundation, coma, hyperventilation, decorticate rigidity
- *Stage IV:* deepening coma, decerebrate rigidity, loss of ocular reflexes, large fixed pupils, divergent eye movements
- *Stage V:* seizures, loss of deep tendon reflexes, flaccidity, respiratory arrest

Treatment and outcome depend on the stage of development at diagnosis and the individual child's symptoms.

Intoxications of the central nervous system

Drug-induced encephalopathies must always be considered a possibility in the child with unexplained neurologic changes. Such encephalopathies may result from accidental ingestion, therapeutic overdosage, intentional overdose, or ingestion of environmental toxins (the most commonly ingested poisons are listed in Table 16-6). About 2 million childhood poisonings that require medical attention occur each year. Approximately 1000 children die each year of poisonings.

High blood levels of lead occur in lead poisoning. If lead poisoning is untreated, lead encephalopathy will result and is responsible for serious and irreversible neurologic damage (Fig. 16-7). Those at great risk are 2- to 3-year-olds and children prone to *pica,* the habitual, purposeful, and compulsive ingestion of nonfood substances, such as clay, dirt, and paint chips. Lead intoxication also may occur from chronic exposure to smelters, sniffing of gasoline, and ingestion of airborne lead.[23]

An estimated 225,000 children in the United States and 4% of children 6 months to 5 years of age have excessive amounts of lead in their blood. Black children have a six times greater incidence of symptoms than white children.

Meningitis

Meningitis refers to the inflammation of the meningeal coverings of the brain. The origin of such inflammation and acute encephalopathy can be bacterial or viral.

Bacterial meningitis

Bacterial meningitis is one of the most serious infections to which infants and children are susceptible. In general, bacterial meningitis affects males more frequently than females and is most prevalent during infancy.[24] Conditions associated with increased incidence of respiratory infection heighten the occurrence of bacterial meningitis.

TABLE 16-5	Major Types of Seizure Disorders Found in Children
Disorder	**Pathology**
Partial seizures	Seizure activity that begins and usually is limited to one part of the left or right hemisphere
Simple	Seizure activity that occurs without loss of consciousness
Complex	Seizure activity that occurs with impairment of consciousness
Generalized seizures	First clinical manifestations indicate that seizure activity starts in or involves both cerebral hemisphere; consciousness may be impaired; manifestations include convulsive activity (tonic-clonic, tonic, or clonic activity) or nonconvulsive activity (absence of seizures)
Unclassified epileptic seizures	Wide variety of abnormal clinical activity, including rhythmic eye movements, chewing, and swimming movements; common in neonatal seizures
Epileptic syndromes	Seizure disorders that display a group of signs and symptoms that occur collectively and characterize or indicate a particular condition
Infantile spasm	Form of epilepsy with episodes of sudden flexion or extension involving the neck, trunk, and extremities; clinical manifestations range from subtle head nods to violent body contractions (jackknife seizures); onset between 3 and 12 mo of age; may be idiopathic or in response to CNS insult; spasms occur in clusters of 5 to 150 times per day; increases with time
Lennox-Gastaut syndrome	Epileptic syndrome with onset early in childhood, 1-5 yr of age; includes various generalized seizures—tonic-clonic, atonic (drop attacks), akinetic, absence, and myoclonic; results in mental retardation and delayed psychomotor developments
Juvenile myoclonic epilepsy	Primary generalized epilepsy of adolescents and young adults; relatively benign with myoclonic jerks of neck, shoulders, and arms; seizures occur singularly or repetitively; generally normal neurologic examination, normal intelligence, and positive family history of seizures
Benign febrile seizures	Brief, self-limited seizures that occur in 3%-4% of children under 5 yr of age; rare before 6 mo or after 5 yr of age; occur with rise in temperature greater than 38° C; accompany an acute respiratory or ear infection; occur during first 24 hr of illness; short (15 min or less), generalized, and predominantly tonic; interictal EEG is normal; do not recur during same infection, and no acute systemic metabolic disorder is present; in complex form, are longer, with focal characteristics, and occur more than once in 24-hr period
Status epilepticus	Continuing or recurring seizure activity in which recovery from the seizure activity is incomplete; unrelenting seizure activity can last 30 min or more; other forms can evolve into status epilepticus; medical emergency that requires immediate intervention

TABLE 16-6	Commonly Ingested Poisons	
Pharmacologic Agents	**Heavy Metals**	**Miscellaneous Agents**
Acetaminophen	Lead	Botulism
Amphetamines	Acute	Carbon monoxide
Anticonvulsants	Chronic	Ethyl alcohol
Antidepressants	Mercury	Organophosphates
Antihistamines	Thallium	Petroleum distillates
Atropine		
Barbiturates		**Venoms**
Methadone		Snake bite
Phencyclidine		Tick paralysis
Salicylates		
Tranquilizers		

From Swaiman, K.F. (1994). Pediatric neurology: Principles and practice (vol. 2, 2nd ed.). St. Louis: Mosby.

Haemophilus influenzae type B is the most common pathogen of bacterial meningitis in children younger than 5 years. Otitis media or sinusitis may be a precursor because the infections almost always are associated with a bacterium in the blood.

The second most common organism is *Neisseria meningitidis* (meningococcus). Approximately 2% to 5% of healthy children are carriers of *N. meningitidis*. The risk of meningitis in day-care center contacts of children with meningococcal disease is 1 per 1000.

The third organism is *Streptococcus pneumoniae*, which is likely to be found in children older than 4 years. Staphylococcal or streptococcal meningitis shows a predilection for children who have had neurosurgery, skull fracture, or a complication of systemic bacterial infection. Infections that originate in the middle ear, sinuses, or mastoid cells also may lead to *S. pneumoniae* in children. In addition, 1 in every 24 children with sickle cell disease develops pneumococcal meningitis by the age of 4 years. *Escherichia coli* and group B β-hemolytic streptococci are the most common causes of meningitis in the newborn period.

Viral meningitis

The hallmark of **viral meningitis,** or aseptic meningitis, is a mononuclear response in the CSF and the presence of normal sugar as well. Viral meningitis may result from a direct infection of a virus, or it may be secondary to disease, such as measles, mumps, herpes, or leukemia.

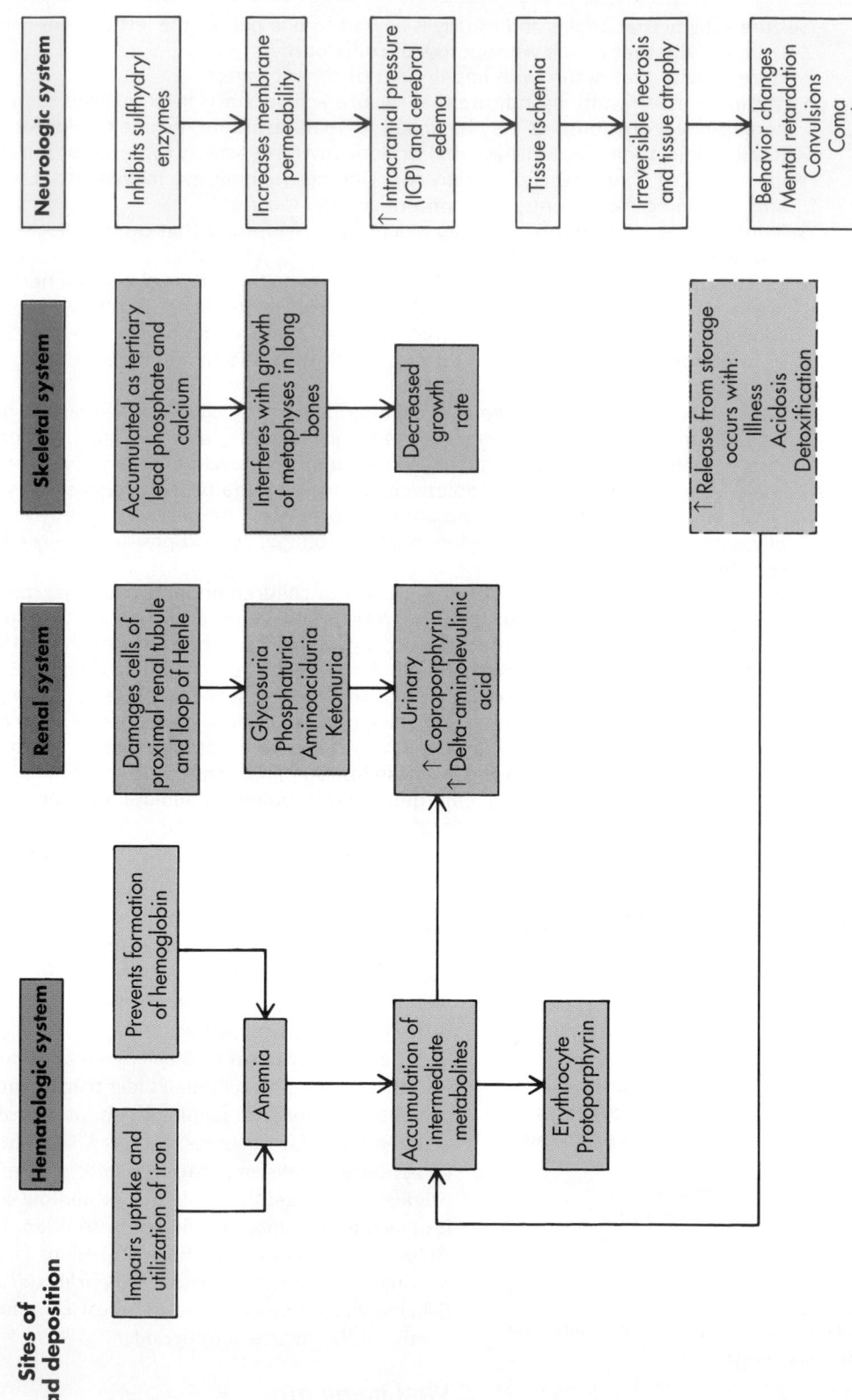

Fig. 16-7 *Systemic effects of increased lead absorption in children.*

Onset of symptoms may be sudden or gradual. Malaise, fever, headache and stiff neck, abdominal pain, and nausea and vomiting are common. Sore throat, chest pain, photophobia, and maculopapular rash can develop also. The child usually recovers spontaneously within 3 to 10 days. Treatment is usually symptomatic.

HUMAN IMMUNODEFICIENCY VIRUS AND CENTRAL NERVOUS SYSTEM INVOLVEMENT

Infants and children have become infected with human immunodeficiency virus (HIV) through a variety of sources, including the placenta, exposure to infected maternal blood and vaginal secretions, and postpartum ingestion of breast milk. Perinatal transmission accounts for approximately 84% of pediatric acquired immunodeficiency syndrome (AIDS) cases in the United States. Infection also can occur from contaminated blood products, although safeguards with blood products have lessened this risk considerably over the past years (see Chapter 7).

The actual incidence of pediatric HIV is not known because no national statistics have been compiled. The Centers for Disease Control and Prevention (CDC) estimate that 10,000 to 20,000 infants and children in the United States currently have HIV. This incidence continues to increase rapidly (see Chapter 7).

A common site for HIV infection in children and infants is the CNS.[25] Many children function well or with minimal delay despite this consideration. Classic signs and symptoms of a progressive encephalopathy may occur throughout the course of illness with a worsening in severity at the end stage of the disease. These include but are not limited to deterioration of fine and gross motor skills, intellectual impairment, language delay and impairment, cognitive and developmental delay, behavioral manifestations (e.g., irritability, lethargy, confusion), and onset of seizures. Infants exposed to the virus during the perinatal period may have acquired microcephaly.

It may be difficult to completely differentiate the impact of HIV infection on the CNS from the impact of prenatal and perinatal exposure. In addition, other insults probably accompany HIV in a young child and affect growth and development, such as drug exposure, prematurity, chronic illness, and a chaotic social atmosphere.[26]

TUMORS
Brain Tumors

Brain tumors are the most common solid tumor and the second most common primary neoplasm in children, second only to leukemia. Overall, brain tumors account for nearly 20% of all childhood cancers, with an annual incidence of 2.4 per 100,000 in the United States; approximately 1500 cases are diagnosed in each year. Brain tumors remain the leading cause of death from disease in children ages 1 to 15 years.[27,28] Gliomas are the most common type of brain tumor in children.

The cause of brain tumors is largely unknown, although genetic, environmental, and immune factors have been implicated in some tumor development. Factors that have been investigated as the cause of brain tumors include familial tendencies, radiation, oncologic viruses, and chemical carcinogens. An important area of study has been the relationship of parental occupation to subsequent brain tumors in offspring. Associations have been found with tumors and parental exposure to hydrocarbons and employment in the aircraft and paper/pulp industries. Alterations in embryologic development also may play a part in the development of childhood brain tumors.

Two thirds of all pediatric brain tumors are found in the posterior fossa (infratentorial) region of the brain, and approximately one third of childhood brain tumors are located in the supratentorial space. Brain tumors can arise from any CNS cell, and tumors are classified by cell type. The types and characteristics of childhood brain tumors are summarized in Table 16-7.

Medulloblastoma, ependymoma, astrocytoma, brain stem glioma, craniopharyngioma, and optic nerve glioma make up approximately 75% to 80% of all pediatric brain tumors. Most brain tumors in children are located in the posterior fossa[29] (Fig. 16-8); treatment strategies and prognosis are listed in Table 16-8.

Signs and symptoms of brain tumors in children vary from generalized and vague to localized and related specifically to the anatomic area. Signs of increased intracranial pressure may occur, including headache, vomiting, lethargy, and irritability. If a young child complains of repeated and worsening headache, a thorough investigation should take place because headache is an uncommon complaint in young children. Headache caused by increased intracranial pressure usually is worse in the morning and gradually improves during the day when the child is upright and venous drainage is enhanced. Frequency of headache and other symptoms worsens as the tumor grows. Irritability or possible apathy and increased somnolence also may result. Like headache, vomiting occurs more commonly in the morning. It frequently is not preceded by nausea and may become projectile, differing from a gastrointestinal disturbance in that the child may be ready to eat immediately after vomiting. Other signs and symptoms include increased head circumference with bulging fontanelle in the child younger than 2 years, cranial nerve palsies, and papilledema. See Box 16-1.

Localized findings relate to the degree of disturbance in physiologic functioning in the area where the tumor is located (see Table 14-12). Infratentorial tumors exhibit localized signs of impaired coordination and balance, including ataxia, gait difficulties, truncal ataxia, and loss of balance. *Medulloblastoma* occurs as an invasive malignant tumor that develops in the vermis of the cerebellum and may extend into the fourth ventricle. *Ependymoma* develops in the

TABLE 16-7   Brain Tumors in Children

Type	Characteristics
Astrocytoma	Arises from astrocytes, often in the cerebellum or lateral hemisphere Slow growing, solid or cystic Often very large before diagnosed Varies in degree of malignancy
Optic nerve glioma	Arises from optic chiasm or optic nerve Slow growing, low-grade astrocytoma
Medulloblastoma (infiltrating glioma)	Often located in cerebellum, extending into fourth ventricle and spinal fluid pathway Rapidly growing malignant tumor Can extend outside CNS
Brain stem glioma	Arises from pons or myeloencephalon Numerous cell types Compresses cranial nerves V through X
Ependymoma	Arises from ependymal cells lining ventricles Circumscribed, solid, nodular tumors
Craniopharyngioma	Arises near pituitary gland, optic chiasm, and hypothalamus Cystic and solid tumors that affect vision, pituitary, and hypothalamic functions

TABLE 16-8   Treatment Strategies for Childhood Brain Tumors

Tumor Type	Treatment and Prognosis
Cerebellar astrocytoma	Surgery; possibly curative Radiation and chemotherapy not proved successful but may delay recurrence Survival rate of more than 5 yr in 50%-75%; if tumor recurs, it does so very slowly
Medulloblastoma	Surgery, primarily as a partial resection to relieve increased intracranial pressure and "debulk" the tumor Radiation as the primary treatment; may include spinal radiation Chemotherapy showing some promise* 35% 5-yr survival rate
Brain stem glioma	Surgery, resection occasionally possible Radiation, primarily palliative treatment Chemotherapy not yet proved beneficial, but new protocols being studied 20%-40% 5-yr survival rate
Ependymoma	Tumor possibly indolent for many years Surgery rarely curative; risk of resecting an infratentorial tumor too great Radiation for palliation (current controversy whether local or craniospinal radiation is best) Chemotherapy used for recurrent disease but with disappointing results
Craniopharyngioma	Surgery possibly successful when a complete resection is performed (partial resection usually requires further treatment) Radiation after partial surgical resection Chemotherapy not commonly used 75%-85% 5-yr survival rate
Optic nerve glioma	Initial treatment controversial Surgery used for diagnosis or relief of hydrocephalus Radiation useful, particularly if the tumor not treated by surgery
Cerebral astrocytoma	Surgery used if resection is possible Radiation useful for all grades of astrocytoma Chemotherapy beneficial in higher grade tumors but further study required

*Reddy, A.T. & Packer, R.J. (1998). Pediatric central nervous system tumors. Current Opinions in Oncology, 10(3), 186-193.

Craniopharyngiomas
- Located adjacent to the sella turcica (structure containing the pituitary gland), often considered to lie supratentorial
- Considered to have benign properties but is life threatening because of its location near vital structures
- 4.9% of brain tumors in children
5%

Optic nerve gliomas
- Most often a low-grade astrocytoma
6%

Cerebral tumors
- Astrocytomas invade surrounding structures but grow slowly
8%
- Ependymomas arise from lining tissue of lateral ventricle
6%

Supratentorial

Brain stem gliomas
- Arise from pons or medulla
- 10% of childhood brain tumors
- Slow growing
- May involve cranial nerves V - X
10%

Infratentorial ependymomas
- Arise from lining tissue of fourth ventricle
- Comprise 13% of childhood brain tumors together with supratentorial ependymomas
13%

Cerebellar astrocytomas
- Most common brain tumor of childhood (20%)
- Slow growing
- Grading system I to IV with I and II less malignant than III and IV
20%

Medulloblastomas
- Arise from cerebellum
- Can invade fourth ventricle, subarachnoid space, and cerebrospinal fluid pathways
- 18% of brain tumors in children
- Fast growing
- Arise from embryonic cerebellum
18%

Infratentorial

Fig. 16-8 *Location of brain tumors in children.*

fourth ventricle and arises from the ependymal cells that line the ventricular system. Because both tumors are located in the posterior fossa region along the midline, presenting signs and symptoms are similar.

In contrast, *cerebellar astrocytomas* are located on the surface of the right or left cerebellar hemisphere and cause unilateral symptoms (occurring on the same side of the tumor), such as head tilt, limb ataxia, and nystagmus when the eyes are turned toward the tumor.

Brain stem gliomas often cause a combination of cranial nerve involvement, cerebellar signs of ataxia, and corticospinal tract dysfunction. Increased intracranial pressure generally does not occur.

The area of the sella turcica, the structure containing the pituitary gland, is the site of several childhood brain tumors; most common of this group is the *craniopharyngioma.* This tumor originates from the pituitary gland or hypothalamus. Usually slow-growing, it may be quite large by the time of diagnosis. Symptoms include headache, seizures, diabetes insipidus, early onset of puberty, and growth delay. Other tumors located in this region of the brain include *optic gliomas.* Tumors that involve the optic tract may cause complete unilateral blindness and hemianopia of the other eye. Optic atrophy is another common finding.

Supratentorial tumors of the cerebral hemispheres in children are uncommon.

Embryonal Tumors
Neuroblastoma

Neuroblastoma is an embryonal tumor originating in neural crest cells that normally give rise to the sympathetic ganglia and the adrenal medulla. Because neuroblastoma involves a defect of embryonal tissue, it most commonly is diagnosed during the first 2 years of life, and 75% are found before the child is 5 years old. Occasionally, these tumors have been diagnosed at birth with metastasis apparent in the placenta. It is seen more commonly in white children (9.6 per million) than in black children (7 per million). Although it accounts for 6% to 8% of pediatric malignancies, neuroblastoma causes 15% of cancer deaths in children.

Neuroblastoma is the most common and immature form of the sympathetic nervous system tumors. Areas of necrosis and calcification often are present in the tumor. More than with any other cancer, neuroblastoma has been associated with spontaneous remission, commonly in infants who have liver, bone marrow, or skin involvement in addition to the primary site.[30]

Although familial tendency has been noted in individual cases, a nonfamilial or sporadic pattern occurs in most children with neuroblastoma. Familial cases of neuroblastoma are considered to have an autosomal dominant pattern of inheritance (mechanisms of inheritance are discussed in Chapter 2).

Clinical Manifestations of Brain Tumors

BOX 16-1

HEADACHE
Recurrent and progressive
In frontal or occipital areas
Worse on arising, less during day
Intensified by lowering head and straining, such as
during bowel movement, coughing, sneezing

VOMITING
With or without nausea or feeding
Progressively more projectile
More severe in morning
Relieved by moving about and changing position

NEUROMUSCULAR CHANGES
Incoordination or clumsiness
Loss of balance (use of wide-based stance, falling, trip-
ping, banging into objects)
Poor fine motor control
Weakness
Hyporeflexia or hyperreflexia
Positive Babinski sign
Spasticity (in child older than 1 year of age)
Paralysis

BEHAVIORAL CHANGES
Irritability
Decreased appetite
Failure to thrive

Fatigue (frequent naps)
Lethargy
Coma

CRANIAL NERVE NEUROPATHY
Cranial nerve involvement varies according to tumor
location
Most common signs
Head tilt
Visual defects (nystagmus, diplopia, strabismus, episodic
"greying out" of vision, and visual field defects)

VITAL SIGN DISTURBANCES
Decreased pulse and respiration
Increased blood pressure
Decreased pulse pressure
Hypothermia or hyperthermia

OTHER SIGNS
Seizures
Cranial enlargement*
Tense, bulging fontanelle at rest*
Nuchal rigidity
Papilledema (edema of optic nerve)

From Wong, D.L. (1997). Whaley and Wong's essentials of pediatric nursing (5th ed.). St. Louis: Mosby.
Present only in infants and young children.

The most common location is in the retroperitoneal region (65% of cases) and most frequently the adrenal
medulla. The tumor is evident as an abdominal mass and
may cause anorexia, bowel and bladder alteration, and
sometimes spinal cord compression.

The second most common location of neuroblastoma is
the mediastinum (area separating the lungs) (15% of cases).
There the tumor may cause dyspnea or infection related to
airway obstruction. Less commonly, neuroblastoma may
arise from the cervical sympathetic ganglion (3% to 4% of
cases). Cervical neuroblastoma often causes Horner syndrome, which consists of miosis (pupil contraction), ptosis
(drooping eyelid), enophthalmos (backward displacement
of the eyeball), and anhidrosis (sweat deficiency).

A number of systemic signs and symptoms are characteristic of neuroblastoma, including weight loss, irritability,
fatigue, and fever. Intractable diarrhea occurs in 7% to 9% of
children and is caused by tumor secretion of a hormone
called *vasoactive intestinal polypeptide (VIP)*.

More than 90% of children with neuroblastoma have increased amounts of catecholamines and associated metabolites in their urine. High levels of urinary catecholamines
and serum ferritin are associated with a poorer prognosis.

Retinoblastoma

Retinoblastoma is a rare congenital eye tumor of young children that originates in the retina of one or both eyes (Fig.
16-9). It demonstrates both an inherited and an acquired
form. The inherited form of the disease generally is diagnosed during the first year of life. The acquired disease most
commonly is diagnosed in children 2 to 3 years of age and
involves unilateral disease.

Approximately 40% of retinoblastomas are inherited as
an autosomal dominant trait with incomplete penetrance.
The remaining 60% are acquired. In the early 1970s, Knud-
son[31] proposed the "two-hit" hypothesis to explain the
occurrence of both hereditary and acquired forms of the disease. This hypothesis predicts that two separate transforming events or "hits" must occur in a normal retinoblast
cell to cause the cancer. Further, it proposes that in the inherited form the first "hit" or mutation occurs in the germ
cell (inherited from either parent) and the mutation is contained in every cell of the child's body. Only a second, random mutation in a retinoblast cell is needed to transform
that cell into cancer. Multiple tumors are observed in the inherited form because these second mutations are likely to
occur in several of the approximately 1 to 2 million

Fig. 16-9 *Retinoblastoma.* Prominent white reflex (caused by retinoblastoma) in dilated pupil of left eye. *(From Damjanov, I. & Linder, J. [1996]. Anderson's pathology [10th ed.]. St. Louis: Mosby.)*

retinoblast cells. In contrast, the acquired form of retinoblastoma requires two independent "hits" or mutations to occur in the same somatic cell (after the egg is fertilized) for transformation to cancer. This is much less likely to happen. Fig.

16-10 illustrates the two-mutation model for these two patterns of mutation.

The primary sign of retinoblastoma is leukokoria, a white pupillary reflex also called *cat's eye reflex,* that is caused by the mass behind the lens (see Fig. 16-9). Other signs and symptoms include strabismus, a red, painful eye, and limited vision.

Because retinoblastoma is a treatable tumor, dual priorities are saving the child's life and restoring useful vision. The prognosis for most children with retinoblastoma is excellent, with a greater than 90% long-term survival.

✓ QUICK CHECK

Why are the principal symptoms of brain tumors in children related to brain stem function?

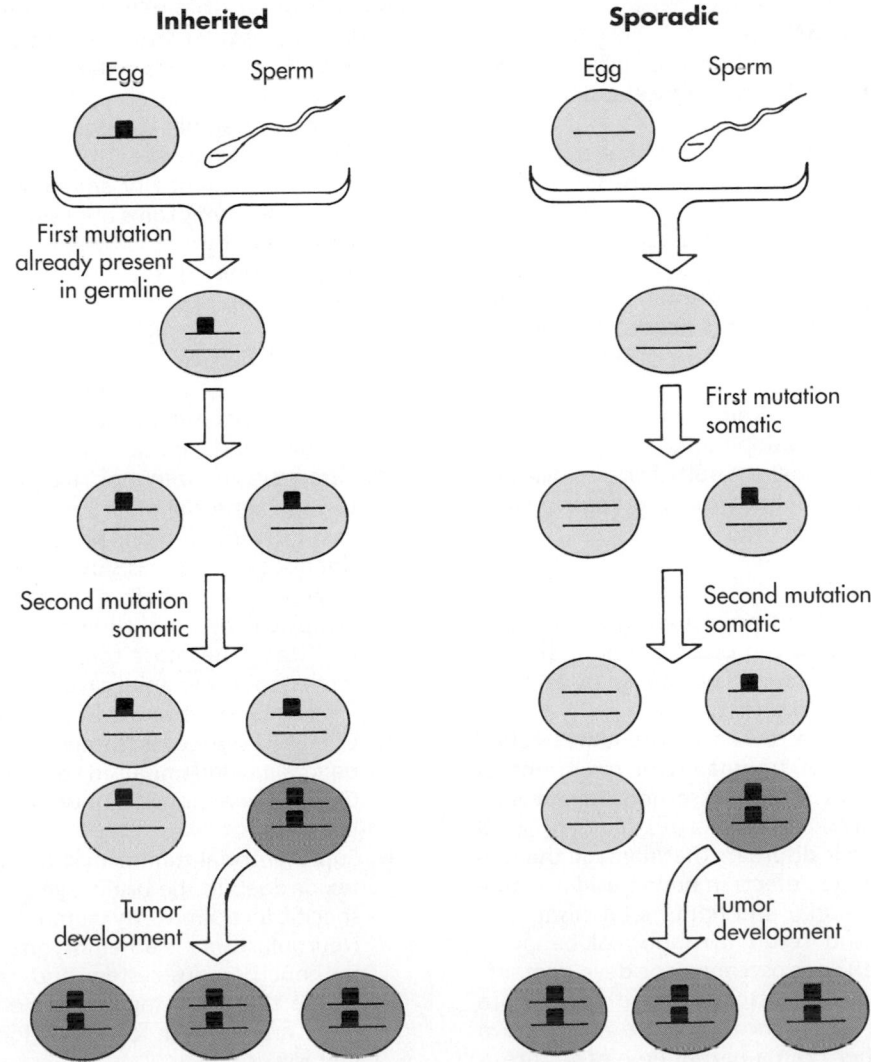

Fig. 16-10 *The two-mutation model of retinoblastoma development.* In inherited retinoblastoma, the first mutation is transmitted through the germline of an affected parent. The second mutation occurs somatically in a retinal cell, leading to development of the tumor. In sporadic retinoblastoma, development of a tumor requires two somatic mutations.

DID YOU UNDERSTAND?

Normal Growth and Development of the Nervous System

1. The central nervous system develops from the neural tube, which is ectodermal in origin. The cranial end of the tube forms the brain, and the spinal cord is formed from the remainder of the tube.
2. The cranial and spinal ganglia form from the neural crest.
3. There are six stages to the development of the nervous system, and disruption of any stage can lead to malfunction of the nervous system.
4. The bones of the skull are joined by sutures, and the wide, membranous junctions of the sutures known as fontanelles close by 20 months of age.
5. Myelin is a sheath that develops around axons to facilitate speed of nerve impulse conduction. Progressive development of reflexes corresponds to normal maturation of nerve tissue.

Structural Malformations

1. Defects of neural tube closure include anencephaly, encephalocele, meningocele, and myelomeningocele.
2. Failure of the vertebrae to close with protrusion of neural tube contents is known as *spina bifida occulta*.
3. Acrania is nearly complete absence of the cranial vault.
4. Premature closure of the cranial sutures causes craniosynostosis and prevents normal skull expansion, resulting in compression of growing brain tissue.
5. Microcephaly is lack of brain growth and retarded mental and motor development.
6. Congenital hydrocephalus results from an overproduction, impaired absorption, or blockage of circulation of cerebrospinal fluid.

Encephalopathies

1. Static encephalopathies are nonprogressive disorders of the brain that can occur during gestation, birth, or childhood and can be caused by endogenous or exogenous factors.
2. Cerebral palsy can be caused by prenatal cerebral hypoxia or perinatal trauma, with symptoms of mental retardation, seizure disorders, or developmental disabilities.
3. Inherited metabolic disorders that damage the nervous system include defects in amino acid metabolism (phenylketonuria) and lipid metabolism (Tay-Sachs disease) and result in abnormal behavior, seizures, and deficient psychomotor development.
4. Seizure disorders are associated with numerous nervous system disorders and more often are a generalized rather than a partial type of seizure.
5. Generalized forms of seizures include tonic-clonic, myoclonic, atonic, akinetic, and infantile spasms.
6. Partial seizures suggest more localized brain dysfunction.

7. Febrile seizures usually are limited to the ages of 6 months to 3 years with a pattern of one seizure per febrile illness.
8. Reye syndrome is associated with influenza B and varicella viruses and symptoms of hypoglycemia, hyperammonemia, and increased serum short-chain fatty acids. Progressive manifestations include lethargy, stupor, rigidity, seizures, and respiratory arrest.
9. Accidental poisonings from a variety of toxins can cause serious neurologic damage.
10. Bacterial meningitis is commonly caused by *Haemophilus influenzae, Neisseria meningitidis,* or *Streptococcus pneumoniae* and may result from respiratory or gastrointestinal infections, with symptoms of fever, headaches, photophobia, seizures, rigidity, and stupor.

Human Immunodeficiency Virus and Central Nervous System Involvement

1. HIV may be transmitted to infants and children through the placenta, by exposure to infected blood or vaginal secretions, or by ingestion of infected breast milk.
2. The incidence of HIV among children is increasing. The classic symptoms are related to progressive encephalopathy.
3. AIDS is one of the 10 leading causes of death among children.

Childhood Tumors

1. Brain tumors are the most common tumors of the nervous system and the second most common type of childhood cancer.
2. Tumors in children most frequently are located below the tentorial plate.
3. Fast-growing tumors produce symptoms early in the disease, whereas slow-growing tumors may become very large before symptoms appear.
4. Symptoms of brain tumors may be generalized or localized. The most common general symptom is increased intracranial pressure (headache, irritability, vomiting, somnolence, bulging of fontanelles).
5. Localized signs of infratentorial tumors in the cerebellum include impaired coordination and balance. Cranial nerve signs occur with tumors in or near the brain stem.
6. Supratentorial tumors may be located near the cortex or deep in the brain. Symptoms depend on the specific location of the tumor.
7. Neuroblastoma is an embryonal tumor of the sympathetic nervous system and can be located anywhere there is sympathetic nervous tissue. Symptoms are related to tumor location and size of metastasis.
8. Retinoblastoma is a congenital eye tumor that has both a hereditary and a nonhereditary form.

KEY TERMS

Acrania, 430
Anencephaly, 428
Arnold-Chiari II malformation, 429
Ataxic cerebral palsy, 432
Bacterial meningitis, 434
Brain stem glioma, 439
Cerebellar astrocytoma, 439
Cerebral palsy, 432
Congenital hydrocephalus, 430
Craniopharyngioma, 439
Craniosynostosis, 430
Cyclopia, 428
Dandy-Walker deformity, 431

Dyskinetic cerebral palsy, 432
Encephalocele, 428
Encephalopathy, 432
Ependymoma, 437
Epilepsy, 434
Fontanelle, 426
Lysosomal storage disease, 432
Macewen sign ("cracked pot" sign), 431
Medulloblastoma, 437
Meningitis, 434
Meningocele, 428
Microcephaly, 430
Myelodysplasia, 428

Myelomeningocele, 429
Neuroblastoma, 439
Optic glioma, 439
Phenylketonuria (PKU), 432
Pica, 434
Retinoblastoma, 440
Reye syndrome, 434
Spastic cerebral palsy, 432
Spina bifida, 430
Spina bifida occulta, 430
Tay-Sachs disease, 433
Viral meningitis, 435

REFERENCES

1. Hobbins, J.C. (1991). Diagnosis and management of neural tube defects today. *New England Journal of Medicine, 324*(10), 690-691.
2. McComb, J.G. (1997). Spinal and cranial neural tube defects. *Seminars in Pediatric Neurology, 4*(3), 192-208.
3. Werler, M.M., Shapiro, S., & Mitchell, A.A. (1993). Periconceptual folic acid exposures and risk of occurrent neural tube defects. *Journal of the American Medical Association, 269*(10), 1257.
4. Marks, J.D. & Koshnood, B. (1998). Epidemiology of common neurosurgical diseases in the neonate. *Neurosurgical Clinics of North America, 9*(1), 63-72.
5. Hall, J.G., Solehdin, F. (1998). Folate and its various ramifications. *Advances in Pediatrics, 45,* 1-35.
5a. Werler, M.M. et al. (1996). Prepregnant weight in relation to risk of neural tube defects. *Journal of American Medical Association, 275*(14), 1089-92.
5b. Wasserman, C.R. et al. (1998). Socioeconomic status, neighborhood social conditions and neural tube defects. *American Journal of Public Health, 88*(11), 674-680.
6. Wiswell, T.E. et al. (1990). Major congenital neurologic malformations. *American Journal of Diseases in Children, 144,* 61-67.
7. Behrman, R.E., Kliegman, R.M., & Arvin, A.M. (1996). *Nelson textbook of pediatrics* (15th ed.). Philadelphia: Saunders.
8. Dias, M.S. & McClone, D.G. (1993). Hydrocephalus in the child with dysraphism. *Neurosurgical Clinics of North America, 4*(4), 715.
9. Reigal, D.J. (1993). Infancy through school years. In F. Rowley-Kelly & D.H. Reigal (Eds.). *Teaching the student with spina bifida.* Baltimore: Brookes.
10. Lollar, D.J. (1993). Learning among children with spina bifida. *Spina Bifida Spotlight* (pp. 1-6). Washington, D.C.: Spina Bifida Association of America.

11. Humphreys, R.P. (1991). Current trends in spinal dysraphism. *Paraplegia, 29*(2), 79.
12. Jackson, P.L. (1996). Hydrocephalus. In P.L. Jackson & J.A. Vessey (Eds.). *Primary care of the child with a chronic condition* (2nd ed.). St. Louis: Mosby.
13. Robertson, P.L. (1998). Pediatric brain tumors. *Primary Care, 25*(2), 323-339.
14. Meberg, A. & Broch, H. (1995). A changing pattern of cerebral palsy: Declining trend for incidence of cerebral palsy in the 20 year period 1970-1989. *Journal of Prenatal Medicine, 23*(50), 359.
15. Dabney, K.W., Lipton, G.E., & Miller, F. (1997). Cerebral palsy. *Current Opinions in Pediatrics 9*(1), 81-88.
16. Fusetti, F. et al. (1998). Structure of tetrameric human phenylanine hydroxylase and its implications for phenyldetonuria. *Journal of Biological Chemistry, 273*(27), 16962-7.
17. Guldberg, P. et al. (1996). Phenylalanine hydrolase gene mutation in the United States: Report from maternal PKU collaborative study. *American Journal of Human Genetics, 59*(1), 84.
18. Osk, F.A. et al. (1994). *Principles of practice of pediatrics* (2nd ed.). Philadelphia: Lippincott.
19. Engel, J. & Pedley, T.A. (1997). *Epilepsy: A comprehensive textbook.* Philadelphia: Lippincott-Raven.
20. Hauser, W.A., Annegers, J.F., Rocca, W.A. (1996). Descriptive epidemiology of epilepsy: Contributions of population-based studies from Rochester. *Mayo Clinic Proceedings, 71*(6), 576-586.
21. Epilepsy Foundation of America. (1999). *Epilepsy facts and figures.* Landover, Md.
22. Ward, M.R. (1997). Reye's syndrome: An update. *Nurse Practitioner, 22*(12), 45-46, 49-50, 52-53.
23. Jackson, R.J. et al. (1998). Preventing childhood lead poisoning: The challenge of change. *American Journal of Preventive Medicine, 14*(3 Suppl.), 84-86.

REFERENCES

24. Booy, R. & Kroll, S. (1994). Bacterial meningitis in children. *Current Opinions in Pediatrics, 6*(1), 29-35.

25. Remington, J.S. & Klein, J.O. (1995). *Infectious diseases of the fetus and newborn infant* (4th ed.). Philadelphia: Saunders.

26. Fahrner, R. (1996). Pediatric HIV infections and AIDS. In P.L. Jackson & J.A. Vessey (Eds.). *Primary care of the child with a chronic condition* (2nd ed.). St. Louis: Mosby.

27. Packer, R.J. (1996). Brain tumors in children. *Current Opinions in Pediatrics, 8*(6), 549-557.

28. Robertson, P.L. (1998). Pediatric brain tumors. *Primary Care, 25*(2), 323-339.

29. Yachnis, A.T. (1997). Neuropathology of pediatric brain tumors. *Seminars in Pediatric Neurology, 4*(4), 282-291.

30. Matthay, K.K. (1997). Neuroblastoma: Biology and therapy. *Oncology (Huntington), 11*(12), 1857-1866.

31. Finger, P.T. (1999). *Retinoblastoma*. Eye Care Foundation.

CHAPTER

17

Mechanisms of Hormonal Regulation

Sue E. Huether

The endocrine system is composed of various glands located throughout the body (Fig. 17-1). These glands can synthesize and release special chemical messengers called hormones. The endocrine system has five general functions: (1) differentiation of the reproductive and central nervous systems in the developing fetus, (2) stimulation of sequential growth and development during childhood and adolescence, (3) coordination of the male and female reproductive systems, which makes sexual reproduction possible, (4) maintenance of an optimal internal environment throughout life, and (5) initiation of corrective and adaptive responses when emergency demands occur. Hormones convey specific regulatory information among cells and organs.

Susan B. Zekauskus, RN, MSN, PNP, contributed to this chapter in the previous edition.

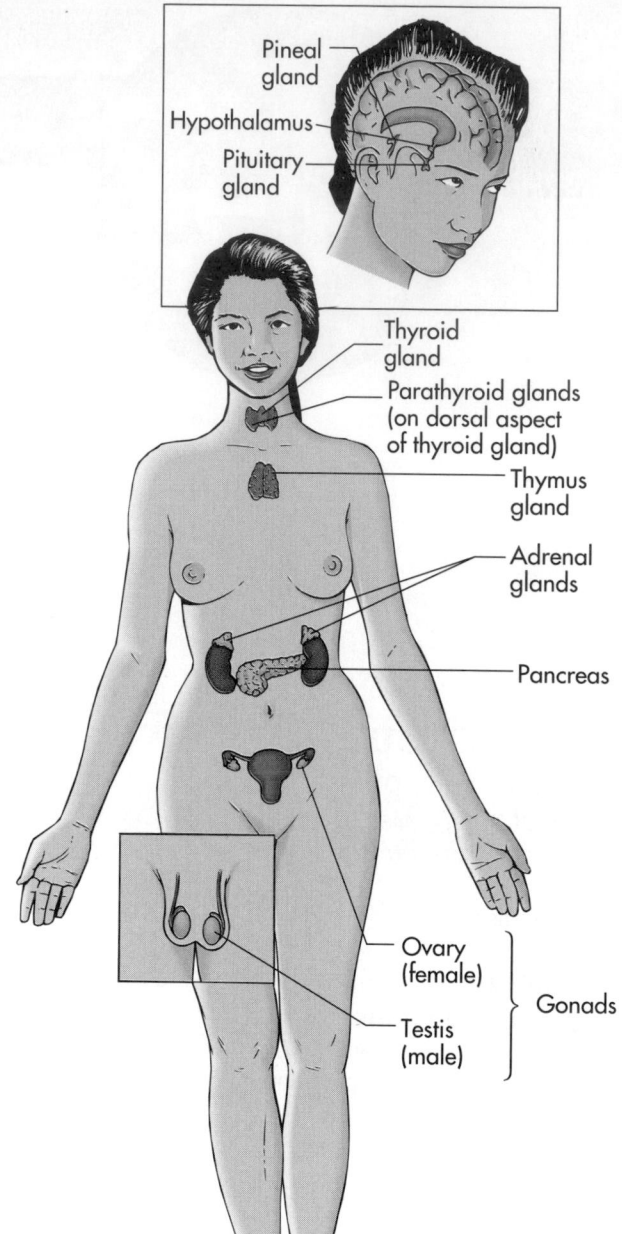

Fig. 17-1 *Principal endocrine glands.* *(From Lindsay, D.T. [1996]. Functional human anatomy. St. Louis: Mosby. By permission of McGraw-Hill Companies, Inc.)*

MECHANISMS OF HORMONAL REGULATION

The endocrine glands respond to specific signals by synthesizing and releasing *hormones* into the circulation, which then trigger intracellular responses. All hormones share certain general characteristics:

1. Have specific rates and patterns of secretion. Three basic secretion patterns are (a) diurnal patterns, (b) pulsatile and cyclic patterns, and (c) patterns that depend on levels of circulating substrates (e.g., calcium, sodium, potassium, or the hormones themselves). Diurnal, pulsatile, and cyclic patterns of hormone release involve consistent patterns of secretion.
2. Operate within feedback systems, either positive or negative, to maintain an optimal internal environment.
3. Affect only target cells with specific receptors for the hormone and then act on these cells to initiate specific cell functions or activities.
4. Are constantly excreted by the kidneys or deactivated by the liver or cellular mechanisms.

Hormones may be classified according to structure, gland of origin, effects, or chemical composition. (Table 17-1 categorizes known hormones by structural category.) The secretion and mechanisms of action of hormones represent an extremely complex system of integrated responses. The endocrine and nervous systems work together to regulate responses to the internal and external environments. Responses are regulated by the secretion of regulatory substances into the bloodstream and the generation of electrical potentials.[1]

Regulation of Hormone Release

Hormones are released either in response to an altered cellular environment or in the maintenance of a regulated level of hormone or other substance. The common processes that regulate endocrine gland secretion include negative feedback, endocrine regulation (a hormone from one endocrine gland controlling another endocrine gland), and neural control.

Hormone secretion may function under one or several regulatory mechanisms. For example, insulin is secreted in response to increased glucose levels (a chemical stimulus); to direct stimulation of the insulin-secreting cells of the pancreas by the autonomic nervous system (a neural stimulus); and to the secretion of cortisol by the adrenal medulla, a form of endocrine regulation.

Feedback systems provide precise monitoring and control of the cellular environment. The most common feedback system, *negative feedback,* occurs because the rising hormone level negates the initiating change that triggered the release of the hormone. For example, if serum calcium levels fall (the initiating change), parathyroid hormone (PTH) secretion is increased. PTH causes an increase in serum calcium. The increase in calcium then decreases PTH secretion, or "turns off" the system, and maintains serum calcium levels (Fig. 17-2). *Positive feedback,* which occurs when hormone secretion continues to trigger additional hormone secretion, is rarely seen in the endocrine system. The feedback loops describe regulation of hormone secretion by hormones themselves (endocrine regulation) (Fig. 17-3).

An example of neural regulation is the release of epinephrine from the adrenal medulla as a result of activation of the sympathetic division of the autonomic nervous system in response to stress. When the stress is removed, the nervous stimulation decreases and less epinephrine is released.

TABLE 17-1	Structural Categories of Hormones				
Proteins	**Glycoproteins**	**Polypeptides**	**Amines**	**Steroids**	**Fatty Acids**
Growth hormone Prolactin Insulin Parathyroid hormone	Folicle-stimulating hormone Luetinizing hormone Thyroid-stimulating hormone	Thyrotropin-releasing hormone Oxytocin Antidiuretic hormone Calcitonin Angiotensin Glucagon Adrenocorticotropic hormone Endorphins Thymosin Melanocyte-stimulating hormone Hypothalamic hormones Lipotropins Somatostatin	Epinephrine Norepinephrine Thyroid hormones (T_4, T_3) Melatonin Vitamin D	Estrogens Progestins (progesterone) Testosterone Mineralocorticoids (aldosterone) Glucocorticoids (cortisol)	Prostaglandins Thromboxanes Prostacyclins Leukotrienes

From Seeley, R.R., Stephens, T.D., & Tate, P. (1995). Anatomy and physiology (3rd ed.). St. Louis: Mosby.

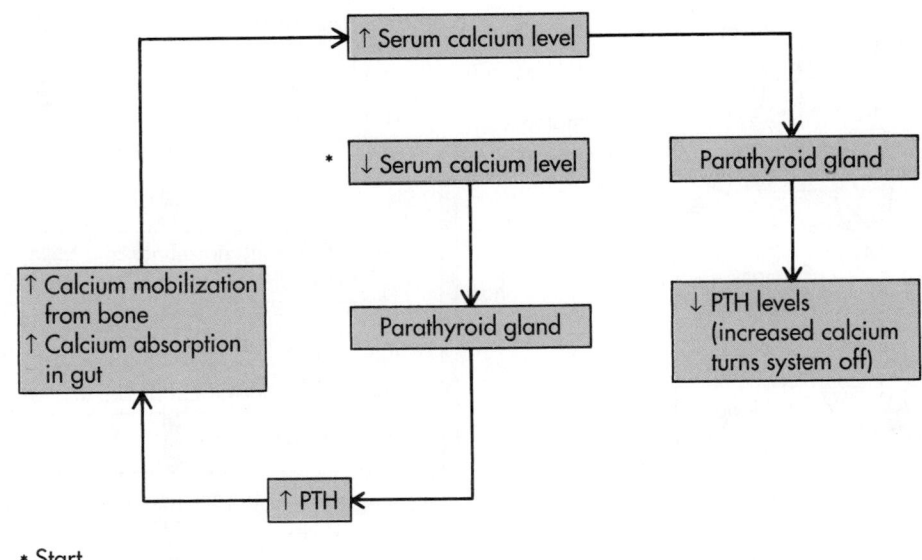

Fig. 17-2 *Negative feedback for calcium regulation.* *PTH,* Parathyroid hormone.

Hormone Transport

Once hormones are released into the circulatory system, they are distributed throughout the body. The protein hormones (insulin, pituitary, hypothalamic, PTH) are water soluble and generally circulate in free (unbound) forms. This process immediately exposes these water-soluble hormones to circulating enzymes, giving them an expected half-life of seconds to minutes. Lipid-soluble hormones are transported bound to plasma proteins. Lipid-soluble hormones can remain in the blood for hours to days. Therefore water-soluble hormones mediate short-acting responses, and lipid solutions mediate more long-acting responses. Water-soluble hormones pass through pores in the walls of capillaries, and lipid-soluble hormones diffuse through the walls of capillaries. Because an equilibrium exists between free hormones and hormones bound to plasma proteins, a significant change in the concentration of binding proteins can affect the concentration of free hormones in the plasma (Table 17-2). Only free hormones can signal a target cell. (Mechanisms of hormone binding are discussed in Chapter 1.)

TABLE 17-2	Binding Proteins, Their Hormones, and Variables That Affect Their Circulating Levels		
Binding Protein	**Hormone**	**Factors That Increase Binding Protein**	**Factors That Decrease Binding Protein**
Corticosteroid-binding globulin	Cortisol Progesterone	Estrogen	Liver disease
Sex hormone–binding globulin	Dihydrotestosterone Testosterone Estradiol	—	Androgens Hypothyroidism Liver disease
Thyroid-binding globulin	T_4 T_3	Estrogen Hyperthyroidism	Testosterone Glucocorticoids Liver disease
Albumin	All lipid-soluble hormones	Estrogen	Liver disease Malnutrition Renal disease

T_4, *Thyroxine;* T_3, *triiodothyronine.*

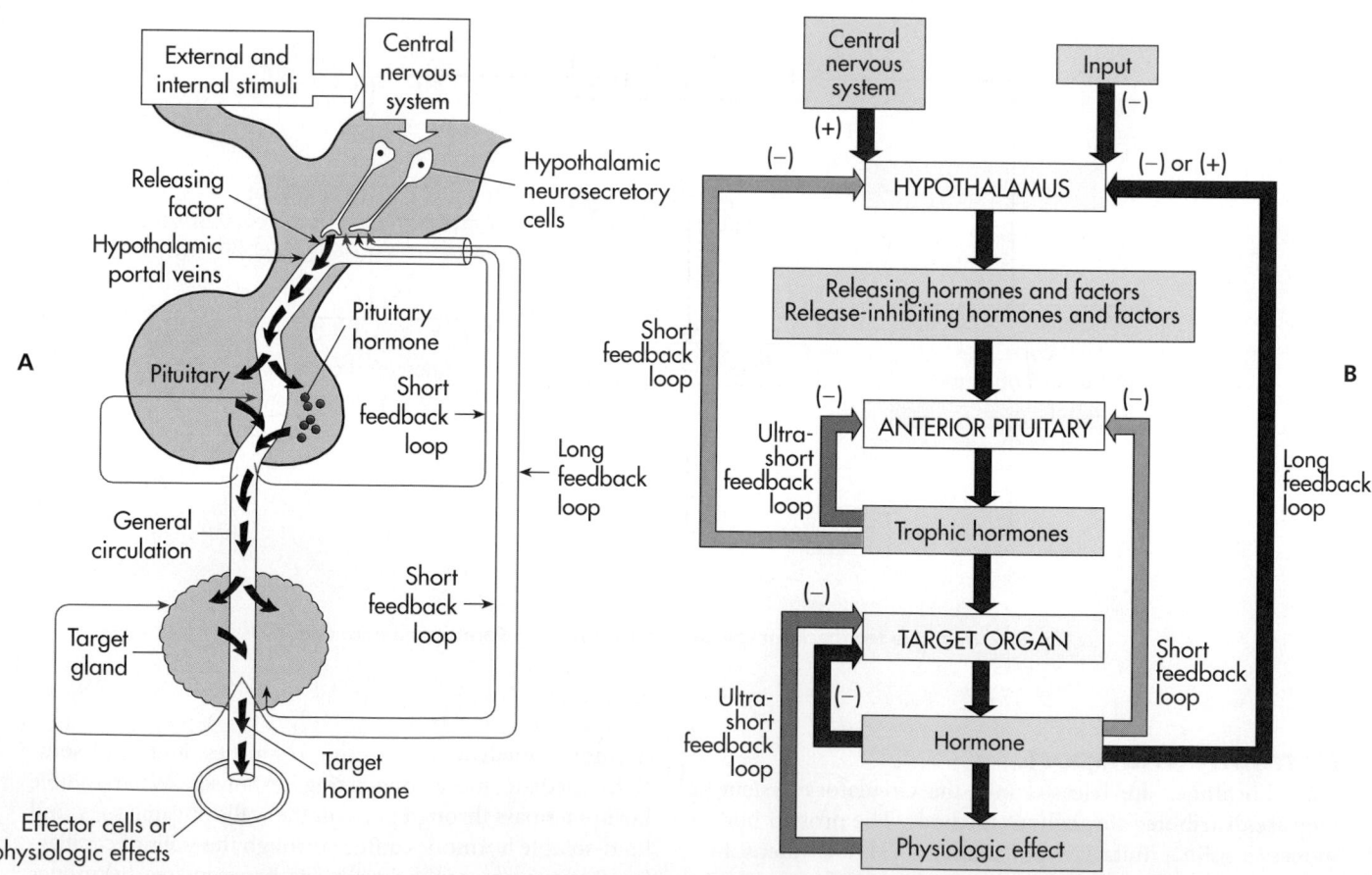

Fig. 17-3 *Feedback loops.* **A,** General model for control and feedback to hypothalamic-pituitary target organ systems. (Blue lines represent negative feedback loops.) **B,** General model for control and negative feedback by hypothalamic-pituitary target organ systems. Negative feedback regulation is possible at three levels: target organ (ultra-short feedback), anterior pituitary (short feedback), and hypothalamus (long feedback).

TABLE 17-3	Types of Hormones, Their Receptors, and Their Mechanisms of Action	
Hormone	**Type of Receptor**	**Mechanism of Action**
Water-soluble hormones		
Glycoproteins, amines, small peptides and proteins (except insulin)	Plasma membrane receptors	Second messenger, cAMP, cGMP, Ca^{++}, others
Insulin	Plasma membrane receptors	Receptor tyrosine kinase, phosphorylation
Lipid-soluble hormones		
Steroid hormones	Nuclear receptors	Nuclear translocation and altered genome transcription
Thyroid hormones (iodothyronines)	Nuclear receptors Cytosolic receptors	Altered genome transcription

cAMP, *Cyclic adenosine monophosphate;* cGMP, *cyclic guanosine monophosphate.*

Mechanisms of Hormone Action

Although a hormone is distributed throughout the body, only those cells with appropriate receptors for that hormone are affected. *Hormone receptors* of the **target cell** have two main functions: (1) to recognize and bind specifically and with high affinity to their particular hormones and (2) to initiate a signal to appropriate intracellular effectors.

The sensitivity of the target cell to a particular hormone is related to the total number of receptors per cell. The more receptors, the more sensitive the cell. Low concentrations of hormone increase the number of receptors per cell; this is called **up regulation.** High concentrations of hormone decrease the number of receptors; this is called **down regulation** (Fig. 17-4). Thus the cell can adjust its sensitivity to the concentration of the signaling hormone.

Hormones affect target cells directly or permissively. **Direct effects** are the obvious changes in cell function that result specifically from stimulation by a particular hormone. **Permissive effects** are less obvious hormone-induced changes that facilitate the maximal response or functioning of a cell. For example, insulin has a direct effect on skeletal muscle cells with insulin receptors, causing increased glucose transport into these cells. Insulin also has a permissive effect on mammary cells, facilitating the response of these cells to the direct effects of prolactin.

If hormones are secreted at higher than physiologic levels or are administered exogenously in high doses, a pharmacologic effect occurs. **Pharmacologic effects** are cell responses seen only at extremely high hormone levels and may not reflect the actions of the hormone at usual or physiologic levels. For example, usual levels of antidiuretic hormone (ADH) affect the renal tubules, increasing water absorption. At higher, or pharmacologic, levels, ADH acts as a vasoconstrictor.

Hormone receptors

Hormone receptors may be located on the plasma membrane or in the intracellular compartment of the target cell. Water-soluble (peptide) hormones, which include the protein hormones and the catecholamines, have a high molecular weight and cannot pass across the cell membrane. They interact or bind with receptors located in or on the cell membrane. Fat-soluble steroid, vitamin D, retinoic acid, and thyroid hormones diffuse freely across the plasma and nuclear membranes and bind with primarily nuclear receptors (Fig. 17-5). (Types of hormones, their corresponding receptors, and the mechanisms by which they affect the cell are summarized in Table 17-3.)

First and second messengers

Receptors for most water-soluble hormones are located in the plasma membranes of cells. The hormone is the *first messenger* and is secreted into the bloodstream, where it interacts with the receptor on the plasma membrane of target cells. The interaction initiates a signal that generates a *second messenger* inside the cell. The second messenger mediates by signaling the effect of the hormone on the target cell, for example, membrane transport, contractile proteins, enzyme activation, protein synthesis, and cellular growth. The second messengers are small molecules, such as cyclic adenosine monophosphate (cAMP). Other second messengers include cyclic guanosine monophosphate (cGMP), inositol triphosphate, calcium or calcium-calmodulin, and the tyrosine kinase system (Fig. 17-6). The receptors on the plasma membrane are continuously synthesized and degraded, so that changes in receptor concentration may occur within hours. In addition, the receptor's affinity for the hormone may vary. Both receptor affinity and receptor con-

Fig. 17-4 *Regulation of target cell sensitivity.* **A,** Low hormone level and *up regulation,* or an increase in number of receptors. **B,** High hormone level and *down regulation,* or a decrease in number of receptors. *(From Thibodeau, G.A. & Patton, K.T. [1999]. Anatomy & physiology [4th ed.]. St. Louis: Mosby.)*

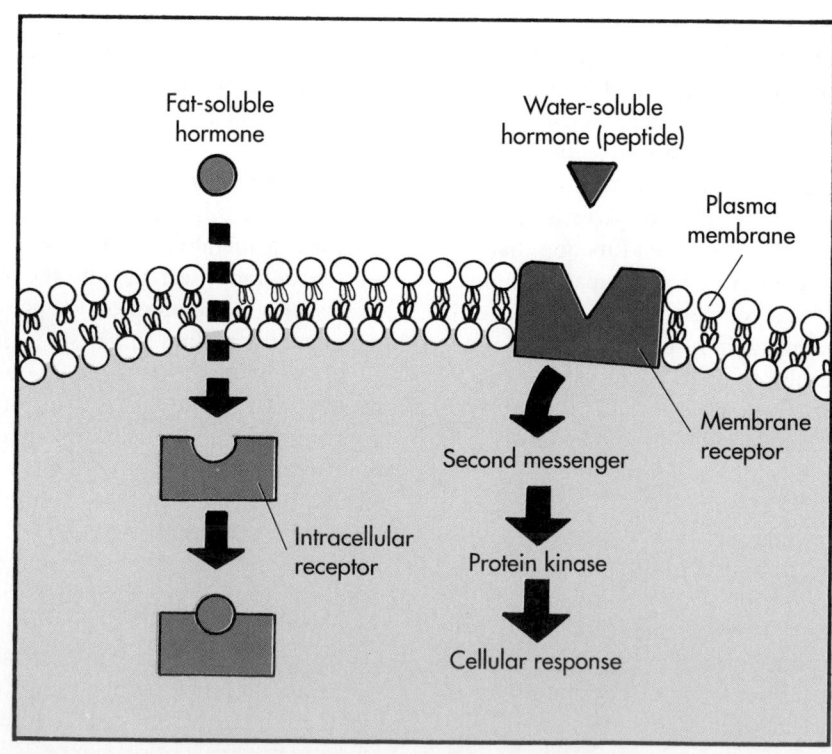

Fig. 17-5 *Hormone binding at target cell.*

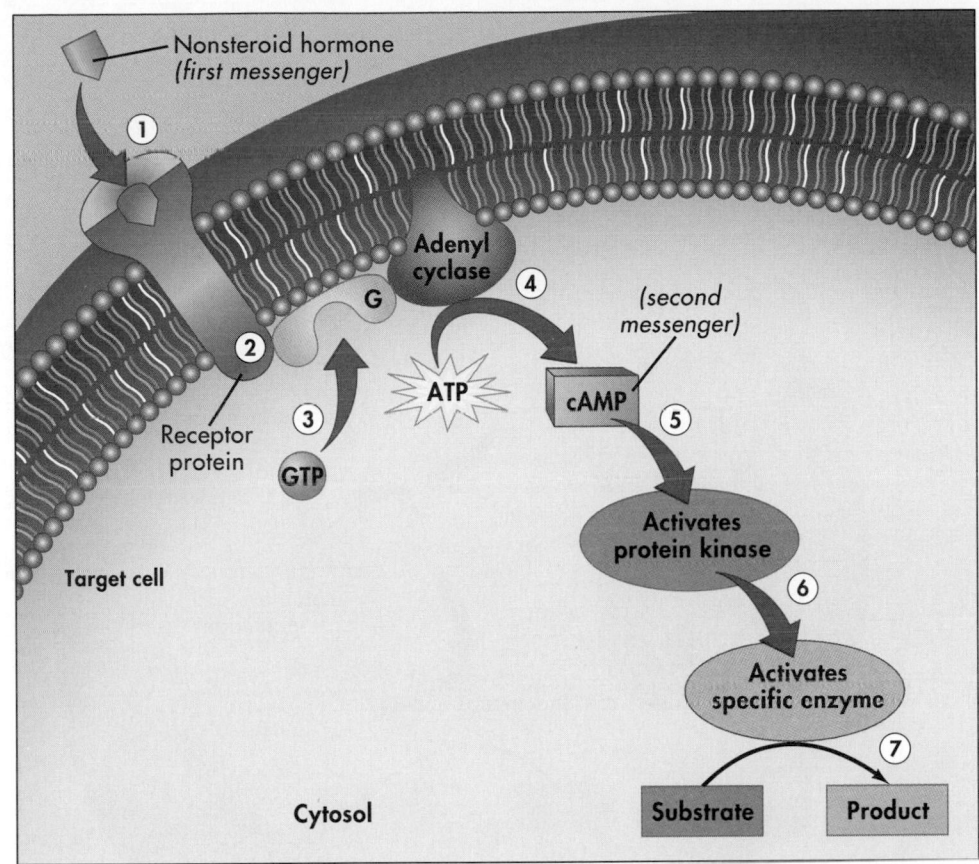

Fig. 17-6 *Example of first- and second-messenger mechanisms.* A nonsteroid hormone *(first messenger)* binds to a fixed receptor in the plasma membrane of the target cell *(1)*. The hormone-receptor complex activates the G protein *(2)*. The activated G protein *(G)* reacts with guanosine triphosphate *(GTP)*, which in turn activates the membrane-bound enzyme adenyl cyclase *(3)*. Adenyl cyclase catalyzes the conversion of adenosine triphosphate *(ATP)* to cyclic adenosine monophosphate (cAMP) *(second messenger, 4)*. cAMP activates protein kinase A *(5)*. Protein kinases activate specific intracellular enzymes *(6)*. These activated enzymes then influence specific cellular reactions, thus producing the target cell's response to the hormone *(7)*. *(From Thibodeau, G.A. & Patton, K.T. [1999].* Anatomy & physiology *[4th ed.]. St. Louis: Mosby.)*

centration are regulated by intracellular and extracellular mechanisms, including the following:

1. Physicochemical environment
   a. pH
   b. Temperature
   c. Calcium concentration
   d. Sodium concentration
2. Urea concentration
   a. Levels of cAMP (a second messenger)
3. Lipid matrix of the plasma membrane
   a. Cholesterol content
   b. Saturation of fatty acid side chains
   c. Polar groups or phospholipids
   d. Alterations of the plasma membrane
4. Circulating levels of hormones
5. Stage of growth and development
6. Diet
7. Exercise
8. Drugs

Hormone-receptor binding increases the intracellular level of second messengers, such as cAMP and cGMP. cAMP activates a protein kinase, which leads to phosphorylation and enzyme activation. cGMP also activates enzymes that direct a number of cellular processes. Consequently both these second messengers direct the actions or products of specific cells.

Inositol triphosphate functions as a second messenger for nonsteroid hormones, such as angiotensin II and gonadotropin-releasing hormone. Hormone receptor binds through a plasma membrane G protein and results in generation of inositol triphosphate. Inositol triphosphate triggers a cascade of chemical reactions that produce the cell's response.

The calcium-calmodulin complex mediates the effects of calcium on intracellular activities, particularly the activation of protein kinases. The calmodulin-dependent protein kinases control intracellular contractile components (myosin, actin), alter plasma membrane permeability to calcium, and

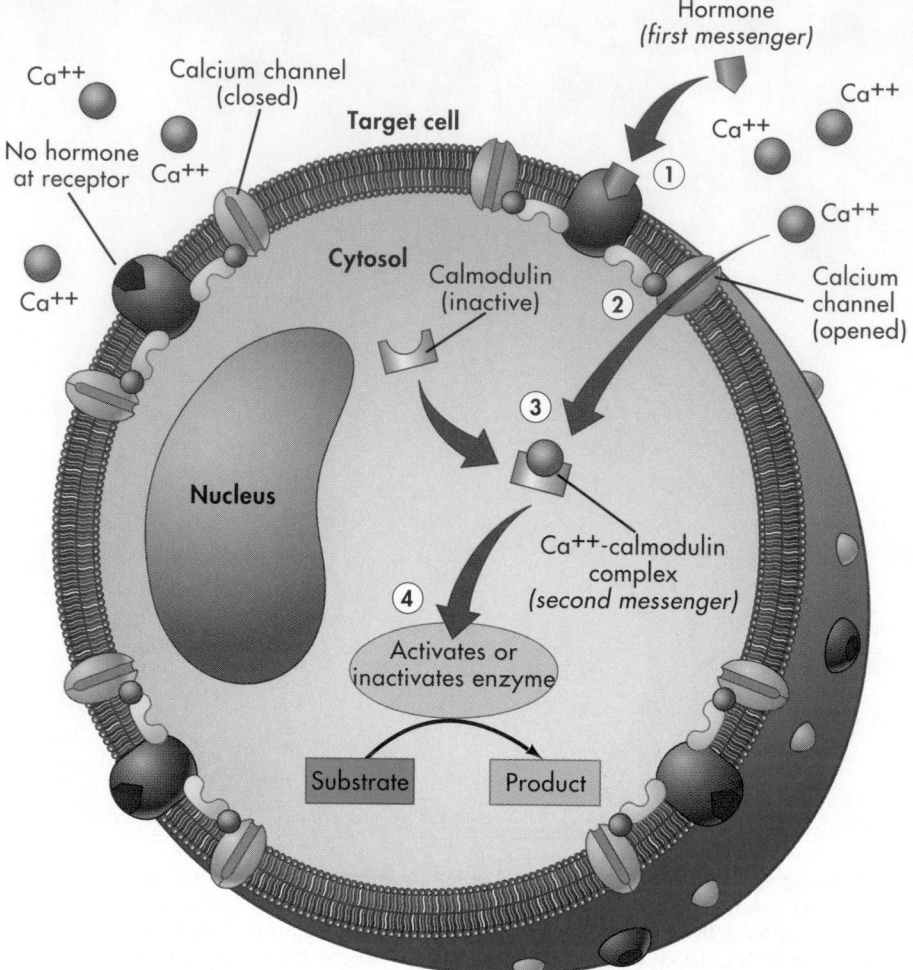

Fig. 17-7 *Calcium-calmodulin as a second messenger.* In this example of a second messenger mechanism, a nonsteroid hormone *(first messenger)* first binds to a fixed receptor in the plasma membrane *(1)*, which activates membrane-bound proteins (G protein, PIP_2) that trigger the opening of calcium channels *(2)*. Calcium ions, which are normally at a higher concentration in the extracellular fluid, diffuse into the cell and bind to a calmodulin molecule *(3)*. The calcium-calmodulin complex thus formed is a second messenger that binds to an enzyme to produce an allosteric effect that promotes or inhibits the enzyme's regulatory effect in the target cell *(4). (From Thibodeau, G.A. & Patton, K.T. [1999].* Anatomy & physiology *[4th ed.] St. Louis: Mosby.)*

regulate intracellular enzyme activity that promotes hormone secretion (Fig. 17-7).

Steroid (lipid-soluble) hormone receptors

The lipid-soluble hormones are steroid hormones (synthesized from cholesterol; include androgens, estrogens, progestins, glucocorticoids, and mineralocorticoids), thyroid hormones, vitamin D, and retinoid. Because these are relatively small, lipophilic, hydrophobic molecules, they can cross the lipid plasma membrane by simple diffusion (see Chapter 1). Receptors for steroid hormones are primarily localized in the nucleus and direct gene expression (Fig. 17-8).[2]

✓ QUICK CHECK

What are hormones? By what mechanisms do they function?

Describe a direct effect and a permissive effect of hormones on cells.

How do first messengers differ from second messengers?

Fig. 17-8 *Steroid hormone mechanism.* According to the mobile receptor hypothesis, lipid-soluble steroid hormone molecules detach from the carrier protein *(1)* and pass through the plasma membrane *(2)*. The hormone molecules then pass into the nucleus where they bind to a mobile receptor to form a hormone-receptor complex *(3)*. This complex then binds to a specific site on a deoxyribonucleic acid *(DNA)* molecule *(4)*, triggering transcription of the genetic information encoded there *(5)*. The resulting messenger ribonucleic acid *(mRNA)* molecule moves to the cytosol, where it associates with a ribosome, initiating synthesis of a new protein *(6)*. This new protein—usually an enzyme or channel protein—produces specific effects on the target cell *(7)*. *(From Thibodeau, G.A. & Patton, K.T. [1999]. Anatomy & physiology [4th ed.]. St. Louis: Mosby.)*

STRUCTURE AND FUNCTION OF THE ENDOCRINE GLANDS
Hypothalamic-Pituitary System

The hormones of the pituitary gland regulate several other endocrine glands and affect diverse body functions. Part of the pituitary gland is directly connected to the brain, and the pituitary gland also is closely related to the nervous system. Some hormones secreted by the pituitary gland act directly on the reproductive system (see Unit 10). Other hormones act in conjunction with the thyroid, adrenal glands, and endocrine pancreas.

The *pituitary gland* is located in the sella turcica (a saddle-shaped depression at the base of the skull). It weighs approximately 0.5 g, except during pregnancy when its weight approaches 1 g. It is composed of two distinctly different lobes: (1) the anterior pituitary, or adenohypophysis; and (2) the posterior pituitary, or neurohypophysis. These two lobes differ in their embryonic origins, cell types, and functional relationship to the hypothalamus.

The anterior pituitary (adenohypophysis) accounts for 75% of the total weight of the pituitary gland. It is composed of three regions: (1) the pars distalis, (2) the pars tuberalis, and (3) the pars intermedia. The *pars distalis* is the major component of the anterior pituitary, the source of the anterior pituitary hormones. The *pars tuberalis* is a thin layer of cells on the anterior and lateral portions of the infundibular

TABLE 17-4	Hormones of the Anterior Pituitary and Their Functions		
Hormone	**Secretory Cell Type**	**Target Organs**	**Functions**
Adrenocorticotropic hormone (ACTH)	Corticotropic	Adrenal gland	Regulates growth and secretion of the adrenal gland, particularly cortisol and the androgenic steroids
Melanocyte-stimulating hormone (MSH)	Melanotropic	Anterior pituitary	Promotes secretion of melanin and lipotropin by anterior pituitary; makes skin darker
Somatotropic hormones			
Growth hormone (GH)	Somatotropic	Muscle, bone, liver	Regulates metabolic processes related to growth and adaptation to physical and emotional stressors, including skeletal growth, muscle growth, increased protein synthesis, increased liver glycogenolysis, increased fat mobilization
		Liver	Induces formation of somatomedins, or insulin-like growth factors (IGFs) that have actions similar to insulin
Prolactin	Lactotropic	Breast	Milk production
Glycoprotein hormones			
Thyroid-stimulating hormone (TSH)	Thyrotropic	Thyroid gland	Increased production and secretion of thyroid hormone Increased iodine uptake
Luteinizing hormone (LH)	Gonadotropic	In women: ovarian follicle	Ovulation, progesterone production
		In men: Leydig cells	Regulates spermatogenesis, testosterone production
Follicle-stimulating hormone (FSH)	Gonadotropic	In women: ovarian follicle	Follicle maturation, estrogen production
		In men: Leydig cells	Spermatogenesis
β-Lipotropin	Corticotropic	Adipose cells	Fat breakdown and release of fatty acids
β-Endorphins	Corticotropic	Adipose cells	Analgesia; may regulate body temperature, food and water intake

stem. The *pars intermedia* lies between the two lobes of the pituitary gland. In the adult the distinct intermediate lobe disappears and individual cells are distributed diffusely throughout the pars distalis and pars nervosa (neural lobe).[3]

The anterior pituitary

The anterior pituitary is composed of two main cell types: (1) the *chromophobes,* which appear to be nonsecretory, and (2) the *chromophils,* which are considered the secretory cells of the adenohypophysis. The chromophils are subdivided into nine secretory cell types, and each cell type secretes a specific hormone or hormones (Table 17-4).

In general, the anterior pituitary hormones are regulated by (1) secretion of hypothalamic peptide hormones or releasing factors, (2) feedback effects of the hormones secreted by target glands, and (3) direct effects of other mediating neurotransmitters. (These are summarized in Fig. 17-3.)

The anterior pituitary secretes tropic hormones, including adrenocorticotropic hormone (ACTH), melanocyte-stimulating hormone (MSH), somatotropic hormones (growth hormone, prolactin), and the glycoprotein hormones (follicle-stimulating hormone, luteinizing hormone

[LH] including the male analog of LH [interstitial cell-stimulating hormone—ICSH], and thyroid-stimulating hormone). Each hormone affects the physiologic function of the specific target organ (see Fig. 17-3 and Table 17-4).

The anterior pituitary hormones are regulated by releasing and inhibiting factors secreted from hypothalamic nuclei. These factors are carried to the anterior pituitary by the hypophysial portal system, which is the primary blood supply to the pituitary gland (Fig. 17-9).

The hypothalamus synthesizes and releases hormones that regulate secretion by other glands, including *prolactin-inhibiting factor (PIF), thyrotropin-releasing hormone (TRH), gonadotropin-releasing* hormone (GnRH), *somatostatin, growth hormone–releasing factor (GRF), corticotropin-releasing hormone (CRH),* and *substance P.* These hormones are summarized in Table 17-5.

The posterior pituitary

The hypothalamic-pituitary unit forms the structural and functional basis for central integration of the neurologic and endocrine systems (Figs. 17-10 and 17-11). The hypothalamus, containing special neurosecretory cells and located at

TABLE 17-5	Hypothalamic Hormones	
Hormone	**Target Tissue**	**Action**
Thyrotropin-releasing hormone (TRH)	Anterior pituitary	Stimulates release of thyroid-stimulating hormones (TSH) Modulates prolactin secretion
Gonadotropin-releasing hormone (GnRH)	Anterior pituitary	Stimulates release of follicle-stimulating hormone (FSH) and luteinizing hormone (LH)
Somatostatin	Anterior pituitary	Inhibits release of growth hormone (GH)
	Gastrointestinal tract	Decreases gastric motility, intestinal secretion, and secretion of TSH, parathyroid hormone, renin, glucagon, and insulin
Growth hormone–releasing factor (GRF)	Anterior pituitary	Stimulates release of GH
Corticotropin-releasing hormone (CRH)	Anterior pituitary	Stimulates release of adrenocorticotropic hormone (ACTH) and β-endorphin
Substance P	Anterior pituitary	Inhibits synthesis and release of ACTH Stimulates secretion of GH, FSH, LH, and prolactin
Prolactin-inhibiting factor (PIF; possibly dopamine)	Anterior pituitary	Inhibits secretion of prolactin
Prolactin-releasing hormone (PRH)	Anterior pituitary	Stimulates secretion of prolactin

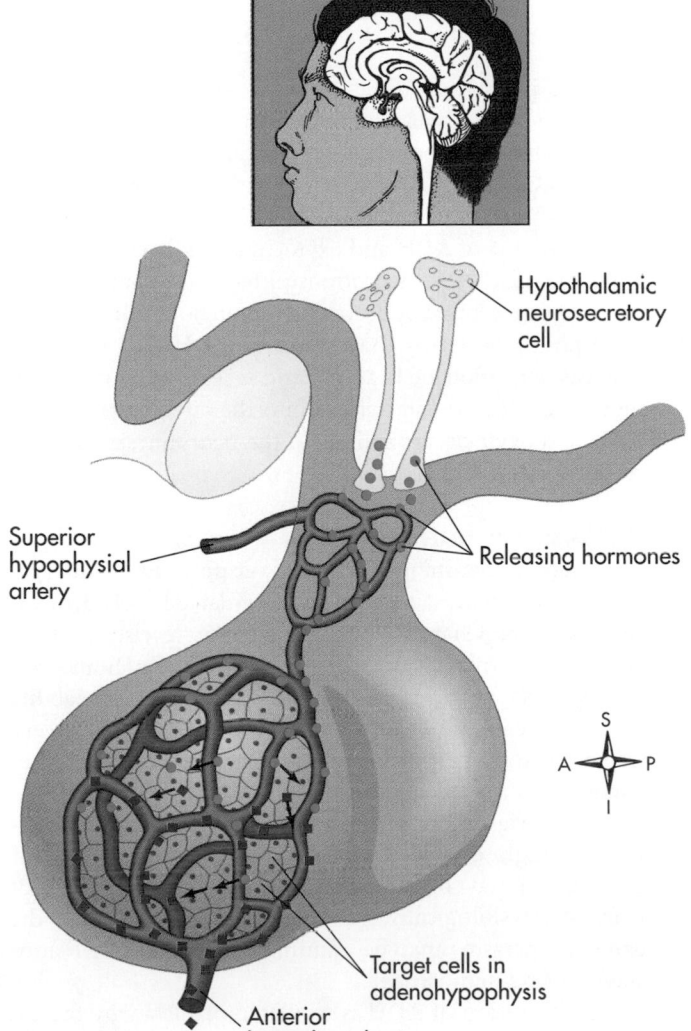

Hypothalamic neurosecretory cell

Superior hypophysial artery

Releasing hormones

S
A ← → P
I

Target cells in adenohypophysis

Anterior hypophysial vein

Fig. 17-9 *Hypophysial portal system.* Neurons in the hypothalamus secrete releasing hormones into veins that carry the releasing hormones directly to the vessels of the adenohypophysis, thus bypassing the normal circulatory route. *(From Thibodeau, G.A. & Patton, K.T. [1999]. Anatomy & physiology [4th ed.]. St. Louis: Mosby.)*

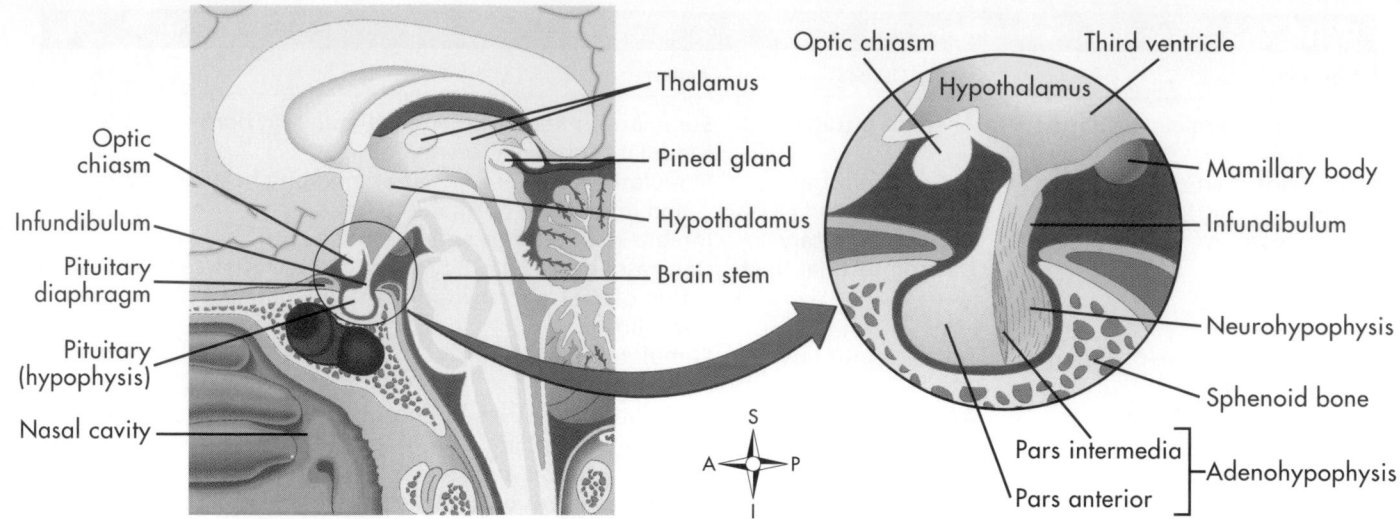

Fig. 17-10 *Location and structure of the pituitary gland (hypophysis).* The pituitary gland is located within the sella turcica of the skull's sphenoid bone and is connected to the hypothalamus by a stalklike infundibulum. The infundibulum passes through a gap in the portion of the dura mater that covers the pituitary (the pituitary diaphragm). The inset shows that the pituitary is divided into an anterior portion, the adenohypophysis, and a posterior portion, the neurohypophysis. The adenohypophysis is further subdivided into the pars anterior and pars intermedia. The pars intermedia is almost absent in the adult pituitary. *(From Thibodeau, G.A. & Patton, K.T. [1999].* Anatomy & physiology *[4th ed.]. St. Louis: Mosby.)*

the base of the brain, is connected to the pituitary gland by a stalklike structure, the **infundibular stem.** The special cells of the hypothalamus are like other neurons in that they have similar electrical properties, organelles, membranes, and synapses. Neurosecretory cells, however, can synthesize and secrete the hypothalamic-releasing hormones and synthesize the hormones of the posterior portion of the pituitary gland.

The embryonic posterior pituitary (neurohypophysis) is derived from the hypothalamus and comprises three parts: (1) the median eminence located at the base of the hypothalamus, (2) the infundibular stem, and (3) the infundibular process, also known as the pars nervosa or neural lobe. The **median eminence** is composed largely of the nerve endings of axons from the ventral hypothalamus. It often is designated as part of the posterior pituitary but contains at least 10 biologically active hypothalamic-releasing hormones, as well as the neurotransmitters dopamine, norepinephrine, serotonin, acetylcholine, and histamine, so it might be more appropriately considered part of the hypothalamus. The infundibular stem contains the axons of neurons that originate in the supraoptic and paraventricular nuclei of the hypothalamus and connects the pituitary gland to the brain. Axons originating in the hypothalamus terminate in the **infundibular process,** which secretes the hormones of the posterior pituitary (see Fig. 17-12).

The posterior pituitary secretes two polypeptide hormones: (1) **antidiuretic hormone (ADH),** also called vasopressin, and (2) oxytocin. These hormones differ by only two amino acids. They are synthesized, along with their binding proteins, the neurophysins, in the supraoptic and paraventricular nuclei of the hypothalamus (Fig. 17-12). They are

packaged in secretory vesicles and are moved down the axons of the infundibular stem to the infundibular process for storage. The posterior pituitary thus can be seen as a storage and releasing site for hormones synthesized in the hypothalamus.

The release of ADH and oxytocin is mediated by cholinergic and adrenergic neurotransmitters. Stimulation of the cholinergic receptors by acetylcholine, angiotensin II, and β-endorphins results in the release of ADH and oxytocin, whereas activation of β-adrenergic receptors inhibits hormone secretion. Before release into the circulatory system, ADH and oxytocin are split from the neurophysins and are secreted in unbound form.

Antidiuretic hormone

The major homeostatic function of the posterior pituitary is the control of plasma osmolality as regulated by ADH, or vasopressin (see Chapter 4). At physiologic levels, ADH increases the permeability of the distal renal tubules and collecting ducts (see Chapter 28). This increased permeability leads to increased water reabsorption and more concentrated urine. Hypercalcemia, prostaglandin E, and hypokalemia can inhibit them.

ADH originally was named *vasopressin* because in extremely high doses it causes vasoconstriction and increased arterial blood pressure. These levels are not reached physiologically, but high doses of ADH (as the drug vasopressin) may be administered to achieve hemostasis during hemorrhage.

The secretion of ADH is regulated primarily by the osmoreceptors of the hypothalamus, located near or in the

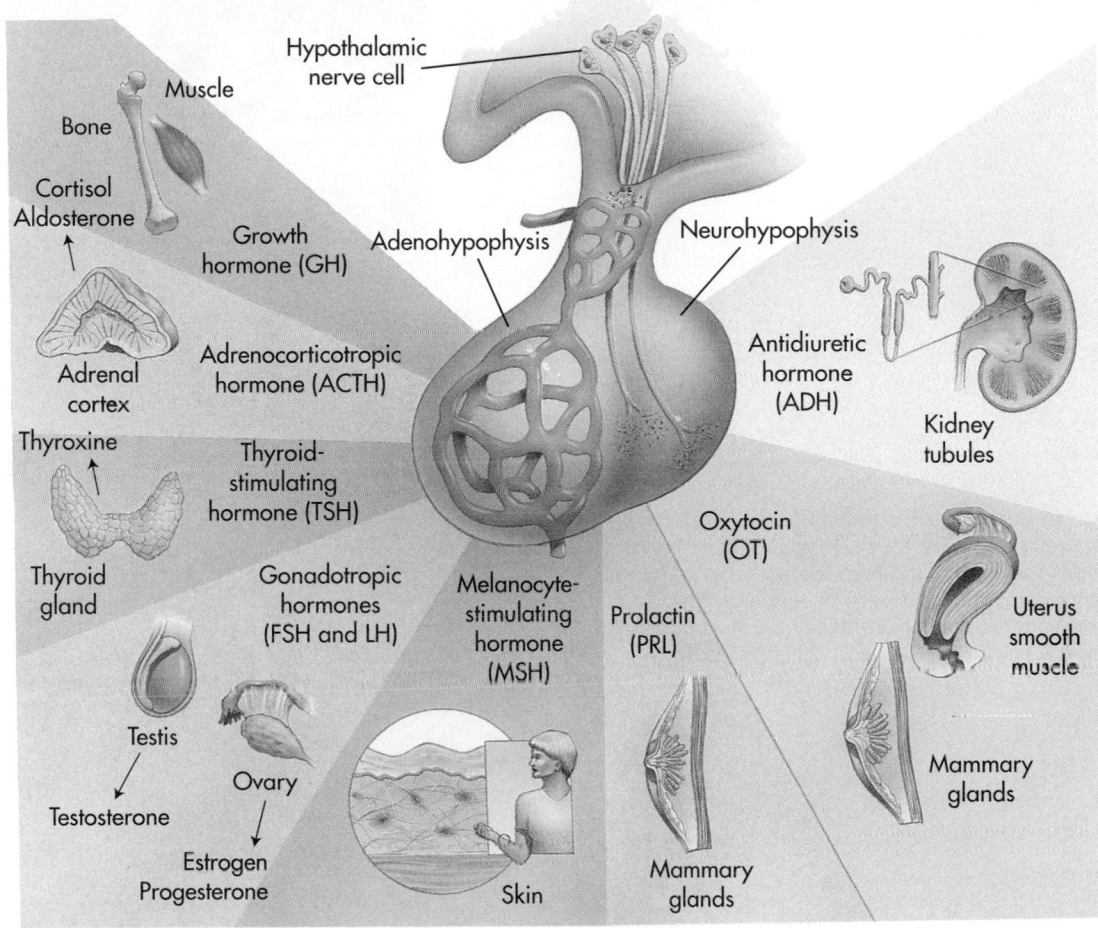

Fig. 17-11 *Anterior pituitary hormones and their target hormones.* Male analog of LH (interstitial cell–stimulating hormone [ICSH]). *(From Thibodeau, G.A. & Patton, K.T. [1999]. Anatomy & physiology [4th ed.]. St. Louis: Mosby.)*

supraoptic nuclei (osmoreceptors are stimulated by increased osmolality). As plasma osmolality increases, the rate of ADH secretion increases.

ADH secretion is increased by changes in intravascular volume, which are monitored by baroreceptors in the left atrium, in the carotid, and in the aortic arches. A volume loss of 7% to 25% stimulates ADH secretion. Stress, trauma, pain, exercise, nausea, nicotine, exposure to heat, and drugs such as morphine also increase ADH secretion. ADH secretion decreases with decreased plasma osmolality, increased intravascular volume, hypertension, and alcohol ingestion. ADH has no direct effect on electrolyte levels.

Oxytocin

Oxytocin is responsible for contraction of the uterus and milk ejection in lactating women and may affect sperm motility in men. In both genders, oxytocin has an antidiuretic effect similar to that of ADH. The function of this hormone is discussed in Chapter 31.

In women, oxytocin is secreted in response to suckling and mechanical distention of the female reproductive tract. Oxytocin binds to its receptors on myoepithelial cells in the mammary tissues and causes contraction of those cells,

which increases intramammary pressure and milk expression ("let-down" reflex).

Oxytocin also acts on the uterus to stimulate contractions. Oxytocin functions near the end of labor to enhance effectiveness of contractions, promote delivery of the placenta, and stimulate postpartum contractions, thereby preventing excessive bleeding.

✓ QUICK CHECK

What is the difference between a releasing hormone and a releasing factor?

What is the action of antidiuretic hormone (ADH)? How is oxytocin similar to ADH?

Thyroid and Parathyroid Glands

The thyroid gland, located in the neck just below the larynx, produces hormones that control the rates of metabolic processes throughout the body. The four parathyroid glands are near the thyroid and function to control serum calcium levels.

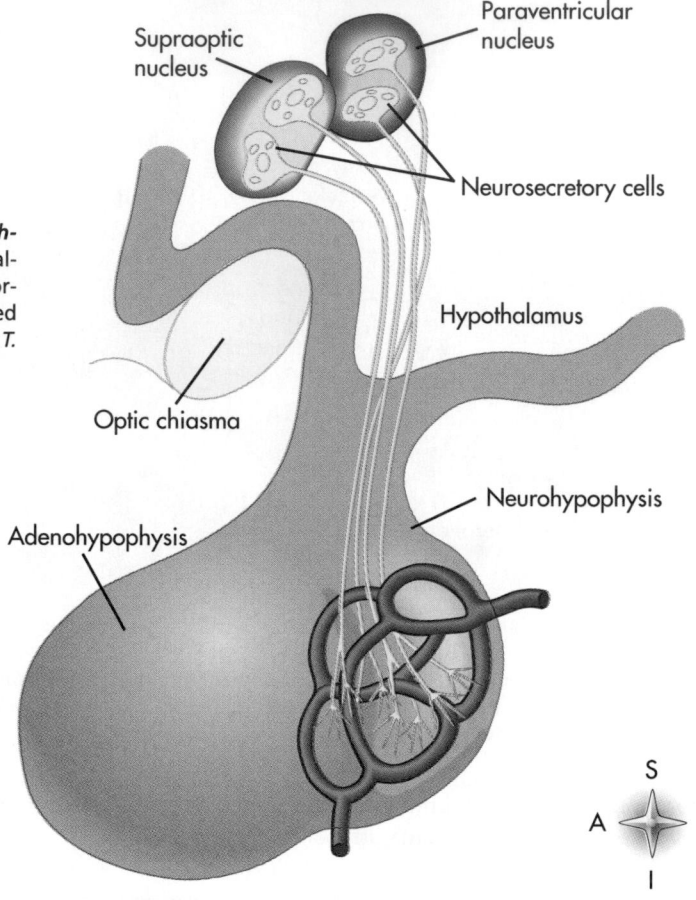

Fig. 17-12 *Relationship of the hypothalamus and neurohypophysis.* Neurosecretory cells have their cell bodies in the hypothalamus and their axon terminals in the neurohypophysis. Thus hormones synthesized in the hypothalamus are actually released from the neurohypophysis. *(From Thibodeau, G.A. & Patton, K.T. [1999]. Anatomy & physiology [4th ed.]. St. Louis: Mosby.)*

Thyroid gland

The two lobes of the **thyroid gland** lie on either side of the trachea, inferior to the thyroid cartilage and joined by the **isthmus** (Fig. 17-13). The normal thyroid gland is not visible on inspection, but it may be palpated on swallowing, which causes it to be displaced upward.

The thyroid gland comprises **follicles** that contain follicular cells that surround a viscous substance called *colloid*. The follicular cells synthesize and secrete the thyroid hormones. Neurons terminate on blood vessels within the thyroid gland and on the follicular cells themselves, so neurotransmitters may directly affect the secretory activity of follicular cells.

Also found in the thyroid are parafollicular, or C, cells. **C cells** secrete various polypeptides, including calcitonin and somatostatin. **Calcitonin,** also called *thyrocalcitonin,* lowers serum calcium levels by direct, rapid, and significant inhibi-

tion of bone-resorbing osteoclasts and promotion of osteoblasts that result in bone formation. (Bone resorption is explained in Chapter 37.) The metabolic consequences of calcitonin deficiency or excess have not yet been identified in humans (Table 17-6). Calcitonin and parathyroid hormone together regulate calcium balance.

Regulation of thyroid hormone secretion

Thyroid hormone is available in the body as either thyroxine (tetraiodothyronine [T_4]) or triiodothyronine (T_3). **Thyroid hormone (TH)** is regulated through a negative feedback loop involving the hypothalamus, the anterior pituitary, and the thyroid gland (see Fig. 17-3). (Fig. 17-13 illustrates the thyroid and parathyroid glands.) Thyrotropin-releasing hormone (TRH), which is synthesized and stored within the hypothalamus, initiates this loop. TRH is released into the hypothalamic-pituitary portal system and circulates to the

TABLE 17-6	Thyroid Gland Hormones and Their Regulation and Functions	
Hormone	**Regulation**	**Functions**

Thyroxine (T_4) and triiodothyronine (T_3)	T_4 and T_3 levels are controlled by TSH
	Released in response to metabolic demand
	Influences on amount secreted
	  Gender
	  Pregnancy
	  Gonadal- and adrenocortical-increased steroids = ↑ levels
	  Exposure to extreme cold = ↑ levels
	  Nutritional state
	  Chemicals
	    GHIH = ↓ levels
	    Dopamine = ↓ levels
	    Catecholamines = ↑ levels
		Regulates protein, fat, and carbohydrate catabolism in all cells
		Regulates metabolic rate of all cells
		Regulates body heat production
		Insulin antagonist
		Maintains growth hormone secretion, skeletal maturation
		Affects CNS development
		Necessary for muscle tone and vigor
		Maintains cardiac rate, force, and output
		Maintains secretion of GI tract
		Affects respiratory rate and oxygen utilization
		Maintains calcium mobilization
		Affects RBC production
		Stimulates lipid turnover, free fatty acid release, and cholesterol synthesis

Calcitonin	Elevated serum calcium—major stimulant for calcitonin
	Other stimulants
	  Gastrin
	  Calcium-rich foods (regardless of serum Ca^{++} levels)
	  Pregnancy
	Lowered serum calcium—suppresses calcitonin release
		Major function
		  Lowers serum calcium by opposing bone-resorbing effects of PTH, prostaglandins, and calciferols by inhibiting osteoclastic activity
		Also lowers serum phosphate levels
		May also decrease calcium and phosphorus absorption in GI tract

From Long, B.C., Phipps, W.J., & Cassmeyer, V.L. (1992). Medical-surgical nursing: A nursing process approach *(3rd ed.)*. St. Louis: Mosby. TSH, *Thyroid-stimulating hormone;* CSN, *central nervous system;* GI, *gastrointestinal;* GHIH, growth hormone–inhibiting hormone; *RBC,* red blood cell; *PTH,* parathyroid hormone.

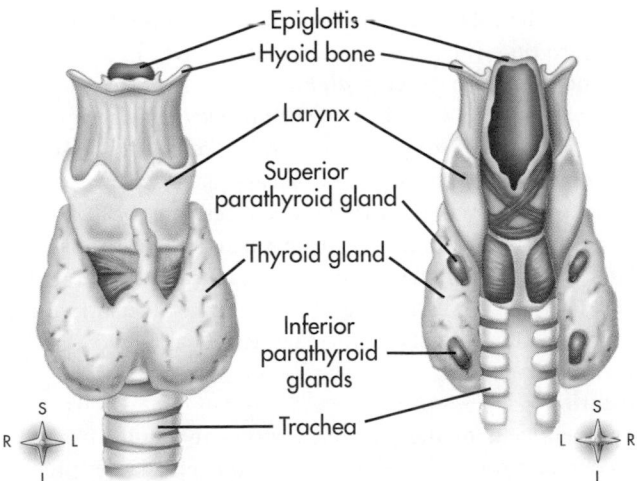

Fig. 17-13 *Thyroid and parathyroid glands.* Note their location to each other and to the larynx and trachea. *(From Thibodeau, G.A. & Patton, K.T. [1999]. Anatomy & physiology [4th ed.]. St. Louis: Mosby.)*

anterior pituitary, where it stimulates the release of thyroid-stimulating hormone (TSH). TRH levels increase with exposure to cold, stress, and decreased levels of thyroxine (T_4).

Thyroid-stimulating hormone (TSH) is a glycoprotein synthesized and stored within the anterior pituitary. Once TSH is secreted by the anterior pituitary, it circulates to bind with receptor sites on the outer side of the thyroid cell's plasma membrane. TSH's effects include (1) an immediate increase in the release of stored thyroid hormone, (2) an increase in iodine uptake and oxidation, (3) an increase in thyroid hormone synthesis, and (4) an increase in the synthesis and secretion of prostaglandins by the thyroid. Thyroid gland hormones and their regulation and function are summarized in Table 17-6.

TH acts on the thyroid gland, the anterior pituitary, and the median eminence to regulate further TH production. It operates in a negative feedback effect to inhibit TRH and TSH, which then decreases TH synthesis and secretion.

Synthesis of thyroid hormone

The thyroid gland produces thyroid hormone (TH) when stimulated by TSH, low serum iodide levels, or drugs interfering with the thyroid gland's uptake of iodide in the blood. The first step in the synthesis of TH is the concentration of iodide (an iodine compound) by the thyroid gland. Because there is an iodine concentration gradient of about 30:1 to 40:1 between the thyroid gland and the blood, iodine is moved by active transport from the extracellular fluid to the thyroid follicular cells. The iodide must be oxidized to iodine, which is facilitated by the enzyme peroxidase inside the follicular cells.

Thyroglobulin, a large glycoprotein synthesized within the follicular cell, is the precursor of thyroid hormones. Uniodinated thyroglobulin is released into the colloid, and iodine combines with tyrosine in the thyroglobulin to form iodotyrosines. Triiodothyronine (T_3) has three iodine molecules, and thyroxine (T_4) has four. Most T_4 is converted to T_3, which acts on the target cell.

Thyroid hormones are transported in the blood in bound and free forms. Most of the TH is transported bound to **thyroxine-binding globulin (TBG)** and to a lesser extent by thyroxine-binding prealbumin. The free form is generally considered to be biologically active, and the bound form serves as a reservoir.

Action of thyroid hormones

TH affects most body tissues by increasing the rate of protein, fat, and glucose metabolism and as a result increases body temperature. Normal linear growth requires TH, as does the central nervous system.

Parathyroid glands

Normally two pairs of small parathyroid glands are present behind the upper and lower poles of the thyroid gland (see Fig. 17-13). Their number may range from two to six.

The parathyroid glands produce **parathyroid hormone (PTH),** a regulator of serum calcium. A decrease in serum ionized calcium stimulates PTH secretion. An increase in serum calcium inhibits PTH secretion. Phosphate, magnesium, and vitamin D levels also affect PTH secretion. An increase in serum phosphate decreases serum calcium and indirectly stimulates PTH secretion. Hypomagnesemia in persons with normal calcium acts as a mild stimulant to PTH secretion; but in persons with hypocalcemia, hypomagnesemia decreases PTH secretion. The overall effect of PTH secretion is to increase serum calcium and decrease serum phosphate.[4] 1,25-Vitamin D promotes calcium and phosphate absorption in the gut, decreases PTH secretion, and promotes bone mineralization. PTH decreases serum phosphate by decreasing renal tubular phosphate reabsorption.

✓ QUICK CHECK

How does the anterior pituitary regulate the thyroid gland?

What form of thyroid hormone is biologically active?

What two organs are the sites of action of parathyroid hormone (PTH)?

HEALTH ALERT
Vitamin D Analogs

The activated form of vitamin D_3 ($1_\alpha25[OH]_2D_3$) has a central role in bone and calcium metabolism as well as inhibiting cell growth. Chemical modifications in the structure of vitamin D_3 have created a new generation of vitamin D analogs with potential therapeutic applications for the treatment of cancer, immune dysfunction, endocrine disorders, and metabolic bone disease. Two analogs have been approved: one for use in the topical treatment of psoriasis (calcipotriene [Dovonex]) and one for secondary hypoparathyroidism in individuals with renal failure (paracalcitol [Zemplar]). Other analogs are being tested for a wide range of clinical disorders.

Data from Brown, A.J. (1998). Vitamin D analogues. American Journal of Kidney Disorders, 32(2, Suppl. 2), S25-S39; Friedrich, M. et al. (1998). Expression of 1,25-dihydroxy vitamin D_3 receptor in breast carcinoma. Journal of Histochemistry and Cytochemistry, 46(11), 1335-1337; Martin, K.J. et al. (1998). Therapy of secondary hyperparathyroidism with 19-nor-1alpha,25-dihydroxvitamin. American Journal of Kidney Disorders, 32(2, Suppl. 2), S61-S66; Verstuyf, A. et al. (1998). Recent developments in the use of vitamin D analogues. Current Opinion in Nephrology and Hypertension, 7(4), 397-403.

Endocrine Pancreas

The **pancreas** is both an endocrine gland that produces hormones and an exocrine gland that produces digestive enzymes. (The exocrine function of the pancreas is discussed in Chapter 34.) The pancreas is located behind the stomach, between the spleen and the duodenum. It houses the **islets of Langerhans.** The islets of Langerhans have three types of hormone-secreting cells: **alpha cells,** which secrete **glucagon; beta cells,** which secrete **insulin; delta cells,** which secrete **gastrin** or **somatostatin;** and **F cells,** which secrete **pancreatic polypeptide.** The alpha and delta cells are located at the periphery of the islet, and beta cells are located in the middle. These hormones regulate much of the carbohydrate, fat, and protein metabolism. (The pancreas is illustrated in Fig. 17-14.) Nerves from both divisions of the autonomic nervous system innervate the pancreatic islets.

Insulin

The beta cells of the pancreas synthesize insulin from the precursor, proinsulin, which is formed from a larger precursor molecule, preproinsulin. Secretion of insulin is regulated by chemical, hormonal, and neural control. Insulin secretion is promoted when blood levels of glucose, amino acids (arginine, lysine), and gastrointestinal hormones (glucagon, gastrin, cholecystokinin, secretin) increase and the beta cells are stimulated parasympathetically. Insulin secretion diminishes in response to low blood levels of glucose (hypoglycemia), high levels of insulin (through negative feedback to the beta cells), and sympathetic stimulation of the alpha cells in the islets. Prostaglandins also may inhibit insulin secretion.

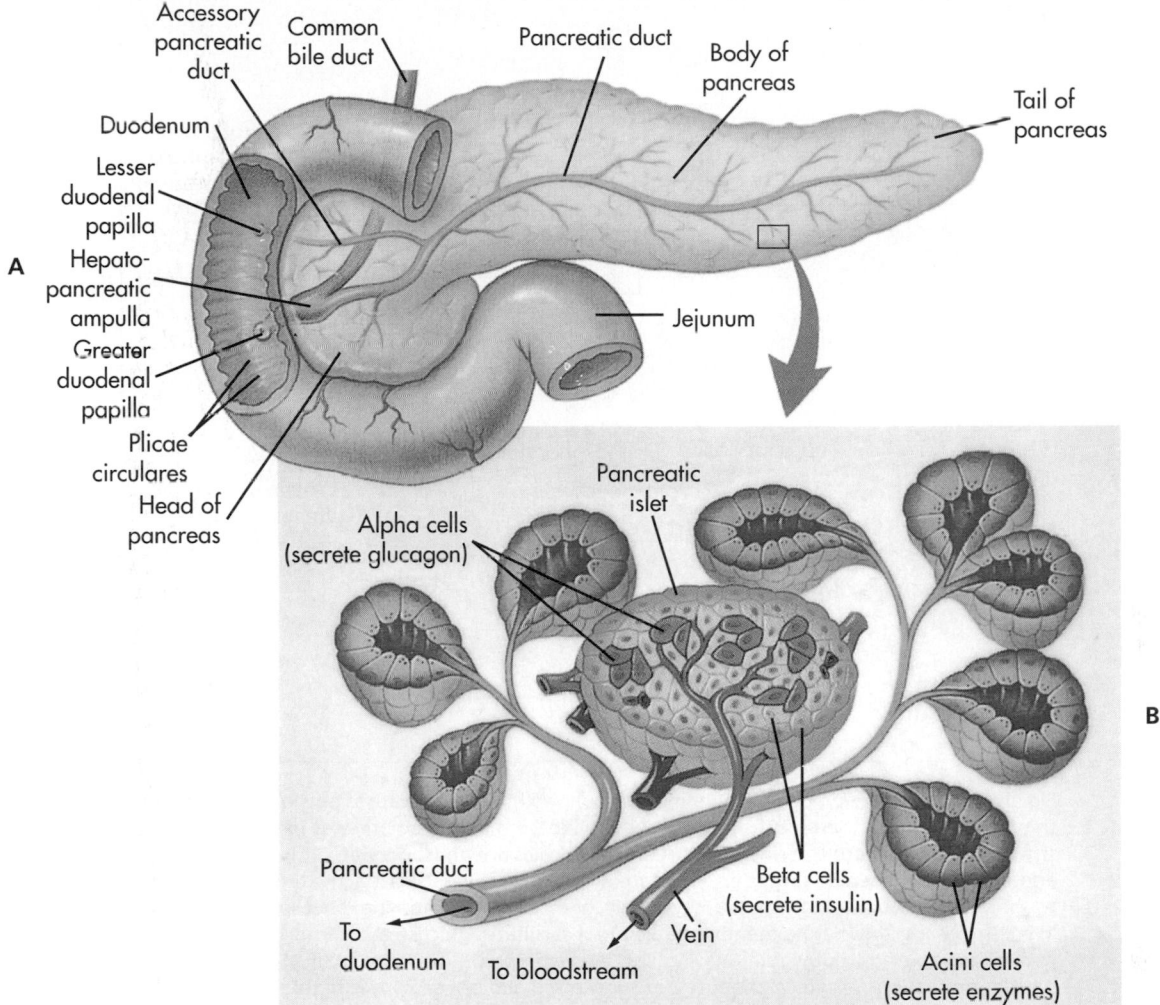

Fig. 17-14 *The pancreas.* A, Pancreas dissected to show main and accessory ducts. The main duct may join the common bile duct, as shown here, to enter the duodenum by a single opening at the major duodenal papilla, or the two ducts may have separate openings. The accessory pancreatic duct is usually present and has a separate opening into the duodenum. **B,** Exocrine glandular cells (around small pancreatic ducts) and endocrine glandular cells of the pancreatic islets (adjacent to blood capillaries). Exocrine pancreatic cells secrete pancreatic juice, alpha endocrine cells secrete glucagon, and beta cells secrete insulin. *(From Thibodeau, G.A. & Patton, K.T. [1999]. Anatomy & physiology [4th ed.]. St. Louis: Mosby.)*

At the target cell, insulin combines with an enzyme-linked plasma membrane receptor, tyrosine kinase. Insulin receptor binding activates tyrosine kinase autophosphorylation and sends a signal to activate glucose transporters and phosphorylate protein kinase.[5] Protein kinase then activates or deactivates target enzymes for glucose metabolism (Fig. 17-15).

Insulin is an anabolic hormone that promotes glucose uptake and the synthesis of proteins, carbohydrates, lipids, and nucleic acids and functions mainly in the liver, muscle, and adipose tissue. The net effect of insulin in these tissues is to stimulate protein and fat synthesis and decrease blood glucose. The brain, red blood cells, kidney, and lens of the eye do not require insulin for glucose transport. Insulin also facilitates the intracellular transport of potassium (K^+),

phosphate, and magnesium. Increased K^+ increases insulin secretion.

Amylin

Amylin is co-secreted with insulin in response to nutrient stimuli. It regulates blood glucose by delaying nutrient uptake and suppressing glucagon secretion after meals.

Glucagon

Glucagon is a catabolic hormone produced by the alpha cells of the pancreas and by cells lining the gastrointestinal tract. Glucagon release is inhibited by high glucose levels and increased by low glucose levels and sympathetic stimulation. Amino acids, such as alanine, glycine, and asparagine, stimulate glucagon secretion.

Fig. 17-15 *Insulin action on cell.* Binding of insulin to its receptor causes autophosphorylation of the receptor, which then itself acts as a tyrosine kinase that phosphorylates insulin receptor substrate (IRS-1). As a result, serine and threonine residues are phosphorylated in other cell proteins and enzymes. Numerous target enzymes are ultimately activated or inactivated, and the result is to shift the metabolism of glucose toward glycogen and pyruvate. The glucose transporter, glut-4, is recruited to the plasma membrane, where it facilitates glucose entry into the cell. The transport of amino acids, potassium, magnesium, and phosphate into the cell is also facilitated. The synthesis of various enzymes is induced or suppressed and cell growth is regulated by signal molecules that modulate gene expression. *mRNAs,* Messenger ribonucleic acids; *DNAs,* deoxyribonucleic acids; *s-s,* disulfide bond; α, alpha unit of insulin receptor; β, beta unit of insulin receptor.

Glucagon acts primarily in the liver and increases blood glucose by stimulating glycogenolysis and gluconeogenesis in muscle and lypolysis in adipose tissue. It is antagonistic to insulin.

Somatostatin

The somatostatin produced by delta cells is essential in carbohydrate, fat, and protein metabolism (homeostasis of ingested nutrients). It is different from hypothalamic somatostatin, which inhibits the release of growth hormone. It is involved in regulating alpha-cell and beta-cell function within the islets by inhibiting secretion of insulin, glucagon, and pancreatic polypeptide.

Pancreatic polypeptide is released by F cells in response to hypoglycemia and protein-rich meals. It inhibits gallbladder contraction and exocrine pancreas secretion.

Adrenal Glands

The *adrenal glands* are paired, pyramid-shaped organs behind the peritoneum and close to the upper pole of each kidney. Each gland is surrounded by a capsule, embedded in fat, and well supplied with blood from the phrenic and renal ar-

teries and the aorta. Venous return on the left is to the renal vein and on the right is to the inferior vena cava.

Each adrenal gland consists of two separate portions—an inner medulla and an outer cortex. These two portions have different embryonic origins, structures, and hormonal functions. In effect, each adrenal gland functions like two separate glands, although there are interrelationships (Fig. 17-16).

The *adrenal cortex,* or outer region of the gland, accounts for 80% of the weight of the adult gland. The cortex is histologically subdivided into the three following zones:

1. The *zona glomerulosa,* the outer layer, which constitutes about 15% of the cortex and primarily produces the mineralocorticoid aldosterone
2. The *zona fasciculata,* the middle layer, which constitutes 78% of the cortex and secretes glucocorticoids: cortisol, cortisone, and corticosterone
3. The *zona reticularis,* the inner layer, which constitutes 7% of the cortex and secretes mineralocorticoids, adrenal androgens and estrogens, and glucocorticoids

The *adrenal medulla,* which accounts for 20% of the gland's total weight, secretes the catecholamines epinephrine

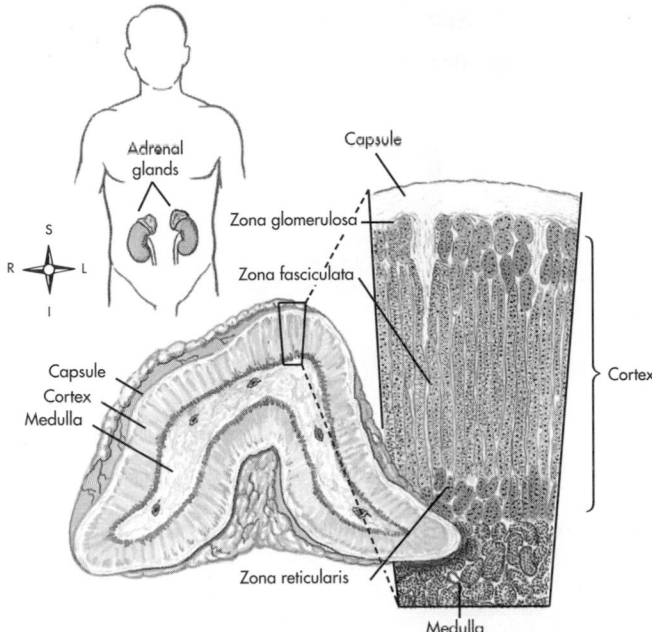

Fig. 17-16 *Structure of the adrenal gland showing cell layers (zonae) of the cortex.* Zona glomerulosa secretes aldosterone. Zona fasciculata secretes abundant amounts of glucocorticoids, chiefly cortisol. Zona reticularis secretes minute amounts of sex hormones and glucocorticoids. *(From Thibodeau, G.A. & Patton, K.T. [1996]. Anatomy & physiology [3rd ed.]. St. Louis: Mosby.)*

(adrenaline), norepinephrine, and dopamine. Both sympathetic and parasympathetic cholinergic fibers innervate the adrenal medulla; the adrenal cortex does not appear to be directly innervated.

Adrenal cortex

The adrenal cortex secretes several steroid hormones, including the glucocorticoids, the mineralocorticoids, and the adrenal androgens and estrogens. These hormones are all synthesized from cholesterol. The cells of the adrenal cortex must be stimulated by **adrenocorticotropic hormone (ACTH)** for cholesterol to be used in steroidogenesis. The best known pathway of steroidogenesis involves the conversion of cholesterol to pregnenolone, which is then converted to the major corticosteroids. The adrenal cortex also contains a high concentration of ascorbic acid and vitamin A.

Glucocorticoids

Functions of the glucocorticoids. The glucocorticoids have metabolic, antiinflammatory, and growth-suppressing effects and influence levels of awareness and sleep patterns.[6] *Glucocorticoids* are steroid hormones that have direct effects on carbohydrate metabolism. They increase blood glucose concentration by promoting gluconeogenesis in the liver and decreasing use of glucose in muscle, adipose tissue, and lymphatic tissue. In extrahepatic tissues the glucocorticoids antagonize insulin and stimulate protein catabolism and inhibit amino acid uptake and protein synthesis. In hepatic tis-

sue, however, glucocorticoids act primarily to stimulate glucose formation and synthesis of enzymes that mediate glucocorticoid effects.

The glucocorticoids act at several sites to inhibit immune and inflammatory reactions (described in Unit 2), such as depressing proliferation of T lymphocytes, including those that produce the antiviral protein interferon; decreasing natural killer cell activity; reversing macrophage activity; decreasing the numbers of eosinophils and fibroblasts; and suppressing the synthesis, secretion, and actions of chemical mediators involved in inflammatory and immune responses. These chemical mediators include interleukins, prostaglandins, leukotrienes, bradykinin, serotonin, and histamine.[7] Glucocorticoids also inhibit bone formation, inhibit ADH secretion, and stimulate gastric acid secretion.

Pathologically high levels of glucocorticoids also increase circulating erythrocytes, leading to polycythemia; increase the appetite; promote fat deposition in the face and cervical areas; increase uric acid excretion; decrease serum calcium levels, possibly by inhibiting gastrointestinal absorption of calcium; suppress the secretion and synthesis of ACTH; and interfere with the action of growth hormone so that somatic growth is inhibited. They also have important "permissive" effects, sensitizing arterioles to the vasoconstrictive effects of norepinephrine.

Glucocorticoids appear to potentiate the effects of catecholamines, thyroid hormone, and growth hormone on adipose tissue. A metabolite of cortisol may act like a barbiturate and depress nerve cell function in the brain, accounting for the noted effects on mood associated with steroid fluctuation in disease or stress.

Cortisol. The most potent naturally occurring glucocorticoid is ***cortisol.*** It is the main secretory product of the adrenal cortex and is needed to maintain life and protect from stress (see Fig. 8-2). Cortisol has a biologic half-life of approximately 90 minutes, with the liver primarily responsible for its deactivation.

Cortisol secretion is regulated primarily by the hypothalamus and the anterior pituitary gland (Fig. 17-17). Corticotropin-releasing hormone (CRH) is produced by several nuclei in the hypothalamus and stored in the median eminence. Once released, CRH travels through the portal vessels to stimulate the production of ACTH, β-lipotropin, γ-lipotropin, endorphins, and enkephalins by the anterior pituitary. ACTH is the main regulator of cortisol secretion and adrenocortical growth.

Three factors appear to be primarily involved in regulating the secretion of ACTH: (1) high circulating levels of cortisol and synthetic glucocorticoids suppress both CRH and ACTH, whereas low cortisol levels stimulate their secretion; (2) diurnal rhythms affect ACTH and cortisol levels (in persons with regular sleep-wake patterns, ACTH peaks 3 to 5 hours after sleep begins and declines throughout the day), and cortisol levels follow a similar pattern; and (3) stress increases ACTH secretion, leading to increased cortisol levels. (Neurologic mechanisms regulating sleep are discussed in Chapter 13.) A form of ACTH (i.e., ir ACTH) is produced by

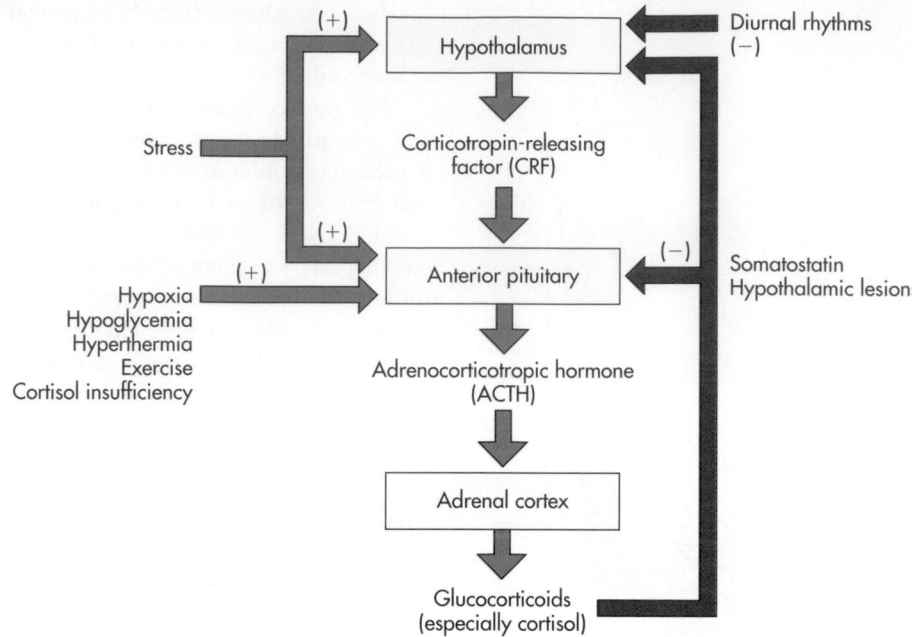

Fig. 17-17 *Feedback control of glucocorticoid synthesis and secretion.*

the cells of the immune system and may account, in part, for integration of the immune and endocrine systems.

Once ACTH is secreted, it binds to specific plasma membrane receptors on the cells of the adrenal cortex and on other extraadrenal tissues. Because both adrenal and extraadrenal tissues have ACTH receptors, a number of effects result from stimulation by ACTH. (These are summarized in Box 17-1.) The most well-known extraadrenal effect is melanocyte stimulation, which causes increased pigmentation.

Once ACTH stimulates the cells of the adrenal cortex, cortisol synthesis and secretion immediately occur. In the healthy person the secretory patterns of ACTH and cortisol are nearly identical. After secretion, most cortisol circulates in bound form attached to albumin but primarily to transcortin. A smaller amount circulates in the free form and diffuses into cells with specific intracellular receptors for cortisol. ACTH is rapidly inactivated in the circulation, and the liver and kidneys remove the deactivated hormone.

Mineralocorticoids: aldosterone

Mineralocorticoid steroids directly affect ion transport by epithelial cells, causing sodium retention and potassium and hydrogen loss. **Aldosterone** is the most potent naturally occurring mineralocorticoid and acts to conserve sodium by increasing the activity of the sodium pump of epithelial cells. (The sodium pump is described in Chapter 1.)

The initial stages of aldosterone synthesis occur in the zona fasciculata and zona reticularis. The final conversion of corticosterone to aldosterone, however, apparently is confined to the zona glomerulosa. Aldosterone synthesis and secretion are regulated primarily by the renin-angiotensin system (described in Chapter 28). Sodium and potassium levels may directly affect aldosterone secretion. ACTH may tran-

Effects of Adrenocorticotropic Hormone   BOX 17-1

ADRENAL
Maintenance of gland size
Depletion of ascorbic acid
Activation of adenylyl cyclase
Conversion of cholesterol to pregnenolone
Maintenance of enzymes active in converting
   pregnenolone to other steroids
Accumulation of cholesterol
Secretion of cortisol and adrenal androgens

EXTRAADRENAL
Melanocyte stimulation
Activation of tissue lipase

siently stimulate aldosterone synthesis but does not appear to be a major regulator of secretion.

Aldosterone secretion is stimulated by angiotensin, which is converted by renin to angiotensin I and then to angiotensins II and III (see Chapter 28), which stimulate aldosterone synthesis. The renin-angiotensin system is activated primarily by sodium and water depletion, increased potassium, and a diminished effective blood volume (Fig. 17-18).[8,9]

When sodium and potassium levels are within normal limits, approximately 50 to 250 mg of aldosterone is secreted daily. Of the secreted aldosterone, 50% to 75% binds to

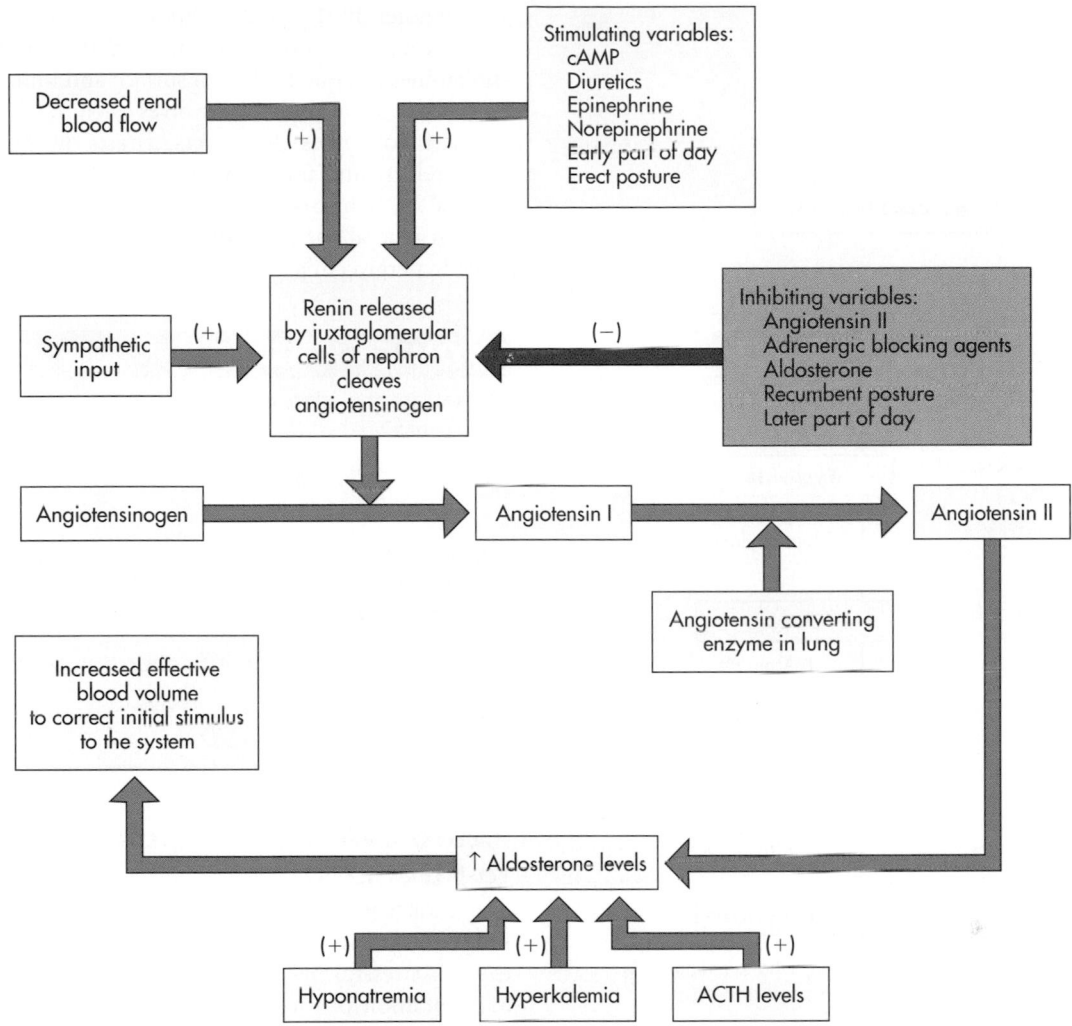

Fig. 17-18 *The feedback mechanisms regulating aldosterone secretion.* *c*AMP, Cyclic adenosine monophosphate; *ACTH*, adrenocorticotropic hormone.

plasma proteins. The large proportion of unbound aldosterone contributes to its rapid metabolic turnover in the liver, its low plasma concentration, and its short half-life (about 15 minutes). Aldosterone is degraded in the liver and is excreted by the kidney.

Aldosterone acts on the distal nephron to increase sodium reabsorption, and it also increases potassium and hydrogen excretion. High levels of aldosterone may result in alkalosis and hypokalemia (see Chapter 4). This renal effect takes 90 minutes to 6 hours. Other effects of aldosterone include enhancement of cardiac muscle contraction and possible stimulation of ectopic ventricular activity, secondary cardiac pacemakers in the ventricles.

Adrenal estrogens and androgens
The healthy adrenal cortex secretes minimal amounts of estrogen and androgens. Some of the weakly androgenic substances secreted by the cortex (dehydroepiandrosterone [DHEA], androstenedione) are converted by peripheral tissues to stronger androgens, such as testosterone, thus accounting for some androgenic effects initiated by the adrenal

cortex. Peripheral conversion of adrenal androgens to estrogens is enhanced in some cases, including aging, obesity, liver disease, and hyperthyroidism.[10] ACTH appears to be the major regulator. The biologic effects and metabolism of the adrenal sex steroids do not vary from those produced by the gonads (see Unit 10).

Adrenal medulla
The adrenal medulla, together with the sympathetic divisions of the autonomic nervous system, is embryonically derived from neural crest cells. Its major products are the catecholamines epinephrine (adrenaline) and norepinephrine (Fig. 17-19), although the medulla is only a minor source of norepinephrine. Epinephrine is 10 times more potent than norepinephrine in exerting metabolic effects.

Adrenal catecholamine secretion is increased by ACTH and the glucocorticoids. The catecholamines apparently directly inhibit their own secretion by decreasing the formation of the tyrosine hydroxylase. Stimuli to adrenal medullary secretion include hypoglycemia, hypoxia, hypercapnia, acidosis, hemorrhage, glucagon, nicotine, pilocarpine, histamine, and angiotensin II. On stimulation of the adrenal medullary cell, cytoplasmic storage granules that contain the catecholamines migrate to the cell surface and undergo exocytosis, a process that probably involves calcium.

Catecholamines have diverse effects on the entire body. Their release and the body's response have been characterized as the fight-or-flight response (see Fig. 8-2 and Table 8-2). In general, the metabolic effects of catecholamines promote hyperglycemia.

Fig. 17-19 *Synthesis of catecholamines.*

Neuroendocrine Response to Stressors

The endocrine system acts together with the nervous and immune systems to respond to stressors. Perception that an event is stressful may be essential to the emotional arousal and initiation of the stress response. Some events, such as bacterial invasion, can activate the stress response without emotional arousal. Details of the stress response are presented in Chapter 8. Methods of hormone measurement are given in Box 17-2.

Methods of Hormone Measurement   BOX 17-2

RADIOIMMUNOASSAY (RIA)
An immunologic technique in which known amounts of antibody and radio-labeled hormone are placed in an assay tube with the unlabeled hormone. The radio-labeled hormone competes chemically with the nonlabeled hormone molecules for binding sites on the antibodies. When increasing amounts of unlabeled hormones are added to the assay, the limited binding sites of the antibody can bind less of the radio-labeled hormone. Therefore the higher the concentration of unlabeled hormone, the fewer the number of radioactive "counts," or labeled hormone, that bind to the fixed concentration of antibody. A quantitative value is established by use of standard reference curves.

ENZYME-LINKED IMMUNOSORBENT ASSAYS (ELISA)
Used to determine circulating hormone levels. The method is similar to that of RIA but is less expensive and easier to conduct. Instead of radio-labeled hormones, an enzyme-labeled hormone is used. The enzyme activity in either the bound or unbound fraction is determined and related to the concentration of the unlabeled hormone.

BIOASSAY
The use of graded doses of hormone in a reference preparation and then comparison of the results with an unknown sample. Bioassays are used more commonly in investigative endocrinology than in clinical laboratories.

▲AGING & *Its Effects on Specific Endocrine Glands*

GENERAL ENDOCRINE CHANGES WITH AGING
Atrophy and weight loss with vascular changes; decreased secretion and clearance of hormones often occurs, variable change in receptor binding and intracellular responses

THYROID
Glandular atrophy, fibrosis, nodularity, and increased inflammatory infiltrates; possible changes in thyroid hormone (TH) difficult to determine because of concurrent disease in elderly persons; may find decreased T₄ secretion and turnover, decline in T₃ (especially in men), diminished thyroid-stimulating hormone (TSH) secretion; reduced response of plasma TSH concentration to thyroid-releasing hormone (TRH) administration (especially in men)

PARATHYROID
Difficult to detect because of decreased calcium intake and circulating vitamin D, as well as blunted response accompanying aging

ADRENAL
Loss of weight in gland with greater proportion of fibrous tissue; decreased metabolic clearance of glucocorticoids and cortisol, thus higher circulating levels of these substances, causing decreased cortisol secretion; dramatic decrease in plasma levels of adrenal androgens and end-products; decreased levels of aldosterone

POSTERIOR PITUITARY
Decrease in size; reduced antidiuretic hormone (ADH) secretion

ANTERIOR PITUITARY
Increased fibrosis and moderate increase in size of gland; decline in growth hormone release

From Timiras, P.S. (1994). Physiological basis of aging and geriatrics (2nd ed.). Boca Raton, Fla.: CRC.

▣ DID YOU UNDERSTAND?

Mechanisms of Hormonal Regulation
1. The endocrine system has diverse functions, including sexual differentiation, growth and development, and continuous maintenance of the body's internal environment.
2. Hormones are chemical messengers synthesized by endocrine glands and released into the circulation.
3. Hormones have specific negative and positive feedback mechanisms. Most hormone levels are regulated by negative feedback, in which hormone secretion raises the level of a specific hormone, ultimately causing secretion to subside.
4. Endocrine feedback is described in terms of short, long, and ultra-short feedback loops.
5. Water-soluble hormones circulate throughout the body in unbound form, whereas lipid-soluble hormones (i.e., steroid and thyroid hormones) circulate throughout the body bound to carrier proteins.
6. Hormones affect only target cells with appropriate receptors and then act on these cells to initiate specific cell functions or activities.
7. Hormones have two general types of effects on cells: (a) direct effects, or obvious changes in cell function, and (b) permissive effects, or less obvious changes that facilitate cell function.
8. Receptors for hormones may be located on the plasma membrane or in the intracellular compartment of a target cell.
9. Water-soluble hormones act as first messengers, binding to receptors on the cell's plasma membrane. The signals initiated by hormone-receptor binding are then transmitted into the cell by the action of second messengers.
10. Lipid-soluble hormones (including steroid and thyroid hormones) may cross the plasma membrane through diffusion. These hormones diffuse directly into the cell nucleus and bind to nuclear receptors.

Structure and Function of the Endocrine Glands
1. The pituitary gland, consisting of anterior and posterior portions, is connected to the central nervous system through the hypothalamus.
2. The hypothalamus regulates anterior pituitary function by secreting releasing hormones and releasing factors into the portal circulation.
3. Hypothalamic hormones include prolactin-inhibiting factor (PIF), which inhibits prolactin secretion; thyrotropin-releasing factor (TRF), which affects release of thyroid hormones; gonadotropin-releasing hormone (GRH), which facilitates release of adrenocorticotropic hormone (ACTH) and endorphins; and substance P, which inhibits ACTH release and stimulates release of a variety of other hormones.
4. The posterior pituitary secretes antidiuretic hormone (ADH), which also is called vasopressin, and oxytocin.
5. ADH controls serum osmolality, increases permeability of the renal tubules to water, and causes vasoconstriction when administered pharmacolog-

Continued

◼ DID YOU UNDERSTAND? —cont'd

Structure and Function of the Endocrine Glands—cont'd

ically in high doses. ADH also may regulate some central nervous system functions.

6. Oxytocin causes uterine contraction and lactation in women and may have a role in sperm motility in men. In both men and women, oxytocin has an antidiuretic effect similar to that of ADH.

7. Hormones of the anterior pituitary are regulated by (a) secretion of hypothalamic-releasing hormones or factors, (b) negative feedback from hormones secreted by target organs, and (c) mediating effects of neurotransmitters.

8. Hormones of the anterior pituitary include ACTH, melanocyte-stimulating hormone (MSH), somatotropic hormones (growth hormone [GH], prolactin), and glycoprotein hormones—follicle-stimulating hormone (FSH), luteinizing hormone (LH), and thyroid-stimulating hormone (TSH).

9. The two-lobed thyroid gland contains follicles, which secrete some of the thyroid hormones, and C cells, which secrete calcitonin and somatostatin.

10. Regulation of thyroid hormone (TH) levels is complex and involves the hypothalamus, anterior pituitary, thyroid gland, and numerous biochemical variables.

11. Thyroid hormone (TH) secretion is regulated by thyroid-releasing hormone through a negative feedback loop that involves the anterior pituitary and hypothalamus.

12. Thyroid-stimulating hormone (TSH), which is synthesized and stored in the anterior pituitary, stimulates secretion of TH by activating intracellular processes, including uptake of iodine necessary for the synthesis of TH.

13. Once secreted, TH acts on the thyroid gland, the anterior pituitary, and the median eminence to regulate further TH production.

14. Synthesis of TH depends on the glycoprotein thyroglobulin, which contains a precursor of TH, tyrosine. Tyrosine then combines with iodine to form precursor molecules of the thyroid hormones thyroxine (T_4) and triiodothyronine (T_3).

15. When released into the circulation, T_3 and T_4 are bound by carrier proteins in the plasma, which store these hormones and provide a buffer for rapid changes in hormone levels. The free form is the active form.

16. Thyroid hormones alter protein synthesis and have a wide range of metabolic effects on proteins, carbohydrates, lipids, and vitamins. TH also affects heat production and cardiac function.

17. The paired parathyroid glands normally are located behind the upper and lower poles of the thyroid. These glands secrete parathyroid hormone (PTH), an important regulator of serum calcium levels.

18. PTH secretion is regulated by levels of ionized calcium in the plasma and by cyclic AMP within the cell.

19. In bone, PTH causes bone breakdown and resorption. In the kidney, PTH increases reabsorption of calcium and decreases reabsorption of phosphorus and bicarbonate.

20. The endocrine pancreas contains the islets of Langerhans, which secrete hormones responsible for much of the carbohydrate metabolism in the body.

21. The islets of Langerhans consist of alpha cells, beta cells, delta cells, and F cells.

22. Alpha cells produce glucagon, which is secreted inversely to blood glucose concentrations.

23. Delta cells secrete somatostatin, which inhibits glucagon and insulin secretion.

24. Beta cells secrete preproinsulin, which is ultimately converted to insulin.

25. F cells secrete pancreatic polypeptide.

26. Insulin is a hormone that regulates blood glucose concentrations and overall body metabolism of fat, protein, and carbohydrates.

27. The paired adrenal glands are situated in the kidneys. Each gland consists of an adrenal medulla, which secretes catecholamines, and an adrenal cortex, which secretes steroid hormones.

28. The steroid hormones secreted by the adrenal cortex are synthesized from cholesterol. These hormones include glucocorticoids, mineralocorticoids, and adrenal androgens and estrogens.

29. Glucocorticoids directly affect carbohydrate metabolism by increasing blood glucose concentration through gluconeogenesis in the liver and by decreasing use of glucose. Glucocorticoids also inhibit immune and inflammatory responses.

30. The most potent naturally occurring glucocorticoid is cortisol, which is necessary for the maintenance of life and for protection from stress. Secretion of cortisol is regulated by the hypothalamus and anterior pituitary.

31. Cortisol secretion is related to secretion of adrenocorticotropic hormone (ACTH), which is stimulated by corticotropin-releasing hormone (CRH). ACTH binds with receptors of the adrenal cortex, which activates intracellular mechanisms (specifically cyclic AMP) and leads to cortisol release.

32. Mineralocorticoids are steroid hormones that directly affect ion transport by epithelial cells, causing sodium retention and potassium and hydrogen loss.

33. Aldosterone is the most potent of the naturally occurring mineralocorticoids. Its primary role is to conserve sodium.

34. Aldosterone secretion is regulated primarily by the renin-angiotensin system and sodium.

35. Aldosterone acts by binding to a site on the cell nucleus and altering protein production within the cell. Its principal site of action is the kidney, where it causes sodium reabsorption and potassium and hydrogen excretion.

36. Androgens and estrogens secreted by the adrenal

▣ DID YOU UNDERSTAND? —cont'd

cortex act in the same way as those secreted by the gonads.

37. The adrenal medulla secretes the catecholamines epinephrine and norepinephrine. Catecholamines are synthesized from the amino acid phenylalanine. Their release is stimulated by sympathetic nervous system stimulation, adrenocorticotropic hormone (ACTH), and glucocorticoids.

38. Catecholamines bind with various target cells and are taken up by neurons or excreted in the urine. They cause a range of metabolic effects characterized as the fight-or-flight response and include hyperglycemia and immune suppression.

39. The endocrine system acts together with the nervous system to respond to stressors.

40. The response to stressors involves (a) activation of the sympathetic division of the autonomic nervous system and (b) activation of the endocrine system.

41. Other hormones that are secreted in response to stress include growth hormone, prolactin, testosterone, antidiuretic hormone (ADH), and insulin.

42. The adrenal glands and the sympathetic neurons that innervate these glands form the sympathoadrenal axis.

KEY TERMS

Adrenal cortex, 462
Adrenal gland, 462
Adrenal medulla, 462
Adrenocorticotropic hormone (ACTH), 463
Aldosterone, 464
Alpha cell, 460
Antidiuretic hormone (ADH), 456
Beta cell, 460
C cell, 458
Calcitonin, 458
Chromophil, 454
Chromophobe, 454
Corticotropin-releasing hormone (CRH), 454
Cortisol, 463
Delta cell, 460
Direct effect, 449
Down regulation, 449
F cell, 460
First messenger, 449
Follicle, 458
Gastrin, 460

Glucagon, 460
Glucocorticoid, 463
Gonadotropin-releasing hormone (GnRH), 454
Growth hormone–releasing factor (GRF), 454
Hormone, 446
Hormone receptor, 449
Infundibular process, 456
Infundibular stem, 456
Insulin, 460
Islet of Langerhans, 460
Isthmus, 458
Median eminence, 456
Mineralocorticoid, 464
Negative feedback, 446
Oxytocin, 457
Pancreas, 460
Pancreatic polypeptide, 460
Parathyroid hormone (PTH), 460
Pars distalis, 453
Pars intermedia, 454
Pars tuberalis, 453

Permissive effect, 449
Pharmacologic effect, 449
Pituitary gland, 453
Positive feedback, 446
Prolactin-inhibiting factor (PIF), 454
Second messenger, 449
Somatostatin, 454, 460
Substance P, 454
Target cell, 449
Thyroglobulin, 460
Thyroid gland, 458
Thyroid hormone (TH), 458
Thyroid-stimulating hormone (TSH), 459
Thyrotropin-releasing hormone (TRH), 454
Thyroxine-binding globulin (TBG), 460
Up regulation, 449
Zona fasciculata, 462
Zona glomerulosa, 462
Zona reticularis, 462

REFERENCES

1. Berne, R.M. & Levy, M.N. (1998). *Physiology* (4th ed.). St. Louis: Mosby.
2. Yamashita, S. (1998). Localization and functions of steroid hormone receptors. *Histology and Histopathology, 13*(1), 255-270.
3. Williams, H.R. & Winson, J.D. (1998). *Williams' textbook of endocrinology* (9th ed.). Philadelphia: Saunders.
4. Jones, G., Strugnell, S.A., & DeLuca, H.F. (1998). Current understanding of the molecular actions of vitamin D. *Physiological Review, 78*(4), 1193-1231.
5. Combettes-Sopuverain, N. & Issad, T. (1998). Molecular basis of insulin action. *Diabetes and Metabolism, 24*(6), 477-489.
6. Steiger, A. et al. (1998). Effects of hormones on sleep. *Hormone Research, 49*(3), 125-130.
7. Wiegers, G.J., & Reul, J.M. (1998). Induction of cytokine receptors by glucocorticoids: Functional and pathological significance. *Trends in Pharmacological Science, 19*(8), 317-321.
8. Bardin, C.W. (1997). *Current therapy in endocrinology and metabolism* (6th ed.). St. Louis: Mosby.
9. Moeller, I. et al. (1998). Bioactive angiotensin peptides. *Journal of Hormones and Hypertension, 12*(5), 289-293.
10. Meikle, W.A., Daynes, R.A., & Araneo, B.A. (1991). Adrenal androgen secretion and biologic effects. *Endocrinology and Metabolism Clinics of North America, 20*(2), 381-400.

CHAPTER

18

Alterations of Hormonal Regulation

Sue E. Huether

Function of the endocrine system involves complex interrelationships and interactions that maintain dynamic steady states and provide growth and reproductive capabilities. Dysfunction was initially described in terms of excessive or insufficient function of the endocrine gland with alterations in hormone levels. These alterations were thought to be caused by either hypersecretion or hyposecretion of the various hormones, leading to abnormal hormone concentrations in the blood. Evidence now shows that dysfunction may result from abnormal receptor function or from altered intracellular response to the hormone-receptor complex.

Check out your CD Companion for chapter-related exercises and answers to the Quick Check questions

MECHANISMS OF HORMONAL ALTERATIONS

Significantly elevated or significantly depressed hormone levels may result from various causes (Fig. 18-1). Feedback systems that recognize the need for a particular hormone may fail to function properly or may respond to inappropriate signals. Dysfunction of an endocrine gland may involve its failure to produce adequate amounts of biologically free or active hormone, or a gland may synthesize or release too much hormone. Once hormones are released into the circulation, they may be degraded at an altered rate or inactivated by antibodies before reaching the target cell. Hormones produced by nonendocrine tissues may cause abnormally elevated hormone levels. This mechanism operates without benefit of the normal feedback system for hormone control, and the ectopic hormone production is said to be autonomous.

Why do target cells fail to respond to hormones? The general types of abnormal target cell responses currently recognized are as follows:

1. *Receptor-associated disorders.* These have been identified primarily in water-soluble hormones, such as insulin. The disorders usually involve a decrease in the number of receptors, leading to decreased or defective hormone-receptor binding; impaired receptor function, resulting in insensitivity to the hormone; presence of antibodies against specific receptors that either reduce available binding sites or mimic hormone action, suppressing or exaggerating target cell response; or unusual expression of receptor function, for example, tumor cells with abnormal receptor activity.

2. *Intracellular disorders.* These involve inadequate synthesis of the second messenger, such as cyclic adenosine monophosphate (cAMP), needed to transduce the hormonal signal into intracellular events. The target cell for water-soluble hormones may have a faulty response to hormone-receptor binding and thus fail to generate the required second messenger, or the cell may respond abnormally to the second messenger if levels of intracellular enzymes or proteins are altered. As a result, the target cell fails to express the usual hormonal effect.

Pathogenic mechanisms affecting target cell response for

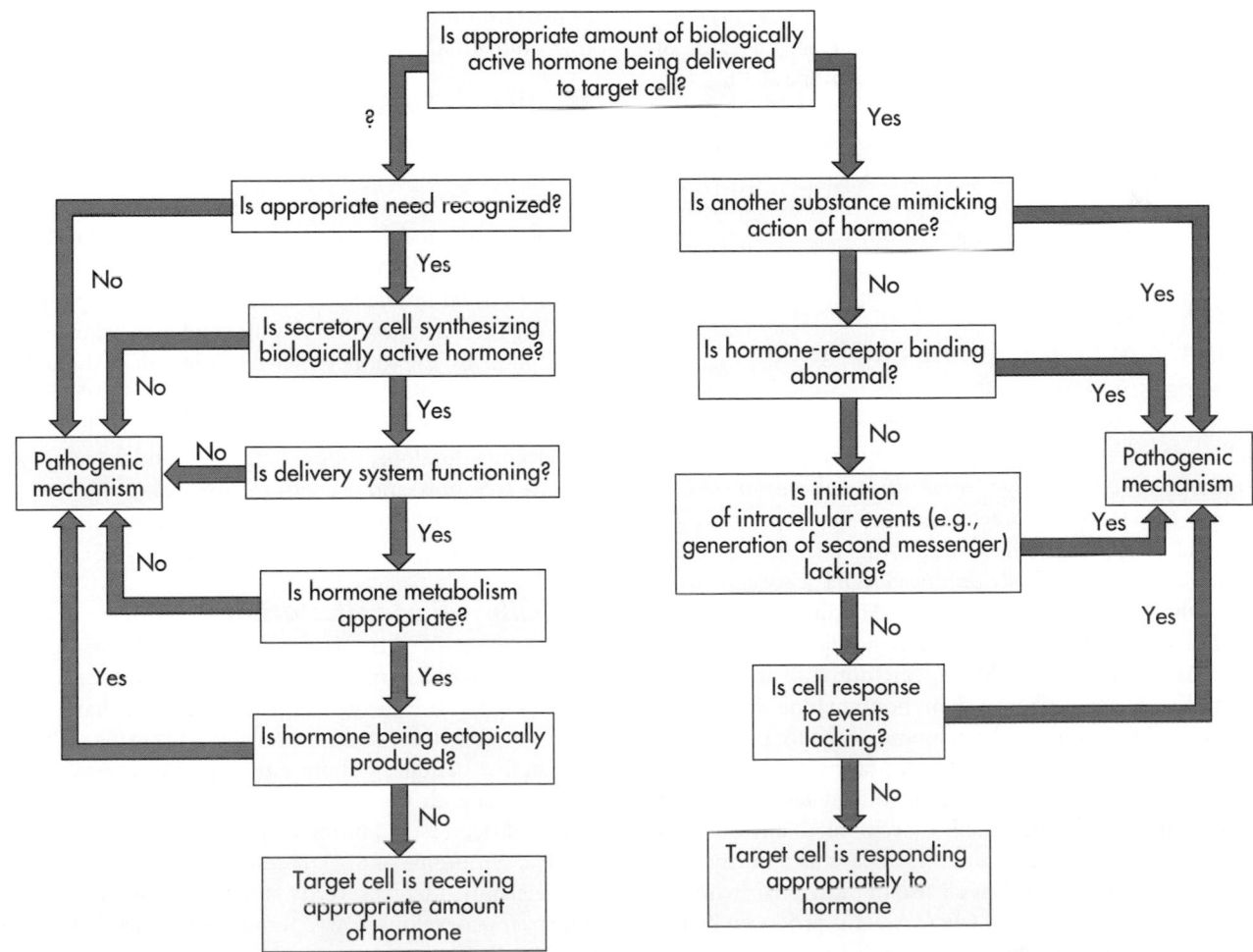

Fig. 18-1 *Hormone delivery to cells.* Phases at which pathogenic mechanisms may develop in delivering appropriate amounts of hormone to the cells.

lipid-soluble hormones either occur less frequently or are recognized less frequently than those affecting water-soluble hormones. The number of intracellular receptors may be decreased, or receptors may have an altered affinity for hormones. The generation of new messenger ribonucleic acid (RNA) may be altered or substrates for new protein synthesis altered, resulting in altered target cell response.

ALTERATIONS OF THE HYPOTHALAMIC-PITUITARY SYSTEM

The most common hypothalamic diseases probably result from interruption in the infundibular stem caused by destructive lesions, rupture after head injury, surgical transection, or stem tumor. Interruption of the physical connections between the hypothalamus and the pituitary causes hypothalamic disease. For example, *diabetes insipidus (antidiuretic hormone insufficiency)* may result, depending on where the infundibular stem is interrupted. The farther away the lesion is from the hypothalamus, the less likely is the occurrence of diabetes insipidus.

Without hypothalamic hormones (Fig. 18-2) women cease to menstruate and men experience impaired spermatogenesis. Adrenocorticotropic hormone (ACTH) response to low serum cortisol levels is decreased because of the absence of corticotropin-releasing hormone (CRH). Hypothalamic hypothyroidism is caused by the absence of thyrotropin-releasing hormone (TRH). Low levels of growth hormone (GH) cause the absence of GH regulatory hormones. Hyperprolactinemia is caused by an absence of usual inhibitory controls of prolactin secretion.

Diseases of the Posterior Pituitary
Syndrome of inappropriate antidiuretic hormone secretion

Diseases of the posterior pituitary are rare and are usually related to abnormal antidiuretic hormone (ADH/ vasopressin) secretion. *Syndrome of inappropriate ADH secretion (SIADH)* is characterized by high levels of ADH without normal physiologic stimuli for its release.[1] The most common cause is ectopically produced ADH, associated with cancer, wherein tumor cells secrete ADH. Tumors associated with SIADH include oat cell adenocarcinoma of the lung (the most common cause of SIADH), carcinoma of the duodenum and pancreas, leukemia, lymphoma, Hodgkin disease, sarcoma, and squamous cell carcinoma of the tongue.

Transient SIADH may follow pituitary surgery, because stored ADH is released in an unregulated fashion. When postoperative fluid volume shifts occur after any surgery, ADH secretion is increased for 5 to 7 days as a normal response to surgery. SIADH is seen also in individuals with infectious pulmonary diseases, where ADH is produced by infected lung tissue[2] or posterior pituitary secretion of ADH is increased in response to a hypoxia-induced decrease in pulmonary perfusion.[3]

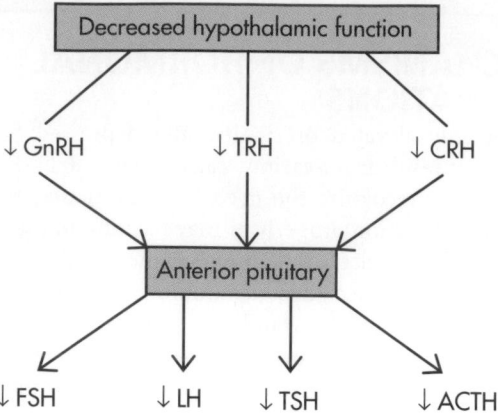

Fig. 18-2 *Loss of hypothalamic hormones.* *GnRH,* Gonadotropin-releasing hormone; *TRH,* thyrotropin-releasing hormone; *CRH,* corticotropin-releasing hormone; *FSH,* follicle-stimulating hormone; *LH,* luteinizing hormone; *TSH,* thyroid-stimulating hormone; *ACTH,* adrenocorticotropic hormone.

Finally, SIADH may be associated with psychiatric disease and various drugs, including hypoglycemic medications (thioridazine), barbiturates, general anesthesia, vincristine, nicotine, morphine, diuretics, synthetic hormones, and selective serotonin reuptake inhibitors (SSRIs). These drugs either simulate ADH release or potentiate circulating ADH.[3]

Pathophysiology

The main features of SIADH are water retention or increases in total body water; solute loss, particularly sodium; and osmotic inactivation of cellular solutes. These features lead to hyponatremia and hypoosmolality. In SIADH, ADH is released continually. Water retention results from the normal action of ADH on the renal tubules and collecting ducts, increasing their permeability to water and increasing water reabsorption by the kidneys. (Renal function is discussed in Chapter 28.)

Extracellular fluid volume expands, and a dilutional hyponatremia develops, suppressing renin and therefore aldosterone secretion, and decreasing proximal tubule reabsorption of sodium. This explains renal sodium loss during hyponatremia.

Clinical Manifestations

A diagnosis of SIADH requires the following signs: (1) serum hypoosmolality and hyponatremia, (2) urine hyperosmolarity (i.e., urine osmolality is greater than expected for the concomitant serum osmolality), (3) urine sodium excretion that matches sodium intake, (4) improvement in hyponatremia with water restriction, and (5) absence of other causes of decreased diluting ability.

The symptoms of SIADH result from hyponatremia and are determined by its severity and sudden onset. Even if hyponatremia develops slowly, serum sodium levels below 110 to 115 mEq/L cause severe and sometimes irreversible neurologic damage. Thirst, impaired taste, anorexia, dyspnea on exertion, fatigue, and dulled sensorium occur when the serum sodium decreases rapidly from 140 to 130 mEq/L. Severe gastrointestinal symptoms, including vomiting and abdominal cramps, occur with a drop in sodium from 130 to 120 mEq/L. With a serum sodium level below 115 mEq/L, confusion, lethargy, muscle twitching, and convulsions may occur. Peripheral edema is absent. Symptoms usually resolve with correction of hyponatremia.

Evaluation and Treatment

Serum electrolyte levels, serum osmolality, urine volume, urine electrolyte levels, and urine osmolality are adequate measures of the presence of SIADH. The treatment of SIADH involves the correction of any underlying causal problems, emergency correction of severe hyponatremia by careful administration of hypertonic saline, and, most important, fluid restriction with careful monitoring. Resolution usually occurs within 3 days, with a 2- to 3-kg weight loss and correction of hyponatremia and salt wasting. Phenytoin may be administered.[4]

Diabetes insipidus

Diabetes insipidus is related to an insufficiency of ADH, leading to hypotonic polyuria and polydipsia. The three forms of diabetes insipidus are as follows[5]:

1. *Neurogenic or central form.* Caused by the absence of ADH; occurs when any organic lesion of the hypothalamus, infundibular stem, or posterior pituitary interferes with ADH synthesis transport or release; lesions include primary brain tumors, hypophysectomy, aneurysms, thrombosis, infections, and immunologic disorders.
2. *Nephrogenic form.* Caused by inadequate response of the renal tubules to ADH, which is usually acquired or may be genetic.[6] Lesions in the collecting tubules are generally related to disorders and drugs that inhibit the generation of cAMP in the tubules, including pyelonephritis, amyloidosis, destructive uropathies, polycystic disease, intrinsic renal disease, lithium carbonate, general anesthetics such as methoxyflurane, and demeclocycline.
3. *Psychogenic form (primary polydipsia).* Caused by extremely large volumes of fluid intake, producing a decreased ADH level.

Pathophysiology

Individuals with diabetes insipidus may have partial to total inability to concentrate urine as a result of chronic polyuria with washout of the medullary concentration gradient (see Chapter 29). Insufficient ADH secretion causes immediate excretion of large volumes of dilute urine, leading to increased plasma osmolality. In conscious individuals, the thirst mechanism is stimulated and induces polydipsia— usually a craving for cold drinks. Some children present with absence of the thirst center and must be encouraged to drink adequate fluid. The urine output varies. With profound ADH deficiency, output may be more than 12 L/day. The urine specific gravity is low. Dehydration develops rapidly without ongoing fluid replacement.

In nephrogenic diabetes insipidus, ADH levels are normal or high but the collecting ducts do not increase their permeability to water in response to ADH. This is related to diseases that irreversibly damage the renal tubules, such as pyelonephritis, polycystic disease, or destructive uropathies. The use of methoxyflurane anesthesia, lithium, or demeclocycline can cause a reversible form of nephrogenic diabetes insipidus.

Diabetes insipidus usually has an acute onset. With neurogenic diabetes insipidus, a classic, three-phase syndrome has been observed related to progressive loss of nerve tissue and with significant diuresis, then antidiuresis, and finally polyuria and polydipsia, reflecting a permanent loss of the ability to secrete adequate amounts of ADH.

Clinical Manifestations

The clinical manifestations of diabetes insipidus include polyuria, nocturia, continuous thirst, polydipsia, low urine specific gravity, low urine osmolality,[7] and high-normal plasma osmolality (300 mOsm/kg H_2O or more). Plasma osmolality is always higher than urine osmolality after 8 hours of water deprivation. Individuals with long-standing diabetes insipidus develop a large bladder capacity and hydronephrosis (see Chapter 29).

Evaluation and Treatment

Water restriction is a useful test because people without diabetes insipidus respond with a rapid decrease in urine volume, whereas persons with diabetes insipidus have no decrease in urine volume or osmolality. Water deprivation tests, or dehydration testing, should be done with careful monitoring because depriving an individual with diabetes insipidus of water can lead to circulatory collapse or hypertonic encephalopathy.

Treatment of neurogenic diabetes insipidus is based on the extent of the ADH deficiency and on age, endocrine and cardiovascular status, and life-style. Some individuals require ADH replacement, but oral hydration often is adequate.

Replacement therapy for symptomatic central or neurogenic diabetes insipidus includes intravascular or, more commonly, intranasal administration of the synthetic vasopressin analog DDAVP (desmopressin). Drugs that potentiate the action of otherwise insufficient amounts of endogenous ADH may be used in individuals with incomplete ADH deficiency.

Diseases of the Anterior Pituitary

Hypopituitarism

Hypopituitarism involves a range of dysfunction from absence of selective pituitary hormones to the complete failure of hormonal functions. Primary hypopituitarism and secondary hypopituitarism are not usually distinguished. Secondary hypopituitarism (resulting from dysfunction of the hypothalamus) is difficult to document because the neurohormonal output of the hypothalamus does not lend itself to measurement.

Pituitary infarction causes hypopituitarism, and infarction may be seen with Sheehan syndrome (postpartum pituitary necrosis), pituitary apoplexy, shock, sickle cell disease, and diabetes mellitus. Other causes of hypopituitarism are head trauma; infections (e.g., meningitis, syphilis, tuberculosis); vascular malformations; surgical ablation related to tumor removal; and, rarely, granulomatous lesions.[8]

Pathophysiology

The pituitary gland is extremely vascular and therefore extremely vulnerable to infarction. The likelihood of infarction is increased when the gland enlarges and becomes more vascular, which occurs during pregnancy. The primary pathologic mechanism in postpartum pituitary infarction is vasospasm of the artery supplying the anterior pituitary. If vasospasm is sustained for more than several hours, tissue necrosis occurs. The pituitary gland may be particularly susceptible because its blood supply, through the portal system, is already partially deoxygenated and, especially in the hyperplastic pituitary of pregnancy, oxygen demands are increased.

Next, edema occurs. The pituitary expands within the fixed confines of the sella turcica, further impeding its blood supply. A second mechanism, which may be involved in Sheehan syndrome (postpartum pituitary infarction), is increased risk for intravascular coagulation. Excessive fibrin is deposited in the pituitary vessels, predisposing to decreased blood supply and infarction.[9]

Clinical Manifestations

The signs and symptoms of hypofunction of the anterior pituitary are highly variable and depend on the affected hormones. In *panhypopituitarism,* when all hormones are absent, the individual suffers from cortisol deficiency, thyroid deficiency, diabetes insipidus, gonadal failure, and loss of secondary sex characteristics. Low GH and somatomedin levels may affect children but generally do not cause symptoms in adults (Fig. 18-3). In addition, postpartum women cannot lactate with decreased or absent prolactin.

ACTH deficiency is a potentially life-threatening disorder, because cortisol is required for functional maintenance. ACTH deficiency usually is encountered with generalized pituitary hypofunction; it rarely occurs as an isolated event. Within 2 weeks of the complete absence of ACTH, symptoms of cortisol insufficiency develop, including nausea, vomiting, anorexia, fatigue, and weakness. The resulting hypoglycemia is caused by increased insulin sensitivity, decreased glycogen reserves, and decreased gluconeogenesis associated with hypocortisolism. In women, adrenal androgen production may cause loss of body hair and decreased libido. ACTH deficiency also limits maximum aldosterone secretion, although the renin-angiotensin system can stimulate some aldosterone secretion. Glomerular filtration rate is decreased, causing decreased urine output. (Renal function is described in Chapter 28.) This may be of some benefit in the individual who has diabetes insipidus, but the polyuria associated with diabetes insipidus worsens after correction of cortisol levels. Frequently, individuals maintain a low

Fig. 18-3 *Hypopituitary dwarfism.* A 4-year-old boy whose height is 25 inches. Girl is also 4 years old and has a normal height of 39 inches. Dwarf has a normal face, as well as head, trunk, and limbs of approximately normal proportions. *(From Brashear, H.R. & Raney, R.B. [1986].* Handbook of orthopaedic surgery *[10th ed.]. St. Louis: Mosby.)*

level of ACTH secretion, so that cortisol replacement is not necessary.

Thyroid-stimulating hormone (TSH) deficiency is rarely seen in isolation but frequently occurs with other pituitary hormone deficiencies. The effects of decreased TSH levels become apparent 4 to 8 weeks after hypothyrotropinemia occurs. Cold intolerance, skin dryness, mild myxedema, lethargy, and decreased metabolic rate occur as with hypothyroidism induced by decreased TSH levels. The symptoms usually are less severe than those of primary hypothyroidism.

The onset of follicle-stimulating hormone (FSH) and luteinizing hormone (LH) deficiencies in women of reproductive age is associated with amenorrhea and an atrophic vagina, uterus, and breasts. In postpubertal males, testicles atrophy and beard growth is stunted. Both men and women experience decreased body hair and diminished libido. FSH and LH deficiencies frequently occur with pressure on the pituitary from other sources, such as tumors. If there is enlargement caused by tumor, symptoms include headache and visual disturbances (blurring and field defects).

Evaluation and Treatment

The diagnostic tests evaluating hypopituitarism must be interpreted together with the individual's signs and symptoms. Radioimmunoassay measures hormone levels, and radiology shows an enlarged sella turcica if a tumor is present. In hypopituitarism, the underlying disorder should be corrected as quickly as possible. Dexamethasone corrects cerebral edema and hypocortisolism. Thyroid and cortisol replacement therapy must be maintained and sex steroid replacement therapy initiated, depending on the individual's needs and desires.

Hyperpituitarism: primary adenoma

Pituitary adenomas usually are benign, slow-growing tumors that arise from cells of the anterior pituitary. Most are microscopic and asymptomatic, found only on postmortem examinations. The cause of pituitary adenomas is not known. The mortality associated with pituitary tumors is usually attributable to alterations in hormone secretion or tissue changes caused by tumor expansion.

Pathophysiology

Local expansion of the adenoma may impinge on the optic chiasma and cause various visual disturbances, depending on the portion of the nerve compressed. If the tumor is malignant, invasion of the oculomotor and trigeminal nerves can occur, with attending symptoms. Extension to the hypothalamus disturbs control of wakefulness, thirst, appetite, and temperature.

The adenomatous tissue secretes the hormone of the cell type from which it arose, without regard to the needs of the body and without benefit of regulatory feedback mechanisms. Because of the pressure exerted by the tumor in the unexpandable skull, those secreting cells that are most sensitive to pressure also may be affected (GH-, FSH-, and LH-secreting cells). The result is hyposecretion of these hormones.

Clinical Manifestations

The clinical manifestations of pituitary adenomas are related to tumor growth and hormone hypersecretion or hyposecretion. Increased tumor size causes headache, fatigue, neck pain or stiffness, and seizures. Visual changes include visual field impairments (frequently beginning in one eye and progressing to the other) and temporary blindness. If the tumor infiltrates other cranial nerves, neuromuscular function is affected.

Hyposecretion of pituitary hormones results in impaired pituitary function. Hyposecretion of GH almost always occurs, but in adults it is clinically asymptomatic. Gonadotropic hyposecretion frequently results in menstrual irregularity in women, decreased libido, and receding secondary sex characteristics in both men and women. If the tumor exerts sufficient pressure, thyroid and adrenal hypofunction may occur, resulting in hypothyroidism and hypocortisolism. Hypersecretion of hormones secreted by the adenoma itself leads to symptoms associated with the particular hormone affected.

Evaluation and Treatment

Diagnosis of pituitary adenoma involves physical and laboratory evaluations, including pertinent hormone assays and radiographic examination of the skull (contrast-enhanced computed tomography [CT]). The goal of treatment is to protect the individual from the effects of tumor growth and to control hormone hypersecretion while minimizing damage to appropriately secreting portions of the pituitary. Surgery and radiation therapy are used also, as appropriate.

> ### ✓ QUICK CHECK
>
> What is the mechanism of receptor-associated hormonal disorder?
>
> Why do individuals with the syndrome of inappropriate antidiuretic hormone (SIADH) secrete concentrated urine?
>
> Why may individuals with a pituitary adenoma develop visual disturbances?

Hypersecretion of growth hormone: acromegaly

Acromegaly is a relatively uncommon disease that occurs in adults exposed to continuously high levels of growth hormone (GH), its target hormone, and insulin-like growth factor 1 (IGF-1). The most common cause of acromegaly is a GH-secreting pituitary adenoma. Acromegaly occurs in adults in their 40s and 50s, although it is often present for years before diagnosis.[10] It is a slowly progressive disease and, if untreated, is associated with a decreased life expectancy. Deaths from acromegaly are apparently caused by hypertension and diabetes mellitus.

Pathophysiology

With a GH-secreting adenoma, the usual GH baseline secretion pattern and sleep-related GH peaks are lost, and a totally unpredictable secretory pattern ensues. With only slight elevations of GH, IGF-1 increases, stimulating growth. In children and adolescents whose epiphyseal plates have not yet closed, the effect of increased GH levels is termed *giantism* (Fig. 18-4). Skeletal growth is excessive, with some individuals becoming 8 or 9 feet tall. In the adult, epiphyseal closure has occurred, and increased amounts of GH and IGF-1 cause connective tissue proliferation and increased cytoplasmic matrix, as well as bony proliferation that results in the characteristic appearance of acromegaly (Fig. 18-5).

GH acts on the renal tubules to increase phosphate reabsorption, leading to mild hyperphosphatemia. The metabolic effects include impaired carbohydrate tolerance and increased metabolic rate. Hyperglycemia results from GH's inhibition of peripheral glucose uptake and increased hepatic glucose production, followed by compensatory hyperinsulinism and, finally, insulin resistance. Diabetes mellitus occurs when the pancreas cannot secrete enough insulin to offset the effects of GH. Coexisting hyperprolactinemia may lead to oligomenorrhea in women and impotence in men.

Fig. 18-4 *Giantism.* A pituitary giant and dwarf contrasted with normal-size men. Excessive secretion of growth hormone by the anterior lobe of the pituitary gland during the early years of life produces giants of this type, whereas deficient secretion of this substance produces well-formed dwarfs. *(From Thibodeau, G.A. & Patton, K.T. [1993]. Anatomy and physiology [2nd ed.]. St. Louis: Mosby.)*

Fig. 18-5 *Acromegaly.* Note large head, forward projection of jaw, and protrusion of frontal bone. *(From Thibodeau, G.A. [1987]. Anatomy and physiology. St. Louis: Mosby.)*

Clinical Manifestations

With connective tissue proliferation, individuals with acromegaly have an enlarged tongue, interstitial edema, enlarged and overactive sebaceous and sweat glands (leading to increased body odor), and coarse skin and body hair. Bony proliferation involves periosteal vertebral growth and enlargement of the bones of the face, hands, and feet (see Fig. 18-5). The lower jaw and forehead also protrude.

Increased IGF-1 levels cause ribs to elongate at the bone-cartilage junction, leading to a barrel-chested appearance and increased proliferation of cartilage in joints. This causes backache, arthralgia, and arthritis, the early manifestations of acromegaly. With bony and soft tissue overgrowth, nerve entrapment occurs, leading to peripheral nerve damage manifested by weakness, muscular atrophy, footdrop, and sensory changes in the hands.

Hypertension and left heart failure are seen in one third to one half of individuals with acromegaly.[11] Because of the space-occupying lesion, central nervous system symptoms of headache, seizure activity, visual disturbances, papilledema, and compression hypopituitarism may occur.[12]

If compression hypopituitarism occurs, gonadotropin secretion may be affected, causing amenorrhea in women and impotence in men. Approximately one third of people with acromegaly have impaired glucose tolerance, and one half of these are diabetic. There is an increased incidence of colon polyps and colon cancer.[13]

Evaluation and Treatment

Diagnosis is confirmed by clinical features of the disease, magnetic resonance imaging (MRI), and elevated levels of GH not suppressed by oral glucose and the presence of IGF-1. The goals of treatment are to normalize or reduce GH secretion, allowing normal pituitary function and relieving or preventing complications related to tumor expansion. The treatment of choice in acromegaly is surgical removal of the GH-secreting adenoma. Radiation therapy may be effective when rapid control of GH levels is not essential, when the individual is not a good surgical candidate, or when hyperfunction persists after subtotal resection. Somatostatin analogs normalize IGF-1 levels.[14]

ALTERATIONS OF THYROID FUNCTION

Thyrotoxicosis

Course of thyrotoxicosis

In *thyrotoxicosis,* thyroid hormones (TH) elicit greater-than-normal responses.[15] Identifying the cause is important in determining treatment and outcome. Hyperthyroidism is a form of thyrotoxicosis in which excess amounts of TH are secreted. Diseases that cause hyperthyroidism include Graves disease, toxic multinodular goiter, thyroid cancer, and increased TSH secretion. Thyrotoxicosis not associated with hyperthyroidism includes subacute thyroiditis, ectopic thyroid tissue, and ingestion of excessive TH. Each condition is associated with a specific pathophysiology and manifestations, and the most commonly occurring ones are described in the following pages. All forms of thyrotoxicosis share some common characteristics.

Clinical Manifestations

The metabolic effects of increased circulating levels of thyroid hormones cause clinical symptoms. The metabolic rate increases with heat intolerance and increased tissue sensitivity to sympathetic stimulation. The major manifestations are summarized in Table 18-1. Minimal or atypical symptoms are common in the elderly population.[16]

Evaluation and Treatment

Elevated serum thyroxine (T_4) and triiodothyronine (T_3) and decreased serum TSH are common in hyperthyroid states. Radioactive iodine is used to test for increased uptake in hyperthyroidism.[17] Treatment is directed at controlling excessive TH production, secretion, or action and employs drug therapy, radioactive iodine therapy, and surgery.

Hyperthyroid conditions

Graves disease

Graves disease is the most common cause of thyrotoxicosis and is the result of stimulation of the thyroid with antibodies against the TSH receptor. The antibodies stimulate the thyroid cells to produce high concentrations of triiodo-L-thyronine (T_3) and L-thyroxine (T_4). The combined action of the antibodies and increased serum levels of TH produce the symptoms of Graves disease: diffuse thyroid enlargement (goiter), ophthalmopathy, dermopathy (pretibial myxedema), and effects on the extremities in various combinations. The incidence is less than 1% in the U.S. population and is more common in women.[18]

The many signs and symptoms of Graves disease can be divided into three components: (1) adrenergic stimulation (tachycardia, palpitations, nervousness, depression, tremor, lid lag, increased systolic blood pressure, increased cardiac contractility); (2) excess thyroid hormone (increased oxygen consumption, metabolic changes in protein metabolism); and (3) immunologic stimulation of diffuse goiter (see Table 18-1).

Two categories of ocular manifestations are associated with Graves disease (Fig. 18-6): (1) functional abnormalities resulting from hyperactivity of the sympathetic division of the autonomic nervous system (lag of the globe on upward gaze and of the upper lid on downward gaze) and (2) infiltrative changes involving the orbital contents with enlargement of the ocular muscles (edema of orbital contents, globe protrusion, paralysis of extraocular muscles, and damage to retina and optic nerve, leading to blindness). These changes result in exophthalmos, periorbital edema, and extraocular muscle weakness leading to diplopia. The individual may experience irritation, pain, lacrimation, photophobia, blurred vision, decreased visual acuity, papilledema, visual field impairment, exposure keratosis, and corneal ulceration. Unfortunately, current treatment for Graves disease does not reverse the ocular changes and is palliative.

Fig. 18-6 *Graves disease.* Note large and protruding eyeballs. *(From Thibodeau, G.A. [1987]. Anatomy and physiology. St. Louis: Mosby.)*

TABLE 18-1	Systemic Effects of Hyperthyroidism	
System	**Manifestations**	**Mechanisms**
Endocrine	Enlarged thyroid gland (97%-99% of cases); systolic or continuous bruit over thyroid; increased cortisol degradation; hypercalcemia and decreased PTH secretion; diminished sensitivity to exogenous insulin	Hyperactivity of the thyroid gland; excess bone resorption leading to hypercalcemia and a disruption of PTH-regulating mechanisms; increased insulin degradation
Reproductive	Oligomenorrhea or amenorrhea in women, impotence and decreased libido in men; increased serum estradiol and estrone but lower than normal levels of free estradiol and estrone	Menstrual cycle alterations that may be related to hypothalamic or pituitary disturbances; increase in sex hormone–binding globulin
Gastrointestinal	Weight loss and an associated increase in appetite; increased peristalsis leading to less formed and more frequent stools; nausea, vomiting, anorexia, abdominal pain; increased use of hepatic glycogen stores and of adipose and protein stores; decrease in serum lipid levels (including triglycerides, phospholipids, cholesterol); changes in vitamin metabolism leading to decrease in tissue stores of vitamins	Increased catabolism leading to the body's inability to meet its metabolic needs; malabsorption; increase in cholesterol excretion in feces and cholesterol conversion to bile salts; impaired conversion of B vitamins to their coenzymes, causing increased need for water-soluble and fat-soluble vitamins
Integumentary	Excessive sweating, flushing, and warm skin; heat intolerance; hair fine, soft, and straight; temporary hair loss; nails that grow away from nail beds, palmar erythema	Hyperdynamic circulatory state
Sensory (eyes)	Ocular manifestations, including elevated upper eyelid leading to decreased blinking and a staring quality; fine tremor of lid; infiltrative ocular changes associated with Graves disease	Overactivity of Müller muscle
Cardiovascular	Increased cardiac output and decreased peripheral resistance; tachycardia at rest; loud heart sounds; supraventricular dysrhythmias	Hypermetabolism and need to dissipate heat
Nervous	Restlessness; short attention span; compulsive movement; fatigue; tremor; insomnia; emotionally labile	Not clearly defined: alterations in cerebral metabolism resulting from excess thyroid hormone
Pulmonary	Dyspnea; reduced vital capacity	Weakness of respiratory muscles

PTH, *Parathyroid hormone.*

Diffuse toxic goiter

The thyroid gland normally enlarges in response to the increased demand for TH that occurs in puberty, pregnancy, iodine deficiency, and immunologic, viral, or genetic disorders. When the condition requiring increased TH resolves, TSH secretion normally subsides and the thyroid gland returns to its original size.

Irreversible changes may occur in some follicular cells, however, so that they now function autonomously. Hyperthyroidism may or may not result from these irreversible changes. Autonomously functioning cells may produce less TH than the body requires. The remainder of the gland then functions to supply the remainder of the body's need, and a euthyroid state is achieved and maintained. If the autonomously functioning cells produce sufficient or excessive TH for the usual body requirement, the remainder of the gland undergoes involution, becoming normal but inactive

tissue. This condition may result in euthyroidism or hyperthyroidism, depending on the amount of TH produced.

Hyperthyroidism can lead to a hypermetabolic state known as thyrotoxicosis or thyrotoxic state. Symptoms usually develop slowly and consist of rapid heart action; tremors; elevated basal metabolic rate; enlarged, multinodular goiter; weight loss; and exophthalmos.

Thyrotoxic crisis

Thyrotoxic crisis (thyroid storm) is a rare but dangerous worsening of the thyrotoxic state, in which death occurs within 48 hours without treatment. The condition may develop spontaneously, but it usually occurs in individuals who have undiagnosed or partially treated Graves disease and are subjected to excessive stress, such as infection, pulmonary or cardiovascular disorders, emotional distress, physical stress, dialysis, plasmapheresis, or inadequate preparation for thyroid surgery.

The systemic symptoms of thyrotoxic crisis include hyperthermia; tachycardia, especially atrial tachydysrhythmias; high-output heart failure; agitation or delirium; and nausea, vomiting, or diarrhea contributing to fluid volume depletion. The symptoms may be attributed to increased β-adrenergic receptors and catecholamines.[19] The treatment is designed (1) to reduce both circulating TH levels by inducing a block of TH synthesis (i.e., propylthiouracil) and thereby reducing their effects to eliminate the precipitating disorder and (2) to provide symptomatic and supportive care.

Hypothyroidism

Deficient production of TH by the thyroid gland results in the clinical state termed *hypothyroidism.* It may be primary or secondary. Primary causes include (1) congenital defects or loss of thyroid tissue after treatment for hyperthyroidism and (2) defective hormone synthesis resulting from autoimmune thyroiditis, endemic iodine deficiency, or antithyroid drugs. Causes of secondary hypothyroidism include (1) insufficient stimulation of the normal gland, causing TSH deficiency from the pituitary or hypothalamus, and (2) peripheral resistance to TH.[20] Hypothyroidism is the most common disorder of thyroid function and occurs more commonly in women.[21]

Fig. 18-7 *Myxedema.* Note edema around eyes and facial puffiness. *(From Thibodeau, G.A. [1987]. Anatomy and physiology. St. Louis: Mosby.)*

HEALTH ALERT

Subclinical Hypothyroidism

Subclinical hypothyroidism (isolated suppression of TSH with normal thyroxine levels) is a condition that occurs in about 5% to 10% of elderly people, particularly women. The causes of subclinical hypothyroidism are similar to those in the general population. Risk factors associated with the condition include cardiovascular effects, hyperlipidemia, and neurologic or emotional effects. Decisions regarding treatment require careful assessment of risks in each individual.

Data from Jackson, I.M. (1998). The thyroid axis and depression. Thyroid, 8(10), 951-956; Mariotti, S. et al. (1998). Thyroid autoimmunity and aging. Experiments in Gerontology, 33(6), 535-541; Samuels, M.H. (1998). Subclinical thyroid disease in the elderly. Thyroid, 8(9), 801-813.

Pathophysiology

In primary hypothyroidism, diminished thyroid tissue leads to decreased production of TH, increased secretion of TSH, and goiter. Secondary hypothyroidism is usually caused by the pituitary's failure to synthesize adequate amounts of TSH. Postpartum pituitary necrosis and a pituitary tumor are the most common causes of secondary hypothyroidism.

Clinical Manifestations

Hypothyroidism generally affects all body systems and occurs insidiously over months or years. The decrease in TH lowers energy metabolism and heat production. The individual develops a low basal metabolic rate, cold intolerance, lethargy, tiredness, and slightly lowered basal body temperature (Table 18-2). The decrease in TH can lead to excessive TSH production and goiter.

The characteristic sign of severe or long-standing hypothyroidism is *myxedema,* which results from the altered composition of the dermis and other tissues. The connective fibers are separated by large amounts of protein and mucopolysaccharide. This complex binds water, producing nonpitting, boggy edema, especially around the eyes, hands, and feet and in the supraclavicular fossae (Fig. 18-7). The tongue and laryngeal and pharyngeal mucous membranes thicken, producing thick, slurred speech and hoarseness.

Evaluation and Treatment

In addition to the clinical symptoms of hypothyroidism,[22] a decrease in serum T_4 and free T_4 is nearly always present. TSH concentration increases from loss of negative feedback from TH. When hypothyroidism is caused by pituitary deficiencies, serum TSH levels and basal metabolic rate (BMR) are decreased. Hormone replacement therapy is the treatment of choice. The restoration of normal TH levels should be timed appropriately; a regimen of hormonal therapy depends on the individual's age, the duration and severity of the hypothyroidism, and the presence of other disorders, particularly cardiovascular disorders.

Hypothyroid conditions

Hypothyroidism results from three relatively rare disorders: acute thyroiditis, subacute thyroiditis, and autoimmune thyroiditis. *Acute thyroiditis* is caused by a bacterial infection of the thyroid gland and is rare. *Subacute thyroiditis* is a non-

TABLE 18-2 Systemic Manifestations of Hypothyroidism

System	Manifestations	Mechanisms
Neurologic	Confusion, syncope, slowed speech and thinking, memory loss; lethargy, headaches, hearing loss, night blindness; slow, clumsy movements; cerebellar ataxia; slow alpha wave activity and loss of amplitude in EEG; decreased tendon reflexes	Decreased cerebral blood flow leading to cerebral hypoxia; reduced intracellular processes caused by decreased beta-adrenergic activity that may be related to a decrease in the number of β-adrenergic receptor sites
Endocrine	Increased TSH production in primary hypothyroidism; enlarged pituitary thyrotropes, increased serum prolactin levels with galactorrhea; decreased rate of cortisol turnover but with normal serum cortisol levels	Impaired TH synthesis or defects in iodide trapping leading to compensatory TSH production; chronic overstimulation of thyrotropes by TRH and by TSH synthesis; stimulation of lactotropes by TRH related to increased prolactin levels; decreased deactivation of cortisol
Reproductive	Anovulation, decreased libido, and a high incidence of spontaneous abortion in women; impotence, decreased libido, and oligospermia in men	Altered metabolism of estrogens and androgens; decreased sex hormone–binding globulin, decreased androgen secretion in men, increased estriol formation in women; low total hormone values but with increased amounts of unbound hormone
Hematologic	Decrease in red cell mass leading to normocytic, normochromic anemia; macrocytic anemia associated with vitamin B_{12} deficiency and inadequate folate or iron absorption in the GI tract	Decreased basal metabolic rate and reduced oxygen requirements, decreased production of erythropoietin, possible relationship between TH and optimal hematologic response to vitamin B_{12}
Cardiovascular	Reduction in stroke volume and heart rate causing lowered cardiac output; increased peripheral vascular resistance to maintain systolic blood pressure; normal response to exercise but with alterations in circulatory system at rest (prolonged circulation time and decreased blood flow to tissues); cool skin and cold tolerance; enlarged heart; decreased intensity of heart sounds and variety of ECG changes (sinus bradycardia, prolonged PR interval, depressed P waves, flattened or inverted T waves, and low-amplitude QRS complexes); cardiac tamponade (although rare)	Decreased metabolic demands and loss of regulatory and rate-setting effects of TH; protein-mucopolysaccharide-rich fluid in the pericardial sac associated with enlarged heart; pericardial effusions associated with heart sounds and ECG changes
Pulmonary	Dyspnea; hypoventilation and carbon dioxide retention, which contribute to myxedema coma; hoarseness	Myxedematous changes in respiratory muscles; pleural effusions associated with dyspnea, although effusions may be asymptomatic
Renal	Decreased renal excretion of water; increased total body water and dilutional hyponatremia; reduced production of erythropoietin	Reduced renal blood flow and glomerular filtration rate; hemodynamic alterations associated with reduced blood flow and filtration; increased total body water related to decreased excretion and mucinous deposits in tissue
Gastrointestinal	Decreased appetite; constipation, weight gain, and fluid retention; decreased absorption of most nutrients; decreased protein metabolism leading to retarded skeletal and soft-tissue growth and slightly positive nitrogen balance; edema; decreased glucose absorption and delayed glucose uptake; increased sensitivity to exogenous insulin; elevated serum lipid values	Reduced intake and reduced peristaltic activity that may progress to fecal impaction; water absorption related to prolonged transit time; fluid retention associated with myxedematous changes; edema associated with high concentrations of exchangeable albumin in the extravascular space caused by increased capillary permeability to proteins; depressed insulin degradation; depressed lipid synthesis and degradation

EEG, *Electroencephalogram;* TSH, *thyroid-stimulating hormone;* TH, *thyroid hormone;* TRH, *thyroid-releasing hormone;* GI, *gastrointestinal;* ECG, *electrocardiogram.*

TABLE 18-2	Systemic Manifestations of Hypothyroidism—cont'd	
System	**Manifestations**	**Mechanisms**
Musculoskeletal	Muscle aching and stiffness; slow movement and slow tendon jerk reflexes; decreased bone formation and resorption, increased bone density; aching and stiffness in joints	Decreased rate of muscle contraction and relaxation contributing to slow movement and reflexes
Integumentary	Coarse, dry, flaky skin; dry, brittle head and body hair; reduced growth of nails and hair; slow wound healing	Reduced sweat and sebaceous gland secretion
	Myxedema	Accumulation of hyaluronic acid, which binds water and causes a puffy appearance
	Cool skin	Decreased circulation to skin

bacterial inflammation of the thyroid often preceded by a viral infection. Both conditions are accompanied by fever, tenderness, and enlargement of the thyroid gland. Symptoms may last for 2 to 4 months, and corticosteroids usually resolve symptoms. *Autoimmune thyroiditis (Hashimoto disease, chronic lymphocytic thyroiditis)* results in destruction of thyroid tissue by circulating thyroid antibodies and infiltration of lymphocytes. Autoimmune thyroiditis also may be caused by an inherited immune defect. Goiter formation is common.

Myxedema coma

A medical emergency, **myxedema coma** is a diminished level of consciousness associated with severe hypothyroidism. Symptoms include hypothermia without shivering, hypoventilation, hypotension, hypoglycemia, and lactic acidosis. Older patients with severe vascular disease and with moderate or untreated hypothyroidism are particularly at risk. The overuse of narcotics or sedatives or an acute illness in hypothyroid individuals can also be causative.

Congenital hypothyroidism

Hypothyroidism in infants occurs when thyroid tissue is absent (thyroid dysgenesis) and with hereditary defects in TH synthesis. Thyroid dysgenesis occurs more frequently in female infants, with permanent abnormalities in 1 of every 4000 live births.[23]

Because TH is essential for embryonic growth, particularly of brain tissue, the infant will be mentally retarded if there is no thyroxine during fetal life. This can be partially reversed if thyroxine is given immediately after birth.

Hypothyroidism at birth involves high birth weight, hypothermia, delay in passing meconium, and neonatal jaundice. Cord blood can be examined in the first days of life for thyroxine and TSH levels. Frequent monitoring of TSH and thyroxine is essential to guide treatment.[24] Treatment is administration of thyroxine.

Without early screening, hypothyroidism may not be evident until after 4 months of age. Symptoms include difficulty eating, hoarse cry, and protruding tongue caused by myxedema of oral tissues and vocal cords; hypotonic muscles of the abdomen with constipation, abdominal protru-

sion, and umbilical hernia; subnormal temperature; lethargy; excessive sleeping; slow pulse; and cold, mottled skin. Skeletal growth is stunted because of impaired protein synthesis, poor absorption of nutrients, and lack of bone mineralization. The child will be dwarfed, with short limbs, if not treated (cretinism) (Fig. 18-8). Dentition is often delayed. Mental retardation varies with the severity of hypothyroidism and the length of delay before treatment is initiated.

Fig.18-8 *An adult cretin.* Note the characteristic facial features, dwarfism (44 inches), absent axillary and scant pubic hair, poorly developed breasts, potbelly, and small umbilical hernia. *(From Schneeberg, N.G. [1970]. Essentials of clinical endocrinology. St. Louis: Mosby.)*

Thyroid carcinoma

Thyroid carcinoma is the most common endocrine malignancy but is relatively rare, with only 13,900 new cases annually and approximately 0.5% of all cancer deaths per year.[25] Iodine deficiency, long-term use of goitrogenic drugs, exposure to ionizing radiation, or a combination of these factors produces thyroid hyperplasia and ultimately malignancy in animals. In about 10% of cases, hyperplasia of the thyroid gland leads to thyroid carcinoma. Exposure to ionizing radiation, especially during childhood, is the most consistent causal factor.

Most individuals with thyroid carcinoma have normal T_3 and T_4 levels and are therefore euthyroid. The cancer is typically discovered as a small thyroid nodule or metastatic tumor in the lungs, brain, or bone. Changes in voice and swallowing and difficulty breathing are related to tumor growth impinging on the trachea or esophagus. Children treated with ionizing radiation for Hodgkin disease have a higher incidence of thyroid cancer in later life.

Diagnosing a thyroid cancer involves (1) measurement of serum thyroid levels, (2) radioisotope scanning, (3) ultrasonography, or (4) needle biopsy. Treatment may include partial or total thyroidectomy, TSH suppression therapy (levothyroxine), radioactive iodine therapy (in iodine-concentrating tumors), postoperative radiation therapy, and chemotherapy (especially in anaplastic carcinoma).[26]

✓ QUICK CHECK

What is thyrotoxicosis?

List three manifestations of Graves disease.

What is myxedema?

ALTERATIONS OF PARATHYROID FUNCTION

Hyperparathyroidism

Hyperparathyroidism is characterized by greater-than-normal secretion of parathyroid hormone (PTH). Hyperparathyroidism is classified as primary, secondary, or tertiary.

 Pathophysiology

Estimates suggest that *primary hyperparathyroidism* occurs in 0.2% to 0.3% of the adult population, with twice as many cases in women. It is generally found in older adults.[27] Because postmenopausal women are at risk for developing osteoporosis, the effects of increased levels of PTH on bone disease can be significant. Most cases of hyperparathyroidism (approximately 80%) result from chief cell adenoma with an increased secretion of PTH.

In primary hyperparathyroidism (Conn disease, primary aldosteronism), PTH secretion is increased and is not under the usual feedback control mechanisms. Gastrointestinal absorption of calcium increases with increased extracellular calcium and reflects the kidney's increased generation of biologically active vitamin D in response to increased PTH levels.[28]

Secondary hyperparathyroidism is a compensatory, although not inevitable, response of the parathyroid glands to chronic hypocalcemia, which can be associated with decreased renal activation of vitamin D (renal failure) (see Chapters 4 and 29). In secondary hyperparathyroidism, secretion of PTH is elevated but PTH cannot achieve normal calcium levels because of kidney failure.

Hyperplasia of the parathyroid glands and loss of sensitivity to circulating calcium levels can cause autonomous secretion of PTH, even with normal calcium levels. This condition is termed *tertiary hyperparathyroidism.* It frequently occurs in individuals with chronic renal failure. Signs and symptoms are similar to those of primary hyperparathyroidism.

Clinical Manifestations

PTH hypersecretion causes hypercalcemia and may be asymptomatic or present with excessive osteoclastic and osteocytic activity, resulting in bone resorption.[29] (Bone resorption is discussed in Chapter 37.) Pathologic changes include pathologic fractures, kyphosis of the dorsal spine, and compression fractures of the vertebral bodies. The increased renal filtration load of calcium leads to hypercalciuria.

Hypercalcemia also affects proximal renal tubular function, causing metabolic acidosis and production of an abnormally alkaline urine. Because calcium and phosphate levels are inversely related, hypercalcemia results in hypophosphatemia (see Chapter 4). Hyperparathyroidism directly results in hyperphosphaturia. The combination of these three variables—hypercalciuria, alkaline urine, and hyperphosphaturia—predisposes the individual to the formation of calcium stones, particularly in the renal pelvis or renal collecting ducts. These may be associated with infections. Both kidney stones and renal infection can lead to impaired renal function. Hypercalcemia also impairs the concentrating ability of the renal tubule by decreasing its response to ADH.

Chronic hypercalcemia of hyperparathyroidism is associated with insulin resistance, necessitating increased insulin secretion to maintain normal glucose levels. Hypercalcemia also affects the muscular, nervous, and gastrointestinal systems, causing fatigue, headache, depression, anorexia, and nausea and vomiting.[30]

Evaluation and Treatment

Hyperparathyroidism is generally diagnosed by excluding all other possible causes of hypercalcemia. A definitive diagnosis must be supported by at least a 6-month history of symptoms associated with hypercalcemia, including kidney stones, hypophosphatemia, hyperchloremia, and increased urinary calcium levels. Tests to document hyperparathyroidism include measurement of serum calcium, phosphorus, magnesium, bicarbonate, chloride, and pH (urinary pH, calcium, hydroxyproline); bone x-ray films and densitometry; catheterization of the thyroid veins to document the source of PTH secretion; and radioimmunoassays.

Treatment involves lowering severely elevated calcium levels, increasing urinary calcium excretion with diuretics, and long-term management of hypercalcemia using drugs that decrease resorption of calcium from bone. Definitive treatment involves the surgical removal of the hyperplastic parathyroid glands.

Hypoparathyroidism

Hypoparathyroidism (abnormally low PTH levels) is most commonly caused by damage to the parathyroid glands during thyroid surgery. A lack of circulating PTH causes depressed serum calcium levels and increased serum phosphate levels. In the absence of PTH, resorption of calcium from bone and regulation of calcium reabsorption from the renal tubules are impaired. Phosphate reabsorption by the renal tubules is therefore increased, causing hyperphosphatemia.

Hypoparathyroidism may also result from hypomagnesemia. Once serum magnesium levels return to normal, PTH secretion does likewise. Hypomagnesemia may be related to chronic alcoholism, malnutrition, malabsorption, increased renal clearance of magnesium caused by the use of aminoglycoside antibiotics or certain chemotherapeutic agents, or prolonged magnesium-deficient parenteral nutritional therapy.

Clinical Manifestations

Symptoms associated with hypoparathyroidism are primarily those of hypocalcemia. Hypocalcemia causes a lowered threshold for nerve and muscle excitation so that a nerve impulse may be initiated by a slight stimulus anywhere along the length of a nerve or muscle fiber. This creates muscle spasms, hyperreflexia, clonic-tonic convulsions, laryngeal spasms, and, in severe cases, death by asphyxiation. Other symptoms of hypocalcemia include dry skin, loss of body and scalp hair, hypoplasia of developing teeth, horizontal ridges on the nails, cataracts, basal ganglia calcifications (which may be associated with a parkinsonian syndrome), and bone deformities, including brachydactyly and bowing of the long bones.

Phosphate retention caused by increased renal reabsorption of phosphate is also associated with hypoparathyroidism. Hyperphosphatemia results from inhibition of the renal enzyme necessary for the conversion of vitamin D to its most active form. This depresses serum calcium levels further by reducing gastrointestinal absorption of calcium.

Evaluation and Treatment

A low serum calcium and high phosphorus level in the absence of renal failure, intestinal disorders, or nutritional deficiencies is diagnostic of hypoparathyroidism. PTH levels are usually normal in primary hypoparathyroidism. Daily doses of PTH can normalize serum and urine calcium levels.[31]

Treatment is directed toward alleviation of the hypocalcemia. In acute states, this involves parenteral administration of calcium, which corrects serum calcium within min-

utes. Maintenance of serum calcium is achieved with pharmacologic doses of an active form of vitamin D and oral calcium. Hypoplastic dentition, cataracts, bone deformities, and basal ganglia calcifications do not respond to the correction of hypocalcemia, but the other symptoms of hypocalcemia are reversible.

✓ **QUICK CHECK**

How does excessive parathyroid hormone (PTH) affect bones?

What are the results of a lack of circulating PTH?

DYSFUNCTION OF THE ENDOCRINE PANCREAS: DIABETES MELLITUS

Diabetes mellitus is not a single disease but a group of disorders with glucose intolerance in common. The term *diabetes mellitus* describes a syndrome characterized by chronic hyperglycemia and other disturbances of carbohydrate, protein, and fat metabolism. The American Diabetes Association classifies four categories of diabetes mellitus[32] (Table 18-3):

1. Type 1 (absolute insulin deficiency)
2. Type 2 (insulin resistance with an insulin secretory deficit)
3. Other specific types
4. Gestational diabetes

The diagnosis of diabetes mellitus is based on clinical manifestations, fasting plasma glucose levels, and glucose tolerance tests (Table 18-4). Because many epidemiologic studies have shown severe cardiovascular disease in individuals with only impaired glucose tolerance (IGT), early screening and detection are important and may be accomplished with plasma screening. IGT is the term used to describe individuals who have plasma glucose levels that are higher than normal but lower than those considered diagnostic for diabetes. IGT results primarily from reduced suppression of hepatic glucose output caused by abnormal pancreatic islet cell function.

Another mechanism used to measure plasma glucose levels over time is the measurement of **glycosylated hemoglobin.** In the normal 120-day life span of the red blood cell, glucose molecules join hemoglobin, forming glycosylated hemoglobin. In an individual with persistent hyperglycemia, increases in the quantities of glycosylated hemoglobins (Hb A_{1c}) are noted. Once a hemoglobin molecule is glycosylated, it remains that way. A buildup of glycosylated hemoglobin within the red cell reflects the average level of glucose to which the cell has been exposed during its life cycle. Measuring glycosylated hemoglobin assesses the effectiveness of therapy by monitoring long-term serum glucose regulation.

For any diagnosis of diabetes mellitus, the goals of therapy are to maintain euglycemia, avoid hypoglycemia, and prevent severe cardiovascular and neurologic complications.

TABLE 18-3 Classification and Characteristics of Diabetes Mellitus

Name	Previous Synonyms	Characteristics
Type 1 diabetes mellitus Absolute insulin deficiency	Insulin-dependent diabetes mellitus (IDDM) Juvenile diabetes Juvenile-onset diabetes Ketosis-prone diabetes Brittle diabetes Idiopathic diabetes	Long preclinical period with abrupt onset of clinical manifestations Individual prone to ketoacidosis Insulin dependent Several syndromes, both primary autoimmune and genetic environment Often affects young people around age of puberty Decrease in size and number of islet cells
Type 2 diabetes mellitus Insulin resistance with an insulin secretory deficiency	Non-insulin-dependent diabetes mellitus (NIDDM) Adult-onset diabetes Maturity-onset diabetes Ketosis-resistant diabetes	Usually not insulin dependent Individual not ketosis prone (but may form ketones under stress) Multiple syndromes: obese, nonobese, and maturity-onset diabetes of the young (MODY) Generally occurs in those over age 40 yr Strong familial pattern being investigated
Other types of diabetes mellitus	Secondary diabetes	Associated with other conditions or syndromes, such as pancreatic disease, hormonal disease, drugs, and chemical agents
Gestational diabetes mellitus (GDM)	Asymptomatic diabetes Chemical diabetes Borderline diabetes Subclinical diabetes Latent diabetes	Glucose intolerance first recognized during pregnancy most likely in the third trimester After pregnancy, glucose may normalize, remain impaired, or progress to diabetes mellitus Occurs in 2% of all pregnancies; 60% will develop diabetes mellitus within 15 yr of gestation

TABLE 18-4 Diagnostic Criteria for Diabetes Mellitus*

Category	Fasting Plasma Glucose	Oral Glucose Tolerance Test		
		1-hr	2-hr	3-hr
Diabetes mellitus	≥126 mg/dl on two occasions and/or Random hyperglycemia and classic symptoms of diabetes >126 mg/dl	≥200 mg dl	≥200 mg/dl	
Impaired fasting glucose	110-125 mg/dl			
Impaired glucose tolerance		≥200 mg/dl	140-200 mg/dl	
Gestational diabetes mellitus	>105 mg/dl on two occasions >105 mg/dl	≥190 mg/dl	≥165 mg/dl	≥145 mg/dl

Recommendations of the American Diabetes Association.

Types of Diabetes Mellitus

Type 1 diabetes mellitus

Although the cause is unknown, *type 1 diabetes mellitus* (previously known as *insulin-dependent diabetes mellitus [IDDM]*) accounts for approximately 10% of all diabetes mellitus in the Western world. Its incidence is increasing in some areas, with other areas showing no change in incidence.[33] Several studies suggest that the incidence and prevalence are higher for whites than for nonwhites, with the highest rate found in Finland and the lowest rate in Japan.[34] Variations oc-

cur, however, even within individual countries. (Table 18-5 summarizes the epidemiology of diabetes mellitus.)

Type 1 diabetes mellitus is thought to be the result of a gene-environment interaction, with the strongest genetic risk markers in the HLA region of chromosome 6. Genetic factors may increase susceptibility to environmental causes of diabetes. There is a 50% concordance rate in twins. Between 10% and 13% of individuals with newly diagnosed type 1 diabetes have a first-degree relative (parent or sibling)

TABLE 18-5	Epidemiology and Etiology of Diabetes Mellitus	
	Type 1 Diabetes: Primary Beta-Cell Defect or Failure	**Type 2 Diabetes: Insulin Resistance With Inadequate Insulin Secretion**
Incidence		
Frequency	One of the most common childhood diseases (10% of all cases of diabetes mellitus) Range from 29.5/100,000 (Finland) to 1.6/100,000 (Japan)	Accounts for most cases ($\approx$90%) Prevalence rate in United States (for age 18 yr and older): 6.6%* Prevalence for Pima Indians (western American Indian group): 39.9%
Change in incidences	Increased incidences in British Isles, Finland, Norway, Denmark, Israel, Germany, and Poland; stable elsewhere	Incidence has risen in United States since 1940
Characteristics		
Age at onset	Peak onset at age 11-13 yr (slightly earlier for girls than for boys) Rare in children younger than 1 yr and adults older than 30 yr	Risk of developing diabetes increases after age 40 yr; in general, incidence increases with age into the 70s; among Pima Indians, incidence peaks between age 40 and 50 yr, then falls
Gender	Similar in males and females	In the United States, more females than males
Racial distribution	Rates for whites 1.5-2 times higher than for nonwhites Higher rates for those of Scandinavian descent than for those of central or southern European descent	Certain racial groups may be more likely to develop type 2 diabetes when exposed to a particular environment Common in migrant groups encountering a different environment (e.g., Polynesians moving from traditional to western life-style) In the United States, risk is highest for American Indians; rates are higher for Pacific Islanders, Japanese, Puerto Ricans, Hispanics, and blacks than for whites
Socioeconomic status	Conflicting data	A disease of the affluent in developing nations but more common among those of lower incomes and less education in the United States
Seasonal distribution	More new cases documented during fall and winter in the northern hemisphere	No known association
Childbirth association	No association documented	Effect of parity on subsequent development of type 2 diabetes varies among different populations
Obesity	Generally normal or underweight	Frequent contributing factor to precipitate type 2 diabetes among those susceptible; a major factor in populations recently exposed to westernized environment Increased risk related to duration, degree, and distribution of obesity
Etiology		
Common theory	*Autoimmune:* genetic and environmental factors, resulting in gradual process of autoimmune destruction in genetically susceptible individuals *Nonautoimmune:* known genetic defects of the beta-cell MODY follow dominant pattern of inheritance with glucokinase gene mutation Strong association with HLA-DR3 and HLA-DR4	Disease results from genetic susceptibility (although the precise gene or genes have not yet been determined) combined with environmental determinants and other risk factors Associated with long-duration obesity

*Data from Brancati, F.L. et al. (1996). Annals of Epidemiology 6(1), 67.
MODY, *Maturity-onset diabetes of the young.*

Continued

TABLE 18-5   Epidemiology and Etiology of Diabetes Mellitus—cont'd

	Type 1 Diabetes: Primary Beta-Cell Defect or Failure	Type 2 Diabetes: Insulin Resistance With Inadequate Insulin Secretion
Etiology—cont'd		
Heredity	Risk to sibling: 5%-10%; risk to offspring: 2%-5% For MODY, risk to siblings and offspring: 50%	Risk to first-degree relative (child or sibling): 10%-15%
Presence of antibody	Islet cell autoantibodies (ICA) and/or autoantibodies to insulin, and autoantibodies to glutamic acid decarboxylase (GAD_{65}) are present in 85%-90% of individuals when fasting hyperglycemia is initially detected	Islet cell antibodies not present
Insulin resistance	Insulin resistance rare	Increased insulin resistance caused by a decrease in number of cell receptor sites and altered cellular metabolism
Insulin secretion	Severe insulin deficiency or no insulin secretion at all	Typically increased at time of diagnosis; may be normal or decreased

with type 1 diabetes. Diagnosis is rare during the first 9 months of life and peaks at 12 years of age.

Historically, type 1 diabetes mellitus has been thought to have an abrupt onset. More recently, however, prospective studies show a distinctive natural history involving genetic susceptibility; a long preclinical period; immunologically mediated destruction of beta cells, eventually leading to insulin deficiency; and hyperglycemia.

Pathophysiology

Type 1 diabetes results from a severe, absolute lack of insulin caused by loss of beta cells Destruction of islet cells is related to genetic susceptibility, autoimmunity, and environmental factors. The autoimmune mechanisms are related to cell and cytokine-mediated injury of beta cells. Frequently (80% to 90% of cases) there are islet cell autoantibodies that participate in damage to islet cells. There are autoantibodies to insulin, and they tend to disappear with time. Autoantibodies are often detected long before symptoms appear. Environmental factors that may trigger autoimmune injury are summarized in Box 18-1.

Hyperglycemia and other symptoms

Before hyperglycemia occurs, 80% to 90% of the insulin-secreting beta cells of the islet of Langerhans must be destroyed. Beta cell abnormalities are present long before the acute clinical onset of type 1 diabetes. Early beta cell destruction may differ from the event that yields clinical symptoms.

Regardless of cause, a disequilibrium of hormones produced by the islets of Langerhans occurs in diabetes mellitus. Both beta cell function and alpha cell function are abnormal, with a lack of insulin and a relative excess of glucagon (produced by alpha cells).

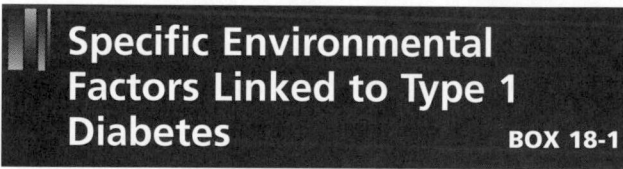

Specific Environmental Factors Linked to Type 1 Diabetes   BOX 18-1

DRUGS AND CHEMICALS
Alloxan
Streptozocin
Pentamidine
Vacor (a rodenticide)

NUTRITIONAL INTAKE
Bovine milk (controversial)
High levels of nitrosamines

VIRUSES
Mumps and coxsackie—type 1 diabetes does occur rarely as a complication of viral infections, but no evidence of substantial relationship exists
Rubella—40% of individuals with congenital rubella infection develop type 1 diabetes later
Cytomegalovirus (CMV)—persistent CMV infections appear to be relevant to pathogenesis of some cases of type 1 diabetes

From Akerblom, H.K. & Knip, M. (1998). Putative environmental factors in type 1 diabetes. Diabetes and Metabolism Review, 14(1), *31-67; Hovi, T. (1998). Molecular epidemiology of enteroviruses with special reference to their potential role in the etiology of insulin-dependent diabetes.* Clinical and Diagnostic Virology, 9(2-3), 89-98.

TABLE 18-6	Clinical Manifestations and Rationale for Type 1 Diabetes Mellitus
Manifestations	**Rationale**
Polydipsia	Because of elevated blood sugar levels, water is osmotically attracted from body cells, resulting in intracellular dehydration and stimulation of thirst in the hypothalamus
Polyuria	Hyperglycemia acts as an osmotic diuretic; the amount of glucose filtered by the glomeruli of the kidney exceeds that which can be reabsorbed by the renal tubules; glycosuria results, accompanied by large amounts of water lost in the urine
Polyphagia	Depletion of cellular stores of carbohydrates, fats, and protein results in cellular starvation and a corresponding increase in hunger
Weight loss	Weight loss occurs because of fluid loss in osmotic diuresis and the loss of body tissue as fats and proteins are used for energy
Fatigue	Metabolic changes result in poor use of food products, contributing to lethargy and fatigue

Hyperglycemia and hyperketonemia are not possible with insulin deficiency alone; glucagon must be present in relative excess. Thus the full metabolic syndrome is caused by both hormones. Relative hyperglucagonemia occurs in every form of diabetes mellitus. The ratio of insulin to glucagon in the portal vein—and not the concentration of each hormone—controls hepatic glucose and fat metabolism. Elevated blood glucose levels fail to suppress the production of glucagon.

Clinical Manifestations

Type 1 diabetes mellitus affects the metabolism of fat, protein, and carbohydrates. Glucose accumulates in the blood and spills into the urine as the renal threshold for glucose is exceeded. In addition, protein and fat breakdown occurs because of the lack of insulin, resulting in weight loss.

Initial clinical manifestations of type 1 diabetes are generally acute, with polyuria, polydipsia, and polyphagia (Table 18-6). Weight loss and wide fluctuations in blood glucose levels occur.

Ketoacidosis is caused by increased metabolism of fats and proteins resulting in high levels of circulating ketones. The pH drops, triggering the buffering systems associated with metabolic acidosis (see Chapter 4). Acetone (a volatile form of ketones) then is blown off, giving the breath a sweet or "fruity" odor. Occasionally, diabetic coma is the initial symptom of the disease.

Evaluation and Treatment

The diagnosis of diabetes is not difficult when the symptoms of polydipsia, polyuria, polyphagia, weight loss, and hyperglycemia are present in fasting and postprandial states.

Currently, treatment regimens are designed to avoid high and low levels of glucose and insulin.[35] Management requires individual planning according to type of disease, age, and activity level, but all individuals require some combination of insulin, meal planning, and exercise. Hemoglobin A_{1c} testing is useful in confirming the diagnosis and in monitoring effectiveness of treatment and preventing complications.[36]

Type 2 diabetes mellitus

Type 2 diabetes mellitus (non-insulin-dependent diabetes mellitus [NIDDM]) is much more common than type 1 and has been rising in incidence since 1940. One case is undiagnosed for each known case in the United States. The condition is more common in native Americans, Hispanics, and blacks. The environment also affects prevalence. Among Polynesians living traditionally, the prevalence is 2.9%, compared with 12% among migrants.[37] It affects people primarily after 40 years of age, many of whom are obese. A gene-environment interaction appears to be responsible.

Pathophysiology

The cause of the common form of type 2 diabetes mellitus is unknown. The genetics of type 2 are complex and not clearly defined. Autoimmune mechanisms are not involved. Individuals with maturity-onset diabetes of youth (MODY), a subset of type 2 diabetes, are normal weight to underweight. MODY is thought to be autosomal dominant because it affects 50% of first-degree relatives.

Insulin resistance is a factor for 60% to 80% of individuals with type 2 diabetes in the Western world. Associated obesity is common. Decreased beta cell responsiveness to plasma glucose levels is noted, along with abnormal glucagon secretion. The islet dysfunction may be caused by a decrease in beta cell mass, abnormal function of the beta cells, alterations in the insulin receptor, or postreceptor events.[38] Levels of insulin may increase to compensate for insulin resistance in peripheral tissues.

Pancreatic changes in individuals with type 2 diabetes mellitus are nonspecific and have been observed to a lesser degree in persons without diabetes. Amyloid of the islets occurs in 10% to 40% of the pancreases from individuals with type 2 diabetes. The extent of amyloid deposits is positively correlated with the age of the individual and the duration and severity of the disease. Amyloid formation is associated with islet cell destruction.[39] In long-standing type 2 diabetes, beta cell mass is decreased by 20% to 40%.[40]

Liver changes are related to elevated serum lipid levels. Fatty pancreatic and hepatic atrophy, although affecting

TABLE 18-7	Clinical Manifestations and Rationale for Type 2 Diabetes Mellitus
Manifestations	**Rationale**
Recurrent infections (e.g., boils and carbuncles; skin infections) and prolonged wound healing	Growth of microorganisms is stimulated by increased glucose levels; impaired blood supply hinders healing
Genital pruritus	Hyperglycemia and glycosuria favor fungal growth; candidal infections, resulting in pruritus, are a common presenting symptom in women
Visual changes	Blurred vision occurs as water balance in the eye fluctuates because of elevated blood glucose levels; diabetic retinopathy may ensue
Paresthesias	Paresthesias are common manifestations of diabetic neuropathies
Fatigue	Metabolic changes result in poor use of food products, contributing to lethargy and fatigue

both those with and those without diabetes, occurs with much greater frequency. These fatty infiltrates may play a role in the development of amyloid deposits in the islets. Although tissue atrophies, fat infiltration may increase the overall size of the liver and pancreas and glycogen vacuoles may be found in the cell nuclei. Ischemia caused by vascular sclerosis may cause the fatty atrophy. Pancreatic fibrosis, occurring in 33% to 66% of individuals with type 2 diabetes, also contributes to loss of beta cell function.

A progressive decrease in the weight and number of beta cells generally occurs in type 2 diabetes, but the cause is unclear. Also, the ratio of alpha cells to beta cells may be completely normal in the individual with type 2 diabetes, and individuals with type 2 diabetes may have plasma and pancreatic insulin levels that are not decreased. This latter finding supports the hypothesis that diabetes is a disorder caused by both insulin and glucagon, so that a deficiency of insulin and an excess of glucagon may be either relative or absolute. An inherited secretory deficiency of the beta cells may also be operative.

The most powerful risk factor for type 2 diabetes is obesity. The risk for developing type 2 diabetes mellitus increases 10 times with severe obesity.[41] Excessive caloric intake predisposes an individual to type 2 diabetes by contributing to obesity.

In obese persons, insulin is less able to facilitate the entry of glucose into the liver, skeletal muscles, and adipose tissue. Multiple theories have been presented to explain this phenomenon,[42] as follows:
1. A decreased number of insulin receptors in the plasma membrane causes decreased insulin binding.
2. Postreceptor events in insulin-sensitive cells are responsible for insulin resistance in obese people.
3. Hyperinsulinemia, which occurs often in the early stages of type 2 diabetes, is a compensatory adaptation to insulin resistance in tissues, so elevated levels of circulating insulin are induced by obesity until the pancreas cannot continue to overproduce insulin.
4. Overeating leads to hyperinsulinemia, which necessitates the development of peripheral insulin resistance to protect against hypoglycemia.

In any event, the mechanism responsible for insulin receptor binding or postreceptor activity may be reversed through weight loss.

Amylin is a hormone co-secreted with insulin of the beta cells. There is a deficiency of amylin in type 1 diabetes that parallels insulin. Problems with glycemic control may be related to altered glucagon control or assimilation of nutrients in relation to amylin deficit. Amyloid deposition may also be related to amylin loss.[43,44]

Clinical Manifestations

Clinical manifestations of type 2 diabetes often are nonspecific. The individual often is overweight and hyperlipidemic. The onset frequently is slow and insidious, making diagnosis difficult. Some of the classic symptoms of diabetes may be present, but more often there will be nonspecific symptoms, such as pruritus, recurrent infections, visual changes, and paresthesias (Table 18-7).

Evaluation and Treatment

Type 2 diabetes is underdiagnosed, but diagnosis uses methods similar to those of type 1 (see p. 487). The goal of treatment is restoration of euglycemia (a normal blood glucose level) and correction of related metabolic disorders. Dietary measures, including the restriction of the total caloric intake, are of primary importance in the overweight individual. As in type 1 diabetes, the ratio of fats, carbohydrates, and protein is important and both cholesterol and saturated fats are restricted. Some research suggests that high-fiber diets also improve diabetic control.[45] As the obese individual loses weight, the body's resistance to insulin often diminishes so that weight loss results in improved glucose tolerance. Hyperglycemic oral medication often is needed for optimal management, and exercise is an essential component of treatment. Insulin therapy is used when oral medications fail to maintain euglycemia.

Gestational diabetes

Gestational diabetes mellitus develops when glucose intolerance appears during pregnancy, and pregnant women at risk should be screened. Risk factors include glycosuria,

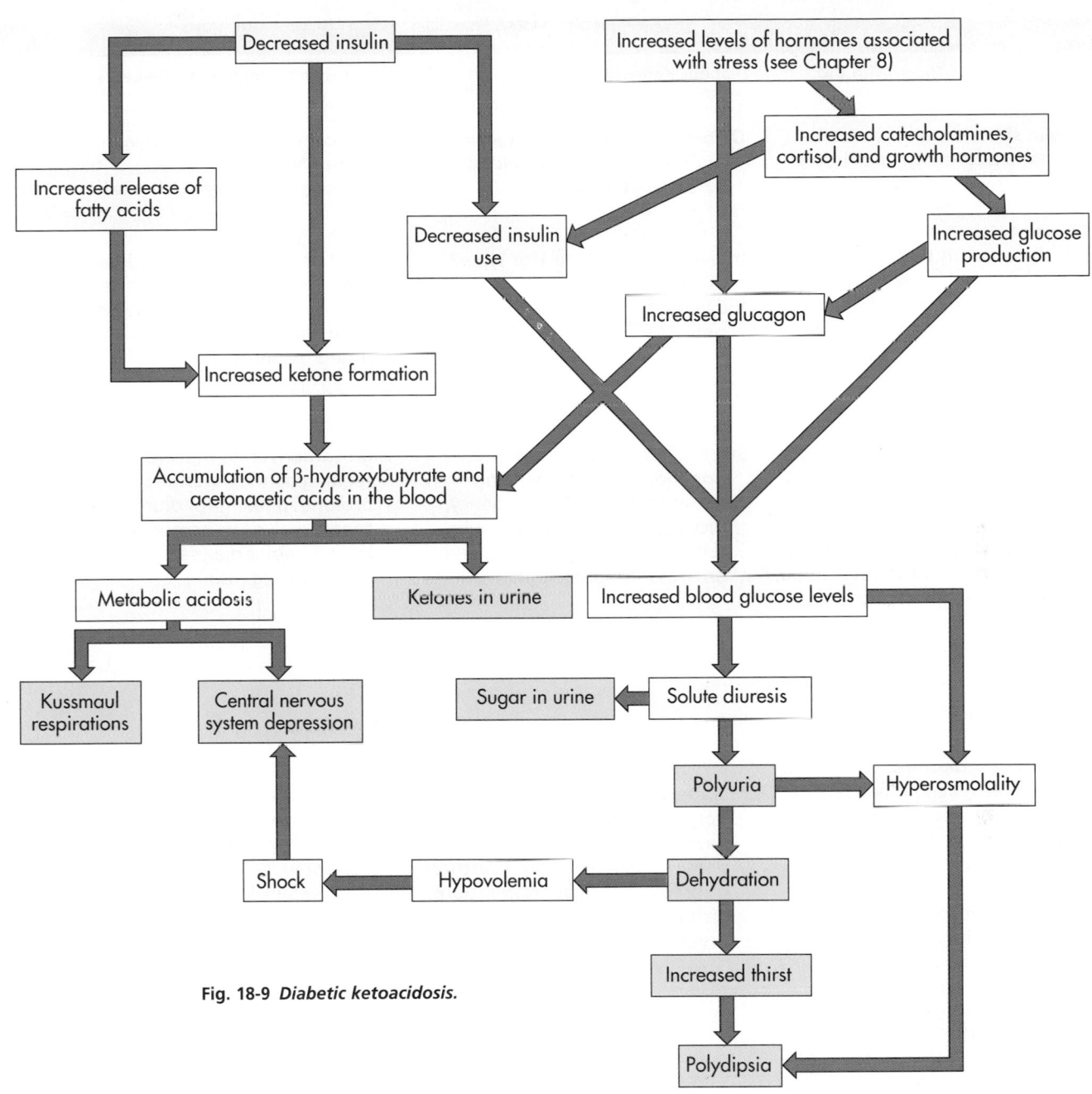

Fig. 18-9 *Diabetic ketoacidosis.*

family history of diabetes, obesity, high maternal age, parity of 5 or more, and a previous complicated pregnancy. Aggressive treatment is required to prevent morbidity and fetal mortality.[46]

Acute Complications of Diabetes Mellitus

The major acute complications of diabetes mellitus are hypoglycemia, diabetic ketoacidosis (Fig. 18-9), and *hyperosmolar nonacidotic diabetes* (see comparison in Table 18-8). In addition, the Somogyi phenomenon and dawn phenomenon may be seen.

Hypoglycemia occurs in more than 90% of cases of type 1 diabetes and is related to insulin treatment. Hypoglycemia in diabetes is sometimes called *insulin shock* or *insulin reac-*

tion. Symptoms result from decreased blood glucose (45 to 60 mg/dl) and neurogenic reactions. Symptoms include pallor, tremor, anxiety, tachycardia, palpitations, diaphoresis, headache, dizziness, irritability, fatigue, poor judgment, confusion, visual disturbances, hunger, seizures, and coma. The treatment is to provide an immediate replacement of glucose. Prevention is achieved with individualized treatment, blood glucose monitoring, and education.

Diabetic ketoacidosis is a serious complication related to a deficiency of insulin and an increase in insulin counterregulatory hormones (catecholamines, cortisol, glucagon, GH). Under these conditions, hepatic glucose production increases and peripheral glucose usage decreases. Fat is mobilized, and ketogenesis is stimulated[47] (see Fig. 18-9).

Nonketotic hyperglycemic hyperosmolar coma is an un-

TABLE 18-8   Common Acute Complications of Diabetes Mellitus

Hypoglycemia in Those With DM	Diabetic Ketoacidosis	Hyperosmolar Nonacidotic Diabetes
Synonyms Insulin shock, insulin reaction from excess exogenous insulin	Diabetic coma syndrome (acidosis, high concentration of blood glucose, dehydration)	Hyperosmolar hyperglycemia nonketotic coma (high concentration of blood glucose with severe dehydration)
Those at risk Individuals with type 1 diabetes Individuals with rapidly fluctuating blood glucose levels Individuals with type 2 diabetes taking oral agents, especially chlorpropamide	Individuals with type 1 or type 2 diabetes Individuals with nondiagnosed diabetes	Elderly or very young individuals with type 2 diabetes, nondiabetics with predisposing factors, those with renal insufficiency, individuals with undiagnosed diabetes
Predisposing factors Excessive insulin or hypoglycemic agent intake; lack of sufficient food intake; excessive physical exercise; abrupt decline in insulin needs (e.g., renal failure; immediately postpartum; some cases of insulin reaction); simultaneous use of insulin-potentiating agents	Stressful situation, such as infection, accident, trauma, emotional stress; insulin deficiency; factors that antagonize insulin, such as steroids, glucagon, and growth hormone; lipolysis	High-carbohydrate diets (e.g., tube feedings; total parenteral nutrition); prolonged mannitol diuresis; peritoneal dialysis or hemodialysis with hyperosmolar dialysate; medications antagonizing insulin
Typical onset Rapid	Slow	Slowest
Presenting symptoms Neurogenic reaction: pallor, sweating, tachycardia, palpitations, hunger, restlessness, anxiety, tremors Cellular malnutrition: fatigue, irritability, headache, loss of concentration, visual disturbances, dizziness, hunger, confusion, transient sensory or motor defects, convulsions, coma, death	Malaise, dry mouth, headache, polyuria, polydipsia, weight loss, nausea, vomiting, pruritus, abdominal pain, lethargy, shortness of breath, Kussmaul respirations, "fruity" or acetone odor to breath	Osmotic diuresis with polyuria, polydipsia, hypovolemia, dehydration (parched lips, poor skin turgor), hypotension, tachycardia, hypoperfusion, weight loss, weakness, nausea, vomiting, abdominal pain, hypothermia, stupor, coma, seizures
Laboratory analysis Serum glucose below 30 mg/dl in newborn (first 2-3 days) and below 55-60 mg/dl in adults	Glucose levels 300-750 mg/dl, reduction in bicarbonate concentration, increased anion gap, increased plasma levels of β-hydroxybutyrate, acetoacetate, and acetone	Glucose levels 600-2000 mg/dl, lack of ketosis, serum osmolarity above 350 mOsm/L, elevated blood urea nitrogen and creatinine

common but significant complication of type 2 diabetes mellitus with a high overall mortality. It occurs more frequently in elderly individuals who have other co-morbidities, including infections or cardiovascular or renal disease. Poor glucose control results in high levels of serum glucose (more than 500 mg/dl) and high serum osmotic pressures that lead to severe dehydration, low blood volume, and low perfusion pressures. Ketosis is less common because

there is enough insulin to prevent lypolysis and protein catabolism. Treatment is controversial but mandates aggressive fluid and electrolyte resuscitation and strict control of serum glucose levels.[48]

The *Somogyi phenomenon* is a unique combination of hypoglycemia during the night with hyperglycemia in the morning hours. The rise in blood glucose occurs because of counterregulatory hormones (epinephrine, GH, corticosteroids), which are stimulated by hypoglycemia during sleep. The waning effect of insulin given the previous evening may also cause hyperglycemia after hypoglycemia independent of or in addition to the effects of counterregulatory hormones. The problem is common in adolescents with type 1 diabetes mellitus and is difficult to identify because it occurs during sleep.[49]

The *dawn phenomenon* is an early morning rise in blood glucose concentration with no hypoglycemia during the night. It occurs more commonly in adolescents with type 1 diabetes and is related to waning of the evening insulin dose. Nocturnal elevations of GH may occur, which decrease metabolism of glucose by muscle and fat. Also, a transient insulin resistance may occur, reflecting a need for increased insulin.[50] The true dawn phenomenon shows a relatively normal blood glucose level until about 3 AM, when the glucose level begins to rise. Periodic monitoring of plasma glucose values in the morning ascertains the need for additional long-acting evening insulin.

Chronic Complications of Diabetes Mellitus

A number of serious complications are associated with any type of long-term diabetes mellitus and include microvascular and macrovascular disease and neuropathies. Most complications are associated with metabolic alterations, primarily hyperglycemia.[51] Strict control of blood glucose significantly reduces complications. Three metabolic events associated with chronic hyperglycemia are involved in the pathogenesis of diabetic complications: nonenzymatic glycosylation, shunting of glucose to the polyol pathway, and activation of protein kinase C.

Hyperglycemia and nonenzymatic glycosylation

Nonenzymatic glycosylation is the reversible attachment of glucose to proteins, lipids, and nucleic acids without the action of enzymes. With recurrent or persistent hyperglycemia, glucose becomes irreversibly bound to collagen and other proteins in blood vessel walls and interstitial tissue; the products of this binding are known as *advanced glycosylation end-products (AGE)*. AGEs have a number of properties that may cause tissue injury or pathologic conditions associated with diabetes:

1. Cross-linking and trapping of proteins, including albumin, low-density lipoprotein (LDL), immunoglobulin, and complement, with thickening of the basement membrane or increased permeability in blood vessels and nerves
2. Binding to cell receptors, such as macrophages, and inducing release of cytokines and growth factors that stimulate cellular proliferation in the glomeruli and smooth muscle of blood vessels
3. Induction of lipid oxidation and oxygen free radicals
4. Inactivation of nitric oxide with loss of vasodilation
5. Procoagulant changes on endothelial cells

Pharmacologic agents, such as aminoguanidine, inhibited AGE formation in experimental trials.

Hyperglycemia and the polyol pathway

Tissues that do not require insulin for glucose transport, such as kidney, red blood cells (RBCs), blood vessels, eye lens, and nerves, use an alternate metabolic pathway for glucose metabolism known as the *polyol pathway.* With hyperglycemia, glucose is shunted to this pathway and is converted to sorbitol (a polyol) by the enzyme aldose reductase. Sorbitol is then converted to fructose by sorbitol dehydrogenase. The accumulation of sorbitol and fructose increases intracellular osmotic pressure and attracts water, leading to cell injury. This is particularly evident in the lens and leads to swelling with visual changes and cataracts. In nerves, sorbitol interferes with ion pumps, damages Schwann cells, and disrupts nerve conduction. RBCs become swollen and stiff and interfere with perfusion.

Aldose reductase inhibitors can slow or prevent some diabetic complications.

Protein kinase C

Protein kinase C (PKC) is an extracellular enzyme that is inappropriately activated in different tissues by hyperglycemia. Various consequences have been observed, including insulin resistance, production of extracellular matrix and cytokines, vascular cell proliferation, enhanced contractility, and increased permeability. These effects may contribute to the macrovascular, microvascular, and neurologic complications of diabetes. D-α-Tocopherol may inhibit PKC activation.[52,53]

Diabetic neuropathies

Diabetic neuropathy is the most common cause of neuropathy in the Western world and is the most common complication of diabetes. The underlying pathologic mechanism includes both metabolic and vascular factors related to hyperglycemia.[54] Advanced glycosylation end-products and increased formation of polyols contribute to nerve degeneration and delayed conduction. Both somatic and peripheral nerve cells show diffuse or focal damage. Sensory deficits and symptoms are more common than motor involvement.

Some neuropathies are progressive, but many, such as painful peripheral neuropathy, mononeuropathy (wristdrop, footdrop), diabetic amyotrophy, diabetic neuropathic cachexia, and visceral manifestations associated with autonomic neuropathy (e.g., delayed gastric emptying, diabetic diarrhea, altered bladder function, orthostatic hypotension), are reversible. Chronic hyperglycemia can also cause cognitive changes.[55] Neuropathy may occur during periods of good glucose control and may be the initial clinical manifestation of diabetes, even without overt glucose intolerance.

Microvascular disease

Thickening of the capillary basement membrane, endothelial hyperplasia, thrombosis, and pericyte degeneration are characteristic of diabetic microangiopathy and emerge over a period of 1 to 2 years. Decreased tissue perfusion eventually results. Although some degree of hyperglycemia is a necessary prerequisite for the vascular changes, no conclusive evidence is available to correlate the basement membrane thickening with the severity of diabetes. The frequency of the lesions appears to be proportional to the duration of the disease (more or less than 10 years) and blood glucose levels. Hypoxia and ischemia of various organs may result from microangiopathy, especially in the retina and kidney. Diagnosis of type 2 diabetes may be delayed until the individual presents with complications related to long-term elevation of blood glucose.

Visual changes

Diabetic retinopathy appears to be a response to retinal ischemia resulting from blood vessel changes and RBC aggregation and is influenced by growth hormone and metabolic control. The prevalence and severity of the retinopathy are strongly related to the age of the individual and duration of the diabetes. Retinopathy develops more rapidly in individuals with type 2 than with type 1 diabetes but is present in the majority of all individuals with diabetes mellitus.[56]

The three stages of retinopathy are *nonproliferative* (stage I), characterized by an increase in retinal capillary permeability, vein dilation, microaneurysm formation, and superficial (flame-shaped) and deep (blot) hemorrhages; *preproliferative* (stage II), a progression of retinal ischemia with areas of poor perfusion that culminate in infarcts; and *proliferative* (stage III), the result of neovascularization and fibrous tissue formation within the retina or optic disc. Traction of the new vessels on the vitreous humor may cause retinal detachment or hemorrhage into the vitreous humor. Macular edema is the leading cause of decreased vision among persons with diabetes. Hard exudates and microaneurysms can result in loss of vision. Blurring of vision also can be a consequence of sorbitol accumulation in the lens and hyperglycemia. Cataract formation and dehydration of the lens, aqueous humor, and vitreous humor reduce visual acuity.

Diabetic nephropathy

Diabetes is the most common cause of end-stage renal disease. AGEs, activation of the polyol pathway, glucose toxicity, and protein kinase C all contribute to renal tissue injury; yet the exact process responsible for destruction of kidneys in diabetes is unknown. The glomeruli are injured by protein denaturation by high glucose levels, hyperglycemia with high renal blood flow, and intraglomerular hypertension exacerbated by systemic hypertension. Renal glomerular changes occur early in diabetes mellitus, occasionally preceding the overt manifestation of the disease. Progressive changes include glomerular enlargement, glomerular basement membrane thickening with proliferation of mesangial cells, and mesangial matrix. This results in diffuse intercapillary glomerulosclerosis and decreased blood flow. Alterations in glomerular membrane permeability occur with loss of negative charge and albuminuria.

Microalbuminuria is the first manifestation of renal dysfunction. Continuous proteinuria generally heralds a life expectancy of less than 10 years. Before proteinuria, no clinical signs or symptoms of progressive glomerulosclerosis are likely to be evident. Later, hypoproteinemia, reduction in plasma oncotic pressure, fluid overload, anasarca (generalized body edema), and hypertension may occur. As renal function continues to deteriorate, individuals with type 1 diabetes may experience hypoglycemia, which necessitates a decrease in insulin therapy. As the glomerular filtration rate drops below 10 ml/min, uremic signs, such as nausea, lethargy, acidosis, anemia, and uncontrolled hypertension,

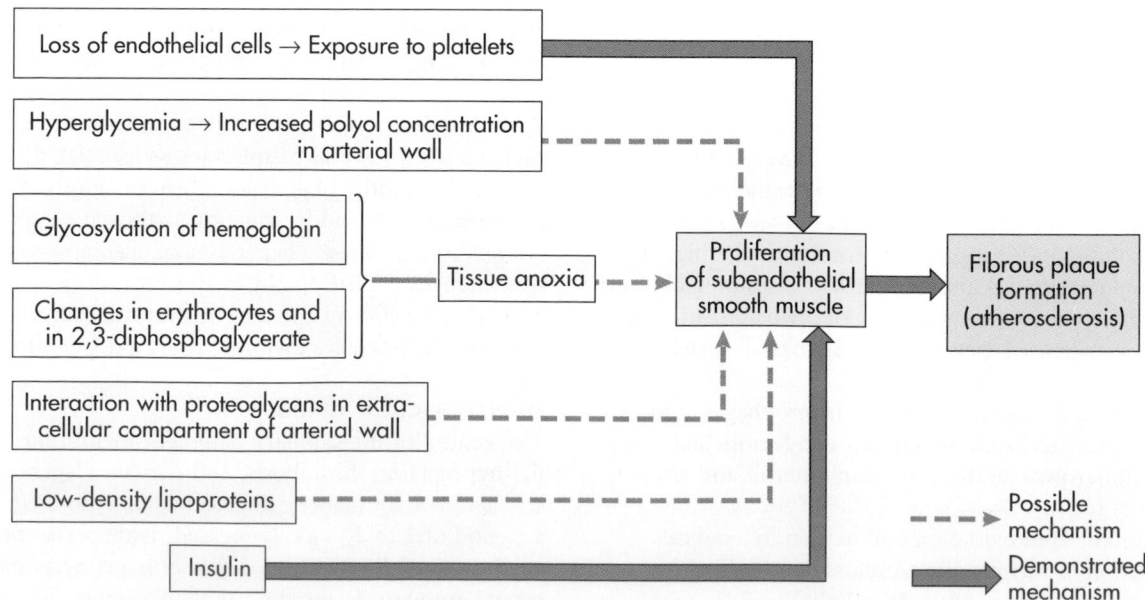

Fig. 18-10 *Diabetes mellitus and atherosclerosis.* Contributing causes of proliferation of subendothelial smooth muscle in arterial wall, resulting in atherosclerosis.

occur (see Chapter 29 for a discussion of renal failure). Impaired kidney function also accelerates retinopathy. Death from renal failure is much more common in individuals with type 1 diabetes mellitus than in those with type 2.

Macrovascular disease

Macrovascular disease causes morbidity and mortality, particularly among individuals with type 2 diabetes mellitus. Unlike microangiopathy, atherosclerotic disease is unrelated to the severity of diabetes and often is present in those with merely an impaired glucose tolerance.[57] (Atherosclerosis is discussed in Chapter 23.) The pathogenesis of atherosclerosis is related to the response to injury. Insulin may directly stimulate atherogenesis with chronic hyperglycemia. Advanced glycosylated end-products attach to cells in the walls of blood vessels and promote changes leading to atherosclerosis (Fig. 18-10).[58]

Lipids may be deposited in the lesions, and triglyceride and serum cholesterol elevations are very common. High-density lipoproteins (HDLs), which tend to protect vessels, are present in only low concentrations in individuals with diabetes. As in the nondiabetic person, the presence of other risk factors, including hypertension, increases vulnerability to atherosclerosis.

Coronary artery disease

The risk of coronary artery disease (CAD) for those with diabetes is higher than for the general population even when hypertension and hyperlipidemia are taken into account. CAD is the most common cause of death in individuals with type 2 diabetes because of insulin resistance, high levels of LDLs and triglycerides, low levels of HDLs, and endothelial cell dysfunction.[59] Mortality is most marked at or before middle age, particularly in women.[60] In general, the prevalence of CAD increases with the duration but not the severity of diabetes.

Myocardial infarction causes death in 20% of those with diabetes. In addition, the incidence of congestive heart failure is higher in individuals with diabetes, even without myocardial infarction. This may be related to the presence of increased amounts of collagen in the ventricular wall, which reduces the mechanical compliance of the heart during filling. Increased platelet adhesion and decreased fibrinolysis promote thrombus formation in persons with diabetes.[61] (Heart disease is described in Chapter 23.)

Stroke

Stroke is twice as common in those with diabetes as in the nondiabetic population.[62] The survival rate for individuals with diabetes after a massive stroke is typically shorter than for nondiabetic individuals. Hypertension is a definite risk factor (see Chapter 23).

Peripheral vascular disease

The increased incidence of peripheral vascular disease (PVD), gangrene, and amputation in the individual with diabetes has been well documented. Many individuals with type 2 diabetes have evidence of PVD at the time of their initial diagnosis.[63] Individuals with diabetes are more likely to have atherosclerosis that appears at a younger age and advances more rapidly than vascular changes in nondiabetic persons. Age, duration of diabetes, genetics, and additional risk factors influence the development of PVD.

Because of occlusions of the small arteries and arterioles, most of the gangrenous changes of the lower extremities occur in patchy areas of the feet and toes.[64] The lesions begin as ulcers and progress to osteomyelitis or gangrene requiring amputation.[65] Significant morbidity and mortality are associated with major amputation.

Infection

The individual with diabetes is at an increased risk for infection throughout the body for at least five reasons:
1. *The senses.* Impaired vision caused by retinal changes and impaired touch caused by neuropathy diminish the prevention of breaks in the skin by decreasing the early warning systems.
2. *Hypoxia.* Once skin integrity is compromised, tissues' susceptibility to infection increases as a result of hypoxia. In addition, the glycosylated hemoglobin in the RBCs impedes the release of oxygen to tissues.
3. *Pathogens.* Some pathogens proliferate rapidly because of increased glucose in body fluids, which provides an excellent source of energy.
4. *Blood supply.* Decreased blood supply results from vascular changes and decreases the supply of white blood cells to the affected area.
5. *White cells.* These cells suffer impaired function, including abnormal chemotaxis and defective phagocytosis.

> ## ✓ QUICK CHECK
>
> What are the major differences between type 1 and type 2 diabetes in relation to insulin?
>
> What are three metabolic alterations related to hyperglycemia that contribute to diabetic complications?
>
> What is the single most important factor in the management of diabetes mellitus?

ALTERATIONS OF ADRENAL FUNCTION
Disorders of the Adrenal Cortex

Disorders of the adrenal cortex are related either to hyperfunction or to hypofunction. Hyperfunction that causes increased levels of circulating cortisol leads to Cushing disease or Cushing syndrome; that which causes increased secretion of adrenal androgens and estrogens leads to virilization or feminization; and that which causes increased levels of aldosterone leads to hyperaldosteronism, which may be primary or secondary. Hypofunction of the adrenal cortex leads to Addison disease, which has a variety of causal factors.

Hypercortical function (Cushing disease, Cushing syndrome)

Cushing syndrome refers to chronic **hypercortisolism** with or without pituitary involvement. *Cushing disease* refers specifically to pituitary-dependent hypercortisolism usually from a pituitary adenoma. Use of exogenous corticosteroids is the most common cause of Cushing syndrome.[66]

Adrenocorticotropic hormone–induced Cushing disease is more common in adults and is two to three times more common in women than in men. Cushing syndrome resulting from ectopic ACTH secretion is more common in older adults, particularly men. Adrenal tumors, rather than pituitary tumors, are more common in children, especially girls. Cushing syndrome can be found in any age but usually occurs between 30 and 50 years of age.

⬛ *Pathophysiology*

Hypercortisolism involving excessive circulating ACTH results from various pathophysiologic alterations, such as (1) dysregulation of hypothalamic or anterior pituitary hormones and (2) autonomous, ectopic ACTH secretion by a tumor outside the pituitary, usually a malignant tumor such as an oat cell carcinoma of the lung. Whatever the cause, two observations consistently apply to individuals with Cushing syndrome: (1) they do not have diurnal or circadian secretion patterns of ACTH and cortisol and (2) they do not increase ACTH and cortisol secretion in response to a stressor.[67] In individuals with ACTH-stimulated hypercorticoadrenalism, secretion of both cortisol and adrenal androgens is increased and cortisol-releasing hormone is inhibited. Hormone-secreting tumors of the adrenal cortex, however, generally secrete only cortisol. When the secretion of cortisol by the tumor exceeds normal cortisol levels, symptoms of hypercortisolism develop.

⬛ *Clinical Manifestations*

Weight gain is the most common feature and results from the accumulation of adipose tissue in the trunk, facial, and cervical areas. These characteristic patterns of fat deposition have been described as "truncal obesity," "moon face," and "buffalo hump" (Figs. 18-11 and 18-12). Transient weight gain from sodium and water retention also may be present.

Glucose intolerance occurs because of cortisol-induced insulin resistance and increased gluconeogenesis and glycogen storage by the liver. Overt diabetes mellitus develops in approximately 20% of individuals with hypercortisolism. Polyuria is a manifestation of hyperglycemia and resultant glycosuria.

Protein wasting is caused by the catabolic effects of cortisol on peripheral tissues. Muscle wasting leads to muscle weakness. In bone, loss of the protein matrix leads to osteoporosis, with pathologic fractures, vertebral compression fractures, bone and back pain, kyphosis, and reduced height. Cortisol interferes with the action of GH in long bones. Children who present with short stature may be experiencing growth retardation related to Cushing syndrome rather than GH deficiency. Bone disease may contribute to hyper-

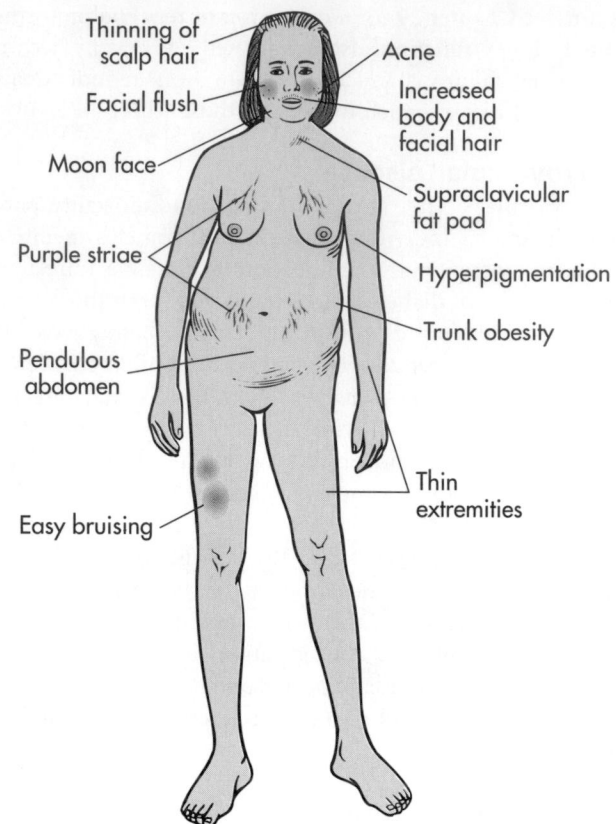

Fig. 18-11 *Symptoms of Cushing disease.*

Labels: Thinning of scalp hair; Facial flush; Moon face; Purple striae; Pendulous abdomen; Easy bruising; Acne; Increased body and facial hair; Supraclavicular fat pad; Hyperpigmentation; Trunk obesity; Thin extremities

calcinuria and resulting renal stones, which are experienced by approximately 20% of individuals with disease. Loss of collagen also leads to thin, weakened integumentary tissues through which capillaries are more visible and which are easily stretched by adipose deposits. Together, these changes account for the characteristic purple striae in the trunk area. Loss of collagenous support around small vessels makes them susceptible to rupture, leading to easy bruising, even with minor trauma. Thin, atrophied skin is also easily damaged, leading to skin breaks and ulcerations.

Hyperpigmentation in Cushing syndrome is associated with very high serum levels of ACTH. The pigmentation involves the mucous membranes, hair, and skin, all of which acquire a characteristic brownish or bronze color.

With elevated cortisol levels, vascular sensitivity to catecholamines is significantly increased, leading to vasoconstriction and hypertension. Mineralocorticoid effects promote sodium retention and hypokalemia. Elevated blood pressure occurs in most individuals with Cushing syndrome. Suppression of the immune system and increased susceptibility to infections also occur.

Approximately 50% of individuals with Cushing syndrome experience alterations in their mental status that range from irritability and depression to severe psychiatric disturbances, such as schizophrenia.[68] Females may experience symptoms of increased adrenal androgen levels, increased hair growth (especially facial hair), acne, and oligomenor-

Fig. 18-12 *Cushing syndrome.* **A,** Preoperatively. **B,** Six months postoperatively. *(From Thibodeau, G.A. [1987].* Anatomy and physiology. *St. Louis: Mosby.)*

rhea. Rarely do androgen levels become high enough to cause changes of the voice, recession of the hairline, and clitoral hypertrophy unless an adrenal carcinoma is involved. Routine laboratory examinations may reveal hyperglycemia, glycosuria, hypokalemia, and metabolic alkalosis.

Evaluation and Treatment

Various laboratory tests must be used to diagnose Cushing syndrome, including urinary free cortisol (17-hydroxycorticosterol) higher than 100 μg/24 hr and plasma cortisol obtained late in the evening higher than 20 μg/dl. A dexamethasone suppression test may be used to confirm the diagnosis and determine the cause.

Without treatment, approximately 50% of individuals with Cushing syndrome die within 5 years of onset as a result of overwhelming infection, suicide, complications from generalized arteriosclerosis, and hypertensive disease. Treatment is specific for the cause of hypercorticoadrenalism and includes medication, radiation, and surgery. Therefore differentiation among pituitary, adrenal, and ectopic causes of the hypercortisolism is essential for effective treatment.

Congenital adrenal hyperplasia

Congenital adrenal hyperplasia results from a deficiency of an enzyme, 21-hydroxylase, that is required for cortisol synthesis. ACTH increases and stimulates adrenal hyperplasia. The 21-hydroxylase deficiency results in masculinization of the female fetus. The adrenal hyperplasia results in salt wasting.

Hyperaldosteronism

Hyperaldosteronism is characterized by excessive aldosterone secretion by the adrenal glands. This can result from a primary adrenal disorder, such as an aldosterone-secreting adenoma, or from excessive stimulation of the normal adrenal cortex by angiotensin, ACTH, or elevated potassium. Hyperaldosteronism may be primary or secondary. In *primary hyperaldosteronism,* excessive secretion of aldosterone is caused by an abnormality of the adrenal cortex. In *secondary hyperaldosteronism,* excessive aldosterone secretion results from an extraadrenal stimulus, most frequently renin-angiotensin.

Primary hyperaldosteronism (Conn disease, primary aldosteronism) presents with hypertension, renal potassium wasting, hypokalemia, and neuromuscular manifestations.[69] The most common cause of primary aldosteronism is a benign, single adrenal adenoma. Adrenal carcinomas and unknown causes account for the remainder of cases. The incidence of primary hyperaldosteronism is estimated to be 1% to 2% of all hypertensive individuals.

Because aldosterone secretion normally is stimulated by the renin-angiotensin system, secondary hyperaldosteronism results from sustained elevated renin release and activation of angiotensin. (Factors that affect renin and aldosterone secretion are summarized in Table 18-9.) This occurs in various situations, including decreased circulating blood volume (e.g., in dehydration, shock, or hypoalbuminemia) and decreased delivery of blood to the kidneys (e.g., renal artery stenosis, heart failure, or hepatic cirrhosis). Here, the

TABLE 18-9	Physiologic Factors Affecting Renin and Aldosterone Secretion	
Factors	Renin Secretion	Aldosterone Secretion
Age	Highest in infants; lowest in the aged	Highest in infants
Menstrual cycle	Highest in luteal phase (see Chapter 17)	Highest in luteal phase
Sodium intake	Increased by salt restriction Decreased by salt loading	Increased by salt restriction Decreased by salt loading
Potassium status	Increased by K^+ depletion	Decreased by K^+ depletion
Posture	Increased with erect posture	Increased with erect posture
Sympathetic nervous stimulation	Increased by catecholamines	Increased through renin secretion
Time of sampling	Highest before noon; lowest in evening	Diurnal rhythm (as for adrenocorticotropic hormone [ACTH])

activation of the renin-angiotensin system and subsequent aldosterone secretion may be seen as compensatory, although in some instances (e.g., congestive heart failure), the increased circulating volume further worsens the condition.

Other causes of secondary hyperaldosteronism are Bartter syndrome, in which the underlying disorder is a renal tubular defect leading to hypokalemia, and renin-secreting tumors of the kidney.

≋ Pathophysiology

In primary hyperaldosteronism, pathophysiologic alterations are caused by excessive aldosterone secretion and the fluid and electrolyte imbalances that ensue. Hyperaldosteronism promotes (1) increased renal sodium and water reabsorption with corresponding hypervolemia (see Chapter 4) and (2) renal excretion of potassium. The extracellular fluid volume overload and suppression of normal feedback mechanisms of renin secretion are characteristic of primary disorders. Edema usually does not occur with primary aldosteronism, because hypervolemia-induced atrial natriuretic factor release results in loss of sodium and water.

In secondary hyperaldosteronism, the effect of increased extracellular volume on renin secretion may vary. If renin secretion is being stimulated by variables other than pressure-initiated cellular changes at the juxtaglomerular apparatus (see Chapter 25), increased circulating blood volume may not decrease renin secretion through feedback mechanisms. This process occurs, for instance, in states of increased estrogen levels.

Potassium secretion is promoted by aldosterone, so that with excessive aldosterone, hypokalemia occurs (see Chapter 4). Hypokalemic alkalosis, changes in myocardial conduction, and skeletal muscle alterations may be seen, particularly with severe potassium depletion. The renal tubules may become insensitive to ADH, thus promoting excessive loss of free water. In this situation, hypernatremia also may occur because water is not able to follow the sodium that is reabsorbed.

≋ Clinical Manifestations

Hypertension and hypokalemia are the hallmarks of hyperaldosteronism. With sustained hypertension, the chronic effects of elevated arterial pressure become evident, for example, left ventricular hypertrophy and progressive arteriosclerosis. Aldosterone-stimulated potassium loss can be substantial, resulting in typical manifestations of hypokalemia. Hypokalemic alkalosis may develop.

≋ Evaluation and Treatment

Various clinical and laboratory measurements are useful in assessing hyperaldosteronism. Tests include the following:
1. Blood pressure: elevated
2. Serum and urinary electrolyte levels: serum sodium is normal or elevated; serum potassium is depressed, but urinary potassium is elevated
3. Serum and urinary levels of aldosterone: increases
4. Aldosterone suppression testing: fludrocortisone acetate (Florinef) is used

Imaging techniques, including CT scans and nuclear magnetic resonance (NMR), may be used to localize an aldosterone-secreting adenoma.

Treatment includes management of hypertension and hypokalemia, as well as correction of any underlying causal abnormalities. If an aldosterone-secreting adenoma is present, it must be surgically removed.[70]

Hypersecretion of adrenal androgens and estrogens

Hypersecretion of adrenal androgens and estrogens may be caused by adrenal tumors, either adenomas or carcinomas, Cushing syndrome, or defects in steroid synthesis. The clinical syndrome that results depends on the hormone secreted, the gender of the individual, and the ages at which the hypersecretion is initiated. Hypersecretion of estrogens causes *feminization,* the development of female sex characteristics. Hypersecretion of androgens causes *virilization,* the development of male sex characteristics (Fig. 18-13).

Fig. 18-13 *Virilization.* Virilization of a young girl by a virilizing tumor of the adrenal cortex. The tumor secretes excess androgens, thereby producing masculinizing adrenogenital syndrome. *(From Thibodeau, G.A. [1987]. Anatomy and physiology. St. Louis: Mosby.)*

The effects of an estrogen-secreting tumor are most evident in males and result in gynecomastia (98% of cases), testicular atrophy, and decreased libido. In female children, such tumors may lead to early development of secondary sex characteristics. The changes caused by an androgen-secreting tumor are more easily observed in females and include excessive face and body hair growth, hirsutism, clitoral enlargement, deepening of the voice, amenorrhea, acne, and breast atrophy. In children, virilizing tumors promote precocious sexual development and bone aging. Treatment of androgen-secreting tumors usually involves surgical excision.

Hypocortical functioning

Hypocortisolism (low levels of cortisol secretion) develops because of either inadequate stimulation of the adrenal glands by ACTH or a primary inability of the adrenals to produce and secrete the adrenocortical hormones. Sometimes there is partial dysfunction of the adrenal cortex, so only synthesis of aldosterone or the adrenal androgens is affected. Hypofunction of the adrenal cortex may affect glucocorticoid or mineralocorticoid secretion or both.

Primary adrenal insufficiency is termed *Addison disease.* It is relatively rare, occurring most often in adults ages 30 to 60 years, although it may appear at any time. Addison disease is caused by autoimmune mechanisms and is more common in women.

🔲 *Pathophysiology*

Addison disease is characterized by elevated serum ACTH levels with inadequate corticosteroid and mineralocorticoid synthesis. The most common cause is idiopathic autoimmune disease. Other causes include familial adrenal insufficiency, amyloidosis, metastatic destruction of the adrenal glands, adrenal hemorrhage, and infections. Before clinical manifestations of hypocortisolism are evident, more than 90% of total adrenocortical tissue must be destroyed.

Idiopathic Addison disease

Idiopathic Addison disease (organ-specific autoimmune adrenalitis) causes adrenal atrophy and hypofunction and is an organ-specific autoimmune disease. Autoantibodies are present in 50% to 70% of individuals with idiopathic Addison disease, and this percentage increases in younger persons and in those with other autoimmune diseases. Apparently, a genetic defect in immune surveillance mechanisms causes a deficiency of immune suppressor cells and this deficiency allows the proliferation of immunocytes directed against specific antigens within the adrenocortical cells.[71]

Idiopathic Addison disease is frequently associated with other autoimmune diseases, especially Hashimoto thyroiditis, pernicious anemia, and idiopathic hypoparathyroidism. In these cases, Addison disease may be inherited as an autosomal recessive trait.[72] (Mechanisms of inheritance are described in Chapter 2.)

The adrenal glands in idiopathic Addison disease are smaller than normal and may be misshapen. Extensive diffuse cortical lymphocytic infiltrate supports the immune component of the disease process.

Secondary hypocortisolism

Secondary hypocortisolism is characterized by low to absent ACTH levels, causing inadequate adrenal stimulation, adrenal atrophy, and ultimately decreased corticosteroidogenesis. The exogenous administration of glucocorticoids for nonendocrine disease causes this form of hypocortisolism. Cortisol-producing endocrine tumors also cause secondary hypocortisolism. The increased glucocorticoid levels suppress ACTH production through normal feedback mechanisms. With decreased ACTH levels, corticosteroid synthesis by the adrenal gland is suppressed but corticosteroid levels remain high because the alteration in cortisol secretion lies outside the regulatory feedback loop. Pituitary hypofunction, as occurs in postpartum pituitary infarction (Sheehan syndrome) and panhypopituitarism, hypophysectomy, or isolated ACTH deficiency, causes inadequate ACTH production and secretion and absence of pituitary responsiveness to normal feedback mechanisms. In all instances of low ACTH levels, adrenal atrophy occurs and endogenous adrenal steroidogenesis is depressed.

TABLE 18-10	Clinical Manifestations and Pathophysiologic Mechanisms of Addison Disease
Clinical Manifestations	**Pathophysiologic Mechanism**
Weakness and easy fatigability that worsens as the day progresses, seen especially after exposure to stressors	Not known, may be related to hypoglycemia, decreased metabolism of proteins
Gastrointestinal disturbances: anorexia, nausea, vomiting, diarrhea, abdominal pain	Not known
Hypoglycemia, manifested by fatigue, mental confusion, apathy, psychosis	Absence of cortisol leads to decreased gluconeogenesis, decreased glycogen storage by liver, decreased metabolism of proteins, increased insulin sensitivity
Hyperpigmentation (seen only in cases of Addison disease with increased ACTH)	Increased secretion of ACTH is accompanied by increased secretion of beta-lipotropin and melanocyte-stimulating hormone; both hormones induce pigment changes in epithelial cells
Vitiligo: white patchy areas of depigmented skin	Autoimmune destruction of melanocytes
Hypotension	Decreased blood volume resulting from hypoaldosteronism causing increased renal sodium losses
Addisonian crisis: severe hypotension and vascular collapse	Combined effects of hypocortisolism, hypoaldosteronism, extracellular volume depletion, and some precipitating stressor (e.g., infection, vomiting, diarrhea)

ACTH, *Adrenocorticotropic hormone.*

Clinical manifestations of secondary hypocortisolism are similar to those of Addison disease, although hyperpigmentation usually does not occur. The renin-angiotensin system usually is normal, so aldosterone and potassium levels also tend to be normal.

Clinical Manifestations

The symptoms of Addison disease are primarily a result of hypocortisolism and hypoaldosteronism. They are summarized in Table 18-10.

Evaluation and Treatment

Serum and urine levels of cortisol, aldosterone, and 17-ketosteroids are all depressed with hypocortisolism. ACTH levels may be increased if there is adrenocortical insufficiency. Because of dehydration, blood urea nitrogen levels and hematocrit levels are increased. Serum glucose is low. Eosinophil and lymphocyte counts frequently are elevated. Hyperkalemia may cause mild alkalosis (see Chapter 4). The ACTH stimulation test may be used to evaluate adrenocortical function.

The treatment of Addison disease involves glucocorticoid and possibly mineralocorticoid replacement therapy, together with dietary modifications. All individuals with hypocortisolism require long-term daily glucocorticoid replacement therapy. With acute stressors, additional cortisol must be administered to approximate the amount of cortisol that might be expected if normal adrenal function were present (approximately 100 to 300 μg/day).

The individual's diet should include at least 150 mEq sodium per day, with sodium intake increased with excessive sweating or diarrhea. Treatment also must include correction of any underlying disorders, such as tuberculosis.

Disorders of the Adrenal Medulla
Tumor of the adrenal medulla

Pheochromocytoma is a catecholamine-producing tumor usually derived from the adrenal medullary cells. Fewer than 10% of these tumors metastasize; if they do, they are usually found in the lungs, liver, bones, or paraaortic lymph glands. Most pheochromocytomas produce norepinephrine, although large tumors secrete both epinephrine and norepinephrine. These tumors are rare (2 to 8 cases per million) and are most common in people in their 40s and 50s, with men and women equally affected.[73]

Pathophysiology

Pheochromocytomas cause excessive production of catecholamines. Other causes of elevated levels of catecholamines include defects in the normal inhibition of tyrosine hydroxylase or defects in the control mechanisms responsible for regulating catecholamine synthesis and release. Approximately 5% of people with pheochromocytomas have no symptoms, apparently because the tumor is nonfunctioning. Such tumors can, however, release catecholamines, especially in response to a stressor.

Clinical Manifestations

The clinical manifestations of a pheochromocytoma are related to the chronic effects of catecholamine secretion and include persistent hypertension associated with flushing, diaphoresis, tachycardia, and palpitations. Hypertension results from increased peripheral vascular resistance and may be sustained or paroxysmal. Headaches appear because of sudden changes in catecholamine levels in the blood, affecting cerebral blood flow. Hypermetabolism may be related to increased thyroid hormone levels resulting from stimulation of the thyroid gland by the catecholamines. Glucose intolerance may occur because of catecholamine-induced inhibition of insulin release by the pancreas. Complaints of warmth, heat intolerance, and weight loss are common despite a normal-to-increased appetite. Other symptoms of catecholamine excess include excessive sweating, palpitations and tachycardia, and gastrointestinal alterations, especially constipation.

An acute episode of hypertension related to hypersecretion of catecholamines may follow specific events, such as exercise, excessive ingestion of tyrosine-containing foods (aged cheese, red wine, beer, yogurt), ingestion of caffeine-containing foods, external pressure on the tumor, and induction of anesthesia. These tumors tend to be extremely vascular and can rupture, causing massive and potentially fatal hemorrhage. Rupture is characterized by a sudden, unexplained decrease in blood pressure; sudden, severe abdominal pain; and a rigid abdomen.

Evaluation and Treatment

A diagnosis of pheochromocytoma is made when increased catecholamine production is demonstrated in the blood or urine. After elevation of urinary or plasma catecholamines is documented, the site of the tumor is determined using radiographic techniques and surgical exploration of the abdomen. Because of the possibility of metastasis, whole-body scanning may be done.

The usual treatment of pheochromocytoma is surgical excision of the tumor. Medical therapy is used to stabilize blood pressure before, during, or after surgery.

✓ QUICK CHECK

What are the symptoms of hyperaldosteronism?

What major diseases are classified as hypocortisolism?

◼ DID YOU UNDERSTAND?

Mechanisms of Hormonal Alterations

1. Abnormalities in endocrine function may be caused by hypersecretion or hyposecretion of hormones, causing alterations in normal hormone levels.
2. Endocrine abnormalities also may be caused by alterations in receptor function through a variety of mechanisms: (a) a decrease in number of receptors, (b) receptor insensitivity to the hormone, (c) antibodies against specific receptors, and (d) general receptor dysfunction.
3. Abnormally high levels of circulating hormones are sometimes caused by hormone release from tissues outside the endocrine system (ectopic foci), which may not respond to normal feedback mechanisms, in which case they are said to function autonomously.

Alterations of the Hypothalamic-Pituitary System

1. Dysfunction in the release of hypothalamic hormones is probably related to interruption of the connection between the hypothalamus and pituitary, the infundibular stem.
2. Disorders of the posterior pituitary include syndrome of inappropriate ADH secretion (SIADH) and diabetes insipidus. SIADH secretion is characterized by abnormally high ADH secretion; diabetes insipidus is characterized by abnormally low ADH secretion.
3. In SIADH, high ADH levels interfere with renal function, leading to hyponatremia and hypoosmolality. SIADH secretion is associated with certain forms of cancer, apparently because of ectopic secretion of ADH by tumor cells.
4. Diabetes insipidus may be neurogenic, caused by insufficient amounts of ADH, or nephrogenic, caused by an inadequate response to ADH. Its principal clinical features are polyuria and polydipsia.
5. Hypopituitarism is dysfunction of the anterior pituitary that causes failure of hormonal functions. Symptoms may be mild to severe.
6. The most common cause of hypopituitarism is pituitary infarction, in which an initiating event leads to circulatory collapse and compensatory vasospasm. Pregnant and postpartum women are most at risk for pituitary infarction.
7. Hyperpituitarism is caused by pituitary adenomas. These are usually benign, slow-growing tumors that arise from cells of the anterior pituitary.
8. Expansion of a pituitary adenoma causes both neurologic and secretory effects. Pressure from the expanding tumor causes hyposecretion of cells, dysfunction of the optic chiasma (leading to visual disturbances), and dysfunction of the hypothalamus and some cranial nerves.
9. Hypersecretion of growth hormone (GH) causes giantism or acromegaly depending on the age at which GH secretion becomes high and unpredictable. Pituitary adenoma is the most common cause of acromegaly.
10. Prolonged, abnormally high levels of GH lead to skeletal growth in children and bone and connective tissue proliferation in adults.

Alterations of Thyroid Function

1. Thyrotoxicosis is a general condition in which thyroid hormone (TH) levels cause greater-than-normal physiologic responses. The condition can be caused by a variety of specific diseases, each of which has its own pathophysiology and course of treatment.
2. In general, hyperthyroidism has a range of en-

Continued

◼ DID YOU UNDERSTAND? —cont'd

Alterations of Thyroid Function—cont'd

docrine, reproductive, gastrointestinal, integumentary, and ocular manifestations. These are caused by increased circulating levels of TH and by stimulation of the sympathetic division of the autonomic nervous system.

3. Graves disease, the most common form of hyperthyroidism, is probably caused by an autoimmune mechanism that overrides normal mechanisms for control of TH secretion.

4. Toxic nodular goiter and toxic multinodular goiter occur when TH-regulating mechanisms and abnormal hypertrophy of the thyroid gland cause hyperthyroidism. Toxic multinodular goiter is caused by independently functioning follicular cells diffused throughout the thyroid gland.

5. Thyrotoxic crisis is a severe form of hyperthyroidism that is often associated with physiologic or psychologic stress. Without treatment, death occurs quickly.

6. Hypothyroidism is caused by deficient production of TH by the thyroid gland. The condition may be primary or secondary, and symptoms depend on the degree of TH deficiency. Common manifestations include decreased energy metabolism, heat production, and myxedema.

7. Acute thyroiditis, a form of hypothyroidism, is inflammation of the thyroid gland, often caused by a bacterium.

8. Subacute thyroiditis, a form of hypothyroidism, is a self-limiting nonbacterial inflammation of the thyroid gland. The inflammatory process damages follicular cells, causing leakage of T_3 and T_4. Hyperthyroidism then is followed by transient hypothyroidism, which is corrected by cellular repair and a return to normal levels in the thyroid.

9. Autoimmune thyroiditis is associated with infiltration or fibrosis of the thyroid, circulating thyroid antibodies, and gradual loss of thyroid function. Autoimmune thyroiditis occurs in those individuals with genetic susceptibility to an autoimmune mechanism that causes thyroid damage and eventual hypothyroidism.

10. Myxedema coma is a severe form of hypothyroidism that may be life threatening without emergency medical treatment.

11. Congenital hypothyroidism is absence of thyroid tissue during fetal development or defects in hormone synthesis.

12. Thyroid carcinoma is a relatively rare cancer. The most consistent causal risk factor associated with thyroid carcinoma is exposure to ionizing radiation, especially in childhood.

Alterations of Parathyroid Function

1. Hyperparathyroidism, which may be primary, secondary, or tertiary, is characterized by greater than normal secretion of parathyroid hormone (PTH).

2. Primary hyperparathyroidism is caused by an interruption of the normal mechanisms that regulate calcium and PTH levels. Manifestations include chronic hypercalcemia, increased bone resorption, and hypercalciuria.

3. Secondary hyperparathyroidism is a compensatory response to hypocalcemia and often occurs with chronic renal failure.

4. Tertiary hyperparathyroidism is associated with hyperplasia of the parathyroid glands and a loss of the regulatory mechanism that governs PTH and calcium levels.

5. Hypoparathyroidism, defined by abnormally low PTH levels, is caused by thyroid surgery or by hereditary mechanisms.

6. The lack of circulating PTH in hypoparathyroidism causes depressed serum calcium levels, increased serum phosphate levels, decreased bone resorption, and eventual hypocalciuria.

Dysfunction of the Endocrine Pancreas: Diabetes Mellitus

1. Diabetes mellitus is a complex syndrome that causes a number of physiologic changes, some of which are metabolic processes and others of which are vascular.

2. A diagnosis of diabetes mellitus is based on elevated plasma glucose concentrations. Classic signs and symptoms are often present as well.

3. The two most common types of diabetes mellitus are type 1 and type 2, also called insulin-dependent diabetes mellitus (IDDM) and non-insulin-dependent diabetes mellitus (NIDDM).

4. Type 1 diabetes mellitus is characterized by loss of beta cells, islet cell antibody, a lack of insulin, and a relative excess of glucagon, which causes improper metabolism of fat, protein, and carbohydrates.

5. Type 1 diabetes mellitus seems to be caused by a gradual process of autoimmune destruction of beta cells in genetically susceptible individuals.

6. In type 1 diabetes mellitus, decreased use of glucose causes glucose accumulation in the blood and subsequent loss in the urine. This in turn causes polyuria and polydipsia resulting from osmotic diuresis.

7. Ketoacidosis, caused by increased levels of circulating ketones without the inhibiting effects of insulin; increased levels of circulating fatty acids; and weight loss are all manifestations of type 1 uncontrolled diabetes mellitus.

8. Type 2 diabetes mellitus is probably caused by genetic susceptibility that is triggered by environmental factors. The most compelling environmental risk factor is obesity.

9. In the obese, insulin has a diminished ability to influence glucose uptake and metabolism.

10. Some insulin production continues in type 2 dia-

DID YOU UNDERSTAND? —cont'd

betes mellitus, but the weight and number of beta cells decrease. There are dysfunctional levels of both insulin and glucagon.

11. Gestational diabetes is glucose intolerance during pregnancy.

12. Acute complications of diabetes mellitus include hypoglycemia, diabetic ketoacidosis, hyperosmolar hyperglycemic nonketotic coma, the Somogyi effect, and the dawn phenomenon.

13. Hypoglycemia is a complication related to insulin treatment.

14. Diabetic ketoacidosis develops when there is an absolute or relative deficiency of insulin and an increase in the insulin counterregulatory hormones of catecholamines, cortisol, glucagon, and growth hormone.

15. Hyperosmolar hyperglycemic nonketotic coma is pathophysiologically similar to diabetic ketoacidosis, although levels of free fatty acids are lower in hyperosmolar nonacidotic diabetes and lack of ketosis indicates that some level of insulin is present.

16. The Somogyi effect is a rebound hyperglycemia. It is treated by decreasing the nocturnal insulin dose to prevent the earlier hypoglycemia episode from occurring.

17. The dawn phenomenon is an early morning rise in glucose levels caused by insulin waning.

18. Chronic sequelae of diabetes mellitus include diabetic neuropathies, microvascular disease (e.g., retinopathy, nephropathy), macrovascular disease (e.g., coronary artery disease, stroke, peripheral vascular disease), and infection.

19. Microangiopathy is caused by thickening of the capillary basement membrane and eventual decreased tissue perfusion affecting the microcirculation.

20. Macrovascular disease associated with diabetes mellitus is probably related to the proliferation of fibrous plaques in the arterial wall and to elevated lipid levels.

21. Incidence of coronary heart disease, peripheral vascular disease, and stroke is greater in those with diabetes than in nondiabetic individuals.

22. Individuals with diabetes are at risk for a variety of infections.

23. Infection may be related to sensory impairment and resulting injury, hypoxia, increased proliferation of pathogens in elevated concentrations of glucose, decreased blood supply associated with vascular damage, and impaired white cell function.

Alterations of Adrenal Function

1. Disorders of the adrenal cortex are related to hyperfunction or hypofunction. No known disorders are associated with hypofunction of the adrenal medulla, but medullary hyperfunction causes clinically defined syndromes.

2. Cortical hyperfunction, or hypercortisolism, causes Cushing syndrome, which may or may not involve the pituitary gland, and Cushing disease, which is hypercortisolism with pituitary involvement.

3. Congenital adrenal hyperplasia results from deficiency of α hydroxylase required for cortisol synthesis.

4. Excessive aldosterone secretion causes hyperaldosteronism, which may be primary or secondary. Primary hyperaldosteronism is caused by an abnormality of the adrenal cortex. Secondary hyperaldosteronism involves an extraadrenal stimulus, often angiotensin.

5. Hyperaldosteronism promotes increased sodium reabsorption, corresponding hypervolemia, increased extracellular volume (which is variable), and hypokalemia related to renal reabsorption of sodium.

6. Hypersecretion of adrenal androgens and estrogens can be a result of adrenal tumors, either adenomas or carcinomas. Hypersecretion of estrogens causes feminization, the development of female sex characteristics. Hypersecretion of androgens causes virilization, the development of male sex characteristics.

7. Hypofunction of the adrenal cortex can affect glucocorticoid or mineralocorticoid secretion or both. Hypofunction can be caused by a deficiency of adrenal-stimulating substance or by a primary deficiency in the gland itself.

8. Hypocortisolism, or low levels of cortisol, is caused by inadequate adrenal stimulation by ACTH or by primary cortisol hyposecretion. Primary adrenal insufficiency is termed *Addison disease.*

9. Addison disease is characterized by elevated ACTH levels with inadequate corticosteroid synthesis and output.

10. Manifestations of Addison disease are related to hypocortisolism and hypoaldosteronism. Symptoms include weakness, fatigability, hypoglycemia and related metabolic problems, lowered response to stressors, vitiligo, and manifestations of hypovolemia and hyperkalemia.

11. Hyperfunction of the adrenal medulla is usually caused by a pheochromocytoma, a catecholamine-producing tumor. Symptoms of catecholamine excess are related to their sympathetic nervous system effects and include hypertension, palpitations, tachycardia, glucose intolerance, excessive sweating, and constipation.

KEY TERMS

Acromegaly, 475
Acute thyroiditis, 479
Addison disease (primary adrenal insufficiency), 497
Advanced glycosylation end-product (AGE), 491
Amylin, 488
Autoimmune thyroiditis (Hashimoto disease, chronic lymphocyte thyroiditis), 481
Congenital adrenal hyperplasia, 495
Cushing disease, 494
Cushing syndrome, 494
Dawn phenomenon, 491
Diabetes insipidus (antidiuretic hormone insufficiency), 472
Diabetes mellitus, 483
Diabetic ketoacidosis, 489
Diabetic neuropathy, 491
Diabetic retinopathy, 492
Feminization, 496
Gestational diabetes mellitus, 488

Giantism, 475
Glycosylated hemoglobin, 483
Graves disease, 477
Hyperaldosteronism, 495
Hypercortisolism, 494
Hyperosmolar nonacidotic diabetes, 489
Hyperparathyroidism, 482
Hypocortisolism, 497
Hypoglycemia, 489
Hypoparathyroidism, 483
Hypopituitarism, 473
Hypothyroidism, 479
Idiopathic Addison disease (organ-specific autoimmune adrenalitis), 497
Myxedema, 479
Myxedema coma, 481
Nonenzymatic glycosylation, 491
Nonketotic hyperglycemic hyperosmolar coma, 489
Panhypopituitarism, 474
Pheochromocytoma, 498
Pituitary adenoma, 475

Polyol pathway, 491
Primary hyperaldosteronism (Conn disease, primary aldosteronism), 495
Primary hyperparathyroidism, 482
Protein kinase C (PKC), 491
Secondary hyperaldosteronism, 495
Secondary hyperparathyroidism, 482
Secondary hypocortisolism, 497
Somogyi phenomenon, 490
Subacute thyroiditis, 479
Syndrome of inappropriate ADH secretion (SIADH), 472
Tertiary hyperparathyroidism, 482
Thyrotoxic crisis (thyroid storm), 478
Thyrotoxicosis, 477
Type 1 diabetes mellitus (insulin-dependent diabetes mellitus [IDDM]), 484
Type 2 diabetes mellitus (non-insulin-dependent diabetes mellitus [NIDDM]), 487
Virilization, 496

REFERENCES

1. Kovacs, L. & Robertson, G.L. (1992). Syndrome of inappropriate antidiuresis. *Endocrinology and Metabolism Clinics of North America, 21*(4), 859-875.
2. Besser, G.M. & Thorner, M.O. (1994). *Clinical endocrinology* (2nd ed.). St. Louis: Mosby.
3. Chan, T.Y. (1997). Drug-induced syndrome of inappropriate antidiuretic hormone secretion: Causes, diagnosis, and management. *Drugs and Aging, 11*(1), 27-44.
4. Gross, P. et al. (1998). The treatment of severe hyponatremia. *Kidney International Supplement, 64,* S6-S11.
5. Baylis, P.H. & Cheetham, T. (1998). Diabetes insipidus. *Archives of Diseases in Children, 79*(1), 84-89.
6. Oksche, A. & Rosenthal, W. (1998). The molecular basis of nephrogenic diabetes insipidus. *Journal of Molecular Medicine, 76*(5), 326-237.
7. Bell, R.N. (1994). Diabetes insipidus. *Critical Care Nursing Clinics of North America, 6*(4), 675-685.
8. Lamberts, S.W., de Herder, W.W., & van der Leyl, A.J. (1998). Pituitary insufficiency. *Lancet, 352*(9122), 127-134.
9. Reid, R.L., Quigley, M.E., & Yen, S.S.C. (1985). Pituitary apoplexy. *Archives of Neurology, 42,* 712-719.
10. Bardin, W.C. (1997). *Current therapy in endocrinology and metabolism.* St. Louis: Mosby.
11. Melmed, S. (1995). Acromegaly. In S. Melmed. *The pituitary.* Cambridge, Mass.: Blackwell Scientific Publications.

12. Ezzat, S. (1997). Acromegaly. *Endocrinology and Metabolism Clinics of North America, 26*(4), 703-723.
13. Felig, P., Baxter, J.D., & Frohman, L.A. (1995). *Endocrinology and metabolism* (3rd ed.). New York: McGraw-Hill.
14. Melmed, S. et al. (1998). Current treatment guidelines for acromegaly. *Journal of Clinical Endocrinology and Metabolism, 83*(8), 2646-2652.
15. Braverman, L.E. & Utiger, R.D. (1991). Introduction to thyrotoxicosis. In S.L. Werner & S.H. Ingbar (Eds.). *The thyroid: A fundamental and clinical text.* Philadelphia: Lippincott.
16. Haddad, G. (1998). Is it hyperthyroidism? You can't always tell from the clinical picture. *Postgraduate Medicine, 104*(1), 42-44, 53-55, 59.
17. Dabon-Almirante, C.L. & Surks, M.I. (1998). Clinical and laboratory diagnosis of thyrotoxicosis. *Endocrinology and Metabolism Clinics of North America, 27*(1), 25-35.
18. McDougall, I.R. (1991). Graves disease. *Medical Clinics of North America, 75*(1), 79-96.
19. Gavin, L.A. (1991). Thyroid crises. *Medical Clinics of North America, 75*(1), 179-193.
20. Williams, R.H. & Wilson, J.D. (1998). *Williams textbook of endocrinology* (9th ed.). Philadelphia: Saunders.
21. Mulder, J.E. (1998). Thyroid disease in women. *Medical Clinics of North America, 82*(1), 103-125.

REFERENCES

22. Zulewiski, H. et al. (1997). Estimation of tissue hypothyroidism by a new clinical score: Evaluation of tissue hypothyroidism by a new clinical score: Evaluation of patient's various grades of hypothyroidism and controls. *Journal of Endocrinology and Metabolism, 82,* 771-776.

23. Klett, M. (1997). Epidemiology of congenital hypothyroidism. *Experimental and Clinical Endocrinology and Diabetes, 105*(Suppl. 4), 19-23.

24. Vogiatzi, M.G. & Kirkland, J.L. (1997). Frequency and necessity of thyroid function tests in neonates and infants with congenital hypothyroidism. *Pediatrics, 100*(3), E6.

25. American Cancer Society (ACS). (1999). *Cancer facts and figures—1999.* Atlanta: The Author.

26. Camargo, C.A. & Kolb, K.O. (1988). Endocrine disorders. In S.A. Schroeder, M.E. Krupp, & L.W. Tierney (Eds.). *Current medical diagnosis and treatment.* Norwalk, Conn.: Langer.

27. Stein, J.H. (1998). *Internal medicine* (5th ed.). St. Louis: Mosby.

28. Horwitz, M.S. & Bilezikian, J.P. (1994). Primary hyperparathyroidism and parathyroid hormone-related protein. *Current Opinions in Rheumatology, 6*(3), 321-328.

29. Mazzuoli, G.F., Erasmo, F., & Pisani, D. (1998). Primary hyperparathyroidism and osteoporosis. *Aging, 10*(30), 225-231.

30. Loh, K.C. et al. (1998). Clinical profile of primary hyperparathyroidism in adolescents and young adults. *Clinical Endocrinology (Oxford), 48*(4), 435-443.

31. Winer, K.K. et al. (1998). A randomized, cross-over trial of once-daily versus twice-daily parathyroid hormone 1-34 in treatment of hypoparathyroidism. *Journal of Endocrinology and Metabolism, 83*(10), 3480-3496.

32. Peters, A.L. & Schriger, D.L. (1998). The new diagnostic criteria for diabetes: The impact on management of diabetes and macrovascular risk factors. *American Journal of Medicine, 105*(1A), 15S-19S.

33. Bennett, P.H. (1997). Epidemiology of diabetes mellitus. In D. Porte & R.S. Sherwin (Eds.). *Diabetes mellitus* (5th ed.). New York: Elsevier.

34. Dahlquist, G. (1998). The aetiology of type 1 diabetes: An epidemiological perspective. *Acta Paediatrics Supplement, 425,* 5-10.

35. Clark, C.M. & Lee, D.A. (1995). Prevention and treatment of the complications of diabetes mellitus. *New England Journal of Medicine, 332*(18), 1210-1217.

36. Peters, A.L., for the Meta-analysis Research Group on the Diagnosis of Diabetes Using Glycated Hemoglobin Levels. (1996). A clinical approach for the diagnosis of diabetes mellitus: An analysis using glycosylated hemoglobin levels. *Journal of the American Medical Association, 276,* 1246-1252.

37. Pickup, J.C. & Williams, C. (1997). *Textbook of diabetes* (2nd ed.). Oxford: Blackwell.

38. Bloomgarden, Z.T. (1998). Insulin resistance: Current concepts. *Clinical Therapy, 20*(2), 216-232.

39. Clark, A. et al. (1991). Autoantibodies to islet amyloid polypeptide in diabetes. *Diabetic Medicine, 8*(7), 668-673.

40. Ferrannini, E. (1998). Insulin resistance versus insulin deficiency in non-insulin-dependent diabetes mellitus: Problems and prospects. *Endocrinology Review, 19*(4), 477-490.

41. Golay, A. & Felber, J.P. (1994). Evolution from obesity to diabetes. *Diabete et Metabolisme, 20*(1), 3-14.

42. Hunter, S.J. & Garvey, W.T. (1998). Insulin action and insulin resistance: Diseases involving defects in insulin receptors, signal transduction, and the glucose transport effector system. *American Journal of Medicine, 105*(4), 331-345.

43. Scherbaum, W.A. (1998). The role of amylin in the physiology of glycemic control. *Experimental and Clinical Endocrinology and Diabetes, 106*(2), 97-102.

44. Young, A. & Denaro, M. (1998). Roles of amylin in diabetes and in regulation of nutrient load [editorial]. *Nutrition, 14*(6), 524-527.

45. Salmeron, J. et al. (1997). Dietary fiber, glycemic load, and risk of non-insulin-dependent diabetes mellitus in women [see Comments]. *Journal of the American Medical Association, 277*(6), 472-477.

46. Salmeron, J. et al. (1997). Dietary fiber, glycemic load, and risk of NIDDM in men. *Diabetes Care, 20*(4), 545-550.

47. Genuth, S.M. (1997). Diabetic ketoacidosis and hyperglycemic hyperosmolar coma. *Current Theories in Endocrinology and Metabolism, 6,* 438-447.

48. Umpierrez, G.E., Khajavi, M., & Kitabachi, A.E. (1996). Review: Diabetic ketoacidosis and hyperglycemic hyperosmolar nonketotic syndrome. *American Journal of Medical Science, 311*(5), 225-233.

49. DeFronzo, R.A. (1998). *Current therapy of diabetes mellitus.* St. Louis: Mosby.

50. Kahn, C.R. & Weir, G.C. (1994). *Joslin's diabetes mellitus* (13th ed.). Philadelphia: Lea & Febiger.

51. Swidan, S.Z. & Montgomery, P.A. (1998). Effect of blood glucose concentrations on the development of chronic complications of diabetes mellitus. *Pharmacotherapy, 18*(5), 961-972.

52. Cooper, M.E. (1998). Pathogenesis, prevention, and treatment of diabetic neuropathy. *Lancet, 352*(19), 213-219.

53. Koya, D. & King, G.L. (1998). Protein kinase C activation in the development of diabetic complications. *Diabetes, 47*(6), 859-866.

54. Wunderlich, R.P. et al. (1998). Pathophysiology and treatment of painful diabetic neuropathy of the lower extremity. *Southern Medical Journal, 91*(10), 894-898.

REFERENCES

55. Mooradian, A.D. (1997). Pathophysiology of central nervous system. *Clinical Neuroscience, 4*(6), 322-326.

56. Dyck, P.J. & Thomas, P.K. (1999). *Diabetic neuropathy* (2nd ed.). Philadelphia: Saunders.

57. Laakso, M. & Lehto, S. (1998). Epidemiology of risk factors for cardiovascular disease in diabetes and impaired glucose tolerance. *Atherosclerosis, 137*(Suppl.), S65-S73.

58. Wautier, J.L. & Guillausseau, P.J. (1998). Diabetes, advanced glycation end-products and vascular disease. *Vascular Medicine, 3*(2), 131-137.

59. Kreisberg, R.A. (1998). Diabetic dyslipidemia. *American Journal of Cardiology, 82*(12A), 67U-73U.

60. Tinker, L.F. (1994). Diabetes mellitus—A priority health care issue for women. *Journal of the American Diabetic Association, 94*(9), 976-985.

61. Carter, A.M. & Grant, P.J. (1997). Vascular homeostasis, adhesion molecules, and macrovascular disease in non-insulin-dependent diabetes mellitus. *Diabetes Medicine, 14*(6), 423-432.

62. McMillan, D.E. (1990). The role of blood flow in diabetic vascular disease. In H. Rifkin & D. Porte (Eds.). *Diabetes mellitus theory and practice* (4th ed.). New York: Elsevier.

63. Fujii, S. (1997). Advances in the understanding of diabetic vascular disease. *Journal of Cardiovascular Risk, 4*(2), 67-69.

64. Diamantopoulos, E.J. et al. (1998). A. Management and outcome of severe diabetic foot infections. *Experimental Clinical Endocrinology and Diabetes, 106*(4), 346-352.

65. Frykberg, R.G. (1998). Diabetic foot ulcers: Current concepts. *Journal of Foot and Ankle Surgery, 37*(5), 440-406.

66. Porterfield, S.P. (1996). *Endocrine physiology.* St. Louis: Mosby.

67. Chabot, V. et al. (1998). Ectopic ACTH Cushing's syndrome: V3 vasopressin receptor but not CRH receptor gene expression in pulmonary carcinoid tumor. *Hormone Research, 50*(4), 226-231.

68. Sonino, N. et al. (1998). Clinical correlates of major depression in Cushing's disease. *Psychopathology, 31*(6), 302-306.

69. Gomez-Sanchez, C.E. (1998). Primary aldosteronism and its variants. *Cardiovascular Research, 37*(1), 8-13.

70. McAlister, F.A. & Lewanczuk, R.Z. (1998). Primary hyperaldosteronism and adrenal incidentaloma: An argument for physiologic testing before adrenalectomy. *Canadian Journal of Surgery, 41*(4), 299-305.

71. Wulffraat, N.M., Drexhage, H.A., & Bottazzo, G.F. (1992). Autoimmune aspects of Addison's disease. In V.H.T. James (Ed.). *The adrenal gland* (2nd ed.). New York: Raven.

72. Soderbergh, A. & Kampe, O. (1996). Adrenal autoantibodies and organ-specific autoimmunity in patients with Addison's disease. *Clinical Endocrinology (Oxford), 45*(4), 453-460.

73. Young, W.F. (1997). Pheochromocytoma and primary aldosteronism: Diagnostic approach. *Endocrinology and Metabolism Clinics of North America, 26*(4), 801-827.

CHAPTER

19

Structure and Function of the Hematologic System

Kathryn L. McCance

Blood cells act as vehicles—cells and chemicals—that travel along the tens of thousands
of miles of blood vessels packed into the human
body. Most cells are red blood cells that, like tanker
trucks, function as carriers; yet, red blood cells also
maneuver more like sports cars, flexing and deforming to squeeze through capillaries smaller than
their own diameters. White blood cells are spherical, larger than red blood cells, and less flexible.
They create more resistance and are much more
likely to create "traffic jams." White blood cells
avoid the small capillaries that red blood cells so ex-
pertly squeeze through. However, disease can
make the white cells "sticky," create traffic jams,
and cause the red cells to lose their cargo. These alterations can lead to difficulties in oxygenation,
acid-base balance, and immune function and, like a
major thoroughfare at rush hour, may alter stream-
line flow.

CHAPTER OUTLINE

COMPONENTS OF THE HEMATOLOGIC SYSTEM
Composition of Blood

Blood consists of various formed elements (cells and proteins) that circulate in the cardiovascular system suspended in plasma, which is approximately 90% water and 10% dissolved substances (solutes). All these elements constitute blood volume, which in adults amounts to about 6 quarts (5.5 L). Approximately 45% to 50% of blood volume consists of formed elements, and the remainder is plasma. The continuous movement of blood keeps the formed elements dispersed throughout the plasma, where they are available to carry out their chief functions: (1) delivery of substances needed for cellular metabolism in the tissues, (2) defense against invading microorganisms and injury, and (3) acid-base balance.

Plasma and plasma proteins

In adults, plasma accounts for 50% to 55% of blood volume (Fig. 19-1). *Plasma* is a complex aqueous liquid containing several organic and inorganic elements (Table 19-1). The concentration of these elements varies depending on diet, metabolic demand, hormones, and vitamins. Plasma differs from serum in that *serum* is plasma that has been altered in the laboratory to remove fibrinogen (a clotting factor) or some other element that is unwanted or unneeded in the sample.

In circulating plasma, the dominant elements by weight (7%) are the *plasma proteins.* These vary in structure and function but can be classified into three major groups, in order by greatest numbers: the *albumins, globulins (immunoglobulins* or gamma [γ-] globulins), and *clotting factors* (chiefly fibrinogen). Whereas immunoglobulins are synthesized by lymphocytes in the lymph nodes and other lymphoid tissues (see Chapter 5 and p. 510), the other plasma proteins are synthesized in the liver.

Albumin (concentration 4 g/dl) is essential for regulating the passage of water and solutes through the capillaries. Because albumin molecules are large and do not diffuse freely through the vascular endothelium, they provide the critical colloid osmotic or oncotic pressure that regulates the passage of water and solutes through the microcirculation (arterioles, capillaries, venules) (see Chapters 1 and 3). Wa-

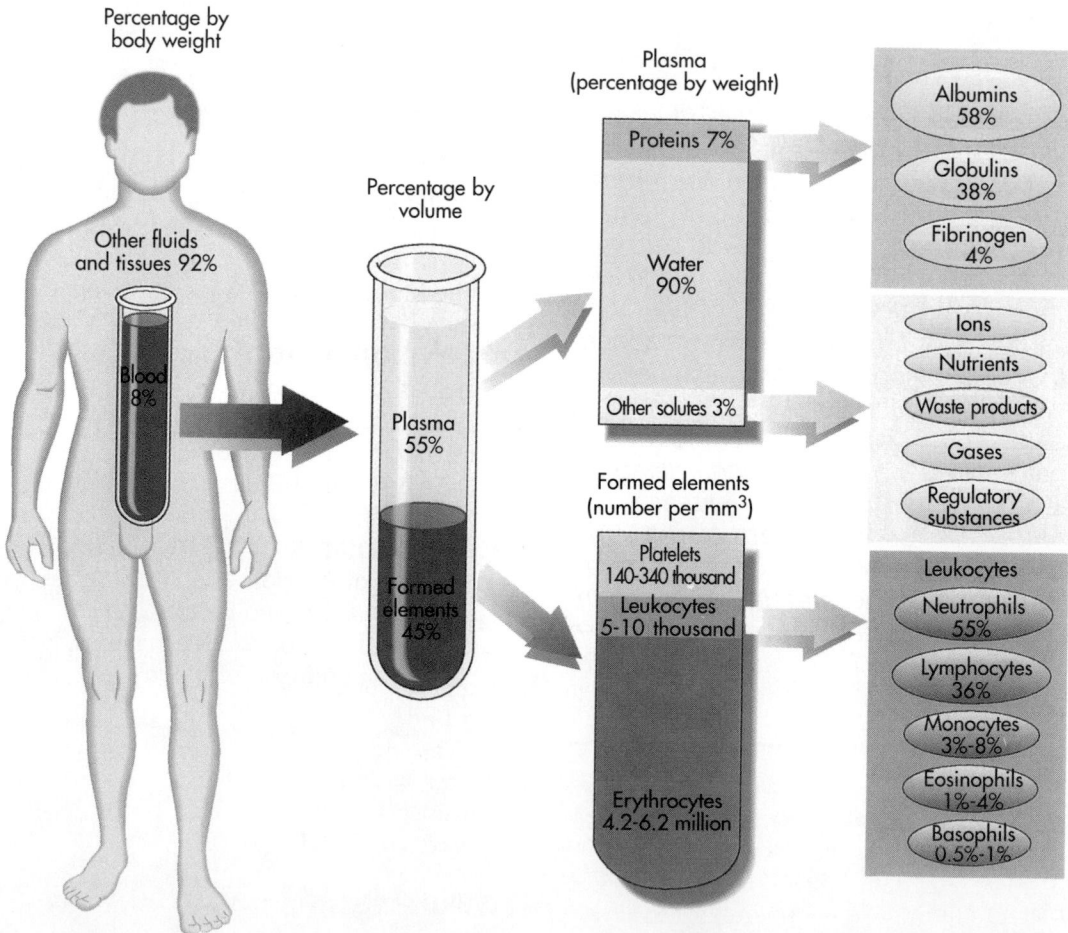

Fig. 19-1 *Composition of whole blood.* Approximate values for the components of blood in a normal adult. *(From Thibodeau, G.A. & Patton, K.T. [1999]. Anatomy & physiology [4th ed.]. St. Louis: Mosby.)*

TABLE 19-1 Organic and Inorganic Components of Arterial Plasma

Constituent	Amount/Concentration	Major Functions
Water	93% of plasma weight	Medium for carrying all other constituents
Electrolytes	Total <1% of plasma weight	Maintain H_2O in extracellular compartment; act as buffers; function in membrane excitability
Na^+	142 mEq/L (142 mM)	
K^+	4 mEq/L (4 mM)	
Ca^{++}	5 mEq/L (2.5 mM)	
Mg^{++}	3 mEq/L (1.5 mM)	
Cl^-	103 mEq/L (103 mM)	
HCO_3^-	27 mEq/L (27 mM)	
Phosphate (mostly HPO_4^{2-})	2 mEq/L (1 mM)	
SO_4^-	1 mEq/L (0.5 mM)	
Proteins	7.3 g/dl (2.5 mM)	Provide colloid osmotic pressure of plasma; act as buffers; bind other plasma constituents (lipids, hormones, vitamins, minerals, etc.); clotting factors; enzymes; enzyme precursors; antibodies (immunoglobulins); hormones; transporters
Albumins	4.5 g/dl	
Globulins	2.5 g/dl	
Fibrinogen	0.3 g/dl	
Transferrin	250 mg/dl	
Ferritin	15-300 mg/L	
Gases		
CO_2 content	22-20 mmol/L plasma	By-product of oxygenation, most CO_2 content is from HCO_3 and acts as a buffer
O_2	Pao_2 80 torr or greater (arterial); Pvo_2 30-40 torr (venous)	Oxygenation
N_2	0.9 ml/dl	By-product of protein catabolism
Nutrients		Provide nutrition and substances for tissue repair
Glucose and other carbohydrates	100 mg/dl (5.6 mM)	
Total amino acids	40 mg/dl (2 mM)	
Total lipids	500 mg/dl (7.5 mM)	
Cholesterol	150-250 mg/dl (4-7 mM)	
Individual vitamins	0.0001-2.5 mg/dl	
Individual trace elements	0.001-0.3 mg/dl	
Iron	50-150 mg/dl	
Waste products		
Urea (BUN)	7-18 mg/dl (5.7 mM)	End-product of protein catabolism
Creatinine (from creatine)	1 mg/dl (0.09 mM)	End-product from energy metabolism
Uric acid (from nucleic acids)	5 mg/dl (0.3 mM)	End-product from protein metabolism
Bilirubin (from heme)	0.2-1.2 mg/dl (0.003-0.018 mM)	End-product of red blood cell destruction
Individual hormones	0.000001-0.5 mg/dl	Functions specific to target tissue

Data from Vander, A.J., Sherman, J.H., & Luchiano, D.S. (1990). Human physiology: The mechanisms of body function. *New York: McGraw-Hill.*

ter and solute particles diffuse out of the arterial portions of the capillaries because blood pressure is greater in arterial than in venous blood vessels. Water and solutes move from tissue cells into the venous portions of the capillaries where the pressures are reversed, oncotic pressure being greater than intravascular pressure or hydrostatic pressure. Albumin also serves as a carrier molecule for both normal components of blood and exogenous agents, such as drugs.

The immunoglobulins, or antibodies, are synthesized by mature lymphocytes called *plasma cells* in the lymphoid organs, chiefly lymph nodes. The immunoglobulins (Ig) include IgA, IgG, IgM, IgD, and IgE. Most of them are critical for defense against infectious microorganisms (see Chapter 5).

The clotting factors promote coagulation and stop bleeding from damaged blood vessels. Fibrinogen is the most plentiful of the clotting factors and is the precursor of the fibrin clot (see p. 521. Other plasma proteins include complement proteins, a group of proteins involved in the immune response, various enzymes and their inhibitors, and specific carriers of such elements as iron and copper. The plasma lipids—triglycerides, phospholipids, cholesterol, and fatty acids—are carried through the blood as complexes with plasma proteins (*lipoproteins*) (see Chapters 1 and 22).

The electrolytes (electrically charged solutes) of the plasma maintain the osmolarity and pH of blood within a physiologic range (see Table 19-1). (Electrolytes are described in Chapters 1 and 3.)

Cellular components of the blood

The cellular elements of the blood are *broadly* classified as *erythrocytes (red blood cells), leukocytes (white blood cells),* and *platelets (thrombocytes).* The components of the blood are listed in Table 19-2.

TABLE 19-2 Cellular Components of the Blood

Cell	Structural Characteristics	Normal Amounts of Circulating Blood	Function	Life Span
Erythrocyte (red blood cell)	Nonnucleated cytoplasmic disk containing hemoglobin	4.2-6.2 million/mm³	Gas transport to and from tissue cells and lungs	80-120 days
Reticulocyte Absolute reticulocyte count		60,000 mm³ 0.5%-2.0% of erythrocytes		
Leukocyte (white blood cell)	Nucleated cell	5000-10,000/mm³	Body defense mechanisms	See below
Lymphocyte	Mononuclear immunocyte	25%-33% of leukocyte count (leukocyte differential)	Humoral and cell-mediated immunity (see Chapter 5)	Days or years depending on type
Monocyte and macrophage	Large mononuclear phagocyte	3%-7% of leukocyte differential	Phagocytosis; mononuclear phagocyte system	Months or years
Eosinophil	Segmented polymorphonuclear granulocyte	1%-4% of leukocyte differential	Phagocytosis, antibody-mediated defense against parasites, allergic reactions, associated with Hodgkin disease, recovery phase of infection	Unknown
Neutrophil	Segmented polymorphonuclear granulocyte	54%-67% of leukocyte differential	Phagocytosis, particularly during early phase of inflammation	4 days
Basophil	Segmented polymorphonuclear granulocyte	0%-0.75% of leukocyte differential	Unknown, but associated with allergic reactions and mechanical irritation	Unknown
Platelet	Irregularly shaped cytoplasmic fragment (not a cell)	140,000-340,000/mm³	Hemostasis after vascular injury; normal coagulation and clot formation/retraction	8-11 days

Erythrocytes

Erythrocytes are the most abundant cells of the blood, occupying approximately 48% of the blood volume in men and about 42% in women. Erythrocytes are primarily responsible for tissue oxygenation. The erythrocyte's cytoplasm consists of a solution containing protein (mostly **hemoglobin [Hb],** which carries the gases) and electrolytes, which regulate diffusion through the cell's plasma membrane. The mature erythrocyte lacks cytoplasmic organelles, so it cannot synthesize protein or carry out oxidative reactions. Because it cannot undergo mitotic division, it lives out its life span (approximately 120 days) in the circulation, dies, and is replaced by a new erythrocyte.

The erythrocyte's size and shape are ideally suited to its function as a gas carrier. It is a small disk with two unique properties: (1) **biconcavity** and (2) **reversible deformability** (Fig. 19-2). The flattened, biconcave shape provides a surface area/volume ratio that is optimal for gas diffusion into and out of the cell. Reversible deformity enables the erythrocyte to squeeze through the microcirculation and then return to normal. During its 120-day life span, the erythrocyte, which

is 8 μm in diameter, repeatedly circulates through splenic sinusoids (see p. 511) and capillaries that are only 2 μm in diameter. To do this, the erythrocyte assumes a torpedo-like shape.

Leukocytes

Leukocytes are white blood cells whose job it is to defend the body against organisms that cause infection and to remove debris, including dead or injured host cells of all kinds (Fig. 19-3). The leukocytes act primarily in the tissues but are transported in the circulation. The average adult has approximately 5000 to 10,000 leukocytes/mm³ of blood.

Leukocytes are classified according to structure as either **granulocytes** or **agranulocytes** and according to function as either **phagocytes** or **immunocytes.** The granulocytes, which include neutrophils, basophils, and eosinophils, are all phagocytes. (Phagocytic action is described in Chapter 7.) Of the agranulocytes, the monocytes and macrophages are phagocytes, whereas the lymphocytes are immunocytes (cells that create immunity; see Chapter 5).

Granulocytes. The granulocytes have many membrane-

Fig. 19-2 *Mature erythrocytes.* Scanning electron micrograph of mature erythrocytes on cell wall. *(Micrograph © 1994, Dennis Kunkel, Ph.D., Micro Vision, Kailua, Hawaii.)*

Fig. 19-3 *Blood cells.* Leukocytes are spherical and have irregular surfaces with numerous extending pili. Leukocytes are the "cotton candy–like" cells in yellow. Erythrocytes are flattened spheres with a depressed center. *(Micrograph © 1993, Dennis Kunkel, Ph.D., Micro Vision, Kailua, Hawaii.)*

bound granules in their cytoplasm. These granules contain enzymes capable of killing microorganisms and catabolizing debris ingested during phagocytosis. The granules also contain powerful biochemical mediators with inflammatory and immune functions. These mediators, along with the digestive enzymes, are released from some granulocytes in response to specific stimuli and from all granulocytes as they reach the end of their natural life span and die. The biochemical mediators have vascular and intercellular effects, and the enzymes participate in the breakdown of free-floating debris from sites of infection or injury. Granulocytes are capable of ameboid movement, by which they migrate through vessel walls (diapedesis) and then to sites where their action is needed.

The ***neutrophil (polymorphonuclear neutrophil [PMN])*** is the most numerous and best understood of the granulocytes (Fig. 19-4). Neutrophils constitute about 55% of the total leukocyte count in adults. Immature neutrophils are called *bands* or *stabs*. Mature neutrophils are called *segmented neutrophils* because of the characteristic appearance of their nucleus.

Neutrophils are the chief phagocytes of early inflammation. Soon after bacterial invasion or tissue injury, neutrophils migrate out of the capillaries and into the inflamed site, where they ingest and destroy microorganisms and debris and then die in 1 or 2 days. The dissolution of dead neutrophils releases digestive enzymes from their cytoplasmic granules. These enzymes dissolve cellular debris and prepare the site for healing.

Eosinophils, which have large, coarse granules, constitute only 1% to 4% of the normal leukocyte count in adults. Like neutrophils, eosinophils are capable of ameboid movement and phagocytosis. Unlike neutrophils, eosinophils in-gest antigen-antibody complexes and are induced by IgE-mediated hypersensitivity reactions to attack parasites. Eosinophils also help to control inflammatory processes. High eosinophil counts in atopic (allergy-prone) individuals experiencing type I allergic reactions, such as asthma or allergic rhinitis, have led researchers to think that eosinophils participate in hypersensitivity reactions to allergens other than parasites (see Chapter 7).

Basophils, which make up less than 1% of the leukocytes, are structurally similar to the mast cells found throughout extravascular tissue (see Fig. 19-4). Like the mast cells, basophils have cytoplasmic granules that contain vasoactive amines (histamine, bradykinin, serotonin) and an anticoagulant (heparin). Their precise function is poorly understood.

Agranulocytes. The agranulocytes—monocytes, macrophages, and lymphocytes—contain *no* lysosomal granules or enzyme-filled digestive vacuoles in their cytoplasm. The digestive vacuoles of the monocytes and macrophages are larger and fewer than those of the granulocytes.

The ***monocytes*** and ***macrophages*** make up the ***mononuclear phagocyte system (MPS),*** formerly called the ***reticuloendothelial system (RES).*** (The MPS is described on p. 512.) Both monocytes and macrophages participate in the immune and inflammatory response, being powerful phagocytes. They also ingest dead or defective host cells, particularly blood cells.

Monocytes are immature macrophages (see Fig. 19-4). After monocytes are formed and released by the bone marrow, they enter the bloodstream and circulate for about 36 hours while maturing into macrophages. Some of the circulating macrophages migrate out of the vessels in response to infection or inflammation. Others migrate to fixed sites in

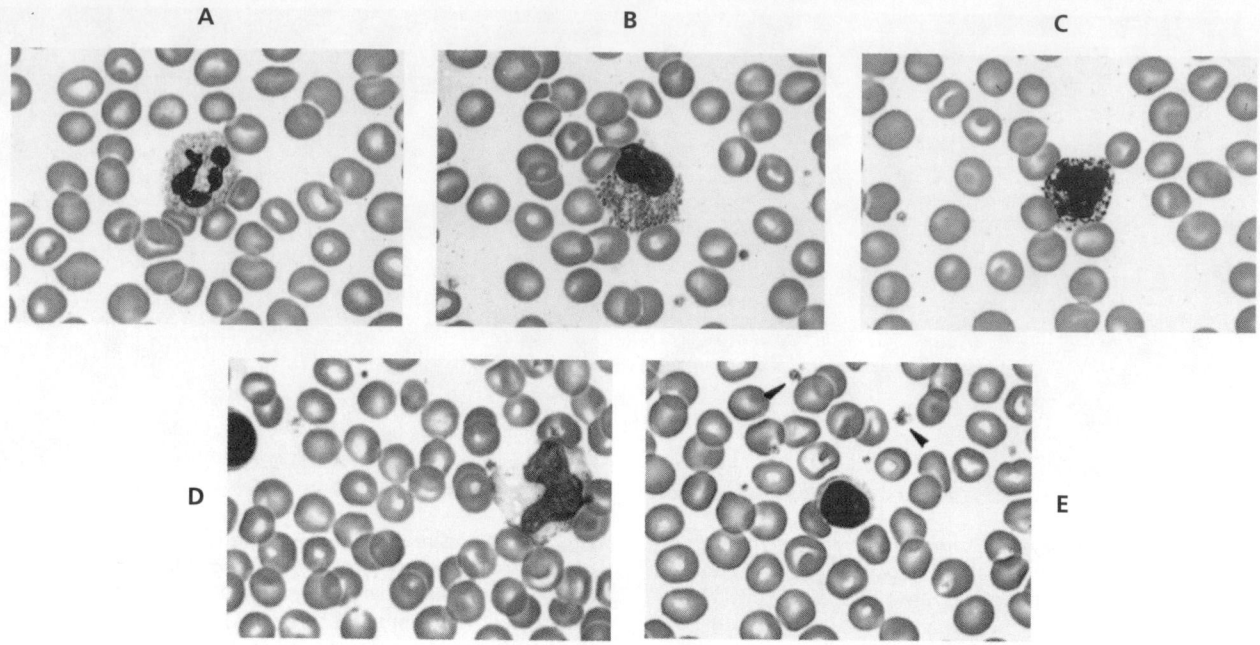

Fig. 19-4 *Leukocytes.* An example of leukocytes in human blood smear. **A,** Neutrophil. **B,** Eosinophil. **C,** Basophil. **D,** Monocyte. **E,** Lymphocyte. *(From Erlandsen, S.L. & Magney, J.E. [1992]. Color atlas of histology. St. Louis: Mosby.)*

the lymphoid tissues of the liver, spleen, lymph nodes, peritoneum, or gastrointestinal tract, where they are active for months or years.

Lymphocytes, which constitute approximately 36% of the total leukocyte count, are the primary cells of the immune response (see Fig. 19-4). Most are located in lymphoid tissues; only a small percentage circulate in the blood. The most important types of lymphocytes are T cells, B cells, and mature B cells (plasma cells). The life span of the lymphocyte can be days, months, or years, depending on its type and subtype. (Lymphocyte function and dysfunction are described in detail in Unit 2.)

Natural killer cells, which resemble lymphocytes, kill some types of tumor cells and some virus-infected cells. The hematopoietic pathway that these cells develop is unknown. These cells are discussed in Chapters 5, 9, and 10.

Platelets

Platelets are not cells, but disk-shaped cytoplasmic fragments essential for blood coagulation and control of bleeding. They lack a nucleus, have no deoxyribonucleic acid (DNA), and are incapable of mitotic division. They do, however, contain cytoplasmic granules capable of releasing biochemical mediators when stimulated by injury to a blood vessel (Fig. 19-5).

There are approximately 140,000 to 340,000 platelets/mulplatelets/mm³ of circulating blood. An additional one third of the body's available platelets are in a reserve pool in the spleen. A platelet lives approximately 10 days and then dies and is removed by macrophages of the MPS, mostly in the spleen. (Platelets are discussed further on p. 521.)

Fig. 19-5 *Scanning electron micrograph of moderately active platelet. (From Bick, R.L. et al. [1993]. Hemostasis and thrombosis. In R.L. Bick. Hematology: Clinical and laboratory practice. St. Louis: Mosby.)*

✓ QUICK CHECK

Why are plasma proteins important to blood volume?

Why are the leukocytes also called granulocytes?

What are the different leukocyte cells?

Compare and contrast granulocytes, agranulocytes, phagocytes, and immunocytes.

Lymphoid Organs

The lymphoid organs, some of which are merely aggregations of lymphoid tissue, are classified as primary or secondary. The *primary lymphoid organs* are the thymus and the bone marrow. The *secondary lymphoid organs* consist of the spleen, lymph nodes, tonsils, and Peyer patches of the small intestine (see Fig. 5-5). All the lymphoid organs link the hematologic and immune systems in that they are sites of residence, proliferation, differentiation, or function of lymphocytes and mononuclear phagocytes (monocytes, macrophages). (The liver, which also has hematologic functions, is primarily a digestive organ and is described in Chapter 33.)

Spleen

The *spleen* is the largest of the secondary lymphoid organs. It is a site of fetal hematopoiesis, its mononuclear phagocytes filter and cleanse the blood, its lymphocytes mount an immune response to blood-borne microorganisms, and it serves as a blood reservoir.

The spleen is a concave, encapsulated organ that weighs about 150 g and is about the size of a fist (see Chapter 5; Fig. 5-5). It is located in the left upper abdominal cavity, curved around a portion of the stomach. Strands of connective tissue (trabeculae) extend throughout the spleen from the splenic capsule, dividing it into compartments that contain masses of lymphoid tissue called *splenic pulp*. The spleen is interlaced with many blood vessels, some of which can distend to store blood.

Blood that circulates through the spleen first encounters the white splenic pulp, which consists of masses of lymphoid tissue containing lymphocytes and macrophages. The white pulp forms clumps around the splenic arterioles and is the chief site of immune and phagocytic function within the spleen. Here blood-borne antigens encounter lymphocytes, initiating the immune response (see Chapter 5).

Some of the blood continues through the microcirculation and enters highly distensible storage areas called *venous sinuses*. Most of the blood, however, oozes through the capillary walls into the principal site of splenic filtration, the red pulp (Fig. 19-6). Here the resident macrophages of the MPS phagocytose old, damaged, or dead blood cells of all kinds (but chiefly erythrocytes), microorganisms, and particles of debris. Hemoglobin from phagocytosed erythrocytes is catabolized, and heme (iron) is stored in the cytoplasm of the macrophages or released back into the blood plasma (see p. 515 and Fig. 19-12). The macrophages also remove certain particulate inclusions from erythrocytes without harming the cells themselves. Blood that filters through the red pulp then moves through the venous sinuses and into the portal circulation.

The venous sinuses (and the red pulp) can store more than 300 ml of blood. Sudden reductions in blood pressure cause the sympathetic nervous system to stimulate constriction of the sinuses and expel as much as 200 ml of blood into the venous circulation, helping to restore blood volume or pressure in the circulation and increasing the hematocrit by as much as 4%.[1]

Fig. 19-6 *Red cells in the spleen.* Transmission electron micrograph of a normal red cell traversing the sinus wall in a human spleen. Note how it must deform to reenter the sinus. *(From Damjanov, I. & Linder, J. [Eds.]. [1996]. Anderson's pathology [10th ed.]. St. Louis: Mosby.)*

The spleen is not necessary for life or for adequate hematologic function. Its absence, however, has several effects that indicate its function. For example, leukocytosis (high levels of circulating leukocytes) often occurs after splenectomy, so the spleen must exert some control over the rate of proliferation of leukocyte cells. Iron levels in the circulation decrease, immune function is diminished, and the blood contains more structurally defective blood cells than normal.

Lymph nodes

Structurally, *lymph nodes* are part of the lymphatic system. Thousands are clustered around the lymphatic veins, which collect interstitial fluid from the tissues and transport it, as lymph, back into the circulatory system near the heart. Functionally, however, lymph nodes are part of the hematologic and immune systems because they are where large numbers of lymphocytes, monocytes, and macrophages develop or function. As the lymph filters through the bean-shaped lymph nodes clustered in the inguinal, axillary, and cervical regions of the body, it is cleansed of foreign particles and microorganisms by the monocytes and macrophages. The microorganisms in lymph stimulate the resident lymphocytes to develop into antibody-producing plasma cells. During an infection, the rate of proliferation of macrophages within the nodes is so great that the nodes enlarge and become tender.

Each lymph node is enclosed in a fibrous capsule (Fig. 19-7), with strands of connective tissue (trabeculae) extending inward, dividing the node into several compartments. Reticular fibers divide the compartments into smaller sections and trap and store large numbers of lymphocytes, monocytes, and macrophages. The node has an outer cortex area and an inner medullary area. Within the cortex are germinal centers, or separate masses of lymphoid tissue. Lymph

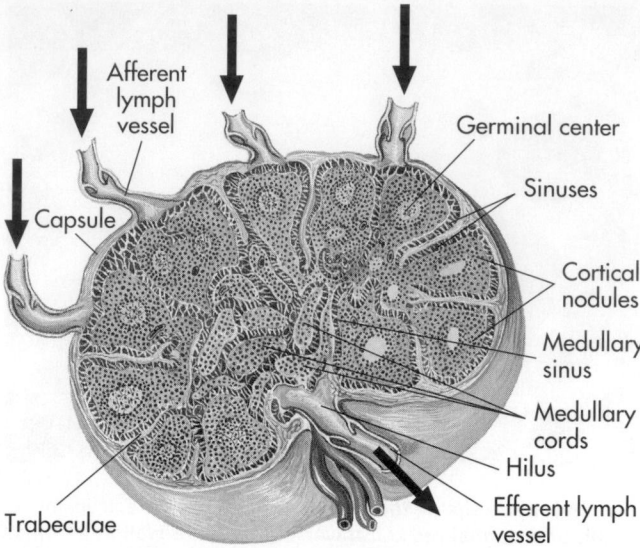

FIG. 19-7 *Cross section of lymph node.* Several afferent valved lymphatics bring lymph to node. A single efferent lymphatic leaves the node at the hilus. Note that the artery and vein also enter and leave at the hilus. Arrows show direction of lymph. *(From Thibodeau, G.A. & Patton, K.T. [1999]. Anatomy & physiology [4th ed.]. St. Louis: Mosby.)*

TABLE 19-3	Mononuclear Phagocyte System (Formerly Called the Reticuloendothelial System)	
Name of Cell	**Location**
Committed stem cells*	Bone marrow
Monoblasts	Bone marrow
Promonoblasts	Bone marrow
Monocytes	Bone marrow and peripheral blood
Macrophages	Tissue
Kupffer cells (inflammatory macrophages)	Liver
Alveolar macrophages	Lung
Histiocytes	Connective tissue
Macrophages	Bone marrow
Fixed and free macrophages	Spleen and lymph nodes
Pleural and peritoneal macrophages	Serous cavities
Microglial cells	Nervous system
Mesangial cells	Kidney
Osteoclasts	Bone
Langerhans cells	Skin
Dendritic cells	Lymphoid tissue

From Halma, C., Daha, M.R., & van-Es-La. (1992). In vivo clearance by the mononuclear phagocyte system in humans: An overview of methods and their interpretation. Clinical Experimental Immunology, *89(10), 1-7; Cotran, R.S. et al. (1994).* Robbins' pathophysiologic basis of disease *(5th ed.). Philadelphia: Saunders.*
Development of blood cells from stem cells in the marrow is discussed on p. 513 and illustrated in Fig. 19-9.

enters the node, slowly filters through its sinuses, and leaves through efferent lymphatic vessels.

The Mononuclear Phagocyte System (MPS)

The MPS consists of a line of cells that originate in the bone marrow, are transported by the bloodstream, and after differentiation to blood monocytes, finally settle in the tissues as mature macrophages. Table 19-3 lists the various names given to macrophages localized in specific tissues.

The cells of the MPS ingest and destroy (by phagocytosis) unwanted materials, such as foreign protein particles, microorganisms, debris from dead or injured cells, defective or injured erythrocytes, and dead neutrophils (see Fig. 6-15). The MPS (mostly in the liver and spleen) is also the main line of defense against bacteria in the bloodstream. In addition, the MPS cleanses the blood of old, injured, or dead erythrocytes, leukocytes, platelets, coagulation products, antigen-antibody complexes, and macromolecules. Recently, the osteoclast cell was classified as a true member of the MPS.[2] Osteoclasts are multinucleated cells specialized for the function of lacunar bone resorption; however, they are also known to have phagocytotic abilities. The osteoclast cell originates from the monocyte cell lineage (see Fig. 19-9). Macrophages also play a role in blood coagulation, wound healing, tissue remodeling, and the control of blood production.

Multiple cell types, including endothelial cells, fibroblasts, and lymphocytes, produce *colony-stimulating factors (CSFs),* which are soluble mediators secreted by cells for the purpose of cell-to-cell communication.[3-5] These factors control the production, maturation, and function of granulocytes and monocyte-macrophages (Table 19-4) and the development of blood cells.

The origin and turnover of all the tissue macrophages named in Table 19-3 are not precisely known. Once monocytes leave the circulation, they do not return. In the tissues, monocytes differentiate into macrophages without dividing and can survive many months or perhaps even years. Under normal circumstances, macrophages show little evidence of mitotic division, but production can be rapidly elevated in response to need, as in infection.

✓ QUICK CHECK

Why is the spleen considered a hematologic organ? Why can humans live without it?

Why are lymph nodes considered part of the hematologic system?

Why is the MPS important for infection control?

TABLE 19-4	Some Examples of Human CSFs	
CSF	**Cell Origin**	**Cell Stimulated**
M-CSF	Macrophage, fibroblast	Macrophage
GM-CSF	T cell, macrophage, fibroblast	Neutrophil, monocyte, macrophage, eosinophil
G-CSF	Macrophage, fibroblast	Neutrophil, eosinophil, basophil
IL-3	T cell	Neutrophil, macrophage
Erythropoietin	Kupffer and peri-tubular kidney cells	Erythrocyte

Morphologic effects of growth factor. Marrow aspirate from a patient receiving granulocyte colony-stimulating factor (G-CSF) showing an early neutrophil response. There is a marked shift toward immaturity in the neutrophils with the majority at the promyelocyte and early myelocyte stages of maturation. (Wright-Giemsa stain.) *(From Damjanov, I. & Linder, J. [Eds.]. [1996]. Anderson's pathology [10th ed.]. St. Louis: Mosby.)*

DEVELOPMENT OF BLOOD CELLS
Hematopoiesis

Blood cell production, termed *hematopoiesis,* occurs in the liver and spleen of the fetus, but after birth it normally occurs only in bone marrow and is known as *medullary hematopoiesis.* This two-stage process involves mitotic division, or **proliferation,** and maturation, or **differentiation.** Each type of blood cell has parent cells, called **stem cells,** that undergo mitosis when they receive specific biochemical signals. The stem cells continue to proliferate until the requisite number of mature daughter cells has entered the circulation.

Hematopoiesis can be divided by activity in the bone marrow by two separate pools: the stem cell pool and the bone marrow pool, with eventual release of mature cells into the peripheral circulation (Fig. 19-8). Investigators propose that in the bone marrow microenvironment a stem cell pool exists where structurally unidentifiable multipotential stem cells (see below) and unipotential committed colony-forming units (CFUs) reside. In addition, there is a bone marrow pool that can be divided into two cell pools: cells that are proliferating and maturing and cells that are stored for later release into the peripheral blood. In the peripheral blood, two pools of cells are also categorized: those circulating and those in storage.[6] Those cells stored around the walls of the blood vessels are often called the **marginating storage pool** (see Fig. 19-8).

Certain blood cells proliferate and differentiate simultaneously. Proliferation usually ceases after a number of doubling divisions, but differentiation continues. Erythrocytes and neutrophils generally mature before entering the blood, but monocytes and other leukocytes do not.

Hematopoiesis continues throughout life, increasing in response to proliferative disease, hemorrhage, hemolytic anemia (in which erythrocytes are destroyed), chronic infection, idiopathic thrombocytopenic purpura (bleeding caused by platelet insufficiency; see Chapter 20), and other disorders that deplete blood cells. In general, long-term stimuli, such as chronic diseases, cause a greater increase in hematopoiesis than acute conditions, such as hemorrhage. Abnormal proliferation of erythrocytes occurs in polycythemia vera, a myeloproliferative disease.

Medullary hematopoiesis can be accelerated by any or all of three mechanisms: (1) conversion of yellow bone marrow, which does not produce blood cells, to red marrow, which does; (2) faster differentiation of daughter cells; and presumably (3) faster proliferation of stem cells. Marrow conversion is stimulated by erythropoietin, the hormone that stimulates erythrocyte production.

In adults, extramedullary hematopoiesis—blood cell production in tissues other than bone marrow—is usually a sign of disease, occurring in pernicious anemia, sickle cell anemia, thalassemia, hemolytic disease of the newborn (erythroblastosis fetalis), hereditary spherocytosis, and certain leukemias. Extramedullary hematopoiesis of apparently normal blood cells has been reported to occur in the spleen, liver, and, less frequently, lymph nodes, adrenal glands, cartilage, adipose tissue, intrathoracic areas, and kidneys.[7]

Stem cell system

The earliest, most primitive ancestor in the **stem cell system** is the **totipotential hematopoietic stem cell (THSC)** (Fig. 19-9). These cells can develop into many types of blood cells and are also called *multipotential stem cells* (see Fig 19-8). One pathway of development leads to various lymphoid tissues, where T and B lymphocytes mature. The other pathway leads to myeloid tissue—the bone marrow. The stem cell of the myeloid pathway is called the **pluripotential stem cell.** It triggers differentiation of (1) neutrophils and monocytes, (2) eosinophils, (3) erythrocytes, and (4) platelets (see Fig. 19-9).

Blood cell production in any pathway requires numerous amplifying cell divisions plus complex maturation changes. Hematopoiesis is partially regulated by the interaction of

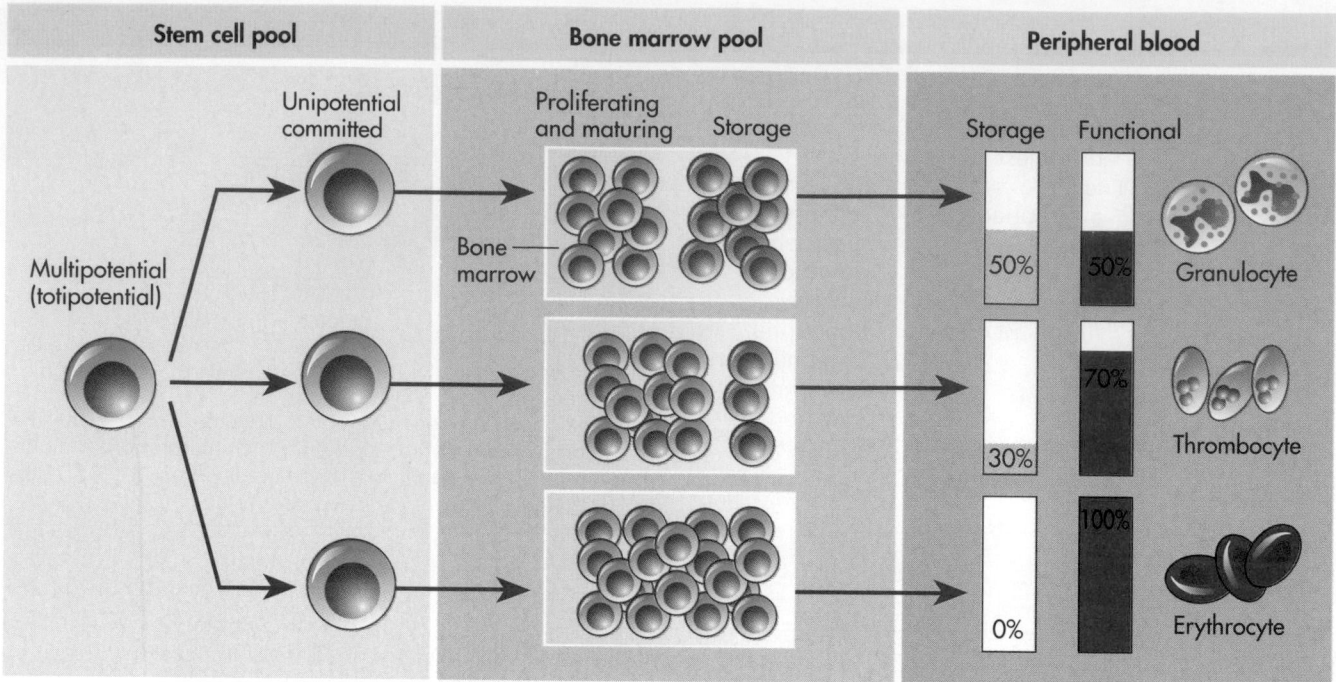

Fig. 19-8 *Hematopoiesis.* Hematopoiesis from the stem cell pool; activity mainly in the bone marrow and in the peripheral blood. *(Modified from Harmening, D.M. [Ed.]. [1997]. Clinical hematology and fundamentals of hemostasis [3rd ed.]. Philadelphia: Davis.)*

hematopoietic growth factors or *colony-stimulating factors (CSFs),* which stimulate the proliferation of progenitor cells and their progeny and initiate the maturation events necessary to produce fully mature cells (see Table 19-4).

Clinical uses of CSFs

Blood granulocyte numbers (e.g., eosinophils, neutrophils, basophils/mast cells) are normally in the range of 4000 to 6000 cells/μl, and susceptibility to infection develops below 1000 cells/μl. During a natural response to a bacterial infection, granulocytes usually rise to 10,000 to 20,000 cells/μl. The CSFs can raise white cell numbers even higher. No advantage, however, is gained from extreme numbers because of the formation of toxic products and tissue damage.[8] CSF treatment can result in shorter periods of intensive nursing and hospitalization such as occurs after bone marrow or stem cell transplantation.

Bone marrow

Bone marrow, also called *myeloid tissue* (*myelos* = marrow), is confined to the cavities of bone. It consists of blood vessels, nerves, mononuclear phagocytes, stem cells, blood cells in various stages of differentiation, and fatty tissue. Adults have two kinds of bone marrow: red, or active (hematopoietic), marrow; and yellow, or inactive, marrow. The large quantities of fat in inactive marrow make it yellow. Not all bones contain active marrow. In adults, active marrow is in the pelvic bones (34%), vertebrae (28%), cranium and mandible (13%), sternum and ribs (10%), and extreme proximal portions of the humerus and femur (4% to 8%).[9]

Inactive marrow predominates in cavities of other bones. (Bones are discussed further in Chapter 36.)

Stem cells in hematopoietic marrow receive the oxygen and nutrients they need for mitosis and maturation from the primary or nutrient arteries of the bones. Branches of these arteries terminate in a capillary network that coalesces into large venous sinuses, which eventually drain into a central vein. Hematopoietic marrow and fat fill the spaces surrounding the network of venous sinuses. Newly produced blood cells traverse narrow openings in the venous sinus walls and thus enter the circulation. Normally, cells do not enter the circulation until they have differentiated to a certain extent, but premature release occurs in certain diseases.

✓ QUICK CHECK

Why is the stem cell system important to hematopoiesis?

Why are some stem cells called multipotential?

Why are CSFs necessary for blood cell proliferation?

Development of Erythrocytes

For almost 100 years it was believed that erythrocytes developed from lymphocytes that were transformed in the spleen. It was not until the 1850s that the bone marrow was accepted as the site of *erythropoiesis.* We now know that erythrocytes are derived from precursor cells called *erythroblasts* (Fig. 19-10). Normal erythroblasts are also called

Stem cells

Totipotential stem cell

Pluripotential stem cell

Myeloid   Lymphoid

Progenitor cells

Proerythroblast   Promyeloblast   Promegalokaryoblast   Prolymphoblast

Differentiating cells in hematopoietic organs

Erythroblast   Myeloblast   Monoblast   Megalokaryoblast   Lymphoid stem cell

Erythrocyte   Granulocyte   Monocyte   Megalokaryocyte   ?

Mature cells in blood

Erythrocyte   Granulocyte   Macrophage   Blood platelets   Natural killer cell

Mast   Osteoclast   B lymphocyte   T lymphocyte

←Antigen→

Eosinophils   Neutrophils   Mast   Basophil   Plasma cell   Activated T cell

Fig. 19-9 *Bone marrow and stem cell systems.* Probable pathways of differentiation, from the totipotential stem cell to mature blood cells.

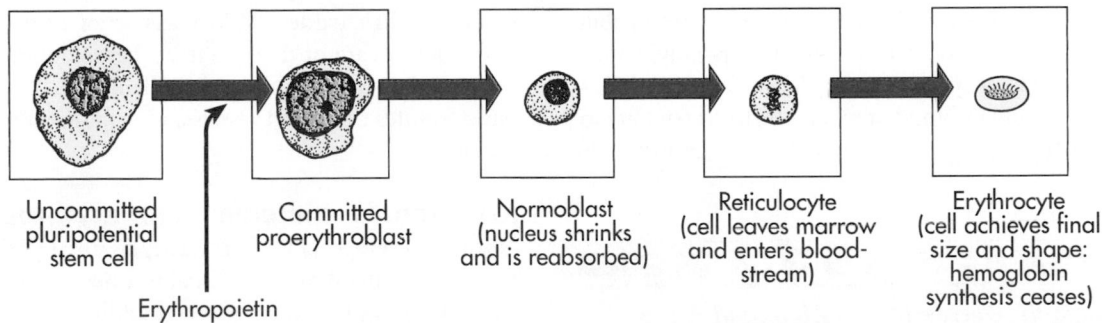

Uncommitted pluripotential stem cell

Committed proerythroblast

Normoblast (nucleus shrinks and is reabsorbed)

Reticulocyte (cell leaves marrow and enters bloodstream)

Erythrocyte (cell achieves final size and shape: hemoglobin synthesis ceases)

Erythropoietin

Fig. 19-10 *Erythrocyte differentiation.* Erythrocyte differentiation from large, nucleated stem cell to small, nonnucleated erythrocyte.

normoblasts, whereas abnormal ones are called ***megaloblasts.*** Erythrocyte development is shown in Fig. 19-10.

Reticulocytes remain in the marrow approximately 1 day and then are released into the venous sinuses. They continue to mature in the bloodstream and may travel to the spleen for several days of additional maturation. The normal reticulocyte count is 1% of the total red blood cell count. Approximately 1% of the body's circulating erythrocyte mass normally is generated every 24 hours. Therefore the reticulocyte count is a useful clinical index of erythropoietic activity and indicates whether new red cells are being produced.

Hemoglobin synthesis

Hemoglobin, the oxygen-carrying protein of the erythrocyte, constitutes approximately 90% of the cell's dry weight. The cytoplasm of a single erythrocyte can contain as many

α₂   β₁

Heme

Heme

β₂   α₁

■ β-polypeptide (globin) chain   ■ α-polypeptide (globin) chain

Fig. 19-11 *Molecular structure of hemoglobin.* Molecule is spherical tetramer weighing approximately 64,500 daltons. It contains a pair of α-polypeptide and a pair of β-polypeptide chains and several heme groups.

as 300 hemoglobin molecules. Hemoglobin enables the blood to transport 100 times more oxygen than could be transported dissolved in plasma alone. Hemoglobin is not one but a family of molecules whose members differ slightly in primary structure. Nonetheless, each member is composed of two pairs of polypeptide chains (the *globins*) and four colorful complexes of iron plus protoporphyrin (the *hemes*) (Fig. 19-11).

Several genes dictate the synthesis of globulin resulting in the formation of a structurally different polypeptide chain (alpha, beta, gamma, delta, epsilon, or zeta [α, β, γ, δ, ε, or ζ]). Hemoglobin A, the most common type of hemoglobin in adults, is composed of two α- and two β-polypeptide chains. Seven different types of hemoglobin have been identified in healthy human blood at all stages, from fetal life to adulthood, testimony to the heterogeneity of the molecule (Table 19-5).

HEALTH ALERT

Hemoglobin Derivatives as Blood Substitute

Recent research on the potential use of hemoglobin derivatives as a blood substitute has revealed that administration of large quantities of free hemoglobin into the circulation results in a variety of toxic side effects. Hemoglobin, like myoglobin, has considerable prooxidant activity; therefore the generation of reactive oxygen free radicals could cause observed toxic reactions. Hemin is known to be very toxic when present in large amounts, and iron could catalyze the formation of hydroxyl radicals (see Chapter 3).

Data from Everse, J. & Hsia, N. (1997). The toxicities of native and modified hemoglobins. Free Radica, Biolog, and Medicine, 22(6), 1075-1099.

Heme is a large, flat, iron-protoporphyrin disk that can carry one molecule of oxygen (O_2). Recall that hemoglobin contains four heme groups; thus it can carry four oxygen molecules. Through a series of complex biochemical reactions, protoporphyrin, a complex four-ringed molecule, is produced and abounds with ferrous iron. It is crucial that the iron be correctly charged. Presence of the reduced ferrous iron (Fe_2^+) allows the formation of normal hemoglobin, which can bind oxygen where it is plentiful (in the lungs) and release it where it is needed (in the tissues). Oxidized ferric iron (Fe_3^{++}) carries an extra positive charge and results in the formation of *methemoglobin,* an unstable type of hemoglobin that cannot bind oxygen. An excess of ferric iron occurs with certain drugs and chemicals, such as nitrates and sulfonamides.

Hemoglobin that is carrying oxygen is called *oxyhemoglobin.* If all four oxygen-binding sites on the oxyhemoglobin's hemes are occupied by oxygen, the molecule is said to be saturated. Oxyhemoglobin that has released its oxygen or is not bound to oxygen for some other reason is called *deoxyhemoglobin (reduced hemoglobin).*

A perplexing question has always been how blood vessels dilate even though red blood cells are filled with a potent vasoconstrictor, hemoglobin. Investigators have long known that nitric oxide from blood vessel walls relaxes and dilates the vessels. Oxygenated hemoglobin was thought to act as a scavenger, rapidly eliminating nitric oxide (chemical synthesized in the lungs and blood vessel walls) from the blood. Yet somehow enough nitric oxide remains to dilate the vessels. Hemoglobin appears to carry its own nitric oxide. In the lungs, nitric oxide combines with hemoglobin's cysteine residue when the oxygen binds to hemoglobin's iron (Fig. 19-12). Blood with the enriched hemoglobin then circulates throughout the body. The nitric oxide on the hemoglobin is part of a chemical group called S-nitrosothiol (SNO). Because the nitric oxide is hidden as part of a thiol, circulating hemoglobin cannot degrade it. As hemoglobin transfers its oxygen to tissue, it also sheds small amounts of nitric oxide, which dilutes the blood vessels and helps get the oxygen into tissues.[10]

Nutritional requirements for erythropoiesis

Normal development of erythrocytes and synthesis of hemoglobin depend on an optimal biochemical state and adequate supplies of the necessary building blocks, including protein, vitamins, and minerals (Table 19-6). If these components are lacking for a prolonged time, erythrocyte production slows and anemia (insufficient numbers of functional erythrocytes) may result (see Chapter 20).

Iron cycle

Approximately 67% of total body iron is bound to heme in erythrocytes and muscle cells, and approximately 30% is stored bound to ferritin or hemosiderin mononuclear phagocytes (i.e., macrophages) and hepatic parenchymal cells. The remaining 3% (less than 1 mg) is lost daily in urine, sweat, bile, and epithelial cells shed from the gut. Iron not lost is continuously recycled, as shown in Fig. 19-13,

TABLE 19-5   Structure of Normal Hemoglobin Molecules

Type of Hemoglobin (Hb)	Identity of Polypeptide Chain	Significance
Hb A	$\alpha_2\beta_2$	92% of adult Hb
Hb A$_{1c}$	$\alpha_2(\beta\text{-NH-glucose})$	5% of adult Hb; increased in diabetes (see Chapter 20)
Hb A$_2$	$\alpha_2\delta_2$	2% of adult Hb; increased in β_2-thalassemia (see Chapter 24)
Hb F	$\alpha_2\gamma_2$	Major fetal Hb from the third through ninth month of gestation; promotes oxygen transfer across platelets; increased in β-thalassemia
Hb Gower 1	ϵ_4 or $\zeta_2\epsilon_2$	Present in early embryo; function unknown
Hb Gower 2	$\alpha_2\epsilon_2$	Present in early embryo; function unknown
Hb Portland	$\zeta_2\gamma_2$	Present in early embryo; function unknown

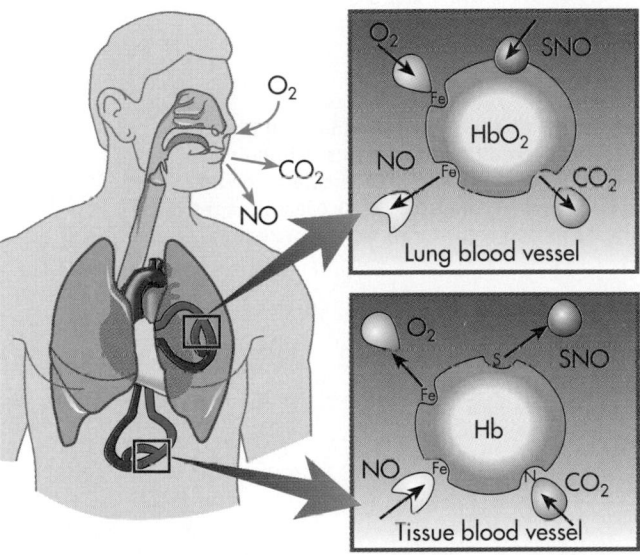

Fig. 19-12 *Hemoglobin (Hb) binding to nitric oxide.* In the lungs, hemoglobin (Hb) binds to nitric oxide (NO) as S-nitrosothiol (SNO). In tissue this SNO is released, and free, circulating NO is bound to a different site for exhalation.

through *transferrin,* a glycoprotein synthesized primarily by the liver but also by tissue macrophages, submaxillary and mammary glands, and ovaries or testes.

Iron for hemoglobin production is delivered to erythroblasts in erythropoietic bone marrow. Once the iron is released into the marrow and incorporated into the erythroblast's mitochondria, the enzyme heme synthetase inserts ferrous iron into protoporphyrin to form heme. Heme then is bound to globin to form hemoglobin. Iron not used in erythropoiesis is stored temporarily as ferritin or hemosiderin and later excreted.

After mature erythrocytes have circulated for 120 days, they are removed from the bloodstream by macrophages of the MPS—chiefly in the spleen. Within the phagolysosomes (digestive vacuoles) of the macrophage, the erythrocyte is catabolized and the iron in hemoglobin is oxidized, forming Fe_3^{+++} (methemoglobin). The heme and globin of methemoglobin dissociate easily, and globin may be reduced to its component amino acids. The iron released by methemoglobin dissociation is stored in the macrophage's cytoplasm as ferritin or hemosiderin or released into the bloodstream, where it is free to bind again to transferrin (see Fig. 19-13). A minute amount of iron is stored in muscle cells by the heme-containing protein myoglobin.

Iron balance is achieved through mechanisms controlling its absorption rather than its excretion. Regulation of iron transport across the plasma membrane of gastrointestinal epithelial cells is related to the cell's iron content and the overall rate of erythropoiesis. If the body's iron stores are low or the demand for erythropoiesis is increased, iron passes rapidly through the epithelial cell and into the plasma, probably by active transport. If body stores are high and erythropoiesis is not increased, iron crosses the epithelial cell's plasma membrane passively and is stored there bound to ferritin. Excretion of iron occurs when the epithelial cells of the intestinal mucosa slough off.

Regulation of erythropoiesis

In healthy humans, the total volume of circulating erythrocytes remains surprisingly constant. The feedback mechanism that maintains an optimal population of erythrocytes is mediated by erythropoietin, which induces the selective proliferation and differentiation of proerythroblasts (see Fig. 19-10). Hemoglobin synthesis begins hours after initial stimulation by erythropoietin.

Erythropoietin is secreted by the kidney in response to tissue hypoxia (Fig. 19-14). It causes a compensatory increase in erythrocyte production if the oxygen content of blood decreases because of anemia, high altitude, or pulmonary disease. The normal steady-state rate of production (2.5 million erythrocytes per second) can increase (to 17 million per second) under anemic or low-oxygen states.[11] The receptors that detect hypoxia are within the kidney, on cells that synthesize and secrete erythropoietin. Thus the body responds to reduced oxygenation of blood in two ways: (1) by increasing intake of oxygen through increased respiration and (2) by increasing the oxygen-carrying capacity of the blood through increased erythropoiesis. Erythropoietin not only stimulates proliferation of stem cells in the marrow but also accelerates maturation of existing erythroblasts.

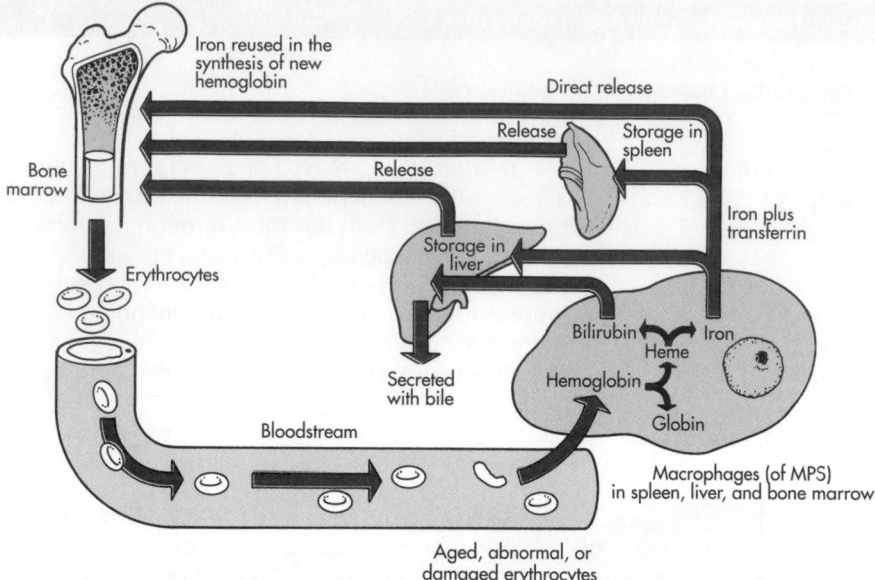

Fig. 19-13 *Iron cycle.* Iron (Fe) released from gastrointestinal epithelial cells circulates in bloodstream associated with its plasma carrier, transferrin. It is delivered to erythroblasts in bone marrow, where most of it is incorporated into hemoglobin. Mature erythrocytes circulate for approximately 120 days, after which they become senescent and are removed by MPS. Macrophages of MPS (mostly in spleen) break down ingested erythrocytes and return iron to bloodstream directly or after storing it as ferritin or hemosiderin.

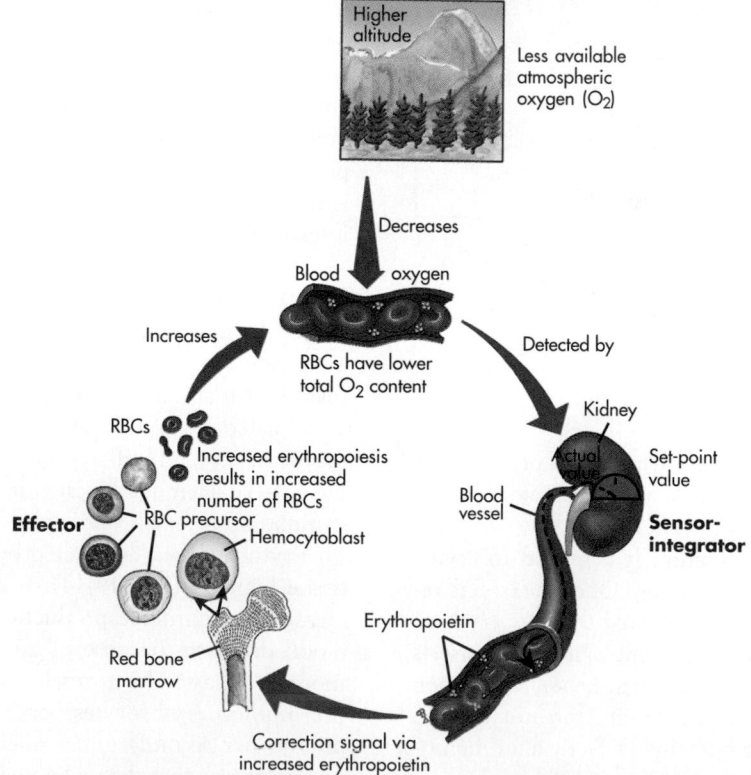

Fig. 19-14 *Role of erythropoietin regulation of red blood cell production and delivery of oxygen.* In addition to decreased oxygen in the atmosphere, other stimulators of erythropoietin release include anemia or decreased population of mature red blood cells (RBCs), decreased hemoglobin synthesis, decreased blood flow, and hemorrhage or excessive bleeding. In response to decreased blood oxygen, the kidneys release erythropoietin, which stimulates erythrocyte production in the bone marrow. *(From Thibodeau, G.A.& Patton, K.T. [1999]. Anatomy & physiology [4th ed.]. St. Louis: Mosby.)*

TABLE 19-6	Nutritional Requirements for Erythropoiesis	
Nutrient	**Role in Erythropoiesis**	**Consequence of Deficiency**
Protein (amino acids)	Structural component of plasma membrane	Decreased strength, elasticity, and flexibility of membrane; hemolytic anemia
	Synthesis of hemoglobin	Decreased erythropoiesis and life span of erythrocytes
Intrinsic factor	Gastrointestinal absorption of vitamin B_{12}	Pernicious anemia
Cobalamin (vitamin B_{12})	Synthesis of DNA, maturation of erythrocytes, facilitator of folate metabolism	Macrocytic (megaloblastic) anemia
Folate (folic acid)	Synthesis of DNA and RNA, maturation of erythrocytes	Macrocytic (megaloblastic) anemia
Vitamin B_6 (pyridoxine)	Heme synthesis, increase folate metabolism?	Hypochromic-microcytic anemia
Vitamin B_2 (riboflavin)	Oxidative reactions	Normochromic-normocytic anemia
Vitamin C (ascorbic acid)	Iron metabolism, acts as a reducing agent to maintain iron in its ferrous (Fe^{++}) form	Normochromic-normocytic anemia
Pantothenic acid	Heme synthesis	Unknown in humans*
Niacin	None, but needed for respiration in mature erythrocytes	Unknown in humans
Vitamin E	Heme synthesis (?); protection against oxidative damage in mature erythrocytes	Hemolytic anemia with increased cell membrane fragility; shortens life span of erythrocytes in individual with cystic fibrosis
Iron	Hemoglobin synthesis	Iron deficiency anemia
Copper	Required for optimal mobilization of iron from tissues to plasma	Hypochromic-microcytic anemia

From Lee, G.R. et al. (1993). Wintrobe's clinical hematology (9th ed.). Philadelphia: Lee & Febiger; Harmening, D.M. (1997). Clinical hematology and fundamentals of hemostasis, (3rd ed.). Philadelphia: Davis.

DNA, *Deoxyribonucleic acid*; RNA, *ribonucleic acid*.

Although pantothenic acid is important for optimal synthesis of heme, experimentally induced deficiency failed to produce anemia or other hematopoietic disturbances.

HEALTH ALERT
Reticulocyte Count

Frequently a clinician needs information about the rate of erythropoiesis to help in making a diagnosis or to prescribe treatment. A reticulocyte count gives this information. Approximately 0.5% to 1.5% of the red blood cells in normal blood at any given time are reticulocytes. A reticulocyte count of less than 0.5% of the red blood cell count usually indicates a slowdown in the process of red blood cell formation. Conversely, a reticulocyte count higher than 1.5% usually indicates an acceleration of red blood cell formation—as occurs, for example, after treatment of anemia.

Understanding how the results of a reticulocyte count can provide useful information on the rate of erythropoiesis is based on an understanding of the process and time (3 to 5 days) that is required to transform a hemopoietic stem cell into a mature red blood cell. Reticulocytes are the final precursors of circulating erythrocytes. Once released in the blood, reticulocytes complete the process of extruding their remaining organelles, which consist chiefly of ribosomes and rough endoplasmic reticulum, and then begin to fully perform their task of oxygen transport as mature erythrocytes.

This test is seldom used alone but, rather, in conjunction with other tests to assist in diagnosis of disease. An increased reticulocyte count may signal an attempt by the body to increase erythrocyte production because of actual blood loss or increased demand, or, perhaps, it may point to atypical myeloid tissue functioning.

Data from Thibodeau, G.A. & Patton, K.T. (1996). Anatomy & physiology (3rd ed., p. 592). St. Louis: Mosby.

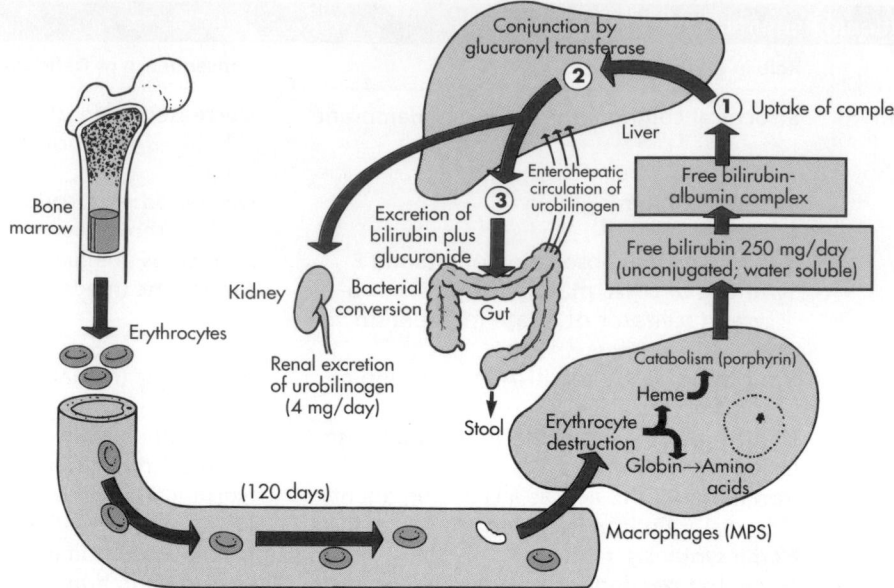

Fig. 19-15 *Metabolism of bilirubin released by heme breakdown.*

Normal destruction of senescent erythrocytes

Although mature erythrocytes lack nuclei, mitochondria, and endoplasmic reticulum, they do have cytoplasmic enzymes capable of glycolysis (anaerobic glucose metabolism) and production of small quantities of adenosine triphosphate (ATP). ATP provides the energy needed to keep the cell alive and its plasma membrane pliable (see Fig. 1-1). Metabolic processes diminish as the erythrocyte ages, so less ATP is available to maintain the functions essential for life. The senescent red cell becomes increasingly fragile and loses its reversible deformability, becoming susceptible to rupture while passing through narrowed regions of the microcirculation.

Aged red cells are selectively sequestered and destroyed by macrophages of the MPS, primarily in the spleen. If the spleen is dysfunctional or absent, macrophages in the liver (Kupffer cells) take over.

Phagocytosis of the erythrocyte is followed by its digestion by proteolytic and lipolytic enzymes within the macrophage. Globin is broken down into amino acids, and iron is recycled (see Fig. 19-13). Porphyrin is reduced to bilirubin, which is transported to the liver, conjugated, and finally excreted in the bile as glucuronide (Fig. 19-15). Bacteria in the intestinal lumen transform conjugated bilirubin into urobilinogen. Although a small portion is reabsorbed, most urobilinogen is excreted in feces.

Conditions causing accelerated erythrocyte destruction increase the load of bilirubin for hepatic clearance, leading to increased serum levels of unconjugated bilirubin and increased urinary excretion of urobilinogen. Gallstones (cholelithiasis) can result from a chronically elevated rate of bilirubin excretion.

✓ QUICK CHECK

Why is the reticulocyte count important?

Why is iron important to erythropoiesis?

Why is erythropoietin significant?

Development of Leukocytes

All leukocytes arise from stem cells in the bone marrow (their pathways of differentiation are shown in Fig. 19-9). The granulocytes (neutrophils, eosinophils, basophils/mast cells) normally mature fully in the marrow and then are released into the bloodstream. The agranulocytes (monocytes, lymphocytes), however, are released into the bloodstream before they undergo their final phase of maturation. The monocytes mature into macrophages within 1 or 2 days of release, and the lymphocytes travel to lymphoid tissues, where they are stimulated to differentiate into T cells or B cells (see Chapter 5).

The bone marrow selectively retains immature granulocytes. Hematopoietic growth factors, including several interleukins, granulocyte-macrophage colony-stimulating factor (GM-CSF), and granulocyte colony-stimulating factor (G-CSF) are required for granulocyte growth and differentiation.

Maintenance of optimal levels of granulocytes and monocytes in the blood depends on the availability of pluripotential stem cells in the marrow, induction of these into committed stem cells, and timely release of new cells from the marrow. The marrow contains a reserve pool that can be rapidly mobilized in response to the body's needs. Once cells are released from the marrow, they join the marginating pool or the circulating pool. The cells in the marginating pool lie along the capillary walls and can move into tissues and mucous membranes. Cells from the circulating pool join the marginating pool to replace the cells that have migrated out of the capillaries. Leukocyte production increases in response to infection, to the presence of steroids, and to reduction or depletion of reserves in the marrow. It is also associated with strenuous exercise, convulsive seizures, heat, intense radiation, increased heart rates, pain, nausea and vomiting, and anxiety.

Development of Platelets

Platelets (thrombocytes) develop from megakaryocytes by endomitosis (see Figs. 19-5 and 19-9), wherein the megakaryocyte undergoes the nuclear phase of cellular division (mitosis) but fails to undergo the cytoplasmic phase (cytokinesis) (see Chapter 1). Without cytokinesis, the cell does not divide into two daughter cells but, rather, expands to accommodate the doubling of its DNA (nuclear) content and breaks up into fragments known as platelets.

An optimal number of platelets and committed platelet precursors (megakaryoblasts) in the bone marrow is maintained by GM-CSF, interleukin-3 (IL-3), IL-11, leukemia inhibitory factor, and thrombopoietin. These factors stimulate committed cells at further stages of differentiation to differentiate faster. Rates of megakaryocyte development, endomitosis, and platelet release are increased. Platelets, once released, circulate for 10 days before they begin to lose their ability to carry out biochemical reactions. Senescent platelets are phagocytosed by neutrophils and monocytes if they are circulating freely or by neutrophils and macrophages if they are part of a clot, or thrombus. They may be removed also by tissue macrophages of the MPS in the liver or spleen.

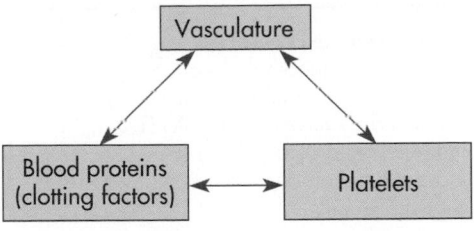

Fig. 19-16 *Three hemostatic compartments.*

MECHANISMS OF HEMOSTASIS

Hemostasis means arrest of bleeding. Mechanisms of hemostasis maintain a relatively steady state of blood volume, pressure, and flow through injured blood vessels. Three equally important anatomic compartments of hemostasis are platelets, blood proteins (clotting factors), and the vasculature (Fig. 19-16). After vascular damage and bleeding, hemostasis involves a complex sequence of events: (1) vasoconstriction (vasospasm), (2) formation of a platelet plug, (3) activation of the coagulation (or clotting) cascade, (4) formation of a blood clot, and (5) clot retraction and clot dissolution (fibrinolysis). All these events involve platelets, clotting factors, and the blood vessels (vasculature).

In general, the relative importance of the hemostatic mechanisms varies with vessel size. Usually, the larger the area of bleeding, the larger the vessel involved (Table 19-7). Sources and types of bleeding are listed in Table 19-7. Vessel vasoconstriction is controlled by local, humoral, and neural factors.

Function of Platelets and Blood Vessels

Platelets must be adequate in number and function to participate optimally in hemostasis. The normal platelet count

TABLE 19-7	Size of Vessel, Sealing Requirements, and Sources and Types of Bleeding			
Vessel	**Size**	**Sealing Requirement**		**Sources and Types of Bleeding**
Capillary	Smallest	Generally direct-sealing		Pinpoint petechial hemorrhage (leakage of blood out of small vessels)
Venule		Mostly fused platelets		Pinpoint petechial hemorrhage (leakage of blood out of small vessels)
Arteriole		Mostly fused platelets		Pinpoint petechial hemorrhage (leakage of blood out of small vessels)
Vein		Vascular contraction, fused platelets, perivascular and intravascular hemostatic factor activation (see Fig. 19-17)		Ecchymosis (large, soft tissue bleeding)
Artery	Largest	Greater vascular contraction, more fused platelets, greater perivascular and intravascular hemostatic factor activation		Rapidly expanding "blowout" hemorrhage

Modified from Harmening, D.M. (Ed.). (1997). Clinical hematology and fundamentals of hemostasis (3rd ed.). Philadelphia: Davis.

I.   Subendothelial exposure
   • Occurs after endothelial sloughing
   • Platelets begin to fill endothelial gaps
   • Promoted by thromboxane A$_2$ (TXA$_2$)
   • Inhibited by prostacyclin I$_2$ (PGI$_2$)
   • Platelet function depends on many factors, especially calcium

II. Adhesion
   • Adhesion between platelet and collagen is promoted by a plasma protein, the von Willebrand factor, that circulates with factor VIII coagulation protein and adenosine diphosphate (ADP)

III. Activation
   • Changes in platelet shape
   • Formation of pseudopods
   • Activation of arachidonic pathway

A

IV. Aggregation
   • Induced by release of TXA$_2$
   • Stabilization of the platelet plug (blood clot) occurs by activation of coagulation factors, thrombin and fibrin
   • Heparin neutralizing factor enhances clot formation

V.   Plug formation

VI. Clot retraction and clot dissolution
   • Clot retraction, using large number of platelets, joins the edges of the injured vessel
   • Clot dissolution is regulated by thrombin and plasminogen activators

Fig. 19-17 *Platelet degranulation.* **A,** Plug formation and clot dissolution.

B   **C**   **D**

Fig. 19-17, cont'd B, After simple endothelial denudation, platelets adhere to the subendothelium in a monolayer fashion. **C,** Platelet-fibrin thrombus formation. **D,** Higher magnification of the thrombus shows a mixture of red cells and platelets incorporated into the fibrin meshwork.. *(B to D from Damjanov, I. & Linder, J. [Eds.]. [1996].* Anderson's pathology *[10th ed.]. St. Louis: Mosby.)*

ranges from 140,000 to 340,000/mm³ depending on the laboratory methods employed. It is unusual for an individual with a platelet count more than 20,000/mm³ to have major hemorrhages.

In hemostasis, platelets adhere to injured vessel walls, undergo granule discharge, and aggregate into clumps or plugs (Fig. 19-17), releasing biochemical mediators. Normally, platelets circulate freely, suspended in plasma. When a vessel is damaged, endothelial sloughing occurs and collagen-containing subendothelial tissue is exposed, attracting platelets out of the plasma within 15 to 20 seconds after injury (see Fig. 19-17). The platelets then undergo dynamic changes in shape from smooth to spiny spheres and pseudopods, exposing receptors on their surfaces. They then degranulate, releasing various potent biochemicals.

Platelets adhere to exposed subendothelial tissues only if the platelets contain sufficient concentrations of calcium to change shape, aggregate, degranulate, and activate arachidonic pathways. Adhesion to the vessel subendothelial layer occurs when the platelet receptor binds to von Willebrand factor (e.g., a plasma protein), bridging the platelet to the injury site (see Fig. 19-17). Erythrocytes apparently increase the rate of platelet adherence by facilitating migration of circulating platelets toward vascular surfaces and by liberating adenosine diphosphate (ADP), which enables platelets to stick to exposed collagen.

Two of the biochemical mediators released by adhered platelets—serotonin and histamine—have immediate effects on smooth muscle in the vascular endothelium, causing an immediate temporary constriction of the injured vessel.[12] (Vasoconstriction is also produced by local reflexes of the nervous system.) Vasoconstriction reduces blood flow and diminishes bleeding. Vasodilation soon follows, permitting the inflammatory response to proceed (see Figs. 23-2 and 23-3).

Other biochemical mediators released by degranulation (also called the *platelet-release reaction*) either promote or inhibit platelet activity and the eventual process of clot formation (see Fig. 19-17). ADP promotes the adherence and subsequent degranulation of nearby platelets by causing their plasma membranes to become ruffled and sticky. The new activated platelets cause a platelet plug to seal the injured endothelium. If the effects of ADP were not counteracted and laminar flow were not sufficient, platelet aggregation could continue indefinitely. This is prevented by two antagonistic prostaglandin derivatives: thromboxane A_2 (TXA_2), produced by platelets; and prostacyclin I_2 (PGI_2), produced by endothelial cells (see Fig. 19-17). TXA_2 causes vasoconstriction and promotes the degranulation of platelets, which then release more ADP. PGI_2 inhibits the effects of TXA_2 by promoting vasodilation and inhibiting platelet degranulation. The net effect of TXA_2 and PGI_2 is to permit platelet aggregation to proceed at the site of injury while preventing adherence to normal vascular endothelium.[13] Heparin-neutralizing factor released by platelets (platelet factor 4) enhances clot formation at the site of injury.

If blood vessel injury is minor, hemostasis is achieved temporarily by the platelet plug, which usually forms within 3 to 5 minutes of injury. Platelet plugs seal the many minute ruptures that occur daily in the microcirculation, particularly in capillaries. With too few platelets, numerous small hemorrhagic areas called *purpuras* develop under the skin and throughout the tissues (see Chapter 20).

Function of Clotting Factors

A *blood clot* is a meshwork of protein strands that stabilizes the platelet plug and traps other cells, such as erythrocytes, phagocytes, and microorganisms (Figs. 19-18 and 19-19).

Fig. 19-18 *Blood clotting mechanism.* **A,** The clotting mechanism involves release of platelet factors at the injury site, formation of thrombin, and trapping of red blood cells (RBCs) in fibrin to form a clot. **B,** An electron micrograph showing entrapped RBCs in a fibrin clot. *(From Thibodeau, G.A. & Patton, K.T. [1999]. Anatomy & physiology [4th ed.]. St. Louis: Mosby.)*

The strands are made of fibrin, which normally is not present in the circulation but, rather, is the end-product of the ***coagulation cascade,*** a series of enzymatic reactions among the clotting factors (Fig. 19-19). According to the cascade theory of coagulation, each coagulation factor is converted to its active form by the preceding factor in a series of chain reactions until fibrin is produced. In effect, soluble clotting factors become insoluble fibrin.

The coagulation cascade is initiated through (1) the intrinsic pathway, activated when Hageman factor (factor XII) in plasma contacts with subendothelial substances exposed by vascular injury; and (2) the extrinsic pathway, activated when tissue thromboplastin, a substance released by damaged endothelial cells, contacts with one of the clotting factors, serum prothrombin conversion factor (factor VII). Both lead to a final common pathway when each has activated factor X (Stuart-Prower factor), and this proceeds to clot formation.

Newer concepts of the coagulation system

Division of the coagulation process into strictly defined extrinsic and intrinsic pathways has been abandoned because the cascade theory has been modified. Newer concepts are denoted by the blue lines in Fig. 19-19. These changes include (1) that factor VIIa of the extrinsic pathway can directly activate factor IX of the intrinsic pathway and (2) that factor VII can be activated by factors XIIa, IXa, Xa, and thrombin. It has therefore been hypothesized that factor VII may be the key regulatory protein that initiates blood coagulation.[6] In addition, tissue factor pathway inhibitor (TFPI) is a newly characterized protein involved in the regulation of hemostasis.[14] For simplicity of presentation, the reader

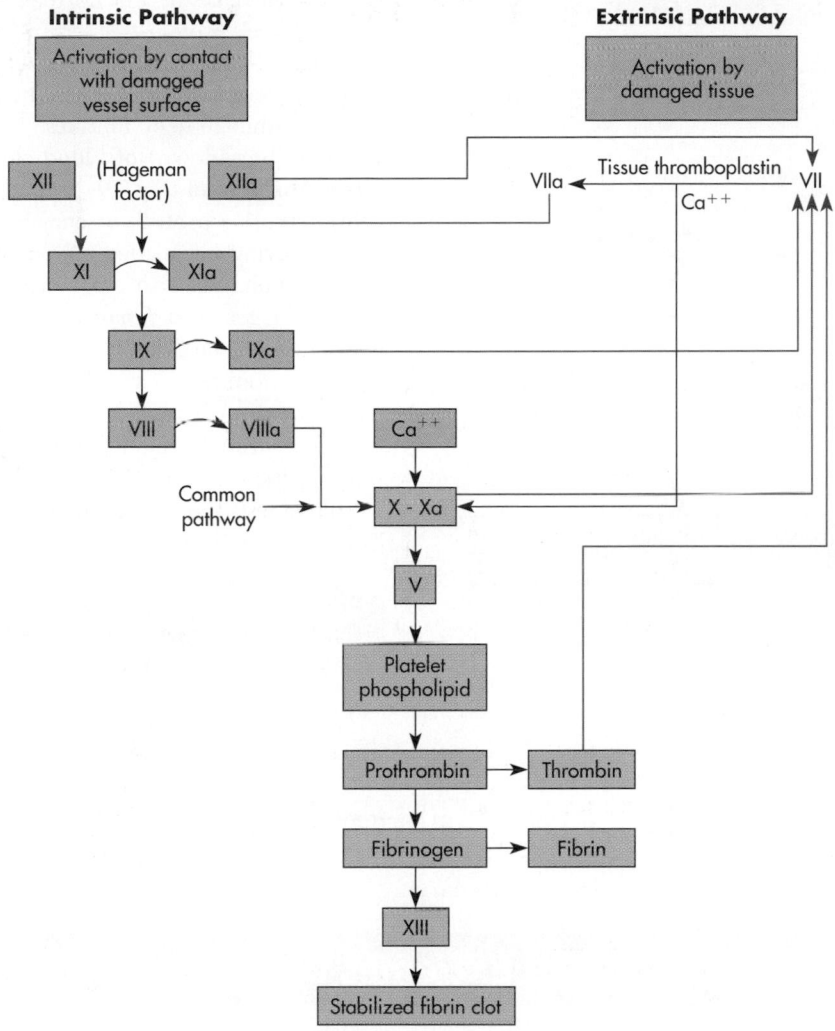

Fig. 19-19 *The "cascade" theory of coagulation.* Recent changes are shown in blue (see text).

should still understand the classic cascade presentation with an awareness of the additional changes. As more information becomes available, the cascade will undoubtedly change.

Control of Hemostatic Mechanisms

The major regulatory events in the clotting processes, including the activation of the clotting factors, the inhibition of these active clotting factors, and the production of circulating anticoagulant proteins, take place on membrane surfaces. The endothelium is a major site of hemostasis. Despite the continual presence of clotting factors and platelets in the circulation, blood normally remains fluid. Two properties of normal vascular endothelium prevent clotting: (1) the smooth texture of the endothelial lining, which prevents adherence of platelets; and (2) the negative charge of protein in the endothelial cells, which repels some negatively charged platelets and clotting factors. Damage to the vascular endothelium destroys both of these properties, enabling

platelets to adhere and initiating the intrinsic pathway of coagulation.

Once activated, coagulation is controlled by anticoagulants, some of which are products of the coagulation cascade itself. For example, once a clot has formed, its fibrin strands absorb 85% to 90% of the thrombin produced at the site. The remaining thrombin is inactivated by antithrombin III. Other anticoagulants, most notably heparin, are produced and secreted locally by tissue mast cells and basophils activated by the injury (see Chapter 6). Heparin not only halts the coagulation cascade but also enhances fibrin's absorption of thrombin in the clot.

Retraction and Lysis of Blood Clots

After a clot is formed, it retracts, or "solidifies." Fibrin strands shorten, becoming denser and stronger, which approximates the edges of the injured vessel wall and seals the site of injury. Retraction is facilitated by the large numbers of platelets trapped within the fibrin meshwork. The

Fig. 19-20 *The fibrinolytic system.*

platelets contract and "pull" the fibrin threads closer together while releasing a factor that stabilizes the fibrin. Contraction expels protein-free serum from the fibrin meshwork (see Fig. 19-18). This process usually begins within a few minutes after a clot has formed, and most of the serum is expressed within 20 to 60 minutes.

Lysis (breakdown) of blood clots is carried out by the *fibrinolytic system* (Fig. 19-20) and is mediated by plasmin (fibrinolysin), a proteolytic enzyme activated by substances present during coagulation and inflammation, such as factor XII, thrombin, and lysosomal enzymes. Plasmin splits fibrin and fibrinogen into *fibrin degradation products (FDPs),* which dissolve the clot. The fibrinolytic system removes clotted blood from tissues and dissolves small clots (thrombi) in blood vessels. A balance between the amounts of thrombin and plasmin in the circulation maintains normal coagulation and lysis. (See Box 19-1.)

Blood tests that reflect chiefly hematologic disorders are listed in Table 19-9.

✓ QUICK CHECK

Why are platelets necessary for stopping bleeding?

Briefly describe the steps in plug formation.

Why does the fibrinolytic system cause clot dissolution?

Hematologic Values at the Extremes of Age   BOX 19-1

Blood cell counts tend to rise above adult levels at birth and then decline gradually throughout childhood. Table 19-8 lists normal ranges during infancy and childhood. The immediate rise in values is the result of accelerated hematopoiesis during fetal life, increased numbers of cells that result from the trauma of birth, and cutting of the umbilical cord.

Average blood volume in the full-term neonate is 85 ml/kg of body weight. The premature infant has a slightly larger blood volume of 90 ml/kg of body weight, with the mean increasing to 150 ml/kg during the first few days after birth. In both full-term and premature infants, blood volume decreases during the first few months. Thereafter the average blood volume is 75 to 77 ml/kg, which is similar to that of older children and adults.

The hypoxic intrauterine environment stimulates erythropoietin production in the fetus and accelerates fetal erythropoiesis, producing polycythemia (excessive proliferation of erythrocyte precursors) of the newborn. After birth, the oxygen from the lungs saturates arterial blood, and more oxygen is delivered to the tissues. In response to the change from a placental to a pulmonary oxygen supply during the first few days of life, levels of erythropoietin and the rate of blood cell formation de-

crease. The very active rate of fetal erythropoiesis is reflected by the large numbers of immature erythrocytes (reticulocytes) in the peripheral blood of full-term neonates. After birth, the number of reticulocytes decreases about 50% every 12 hours, so it is rare to find an elevated reticulocyte count after the first week of life. During this period of rapid growth the rate of erythrocyte destruction is greater than that in later childhood and adulthood. In full-term infants, normal erythrocyte life span is 60 to 80 days; in premature infants, it may be as short as 20 to 30 days; and in children and adolescents, it is the same as that in adults—120 days.

In premature infants, the postnatal fall in hemoglobin and hematocrit values is more marked than in the full-term infant. In the preschool and school-age child, hemoglobin, hematocrit, and red blood cell counts gradually rise. Metabolic processes within the erythrocytes of neonates differ significantly from those of erythrocytes in the normal adult. The relatively young population of erythrocytes in the newborn consumes greater quantities of glucose than do erythrocytes in adults.

The lymphocytes of children tend to have more cytoplasm and less compact nuclear chromatin than do the lymphocytes of adults. A possible explanation is that children tend to have more frequent viral infec-

Values at the Extremes of Age—cont'd   BOX 19-1

tions, which are associated with atypical lymphocytes. Even minor infections, in which the child fails to exhibit clinical manifestations of illness, and administration of immunizations may result in lymphocyte changes.

The lymphocyte count is high at birth and continues to rise during the first year of life; then it steadily declines until lower adult values are reached. It is unknown whether these developmental variations are physiologic or a pathologic response to frequent viral infection and immunizations in children.

At birth, the neutrophil count is very high and rises during the early days of life. After 2 weeks, neutrophil counts fall to within or below normal adult ranges. By approximately 4 years of age the neutrophil count is the same as that of an adult.

Eosinophil count is high in the first year of life and is higher in children than in teenagers or adults. Monocyte counts are high in the first year of life and then decrease to adult levels. Platelet counts in full-term neonates are comparable with platelet counts in adults and remain so throughout infancy and childhood.

Blood composition changes little with age. Erythrocyte life span is normal, although erythrocytes are replenished more slowly after bleeding, probably because of iron depletion. Total serum iron, total iron-binding capacity, and intestinal iron absorption are all decreased in elderly persons. Iron deficiency is often responsible for the low hemoglobin levels noted in elderly persons. The plasma membranes of erythrocytes become increasingly fragile, with portions lost, presumably because of physical trauma inflicted during circulation.

Lymphocyte function decreases with age (see Chapters 5 and 6), causing changes in cellular immunity with some decline in T cell function. The humoral immune system is less able to respond to antigenic challenge.

No changes in platelet numbers or structure have been observed in elderly persons, yet evidence shows that platelet adhesiveness probably increases. Although fibrinogen levels and factors V, VII and IX tend to be increased in elderly people, evidence about hypercoagulability is inconclusive.

TABLE 19-8   Hematologic Values During Infancy and Childhood

				Differential Counts					
Age	Hemoglobin (g/dl):Mean	Hematocrit (%):Mean	Reticulocytes (%):Mean	Leukocytes (WBC/mm³): Mean	Neutrophils (%):Mean	Lymphocytes (%):Mean	Eosinophils (%):Mean	Monocytes (%):Mean	Platelets (10³/mm³)
Cord blood	16.8	55	5.0	18,000	61	31	2	6	290
2 wk	16.5	50	1.0	12,000	40	48	3	9	252
3 mo	12.0	36	1.0	12,000	30	63	2	5	140-340
6 mo-6 yr	12.0	37	1.0	10,000	45	48	2	5	140-340
7-12 yr	13.0	38	1.0	8000	55	38	2	5	140-340
Adult	13.0	40	1.0	8000	55	35	2	5	140-340
Female	14	41	0.8-4.1	7400	54-62	25-33	1-4	3-7	140-340
Male	16	47	0.8-2.5	7400	54-62	25-33	1-4	3-7	140-340

TABLE 19-9   Blood Tests for Hematologic Disorders

Cell Type and Test	Property Evaluated by Test	Possible Hematologic Cause of Abnormal Findings
Erythrocyte		
Red cell count	Number (in millions) of erythrocytes/µl of blood	Altered erythropoiesis, anemias, hemorrhage, Hodgkin disease, leukemia
Mean corpuscular volume	Size of erythrocytes	Anemias, thalassemias
Mean corpuscular hemoglobin (MCH)	Amount of hemoglobin in each erythrocyte (by weight)	Anemias, hemoglobinopathy
Mean corpuscular hemoglobin concentration (MCHC)	Concentration of hemoglobin in each erythrocyte (percentage of erythrocyte occupied by hemoglobin)	Anemias, hereditary spherocytosis
Hemoglobin determination	Amount of hemoglobin (by weight)/dl of blood	Anemias

Data from Byrne, C.J. et al. Laboratory tests: Implications for nursing care. Menlo Park, Calif.: Addison-Wesley; Bick, R.L. et al. (1993). Hematology: Clinical and laboratory practice. St. Louis: Mosby.

NOTE: *See Fig. 19-19 for information about clotting factors and their sequence of activation in the coagulation cascade.*

Continued

TABLE 19-9	Blood Tests for Hematologic Disorders—cont'd	
Cell Type and Test	**Property Evaluated by Test**	**Possible Hematologic Cause of Abnormal Findings**
Erythrocyte—cont'd		
Hematocrit determination	Percentage of a given volume of blood that is occupied by erythrocytes	Hemorrhage, polycythemia, erythrocytosis, anemias, leukemia
Reticulocyte count	Number of reticulocytes/μl of blood (also expressed as percentage of reticulocytes in total red cell count)	Hyperactive or hypoactive bone marrow function
Erythrocyte osmotic fragility test	Cellular shape (biconcavity), structure of plasma membrane	Anemias, hemolytic disease caused by ABO or Rh incompatibility, Hodgkin disease, polycythemia vera, thalassemia major
Hemoglobin electrophoresis	Relative percentage of different types of hemoglobin in erythrocytes	Sickle cell disease, sickle cell trait, hemoglobin C disease, hemoglobin C trait, thalassemias
Sickle cell test	Presence of hemoglobin S in erythrocytes	Sickle cell trait, sickle cell anemia
Glucose-6-phosphate dehydrogenase (G6PD) deficiency test	Deficiency of G6PD in erythrocytes	Hemolytic anemia
Hemoglobin metabolism		
Serum ferritin determination	Depletion of body iron (potential deficiency of heme synthesis)	Iron deficiency anemias
Total iron-building capacity (TIBC)	Amount of iron in serum plus amount of transferrin available in serum (μg/dl)	Hemorrhage, iron deficiency anemia, hemochromatosis, hemosiderosis, iron overload, anemias, thalassemia
Transferrin saturation	Percentage of transferrin that is saturated with iron	Acute hemorrhage, hemochromatosis, hemosiderosis, sideroblastic anemia, iron deficiency anemia, iron overload, thalassemia
Porphyrin analysis (protoporphyrin analysis)	Concentration of protoporphyrin in erythrocytes (μg/dl); an indicator of iron-deficient erythropoiesis	Megaloblastic anemia, congenital erythropoietic porphyria
Direct antiglobulin test (DAT)	Antibody binding to erythrocytes	Hemolytic disease of the newborn, autoimmune hemolytic anemia, drug-induced hemolytic anemia, transfusion reaction
Antibody screen (indirect Coombs test)	Detection of antibodies to erythrocyte antigens (other than the ABO antigens)	Same as for DAT
Leukocytes: differential white cell count (absolute number of a type of leukocyte/μl of blood)	See below	See below
Neutrophil count	Neutrophils/μl	Myeloproliferative disorders, hematopoietic disorders, hemolysis, infection
Lymphocyte count	Lymphocytes/μl	Infectious lymphocytosis, infectious mononucleosis, hematopoietic disorders, anemias, leukemia, lymphosarcoma, Hodgkin disease
Plasma cell count	Plasma cells/μl	Infectious mononucleosis, lymphocytosis, plasma cell leukemia
Monocyte count	Monocytes/μl	Hodgkin disease, infectious mononucleosis, monocytic leukemia, non-Hodgkin lymphoma, polycythemia vera

TABLE 19-9	Blood Tests for Hematologic Disorders—cont'd	
Cell Type and Test	**Property Evaluated by Test**	**Possible Hematologic Cause of Abnormal Findings**
Eosinophil count	Eosinophils/μl	Hematopoietic disorders
Basophil count	Basophils/μl	Chronic myelogenous leukemia, hemolytic anemias, Hodgkin disease, polycythemia vera
Platelets and clotting factors		
Platelet count	Number of circulating platelets (in thousands)/μl of blood	Anemias, multiple myeloma, myelofibrosis, polycythemia vera, leukemia, disseminated intravascular coagulation (DIC), hemolytic disease of the newborn, idiopathic thrombocytopenic purpura, transfusion reaction, lymphoproliferative disorders
Bleeding time	Duration of bleeding following a standardized superficial puncture wound of the skin, integrity of the platelet plug, measured in minutes following puncture	Leukemia, anemias, DIC, fibrinolytic activity, purpuras, hemorrhagic disease of the newborn, infectious mononucleosis, multiple myeloma, clotting factor deficiencies, thrombasthenia, thrombocytopenia, von Willebrand disease
Clot retraction test	Platelet number and function, fibrinogen quantity and use, measured in hours required for expression of serum from a clot incubated in a test tube	Acute leukemia, aplastic anemia, factor XIII deficiency, increased fibrinolytic activity, Hodgkin disease, hyperfibrinogenemia or hypofibrinogenemia, idiopathic thrombocytopenic purpura, multiple myeloma, polycythemia vera, secondary thrombocytopenia, thrombasthenia
Platelet adhesion studies	Ability of platelets to adhere to foreign surfaces	Anemia, macroglobulinemia, Bernard-Soulier syndrome, multiple myeloma, myeloid metaplasia, plasma cell dyscrasias, thrombasthenia, thrombocytopathy, von Willebrand disease
Platelet aggregation tests	Ability of platelets to adhere to one another	Afibrinogenemia, Bernard-Soulier syndrome, thrombasthenia, hemorrhagic thrombocythemia, myeloid metaplasia, plasma cell dyscrasias, platelet release defects, polycythemia vera, preleukemia, sideroblastic anemia, von Willebrand disease, Waldenström macroglobulinemia, hypercoagulability
Whole blood clotting time (Lee-White coagulation time)	Overall ability of blood to clot, as measured in minutes in a test tube	Afibrinogenemia, clotting factor deficiencies, excessive fibrinolysis, hemorrhagic disease of the newborn, hypofibrinogenemia, hypoprothrombinemia, leukemia
Circulating anticoagulants (immunoglobulin G [IgG] antibodies that inhibit coagulation)	Presence of antibodies that neutralize clotting factors and inhibit coagulation, as indicated by prolonged clotting time, prothrombin time, or partial thromboplastin time	Afibrinogenemia, presence of fibrin-fibrinogen degradation products, macroglobulinemia, multiple myeloma, DIC, plasma cell dyscrasias
Partial thromboplastin time (PTT)	Effectiveness of clotting factors (except factors VII and VIII), effectiveness of intrinsic pathway of coagulation cascade, as measured by a test tube (in seconds)	Presence of circulating anticoagulants, DIC, clotting factor deficiencies, excessive fibrinolysis, hemorrhagic disease of the newborn, hypofibrinogenemia and afibrinogenemia, prothrombin deficiency, von Willebrand disease, acute hemorrhage

Continued

TABLE 19-9	Blood Tests for Hematologic Disorders—cont'd	
Cell Type and Test	Property Evaluated by Test	Possible Hematologic Cause of Abnormal Findings
Platelets and clotting factors—cont'd		
Prothrombin time	Effectiveness of activity of prothrombin, fibrinogen, and factors V, VII, and X; effectiveness of vitamin K-dependent coagulation factors of the extrinsic and common pathways of the coagulation cascade as measured in a test tube (in seconds)	Hypofibrinogenemia, dysfibrinogenemia, and afibrinogenemia; presence of circulating anticoagulants; DIC; deficiency of factors V, VII, or X; presence of fibrin degradation products, increased fibrinolytic activity, hemolytic jaundice, hemorrhagic disease of the newborn; acute leukemia, polycythemia vera, prothrombin deficiency, multiple myeloma
Thrombin time	Quantity and activity of fibrinogen as measured in a test tube (in seconds)	Hypofibrinogenemia, dysfibrinogenemia, and afibrinogenemia; presence of circulating anticoagulants; hemorrhagic disease of the newborn, polycythemia vera; increase in fibrinogen-fibrin degradation products; increased fibrinolytic activity
Fibrinogen assay	Amount of fibrinogen available for fibrin formation	Acute leukemia, congenital hypofibrinogenemia or afibrinogenemia, DIC, increased fibrinolytic activity, severe hemorrhage
Fibrin-fibrinogen degradation products (fibrin-fibrinogen split products)	Fibrinogenic activity as measured by levels of fibrin-fibrinogen degradation products (in μg/ml of blood)	Transfusion reactions, DIC, internal hemorrhage in the newborn, deep vein thrombosis, pulmonary embolism

☐ DID YOU UNDERSTAND?

Components of the Hematologic System

1. Blood consists of a variety of formed elements: about 90% water and 10% solutes. In adults the total blood volume is approximately 5.5 L.
2. Plasma, a complex aqueous liquid, contains three major groups of plasma proteins: (a) albumins, (b) globulins, and (c) clotting factors.
3. The cellular elements of blood are the erythrocytes, leukocytes, lymphocytes, and platelets.
4. Erythrocytes are the most abundant cells of the blood, occupying approximately 48% of the blood volume in men and approximately 42% in women. Erythrocytes are responsible for tissue oxygenation.
5. Leukocytes are fewer in number than erythrocytes and constitute approximately 5000 to 10,000 cells/mm³ of blood. Leukocytes defend the body against infection and remove dead or injured host cells.
6. Leukocytes are classified as either granulocytes (neutrophils, basophils, eosinophils) or agranulocytes (monocytes/macrophages, lymphocytes).
7. Platelets are not cells, but disk-shaped cytoplasmic fragments. Platelets are essential for blood coagulation and control of bleeding.
8. The lymphoid organs are classified as primary (thymus and bone marrow) or secondary (spleen, lymph nodes, tonsils, Peyer patches of the small intestine).
9. The lymphoid organs are sites of residence, proliferation, differentiation, or function of lymphocytes and mononuclear phagocytes.
10. The spleen is the largest of the secondary lymphoid organs and functions as the site of fetal hematopoiesis, filters and cleanses the blood, and is a reservoir for lymphocytes and other blood cells.
11. The lymph nodes are the site of development or activity of large numbers of lymphocytes, monocytes, and macrophages.
12. The mononuclear phagocyte system (MPS), previously called the *reticuloendothelial system (RES)*, is composed of monoblasts, promonocytes, and monocytes in bone marrow, monocytes in peripheral blood, and macrophages in tissue.
13. The MPS is the main line of defense against bacteria in the bloodstream and cleanses the blood by removing old, injured, or dead blood cells; antigen-antibody complexes; and macromolecules.

Development of Blood Cells

1. Hematopoiesis, or blood cell production, occurs in the liver and spleen of the fetus and in the bone marrow after birth.

DID YOU UNDERSTAND? —cont'd

2. Hematopoiesis involves two stages: (a) proliferation and (b) differentiation, or maturation. Each type of blood cell has parent cells called *stem cells.*

3. Hematopoiesis continues throughout life to replace blood cells that grow old and die, are killed by disease, or are lost through bleeding.

4. Bone marrow consists of blood vessels, nerves, mononuclear phagocytes, stem cells, blood cells in various stages of differentiation, and fatty tissue.

5. Hemoglobin, the oxygen-carrying protein of the erythrocyte, enables the blood to transport 100 times more oxygen than could be transported dissolved in plasma alone.

6. Erythropoiesis depends on the presence of vitamins (especially vitamin B_{12}, folate vitamin, vitamin B_6, riboflavin, pantothenic acid, niacin, ascorbic acid, and vitamin E).

7. Regulation of erythropoiesis is mediated by erythropoietin. Erythropoietin is secreted by the kidneys in response to tissue hypoxia and causes a compensatory increase in erythrocyte production if the oxygen content of the blood decreases because of anemia, high altitude, or pulmonary disease.

8. Maintenance of optimal levels of granulocytes and monocytes in the blood depends on the availability of pluripotential stem cells in the marrow, induction of these into committed stem cells, and timely release of new cells from the marrow.

9. Specific humoral CSFs are necessary for the adequate growth of myeloid, erythroid, lymphoid, and megakaryocytic lineages.

10. Platelets develop from megakaryocytes by a process called *endomitosis.* In endomitosis, the megakaryocytes undergo mitosis but not cytokinesis; thus the cell does not divide into two daughter cells.

Mechanisms of Hemostasis

1. Hemostasis, or arrest of bleeding, involves (a) vasoconstriction (vasospasm), (b) formation of a platelet plug, (c) activation of the clotting cascade, (d) formation of a blood clot, and (e) clot retraction and clot dissolution.

2. Two properties of normal vascular endothelium prevent clotting: (a) the smooth texture of the endothelial lining that prevents adherence of platelets and (b) the negative charge of protein in the endothelial cells that repels some negatively charged platelets and clotting factors.

3. Lysis of blood clots is the function of the fibrinolytic system. Plasmin, a proteolytic enzyme, splits fibrin and fibrinogen into fibrin degradation products that dissolve the clot.

⚠ AGING AND THE HEMATOLOGIC SYSTEM

1. Blood composition changes little with age. A delay in erythrocyte replenishment may occur after bleeding, presumably because of iron deficiency.

2. Lymphocyte function appears to decrease with age. Particularly affected is a decrease in cellular immunity.

3. Platelet adhesiveness probably increases with age.

KEY TERMS

Agranulocyte, 508
Albumin, 506
Basophil, 509
Biconcavity, 508
Blood clot, 523
Bone marrow (myeloid tissue), 514
Clotting factor, 506
Coagulation cascade, 524
Colony-stimulating factor (CSF), 512, 514
Deoxyhemoglobin (reduced hemoglobin), 516
Differentiation (maturation), 513
Eosinophil, 509
Erythroblast, 514
Erythrocyte (red blood cell [RBC]), 507
Erythropoiesis, 514
Fibrin degradation product (FDP), 526
Fibrinolytic system, 526
Globin, 516
Globulin (immunoglobulin), 506

Granulocyte, 508
Hematopoiesis, 513
Hematopoietic growth factor, 514
Heme, 516
Hemoglobin (Hb), 508
Hemostasis, 521
Immunocyte, 508
Leukocyte (white blood cell), 507
Lipoprotein, 507
Lymph node, 511
Lymphocyte, 510
Macrophage, 509
Marginating storage pool, 513
Megaloblast, 515
Methemoglobin, 516
Monocyte, 509
Mononuclear phagocyte system (MPS) (reticuloendothelial system [RES]), 509
Natural killer cells, 510
Neutrophil (polymorphonuclear neutrophil [PMN]), 509

Normoblast, 515
Oxyhemoglobin, 516
Phagocyte, 508
Plasma, 506
Plasma protein, 506
Platelet (thrombocyte), 507
Pluripotential stem cell , 513
Primary lymphoid organ, 511
Proliferation (mitotic division), 513
Reticulocyte, 515
Reversible deformability, 508
Secondary lymphoid organ, 511
Serum, 506
Spleen, 511
Stem cell, 513
Stem cell system, 513
Totipotential hematopoietic stem cell (THSC) (multipotential stem cell), 513
Transferrin, 517

REFERENCES

1. Guyton, A.C. & Hall, J.E. (1997). *Human physiology and mechanisms of disease* (6th ed.). Philadelphia: Saunders.
2. Wang, W. et al. (1997). Osteoclasts are capable of particle phagocytosis and bone resorption. *Journal of Pathology, 182*(1), 92-98.
3. Ketley, N.J. & Newland, A.C. (1997). Haemopoietic growth factors. *Postgraduate Medical Journal, 73*(858), 215-221.
4. Rameshwar, P., Poddar, A., & Gascon, P. (1997). Hematopoietic regulation mediated by interactions among the neurokinins and cytokines. *Leukemia and Lymphoma, 28*(1-2), 1-10.
5. Veiby, O.P., Mikhail, A.A., & Snodgrass, H.R. (1997). Growth factors and hematopoietic stem cells. *Hematologic and Oncologic Clinics of North America, 11*(6), 1173-1184.
6. Harmening, D.M. (Ed.). (1997). *Clinical hematology and fundamentals of hemostasis* (3rd ed.). Philadelphia: Davis.
7. Lee, G.R. et al. (1993). *Wintrobe's clinical hematology* (9th ed.). Philadelphia: Lea & Febiger.
8. Metcalfe, D. (1994). Thrombopoietin—At last. *Nature, 369,* 519-520.
9. Russell, W.J. et al. (1966). Active bone marrow distribution in the adult. *British Journal of Radiology, 39,* 735.
10. Jai, L., Bonaventura, J., & Stamler, J.S. (1996). S-nitrosohaemoglobin: A dynamic activity of blood involved in vascular control. *Nature, 380*(6571), 221.
11. Goldwasser, E. (1990). Erythropoietin: Molecular and cellular biology. In J. Spivak, W. Drohan, & D. Dooley (Eds.). *Hematopoietic growth factors in transfusion medicine.* New York: Wiley.
12. de Sauvage, F.J. et al. (1994). Stimulation of megakaryocytopoiesis and thrombopoiesis by the c-Mpl ligand. *Nature, 369*(6481), 533-538.
13. Fischbach, D. & Fogdall, R. (1981). *Coagulation, the essentials.* Baltimore: Williams & Wilkins.
14. Rosenson, R.S. & Lowe, G.D. (1998). Effects of lipids and lipoproteins on thrombosis and rheology. *Atherosclerosis, 140*(2), 271-280.

CHAPTER

20

Alterations of Hematologic Function

Thom J. Mansen and Kathryn L. McCance

Alterations of erythrocyte function involve either insufficient or excessive numbers of erythrocytes in the circulation or normal numbers of cells with abnormal components. Anemias are conditions in which there are too few erythrocytes or an insufficient volume of erythrocytes in the blood. Polycythemias are conditions in which erythrocyte numbers or volume is excessive. Each of these two conditions has many causes, explaining why each has so many names. Anemia and polycythemia are not diseases per se, but rather they are pathophysiologic manifestations of a variety of disease states.

Many disorders involving leukocytes range from purely reactive alterations, such as leukocytosis, to proliferative disorders, such as leukemia. An event of importance to hematology has been its increasing relationship with oncology. Many hematologic disorders are malignancies, and many nonhematologic malignancies metastasize to bone marrow. Thus a large portion of this chapter is devoted to malignant disease.

Because the only role of clotting (hemostasis) is to stop bleeding, this interesting self-regulatory system obviously is essential to survival. Remarkable is the fact that blood clots when shed and normally does not clot within blood vessels. Platelets—through a renaissance of research interest—are known to have roles in clotting, wound healing, inflammation, and phagocytosis of foreign matter. They also play deleterious roles, however, in the pathogenesis of many diseases. In addition, this chapter covers various clotting factors and their control systems.

ALTERATIONS OF ERYTHROCYTE FUNCTION

Strictly speaking, *anemia* is a reduction in the total number of circulating erythrocytes or a decrease in the quality or quantity of hemoglobin. The causes of anemia are (1) altered production of erythrocytes, (2) blood loss, (3) increased erythrocyte destruction, or (4) a combination of all three.

Classification of Anemias

Anemias are classified by their causes or by the changes that occur in the size and shape of the erythrocyte. The most common classification of anemias is based on the changes that affect the cell's size and hemoglobin content (Table 20-1). Terms that end with "cytic" refer to cell size, and those that end with "chromic" refer to hemoglobin content. Other terms that might indicate changes in the erythrocyte associated with anemias are *anisocytosis* (various sizes) and *poikilocytosis* (various shapes).

Clinical Manifestations of Anemias

The symptoms of anemia vary, depending on the body's ability to compensate for the reduced oxygen-carrying capacity of the blood. Anemia that is mild and starts gradually is usually easier to compensate for and may cause problems for the individual only during physical exertion. Compensation generally involves the cardiovascular, respiratory, and hematologic systems (Fig. 20-1). Laboratory tests for various anemias are described in Box 20-1.

In the presence of decreased red blood cells, the consistency and volume of blood are reduced. To compensate, interstitial fluid moves into the blood vessels and the amount of plasma increases. This maintains an adequate blood vol-

---

TABLE 20-1   Morphologic Classification of Anemias

Morphology and Cause of Reduced Oxygen-Carrying Capacity of the Blood	Name and Mechanism of Anemic Condition	Primary Cause of Associated Disorder
Macrocytic-normochromic anemia: large, abnormally shaped erythrocytes but normal hemoglobin concentrations	Pernicious anemia: lack of vitamin B_{12} (cobalamin) for erythropoiesis; abnormal DNA and RNA synthesis in the erythroblast; premature cell death	Congenital or acquired deficiency of intrinsic factor (IF); genetic disorder of DNA synthesis
	Folate deficiency anemia: lack of folate for erythropoiesis; premature cell death	Dietary folate deficiency
Microcytic-hypochromic anemia: small, abnormally shaped erythrocytes and reduced hemoglobin concentration	Iron deficiency anemia: lack of iron for hemoglobin production; insufficient hemoglobin	Chronic blood loss; dietary iron deficiency, disruption of iron metabolism or iron cycle (see Chapter 19)
	Sideroblastic anemia: dysfunctional iron uptake by erythroblasts and defective porphyrin and heme synthesis	Congenital dysfunction of iron metabolism in erythroblasts, acquired dysfunction of iron metabolism as a result of drugs or toxins
	Thalassemia: impaired synthesis of α- or β-chain of hemoglobin A; phagocytosis of abnormal erythroblasts in the marrow	Congenital genetic defect of globin synthesis
Normocytic-normochromic anemia: destruction or depletion of normal erythroblasts or mature erythrocytes	Aplastic anemia: insufficient erythropoiesis	Depressed stem cell proliferation resulting in bone marrow aplasia
	Posthemorrhagic anemia: blood loss	Acute or chronic hemorrhage that stimulates increased erythropoiesis, which eventually depletes body iron
	Hemolytic anemia: premature destruction (lysis) of mature erythrocytes in the circulation	Any condition that increases fragility of erythrocytes
	Sickle cell anemia: abnormal hemoglobin synthesis, abnormal cell shape with susceptibility to damage, lysis, and phagocytosis	Congenital dysfunction of hemoglobin synthesis
	Anemia of chronic inflammation (disease): abnormally increased demand for new erythrocytes	Chronic infection or inflammation; malignancy

DNA, Deoxyribonucleic acid; RNA, ribonucleic acid.

ume, but the viscosity (thickness) of the blood is decreased. The "diluted" blood flows faster and more turbulently than normal blood, causing a hyperdynamic circulatory state. Cardiac manifestations associated with this hyperdynamic state are an increased heart rate, which may lead to cardiac dilation, and heart valve insufficiency if the underlying anemic condition is not corrected.

Hypoxia, which results from the reduced oxygen-carrying capacity of the blood, causes dilation of arterioles, capillaries, and venules, increasing the flow of blood through them and further contributes to cardiac manifestations. Increased peripheral blood flow and venous return promote an increase in heart rate and stroke volume in an effort to meet normal oxygen demand and prevent cardiopulmonary congestion. All of these mechanisms may lead to heart failure.

Tissue demand for oxygen affects the rate and depth of breathing and the release of oxygen from hemoglobin. Re-

lease of oxygen from hemoglobin is increased to meet tissue demands for oxygen with a concomitant increase in ventilatory rate and depth to bring in more oxygen to oxygenate the blood. The combination of all these compensatory mechanisms may cause individuals to experience shortness of breath (dyspnea), a rapid and pounding heartbeat, dizziness, and fatigue. In mild, chronic cases, symptoms might be present only when there is an increased demand for oxygen (e.g., physical exertion), but in severe cases, symptoms may be experienced even at rest.

Manifestations of anemia may be seen in other parts of the body. The skin, mucous membranes, lips, nail beds, and conjunctivae become either pale because of reduced hemoglobin concentration or yellowish (jaundiced) because of accumulation of end-products of red cell *hemolysis* (destruction) if this is a cause of anemia. Decreased oxygen delivery to the skin results in impaired healing and loss of elasticity,

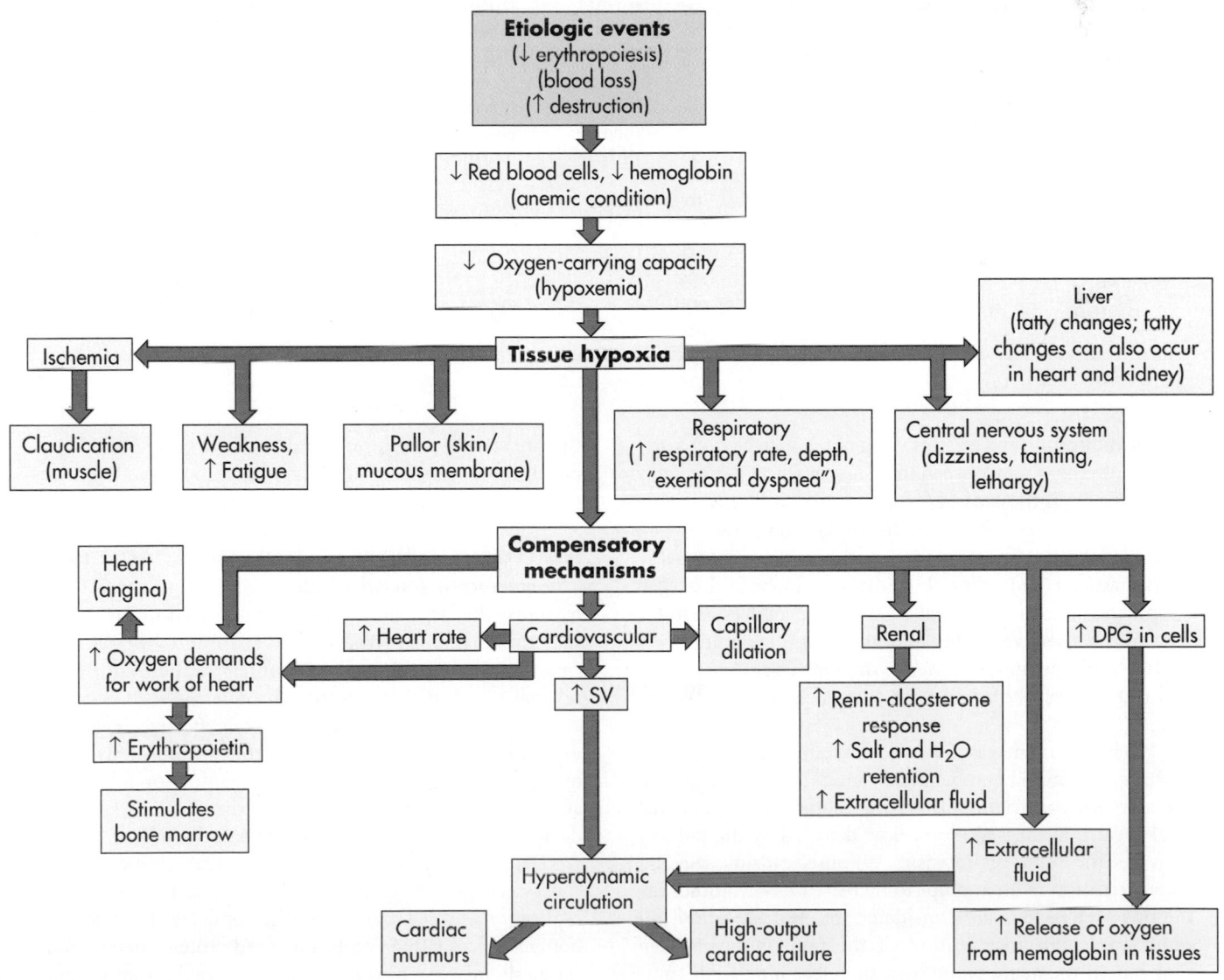

Fig. 20-1 *Progression and manifestations of anemia. SV,* Stroke volume; *DPG,* disphosphatidyl-glycerol.

Laboratory Tests for Various Anemias   BOX 20-1

Test	Pernicious Anemia	Folate Deficiency Anemia	Iron Deficiency Anemia	Sideroblastic Anemia	Aplastic Anemia	Posthemorrhagic Anemia	Hemolytic Anemia	Anemia of Chronic Inflammation
Hemoglobin	Low	Low	Low	Low	Low or normal	Normal or low	Low	Low
Hematocrit	Low	Low	Low	Low	Low or normal	Normal or low	Low	Low
Reticulocyte count	Low	Low	Normal or slightly high or low	Normal or slightly high	Low	Increased	High	Normal
Mean corpuscular volume (MCV)	High	High	Low	Low	Normal or slightly high	Slightly low	Normal or high	Normal or low
Plasma iron	High	High	Low	High	High	Normal	Normal or high	Low
Total iron-binding capacity	Normal	Normal	High	Normal	Normal	Normal	Normal	Low
Ferritin	High	High	Low	High	Normal	Normal	Normal	Normal
Serum B_{12}	Low	Normal	Normal	Normal	Normal	Normal	Normal	Normal
Folate	Normal	Low	Normal	Normal	Normal	Normal	Normal	Normal
Bilirubin	Slightly high	Slightly high	Normal	High	Normal	Normal	Slightly high	Normal
Free erythrocyte protoporphyrin	Normal	Normal	High	Increased or normal	High	Normal	Normal	Normal or slightly high
Transferrin	Slightly high	Slightly high	Low	High	Normal	Normal	Normal	Slightly low

as well as thinning and early graying of the hair. Nervous system involvement may be seen in instances where a deficiency of vitamin B_{12} is the cause. Myelin degeneration occurs causing a loss of nerve fibers in the spinal cord, resulting in paresthesias (numbness), gait disturbances, extreme weakness, spasticity, and reflex abnormalities. Decreased oxygen supply to the gastrointestinal tract often produces abdominal pain, nausea, vomiting, and anorexia. Low-grade fever (<101° F) occurs in some anemic individuals and may result from the release of leukocyte pyrogens from ischemic tissues.

When the anemia is severe or acute in onset (i.e., hemorrhage), the initial compensatory mechanism is peripheral blood vessel constriction, diverting blood flow to essential vital organs. Decreased blood flow detected by the kidneys activates the renin-angiotensin response, causing salt and water retention in an attempt to increase blood volume. Situations such as this are considered an emergency and require immediate intervention of the underlying problem that caused the acute blood loss; therefore long-term compensatory mechanisms do not develop.

Anemias that develop slowly also require treatment of

the underlying condition and associated symptoms. Therapies include transfusions, dietary corrections, and administration of supplemental vitamins or iron.

Macrocytic-Normochromic Anemias

The *macrocytic (megaloblastic) anemias* are characterized by unusually large stem cells (megaloblasts) in the marrow that mature into erythrocytes that are unusually large in size (macrocytic). The hemoglobin content in these large cells is normal and classified as normochromic.

These anemias are the result of ineffective erythrocyte deoxyribonucleic acid (DNA) synthesis, commonly caused by deficiencies of vitamin B_{12} (cobalamin) or folate (folic acid). These defective erythrocytes die prematurely, which decreases their numbers in the circulation, causing anemia.

Defective DNA synthesis in megaloblastic anemias causes cell growth to proceed at unequal rates with DNA replication and cell division blocked or delayed. However, ribonucleic acid (RNA) replication and protein (hemoglobin) synthesis proceed normally. The end result is an overproduction of hemoglobin during delayed cellular division, creating a larger than normal erythrocyte.

Fig. 20-2 *Appearance of red blood cells in various disorders.* **A,** Normal blood smear. **B,** Hypochromic-microcytic anemia (iron deficiency). **C,** Macrocytic anemia (pernicious anemia). **D,** Macrocytic anemia in pregnancy. **E,** Hereditary elliptocytosis. **F,** Myelofibrosis (teardrop). **G,** Hemolytic anemia associated with prosthetic heart valve. **H,** Microangiopathic anemia. **I,** Stomatocytes. **J,** Spherocytes (hereditary spherocytosis). **K,** Sideroblastic anemia; note the double population of red blood cells. **L,** Sickle cell anemia. **M,** Target cells (after splenectomy). **N,** Basophil stippling in case of unexplained anemia. **O,** Howell-Jolly bodies (after splenectomy). *(From Wintrobe, M.M. et al. [1981]. Clinical hematology [8th ed.]. Philadelphia: Lea & Febiger.)*

Fig. 20-3 *Bone marrow aspirate from individual with pernicious anemia.* Bone marrow aspirate smear from an individual with megaloblastic red cell precursors and giant metamyelocytes. The chromatin in the red blood cell nuclei is more dispersed than in normal red cell precursors at comparable stages of maturation; the giant metamyelocytes have dispersed nuclear chromatin in contrast to normal metamyelocytes, which have condensed chromatin (Wright-Giemsa stain). *(From Damjanov, I. & Linder, J. [Eds.]. [1996]. Anderson's pathology [10th ed.]. St. Louis: Mosby.)*

Pernicious anemia

Pernicious anemia, the most common type of megaloblastic anemia, is a chronic condition caused by malabsorption of vitamin B_{12} (Fig. 20-2, *C*). The term *pernicious* means highly injurious or destructive and reflects the fact that this condition was once fatal. Pernicious anemia is most common in late adult life and rare in individuals younger than 30 years, unless it is congenital, which usually occurs before 2 years of age. Pernicious anemia is most common among Scandinavian, English, and Irish peoples. In the United States, both genders appear to be equally affected.

≡ *Pathophysiology*

Pernicious anemia is caused by defective gastric secretion of intrinsic factor (IF), which is needed for absorption of vitamin B_{12}. Vitamin B_{12} is necessary for nuclear maturation and DNA synthesis in red blood cells. Deficiency of IF may be congenital or may be the result of adult-onset atrophy of the gastric mucosa in which the parietal cells are destroyed and all secretions of the stomach—hydrochloric acid, pepsin, and IF—are deficient. Gastric atrophy may be caused by type A chronic gastritis, an autoimmune disorder, but it may also be caused by heavy alcohol ingestion, hot tea, and cigarette smoking. Complete or partial removal of the stomach (gastrectomy) may also cause IF deficiency and result in pernicious anemia. Individuals with chronic gastritis are also at risk for the development of gastric cancer and must be followed regularly to prevent this condition.

Pernicious anemia affects both red cell and white cell precursors in bone marrow. Platelet precursors are less affected. The number and size of all developing blood cells increase, and enormous white cells with large and unusually shaped nuclei are present (Fig. 20-3). Alterations in blood cell development and maturation depend on the extent of B_{12} deficiency and other associated metabolic causes leading to anemia.

≡ *Clinical Manifestations*

Pernicious anemia develops slowly, so by the time treatment is sought it is usually severe. Early symptoms, which are nonspecific, vague, and often ignored, include infections, mood swings, and gastrointestinal, cardiac, or kidney ailments. When the hemoglobin has decreased significantly (7 to 8 g/dl), the individual experiences the classic symptoms of anemia: weakness, fatigue, paresthesias of feet and fingers, difficulty walking, loss of appetite, abdominal pain, weight loss, and a sore tongue that is smooth and beefy red. The skin may become "lemon yellow," caused by a combination of pallor and jaundice.

≡ *Evaluation and Treatment*

Evaluation is based on blood tests (see Box 20-1), bone marrow aspiration, clinical manifestations, and the Schilling test. In this test, cobalamin absorption is measured indirectly by administering radioactive cobalamin and measuring its excretion in the urine.

Untreated pernicious anemia is fatal, usually because of heart failure. With replacement therapy using vitamin B_{12}, mortality has decreased significantly. Vitamin B_{12} must be administered by injection since there is no IF in the stomach to allow for absorption of orally administered supplements. Relapses are usually caused by noncompliance with prescribed therapy. Pernicious anemia is not curable; therefore treatment must be continued throughout the individual's lifetime.

Folate deficiency anemias

The vitamin folate (folic acid) is essential for RNA and DNA synthesis within the erythrocyte, making it important for cell development and maturation. Humans are totally dependent on dietary intake, and folate's absorption from the upper small intestine is not mediated by any other element (i.e., IF). Folate circulates through and is stored in the liver. Folate deficiency occurs more frequently than B_{12} deficiency, particularly in persons with alcoholism and other individuals who are malnourished because of fad diets or diets low in vegetables.

Clinical manifestations are similar to those of pernicious anemia, except for the lack of neurologic symptoms. Evaluation is based on blood tests, measurement of serum folate levels, and presenting signs and symptoms. Treatment requires administration of oral folate preparations until adequate blood levels are obtained and manifestations are reduced or eliminated. Recent research also indicates that folate is essential for reducing blood levels of homocysteine, which has been recently recognized as a risk factor for the development of coronary artery disease.

Microcytic-Hypochromic Anemias

The *microcytic-hypochromic anemias* are characterized by abnormally small erythrocytes that contain abnormally reduced amounts of hemoglobin (Fig. 20-2, *B*). Hypochromia occurs even in cells of normal size.

Microcytic-hypochromic anemia can result from (1) disorders of iron metabolism, (2) disorders of porphyrin and heme synthesis, or (3) disorders of globin synthesis. Specific conditions include iron deficiency anemia, sideroblastic anemia, and thalassemia.

Iron deficiency anemia

Pathophysiology

Iron deficiency anemia (IDA) is the most common type of anemia throughout the world. Causes of anemia in developing countries include hookworm infestations and possibly inadequate intake; however, this cause is being reevaluated. Low levels of iron are hypothesized to be an adaptive defense mechanism to increased exposure to pathogens. Survival of pathogens depends on iron; thus with decreased levels of iron available, they die.

In developed countries, pregnancy and a continuous loss of blood are the most common causes. A blood loss of 2 to 4 ml/day (1 to 2 mg of iron) is enough to cause IDA. In men, bleeding may result from ulcers, hiatal hernia, esophageal varices, cirrhosis, hemorrhoids, ulcerative colitis, or cancer. In women, menorrhagia (profuse menstruation) and pregnancy cause primary IDA. Both genders may develop IDA from (1) use of medications that cause gastrointestinal bleeding; (2) surgical procedures that decrease stomach acidity, intestinal transit time, and absorption; (3) insufficient dietary intake of iron; and (4) eating disorders such as pica—the craving and eating of nonnutritional substances. Iron deficiency is common in children younger than 2 years of age because of the significant requirements for growth.[1,2]

IDA develops slowly through three overlapping stages. In stage I, the body's iron stores for red cell production are depleted. In stage II, insufficient iron is transported to the marrow and altered red cell production begins. Stage III begins when the hemoglobin-deficient red cells enter the circulation and replace normal erythrocytes that have grown old and have been destroyed. The manifestations of IDA appear in stage III when there is insufficient iron supply and diminished hemoglobin synthesis.

Clinical Manifestations

The onset of symptoms of this anemia is gradual, and individuals usually do not seek medical attention until hemoglobin levels drop to 7 or 8 g/dl. Early symptoms are nonspecific and include fatigue, weakness, shortness of breath, and pale ear lobes, palms, and conjunctiva (Fig. 20-4).

As the condition progresses and becomes more severe, structural and functional changes also occur in epithelial tissue. The fingernails become brittle, thin, and spoon shaped or concave (Fig. 20-5). Tongue papillae may atrophy and cause soreness along with redness and burning (Fig. 20-6).

Fig. 20-4 *Pallor and iron deficiency.* Pallor of the skin, mucous membranes, and palmar creases in an individual with hemoglobin of 9 g/dl. Palmar creases become as pale as the surrounding skin when the hemoglobin level approaches 7 g/dl. *(From Hoffbrand, A.V. & Pettit, J.E. [1988]. Sandoz atlas of clinical hematology. London: Gower Medical.)*

Fig. 20-5 *Koilonychia.* The nails are concave, ridged, and brittle. *(From Hoffbrand, A.V. & Pettit, J.E. [1988]. Sandoz atlas of clinical hematology. London: Gower Medical.)*

Fig. 20-6 *Glossitis.* Tongue of individual with iron deficiency anemia has bald, fissured appearance caused by loss of papillae and flattening. *(From Hoffbrand, A.V. & Pettit, J.E. [1988]. Sandoz atlas of clinical hematology. London: Gower Medical.)*

These changes can be reversed within 1 to 2 weeks of iron replacement. The corners of the mouth become dry and sore (angular stomatitis), and an individual may experience difficulty with swallowing because of a "web" that develops from mucus and inflammatory cells at the opening of the esophagus. These lesions may develop into cancer.

Iron is also a component of many other enzymes in the body, and lack of iron alters other physiologic processes. Individuals with IDA also exhibit gastritis, neuromuscular changes, irritability, headache, numbness, tingling, and vasomotor disturbances. Gait disturbances are rare. In the elderly population, mental confusion, memory loss, and disorientation may be overlooked as "normal" age-related changes.

Evaluation and Treatment

Evaluation is based on clinical manifestations and laboratory tests (see Box 20-1). Iron stores are measured directly, by bone marrow biopsy, or indirectly, by tests that measure serum ferritin, transferrin saturation, or total iron-binding capacity. A sensitive indicator of heme synthesis is the amount of free erythrocyte protoporphyrin (FEP) within erythrocytes.

The first step in treatment of IDA is to find and eliminate, or rule out, sources of bleeding. Iron replacement is very effective, and results are generally seen within the first month of therapy. A reliable indicator of the response to therapy is an increase in reticulocytes.

Sideroblastic anemia

Sideroblastic anemias (SAs) are a heterogeneous group of disorders characterized by anemia of varying severity as a result of inefficient iron uptake, which results in abnormal hemoglobin synthesis. Diagnosis of SA is based on the presence of ringed sideroblasts in the bone marrow, which are red cells that contain iron granules that have not been synthesized into hemoglobin but instead are arranged in a circle around the nucleus. Individuals with SA also have increased tissue levels of iron.

Pathophysiology

Sideroblastic anemias may be acquired or hereditary. The hereditary form is very rare, with almost all reported cases occurring in males, supporting a recessive X-linked transmission; however, autosomal transmission affecting females has been reported. Primary acquired SA is less common than secondary and is usually found in elderly persons. Specific causes of primary acquired SA are unknown. One proposed cause is a deficiency or reduced activity of certain enzymes that control heme synthesis. Another viewpoint is that there is some deficiency within the mitochondria themselves, related to iron metabolism disrupting mitochondrial function and, ultimately, heme synthesis.

Secondary SA is most often the result of drugs or toxins (i.e., ethanol, chloramphenicol, isoniazid, phenylbutazone, antineoplastics, lead, radiation). Chromosome damage from these agents appears to be the basis for development of the anemia. Altered erythropoiesis in the marrow results from this type of damage.

Clinical Manifestations

Along with the cardiovascular and respiratory manifestations common to all anemias, individuals with SA may show signs of iron overload, including mild to moderate enlargement of the liver (hepatomegaly) and spleen (splenomegaly); however, liver function remains normal or only mildly affected. Occasionally the skin may become abnormally colored (bronze-tinted). The iron overload *(hemosiderosis)* associated with SA may result in heart rhythm disturbances, which are a major complication, but fortunately they are quite uncommon and occur generally late in the course of the disease. Individuals with acquired SA usually display mild symptoms.

Evaluation and Treatment

Initially, SA may be mistaken for deficiency of stem cells in the marrow *(hypoplastic anemia)* or iron deficiency anemia. (Laboratory findings are listed in Box 20-1.) The diagnosis of SA is established by bone marrow biopsy, which demonstrates packed erythrocyte stem cells and mononuclear phagocytes that contain large amounts of iron as hemosiderin. The presence of sideroblasts confirms the diagnosis.

Treatment and management of secondary SA involve identification and removal of the causative agent. In primary SA, transfusions may be necessary to relieve the associated symptoms and pyridoxine therapy may be beneficial for some individuals. Iron is rarely given, and multiple transfusions may result in iron overdose. Sideroblastic anemia may convert to *myelodysplastic syndrome* with the possibility of developing acute myeloblastic leukemia. Death may result from infections, bone marrow failure, liver failure, or heart rhythm disturbances.

HEALTH ALERT

Increased Iron Levels and Heart Disease in Men

Although iron is an essential element for adequate erythrocyte development, recent studies in Finland suggest a relationship between increased levels of iron and heart disease in men. This relationship is still viewed with caution, however. The most recent study, using more refined techniques, found that men with the lowest ratio of transferrin receptors to ferritin had the most iron in their bodies and the greatest risk of heart attack. The proposed mechanism contributing to heart attacks is iron's combining with oxygen that promotes low-density lipoprotein (LDL) oxidation and the formation of free radicals that then damage coronary arteries and facilitate atherosclerosis. The American Heart Association states that more research needs to be done and that iron is still an important nutrient for women and children.

From American Heart Association. (1998). American Heart Association meeting report: Research supports link between iron levels and heart disease (NR 97-4598 SS97/Salonen). (available at http://www.americanheart.org/Whats News/AHA News Releases/ NR2658.html); Findlay, S., Podolsky, D., & Silberner, J. (1992). U.S. News & World Report (pp. 61-68), September 21.

Normocytic-Normochromic Anemias

In *normocytic-normochromic anemias (NNAs),* erythrocytes are relatively normal in size and hemoglobin content but insufficient in number. These anemias do not share any common cause, pathologic mechanism, or morphologic characteristics. They are less common than the macrocytic-normochromic and the microcytic-hypochromic anemias.

TABLE 20-2	Normocytic-Normochromic Anemias		
Anemia	**Pathophysiology**	**Clinical Manifestations**	**Evaluation and Treatment**
Aplastic	Rare; may result from infiltrative disorders of bone marrow; autoimmune diseases, renal failure; splenic dysfunction; cobalamin or folate deficiency; parvovirus infection; or exposure to radiation, drugs, and toxins; may also be congenital Seed or stem cell deficiency theory proposes that common stem cell population is altered so it cannot proliferate or differentiate Microenvironmental deficiency theory proposes that stem cell environment is altered to inhibit erythropoiesis Outcome ranges from death (marrow unable to recover from insult) to minimal manifestations with life span of additional years	Classic cardiovascular and respiratory manifestations With damaged or deficient stem cells of platelets and leukocytes, thrombocytopenia, hemorrhage into the tissues, leukopenia, and infection may result	Bone marrow biopsy determines whether anemia is caused by pure red cell aplasia or hypoplasia Must treat underlying disorder or prevent further exposure to causative agent Blood transfusions, marrow transplant, and pharmacologic stimulation of bone marrow function are treatment options
Posthemorrhagic	Caused by sudden blood loss with normal iron stores	Often obscured by cardiovascular manifestations of acute hemorrhage Severe shock, lactic acidosis, and death can occur if blood loss exceeds 40%-50% of plasma volume	Restoration of blood volume needed by intravenous administration of saline, dextran, albumin, or plasma Transfusion of whole blood also required occasionally
Hemolytic	May be acquired or hereditary Acquired: caused by infection, systemic disease, drugs or toxins, liver disease, kidney disease, abnormal immune responses Hereditary: caused by abnormalities of the RBC membrane or cytoplasmic contents (cellular); present at birth Hemolysis occurs in blood vessels or lymphoid tissues that filter blood (e.g., spleen, liver) Erythrocytes become rigid, slowing their passage and making them vulnerable to phagocytosis Types: warm antibody disease (mediated by IgG antibody specific for erythrocyte antigens), cold antibody disease (mediated by IgM), and drug induced	Splenomegaly, jaundice, aplastic hemolytic or megaloblastic crises can develop with viral infection With severe disease, bones become deformed and pathologic fractures occur Cardiovascular and respiratory manifestations correspond with severity of anemia	Blood and bone marrow studies Erythroid hyperplasia is found in marrow and blood smears Treatment of acquired disease involves removing the cause or treating the underlying disorder Other forms of treatment are transfusions, splenectomy, and steroids or folate

RBC, *Red blood cells;* AIDS, *acquired immunodeficiency syndrome;* SLE, *systemic lupus erythemotosus.*

Continued

TABLE 20-2	Normocytic-Normochromic Anemias—cont'd		
Anemia	**Pathophysiology**	**Clinical Manifestations**	**Evaluation and Treatment**
Anemia of chronic inflammation	Associated with chronic infections, such as AIDS, chronic noninfectious inflammatory diseases, such as rheumatoid arthritis, SLE, and malignancies Causes are decreased erythrocyte life span; failure of mechanisms of compensatory erythropoiesis; and disturbance of the iron cycle	Manifestations fewer and milder than most other anemias Generally disability caused by chronic disease limits physical activity so hemoglobin levels adequate; if they drop, signs of iron deficiency anemia develop	Blood tests reveal iron deficiency in marrow despite normal or increased iron stores elsewhere No treatment is needed unless anemia becomes symptomatic Erythropoietin may be used

RBC, *Red blood cells;* AIDS, *acquired immunodeficiency syndrome;* SLE, *systemic lupus erythemotosus.*

Four distinct anemic conditions—aplastic anemia, posthemorrhagic anemia, hemolytic anemia, and anemia of chronic inflammation—exemplify the diversity of the NNA characteristics and are summarized in Table 20-2. Sickle cell anemia is another category of NNA and is discussed in Chapter 21.

✔ QUICK CHECK

How do cell size and content determine classification of anemia?

Why is iron important to hemoglobin synthesis, and why is iron deficiency related to anemia?

Why can an individual with "normal" cell parameters still develop an anemia?

MYELOPROLIFERATIVE RED CELL DISORDERS (POLYCYTHEMIA VERA)

Hematologic dysfunction may result from an overproduction of cells, as well as a deficiency. One or more marrow elements may be produced in excess, responding to exogenous (radiation, drugs) or endogenous (physiologic compensatory response, immune disorder) signals. An excess of red cells produces a group of disorders classified as polycythemia (Table 20-3). *Polycythemia vera (PV)* is an unusual myeloproliferative disease that causes *erythrocytosis*—excessively large numbers of erythrocytes in the blood.

⇒ *Pathophysiology*

Polycythemia vera (PV) is considered a neoplastic disorder caused by an insidious excessive proliferation of erythrocyte precursors in the marrow. There is also an increase in circulating platelets and granulocytes, which suggests that PV is caused by an abnormality of the pluripotential stem cell.

There are essentially two types of PV—*relative* and *absolute*. Relative PV is characterized by hemoconcentration of the blood that is frequently seen with dehydration. Treatment requires rehydration and causes no further complications. Absolute PV consists of two types: primary and secondary. Absolute primary PV is relatively rare and predominantly occurs in white men between 40 and 60 years of age who are of European Jewish descent. Rarely is PV seen in children or multiple members of a single family.

Secondary absolute polycythemia is more common and is essentially a physiologic response to hypoxia. Individuals who live at high altitudes (10,000 feet or above), smokers, and those with congestive heart failure or chronic obstructive pulmonary disease frequently have higher red cell counts. Abnormal types of hemoglobin and increased secretion of erythropoietin associated with certain renal tumors may also cause secondary absolute PV.

⇒ *Clinical Manifestations*

Clinical manifestations of PV are caused by increased blood cellularity, which increases blood viscosity, causing clogging and occlusion of blood vessels. Tissue injury (ischemia) and death (infarction) may be the outcome of blood vessel blockage and occur about 40% of the time. Circulatory alterations caused by the thick, sticky blood also give rise to other manifestations, such as plethora (ruddy, red color of the face, hands, feet, ears, and mucous membranes), engorgement of retinal and cerebral veins, and liver and spleen enlargement. Other symptoms may include headache, drowsiness, confusion, depression, and visual disturbances. The increased blood volume increases blood pressure, and the individual may develop cardiac angina. Gastric ulcers also may develop.

A unique feature of PV is the development of intense, painful itching that appears to be exacerbated by heat and relieved by cooling. The itching is generally not responsive to antihistamines even though it is thought to be related to mast cell accumulation of the skin.

TABLE 20-3	Disorders Classified as Polycythemia	
Type of Polycythemia	**Mechanism of Increased Erythropoiesis**	**Cause or Associated Disorder**
Primary polycythemia (polycythemia vera)	Excessive proliferation of erythroid precursors in marrow; increased sensitivity of pluripotential stem cell to erythropoietin	Unknown
Secondary polycythemia	Physiologic increase in erythropoietin secretion by the kidneys in response to underlying systemic disorder	Tissue hypoxia caused by cardiopulmonary disorders (chronic obstructive pulmonary disease, congestive heart failure), decreased barometric pressure, cardiovascular malformations causing mixing of arterial and venous blood, methemoglobinemia, carboxyhemoglobinemia, smoking, obesity
	"Nonphysiologic"* increase in erythropoietin secretion	Renal disorders, cerebellar hemangioblastomas, hepatoma (liver tumor), ovarian carcinoma, uterine leiomyoma, pheochromocytoma, adrenocortical hypersecretion
Familial polycythemia	Genetically induced increase in erythroid precursors of the marrow Abnormal Hb with increased oxygen affinity Decreased 2,3-DPG Increased sensitivity of stem cells to erythropoietin Increased erythropoietin in secretion	Genetic defect

Hb, *Hemoglobin;* 2,3-DPG, *2,3-diphosphoglycerate.*
Nonphysiologic means that there is no obvious physiologic explanation for hypersecretion of erythropoietin.

Evaluation and Treatment

Blood tests and laboratory findings (characterized by an absolute increase in red blood cells and in total blood volume) establish the diagnosis. There may also be associated increases in white blood cells and platelets. A bone marrow examination may be done; however, it cannot definitively confirm the diagnosis. Treatment of PV consists of reducing erythrocytosis and blood volume, controlling symptoms, and preventing clogging and clotting of the blood vessels. Phlebotomy, or removal of blood from the circulation (approximately 300 to 500 ml), is used to decrease erythrocytes and blood volume. Smokers are urged to quit, and individuals with congestive heart failure and chronic obstructive pulmonary disease are placed on appropriate drug intervention.

Without proper treatment, 50% of individuals with PV die within 18 months of the onset of initial symptoms. The main cause of death is thrombosis or hemorrhage. A significant potential outcome of PV is the conversion to acute myeloid leukemia (AML), which occurs spontaneously in 10% of individuals. AML is generally resistant to conventional therapy. Conversion to AML is thought to be related to treatment methods using cytotoxic agents. Although PV is a chronic disorder, appropriate therapy results in remissions and prevention of significant pathologic outcomes.

ALTERATIONS OF LEUKOCYTE FUNCTION

Leukocyte function is affected if too many or too few white cells are present in the blood or if the cells that are present are structurally or functionally defective. Disorders can be either quantitative or qualitative. Quantitative disorders can result from bone marrow activity or premature destruction of cells in the circulation. However, many disorders originate in the circulation or lymphoid organs in response to invasion by infectious microorganisms.

Most qualitative disorders are the result of altered leukocyte function in mechanisms of self-defense. The phagocytic cells (granulocytes, monocytes, macrophages) may lose their ability to act as effective phagocytes, and the lymphocytes may lose their ability to respond to antigens. (Disruptions of inflammatory and immune processes caused by leukocyte disorders are described in Chapter 7.) Other leukocyte alterations are hematologic defects, including infectious mononucleosis and cancers of the blood—leukemia and multiple myeloma.

Quantitative Alterations of Leukocytes

Quantitative alterations are an increased or decreased number of leukocytes in the blood. An increase in numbers of leukocytes in the blood is known as *leukocytosis,* and a decreased number is *leukopenia.* Usually a specific type of white blood cell is affected in either of these conditions.

Leukocytosis is a normal protective response to physiologic stressors, such as invading microorganisms, strenuous exercise, emotional changes, temperature changes, anesthesia, surgery, pregnancy, and some drugs, hormones, and toxins. It also is caused by pathologic conditions, such as malignancies and hematologic disorders. Leukopenia is never a normal response condition, nor is it ever considered beneficial. As the leukocyte count falls to less than 1000/mm³ the risk of infection increases drastically. With counts below 500/mm³, the possibility for life-threatening infections is high. Leukopenia can be caused by radiation, anaphylactic shock, systemic lupus erythematosus, and certain chemotherapeutic agents.

Granulocytes and monocytes

Increased levels of circulating granulocytes (neutrophils, eosinophils, basophils) and monocytes are chiefly a physiologic response to infection. Increases can occur also as a result of myeloproliferative disorders (polycythemia vera, chronic myelocytic leukemia [CML]) that increase stem cell proliferation in the bone marrow.

Decreases occur when infectious processes "use up" the circulating granulocytes and monocytes by pulling them out of the circulation and into infected tissues faster than they can be replaced. Decreases can be caused also by disorders that suppress marrow function.

Granulocytosis begins when stored blood cells are released. *Neutrophilia* is another term that may be used to describe *granulocytosis* because neutrophils are the most numerous of the granulocytes (Table 20-4). Neutrophilia is seen in the early stages of infection or inflammation. Specific conditions associated with neutrophilia are identified in Table 20-4.

As the mature neutrophils are used up in fighting the infection, the requirement for new neutrophils increases. To meet this need, the bone marrow releases immature neutrophils (and other leukocytes) into the blood. Premature release of the immature cells is responsible for the phenomenon known as a *shift-to-the-left* or *leukemoid reaction.* This refers to the microscopic detection of disproportionate numbers of immature leukocytes in smears of peripheral blood. To understand this phenomenon, visualize cellular differentiation, maturation, and release as progressing from left to right instead of up and down as shown in Fig. 19-9. The early release of immature white cells prevents the completion of the sequence and shifts the action toward the left side of the diagram. As the infection or inflammation subsides, the demand for leukocytes also decreases and the normal progression of differentiation and maturation resumes; thus a *shift-to-the-right,* or back to normal, occurs, which replenishes circulating granulocytes.

Circulating neutrophils are reduced in *neutropenia.* Clinically, neutropenia exists when the neutrophil count is less than 2000/mm³. Reduction in neutrophils occurs in severe prolonged infections when production of granulocytes cannot keep up with demand.

In the absence of overwhelming infection, other causes of neutropenia include hematologic, immunologic/inflammatory, nutritional/metabolic, and infectious disorders; neutropenia may become chronic with serial absolute neutrophil counts less than 500/mm³ that may last for months to years.[3] Hematologic disorders that affect bone marrow function cause ineffective or defective neutrophil production, and disorders associated with immune and inflammatory dysfunctions cause decreased neutrophil survival. Abnormal neutrophil distribution and sequestration are associated with hypersplenism and pseudoneutropenia, which can be caused by starvation and anorexia nervosa. Viral infections (human immunodeficiency virus [HIV], Epstein-Barr virus [EBV]), as well as chemotherapy and other toxic drugs received for cancer treatment and transplantation, may also cause neutropenia.

If neutrophils are drastically reduced (<500/mm³) and the entire granulocyte count is extremely low, *granulocytopenia* or *agranulocytosis* results. Usually, when this occurs, hematopoiesis is arrested in the bone marrow or cell destruction increases in the circulation. Chemotherapeutic agents used to treat hematologic and other malignancies cause bone marrow suppression. (Other drugs causing agranulocytosis are listed in Table 20-5.) Although drug-induced agranulocytosis is rare, mortality is 10% to 48%.[4] Clinical manifestations of agranulocytosis include infection (particularly of the respiratory system), general malaise, septicemia, fever, tachycardia, and ulcers in the mouth and colon. If untreated, sepsis results in death within 3 to 6 days. Other conditions associated with neutropenia are identified in Table 20-4.

Eosinophilia is an absolute increase in the total numbers of circulating eosinophils. Allergic disorders associated with asthma, hay fever, and drug reactions frequently cause eosinophilia. During the hypersensitivity reaction, eosinophilic chemotaxic factor of anaphylaxis (CTF-A) and histamine are released from mast cells, attracting eosinophils to the area. Areas with abundant mast cells, such as the respiratory and gastrointestinal tracts, are commonly affected. Eosinophilia may also occur in dermatologic disorders, eosinophilia-myalgia syndrome, and parasitic invasion. Other conditions that cause eosinophilia are detailed in Table 20-4.

Eosinopenia, a decrease in circulating eosinophils, generally is caused by migration of eosinophils into inflammatory sites. It may be seen in Cushing syndrome and as a result of stress caused by surgery, shock, trauma, burns, or mental distress. Other conditions that cause eosinopenia are detailed in Table 20-4.

Basophilia is quite rare and generally is seen as a response to inflammation and immediate hypersensitivity reactions. Basophils contain histamine that is released during an allergic reaction. Increased basophils are seen in myelo-

TABLE 20-4	Other Conditions Associated With Neutrophils, Eosinophils, Basophils, Monocytes, and Lymphocytes	
Condition	**Cause**	**Example**
Neutrophil		
Neutrophilia (granulocytosis)	Inflammations or tissue necroses	Surgery, burns, MI, pneumonitis, rheumatic fever, rheumatoid arthritis
	Infections	Gram-positive (staphylococci, streptococci, pneumococci), gram-negative (Escherichia coli, Pseudomonas species)
	Physiologic	Exercise, extreme heat or cold, third-trimester pregancy, emotional distress
	Hematologic	Acute hemorrhage, hemolysis, myeloproliferative disorder, CGL
	Drugs or chemicals	Epinephrine, steroids, heparin, histamine, endotoxin
	Metabolic	Diabetes (acidosis), eclampsia, gout, thyroid storm
	Neoplasms	Liver, GI tract, bone marrow
Neutropenia	Decreased marrow production	Radiation, chemotherapy, leukemia, aplastic anemia, abnormal granulopoiesis
	Increased destruction	Splenomegaly, hemodialysis, immune reaction
	Infections	Gram-negative (typhoid), viral (influenza, hepatitis B, measles, mumps, rubella), severe infections, protozoal infections (malaria)
Eosinophil		
Eosinophilia	Allergies	Asthma, hay fever, drug sensitivity
	Infections	Parasites (trichinosis, hookworm), chronic (fungal, leprosy, TB)
	Malignancies	CML, lung, stomach, ovary, Hodgkin disease
	Dermatoses	Pemphigus, exfoliative dermatitis (drug-induced)
	Drugs	Digitalis, heparin, streptomycin, tryptophan (eosinophilia-myalgia syndrome), penicillins, propranolol
Eosinopenia	Stress responses	Trauma, shock, burns, surgery, mental distress
	Drugs	Steroids (Cushing syndrome)
Basophil		
Basophilia	Inflammations	Infection (measles, chickenpox), hypersensitivity reaction (immediate)
	Hematologic	Myeloproliferative disorders (CML, polycythemia vera, Hodgkin disease, hemolytic anemia)
	Endocrine	Myxedema, antithyroid therapy
Basopenia	Physiologic	Pregnancy, ovulation, stress
	Endocrine	Graves disease
Monocyte		
Monocytosis	Infections	Bacterial (SBE, TB), recovery phase of infection
	Hematologic	Myeloproliferative disorders, Hodgkin disease, agranulocytosis
	Physiologic	Normal newborn
Monocytopenia	Rare	
Lymphocyte		
Lymphocytosis	Physiologic	4 mo to 4 yr
	Acute infections	Infectious mononucleosis, CMV infection, pertussis, hepatitis, mycoplasma pneumonia, typhoid
	Chronic infections	Congenital syphilis, tertiary syphilis
	Endocrine	Thyrotoxicosis, adrenal insufficiency
	Malignancies	ALL, CLL, lymphosarcoma cell leukemia
Lymphocytopenia	Immunodeficiency syndromes	AIDS, agammaglobulinemia
	Lymphocyte destruction	Steroids (Cushing syndrome), radiation, chemotherapy Hodgkin disease CHF, renal failure, TB, SLE, aplastic anemia

MI, *Myocardial infarction;* CGL, *chronic granulocytic leukemia;* GI, *gastrointestinal;* CML, *chronic myelogenous leukemia;* TB, *tuberculosis;* SBE, *subacute bacterial endocarditis;* CMV, *cytomegalovirus;* ALL, *acute lymphocytic leukemia;* CLL, *chronic lymphocytic leukemia;* AIDS, *acquired immunodeficiency syndrome;* CHF, *congestive (left) heart failure;* SLE, *systemic lupus erythematosus.*

TABLE 20-5	Examples of Drugs Associated With Neutropenia and Agranulocytosis	
Drug Group	**Neutropenia**	**Agranulocytosis**
Analgesics, sedatives, antiinflammatory agents	Gold compounds; phenylbutazone; indomethacin	Phenacetin; barbiturates; aminopyrine; dipyrone
Antibiotics	Cephalosporins; semisynthetic penicillins	Sulfonamides; chloramphenicol; methicillin
Antithyroid agents	Methimazole	Propylthiouracil
Psychotropic agents	Tricyclic antidepressants	Phenothiazine
Anticonvulsant agents	Trimethadione, primidone, phenytoin	Phenytoin
Antidysrhythmic agents	Procainamide; quinidine, propranolol, methyldopa	

proliferative disorders, such as chronic myeloid leukemia and myeloid metaplasia. Other conditions that are associated with basophilia are listed in Table 20-4.

Basopenia is seen in hyperthyroidism, acute infection, and long-term therapy with steroids. Other conditions associated with basopenia are listed in Table 20-4.

Monocytosis, an increase in monocytes, is often transient and correlates poorly with disease states. It is usually associated with neutropenia during bacterial infections, particularly in the late stages or recovery stage, when monocytes are needed to phagocytize surviving microorganisms and debris. Increased monocytes also may indicate marrow recovery from agranulocytosis. Monocytosis is often seen in chronic infections such as tuberculosis (TB) and subacute bacterial endocarditis (SBE). Other conditions associated with monocytosis are identified in Table 20-4. *Monocytopenia,* a decrease in monocytes, is rare but has been identified with hairy cell leukemia and prednisone therapy.

Lymphocytes

The quantity of lymphocytes is altered when they are activated by antigenic stimuli, usually microorganisms (see Chapter 5). *Lymphocytosis* is rare in acute bacterial infections and is seen most commonly in acute viral infections, particularly those caused by the Epstein-Barr virus (EBV)—a causative agent in infectious mononucleosis. Other specific disorders associated with lymphocytosis are listed in Table 20-4

Lymphocytopenia may be attributed to (1) abnormalities of lymphocyte production associated with neoplasias and immune deficiencies and (2) destruction by drugs, viruses, or radiation. It may also occur in individuals for no apparent reason. Conditions associated with lymphocytopenia are identified in Table 20-4. The lymphocytopenia associated with heart failure and other acute illnesses may be caused by elevated levels of cortisol. The most recent condition in which lymphocytopenia is a major problem is acquired immunodeficiency syndrome (AIDS). The lymphocytopenia associated with this condition is caused by the HIV virus, which destroys T-helper lymphocytes. (For a detailed discussion of AIDS, see Chapter 7.)

Infectious Mononucleosis

Infectious mononucleosis (IM) is an acute infection of B lymphocytes (B cells). The most common agent is the Epstein-Barr virus (EBV); however, cytomegalovirus (CMV) and other viruses, as well as the bacterium *Toxoplasma gondii,* have been identified as causing symptoms resembling IM.[5]

IM usually affects young adults between the ages of 15 and 35 years, with peak incidences between 15 and 19 years. Transmission is by close personal contact, with kissing being most closely identified with the condition, hence the term *kissing disease.* Initially there is widespread invasion of the B lymphocytes located in the mouth, nose, and throat, which possess receptor sites for the EBV.

Unaffected B cells produce antibodies against the virus, and T lymphocytes (T cells) assist the B cell response of attacking the virus directly (see Chapter 5). The production of B and T cell clones and the process of removing dead and damaged leukocytes are largely responsible for the swelling of lymphoid tissues (lymph nodes, spleen, tonsils, and occasionally, liver). Sore throat and fever, two initial manifestations of IM, are caused by inflammation at the site of viral entry—the mouth and throat.

The incubation period for IM is approximately 30 to 50 days. Early flulike symptoms, such as headache, malaise, and fatigue, appear during the first 3 to 5 days, varying in severity for the next 7 to 20 days. At the time of diagnosis, the individual commonly presents with the classic triad of symptoms: fever, sore throat, and enlargement of the cervical lymph nodes. As the condition progresses, generalized lymph node enlargement may also develop. Enlargement of the spleen and liver may be present, although it is not as common as lymph node enlargement.[6] Rarely, other organ systems may be involved. Neurologic system manifestations may include encephalitis, meningitis, Guillian-Barré syndrome, and Bell palsy. Ocular manifestations may include eyelid and periorbital edema, dry eyes, keratitis, uveitis, and conjunctivitis. Pulmonary involvement is very rare, although incidences of pneumonia and respiratory failure have been documented; however, they are most likely to develop in immunocompromised individuals.

IM is usually self-limiting, and recovery occurs in a few weeks. Treatment consists of rest and alleviation of symptoms with analgesics and antipyretics. Acyclovir has been used in immunocompromised individuals but is not considered standard therapy. IM and EBV infection were thought to be associated with chronic fatigue syndrome, but that is no longer thought to be true.

Laboratory findings include increased relative and absolute lymphocyte and monocyte counts, with 10% to 20% atypical forms. In the first week the leukocyte count may be normal or slightly low, secondary to mild neutropenia. After the first week, the leukocyte count increases to 10,000/μl to 20,000/mm³ and stays at this level for 4 to 8 weeks. Platelet counts are low (<140,000/mm³). Serologic tests (e.g., Monospot agglutination test) are necessary to diagnose EBV infection.

✓ QUICK CHECK

Explain the relationship between early release of premature white blood cells and a "shift-to-the-left."

Leukemias

Leukemia is a malignant disorder of the blood and blood-forming organs causing an accumulation of dysfunctional cells and a loss of cell division regulation. The common pathologic feature of all forms of leukemia is an uncontrolled proliferation of leukocytes, causing an overcrowding of bone marrow and decreased production and function of normal hematopoietic cells.

The classification of leukemia has become increasingly complex and is based on (1) the type of cell involved (either myeloid or lymphoid) and (2) the point in the cellular development process when maturation is arrested, which identifies the two major forms of leukemia (acute or chronic). Further classification of leukemia, which was developed in 1976, is based on structure, number of cells, genetics, identification of surface markers, and histochemical staining that provides significant therapeutic prognostic information.

Acute leukemia represents an early arrest in cell development and is characterized by undifferentiated cells, usually a blast cell. The onset of disease is abrupt and rapid. Disease progression results in a short survival time. In chronic leukemia, the predominant cell appears mature but does not function normally. The onset of the disease is gradual, and the prolonged clinical course results in a relatively longer survival time. Over the past 2 decades, remission induction rate and survival have increased. This progress is the result of more effective chemotherapeutic agents, improved blood product and antimicrobial support, and specialized nursing care. Chemotherapy and bone marrow transplants have significantly increased the survival time for individuals with acute leukemia.[7,8]

Leukemia occurs with varying frequencies at different ages and is more common in adults (about 27,900 cases/yr) than in children (2300 cases/yr).[8] Acute lymphoblastic leukemia (ALL) is the most common type in children and accounts for more than half of all cases (1500), with males having a slightly higher risk than females.[9] Acute myelogenous leukemia (AML) (approximately 10,100 cases/yr) and chronic lymphocytic leukemia (CLL) (approximately 7800 cases/yr) are the most common types in adults.[8] The countries with the highest overall incidence are the United States, Canada, Sweden, and New Zealand.

⬛ *Pathophysiology*

Leukemias are considered clonal disorders in that a single progenitor cell undergoes transformation.[10] An interesting paradox is that leukemic cells apparently divide more *slowly* and take longer to synthesize DNA than other blood precursors. Acute leukemia therefore is not caused by rapid cellular proliferation but is, instead, caused by the blocking of blood cell precursors. Leukemic cells accumulate relentlessly in most affected individuals, and they compete with normal cellular proliferation. Thus acute leukemia is a disorder of both accumulation and proliferation.

Although the exact cause of leukemia is unknown, it is clear that causal risk factors along with a genetic predisposition can alter nuclear DNA, producing a leukemic cell that does not mature and respond to normal regulatory mechanisms. More than 30 different, structurally abnormal chromosomes have been identified and are reported in 40% to 50% of individuals with acute leukemia.[11] It appears that certain chromosomes are repeatedly more involved than others and that a mutation in a single cell gives rise to some leukemias.

Genetic mechanisms remain unclear; however, there is a statistically significant tendency for leukemia to recur in families. There also appears to be an increased incidence of leukemia in association with other hereditary abnormalities such as Down syndrome, Fanconi anemia, and congenital X-linked agammaglobulinemia.

Acute leukemia may also develop from acquired disorders and include chronic myelocytic leukemia (CML), polycythemia vera, myelofibrosis, Hodgkin disease, multiple myeloma, ovarian cancer, chronic lymphocytic leukemia (CLL), and sideroblastic anemia. Large doses of ionizing radiation result in an increased incidence of myelogenous leukemia. Viruses are known to cause leukemia in certain animals but have not yet been proved to cause leukemia in human beings. Drugs that cause bone marrow depression (e.g., chloramphenicol, phenylbutazone, and certain alkylating agents, such as cyclophosphamide [Cytoxan]) also can predispose an individual to leukemia. Acute myelogenous leukemia (AML) is the most frequently reported secondary cancer after high doses of chemotherapy for Hodgkin disease, multiple myeloma, ovarian cancer, non-Hodgkin lymphoma, and breast cancer.

In some cases, leukemia develops in the most primitive blood precursors—pluripotential stem cells—which give rise to all other blood cells (Fig. 20-7). The leukemia blasts,

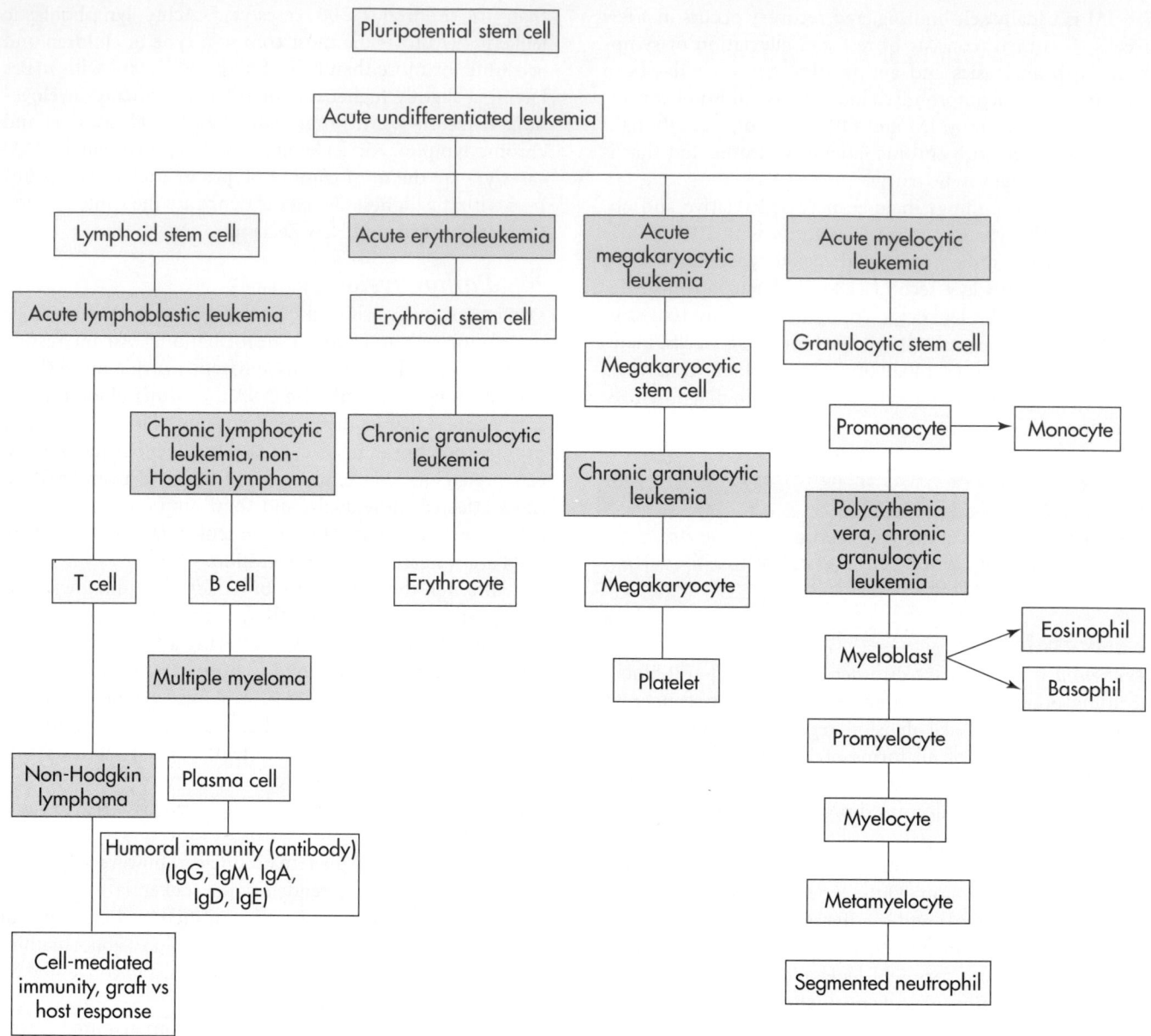

Fig. 20-7 *Cell-specific leukemias.* Differentiation pathways of blood-forming cells and reported sites of block resulting in cell-specific leukemias. *Ig,* Immunoglobulin.

or precursor cells, literally "crowd out" the marrow and cause cellular proliferation of the other cell lines to cease. Normal granulocytic-monocytic, lymphocytic, erythrocytic, and megakaryocytic stem cells cease to function, resulting in *pancytopenia* (a reduction in all cellular components of the blood). Transformation also may occur specifically in the granulocyte-monocyte series and not in the erythrocyte maturation pathway.

Acute leukemias

About 80% of acute lymphoblastic leukemias (ALLs) arise from the B cell line, and about 15% to 20% of all ALL cases arise from T cell lineage. A very small percentage of ALL cases have neither B nor T cell origination and are called *null*

cell. Mortality for acute leukemias varies. North America and Scandinavian countries have the highest mortality; Eastern European countries, Asia (except Japan), and Central America have the lowest mortality. Japan's higher mortality is the result of atomic bombs. Blacks have consistently shown a lower mortality than whites.

Leukemia is seen in both genders and in all ages, with the incidence curve rising steeply in individuals older than 50 years. The 5-year survival rate for those with leukemia is 38%, largely because of poor survival rates of individuals with certain types of leukemia (e.g., acute myelocytic). Over the past 30 years, survival rates for those with ALL, especially children, have increased dramatically (from 4% to 73%), mostly because of chemotherapy.

Clinical Manifestations

The clinical manifestations of all varieties of acute leukemia are generally similar. Mechanisms associated with common manifestations are summarized in Table 20-6. Signs and symptoms related to bone marrow depression include fatigue caused by anemia, bleeding resulting from thrombocytopenia, and fever caused by infection.

Anorexia is associated with weight loss, diminished sensitivity to sour and sweet tastes, wasting of muscle, and difficulty swallowing. The leukemic individual often experiences abdominal pain and tenderness and also breast tenderness.

Neurologic manifestations may be caused by either leukemic infiltration or cerebral bleeding. Headache, vomiting, papilledema, facial palsy, blurred vision, auditory disturbances, and meningeal irritation can occur if leukemic cells infiltrate the cerebral or spinal meninges. Because chemotherapeutic agents do not pass the blood-brain barrier, leukemia cells can grow more easily.

Evaluation and Treatment

Because leukemia frequently is confused with other conditions, early detection is difficult. Persistent symptoms need intensive medical investigation. The diagnosis is made through blood tests and examination of bone marrow.

Chemotherapy, used in various combinations, is the treatment of choice for leukemia. Supportive measures include blood transfusions, antibiotics, antifungals, and antivirals. Bone marrow transplantation using both allogeneic (other than from twins) and autologous (self) marrow is now being used successfully in the treatment of leukemia in individuals younger than 50 years.

Improved survival rates (80% to 90% complete remission, with long-term survival of 30% to 40%) in individuals with acute leukemia have occurred over the past 3 decades.[12] Factors influencing increased survival rate include the use of combined and multimodality treatment methods, improved supportive services such as blood banking and nutritional support, and antimicrobial treatment. Hematopoietic growth factors have also speeded up neutrophil recovery in myeloablative therapy and bone marrow transplant.[12]

Chronic leukemias

The two main types of chronic leukemia are (1) myelocytic (CML) and (2) lymphocytic (CLL). Unlike cells in acute leukemia, chronic leukemic cells are well differentiated and can be readily identified. Individuals with chronic leukemia have a longer life expectancy, usually extending several years from the time of diagnosis.

Pathophysiology and Clinical Manifestations

Chronic leukemia advances slowly and insidiously, generally unknown to the individual until symptoms appear. When symptoms do appear, they include splenomegaly, extreme fatigue, weight loss, night sweats, and low-grade fever.

The incidence of chronic myelocytic leukemia (CML) is

Fig. 20-8 *Philadelphia chromosome.* Schema of the Philadelphia (Ph) translocation (+) seen in chronic myelocytic leukemia. The Ph¹ chromosome results from an exchange of materials between chromosomes 9 and 22, that is, t(9;22)(q34;q11). Because chromosome 22 gives up much more of its long arm than that translocated to it from chromosome 9, chromosome 22 becomes much abbreviated and is known as Ph¹. *(From Damjanov, I. & Linder, J. [Eds.]. [1996]. Anderson's pathology [10th ed.]. St. Louis: Mosby.)*

approximately 1 per 100,000 people. CML is a group of diseases called *myeloproliferative disorders,* which also includes polycythemia vera, primary thrombocytosis, and idiopathic myelofibrosis (invasion of bone marrow by fibrous tissue).

The presence of the Philadelphia chromosome is a diagnostic marker for CML (Fig. 20-8). The Philadelphia chromosome results from a reciprocal translocation between the long arms of chromosomes 9 and 22 and can be demonstrated in all blood cell precursors, meaning that the disease originates in a progenitor stem cell[13] (see Chapter 2). With such strong evidence that CML begins in a stem cell, it is not clear why myeloid cells predominate. The median age for persons with Philadelphia chromosome-positive CML is 40 to 45 years. Identifying the Philadelphia chromosome allows the clinician to follow the transformation process, which occurs in erythroid, megakaryocytic, and macrophage cell lines. Although structural cellular abnormalities are not readily identified, absent or low levels of the enzyme neutrophil alkaline phosphatase, along with decreased phagocytic capabilities, indicate that cells fail to differentiate normally. There is no known specific cause for CML except exposure to ionizing radiation.[14]

The presence of the Philadelphia chromosome in all three cell lines apparently has no detrimental effect on the development and function of erythrocytes and platelets. CML is divided into two stages: chronic and terminal. The chronic stage is characterized by excessive proliferation and accumulation of mature granulocytes and precursors. Splenomegaly is prominent and more painful, and lymphadenopathy generally is not present. Liver function is rarely altered in spite of enlargement. Hyperuricemia is common

TABLE 20-6 Clinical Manifestations and Related Pathophysiology in Leukemia

Clinical Manifestations	Laboratory Abnormalities	Cause	Comments
Anemia	Either a decrease or normal number of erythroblasts; key is the relative *proportion* of erythroblasts to total count (decreased in anemia)	Decreased RBC production may be caused by decreased stem cell input or ineffective erythropoiesis or both	In acute leukemia, anemia is usually present from the beginning, often the first symptom noticed, and severe; mild form without symptoms is common in CML and CLL; hemorrhage common in acute forms, occasional in CML, but rare in CLL
Bleeding (purpura, petechiae, ecchymosis, hemorrhage)	Decreased and possibly abnormal platelets	Reduction in megakaryocytes leading to thrombocytopenia	Bleeding more common in acute than in chronic leukemia
Infection	Infection is likely with an AGC below 500/mm³ (AGC is the proportion of neutrophils and bands to the total white blood cell count)	Infections are caused by organisms endogenous to the host or present in the environment; gram-negative bacilli; granulocytopenic persons have an impaired inflammatory response; immunodeficiency resulting from chemotherapy, corticosteroids, and the disease process contributes to the infection	Major sites of infection: the oral cavity, throat, lower colon, urinary tract, lungs, and skin; prevention of infection focuses on restoration of host defenses, decreasing invasive procedures, and reducing colonization of organisms
Weight loss	Decreased 24-hr urinary creatinine excretion; hypoalbuminemia	Condition can be attributed to pain, depression, chemotherapy, radiation therapy, some unknown circulating inhibitor, and alterations in taste	Causes of weight loss are poorly understood
Bone pain	Frequently no radiographic evidence of bone problems	Result of bone infiltration by leukemic cells or intramedullary infection	If combination drug regimens are ineffective, radiation therapy is used
Liver, spleen, and lymph node enlargement	Biopsy abnormal for liver and spleen	Leukemic cell infiltration causes splenic, hepatic, and lymph node enlargement; lymph nodes also undergo leukemia proliferation as in CLL	
Elevated uric acid	Normal excretion of uric acid is 300-500 mg/day; the leukemic individual can excrete 50 times more	Uric acid is a normal byproduct of protein catabolism; nucleic acid catabolism is accelerated in the leukemic individual; urate precipitation in the leukemic individual is increased from dehydration caused by anorexia or fever and drug therapy	Hyperuricemia is present in both acute leukemia and CML; increasing urine pH or decreasing acid production with the drug allopurinol

RBC, *Red blood cell;* CML, *chronic myelocytic leukemia;* CLL, *chronic lymphocytic leukemia;* AGC, *absolute granulocyte count.*

and produces gouty arthritis. Infections, fever, and weight loss are also frequently seen. The terminal stage begins 30 to 40 months later and is characterized by rapid and progressive leukocytosis with an increase in basophils. In the later stages of the terminal phase, which now resembles AML, blast cells or promyelocytes predominate and the individual experiences a "blast crisis." Survival after the onset of the terminal phase is approximately 3 months.

Chronic lymphocytic leukemia (CLL) predominantly involves malignant transformation of B cells; rarely (<5% of cases) are T cells involved. The malignant transformation is thought to be caused by failure of the normal mechanisms of programmed cell destruction (apoptosis), so that these cells have an extended life, thus the chronic nature of the disease.[15] These cells also fail to function effectively in stimulating the production of immunoglobulins and the stimulation of helper T cells activity. These particular mechanisms are currently under investigation.[16]

Humoral immunity suppression is the most significant effect in CLL. Individuals are at risk for infections commonly fought by B cell immunoglobulins and for the development of autoimmune diseases that result in secondary cancers. Anemia, thrombocytopenia, and neutropenia are typically present with overt CLL. Invasion of most organs by leukemic cells is uncommon, but infiltration of lymph nodes, liver, spleen, and salivary glands is demonstrated. Central nervous system involvement and elevated blood levels of calcium are rare, whereas elevated levels of lactic dehydrogenase (LDH) and uric acid are common.

Evaluation and Treatment

State-of-the-art treatment for CML does not cure the disease, prevent blastic transformation, or prolong the average survival time. Therapeutic approaches include bone marrow transplantation (BMT), biologic response modifiers, and combination chemotherapy.[17] Compared with biologic response modifiers and combination chemotherapy, BMT appears to more significantly increase the survival time. When to begin treatment for CLL is difficult to determine and is related to the degree of symptoms when started. Treatment consists of alkylating agent and/or purine analog chemotherapy. Steroids and, later, splenectomy may also be used to control leukocytosis and cytopenias. Radiation therapy may be used to alleviate lympadenopathy. Late stages of the disease require combination chemotherapy.

✓ QUICK CHECK

Why is infection a major problem in leukemia?

Compare and contrast the two types of chronic leukemia.

What is the significance of the Philadelphia chromosome, and how is it related to leukemia?

Multiple Myeloma

Multiple myeloma is a B cell cancer associated with mature plasma cell structure and function and the production of an abnormal immunoglobulin. Recent studies support early B lymphocytes, such as hematopoietic stem cells in the bone marrow, as the origin of myeloma. These early abnormal cells leave the marrow and move through the circulation to extramedullary sites, probably lymph nodes, which are required for further development.[18] They then return to the bone marrow or other soft tissue sites, aided by cell adhesion molecules, for further expansion and maturation.[19] Cytokines, particularly interleukin-6 (IL-6), have been identified as major factors that promote the growth and survival of multiple myeloma cells.[20] (Lymphocytes and cytokines are described in Chapter 5.) Multiple myeloma is characterized by multiple malignant tumor masses of plasma cells scattered throughout the skeletal system and sometimes in soft tissue.

The reported incidence of multiple myeloma has doubled in the past 2 decades, probably because of more sensitive testing used for diagnosis. In 1999 the number of new cases in the United States was 13,700.[8] Multiple myeloma occurs in all races, but the incidence rate in blacks (7 to 10 per 100,000) is at least twice that of whites (3 to 4 per 100,000). It rarely occurs before the age of 40 years, and it then increases in incidence, peaking during the seventh decade for women and the eighth decade for men. It is also more common in men.

Exact causes are unknown, but genetics are strongly suspected because tumors occur in specific strains of mice and in human siblings and close relatives. Chronic stimulation of the mononuclear phagocyte system by chemicals, bacteria, and viral agents has also been suggested as a possible cause but is not supported by recent studies.[21]

HEALTH ALERT
Multiple Myeloma and Farming

A series of analyses of peer-reviewed studies of multiple myeloma and farming have been performed. Consistently found is an association between multiple myeloma and farming. Exposures commonly experienced by farmers and thought to contribute to the occurrence of multiple myeloma include infections, microorganisms, solvents, and pesticides.

Data from Khuder, S.A. & Mutgi, A.B. (1997). Meta-analysis of multiple myeloma and farming. American Journal of Industrial Medicine, 32(5), 510-516.

Pathophysiology

Malignant plasma cells arise from one clone of B cells that produce abnormally large amounts of one class of immunoglobulin (usually IgG, occasionally IgA, and rarely IgM, IgD, or IgE). This abnormal immunoglobulin is called

Fig. 20-9 *Multiple (plasma cell) myeloma.* **A,** Roentgenogram of femur showing extensive bone destruction caused by tumor. Note absence of reactive bone formation. **B,** Gross specimen from same individual; myelomatous sections appear as dark granular sections. *(From Kissane, J.M. [Ed.]. [1990]. Anderson's pathology [9th ed.]. St. Louis: Mosby.)*

the *M-protein.* In excessive amounts, M-protein causes ineffective antibody production and thus is responsible for many of the clinical manifestations of the disease. Bence Jones proteins, the light chain of immunoglobulin molecules, are present in the urine and contribute to damage to renal tubular cells.

Multiple myeloma becomes evident as diffuse destructive bone lesions (Fig. 20-9). The bones most commonly affected, in decreasing order of frequency, are the vertebrae, ribs, skull, pelvis, femur, clavicle, and scapula.[22,23] The plasma cells secrete osteoclastic activating factors, which progressively destroy cortical bone. (Bone structures are described in Chapter 36.)

Clinical Manifestations

Clinical manifestations result from (1) infiltration and destruction of organs, particularly bone, by the neoplastic plasma cells and (2) M-protein consisting of an excess of immunoglobulins with altered physiologic properties and immune function. Infiltration of bones by malignant plasma cells and resultant destruction of bone tissue cause pain, the most common presenting symptom, and pathologic fractures. Hypercalcemia resulting from bone breakdown contributes to renal disease and may cause confusion, lethargy, and weakness.

The major complication is repeated infections caused by suppressed humoral (antibody-mediated) immune response. Cell-mediated (T cell) function is relatively normal.

Humoral immune function is suppressed by unknown factors secreted by malignant plasma cells. Renal insufficiency and failure, another cause of death, result from Bence Jones proteinuria.

Evaluation and Treatment

Diagnosis of multiple myeloma is made by radiographic and laboratory studies and biopsy of a lesion. Chemotherapy, radiation therapy, plasmapheresis (exchange), and marrow transplant have been used for treatment. Individuals with multiple bone lesions, if untreated, rarely survive more than 6 to 12 months. With chemotherapy and aggressive management of complications, the prognosis can improve significantly, with a median survival of 24 to 30 months and a 10-year survival rate of 3%.

ALTERATIONS OF LYMPHOID FUNCTION

Lymphadenopathy

Normally, lymph nodes are discrete and not palpable. Lymphadenopathy is characterized by enlarged lymph nodes that are palpable and often tender (Fig. 20-10). Localized lymphadenopathy usually indicates drainage from an area of inflammation. Generalized lymphadenopathy, associated with infection, occurs less often and is generally seen in the presence of malignant or nonmalignant disease. Lymphadenopathy is of more significance in adult disease than in children.

Lymph node enlargement is caused by an increase in size and number of its germinal centers, proliferation of lymphocytes and monocytes (immature phagocytes), or invasion by malignant cells. Palpable nodes, however, may only indicate a reaction to minor trauma or infection of a specific structure. The location and size of the enlarged nodes are important factors in diagnosing the cause of the lymphadenopathy, as are the individual's age, gender, and geographic location. Generalized lymphadenopathy occurs with non-Hodgkin lymphomas, chronic lymphocytic leukemia, histiocytoses, and disorders that produce lymphocytosis. In general, lymphadenopathy results from four types of conditions: (1) neoplastic disease, (2) immunologic or inflammatory conditions, (3) endocrine disorders, or (4) lipid storage diseases. Diseases of unknown cause, including autoimmune diseases and reactions to drugs, also may lead to generalized lymphadenopathy.

QUICK CHECK

Describe the relationship between plasma cell malignancy and the development of infection in multiple myeloma.

Describe the features of a clonal disorder. Give an example.

How is lymphadenopathy related to infection?

Malignant Lymphomas

Lymphomas consist of a diverse group of malignant neoplasms that develop from the proliferation of lymphocytes, histiocytes, and their precursors and derivatives in lymphoid tissue; they exhibit a wide variety of clinical and histologic patterns. Within the broad classification of malignant lymphomas there are two categories based on histologic differences—Hodgkin disease (HD) and non-Hodgkin lymphoma (NHL). Bone marrow involvement is more prevalent in NHL than in HD.

Malignant lymphomas are the fifth most common cause of death from cancer in the United States. Incidence rates differ with respect to age, gender, geographic location, and socioeconomic class. In 1998, approximately 64,000 cases, including 7200 cases of HD and 56,800 cases of NHL, were expected to be diagnosed. Since the 1970s, incidence rates for NHL have increased over 65%. A large portion of the increase had been attributed to lymphomas developing in association with immunodeficiencies, including AIDS and organ transplants.[8,24] Incidence of HD has declined over the same time period, especially among elderly persons.

Hodgkin disease

Pathogenesis

Hodgkin disease (HD) is distinguished from other lymphomas by the presence of *Reed-Sternberg (RS) cells* (Fig. 20-11). It is widely accepted that the RS cells or their variant

Fig. 20-10 *Lymphadenopathy.* Individual with lymphocyte leukemia with extreme but symmetric lymphadenopathy. *(Courtesy Dr. A.R. Kagan, Los Angeles. From del Regato, J.A., Spjut, H.J., & Cox, J.D. [1985]. Cancer: Diagnosis, treatment, and prognosis [6th ed.]. St. Louis: Mosby.)*

represents the malignant transformation of cells, although the exact mechanisms triggering the transformation remain uncertain.[25] The RS cells are necessary for the diagnosis of HD; however, they are not specific to HD. In rare instances, cells resembling them can be found in benign illnesses, as well as other forms of neoplasia, including NHL, solid tissue cancers, and infectious mononucleosis. Hodgkin disease arises in a single node of a chain of nodes and spreads characteristically to anatomically contiguous nodes.

Attempts to understand the development of the neoplastic cell of HD have remained inconclusive. The origin of the RS cell may differ for various subtypes of the disease, such as activated lymphoid cells with features of B cell, T cell, or monocytic cell lines. There is evidence of proto-oncogene involvement in the transformation to RS cells or their variants. The transformed cells secrete and release specific cytokines that result in accumulation of inflammatory cells and produce the local and systemic effects.[25] The four types of HD (Table 20-7) are based on the appearance of the nonmalignant cells involved and the specific type of cytokine involved.

The incidence of HD is approximately 2.6/100,000 males and 2.2/100,000 females. The incidence is greater in whites than blacks, with Denmark, the Netherlands, and

Fig. 20-11 *Lymph nodes.* **A,** Lymphocytes and histiocytes of Hodgkin disease, nodular type. Large nodules with small, round lymphocytes, histiocytes, and scattered lymphocyte and histiocyte cells. **B,** Diagnostic Reed-Sternberg cell. A large multinucleated or multilobed cell with inclusion body–like nucleoli surrounded by a halo of clear nucleoplasm. *(From Damjanov, I. & Linder, J. [Eds.]. [1996]. Anderson's pathology [10th ed.]. St. Louis: Mosby.)*

TABLE 20-7	Subtypes of Hodgkin Disease	
Subtype	**Incidence**	**Clinical Presentation**
Lymphocyte predominance	Found in all ages but more common in adults than children Incidence in males exceeds that in females	Peripheral node involvement Spares the mediastinum Usually localized at diagnosis Survival is long with or without treatment Late relapses common
Nodular sclerosing	Found in all ages but most common in adolescents and young adults Incidence in females equals or exceeds that in males	Mediastinal involvement Stage and bulk of disease have prognostic significance
Mixed cellularity	Common in adults Incidence in males exceeds that in females	Stage more advanced than in nodular sclerosis and lymphocyte predominance subtypes Involves lymph nodes, spleen, liver, or marrow
Lymphocyte depletion	Least common variant Most common type in elderly persons, human immunodeficiency virus (HIV)-positive individuals, and persons in nonindustrialized countries	Abdominal lymphadenopathy; spleen, liver, and bone marrow involvement, without peripheral lymphadenopathy Stage is more advanced at diagnosis

the United States having the highest incidence; Japan and Australia have the lowest incidence. The overall incidence is lower in economically disadvantaged countries, but proportionately there is a higher incidence in the elderly population. HD peaks at two different times—during the second and third decades of life and later during the sixth and seventh decades. There is evidence to suggest that three distinct types of HD exist related to the age when diagnosed— a childhood form (<14 years old), a young adult form (15 to 34 years old), and an older form (55 to 74 years old).[25] The box on the right summarizes the risk factors for development of HD.

RISK FACTORS

HODGKIN DISEASE
- Family history
- Association with human leukocyte antigens (HLA: A1, B5, B18, B27, and DR5)
- Smaller family size?
- Increased education of mother?
- Prior tonsillectomy or appendectomy
- Wood working
- High socioeconomic status

Fig. 20-12 *Hodgkin disease and enlarged cervical lymph node.* Typical enlarged cervical lymph node in the neck of a 35-year-old woman with Hodgkin disease. *(From del Regato, J.A., Spjut, H.J., & Cox, J.D. [1985]. Cancer: Diagnosis, treatment, and prognosis [6th ed.]. St. Louis: Mosby.)*

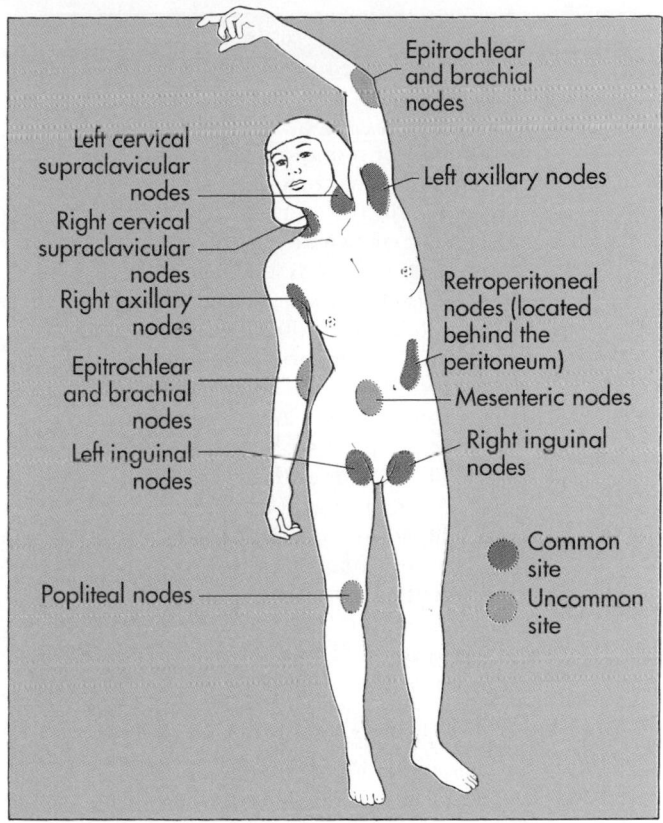

Fig. 20-13 *Common and uncommon involved lymph node sites for Hodgkin disease.*

Clinical Manifestations

Many characteristic features of HD can be explained by the complex action of cytokines and other growth factors that are expressed by the malignant cells causing other malignant and nonmalignant lymph cells to proliferate. An enlarged, painless mass in the neck is often the first sign of HD (Fig. 20-12). The discovery of an asymptomatic mediastinal mass on routine chest x-ray is not uncommon. The cervical, axillary, inguinal, and retroperitoneal lymph nodes are commonly affected in HD (Fig. 20-13). Local symptoms caused by pressure and obstruction are the result of the lymphadenopathy.

Intermittent fever, without other symptoms of infection, and drenching night sweats are relatively common. These constitutional symptoms and weight loss have been associated with a poor prognosis. The Cotswold staging classification system is used for HD (Table 20-8) and is based on medical history, examination (presence of symptoms and palpable lymph nodes), and other radiologic and hematologic results. This system is able to establish a correlation between anatomic extent of the disease and prognosis.

Although HD rarely arises in the lung, mediastinal and hilar node adenopathy can cause secondary involvement of the trachea, bronchi, pleura, or lungs. Retroperitoneal nodes can involve vertebral bodies and nerves and can cause dis-

placement of ureters. Spinal cord involvement is more common in the dorsal and lumbar regions than in the cervical region. Although uncommon, skin manifestations include psoriasis, causing itching and scratching.

As a result of direct invasion from mediastinal lymph nodes, pericardial involvement can cause pericardial friction rub, pericardial effusion, and engorgement of neck veins. The gastrointestinal tract and urinary tract are rarely involved. Anemia is frequently found in individuals associated with a low serum iron and iron-binding capacity. Other laboratory findings include elevated sedimentation rate, leukocytosis, and eosinophilia. With advanced stages of HD, leukopenia occurs.

Splenic involvement in HD depends on the type (Box 20-2). The spleen is involved in 60% of cases of mixed cellularity and lymphocytic types. Only 34% of cases reveal splenic involvement with lymphocyte predominance and nodular sclerosis types.

Evaluation and Treatment

Because of the variability in symptoms, early definitive detection may be difficult. Asymptomatic lymphadenopathy can progress undetected for several years. Careful evaluation, including chest x-ray films, lymphangiography, and biopsy, should be carried out for individuals with fever of

TABLE 20-8	Cotswold Staging Classification System
Stage	**Criteria**
I	Involvement of a single lymph node region or lymphoid structure (i.e., spleen, thymus, Waldeyer ring)
II	Involvement of two or more lymph node regions on the same side of the diaphragm (the mediastinum is a single site, hilar lymph nodes are lateralized); the number of anatomic sites should be indicated by a suffix (i.e., II$_3$)
III	Involvement of lymph node regions or structures on both sides of the diaphragm Stage III$_1$: with or without splenic hilar, celiac, or portal nodes Stage III$_2$: with paraaortic, iliac, mesenteric nodes

IV	Involvement of extranodal site(s) beyond that designated "E"
	Modifying characteristics
	A: no symptoms
	B: fever, drenching sweats, weight loss
	X: bulky disease
	   >$^1/_3$ widening of mediastinum
	   >10-cm maximum dimension of nodal mass
	E: involvement of a single extranodal site contiguous or proximal to known nodal site
	CS: clinical stage
	PS: pathologic stage

Data from Lister, T.A. & Crowther, D. (1990). Seminars in Oncology 17, 696.

Classification of Hodgkin Disease
BOX 20-2

Lymphocyte predominant
  Diffuse pattern
  Nodular pattern
Mixed cellularity
Nodular sclerosis*
Lymphocyte depleted

*Most common type (40% to 80%).

TABLE 20-9	Clinical Differences Between Non-Hodgkin Lymphoma and Hodgkin Disease	
Characteristic	**Non-Hodgkin Lymphoma**	**Hodgkin Disease**
Nodal involvement	Multiple peripheral nodes	Localized to single axial group of nodes (i.e., cervical, mediastinal, paraaortic)
	Mesenteric nodes and Waldeyer ring commonly involved	Mesenteric nodes and Waldeyer ring rarely involved
Spread	Noncontiguous	Orderly spread by contiguity
B* symptoms	Uncommon	Common
Extranodal involvement	Common	Rare
Extent of disease	Rarely localized	Often localized

*Fever, weight loss, night sweats.

unknown origin; 75% of individuals diagnosed with HD are cured. Irradiation, chemotherapy, monoclonal antibodies, and bone marrow transplantation have been responsible for the increasingly successful treatment of HD.

Non-Hodgkin lymphoma

Pathophysiology
Non-Hodgkin lymphoma (NHL) is a generic term for a wide spectrum of disorders characterized by the malignant transformation of the lymphoid system, differentiated from HD by lack of RS cells and other cellular changes not characteristic of HD. The malignant transformation affects different developmental and functional systems of the lymph system.

The diversity of characteristics associated with NHL suggests that there are a wide variety of causes, which include viral infections, immune disorders, and genetic abnormalities. Environmental factors, along with exposure to chemicals, have also been suspected of causing NHL, and recently *Helicobacter pylori* has been implicated.[24]

Clinical Manifestations
Clinical manifestations of NHL usually start out as localized or generalized lymphadenopathy, similar to HD. Differences in clinical features are noted in Table 20-9. The cervical, axillary, inguinal, and femoral chains are the most frequently affected sites. Generally, the swelling is painless and the nodes have enlarged and transformed over a period of months or years. Extranodal sites of involvement are the nasopharynx, gastrointestinal tract, bone, thyroid, testes, and soft tissue. Some individuals have retroperitoneal and abdominal masses with symptoms of abdominal fullness, back pain, ascites (fluid in the peritoneal cavity), and leg swelling.

Evaluation and Treatment
Individuals with NHL can survive for long periods. Survival with nodular lymphoma ranges up to 15 years. Individuals

Fig. 20-14 *Burkitt lymphoma.* Burkitt lymphoma involving the jaw in young African boy. *(Courtesy Dr. J.N.P. Davies, Albany, N.Y. From del Regato, J.A., Spjut, H.J., & Cox, J.D. [1985]. Cancer: Diagnosis, treatment, and prognosis [6th ed.]. St. Louis: Mosby.)*

with diffuse disease generally do not survive as long. Many investigators believe that more aggressive treatment increases the cure rate. Autologous marrow transplantation is now proposed for recurrent disease when no curative regimen exists and for persons with poor-risk lymphomas. High-grade NHL is seen with increasing frequency in persons with AIDS and has an extremely poor prognosis.

Burkitt lymphoma

Burkitt lymphoma is a tumor with unique clinical and epidemiologic features. It occurs in children from east-central Africa and New Guinea and involves primarily the jaw and facial bones (Fig. 20-14). Epstein-Barr virus (found in nasopharyngeal secretions) is associated with Burkitt lymphoma in African children.

The American type of Burkitt lymphoma usually involves the abdomen and is characterized by extensive marrow replacement. The affected cell is a B cell that undergoes cancerous transformation and progression. The African variety has been successfully treated with radiotherapy and cyclophosphamide. The American type is more resistant to treatment.

ALTERATIONS OF SPLENIC FUNCTION

In the past, *splenomegaly* (enlargement of the spleen) has been identified with various disease states. It is now recog-

nized that splenomegaly is not necessarily pathologic, because an enlarged spleen may be present in certain individuals without any evidence of disease. Splenomegaly may be, however, one of the first physical signs of underlying conditions, and its presence should not be ignored. In conditions where splenomegaly is present, the normal functions of the spleen may become overactive and produce a condition known as *hypersplenism.*

Current criteria for hypersplenism include (1) anemia, leukopenia, thrombocytopenia, or combinations of these; (2) cellular bone marrow; (3) splenomegaly; and (4) improvement after splenectomy.[26] It is recognized that individuals may present with problems without having met all the above clinical criteria; therefore the relevance and significance of hypersplenism are still uncertain.

Overactivity of the spleen results in hematologic alterations that affect all blood components. Sequestering of red cells, white cells, and platelets in the spleen results in a reduction of all circulating blood cells. In addition, the sequestered red cells are exposed to splenic conditions that accelerate their destruction, further contributing to the decreased red cell concentration. The extent of red cell destruction depends on the degree of splenomegaly.[26] These combined activities result in an anemia.

The white cells and platelets are also affected by sequestering, although not to the same degree as the red cell. Again, the size of the spleen is the determining factor in the amount of cells sequestered.

Specific diseases and their particular conditions related to the various classifications of splenomegaly are detailed in Box 20-3. Different pathologic processes that produce splenomegaly will be briefly described.

Acute inflammatory or infectious processes cause splenomegaly because of increased demand for defensive activities. An acutely enlarged spleen secondary to infection may become so filled with erythrocytes that its natural rubbery resilience is lost and it becomes fragile and vulnerable to blunt trauma.[1] Traumatic rupture of the spleen is a complication in individuals with infectious mononucleosis.[27]

Congestive splenomegaly is accompanied by ascites, portal hypertension, and esophageal varices and is most commonly seen in hepatic cirrhosis. Splenic hyperplasia develops in any disorder in which splenic workload is increased and is most commonly associated with various types of anemias (hemolytic) and chronic myeloproliferative disorders (i.e., polycythemia vera).

Infiltrative splenomegaly is caused by engorgement of the splenic macrophages with indigestable materials associated with various "storage diseases." Tumors and cysts are neoplastic disorders that cause actual growth of the spleen. Metastatic tumors of the spleen are rare and may result from skin, lungs, breast, and cervical primary sites.[26]

Treatment for hypersplenism is splenectomy; however, it may not always be indicated. It is generally beneficial to perform a splenectomy when the spleen is causing destruction of the red cells; it is not performed when the spleen is caus-

Diseases Related to Classification of Splenomegaly   BOX 20-3

INFLAMMATION OR INFECTIONS
1. Acute
   a. Viral (hepatitis, infectious mononucleosis, cytomegalovirus)
   b. Bacterial (salmonella, gram negative)
   c. Parasite (typhoid)
2. Subacute or chronic
   a. Bacterial (subacute bacterial endocarditis, tuberculosis)
   b. Parasite (malaria)
   c. Fungal (histoplasmosis)
   d. Felty syndrome
   e. Systemic lupus erythematosus
   f. Rheumatoid arthritis

CONGESTIVE
1. Cirrhosis
2. Heart failure
3. Portal vein obstruction (portal hypertension)
4. Splenic vein obstruction

INFILTRATIVE
1. Gaucher disease
2. Amyloidosis
3. Diabetic lipemia

TUMORS OR CYSTS
1. Malignant
   a. Polycythemia rubra vera
   b. Thrombocytopenia
   c. Chronic leukemia (chronic myelocytic leukemia, chronic lymphocytic leukemia)
   d. Hodgkin disease
   e. Acute leukemia
   f. Metastatic solid tumors
2. Nonmalignant: hemartoma
3. Cysts
   a. True: lymphangiomas, hemangiomas, epithelial, endothelial
   b. False: hemorrhagic, serous, inflammatory

---

ing favorable effects, such as antibody production and hematopoiesis.[26] Splenectomy for splenic rupture is no longer considered mandatory in light of the possibility of overwhelming sepsis after removal. Repair of the ruptured spleen should be considered before deciding to remove the spleen.

> ✓ **QUICK CHECK**
>
> Contrast the principal features of Hodgkin disease with those of non-Hodgkin lymphoma.
>
> What is Burkitt lymphoma?
>
> Identify the major causes of splenomegaly. How does it differ from hypersplenism?

ALTERATIONS OF PLATELETS AND COAGULATION
Disorders of Platelet Function

Quantitative or qualitative abnormalities of platelets can interrupt normal blood coagulation and prevent hemostasis. The quantitative abnormalities are thrombocytopenia, a decrease in the number of circulating platelets, and thrombocythemia, an increase in the number of platelets. Qualitative disorders affect the structure or function of individual platelets and can coexist with the quantitative disorders. Qualitative disorders usually prevent platelet adherence and aggregation, preventing formation of a platelet plug.

Thrombocytopenia

Thrombocytopenia is defined as a platelet count below 100,000/mm³ of blood. A count of 50,000/mm³ or less increases the potential for hemorrhage associated with minor trauma. Spontaneous bleeding can occur with counts between 10,000/mm³ and 15,000/mm³, which result in petechiae, ecchymoses, larger purpuric spots, or frank bleeding from mucous membranes.[28] Severe bleeding results if the count is below 10,000/mm³ and can be fatal if it occurs in the gastrointestinal tract, respiratory system, or central nervous system.

Thrombocytopenia is often secondary to other conditions present in the body, either acquired or congenital. The acquired states are more common and include such conditions as acute viral infections (EBV, rubella, CMV, and HIV). Thrombocytopenia may also accompany nutritional deficiency states associated with vitamin B₁₂, folic acid, and iron. Bone marrow replacement and bone marrow hypoplasia (aplastic anemia) may also precipitate thrombocytopenia. Drugs (thiazides, estrogens, quinine-containing medications, chemotherapy) and toxins (ethanol, cocaine) are also implicated as causing thrombocytopenia.

Heparin is identified as the most common cause of drug-induced thrombocytopenia. Approximately 5% of individuals treated with heparin develop heparin-induced thrombocytopenia (HIT).[29] Some individuals have been known to develop paradoxical thrombosis, which consists of white platelet aggregates, a condition known as *white clot syndrome.* If this condition is not recognized and treated, intravascular aggregation of platelets can cause rapid development of multiple thrombotic disease and lead to arterial, venous, cerebral, and pulmonary thrombosis and acute myocardial infarction. The individual may have gangrene in an upper or lower extremity or signs and symptoms of pulmonary emboli and stroke.

Thrombocytopenia is also secondary to altered platelet distribution or destruction, which is associated with congestive hypersplenism described on p. 557.

Thrombocytopenia is also caused by increased platelet destruction. *Immune thrombocytopenic purpura (ITP)* is the major cause of platelet destruction in this category. IgG has been identified as the primary antibody that adheres to the platelet, initiating the immune destruction of the platelet. The majority of the destruction of platelets takes place in the spleen when the antibody-bound platelet comes in contact with the mononuclear phagocyte cells of the spleen.

ITP is a common disease in adults and is frequently a chronic condition more prevalent in females. The incidence is highest in the young adult group (20 to 40 years old), but ITP is found in all age categories. Initial manifestations range from minor problems (development of petechiae and purpura) over the course of several days to major hemorrhage from mucosal sites (epistaxis, hematuria, menorrhagia, bleeding gums). Rarely will an individual present with intracranial bleeding or other sites of internal bleeding.

Diagnosis of ITP is based on a history of bleeding symptoms and associated symptoms (weight loss, fever, headache). Risk factors are also identified (HIV infection), and medications are screened for a potential cause of ITP, as well as any family history of bleeding. Physical examination signs are also evaluated for types of bleeding, location, and severity of bleeding. In addition, evidence of other infections (bacterial, HIV) and thrombosis is assessed.

Initial therapy for ITP is infusion of glucocorticoids (prednisone), which prevents further destruction of platelets. Splenectomy is also considered in individuals who may not respond to prednisone therapy; however, splenectomy is not without risks, and approximately 10% to 20% of individuals who undergo a splenectomy require further treatment.[30]

Thrombocytopenia is also a manifestation of the thrombotic microangiopathy identified as *thrombotic thrombocytopenia purpura (TTP)*. In this condition, platelets aggregate and cause occlusion of arterioles and capillaries within the microcirculation. Platelet aggregation occurs without the activation of the coagulation cascade.[28] TTP is clinically related to other thrombotic microangiopathic conditions, including hemolytic uremic syndrome, malignant hypertension, preeclampsia, and pregnancy-induced HELLP (Hemolysis, Elevated Liver enzymes, Low Platelet count) syndrome.

TTP is more common in females and occurs in mid to late adulthood with the peak incidence in the 40s. It is rarely seen in infants and elderly persons.[31] Early diagnosis and treatment are important since it may prove fatal if left untreated. Plasma exchange with fresh frozen plasma is the treatment of choice. Steroids have not been beneficial in treatment of TTP.[28]

Thrombocythemia

Thrombocythemia (also called thrombocytosis) is defined as a platelet count greater than 400,000/mm³ of blood. Thrombocythemia may be primary or secondary and is usually asymptomatic until the count exceeds 1 million/mm³. At this point, intravascular clot formation (thrombosis), hemorrhage, or other abnormalities can occur.

Transient thrombocythemia is a normal, physiologic response to stress, infection, trauma, exercise, and ovulation. Abnormal thrombocythemia is caused by accelerated platelet production in the bone marrow.

Primary thrombocythemia is a myeloproliferative condition in which platelets are produced in greater numbers than normal, which leads to platelet counts in excess of 600,000/mm³.

The precise mechanism causing thrombocythemia is not clearly identified. The platelets of affected individuals appear to have a normal survival time, and current evidence suggests that the disorder is caused by increased megakaryocyte production that originates at the pluripotential hematopoietic stem cell. Thrombosis of the microvasculature is present in the majority of instances, frequently associated with the fingers and toes. Other manifestations of the condition include neurologic symptoms, with headache being the most common symptom; other neurologic symptoms are paresthesias and transient ischemic attacks (TIAs). Hemorrhagic manifestations are often seen in these individuals, with the primary site of bleeding being the gastrointestinal tract, which may be mistaken for a duodenal ulcer.

Treatment of primary thrombocythemia is problematic and not well delineated. The degree of platelet reduction to reduce morbidity is not well established.

Secondary thrombocytosis occurs after splenectomy because platelets that normally would be stored in the spleen remain in circulating blood. The increase in platelets may be gradual, with thrombocytosis not occurring for up to 3 weeks after splenectomy. Secondary thrombocytosis (reactive thrombocytosis) also may occur as a moderate rise in the platelet count that resolves with treatment of the underlying condition, such as rheumatoid arthritis and cancers.

Alterations of Platelet Function

Qualitative alterations in platelet function are presented when an individual demonstrates an increased bleeding time in the presence of a normal platelet count. Qualitative alterations may be acquired or congenital. Congenital alterations are quite rare and may be categorized into four types: (1) disorders of platelet adhesion, (2) disorders of platelet aggregation, (3) disorders of platelet secretion, and (4) disorders of platelet procoagulant activity.[32] Acquired disorders of platelet function are more common than the congenital disorders and may be categorized into three principal causes:

Drugs Known to Affect Platelet Functions*† BOX 20-4

Nonsteroidal antiinflammatories
   Acetylsalicylic acid (ASA)
   Ibuprofen
   Naproxen
   Indomethacin
B-Lactam antibiotics
   Penicllin G (all penicillin derivatives ending in "cillin")
   Cephalosporins
Cardiovascular drugs
   Nitroglycerin
   Propranolol
   Nifedipine
   Verapamil
   Quinidine
   Diltiazem
Psychotropic drugs
   Tricyclic antidepressants: imipramine
   Phenothiazines: chlorpromazine, promethazine
Anesthetics
   Local: lidocaine, procaine
   General: halothane
Antihistamines
   Diphenhydramine
Food additives or foods
   Ethanol
   Cumin
   Turmeric
   Clove

Of these drugs and agents, only ASA causes significantly increased bleeding time. Other drugs affect platelet aggregation or bleeding time.
†*Generic drug names used in this box.*

(1) drugs, (2) systemic conditions, and (3) hematologic alterations.

Multiple drugs are known to affect platelet function (Box 20-4). Of this vast array of drugs, aspirin is the only known drug specifically used for its antithrombotic activity.[33] Systemic disorders of the affected platelet function are identified as chronic renal disease, cardiopulmonary bypass surgery, and antiplatelet antibodies associated with autoimmunity disorders. Hematologic disorders that cause platelet dysfunction are chronic myeloproliferative disorders, leukemias and myelodysplastic syndromes, and dysproteinemias.

Disorders of Coagulation

Disorders of coagulation are usually caused by defects or deficiencies of one or more of the clotting factors. (Normal function of the clotting factors is described in Chapter 19.) Qualitative or quantitative abnormalities prevent the enzymatic reactions by which clotting factors are normally transformed from circulating plasma proteins to a stable fibrin clot (see Fig. 19-18).

Some clotting factor defects are inherited and involve a single factor, such as the hemophilias and von Willebrand disease, caused by deficiencies of clotting factors (see p. 523). Other coagulation defects are acquired and tend to result from deficient synthesis of clotting factors by the liver. Causes include liver disease and dietary deficiency of vitamin K.

Other coagulation disorders are attributed to pathologic conditions that trigger coagulation inappropriately, engaging the clotting factors and causing detrimental clotting within blood vessels. For example, any cardiovascular abnormality that alters normal blood flow by speeding it up, slowing it down, or obstructing it can create conditions in which coagulation proceeds within the vessels. In ***thromboembolic disease,*** blood clots obstruct blood vessels. Coagulation is also stimulated by the presence of tissue thromboplastin, which is released by damaged or dead tissues. Therefore conditions in which tissue decay or damage releases a great deal of tissue thromboplastin, as in complications of pregnancy, including death of the fetus and placental decay within the mother, can cause widespread and possibly fatal intravascular coagulation. Vasculitis, or inflammation of the blood vessels, along with damage to inflamed vessels causes platelet activation, which in turn activates the coagulation cascade. In extensive or prolonged vasculitis, blood clot formation can overcome mechanisms that normally control clot formation and breakdown, leading to clogging of the vessels. In each of these acquired conditions, normal hemostatic function proves detrimental to the body by consuming coagulation factors excessively or by overwhelming normal control of clot formation and breakdown (fibrinolysis) (see Fig. 19-20).

Impaired hemostasis

Impaired hemostasis, or the inability to promote coagulation and the development of a stable fibrin clot, is commonly associated with liver dysfunction, caused by either specific liver disorders or lack of vitamin K.

Vitamin K deficiency

Vitamin K, a fat-soluble vitamin, is necessary for the synthesis of normal prothrombin; the procoagulant factors II, VII, IX, and X; and the anticoagulant factors (proteins C and S). Parenteral administration of vitamin K is the treatment of choice and usually results in correction of the deficiency. Fresh frozen plasma may also be administered and is usually reserved for individuals with life-threatening hemorrhages or who require emergency surgery.

Liver disease

Individuals who have liver disease present with a broad range of hemostatic derangements that may be characterized by defects in the clotting or fibrinolytic system and by platelet function.[34] The usual sequence of events is an initial reduction in clotting factors, which parallels the degree of parenchymal cell damage or destruction. Factor VII is the first to decline because of its rapid turnover, followed by declines in factors II and X. Factor IX levels are less affected and do not decline until the liver destruction is well advanced. Protein C levels decline early, similar to levels of factor VII, and protein S levels decline in the later stages of liver disease. Declines of factor V are of special importance because factor V plasma levels appear to be a direct reflection of liver cell damage.[34]

Other alterations in hemostasis in liver disease include increased fibrinolytic activity, which may be primary in origin or a reflection of disseminated intravascular coagulation (DIC). This increased fibrinolysis results from increased levels and impaired clearance of fibrinolytic activators and decreased levels of inhibitors, such as alpha$_2$- (α_2) antiplasmin.

Thrombocytopenia and thrombocytopathies are also seen in liver disease. Thrombocytopenia is related to splenomegaly, which often accompanies liver disease and is associated with portal hypertension. Splenic pooling of platelets is the major cause of thrombocytopenia. Thrombocytopathies are associated with elevated levels of fibrin split products, ethanol, or drugs.

Treatment of hemostasis alterations in liver disease must be comprehensive to cover all aspects of alterations related to platelet, clotting, and fibrinolytic dysfunctions. Fresh frozen plasma administration is the treatment of choice; however, not all individuals tolerate the volume needed to adequately replace all deficient factors. Alternative modalities include the addition of exchange transfusions and platelet concentration to fresh frozen plasma administration.

Consumptive thrombohemorrhagic disorders

Consumptive thrombohemorrhagic disorders are a heterogeneous group of conditions that manifest the entire range of hemorrhagic and thrombotic pathologic findings.[35] The symptoms of these disorders also range from the subtle to the devastating and are generally considered to be intermediary disease processes that complicate a vast number of primary disease states. These disorders have also been characterized by confusion and controversy related to their diagnosis, treatment, and management. No one definition is capable of covering all the possible varieties of these disorders; however, DIC is the most common term used in the clinical setting to describe a pathologic condition that is associated with hemorrhage and thrombosis.

Disseminated intravascular coagulation

Disseminated intravascular coagulation (DIC) is an acquired clinical syndrome whose manifestations result from increased protease activity in the blood because of unregulated release of thrombin with subsequent fibrin formation and accelerated fibrinolysis. DIC may be localized to one specific organ or generalized, involving multiple organs.[36] The clinical course of DIC is largely determined by the intensity of the stimulus and the status of the endothelium, liver, and bone marrow.[37]

Bick[38] provides the following clear definition of DIC: "a systemic thrombohemorrhagic disorder seen in association with well-defined clinical situations and laboratory evidence of (1) procoagulant activation, (2) fibrinolytic activation,

(3) inhibitor consumption, and (4) biochemical evidence of end-organ damage or failure" (p. 521).

DIC is associated with a wide variety of clinical conditions, specifically those that activate the clotting cascade. Significant clinical conditions that facilitate procoagulant activity are (1) arterial hypotension, frequently accompanying shock; (2) hypoxemia; (3) acidemia; and (4) stasis of capillary blood flow.[36] Each of these conditions can promote the development of DIC by causing one or more of the following pathologic mechanisms: (1) endothelial damage, (2), tissue damage, and (3) direct activation of factor X.[36]

Endothelial damage exposes the negatively charged basement membrane, which then becomes a hemostatically active vascular surface and activates Hageman factor (XII). Specific substances that have been identified as damaging agents are endotoxins associated with gram-negative sepsis, the cytokines interleukin-1 and tumor necrosis factor, and neutrophil proteases that are associated with the inflammatory process.

Infection is the most common cause of DIC, with approximately 10% to 20% of individuals with gram-negative sepsis manifesting symptoms of DIC (see Risk Factors box). Gram-positive microorganisms have also been implicated as a cause of DIC along with fungi, protozoans (malaria), and viruses (flu, herpes). Hypoxia and low blood flow states associated with cardiopulmonary arrest can also damage the endothelium and activate the intrinsic clotting cascade, triggering DIC.

RISK FACTORS

ACUTE DISSEMINATED INTRAVASCULAR COAGULATION (DIC)
- Obstetric accidents
- Amniotic fluid embolism
- Eclampsia
- Intravascular hemolysis
- Transfusion reactions
- Bacteremia
- Gram-negative (endotoxin)
- Gram-positive (mucopolysaccharides)
- Viremias
- Cytomegalovirus (CMV)
- Hepatitis
- Varicella
- Metastatic malignancy
- Leukemia
- Burns
- Traumatic crush injuries and tissue necrosis
- Liver disease
- Obstructive jaundice
- Acute liver failure
- Vascular disorders
- Arterial hypotension secondary to shock
- Prosthetic devices
- Aortic balloon

Modified from Bick, R.L et al. (1993). Hematology: Clinical and laboratory practice. *St. Louis: Mosby.*

DIC is also precipitated by direct tissue damage and the subsequent exposure to tissue factor (TF). Release of TF occurs in a variety of clinical conditions, particularly when there is a breakdown of the normal tissue structure, such as occurs in ischemia and necrosis, surgical manipulation, and crushing injury. In instances of tissue damage there is also injury to the endothelium, which complicates the situation and also predisposes to the development of DIC.

In addition to endothelial or tissue damage, DIC may be precipitated by direct proteolytic activation of factor X. This has also been described as thrombin mimicry[39] and is the result of proteases directly converting fibrinogen to fibrin. These proteases may come from snake venom, tumor cells, or the pancreas and liver and are released during bouts of pancreatitis and various stages of liver disease. Direct proteolytic activity appears not to depend on any type of damage either to the endothelium or tissue.

Miscellaneous causes of DIC have been identified, most notably blood transfusion. Transfused blood dilutes the clotting factors, as well as circulating, naturally occurring antithrombins. Antibody-antigen reactions are also responsible for the development of DIC after anaphylaxis.

The pathophysiology of DIC is shown in Fig. 20-15. DIC is initiated by one of the above-described mechanisms activating either the intrinsic or extrinsic clotting cascade; however, it appears that the extrinsic system is dominant. In the majority of situations, it is damage or injury to either tissue or epithelium that precipitates DIC. The normal physiologic response to damage is the release of tissue factor, which then complexes with factor VII and directly generates the enzymatic components of the tenascin and prothrombinase complexes that are necessary for the synthesis of thrombin.[40]

The amount of thrombin that enters the systemic circulation during DIC exceeds the ability of the body's naturally occurring antithrombins (proteins C and S, and antithrombin III [AT-III]) to regulate it. In the presence of damaged epithelium, there is uninhibited thrombin activity, which causes unrestricted clot formation. As a result of widespread and diffuse clotting activity, the clotting factors are consumed and hemorrhage ensues. This leads to the primary pathophysiologic paradox of DIC—thrombosis in the presence of hemorrhage.

Once clotting occurs, the fibrinolytic pathway is activated, which acts to degrade the clot that has formed. After the coagulation and fibrinolytic systems have been activated, large amounts of circulating prothrombin and plasminogen are converted to thrombin and plasmin.[41]

The obstruction that results from circulatory deposition of thrombin and clot formation interferes with blood flow and causes widespread organ hypoperfusion that can result in ischemia, infarction, and necrosis, further potentiating and complicating the existing DIC process and causing multiple organ dysfunction and failure.[36] (Multisystem organ dysfunction and failure are discussed further in Chapter 23).

The thrombin-induced platelet aggregation, which occurs early in the clotting cascade, initially plays a role in the

Clinical Manifestations Associated With Disseminated Intravascular Coagulation (DIC) BOX 20-5

INTEGUMENTARY SYSTEM
Widespread hemorrhage and vascular lesions
Oozing from puncture sites, incisions, mucous membranes
Acrocyanosis (irregular-shaped cyanotic patches)
Gangrene

CENTRAL NERVOUS SYSTEM
Subarachnoid hemorrhage
Altered state of consciousness (slight confusion to convulsions and coma)

GASTROINTESTINAL SYSTEM
Occult bleeding to massive gastrointestinal bleeding
Abdominal distention
Malaise
Weakness

PULMONARY SYSTEM
Pulmonary infarctions
ARDS*
Cyanosis
Tachypnea
Hypoxemia

RENAL SYSTEM
Hematuria
Oliguria
Renal failure

Modified from Bailes, B.K. (1992). Disseminated intravascular coagulation, AORN Journal, 55(22), 517-529.
*ARDS, Adult respiratory distress syndrome.

microcirculatory coagulation and obstruction. Eventually the platelets are consumed causing a thrombocytopenia that increases the risk for further bleeding.

Plasmin, a potent proteolytic enzyme that digests fibrin and fibrinogen, is present in higher than normal amounts in DIC. The main role of plasmin is to degrade or digest the fibrin clot. As fibrin is degraded by plasmin, fibrin degradation products (FDPs) are released into the circulation. High concentrations of FDPs, which are potent anticoagulants, further contribute to the bleeding manifestations of DIC.

The positive feedback loop that perpetuates the cycle of thrombosis and hemorrhage persists until the underlying cause of the DIC is removed or appropriate therapeutic interventions are used.

Clinical signs and symptoms of DIC present a wide spectrum of possibilities (Box 20-5). Initial signs of acute DIC

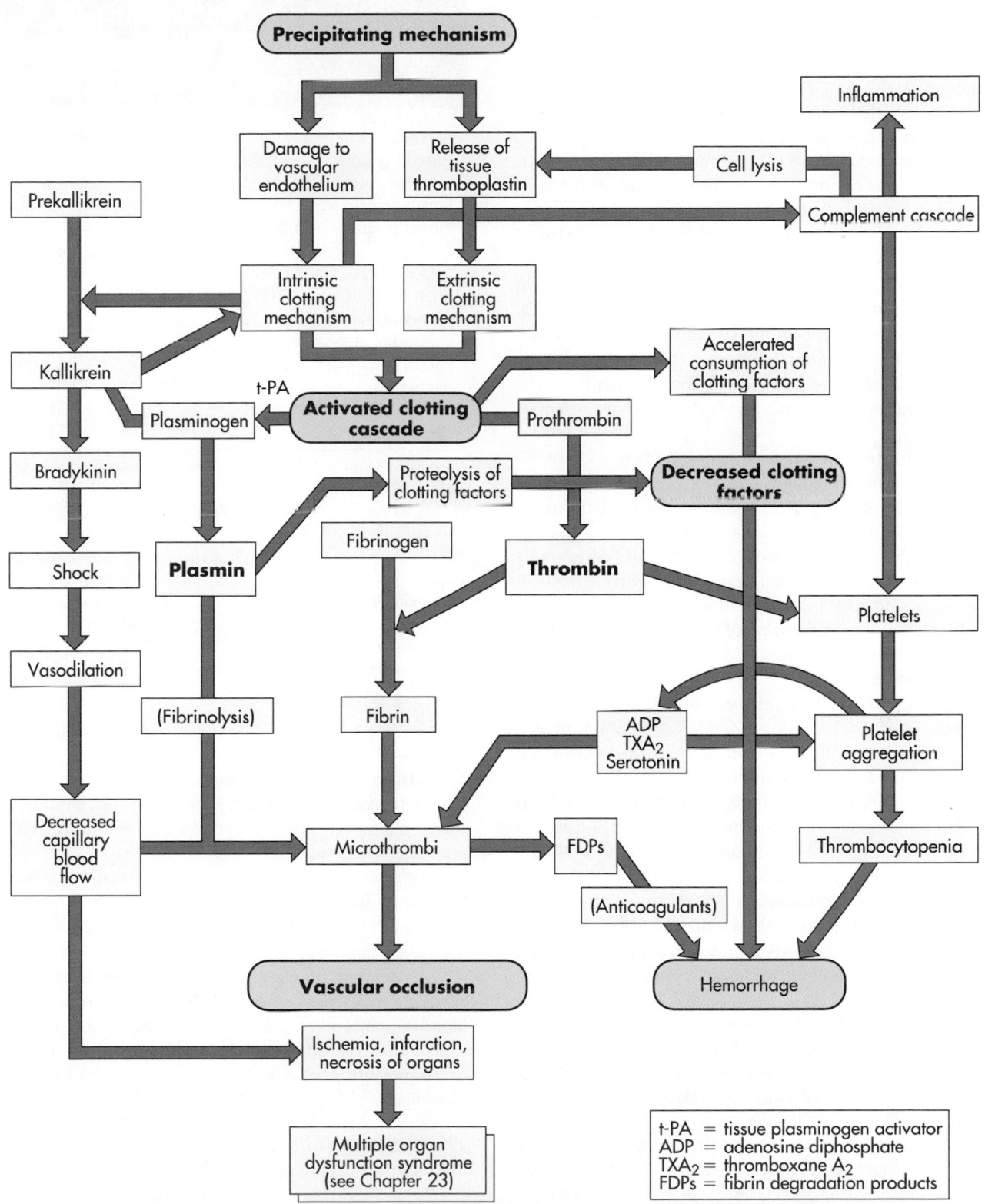

Fig. 20-15 *Pathophysiology of disseminated intravascular coagulation (DIC).* The coagulation cascade is activated if sufficient amounts of specific substances are released into the blood. If the linings of the blood vessels are damaged, the substance released by the injured endothelium initiates the intrinsic pathway for coagulation (see Chapter 19). If tissues anywhere in the body are dead, their decay releases tissue thromboplastin into the blood, initiating the extrinsic pathway of coagulation.

are related to rapid development of hemorrhaging (oozing) from venipuncture sites, arterial lines, or surgical wounds or development of ecchymotic lesions (purpura, petechiae) and hematomas. Other sites of bleeding include the eyes (sclera, conjunctiva), the nose, and the gums. Most individuals with DIC demonstrate bleeding at three unrelated sites, and any combination may be observed.[38]

Manifestations of thrombosis are not always as evident, even though it is often the first pathologic alteration to occur. Organ systems that are susceptible to microvascular thrombosis associated with dysfunction include the cardiovascular, pulmonary, central nervous, renal, and hepatic systems. Changes in level of consciousness, behavior, and mentation, confusion, seizure activity, oliguria, hematuria, hypoxia, hypotension, hemoptysis, chest pain, and tachycardia are manifestations associated with thrombosis of the organs. Hemorrhaging into closed compartments of the body can also occur and may preclude the development of shock.

Cutaneous microvascular occlusion leads to focal infection and necrosis of the digits and may result in gangrene of the upper or lower extremities. Manifestations to be aware of include pale mottled skin and the development of cyanosis.

Individuals with chronic or low-grade DIC do not present with the overt manifestations of hemorrhaging and thrombosis and may be described as having compensated DIC.[38] The major manifestation of this type of DIC is an increased turnover and decreased survival time of the components of hemostasis.

The diagnosis of DIC is primarily based on clinical manifestations with confirmation provided by laboratory evidence. Although no one laboratory test exists to confirm the existence of DIC, data from multiple tests, collaborated with clinical manifestations, provide appropriate information to establish the diagnosis. These tests are identified and the results of the presence of DIC are summarized in Box 20-6.

Treatment of DIC is directed toward (1) removal of the underlying pathologic condition, (2) restoration of an appropriate balance between coagulation and fibrinolysis, and (3) maintaining organ viability.[36] Removal of the underlying pathologic condition is the initial intervention in the treatment phase.

Restoration of balance between the coagulation factors is more difficult to attain. Heparin has been used frequently in this manner; however, its use is controversial and only indicated in certain types of situations related to DIC. Its use seems to be effective in DIC caused by a retained dead fetus and acute promyelocytic leukemia. Heparin is also indicated when organ function is compromised by microthrombi or there is a risk of losing an extremity because of vascular occlusion. Heparin is contraindicated for use in DIC that is precipitated by septic shock or where there is evidence of postoperative bleeding, peptic ulcer, or central nervous system bleeding.

Other drugs that are used to restore the balance of coagulation factors fall into the category of replacement therapy. Replacement therapy for deficient coagulation factors,

Laboratory Tests for Disseminated Intravascular Coagulation (DIC) BOX 20-6

Test	Result*
Bleeding time	>7 min
Platelet count	<130,000†
Plasma fibrinogen levels	<195 mg/dl
Fibrin degradation products (FDPs)	>10 µg/ml
Activated partial thromboplastin time (APTT)	>36 sec
Prothrombin time (PT)	>12 sec
One-stage factor assays‡ (extrinsic coagulation system)	
Factor II	<25 µg/ml
Factor V	<50%
Factor VII	<65%
Factor X	<45%

Data from Bailes, B.K. (1992). Disseminated intravascular coagulation. AORN Journal, 55(2), 517-529; Coffin, C.M. (1989). Potentially catastrophic bleeding disorders: Approaches to diagnosis and management. Bleeding Disorders, 85(3), 217-225.

*Results may vary depending on the laboratory and measurements used.

†In endotoxin-induced DIC, platelets decrease earlier than fibrinogen level; in other causes of DIC, fibrinogen levels fall earlier.

‡One-stage factor assay may be used when APTT and PT are done to determine deficiencies of specific factors.

platelets, and other coagulation elements is gaining importance as a treatment modality. Their use is not without controversy, however, since a major concern with using replacement therapy is "adding fuel to the fire."

Antithrombin III (AT-III) has just been approved for clinical use in the United States and is also a controversial treatment.[36] It is used to attempt to correct coagulation abnormalities and prevent thrombotic complications.

Maintenance of organ viability is treated primarily with adequate fluid replacement to sustain adequate circulating blood volume and maintain optimal tissue and organ perfusion. Fluid resuscitation may also be required to restore blood pressure, cardiac output, and urine output to normal parameters.

Thromboembolic disease

Abnormal clots may occur occasionally within the vascular system. If the clot is stationary or adheres to the vessel wall, it is called a **thrombus** (Fig. 20-16). Thrombi are composed of fibrin and blood cells. Thrombi that form in the arterial system do so under conditions of high blood flow and are composed mostly of platelet aggregates held together by fibrin strands. Venous thrombi form in conditions of low flow and are composed mostly of red cells with larger amounts of fibrin and very few platelets.[42]

Fig. 20-16 *Thrombus.* Thrombus arising in valve pocket at upper end of superficial femoral vein. Postmortem clot on the right is shown for comparison. *(From McLachlin, J. & Paterson, J.C. [1951]. Some basic observations on venous thrombosis and pulmonary embolism.* Surgery, Gynecology, & Obstetrics, 93, 1-8.)

A thrombus may block blood flow within a vessel that supplies nutrients to tissues that are critical to survival, such as the heart, brain, or lungs. A thrombus has the potential to break away from the vessel wall and travel within the bloodstream to a distant site.

An intravascular clot that floats within the blood is called an *embolus.* The mobile embolus travels within the bloodstream until it comes to a point that is smaller than itself and lodges within the vasculature. Once it becomes lodged, it effectively blocks blood flow into the distal portions of the circulatory system; thus the tissues and organs that depend on delivery of blood from that particular section of the circulatory system are deprived of blood. Once deprived of an adequate blood supply, these tissues and organs sustain injury or death.

Prethrombotic conditions predispose an individual to the development of thrombi. These prethrombotic states, in general, are caused by hypercoagulability within the vasculature. Hypercoagulability may be attributable to hereditary or acquired causes.

Acquired hypercoagulability and thrombosis

The acquired hypercoagulable states are caused mostly by conditions that promote venous stasis. The most common clinical states that predispose to thromboembolic phenomena are major surgery (orthopedic), acute myocardial infarction, congestive heart failure limb paralysis, spinal injury, malignancy, advanced age, the postpartum period, and bed rest longer than 1 week.[43] During these clinical states, the body is at greatest risk for the development of thrombi be-

cause of predisposing factors that exist that promote thrombus formation. These factors are referred to as the **Virchow triad** and are (1) injury to the blood vessel endothelium, (2) abnormalities of blood flow, and (3) hypercoagulability of the blood.[?]

Endothelial injury to blood vessels occurs as a result of atherosclerosis (plaque deposits on arterial walls). Atherosclerosis initiates platelet adhesion, aggregation, and formation of a thrombus that resembles a platelet plug. Other causes of vessel endothelial injury may be related to hemodynamic alterations associated with hypertension and turbulent blood flow that occurs in other arterial disorders. Injury may also occur in the presence of radiation injury, exogenous chemical agents (cigarette toxins), endogenous agents (cholesterol), bacterial toxins or endotoxins, or immunologic complex deposits. Whatever the precipitating cause of endothelial injury, it is a potent thrombogenic agent.[2]

Several abnormalities of blood flow can cause thrombus formation. In arterial vessels, thrombosis occurs in conditions of rapid flow. Changes that create turbulence or change the rate of blood flow promote thrombus enlargement that can ultimately occlude the vessel. In veins, slow blood flow contributes to thrombosis, which becomes more severe with further slowing or stagnation. The slower the flow, the greater the quantity of activated clotting factors that remain in close proximity in the vessels. This is the mechanism by which thrombosis occurs in conditions of venous stasis.

Hypercoagulability of the blood may be described as an alteration of the blood that in some way predisposes to thrombus formation. This is a rare cause of thrombosis. Hypercoagulability may result from primary or secondary causes. Primary causes are the congenital conditions related to proteins C and S, and AT-III deficiencies. Secondary causes are those that occur in a variety of clinical conditions previously identified at the beginning of this section. It is not well understood what causes hypercoagulability of blood in these particular conditions. Hypercoagulability is known to increase with age, particularly after 45 years of age. Increased platelet activity is also thought to play a significant role in promoting a hypercoagulable state.

Whether episodes of thromboembolism are life threatening depends on the site of vessel occlusion. Therapy consists of removal or breakdown of the clot and supportive measures. Anticoagulant therapy is effective in treating or preventing venous thrombosis; it is not useful in treating or preventing arterial thrombosis. Parenteral heparin is the major anticoagulant used to treat thromboembolism. Oral coumarin drugs are also widely used, particularly for outpatients.

More aggressive therapy may be indicated for such conditions as pulmonary embolism, coronary thrombosis, or thrombophlebitis. Streptokinase or t-PA (tissue plasminogen activator) activate the fibrinolytic system and are administered to accelerate the lysis of known thrombi. Thrombolytic therapy has limited uses and is prescribed with a high degree of caution because it can cause hemorrhagic complications.

✓ **QUICK CHECK**

Identify the three pathologic causes of DIC, and describe the manifestations associated with it.

Compare and contrast thrombocytopenia with thrombocytosis.

Why does vitamin K deficiency predispose an individual to coagulation disorder?

Compare and contrast a thrombus with an embolus.

How does Virchow triad promote the development of a thrombus?

☐ DID YOU UNDERSTAND?

Alterations of Erythrocyte Function

1. Anemia is generally defined as a reduction in the number or volume of circulating red cells or an alteration in hemoglobin.
2. Anemias can be classified according to (a) erythrocyte size, (b) concentration of hemoglobin, (c) cause of low blood count, or (d) the kinetics of why constant and adequate numbers of mature erythrocytes are not maintained in the circulation.
3. Clinical manifestations of anemia can be found in all organs and tissues throughout the body. Decreased oxygen delivery to tissues can cause fatigue, dyspnea, syncope, angina, compensatory tachycardia, and organ dysfunction.
4. Macrocytic (megaloblastic) anemias are most commonly caused by deficiency of vitamin B_{12}. Pernicious anemia can be fatal unless vitamin B_{12} replacement is given.
5. Microcytic-hypochromic anemias are characterized by abnormally small red cells with insufficient hemoglobin content. The most common cause is iron deficiency.
6. Iron deficiency anemia usually develops slowly, with gradual insidious onset of symptoms. Fatigue, weakness, dyspnea, alteration of various epithelial tissues, and vague neuromuscular complaints result.
7. Iron deficiency anemia is usually a result of a chronic blood loss or poor nutritional intake. Once the source of blood loss is identified and corrected, iron replacement therapy can be initiated. Elevated reticulocyte count is a good index of response to iron therapy.
8. Sideroblastic anemia results from impaired iron metabolism and abnormal sequestration of iron. Treatment varies depending on the cause.
9. Normocytic-normochromic anemias are characterized by insufficient numbers of normal erythrocytes. Included in this category are aplastic, posthemorrhagic, and hemolytic anemia and anemia of chronic inflammation.
10. In aplastic anemia erythrocyte stem cells are underdeveloped, defective, or absent. Unless the cause is determined, bone marrow aplasia results in death.
11. Sudden blood loss results in a normocytic-normochromic anemia. Restoration of blood volume by plasma expanders or transfusions may diminish subjective symptoms of anemia. Hemoglobin restoration may take 6 to 8 weeks.
12. Premature destruction of erythrocytes (hemolytic anemia) may be acquired or hereditary. Of the acquired forms, autoimmune reaction and drug-induced hemolysis are the most common.
13. Anemia of chronic inflammation is associated with chronic infections, chronic inflammatory diseases, and malignancies.

Myeloproliferative Red Cell Disorders (Polycythemia Vera)

1. Polycythemia vera is characterized by excessive proliferation of erythrocyte precursors in the bone marrow. Signs and symptoms result directly from increased blood volume and viscosity. Therapeutic phlebotomy to remove excessive blood volume and use of radioactive phosphorus have been helpful in decreasing the excessive red cell pool.

Alterations of Leukocyte Function

1. Quantitative alterations of leukocytes (too many or too few) can be caused by bone marrow dysfunction or premature destruction of cells in the circulation.
2. Many quantitative changes in leukocytes occur in response to invasion by microorganisms.
3. Leukocytosis is a condition in which the leukocyte count is higher than normal and is usually a response to stress and invasion of microorganisms.
4. Leukopenia is a condition in which the leukocyte count is lower than normal and is caused by pathologic conditions, such as malignancies and hematologic disorders.
5. Granulocytosis (particularly as a result of neutrophilia) occurs in response to infection.
6. When the demand for neutrophils exceeds the supply in the circulation, the marrow releases immature cells, causing a shift-to-the-left.
7. Eosinophilia results most commonly from parasitic invasion and ingestion or inhalation of toxic foreign particles.
8. Basophilia is seen in hypersensitivity reactions because of the high content of histamine and subsequent release.
9. Monocytosis occurs during the late or recuperative phase of infection when macrophages (mature monocytes) phagocytose surviving microorganisms and debris.
10. Granulocytopenia, a condition resulting in a decrease in neutrophils, can be a life-threatening con-

▣ DID YOU UNDERSTAND? —cont'd

dition if sepsis occurs; it is often caused by chemotherapeutic agents, severe infection, and radiation.

11. The common pathologic feature of all forms of leukemia is an uncontrolled proliferation of leukocytes.

12. All leukemias can be designated as (a) lymphocytic, (b) myelocytic or myelogenous, or (c) monocytic. The acute leukemias are divided into two major types: acute myelogenous leukemia (AML) and acute lymphoblastic leukemia (ALL).

13. The two principal types of chronic leukemia are chronic myelocytic leukemia (CML, sometimes also called granulocytic [CGL]) and chronic lymphocytic leukemia (CLL).

14. Although the exact cause of leukemia is unknown, it is considered a clonal disorder. A high incidence of acute leukemias and CLL is reported in certain families, suggesting a genetic predisposition.

15. In leukemia, blasts (precursor cells) "crowd out" the marrow and cause cellular proliferation of the other cell lines to cease.

16. The major clinical manifestations of leukemia include fatigue caused by anemia, bleeding caused by thrombocytopenia, fever secondary to infection, anorexia, and weight loss.

17. Chemotherapy is the treatment of choice for leukemia. Acute leukemias are associated with an increasing survival rate of 80% to 90%, with long-term survival of 30% to 40%. Chronic leukemias are associated with a longer life expectancy.

18. Chronic leukemias progress differently from acute leukemias, advancing slowly and without warning.

19. Multiple myeloma is a neoplasm of B cells (immature plasma cells) and mature plasma cells. It is characterized by multiple malignant tumor masses of plasma cells scattered throughout the skeletal system and sometimes in soft tissue.

20. The exact cause of multiple myeloma is unknown, but genetic factors and chronic stimulation of the mononuclear phagocyte system by bacteria, viral agents, and chemicals have been suggested.

21. The major clinical manifestations for multiple myeloma include recurrent infections caused by suppression of the humoral immune response and renal disease as a result of Bence Jones proteinuria.

22. Chemotherapy is the treatment of choice for multiple myeloma. Survival is still only 2 to 3 years with chemotherapy, however.

Alterations of Lymphoid Function

1. The number of lymphocytes is decreased (lymphocytopenia) in most acute infections and in some immunodeficiency syndromes.

2. Lymphocytosis occurs in viral infections (infectious mononucleosis and infectious hepatitis, in particular), leukemia, lymphomas, and some chronic infections.

3. Infectious mononucleosis is an acute infection of B lymphocytes most commonly associated with the Epstein-Barr virus (EBV) (a type of herpesvirus).

4. Two of the earliest manifestations of infectious mononucleosis are sore throat and fever caused by inflammation at the site of viral entry.

5. Most cases of EBV infectious mononucleosis include fever lasting 7 to 10 days, sore throat, and enlargement and tenderness of the cervical lymph nodes.

6. Lymphomas are tumors of primary lymphoid tissue (thymus, bone marrow) or secondary lymphoid tissue (lymph nodes, spleen, tonsils, intestinal lymphoid tissue). The two major types of malignant lymphomas are Hodgkin disease and non-Hodgkin lymphoma.

7. Distinctive abnormal chromosomes are present in multiple cells of the lymph nodes of an individual with Hodgkin disease. The abnormal cell is called the Reed-Sternberg cell.

8. A virus might be involved in the pathogenesis of Hodgkin disease. Some familial clustering suggests an unknown genetic mechanism.

9. An enlarged, painless mass or swelling, most commonly in the neck, is an initial sign of Hodgkin disease. Local symptoms are produced by lymphadenopathy, usually caused by pressure or obstruction.

10. Treatment of Hodgkin disease includes radiation therapy and chemotherapy. A cure is possible regardless of stage of Hodgkin disease; however, individuals treated with chemotherapy who relapse in less than 2 years have a poor prognosis.

11. The cause of lymph node enlargement and cancerous transformation in non-Hodgkin lymphoma is unknown. Immunosuppressed persons have a higher incidence of non-Hodgkin lymphoma, suggesting an immune mechanism.

12. Generally, with non-Hodgkin lymphoma, the swelling of lymph nodes is painless and the nodes have enlarged and transformed over a period of months or years.

13. Individuals with non-Hodgkin lymphoma can survive for long periods. Treatment is with chemotherapy.

14. Burkitt lymphoma involves the jaw and facial bones and occurs in children from east-central Africa and New Guinea.

Alterations of Splenic Function

1. Splenomegaly (enlargement of the spleen) may be considered normal in certain individuals, but its presence should not be ignored.

2. Splenomegaly results from (a) acute inflammatory or infectious processes, (b) congestive disorders, (c) infiltrative processes, and (d) tumors or cysts.

3. Hypersplenism results from splenomegaly and overactivity of the spleen.

Continued

■ DID YOU UNDERSTAND? —cont'd

Alterations of Platelets and Coagulation

1. Thrombocytopenia is characterized by a platelet count below 100,000 platelets/mm³ of blood; a count below 50,000/mm³ increases the potential for hemorrhage associated with minor trauma.

2. Thrombocytopenia exists in primary or secondary forms.

3. Thrombocytopenia is commonly associated with autoimmune diseases and viral infections; bacterial sepsis with DIC also results in thrombocytopenia.

4. Thrombocythemia is characterized by a platelet count more than 400,000 platelets/mm³ of blood and is symptomatic when the count exceeds 1,000,000/mm³, at which time the risk for intravascular clotting (thrombosis) is high.

5. Thrombocythemia is caused by accelerated platelet production in the bone marrow.

6. Qualitative alterations in normal platelet adherence or aggregation prevent platelet plug formation and may result in prolonged bleeding times.

7. Platelet dysfunction results from changes in the cellular contents and integrity.

8. Disorders of coagulation are usually caused by defects or deficiencies of one or more clotting factors.

9. Pathologic conditions can trigger coagulation, inappropriately using up the clotting factors and causing detrimental clotting within blood vessels.

10. Coagulation is impaired when there is a deficiency

of vitamin K because of insufficient production of prothrombin and clotting factors II, VII, IX, and X.

11. Liver disease accounts for a pattern of hemostatic derangement caused by a disruption of the synthesis of clotting factors.

12. Disseminated intravascular coagulation (DIC) is a complex syndrome resulting from a variety of clinical conditions that increase protease activity in the blood with fibrin formation and accelerated fibrinolysis.

13. DIC is characterized by a cycle of intravascular clotting followed by active bleeding because of the consumption of coagulation factors and platelets and diffuse fibrinolysis.

14. Thromboembolic disease results from a fixed (thrombus) or moving (embolus) clot that blocks flow within a vessel, denying nutrients to tissues distal to the occlusion; death can result when clots obstruct blood flow to the heart, brain, or lungs.

15. Hypercoagulability is the result of deficient anticoagulation proteins. Secondary causes are conditions that promote venous stasis.

16. The term *triad of Virchow* refers to three factors that can cause thrombus formation: (a) loss of integrity of the vessel wall, (b) abnormalities of blood flow, and (c) alterations in the blood constituents.

KEY TERMS

Agranulocytosis, 544
Anemia, 534
Anisocytosis, 534
Basopenia, 546
Basophilia, 544
Burkitt lymphoma, 557
Consumptive thrombohemorrhagic disorder, 561
Disseminated intravascular coagulation (DIC), 561
Embolus, 565
Eosinopenia, 544
Eosinophilia, 544
Erythrocytosis, 542
Granulocytopenia, 544
Granulocytosis, 544
Hemolysis, 535
Hemosiderosis, 540
Hodgkin disease (HD), 553
Hypersplenism, 557
Hypoplastic anemia, 540

Immune thrombocytopenic purpura (ITP), 559
Impaired hemostasis, 560
Infectious mononucleosis (IM), 546
Iron deficiency anemia (IDA), 539
Leukemia, 547
Leukocytosis, 544
Leukopenia, 544
Lymphocytopenia, 546
Lymphocytosis, 546
Macrocytic (megaloblastic) anemia, 536
Microcytic-hypochromic anemia, 539
Monocytopenia, 546
Monocytosis, 546
M-protein, 552
Multiple myeloma, 551
Myelodysplastic syndrome, 540
Neutropenia, 544
Neutrophilia, 544
Non-Hodgkin lymphoma (NHL), 556

Normocytic-normochromic anemia (NNA), 540
Pancytopenia, 548
Pernicious anemia, 538
Poikilocytosis, 534
Polycythemia vera (PV), 542
Primary thrombocythemia, 559
Reed-Sternberg (RS) cell, 553
Shift-to-the-left (leukemoid reaction), 544
Shift-to-the-right, 544
Sideroblastic anemia (SA), 540
Splenomegaly, 557
Thrombocytopenia, 558
Thromboembolic disease, 560
Thrombotic thrombocytopenia purpura (TTP), 559
Thrombus, 564
Virchow triad, 565
White clot syndrome, 558

REFERENCES

1. Booth, I.W. & Aukett, M.A. (1997). Iron deficiency anaemia in infancy and early childhood. *Archives of Disease in Childhood, 76*(6), 549-553.
2. Childs, F. et al. (1997). Dietary education and iron deficiency anaemia in the inner city. *Archives of Disease in Childhood, 76*(2), 144-147.
3. Welte, K. & Dale, D. (1996). Pathophysiology and treatment of severe chronic neutropenia. *Annals of Hematology, 72*(4), 158-165.
4. Julia, A. et al. (1991). Drug induced agranulocytosis: Prognostic factors in a series of 168 episodes. *British Journal of Haematology, 70*, 366.
5. Betts, R.F. (1990). Mononucleosis syndromes. In W.J. Williams et al. (Eds.). *Hematology* (4th ed.). New York: McGraw-Hill.
6. Schaller, R.J. & Counselman, F.L. (1995). Infectious mononucleosis in young children. *American Journal of Emergency Medicine 13*(4), 438.
7. Sandler, D.P. & Ross, J.A. (1997). Epidemiology of acute leukemia in children and adults. *Seminars in Oncology 24*(1), 3-16.
8. American Cancer Society. (1999). *Cancer facts & figures.* New York: The Author.
9. Pui, C.H. (1997). Acute lymphoblastic leukemia. *Pediatric Clinics of North America, 44*(4), 831-846.
10. Fialdow, P.J., Jannsen, J.W.G., & Bertram, C.R. (1991). Clonal remission in adult non-lymphocytic leukemia: Evidence for a multistep pathogenesis of the malignancy. *Blood, 77*, 1415.
11. Caliguri, M.A., Strout, M.P., & Cilliland, D.G. (1997). Molecular biology of acute myeloid leukemia. *Seminars in Oncology, 24*(1), 32-44.
12. Laport., G.F. & Larson, R.A. (1997). Treatment of acute lymphoblastic leukemia. *Seminars in Oncology, 24*(1), 70-82.
13. Verfaille, C.M. (1998). Biology of myelogenous leukemia. *Hematology/Oncology Clinics of North America, 12*(1), 1-29.
14. Kantarjian, H.M. et al. (1998). Clinical course and therapy of chronic myelogenous leukemias with interferon alpha and chemotherapy. *Hematology/Oncology Clinics of North America, 12*(1), 34-80.
15. Reed, J.C. (1998). Molecular biology of chronic lymphocytic leukemia. *Seminars in Oncology, 25*(1), 11-18.
16. Bartik, M.M., Welker, D., & Kay, N.E. (1998). Impairments in immune function in B cell chronic lymphocytic leukemia. *Seminars in Oncology, 25*(1), 27-33.
17. Hehlmann, R. et al. (1992). Chronic myelogenous leukemia: Recent developments in prognostic evaluation and chemotherapy. *Leukemia, 6*(Suppl. 3), 110S.
18. Epstein, J. (1992). Myeloma phenotype: Clues to disease origin and manifestations. *Hematology/Oncology Clinics of North America, 6*(2), 249.

19. Teoh, G. & Anderson, C. (1997). Interaction of tumor and host cells with adhesion and extracellular matrix molecules in the development of multiple myeloma. *Hematology/Oncology Clinics of North America, 11*(1), 1-26.
20. Mishimoto, N. et al. (1997). Myeloma biology and therapy: Present status and future developments. *Hematology/Oncology Clinics of North America, 11*(1), 159-172.
21. Doody, M.M. et al. (1992). Leukemia, lymphoma, and multiple myeloma following selected medical conditions. *Cancer Causes and Control, 5*, 449.
22. Boccadoro, M. & Pileri, A. (1997). Diagnosis, prognosis, and standard treatment of multiple myeloma. *Hematology/Oncology Clinics of North America, 11*(1), 111-132.
23. Bataille, R.S., Manolagas, S.C., & Berensen, J. (1997). Pathogenesis and management of bone lesions in multiple myeloma. *Hematology/Oncology Clinics of North America, 11*(2), 349-362.
24. Yarbro, C.H. & McFadden, M.E. (1997). Malignant lymphomas. In S.L. Groenwald et al. (Eds.). *Cancer nursing: Principles and practice* (pp. 1319-1333). Boston: Jones & Bartlett.
25. Hudson, M.H. & Donaldson, S.S. (1997). Hodgkin's disease. *Pediatric Clinics of North America, 44*(4), 891-906.
26. Athens, J.W. (1993). Disorders primarily involving the spleen. In G.R. Lee et al. (Eds.). *Wintrobe's clinical hematology.* Philadelphia: Lea & Febiger.
27. Bailey, R.E. (1994). Diagnosis and treatment of infectious mononucleosis. *American Family Physician, 49*(4), 879.
28. Rutherford, C.J. & Frankel, E.P. (1994). Thrombocytopenia: Issues in diagnosis and therapy. *Medical Clinics of North America, 78*(3), 555.
29. Walenga, J.M. & Bick, R.L. (1998). Heparin induced thrombocytopenia, paradoxical thromboembolism, and other side effects of heparin therapy. *Medical Clinics of North America, 82*(3), 635-658.
30. Bussell, J. & Clines, D. (1995). Immune thrombocytopenia purpura, neonatal alloimmune thrombocytopenia, and post-transfusion purpura. In R. Hoffman et al. (Eds.). *Hematology: Basic principles and practice.* New York: Churchill Livingstone.
31. Moake, J.L. (1995). Thrombotic thrombocytopenia and the hemolytic uremic syndrome. In R. Hoffman et al. (Eds.). *Hematology: Basic principles and practice.* New York: Churchill Livingstone.
32. Bennett, J.S. (1995). Hereditary disorders of platelet function. In R. Hoffman et al (Eds.). *Hematology: Basic principles and practice.* New York: Churchill Livingstone.

REFERENCES

33. George, J.N., & Shattil, S.J. (1995). Acquired disorders of platelet function. In R. Hoffman et al (Eds.). *Hematology: Basic principles and practice.* New York: Churchill Livingstone.

34. Mammen, E.F. (1994). Coagulation defects in liver disease. *Medical Clinics of North America, 78*(3), 545.

35. Marder, V.J. et al. (1994). Consumptive thrombohemorrhagic disorders. In R.W. Colman et al. (Eds.). *Hemostasis and thrombosis: Basic principles and clinical practice.* Philadelphia: Saunders.

36. Bell, T.N. (1996). Coagulation and disseminated intravascular coagulation. In V.H. Secor (Ed.). *Multiple organ dysfunction and failure.* St. Louis: Mosby.

37. Williams, E.C., & Mosher, D.F. (1995). Disseminated intravascular coagulation. In R. Hoffman et al. (Eds.). *Hematology: Basic principles and practice.* New York: Churchill Livingstone.

38. Bick, R.L. (1996). Disseminated intravascular coagulation: Objective clinical and laboratory diagnosis, treatment, and assessment of therapeutic response. *Seminars in Thrombosis and Hemostasis, 22*(1), 69-88.

39. Johnson, P.C. (1996). Disseminated intravascular coagulation. In D.E. Fry (Ed.). *Multiple system organ failure.* St. Louis: Mosby.

40. Baglin, T. (1996). Disseminated intravascular coagulation: Diagnosis and treatment. *British Medical Journal, 312,* 683.

41. Bailes, B.K. (1992). Disseminated intravascular coagulation. *Journal of the American Operating Room Nurses, 55*(2), 517.

42. Hirsch, J. et al. (1994). Overview of the thrombotic process and its therapy. In R.W. Coleman et al. (Eds.). *Hemostasis and thrombosis: Basic principles and clinical practice.* Philadelphia: Lippincott.

43. Freed, J. (1990). Hypercoagulability: Should every patient with venous thrombosis be tested? *Postgraduate Medicine, 90,* 157.

CHAPTER

21

Alterations of Hematologic Function in Children

Nancy E. Kline and Kathryn L. McCance

A mong the diseases that affect erythrocytes are acquired disorders, such as iron deficiency anemia and hemolytic disease of the newborn, and inherited disorders, such as glucose-6-phosphate dehydrogenase deficiency, sickle cell disease, and the thalassemias.

Childhood disorders of coagulation and platelets include inherited hemorrhagic diseases, such as the hemophilias, and antibody-mediated hemorrhagic diseases, including idiopathic thrombocytopenic purpura. Finally, leukocyte disorders, such as leukemia and the lymphomas (both non-Hodgkin lymphoma and Hodgkin disease) are discussed.

Kathleen Hardin Mooney, RN, PhD, contributed to this chapter in the previous edition.

DISORDERS OF ERYTHROCYTES

Anemia is the most common blood disorder in children. Like the anemias of adulthood, the anemias of childhood are caused by ineffective erythropoiesis or premature destruction of erythrocytes. The most common cause of insufficient erythropoiesis is iron deficiency, which may result from insufficient dietary intake or chronic loss of iron caused by bleeding. The *hemolytic anemias* of childhood may be divided into (1) disorders that result from premature destruction caused by intrinsic abnormalities of the erythrocytes and (2) disorders that result from damaging extraerythrocytic factors. The hemolytic anemias are either inherited or acquired.

The most dramatic form of acquired congenital hemolytic anemia is *hemolytic disease of the newborn (HDN),* also termed *erythroblastosis fetalis.* HDN is an alloimmunity (isoimmunity) disease in which maternal blood and fetal blood are antigenically incompatible, causing the mother's immune system to produce antibodies against fetal erythrocytes. Fetal erythrocytes attacked by (i.e., bound to) maternal antibodies are recognized as foreign or defective by the fetal mononuclear phagocyte system and are removed from the circulation by phagocytosis, usually in the fetal spleen. (For a complete discussion of HDN, see discussion that follows.) Other acquired hemolytic anemias—some of which begin in utero—include those caused by infections or the presence of toxic chemicals.

The inherited forms of hemolytic anemia result from intrinsic defects of the child's erythrocytes, any of which can lead to erythrocyte removal by the mononuclear phagocyte system. Structural defects include abnormal cellular size or shape and abnormalities of plasma membrane structure (spherocytosis). Intracellular defects include enzyme deficiencies, the most common of which is *glucose-6-phosphate dehydrogenase (G6PD) deficiency,* and defects of hemoglobin synthesis, which manifest as sickle cell disease or thalassemia, depending on which component of hemoglobin is defective. These and other causes of childhood anemia are listed in Table 21-1.

Acquired Disorders

Iron deficiency anemia

Iron deficiency anemia is the most common blood disorder of infancy and childhood, with the highest incidence occurring between 6 months and 2 years of age. Incidence is not related to gender or race, but socioeconomic factors are important because they affect nutrition. Iron deficiency anemia is common in children because they need an extremely high amount of iron for normal growth to occur.

Between 4 years of age and the onset of puberty, dietary iron deficiency is uncommon. During adolescence, however, it is relatively common, especially in menstruating females. Rapid growth, together with the average teenager's dietary habits, causes iron depletion.

Pathophysiology

Blood loss is a common cause of iron deficiency anemia in childhood. Chronic iron deficiency anemia from occult (hidden) blood loss may be caused by a gastrointestinal lesion, parasitic infestation, or hemorrhagic disease. As many as one third of infants with severe iron deficiency anemia have chronic intestinal blood loss induced by exposure to a heat-labile protein in cow's milk. Such exposure causes an inflammatory gastrointestinal reaction that damages the mucosa and results in diffuse hemorrhage.

Clinical Manifestations

The symptoms of mild anemia—lethargy and lassitude—usually are not present or detectable in infants and young children, who are unable to describe these symptoms. Therefore parents generally do not note any change in the child's behavior or appearance until moderate anemia has developed. General irritability, decreased activity tolerance, weakness, and lack of interest in play are nonspecific indications of anemia. When the hemoglobin determination falls below 5 g/dl, pallor, anorexia, tachycardia, and systolic murmurs may occur.

Other symptoms and signs include splenomegaly, widened skull sutures, decreased physical growth and developmental delays, pica (a behavior in which nonfood substances are eaten), and altered neurologic and intellectual functions, especially those involving attention span, alertness, and learning ability.

Evaluation and Treatment

The most definitive test for differentiating iron deficiency from other microcytic states is the absence of iron stores in the bone marrow. However, measurement of serum ferritin iron concentration, transferrin saturation, iron-binding capacity, and, more recently, serum transferrin receptors may prevent proceeding to actual bone marrow evaluation.[1] Evaluation and treatment of iron deficiency anemia in children are similar to those in adults. Dietary modification is required to prevent recurrences of iron deficiency anemia.

Hemolytic disease of the newborn

The most common cause of hemolytic anemia in newborns is alloimmune disease (HDN). HDN can occur only if antigens on fetal erythrocytes differ from antigens on maternal erythrocytes. Maternal-fetal incompatibility exists if mother and fetus differ in ABO blood type or if the fetus is Rh-positive and the mother is Rh-negative. Some minor blood antigens may also be involved. (The antigenic properties of erythrocytes are described in Chapter 5.)

ABO incompatibility occurs in about 20% to 25% of all pregnancies, but only 1 in 10 cases of ABO incompatibility results in HDN. Rh incompatibility occurs in fewer than 10% of pregnancies and rarely causes HDN in the first incompatible fetus. Even after five or more pregnancies, only 5% of women have babies with hemolytic disease. Usually erythrocytes from the first incompatible fetus cause the

TABLE 21-1	Anemias of Childhood
Cause	**Anemic Condition**
Deficient erythropoiesis or hemoglobin synthesis	
Decreased stem cell population in marrow (congenital or acquired pure red cell aplasia)	Normocytic-normochromic anemia
Decreased erythropoiesis despite normal stem cell population in marrow (infection, inflammation, cancer, chronic renal disease, congenital dyserythropoiesis)	Normocytic-normochromic anemia
Deficiency of a factor or nutrient needed for erythropoiesis	
Cobalamin (vitamin B_{12}), folate	Megaloblastic anemia
Iron	Microcytic-hypochromic anemia
Increased or premature hemolysis	
Alloimmune disease (maternal-fetal Rh, ABO, or minor blood group incompatibility)	Hemolytic disease of the newborn (HDN)
Autoimmune disease (idiopathic autoimmune hemolytic anemia, symptomatic systemic lupus erythematosus, lymphoma, drug-induced autoimmune processes)	Autoimmune hemolytic anemia
Inherited defects of plasma membrane structure (spherocytosis, elliptocytosis, stomatocystosis) or cellular size or both (pyknocytosis)	Hemolytic anemia
Infection (bacterial sepsis, congenital syphilis, malaria, cytomegalovirus infection, rubella, toxoplasmosis, disseminated herpes)	Hemolytic anemia
Intrinsic and inherited enzymatic defects (deficiencies) of glucose-6-phosphate dehydrogenase [G-6-PD], pyruvate kinase, 5'-nucleotidase, glucose phosphate isomerase)	Hemolytic anemia
Inherited defects of hemoglobin synthesis	Sickle cell anemia Thalassemia
Disseminated intravascular coagulation (see Chapter 20)	Hemolytic anemia
Galactosemia	Hemolytic anemia
Prolonged or recurrent respiratory or metabolic acidosis	Hemolytic anemia
Blood vessel disorders (cavernous hemangioma, large vessel thrombus, renal artery stenosis, severe coarctation of the aorta)	Hemolytic anemia

mother's immune system to produce antibodies that affect the fetuses of subsequent incompatible pregnancies. Only one in three cases of HDN is caused by Rh incompatibility; most cases are caused by ABO incompatibility.

Pathophysiology

HDN will result (1) if the mother's blood contains preformed antibodies against fetal erythrocytes or produces them on exposure to fetal erythrocytes, (2) if sufficient amounts of antibody (usually immunoglobulin G [IgG]) cross the placenta and enter fetal blood, and (3) if IgG binds with sufficient numbers of fetal erythrocytes to cause widespread antibody-mediated hemolysis or splenic removal. (Antibody-mediated cellular destruction is described in Chapter 5.)

Maternal antibodies may be formed against type B erythrocytes if the mother is type A or against type A if the mother is type B. Usually, however, the mother is type O and the fetus is A or B. ABO incompatibility can cause HDN even if fetal erythrocytes do not escape into the maternal circulation during pregnancy. This occurs because the blood of most adults already contains anti-A or anti-B antibodies, which are produced on exposure to certain foods or infection by gram-negative bacteria. (Anti-O antibodies do not exist because type O erythrocytes are not antigenic.) Therefore IgG against type A or B erythrocytes usually is preformed in maternal blood and can enter the fetal circulation throughout the first incompatible pregnancy.

Anti-Rh antibodies, on the other hand, are formed only in response to the presence of incompatible (Rh-positive) erythrocytes in the blood of an Rh-negative mother. Sources of exposure include fetal blood that is mixed with the mother's blood at the time of delivery, transfused blood, and, rarely, previous sensitization of the mother by her own mother's incompatible blood (Fig. 21-1).

The first Rh-incompatible pregnancy generally presents no difficulties because very few fetal erythrocytes cross the placental barrier during gestation. When the placenta detaches at birth, however, a large number of fetal erythrocytes usually enter the mother's bloodstream. If the mother is Rh-negative and the fetus is Rh-positive, the mother produces anti-Rh antibodies. Anti-Rh antibodies persist in the bloodstream for a very long time, and if the next offspring is Rh-positive, the mother's anti-Rh antibodies can enter the fe-

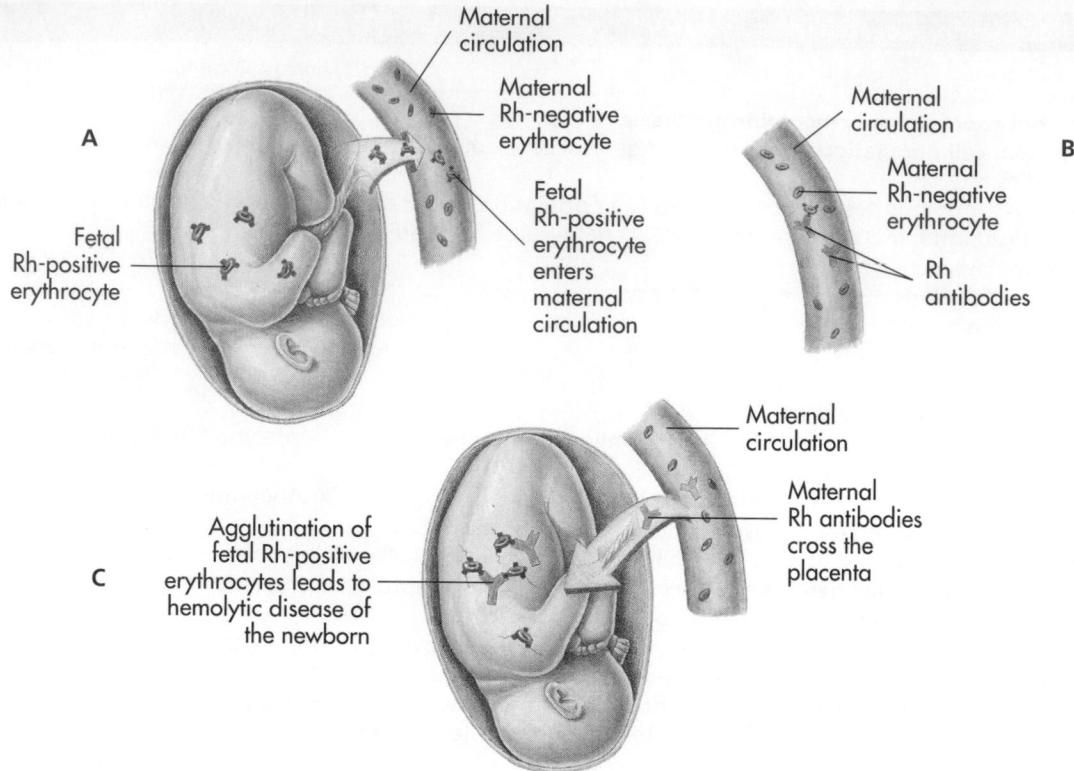

Fig. 21-1 *Hemolytic disease of the newborn (HDN).* **A,** Before or during delivery, Rh-positive erythrocytes from the fetus enter the blood of an Rh-negative woman through a tear in the placenta. **B,** The mother is sensitized to the Rh antigen and produces Rh antibodies. Because this usually happens after delivery, there is no effect on the fetus in the first pregnancy. **C,** During a subsequent pregnancy with an Rh-positive fetus, Rh-positive erythrocytes cross the placenta, enter the maternal circulation, and stimulate the mother to produce antibodies against the Rh antigen. The Rh antibodies from the mother cross the placenta, using agglutination and hemolysis of fetal erythrocytes, and HDN develops. *(Modified from Seeley, R.R., Stephens, T.D., & Tate, P. [1995]. Anatomy and physiology [3rd ed.]. St. Louis: Mosby.)*

tus's bloodstream and destroy the erythrocytes. Antibodies against Rh antigen D are of the IgG class and easily cross the placenta.

IgG-coated fetal erythrocytes usually are destroyed in the spleen. As hemolysis proceeds, the fetus becomes anemic. Erythropoiesis accelerates, particularly in the liver and spleen, and immature nucleated cells (erythroblasts) are released into the bloodstream (hence the name *erythroblastosis fetalis*). The degree of anemia depends on the length of time the antibody has been in the fetal circulation, antibody concentration, and the ability of the fetus to compensate for increased hemolysis. Unconjugated (indirect) bilirubin, which is formed during breakdown of hemoglobin, is transported across the placental barrier into the maternal circulation and is excreted by the mother. Hyperbilirubinemia occurs in the neonate after birth because excretion of lipid-soluble unconjugated bilirubin through the placenta no longer is possible.

The pathophysiologic effects of HDN are more severe in Rh incompatibility than in ABO incompatibility. ABO incompatibility may resolve after birth without life-threatening complications. Maternal-fetal incompatibility in which a

mother with type O blood has a child with type A or B blood usually is so mild that it does not require treatment.

Rh incompatibility is more likely than ABO incompatibility to cause severe or even life-threatening anemia, death in utero, or damage to the central nervous system. Severe anemia alone can cause death as a result of cardiovascular complications. Extensive hemolysis also results in increased levels of unconjugated bilirubin in the neonate's circulation. If bilirubin levels exceed the liver's ability to conjugate and excrete bilirubin, some of it is deposited in the brain, causing cellular damage and eventually, if the neonate does not receive exchange transfusions, death.

Fetuses that do not survive anemia in utero usually are stillborn, with gross edema in the entire body, a condition called **hydrops fetalis.** Death can occur as early as 17 weeks' gestation and results in spontaneous abortion.

Clinical Manifestations

Neonates with mild HDN may appear healthy or slightly pale, with slight enlargement of the liver or spleen. Pronounced pallor, splenomegaly, and hepatomegaly indicate severe anemia, which predisposes the neonate to cardiovas-

TABLE 21-2	Inheritance of Sickle Cell Disease	
Hemoglobin Inherited From First Parent	**Hemoglobin Inherited From Second Parent**	**Form of Sickle Cell Disease in Child**
Hb S (an abnormal hemoglobin)	Hb S	Sickle cell anemia: homozygous inheritance in which the child's hemoglobin is mostly Hb S, with the remainder Hb F (fetal hemoglobin)
Hb S	Defective or insufficient alpha or beta chains of Hb A (alpha- or beta-thalassemia)	Sickle cell–thalassemia disease (heterozygous inheritance of Hb S and alpha- or beta-thalassemia)
Hb S	Hb C or D (both abnormal hemoglobins)	Sickle cell–hemoglobin C (or D) disease (heterozygous inheritance of hemoglobin S and either C or D)
Hb S	Normal hemoglobins (mostly Hb A)	Sickle cell trait, the carrier state (heterozygous inheritance of Hb S and normal hemoglobin)

cular failure and shock. Life-threatening Rh incompatibility is rare today, largely because of the routine use of Rh immunoglobulin.

Because the maternal antibodies remain in the neonate's circulatory system after birth, erythrocyte destruction can continue. This causes **hyperbilirubinemia** and **icterus neonatorum (neonatal jaundice)** shortly after birth. Without replacement transfusions, in which the child receives Rh-negative erythrocytes, the bilirubin is deposited in the brain, a condition termed **kernicterus.** Kernicterus produces cerebral damage and usually causes death (**icterus gravis neonatorum**). Infants who do not die may have mental retardation, cerebral palsy, or high-frequency deafness.

Evaluation and Treatment

Routine evaluation of fetuses at risk for HDN (i.e., fetuses resulting from Rh- or ABO-incompatible matings) includes the Coombs test. The indirect Coombs test measures antibody in the mother's circulation and indicates if the fetus is at risk for HDN. The direct Coombs test measures antibody already bound to the surfaces of fetal erythrocytes and is used primarily to confirm the diagnosis of antibody-mediated HDN. A recent advancement in the early diagnosis of HDN is the access to the fetal circulation directly through intravenous umbilical cord sampling.

The key to treatment of HDN resulting from Rh incompatibility lies in prevention (immunoprophylaxis). One of the success stories of immunology has been the results obtained with Rh immune globulin (RhoGAM), a preparation of antibody against Rh antigen D. If an Rh-negative woman is given Rh immune globulin within 72 hours of exposure to Rh-positive erythrocytes, she will not produce antibody against the D antigen, and the next Rh-positive baby will be protected.

If antigenic incompatibility of the mother's erythrocytes is not discovered in time to administer prophylactic immune globulin (RhoGAM) and a child is born with HDN, treatment consists of exchange transfusions in which the neonate's blood is replaced with new Rh-positive blood that is not contaminated with anti-Rh antibodies. Phototherapy also is used to reduce the toxic effects of unconjugated bilirubin.

Inherited Disorders
Sickle cell disease

Sickle cell disease is a group of disorders characterized by the production of abnormal **hemoglobin S (Hb S)** within the erythrocytes. Hb S is formed by a genetic mutation in which one amino acid (valine) replaces another (glutamic acid) (Fig. 21-2). Hb S, the so-called sickle hemoglobin, reacts to deoxygenation and dehydration by solidifying and stretching the erythrocyte into an elongated sickle shape, producing hemolytic anemia.

Sickle cell disease is an inherited, autosomal recessive disorder expressed as sickle cell anemia, sickle cell–thalassemia disease, or sickle cell–hemoglobin C disease, depending on mode of inheritance (Table 21-2). (See Chapter 2 for a discussion of genetic inheritance of disease.) *Sickle cell anemia,* a homozygous form, is the most severe. *Sickle cell–thalassemia* and *sickle cell–Hb C disease* are heterozygous forms in which the child simultaneously inherits another type of abnormal hemoglobin from one parent. *Sickle cell trait,* in which the child inherits Hb S from one parent and normal hemoglobin (Hb A) from the other, is a heterozygous carrier state that rarely has clinical manifestations. All forms of sickle cell disease are lifelong conditions and have no known cure.

Sickle cell disease tends to occur in persons with origins in equatorial countries, particularly central Africa, the Near East, the Mediterranean area, and parts of India. In the United States, sickle cell disease is most common in blacks, with a reported incidence ranging from 1:400 to 1:500 live births. In the general population the risk of two black parents having a child with sickle cell anemia is 0.7%. Sickle cell–hemoglobin C disease is less common (1 in 800 births), and sickle cell–thalassemia occurs in 1 in 1700 births.

Sickle cell trait occurs in 7% to 13% of African Americans, whereas its incidence among East Africans may be as high as 45%. The sickle cell trait may provide protection

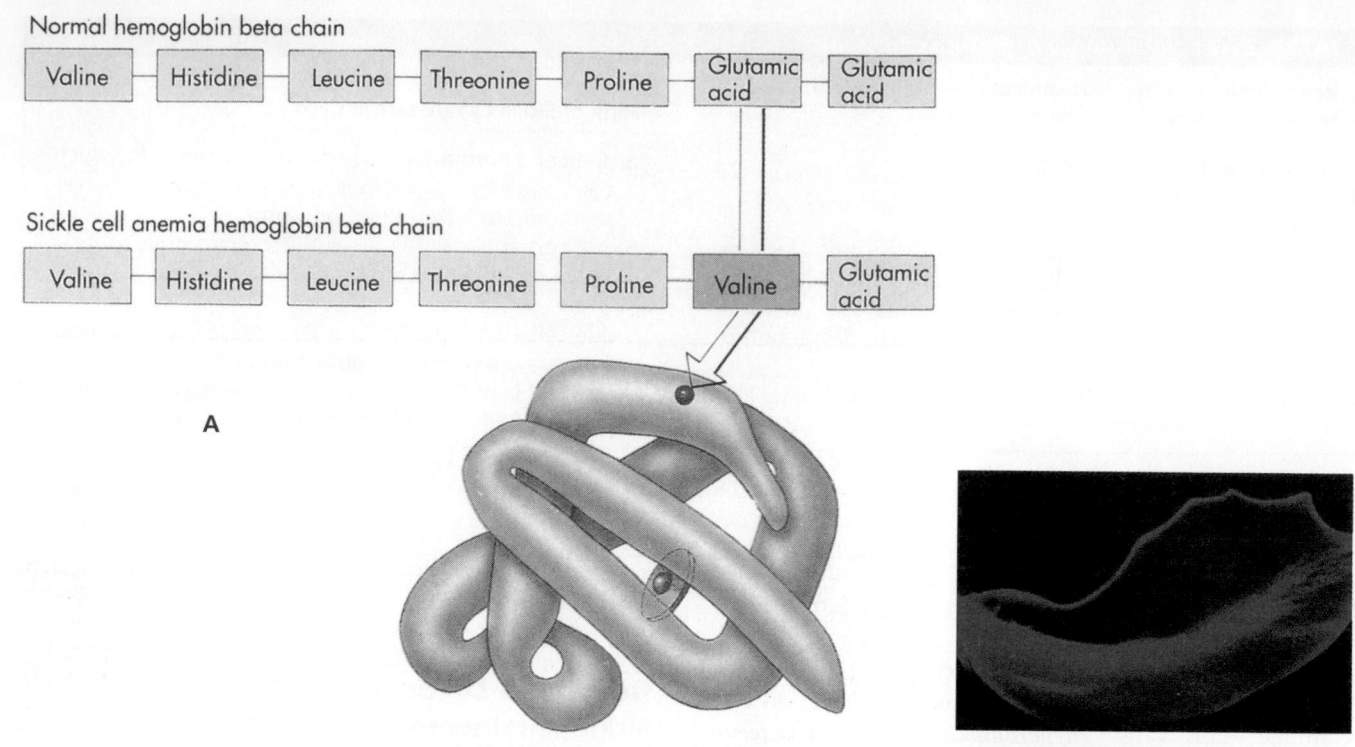

Fig. 21-2 *Sickle cell hemoglobin.* **A,** Sickle cell hemoglobin is produced by a recessive allele of the gene encoding the beta chain of the protein hemoglobin. It represents a single amino acid change from glutamic acid to valine at the sixth position of the chain. In the folded beta-chain molecule, the sixth position contacts the alpha chain and the amino acid change causes the hemoglobins to aggregate into long chains, altering the shape of the cell. **B,** Characteristic shape of sickled red blood cell (or cells). *(A from Raven, P.H. & Johnson, G.B. [1993]. Biology [3rd ed.]. Boston: Times Mirror Higher Education Group. By permission of McGraw-Hill; B from Miale, J.B. [1982]. Laboratory medicine: Hematology [6th ed.]. St. Louis: Mosby, courtesy Dr. M. Bessis.)*

against lethal forms of malaria, a genetic advantage to carriers who reside in endemic regions for malaria (Mediterranean and African zones) but no advantage to carriers living in the United States.

Pathophysiology

Hemoglobin S is soluble and usually causes no problem when properly oxygenated. When oxygen tension decreases, the single amino acid substitution in the beta-globin chain of Hb S polymerizes, forming abnormal fluid polymers. As these polymers realign, they cause the red cell to deform into the sickle shape.[2,3] Sickling depends on the degree of oxygenation, pH, and dehydration of the individual. A decrease in oxygenation (hypoxemia) and pH, as well as dehydration, increases sickling. Deoxygenation is probably the most important variable in determining the occurrence of sickling.[4] Sickle-trait cells sickle at oxygen tensions of about 15 mm Hg, whereas those from an individual with sickle cell disease begin to sickle at about 40 mm Hg. Sickled erythrocytes tend to plug the blood vessels, increasing viscosity of the blood, which slows circulation and causes vascular occlusion, pain, and organ infarction. Viscosity increases the time of exposure to less oxygenation, promoting further sickling. Sickled cells undergo hemolysis in the spleen or become sequestered there, causing blood pooling and infarction of splenic vessels. The anemia that follows triggers erythropoiesis in the marrow and, in extreme cases, in the liver.

Sickling usually is not permanent; most sickled erythrocytes regain a normal shape after reoxygenation and rehydration. Irreversible sickling is caused by irreversible plasma membrane damage caused by sickling. In persons with sickle cell anemia, in which the erythrocytes contain a high percentage of Hb S (75% to 95%), up to 30% of the erythrocytes can become irreversibly sickled. Occasionally, irreversible sickling occurs in sickle cell disease but not in the carrier state (sickle cell trait). Sickling can also be triggered by increased plasma osmolality, decreased plasma volume, and low environmental temperature.

Clinical Manifestations

When sickling occurs, the general manifestations of hemolytic anemia—pallor, fatigue, jaundice, and irritability—sometimes are accompanied by acute manifestations called *crises.* Extensive sickling can precipitate the following four types of crises:

1. ***Vasoocclusive crisis (thrombotic crisis).*** This begins with sickling in the microcirculation. As blood flow is obstructed by sickled cells, vasospasm occurs and a "logjam" effect blocks all blood flow through the vessel. Unless the process is reversed, thrombosis and infarction (death

caused by lack of oxygen) of local tissue follow. Vasoocclusive crisis is extremely painful and may last for days or even weeks, with an average duration of 4 to 6 days. The frequency of this type of crisis is variable and unpredictable.

2. *Sequestration crisis.* Large amounts of blood become acutely pooled in the liver and spleen. This type of crisis is seen only in the young child. Because the spleen can hold as much as one fifth of the body's blood supply at one time, up to 50% mortality has been reported, with death caused by cardiovascular collapse.

3. *Aplastic crisis.* Profound anemia is caused by diminished erythropoiesis despite an increased need for new erythrocytes. In sickle cell anemia, erythrocyte survival is only 10 to 20 days. Normally a compensatory increase in erythropoiesis (five to eight times normal) replaces the cells lost through premature hemolysis. If this compensatory response is compromised, aplastic crisis develops in a very short time.

4. *Hyperhemolytic crisis.* Although unusual, this may occur in association with certain drugs or infections.

The clinical manifestations of sickle cell disease usually do not appear until the infant is at least 6 months old, at which time the postnatal decrease in Hb F causes concentrations of Hb S to rise (Fig. 21-3). Infection is the most frequent cause of death because of sickle cell disease. Sepsis and meningitis develop in as many as 10% of children with sickle cell anemia during the first 5 years of life, with a mortality of 25%. Survival time is unpredictable, but many individuals die in their twenties.

Sickle cell–Hb C disease is usually milder than sickle cell anemia. The main clinical problems are related to vasoocclusive crises and are believed to result from higher hematocrit values and viscosity. In older children, sickle cell retinopathy, renal necrosis, and aseptic necrosis of the femoral heads occur along with obstructive crises.

Sickle cell–thalassemia has the mildest clinical manifestations of all the sickle cell diseases. The normal hemoglobins, particularly Hb F, inhibit sickling. In addition, the erythrocytes tend to be small (microcytic) and to contain relatively little hemoglobin (hypochromic), making them less likely to occlude the microcirculation, even when in a sickled state.

Evaluation and Treatment

The sickle cell trait does not affect life expectancy or interfere with daily activities. However, on rare occasions, severe hypoxia caused by shock, vigorous exercising at high altitudes, flying at high altitudes in unpressurized aircraft, or undergoing anesthesia is associated with vasoocclusive episodes in persons with sickle cell trait. These cells form an ivy shape instead of a sickle shape.

The parents' hematologic history and clinical manifestations may suggest that a child has sickle cell disease, but hematologic tests are necessary for diagnosis. If the sickle solubility test confirms the presence of Hb S in peripheral blood, hemoglobin electrophoresis provides information

about the amount of Hb S in erythrocytes. Prenatal diagnosis can be made after chorionic villus sampling as early as 8 to 10 weeks' gestation or amniotic fluid analysis at 15 weeks' gestation. Newborn screening for sickle cell disease should be performed according to state law.

Treatment of sickle cell disease consists of supportive care aimed at preventing consequences of anemia and avoiding crises. Genetic counseling and psychologic support are important for the child and family.

HEALTH ALERT

Hydroxyurea Treatment for Severe Sickle Cell Disease

Hydroxyurea is an antimetabolite that inhibits deoxyribonucleic acid (DNA) synthesis and causes an increase in the synthesis of hemoglobin F. Early clinical trials of hydroxyurea in adult patients with severe sickle cell disease revealed an increase in hemoglobin F and a significant reduction in vasoocclusive crises. Similar results have been reported in children. Median hemoglobin F concentration increased from 4.65% to 15.34%, and the number of hospital days decreased from 15.2 to 1.8 in 16 of 22 patients treated for 6 months. Hydroxyurea is well tolerated, with the most common side effect being myelosuppression.

Data from Ferster, A. et al. (1996). Hydroxyurea for treatment of severe sickle cell anemia: A pediatric clinical trial. Blood, 88, 1960-1964.

Thalassemias

The alpha- and beta-thalassemias are inherited autosomal recessive disorders that cause an impaired rate of synthesis of one of the two chains—alpha or beta—of adult hemoglobin (Hb A). The disorder was named *thalassemia,* which is derived from the Greek word for *sea,* because it was discovered initially in persons with origins near the Mediterranean Sea. Beta-thalassemia, in which synthesis of the beta-globin chain is slowed or defective, is prevalent among Greeks, Italians, and some Arabs and Sephardic Jews. Alpha-thalassemia, in which the alpha chain is affected, is most common among Chinese, Vietnamese, Cambodians, and Laotians. Both alpha and beta thalassemias are common among blacks.

Both alpha- and beta-thalassemias are referred to as major or minor, depending on how many of the genes that control alpha- or beta-chain synthesis are defective and whether the defects are inherited homozygously (thalassemia major) or heterozygously (thalassemia minor). Pathophysiologic effects range from mild microcytosis to death in utero, depending on the number of defective genes and mode of inheritance. The anemic manifestation of thalassemia is microcytic-hypochromic hemolytic anemia.

Pathophysiology

The fundamental defect in beta-thalassemia is the uncoupling of alpha- and beta-chain synthesis. Beta chain production is depressed—moderately in the heterozygous form,

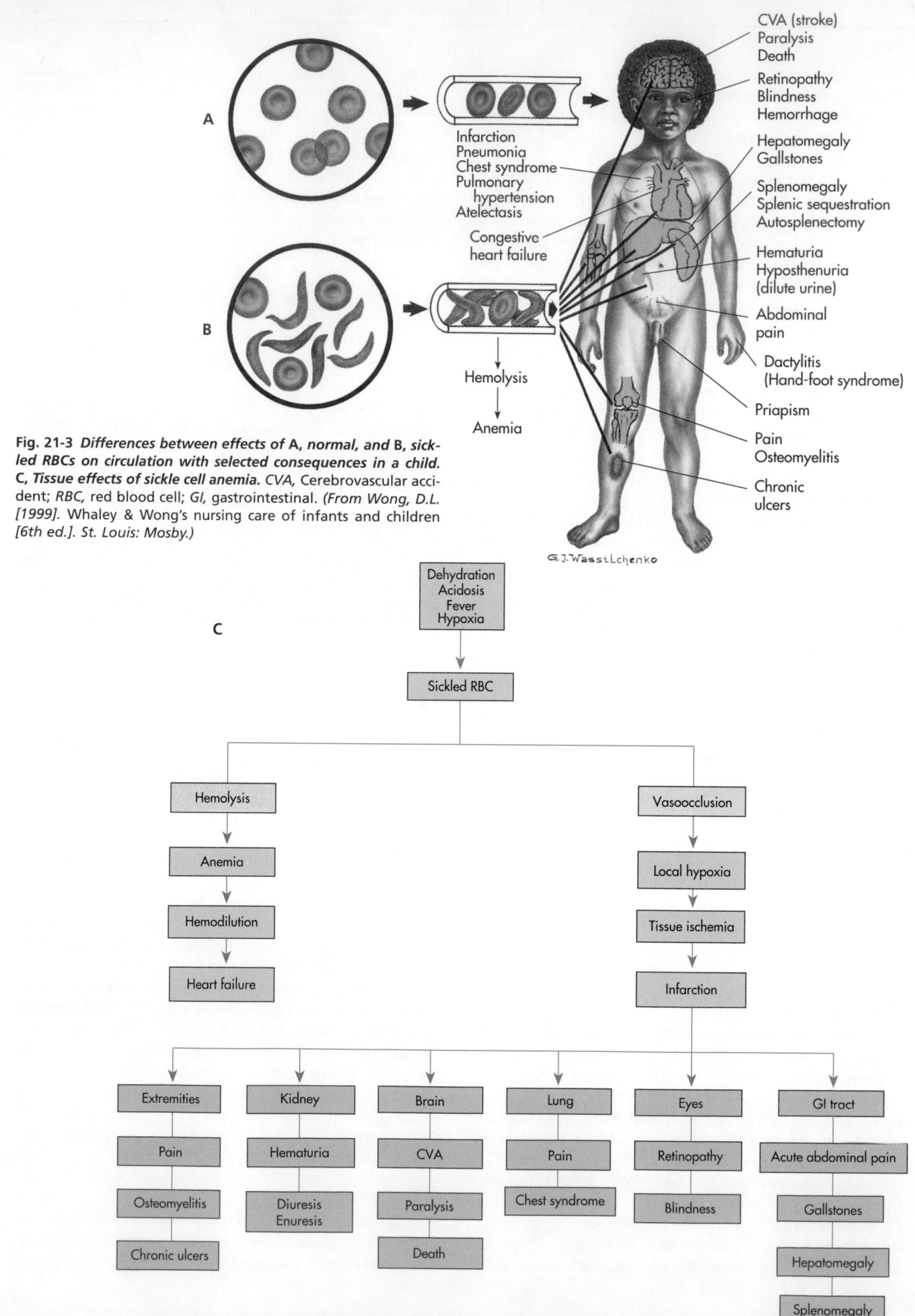

Fig. 21-3 *Differences between effects of A, normal, and B, sickled RBCs on circulation with selected consequences in a child. C, Tissue effects of sickle cell anemia. CVA, Cerebrovascular accident; RBC, red blood cell; GI, gastrointestinal. (From Wong, D.L. [1999]. Whaley & Wong's nursing care of infants and children [6th ed.]. St. Louis: Mosby.)*

beta-thalassemia minor, and severely in the homozygous form, *beta-thalassemia major* (also called *Cooley anemia*). This results in erythrocytes having a reduced amount of hemoglobin and accumulations of free alpha chains. The free alpha chains are unstable and easily precipitate in the cell. Most erythroblasts that contain precipitates are destroyed by mononuclear phagocytes in the marrow, resulting in ineffective erythropoiesis and anemia. Some of the precipitate-carrying cells do mature and enter the bloodstream, but they are destroyed prematurely in the spleen, resulting in mild hemolytic anemia.

There are four forms of alpha-thalassemia: (1) *alpha-trait* (the carrier state), in which a single alpha chain–forming gene is defective, (2) *alpha-thalassemia minor,* in which two genes are defective, (3) *hemoglobin H disease,* in which three genes are defective, and (4) *alpha-thalassemia major,* a fatal condition in which all four alpha-forming genes are defective. Death is inevitable because alpha chains are absent and oxygen cannot be released to the tissues.

Clinical Manifestations

Beta-thalassemia occurs more commonly than does alpha-thalassemia. Occasionally, synthesis of gamma or delta polypeptide chains is defective, resulting in gamma- or delta-thalassemia. (Hemoglobin chains are described in Chapter 19.)

Beta-thalassemia minor causes mild to moderate microcytic-hypochromic anemia, mild splenomegaly, bronze coloring of the skin, and hyperplasia of the bone marrow. The degree of reticulocytosis depends on the severity of the anemia and results in skeletal changes (Fig. 21-4). Hemolysis of immature (and therefore fragile) erythrocytes may cause a slight elevation in serum iron and indirect bilirubin levels. Persons with beta-thalassemia minor are usually asymptomatic.

Persons with beta-thalassemia major may become quite ill. Anemia is severe and results in a significant cardiovascular burden with high-output congestive heart failure. In the past, death resulted from cardiac failure. Today, blood transfusions can increase life span by 1 to 2 decades and death usually is caused by hemochromatosis (from transfusions). Liver enlargement occurs as a result of progressive hemosiderosis, whereas enlargement of the spleen is caused by extramedullary hemopoiesis and increased destruction of red blood cells (Fig. 21-5). Growth and maturation are retarded, and a characteristic chipmunk deformity develops on the face, caused by expansion of bones to accommodate hyperplastic marrow.

Persons who inherit the mildest form of alpha-thalassemia (the alpha trait) usually are symptom free or have mild microcytosis. Alpha-thalassemia minor has clinical manifestations that are virtually identical to those of beta-thalassemia minor: mild microcytic-hypochromic reticulocytosis, bone marrow hyperplasia, increased serum iron concentrations, and moderate splenomegaly.

Signs and symptoms of alpha-thalassemia major are similar to those of beta-thalassemia major, but milder. Mod-

Fig. 21-4 *A 20-year-old Pakistani with beta thalassemia demonstrating mild frontal bossing of the right forehead, mild maxillary prominence, and short stature (145 cm). (From Wong, D.L. [1999]. Whaley & Wong's nursing care of infants and children [6th ed.]. St. Louis: Mosby.)*

erate microcytic-hypochromic anemia, enlargement of the liver and spleen, and bone marrow hyperplasia are evident.

Alpha-thalassemia major causes hydrops fetalis and fulminant intrauterine congestive heart failure. In addition to edema and massive ascites, the fetus has a grossly enlarged heart and liver. Diagnosis usually is made postmortem. Prenatal screening for this disorder can be performed by use of chorionic villus sampling. These cells can be analyzed, and a DNA genetic map can be constructed and evaluated for the abnormalities characteristic of hydrops fetalis.

Both alpha- and beta-thalassemia major are life threatening. Children with thalassemia major generally are weak, fail to thrive, show poor development, and experience cardiovascular compromise with high-output failure secondary to anemia. Untreated, they will die by 5 to 6 years of age.

Evaluation and Treatment

Evaluation of thalassemia is based on familial disease history, clinical manifestations, and blood tests. Peripheral

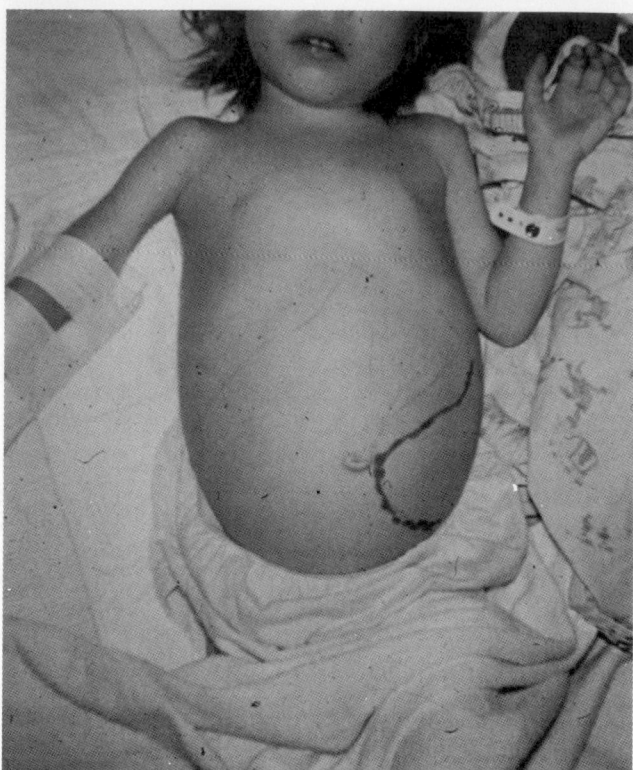

Fig. 21-5 *A child with beta thalassemia major who has severe splenomegaly.* (From Jorde, L.B. et al. [1999]. Medical genetics [2nd ed.]. St. Louis: Mosby.)

blood smears that show microcytosis and hemoglobin electrophoresis that demonstrates diminished amounts of alpha or beta chains are used to make the diagnosis. Analysis of fetal DNA from withdrawn amniotic fluid is used as a screening test to detect hydrops fetalis (alpha-thalassemia major). Newborn screening for thalassemia should be done according to state law.

Persons who are silent carriers or have thalassemia minor generally have few if any symptoms and require no specific treatment. Therapies to support and prolong life are necessary, however, for thalassemia major. There is no cure for either condition. For both symptom-free carriers and those with the disease, prenatal diagnosis and genetic counseling may be the most important therapeutic measures that can be offered.

✓ QUICK CHECK

Why do clinical manifestations of sickle cell disease not appear until the infant is at least 6 months old?

Why is Rh incompatibility rare today?

Why do children with thalassemia major develop cardiovascular complications?

DISORDERS OF COAGULATION AND PLATELETS
Inherited Hemorrhagic Disease
Hemophilias

Awareness of a serious bleeding disorder in males was documented nearly 2000 years ago in the Babylonian Talmud, which exempted from the rite of circumcision those boys having male relatives prone to excessive bleeding. In 1803 the first description of this disorder appeared in the medical literature, where it was noted to be X-linked in nature and associated with joint bleeding and crippling.

Table 21-3 lists the coagulation factors that are associated with clinical bleeding. Until 1952 the term *hemophilia* was reserved for deficiency of factor VIII (antihemophilic factor). Since that time two additional coagulation proteins, factor IX (plasma thromboplastin component [PTC]) and factor XI (plasma thromboplastin antecedent [PTA]), have been identified and their deficiency has been associated with similar clinical manifestations. Congenital deficiencies of these three plasma clotting factors—VIII, IX, and XI—account for 90% to 95% of the hemorrhagic bleeding disorders collectively called hemophilia. Table 21-3 lists coagulation disorders in children, and the major types of hemophilia are summarized in Table 21-4.

▰ *Pathophysiology*

Two types of defects dominate the hereditary defects of hemophilia to date: gene deletions and point mutations (base pair substitutions). Both types of genetic defects are associated with severe hemophilia A, in which no factor VIII circulates in the blood. To date, about 50 deletion mutations in the gene for factor VIII have been identified at the molecular level and about 34 independent deletion mutations in the factor IX gene have been found to be the cause of hemophilia B.[5,6] The molecular defect that leads to hemophilia is identical among members of a given family; however, the deletional mutation has been unique in each family studied.[5]

Point mutations, in which a single base in the DNA is mutated to another base, represent a second type of mutation that causes hemophilia. When a point mutation gives rise to a de novo stop codon (nonsense mutation), translation of the protein ceases and a shortened version of the protein is synthesized. Usually the protein is destroyed intracellularly and never reaches the plasma. This type of defect is associated with severe hemophilia, that is, with coagulant activity levels below 1%.[5] Point mutations in which one amino acid is substituted for another can cause phenotypes of varying severity. The mutation of an important amino acid can destroy protein function, activation, or folding; inhibit intracellular processing; or cause protein clearance.[5] Unlike deletional mutations, point mutations at the same site have been recorded in different families with hemophilia.

Not all coagulation disorders are discussed in this chapter because some are extremely rare (congenital dysfibrinogenemias), whereas others have no clinical significance (e.g.,

TABLE 21-3	Coagulation Disorders in Children			
Factor (Deficiency)	Genetics	Frequency in Population (per 10⁶)	Disorder	
I (fibrinogen)	AR	0.1	Afibrinogenemia, hypofibrinogenemia	
II (prothrombin)	AR	0.1	Hypoprothrombinemia	
III (thromboplastin)				
IV (Ca⁺⁺)				
V	AR	0.1	Parahemophilia, factor V deficiency	
VII	AR	0.1	Factor VII deficiency	
VIII (AHF)	X-R	30-40	Hemophilia A, classic hemophilia; von Willebrand disease	
IX (PTC)	X-R	3-4	Hemophilia B, Christmas disease	
X	AR	0.1	Factor X deficiency	
XI (PTA)	AR	1	Hemophilia C, PTA deficiency	
XII	AR	0.1	Hageman trait	
XIII	AR	0.1	Factor XIII deficiency	

Modified from Kelley, V.S. (1983). Practice of pediatrics (vol. 5). New York: Harper & Row.
AR, *Autosomal recessive;* X-R, *X-linked recessive;* AHF, *antihemophilic factor,* PTC, *plasma thromboplastin component;* PTA, *plasma thromboplastin antecedent.*

TABLE 21-4	The Hemophilias
Type	Description
Hemophilia A (classic hemophilia)	Caused by factor VIII deficiency; most common of hemophilias; inherited as X-linked recessive disorder; factor VIII gene has been mapped to the distal arm of X chromosome and clones; affects males and is transmitted by females; 1:10,000 male births; occurs with varying degrees of severity
Hemophilia B (Christmas disease)	Caused by factor IX deficiency; transmitted as X-linked recessive trait; clinically indistinguishable from factor VIII deficiency, however, less severe than hemophilia A (the IX gene has also been cloned); occurs with varying degrees of severity
Hemophilia C	Caused by factor IX deficiency; inherited as an autosomal recessive disease; occurs equally in males and females; bleeding is usually less severe than with A or B
von Willebrand disease	Also caused by factor VIII deficiency; results from an inherited autosomal dominant trait encoded by a gene on chromosome 12; has variable clinical manifestations and hematologic findings; infusion of plasma causes factor VIII activity to increase

Hageman factor deficiency, a condition in which profound laboratory deficiency of factor XII has absolutely no clinical effects on the child).

Clinical Manifestations

Although abnormal bleeding may occur in the newborn period, particularly after circumcision, spontaneous bleeding as a result of hemophilia is infrequent during the first year of life. There is no transfer of maternal clotting factor to the fetus, yet many boys with hemophilia are circumcised without excessive bleeding. Normal hemostasis is achieved in these infants because clotting is activated through the extrinsic coagulation cascade.

During the first year, spontaneous bleeding often is minimal but hematoma formation may result from injections and from firm holding (e.g., under the arms). Easy bruising or hemarthrosis (bleeding into joints) or both occur with ambulation. By age 3 to 4 years, 90% of children with hemophilia have had episodes of persistent bleeding from relatively minor traumatic lacerations (e.g., to the lip or tongue). This usually is the first clinical manifestation of hemophilia. Hemorrhage into the elbows, knees, and ankles causes pain, limits joint movement, and predisposes the child to degenerative joint changes. Spontaneous hematuria and epistaxis are troublesome but minor complications.

Recurrent bleeding, both spontaneous and after minor trauma, is a lifelong problem. Many affected persons experience phases or cycles of spontaneous bleeding episodes. Mechanisms that cause this phenomenon are unknown. Intracranial hemorrhage and bleeding into the tissues of the neck or abdomen constitute life-threatening emergencies.

Evaluation and Treatment

Although laboratory tests are of primary value in the evaluation of hemorrhagic disorders, the history and physical assessment also are very important. The three phases of coag-

Laboratory Tests of the Three Phases of Coagulation   BOX 21-1

Test	Phase	Significance
Thrombin time	III	Measures fibrinogen; usually elevated first because without fibrinogen, blood cannot clot
Prothrombin	II	A decrease indicates a deficiency of factors II, V, VII, or X; also used to monitor warfarin sodium (Coumadin) therapy
Activated partial thromboplastin time (PTT or APTT)	I	Assesses for factors XII, XI, IX, and VIII; also used to monitor heparin therapy

ulation can be individually assessed by simple, reliable tests (Box 21-1).

The recent cloning of the factor VIII gene and the purification of the recombinant factor VIII have resulted in factor VIII products that minimize the risk of transmission of viral infection (e.g., human immunodeficiency virus [HIV], hepatitis) and are potentially less expensive than plasma-derived factor VIII. Unfortunately, those individuals with hemophilia who were treated before current purification techniques may have been exposed to HIV. Currently, it is estimated that half of the 20,000 hemophiliacs in the United States have contracted HIV from blood products.

The prognosis for children with hemophilia is promising. Programs of comprehensive care and home treatment have improved the quality of life for those with hemophilia and enhanced their general physical capabilities.

Antibody-Mediated Hemorrhagic Disease

The antibody-mediated hemorrhagic diseases are a group of disorders caused by the immune response. Antibody-mediated destruction of platelets or antibody-mediated inflammatory reactions to allergens damage blood vessels and cause seepage into tissues. The thrombocytopenic purpuras may be intrinsic or idiopathic, or they may be transient phenomena transmitted from mother to fetus. The inflammatory, or "allergic," purpuras, although rare, occur in response to allergens in the blood. All these disorders first appear during infancy or childhood.

Idiopathic thrombocytopenic purpura

Acute *idiopathic thrombocytopenic purpura (ITP; autoimmune [primary] thrombocytopenic purpura)* is the most common disorder of platelet consumption. Antiplatelet antibodies bind to the plasma membranes of platelets, causing platelet sequestration and destruction by mononuclear phagocytes in the spleen and other lymphoid tissues at a rate that exceeds the ability of the bone marrow to produce them.

Pathophysiology

In approximately 70% of cases of ITP, there is an antecedent viral disease (e.g., cytomegalovirus [CMV], Epstein-Barr virus [EBV], parvovirus, or respiratory infection) that precedes the eruption of petechiae or purpura by 1 to 3 weeks. High levels of IgG have been found bound to platelets and may represent immune complexes on the platelet surface.[7]

Clinical Manifestations

Bruising and a generalized petechial rash often occur with acute onset. Asymmetric bruising is typical and is found most frequently on the legs and trunk. Hemorrhagic bullae of the gums, lips, and other mucous membranes may be prominent, and epistaxis (nose bleeding) may be severe and difficult to control. Otherwise, the child appears well. The acute phase lasts 1 to 2 weeks, but thrombocytopenia often persists. Although the incidence is less than 1%, intracranial hemorrhage is the most serious complication of ITP. In some cases the onset is more gradual, and clinical manifestations consist of moderate bruising and a few petechiae.

Evaluation and Treatment

Laboratory examination reveals a low platelet count, and the few platelets observed on a smear are large, reflecting increased bone marrow production. The Ivy bleeding time is prolonged. Bone marrow aspiration reveals normal or increased megakaryocytes and normal erythrocytes and granulocytes.

Even without treatment, the prognosis for children with ITP is excellent. Seventy-five percent recover completely within 3 months. After the initial acute phase, spontaneous clinical manifestations subside. By 9 to 12 months after onset, 80% to 90% of affected children have regained normal platelet counts.[8]

✓ QUICK CHECK

List the major disorders of coagulation and platelets found in children.

How do gene deletions differ from point mutations?

Why are persons with hemophilia at risk for developing degenerative joint changes?

Describe idiopathic thrombocytopenic purpura (ITP).

NEOPLASTIC DISORDERS

Leukemia and Lymphoma

Leukemia, cancer of the blood-forming tissues, is the most common malignancy of childhood, representing approximately 33% of all childhood cancers. Childhood lymphoma, or cancer of the lymphoid system (primarily lymph nodes), is the third most common malignant neoplasm of children in the United States, representing approximately 11% of all childhood cancers. (See Chapter 20 for a discussion of leukemia in adults.) Box 21-2 defines the major classifications of leukemia.

Leukemia

From 80% to 85% of leukemias in children are acute lymphoblastic leukemia (ALL) or acute undifferentiated leukemia (AUL). The remaining 15% to 20% are acute nonlymphocytic leukemias (ANLLs) (which include myeloblastic, promyelocytic, monocytic, and myelomonoblastic) and the very rare red blood cell leukemia, erythroleukemia. Because the vast majority of ANLL cases involve the myeloblastic cell, many experts refer to the disease as AML (acute myelogenous leukemia). Leukemia accounts for 25% of cases of cancer in black children and 34% of cases of cancer in white children. Approximately 2300 new cases are diagnosed each year in the United States. Of those 2300 children, 1500 are diagnosed with ALL.[9] Both a juvenile form and an adult form of chronic myelocytic leukemia (CML) develop in children, but this condition (CML) is uncommon and accounts for only 2% of all leukemias in childhood. Chronic lymphocytic leukemia (CLL) is virtually nonexistent in children.

The peak incidence for childhood ALL is approximately 4 years of age. Acute leukemia is nearly twice as common in white children as in nonwhite children (4.2:100,000 versus 2.4:100,000, respectively). Childhood ALL also is more common in boys than in girls (1.3:1.0).

Pathogenesis

Investigations into the causes of childhood leukemia have focused on genetic susceptibility, environmental factors, and viral infections. Observations of a familial tendency and links with a number of inherited disorders have implicated genetic factors in the origin of leukemia.

Inherited diseases that predispose a child to leukemia (both ALL and ANLL) include Down syndrome (1:74 chance before the age of 10 years), Fanconi anemia (1:12 chance before the age of 21 years), Bloom syndrome (1:8 chance before the age of 26 years), and ataxia-telangiectasia (1:8 chance before the age of 25 years).[9] Leukemia also has been associated with known genetic diseases, such as congenital agammaglobulinemia. ANLL in children sometimes is associated with loss or deletion of chromosome 7.[10] ANLL can develop from preexisting myeloproliferative disorders that also are preleukemia syndromes. When these disorders progress to ANLL, an insidious pattern of leukemic dysfunction usually is revealed.

General Classifications of Leukemia   BOX 21-2

Lympho	Leukemia involving the lymphoid tissue and the lymphatic system (e.g., lymphatic vessels, lymph nodes, spleen, thymus)
Myelo	Those of bone marrow (myeloid) origin
Blastic and acute	Those involving immature cells
Cytic and chronic	Those involving mature cells

Modified from Wong, D.L. (1997). Whaley & Wong's essentials of pediatric nursing (5 ed.). St. Louis: Mosby.

Most research on environmental factors as etiologic agents has centered on exposure to ionizing radiation. Atomic bomb survivors have been shown to have an increased risk for leukemia. The degree of risk depends on the distance from the epicenter. The peak incidence period is 4 to 8 years after exposure to the radiation. Whereas ANLL most often develops in adults who are exposed to radiation, ALL is more likely to develop in children. The therapeutic use of x-rays for thymic enlargement in children also has been linked to subsequent development of ALL in children.[11] In a more recent study, no increased risk of childhood leukemia was found in children who had received small doses of radiation from diagnostic x-rays.[12] Radiation exposure during the prenatal period is, however, associated with a marked risk of development of pediatric leukemia.[13] Although most studies of radiation exposure have focused on artificial radiation sources, there is considerable interest in natural background radiation, particularly the possible role of radon exposure in subsequent childhood and adult cancers. Studies continue in this area.[14] Electromagnetic field (EMF) exposure from power poles and small appliances has not been demonstrated to be a causative factor in acute leukemias.[15] No evidence suggests a chemical or drug association in childhood leukemia.

Leukemic clusters that represent a greater number of leukemia cases occurring in a particular geographic location have raised speculation about environmental factors and infectious patterns of transmission. Careful follow-up, however, has failed to document the abnormal clustering. Explanations for this phenomenon therefore are statistical artifact and coincidence. However, one reported leukemic cluster in the town of Woburn, Massachusetts, has been linked to possible water supply contamination by chemicals from factory waste.[16]

Viruses clearly have been known to cause leukemia in a number of animals, including cats, fowl, and mice. Scientists have linked retroviruses with several adult cancers, but retroviruses have not been linked with childhood leukemia.

Gibson and colleagues[17] reported findings that indicate the interaction of multiple factors in the cause of childhood leukemia. Children exposed to four specific factors had a

4.64 times greater risk for development of leukemia than did children who had not experienced similar exposures. The four factors are (1) radiation of the mother before conception, (2) prenatal radiation of the child, (3) maternal history of miscarriages, and (4) early viral illness in the child. These, along with other evidence, strongly suggest that childhood leukemia is likely to be the result of a multiple interaction between hereditary or genetic predisposition and environmental influences.[18] This interaction is called *ecogenetics* and focuses on the genetic variations that occur in relation to environmental factors.

Clinical Manifestations

The onset may be abrupt or insidious, but the most common symptoms reflect the consequence of bone marrow failure: decreased red blood cells and platelets and changes in white blood cells. Pallor, fatigue, petechiae, purpura, bleeding, and fever generally are present. Approximately 45% of children have a hemoglobin level below 7 g/dl. If acute blood loss occurs, characteristic symptoms of tachycardia, air hunger, restlessness, and thirst may be present. Epistaxis frequently occurs in children with severe thrombocytopenia.

Fever is usually present as a result of (1) infection associated with the decrease in functional neutrophils and (2) hypermetabolism associated with the ongoing rapid growth and destruction of leukemic cells. White blood cell counts greater than 200,000/mm³ can cause leukostasis, an intravascular clumping of cells that results in infarction and hemorrhage, usually in the brain and lung.

Renal failure as a result of hyperuremia (high uric acid levels) can be associated with ALL, particularly at diagnosis or during active treatment. Extramedullary invasion with leukemic cells can occur in nearly all body tissue. The central nervous system (CNS) is a common site of infiltration of extramedullary leukemias, although fewer than 10% of children with ALL have CNS involvement at diagnosis. CNS infiltration manifests later in the course of the disease. The most common symptoms of CNS involvement relate to increased intracranial pressure, causing early morning headaches, nausea, vomiting, irritability, and lethargy.

Gonadal involvement, with testicular and ovarian infiltration, has been demonstrated in postmortem examination in 57% and 35% of children, respectively. Leukemic infiltration into bones and joints is common. Reports of bone or joint pain actually lead to the diagnosis of leukemia in some children. In most children, bone pain is characterized as migratory, vague, and without areas of swelling or inflammation. If joint pain is the primary symptom and some swelling is associated with the pain, however, misdiagnoses of rheumatoid arthritis and rheumatic fever have occurred.

Other organs reported to be sites of leukemic invasion include the kidneys, heart, lungs, thymus, eyes, skin, and gastrointestinal tract. Skin involvement is more common in ANLL than in ALL. Children with leukemia usually have had symptoms for only 1 week before diagnosis.

Fig. 21-6 *Monoblasts from acute monoblastic leukemia.* Monoblasts in a marrow smear from a patient with acute monoblastic leukemia. The monoblasts are larger than myeloblasts and usually have abundant cytoplasm, frequently with delicate scattered azurophilic granules. *(From Damjanov, I. & Linder, J. [Eds.]. [1996]. Anderson's pathology [10th ed.]. St. Louis: Mosby.)*

Evaluation and Treatment

Although blood test results can raise the clinician's suspicion of leukemia, a bone marrow aspiration is required to establish the diagnosis. The **blast cell** is the hallmark of acute leukemia (Fig. 21-6). This relatively undifferentiated cell is characterized by diffusely distributed nuclear chromatin, with one or more nucleoli and basophilic cytoplasm. Healthy children have fewer than 5% blast cells in the bone marrow and none in the peripheral blood. In ALL, the bone marrow often is replaced by 80% to 100% blast cells, with a reduction in normal developing red blood cells and granulocytes. Occasionally, the marrow appears hypocellular, making the diagnosis difficult to differentiate from aplastic anemia. When this occurs, bone marrow biopsy or biopsy of extramedullary sites is necessary to confirm the diagnosis.

Combination chemotherapy, with or without radiation therapy to localized sites, such as the CNS, is the treatment of choice for acute leukemia. In ALL, identification of various risk groups has led to the development of different intensities of drug protocols. Thus treatment is tailored specifically for a particular risk group. The 5-year relative survival rate for ALL is about 80%.[19]

Lymphomas

Non-Hodgkin lymphoma (NHL) and Hodgkin disease comprise approximately 11% of all childhood cancer. Approximately 750 cases of childhood lymphoma are diagnosed in the United States annually.[20] Either group of diseases is rare before the age of 5 years, and the relative incidence increases throughout childhood. Boys are more likely to be diagnosed with a malignant lymphoma than are girls. At particular risk are children with inherited or acquired immunodeficiency syndromes, who have increased rates of lymphoreticular cancers that range between 100 and 10,000 times the rate of normal children. The cancers are most commonly NHLs.[21] Children who are artificially immunosuppressed after organ transplantation, especially if cyclosporine is the immunosuppressive agent, also are at increased risk for lymphomas.

Non-Hodgkin lymphoma

Generally, most classification systems divide NHL into two categories—nodular or diffuse—on the basis of cellular pattern. Whereas one half of all adults with NHL have a nodular form of the disease, children rarely demonstrate this pattern. Nodular disease represents a less aggressive form of lymphoma. Almost without exception, childhood NHL becomes evident as a diffuse disease and can be further subdivided into three groups: (1) large cell (histiocytic), (2) lymphoblastic, and (3) small noncleaved cell (Burkitt or non-Burkitt lymphoma). Large cell NHL often involves chromosomal translocations. Disease sites commonly involve extranodal sites, such as brain, lung, bone, and skin. Lymphoblastic NHL also shows chromosomal translocations, particularly chromosomes 7 and 14. Disease sites commonly include the mediastinum and peripheral lymph nodes. Small noncleaved cell NHL involves chromosome translocations of 8 and 14. Children with small noncleaved cell NHL commonly have intraabdominal disease at diagnosis.

As in ALL, immunophenotyping is an important part of the classification of childhood NHL. Almost 45% of cases of the disease in children originate from T cells; an equal number originate from B cells. The remaining group, which represents less than 10% of childhood NHLs, is classified as non-T, non-B.

⊞ *Pathogenesis*

Viral etiology is suggested, with the strongest correlation between the Epstein-Barr virus and African Burkitt lymphoma. The relationship outside Africa is weak, however, even though the tumor is histopathologically and clinically indistinguishable. Chronic immunostimulation also has been suggested as a factor in the development of lymphomas because these diseases are seen more frequently when chronic persistent antigenic stimulation occurs from infection, such as malaria or intestinal parasites. Genetic susceptibility also may play a role in the process of malignant transformation. There is increased evidence of NHL in children with congenital immunodeficiency syndromes, such as Wiskott-Aldrich syndrome, ataxia-telangiectasia, and Bloom syndrome. Children with acquired immunodeficiency syndrome (AIDS) also are at greater risk for NHL.[21]

⊞ *Clinical Manifestations*

NHL has been found to arise from any lymphoid tissue. Signs and symptoms therefore are specific for the site involved. Because childhood NHL is a rapidly progressive disease, symptoms generally are present only a few weeks before diagnosis is made. Rapidly enlarging lymphoid tissue and

painless lymphadenopathy are common with abdominal sites of involvement, usually representing a gastrointestinal origin for the disease. Symptoms often include abdominal pain and vomiting, but a palpable mass is not always present. Most children with abdominal symptoms have diffuse, small noncleaved cell NHL (Burkitt or non-Burkitt) of B cell origin. If the tumor recurs, it appears again in the abdomen before distant spread.

The other common site of childhood NHL is the chest region. An anterior mediastinal mass, with or without pleural effusion, often is present. If the mass is large enough, respiratory compromise, tracheal compression, and superior vena cava syndrome may arise, which constitute a medical emergency. Children with anterior mediastinal involvement often are male adolescents and usually have diffuse lymphoblastic lymphoma of T cell origin. This often evolves into extensive bone marrow involvement and is considered to be an overt leukemic phase, therefore referred to as *leukemic transformation*. CNS involvement and testicular infiltration often occur.

CNS involvement is common. A relatively small number (10% to 20%) of children with NHL have lymphoid tissue involvement of the head and neck (Waldeyer ring, nasopharynx, sinuses). Signs and symptoms include tonsillitis, sinusitis, and a painless nasopharynx mass. In African Burkitt lymphoma, involvement of facial bones, particularly the jaw, is common.

⊞ *Evaluation and Treatment*

Diagnosis is made by biopsy of disease sites, usually the involved lymph nodes, tonsils, bone marrow, spleen, liver, bowel, or skin. Most children with NHL are cured of the disease. Optimal treatment is still being developed, but combination chemotherapy, with or without radiation therapy for prevention of CNS involvement, is being used successfully.[22]

Children with advanced small noncleaved cell lymphoma of the abdomen have the poorest prognosis. Although remission occurs in more than 90% of these children, most experience subsequent relapses. Even in the presence of advanced lymphoblastic lymphoma, however, 60% to 80% of children can be cured. Overall, children with localized disease have a 90% survival rate and those with advanced disease have a 60% to 70% survival rate.[22]

Hodgkin disease

Although the etiologic agent for **Hodgkin disease,** a lymphoma, has not been identified in children, an infectious mode of transmission, particularly focused on viruses, has been implicated. Many persons with Hodgkin disease have high Epstein-Barr virus titers. At this time, however, the evidence is not sufficient to link an Epstein-Barr virus infection to Hodgkin disease.

Genetic susceptibility has been suggested because observations show that siblings have a sevenfold increase in risk, particularly siblings of the same sex. In general, Hodgkin

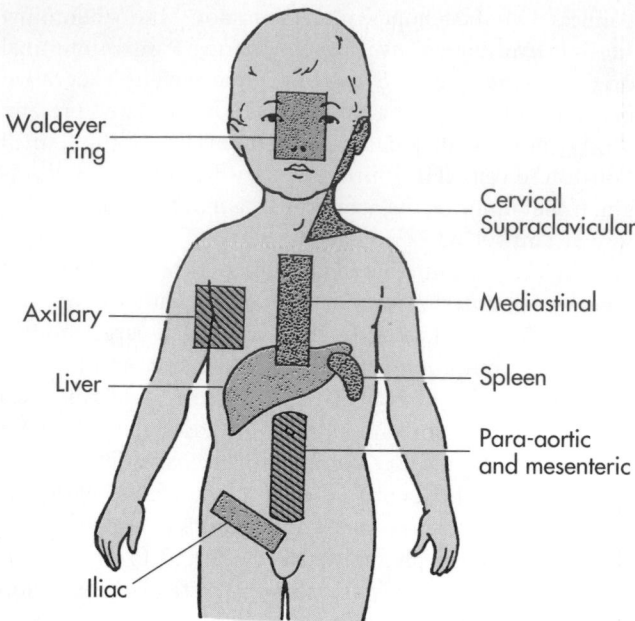

Waldeyer ring

Cervical Supraclavicular

Axillary

Mediastinal

Liver

Spleen

Para-aortic and mesenteric

Iliac

Fig. 21-7 *Main areas of lymphadenopathy and organ involvement in Hodgkin disease. (From Wong, D.L. [1999.] Whaley & Wong's nursing care of infants and children [6th ed.]. St. Louis: Mosby.)*

disease is more common in males—in childhood, 60% of all cases occur in males.

Hodgkin disease is rare in childhood. It occurs only infrequently in children younger than 2 years, and few cases are observed before the age of 5 years. A gradual rise in incidence occurs through the age of 11 years, with a marked increase through adolescence that continues into the thirties. The annual incidence of Hodgkin disease in the United States is 4:1,000,000 in children younger than 15 years.

Painless adenopathy in the lower cervical chain, with or without fever, is the most common symptom in children. Other lymph nodes and organs may also be involved (Fig. 21-7). Mediastinal involvement can cause pressure on the trachea or bronchi, leading to airway obstruction. Extranodal primary sites in Hodgkin disease are rare. Initial symptoms consist of anorexia, malaise, and lassitude. Intermittent fever is present in 30% of children, and weight loss also may accompany these symptoms. Hodgkin disease has a well-defined staging system that considers extent and location of disease and the presence of fever, weight loss, or night sweats at diagnosis. Treatment for Hodgkin disease includes chemotherapy and radiation therapy. For many years the standard chemotherapy was a regimen of *m*echlorethamine, Oncovin (vincristine), *p*rocarbazine, and *p*rednisone (MOPP). However, these drugs can cause permanent sterility. A new drug combination consisting of *A*driamycin (doxorubicin), *b*leomycin, *v*inblastine, and *d*acarbazine (ABVD) has been shown to be superior to MOPP; it is less toxic and requires 6 to 8 months of treatment rather than the traditional 12 months of MOPP treatment. The survival rate for children with Hodgkin disease is very high. Most children are seen initially with limited disease and have a 90% survival rate. Even children who are first seen with advanced disease have a 70% to 80% survival rate.[23]

✓ QUICK CHECK

List the childhood leukemias in order of rate of incidence.

Why do children with leukemia experience bone or joint pain?

Why do some children with non-Hodgkin lymphoma (NHL) develop respiratory compromise?

▣ DID YOU UNDERSTAND?

Disorders of Erythrocytes

1. Iron deficiency anemia is the most common blood disorder of infancy and childhood; the highest incidence occurs between 6 months and 2 years of age.

2. Hemolytic disease of the newborn (HDN) results from incompatibility between the maternal and the fetal blood, which may involve differences in Rh factors or blood type (ABO). Maternal antibodies enter the fetal circulation and cause hemolysis of fetal erythrocytes. Because the immature liver is unable to conjugate and excrete the excess bilirubin that results from the hemolysis, icterus neonatorum or kernicterus or both can develop. Kernicterus, which also may result from other causes, causes increased breakdown of red blood cells or decreased liver output of enzymes.

3. Infections of the newborn, often acquired by the mother and transmitted to the infant, may result in hemolytic anemia.

4. Sickle cell disease is a genetically determined defect of hemoglobin synthesis inherited by an autosomal recessive transmission and causing a change in the shape of a red blood cell that results in decreased oxygen or hydration. It is most common among Africans and those of Mediterranean descent.

5. The thalassemias are a heterogeneous group of hereditary hypochromic anemias of varying severity. Basic genetic defects include abnormalities of messenger-RNA processing or deletion of genetic materials, resulting in a decrease in the chains for hemoglobin.

☑ DID YOU UNDERSTAND? —cont'd

Disorders of Coagulation and Platelets

1. Hemophilia is a condition characterized by impairment of the coagulation of blood and subsequent tendency to bleed. The classic disease is hereditary and limited to males, being transmitted through the female to the second generation. Many similar conditions attributable to the absence of various clotting factors are now recognized.
2. The acquired antibody-mediated hemorrhagic diseases include idiopathic thrombocytopenic purpura (ITP), transient neonatal thrombocytopenia, and autoimmune vascular purpura.
3. ITP, the most common of the childhood thrombocytopenic purpuras, is a disorder of platelet consumption in which antiplatelet antibodies bind to the plasma membranes of platelets. This results in platelet sequestration and destruction by mononuclear phagocytes at a rate that exceeds the ability of the bone marrow to produce them.

Neoplastic Disorders

1. The childhood leukemias include, in order of their rate of incidence, acute lymphoblastic, acute non-lymphoblastic, and the very rare chronic myelocytic leukemia.
2. Although the cause of childhood leukemia is not known, it is probably the result of multiple interactions between hereditary or genetic predisposition and environmental influences.
3. Acute lymphoblastic leukemia is a potentially curable disease, with about 80% of cases cured.
4. The lymphomas of childhood are non-Hodgkin lymphoma and Hodgkin disease.
5. The origin of non-Hodgkin lymphoma is unknown. Factors that have been implicated include defective host immunity, a viral agent, chronic immunostimulation, and genetic predisposition.
6. Non-Hodgkin lymphoma has a favorable prognosis, with a 60% to 80% rate of cure.
7. Hodgkin disease is thought to be caused by a yet unidentified etiologic agent.
8. Hodgkin disease is a readily curable disease with survival statistics similar to those of adults.

KEY TERMS

REFERENCES

1. Kline, N.E. (1996). A practical approach to the child with anemia. *Journal of Pediatric Healthcare, 10,* 99-105.
2. Bunn, H.F. (1997). Pathogenesis and treatment of sickle cell disease. *New England Journal of Medicine, 337*(11), 762-769.
3. Harmening, D.M. (1997). *Clinical hematology and fundamentals of hemostasis* (3rd ed.). Philadelphia: Davis.
4. Holuchi, K., Onyike, A.E., & Osterhout, M.L. (1996). Sickling in vitro of reticulocytes from patients with sickle cell disease. *Experimental Hematology, 24,* 68-76.
5. Furie, B. & Furie, B.C. (1992). Molecular and cellular biology of blood coagulation. *New England Journal of Medicine, 326*(12), 800-806.
6. Jorde, L.B. et al. (1999). *Medical genetics* (2nd ed.). St. Louis: Mosby.
7. Olee, T. et al. (1997). Generation and analysis of an IgG anti-platelet autoantibody reveals unusual molecular features. *British Journal of Hematology, 96,* 836-845.
8. Beardsley, D.S. & Nathan, D.G. (1998). Platelet abnormalities in infants and children. In S.H. Orkin (Ed.). *Nathan and Oski's hematology of infancy and childhood* (5th ed.). Philadelphia: Saunders.

REFERENCES

9. Gurney, J. et al. (1995). Incidence of cancer in children in the U.S.: Sex-, race-, and 1-year age-specific rates by histologic type. *Cancer, 75,* 2186-2189.

10. Golub, T.R., Weinstein, J.H., & Grier, H.E. (1997). Acute myelogenous leukemia. In P.A. Pizzo & D.G. Poplack (Eds.). *Principles and practice of pediatric oncology* (3rd ed.). Philadelphia: Lippikncott-Raven.

11. Murray, R., Heckel, P., & Hempelmann, L. (1959). Leukemia in children exposed to ionizing radiation. *New England Journal of Medicine, 261,* 585-589.

12. Baverstam, U. & Holmberg, M. (1989). Are low doses of radiation leukemogenic in children? *Leukemia Research, 13*(7), 515-517.

13. Wakford, R. (1995). The risk of childhood cancer from intrauterine and preconceptional exposure to ionizing radiation. *Environmental Health Perspectives, 10*(3), 1018-1025.

14. Henshaw, D.L., Eatough, J.P., & Richardson, R.B. (1990). Radon as a causative factor in induction of myeloid leukemia and other cancers. *Lancet, 355,* 100-112.

15. Linet, M.S. et al. (1997). Residential exposure to magnetic fields and acute lymphoblastic leukemia in children. *New England Journal of Medicine, 337,* 1-7.

16. Lagakos, S.W., Wessen, B.J., & Zelen, M. (1986). An analysis of contaminated well water and health effects in Woburn, Massachusetts. *Journal of the American Statistical Association, 81,* 583-596.

17. Gibson, R.W. et al. (1968). Leukemia in children exposed to multiple risk factors. *New England Journal of Medicine, 279,* 906-909.

18. Plon, S.E. & Peterson, L.E. (1997). Childhood cancer, heredity, and the environment. In P.A. Pizzo & D.G. Poplack (Eds.). *Principles and practice of pediatric oncology* (3rd ed.). Philadelphia: Lippincott-Raven.

19. American Cancer Society. (1999). *Cancer facts and figures—1999.* New York: Author.

20. Reis, L.A., Miller, R.W., & Smith, M. (1994). Cancer in children (ages 0-14 and ages 0-19) (Pub. #94-2789). In B. Miller, L.A. Reis, & B. Hankey (Eds.). *SEER Cancer Statistics Review 1973-1991.* Bethesda, Md.: U.S. Department of Health and Human Services, National Institute of Health.

21. Mueller, B.U. & Pizzo, P.A. (1997). Pediatric AIDS and childhood cancer. In P.A. Pizzo & D.G. Poplack (Eds.). *Principles and practice of pediatric oncology* (3rd ed.). Philadelphia: Lippincott-Raven.

22. Shad, A. & Magrath, I. (1997). Malignant non-Hodgkin's lymphoma in children. In P.A. Pizzo & D.G. Poplack (Eds.). *Principles and practice of pediatric oncology* (3rd ed.). Philadelphia: Lippincott-Raven.

23. Kornblith, A.B. et al. (1992). Comparison of psychosocial adaptation and sexual function of survivors of advanced Hodgkin disease treated by MOPP, ABVD, or MOPP alternating with ABVD. *Cancer, 70*(10), 2508-2516.

CHAPTER 22

Structure and Function of the Cardiovascular and Lymphatic Systems

Kathryn L. McCance

The function of the circulatory system is quite simple: to deliver oxygen, nutrients, and other substances to all the body's cells and to remove the waste products of cellular metabolism. Delivery and removal are achieved by a wonderfully complex array of tubing (the blood vessels) connected to a pump (the heart). The heart pumps blood continuously through the blood vessels with cooperation from other systems, particularly the nervous and endocrine systems, which are intrinsic regulators of the heart and blood vessels. Nutrients and oxygen are supplied by the digestive and respiratory systems; gaseous wastes of cellular metabolism are blown off by the lungs; and other wastes are removed by the kidneys.

THE CIRCULATORY SYSTEM

The heart pumps blood through two separate circulatory systems: one to the lungs and one to all other parts of the body. Structures on the right side of the heart, or *right heart,* pump blood through the lungs. This system is termed the *pulmonary circulation.* The left side of the heart, or *left heart,* sends blood throughout the *systemic circulation,* which supplies all of the body except the lungs (Fig. 22-1). These two systems are serially connected; thus the output of one becomes the input of the other.

Arteries carry blood flow from the heart to all parts of the body, where they branch into increasingly smaller vessels and ultimately become a fine meshwork of capillaries. Capillaries allow the closest contact and exchange between the blood and the interstitial space, or interstitium—the environment in which the cells live. Veins channel blood flow from capillaries in all parts of the body back to the heart. The plasma passes through the walls of the capillaries into the interstitial space. This fluid is eventually returned to the cardiovascular system by vessels of the lymphatic system.

THE HEART

The adult heart weighs less than 1 pound (2.2 kg) and is about the size of a fist. It lies obliquely (diagonally) in the *mediastinum,* an area above the diaphragm and between the lungs. Heart structures can be described with respect to three general categories of function:

1. *Structural support of heart tissues and circulation of pulmonary and systemic blood through the heart.* This includes the heart wall and fibrous skeleton, which enclose and support the heart and divide it into four chambers; the valves that direct flow through the chambers; and the great vessels that conduct blood to and from the heart.
2. *Maintenance of heart cells.* This comprises vessels of the coronary circulation—the arteries and veins that serve the metabolic needs of all the heart cells—and the lymphatic vessels of the heart.
3. *Stimulation and control of heart action.* Among these structures are the nerves and specialized muscle cells that direct the rhythmic contraction and relaxation of the heart muscles, propelling blood throughout the pulmonary and systemic circulatory system.

Structures That Direct Circulation Through the Heart
The heart wall

The heart wall has three layers—the pericardium, myocardium, and endocardium (Fig. 22-2). The *pericardium* is a double-walled membranous sac that encloses the heart and (1) prevents displacement of the heart during gravitational acceleration or deceleration, (2) is a physical barrier that protects the heart against infection and inflammation from the lungs and pleural space, and (3) contains pain receptors and mechanoreceptors to elicit reflex changes in blood pres-

sure and heart rate. The two layers of the pericardium are the parietal and the visceral pericardia (Fig. 22-2). These are separated by a fluid-containing space called the *pericardial cavity.* The *pericardial fluid* (10 to 30 ml), which is secreted by cells of the mesothelium, lubricates the membranes that line the pericardial cavity, enabling them to slide over one another with a minimum of friction as the heart beats. The amount and character of the pericardial fluid are altered if the pericardium is inflamed (see Chapter 23)

The thickest layer of the heart wall, the *myocardium,* is composed of cardiac muscle and is anchored to the heart's fibrous skeleton. The thickness of the myocardium varies tremendously in the various heart chambers and is related to the amount of resistance the muscle must overcome to pump blood from that chamber. The internal lining of the myocardium, the *endocardium,* comprises connective tissue and squamous cells (see Fig. 22-2). This lining is continuous with the endothelium that lines all the arteries, veins, and capillaries of the body, creating a continuous, closed circulatory system.

Chambers of the heart

The heart has four chambers: the *left atrium,* the *right atrium,* the *right ventricle,* and the *left ventricle.* (Blood flow through these chambers is illustrated in Fig. 22-3.) The atria are smaller than the ventricles and have thinner walls. The ventricles have a thicker myocardial layer and constitute much of the bulk of the heart. The ventricles are formed by a continuum of muscle fibers originating from the fibrous skeleton at the base of the heart.[1]

The two atria have thin walls because they are low-pressure chambers that serve as storage units and conduits for blood rather than pumps that must forcefully eject blood. The ventricles must propel blood all the way through the pulmonary or systemic circulation and so must be strong enough to pump against pressures throughout these systems. The mean pulmonary capillary pressure, or force favoring movement of fluid out of the pulmonary capillaries into the interstitium, is only 15 mm Hg. In comparison, the mean arterial pressure is about 92 mm Hg. Pressure is greatest in the systemic circulation, which is driven by the left ventricle. This explains why the left ventricle's myocardium is several times thicker than that of the right ventricle.

The right ventricle is shaped like a crescent, or triangle, enabling a bellowslike action that efficiently ejects large volumes of blood through a very small valve into the low-pressure pulmonary system. The left ventricle is larger and bullet shaped, helping it to eject blood through a relatively large valve opening into the high-pressure systemic circulation.

The septal membrane separates the right and left sides of the heart and prevents blood from crossing over. The atria are separated by the interatrial septum, and the ventricles by the interventricular septum. Indentations of the endocardium form valves that separate the atria from the ventricles and the ventricles from the aorta and pulmonary arteries.

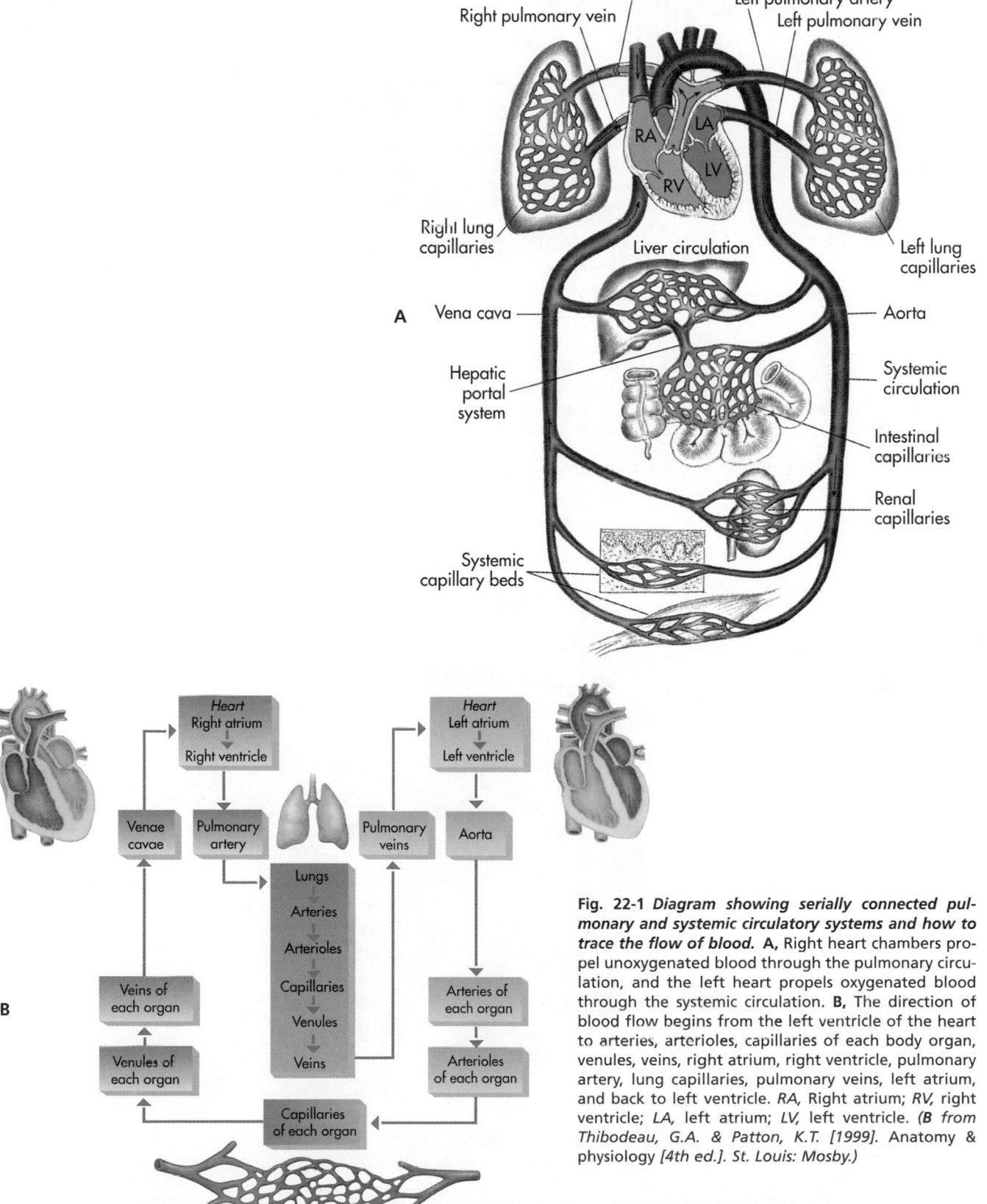

Fig. 22-1 *Diagram showing serially connected pulmonary and systemic circulatory systems and how to trace the flow of blood.* **A,** Right heart chambers propel unoxygenated blood through the pulmonary circulation, and the left heart propels oxygenated blood through the systemic circulation. **B,** The direction of blood flow begins from the left ventricle of the heart to arteries, arterioles, capillaries of each body organ, venules, veins, right atrium, right ventricle, pulmonary artery, lung capillaries, pulmonary veins, left atrium, and back to left ventricle. *RA,* Right atrium; *RV,* right ventricle; *LA,* left atrium; *LV,* left ventricle. *(B from Thibodeau, G.A. & Patton, K.T. [1999]. Anatomy & physiology [4th ed.]. St. Louis: Mosby.)*

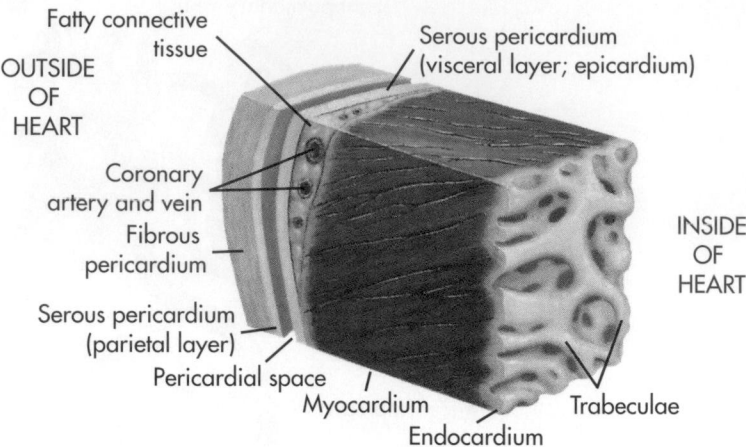

Fatty connective tissue

OUTSIDE OF HEART

Serous pericardium (visceral layer; epicardium)

Coronary artery and vein

Fibrous pericardium

INSIDE OF HEART

Serous pericardium (parietal layer)

Pericardial space

Myocardium

Endocardium

Trabeculae

Fig. 22-2 *Wall of the heart.* This section of the heart wall shows the fibrous pericardium, the parietal and visceral layers of the serous pericardium (with the pericardial space between them), the myocardium, and the endocardium. Note the fatty connective tissue between the visceral layer of the serous pericardium (epicardium) and the myocardium. Note also that the endocardium covers beamlike projections of myocardial muscle tissue, called *trabeculae.* *(From Thibodeau, G.A. & Patton, K.T. [1999].* Anatomy & physiology *[4th ed.]. St. Louis: Mosby.)*

Right pulmonary artery

TO LUNG

FROM LUNG

Superior vena cava (from head and arms)

Pulmonary semilunar valve

Right atrium

Tricuspid valve

Chordae tendineae

Right ventricle

Inferior vena cava (from trunk and legs)

Aortic arch

Left pulmonary artery

TO LUNG

Pulmonary trunk

Left atrium

Branches of left pulmonary vein

FROM LUNG

Aortic semilunar valve

Mitral valve

Left ventricle

Interventricular septum

Myocardium (heart muscle)

Papillary muscle

Descending aorta

Fig. 22-3 *Structures that direct blood flow through the heart.* Arrows indicate path of blood flow through chambers, valves, and major vessels. *(Modified from Thibodeau, G.A. [1987].* Anatomy & physiology. *St. Louis: Mosby.)*

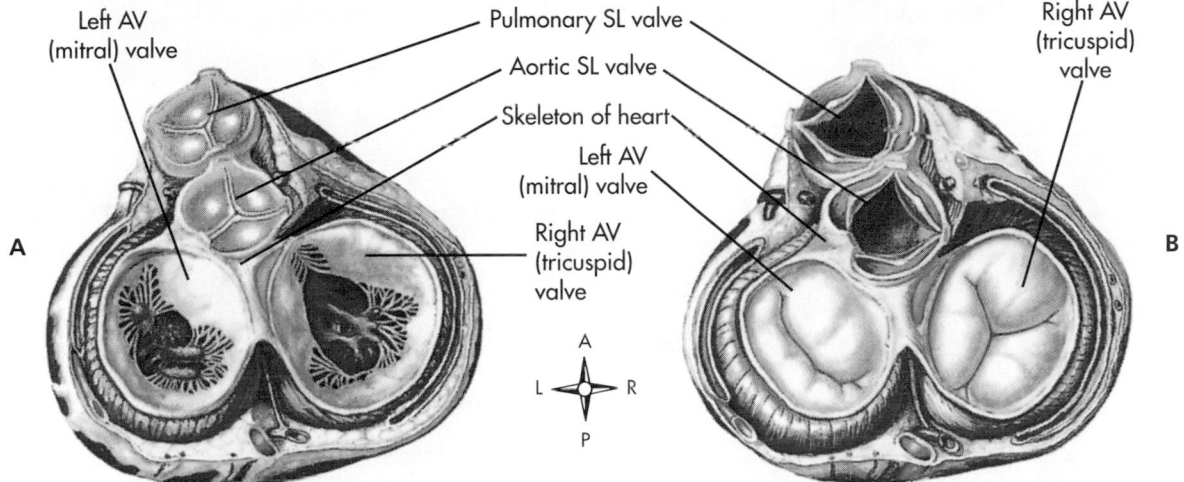

Fig. 22-4 *Structure of the heart valves.* **A,** The heart valves in this drawing are depicted as viewed from above (looking down into the heart). Note that the semilunar *(SL)* valves are closed and the atrioventricular *(AV)* valves are open, as when the atria are contracting. **B** is similar to **A** except that the semilunar valves are open and the atrioventricular valves are closed, as when the ventricles are contracting. *(From Thibodeau, G.A. & Patton, K.T. [1999]. Anatomy & physiology [4th ed.]. St. Louis: Mosby.)*

Fibrous skeleton of the heart

Four rings of dense fibrous connective tissue provide a firm anchorage for the attachments of the atrial and ventricular musculature, as well as the valvular tissue (Fig. 22-4). The fibrous rings are adjacent and form a central, fibrous supporting structure collectively termed the *annuli fibrosi cordis.*

Valves of the heart

One-way blood flow through the heart is ensured by the four heart valves. The coordinated actions of the *atrioventricular* (mitral and tricuspid) and *semilunar* (pulmonary and aortic) *valves* are shown in Figs. 22-3 and 22-4.

The heart valve openings are guarded by flaps of tissue called *leaflets* or *cusps,* which are attached to the papillary muscles by the *chordae tendineae cordis* (see Fig. 22-3). The *papillary muscles* are extensions of the myocardium that pull the cusps together and downward at the onset of ventricular contraction, thus preventing their backward expulsion into the atria.

The right atrioventricular valve is called the *tricuspid valve* because it has three cusps. The left atrioventricular valve is a bicuspid (two-cusp) valve called the *mitral valve.* The tricuspid and mitral valves function as a unit because the atrium, fibrous rings, valvular tissue, chordae tendineae, papillary muscles, and ventricular walls are connected. Collectively, these six structures are known as the *mitral and tricuspid complex.* Damage to any one of the complex's six components can alter function significantly.

The great vessels

Blood moves in and out of the heart through several large vessels (see Fig. 22-3). The right heart receives venous blood

from the systemic circulation through the *superior* and *inferior venae cavae,* which enter the right atrium. Blood leaves the right ventricle and enters the pulmonary circulation through the *pulmonary artery.* This artery divides into right and left branches to transport unoxygenated blood from the right heart to the right and left lungs. The pulmonary arteries branch further into the pulmonary capillary bed, where oxygen and carbon dioxide exchange occurs.

The four *pulmonary veins,* two from the right lung and two from the left lung, carry oxygenated blood from the lungs to the left side of the heart. The oxygenated blood moves through the left atrium and ventricle and out into the *aorta,* which delivers it to systemic vessels that supply the body.

Blood flow during the cardiac cycle

The pumping action of the heart consists of contraction and relaxation of the myocardial layer of the heart wall. Each contraction and the relaxation that follows it constitute one *cardiac cycle.* (Blood flow through the heart during a single cardiac cycle is illustrated in Fig. 22-5.) During relaxation, termed *diastole,* blood fills the ventricles. The contraction that follows, termed *systole,* propels the blood out of the ventricles and into the circulation. Contraction of the left ventricle is slightly earlier than contraction of the right ventricle.

The phases of the cardiac cycle can be identified on initiation of ventricular myocardial contraction (Figs. 22-6 and 22-7). As blood is pushed through the heart, it is mixed by passing through the strands of the *trabeculae carneae.* Expulsion of blood from the ventricles marks the end of one cardiac cycle.

Diastole

Systole

Fig. 22-5 *Blood flow through the heart during a single cardiac cycle.* **A,** During diastole, blood flows into atria, atrioventricular valves are pushed open, and blood begins to fill ventricles. Atrial systole squeezes any blood remaining in atria out into ventricles. **B,** During ventricular systole, ventricles contract, pushing blood out through semilunar valves into pulmonary artery (right ventricle) and aorta (left ventricle). *(Modified from Thibodeau, G.A. & Patton, K.T. [1996]. Anatomy & physiology [3rd ed.]. St. Louis: Mosby.)*

✓ QUICK CHECK

Why are the two separate circulatory systems said to be "serially connected"?

Why does the thickness of the myocardium vary tremendously in the different heart chambers?

Trace blood flow through the heart during a single cardiac cycle.

Normal intracardiac pressures
Normal intracardiac pressures are shown in Figs. 22-6 and 22-8.

Structures That Support Cardiac Metabolism: The Coronary Vessels
The blood within the heart chambers does not supply oxygen and other nutrients to the cells of the heart. Like all other organs, including the lungs, heart structures are nourished by vessels of the systemic circulation. The branch of the systemic circulation that supplies the heart is termed the *coronary circulation* and consists of *coronary arteries,*

which receive blood through openings in the aorta called the *coronary ostia,* and the *cardiac veins,* which empty into the right atrium through the opening of a large vein called the *coronary sinus* (Fig. 22-9). (Regulation of the coronary circulation, which is similar to regulation of flow through systemic and pulmonary vessels, is described elsewhere.)

Coronary arteries
The *right coronary artery* and the *left coronary artery* (see Fig. 22-9) traverse the epicardium, myocardium, and endocardium and branch to become arterioles and then capillaries. Their main branches are outlined in Box 22-1.

Collateral arteries
The collateral arteries are really connections, or anastomoses, between two branches of the same or the opposite coronary artery. The epicardium contains more collateral vessels than the endocardium. The function of the collateral circulation seems to be to protect the heart. Gradual coronary occlusion results in the growth of coronary collaterals. The collateral circulation is responsible for supplying blood and oxygen to the myocardium that has been deprived of oxygen following severe narrowing and reduced vasoelastic

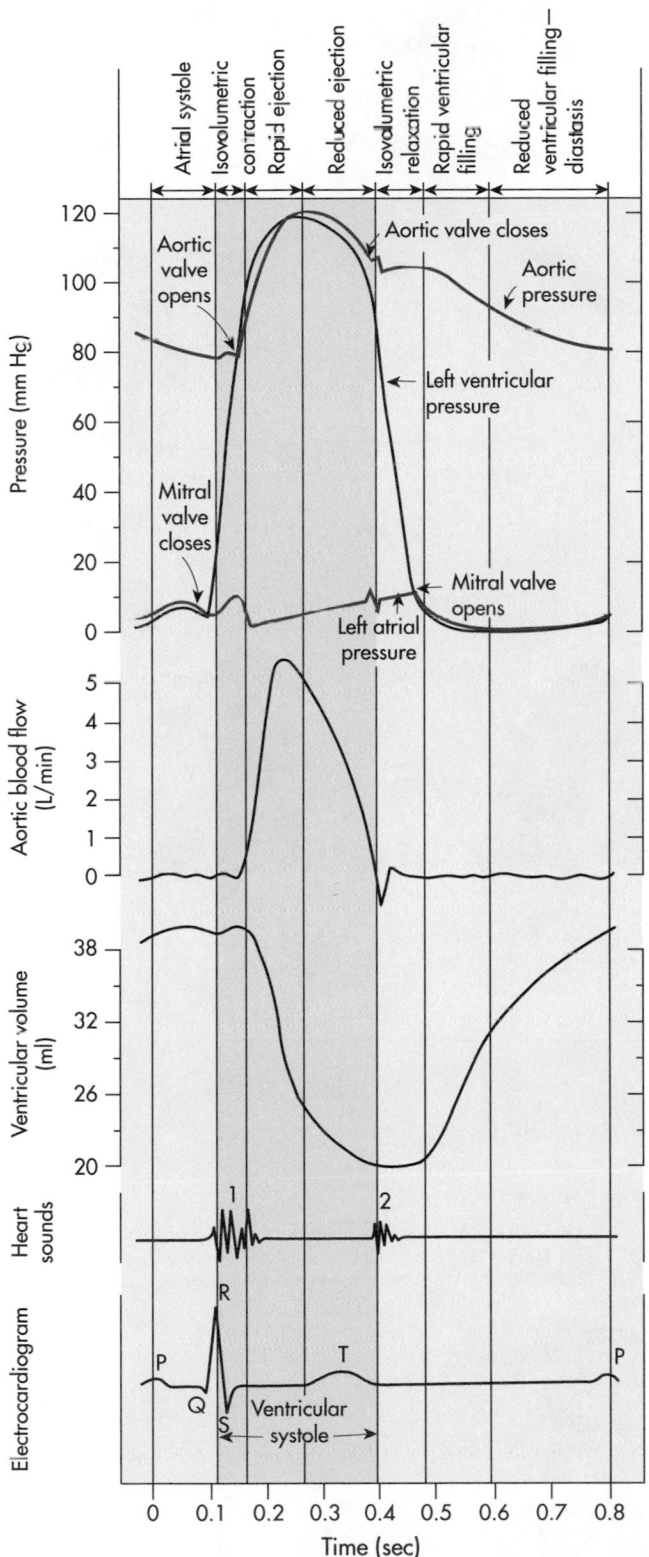

Fig. 22-6 *Major phases of cardiac cycle.* This chart summarizes several diagrams of heart function (cardiac pumping cycle, blood pressure, blood flow, volume, heart sounds, and electrocardiogram [ECG]), all adjusted to the same time scale. *(From Berne, R.M. & Levy, M.N. [Eds.]. [1990]. Principles of physiology. St. Louis: Mosby.)*

Main Branches of the Coronary Arteries   BOX 22-1

Left coronary artery. Arises from single ostium behind left cusp of aortic semilunar valve; ranges from a few millimeters to a few centimeters long; passes between left arterial appendage and pulmonary artery and generally divides into two branches—the left anterior descending artery and the circumflex artery; other branches distributed diagonally across the free wall of the left ventricle

Left anterior descending artery (or anterior interventricular artery). Delivers blood to portions of left and right ventricles and much of interventricular septum; travels down the anterior surface of interventricular septum toward apex of the heart

Circumflex artery. Travels in a groove *(coronary sulcus)* that separates left atrium from left ventricle and extends to left border of heart; supplies blood to left atrium and lateral wall of left ventricle; often branches to posterior surfaces of left atrium and left ventricle

Right coronary artery. Originates from an ostium behind the right aortic cusp, travels behind the pulmonary artery and extends around the right heart to the heart's posterior surface, where it branches to atrium and ventricle; three major branches are conus (supplies blood to upper right ventricle), right marginal branch (travels right ventricle to the apex), and posterior descending branch (lies in posterior interventricular sulcus and supplies smaller branches to both ventricles)

function of a major coronary artery.[2] In response to flow, stress, and pressure, collateral vessels are restructured and remodeled. The remodeling implies synthesis and degradation of extracellular matrix components in the vessel wall.

Coronary capillaries

The heart has an extensive capillary network, with approximately 3300 capillaries per square millimeter (ca/mm²) or about one capillary per muscle cell (muscle fiber).[3] Blood travels from the arteries to the arterioles and then into the capillaries, where exchange of oxygen and other nutrients takes place. Any alteration of the cardiac muscles dramatically affects blood flow in the capillaries.

Coronary veins and lymphatic vessels

After passing through the extensive capillary network, blood from the coronary arteries drains into the cardiac veins, which travel alongside the arteries. Most of the venous drainage of the heart occurs through veins in the visceral pericardium. The veins then feed into the *great cardiac vein* (see Fig. 22-9) and coronary sinus on the posterior surface of the heart, between the atria and ventricles, in the coronary

Fig. 22-7 *The phases of the cardiac cycle. 1,* Atrial systole. *2,* Isovolumetric ventricular contraction. Ventricular volume remains constant as pressure increases rapidly. *3,* Ejection. *4,* Isovolumetric ventricular relaxation. Both sets of valves are closed, and the ventricles are relaxing. *5,* Passive ventricular filling. The atrioventricular (AV) valves are forced open, and the blood rushes into the relaxing ventricles. *(From Thibodeau, G.A. & Patton, K.T. [1999].* Anatomy & physiology *[4th ed.]. St. Louis: Mosby.)*

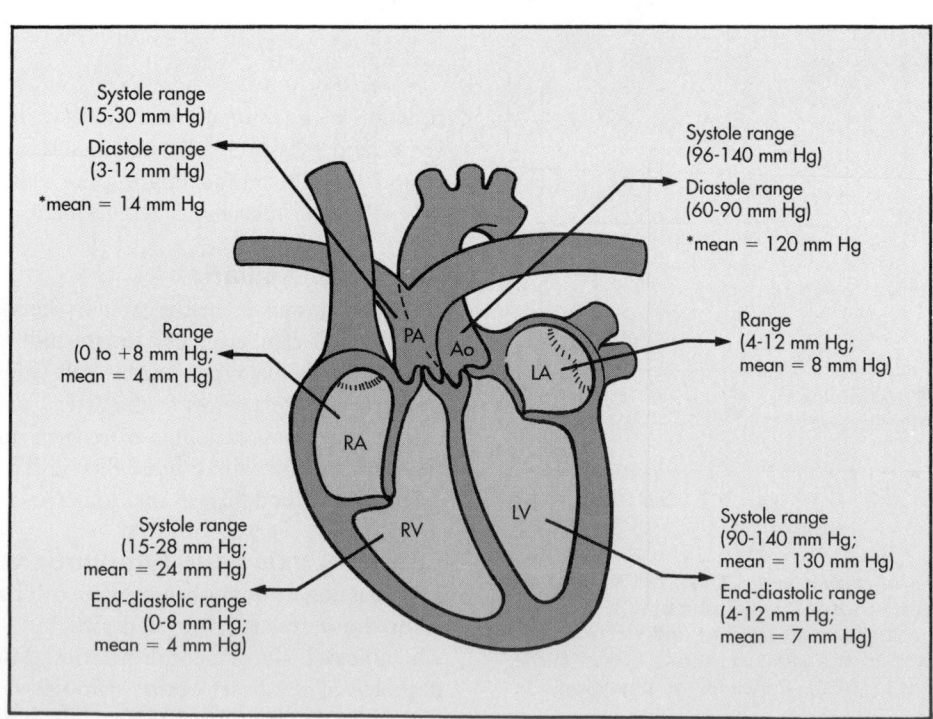

Fig. 22-8 *Normal intracardiac pressures. RA,* Right atrium; *LA,* left atrium; *RV,* right ventricle; *LV,* left ventricle; *PA,* pulmonary artery; *Ao,* aorta. *Main mean pressure.

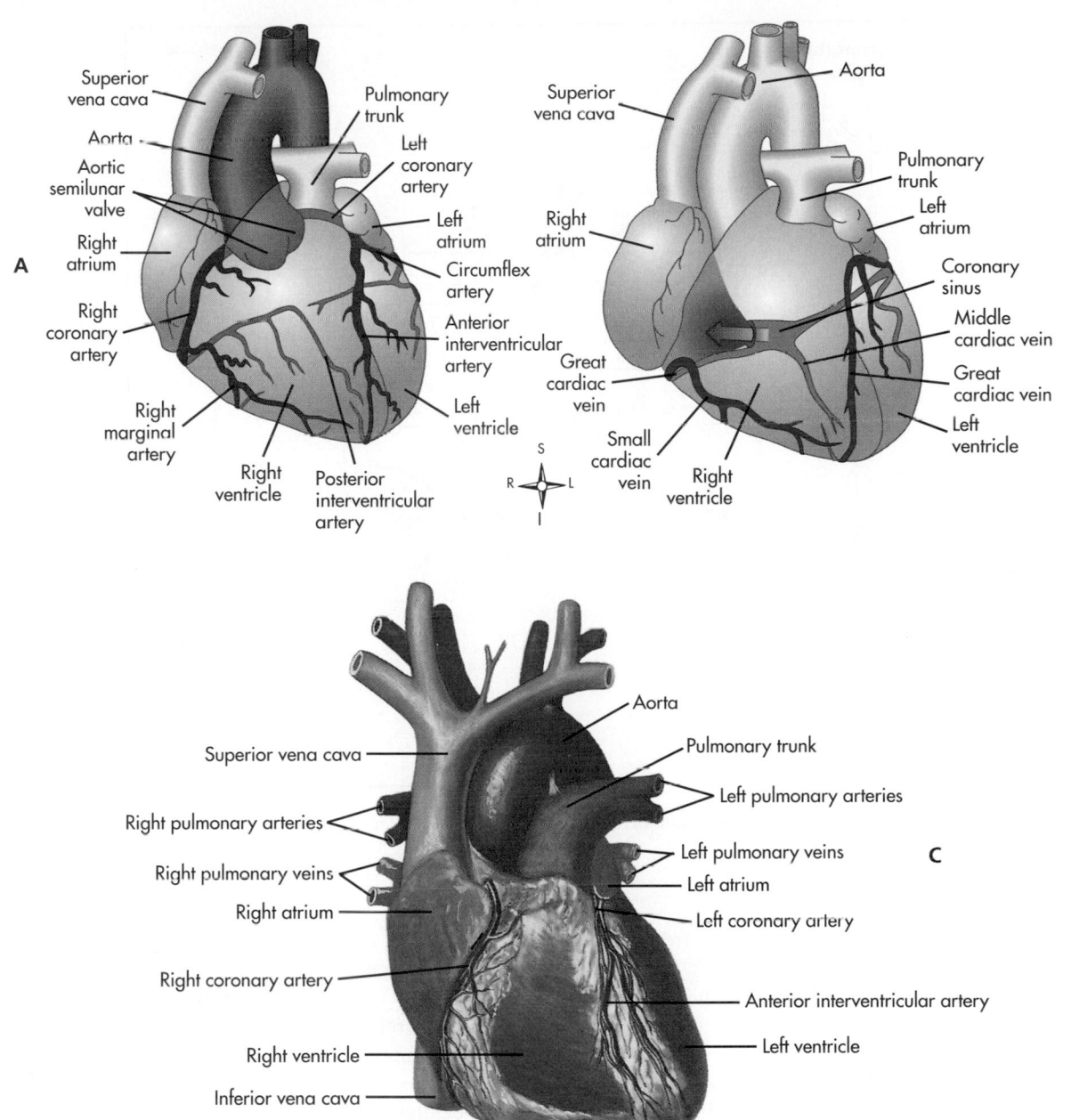

Fig. 22-9 *Coronary circulation.* A, Arteries. **B,** Veins. Both **A** and **B** are anterior views of the heart. Vessels near the anterior surface are more darkly colored than vessels of the posterior surface seen through the heart. **C,** View of the anterior (sternocostal) surface. (*A and B modified from Thibodeau, G.A. & Patton, K.T. [1999]. Anatomy & physiology [4th ed.]. St. Louis: Mosby; C from Seeley, R.R., Stephens, T.D., & Tate, P. [1995]. Anatomy and physiology [3rd ed.]. St. Louis: Mosby.)*

sulcus. Venous coronary blood empties into the right atrium from the coronary sinus. Blood from the left ventricular walls is generally drained through the coronary sinus and its tributaries, which together form the largest system of coronary veins. The great cardiac vein primarily drains the anterior surface of the heart. The *posterior vein of the left ventricle,* the largest on the posterior surface of the heart, branches from the coronary sinus and accompanies the circumflex artery.

The myocardium has an extensive system of lymphatic vessels. With cardiac contraction, the lymphatic vessels drain fluid to lymph nodes in the anterior mediastinum that eventually empty into the superior vena cava. The lymphatics are important for protecting the myocardium against injury. (The lymphatic vessels are described on p. 622.)

Structures That Control Heart Action

The continuous, rhythmic repetition of the cardiac cycle (systole and diastole) depends on the transmission of electrical impulses, termed *cardiac action potentials,* through the myocardium. (Action potentials are described in Chapters 1 and 4.) The muscle fibers of the myocardium are

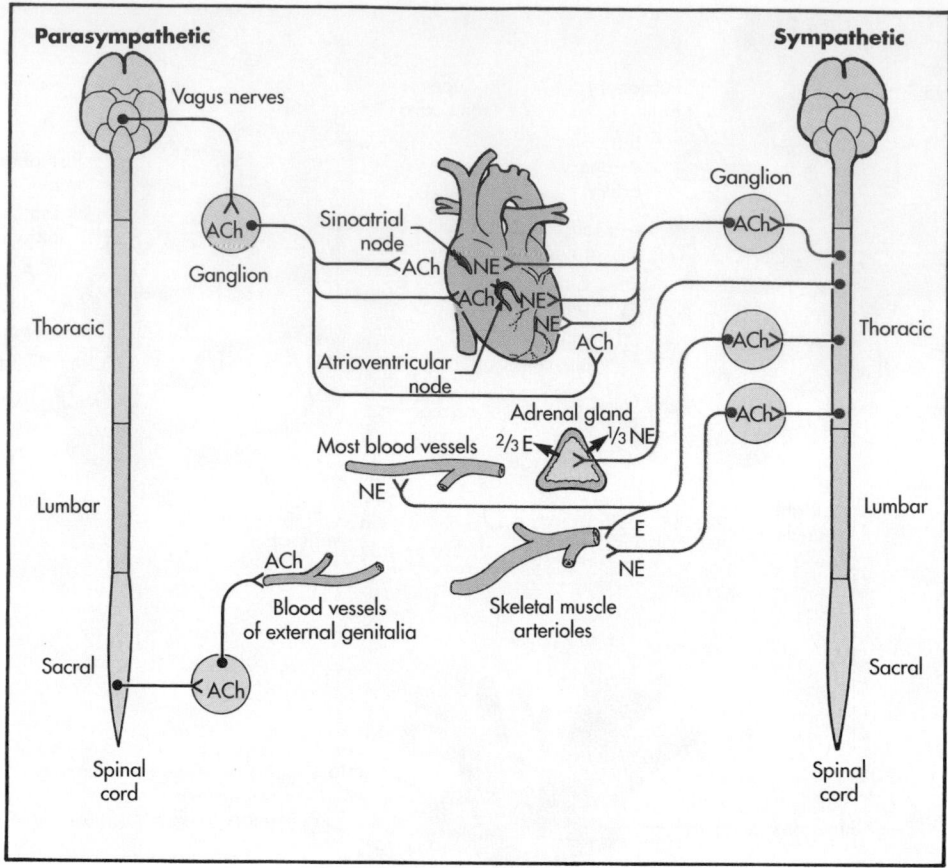

Fig. 22-10 *Autonomic innervation of cardiovascular system. ACh,* Acetylcholine; *NE,* norepi-nephrine; *E,* epinephrine.

uniquely joined so that action potentials pass from cell to cell very rapidly and efficiently.

The myocardium also contains its own ***conduction system***—specialized cells that enable it to generate and transmit action potentials without stimulation from the nervous system. These cells are concentrated at certain sites in the myocardium called ***nodes.*** Although the heart is innervated by the autonomic nervous system (both sympathetic and parasympathetic fibers), neural impulses are not needed to maintain the cardiac cycle. Thus the heart will beat in the absence of any nervous connection. The cardiac cycle is stimulated by the nodes of specialized cells and "fine tuned" as needed by the autonomic fibers. The sympathetic and parasympathetic nerves affect the speed of the cardiac cycle (***heart rate,*** or beats per minute) and the diameter of the coronary vessels (Fig. 22-10).

Heart action is also influenced by substances delivered to the myocardium in coronary blood. Nutrients and oxygen are needed for cellular survival and normal function, whereas hormones and biochemicals affect the strength and duration of myocardial contraction and the degree and duration of myocardial relaxation.

The conduction system

Normally electrical impulses arise in the ***sinoatrial node (SA node, sinus node),*** which is often called the *pacemaker of the*

heart. The SA node is located at the junction of the right atrium and superior vena cava, just above the tricuspid valve (Fig. 22-11). The SA node's ***P cells,*** so called because they are pale and primitive appearing, are assumed to be the site of impulse formation.[4]

In the resting adult the SA node generates about 75 action potentials per minute. Each one travels rapidly from cell to cell and through special pathways in the atrial myocardium, causing both atria to contract, beginning systole. Ventricular contraction is delayed because the fibrous skeleton of the heart interrupts cell-to-cell transmission of the electrical impulses. The action potential is transmitted from the atrial to the ventricular myocardium through fibers of the conduction system, traveling first to the ***atrioventricular node (AV node),*** then to the ***bundle of His (atrioventricular bundle, common bundle),*** and finally through the ***bundle branches*** of the interventricular septum to Purkinje fibers in the heart wall (see Fig. 22-11).

The AV node is located in the right atrial wall above the tricuspid valve and anterior to the ostium of the coronary sinus. Behind it are numerous autonomic ganglia, presumably vagal (parasympathetic).[5] These ganglia may serve as receptors for the vagus nerve and cause slowing of the cardiac cycle.

Conducting fibers from the AV node converge to form the bundle of His, a triangle within the posterior border of the interventricular septum. The two lower ends of the tri-

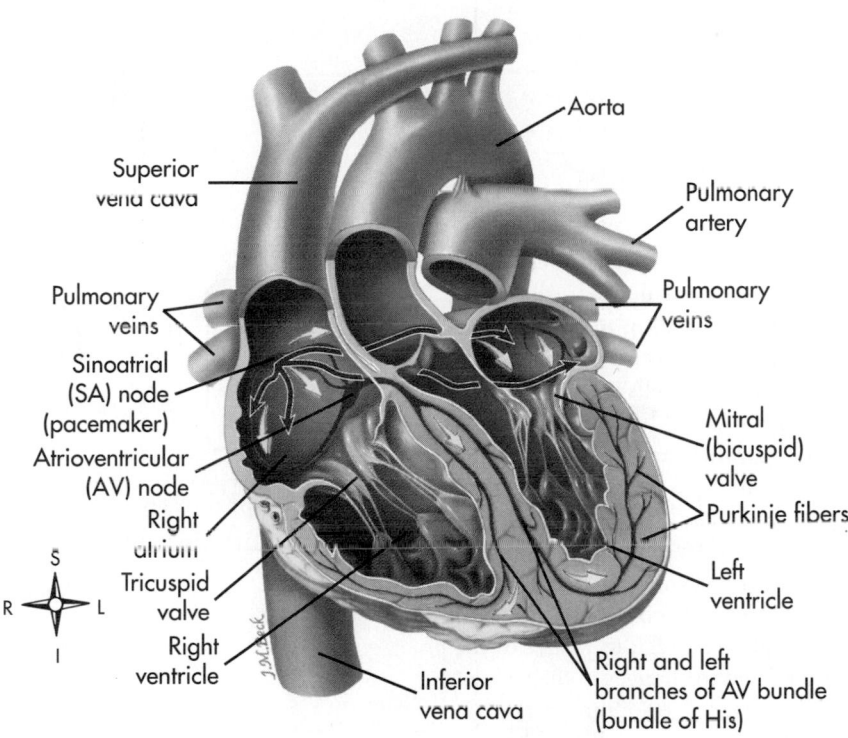

Fig. 22-11 *Conduction system of heart.* Specialized cardiac muscle cells in the wall of the heart rapidly conduct an electrical impulse throughout the myocardium. The signal is initiated by the sinoatrial (SA) node (pacemaker) and spreads to the rest of the atrial myocardium and to the atrioventricular (AV) node. The AV node then initiates a signal that is conducted through the ventricular myocardium by way of the atrioventricular bundle (of His) and Purkinje fibers. *(Modified from Thibodeau, G.A. & Patton, K.T. [1996].* Anatomy & physiology *[3rd ed.]. St. Louis: Mosby.)*

angle give rise to the right and left bundle branches. The *right bundle branch (RBB)* is thin and travels without much branching to the right ventricular apex. Because of its thinness and relative lack of branches, the RBB is susceptible to interruption by damage to the endocardium.

The *left bundle branch (LBB)* arises perpendicularly from the bundle of His and, in some hearts, divides into two branches, or fascicles. The left anterior bundle branch (LABB) passes the left anterior papillary muscle and the base of the left ventricle and crosses the aortic outflow tract. Damage to the aortic valve or the left ventricle can interrupt this branch. The left posterior bundle branch (LPBB) travels posteriorly, crossing the left ventricular inflow tract to the base of the left posterior papillary muscle. This branch spreads diffusely through the posterior inferior left ventricular wall. Blood flow through this portion of the left ventricle is relatively nonturbulent, so the LBB is somewhat protected from injury caused by wear and tear.

The *Purkinje fibers* are the terminal branches of the RBB and LBB. They extend from the ventricular apexes to the fibrous rings and penetrate the heart wall to the outer myocardium. P cells are also found among the Purkinje fibers.

Bachmann bundle, the middle internodal pathway, and the posterior internodal pathway apparently connect the right and left atria and the SA node and the AV node.[1,6-9]

✓**QUICK CHECK**

Why are collateral vessels important to heart function?

Does the SA node control heart action? Why?

Trace the route of an action potential originating from the SA node.

Why are the left and right coronary vessels considered the major coronary vessels?

Propagation of cardiac action potentials

Electrical activation of the muscle cells, termed *depolarization,* is caused by the movement of electrically charged solutes (ions) across cardiac cell membranes. Deactivation, called *repolarization,* occurs the same way. (Movement of ions across cell membranes is described in Chapter 1; electrical activation of muscle cells is described in Chapter 36.)

TABLE 22-1	Intracellular and Extracellular Ion Concentrations in the Myocardium	
Ion	Intracellular Concentration	Extracellular Concentration
Sodium (Na⁺)	15 mM	145 mM
Potassium (K⁺)	150 mM	4 mM
Chloride (Cl⁻)	5 mM	120 mM
Calcium (Ca⁺⁺)	10^{-7} M	2 mM

mM, *Millimoles per kilogram;* M, *moles per kilogram.*

When ions move into and out of the cell, an electrical (voltage) difference across the cell membrane, called the *membrane potential,* is created. The resting membrane potential of myocardial cells is between −80 and −90 millivolts (mV), whereas that of SA and AV node cells is –60 mV. During depolarization, the inside of the cell becomes less negatively charged. In cardiac cells the difference between resting membrane potential (in millivolts) and the decreased negative charge caused by depolarization is the cardiac action potential. Table 22-1 summarizes the intracellular and extracellular ionic concentrations of cardiac muscle. Hence, drugs that block (e.g., calcium) have profound effects on the action potential and can alter heart rate. The various phases of the cardiac action potential are related to changes in the permeability of the cell membrane, primarily to sodium and potassium. Threshold is the point at which the cell membrane's selective permeability to sodium and potassium is temporarily disrupted, leading to depolarization.

A **refractory period,** during which no new cardiac action potential can be initiated by a stimulus, follows depolarization. This effective or absolute refractory period corresponds to the time needed for the reopening of channels that permit sodium and calcium influx. A relative refractory period occurs near the end of repolarization, following the effective refractory period. During this time the membrane can be depolarized again but only by a greater-than-normal stimulus. Abnormal refractory periods as a result of disease can cause abnormal heart rhythms or dysrhythmias, including ventricular fibrillation and cardiac arrest (see Chapter 23).

The normal electrocardiogram. The normal electrocardiogram is recorded from electrical activity transmitted by skin electrodes, that is, the sum of all the cardiac action potentials (Fig. 22-12). The **P wave** represents atrial depolarization. The **PR interval** is a measure of time from the onset of atrial activation to the onset of ventricular activation (normally

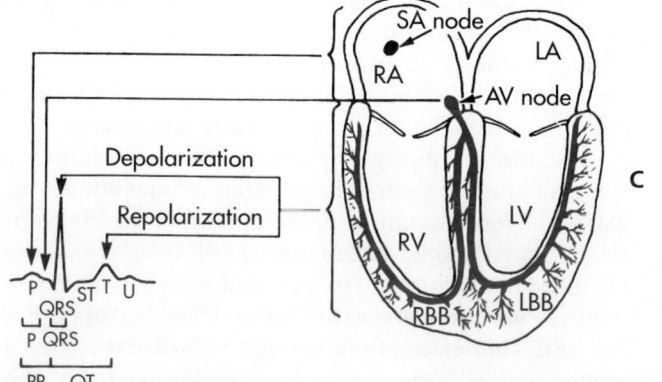

Fig. 22-12 *Electrocardiogram (ECG) and cardiac electrical activity.* **A,** Normal ECG. Depolarization and repolarization. **B,** ECG intervals among P, QRS, and T waves. **C,** Schematic representation of ECG and its relationship to cardiac electrical activity. *RA,* Right atrium; *LA,* left atrium; *RV,* right ventricle; *LV,* left ventricle; *RBB,* right bundle branch; *LBB,* left bundle branch. (*A and B from Thibodeau, G.A. & Patton, K.T. [1993]. Anatomy and physiology [2nd ed.]. St. Louis: Mosby;* **C** *from Thibodeau, G.A. [1987]. Anatomy & physiology. St. Louis: Mosby.)*

0.12 to 0.20 second). The PR interval represents the time necessary to travel from the sinus node through the atrium, AV node, and His-Purkinje system to activate ventricular myocardial cells. The **QRS complex** represents the sum of all ventricular muscle cell depolarizations. The configuration and amplitude of the QRS complex vary considerably among individuals. The duration is normally between 0.06 and 0.10 second. During the **ST interval** the entire ventricular myocardium is depolarized. The **QT interval** is sometimes called the "electrical systole" of the ventricles. It lasts about 0.4 second but varies inversely with the heart rate.

Automaticity. **Automaticity,** or the property of generating spontaneous depolarization to threshold, enables the SA and AV nodes to generate cardiac action potentials without any stimulus. Cells capable of spontaneous depolarization are called **automatic cells.** Those of the cardiac conduction system can stimulate the heart to beat even when it is removed from the body. Spontaneous depolarization is possible in automatic cells because the membrane potential does not "rest" during return to the resting membrane potential. Instead, it slowly creeps toward threshold during the diastolic phase of the cardiac cycle. Because threshold is approached during diastole, return to the resting membrane potential in automatic cells is called **diastolic depolarization.** The electrical impulse normally begins in the SA node because its cells depolarize more rapidly than other automatic cells.

Rhythmicity. **Rhythmicity** is the regular generation of an action potential by the heart's conduction system. The SA node sets the pace because normally it has the fastest rate. The SA node depolarizes spontaneously 60 to 100 times per minute. If the SA node is damaged, the AV node will become the heart's pacemaker at a rate of about 40 to 60 spontaneous depolarizations per minute. Eventually, however, conduction cells in the atria usually take over from the AV node. Purkinje fibers are capable of spontaneous depolarization, but at a rate of only 30 to 40 beats/min.

✓ QUICK CHECK

Why does the myocardial cell become less negatively charged during depolarization?

Why is the normal electrocardiogram composed of five waves—P, Q, R, S, and T?

Why is spontaneous depolarization possible in some cardiac cells?

Cardiac innervation

Although the heart's nodes and conduction system generate cardiac action potentials independently, the autonomic nervous system influences the *rate* of impulse generation (firing), depolarization, and repolarization of the myocardium and the strength of atrial and ventricular contraction. Autonomic neural transmission produces changes in the heart and circulatory system faster than metabolic or humoral agents (see Fig. 22-10). Speed is important, for example, in

stimulating the heart to increase its pumping action during times of stress or fear—the so-called *fight-or-flight response.* Although increased delivery of oxygen, glucose, hormones, and other blood-borne factors sustains increased cardiac activity, the rapid initiation of increased activity depends on the sympathetic and parasympathetic fibers of the autonomic nervous system.

Sympathetic and parasympathetic nerves

Sympathetic nerve fibers innervate all parts of the atria and ventricles. Parasympathetic fibers from the vagus nerve innervate these structures plus the SA and AV nodes (see Fig. 22-10). Strong vagal stimulation can block cardiac action potentials transmitted from the atria. Sympathetic nerves can also shorten the conduction time through the AV node and increase the rhythmicity of the AV pacemaker fibers.

Sympathetic nervous activity enhances myocardial performance. Neurally released norepinephrine or circulating catecholamines interact with β-adrenergic receptors on the cardiac cell membranes. The overall effect is an increased influx of Ca^{++}, which increases the contractile strength of the heart. In addition, sympathetic nervous activity increases heart rate, whereas parasympathetic (vagal) activity decreases heart rate. The vagus nerve releases acetylcholine. In the heart, receptors for these neurotransmitters are found in the myocardium and in the coronary vessels. When the autonomic nervous system is active, the vagal effects usually dominate.

Myocardial cells

The cells of cardiac muscle (the myocardium) and of muscle that makes voluntary movement possible (skeletal muscle) are nearly identical in structure, function, and microscopic appearance. (The properties of skeletal muscle are described in detail in Chapter 36.) Both types of muscle tissue are composed of long, narrow fibers that contain bundles of longitudinally arranged myofibrils; a nucleus (cardiac muscle) or many nuclei (skeletal muscle); mitochondria; an internal membrane system (the sarcoplasmic reticulum); cytoplasm (sarcoplasm); and a plasma membrane (the sarcolemma), which encloses the cell. Cardiac and skeletal muscle cells also have an "external" membrane system made up of transverse tubules (T tubules) formed by invaginations of the sarcolemma. The sarcoplasmic reticulum forms a network of channels that surrounds the muscle fiber.

Because the myofibrils in both cardiac and skeletal fibers are made up of alternating light and dark bands of protein, the fibers appear striped, or striated. The dark and light bands of the myofibrils are called *sarcomeres* and are normally between 1.6 and 2.2 μm long. Length determines the limits of myocardial stretch at the end of diastole and subsequently the force of contraction during systole.

Differences between cardiac and skeletal muscle reflect heart function. Cardiac cells are arranged in branching networks throughout the myocardium, whereas skeletal muscle cells tend to be arranged in parallel units throughout the length of the muscle. Cardiac fibers have only one nucleus, whereas skeletal muscle cells have many nuclei. Other differences enable cardiac fibers to (1) transmit action potentials quickly from cell to cell, (2) maintain high levels of energy synthesis, and (3) gain access to more ions, particularly sodium and potassium, in the extracellular environment.

First, electrical impulses are transmitted rapidly from cardiac fiber to cardiac fiber because the network of fibers is connected at **intercalated disks,** which are thickened portions of the sarcolemma. The intercalated disks contain two junctions: desmosomes, which attach one cell to another; and gap junctions, which allow the electrical impulse to spread from cell to cell (see Chapter 1). Together, these junctions provide a low-resistance pathway for impulse propagation.

Second, unlike skeletal muscle, the heart cannot rest and is in constant need of energy compounds such as adenosine triphosphate (ATP). Therefore the cytoplasm surrounding the bundles of myofibrils in each cardiac muscle cell contains a superabundance of mitochondria (25% of the cellular volume). Cardiac muscle cells have more mitochondria than do skeletal muscle cells to provide the necessary respiratory enzymes for aerobic metabolism and supply quantities of ATP sufficient for the constant action of the myocardium.

Third, cardiac fibers contain more T tubules than do skeletal muscle fibers. This gives each myofibril in the myocardium ready access to molecules needed for the continuous transmission of action potentials, which involves transport of sodium and potassium through the walls of the T tubules. Because the T tubule system is continuous with the extracellular space and the interstitial fluid, it facilitates the rapid transmission of the electrical impulses from the surface of the sarcolemma to the myofibrils inside the fiber. This activates all the myofibrils of one fiber simultaneously. The sarcoplasmic reticulum is located around the myofibrils. When an action potential is transmitted through the T tubules, it induces the sarcoplasmic reticulum to release its stored calcium, which activates the contractile proteins, actin and myosin.

Actin, myosin, and the troponin-tropomyosin complex

The thick filaments of **myosin** constitute the central dark band called the **anisotropic,** or **A, band** (Fig. 22-13). The myosin molecule resembles a golf club with two large bulbous heads protruding from one end of a straight shaft (Fig. 22-14, *A*). The bilobed heads contain an actin-binding site and a site of ATPase activity. A thick filament contains about 200 myosin molecules bundled together with the heads of the molecules (called *cross-bridges*) facing outward (see Fig. 22-14, *A*). The actin molecules are part of the thin filaments (Fig. 22-14, *B*). The light bands are called **isotropic,** or **I, bands** (see Fig. 22-13). The thin filaments of actin appear light and extend from the **Z line,** a dense fibrous line that crosses the center of each I band. The area from one dark Z line to an adjacent Z line is the sarcomere. In the center of the sarcomere is the H zone, a somewhat less dense region. A thin, dark **M line** travels the center of the H zone. A single

Fig. 22-13 *Sarcomere.* **A,** Electron photomicrograph of sarcomere. **B,** Schematic of location and interaction of actin and myosin. *(Modified from Thibodeau, G.A. & Patton, K.T. [1996]. Anatomy & physiology [3rd ed.]. St. Louis: Mosby.)*

tropomyosin molecule (a relaxing protein) lies alongside seven actin molecules. Troponin, another relaxing protein, associates with the tropomyosin molecule, forming the **troponin-tropomyosin complex** (Fig. 22-15). The troponin complex itself has three components. **Troponin T** aids in the binding of the troponin complex to actin and tropomyosin; **troponin I** inhibits the ATPase of actomyosin; and **troponin C** contains binding sites for the calcium ions involved in contraction.

Myocardial metabolism

Cardiac muscle, like other muscle tissue, depends on the constant production of ATP for energy. ATP is produced within the mitochondria mainly from glucose, fatty acids, and lactate. If the myocardium is inadequately perfused because of coronary artery disease, anaerobic metabolism becomes an essential source of energy (see Chapter 1). The energy produced by metabolic processes is used for muscle contraction and relaxation, electrical excitation, membrane transport, and synthesis of large molecules. Normally, the amount of ATP produced supplies sufficient energy to pump blood throughout the system.

Cardiac work is often expressed in terms of **myocardial oxygen consumption (MV̇O₂),** which correlates closely with total cardiac energy requirements. MV̇O₂ is determined by the following three major factors: (1) amount of wall stress during systole, which can be estimated by measuring the sys-

Fig. 22-14 *Structure of myosin.* **A,** Each myosin molecule is a coil of two chains wrapped around one another. At the end of each chain is a globular region, much like a golf club, called the *head.* Myosin molecules usually are combined into filaments, which are stalks of myosin from which the heads protrude. **B,** Actin microfilament. *(From Raven, P.H. & Johnson, G.B. [1995]. Understanding biology [3rd ed.]. Dubuque, Iowa: Brown.)*

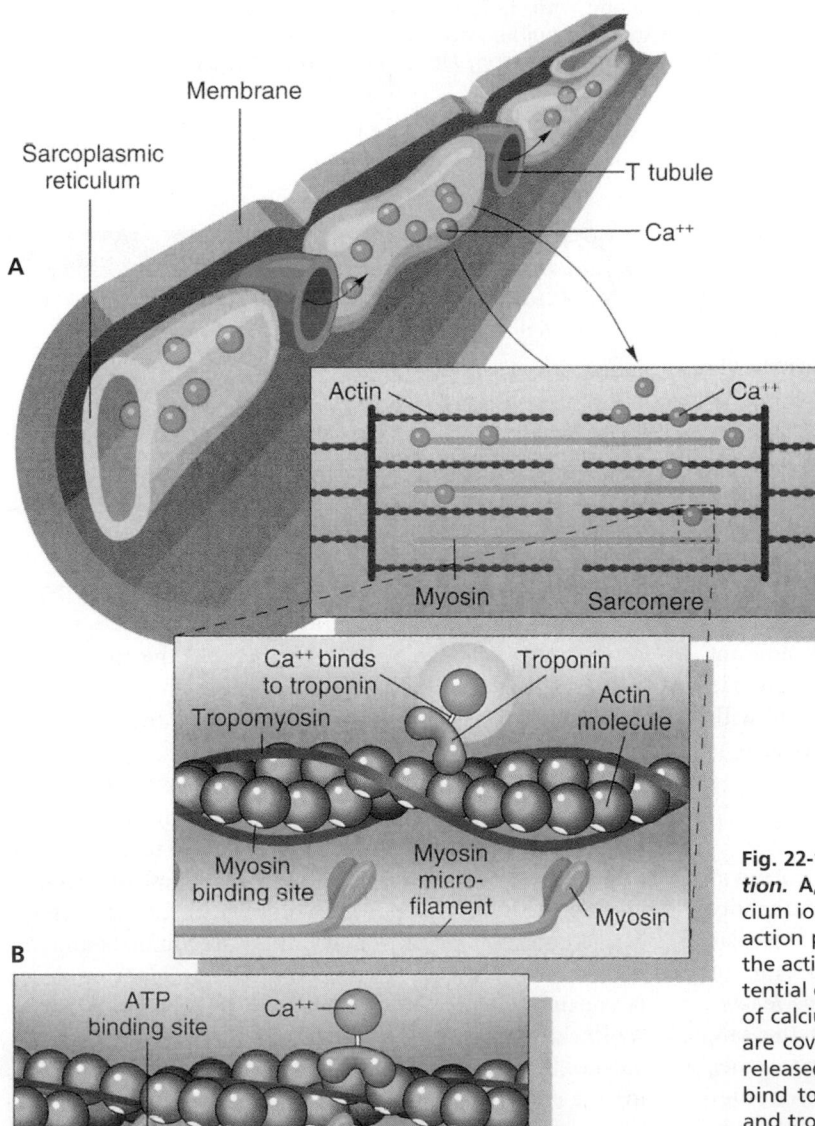

Fig. 22-15 *Myofilaments and mechanisms of muscle contraction.* **A,** Thin and thick myofilaments. In resting muscle, calcium ions are stored in the sarcoplasmic reticulum. When an action potential reaches the muscle cell, the T tubules carry the action potential deep into the sarcoplasm. The action potential causes the sarcoplasmic reticulum to release the store of calcium ions. **B,** In resting muscle the myosin binding sites are covered by troponin and tropomyosin. The calcium ions released into the sarcoplasm as a result of action potential bind to the troponin. This binding causes the tropomyosin and troponin to move out of the way of the myosin binding sites, leaving the myosin heads free to bind to the actin microfilament. *ATP,* Adenosine triphosphate. *(From Raven, P.H. & Johnson, G.B. [1995]. Understanding biology [3rd ed.]. Dubuque, Iowa: Brown.)*

Fig. 22-16 *Cross-bridge theory of muscle contraction.* **A,** Each myosin cross-bridge in the thick filament moves into a resting position after an adenosine triphosphate (ATP) molecule binds and transfers its energy. **B,** Calcium ions released from the sarcoplasmic reticulum bind to troponin in the thin filament, allowing tropomyosin to shift from its position blocking the active sites of actin molecules. **C,** Each myosin cross-bridge then binds to an active site on a thin filament, displacing the remnants of ATP hydrolysis—adenosine diphosphate (ADP) and inorganic phosphate (P_i). **D,** The release of stored energy from step A provides the force needed for each cross-bridge to move back to its original position, pulling actin along with it. Each cross-bridge will remain bound to actin until another ATP molecule binds to it and pulls it back into its resting position, **A.** *(From Thibodeau, G.A. & Patton, K.T. [1999]. Anatomy & physiology [4th ed.]. St. Louis: Mosby.)*

tolic blood pressure; (2) duration of systolic wall tension, which is measured indirectly by the heart rate; and (3) contractile state of the myocardium, for which no clinical measurement exists.

The oxygen supply to the myocardium is delivered exclusively by the coronary arteries. From 70% to 75% of the oxygen from the coronary arteries is used immediately by cardiac muscle, leaving little oxygen in reserve. Any increased energy needs can be met only by increasing coronary blood flow. When oxygen content decreases, the local concentration of metabolic factors increases. One of these, adenosine, dilates coronary arterioles, increasing coronary blood flow. Oxygen content of the blood cannot be increased under normal atmospheric conditions, nor can the amount of O_2 extracted from the blood be appreciably increased from the resting level. $M\dot{V}O_2$ can increase several-fold with exercise and decrease moderately under conditions such as hypotension and hypothermia.[1]

Myocardial contraction and relaxation

Myocardial contractility is a change in developed tension at a given resting fiber length. In functional terms, contractility is the ability of the heart muscle to shorten. On a molecular basis, thin filaments of actin slide over thick filaments of myosin, according to the *cross-bridge theory of muscle contraction.* Anatomically, contraction occurs when the sarcomere shortens so adjacent Z lines move closer together (Fig. 22-16). The A band width, including thick myosin filaments, is unchanged, with the movement coming from the long sets of filaments. The degree of shortening depends on how much the thin filaments overlap the thick filaments.

✓ **QUICK CHECK**

What features distinguish myocardial cells from skeletal cells?

Describe the interactions of actin, myosin, and the troponin-tropomyosin complex in controlling heart function.

What are cross-bridges?

Calcium and excitation-contraction coupling

Excitation-contraction coupling is the process by which an action potential in the plasma membrane of the muscle fiber triggers the cycle, leading to cross-bridge activity and contraction. Activation of this cycle depends on the availability of calcium.

Calcium is stored in the tubule system and the sarcoplasmic reticulum. It enters the myocardial cell from the interstitial fluid after electrical excitation, which increases membrane permeability to calcium. Two types of calcium channels (L-type, T-type) are identified in cardiac tissues. The L-type, or long-lasting, channels predominate and are the channels blocked by *calcium channel—blocking drugs* (verapamil, nifedipine, diltiazem). The T-type, or transient, channels are much less abundant in the heart and are not blocked by calcium channel-blocking drugs.[1] Calcium entering the cell triggers the release of calcium from the storage sites, particularly the sarcoplasmic reticulum. Calcium then diffuses toward the myofibrils and binds with troponin.

The calcium-troponin complex interaction facilitates the

Fig. 22-17 *Frank-Starling law of the heart.* Relationship between length and tension in heart. End-diastolic volume determines end-diastolic length of ventricular muscle fibers and is proportional to tension generated during systole, as well as to cardiac output, stroke volume, and stroke work. A change in myocardial contractility causes the heart to perform on a different length-tension curve. *A,* Increased contractility; *B,* normal contractility; *C,* heart failure or decreased contractility. (See text.)

contraction process. In the resting state, troponin I is bound to actin and the tropomyosin molecule covers the sites where the myosin heads bind to actin. Therefore interaction between actin and myosin is prevented. Calcium binding to troponin inhibits troponin C (which enhances troponin I—actin binding) and causes tropomyosin to move away, consequently uncovering the binding sites on the myosin heads. Myosin and actin can now form cross-bridges, and ATP can be dephosphorylated to adenosine diphosphate (ADP). Under these circumstances, sliding of the thick and thin filaments can occur, and the muscle contracts.

HEALTH ALERT

New Markers of Myocardial Injury

Troponin I and troponin T have recently been promoted as new markers of myocardial injury. The markers specifically help determine prognosis in individuals who have unstable chest pain (angina).

Data from Luscher, M.S. et al. (1997). Applicability of cardiac troponin T and I for early risk stratification in unstable coronary artery disease. Circulation, 96(8), 2578-2585.

Myocardial relaxation

Adequate relaxation is just as vital to optimal cardiac function as contraction; and calcium, troponin, and tropomyosin also facilitate relaxation. After contraction, free calcium ions are actively pumped out of the cell back into the interstitial fluid or reaccumulated in the sarcoplasmic reticulum and stored. Troponin releases its bound calcium. The tropomyosin complex blocks the active sites on the actin molecule, preventing cross-bridges with the myosin heads.

Factors Affecting Cardiac Performance

The following four factors affect cardiac performance directly:

1. *Preload:* pressure generated at the end of diastole; depends on both the heart and the vascular system
2. *Afterload:* resistance to ejection during systole; depends on both the heart and the vascular system
3. *Heart rate:* a characteristic of cardiac tissue per se and subject to neural and humoral influence
4. *Myocardial contractility:* another cardiac tissue characteristic that is influenced by neural and humoral mechanisms

To understand the factors affecting cardiac performance, it is first necessary to understand two physical laws that explain the mechanisms of heart action: the Frank-Starling law of the heart and Laplace law.

Frank-Starling law of the heart

The *Frank-Starling law of the heart,* or length-tension relationship of cardiac muscle, relates resting sarcomere length, expressed as the volume of blood in the heart at the end of diastole, or **end-diastolic volume,** to tension generation, described as development of left ventricular pressure. Thus the volume of blood in the heart at the end of diastole (the length of its muscle fibers) is directly related to the force of contraction during the next systole. It is common to use preload (i.e., filling pressure) as an index of ventricular volume.

The mechanical function of the heart is characterized by a number of length-tension curves (Fig. 22-17). Factors that increase contractility cause the heart to operate on a higher length-tension curve (curve A). Heart failure (curve C) is characterized by a lower length-tension curve (see Chapter 23). The relationship between stretch and contraction can be compared with that of a rubber band. To a certain point, the more the rubber band is stretched, the farther it will fly when one end is released. Beyond that point, however, the rubber band will break.

The cross-bridge theory partially accounts for the length-tension mechanism of cardiac muscle. According to the Frank-Starling law, the longer the initial resting length of the cardiac muscle fiber (optimal length is between 2.2 μm and 2.4 μm), the greater the strength of contraction. At 2.2 μm there is an optimal number of active cross-bridges between actin and myosin. If the fibers are stretched beyond 2.2 μm to 2.4 μm, the force of contraction decreases because actin and myosin become partially disengaged, disrupting many of the cross-bridges. Excessive stretching, to about 3.65 μm, causes actin and myosin to become completely disengaged and causes developed tension (force of contraction) to drop to zero. Heart failure occurs when it takes higher and higher filling pressures to accomplish normal contractile force.

Laplace law

In **Laplace law,** wall tension is related directly to the product of intraventricular pressure and internal radius and inversely to the wall thickness. The amount of tension generated in the wall of the ventricle (or any chamber or vessel) to produce a given intraventricular pressure depends on the size (radius and wall thickness) of the ventricle. The law of Laplace is useful for understanding aneurysm formation, distensibility in blood vessels, and the effects of ventricular dilation on myocardial contraction, an important factor in heart failure.

Preload

Left ventricular **preload** is the pressure generated in the left ventricle at the end of diastole, or left ventricular **end-diastolic pressure.** It is determined by end-diastolic volume, which according to the Frank-Starling law, stretches the cardiac muscle fibers that in turn develop tension, or force, for contraction. Within a physiologic range of muscle stretching, increased preload increases cardiac output (volume of blood pumped per minute; Fig. 22-18). Pressure changes are important because increased left ventricular filling pressures "back up" into the pulmonary circulation, where they force plasma out through vessel walls, causing fluid to accumulate in lung tissues (pulmonary edema; see Chapter 26).

Afterload

Left ventricular **afterload** is the resistance or impedance to ejection of blood from the left ventricle. It is the load the muscle must move after it starts to contract. Aortic systolic pressure is a good index of afterload. Low aortic pressures (decreased afterload) enable the heart to contract more rapidly, whereas high aortic pressures (increased afterload) slow contraction and cause higher work loads against which the heart must function so it can eject less blood. Pressure in the ventricle must exceed aortic pressure before blood can be pumped out during systole. The lighter the afterload, the faster the contraction; the heavier the afterload, the slower the contraction.

Afterload is also related to extent of shortening. Increases in aortic pressure, with a constant preload, result in decreased blood pumped by the left ventricle. Decreased aortic pressure allows the left ventricle to pump a larger volume.

Heart rate

The average heart rate in normal adults is about 70 beats/min. This diminishes by 10 to 20 beats/min during sleep and can accelerate to more than 100 beats/min during muscular activity or emotional excitement. In well-conditioned athletes at rest the heart rate is normally about 50 to 60 beats/min. In highly trained or elite athletes the resting heart rate can be below 50 beats/min. Highly trained athletes have a lower resting heart rate, greater stroke volume, and lower peripheral resistance in active muscles than they had before training. The low resting heart rate is the result of an increased vagal stimulation and lower sympathetic stimulation.[1] The lowered peripheral resistance is attributed to the increased number of arterioles in skeletal muscle. The decrease in peripheral resistance increases the venous return, causing the cardiac output to increase.[1] As the resting heart rate falls in individuals during physical training, the end-diastolic fiber length of the ventricles increases, since the longer duration of diastole results in greater filling. The increased end-diastolic fiber length increases stroke volume, which helps to compensate for the decreased heart rate. Neural factors, including neural reflexes, hormones, and chemicals, all influence heart rate.

Cardiovascular control centers in the brain

The **cardiovascular control center** is in the brain stem in the medulla, with secondary areas in the hypothalamus, cerebral cortex, thalamus, and complex networks of exciting or inhibiting interneurons (connecting neurons) throughout the brain. The hypothalamic centers regulate cardiovascular responses to changes in temperature; the cerebral cortex centers adjust cardiac reaction to a variety of emotional states; and the medullary control center regulates heart rate and blood pressure.

The nerve fibers from the cardiovascular control center synapse with autonomic neurons. When the parasympathetic nerves to the heart are stimulated, the sympathetic nerves to the heart, arterioles, and veins are usually inhibited. Because parasympathetic excitation and simultaneous sympathetic inhibition generally depress cardiac function (e.g., decrease the heart rate), these interneurons are often referred to as the **cardioinhibitory center.**[10] Excitation occurs with parasympathetic inhibition and sympathetic stimulation, and these interneurons are collectively called the **cardioexcitatory center.**[10] Therefore heart rate can be slowed by (1) inhibition of sympathetic stimulation of the SA node and (2) activation of parasympathetic stimulation of the SA node; and it can be increased by (1) activation of sympathetic nerves and (2) inhibition of parasympathetic nerves.

The resting heart rate in healthy individuals is primarily

Fig. 22-18 *Factors affecting cardiac performance.* Cardiac output, which is amount of blood (in liters) ejected by the heart per minute, depends on heart rate (beats per minute) and stroke volume (milliliters of blood ejected during ventricular systole).

under the control of parasympathetic stimulation. Parasympathetic effects from the vagus nerves override sympathetic effects in the SA node. Interruption of the vagus nerves causes significant tachycardia (abnormally fast heart rate) because the inhibitory parasympathetic influence is lost.

Neural reflexes

The **Bainbridge reflex** causes the heart rate to increase after intravenous infusions of blood or other fluid. The magnitude of the change in heart rate depends on the initial heart rate. If the initial rate is slow, intravenous infusion usually accelerates it, but if the initial rate is rapid, infusions will usually slow it down.[1]

The **baroreceptor reflex** facilitates blood pressure changes and heart rate changes. It is mediated by tissue pressure receptors (pressoreceptors) in the aortic arch and carotid arteries. The pressoreceptors increase their rate of discharge, sending neural impulses over the glossopharyngeal nerve (ninth cranial nerve) and through the vagus nerve to the cardiovascular control centers in the medulla. These centers increase parasympathetic activity and decrease sympathetic activity, causing blood vessels to dilate and heart rate to decrease. Responses to the baroreceptor reflex return the blood pressure to its previous level, which may or may not be normal. The higher the blood pressure, the greater the reflexive decrease in heart rate. If blood pressure is decreased, the baroreceptor reflex accelerates heart rate and causes vessels to constrict, raising blood pressure back toward normal.

Neural receptors in the lungs cause heart rate to increase during inspiration and decrease during expiration. The vagal fibers are stretched in inspiration and inhibit the car-

dioinhibitory center of the medulla. This allows unopposed sympathetic acceleration of heart rate.

Hormones and biochemicals

Hormones and biochemicals affect the arteries, arterioles, venules, capillaries, and contractility of the myocardium. Norepinephrine increases heart rate, enhances myocardial contractility, and constricts blood vessels. Epinephrine dilates vessels of the liver and skeletal muscle and also causes an increase in myocardial contractility. Some adrenocortical hormones, such as hydrocortisone, potentiate the effects of these catecholamines.

Thyroid hormones enhance sympathetic activity, promoting increased cardiac output. A decrease in growth hormone, as well as thyroid and adrenal hormones, results in bradycardia (heart rate below 60 beats/min), reduced cardiac output, and low blood pressure.

Myocardial contractility

Stroke volume, or the volume of blood ejected per beat during systole, depends on the *force* of contraction, which depends on myocardial contractility, or the degree of myocardial fiber shortening. Two major factors determine the force of contraction: (1) changes in the stretching of the ventricular myocardium caused by changes in ventricular volume (preload) and (2) alterations in the sympathetic activation of the ventricles. Increased blood flow from the veins into the heart distends the ventricle by increasing preload, which increases the stroke volume and, subsequently, cardiac output. Increased output then causes increased venous return, atrial volume and pressure, and eventually increased end-diastolic volume and stroke volume.

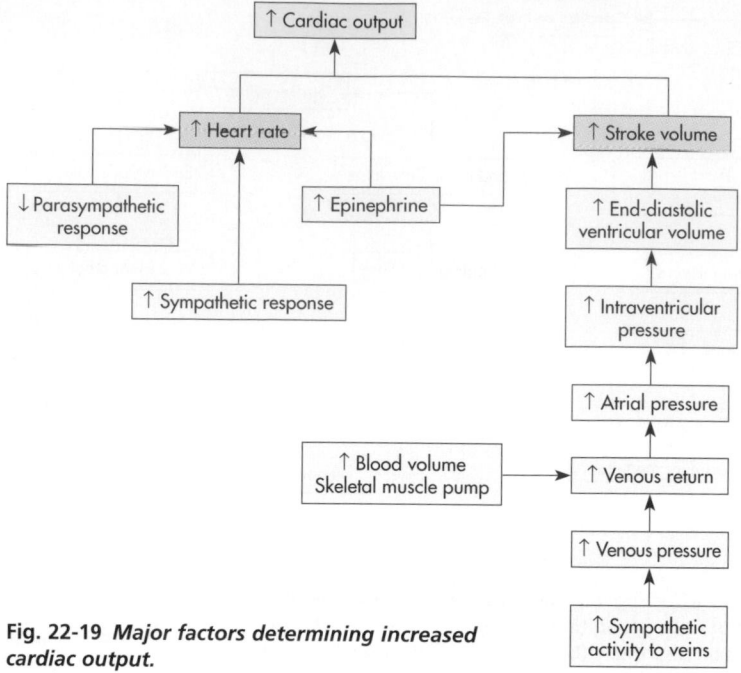

Fig. 22-19 *Major factors determining increased cardiac output.*

Factors affecting contractility are called ***inotropic agents.*** Positive inotropic agents increase the velocity of myocardial contraction and stroke volume and include excess thyroid hormone, epinephrine, norepinephrine, dopamine or isoproterenol infusion, and calcium salt infusion. The negative inotropic agents decrease the velocity of myocardial contraction and the stroke volume and include alcohol, procainamide, quinidine, and propranolol.

Myocardial contractility is also affected by oxygen and carbon dioxide levels (tensions) in the coronary blood. With severe hypoxemia (arterial oxygen saturation less than 50%), contractility is decreased. With less severe hypoxemia (saturation more than 50%), contractility is stimulated. Moderate degrees of hypoxemia may increase contractility by enhancing the myocardial response to circulating catecholamines.[1]

Factors determining cardiac output

Cardiac output is the volume of blood flowing through either the systemic or the pulmonary circuit per minute and is expressed in liters per minute. Heart rate is multiplied by stroke volume to determine cardiac output. The volume to which the ventricle fills is determined by the ventricular filling pressure and the ventricle's compliance. The filling pressures of the ventricles are the ***right*** and ***left atrial pressures,*** respectively. Normal cardiac output is about 5 L/min for a resting adult. A summary of the major factors that determine cardiac output is presented in Fig. 22-19. (Also see preceding discussions of heart rate and myocardial contractility [stroke volume].)

The ventricle does not eject all the blood it contains; the amount ejected is called the ***ejection fraction,*** or the stroke volume divided by the end-diastolic volume. The end-

diastolic volume of the normal ventricle is about 70 to 80 ml/m^2; the normal ejection fraction of the resting heart is about 60% to 75%.[11] The ejection fraction is increased by factors that increase contractility (e.g., sympathetic nervous system activity). A decrease in ejection fraction is a hallmark of ventricular failure.[11] The effects of aging on cardiovascular function are summarized in the Aging box.

✓ QUICK CHECK

Why is sympathetic activity important to cardiac output?

Why is the Frank-Starling law of the heart important to understand heart failure?

What are the important factors regulating cardiac performance?

THE SYSTEMIC CIRCULATION

The arteries and veins of the systemic circulation are illustrated in Fig. 22-20. Blood from the left side of the heart flows through the aorta and into the systemic arteries. The ***arteries*** branch into small ***arterioles,*** which branch further into the smallest vessels, the ***capillaries,*** where nutrient exchange between the blood and tissues occurs. Blood from the capillaries then enters tiny ***venules*** that join together to form the larger veins, which return venous blood to the right heart. ***Peripheral vascular system*** is an imprecise term used to describe the part of the systemic circulation that supplies the skin and the extremities, particularly the legs and feet.

⚠ AGING & *Cardiovascular Function*

Determinant	Resting Cardiac Performance	Exercise Cardiac Performance
Cardiac output	Unchanged or slightly decreased in women only	Declines because of a decrease in heart rate and stroke volume
Heart rate	Slight decrease	Increases less than in younger people, possibly because of decreased cardiovascular response to catecholamines; overall slight decrease
Stroke volume	Slight increase	Slight increase
Ejection fraction	Unchanged	Increases more from rest to exercise in younger people than in older people
Afterload	Increased	Uncertain
End-diastolic volume	Unchanged	Smaller for women
End-systolic volume	Unchanged	Lesser increase
Contraction	Increased because of prolonged relaxation	Decreases with vigorous exercise*
Cardiac dilation	No change	Increases at end diastole and end systole
V̇O₂ max	Not applicable	Declines because of a decline in skeletal muscle mass
Size of ventricle	Hypertrophy secondary to loss of cells and impedance to ventricular ejection	Uncertain
Large arteries	Stiffen with age	Uncertain

Data from Gerstenblith, G. & Lakatta, E.G. (1995). Aging and the cardiovascular system. In J.T. Willerson & J.N. Cohn (Eds.). Cardiovascular medicine. New York: Churchill Livingstone; Weisfeldt, M. (1998). Aging changes in the cardiovascular system and response to stress. American Journal of Hypertension 11(3 Pt 2), 415-455.
*As measured by end-systolic volume/systolic blood pressure (ESV/SBP), an index of contractility.

Structure of Blood Vessels

Blood vessel walls are composed of three layers: (1) the *tunica intima* (innermost, or *intimal, layer*), (2) the *tunica media* (middle, or *medial, layer*), and (3) the *tunica externa* or *adventitia* (outermost, or external, layer). These structures are illustrated in Fig. 22-21. Blood vessel walls vary in thickness depending on the thickness or absence of one or more of these three layers. Cells of the larger vessels are nourished by the *vasa vasorum,* small vessels located in the tunica externa.

Arterial vessels

Arterial walls are composed of elastic connective tissue, fibrous connective tissue, and smooth muscle. *Elastic arteries* have a very thick tunica media with more elastic fibers than smooth muscle fibers. Examples include the aorta and its major branches and the pulmonary trunk. Elasticity allows the vessel to stretch as blood is ejected from the heart during systole. During diastole, elasticity promotes recoil of the arteries, maintaining blood pressure within the vessels.

Muscular arteries are medium-size and small arteries and are farther from the heart than the elastic arteries. They contain more muscle fibers than the elastic arteries because they need less stretch and recoil. The muscular arteries distribute blood to arterioles throughout the body and help control blood flow because their smooth muscle can be stimulated to contract or relax. Contraction narrows the vessel *lumen* (the internal cavity of the vessel), which diminishes flow through the vessel *(vasoconstriction).* When the smooth muscle layer relaxes, more blood flows through the vessel lumen *(vasodilation).*

An artery becomes an arteriole where the diameter of its lumen narrows to less than 0.5 mm. The arterioles are composed almost exclusively of smooth muscle and regulate the flow of blood into the capillaries by vasoconstriction, which retards the flow of blood into the capillaries, and vasodilation, which permits blood to enter the capillaries freely (Fig. 22-22). The thick smooth muscle layer of the arterioles is a major determinant of the resistance blood encounters as it flows through the systemic circulation.

The capillary network is composed of connective channels, or thoroughfares, called *metarterioles,* and "true" capillaries (Fig. 22-23). The capillaries branch from the metarterioles, meeting at a ring of smooth muscle called the *precapillary sphincter.* As the sphincters contract and relax, they regulate blood flow through the capillaries. Appropriately stimulated, the precapillary sphincters help to maintain arterial pressure and regulate selective flow to vascular beds.

The capillary walls are very thin, making possible the rapid exchange of substrates, metabolites, and special products (e.g., hormones) between the blood and the interstitial fluid, from which they are taken up by the cells. A single endothelial cell may form the entire vessel wall if the capillary has no tunica media or tunica externa. In some capillaries, the endothelial cells contain oval windows or pores termed *fenestrations,* which are generally covered by a thin diaphragm.

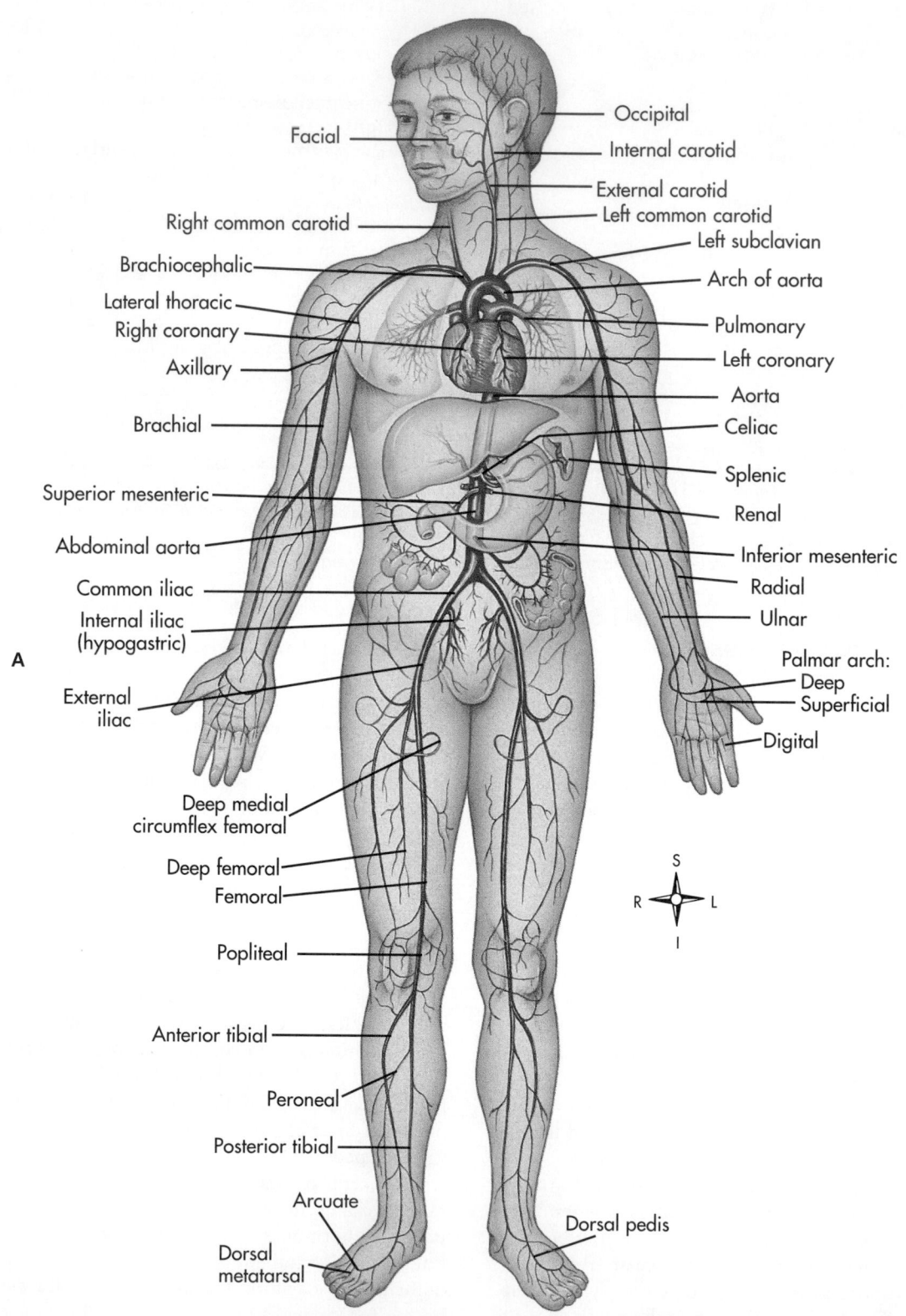

Facial

Occipital

Internal carotid

External carotid

Right common carotid

Left common carotid

Left subclavian

Brachiocephalic

Arch of aorta

Lateral thoracic

Pulmonary

Right coronary

Left coronary

Axillary

Aorta

Brachial

Celiac

Splenic

Superior mesenteric

Renal

Abdominal aorta

Inferior mesenteric

Common iliac

Radial

Internal iliac
(hypogastric)

Ulnar

Palmar arch:
Deep
Superficial

A

External
iliac

Digital

Deep medial
circumflex femoral

Deep femoral

Femoral

Popliteal

Anterior tibial

Peroneal

Posterior tibial

Arcuate

Dorsal pedis

Dorsal
metatarsal

Fig. 22-20 *Circulatory system.* **A,** Principal arteries of body.

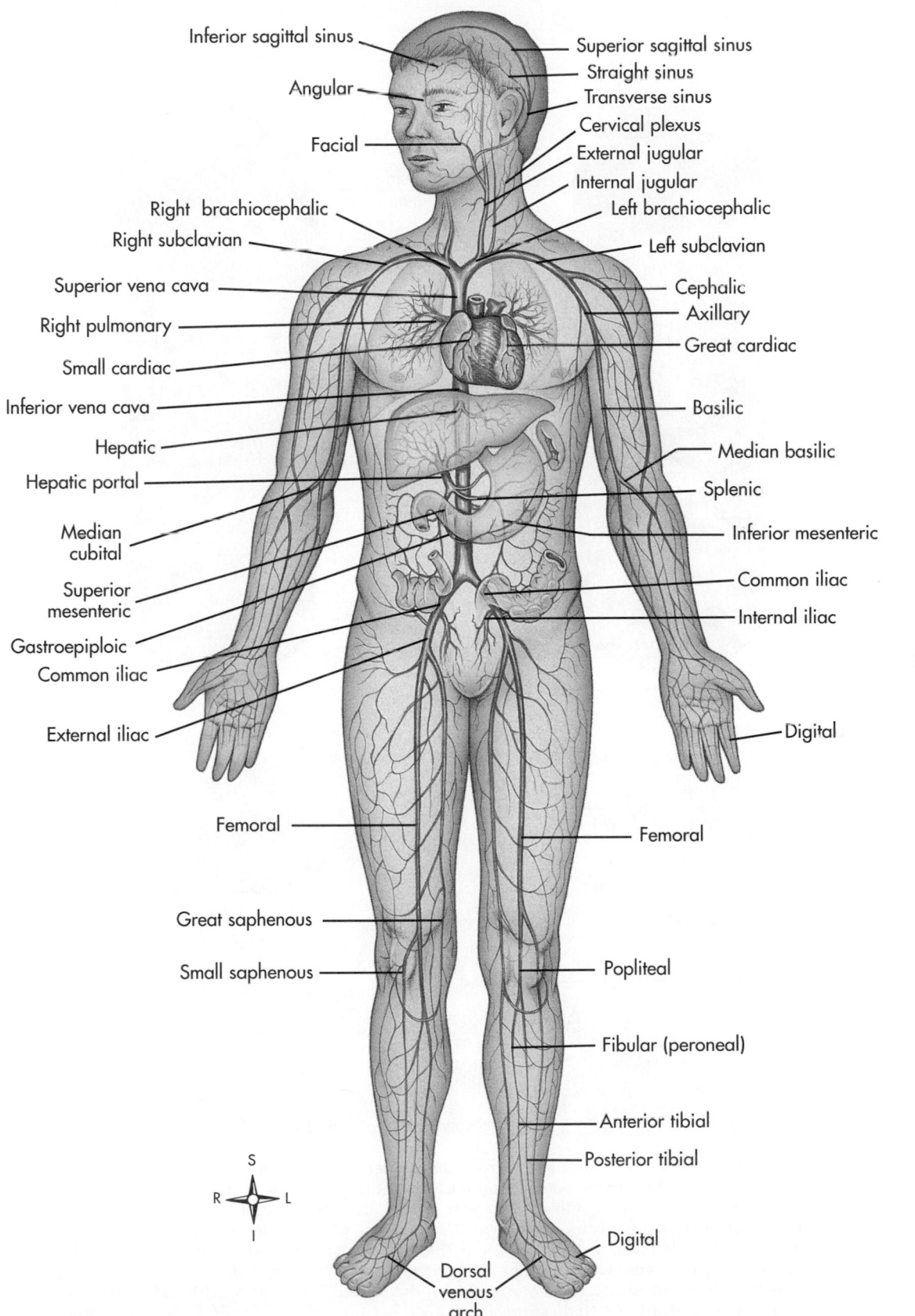

Inferior sagittal sinus
Angular
Facial
Right brachiocephalic
Right subclavian
Superior vena cava
Right pulmonary
Small cardiac
Inferior vena cava
Hepatic
Hepatic portal
Median cubital
Superior mesenteric
Gastroepiploic
Common iliac
External iliac
Femoral
Great saphenous
Small saphenous

Superior sagittal sinus
Straight sinus
Transverse sinus
Cervical plexus
External jugular
Internal jugular
Left brachiocephalic
Left subclavian
Cephalic
Axillary
Great cardiac
Basilic
Median basilic
Splenic
Inferior mesenteric
Common iliac
Internal iliac
Digital
Femoral
Popliteal
Fibular (peroneal)
Anterior tibial
Posterior tibial
Digital
Dorsal venous arch

S
R — L
I

B

Fig. 22-20, cont'd B, Principal veins of body. *(From Thibodeau, G.A. & Patton, K.T. [1999]. Anatomy & physiology [4th ed.]. St. Louis: Mosby.)*

Fig. 22-21 *Schematic drawings and micrograph of artery and vein.* **A,** Shown are the comparative thickness of three coats: outer coat (tunica adventitia), muscle coat (tunica media), and lining of endothelium (tunica intima). Note that muscle and outer coats are much thinner in veins than in arteries and that veins have valves. **B,** Micrograph of a cross section of tissue containing both an artery *(left)* and a vein *(right).* Note the thickness of the smooth muscle (tunica media) in the artery compared with the vein. *(A modified from Thompson, J.M. et al. [1997]. Mosby's clinical nursing [4th ed.]. St. Louis: Mosby; B from Thibodeau, G.A. & Patton, K.T. [1999]. Anatomy & physiology [4th ed.]. St. Louis: Mosby.)*

Capillary

Arteriole

Precapillary
sphincters

Fig. 22-22 *Capillary wall.* Capillaries have a wall composed of only a single layer of flattened cells, whereas the walls of the larger vessels also have smooth muscle. *(From Thibodeau, G.A. & Patton, K.T. [1999]. Anatomy & physiology [4th ed.]. St. Louis: Mosby.)*

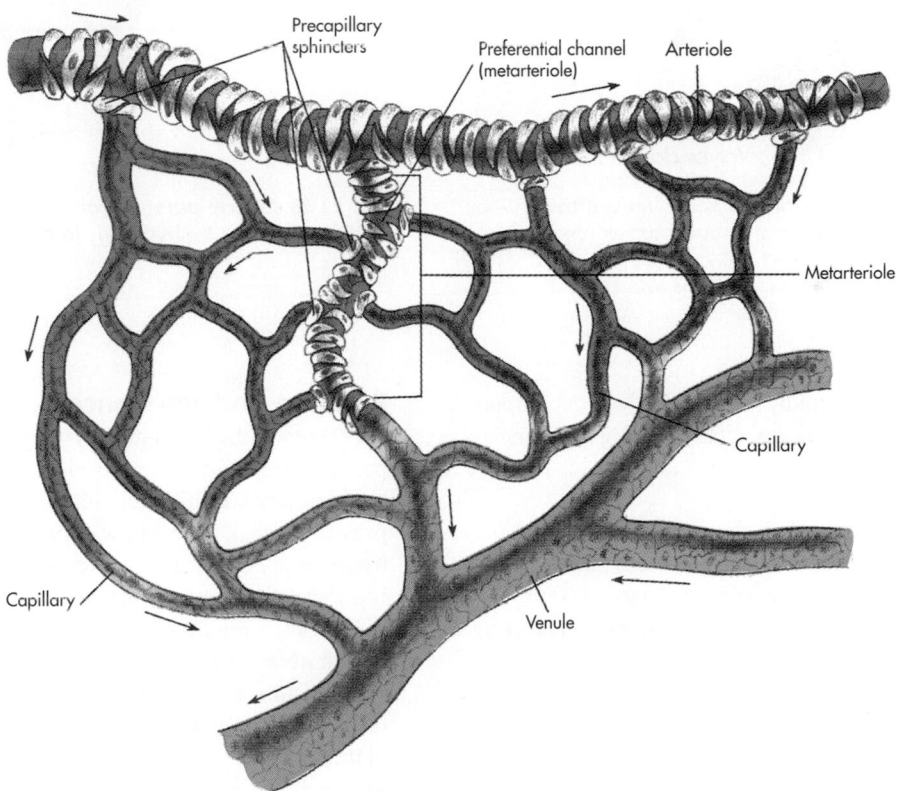

Precapillary
sphincters

Preferential channel
(metarteriole)

Arteriole

Metarteriole

Capillary

Capillary

Venule

Fig. 22-23 *Capillary network.* Blood enters network as arterial blood and exits as venous blood.

Substances pass between the capillary lumen and the interstitial fluid (1) through junctions between endothelial cells, (2) through fenestrations in endothelial cells, (3) in vesicles moved by active transport across the endothelial cell membrane, or (4) by diffusion through the endothelial cell membrane. A single capillary may be only 0.5 to 1 mm in length and 0.01 mm in diameter, but the capillaries are so numerous that their total surface area may be more than 600 m^2, or larger than 100 football fields.

Control of vessel contraction or relaxation: vasomotion

The endothelium is a source of substances that promote contraction or relaxation, *vasomotion,* of the vascular smooth muscle. *Prostacyclin,* a prostaglandin formed in the endothelium from arachidonic acid, can relax vascular smooth muscle through increases in cyclic adenosine monophosphate (cAMP). Prostacyclin inhibits platelet adherence to the endothelium, thereby preventing intravascular clot formation.

Endothelial-derived relaxing factor (EDRF), now identified as *nitric oxide (NO),* is produced and released by stimulation of the endothelial cells. NO activates second messengers in the vascular smooth muscle, producing relaxation. NO is also known as an antithrombotic agent in the vasculature.

The endothelium also can produce an *endothelial-derived contracting factor (EDCF),* a vasoconstrictor, yet little is known about its function. Apparently it is not *endothelin,* a potent vasoconstrictor protein that has been isolated from endothelial cells. The endothelium also secretes an-

Fig. 22-24 *Valves of vein.* Pooled blood is moved toward heart as valves are forced open by pressure from volume of blood downstream. *(From Thibodeau, G.A. & Patton, K.T. [1999]. Anatomy & physiology [4th ed.]. St. Louis: Mosby.)*

Fig. 22-25 *Muscle pump. (From Thibodeau, G.A. & Patton, K.T. [1999].* Anatomy & physiology *[4th ed.]. St. Louis: Mosby.)*

giotensin (see p. 618). A rapidly growing body of data supports the concept of endothelin as a paracrine-acting hormone.[12,13]

Veins

The smallest venules closest to the capillaries have an inner lining, composed of the endothelium of the tunica intima and surrounded by fibrous tissue. The largest venules are surrounded by a few smooth muscle fibers constituting a thin tunica media.

Compared with arteries, *veins* are thin walled and fibrous and have a larger diameter (see Fig. 22-21). Veins also are more numerous than arteries. In veins the tunica externa has less elastic tissue than in arteries so veins do not recoil after distention as quickly as arteries. Like arteries, veins receive nourishment from the tiny vasa vasorum. Some veins, most commonly in the lower limbs, contain valves to regulate the one-way flow of blood toward the heart (Fig. 22-24). These valves are folds of the tunica intima and resemble the semilunar valves of the heart. When a person stands up, contraction of the skeletal muscles of the legs compresses the deep veins of the legs and assists the flow of blood toward the heart. This important mechanism of venous return is called the *muscle pump* (Fig. 22-25).

Factors Affecting Blood Flow

Blood flow is the amount of fluid moved per unit of time and is usually expressed as liters or milliliters per minute (ml/min) or cubic centimeters per second (cm³/sec). Flow is regulated by the same physical properties that govern the movement of simple fluids in a closed, rigid system, that is, pressure, resistance, velocity, turbulent versus laminar flow, and compliance.

Pressure and resistance

Pressure in a liquid system is the force exerted on the liquid per unit area and is expressed as dynes per square centimeter (dyn/cm²), millimeters of mercury (mm Hg), or units of pressure (torr). Blood flow depends partly on the difference between pressures in the arterial and venous vessels supplying the organ. Fluid moves from the arterial "side" of the capillaries, a region of greater pressure, to the venous side, a region of lesser pressure.

Resistance is the opposition to force. In the cardiovascular system, most opposition to blood flow is provided by the diameter and length of the blood vessels themselves. Therefore changes in blood flow through an organ result from changes in the vascular resistance within the organ. Resistance in a vessel is inversely related to blood flow; that is, increased resistance leads to decreased blood flow. *Poiseuille law* shows the relationship among blood flow, pressure, and resistance:

$$Q = \frac{\delta P}{R}$$

where Q = blood flow, δP = the pressure difference ($P_1 - P_2$), and R = resistance. Resistance to flow cannot be measured directly, but it can be calculated if the pressure difference and flow volumes are known.

Blood flow varies inversely with the viscosity of the fluid. Thick fluids move more slowly and experience greater resistance to flow than thin fluids. Blood that contains a high percentage of red cells is more viscous. This relationship is expressed as the hematocrit—the ratio of the volume of red

Fig. 22-26 *Lumen diameter, blood flow, and resistance.* **A,** Effect of lumen diameter on flow through vessel. *d,* Diameter. **B,** Blood flows with great speed in the large arteries. However, branching of arterial vessels increases the total cross-sectional area of the arterioles and capillaries, reducing the flow rate. When capillaries merge into venules and venules merge into veins, the total cross-sectional area decreases, causing the flow rate to increase. *(B from Thibodeau, G.A. & Patton, K.T. [1999]. Anatomy & physiology [4th ed.]. St. Louis: Mosby.)*

blood cells to the volume of whole blood. A high hematocrit reduces flow through the blood vessels, particularly the *microcirculation* (arterioles, capillaries, venules). Conditions in which the hematocrit is elevated, for example, dehydration, cyanotic congenital heart disease, or polycythemia, can lead to increased cardiac work as a result of increased vascular resistance.

The viscosity of blood also increases if blood flow becomes very slow or stagnates *(anomalous viscosity).* This is generally not significant unless cardiac output is low as in shock. (Shock is described in Chapter 23.)

Poiseuille formula for resistance to fluid flow through a tube takes into account the length of the tube, the viscosity of the fluid, and the radius of the tube's lumen. Resistance (R) is proportional to a constant ($8/\pi$), the viscosity of the blood (η), and the length of the vessel (l), and it is inversely proportional to the fourth power of the lumen's radius (v_4).[1] Because this relationship was derived using straight, rigid tubes with steady, streamlined flow, it cannot be applied *directly* to the vascular system, but it is a useful model of vascular resistance.

The most important factor determining resistance *in a single vessel* is the caliber of the vessel's lumen, expressed in Poiseuille formula as its radius and in Fig. 22-26 as its diameter. Small changes in the lumen's radius lead to large changes in vascular resistance.

Generally, resistance to flow is greater in longer tubes because resistance increases with length. Blood flowing through the distributing arteries, beginning with branches off the aorta and ending at arterioles in the capillary bed, encounters more resistance than blood flowing through the

capillary bed itself, where flow is distributed among many short, tiny branches arranged in parallel.

Resistance to flow through a system of vessels, or *total resistance,* depends not only on characteristics of individual vessels but also on whether the vessels are arranged in series or in parallel (Fig. 22-27). For vessels arranged in series, total resistance equals the sum obtained by adding all the individual resistances calculated using the Poiseuille formula. For vessels arranged in parallel, total resistance equals the sum of the reciprocals ($1/R$) of the individual resistances.

Total resistance is related to the total cross-sectional area of a system of vessels in parallel and to the number of vessels in parallel that make up the total cross-sectional area. The larger the total cross-sectional area, as in the capillary system, the lower the resistance. However, if a cross-sectional area is made up of a very large number of parallel vessels, the overall resistance will be greater than it would be if the cross-sectional area were made up of only two or three parallel vessels. Therefore resistance is greater in smaller vessels than in larger vessels. The total cross-sectional area of the arteriolar system is greater than that of the arterial system, yet the greater number of arterioles arranged in parallel leads to great resistance to flow in the arteriolar system. Although the capillary system has a larger number of vessels in parallel than the arteriolar system, the total cross-sectional area is greater, resulting in lower resistance overall through the capillary system. The relationship between flow and cross-sectional area has physiologic significance. Despite the narrow diameter of each vessel (which normally increases resistance), total resistance in any capillary bed is relatively

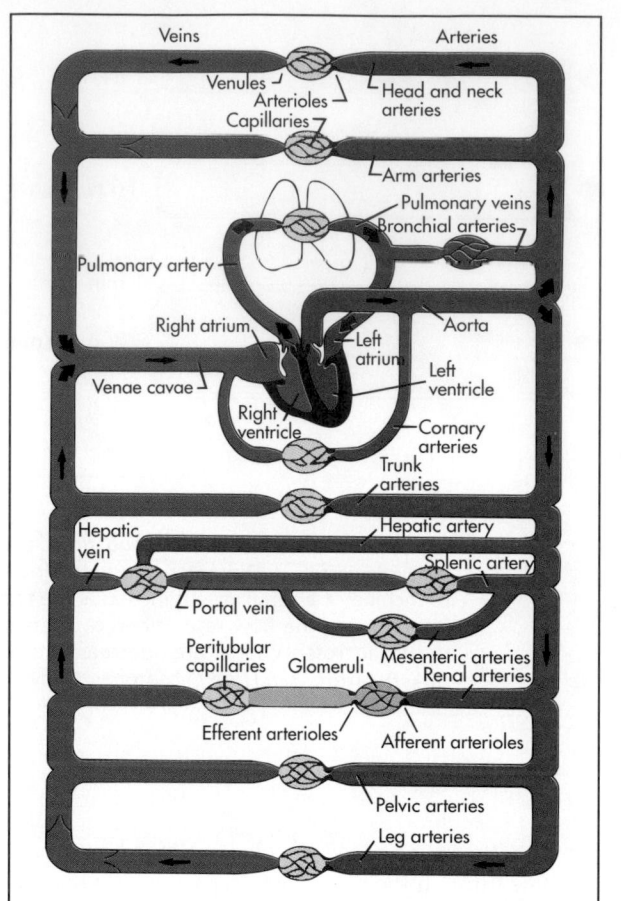

Fig. 22-27 *Schematic diagram of the parallel and series arrangement of the vessels composing the circulatory system.* **A,** Resistance in blood vessels arranged in series or parallel. *R,* Resistance in an individual vessel. **B,** The capillary beds are represented by thin lines connecting the arterioles (on the right) and the veins (on the left). The crescent-shaped thickenings proximal to the capillary beds represent the arterioles (resistance vessels). *(B from Berne, R.M. & Levy, M.N. [1992]. Cardiovascular physiology [6th ed.]. St. Louis: Mosby.)*

low. This, plus the slow velocity of flow in each vessel, promotes optimal capillary-tissue exchange.

Neural control of total peripheral resistance

Total resistance in the systemic circulation, sometimes called *total peripheral resistance,* is determined primarily by change in the diameter of the arterioles. Reflex control of total cardiac output and peripheral resistance includes (1) sympathetic stimulation of heart, arterioles, and veins; and (2) parasympathetic stimulation of the heart only.

The autonomic nervous system is monitored by the cardiovascular control center in the brain (see p. 606). The hypothalamic centers regulate vascular (and cardiac) responses to changes in temperature. When the body's core temperature exceeds normal, the hypothalamus reflex initiates dilation of arterioles and veins in the skin. This causes shunting of blood to the skin, where heat is lost from sweating, radiation, conduction, or convection. When body core temperature decreases below normal, surface vessels constrict, shunting blood to the vital organs. Vasoconstriction is regulated by an area of the brain stem that maintains a constant (tonic) output of norepinephrine from sympathetic fibers in the peripheral arterioles. This tonic activity is essential for maintenance of blood pressure.

During exercise and stress, the sympathetic fibers that stimulate vasodilation of skeletal muscle arterioles are

thought to be under the direct control of the cerebral cortex and hypothalamus and *not* the medullary centers.[14] Information about pressure and resistance is sensed by neural receptors (baroreceptors, chemoreceptors) in arterial walls and delivered to the medullary centers.

Baroreceptors

Major stretch receptors (baroreceptors) are located in the aorta and in the carotid sinus (Fig. 22-28). They respond to changes in smooth muscle fiber length by altering their rate of discharge and supply sensory information to the cardiovascular center that regulates blood pressure. The net effect of this major blood pressure–regulating reflex is to reduce blood pressure to normal by decreasing cardiac output (heart rate and stroke volume) and peripheral resistance. (Postural changes and the baroreceptor reflex are discussed in Chapter 23.)

Arterial chemoreceptors

Specialized areas within the aortic and carotid arteries are sensitive to concentrations of oxygen, carbon dioxide, and hydrogen ions (pH) in the blood. These chemoreceptors are most important for the control of respiration but also transmit impulses to the medullary cardiovascular centers that regulate blood pressure. If arterial oxygen concentration or pH falls, a reflexive increase in blood pressure occurs, whereas

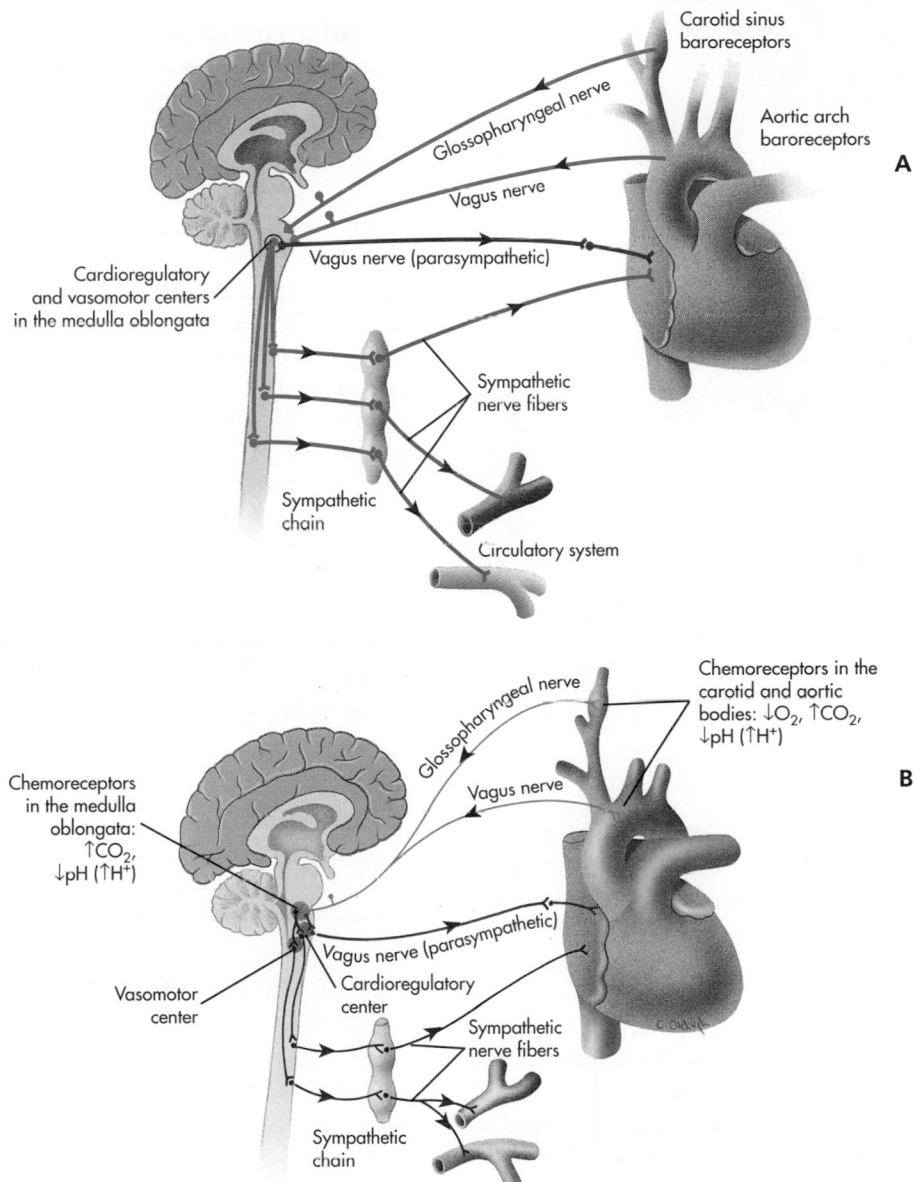

Fig. 22-28 *Baroreceptors and chemoreceptor reflex control of blood pressure.* A, Baroreceptor reflexes. Baroreceptors located in the carotid sinuses and aortic arch detect changes in blood pressure. Action potentials are conducted to the cardioregulatory and vasomotor centers. The heart rate can be decreased by the parasympathetic system; the heart rate and stroke volume can be increased by the sympathetic system. The sympathetic system also can constrict or dilate blood vessels. **B,** Chemoreceptor reflexes. Chemoreceptors located in the medulla oblongata and in the carotid and aortic bodies detect changes in blood oxygen, carbon dioxide, or pH. Action potentials are conducted to the medulla oblongata. In response, the vasomotor center can cause vasoconstriction or dilation of blood vessels by the sympathetic system, and the cardioregulatory center can cause changes in the pumping activity of the heart through the parasympathetic and sympathetic systems. *(From Seeley, R.R., Stephens, T.D., & Tate, P. [1995]. Anatomy and physiology [3rd ed]. St. Louis: Mosby.)*

Fig. 22-29 *Laminar and turbulent blood flow.* **A,** Laminar flow. Fluid flows in long, smooth-walled tubes as if it is composed of a large number of concentric layers. **B,** Turbulent flow. Turbulent flow is caused by numerous small currents flowing crosswise or oblique to the long axis of the vessel, resulting in flowing whorls and eddy currents. *(From Seeley, R.R., Stephens, T.D., & Tate, P. [1995]. Anatomy and physiology [3rd ed]. St. Louis: Mosby.)*

an increase in carbon dioxide causes a decrease in blood pressure. The major chemoreceptive reflex is the result of alterations in arterial oxygen concentration with only minor effects resulting from altered pH or carbon dioxide levels.

Velocity
Blood velocity is the *distance* blood travels in a unit of time, usually centimeters per second (cm/sec). It is directly related to blood flow (*amount* of blood moved per unit of time) and inversely related to the cross-sectional area of the vessel in which the blood is flowing. As blood moves from the aorta to the capillaries, the total cross-sectional area of the vessels increases and velocity of flow decreases.

Laminar versus turbulent flow
Normally, blood flow through the vessels is *laminar,* meaning that concentric layers of molecules move "straight ahead." Each concentric layer flows at a different velocity (Fig. 22-29). The cohesive attraction between the fluid and the vessel wall prevents the molecules of blood that are in contact with the wall from moving. The next thin layer of blood is able to slide slowly past the stationary layer and so on until, at the center, the blood velocity is greatest. Large vessels have room for a large center layer; therefore they have less resistance to flow and greater flow and velocity than smaller vessels.

Where flow is obstructed, the vessel turns, or blood flows

over rough surfaces, the flow becomes *turbulent,* with whorls or eddy currents that produce noise, causing a murmur to be heard on auscultation. Resistance increases with turbulence.

Vascular compliance
Vascular compliance is the increase in volume a vessel can accommodate for a given increase in pressure. Compliance depends on the ratio of elastic fibers to muscle fibers in the vessel wall. The elastic arteries are more compliant than the muscular arteries, and the veins are more compliant than either type of artery, and they can serve as storage areas for the circulatory system.

Compliance determines a vessel's response to pressure changes. For example, with a very small increase in pressure, a large volume of blood can be accommodated by the venous system. In the less compliant arterial system, where smaller volumes and higher pressures are normal, small variations in pressure cause little or no change in the volume of blood within the arterial vessels.

Stiffness is the opposite of compliance. Several conditions and disorders can cause stiffness, with the most common being arteriosclerosis (see Chapter 23).

✓ QUICK CHECK

Why is the muscle pump important to venous blood flow?

How does lumen diameter affect blood flow through vessels?

Why does total cross-sectional area in the capillary system lower the resistance to flow?

Regulation of Blood Pressure
Arterial pressure
Arterial pressure is constantly regulated to maintain tissue *perfusion,* or blood supply to the capillary beds, during a wide range of physiologic conditions, including changes in body position, muscular activity, and circulating blood volume. The *mean arterial pressure (MAP),* which is the average pressure in the arteries throughout the cardiac cycle, depends on the elastic properties of the arterial walls and the *mean* volume of blood in the arterial system. MAP can be approximated from the measured values of the systolic (Ps) and diastolic (Pd) pressures as follows: MAP = Pd + 1/3(Ps − Pd, or pulse pressure). The major factors and relationships that regulate arterial blood pressure are summarized in Fig. 22-30. Table 22-2 summarizes factors that affect both mean arterial pressure and capillary flow.

Antidiuretic hormone, renin-angiotensin system, atrial natriuretic hormone, and insulin
Blood pressure can be influenced by factors that change the total volume of blood in the circulatory system. Recall that

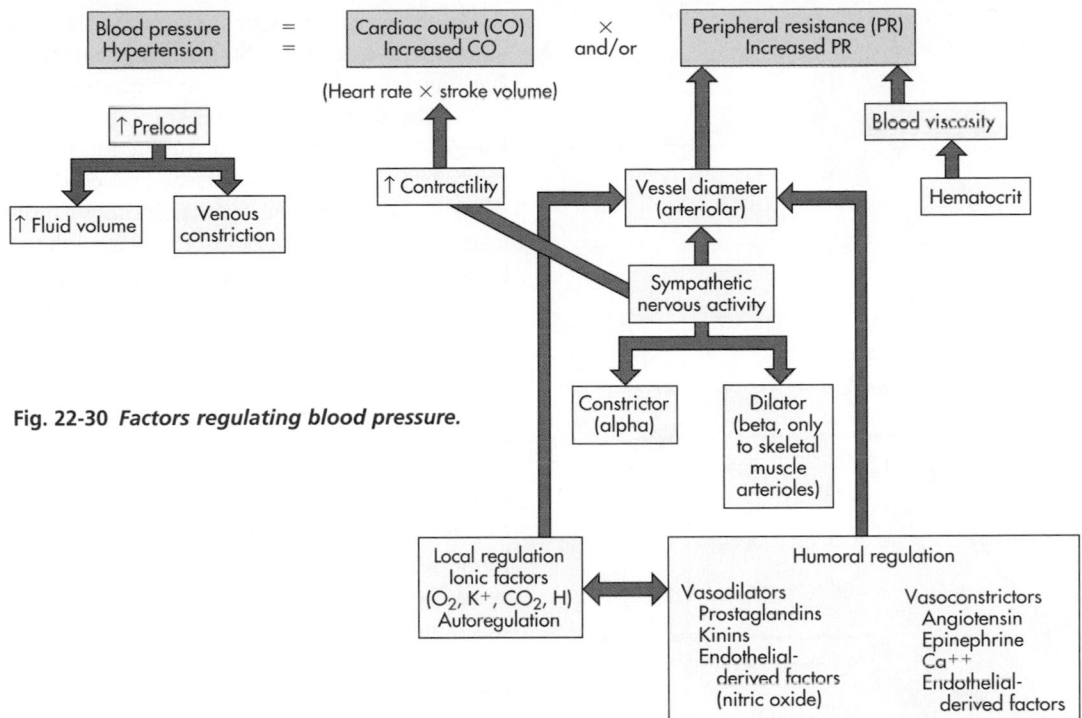

Fig. 22-30 *Factors regulating blood pressure.*

ADH (antidiuretic hormone) is released by the posterior pituitary and causes reabsorption of water by the kidney. With reabsorption, the blood plasma volume will increase, increasing blood pressure (Fig. 22-31) (see also Chapters 4 and 17).

Renin is an enzyme synthesized and secreted by the juxtaglomerular cells of the kidney. It has also been found in the adrenal cortex, salivary gland, prolactin-producing and luteinizing hormone–producing cells of the pituitary, arterial smooth muscle cells in the vascular endothelial cell, brain, and myocardium.[15] Factors that control renin release include the following:

1. A drop in blood pressure (e.g., the renal artery)
2. A decrease in the amount of sodium delivered to the kidney (although recent evidence indicates a role for chloride in regulating renin secretion)[15]
3. β-adrenergic stimuli (increase renin release)
4. β-adrenergic inhibitors (decrease renin release)
5. Angiotensin II (reduces renin release)
6. Low potassium concentrations in plasma (increase renin release)

Once in the circulation, renin splits off a polypeptide from angiotensinogen to generate *angiotensin I.* This is converted by an enzyme, angiotensin-converting enzyme (ACE), to *angiotensin II,* a powerful vasoconstrictor that stimulates the secretion of *aldosterone* from the adrenal gland (see Figs. 22-31 and 17-18). Angiotensin II is now considered a growth promoter in cardiovascular tissues, resulting in vascular hypertrophy and progression of hypertension. Aldosterone causes reabsorption of sodium in the kidneys. In addition, angiotensin II causes some sodium re-

TABLE 22-2	Factors That Affect Mean Arterial Pressure and Capillary Flow	
	Mean Arterial Pressure	**Capillary Flow**
Peripheral resistance*		
Increased	Increased	Decreased
Decreased	Decreased	Increased
Heart rate†		
Increased	Increased	Increased
Decreased	Decreased	Decreased
Stroke volume‡		
Increased	Increased	Increased
Decreased	Decreased	Decreased

From Little, R.C. (1985). Physiology of the heart and circulation (3rd ed.). St. Louis: Mosby.
*Cardiac output constant.
†Peripheral resistance and stroke volume constant.
‡Peripheral resistance and heart rate constant.

tention in the kidneys and suppresses renin secretion from the juxtaglomerular cells.[15,16]

This kidney-based renin-angiotensin system serves as an important regulatory loop. For example, decreases in blood pressure or sodium delivery to the kidneys (macula densa), as might occur after hemorrhage or extracellular volume deficits (dehydration), stimulate secretion of renin, which

Posterior pituitary

ADH

ANH

(Vasoconstriction)

Adrenal cortex

Angiotensin II (ACE)

Aldosterone

Angiotensin I

Renin

Angiotensinogen

Kidney

Fluid and Na+ loss from ANH (urine)

Fig. 22-31 *Three mechanisms that influence total plasma volume.* The antidiuretic hormone (ADH) mechanism and renin-angiotensin and aldosterone mechanisms tend to increase water retention and thus increase total plasma volume. The atrial natriuretic hormone (ANH) mechanism antagonizes these mechanisms by promoting water loss and thus promoting a decrease in total plasma volume. *ACE,* Angiotensin converting enzyme. *(Modified from Thibodeau, G.A. & Patton, K.T. [1999].* Anatomy & physiology *[4th ed.]. St. Louis: Mosby.)*

forms angiotensin I, which is converted to angiotensin II, and restores blood pressure. Sodium retention also results from increased secretion of aldosterone. Overall, the renin-angiotensin system is activated after volume depletion or hypotension, or both, and is suppressed after volume repletion and hypertension. Basic knowledge of the renin-angiotensin system has advanced. In the past 10 years one of the most important advances is knowledge of a *tissue-based* renin-angiotensin system that can be independently regulated from the circulation. New data on the role of the tissue renin-angiotensin system are redefining our understanding of the pathophysiology of hypertension and other vascular disorders. The tissue renin-angiotensin system is activated in response to tissue injury.[17,18] This system is involved in maladaptive alterations, such as ventricular and vascular remodeling, alterations in renal function, and atherosclerosis[18] (see Chapter 23). Particularly significant is an increased recogni-

tion of the role of angiotensin II in these processes. Angiotensin II has two subtypes of receptors, AT1 and AT2. Both subtypes, AT1 and AT2, are expressed in human hearts. AT1 is also found on vascular smooth muscle and endothelial cells, nerve endings, and conduction tissues. AT2 has, so far, been found in fibrous tissue and endothelial cells. AT1 mediates myocyte hypertrophy, fibroblast proliferation, collagen synthesis, smooth muscle cell growth, endothelial adhesion molecule expression, and catecholamine synthesis.[19] Therefore treatments such as angiotensin-converting enzyme (ACE) inhibitors and angiotensin receptor (ATR) antagonists that inhibit mostly AT1 receptors are a main target in preventive and reparative strategies in cardiovascular diseases.

Another mechanism that can change blood plasma volume and, therefore, blood pressure is the *atrial natriuretic hormone* or factor *(ANH)* (see Fig. 22-31). ANH is a hormone secreted from cells in the right atrium when right atrial blood pressure increases. ANH inhibits antidiuretic hormone by increasing urine sodium loss, leading to the formation of a large volume of dilute urine that decreases blood volume and blood pressure.

In vitro studies demonstrate that *insulin* has direct vascular actions that contribute to both vascular protection and injury. The vascular protection and injury properties are summarized in Box 22-2. More attention is being given to insulin resistance as a cause of atherosclerosis because persons with type II diabetes have a threefold increased risk of coronary artery disease and persons with prediabetes, without chronic hyperglycemia, have a twofold increased risk.[20,21]

Venous pressure

The main determinants of venous blood pressure are (1) the volume of fluid within the veins and (2) the compliance (distensibility) of the vessel walls. The venous system accommodates approximately 60% of the total blood volume at any given moment, with venous pressure averaging less than 10 mm Hg. The arteries accommodate about 15% of the total blood volume, with an average arterial pressure (blood pressure) of about 100 mm Hg.[14]

The sympathetic nervous system controls compliance. The walls of the veins are highly innervated by sympathetic fibers that, when stimulated, cause venous smooth muscle to contract and increase muscle tone. This stiffens the wall of the vein, which reduces distensibility and increases blood pressure, forcing more blood through the veins and into the right heart.

Two other mechanisms that increase venous pressure and venous return to the heart are (1) the skeletal muscle pump and (2) the respiratory pump. During skeletal muscle contraction, the veins within the muscles are partially compressed, causing decreased venous capacity and increased return to the heart. The respiratory pump acts during inspiration, when the veins of the abdomen are partially compressed by the downward movement of the diaphragm. Increased abdominal pressure moves blood toward the heart.

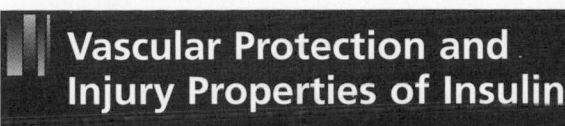

Vascular Protection and Injury Properties of Insulin

BOX 22-2

PROTECTION

Insulin increases endothelial cell production of nitric oxide.

Nitric oxide (NO) (in vitro) inhibits growth of vascular smooth muscle cells.

NO decreases the inflammatory reaction by inhibiting the expression of adhesion molecules, inhibiting the activity of proinflammatory cytokines (e.g., TNF-α, monocyte chemoattractant protein-1 MCP-1]). Thus NO decreases the binding of monocytes/macrophages to the vessel wall. NO also inhibits the thrombotic process by preventing platelet adhesion and enhancing the effect of prostacyclin to inhibit platelet aggregation.

INJURY

Insulin slightly increases growth of vascular smooth muscle cells (VSMCs).

Insulin increases the effect of platelet-derived growth factor.

Insulin resistance is likely more important to the atherogenesis process than *hyperinsulinemia,* and insulin resistance likely disrupts the balance between vasoprotective effects mediated by NO and the atherogenic effects involving VSMC growth and migration, stimulating plasminogen activator inhibitor-1 and increasing clot formation.

Data from Loscalzo, J. (1992). Antiplatelet and antithrombotic effects of organic nitrates. American Journal of Cardiology, 70, 18B-22B; Fagan, T.C. & Deedwania, P.C. (1998). The cardiovascular dysmetabolic syndrome. American Journal of Medicine, 105(1A), 77S-82S; Hsueh, W.A. & Law, R.E. (1998). Cardiovascular risk continuum: Implications of insulin resistance and diabetes. American Journal of Medicine, 105(1A), 4S-14S; Randomski, M.W. & Moncada, S. (1993). The biological and pharmacological role of nitric oxide in platelet function. Advances in Experimental Medicine and Biology, 344, 251-264; Zeiher, A.M. et al. (1995). Nitric oxide modulates the expression of monocyte chemoattractant protein-1 in cultured human endothelial cells. Circulation Research, 76, 980-986.

Regulation of the Coronary Circulation

Flow of blood in the coronary circulation is directly proportional to the perfusion pressure and inversely proportional to the vascular resistance of the bed. **Coronary perfusion pressure** is the difference between pressure in the aorta and pressure in the coronary vessels of the right atrium. Aortic pressure is the driving pressure that perfuses vessels of the myocardium. Vasodilation and vasoconstriction normally maintain coronary blood flow despite stresses imposed by the constant contraction and relaxation of the heart muscle and despite shifts (within a physiologic range) of coronary perfusion pressure.

Several anatomic factors influence coronary blood flow. The aortic valve cusps obstruct coronary blood flow by pushing against the openings of the coronary arteries during systole. Also during systole, the coronary arteries are compressed by ventricular contraction. The resulting **systolic compressive effect** is particularly evident in the subendocardial layers of the left ventricular wall and can greatly decrease coronary blood flow. Therefore most coronary blood flow in the left ventricle occurs during diastole. During the period of systolic compression, when flow is slowed or stopped, oxygen is supplied by **myoglobin,** a protein present in heart muscle that binds oxygen during diastole and then releases it when blood levels of oxygen fall during systole.[22]

Autoregulation

Autoregulation (automatic self-regulation) enables individual vessels to regulate blood flow by altering their own arteriolar resistances. Autoregulation in the coronary circulation maintains constant blood flow at perfusion pressures (mean arterial pressure) between 60 and 180 mm Hg, provided that other influencing factors are held constant. Thus autoregulation ensures constant coronary blood flow despite shifts in the perfusion pressure within the stated range.

The mechanism of autoregulation is not known, but two explanations have been proposed. The **myogenic hypothesis** proposes that autoregulation originates in vascular smooth muscle, presumably of the arterioles, as a response to an increase in arterial pressure. Smooth muscle stretches in response to an increase in perfusion pressure. The stretching eventually stimulates contraction of the smooth muscles, which increases vascular resistance. Initially, coronary blood flow increases with the abrupt distention of the blood vessels. The return of more normal flow follows constriction of the arterioles. This mechanism also works in the opposite direction; that is, vasodilation is stimulated by decreased arterial pressure.[22] This follows the law of Laplace.

The **metabolic hypothesis** of autoregulation proposes that autoregulation of coronary vessels originates in the myocardium. The stimulus is a drop in coronary perfusion pressure or an increase in the metabolic needs of the myocardium (e.g., because of strenuous exercise). With an increased myocardial oxygen requirement, myocardial cells release substances that promote vasodilation. The best known of these substances is adenosine, a potent vasodilator released in response to a decrease in myocardial oxygenation. Low coronary blood flow, hypoxemia, or increased metabolic activity of the heart can all increase the heart muscle's need for oxygen.[1,23] An increased concentration of adenosine in the interstitial fluid decreases the resistance of the coronary arterioles and increases blood flow. Perfusion strongly correlates with the amount of adenosine released.[23] When coronary perfusion pressure is increased, the increased flow washes out the vasodilatory substances. As the dilators are washed out, vasoconstriction occurs and returns flow toward normal.[22]

Autonomic regulation

Stimulation of the sympathetic nerves to the heart causes a marked increase in coronary blood flow, even though it also causes vasoconstriction of the coronary vessels. Why? The increased coronary flow is the result of acceleration of heart rate and enhancement of myocardial contractility (more forceful systole). Although the longer, forceful myocardial contraction and the tachycardia (heart rate more than 100 beats/min) tend to restrict coronary flow, the increased myocardial metabolism tends to counteract these factors by dilating the coronary arterioles.[24] Therefore the net effect of sympathetic stimulation is to increase coronary blood flow.

Although the coronary vessels themselves contain sympathetic (α- and β-adrenergic) and parasympathetic neural receptors, coronary blood flow is regulated locally through metabolic autoregulation. Metabolic autoregulation overrides neurogenic influences.[1,11]

✓ QUICK CHECK

Why is capillary flow increased with increased mean arterial pressure?

Why is angiotensin significant in blood flow?

Identify the factors regulating blood pressure.

Why is atrial natriuretic hormone (ANH) important in regulating blood volume and blood pressure?

THE LYMPHATIC SYSTEM

The lymphatic system is a special vascular system that picks up excess tissue fluid and returns it to the bloodstream (Fig. 22-32). Normally, fluid is forced out of the blood at the arterial end of the capillary bed and is reabsorbed into the bloodstream at the venous end. However, capillary outflow exceeds venous reabsorption by about 3 L/day so some fluid lags behind in the interstitium. To maintain sufficient blood volume in the cardiovascular system, this fluid must eventually rejoin the bloodstream; this is the function of the lymphatic system.

The components of the lymphatic system are the lymphatic vessels and the lymph nodes (Fig. 22-33). (Lymph nodes and lymphoid tissues are described in Chapters 5 and 7.) In this pumpless system a series of valves ensures one-way flow of the excess interstitial fluid (now called lymph) toward the heart. The lymphatic capillaries are closed at the ends, as shown in Fig. 22-34.

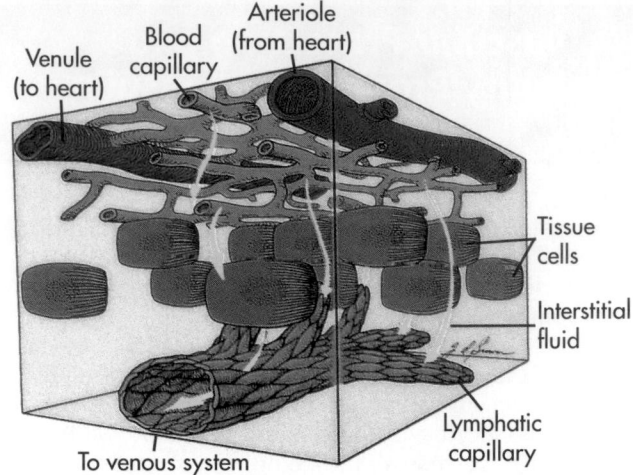

Fig. 22-32 *Role of the lymphatic system in fluid balance.* Fluid from plasma flowing through the capillaries moves into interstitial spaces. Although much of this interstitial fluid is either absorbed by tissue cells or reabsorbed by capillaries, some of the fluid tends to accumulate in the interstitial spaces. As this fluid builds up, it tends to drain into lymphatic vessels that eventually return the fluid to the venous blood. *(From Thibodeau, G.A. & Patton, K.T. [1999]. Anatomy & physiology [4th ed.]. St. Louis: Mosby.)*

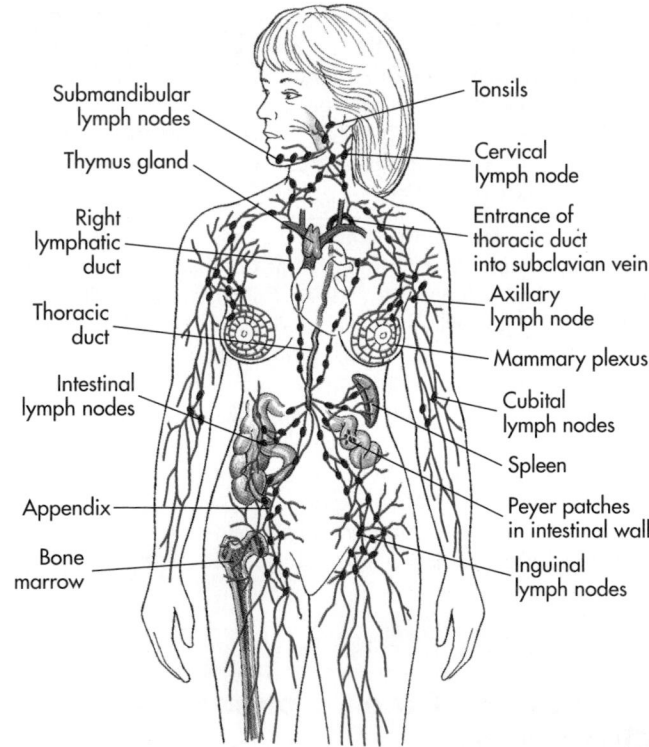

Fig. 22-33 *Schematic representation of lymphatic vessels, larger lymphatic trunks, and lymph nodes. (Modified from Seeley, R.R., Stephens, T.D., & Tate, P.T. [1995]. Anatomy & physiology. [3rd ed.]. St. Louis: Mosby.)*

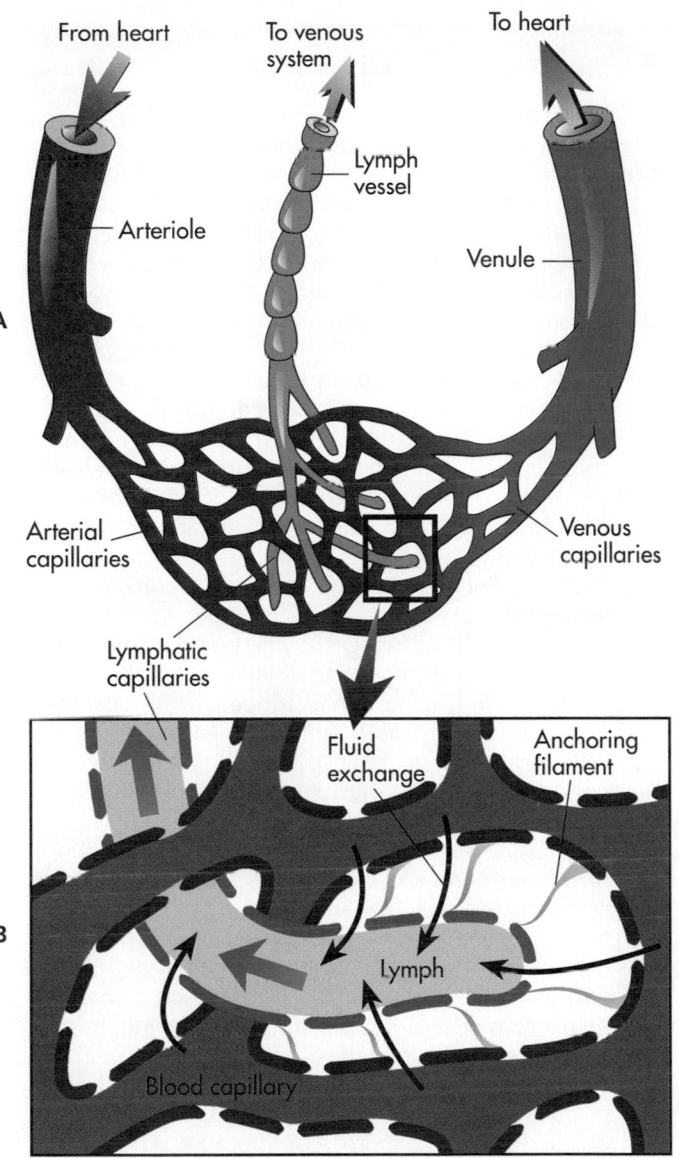

Fig. 22-34 *Lymphatic capillaries.* A, Schematic representation of lymphatic capillaries. **B,** Anatomic components of microcirculation.

Lymph consists primarily of water and small amounts of dissolved proteins, mostly albumin, that are too large to be reabsorbed into the less permeable blood capillaries. Once within the lymphatic system, lymph travels through larger vessels called *lymphatic venules* and *lymphatic veins.* The lymphatic vessels run alongside the arteries and veins and eventually drain into one of two large ducts in the thorax—the right lymphatic duct and the thoracic duct. The *right lymphatic duct* drains lymph from the right arm and the right side of the head and thorax, whereas the larger *thoracic duct* receives lymph from the rest of the body (see Fig. 22-33). The right lymphatic duct and the thoracic duct drain lymph into the right and left subclavian veins, respectively.

The lymphatic veins are thin walled like the veins of the cardiovascular system. In the larger lymphatic veins, endothelial flaps form valves similar to those in the circulatory veins (see Fig. 22-24). The valves permit lymph to flow in only one direction because lymphatic vessels are compressed intermittently by contraction of skeletal muscles, pulsatile expansion of an artery in the same sheath, and contraction of the smooth muscles in the walls of the lymphatic vessel.

As lymph is transported toward the heart, it is filtered through thousands of bean-shaped *lymph nodes* clustered along the lymphatic vessels (see Fig. 22-34). Lymph enters the node through several *afferent lymphatic vessels,* filters through the sinuses in the node, and leaves by way of *efferent lymphatic vessels.* Lymph flows slowly through the node, which facilitates the phagocytosis of foreign substances within the node and prevents them from reentering the bloodstream. (Phagocytosis is described in Chapter 6.)

✓ QUICK CHECK

Why is the lymphatic system considered a circulatory system?

Why are lymph nodes important?

What are some important changes in the cardiovascular system in elderly persons?

DID YOU UNDERSTAND?

The Circulatory System
1. The circulatory system is the body's transport system. It delivers oxygen, nutrients, metabolites, hormones, neurochemicals, proteins, and blood cells through the body and carries metabolic wastes to the kidneys and lungs for excretion.
2. The circulatory system consists of the heart and blood vessels and is made up of two separate, serially connected systems: the pulmonary circulation and the systemic circulation.
3. The pulmonary circulation is driven by the right side of the heart; its function is to deliver blood to the lungs for oxygenation.
4. The systemic circulation is driven by the left side of the heart, and its function is to move oxygenated blood throughout the body.
5. The lymphatic vessels collect fluids from the interstitium and return the fluids to the circulatory system.

The Heart
1. The heart consists of four chambers (two atria and two ventricles), four valves (two atrioventricular valves and two semilunar valves), a muscular wall, a fibrous skeleton, a conduction system, nerve fibers, systemic vessels (the coronary circulation),

Continued

☐ DID YOU UNDERSTAND? —cont'd

The Heart—cont'd

    and openings where the great vessels enter the atria and ventricles.

2. The heart wall, which encloses the heart and divides it into chambers, is made up of three layers: the pericardium (outer layer), the myocardium (muscular layer), and the endocardium (inner lining).

3. The myocardial layer of the two atria, which receive blood entering the heart, is thinner than the myocardial layer of the ventricles, which have to be stronger to squeeze blood out of the heart.

4. The right and left sides of the heart are separated by portions of the heart wall called the *interatrial septum* and the *interventricular septum.*

5. Unoxygenated (venous) blood from the systemic circulation enters the right atrium through the superior and inferior venae cavae. From the atrium the blood passes through the right atrioventricular (tricuspid) valve into the right ventricle. In the ventricle the blood flows from the inflow tract to the outflow tract and then through the pulmonary semilunar valve (pulmonary valve) into the pulmonary artery, which delivers it to the lungs for oxygenation.

6. Oxygenated blood from the lungs enters the left atrium through the four pulmonary valves (two from the left lung and two from the right lung). From the left atrium, the blood passes through the left atrioventricular valve (mitral valve) into the left ventricle. In the ventricle the blood flows from the inflow tract to the outflow tract and then through the aortic semilunar valve (aortic valve) into the aorta, which delivers it to systemic arteries of the entire body.

7. The heart valves ensure the one-way flow of blood from atrium to ventricle and from ventricle to artery.

8. Oxygenated blood enters the coronary arteries through an opening in the aorta, and unoxygenated blood from the coronary veins enters the right atrium through the coronary sinus.

9. The pumping action of the heart consists of two phases: diastole, during which the myocardium relaxes and the chambers fill with blood, and systole, during which the myocardium contracts, forcing blood out of the ventricles. A cardiac cycle consists of one systolic contraction and the diastolic relaxation that follows it. Each cardiac cycle constitutes one "heartbeat."

10. The conduction system of the heart generates and transmits electrical impulses (cardiac action potentials) that stimulate systolic contractions. The autonomic nerves (sympathetic and parasympathetic fibers) can adjust heart rate and systolic force, but they do not stimulate the heart to beat.

11. The normal electrocardiogram is the sum of all action potentials. The P wave represents atrial depolarization; the QRS complex is the sum of all ventricular cell depolarizations. The ST interval occurs when the entire ventricular myocardium is depolarized.

12. Cardiac action potentials are generated by the sinoatrial node at the rate of about 75 impulses per minute. The impulses can travel through the conduction system of the heart, stimulating myocardial contraction as they go.

13. Cells of the cardiac conduction system possess the properties of automaticity and rhythmicity. Automatic cells return to threshold and depolarize rhythmically without outside stimulus. The cells of the sinoatrial node depolarize faster than other automatic cells, making it the natural pacemaker of the heart. If the sinoatrial node is disabled, the next fastest pacemaker, the atrioventricular node, takes over.

14. Each cardiac action potential travels from the sinoatrial node to the atrioventricular node to the bundle of His (atrioventricular bundle), through the bundle branches, and finally to the Purkinje fibers. There the impulse is stopped. It is prevented from reversing its path by the refractory period of cells that have just been polarized. The refractory period ensures that diastole (relaxation) will occur, thereby completing the cardiac cycle.

15. Adrenergic receptor number, type, and function govern autonomic (sympathetic) regulation of heart rate, contractile force, and the dilation or constriction of coronary arteries. The presence of specific receptors (α_1, α_2; β_1, β_2) in the myocardium and coronary vessels determines the effects of the neurotransmitters norepinephrine and epinephrine.

16. Unique features that distinguish myocardial cells from skeletal cells enable myocardial cells to transmit action potentials faster (through intercalated disks), synthesize more ATP (because of a large number of mitochondria), and have readier access to ions in the interstitium (because of an abundance of transverse tubules). These combined differences enable the myocardium to work constantly, which skeletal muscle is not required to do.

17. Cross-bridges between actin and myosin enable contraction. Calcium and its interaction with the troponin complex facilitate the contraction process. With troponin release of calcium, myocardial relaxation begins.

18. Cardiac performance is affected by preload, afterload, heart rate, and myocardial contractility.

19. Preload, or pressure generated in the ventricles at the end of diastole, depends on the amount of blood in the ventricle. Afterload is the resistance to ejection of the blood from the ventricle. Afterload depends on pressure in the aorta.

20. Heart rate is determined by the sinoatrial node and by components of the autonomic nervous system, including cardiovascular control centers in the brain, neuroreceptors in the atria and aorta, hormones, and catecholamines (epinephrine, norepinephrine).

21. Contractility is the potential for myocardial fiber shortening during systole. It is determined by the amount of stretch during diastole (i.e., preload) and by sympathetic stimulation of the ventricles.

22. The Frank-Starling law of the heart states that the myocardial stretch determines the force of myocardial contraction (the greater the stretch, the stronger the contraction).

23. Laplace law states that the amount of contractile force generated within a chamber depends on the radius of the chamber and the thickness of its wall (the smaller the radius and the thicker the wall, the greater the force of contraction).

The Systemic Circulation

1. Blood flows from the left ventricle into the aorta and from the aorta into arteries that eventually branch into arterioles and capillaries, the smallest of the arterial vessels. Oxygen, nutrients, and other substances needed for cellular metabolism pass from the capillaries into the interstitium, where they are available for uptake by the cells. Capillaries also absorb products of cellular metabolism from the interstitium.

2. Venules, the smallest veins, receive capillary blood. From the venules, the venous blood flows into larger and larger veins until it reaches the venae cavae, through which it enters the right atrium.

3. Vessel walls consist of three layers: the tunica intima (inner layer), the tunica media (middle layer), and the tunica externa (the outer layer).

4. Layers of the vessel wall differ in thickness and composition from vessel to vessel, depending on the vessel's size and location within the circulatory system. In general, the tunica media of arteries close to the heart contains a greater proportion of elastic fibers because these arteries must be able to distend during systole and recoil during diastole. Distributing arteries farther from the heart contain a greater proportion of smooth muscle fibers because these arteries must be able to constrict and dilate to control blood pressure and volume within specific capillary beds.

5. Blood flow into the capillary beds is controlled by the contraction and relaxation of smooth muscle bands (precapillary sphincters) at junctions between metarterioles and capillaries. The endothelium is probably a source of prostaglandins that control vasomotion.

6. Blood flow through the veins is assisted by the contraction of skeletal muscles (the muscle pump), and backflow in the lower body is prevented by one-way valves, particularly in the deep veins of the legs.

7. Blood flow is affected by blood pressure; resistance to flow within the vessels; blood consistency (which affects velocity); anatomic features that may cause turbulent or laminar flow; and compliance (distensibility) of the vessels.

8. Poiseuille law describes the relationship of blood flow, pressure, and resistance as the difference between pressure at the inflow end of the vessel and pressure at the outflow end divided by resistance within the vessel.

9. According to Poiseuille formula, resistance depends on the vessel's length and radius and on the viscosity of the blood. The greater the vessel's length and the blood's viscosity and the narrower the radius of the vessel's lumen, the greater the resistance within the vessel.

10. Total peripheral resistance, or the resistance to flow within the entire systemic circulatory system, depends on the combined lengths and radii of all the vessels within the system and on whether the vessels are arranged in series (greater resistance) or in parallel (lesser resistance).

11. Poiseuille law and Poiseuille formula are based on physical laws governing the behavior of fluids in a straight tube. In the body, blood flow is also influenced by neural stimulation (of vasoconstriction or vasodilation) and by autonomic features that cause turbulence within the vascular lumen (e.g., protrusions from the vessel wall, twists and turns, bifurcations).

12. Arterial blood pressure is influenced and regulated by factors that affect cardiac output (heart rate, stroke volume), total resistance within the system, and blood volume.

13. Venous blood pressure is influenced by blood volume within the venous system and compliance of the venous walls.

14. Blood flow through the coronary circulation is governed not only by the same principles as flow through other vascular beds but also by adaptations dictated by cardiac dynamics. First, blood flows into the coronary arteries during diastole rather than systole, because during systole, the cusps of the aortic semilunar valve block the openings of the coronary arteries. Second, systolic contraction inhibits coronary artery flow by compressing the coronary arteries.

15. Autoregulation enables the coronary vessels to maintain optimal perfusion pressure despite systolic effects, and myoglobin in heart muscle stores oxygen for use during the systolic phase of the cardiac cycle.

The Lymphatic System

1. The vessels of the lymphatic system run in the same sheaths with the arteries and veins.

2. Lymph (interstitial fluid) is absorbed by lymphatic venules in the capillary beds and travels through ever larger lymphatic veins until it is emptied through the right or left thoracic duct into the right or left subclavian vein.

3. As lymph travels toward the thoracic ducts, it is filtered by thousands of lymph nodes clustered around the lymphatic veins. The lymph nodes are sites of immune function.

KEY TERMS

A band, 602
Afferent lymphatic vessel, 623
Afterload, 606
Aldosterone, 619
Angiotensin I, 619
Angiotensin II, 619
Anisotropic band, 602
Anomalous viscosity, 615
Aorta, 593
Arteriole, 608
Artery, 608
Atrial natriuretic hormone (ANH), 620
Atrioventricular node (AV node), 598
Atrioventricular valve, 593
Automatic cell, 601
Automaticity, 601
Autoregulation, 621
Bachmann bundle, 599
Bainbridge reflex, 607
Baroreceptor reflex, 607
Blood flow, 614
Blood velocity, 618
Bundle branch, 598
Bundle of His (atrioventricular bundle, common bundle), 598
Calcium channel–blocking drug, 604
Capillary, 608
Cardiac action potential, 597
Cardiac cycle, 593
Cardiac output, 608
Cardiac vein, 594
Cardioexcitatory center, 606
Cardioinhibitory center, 606
Cardiovascular control center, 606
Chordae tendineae cordis, 593
Conduction system, 598
Coronary artery, 594
Coronary circulation, 594
Coronary ostium, 594
Coronary perfusion pressure, 621
Coronary sinus, 594
Cross-bridge theory of muscle contraction, 604

Depolarization, 599
Diastole, 593
Diastolic depolarization, 601
Efferent lymphatic vessel, 623
Ejection fraction, 608
Elastic artery, 609
End-diastolic pressure, 606
End-diastolic volume, 605
Endocardium, 590
Endothelial-derived contracting factor (EDCF), 613
Endothelial-derived relaxing factor (EDRF; nitric oxide), 613
Excitation-contraction coupling, 604
Fenestration, 609
Frank-Starling law of the heart, 605
Great cardiac vein, 595
Heart rate, 598
I band, 602
Inferior vena cava, 593
Inotropic agent, 608
Insulin, 620
Intercalated disk, 602
Isotropic band, 602
Laminar flow, 618
Laplace law, 606
Left atrial pressure, 608
Left atrium, 590
Left bundle branch (LBB), 599
Left coronary artery, 594
Left heart, 590
Left ventricle, 590
Lumen, 609
Lymph, 623
Lymph node, 623
Lymphatic vein, 623
Lymphatic venule, 623
M line, 602
Mean arterial pressure (MAP), 618
Mediastinum, 590
Metabolic hypothesis, 621
Metarteriole, 609
Microcirculation, 615

Mitral and tricuspid complex, 593
Mitral valve (left atrioventricular valve, bicuspid valve), 593
Muscle pump, 614
Muscular artery, 609
Myocardial contractility, 604
Myocardial oxygen consumption ($M\dot{V}O_2$), 602
Myocardium, 590
Myogenic hypothesis, 621
Myoglobin, 621
Myosin, 602
Nitric oxide (NO), 613
Node, 598
P cell, 598
P wave, 600
Papillary muscle, 593
Perfusion, 618
Pericardial cavity, 590
Pericardial fluid, 590
Pericardium, 590
Peripheral vascular system, 608
Poiseuille formula, 615
Poiseuille law, 614
Posterior vein of the left ventricle, 597
PR interval, 600
Precapillary sphincter, 609
Preload, 606
Pressure, 614
Prostacyclin, 613
Pulmonary artery, 593
Pulmonary circulation, 590
Pulmonary vein, 593
Purkinje fiber, 599
QRS complex, 601
QT interval, 601
Refractory period, 600
Renin, 619
Repolarization, 599
Resistance, 614
Rhythmicity, 601
Right atrial pressure, 608
Right atrium, 590

KEY TERMS

Right bundle branch (RBB), 599
Right coronary artery, 594
Right heart, 590
Right lymphatic duct, 623
Right ventricle, 590
Semilunar valve, 593
Sinoatrial node (SA node, sinus node), 598
ST interval, 601
Stroke volume, 607
Superior vena cava, 593
Systemic circulation, 590

Systole, 593
Systolic compressive effect, 621
Thoracic duct, 623
Total resistance, 615
Trabeculae carneae, 593
Tricuspid valve (right atrioventricular valve), 593
Troponin C, 602
Troponin I, 602
Troponin T, 602
Troponin-tropomyosin complex, 602
Tunica externa (adventitial layer), 609

Tunica intima (intimal layer), 609
Tunica media (medial layer), 609
Turbulent flow, 618
Vasa vasorum, 609
Vascular compliance, 618
Vasoconstriction, 609
Vasodilation, 609
Vasomotion, 613
Vein, 614
Venule, 608
Z line, 602

REFERENCES

1. Berne, R.M. & Levy, M.N. (1996). *Principles of pathophysiology* (2nd ed.). St. Louis: Mosby.

2. Tyagi, S.C. (1997). Vasculogenesis and angiogenesis: Extracellular matrix remodeling in coronary collateral arteries and the ischemic heart. *Journal of Cellular Biochemistry, 65*(3), 388-394.

3. Underhill, S.L. et al. (Eds.). (1982). *Cardiac nursing.* Philadelphia: Lippincott.

4. DeHaan, R.L. (1965). Development of pacemaker tissue in the embryonic heart. *Annals of the New York Academy of Sciences, 127,* 7.

5. James, T.N. (1968). The coronary circulation and conduction system in acute myocardial infarction. *Progressive Cardiovascular Disease, 10,* 410.

6. Katz, A.M. (1977). *Physiology of the heart.* New York: Raven.

7. Soderstrom, M. (1948). Myocardial infarction and mitral thrombosis in the atria of the heart. *Acta Medica Scandinavian Supplementum, 132*(217), 114.

8. Thorel, C. (1909). Vorlarifig mittelung uber eine besondere muskel ver bindung zwischen der cava superior und dem hisschen bundel. *Munich Med Wochenschrift, 56,* 2159.

9. Wenckebach, K.F. (1908). Bietrage zur kenntnis der mengchlinhen hertztatigkeit. *Archives of Anatomy and Physiology, 3,* 53.

10. Little, R.C. (1985). *Physiology of the heart and circulation* (3rd ed.). St. Louis: Mosby.

11. Schlant, R.C. & Sonnenblick, E.H. (1990). Normal physiology of the cardiovascular system. In J.W. Hurst et al. (Eds.). *The heart: Arteries and veins* (7th ed.). New York: McGraw-Hill.

12. Hocher, B. et al. (1997). The paracrine endothelin system: Pathophysiology and implications in clinical medicine. *European Journal of Clinical Chemistry and Clinical Biochemistry, 35*(3), 175-189.

13. Ortega-Mateo, A. & de-Artinano, A.A. (1997). Highlights on endothelins: A review. *Pharmacological Research, 36*(5), 339-351.

14. Vander, A.J., Sherman, J.H., & Luciano, D.S. (1990). *Human physiology: The mechanisms of body function* (5th ed.). New York: McGraw-Hill.

15. Re, R.N. (1987). The renin-angiotensin systems. In E.D. Frohlich (Ed.). Essential hypertension. *Medical Clinics of North America, 71*(5).

16. Re, R. et al. (1978). Inhibition of angiotensin-converting enzyme for diagnosis of renal artery stenosis. *New England Journal of Medicine, 298*(11), 582-586.

17. Dietz, R. et al. (1998). Angiotensin II and coronary artery disease, congestive heart failure, and sudden cardiac death. *Basic Research in Cardiology, 93*(Suppl. 2), 101-108.

18. Gibbons, G.H. (1998). The pathophysiology of hypertension: The importance of angiotensin II in cardiovascular remodeling. *American Journal of Hypertension, 11*(11 Pt 2), 177S-181S.

19. Regitz-Zagrosek, V., Fielitz, J., & Fleck, E. (1998). Myocardial angiotensin receptors in human hearts. *Basic Research in Cardiology Supplement, 2,* 37-42.

20. Fagan, T.C. & Deedwania, P.C. (1998). The cardiovascular dysmetabolic syndrome. *American Journal of Medicine, 105*(1A), 77S-82S.

21. Hsueh, W.A. & Law, R.E. (1998). Cardiovascular risk continuum: Implications of insulin resistance and diabetes. *American Journal of Medicine, 105*(1A), 4S-14S.

22. Sparks, H.V. & Rooke, T.W. (1987). *Essentials of cardiovascular physiology.* Minneapolis: University of Minnesota Press.

23. Berne, R.M. (1980). The role of adenosine in the regulation of coronary blood flow. *Circulation Research, 47,* 807.

24. Berne, R.M. & Levy, M.N. (Eds.). (1993). *Physiology* (3rd ed.). St. Louis: Mosby.

www.mosby.com/MERLIN/Huether

CHAPTER

23

Alterations of Cardiovascular Function

Valentina L. Brashers, Stephanie J. Richardson,
Sheryl S. Davey, and Kathryn L. McCance

In the past, pathophysiology of the heart empha-sized coronary artery disease (CAD) or congenital heart diseases. Today emphasis is on reperfusion (reoxygenation) injury, myocardial hypertrophy, in-jury to the endothelium as the initiating event in the pathogenesis of cardiovascular disease, and those diseases requiring cardiac transplants.

CHAPTER OUTLINE

 Check out your CD Companion for chapter-related exercises and answers to the Quick Check questions

DISEASES OF THE ARTERIES AND VEINS

Arteriosclerosis

Arteriosclerosis is a chronic disease of the arterial system characterized by abnormal thickening and hardening of the vessel walls. Smooth muscle cells and collagen fibers migrate into the tunica intima, causing it to stiffen and thicken, gradually narrowing the arterial lumen (Fig. 23-1). Changes in lipid, cholesterol, and phospholipid metabolism within the tunica intima also contribute to arteriosclerosis. Although these changes may be part of normal aging, pathophysiologic conditions such as high blood pressure, insufficient perfusion of tissues, or weakening and outpouching of arterial walls can be exacerbated.

Atherosclerosis

Atherosclerosis is a form of arteriosclerosis in which soft deposits of intraarterial fat and fibrin on the vessels walls harden over time. Atherosclerosis is not a single disease entity. It can take several forms, depending on the anatomic location, age, genetic and physiologic status, and risk factors to which the individual is exposed. It is the leading contributor to coronary artery and cerebrovascular disease. (Atherosclerosis of the coronary arteries is described on p. 643; atherosclerosis of the cerebral arteries is described in Chapter 15.)

Pathophysiology

Atherosclerosis begins with injury to the endothelial cells that line artery walls.[1,2] Possible causes of **endothelial injury** include smoking, hypertension, diabetes (insulin resistance), hyperhomocystinemia, hyperdyslipidemia, autoimmune phenomena, and infection (e.g., chlamydia) (see Health Alert box). Injured endothelial cells become inflamed and cannot make normal amounts of antithrombic and vasodilating cytokines (Figs. 23-2 and 23-3). Macrophages adhere to the injured endothelium and release enzymes and toxic oxygen radicals that further injure the vessel wall and result in oxidation (e.g., addition of oxygen) of low-density lipoprotein (LDL). Oxidized LDL is engulfed by macrophages, which then penetrate into the intima of the vessel. These lipid-laden macrophages are now called **foam cells,**

and when they accumulate in significant amounts, they form a lesion called a **fatty streak** (Fig. 23-4). These lesions can be found in the walls of arteries of most people, even young children.[3] Once formed, fatty streaks produce more toxic oxygen radicals and cause immunologic and inflammatory changes resulting in progressive damage to the vessel wall. Treatment that lowers LDL may reverse this process.

HEALTH ALERT

Insulin Resistance and Cardiovascular Disease

The association of diabetes with increased risk for cardiovascular diseases, such as hypertension, hyperdyslipidemia, atherosclerosis, and ischemic heart disease, has been evident to researchers for many years. More recently, investigators have been exploring the role of insulin resistance, even in the absence of clinical diabetes, in the pathogenesis of these diseases. Studies show that insulin resistance is common in individuals with hypertension and atherosclerotic vascular disease and is associated with endothelial cell dysfunction, structural changes in vessel walls, abnormal vasoconstriction, smooth muscle proliferation, and salt sensitivity. Exercise, proper diet, and the use of angiotensin II inhibitors can all reduce insulin resistance and are linked to decreased risk for these cardiovascular diseases. Although no direct cause-and-effect relationship has been defined, this area of investigation may lead to improved methods of cardiovascular disease prevention and management. (Also see pp. 620-621.)

Data from Fagan, T.C. & Deedwania, P.C. (1998). The cardiovascular dysmetabolic syndrome. American Journal of Medicine, 105(1A), 77S-82S; Fuenmayor, N., Moreira, E., & Cubeddu, L.X. (1998). Salt sensitivity is associated with insulin resistance in essential hypertension. American Journal of Hypertension, 11(4, Pt.1), 397-402; Hsueh, W.A. & Law, R.E. (1997). Pharmacological treatment and mechanisms of insulin resistance. Impact on vascular smooth muscle cells, blood pressure, and lipids. Annals of the New York Academy of Sciences, 827, 170-177; Hsueh, W.A. & Law, R.E. (1998). Cardiovascular risk continuum: Implications of insulin resistance and diabetes. American Journal of Medicine, 105(1A), 4S-14S; Suzuki, M. et al. (1996). Mechanisms and clinical implication of insulin resistance syndrome. Diabetes, 45(Suppl. 3), S52-S54.

Fig. 23-1 *Arteriosclerosis.* **A,** Cross section of a normal artery and an artery altered by disease. **B,** A small artery in the myocardium is occluded by a mass of blue-staining platelets, yellow-staining red cells, and cholesterol bodies. *(B from Damjanov, I. & Linder, J. [Eds.]. [1996]. Anderson's pathology [10th ed.]. St. Louis: Mosby.)*

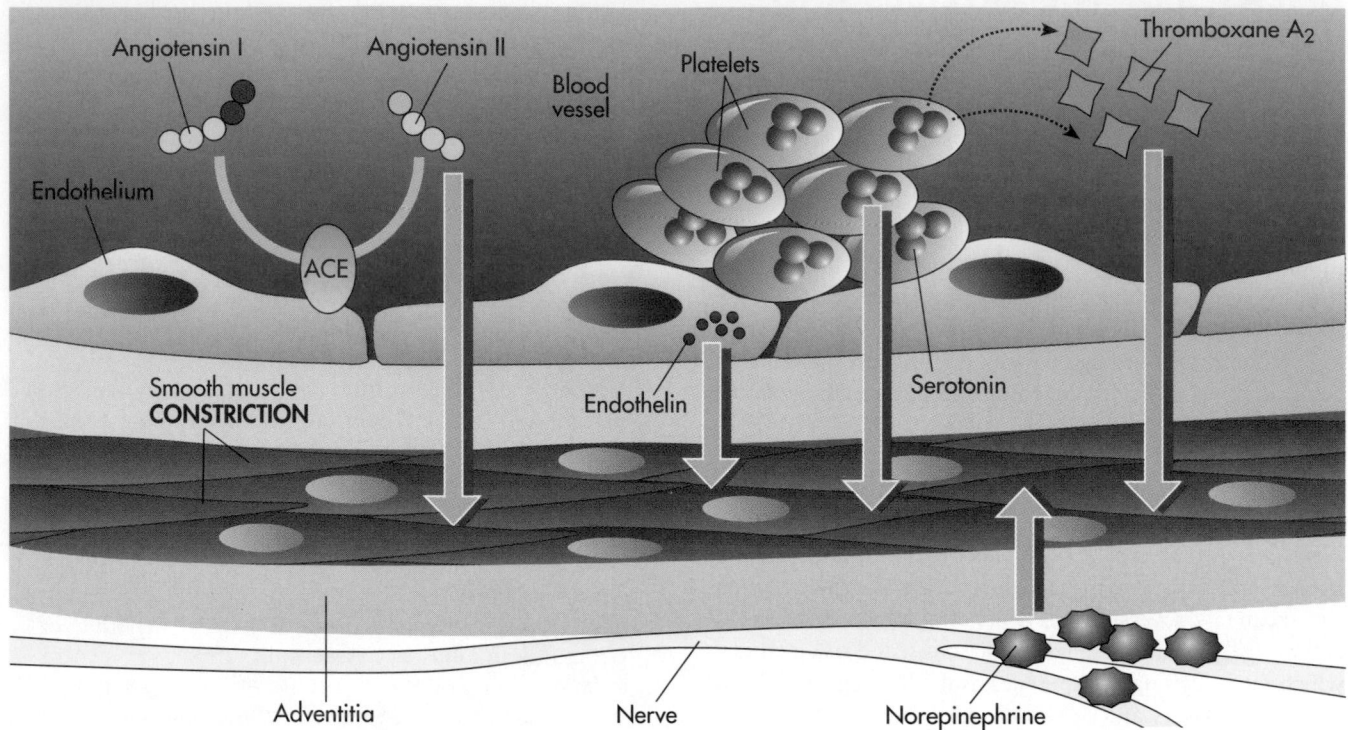

Fig. 23-2 *The endothelium regulates vasomotion (constriction and dilation) and platelet aggregation by releasing a variety of constricting and dilating substances.* Constricting factors include arachidonic acid metabolites, such as thromboxane A_2 (which aspirin inhibits), and a potent amino acid peptide called *endothelin*. The endothelium also converts angiotensin I into angiotensin II by the membrane-bound angiotensin-converting enzyme that also metabolizes the endogenous endothelium-dependent vasodilator, bradykinin. *(Modified from Stern, S. [Ed.]. [1998]. Silent myocardial ischemia. St. Louis: Mosby.)*

At this point, smooth muscle cells proliferate, produce collagen, and migrate over the fatty streak forming a *fibrous plaque* (see Fig. 23-4). This results in further endothelial cell dysfunction, necrosis of underlying vessel tissue, and narrowing of the vessel lumen as the lesion protrudes out from the wall. Vessel obstruction can become significant enough to reduce blood flow to distal tissues, especially during exercise. As the plaque continues to develop, it can ulcerate or rupture, resulting in platelet adherence to the lesion. This is now referred to as a *complicated lesion* (see Fig. 23-4). Platelet adherence to the plaque can initiate the coagulation cascade and result in rapid thrombus formation with complete vessel occlusion causing tissue ischemia and infarction. Efforts to prevent this process include antiplatelet medications, such as aspirin, and the new platelet glycoprotein IIb/IIIa receptor antagonists.[4]

Atherosclerotic lesions generally cause no symptoms until 60% or more of the tissue's blood supply is occluded. If plaque formation occurs slowly, collateral arteries may develop.

Clinical Manifestations

Atherosclerosis presents with symptoms and signs that result from inadequate perfusion of tissues because of obstruction of the vessels that supply them. Early in the course of the dis-

ease, partial vessel obstruction may lead to transient ischemic events, often associated with exercise or stress. As the lesion becomes complicated, increasing obstruction with superimposed thrombosis may result in tissue infarction. CAD caused by atherosclerosis is the major cause of myocardial ischemia and is one of the most important health issues in the United States (see p. 643). Atherosclerotic obstruction of the vessels supplying the brain is the major cause of stroke. Similarly, any part of the body may become ischemic when its blood supply is compromised by atherosclerotic lesions. Often, more than one vessel will become involved with this disease process such that an individual may present with symptoms from several ischemic tissues at the same time, and disease in one area may indicate that the individual is at risk for other ischemic complications elsewhere. Finally, diffuse atherosclerotic disease may elevate the total systemic vascular resistance and cause hypertension.

Evaluation and Treatment

In evaluating individuals for the presence of atherosclerosis, a complete health history, including risk factors, and physical examination, including laboratory data, are considered. Judicious use of x-ray films, electrocardiography, ultrasonography, nuclear scanning, and angiography may be necessary to identify affected vessels, particularly coronary vessels.

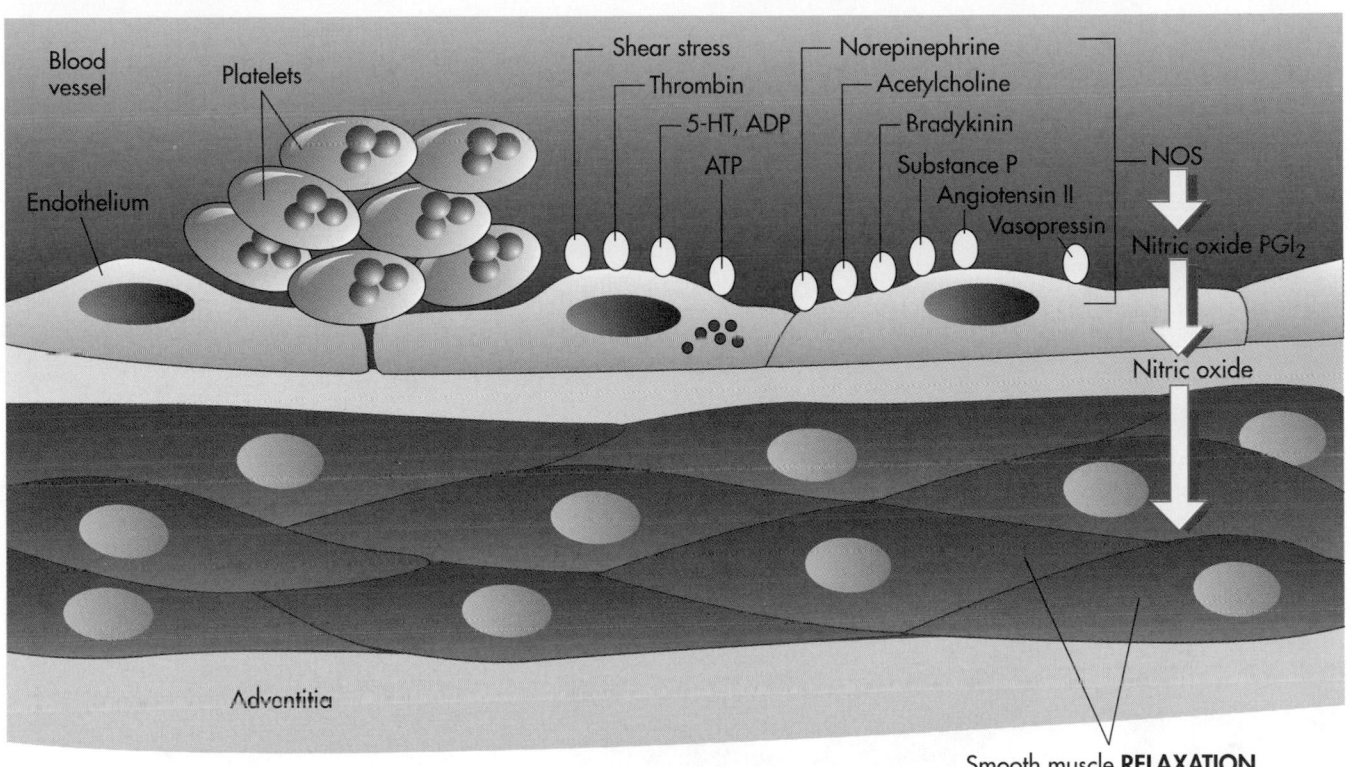

Fig. 23-3 *Factors causing endothelium-dependent vasodilation.* A variety of exogenous pharmacologic substances, platelet-derived factors, and shear stress can promote release of nitric oxide by stimulating nitric oxide synthase (NOS). Prostacyclin (PGI$_2$) causes relaxation of vascular smooth muscle cells by a cyclic adenosine monophosphate (AMP)-dependent mechanism, and both nitric oxide and PGI$_2$ inhibit platelet aggregation. *5-HT,* Serotonin; *ADP,* adenosine diphosphate; *ATP,* adenosine triphosphate. *(Modified from Stern, S. [Ed.]. [1998].* Silent myocardial ischemia. *St. Louis: Mosby.)*

HEALTH ALERT

Noninvasive Techniques Can Detect Blocked Arteries

New studies suggest that new techniques can detect blocked arteries before a myocardial infarction occurs. Investigators used an ultrafast computed tomography (CT) scan and an intravenous contrast medium dye. The sensitivity for detection of stenosis obstructing at least 50% of the lumen was 77%. In the left main, left anterior descending, left circumflex, and right anterior descending coronary arteries, the sensitivities were 100%, 82%, 83%, and 60%, respectively. Noninvasive technology is promising, especially for detecting disease in the left main and left anterior descending coronary arteries.

Data from Rensing, J.B. et al. (1998). Intravenous coronary angiography by electron beam computed tomography: A clinical evaluation. Circulation, 98, *2509-2512; Achenbach, S., Moshage, W., & Ropers, D. (1997). Noninvasive, three-dimensional visualization of coronary artery bypass grafts by electron beam tomography.* American Journal of Cardiology, 79(7), *856-861.*

The primary goal in the management of atherosclerosis is to restore adequate blood flow to the affected tissues. If an individual has presented with acute ischemia (e.g., myocardial infarction, stroke), interventions are specific to the diseased area and are discussed under those topics. In situations where the disease process does not require immediate intervention, management focuses on removing the initial causes of vessel damage and preventing lesion progression. This includes exercise, smoking cessation, and control of hypertension and diabetes where appropriate while reducing LDL cholesterol by diet or medications or both.

Fat intake should be reduced to less than 30% of daily calorie consumption, with no more than 10% saturated fats, no more than 10% polyunsaturated fats, and 10% to 15% monounsaturated fats. Monounsaturated fats reduce atherogenesis while avoiding the problems of polyunsaturated fats with production of free radicals. Daily cholesterol intake must be reduced to 250 to 300 mg.

The National Cholesterol Education Program (NCEP) Expert Panel[5] has recommended target total blood cholesterol levels of less than 200 mg/dl with LDLs less than 130 mg/dl and high-density lipoproteins (HDLs) more than 35 mg/dl. Drugs that decrease lipidemia are prescribed only if serum lipoproteins are not reduced by a reasonable trial of dietary modification or if lipid levels are dangerously ele-

Fig. 23-4 *Progression of atherosclerosis.* **A,** Damaged endothelium. **B,** Diagrams of fatty streak and lipid core formation; diagram of oxidized LDL (i.e., combining of oxygen free radicals with LDL). **C,** Diagram of fibrous plaque; micrograph of fibrous plaques (fibrolipid) in human aorta. Raised plaques are visible: some are yellow; others are white. One plaque is complicated by red thrombus deposition. **D,** Diagram of complicated lesion; micrograph of coronary thrombus: thrombus is red; collagen is blue. *LDL,* Low-density lipoprotein. *(Micrographs and diagrams of lipid formation and foam cell formation from Damjanov, I. & Linder, J. [Eds.]. [1996]. Anderson's pathology [10th ed.]. St Louis: Mosby.)*

TABLE 23-1	Classification of Blood Pressure for Adults Age 18 Years or Older	
Category	Systolic (mm Hg)	Diastolic (mm Hg)
Optimal	<120	<80
Normal	<130	<85
High normal	130-139	85-89
Hypertension		
Stage 1 (mild)	140-159	90-99
Stage 2 (moderate)	160-179	100-109
Stage 3 (severe)	≥180	≥110

From Anonymous. (1997). The sixth report of the Joint National Committee on Prevention, Detection, Evaluation, and Treatment of High Blood Pressure. Archives of Internal Medicine, 157, 2413-2446.

vated in an individual who will require a considerable time for significant dietary change and weight reduction.

Hypertension

Hypertension is consistent elevation of systemic arterial blood pressure. Approximately 50 million Americans, including 2.8 million children ages 6 to 17 years, have hypertension. Individuals are diagnosed as having hypertension when the average of two or more diastolic blood pressure measurements made on three consecutive clinical visits is 90 mm Hg or higher or when the average systolic blood pressure measurements made on three consecutive visits is greater than 140 mm Hg. The new classification presented in Table 23-1 describes stages of blood pressure.[6] "Optimal" blood pressure is associated with the lowest cardiovascular risk, whereas those who fall into the "high normal" category are at significant risk of developing hypertension unless lifestyle modification is initiated. All stages of hypertension are associated with increased risk of cardiovascular disease events. Stage 1, previously termed *mild,* is the most common form of high blood pressure in the adult population. All stages of hypertension need effective long-term therapy.[6]

Hypertension is caused by increases in cardiac output, total peripheral resistance, or both. (The many factors affecting cardiac output and peripheral resistance are described in Chapter 22; see Figs. 22-19 and 22-27.) Cardiac output is increased by conditions that increase heart rate or stroke volume, whereas peripheral resistance is increased by factors that increase blood viscosity or reduce vessel diameter, particularly of the arterioles.

Individuals may have combined systolic and diastolic hypertension or isolated systolic hypertension. Most cases of combined systolic and diastolic hypertension are diagnosed as *primary hypertension* (also called *essential* or *idiopathic* hypertension). From 92% to 95% of hypertensive individuals have primary disease. *Secondary hypertension* is caused by altered hemodynamics associated with a primary disease, such as arteriosclerosis. This form of hypertension accounts for only 5% to 8% of cases. *Isolated systolic hypertension* is elevated systolic blood pressure accompanied by normal di-

astolic blood pressure (below 90 mm Hg). It is a manifestation of increased cardiac output, rigidity of the aorta, or both.

The prevalence of hypertension increases with age, is higher for blacks than for whites, and in both whites and blacks is higher in less educated than more educated people.[7] In young adulthood and early middle age, hypertension prevalence is higher for men than women; thereafter, the reverse is true.[6]

Factors associated with primary hypertension

A combination of genetic and environmental factors may be responsible for primary hypertension (see Risk Factor box). Genetic predisposition to hypertension is thought to be polygenic, with inherited defects in renal sodium excretion, cell membrane sodium or calcium transport, and sympathetic response to neurogenic hormones.[8,9] Many risk factors for primary hypertension are also risk factors for other cardiovascular disorders, several of which are often found together.

RISK FACTORS

PRIMARY HYPERTENSION
- Family history
- Advancing age
- Cigarette smoking
- Obesity
- Heavy alcohol consumption
- Gender (men <50 years; women >50 years)
- Black race
- High dietary sodium intake
- Low dietary intake of potassium, calcium, magnesium
- Glucose intolerance

Although populations with high dietary sodium intake have a high incidence of hypertension, low dietary potassium, calcium, and magnesium intakes are also risk factors.[6,10,11] The nicotine in cigarette smoke is a vasoconstrictor that can acutely elevate both systolic and diastolic blood pressure. Habitual smoking is associated with an increased incidence of severe hypertension and myocardial hypertrophy resulting from hypertension.[12] The incidence of hypertension is also higher among heavy drinkers of alcohol (more than three drinks per day) than among abstainers, but moderate drinkers (two to four drinks per week) appear to have lower blood pressures, as well as lower cardiovascular mortality, than either abstainers or heavy drinkers.[13]

Pathophysiology

Chronic hypertension damages the walls of systemic blood vessels. Prolonged vasoconstriction and high pressures within these vessels, particularly the arteries and arterioles, stimulate thickening and strengthening to withstand the stress. Arterial smooth muscle undergoes hypertrophy (cellular enlargement) and hyperplasia (cellular proliferation). Eventually, the lumens of the tunica intima and tunica media narrow permanently.

Fig. 23-5 *Summary of pathophysiology of hypertension.*

Hypertensive injury of vessel walls also stimulates the biochemical mediators of inflammation (histamine, leukotrienes, prostaglandins) to increase the permeability of the vascular endothelium. As permeability increases, sodium, calcium, water, plasma proteins, and other blood-borne (humoral) substances enter vessel walls, causing further thickening and, in the case of calcium, increasing responsiveness to stimuli, causing smooth muscle contraction (i.e., vasoconstriction) (Fig. 23-5).

In the coronary vessels, hypertension causes or aggravates other conditions (e.g., atherosclerosis) that diminish vessel size. Therefore hypertension combined with CAD increases the risk of coronary artery occlusion and myocardial infarction.

Primary hypertension

Primary hypertension is the result of an extremely complicated interaction of genetics and the environment mediated by a host of neurohumoral effects. Current theories of the pathogenesis include (1) increases in blood volume, (2) increased activity of the sympathetic nervous system, (3) increased activity of the renin-angiotensin-aldosterone (RAA) system, (4) water and sodium retention by the kidneys, and (5) hormonal inhibition of sodium-potassium transport across cell walls in the kidneys and blood vessels. Any or all of these mechanisms may play a role.

Fig. 23-6 illustrates the *hemodynamic hypothesis of onset*. This attributes the onset of hypertension to fluid overload. Early primary hypertension consists of a series of cardiovascular adjustments to increased blood volume. First, cardiac output increases to handle the increased volume of blood circulating through the heart. As the systemic arteries sense the volume increase, their autoregulatory mechanisms try to slow things down by causing vasoconstriction. Because blood volume remains high, the increase in total peripheral resistance caused by vasoconstriction leads to hypertension. If this scenario persists, the increase in peripheral resistance becomes fixed, hypertension is established, and vascular damage begins.

The sympathetic nervous system has been implicated in both the development and the maintenance of high blood pressure and plays a role in hypertensive end-organ damage.[14] Overstimulation of the α- and β-adrenergic receptors results in vasoconstriction and increased cardiac output, thus raising the blood pressure.

The renin-angiotensin-aldosterone system plays an important role in blood pressure regulation by moderating vascular tone and influencing salt and water retention by the kidneys (see pp. 618-620). Further, angiotensin II mediates arteriolar remodeling, which is structural change in the vessel wall that results in permanent increases in peripheral resistance. Overactivity of this system has been associated with polymorphisms and has been implicated as an important cause of primary hypertension.[15] Finally, angiotensin II is associated with end-organ effects of hypertension, including atherosclerosis, renal disease, and cardiac hypertrophy.[16-18]

One probable contributor to primary hypertension in many individuals is a defect in sodium excretion by the kidneys. This defect means that the kidney requires a high level of arterial pressure to stimulate it to excrete sodium and water; this has been described as a shift in the pressure-natriuresis relationship. Several mediators play roles in the abnormal response to blood pressure by the kidney, including atrial natriuretic peptide, catecholamines, angiotensin II, prostaglandins, and nitric oxide.[19] The defect in renal sodium excretion is aggravated by dietary sodium intake of more than 60 mEq/day (Fig. 23-7).

Another mechanism of sodium retention is thought to be an interruption of the sodium-potassium pump, which normally governs the transport of sodium and potassium across cell membranes (see Chapters 1 and 4). In individuals with this defect, a humoral factor is thought to inhibit sodium excretion from cells, causing intracellular sodium to accumulate but also leading to increases of intracellular calcium. Because intracellular calcium promotes smooth muscle contractility, extra calcium in vascular smooth muscle

Fig. 23-6 *Primary hypertension.* Hemodynamic events of early primary hypertension *(thin arrows)* and established primary hypertension *(thick arrows)*. Genetic factors may cause defects in renal excretion of sodium, vascular tone, and structural regulation of vascular size. Environmental factors, such as increased sodium intake (and low intake of magnesium, calcium, and potassium), potentiate the effects of genetic factors. The resultant increase in cardiac output and peripheral resistance contributes to hypertension (see text for further discussion). *ECF,* Extracellular fluid.

Fig. 23-7 *Two related mechanisms of sodium-induced primary hypertension. ECF,* Extracellular fluid.

cells increases vascular reactivity, producing vasoconstriction with increased peripheral resistance and hypertension. The cellular events related to sodium-induced hypertension are summarized in Fig. 23-7.

✓ **QUICK CHECK**

Define arteriosclerosis, and briefly describe characteristic changes.

How is the renal system involved in primary hypertension?

Describe the hemodynamic hypothesis of onset for hypertension.

Secondary hypertension

Secondary hypertension is caused by a systemic disease process that raises peripheral vascular resistance or cardiac output. Examples include renal vascular or parenchymal disease, adrenocortical tumors, adrenomedullary tumors (pheochromocytoma), and drugs (oral contraceptives, corticosteroids, antihistamines). If the cause is identified and removed before permanent structural changes occur, blood pressure returns to normal.

Isolated systolic hypertension

Elevations of systolic pressure alone are usually caused by increases in cardiac output, total peripheral vascular resistance, or both. Isolated systolic hypertension caused by increased cardiac output can be secondary to dysfunction of the aortic semilunar valve (aortic valve insufficiency), any abnormal opening between heart chambers (arteriovenous fistula, patent ductus arteriosus; see Chapter 25), thyrotoxic crisis (thyroid storm), Paget disease of the bone, and

TABLE 23-2	Pathologic Effects of Sustained, Complicated Primary Hypertension	
Site of Injury	**Mechanism of Injury**	**Potential Pathologic Effect**
Heart		
Myocardium	Increased work load combined with diminished blood flow through coronary arteries	Left ventricular hypertrophy, myocardial ischemia, left heart failure
Coronary arteries	Accelerated atherosclerosis (coronary artery disease)	Myocardial ischemia, myocardial infarction, sudden death
Kidneys	Renin and aldosterone secretion stimulated by reduced blood flow	Retention of sodium and water, leading to increased blood volume and perpetuation of hypertension
	Reduced oxygen supply	Tissue damage that compromises filtration
	High pressures in renal arterioles	Nephrosclerosis leading to renal failure
Brain	Reduced blood flow and oxygen supply; weakened vessel walls	Transient ischemic attacks, cerebral thrombosis, aneurysm, hemorrhage
Eyes (retinas)	Reduced blood flow	Retinal vascular sclerosis
Aorta	High arteriolar pressure	Exudation, hemorrhage
		Dissecting aneurysm (see p. 639)
Arterial vessels of lower extremities	Weakened vessel wall	Intermittent claudication, gangrene

beriberi. Rigidity of the aorta is the chief vascular cause of isolated systolic hypertension.

Isolated systolic hypertension is most common in the elderly population, where the aortic rigidity is caused by arteriosclerosis, which increases total peripheral vascular resistance. Changes associated with aging alter the aortic valve so that increased cardiac output is needed to maintain blood flow into the systemic circulation.

Complicated hypertension

Complicated hypertension is sustained primary hypertension that has pathologic effects beyond hemodynamic alterations and fluid and electrolyte imbalances. Complicated hypertension commonly compromises the structure and function of the vessels themselves: the heart, aorta, kidneys, eyes, brain, and lower extremities. The two major mechanisms of tissue damage are ischemia and edema. Ischemia deprives tissues of the oxygen and nutrients needed for survival and function. Leakage of fluids into the interstitial space, and even hemorrhage, are caused by high pressures in the vessels. The heart is particularly susceptible to injury because although high cardiac output is stimulating myocardial hypertrophy, vasoconstriction is diminishing blood flow through the coronary arteries. The pathophysiology of complicated hypertension is summarized in Table 23-2.

Cardiovascular complications include left ventricular hypertrophy, angina pectoris, left heart failure (congestive heart failure), coronary artery disease, myocardial infarction, and sudden death. Vascular complications include the formation, dissection, and rupture of aneurysms (outpouchings in vessel walls); intermittent claudication (severe pain during walking); and gangrene resulting from vessel occlusion. Possible renal complications are parenchymal damage, nephrosclerosis, renal arteriosclerosis, and renal insufficiency or failure.

Malignant hypertension (rapidly progressive hypertension in which diastolic pressure is usually above 140 mm Hg) can cause encephalopathy, a profound cerebral edema that disrupts cerebral function and causes loss of consciousness. High arterial pressure renders the cerebral arterioles incapable of regulating blood flow to the cerebral capillary beds. Capillary permeability is increased by high hydrostatic pressures in the capillaries, which causes vascular fluid to exude into the interstitial space. If blood pressure is not reduced, cerebral edema and cerebral dysfunction increase until death occurs. Organ damage resulting from malignant hypertension is life threatening. Besides encephalopathy, malignant hypertension can cause papilledema, cardiac failure, uremia, retinopathy, and cerebrovascular accident.

Clinical Manifestations

The early stages of hypertension have no clinical manifestations other than elevated blood pressure. Most important, there are no signs and symptoms to cause the individual to seek health care; thus hypertension is called a silent disease. Some hypertensive individuals never have signs, symptoms, or complications, whereas others become very ill, and hypertension can be a cause of death. Still other individuals have anatomic and physiologic damage caused by past hypertensive disease, despite current blood pressures within normal ranges.

The chance of developing primary hypertension increases with age, over and above the natural rise in blood pressure associated with aging. In individuals at risk for primary hypertension, the factors leading to development of hypertension accumulate during the first 2 or 3 decades of life. Although hypertension is usually thought to be an adult health problem, it is important to remember that hypertension does occur in children and is being diagnosed with increasing frequency.[20] Usually, however, increased peripheral resistance and early hypertension develop in the second, third, and fourth decades of life. If elevated blood pressure is not detected and treated, it becomes established and may begin to accelerate atherosclerosis when the individual is 30 to 50 years of age. This sets the stage for the complications of hypertension that begin to appear during the fourth, fifth, and sixth decades of life.

Most clinical manifestations of hypertensive disease are caused by complications that damage organs and tissues outside the vascular system. Besides elevated blood pressure, the signs and symptoms therefore tend to be specific for the organs or tissues affected. Evidence of heart disease, renal insufficiency, central nervous system dysfunction, impaired vision, impaired mobility, vascular occlusion, or edema can all be caused by sustained hypertension.

Evaluation and Treatment

Diagnostic tests for suggested hypertension include repeated blood pressure measurements (or 24-hour blood pressure monitoring in selected individuals), complete blood count, urinalysis, biochemical blood profile (plasma glucose, sodium, potassium, calcium, magnesium, creatinine, cholesterol, triglycerides), and an electrocardiogram. Individuals who have elevated blood pressure are assumed to have primary hypertension unless their history, physical examination, or initial diagnostic screening indicates secondary hypertension.

HEALTH ALERT

Potassium, Calcium, and Magnesium Supplementation in the Management of Hypertension

Potassium, calcium, and magnesium are important cations that influence renal sodium excretion and vascular tone. Decreased extracellular levels of potassium and magnesium have been shown to increase cytoplasmic free calcium in arteriolar smooth muscle cells, which causes increased phosphorylation of myosin light chains, locking them in the contractile state. Recent studies have confirmed that increased dietary intake of potassium, calcium, and magnesium can reduce blood pressure in many individuals, even if sodium intake is restricted. Adequate intake of these minerals is now included in recent guidelines for the management of hypertension.

Data from Kawano, Y. et al. (1998). Effects of magnesium supplementation in hypertensive patients: Assessment by office, home, and ambulatory blood pressures. Hypertension, 32(2), 260-265; *Martens, J.R. & Gelband, C.H. (1998). Ion channels in vascular smooth muscle: Alterations in essential hypertension.* Proceedings of the Society for Experimental Biology and Medicine, 218(3), 192-203; *McCarron, D.A. (1997). Role of adequate dietary calcium intake in the prevention and management of salt-sensitive hypertension.* American Journal of Clinical Nutrition, 65(Suppl.), 712S-716S; *Nurminen, M.L., Korpela, R., & Vapaatalo, H. (1998). Dietary factors in the pathogenesis and treatment of hypertension.* Annals of Medicine, 30(2), 143-150.

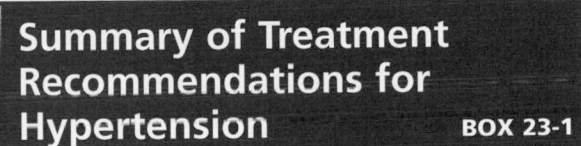

Summary of Treatment Recommendations for Hypertension   BOX 23-1

LIFE-STYLE MODIFICATIONS
Weight reduction
Moderation of alcohol intake
Regular physical activity
Reduction of sodium intake
Smoking cessation
↓

INADEQUATE RESPONSE
↓

CONTINUE LIFE-STYLE MODIFICATIONS
INITIAL PHARMACOLOGIC SELECTION
Diuretics or β blockers are preferred because reduction in morbidity and mortality has been shown
Angiotensin converting enzyme (ACE) inhibitors, angiotensin II receptor blockers, calcium antagonists, α-receptor blockers, and α-β blockers should be used in specific populations, such as persons with diabetes, heart failure, or myocardial infarction
↓

INADEQUATE RESPONSE
↓

↑Drug dosage *or* substitute another drug *or* add second agent from different class
↓   ↓
↓

INADEQUATE RESPONSE
Add second or third agent and/or diuretic if not already prescribed

From Anonymous. (1997). The sixth report of the Joint National Committee on Prevention, Detection, Evaluation, and Treatment of High Blood Pressure. Archives of Internal Medicine, 157, 2430.

Treatment of primary hypertension depends on its severity. Box 23-1 presents a summary of new guidelines for treatment. Life-style modification is also very important in preventing hypertension for those individuals who fall into the "high normal" category.[6]

Orthostatic (Postural) Hypotension

The term ***orthostatic (postural) hypotension*** refers to a decrease in both systolic and diastolic arterial blood pressure on standing. When a normal individual stands up, the gravitational changes on the circulation are compensated for by such mechanisms as reflex arteriolar and venous constriction, increased heart rate, and mechanical factors, such as the closure of valves in the venous system, pumping of the leg muscles, and a decrease in intrathoracic pressure. The normally increased sympathetic activity during upright posture is mediated through a stretch receptor (baroreceptor) reflex that responds to shifts in volume caused by postural changes. This reflex promptly increases heart rate and constricts the systemic arterioles. Thus arterial blood pressure is maintained.

Orthostatic hypotension is often accompanied by dizziness, blurring or loss of vision, and syncope or fainting caused by insufficient vasomotor compensation and reduction of blood flow through the brain. This occurs because the normal or compensatory vasoconstrictor response to standing is thus replaced by a marked vasodilation and blood pooling in the muscle vasculature, as well as in the splanchnic and renal beds.

Orthostatic hypotension may be acute and temporary or chronic. *Acute orthostatic hypotension* is caused when the normal regulatory mechanisms are sluggish as a result of (1) anatomic variation, (2) altered body chemistry, (3) drug action (e.g., antihypertensives, antidepressants), (4) prolonged immobility caused by illness, (5) starvation, (6) physical exhaustion, (7) any condition that produces volume depletion (e.g., massive diuresis, potassium or sodium depletion), or (8) venous pooling (e.g., pregnancy, extensive varicosities of the lower extremities). Elderly persons are particularly susceptible to this type of orthostatic hypotension.[21]

Chronic orthostatic hypotension may be (1) secondary to a specific disease or (2) idiopathic or primary. The diseases that cause secondary orthostatic hypotension are endocrine disorders (e.g., adrenal insufficiency, diabetes mellitus), metabolic disorders (e.g., porphyria), or diseases of the central or peripheral nervous system (e.g., intracranial tumors, cerebral infarcts, Wernicke encephalopathy, peripheral neuropathies).

The term *idiopathic,* or *primary, orthostatic hypotension* implies no known initial cause. Some define the disorder as a separate entity, whereas others suggest it is a part of a generalized degenerative central nervous system disease. It affects men more often than women and usually occurs between the ages of 40 and 70 years. In addition to cardiovascular symptoms, impotence and bowel and bladder dysfunction are often found in this type.

Although no curative treatment is available for idiopathic orthostatic hypertension, it can often be adequately managed with a combination of nondrug and drug therapies. In the secondary form, syncope ceases when the underlying disorder is corrected.

Aneurysm

An *aneurysm* is a localized dilation or outpouching of a vessel wall or cardiac chamber. The law of Laplace discussed in detail in Chapter 22 can provide an understanding of the hemodynamics of an aneurysm. Presumably, a ventricular wall aneurysm forms when intraventricular tension stretches the noncontracting infarcted muscle. The stretching produces infarct expansion, a weak and thin layer of necrotic muscle, and fibrous tissue that bulges with each systole. With time, the aneurysm becomes more fibrotic but continues to bulge with each systole, thus acting as a reservoir for some of the stroke volume.

Fig. 23-8 *Aneurysms.* **A,** Abdominal aortic atherosclerotic aneurysm. **B,** In a long-axis view of the left ventricle there is a large, thin-walled apical aneurysm that does not contain thrombus. *(From Damjanov, I. & Linder, J. [Eds.]. [1996].* Anderson's pathology *[10th ed.]. St. Louis: Mosby.)*

The aorta is particularly susceptible to aneurysm formation because of constant stress on the vessel wall and the absence of penetrating vasa vasorum in the adventitial layer. Three fourths of all aneurysms occur in the abdominal aorta (Fig. 23-8). Atherosclerosis is the most common cause of aneurysms because plaque formation erodes the vessel wall. Arteriosclerosis and hypertension are found in more than half of all individuals with aneurysms. Syphilis and other infections also can cause aortic aneurysms.

True aneurysms involve all three layers of the arterial wall and are best described as a weakening of the vessel wall. Most are fusiform and circumferential (Fig. 23-9). *False aneurysms* and *saccular aneurysms* are usually the result of trauma. Dissection of the layers of the arterial wall occurs so that blood is contained at the point of aneurysm by the adventitial layer (dissecting saccular aneurysm) or by a clot (false aneurysm).

Aortic aneurysms can be very painful. Symptoms of dysphagia (difficulty swallowing) and dyspnea (breathlessness) are caused by the pressure of a large volume of blood on surrounding organs. An aneurysm that impairs flow to an extremity causes symptoms of ischemia. Cerebral aneurysms, which frequently occur in the circle of Willis, are associated

Fig. 23-9 *Longitudinal sections showing types of aneurysms.* The fusiform circumferential and fusiform saccular aneurysms are true aneurysms, caused by weakening of the vessel wall. False and saccular aneurysms involve a break in the vessel wall, usually caused by trauma.

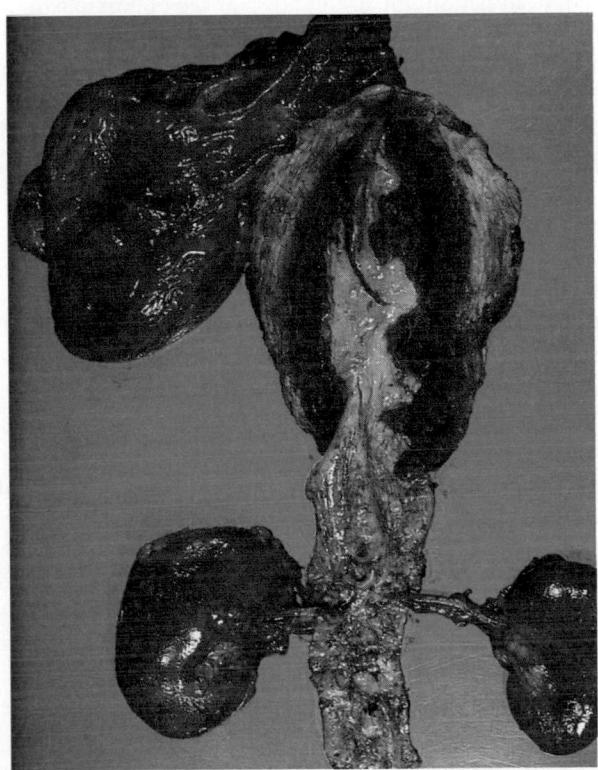

Fig. 23-10 *Dissecting aneurysm of thoracic aorta. (From Damjanov, I. & Linder, J. [Eds.]. [1996]. Anderson's pathology [10th ed.]. St. Louis: Mosby.)*

with signs and symptoms of increased intracranial pressure. Signs and symptoms of stroke occur when cerebral aneurysms leak. (Cerebral aneurysms are described in Chapter 15.)

Medical treatment of aneurysms includes reducing blood pressure and circulating blood volume. Smoking cessation is part of the treatment, because cigarette smoking is associated with a more rapid increase in the size of thoracic aortic aneurysm.[22,23] Beta blockade can be very successful in preventing the enlargement of an abdominal aortic aneurysm.[24]

Surgical treatment of aneurysms larger than 5 cm in diameter is replacement with a prosthetic graft.[25] If the weakness or separation of vascular layers spreads, the aneurysm becomes a ***dissecting aneurysm*** (Fig. 23-10). Dissecting aneurysms and leaking aneurysms require emergency treatment and carry a postoperative mortality of 68%.[26] Leaking cerebral aneurysms, especially those associated with vascular spasms as a compensatory mechanism, are treated with clot-stabilizing drugs and a number of clinical measures designed to reduce intracranial pressure and induce hemodynamic stability before surgical intervention.

Thrombus Formation

A ***thrombus*** is a blood clot that remains attached to a vessel wall (see Figs. 20-16 and 23-12). A detached thrombus is a ***thromboembolus.*** Thrombi tend to develop wherever intravascular conditions promote activation of the coagulation, or clotting, cascade (e.g., intimal irritation, roughening, inflammation [including surgical procedures], traumatic injury, infection, low blood pressures or obstructions that cause blood stasis and pooling within the vessels). (Mechanisms of coagulation are described in Chapter 19.) In the arteries, activation of the coagulation cascade is usually caused by roughening of the tunica intima by atherosclerosis. Invasion of the tunica intima by an infectious agent also roughens the normally smooth lining of the artery, causing platelets to adhere readily. An anatomic change in an artery can stimulate thrombus formation, particularly if the change results in a pooling of arterial blood. In the veins, thrombus formation is more often associated with inflammation (phlebitis), a condition termed *thrombophlebitis.* Thrombi also form on heart valves altered by calcification or bacterial vegetation. Valvular thrombi are most commonly associated with inflammation of the endocardium (endocarditis) and rheumatic heart disease. Shock (circulatory failure), particularly shock resulting from septicemia, can also activate the intrinsic and extrinsic pathways of coagulation. The im-

TABLE 23-3	Types of Emboli
Type	**Characteristics**
Arteries	
Arterial thromboem-bolism	Dislodged thrombus; source is usually from the heart; most common sites of obstruction are lower extremities (femoral and popliteal arteries), coronary arteries, and cerebral vasculature
Venous	
Venous thromboem-bolism	Dislodged thrombus; source is usually from the lower extremities; obstructs branches of the pulmonary artery
Air embolism	A bolus of air displaces blood in the vasculature; source usually room air entering circulation through IV lines; trauma to the chest also may allow air from lungs to enter vascular space
Amniotic fluid em-bolism	A bolus of amniotic fluid; extensive intraabdominal pressure attending labor and delivery can force amniotic fluid into bloodstream of mother; introduces antigens, cells, and protein aggregates that trigger inflammation, coagulation, and immune responses
Bacterial embolism	Aggregates of bacteria in bloodstream; source is subacute bacterial endocarditis of abscess
Fat embolism	Globules of fat floating in the bloodstream associated with trauma to long bones; affect the lungs in particular
Foreign matter	Small particles or fibers introduced during trauma or through an IV or intraarterial line; coagulation cascade is initiated and thromboemboli form around the particles

paired cellular metabolism that occurs with all types of shock activates the extrinsic pathway of coagulation, whereas blood stasis caused by very low blood pressures activates the intrinsic pathway.

Arterial thrombi may grow large enough to occlude the artery, causing ischemia in tissue supplied by the artery. In addition, the thrombus may dislodge and become a thromboembolus that can occlude flow into a distal systemic vascular bed. Venous thrombi can make it more difficult for blood to drain from distal venous beds (especially in the legs), resulting in edema. Venous thrombi can also embolize; these clots travel to the pulmonic vascular bed.

Pharmacologic treatment involves the administration of heparin, warfarin derivatives, or thrombolytics. Thrombin inhibitors, such as hirudin, are being investigated as anticoagulants. A balloon-tipped catheter can also be used to remove or compress an arterial thrombus. Various combinations of drug and catheter therapies are sometimes used concurrently.

Embolism

Embolism is the obstruction of a vessel by an *embolus*—a bolus of matter circulating in the bloodstream. The embolus may consist of a dislodged thrombus; an air bubble; an aggregate of amniotic fluid; an aggregate of fat, bacteria, or cancer cells; or a foreign substance. An embolus travels in the bloodstream until it reaches a vessel through which it cannot fit. No matter how tiny it is, an embolus will eventually lodge in a systemic or pulmonary vessel determined by its source. Pulmonary emboli originate on the venous side (mostly from the deep veins of the legs) of the systemic circulation or in the right heart; systemic (or arterial) emboli most commonly originate in the left heart and are associated with

thrombi after myocardial infarction, valvular disease, left heart failure, endocarditis, and dysrhythmias.

Embolism causes ischemia or infarction in tissues distal to the obstruction. Embolism of a central organ causes organ dysfunction and pain. Infarction and subsequent necrosis of a central organ are life threatening, not only because of organ dysfunction but also because of sepsis. Embolism of a coronary or cerebral artery is an immediate threat to life if the embolus severely obstructs a major vessel. Occlusion of a coronary artery will cause a myocardial infarction (see p. 648), whereas occlusion of a cerebral artery causes a stroke (see Chapter 15). The types of emboli are summarized in Table 23-3.

Peripheral Arterial Disease
Thromboangiitis obliterans (Buerger disease)

Thromboangiitis obliterans (Buerger disease), which tends to occur in young men who are heavy cigarette smokers, is an inflammatory disease of the peripheral arteries accompanied by thrombi and sometimes vasospasm of arterial segments. These disorders can eventually occlude and obliterate (render physiologically useless) portions of small and medium-sized arteries in the feet and sometimes in the hands. The incidence of Buerger disease has been steadily declining, probably because of a decrease in cigarette smoking in men.[27] Buerger disease has been associated with cerebrovascular disease (stroke)[28] and rheumatic symptoms (joint pain).[29,30] There is evidence that this disease is carried on the HLA gene.[29]

In Buerger disease, peripheral vessels are less responsive to acetylcholine, which normally causes vasodilation.[31] Although collateral vessels develop in Buerger disease, they are inadequate to supply the extremities with blood. These collateral vessels have a characteristic corkscrew shape, believed to be a result of dilated vasa vasorum in the affected artery.[32]

The chief symptom of thromboangiitis obliterans is pain and tenderness of the affected part. Clinical manifestations are caused by sluggish blood flow and include rubor (redness of the skin), which is caused by dilated capillaries under the skin, and cyanosis, which is caused by blood that remains in the capillaries after its oxygen has diffused into the interstitium. Chronic ischemia causes the skin to thin and become shiny, and it causes the nails to become thickened and malformed. In advanced disease, ischemia resulting from vessel obliteration can cause gangrene, necessitating amputation in up to 23% of all cases.[33]

The most important part of treatment is cessation of cigarette smoking. If smoking continues, the likelihood of recurrence of the disease and amputation is high.[30,34] All other measures are aimed at improving circulation to the foot or hand. Vasodilators are prescribed to alleviate vasospasm, and exercises are taught that use gravity to improve blood flow. If vasospasm persists, sympathectomy may be performed. Sympathectomy is successful in up to 87% of all cases.[34]

HEALTH ALERT
Smoking and Rise of Disease in Women

Although reduced rates of smoking have led to a corresponding decrease in diseases such as lung cancer and Buerger disease for men, these diseases are on the rise in women—probably because more women take up smoking each year than men.

Raynaud phenomenon and disease

Raynaud phenomenon and *Raynaud disease* both are characterized by attacks of vasospasm in the small arteries and arterioles of the fingers and, less commonly, the toes. Although the clinical manifestations of the phenomenon and the disease are the same, their causes differ.

Raynaud phenomenon is secondary to systemic diseases, particularly collagen vascular disease (scleroderma), pulmonary hypertension, thoracic outlet syndrome, myxedema trauma, serum sickness, or long-term exposure to environmental conditions, such as cold or vibrating machinery in the workplace.[35] Raynaud disease, however, is a primary vasospastic disorder of unknown origin. It tends to affect young women and to consist of vasospastic attacks triggered by brief exposure to cold or by emotional stress. Genetic predisposition may play a role in its development.

The clinical manifestations of the vasospastic attacks of either disorder are changes in skin color and sensation caused by ischemia. Vasospasm occurs with varying frequency and severity and causes pallor, numbness, and the sensation of cold in the digits. Attacks tend to be bilateral, and manifestations usually begin at the tips of the digits and progress to the proximal phalanges. Sluggish blood flow resulting from ischemia may cause the skin to appear cyanotic. Rubor, throbbing, and paresthesias follow. Skin color returns

to normal after the attack, but frequent, prolonged attacks interfere with cellular metabolism, causing the skin of the fingertips to thicken and the nails to become brittle. In severe, chronic Raynaud phenomenon or disease, ischemia can eventually cause ulceration and gangrene.

Treatment for Raynaud phenomenon consists of removing the stimulus or treating the primary disease process. Treatment of Raynaud disease is limited to prevention or alleviation of vasospasm itself, because no underlying disorder has been identified. Stimuli that trigger attacks (e.g., cold, emotional stress) are avoided, and cigarette smoking is stopped to eliminate the vasoconstricting effects of nicotine. If attacks of vasospasm become frequent or prolonged, vasodilators and rauwolfia alkaloids, such as reserpine, are administered. Calcium blockers also may be tried to decrease vasospasm caused by vascular reactivity from calcium influx.

✓ QUICK CHECK

Describe the two ways shock can lead to thrombus formation.

Trace the path of an embolism that dislodges from the saphenous vein.

Trace the path of an embolism that dislodges from the left atrium.

Compare the physical manifestations of Buerger disease and Raynaud disease.

Sympathectomy is the next line of treatment. If ischemia leads to ulceration and gangrene, amputation is necessary.

Diseases of the Veins
Varicose veins and chronic venous insufficiency

A *varicose vein* is a vein in which blood has pooled, producing distended, tortuous, and palpable vessels. Causes include (1) trauma to the saphenous veins that damages one or more valves or (2) gradual venous distention caused by a combination of standing for long periods, which diminishes the action of the muscle pump, and the pull of gravity on blood within the legs (see Fig. 22-25 for the muscle pump).

Veins are thin-walled, highly distensible vessels with valves to prevent backflow and pooling of blood. If a valve is damaged, a section of the vein is subjected to the pressure of a larger volume of blood under the influence of gravity. The vein swells, and increased hydrostatic pressure pushes plasma through the stretched vessel wall, causing edema of surrounding tissues.

Venous distention can develop over time in individuals who habitually stand for long periods, wear constricting garments, or cross the legs at the knees. Eventually the pressure in the vein damages venous valves, rendering them incompetent and unable to maintain normal venous pressure. Hydrostatic pressure increases, further distending the vein and making it tortuous; edema then develops in the extremity.

Fig. 23-11 *Venous stasis ulcer.* *(From Rosai, J. [1989]. Ackerman's surgical pathology [7th ed., vol. 2]. St. Louis: Mosby.)*

Fig. 23-12 *Multiple venous thrombi.* *(From Rosai, J. [1989]. Ackerman's surgical pathology [7th ed., vol. 2]. St. Louis: Mosby.)*

Chronic venous insufficiency (CVI) is inadequate venous return over a long period. CVI affects about 5% of adults in developing countries.[36] It causes pathologic changes as a result of ischemia in the vasculature, skin, and supporting tissues. Symptoms include chronic pooling of blood in the veins of the lower extremities and hyperpigmentation of the skin of the feet and ankles. Edema in these areas may extend to the knees.

Circulation to the extremities becomes so sluggish that the metabolic demands of the cells for oxygen, nutrients, and waste removal are barely met.[37,38] Any trauma or pressure can therefore lower the oxygen supply and cause cell death and necrosis (venous stasis ulcers) (Fig. 23-11). *Venous stasis ulcers* have a recurrence rate that ranges from 29% to 59%, even with optimal nonsurgical treatment.[39,40] Infection can occur because poor circulation impairs the delivery of the cells and biochemicals for the immune and inflammatory responses. This same sluggish circulation makes infection following reparative surgery a significant risk.[41] Contact allergies that develop in this population and the presence of HLA antigens in the ulcerated tissue suggest that a defective inflammatory response involving mast cells, Langerhans cells, and local growth factor contributes to the generation of venous stasis ulcers.[42]

Treatment of varicose veins and CVI begins conservatively and progresses as needed to surgical saphenous vein stripping. Excellent wound healing results have followed noninvasive treatments, such as compression stockings,[40,43] physical exercise, and low-frequency ultrasound.[44]

Thrombus formation in veins

The process of thrombus formation in the veins is the same as that of thrombus formation in the arteries. Venous thrombi are more common than arterial thrombi, however, because flow and pressure are lower in the veins than in the arteries (Fig. 23-12). With aging, in particular, the deep veins in the lower extremities become susceptible to thrombus formation, particularly if the individual is on long-term bed rest or wears constrictive clothing.

The inflammatory response triggered by the clotting cascade causes extreme tenderness, swelling, and redness in the area where the thrombus forms.[45] The major danger associated with deep venous thrombosis is that a portion of the thrombus will embolize to the lungs (pulmonary embolus, see Chapter 26).

The clinical manifestations of deep venous occlusion are often very subtle, with few symptoms or findings on physical examination. Prevention is important in at-risk individuals and includes early ambulation and prophylactic anticoagulation. If thrombosis does occur, diagnosis is confirmed by Doppler ultrasonography and management consists of anticoagulation with heparin (low-molecular weight heparin) and warfarin.[46]

Superior vena cava syndrome

Superior vena cava syndrome (SVCS) is a progressive occlusion of the superior vena cava (SVC) that leads to venous distention in the upper extremities and head. Causes include bronchogenic cancer (75% of cases), followed by lymphomas (15%), and metastasis of other cancers (7%). The right main stem bronchus abuts the SVC so that cancers occurring in this bronchus may press on the SVC. The SVC is also a relatively low-pressure vessel that lies in the closed thoracic compartment; therefore tissue expansion can easily compress the SVC. Finally, the SVC is surrounded by lymph nodes and lymph chains that commonly become involved in thoracic cancers and compress the SVC during tumor growth. Because onset of SVCS is slow, collateral venous drainage to the azygous vein usually has time to develop. Chronic cases of SVCS have also been attributed to arteriovenous shunt lesions, lymphadenopathy in cystic fibrosis, and goiter.[47,48] Acute cases of SVCS have been attributed to pacemaker implantation, long-term indwelling central venous catheters, and pleural effusion.[49]

Clinical manifestations of SVCS are edema and venous distention in the upper extremities and face, including the ocular beds. Cerebral and central nervous system edema may cause headache, visual disturbance, and impaired consciousness. The skin of the face and arms is purple and taut, and capillary refill time is prolonged. Respiratory distress may be present because of edema of bronchial structures or compression of the bronchus by a carcinoma. In infants, SVCS can lead to hydrocephalus.[50]

Treatment of SVCS is usually delayed for 24 hours to determine its cause. Because of its slow onset and the development of collateral venous drainage, SVCS is generally not a vascular emergency, but it is an oncologic emergency.[51] Treatment consists of radiation therapy and the administration of diuretics, steroids, and anticoagulants, as necessary.[52,53] Surgical treatment includes stent or graft placement and provides more rapid relief than medical management.[54-56]

Coronary Artery Disease, Myocardial Ischemia, and Myocardial Infarction

Coronary artery disease (CAD), myocardial ischemia, and myocardial infarction form a pathophysiologic continuum that impairs the pumping ability of the heart by depriving the heart muscle of blood-borne oxygen and nutrients. The earliest lesions of the continuum are those of *coronary artery disease*—any vascular disorder that narrows or occludes the coronary arteries; the most common cause of coronary obstruction is atherosclerosis (Fig. 23-13). CAD can diminish the myocardial blood supply until deprivation impairs myocardial metabolism enough to cause *ischemia,* a local state in which the cells are temporarily deprived of blood supply. They remain alive but cannot function normally. Persistent ischemia or the complete occlusion of a coronary artery causes *infarction,* or death, of the deprived myocardial tissue. Infarction constitutes the often-fatal event known as a *heart attack.*

Development of coronary artery disease

In the United States, CAD causes more than 700,000 myocardial infarctions per year. Despite a dramatic decline in mortality in the past decade, CAD causes one third of all deaths in the United States.[57] In the 1960s researchers began to identify risk factors that contribute to the onset and escalation of CAD. The factors were classified as either modifiable or nonmodifiable. The nonmodifiable risk factors refer to variables that cannot be altered by persons wishing to decrease their risk of cardiovascular disease. The role that some of the modifiable risk factors play in precipitating or exacerbating cardiovascular disease is controversial.[58] Dyslipidemia (e.g., hypercholesterolemia), hypertension, and cigarette smoking have, however, been identified objectively as most predictive of CAD.[59] Newer studies suggest that hyperhomocystinemia is also an important modifiable risk factor (see Table 23-4 and Health Alert box).[60,61] Several important risk factors are summarized in Table 23-4.

Fig. 23-13 *Atherosclerosis.* **A,** Concentric coronary plaque. The lumen is central. There are multiple, new small blood vessels within the plaque, the late result of disruption. **B,** Cell types in fibrolipid plaque. The plaque cap (brownish) contains numerous enlongated, smooth muscle cells; some contain lipid. Macrophages are clustered on the edge of the core. *(From Damjanov, I. & Linder, J. [Eds.]. [1996]. Anderson's pathology [10th ed.]. St. Louis: Mosby.)*

HEALTH ALERT

Homocysteine and Heart Disease

Dietary deficiencies of folate, B_6, and B_{12} can result in increased levels of homocysteine in the blood. Hyperhomocystinemia has been found to be an important risk factor for coronary artery disease. Mechanisms by which hyperhomocystinemia may contribute to atherogenesis include endothelial cell injury, increased smooth muscle proliferation, increased platelet aggregation, and abnormalities of fibrinolysis. Administration of folate (400-1000 μg/day) can reduce homocysteine levels and coronary risk.

Data from Rimm, E.B et al. (1998). Folate and vitamin B_6 from diet and supplements in relation to risk of coronary heart disease among women. Journal of the American Medical Association, 279(5), *359-364; Stein, J.N. & McBride, P.E. (1998). Hyperhomocystinemia and atherosclerotic vascular disease: Pathophysiology, screening, and treatment.* Archives of Internal Medicine, 158(12), *1301-1306; Wald, N.J. et al. (1998). Homocysteine and ischemic heart disease: Results of a prospective study with implications regarding prevention.* Archives of Internal Medicine, 158(8), *862-867; Welch, G.N. & Lascalzo, J. (1998). Homocysteine and atherothrombosis.* New England Journal of Medicine, 388(15), *1042-1050.*

TABLE 23-4	Risk Factors Associated With the Development of Coronary Artery Disease
Type	**Characteristics**
Hyperlipidemia	May develop as a result of high dietary fat intake, especially saturated fats and trans-fatty acids, systemic disease (pancreatitis, diabetes mellitus, hypothyroidism, nephrosis, systemic lupus erythematosus), and genetic defects (familial dyslipoproteinemias)
Hypertension	Elevated blood pressure can precipitate or exacerbate atherosclerotic process by causing trauma to arterial walls; then atherogenic plaques stiffen, narrowing arterial walls and increasing peripheral resistance and myocardial work load
Cigarette smoking	Of annual mortality from coronary artery disease, 30% traceable to cigarette smoking; nicotine stimulates catecholamine release, increasing heart rate and peripheral vascular constriction, and therefore blood pressure, cardiac work load, and oxygen demand
Diabetes mellitus	Often associated with increased lipid levels, obesity, and hypertension; glucose intolerance rises sharply; insulin resistance contributes to arterial damage
Genetic predisposition	Coronary-prone families account for 50% of early (under age 55 yr for men and under 70 yr for women) coronary disease; serum cholesterol level one of most predictive risk factors for coronary heart disease, with cholesterol risk factor (familial hypercholesterolemia) considered the most important genetic contribution; familial hypertension also significant
Obesity	Pattern of fat distribution significant; upper body obesity indicates greater risk of cardiovascular disease than lower body obesity; also predisposes individual to hypertension, hyperlipidemias, and impaired glucose tolerance; with increased obesity, heart enlarges, with increased oxygen consumption and work load
Sedentary life-style	Physical exercise may delay or prevent development of coronary artery disease by reducing blood pressure, decreasing the urge to smoke and eat, improving carbohydrate metabolism, and improving psychologic outlook; conversely, sedentary life-style predisposes to coronary artery disease
Estrogen deficiency	Mortality is reduced in women receiving estrogen replacement after menopause; estrogen-containing oral contraceptives may increase risk in premenopausal women; added risk to those who smoke while using contraceptives
Heavy alcohol consumption	Alcohol increases body weight, triglyceride levels, and systolic blood pressure and may impair left ventricular function; direct cardiotoxic effect with excessive alcohol results in collagen accumulation, diminished nucleic acid pools, and loss of membrane transport systems
Gender	Incidence is greater in males than premenopausal women; after menopause the incidence is about the same; gender differences appear to be attributable to differences in circulating estrogens and androgenic hormones; low HDL levels appear to be riskier for women than high LDL levels; the male pattern of obesity—gaining weight in the abdomen—puts women at higher risk (waist/hip ratio >0.8), and diabetes appears to be riskier in women than men
Personality	Persons with suppressed or expressed hostility are more likely to develop coronary heart disease
Hyperhomocystinemia	Genetic or dietary cause (inadequate folate intake); increased serum levels of homocysteine can damage coronary artery endothelium and are strongly correlated with risk for coronary artery disease
Unknown	Sustained activation of the renin-angiotensin system

HDL, *High-density lipoprotein;* LDL, *low-density lipoprotein.*

Myocardial ischemia

Pathophysiology

The coronary arteries normally supply blood flow sufficient to meet the demands of the myocardium as it labors under varying work loads. Oxygen is extracted from these vessels with maximal efficiency. If needs are not met, healthy coronary arteries can dilate to increase the flow of oxygenated blood to the myocardium. Various pathologic mechanisms can interfere with blood flow through the coronary arteries, giving rise to myocardial ischemia. Narrowing of a major coronary artery by more than 50% impairs blood flow enough to hamper cellular metabolism when myocardial demand increases (see Fig. 23-13).

The most common cause of myocardial ischemia is atherosclerosis. Plaques form in the arterial system and occlude vessels, depriving the myocardium of oxygen and nutrients. Thrombi may form in the coronary arteries as a result of ulceration of atherosclerotic plaques. The growing mass of plaque, platelets, fibrin, and cellular debris eventually can

Fig. 23-14 *Cycle of ischemic events.*

narrow the lumen enough to impede blood flow (see Fig. 23-4).[62,63] Platelet aggregations release the prostaglandin thromboxane A₂, a potent vasoconstrictor that can cause spasm of the coronary arteries and promote platelet aggregation, resulting in a vicious positive feedback cycle of vasoconstriction and platelet buildup in the vessel walls.

Myocardial ischemia develops if the flow or oxygen content of coronary blood is insufficient to meet the metabolic demands of myocardial cells. Imbalances between blood supply and myocardial demand can result from conditions reducing supply (e.g., hemodynamic factors, such as increased resistance in coronary vessels, hypotension, or decreased blood volume; cardiac factors, such as decreases of diastolic filling time, increases in heart rate, or valvular incompetence; hematologic factors, such as the oxygen content of the blood; or systemic disorders that reduce blood flow or the availability of oxygen) or increasing demand (e.g., high systolic blood pressure; increased ventricular volume; increased thickness of the myocardium; increased heart rate resulting from exercise, stress, hyperthyroidism, anemia, or hyperviscosity of the blood; conditions that heighten the myocardium's contractile response). Ischemia occurs if demand exceeds supply and develops within 10 seconds of coronary occlusion. After several minutes, the heart cells lose the ability to contract, thus hampering pump function and depriving the myocardium of a glucose source necessary for aerobic metabolism. Anaerobic processes take over, and lactic acid accumulates. Cardiac cells remain viable for approximately 20 minutes under ischemic conditions. If blood flow is restored, aerobic metabolism resumes, contractility is restored, and cellular repair begins. If perfusion is not restored, then myocardial infarction occurs (Fig. 23-14).[63]

▆ *Clinical Manifestations*

Angina pectoris is chest pain caused by myocardial ischemia. The discomfort is usually transient, lasting approximately 3 to 5 minutes. If blood flow is restored, no permanent change or damage results.

Angina pectoris is typically experienced as substernal chest discomfort, ranging from a sensation of heaviness or pressure to moderately severe pain. Individuals often describe the sensation by clenching a fist over the left sternal border. Discomfort may radiate to the neck, lower jaw, left arm, and left shoulder, or, occasionally, to the back or down the right arm. Discomfort is commonly mistaken for indigestion. The pain is presumably caused by the buildup of lactic acid or abnormal stretching of the ischemic myocardium that irritates myocardial nerve fibers. These afferent sympathetic fibers enter the spinal cord from levels C3 to T4, accounting for the variety of locations and radiation patterns of anginal pain. Pallor, diaphoresis, and dyspnea may be associated with the pain.

There are three types of angina:

1. *Stable angina.* Caused by luminal narrowing and hardening of the arterial walls, so that affected vessels cannot dilate in response to increased myocardial demand associated with physical exertion or emotional stress. The pain is usually relieved by rest and nitrates; lack of relief indicates individual may be developing infarction.

2. *Unstable angina.* Indicates advanced ischemic heart disease and is seldom predictable. Onset and course of unstable angina differ with each attack; attacks increase in frequency and duration with time, often occurring at rest, when ischemia is caused by thrombi forming transiently over atherosclerotic lesions, resulting in inadequate oxygenation. May be a manifestation of impending infarction.[64]

3. *Prinzmetal angina.* Chest pain attributable to transmural ischemia of myocardium that occurs unpredictably and almost exclusively at rest. Pain is caused by vasospasm of one or more major coronary arteries with or without associated atherosclerosis. The pain frequently occurs at night during rapid-eye-movement sleep and may have a cyclic pattern of occurrence. The angina may result from hyperactivity of sympathetic nervous system, increased calcium flux in arterial smooth muscle, or impaired production or release of prostaglandin or thromboxane.

Fig. 23-15 A, *Baseline.* B, *Transient total occlusion of left anterior descending branch of the left coronary artery after mental stress.* C, *After nitrates and nifedipine, artery reopened to same diameter as baseline.* *(From Stern, S. [Ed.] [1998].* Silent myocardial ischemia. *St. Louis: Mosby.)*

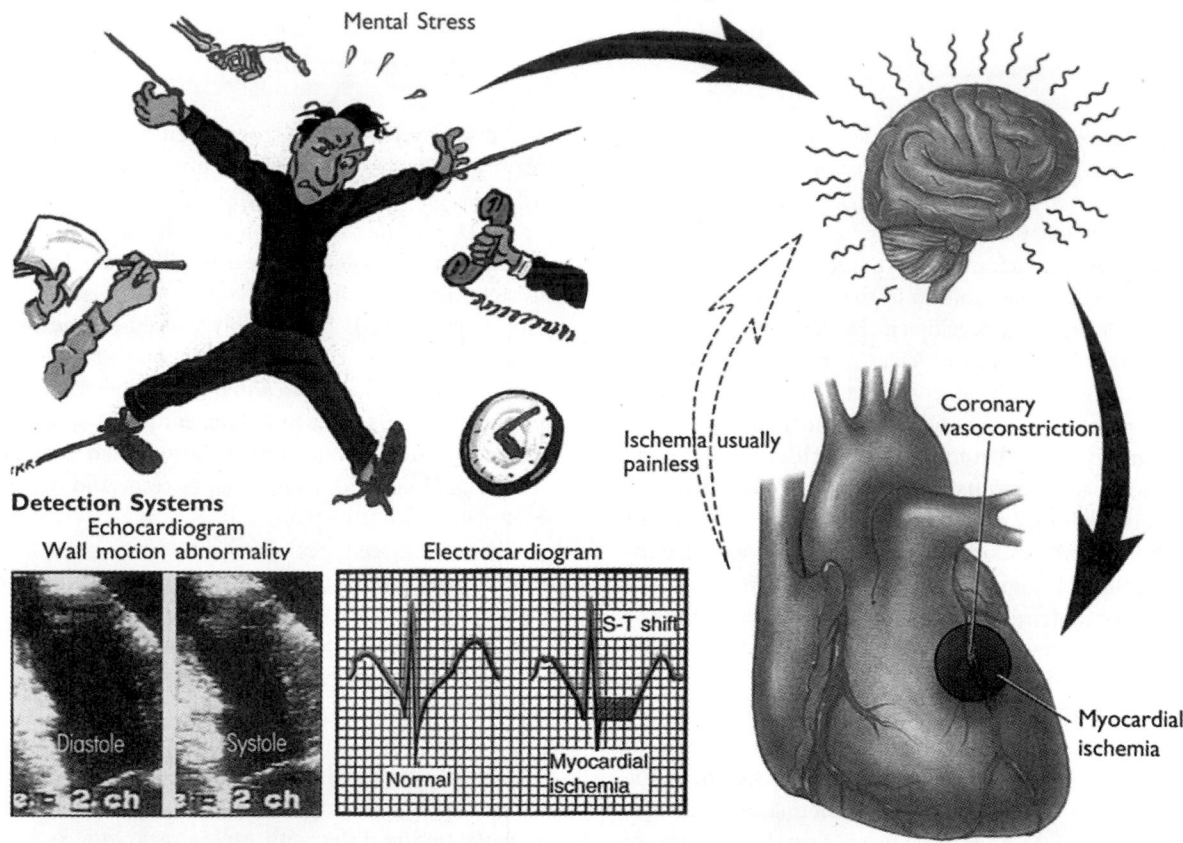

Fig. 23-16 *The ischemic cost of aggravation.* Linkages among daily mental and emotional stimuli, brain activity, and coronary and myocardial physiology. *(From Papodemetrion, V. et al. [1996].* Transient coronary occlusion with mental stress. American Heart Journal, 132, *1299-1301.)*

Silent ischemia and mental stress–induced ischemia

Myocardial ischemia often does not cause detectable symptoms such as angina. Ischemia can be totally asymptomatic and referred to as *silent ischemia.* In addition, myocardial ischemia can be silent in the majority of episodes in individuals who also experience angina.[65] Recent studies have addressed the pathophysiologic differences between silent and symptomatic ischemia. One proposed mechanism for the absence of angina in silent myocardial ischemia is the presence of a global or regional abnormality in left ventricular symptomatic afferent innervation. Such abnormality might occur as part of a metabolic dysfunction in diabetes mellitus, following surgical denervation during coronary artery bypass grafting (CABG) or cardiac transplantation, or following ischemic local nerve injury by myocardial infarction.[65-67]

Another area that is receiving renewed interest is the lack of angina, even though an artery is occluded, in some individuals during mental stress (Figs. 23-15 to 23-17).[68] Older studies have documented that although some individuals

Fig. 23-17 *Pathophysiologic model of the effects of acute stress as a trigger of cardiac clinical events, including myocardial ischemia in patients with coronary artery disease.* Acting via the central and autonomic nervous systems, stress can produce a cascade of physiologic responses that may lead to myocardial ischemia, potentially fatal dysrhythmia, plaque rupture, or coronary thrombosis. *VF,* Ventricular fibrillation; *VT,* ventricular tachycardia; *MI,* myocardial infarction; *LV,* left ventricular. *(From Krantz, D.S. et al. [1996]. Mental stress as a trigger of myocardial ischemia and infarction. In P.C. Deedwania & G.H. Tofler [Eds.]. Triggers and timing of cardiac events. [2nd ed.]. London: Saunders.)*

(94%) had angina during treadmill exercise, only 33% had angina during a mental stress–induced hypoperfusion.[69] Rozansky and colleagues[70] documented myocardial ischemia by radionuclide angiography (RNA) during mental stress, the majority of which cases (83%) were silent. They also noted a smaller increase in heart rate during mental stress than during exercise, although the systolic blood pressure response was comparable and the diastolic blood pressure response was even greater with mental stress.[65] These observations, confirmed in similar studies,[71,72] suggest that the increases in blood pressure induced by mental stress, and increases in myocardial oxygen demand, may play a role in the pathophysiology of mental stress–induced myocardial ischemia.[65]

Silent myocardial ischemia is very prevalent in individuals with a variety of acute and chronic coronary syndromes. Silent ischemia is detected with greater sensitivity and specificity with stress radionuclide imaging than by exercise electrocardiogram testing alone.[65]

▆ Evaluation and Treatment

Physical examination may disclose extra, rapid heart sounds (left ventricular gallop or S_3), indicating impaired left ventricular function during ischemia. The presence of xanthelasmas (small fat deposits) around the eyelids or arcus senilis of the eyes (a yellow lipid ring around the cornea) suggests dyslipidemia and possible atherosclerosis.

Electrocardiography is a critical tool for the diagnosis of myocardial ischemia. Because many individuals have normal electrocardiograms when there is no pain, diagnosis requires that electrocardiography be performed during an attack of angina. Transient ST segment depression and T wave inversion are characteristic signs of subendocardial ischemia. ST elevation, indicative of transmural ischemia, is seen in individuals with Prinzmetal angina (Fig. 23-18). The electrocardiogram can also indicate which coronary artery is involved. Exercise stress testing is useful in differentiating angina from other types of chest pain, as well as detecting ischemic changes that occur in the absence of anginal pain.

Radioisotope imaging with thallium-201 is another technique used to diagnose CAD. Active-transport mechanisms (the Na-K-ATPase system) cause thallium to enter myocardial cells. An area of myocardial infarction appears as a region of diminished or no activity (a "cold spot"). Defects that are absent at rest but can be induced by exercise represent ischemia. A newer test, called SPECT (single photon emission computerized tomography), is even more effective at identifying ischemia and estimating coronary risk.[73]

Coronary angiography helps determine the anatomic extent of CAD. The procedure is expensive and carries some risk; thus it is used primarily to evaluate for possible percutaneous transluminal coronary angioplasty (PTCA) or coronary artery bypass graft (CABG) surgery for individuals whose noninvasive studies suggest severe disease.

The primary aim of therapy for myocardial ischemia and angina is to reduce myocardial oxygen consumption by favorably altering its various determinants. The factors most amenable to pharmacologic manipulation are blood pressure, heart rate, contractility, and left ventricular volume. Drugs used include nitrates, β-adrenergic blocking agents, calcium channel blockers (verapamil, nifedipine, diltiazem),

Fig. 23-18 *Electrocardiogram (ECG) and ischemia.* **A,** Normal ECG. **B,** Electrocardiographic alterations associated with ischemia.

and antiplatelet agents (aspirin, sulfinpyrazone, dipyridamole, or the new platelet glycoprotein IIb/IIIa receptor antagonists).[74,75] Unstable angina suggests a high likelihood of impending infarction and requires admission to the hospital. Management includes anticoagulation and consideration for emergent PTCA or surgery.

Percutaneous transluminal coronary angioplasty (PTCA) is a procedure whereby stenotic (narrowed) coronary vessels are dilated with a balloon dilation catheter. It is generally used to treat single-vessel disease but can be effective with multiple-vessel disease or stenosis of a coronary artery or a venous bypass graft. Restenosis of the artery is the major complication of this procedure; the placement of a coronary artery stent can reduce this risk.[76]

Ischemic heart disease can be surgically treated by a coronary artery bypass graft (CABG) usually using the saphenous vein from the thigh. A technique using the left internal mammary artery (LIMA) has shown promise for significant improvement in long-term graft patency.

✓ QUICK CHECK

What causes varicose veins?

Why does damage to a valve of a vein increase development of a varicose vein?

Why do hypertension and increased cholesterol increase the development of coronary artery disease?

Discuss the relationships among myocardial ischemia, angina, and silent ischemia.

Myocardial infarction

Myocardial infarction is the irreversible hypoxia and cellular death of myocardial cells caused by prolonged ischemia. The incidence of myocardial infarction increases sharply with advancing age, with a marked male predominance.[77] Women lag behind men in incidence by about 20 years, but this gap in incidence closes with advancing age. The incidence increases substantially beyond age 45 years in men and 55 years in women. In men, the annual myocardial infarction rate under age 65 years (6 per 1000) more than doubles to 13 per 1000 after that age. Myocardial infarctions are sometimes silent and considered "unrecognized" *(silent heart attack).* About half of the unrecognized myocardial infarctions in men are completely silent, whereas only one third are silent in women.[77,78] A large portion of myocardial infarctions are atypical, such that neither the person nor practitioner even considers the possibility.[77] Possibilities that are considered include gallstones, hiatus hernia, cervical arthritis, or peptic ulcer.[77] Long-term angina pectoris precedes myocardial infarction about 20% of the time, and when the myocardial infarction is silent or unrecognized, only 5% are preceded by long-term angina.[77]

Acute myocardial infarction can be considered the end point of the coronary artery disease–myocardial ischemia continuum. Prolonged, unrelieved ischemia that interrupts the blood supply to the myocardium results in an acute coronary event. Unlike the temporary ischemia that causes angina and reversible cellular injury, the prolonged ischemia that causes infarction leads to irreversible hypoxia and cellular death (Fig. 23-19).

Assuming myocardial infarction is on a continuum with the ischemic attacks of angina, hypoxia could result from

Fig. 23-19 *Plaque disruption and myocardial infarction.* **A,** Plaque disruption. The cap of the lipid-rich plaque has become torn with the formation of a thrombus, mostly inside the plaque. **B,** Myocardial infarction. This infarct is 6 days old. The center is yellow and necrotic with a hemorrhagic red rim. The responsible artery occlusion is probably in the right coronary artery. The infarct is on the posterior wall. *(From Damjanov, I. & Linder, J. [Eds.]. [1996].* Anderson's pathology *[10th ed.]. St. Louis: Mosby.)*

long-term obstruction by atherosclerotic plaques, hemorrhage into a plaque, embolism caused by thrombi or atheromatous material, or coronary spasm. Thrombus formation resulting from abnormal platelet aggregation seems to be the most likely cause of eventual arterial occlusion. Evidence indicates that the fissuring and rupturing of atherosclerotic plaques stimulate platelet aggregation, platelet-thrombus formation, and abnormal vasomotor tone on the plaque location.[62,63] Substances such as serotonin, thromboxane A_2, adenosine diphosphate (ADP), adenosine triphosphate (ATP), platelet-activating factor (PAF), and platelet-activated growth factor contribute to acute myocardial infarction.

Pathophysiology
Cellular injury
Cardiac cells can withstand ischemic conditions for about 20 minutes before cellular death takes place. After only 30 to 60 seconds of hypoxia, electrocardiographic changes are visible. Yet even if cells are metabolically altered and nonfunctional, they can remain viable if blood flow returns within 20 minutes.

After 8 to 10 seconds of decreased blood flow, the affected myocardium becomes cyanotic and cooler. Myocardial oxygen reserves are used very quickly (within about 8 seconds) after complete cessation of coronary flow. Glycogen stores decrease as anaerobic metabolism begins. Unfortunately, glycolysis can supply only 65% to 70% of the total myocardial energy requirement and produces much less ATP than aerobic processes. Hydrogen ions and lactic acid accumulate. Because myocardial tissues have poor buffering capabilities and myocardial cells are very sensitive to low cellular pH, accumulation of these products further compromises the myocardium. Acidosis may make the myocardium

more vulnerable to the damaging effects of lysosomal enzymes and may suppress impulse conduction and contractile function, thereby leading to heart failure.

Oxygen deprivation also is accompanied by electrolyte disturbances, specifically loss of potassium, calcium, and magnesium from cells. Myocardial cells deprived of necessary oxygen and nutrients lose contractility, thereby diminishing the pumping ability of the heart. Normally, the myocardium takes up varying quantities of catecholamines (epinephrine, norepinephrine). Significant arterial occlusion causes the myocardial cells to release catecholamines, predisposing the individual to serious imbalances of sympathetic and parasympathetic function, irregular heartbeats (dysrhythmia), and heart failure. Catecholamines mediate the release of glycogen, glucose, and stored fat from body cells. Therefore plasma concentrations of free fatty acids and glycerol rise within 1 hour after the onset of acute myocardial infarction. Excessive levels of free fatty acids can have a harmful detergent effect on cell membranes. Norepinephrine elevates blood sugar levels through stimulation of liver and skeletal muscle cells and suppresses pancreatic β-cell activity, which reduces insulin secretion and elevates blood glucose further. Not surprisingly, hyperglycemia is noted approximately 72 hours after an acute myocardial infarction.

Cellular death
After about 20 minutes of myocardial ischemia, irreversible hypoxic injury causes cellular death and tissue necrosis. This results in the release of certain intracellular enzymes through the damaged cell membranes into the interstitial spaces. The lymphatics pick up the enzymes and transport them into the bloodstream, where they can be detected by serologic tests.

Fig. 23-20 *Myocardial infarction.* **A,** Local infarct confined to one region. **B,** Massive large infarct caused by occlusion of three coronary arteries. *(From Damjanov, I. & Linder, J. [Eds.]. [1996]. Anderson's pathology [10th ed.]. St. Louis: Mosby.)*

Structural and functional changes

Myocardial infarction results in both structural and functional changes of cardiac tissues (Fig. 23-20). Gross tissue changes at the area of infarction may not become apparent for several hours, despite almost immediate onset (within 30 to 60 seconds) of electrocardiographic changes. Cardiac tissue surrounding the area of infarction also undergoes changes that can be categorized into (1) *myocardial stunning*—a temporary loss of contractile function that persists for hours to days after perfusion has been restored; (2) *hibernating myocardium*—tissue that is persistently ischemic and undergoes metabolic adaptation to prolong myocyte survival until perfusion can be restored; and (3) *myocardial remodeling*—a process mediated by angiotensin II that causes myocyte hypertrophy and loss of contractile function in the areas of the heart distant from the site of infarction. All these changes can be limited through rapid restoration of coronary flow and the use of angiotensin converting enzyme (ACE) inhibitors.[79,80]

The severity of functional impairment depends on the size of the lesion and the site of infarction. Functional changes can include (1) decreased cardiac contractility with abnormal wall motion, (2) altered left ventricular compliance, (3) decreased stroke volume, (4) decreased ejection fraction, (5) increased left ventricular end-diastolic pressure, and (6) sinoatrial node malfunction. Life-threatening dysrhythmias and heart failure often follow myocardial infarction.

Repair

Myocardial infarction causes a severe inflammatory response that ends with wound repair (see Chapter 6). Damaged cells undergo degradation, fibroblasts proliferate, and scar tissue is synthesized. Many cell types, hormones, and nutrient substrates must be available for optimal healing to proceed. Within 24 hours, leukocytes infiltrate the necrotic area, and proteolytic enzymes from scavenger neutrophils

degrade necrotic tissue. A pseudodiabetic state often develops as catecholamines released from damaged cells stimulate release of glucose and free fatty acids. By the second week, insulin secretion increases to mobilize glucose from the repair processes. The collagen matrix that is deposited is initially weak, mushy, and vulnerable to reinjury. Unfortunately it is at this time in the recovery period (10 to 14 days after infarction) that individuals feel more like increasing activities and may stress the newly formed scar tissue. After 6 weeks the necrotic area is completely replaced by scar tissue, which is strong but cannot contract and relax like healthy myocardial tissue.

Clinical Manifestations

The first symptom of acute myocardial infarction is usually sudden, severe chest pain. The pain is similar to angina pectoris but more severe and persistent and is not relieved by nitrates. It may be described as heavy and crushing, such as a "truck sitting on my chest." Radiation to the neck, jaw, back, shoulder, or left arm is common. Some individuals, especially those who are elderly or have diabetes, experience no pain, thereby having a "silent" infarction. Infarction often stimulates a sensation of unrelenting indigestion. Nausea and vomiting may occur because of reflex stimulation of vomiting centers by pain fibers. Vasovagal reflexes from the area of the infarcted myocardium may also affect the gastrointestinal tract. Catecholamine release results in sympathetic stimulation, producing diaphoresis and peripheral vasoconstriction that cause the skin to become cool and clammy. Fever may develop in the first 24 hours and persist for 1 week because of inflammatory activity within the myocardium.

Various cardiovascular changes are found on physical examination:

1. Blood pressure initially decreases.
2. The sympathetic nervous system is reflexively activated to compensate, resulting in a temporary increase in heart rate and blood pressure.

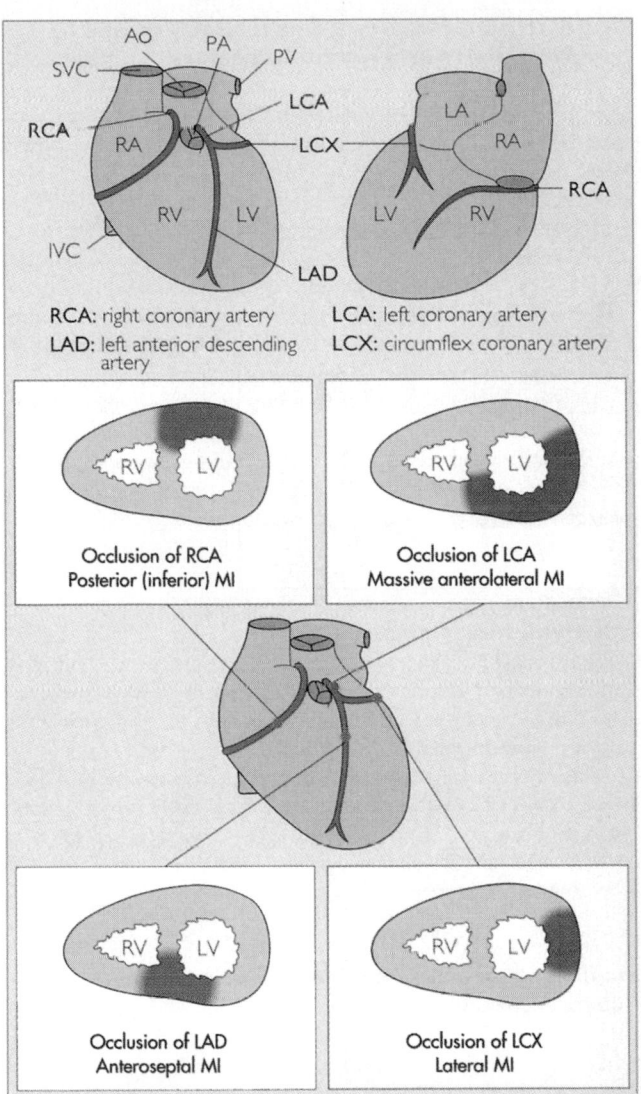

Fig. 23-21 *Site of myocardial infarction (MI) and vessel involvement. Ao,* Aorta; *PA,* pulmonary artery; *PV,* pulmonary vein; *LV,* left ventricle; *RV,* right ventricle; *IVC,* inferior vena cava; *RA,* right atrium; *SVC,* superior vena cava; *LA,* left atrium. *(Modified from Stevens, A. & Lowe, J. [1995]. Pathology. St. Louis: Mosby.)*

3. Abnormal extra heart sounds reflect left ventricular dysfunction.
4. Pericardial friction rub (roughened membranes rubbing against each other) and cardiac murmurs may result from inflammation.

Laboratory data reveal leukocytosis and elevated sedimentation rate, both of which indicate inflammation. The individual's blood sugar is usually elevated, and the glucose tolerance level may remain abnormal for several weeks. Hypoxemia develops, particularly in individuals not given supplemental oxygen.[81]

A transient rise in plasma enzyme levels can confirm the occurrence of myocardial infarction and indicate its severity. The enzymes released by myocardial cells include creatine kinase (CK), lactic dehydrogenase (LDH), and, to a lesser extent, aspartate aminotransferase (AST). These enzymes exist in several different active molecular forms called *isoenzymes,* which are present in different amounts within particular tissues. If serologic tests show abnormally high levels of isoenzymes associated with cardiac tissue (CK-MB, LDH-1), acute myocardial infarction has probably occurred. Of the three isoenzymes, CK-MB is most specific for myocardial infarction, although its level may also increase in individuals with other conditions. A new assay based on monoclonal antibodies against troponin I may be a more specific marker for myocardial injury than CK-MB.[82,83] Serum precursor protein rises before other serum markers (CK, CK-MB, myoglobin) and may become an important assay for the prediction of imminent myocardial infarction.[84] Elevation of CK-MB, LDH-1, and AST will be noted at characteristic times. The higher the serum concentration of CK-MB, the more extensive the tissue damage that has occurred. Blood is drawn for enzyme determinations as soon as possible after the onset of symptoms and for serial enzyme levels every 4 hours for three additional measurements. If these consecutive measurements reveal no significant enzyme elevation, then myocardial infarction is ruled out.

Myocardial infarction can occur in various regions of the heart wall and may be described as anterior, inferior, posterior, lateral, subendocardial, endocardial, subepicardial, epicardial, intramural, or transmural, depending on the anatomic location and extent of tissue damage from infarction (Fig. 23-21). Twelve-lead electrocardiograms (ECGs) help to localize the affected area through identification of Q waves and changes in ST segments and T waves (Fig. 23-22). The infarcted myocardium is surrounded by a zone of hypoxic injury, which may progress to necrosis or return to normal. Infarcted tissue is electrically silent and does not contribute to the ECG. Transmural infarcts are large enough to create inscription of a Q wave on the ECG (Q wave infarction). Small infarcts are usually subendocardial and do not create a Q wave (non–Q wave infarction). Adjacent to the zone of hypoxic injury is a zone of reversible ischemia. Ischemic and injured myocardial tissue causes ST and T wave changes. As the myocardium heals, the ST segment and T waves gradually return to normal, but abnormal Q waves generally persist.

Radionucleotide imaging with thallium-201 can provide a diagnostic picture in individuals with acute or healed myocardial infarction. Technetium-99m pyrophosphate is also taken up by areas of myocardial infarction, which appear as "hot spots." Unfortunately, the area of infarction must be large enough to visualize the hot spot, and the scan may remain positive for many months after infarction.

Although the incidence of sudden cardiac death is decreasing, about 350,000 to 400,000 people in the United States alone present with sudden cardiac death annually.[85] Silent ischemia presents probably 70% of all ischemic crises, and this percentage may be greater if the silent ischemia of totally asymptomatic individuals is considered.[85] Sudden cardiac death is a multifactorial problem. Risk factors for sudden death are related to three factors: ischemia, left ven-

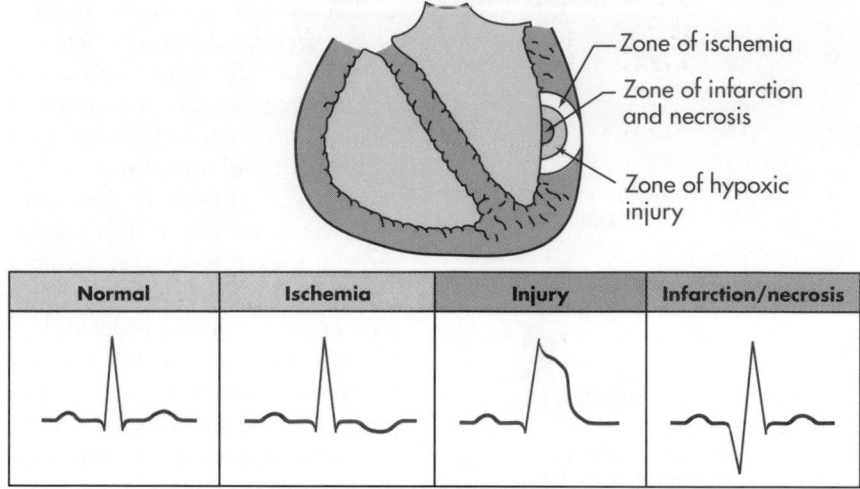

Fig. 23-22 *Electrocardiographic alterations associated with the three zones of myocardial infarction.*

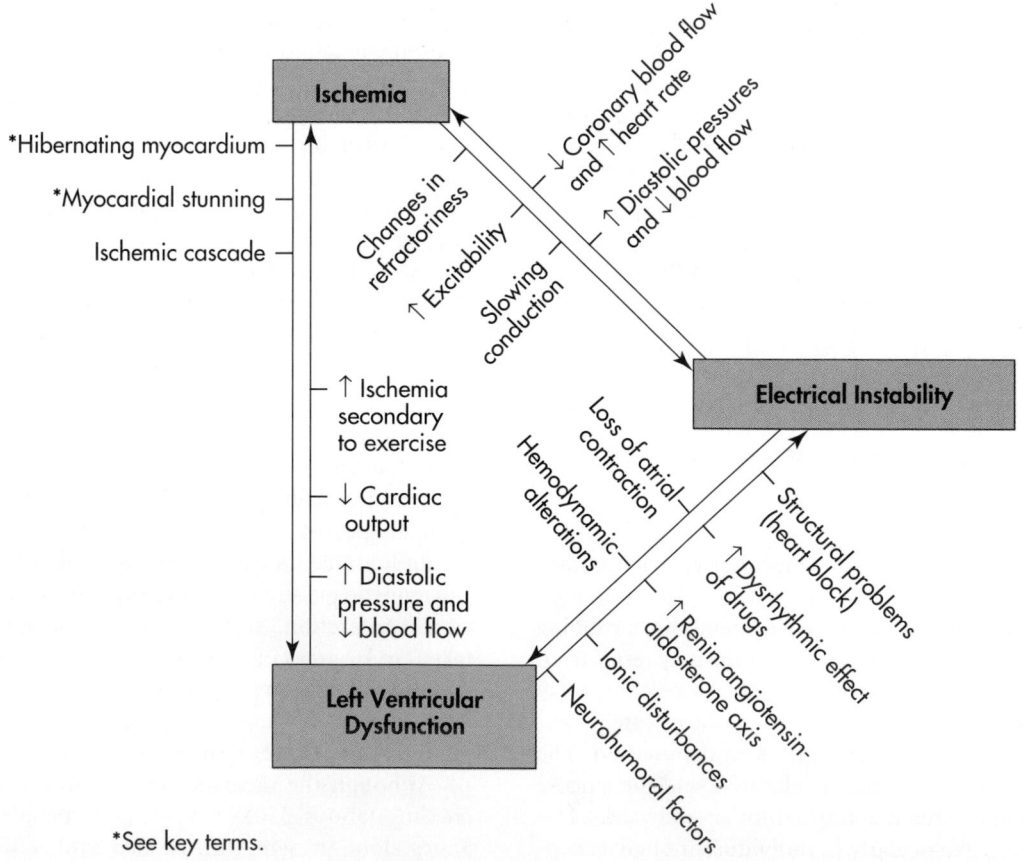

*See key terms.

Fig. 23-23 *Three interacting factors related to sudden cardiac death.* The three factors are ischemia, left ventricular dysfunction, and electrical instability. (*See Key terms.)

TABLE 23-5	Complications With Myocardial Infarctions
Type	**Characteristics**
Dysrhythmias	Disturbances of cardiac rhythm that affect 90% of cardiac infarction patients
	Caused by ischemia, hypoxia, autonomic nervous system imbalances, lactic acidosis, electrolyte abnormalities, alterations of impulse conduction pathways or conduction abnormalities, drug toxicity, or hemodynamic abnormalities
Left ventricular failure (congestive heart failure)	Characterized by pulmonary congestion, reduced myocardial contractility, and abnormal heart wall motion
	Cardiogenic shock can develop
Inflammation of the pericardium (pericarditis)	Includes pericardial friction rubs
	Frequently noted 2 to 3 days later and associated with anterior chest pain that worsens with respiratory effort
Dressler postinfarction syndrome	Essentially a delayed form of pericarditis that occurs 1 wk to several months after acute MI
	Thought to be immunologic response to necrotic myocardium and marked by pain, fever, friction rub, pleural effusion, and arthralgias
Organic brain syndrome	Occurs if blood flow to brain is impaired secondary to MI
	Transient ischemic attacks or cerebrovascular accident may occur if thromboemboli break loose in coronary arteries or cardiac valves
Rupture of heart structures	Caused by necrosis of tissue in or around papillary muscles
	Affects papillary muscles of chordae tendinae cordis
	Predisposing factors include thinning of wall, poor collateral flow, shearing effect of muscular contraction against stiffened necrotic area, marked necrosis at terminal end of blood supply and aging of myocardium with laceration of myocardial microstructure
Rupture of wall of infarcted ventricle	Can be caused by aneurysm formation when pressure becomes too great
	Left ventricular aneurysm is late (month to years) complication of MI
Infarctions around septal structures	Occur in those structures that separate heart chambers and lead to septal rupture
	Associated with audible, harsh cardiac murmurs, increased left ventricular end-diastolic pressure, and decreased systemic blood pressure
Systemic thromboembolism	Commonly found in postmortem examinations of individuals dying of MI
	May disseminate from debris and clots that collect inside dilated aneurysmal sacs or from infarcted endocardium
	Especially common are pulmonary emboli and deep venous thrombi of legs
	Reduced incidence associated with early mobilization and prophylactic anticoagulation therapy
Sudden death	Dysrhythmias frequently causative, particularly ventricular fibrillation
	Knowledge of CPR has increased survival
	Risk of death increased by age more than 65 yr, previous angina pectoris, hypotension or cardiogenic shock, acute systolic hypertension at time of admission, diabetes mellitus, dysrhythmias or conduction defects, and previous MI

MI, *Myocardial infarction;* CPR, *cardiopulmonary resuscitation.*

tricular dysfunction, and electrical instability. These factors interact with each other (Fig. 23-23).

Complications

The number and severity of postinfarction complications depend on the location and extent of necrosis, the individual's physiologic condition before the infarction, and the availability of swift therapeutic intervention. Table 23-5 lists the most common complications.

Evaluation and Treatment

The diagnosis of acute myocardial infarction is made on the basis of history, physical examination, ECG, serial enzyme alterations, and radionucleotide or ultrasound imaging. Acute myocardial infarction requires admission to the hospital, often directly into a coronary care unit. The individual should be placed on supplemental oxygen and given an aspirin immediately (ticlopidine if allergic to aspirin). Pain relief is of utmost importance and involves the use of sublingual nitroglycerin or morphine sulfate. Continuous monitoring of cardiac rhythms and enzymatic changes is essential, because the first 24 hours after onset of symptoms is the time of highest risk for sudden death. Individuals who are in shock require aggressive fluid resuscitation and possible emergent invasive procedures (see p. 684).

If the individual is diagnosed within a few hours of the onset of pain and has no contraindications, thrombolytic therapy with tissue plasminogen activator (t-PA) should be administered. This is followed by heparin infusion. Additional therapies that should be considered include emergent PTCA, angiotensin converting enzyme (ACE) inhibitors, and β blockers.[86-88]

Bed rest, followed by gradual return to activities of daily living, reduces the myocardial oxygen demands of the compromised heart. Individuals not receiving thrombolytic or heparin infusion must receive deep venous thrombosis prophylaxis as long as their activity is significantly limited. Stool softeners are given to eliminate the need for straining, which can precipitate bradycardia and can be followed by increased venous return to the heart, causing possible cardiac overload. Education on diet, caffeine, smoking cessation, exercise, and other aspects of risk factor reduction is crucial for secondary prevention of recurrent myocardial ischemia.

✓ QUICK CHECK

Describe the coronary artery disease–myocardial ischemia continuum.

Describe the pathophysiology of a myocardial infarction.

What complications are associated with the period after infarction?

DISORDERS OF THE HEART WALL
Disorders of the Pericardium

Pericardial disease is often a localized manifestation of another disorder, such as infection (bacterial, viral, fungal, rickettsial, or parasitic); trauma or surgery; neoplasm; or a metabolic, immunologic, or vascular disorder (uremia, rheumatoid arthritis, systemic lupus erythematosus, periarteritis nodosa). The pericardial response to injury from these diverse causes may consist of acute pericarditis, pericardial effusion, or constrictive pericarditis.[89]

Acute pericarditis

Although the cause is frequently unknown, *acute pericarditis* (acute inflammation of the pericardium) is commonly caused by infection (viral or bacterial), uremia, neoplasm, myocardial infarction, surgery, or trauma.[89] The pericardial membranes become inflamed and roughened, and an exudate may develop (Fig. 23-24).

Symptoms include sudden onset of severe chest pain that worsens with respiratory movements. Although the pain may radiate to the back, it is generally felt in the anterior chest and may be confused initially with the pain of acute myocardial infarction. Individuals with acute pericarditis also report dysphagia, restlessness, irritability, anxiety, weakness, and malaise.

Physical examination often discloses low-grade fever and sinus tachycardia. Friction rub, a short, scratchy, grating sensation similar to the sound of sandpaper, may be heard at the cardiac apex and left sternal border and is diagnostic for pericarditis. The rub is caused by the roughened pericardial membranes rubbing against each other. Friction rubs are not always present and may be intermittently heard and transient. Electrocardiographic changes may reflect inflammatory processes through PR segment depression and diffuse ST segment elevation without Q waves.[90]

Fig. 23-24 *Acute pericarditis.* Note shaggy coat of fibers covering surface of heart. *(From Anderson, W.A.D. & Scotti, T.M. [1980]. Synopsis of pathology [10th ed.]. St. Louis: Mosby.)*

Fig. 23-25 *Exudate of blood in the pericardial sac from rupture of aneurysm. (From Anderson, W.A.D. & Scotti, T.M. [1980].* Synopsis of pathology *[10th ed.]. St. Louis: Mosby.)*

Treatment for uncomplicated acute pericarditis consists of relieving symptoms. Exploration of the underlying cause is important. If pericardial effusion develops, aspiration of the excessive fluid may be necessary. Acute pericarditis is usually self-limiting but occasionally may progress to chronic constrictive pericarditis.[89]

Pericardial effusion

Pericardial effusion—the accumulation of fluid in the pericardial cavity—can occur in all forms of pericarditis. The fluid may be a transudate, such as the serous effusion that develops with left heart failure, overhydration, or hypoproteinemia. More often, however, the fluid is an exudate, which reflects pericardial injury and inflammation (Fig. 23-25).

(Types of exudate are described in Chapter 6.) If the fluid is serosanguineous, the underlying cause is likely to be tuberculosis, neoplasm, uremia, or radiation. Idiopathic serosanguineous (cause unknown) effusion is possible, however. Effusions of frank blood are generally related to aneurysms, trauma, or coagulation defects. If chyle leaks from the thoracic duct, it may enter the pericardium and lead to cholesterol pericarditis.

Pericardial effusion, even in large amounts, is not necessarily clinically significant, except that it indicates an underlying disorder, such as systemic lupus erythematosus. If the fluid creates sufficient pressure to cause cardiac compression, a serious condition known as *tamponade* exists. If an effusion develops gradually, the pericardium can stretch to accommodate large quantities of fluid without compressing the heart. If the fluid accumulates rapidly, however, even a small amount (50 to 100 ml) may cause serious tamponade. The danger is that pressure exerted by the pericardial fluid eventually will equal diastolic pressure within the heart chambers. The first structures to be affected by tamponade are the right atrium and ventricle, where diastolic pressures are normally lowest. Compression by pericardial fluid interferes with right atrial filling during diastole, resulting in increased venous pressure, systemic venous congestion, and signs and symptoms of right heart failure (distention of the jugular veins, edema, hepatomegaly). Decreased atrial filling leads to decreased ventricular filling, decreased stroke volume, and reduced cardiac output. Life-threatening circulatory collapse may occur.

The most significant clinical finding is pulsus paradoxus, in which arterial blood pressure during expiration exceeds arterial pressure during inspiration by more than 10 mm Hg. Pulsus paradoxus indicates tamponade and reflects impairment of diastolic filling of the left ventricle plus reduction of blood volume within all four cardiac chambers. Presence of a large pericardial effusion or tamponade magnifies the normally insignificant effect of inspiration on intracardiac flow and volume.

Other clinical manifestations of pericardial effusion are distant or muffled heart sounds, poorly palpable apical pulse, dyspnea on exertion, and dull chest pain. A chest x-ray film may disclose a "water-bottle" configuration of the cardiac silhouette. An echocardiogram can detect an effusion as small as 20 ml.

Treatment of pericardial effusion or tamponade generally consists of pericardiocentesis (aspiration of excessive pericardial fluid). Persistent pain may be treated with analgesics, antiinflammatory medications, or steroids. Surgery may be required if the underlying cause of tamponade is trauma or aneurysm.

Individuals with acute pericarditis secondary to certain underlying conditions may have pericardial effusion. This manifestation is common in (1) individuals with uremia who are in need of dialysis and have fluid overload and left ventricular failure; (2) individuals who have lymphoma or breast cancer or who are receiving radiation therapy; (3) individuals who are taking drugs such as procainamide and minoxidil; and (4) individuals who have undergone surgery

Fig. 23-26 *Constrictive pericarditis.* Note band of calcified tissue that constricts heart. (Measurement in centimeters.) *(From Kissane, J.M. [Ed.]. [1990]. Anderson's pathology [9th ed.]. St. Louis: Mosby.)*

that involved an incision of the heart wall. If an effusion is neoplasm induced, chemotherapeutic agents may be injected into the pericardial space. Tetracycline also may be injected into the pericardium to induce pericardial sclerosis and prevent further fluid accumulation.[89,91]

Constrictive pericarditis

Constrictive pericarditis (chronic pericarditis) was synonymous with tuberculosis years ago (Fig. 23-26). Currently in the United States, this form of pericardial disease is either idiopathic or associated with radiation exposure, rheumatoid arthritis, uremia, or coronary artery bypass graft. In constrictive pericarditis, fibrous scarring with occasional calcification of the pericardium causes the visceral and parietal pericardial layers to adhere, obliterating the pericardial cavity. The fibrotic lesions encase the heart in a rigid shell. Like tamponade, constrictive pericarditis compresses the heart and eventually reduces cardiac output. Unlike tamponade, however, constrictive pericarditis always develops gradually.

Symptoms tend to be exercise intolerance, dyspnea on exertion, fatigue, and anorexia. Clinical assessment shows weight loss, edema, distention of the jugular vein, and hepatic congestion. Restricted ventricular filling may cause a pericardial knock (early diastolic sound).

Electrocardiographic findings include T wave inversions and atrial fibrillation. An echocardiogram may suggest evidence of nonspecific pericardial thickening. Computed tomography is best able to detect constrictive processes. Chest x-ray films frequently disclose prominent pulmonary vessels and calcification of the pericardium.

Initial treatment for constrictive pericarditis is pharmacologic and dietary. Digitalis glycosides, diuretics, and sodium restriction are often prescribed. If these modalities

TABLE 23-6	Effects of Cardiomyopathies on Circulation Through the Heart		
	Type of Cardiomyopathy		
Effect	**Dilated**	**Hypertrophic**	**Restrictive**
Hemodynamic			
Cardiac output	Decreased	Normal	Normal or decreased
Stroke volume	Decreased	Normal or increased	Decreased
Ventricular filling pressure	Increased	Normal or increased	Increased
Ejection fraction	Decreased	Increased	Normal or decreased
Inflow resistance	Normal	Increased	Increased
Outflow tract obstruction	None	Increased	None
Formation of intracardiac thrombi	Increased	None	Increased
Structural or functional			
Chamber size	Increased	Normal or decreased	Decreased or normal
Myocardial mass	Increased	Increased	Normal or increased
Endocardial thickness	Normal or increased	Increased	Increased
Contractility	Decreased	Increased or decreased	Normal or decreased
Mitral valve competence	Decreased	Decreased	Decreased

Data from DeSanctis, R.W. (1990). Cardiomyopathies. Scientific American Medicine, 1(1-XIV), 1-23; Wenger, N.K., Ablemann, W.H., & Roberts, W.C. (1990). Cardiomyopathy and specific heart muscle disease. In J.W. Hurst et al. (Eds.). The heart, arteries, and veins (7th ed.). New York: McGraw-Hill.

are unsuccessful, surgical excision of the restrictive pericardium is indicated.

Disorders of the Myocardium: The Cardiomyopathies

The *cardiomyopathies* are a diverse group of diseases that primarily affect the myocardium itself and are not secondary to the usual cardiovascular disorders. They may, however, be secondary to infectious disease, exposure to toxins, systemic connective tissue disease, infiltrative and proliferative disorders, or nutritional deficiencies. However, most cases are idiopathic; that is, their cause is unknown. The cardiomyopathies are categorized as dilated (formerly, congestive), hypertrophic, or restrictive, depending on their physiologic effects on the heart (Fig. 23-27 and Tables 23-6 and 23-7).[92]

✓ QUICK CHECK

Why does pericarditis develop?

What are the cardiomyopathies? List the major disorders.

Briefly describe the pathophysiologic effects of the cardiomyopathies.

Disorders of the Endocardium
Valvular dysfunction

Disorders of the endocardium, the innermost lining of the heart wall, damage the heart valves, which are composed of endocardial tissue. Endocardial damage can be either congenital or acquired. The acquired forms cause inflammatory, ischemic, traumatic, degenerative, or infectious alterations of valvular structure and function.[93,94] The usual cause of acquired valvular dysfunction is inflammation of the endo-

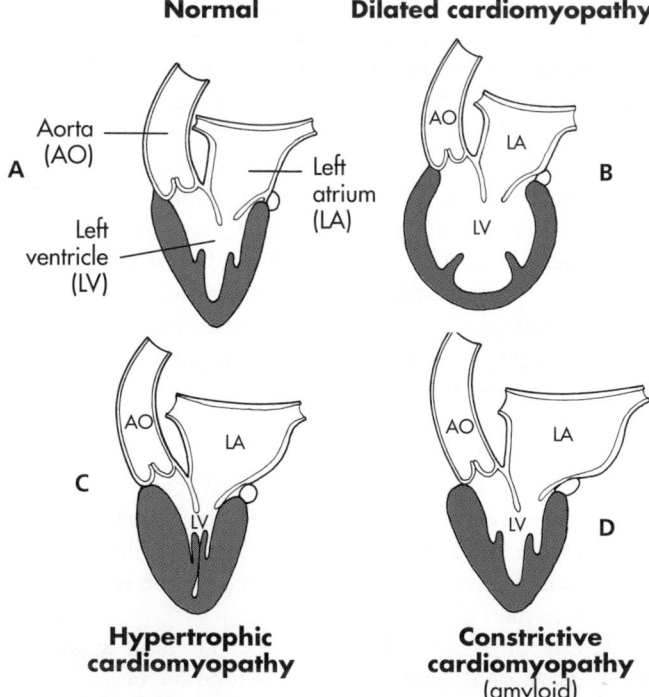

Fig. 23-27 *Diagram showing major distinguishing pathophysiologic features of the three types of cardiomyopathy.* **A,** The normal heart. **B,** In the dilated type of cardiomyopathy, the heart has a globular shape and the largest circumference of the left ventricle is not at its base but midway between apex and base. **C,** In the hypertrophic type, the wall of the left ventricle is greatly thickened; the left ventricular cavity is small, but the left atrium may be dilated because of poor diastolic relaxation of the ventricle. **D,** In the restrictive (constrictive) type, the left ventricular cavity is of normal size, but, again, the left atrium is dilated because of the reduced diastolic compliance of the ventricle. *(From Kissane, J.M. [Ed.]. [1990]. Anderson's pathology [9th ed.]. St. Louis: Mosby.)*

TABLE 23-7	Pathophysiologic Effects of the Cardiomyopathies		
	Type of Cardiomyopathy		
Pathophysiology	**Dilated**	**Hypertrophic**	**Restrictive**
Major symptoms	Fatigue, weakness, palpitations	Dyspnea, angina pectoris, fatigue, dizziness (syncope), palpitations	Dyspnea, fatigue
Cardiomegaly	Moderate to marked	Mild to moderate	Mild
Hypertrophy	Left ventricular myocardium	Left ventricular myocardium and interventricular septum	Left ventricular myocardium
Alterations of chamber volume	Volume increased	Volume decreased, particularly in left ventricle	Volume normal to decreased
Alterations of chamber compliance	Compliance increased	Compliance decreased, particularly in left ventricle	Compliance decreased, particularly in left ventricle
Alterations of systolic function (myocardial contractility)	Contractility decreased in left ventricle	Contractility increased or vigorous	None
Valvular incompetence	Atrioventricular valves, particularly mitral	Mitral valve	Atrioventricular valve
Conduction defects	Intraventricular	Nonspecific	Atrioventricular
Dysrhythmias	Sinoatrial tachycardia; atrial and ventricular dysrhythmias	Atrial and ventricular dysrhythmias	Tachydysrhythmias
Thromboembolism	Systemic or pulmonary	Systemic or pulmonary	Systemic or pulmonary
Associated conditions	Alcoholism, pregnancy, infection, nutritional deficiency, exposed to toxins	Possible inherited defect of muscle growth and development	Infiltrative disease
Eventual cardiovascular event	Left heart failure	Left heart failure	Right heart failure

cardium secondary to acute rheumatic fever or infectious endocarditis (see p. 660). Structural alterations of the heart valves lead to stenosis, incompetence, or both.

In *valvular stenosis,* the valve orifice is constricted and narrowed, so blood cannot flow forward and the work load of the cardiac chamber "in front" of the diseased valve is increased (Fig. 23-28). Pressure (intraventricular or atrial) rises in the chamber to overcome resistance to flow through the valve, causing the myocardium to work harder and producing myocardial hypertrophy.

In *valvular regurgitation* (also called *insufficiency* or *incompetence*), the valve leaflets, or cusps, fail to shut completely, permitting blood flow to continue even when the valve is supposed to be closed (see Fig. 23-28). During systole, some blood leaks back into the atrial chamber "upstream." Valvular regurgitation increases the volume of blood the heart must pump and increases the work load of both atrium and ventricle. Valvular incompetence causes cardiomegaly. Increased volume leads to chamber dilation, and increased work load leads to hypertrophy. Although all four heart valves may be affected, those of the left heart (mitral and aortic semilunar valves) are far more commonly affected than those of the right heart (tricuspid and pulmonic semilunar valves).

Valvular dysfunction stimulates chamber dilation and myocardial hypertrophy, both of which are compensatory mechanisms intended to increase the pumping capability of the heart. Eventually, myocardial contractility is diminished, the ejection fraction is reduced, diastolic pressure increases, and the ventricles fail from overwork. Depending on the severity of the valvular dysfunction and the capacity of the heart to compensate, valvular alterations cause a range of symptoms and some degree of incapacitation (Table 23-8). Valvular dysfunction is treated with cardiac glycosides, diuretics, dietary salt restriction, and antibiotics until prosthetic valve replacement becomes necessary.

Stenosis

Aortic stenosis. Aortic stenosis has three common causes: (1) inflammatory damage caused by rheumatic heart disease, (2) congenital malformation (see Chapters 2 and 24), and (3) degeneration resulting from calcification (see Chapter 3). The orifice of the aortic semilunar valve narrows, causing diminished blood flow from the left ventricle into the aorta (see Fig. 23-28). Outflow obstruction increases pressure within the left ventricle as it tries to eject blood through the narrowed opening.

Aortic stenosis tends to develop gradually. Clinical manifestations include decreased stroke volume, reduced systolic blood pressure, and narrowed pulse pressure (difference between systolic and diastolic pressure). Heart rate is often slow, and pulses are faint. Resistance to flow gives rise to a

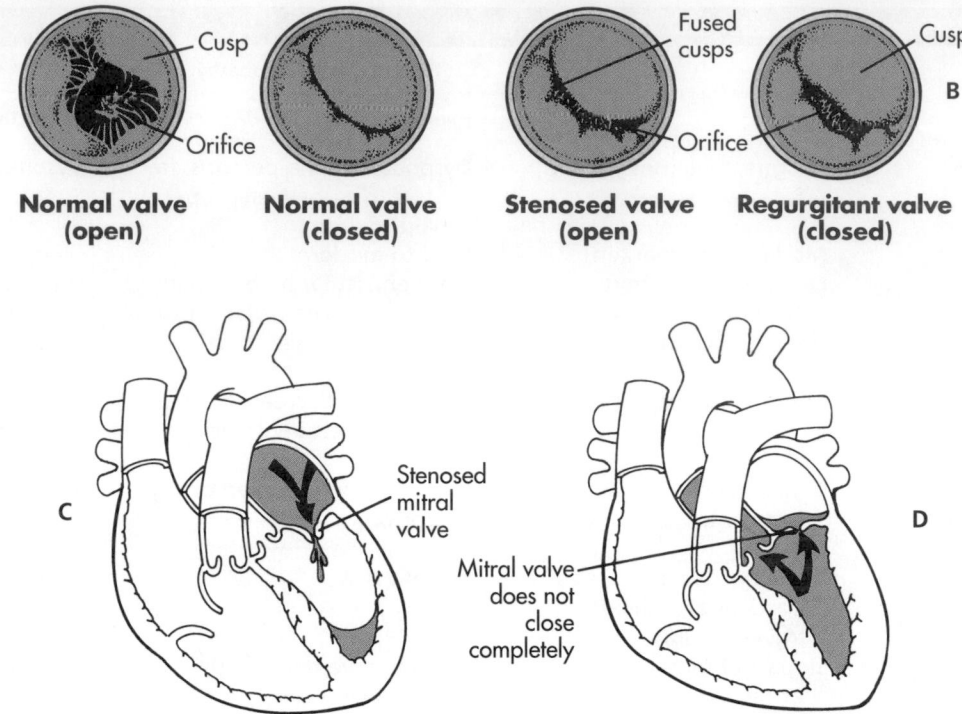

Fig. 23-28 *Valvular stenosis and regurgitation.* **A,** Normal position of the valve leaflets, or cusps, when the valve is open and closed. **B,** Open position of a stenosed valve (*left*) and open position of a closed regurgitant valve (*right*). **C,** Hemodynamic effect of mitral stenosis. The stenosed valve is unable to open sufficiently during left atrial systole, inhibiting left ventricular filling. **D,** Hemodynamic effect of mitral regurgitation. The mitral valve does not close completely during left ventricular systole, permitting blood to reenter the left atrium.

crescendo-decrescendo systolic heart murmur. Left ventricular hypertrophy develops to compensate for the increased work load. Eventually, hypertrophy increases myocardial oxygen demand, which the coronary arteries may be unable to meet. Then ischemia may cause attacks of angina. Untreated aortic stenosis can lead to dysrhythmias, myocardial infarction, and heart failure. Most symptoms of aortic stenosis are attributable to diminished stroke volume, which results in diminished tissue perfusion.

Mitral stenosis. **Mitral stenosis** impairs the flow of blood from the left atrium to the left ventricle. Mitral stenosis is most commonly caused by acute rheumatic fever or bacterial endocarditis, although uncommonly it can be congenital. Narrowing of the orifice occurs as inflammatory lesions in the valvular leaflets heal (Fig. 23-29). Scarring causes the leaflets to become fibrous and fused, and the chordae tendineae cordis become shortened.

As in aortic stenosis, impedance to blood flow results in incomplete emptying of the left atrium and elevated atrial pressure as the chamber tries to force blood through the stenotic valve. Continued increases in left atrial volume and pressure cause chamber dilation and hypertrophy. The risk of developing atrial dysrhythmias (especially fibrillation) and dysrhythmia-induced thrombi is high. As mitral stenosis progresses, symptoms of decreased cardiac output occur, especially during exertion. Continued elevation of left atrial

Fig. 23-29 *Mitral stenosis with classic "fish mouth" orifice.* *(From Stevens, A. & Lowe, J. [1995]. Pathology. St. Louis: Mosby.)*

pressure and volume causes pressure to rise in the pulmonary circulation. If untreated, chronic mitral stenosis develops into pulmonary hypertension, edema, and right ventricular failure.

Atrial enlargement is demonstrated by chest x-ray films and electrocardiography. Blood flow through the stenotic valve gives rise to a rumbling decrescendo diastolic murmur.

TABLE 23-8   Clinical Manifestations of Valvular Stenosis and Regurgitation

Manifestation	Aortic Stenosis	Mitral Stenosis	Aortic Regurgitation	Mitral Regurgitation	Tricuspid Regurgitation
Cardiovascular outcome*	Left ventricular failure	Right ventricular failure	Left heart failure	Left heart failure	Right heart failure
General symptoms	Fatigue	Fatigue, weakness	Fatigue, weakness	Fatigue, weakness	Peripheral edema (with heart failure)
Respiratory effects	Dyspnea on exertion	Dyspnea on exertion, orthopnea, paroxysmal nocturnal dyspnea, predisposition to respiratory infections, hemoptysis, pulmonary hypertension, and edema	Dyspnea with effort	Dyspnea; occasional hemoptysis	Dyspnea
Central nervous system effects	Syncope, especially on exertion	Neural deficits only associated with emboli (e.g., hemiparesis)	Syncope	None	None
Gastrointestinal effects	None	Ascites; hepatic angina with hepatomegaly	None	None	Ascites, hepatomegaly (with heart failure)
Pain	Angina pectoris	Chest pain	Chest pain (anginal)	None	Palpitations
Heart rate, rhythm	Bradycardia, dysrhythmias (with heart failure)	Palpitations (atrial fibrillation)	Palpitations, water-hammer pulse	Palpitations	Atrial fibrillations
Heart sounds	Systolic murmur	Diastolic murmur, accentuated first heart sound, opening snap	Diastolic and systolic murmurs	Murmur throughout systole	Murmur throughout systole
Most common cause	Congenital, rheumatic fever	Rheumatic fever	Bacterial endocarditis; aortic root disease	Floppy valve; coronary artery disease	Congenital

Data from Braunwald, E. (Ed.). (1997). Heart disease: A textbook of cardiovascular medicine (5th ed.). Philadelphia: Saunders; Carabello, B.A. & Crawford, F.A. (1997). Medical progress! Valvular heart disease. New England Journal of Medicine, 337, 32-41.
*If disease not treated.

The first heart sound (S_1) is often accentuated and somewhat delayed because of increased left atrial pressure. Other signs and symptoms are generally those of pulmonary congestion and right heart failure.

Regurgitation

Aortic regurgitation. **Aortic regurgitation** is caused by an acute or chronic lesion of rheumatic fever, bacterial endocarditis, syphilis, hypertension, connective tissue disorders (e.g., Marfan syndrome), or atherosclerosis. The hemodynamic repercussions depend on the size of the "leak." During systole, blood is ejected from the left ventricle into the aorta. If the aortic semilunar valve is affected, some of the ejected blood flows back into the left ventricle. Volume overload occurs in the ventricle because it receives blood from the left atrium during diastole and blood from the aorta during systole. Over time, the end-diastolic volume of the left ventricle

increases and myocardial fibers stretch to accommodate the extra fluid. Compensatory dilation permits the left ventricle to increase its stroke volume and maintain cardiac output. Ventricular dilation and hypertrophy eventually cannot compensate for aortic incompetence, and heart failure develops.

Clinical manifestations include widened pulse pressure resulting from increased stroke volume and backflow. Turbulence across the aortic valve during diastole produces a characteristic murmur. Large stroke volume and rapid runoff of blood from the aorta cause prominent carotid pulsations and throbbing peripheral pulses (water-hammer pulse). Other symptoms are usually associated with heart failure that occurs when the ventricle can no longer enlarge. Dysrhythmias and endocarditis are common complications of aortic regurgitation.

Mitral regurgitation. **Mitral regurgitation,** unlike mitral stenosis, has various causes, including mitral valve prolapse, rheumatic heart disease, infective endocarditis, CAD, connective tissue diseases (Marfan syndrome), and congestive cardiomyopathy. Mitral regurgitation permits backflow of blood from the left ventricle into the left atrium during ventricular systole, giving rise to a loud pansystolic (throughout systole) murmur that radiates into the back and axilla. The left ventricle becomes dilated and hypertrophied to maintain adequate cardiac output, despite increased volume from the left atrium. The volume of backflow reentering the left atrium gradually increases, causing atrial dilation. As the left atrium enlarges, the valve structures stretch and become deformed, leading to further backflow. As mitral valve regurgitation progresses, left ventricular function may become impaired to the point of failure. Eventually, increased atrial pressure also causes pulmonary hypertension and failure of the right ventricle. Mitral incompetence is usually well tolerated—often for years—until ventricular failure occurs. Most clinical manifestations are caused by heart failure.

Tricuspid regurgitation. Tricuspid regurgitation is more common than tricuspid stenosis and is usually associated with failure and dilation of the right ventricle secondary to high blood pressure in the pulmonary circulation or right ventricle. Rheumatic heart disease and infective endocarditis are less common causes. Tricuspid valve incompetence leads to volume overload in the right ventricle, increased systemic venous blood pressure, and right heart failure. Pulmonic semilunar valve dysfunction can have the same consequences as tricuspid valve dysfunction.

Mitral valve prolapse syndrome

In ***mitral valve prolapse syndrome (MVPS)*** the anterior and posterior cusps of the mitral valve billow upward (prolapse) into the atrium during systole (Fig. 23-30). The cusps are enlarged, thickened, and scalloped, possibly secondary to collagenous abnormalities, and the chordae tendineae cordis may be elongated, permitting the valve cusps to stretch upward. Mitral regurgitation occurs if the ballooning valve permits blood to leak into the atrium.

Mitral valve prolapse is the most common valve disorder in the United States.[94] It tends to be most prevalent in young women. Recent studies suggest an autosomal dominant inheritance pattern. Because mitral valve prolapse is often associated with other inherited connective tissue disorders (Marfan syndrome, Ehlers-Danlos syndrome, osteogenesis imperfecta), it may result from a genetic or environmental disruption of valvular development during the fifth or sixth week of gestation. There also may be a relationship between symptomatic mitral valve prolapse and hyperthyroidism.

Many cases of mitral valve prolapse are completely asymptomatic. Cardiac auscultation on routine physical examination may disclose a regurgitant murmur or midsystolic click in an otherwise healthy individual, or echocardiography may demonstrate the condition in the absence of auscultatory findings. Symptomatic mitral valve prolapse can cause palpitations related to dysrhythmias, tachycardia, light-headedness, syncope, fatigue (especially in the morn-

ing), lethargy, weakness, dyspnea, chest tightness, hyperventilation, anxiety, depression, panic attacks, and atypical chest pain. Many symptoms are vague and puzzling and are unrelated to the degree of prolapse. Mitral valve prolapse was once considered a psychiatric malady. Recent research has suggested that individuals with mitral valve prolapse have an autonomic dysfunction in which inordinate quantities of catecholamines are produced, with or without adrenergic stimulation.[94] This finding could explain why mitral valve prolapse causes such a variety of subjective complaints.

Its high incidence rate suggests that mitral valve prolapse may be a normal variant rather than a pathologic entity. Although severe sequelae, such as chorda rupture, ventricular failure, systemic emboli, and sudden death, are possible, the disorder is actually associated with minimal mortality and morbidity. Most individuals experience no physical limitations. In fact, the psychologic effects of chest pain and knowledge of the diagnosis may be more disabling than the disease itself.

Evaluation of mitral valve prolapse includes physical assessment and laboratory evaluation. Echocardiography is the procedure of choice for diagnosing the disorder. Cardiac angiography is rarely necessary to confirm the diagnosis.

Management is matched to the degree of mitral regurgitation. If regurgitation is present, antibiotic prophylaxis for infective endocarditis is given before invasive procedures, but physical activities are not restricted. Occasionally β blockers are needed to alleviate syncope, severe chest pain, or palpitations. Hypovolemia (resulting from diuretics or donating blood) is avoided because it can decrease ventricular volume, thereby increasing stress on the prolapsed mitral valve. Surgical repair or valve replacement may be required.[94]

Acute rheumatic fever and rheumatic heart disease

Rheumatic fever is a diffuse, inflammatory disease caused by a delayed immune response to infection by the group A β-hemolytic streptococcus. In its acute form, rheumatic fever is a febrile illness characterized by inflammation of the joints, skin, nervous system, and heart. If untreated, rheumatic fever can cause scarring and deformity of cardiac structures, resulting in ***rheumatic heart disease.***

The incidence of acute rheumatic fever declined in the United States during the 1960s, 1970s, and early 1980s because of medical and socioeconomic improvements, as well as changes in the virulence of group A streptococci.[95,96] A resurgence of rheumatic fever, especially in the intermountain western regions of the United States, occurred from 1984 through 1992.[95] Recent outbreaks in Utah and Pennsylvania corresponded with the reappearance of highly virulent strains. Because crowding and poor hygiene are environmental risk factors for acute rheumatic fever, the disease continues to be a major cause of death and disability for underprivileged populations.

The acute disease occurs most frequently in children between the ages of 5 and 15 years. Only 3% of those with pharyngeal streptococcal infection will acquire acute rheumatic

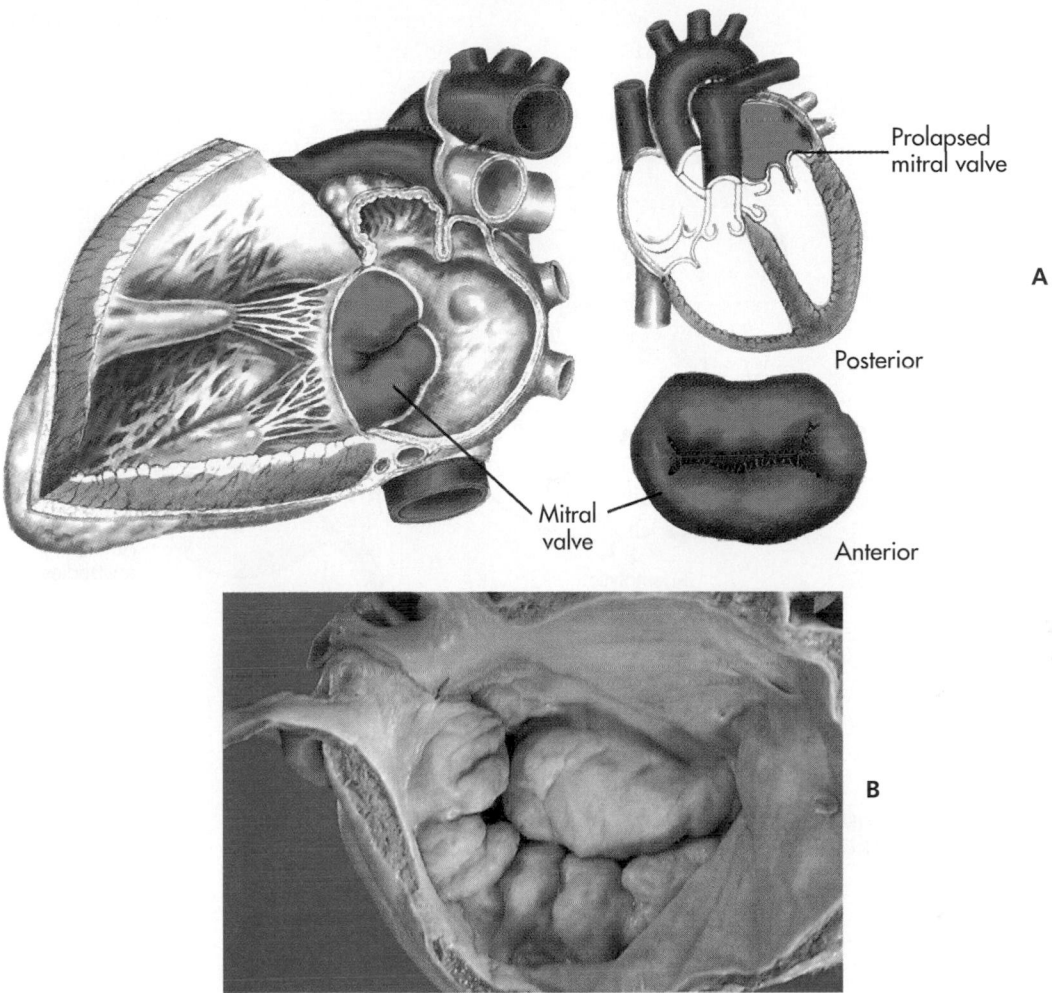

Fig. 23-30 *Mitral valve prolapse.* **A,** Normal mitral valve (*lower right*) and prolapsed mitral valve (*left*). Prolapse permits the valve leaflets to billow back into the atrium during left ventricular systole. The billowing causes the leaflets to part slightly, permitting regurgitation into the atrium. **B,** Looking down into the mitral valve, the ballooning of the leaflets is seen. *(B from Stevens, J. & Lowe, J. [1995]. Pathology. St. Louis: Mosby.)*

fever. Appropriate antibiotic therapy given within the first 9 days of infection usually prevents rheumatic fever.

The incidence of rheumatic fever tends to run in families, lending support to the concept of genetic predisposition, perhaps involving an abnormal immune response to antigens expressed by the bacterial membrane. Individuals who have experienced one attack of acute rheumatic fever are more susceptible than the general population to recurrent attacks.

Pathophysiology

Acute rheumatic fever can develop *only* as a sequel to pharyngeal infection by group A β-hemolytic streptococcus. Streptococcal skin infections do not progress to acute rheumatic fever, although both skin and pharyngeal infections can cause acute glomerulonephritis.[95] Acute rheumatic fever probably affects the heart, joints, central nervous system, and skin through an abnormal humoral and cell-mediated immune response to group A streptococcal cell membrane antigens (Fig. 23-31). These antigens can bind to receptors on heart, muscle, and brain cells and have an affinity for membrane receptors within synovial joints, where they trigger an autoimmune response.

Diffuse, proliferative, and exudative inflammatory lesions develop in the connective tissues, especially in the heart, joints, and skin. The inflammation may subside before treatment, leaving behind damage to the heart valves and increasing the individual's susceptibility to recurrent acute rheumatic fever after any subsequent streptococcal infections. Repeated attacks of acute rheumatic fever cause chronic proliferative changes in the previously mentioned organs as a result of scarring, granulomas, and thromboses.

Approximately 10% of individuals with rheumatic fever develop rheumatic heart disease. It begins as ***carditis,*** or inflammation of the heart, called rheumatic heart disease. Rheumatic heart disease (RHD) continues to be a common health problem in the developing world, causing morbidity and mortality among both children and adults.[95,96] Even

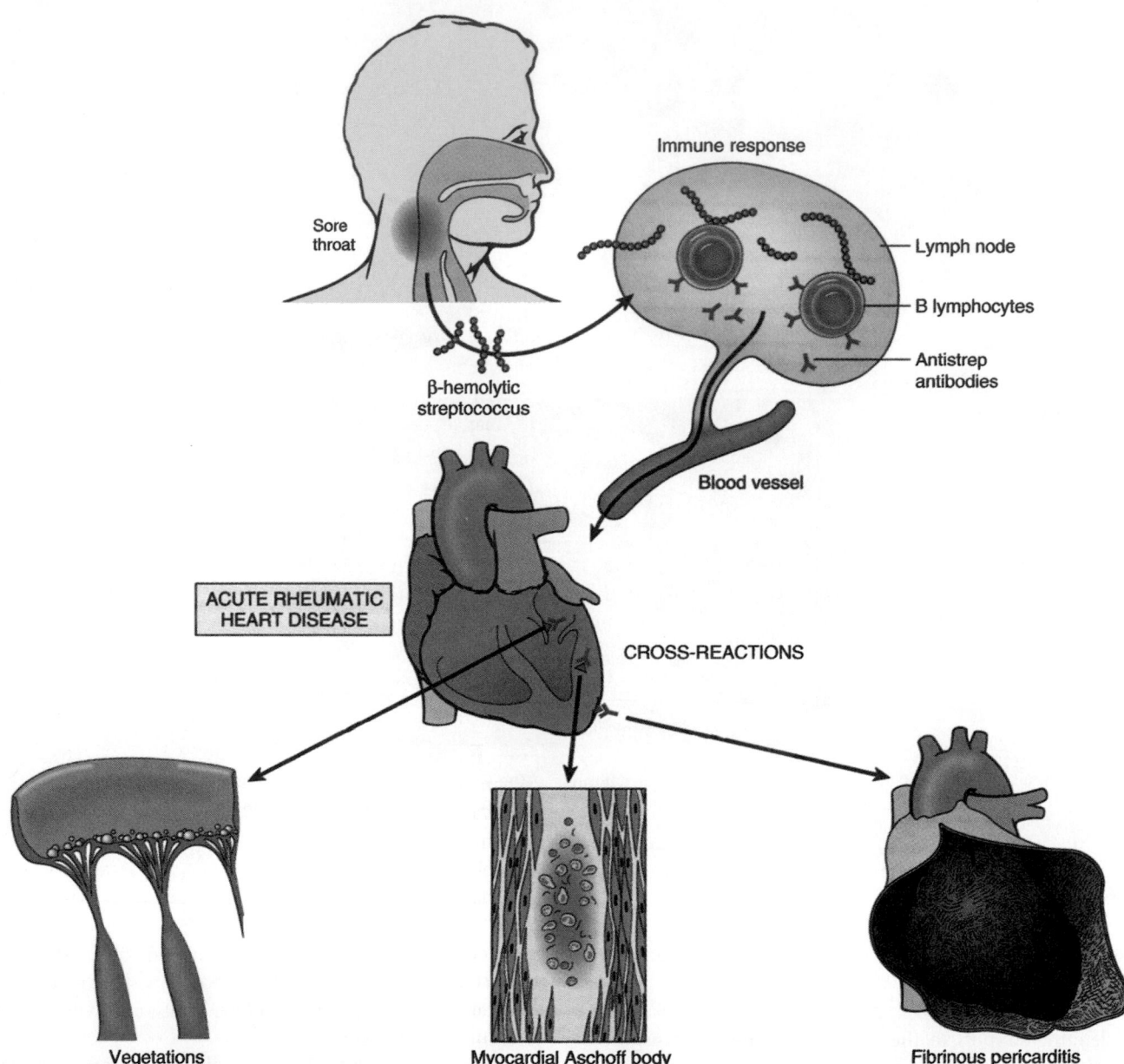

Immune response

Sore
throat

Lymph node

B lymphocytes

Antistrep
antibodies

β-hemolytic
streptococcus

Blood vessel

**ACUTE RHEUMATIC
HEART DISEASE**

CROSS-REACTIONS

Vegetations

Myocardial Aschoff body

Fibrinous pericarditis

Fig. 23-31 *Pathogenesis and structural alterations of acute rheumatic heart disease.* Beginning usually with a sore throat, rheumatic fever can develop only as a sequel to pharyngeal infection by group A β-hemolytic streptococcus. Suspected as a hypersensitivity reaction it is proposed that antibodies directed against the M proteins of certain strains of streptococci cross-react with tissue glycoproteins in the heart, joints, and other tissues. The exact nature of cross-reacting antigens has been difficult to define, but it appears that the streptococcal infection causes an autoimmune response against self-antigens. Inflammatory lesions are found in various sites; the most distinctive within the heart are called *Aschoff bodies.* The chronic sequelae result from progressive fibrosis because of healing of the inflammatory lesions and the changes induced by valvular deformities. *(From Cotran, R.S., Kumar, V., & Collins, T. [1999]. Robbin's pathologic basis of disease [6th ed.]. Philadelphia: Saunders.)*

Fig. 23-32 *Mitral stenosis.* Mitral stenosis and clumps of vegetation *(V)* containing platelets and fibrin. Mitral leaflets are thickened and fused and have clumps of vegetation containing platelets and fibrin. *(From Stevens, A. & Lowe, J. [1995]. Pathology. St. Louis: Mosby.)*

mild cases of rheumatic fever can cause carditis in all three layers of the heart wall. The primary lesion usually involves the endocardium, which lines the heart chambers and includes the heart valves. Endocardial inflammation causes swelling of the valve leaflets, with secondary erosion along the lines of leaflet contact. Small, beadlike clumps of vegetation containing platelets and fibrin are deposited on eroded valvular tissue and on the chordae tendineae cordis (Fig. 23-32). These lesions can become progressively adherent. Scarring and shortening of the involved structures occur over time. The valves lose their elasticity, and the leaflets may adhere to each other.

If inflammation penetrates the myocardium, localized fibrin deposits develop that are surrounded by areas of necrosis. These fibrinoid necrotic deposits are called *Aschoff bodies.* Pericardial inflammation is usually characterized by serofibrinous effusion within the pericardial cavity. Cardiomegaly and left heart failure may occur during episodes of untreated acute or recurrent rheumatic fever. Conduction defects and atrial fibrillation are frequently associated with rheumatic heart disease.[96]

Clinical Manifestations

Many common clinical manifestations of acute rheumatic fever—fever, lymphadenopathy, arthralgia, nausea, vomiting, epistaxis (nose bleed), abdominal pain, and tachycardia—are associated with other disorders as well and are therefore not diagnostic of the disease. The major specific manifestations of acute rheumatic fever are carditis, acute migratory polyarthritis, chorea, and erythema marginatum, which may occur singly or in combination 1 to 5 weeks after streptococcal infection of the pharynx.

Carditis. The earliest cardiac manifestation of acute rheumatic fever may be a previously undetected murmur caused by mitral or aortic semilunar valve dysfunction.

Chest pain is caused by pericardial inflammation. Pericardial effusion produces an audible friction rub. Extra heart sounds, heart block (see p. 669), atrial fibrillation, and a prolonged PR interval are frequently associated with chronic rheumatic heart disease.

Polyarthritis. The classic presenting manifestation of acute rheumatic fever is acute migratory polyarthritis (inflammation of more than one joint). Although all the synovial joints may be involved, the large joints of the extremities are most frequently affected. Two or more joints are usually involved simultaneously or in succession. Exudative synovitis causes heat, redness, swelling, severe pain, and tenderness, but no permanent disability. Palpable subcutaneous nodes often develop over bony prominences and along extensor tendons. They do not interfere with joint function and often go unnoticed.

Chorea. Sydenham chorea, or St. Vitus dance, is a disorder of the central nervous system characterized by sudden, aimless, irregular, involuntary movements. (Chorea is described in Chapter 14.) It is more common in girls than in boys and may occur several months after the streptococcal infection. The chorea is self-limiting, running its course within weeks or months, and has no permanent neural sequelae.

Erythema marginatum. Erythema marginatum is a distinctive truncal rash that often accompanies acute rheumatic fever. It consists of nonpruritic, pink, erythematous macules that never occur on the face or hands. The rash is transitory and may change in appearance within minutes or hours. Heat (e.g., bathing) darkens the rash. The macules may fade in the center and be mistaken for ringworm.

Evaluation and Treatment

When correlated with physical assessment findings, laboratory values lend significant support to the diagnosis of acute rheumatic fever. A positive throat culture for group A β-hemolytic streptococci can be an important finding when associated with certain physical signs. Cultures may be negative when the rheumatic attack begins, however. Documented recent scarlet fever is another potentially strong diagnostic aid to acute rheumatic fever, but diagnosis of scarlet fever may depend on a positive throat culture and may be difficult to distinguish from other disorders associated with a similar rash. Most strains of group A β-hemolytic streptococcus produce a hemolytic factor called *streptolysin O.* Antibodies against this hemolytic factor increase as the individual's immune system fights the disease. Antistreptolysin O antibody titers greater than 250 Todd units in adults and 333 Todd units in children are considered elevated and diagnostic. Several other antibody tests are sensitive prognosticators of streptococcal infection, including antideoxyribonucleotidase (anti-DNase B), antihyaluronidase, and antistreptozyme (ASTZ).

Elevated white blood cell count, erythrocyte sedimentation rate, and C-reactive protein indicate inflammation. All three are usually increased at the time cardiac or joint symptoms begin to appear. They are more useful in identifying an acute inflammatory process and suggesting prognosis than

TABLE 23-9	Jones Criteria (Updated) Used for Diagnosis of Initial Attack of Rheumatic Fever
Criteria	**Description**
Major manifestations	Carditis, polyarthritis, chorea, erythema marginatum, subcutaneous nodules
Minor manifestations	Clinical: arthralgia, fever; laboratory: elevated C-reactive protein; electrocardiographic: prolonged PR interval
Supporting evidence of streptococcal infection	Increased titer of streptococcal antibodies: antistreptolysin O (ASO), other; positive throat culture for group A *Streptococcus*

Guidelines for the diagnosis of rheumatic fever. Jones Criteria, 1992 update. Special Writing Group of the Committee on Rheumatic Fever, Endocarditis, and Kawasaki Disease of the Council on Cardiovascular Disease in the Young of the American Heart Association. Journal of the American Medical Association, 268(15), 2069-2073.

in diagnosing acute rheumatic fever. The levels of these tests decrease as the inflammatory process resolves.

In 1944 the Jones criteria (Table 23-9) were established to assist in the diagnosis of acute rheumatic fever. The criteria have been modified several times by the American Heart Association, most recently in 1965.[97] No single laboratory test, sign, or symptom is definitive of acute rheumatic fever, but certain combinations of criteria indicate that acute disease is probably present.

Therapy for acute rheumatic fever is aimed at eradicating the streptococcal infection and involves a 10-day regimen of oral penicillin or erythromycin administration. Salicylates are used as antiinflammatory agents for both rheumatic carditis and arthritis. Serious carditis may require adding cardiac glycosides, corticosteroids, diuretics, and bed rest to the regimen. Surgical repair of damaged valves may be needed in chronic recurrent rheumatic fever/carditis. Active disease is considered resolved when (1) the murmur has disappeared or cardiac status becomes stable, (2) major manifestations are no longer present, (3) the individual is afebrile, and (4) the erythrocyte sedimentation rate is normal or stabilized. This may take 1 to 6 months.

Research suggests that a rheumatic recurrence will develop in 50% to 65% of children with known rheumatic fever if they have another group A streptococcal infection. Recurrence rates decline with the length of time elapsed since the last infection. To prevent recurrence of acute rheumatic fever, continuous prophylactic antibiotic therapy is necessary.[95,96]

✓ QUICK CHECK

Compare the effect of aortic stenosis with mitral stenosis on the left ventricle and atrium.

Describe aortic regurgitation, mitral regurgitation, and tricuspid regurgitation.

Why is mitral valve prolapse considered an inherited disorder?

Why does inflammation predispose to rheumatic heart disease?

Infective endocarditis

Infective endocarditis is a general term used to describe inflammation of the endocardium—especially the cardiac valves. Causal agents include bacteria, viruses, fungi, rickettsiae, and parasites, but bacterial infection, particularly by streptococci or staphylococci, is most common. Infective carditis was once a lethal disease, but morbidity and mortality diminished significantly with the advent of antibiotics and improved diagnostic techniques (see Risk Factors box). It is relatively rare (3 to 4 cases per 100,000 population per year).[98]

▌RISK FACTORS

INFECTIVE CARDITIS
- Acquired valvular heart disease (especially mitral valve prolapse)
- Implantation of prosthetic heart valves
- Congenital lesions associated with highly turbulent flow (e.g., ventricular septal defect)
- Previous attack of infective endocarditis
- Male gender
- Intravenous drug abuse
- Long-term indwelling catheterization (e.g., for pressure monitoring, feeding, hemodialysis)
- Recent cardiac surgery

 Pathophysiology

The pathogenesis of infective endocarditis requires at least three critical elements (Fig. 23-33). First, the endocardium (e.g., heart valve) must be "prepared," usually by endothelial damage, for microorganism colonization. Second, bloodborne microorganisms must adhere to the damaged endocardial surface. Third, the adherent microorganisms must proliferate and promote the propagation of infective endocardial vegetation.

Endocardial damage exposes the endothelial basement membrane, which contains a type of collagen that attracts platelets and thereby stimulates thrombus formation on the membrane. This causes an inflammatory reaction (*nonbacterial thrombotic endocarditis*). Infective endocarditis cannot develop unless microorganisms gain access to the blood-

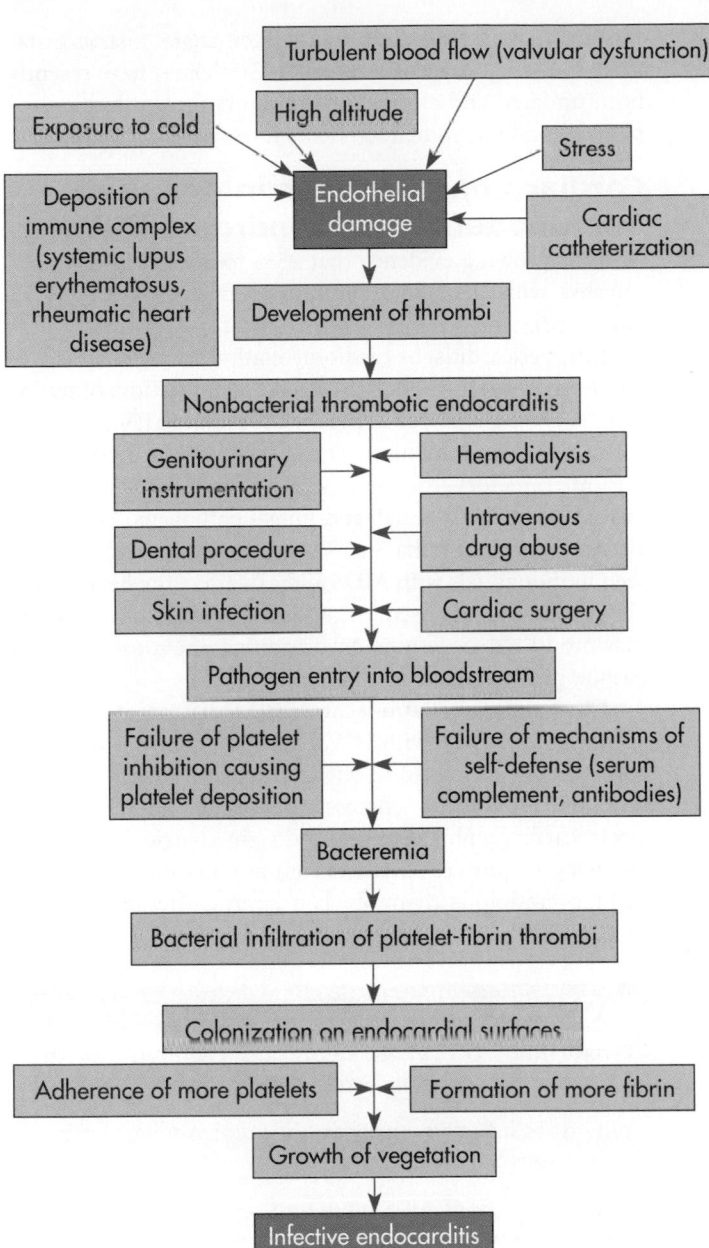

Fig. 23-33 *Pathogenesis of infective endocarditis.*

stream. They may enter the bloodstream during minor procedures, such as dental cleaning or bladder catheterization, or they may spread from uncomplicated upper respiratory or skin infections.

Adherence of microorganisms to the endocardial surface is facilitated by the coexistence of nonbacterial thrombotic endocarditis. However, bacteremia can cause infective endocarditis even on healthy, intact endocardium.[98]

Once the endocardial surface is colonized, infected vegetation forms (Fig. 23-34). Bacteria may accelerate fibrin formation by activating the clotting cascade. Although endocardial tissue is constantly bathed in antibody-containing blood and is surrounded by scavenging monocytes and polymorphonuclear leukocytes, bacterial colonies are inaccessible to host defenses because they are embedded in the protective fibrin clots. The lesions can form anywhere on the endocardium but usually occur on the endocardial surfaces of heart valves and surrounding structures.

Clinical Manifestations

Infective endocarditis may be acute, subacute, or naggingly chronic. It causes varying degrees of valvular dysfunction and may be associated with manifestations involving several organ systems (lungs, eyes, kidneys, bones, joints, central nervous system), making diagnosis exceedingly difficult. The "classic" findings of fever, cardiac murmur, and petechial lesions of the skin, conjunctiva, and oral mucosa are not always present.

Signs and symptoms of infective endocarditis are caused by infection and inflammation, systemic spread of microemboli, and immune complex deposition. A history of fever, anorexia, weight loss, back pain, and night sweats; a new or

Fig. 23-34 *Bacterial endocarditis of mitral valve.* Lesion in combination with old rheumatic valvulitis. *(From Kissane, J.M. [Ed.]. [1990]. Anderson's pathology [9th ed.]. St. Louis: Mosby.)*

significantly changed cardiac murmur; petechiae; positive blood cultures; elevated erythrocyte sedimentation rate; and urine abnormalities make the diagnosis quite clear. Sudden onset of severely debilitating symptoms indicates acute disease.

If infective endocarditis extends farther into the heart wall and invades the conduction system, electrocardiography may show a prolonged PR interval, left bundle branch block, or complete heart block (see p. 669). Emboli may travel to the coronary arteries and cause an acute myocardial infarction.

🟰 *Evaluation and Treatment*

Transesophageal echocardiography is useful for diagnosing infective endocarditis and predicting the prognosis, especially in cases where blood cultures are negative.[99] If peripheral emboli are suggested, organ scans can be performed to confirm their presence. Antimicrobial therapy is generally given for 4 to 6 weeks, beginning with intravenous and ending with oral administration. In some cases, two different antibiotics are given simultaneously to eliminate the offending microorganism and prevent the development of drug resistance. Penicillin and streptomycin are commonly used to treat infective endocarditis. Vancomycin in combination with an aminoglycoside is used in penicillin-allergic individuals. Other drugs may be necessary to treat left heart failure secondary to valvular dysfunction.

Current trends in therapy indicate that mortality in medication-resistant endocarditis can be reduced with surgical valve replacement.[100,101] Unfortunately, the presence of an artificial valve is itself a significant risk factor for infective endocarditis. Valve failure and valve-induced embolization are known consequences of prosthetic valve placement.

Individuals who are known to be at risk for infective endocarditis can avoid the disease by taking antibiotics before and after any procedure that carries the risk of transient bac-

teremia (e.g., dental cleaning, genitourinary instrumentation, open cardiovascular surgery). Guidelines have recently been updated and clearly list indicators for antibiotic prophylaxis and recommended doses for specific procedures.[102]

Cardiac Complications in Acquired Immunodeficiency Syndrome (AIDS)

There is growing evidence that 25% to 50% of individuals infected with the human immunodeficiency virus (HIV) have cardiac involvement consisting of myocarditis, endocarditis, pericarditis, or cardiomyopathy.[103] Cardiac involvement can result from the HIV itself, inflammation, other infections, malignancy, or drugs. In addition to HIV infection, the cardiac involvement may be induced by the accompanying inflammatory response or by various bacterial, viral, protozoan, mycobacterial, and fungal pathogens. Malignancies, such as lymphoma and Kaposi sarcoma, are frequently seen in individuals with AIDS and can affect the heart. Anti-HIV drugs or drugs used to combat opportunistic infections may produce toxic lesions. Myocarditis is the most common pathologic finding.

Clinical manifestations of cardiac disease are seen in about 10% of those with HIV. Left heart failure is the most common and is related to left ventricular dilation and dysfunction. Pericardial effusion, ventricular dysrhythmias, electrocardiographic changes, and right ventricular dilation and hypertrophy are other less common findings. Treatment includes antibiotic therapy when appropriate and relief of symptoms.

✓ QUICK CHECK

What three critical elements are required for the pathogenesis of infective endocarditis?

Why does infective endocarditis involve several organ systems?

What affect does AIDS have on the heart?

MANIFESTATIONS OF HEART DISEASE
Dysrhythmias

A *dysrhythmia,* or *arrhythmia,* is a disturbance of heart rhythm. Normal heart rhythms are generated by the sinoatrial (SA) node and travel through the heart's conduction system, causing the atrial and ventricular myocardium to contract and relax at a regular rate that is appropriate to maintain circulation at various levels of physical activity (see Chapter 22). Dysrhythmias range in severity from occasional "missed" or rapid beats to serious disturbances that impair the pumping ability of the heart, contributing to heart failure and death. Dysrhythmias can be caused by either an abnormal rate of impulse generation (Table 23-10) by the SA node or other pacemaker or the abnormal conduction of impulses (Table 23-11) through the heart's conduction system, including the myocardial cells themselves.

TABLE 23-10	Disorders of Impulse Formation			
Type	**Electrocardiogram**	**Effect**	**Pathophysiology**	**Treatment**
Sinus bradycardia	P rate 60 or less PR interval normal QRS for each P	Increased preload Decreased mean arterial pressure	Hyperkalemia: slows depolarization Vagal hyperactivity: unknown Digoxin toxicity common Late hypoxia: lack of adenosine triposphate (ATP)	If hypotensive, treat cause and support Follow with sympathomimetics, cardiotonics, and pacer Vagolytics
Simple sinus tachycardia	P rate 100-150 PR interval normal QRS for each P	Decreased filling times Decreased mean arterial pressure Increased myocardial demand	Catecholamines: rise in resting potential, calcium influx Fever: unkown Early failure and lung disease; hypoxic cell metabolism Hypercalcemia	Oxygen, bed rest Calcium blockers
Premature atrial contractions (PACs) or beats*	Early P waves that may have changed morphology PR interval normal QRS for each P	Occasional decreased filling time and mean arterial pressure	Electrolyte disturbances: decrease all phases Hypoxia and elevated preload: cell membrane disturbances Hypercalcemia	Treat underlying cause Digoxin
Sinus dysrhythmia	Rate varies P-P regularly irregular, short with inspiration, long with exhalation PR interval normal QRS for each P	Variable filling times Variable mean arterial pressures Variable oxygen demand	Unknown Common in young children and young adults	None
Atrial tachycardia (includes premature atrial tachycardia if onset is abrupt)	P rate 151-250 P morphology may differ from sinus P PR interval normal P/QRS ratio variable	Decreased filling time Decreased mean arterial pressure Increased myocardial demand	Same as PACs: leads to increased atrial automaticity, atrial reentry Digoxin toxicity: common	Control ventricular rate Digoxin, calcium blockers, vagus stimulation Pace to override
Atrial flutter*	P rate 251-300, morphology may vary from sinus P PR interval usually not observable P/QRS ratio variable	Decreased filling time Decreased mean arterial pressure	Same as atrial tachycardia Aging	Same as atrial tachycardia Synchronous cardioversion
Atrial fibrillation*	P rate >300 and usually not observabe No PR interval QRS rate variable and rhythm irregular	Same as atrial flutter	Same as atrial tachycardia Aging	Same as atrial tachycardia
Idiojunctional rhythm	P absent or independent QRS normal, rate 41-59, regular	Decreased cardiac output from loss of atrial contribution to ventricular preload Decreased mean atrial pressure as a result of bradycardia	Atrial and sinus bradycardia, standstill, or block	Same as sinus bradycardia

Most common in adults.
†*Life-threatening in adults.*

Continued

TABLE 23-10	Disorders of Impulse Formation—cont'd			
Type	Electrocardiogram	Effect	Pathophysiology	Treatment
Junctional brady-cardia	P absent or independent QRS normal, rate 40 or less	Same as idiojunctional rhythm	Same as idiojunctional rhythm Vagal hyperactivity	Same as sinus bradycardia
Premature junctional contractions (PJCs) or beats	Early beats without P waves QRS morphology normal	Decreased cardiac output from loss of atrial contribution to ventricular preload for that beat	Hyperkalemia (5.4-6 mEq/L) Hypercalcemia, hypoxia, and elevated preload (see PACs)	Same as PAC
Accelerated junctional rhythm	P absent or independent QRS morphology normal, rate 60-99	Decreased cardiac output from loss of atrial contribution to ventricular preload	Same as PJCs	Same as PAC
Junctional tachy-cardia	P absent or independent QRS morphology normal, rate 100 or more	Decreased cardiac output from loss of atrial contribution to ventricular preload Increased myocardial demand because of tachycardia	Same as PJCs	Same as PAC
Idioventricular rhythm†	P absent or independent QRS >0.11 and rate 20-39	Same as idiojunctional rhythm	Sinus, atrial, and junctional bradycardia, standstill, or block	Same as sinus bradycardia
Ventricular brady-cardia†	P absent or independent QRS >0.11 and rate 60-21	Same as idiojunctional rhythm	Same as idiojunctional rhythm	Same as sinus bradycardia
Agonal rhythm/electro-mechanical dis-sociation†	P absent or independent QRS >0.11 and rate 20 or less	Absent or barely present cardiac output and pulse Not compatible with life	Depolarization and contraction not coupled: electrical activity present with little or no mechanical activity Usually caused by profound hypoxia	Vigorous pharmacology aimed at restoring rate and force Usually ineffective May attempt to pace
Ventricular stand-still or asystole†	P absent or independent QRS absent	No cardiac output Not compatible with life	Profound ischemia, hyperkalemia, acidosis	Same as agonal rhythm, including electrical defibrillation
Premature ventricular contractions (PVCs) or depolarizations*	Early beats with P waves QRS occasionally opposite in deflection from usual QRS	Same as premature junctional contractions	Same as PJCs, including aging and induction of anesthesia Impulse originates in cell outside normal conduction system and spreads through intercalated disks	Pharmacology to change thresholds, refractory periods; reduce myocardial demand, increase supply Removal of cause
Accelerated ventricular rhythm	P absent or independent QRS >0.11 and rate 41-99	Same as accelerated junctional rhythm	Same as PVCs	Same as PVCs

*Most common in adults.
†Life-threatening in adults.

TABLE 23-10 Disorders of Impulse Formation—cont'd

Type	Electrocardiogram	Effect	Pathophysiology	Treatment
Ventricular tachy-cardia†	P absent or independent QRS >0.11 and rate 100 or more	Same as junctional tachycardia	Same as PVCs	Same as PVCs, including electrical cardioversion
Ventricular fibrillation†	P absent QRS >300 and usually not observable	Same as ventricular standstill	Same as PVCs Rapid infusion of potassium	Same as PVCs, including electrical defibrillation

Most common in adults.
†Life-threatening in adults.

TABLE 23-11 Disorders of Impulse Conduction

Type	ECG	Effect	Pathophysiology	Treatment
Sinus block	Occasionally absent P, with loss of QRS for that beat	Occasional decrease in cardiac output Increase in preload for the following beat	Local hypoxia, scarring of intraatrial conduction pathways, electrolyte imbalances Increased atrial preload	Conservative Usually do not progress in severity Pharmacologic treatment includes vagolytics, sympathomimetics, pacing
First-degree block*	PRI > 0.2 sec	None	Same as sinus block Hyperkalemia (>7 mEq/L) Hypokalemia (<3.5 mEq/L) Formation of myocardial abscess in endocarditis	Conservative Discovery and correction of cause
Second-degree block, Mobitz I, or Wenckebach*	Progressive prolongation of PRI until one QRS is dropped Pattern of prolongation resumes	Same as sinus block	Hypokalemia (<3.5 mEq/L) Faulty cell metabolism in AV node Severity increases as heart rate increases Supports theory that AV node is fatiguing Digoxin toxicity, β blockade CAD, MI, hypoxia, increased preload, valvular surgery and disease, diabetes	Same as sinus block
Second-degree block or Mobitz II	Same as sinus block	Same as sinus block	Hypokalemia (<3.5 mEq/L) Faulty cell metabolism below AV node Antidysrhythmics, tricyclic antidepressants CAD, MI, hypoxia, increased preload, valvular surgery and disease, diabetes	More aggressively than Mobitz I, since can progress to type III Pacemaker after pharmacologic treatment

AV, *Atrioventricular;* CAD, *coronary artery disease;* MI, *myocardial infarction;* RBBB, *right bundle branch block;* LBBB, *left bundle branch block;* CHR, *congestive heart failure;* MR, *mitral regurgitation;* PRI, *PR interval.*
Most common in adults.
†Life-threatening in adults.

Continued

TABLE 23-11	Disorders of Impulse Conduction—cont'd			
Type	**ECG**	**Effect**	**Pathophysiology**	**Treatment**
Third-degree block†	P waves present and independent of QRS No observed relationship between P and QRS Always AV dissociation	Same as idiojunctional rhythm	Hypokalemia (<3.5 mEq/L) Faulty cell metabolism low in bundle of His MI, especially inferior wall, as nodal artery interrupted; results in ischemia of AV node	Pharmacologic unit pacemaker inserted Temporary pacing if caused by inferior MI, since ischemia usually resolves
Atrioventricular dissociation	P waves present and independent of QRS, but not always because of block (e.g., ventricular tachycardia) AV dissociation not always third-degree block	Decreased cardiac output from loss of atrial contribution to ventricular preload Variable effect on myocardial demand, depending on ventricular rate	May result from third-degree block or accelerated junctional or ventricular rhythm or be caused by sinus, atrial, and junctional bradycardias	Treat according to cause Pacemaker or reducing rate of AV or ventricular discharge, or increasing rate of sinus or AV node discharge
Ventricular block	QRS > 0.11 sec R-S-R' in V_1, V_2, V_5, V_6	None	Faulty cell metabolism in right and left bundle branches RBBB more common than LBBB because of dual blood supply to left bundle branch CHR, MR, especially anterior MI, because of infarct of fascicles Left anterior hemiblock more common than left posterior hemiblock, since posterior fascicles have dual blood supply	Isolated RBBB or LBBB or hemiblock not treated If acute and/or associated with acute anterior MI, treated with permanent pacer and vigorous pharmacology
Aberrant conduction	QRS > 0.11 sec	None, unless ventricular rate abnormalities present*	Conduction of impulse through intercalated disks, since conduction system transiently blocked because of hypoxia, electrolyte imbalances, digoxin toxicity, excessively rapid rates of discharge	Correct underlying cause

AV, *Atrioventricular*; CAD, *coronary artery disease*; MI, *myocardial infarction*; RBBB, *right bundle branch block*; LBBB, *left bundle branch block*; CHR, *congestive heart failure*; MR, *mitral regurgitation*; PRI, *PR interval*.
*Most common in adults.
†Life-threatening in adults.

Heart Failure
Types

Heart failure is a general term used to describe several types of cardiac dysfunction that result in inadequate perfusion of tissues with vital blood-borne nutrients. Most causes of heart failure result from dysfunction of the left ventricle (systolic and diastolic heart failure). The right ventricle also may be dysfunctional, especially in pulmonary disease (right ventricular failure). Finally, some conditions cause inadequate perfusion despite normal or elevated cardiac output (high-output failure).

TABLE 23-11   Disorders of Impulse Conduction—cont'd

Type	ECG	Effect	Pathophysiology	Treatment
Preexcitation syndromes (Wolff-Parkinson-White and Lown-Ganong-Levine)	P present with QRS for each P PRI < 0.12 and WRS > 0.11 because of presence of delta wave in PRI	None	Congenital presence of accessory pathways (bundle of Kent and fiber of Mahaim) that conduct very rapidly and bypass the AV node, causing early ventricular depolarization in relation to atrial depolarization Prone to tachycardias and atrial fibrillation that can result in very rapid ventricular rates (reason unknown)	Aimed at lining up refractory periods of accessory pathway and AV node to prevent reentry May slow rate with drug therapy May surgically cut pathways

AV, *Atrioventricular;* CAD, *coronary artery disease;* MI, *myocardial infarction;* RBBB, *right bundle branch block;* LBBB, *left bundle branch block;* CHR, *congestive heart failure;* MR, *mitral regurgitation;* PRI, *PR interval.*
*Most common in adults.
†Life-threatening in adults.

HEALTH ALERT

Angiotensin II Receptor Blockers: The New Antihypertensive Medications

Angiotensin II plays an important role in the pathophysiology of a number of important cardiovascular diseases, including hypertension, atherosclerosis, myocardial infarction, and congestive heart failure. This hormone is made both systemically (the renin-angiotensin-aldosterone system) and locally by vascular endothelial cells, smooth muscle cells, myocytes, and other cells throughout the body. Some deleterious effects of antiogensin II include increased vascular tone, vascular remodeling, ischemic myocardial remodeling, and ventricular hypertrophy. Angiotensin converting enzyme (ACE) inhibitors block the systemic production of angiotensin II and have been found to be effective in treating many of these problems, but they may have side effects (cough, angioedema). In addition, they may not adequately block the effects of locally produced angiotensin II. A new class of drugs blocks angiotensin II receptors (there are two types; the drugs discussed here block the AT1 receptor) and may be more effective in treating these conditions with fewer side effects. Numerous studies are underway to determine the role of these drugs in treating cardiovascular disease.

Data from Burrell, L.M. (1997). A risk-benefit assessment of losartan potassium in the treatment of hypertension. Drug Safety, 16(1), 56-65; *Goldsmith, D.J. (1997). Angiotensin receptor antagonists.* Lancet, 349(9060), 1255; *Goodfriend, T.L., Elliott, M.E., & Catt, K.J. (1996). Angiotensin receptors and their antagonists.* New England Journal of Medicine, 334(25), 1649-1654; *Kassler-Taub, K. et al. (1998). Comparative efficacy of two angiotensin II receptor antagonists, irbesartan and losartan, in mild-to-moderate hypertension. Irbesartan-Losartan Study Investigators.* American Journal of Hypertension, 11(4, Pt. 1), 445-453; *Simon, T.A. et al. (1998). Safety of irbesartan in the treatment of mild to moderate systemic hypertension.* American Journal of Cardiology, 1582(2), 179-182.

Left heart failure (congestive heart failure)

Left heart failure is commonly called *congestive heart failure* and can be further categorized as systolic heart failure or diastolic heart failure. Synonyms for these terms are systolic ventricular dysfunction and diastolic ventricular dysfunction. These two types of heart failure can occur together in one individual or singly.

Systolic heart failure is defined as an inability of the heart to generate an adequate cardiac output to perfuse vital tissues. Cardiac output depends on the heart rate and stroke volume. Stroke volume is influenced by three major determinants: contractility, preload, and afterload (see Chapter 22).

Contractility is reduced by diseases that disrupt myocyte activity. Myocardial infarction is the most common cause of decreased contractility, and other causes include myocarditis and cardiomyopathies. Myocardial ischemia results in a process called **ventricular remodeling**, which causes progressive myocyte contractile dysfunction over time (Box 23-2). When contractility is decreased, stroke volume falls and left ventricular end-diastolic volume (LVEDV) increases. This increase causes dilation of the heart and an increase in preload (Fig. 23-35).

Ventricular Remodeling in Ischemic Heart Disease and Hypertension: The Role of Angiotensin II and Catecholamines in Heart Failure   BOX 23-2

The myocardium near areas of infarction in individuals with coronary disease has been found to undergo cellular changes with hypertrophy, production of abnormal contractile proteins, and collagen deposition between myocytes. This process is called *ventricular remodeling*. Similar changes occur in the myocardium of individuals with significant hypertension. Investigators have implicated angiotensin II and catecholamines as the likely neurohumoral agents responsible for these effects. The overall result of these abnormalities is progressive loss of myocardial contractile function and increased likelihood of left heart failure as a complication of ischemic heart disease and hypertension. Trials of angiotensin-converting enzyme (ACE) inhibitors and β blockers in myocardial infarction and systolic left heart failure have consistently resulted in improved myocardial contractility and survival. These agents are now an integral part of the management of myocardial infarction and left heart failure.

Data from Paul, S. (1995). The pathophysiologic process of ventricular remodeling: From infarct to failure. Critical Care Nurse Quarterly, 18, 7; *Pratt, N.G. (1995). Pathophysiology of heart failure: Neuroendocrine response.* Critical Care Nurse Quarterly, 18, 22; *Sackner-Bernstein, J.D. & Mancini, D.M. (1995). Rationale for treatment of patients with chronic heart failure with adrenergic blockade.* Journal of the American Medical Association, 274, 1462; *Williams, R.R et al. (1995). Guidelines for evaluation and management of heart failure.* Journal of the American College of Cardiology, 26, 1376; *Yoshikawa, T. et al. (1996). Early reduction of neurohumoral factors plays a key role in mediating the efficacy of beta-blocker therapy for congestive heart failure.* American Heart Journal, 131, 329.

Preload, or LVEDV, increases with decreased contractility (see above) or an excess of plasma volume (intravenous fluid administration, renal failure, mitral valvular disease). Increases in LVEDV can actually improve cardiac output, but as preload continues to rise, it causes a stretching of the myocardium that eventually can lead to dysfunction of the sarcomeres and decreased contractility (Fig. 23-36).

Increased afterload is most commonly a result of increased peripheral vascular resistance (PVR), such as that seen with hypertension (Fig. 23-37); it can also be the result of aortic valvular disease. With increased PVR, there is resistance to ventricular emptying and more work load for the left ventricle, which responds with hypertrophy of the myocardium. Hypertrophy results in an increase in oxygen demand by the thickened myocardium and leads to changes in the myocytes themselves, also called *ventricular remodeling*. In addition, hypertrophy results in the deposition of collagen between the myocytes; this can disrupt the integrity of the muscle, decrease contractility, and make the ventricle more likely to dilate and fail.[104]

As cardiac output falls, renal perfusion diminishes with activation of the renin-angiotensin-aldosterone system, which acts to increase PVR and plasma volume, thus increasing afterload and preload further. In addition, baroreceptors in the central circulation detect the decrease in perfusion and stimulate the sympathetic nervous system to cause yet more vasoconstriction and the hypothalamus to produce antidiuretic hormone. It is believed that angiotensin and the catecholamines not only disturb cardiac hemodynamics but also are directly cardiotoxic. The neurohumoral aspects of left heart failure suggest that treatment must include angiotensin and sympathetic inhibition to prevent long-term damage to the myocardium.[105,106] This vicious cycle of decreasing contractility, increasing preload, and increasing afterload causes progressive worsening of left heart failure (Fig. 23-38).

The clinical manifestations of left heart failure are the result of pulmonary vascular congestion and inadequate perfusion of the systemic circulation. Individuals experience dyspnea, orthopnea, cough of frothy sputum, fatigue, decreased urine output, and edema. Physical examination often reveals pulmonary edema (cyanosis, rales, pleural effusions), hypotension or hypertension, an S_3 gallop, and evidence of underlying CAD or hypertension. The diagnosis is made with echocardiography revealing decreased cardiac output and cardiomegaly; some people may need invasive catheterization to document underlying coronary disease.

Management of systolic left heart failure is aimed at interrupting the worsening cycle of decreasing contractility, increasing preload, and increasing afterload. The **acute onset of left (congestive) heart failure** is most often the result of acute myocardial ischemia and must be managed in conjunction with managing the underlying coronary disease (see p. 647). Oxygen, nitrate, and morphine administration improves myocardial oxygenation and helps relieve coronary spasm while lowering preload through systemic venodilation. Intravenous inotropic drugs, such as dopamine or dobutamine, increase contractility and can help raise the blood pressure in hypotensive individuals. Diuretics reduce preload, and ACE inhibitors reduce both preload and afterload by decreasing aldosterone levels and reducing PVR. Short-acting intravenous β blockers also have been found to reduce mortality in selected people. Finally, individuals with severe systolic failure may benefit from acute coronary bypass or percutaneous transluminal coronary angioplasty (PTCA). These people are frequently supported with the intraaortic balloon pump (IABP) until they can be taken safely to the operating room; the IABP is positioned in the aorta just distal to the aortic valve and is inflated during diastole to improve coronary perfusion and deflated during systole to reduce afterload.

Management of **chronic left heart failure** also relies on increasing contractility and reducing preload and afterload. The inotropic drug of choice in chronic systolic heart failure

```
                    ↑ Systemic vascular
                         resistance
                              │
                              ▼
┌──────────────┐      ┌──────────────────┐      ┌──────────────┐
│ Peripheral   │─────▶│ ↑ Force of LV    │─────▶│ Coronary     │
│ artery       │      │   contraction    │      │ artery       │
│ constriction │      └──────────────────┘      │ constriction │
└──────────────┘              │                  └──────────────┘
       ▲                      ▼                          │
       │              ┌──────────────────┐               ▼
       │              │ ↑ LV oxygen      │       ┌──────────────┐
┌──────────────┐      │   demand         │       │ ↓ Oxygen     │
│ Epinephrine  │      └──────────────────┘       │   supply     │
│ release      │──────────────│──────────┐       └──────────────┘
└──────────────┘              ▼          │               │
       │               ┌─────────────┐◀──┴───────────────┘
       │               │ LV hypoxia  │◀──────────────┐
       ▼               └─────────────┘               │
┌──────────────────┐          ▲                      │
│ ↓ Systemic blood │◀─┌──────────────────┐           │
│   pressure       │  │ ↓ Force of LV    │           │
└──────────────────┘  │   contraction    │           │
    │       │         └──────────────────┘           │
    ▼       ▼                 │                       │
┌─────┐ ┌──────────────┐      ▼                       │
│ ADH │ │ ↓ Renal      │  ┌──────────┐                │
└─────┘ │ blood flow   │  │ ↑ LVEDP  │                │
   │    └──────────────┘  └──────────┘                │
   │         │                 │                      │
   │         ▼                 ▼                       │
   │    ┌─────────┐      ┌──────────────┐             │
   │    │ Renin   │─────▶│ ↑ LV preload │◀────────────┘
   │    └─────────┘      └──────────────┘
   │         │                 │
   │         ▼                 ▼
   │  ┌──────────────┐   ┌──────────────┐
   │  │ Angiotensin  │   │ ↑ LA preload │
   │  └──────────────┘   └──────────────┘
   │         │                 │
   │         ▼                 ▼
   │  ┌──────────────┐   ┌─────────────────┐
   │  │ Aldosterone  │   │ Pulmonary edema │
   │  └──────────────┘   └─────────────────┘
   │         │                 │
   ▼         ▼                 ▼
┌──────────────────┐   ┌──────────────────┐
│ Sodium and water │──▶│ ↑ Pulmonary      │
│ retention        │   │   vascular       │
└──────────────────┘   │   resistance     │
        │              └──────────────────┘
        ▼                      │
┌──────────────────┐           ▼
│ Peripheral edema │     ┌──────────────┐
└──────────────────┘     │ RV failure   │
                         └──────────────┘
                                │
                                ▼
                         ┌──────────────┐
                         │ ↑ RV preload │
                         └──────────────┘
```

Fig. 23-35 *Left heart failure (congestive heart failure) from elevated systemic vascular resistance.* Left heart failure leads to right heart failure. Systemic vascular resistance and preload are exacerbated by renal and adrenal mechanisms. *LV,* Left ventricular; *LVEDP,* left ventricular end-diastolic pressure; *LA,* left atrial; *ADH,* antidiuretic hormone; *RV,* right ventricular.

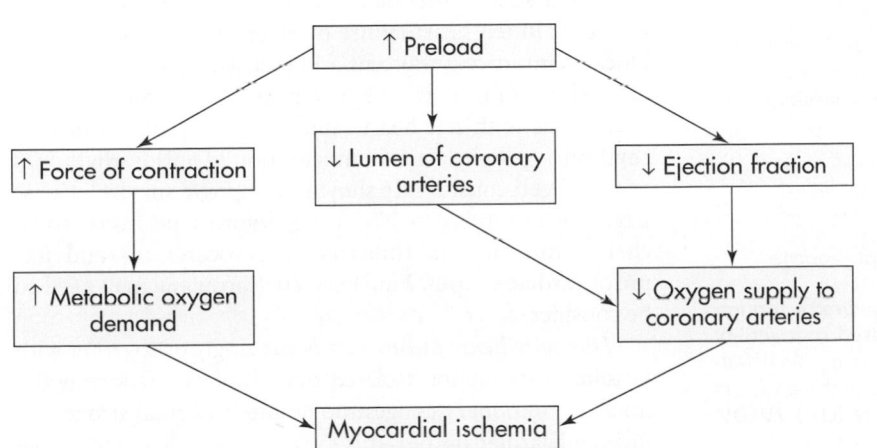

Fig. 23-36 *The effect of elevated preload on myocardial oxygen supply and demand.*

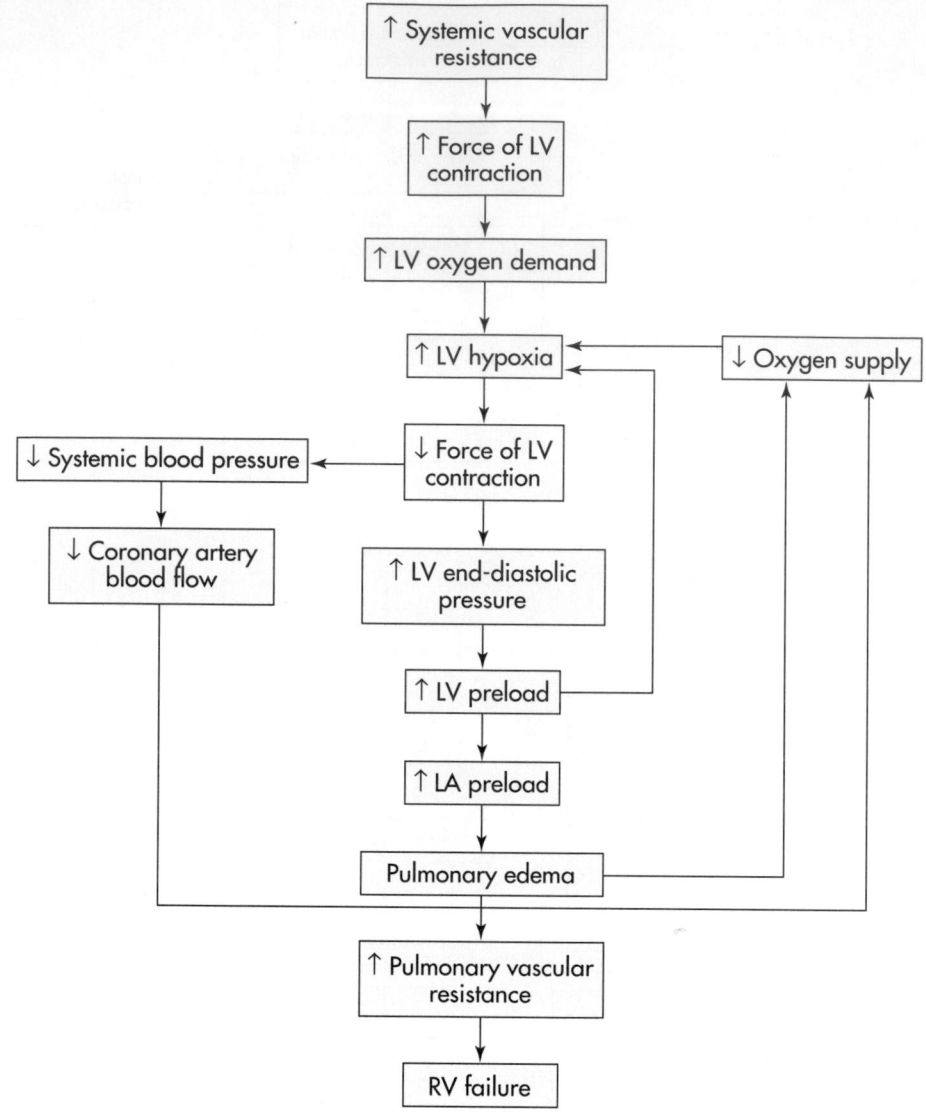

Fig. 23-37 *Left heart failure resulting from systemic hypertension.* Left heart failure leads to right heart failure. *LV,* Left ventricular; *LA,* left atrial; *RV,* right ventricular.

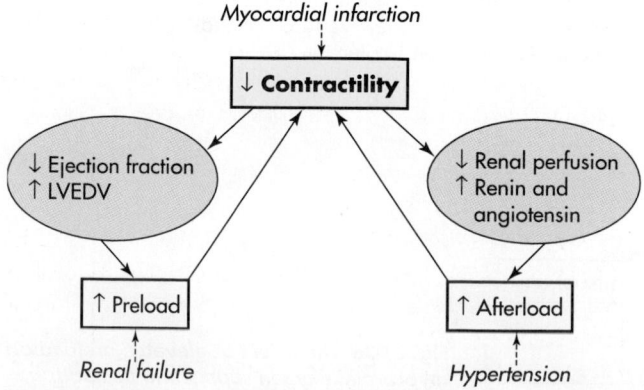

Fig. 23-38 *The vicious cycle of systolic heart failure.* Although the initial insult may be one of primary decreased contractility (e.g., myocardial infarction), increased preload (e.g., renal failure), or increased afterload (e.g., hypertension), all three factors play a role in the progression of left heart failure (LHF). *LVEDV,* Left ventricular end-diastolic volume.

is digoxin. Studies have confirmed its safety and efficacy in treating symptomatic left heart failure.[107] Salt restriction and diuretics are effective in reducing preload. ACE inhibitors reduce preload and afterload and have been shown to reduce mortality in left heart failure by as much as 30%.[108,109] Beta blockers improve symptoms and increase survival but must be used carefully to avoid hypotension.[110,111] Although many individuals with left heart failure die suddenly from dysrhythmias, prophylactic administration of antidysrhythmics has not been consistently shown to improve survival. Coronary bypass surgery or PTCA may improve perfusion to ischemic myocardium (hibernating myocardium) and improve cardiac output. Finally, heart transplant may need to be considered.

Diastolic heart failure can occur singly or together with systolic heart failure. Isolated diastolic heart failure is defined as pulmonary congestion despite a normal stroke volume and cardiac output. It is the cause of 25% to 40% of all

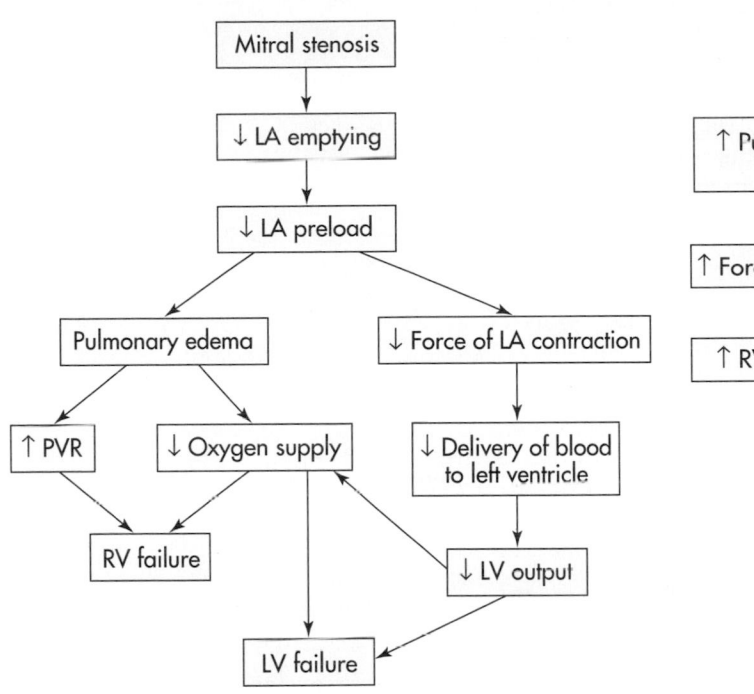

Fig. 23-39 *Left atrial failure caused by mitral stenosis.* *LA,* Left atrial; *PVR,* pulmonary vascular resistance; *LV,* left ventricular.

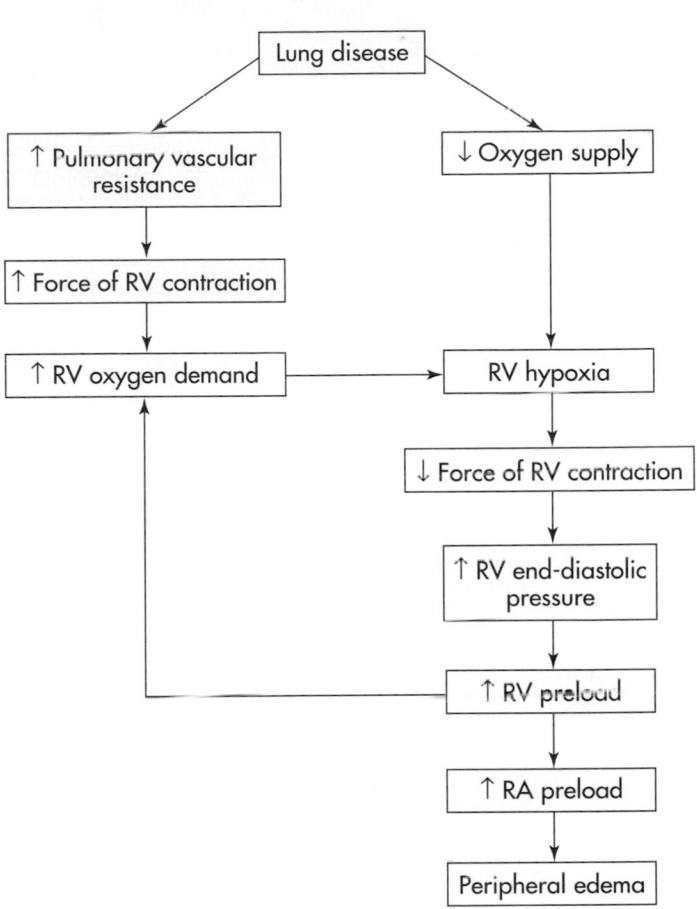

Fig. 23-40 *Right heart failure (cor pulmonale) caused by lung disease.* *RV,* Right ventricular; *RA,* right atrial.

cases of left heart failure. It results from decreased compliance of the left ventricle and abnormal diastolic relaxation such that a normal LVEDV results in an increased left ventricular end-diastolic pressure (LVEDP).[112] This pressure is reflected back into the pulmonary circulation and results in pulmonary edema. The major causes of diastolic dysfunction include hypertension-induced myocardial hypertrophy and myocardial ischemia with resultant ventricular remodeling. Other causes include aortic valvular disease, mitral valve disease (Fig. 23-39), and cardiomyopathies.

Individuals with diastolic dysfunction present with dyspnea on exertion, fatigue, evidence of pulmonary edema (rales on auscultation, pleural effusions), and evidence of underlying coronary disease, hypertension, or valvular disease. Diagnosis is initially made by echocardiography, which demonstrates poor ventricular filling with normal ejection fractions. Precise measurements of pressures require catheterization. Management is aimed at improving ventricular relaxation and prolonging diastolic filling times to reduce diastolic pressure. Calcium channel blockers, β blockers, and ACE inhibitors have all been used with varying success.[112] An innovative surgical technique that involves the transplantation of a portion of the latissimus dorsi muscle into the wall of the noncompliant left ventricle (dynamic cardiomyoplasty) is being tried with some early success.[113]

Right heart failure

Right heart failure can result from left heart failure caused by an increase in left ventricular filling pressure that is reflected back into the pulmonary circulation. As pressure in the pulmonary circulation rises, the resistance to right ventricular emptying increases (Fig. 23-40). The right ventricle

is poorly prepared to compensate for this increased workload and will dilate and fail. When this happens, pressure will rise in the systemic venous circulation, resulting in peripheral edema and hepatosplenomegaly. Treatment relies on management of the left ventricular dysfunction as just outlined. When right heart failure occurs in the absence of left heart failure, it is caused most commonly by diffuse hypoxic pulmonary disease such as chronic obstructive pulmonary disease (COPD), cystic fibrosis, and adult respiratory distress syndrome (ARDS). The mechanisms for this type of right ventricular dysfunction (*cor pulmonale*) are discussed in Chapter 26.

High-output failure

High-output failure is the inability of the heart to adequately supply the body with blood-borne nutrients, despite adequate blood volume and normal or elevated myocardial contractility. In high-output failure, the heart increases its output but the body's metabolic needs are still not met. Common causes of high-output failure are anemia, septicemia, hyperthyroidism, and beriberi (Fig. 23-41).

Anemia decreases the oxygen-carrying capacity of the blood. Metabolic acidosis occurs as the body's cells switch to anaerobic metabolism (see Chapter 4). In response to metabolic acidosis, heart rate and stroke volume increase in an at-

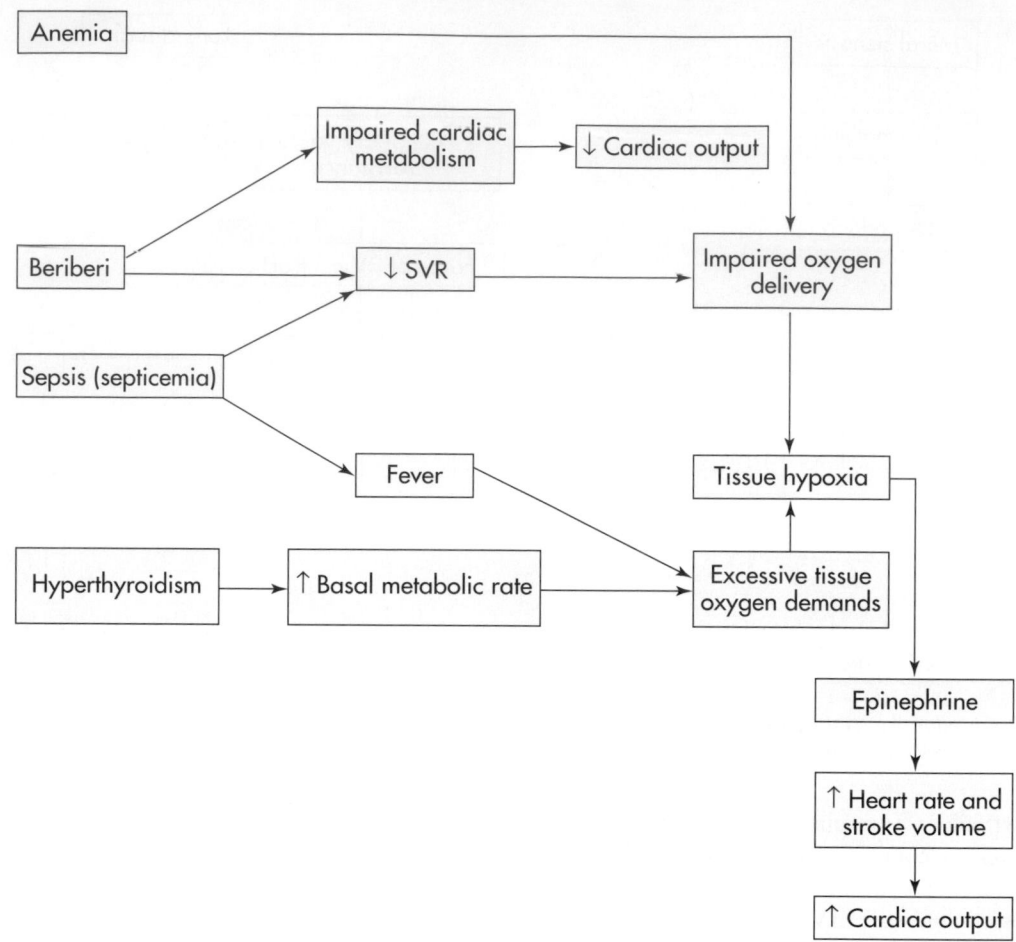

Fig. 23-41 *High-output failure.* *SVR,* Systemic vascular resistance.

tempt to circulate blood faster. If anemia is severe, however, even maximum cardiac output does not supply the cells with enough oxygen for metabolism.

In septicemia, disturbed metabolism, bacterial toxins, and the inflammatory process cause systemic vasodilation and fever. Faced with a lowered systemic vascular resistance (SVR) and an elevated metabolic rate, cardiac output increases to maintain blood pressure and prevent metabolic acidosis. In overwhelming septicemia, however, the heart may not be able to raise its output enough to compensate for vasodilation. Body tissues show signs of inadequate blood supply despite a very high cardiac output.

Hyperthyroidism accelerates cellular metabolism through the actions of elevated levels of thyroxine from the thyroid gland. This may occur chronically (thyrotoxicosis) or acutely (thyroid storm). Because the body's demand for oxygen threatens to cause metabolic acidosis, cardiac output increases. If blood levels of thyroxine are high and the metabolic response to thyroxine is quite vigorous, even an abnormally elevated cardiac output may be inadequate.

In the United States, beriberi (thiamine deficiency) usually is caused by malnutrition secondary to chronic alcoholism. Beriberi actually causes a mixed type of heart failure. Thiamine deficiency impairs cellular metabolism in all tissues, including the myocardium. In the heart, impaired cardiac metabolism leads to insufficient contractile strength. In blood vessels, thiamine deficiency leads mainly to peripheral vasodilation, which decreases SVR. Heart failure ensues as decreased SVR triggers increased cardiac output, which the impaired myocardium is unable to deliver. The strain of demands for increased output in the face of impaired metabolism may deplete cardiac reserves until low-output failure begins.

✓ QUICK CHECK

Why are changes in LVEDV important for left heart failure?

What is ventricular remodeling?

What is the vicious cycle of systolic heart failure?

SHOCK

In *shock* the cardiovascular system fails to perfuse the tissues adequately, resulting in widespread impairment of cellular metabolism. Because tissue perfusion can be disrupted by any factor that alters heart function, blood volume, or blood pressure, shock has many causes and various clinical manifestations. Ultimately, however, shock progresses to organ failure and death, unless compensatory mechanisms reverse the process or clinical intervention succeeds. Untreated severe shock overwhelms the body's compensatory mechanisms through positive feedback loops that initiate and maintain a downward physiologic spiral.

Subjective complaints in shock are usually nonspecific and may not be particularly helpful to the clinician. The individual may report feeling sick, weak, cold, hot, nauseated, dizzy, confused, afraid, thirsty, and short of breath. Observable and measurable signs and symptoms are often conflicting in nature. Hypotension, characterized by a mean arterial pressure below 60 mm Hg, is common to almost all shock states.[114,115] Cardiac output and urinary output are usually— but not always—decreased. Respiratory rate is usually increased. Variable indicators of shock include alterations of heart rate, core body temperature, skin temperature, systemic vascular resistance (SVR), and skin color. Dyspnea, diaphoresis, and altered sensorium may be obvious.

Impairment of Cellular Metabolism

The final common pathway in shock of any type is impairment of cellular metabolism. Fig. 23-42 illustrates the pathophysiology of shock at the cellular level.

Impairment of oxygen use

Without oxygen, the cell shifts from aerobic to anaerobic metabolism. Anaerobic metabolism is a less efficient method of extracting energy from carbon bonds, and the cell begins to use its stores of adenosine triphosphate (ATP) faster than stores can be replaced. Without ATP, the cell cannot maintain an electrochemical gradient across its selectively permeable membrane. Specifically, the cell cannot operate the sodium-potassium pump. Sodium and chloride accumulate inside the cell, and potassium exits. Cells of the nervous system and myocardium are profoundly and immediately affected. The resting potentials of these cells are reduced, and action potentials decrease in amplitude. Various clinical manifestations of impaired central nervous system and myocardial function result.

As sodium moves into the cell, water follows. Throughout the body, the water drawn from the interstitium into the cells is "replaced" by water that is, in turn, drawn out of the vascular space. This decreases circulatory volume. Within the cells, water causes cellular edema that disrupts cellular membranes, releasing lysosomal enzymes that injure the cells internally and leak into the interstitium.

Three positive feedback loops further impair oxygen use: (1) activation of the clotting cascade, (2) decreased circulatory volume, and (3) lysosomal enzyme release. The clotting cascade activates the inflammatory response and also accounts for common complications of shock, such as renal failure, adult respiratory distress syndrome, and disseminated intravascular coagulation. Decreased circulatory volume causes the second positive feedback loop and magnifies decreased tissue perfusion in all types of shock. Lysosomal enzymes, the third positive feedback loop, not only injure the cell that released them, but also injure adjacent cells. By

damaging the mechanisms of surrounding cells, lysosomal enzymes extend areas of impaired metabolism and cellular injury.

In addition to decreasing ATP stores, anaerobic metabolism affects the pH of the cell and metabolic acidosis develops. A compensatory mechanism enables cardiac and skeletal muscles to use lactic acid as a fuel source, but only for a limited time.

The decreasing pH of the cell that is functioning anaerobically has serious consequences. Enzymes necessary for cellular function dissociate under acid conditions. Enzyme dissociation stops cell function, repair, and division. As lactic acid is released systemically, blood pH drops, reducing the oxygen-carrying capacity of the blood (see Chapter 4). Therefore less oxygen is delivered to the cells. Further acidosis triggers the release of more lysosomal enzymes because the low pH disrupts lysosomal membrane integrity.

Impairment of glucose use

Impaired glucose use can be caused by either impaired glucose delivery or impaired glucose uptake by the cells (see Fig. 23-42). The reasons for inadequate glucose delivery are the same as those enumerated for inadequate oxygen delivery. In addition, in septic and anaphylactic shock, glucose metabolism may be increased or disrupted because of fever or bacteria, and glucose uptake can be prevented by the presence of vasoactive toxins, endotoxins, histamine, and kinins.

Some compensatory mechanisms activated by shock contribute to decreased glucose uptake by the cells. High serum levels of cortisol, thyroid hormone, and catecholamines account for hyperglycemia and insulin resistance, tachycardia, increased SVR, and increased cardiac contractility. Cells shift to glycogenolysis, gluconeogenesis, and lipolysis to generate fuel for survival (see Chapter 1). Except in the liver, kidneys, and muscles, the body's cells have extremely limited stores of glycogen. In fact, total body stores can fuel the metabolism for only about 10 hours. The depletion of fat and glycogen stores is not itself a cause of organ failure, but the energy costs of glycogenolysis and lipolysis are considerable and contribute to the cells' failure.

The depletion of protein is, however, a cause of organ failure. When gluconeogenesis causes proteins to be used for fuel, these proteins are no longer available to maintain cellular structure, function, repair, and replication. The breakdown of protein occurs in starvation states, hyperdynamic metabolic states, and septic shock. The breakdown of protein into amino acids that occurs with septicemia is called *septic autocannibalism*. During anaerobic metabolism, protein breakdown liberates alanine, which is converted to pyruvate. In sepsis, pyruvic acid is changed into lactic acid, and a positive feedback loop is formed.

As proteins are broken down anaerobically, ammonia and urea are produced. Ammonia is toxic to living cells. Uremia develops, and uric acid further disrupts cellular metabolism.

Proteins are broken down preferentially. Serum albumin and other plasma proteins are consumed for fuel first. Serum protein consumption decreases capillary osmotic pressure

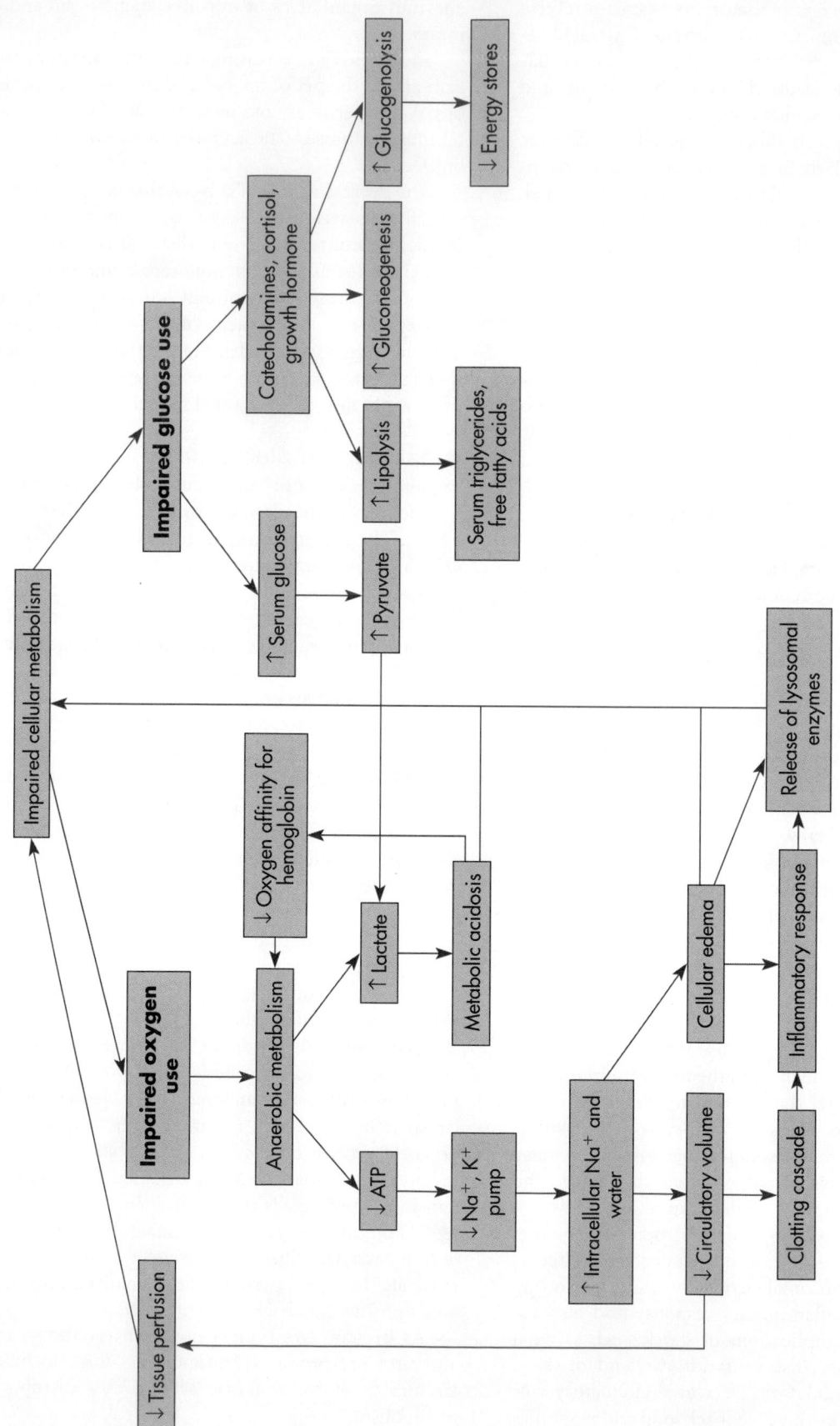

Fig. 23-42 *Impaired cellular metabolism in shock.* *ATP,* Adenosine triphosphate.

and contributes to the development of interstitial edema, creating another positive feedback loop that decreases circulatory volume. In septic shock, plasma protein breakdown includes breakdown of immunoglobulins, thereby impairing immune system function when it is most needed.

Muscle wasting caused by protein breakdown weakens skeletal and cardiac muscle. Skeletal muscle wasting impairs the muscles that facilitate breathing. Muscle wasting therefore alters the actions of both heart and lungs. The delivery of oxygen and glucose to the cells is directly reduced, as is the removal of waste products, forming another positive feedback loop.

A final outcome of impaired cellular metabolism is the buildup of metabolic end-products in the cell and interstitial spaces. Waste products are toxic to the cells and further disrupt cellular function and membrane integrity. Once a sufficiently large number of cells from vital organs have damage to cellular membranes, leakage of lysosomal enzymes, and ATP depletion, shock can be irreversible.[114]

Types of Shock

Shock can be classified by cause, by principal pathophysiologic process, or by clinical manifestations. Classification by cause is perhaps the most useful because it suggests the principal pathophysiologic process and focuses on the underlying disorder, which must be treated to prevent the irreversible impairment of cellular metabolism. Shock is classified by cause as cardiogenic (caused by heart failure), hypovolemic (caused by insufficient intravascular fluid volume), neurogenic (caused by neural alterations of vascular smooth muscle tone), anaphylactic (caused by immunologic processes), or septic (caused by infection).

Cardiogenic shock

Cardiogenic shock results from heart failure from any cause. Most cases of cardiogenic shock follow myocardial infarction, but shock also can follow left heart failure, myocardial ischemia, myocardial or pericardial infections, and heart failure resulting from drug toxicity. Cardiogenic shock is unresponsive to treatment, with a mortality of more than 70% reported. Mortality improves with the use of percutaneous coronary angioplasty and thrombolytic/aspirin therapy.[116-119] The pathophysiology of cardiogenic shock is shown in Fig. 23-43.

The clinical manifestations of cardiogenic shock are caused by widespread impairment of cellular metabolism.

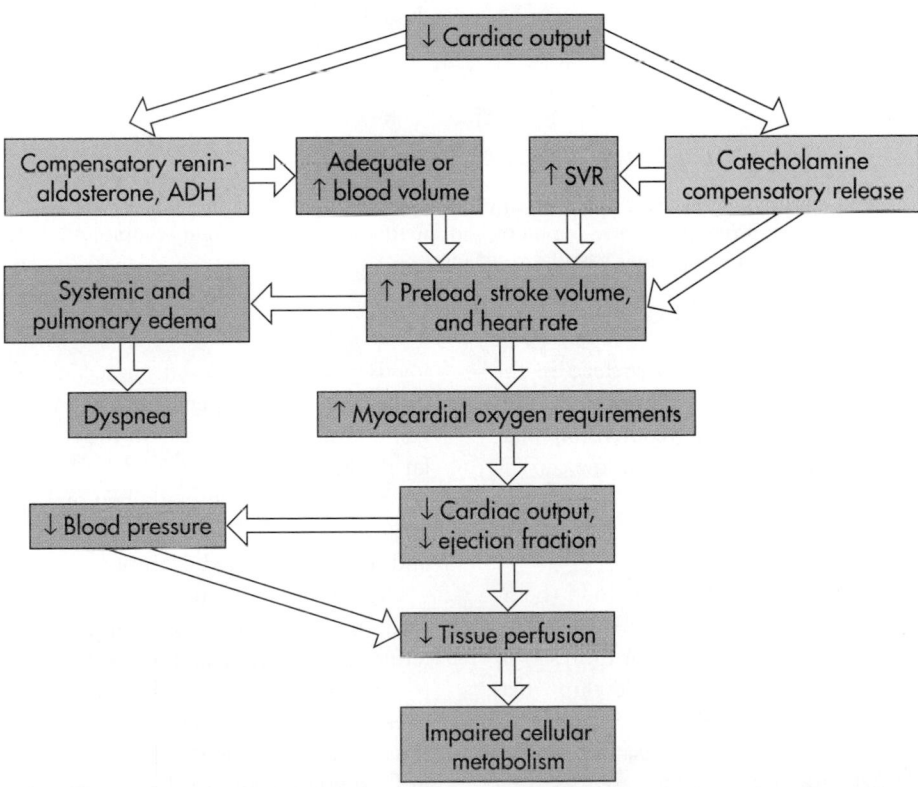

Fig. 23-43 *Cardiogenic shock.* Shock becomes life threatening when compensatory mechanisms *(in blue)* cause increased myocardial oxygen requirements. Renal and hypothalamic adaptive responses (i.e., renin-angiotensin-aldosterone and antidiuretic hormone [ADH]) maintain or increase blood volume. The adrenal gland releases catecholamines (e.g., mostly epinephrine, some norepinephrine), causing vasoconstriction and increases in contractility and heart rate. These adaptive mechanisms, however, increase myocardial demands for oxygen and nutrients. These demands further strain the heart, which can no longer pump an adequate volume, resulting in shock and impaired metabolism. *SVR,* Systemic vascular resistance.

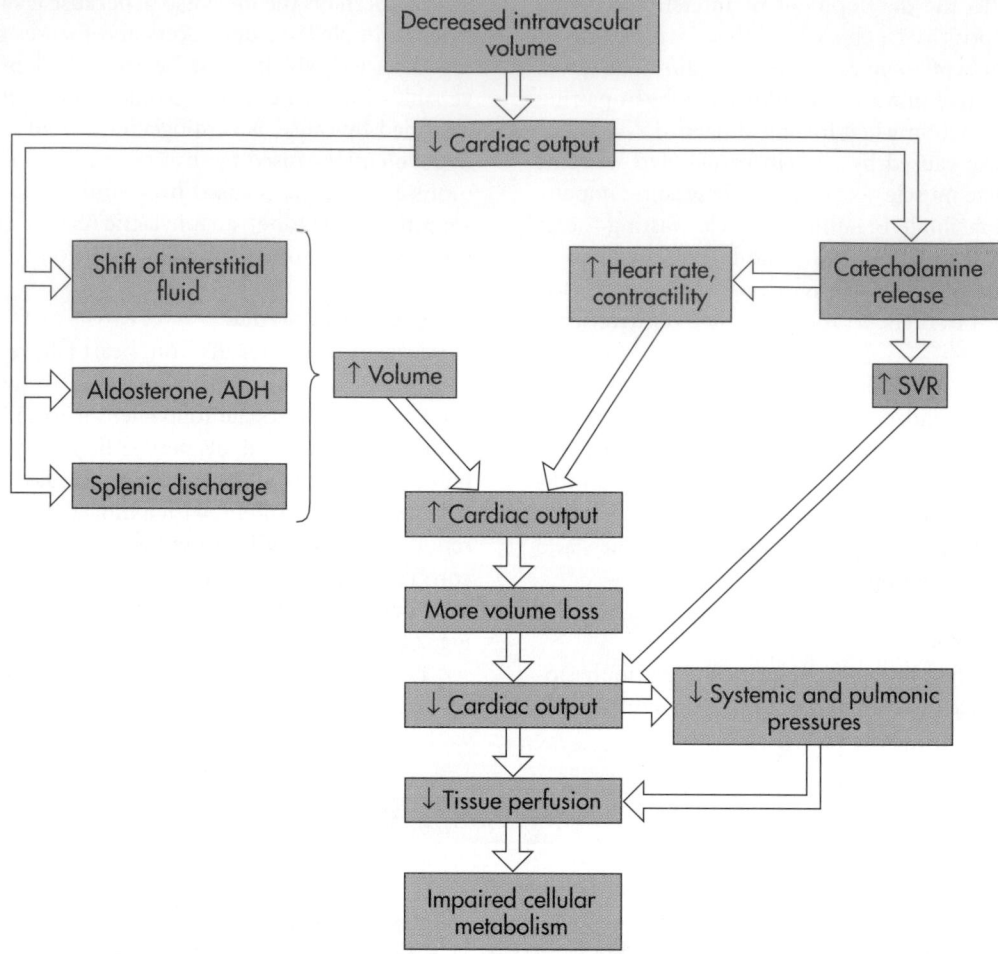

Fig. 23-44 *Hypovolemic shock.* This type of shock becomes life threatening when compensatory mechanisms *(in purple)* are overwhelmed by continued loss of intravascular volume. *ADH,* Antidiuretic hormone; *SVR,* systemic vascular resistance.

They include impaired mentation, elevated preload in the systemic and pulmonary vasculature, systemic and pulmonary edema, dusky skin color, marked hypotension, oliguria, ileus, and dyspnea. Elevated preloads and low cardiac output are manifestations of heart failure.

Hypovolemic shock

Hypovolemic shock is caused by loss of whole blood (hemorrhage), plasma (burns), or interstitial fluid (diaphoresis, diabetes mellitus, diabetes insipidus, emesis, or diuresis) in large amounts. Hypovolemic shock begins to develop when intravascular volume has decreased by about 15%.

Hypovolemia is offset initially by compensatory mechanisms (Fig. 23-44). Heart rate and SVR increase, boosting both cardiac output and tissue perfusion pressures. Interstitial fluid moves into the vascular compartment. The liver and spleen add to blood volume by disgorging stored red blood cells and plasma. In the kidneys, renin stimulates aldosterone release and the retention of sodium (and hence water), whereas ADH from the posterior pituitary gland increases water retention. However, if the initial fluid or blood loss is great or if loss continues, compensation fails, resulting in decreased tissue perfusion. As in cardiogenic shock, oxygen and nutrient delivery to the cells is impaired and cellular metabolism fails.

Mortality for traumatic hemorrhagic shock ranges from 10% to 31%. Fluid replacement is the treatment of choice and must be initiated promptly.

The clinical manifestations of hypovolemic shock include high SVR, poor skin turgor, thirst, oliguria, low systemic and pulmonary preloads, rapid heart rates, thready pulse, and mental status deterioration. The differences between the signs and symptoms of hypovolemic shock and those of cardiogenic shock are mainly caused by differences in fluid volume and cardiac muscle health.

Neurogenic shock

Neurogenic shock (sometimes called *vasogenic shock*) is a widespread and massive vasodilation that results from parasympathetic overstimulation or sympathetic understimulation (Fig. 23-45) (see Chapter 22). The loss of vascular tone results in "relative hypovolemia." Blood volume has

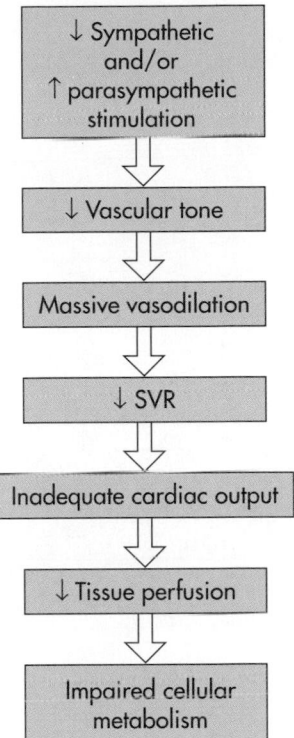

Fig. 23-45 *Neurogenic shock. SVR,* Systemic vascular resistance.

not changed, but the amount of space containing the blood has increased, so that SVR decreases drastically, meaning that pressure in the vessels is inadequate to drive nutrients across capillary membranes to the cells. As with other types of shock, this leads to impaired cellular metabolism.

Neurogenic shock can be caused by any factor that stimulates parasympathetic or inhibits sympathetic stimulation of vascular smooth muscle. Trauma to the spinal cord or medulla and conditions that interrupt the supply of oxygen or glucose to the medulla can cause neurogenic shock by interrupting sympathetic activity. Depressive drugs, anesthetic agents, and severe emotional stress and pain are other causes.

The clinical hallmark of neurogenic shock is a very low SVR, along with indicators of excessive parasympathetic activity. Bradycardia is the most obvious manifestation, especially in the early stages. Fainting occurs if blood pressure decreases to the point that cerebral metabolism is not sufficient to support consciousness.

Anaphylactic shock

Anaphylactic shock results from a widespread hypersensitivity reaction known as anaphylaxis. The basic physiologic alteration is the same as that of neurogenic shock: vasodilation, *peripheral pooling,* and relative hypovolemia, leading to decreased tissue perfusion and impaired cellular metabolism (Fig. 23-46). Anaphylactic shock is often more severe than other types of normovolemic shock because the hypersensitivity reaction that triggers vasodilation has other pathophysiologic effects that rapidly involve the entire body.

Anaphylactic shock begins as an allergic reaction to an allergen. Some allergens known to cause these reactions are insect venoms, pollens, shellfish, penicillin, and animal sera. Once in the body, the allergen binds to immunoglobulin E (IgE) antibody, initiating degranulation of mast cells. This provokes an extensive immune and inflammatory response, including vasodilation and increased vascular permeability, resulting in peripheral pooling and tissue edema. Extravascular effects include constriction of extravascular smooth muscle, often causing respiratory difficulty because it affects smooth muscle layers in airway walls (e.g., the larynx and bronchioles; see Chapter 26).

The onset of anaphylactic shock is usually sudden, and progression to death can occur within minutes unless emergency treatment is given. The first manifestations may be anxiety, difficulty breathing, gastrointestinal cramps, edema, hives (urticaria), and sensations of burning or itching of the skin. A precipitous fall in blood pressure occurs and is followed by impaired mentation. Other signs include decreased SVR, with high or normal cardiac output, and oliguria. Treatment begins with removal of the antigen (if possible). Epinephrine is administered to cause vasoconstriction and reverse airway constriction. Volume expanders (e.g., lactated Ringer solution) are given intravenously to reverse the relative hypovolemia, and antihistamines, cromolyn sodium, and corticosteroids are given to stop the inflammatory reaction.[120]

✓ QUICK CHECK

Describe the mechanisms operative in shock.

Why does myocardial infarction often cause cardiogenic shock?

How is hypovolemic shock manifested?

Why is anaphylactic shock considered a medical emergency?

Septic shock

Septic shock is one component of a continuum of progressive dysfunction called the *systemic inflammatory response syndrome (SIRS).* The syndrome begins with an infection that progresses to bacteremia, then sepsis, then severe sepsis, then septic shock, and then multiple organ dysfunction syndrome (MODS). Consensus about definitions of each component was achieved in 1992,[121] and definitions are presented in Table 23-12.

The incidence of sepsis in the United States is between 300,000 and 500,000 cases annually.[122-124] Septic shock, a common cause of death of individuals in intensive care units, has a mortality in the United States from 20%[122] to as high as 80%[122,125,126] and can be caused by any class of microorganism. Although 2 decades ago gram-negative bacteria were by far the most frequent microorganisms to cause septic shock, gram-positive bacteria now have become the most common isolates.[127] Septic shock also can be caused by

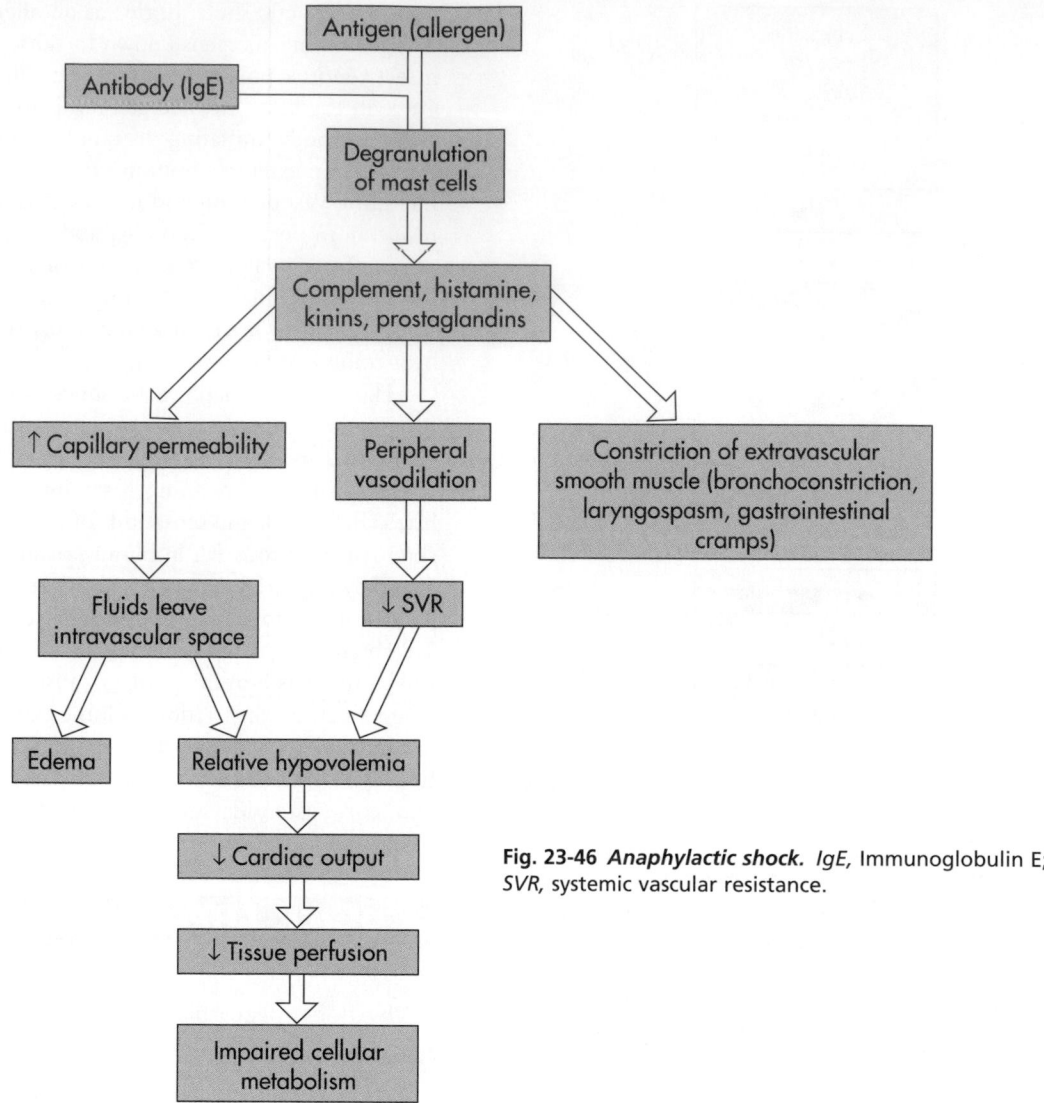

Fig. 23-46 *Anaphylactic shock.* *IgE,* Immunoglobulin E; *SVR,* systemic vascular resistance.

fungi and viruses.[122,123] Prognosis is significantly affected by the source and virulence of the infectious microorganism.

Septic shock begins with a nidus of infection that may be readily discernible or extremely difficult to locate (Fig. 23-47). Bacteria then enter the bloodstream to produce bacteremia in one of two ways: (1) directly from the site of infection or (2) from toxic substances released by the bacteria directly into the bloodstream. These toxic substances, which act as triggering molecules in the septic syndrome, include endotoxins produced by gram-negative microorganisms and exotoxins produced by gram-positive microorganisms.

The triggering molecules cause the host to initiate a nonspecific, first-line defensive response using phagocytic cells (macrophages, monocytes, neutrophils) and the complement cascade. Shortly after this response, a specific immune response is initiated with the release of primary mediators (tumor necrosis factor, interleukin-1, anaphylatoxin C5a). Release of these mediators triggers intense cellular responses and subsequent release of secondary mediators, including cytokines, complement fragments, prostaglandins, platelet-

activating factor, oxygen-free radicals, nitric oxide, and proteolytic enzymes. Chemotaxis, activation of granulocytes, and reactivation of the phagocytic cells and the inflammatory cascades result. The host frequently progresses from septic shock to MODS following the release of secondary mediators.[128] (Chapter 6 discusses the description and function of inflammatory cells and mediators.)

Clinical manifestations of septic shock are low arterial pressure, low SVR from vasodilation, systemic edema, and an alteration in oxygen extraction by all cells. Tachycardia causes cardiac output to remain normal or become elevated, although myocardial contractility is reduced. Temperature instability is present, ranging from hyperthermia to hypothermia. Effects on other organ systems may result in deranged renal function, gastrointestinal mucosa changes that result in release of bacteria from the gut into the bloodstream, jaundice, clotting abnormalities, deterioration of mental status, and adult respiratory distress syndrome.

Present treatment is symptomatic and supportive. It includes multiple drug antibacterial therapy, removal of the

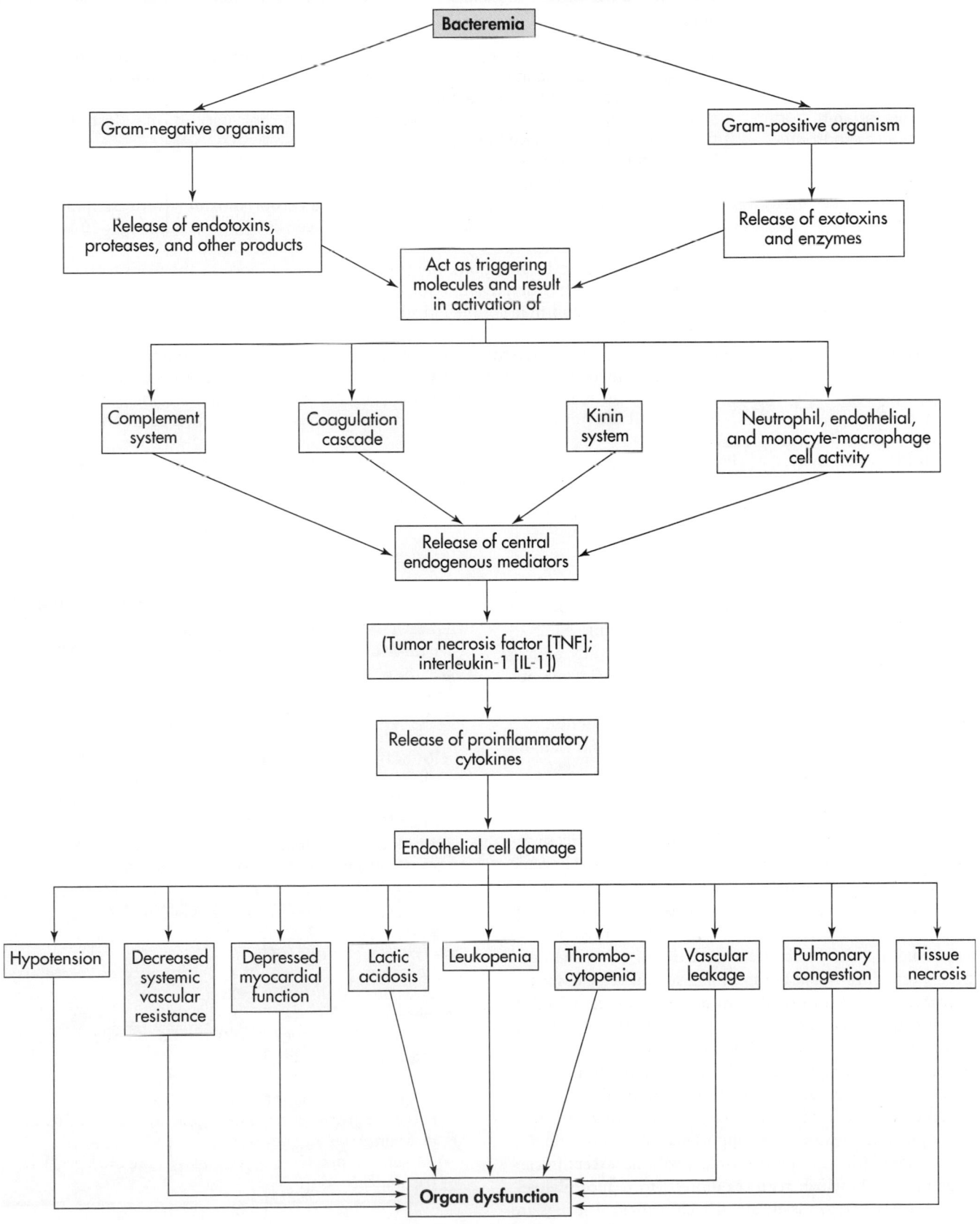

Fig. 23-47 *Septic shock cascade.*

TABLE 23-12	Causes and Definitions of Septic Shock
Cause	**Definition**
Infection	Microbial phenomenon characterized by an inflammatory response to the presence of microorganisms or the invasion of normally sterile host tissue by those microorganisms
Bacteremia	Presence of viable bacteria in the blood
Systemic inflammatory response syndrome	A systemic inflammatory response to a variety of severe clinical insults manifested by two or more of the following signs: Temperature >38° C or <36° C Heart rate >90 beats/min Respiratory rate >20 breaths/min or arterial blood carbon dioxide level <32 mm Hg White blood cell count >12,000 cells/mm³, <4000 cells/mm³, or containing <10% immature forms (bands)
Sepsis	The systemic response to infections manifested by two or more of the signs listed above
Severe sepsis	Sepsis associated with organ dysfunction, hypoperfusion, or hypotension; hypoperfusion and percussion abnormalities may include but are not limited to lactic acidosis, oliguria, or an acute alteration in mental status
Septic shock	Sepsis with hypotension (systolic blood pressure <90 mm Hg or a reduction >40 mm Hg from baseline in the absence of other causes for hypotension; this occurs despite adequate fluid resuscitation, along with the presence of perfusion abnormalities that may include but are not limited to lactic acidosis, oliguria, or an active alteration in mental status)
Multiple organ dysfunction syndrome	Presence of altered organ function in an acutely ill individual such that homeostasis cannot be maintained without intervention

From American College of Chest Physicians/Society of Critical Care Medicine Consensus Conference Committee. (1992). Critical Care Medicine, *20(6), 864.*

source of infection if one is found, fluid resuscitation, and vasoactive medications to improve hemodynamic parameters. Many experimental treatments are under study, among them nonsteroidal antiinflammatory drugs, naloxone administration, and mediator inhibitors. Among the most promising of the latter is nitric oxide synthase inhibitor.[115,124] Because the septic syndrome is incompletely understood, recommended treatment continues to evolve.

Treatment for Shock

The first treatment for shock is to discover and correct or remove the underlying cause. Thus treatment for cardiogenic shock begins with treatment of heart failure or at least enhancement of cardiac output. If hypovolemia is the cause of shock, hemorrhage and other causes of fluid loss must be stopped. In neurogenic shock as a result of spinal cord trauma, stabilization of the spine and surrounding tissue is a beginning, and pain usually can be decreased to a level at which neurally mediated decreases of SVR cease. The initial treatment for anaphylactic shock is to remove or neutralize the antigen. Treatment for septic shock begins with eradication of the infective agent, usually with antibiotics.

After the underlying cause or condition is corrected as far as possible, treatment is supportive. Intravenous fluid is administered to expand intravascular volume, except in cardiogenic shock, which requires diuresis to reduce preload. Supplemental oxygen is always given. Cardiotonic drugs are given early in cardiogenic shock and later in other forms of shock. Trials of antiinflammatory drugs and other specific anticytokine therapies have so far proven ineffective for sep-

RISK FACTORS

INFLAMMATORY MEDIATORS CONTRIBUTING TO SEPTIC SHOCK

The Interleukins
- Released by macrophages in septic shock in response to bacterial toxins
- Net effect: produce fever, vasodilation and hypotension, edema, and elevated white blood count

Tumor Necrosis Factor
- Produced from macrophages, natural killer cells, and mast cells in response to endotoxin and interleukins
- Net effect: generates same symptoms of septic shock that interleukins do, thus is redundant

Platelet-Activating Factor
- Released from mononuclear phagocytes, platelets, and some endothelial cells in response to endotoxin
- Net effect: generates symptoms of shock as do interleukins and tumor necrosis factor but may also initiate multiple organ failure

Myocardial Depressant Factor
- Secreted from white blood cells in response to endotoxin
- Net effect: produces myocardial depression and ventricular dilation

HEALTH ALERT

Specific Therapies for Sepsis?

For several years investigational therapies for the treatment of sepsis have focused on inhibition of proinflammatory mediators, such as endotoxin and cytokines. A large number of these antiinflammatory approaches have failed, suggesting that the hypothesis on which the trials were based was flawed. A new hypothesis has recently been presented that extends the concept of the pathologic condition of sepsis to include a compensatory antiinflammatory syndrome. In other words, there is an oscillation of proinflammatory and antiinflammatory mediators in SIRS. Agents to control the antiinflammatory process have also been tested and so far have been disappointing. The problem of modulating mediators that have opposing functions and are released at different times during the clinical course of sepsis makes development of specific mediator-inhibition therapy for SIRS very difficult. Therefore, in the near future, the treatment of SIRS will continue to be supportive.

Data from Ace, B.A. (1997). Multiple organ failure, multiple organ dysfunction syndrome, and systemic inflammatory response syndrome. Archives of Surgery, *132(7), 603-707; Baue, A.E. (1996). Clinical trials of new and novel therapeutic agents.* World Journal of Surgery, *20, 493-498; Bone, R.C., Grodzin, C.J., & Balk, R.A. (1997). Sepsis: A new hypothesis for pathogenesis of the disease process.* Chest, *112(7), 235-243; Chernow, B. (1996). Back to the drawing board.* Critical Care Medicine, *24(7), 1097-1098.*

tic shock, but numerous investigations continue into novel therapeutic interventions.[129-131]

Once positive feedback loops are established, intervention in shock is difficult. Prevention and very early treatment offer the best prognosis.

✓ QUICK CHECK

Why is severe hypotension common to all types of shock?

How is glucose use impaired in shock?

Why is correction of the underlying problem the most important treatment for all kinds of shock?

Multiple Organ Dysfunction Syndrome

Multiple organ dysfunction syndrome (MODS) is the progressive dysfunction of two or more organ systems resulting from an uncontrolled inflammatory response to a severe illness or injury. The organ dysfunction can progress to organ failure and death (Fig. 23-48). Although sepsis and septic shock are the most common causes, MODS can be initiated by any severe injury or disease process that activates a massive systemic inflammatory response in the host. Clinical in-

fection is not necessary for its development. Other common triggers are severe trauma, burns, acute pancreatitis, major surgery, circulatory shock, adult respiratory distress syndrome, and necrotic tissue.

MODS is a relatively new diagnosis, first recognized as a distinct clinical syndrome in the mid-1970s.[132,133] Today MODS is the most common cause of mortality in intensive care units.[134-136] Mortality for individuals with MODS is between 50% and 90%,[137-139] and it approaches 100% if there is failure of three or more organs.[140] Moreover, mortality has not improved over the past 20 years.[141] People at greatest risk for developing MODS are elderly individuals and persons with significant tissue injury or preexisting disease (see Risk Factors box).[142,143]

⏐RISK FACTORS

DEVELOPMENT OF MODS

- Age >65 years
- Baseline organ dysfunction (e.g., renal insufficiency)
- Bowel infarction
- Coma on admission
- Corticosteroids
- Inadequate, delayed resuscitation
- Malnutrition
- Multiple blood transfusions (>6 units/12 hr)
- Persistent infectious focus
- Preexisting chronic disease (e.g., cancer, diabetes)
- Presence of hematoma
- Significant tissue injury

⇛ Pathophysiology

As a result of the initiating insult (sepsis, injury, or disease), the neuroendocrine system is activated with the release of the stress hormones cortisol, epinephrine, and norepinephrine into the bloodstream (see Chapter 8). The sympathetic nervous system is stimulated to compensate for complications resulting from the injury, such as fluid loss and hypotension. Vascular endothelial damage occurs as a direct result of injury or from damage by bacterial toxins and inflammatory mediators released into the circulation. The vascular endothelium becomes permeable, allowing fluid and protein to leak into the interstitial spaces, contributing to hypotension and hypoperfusion. When the endothelium is damaged, platelets and tissue thromboplastin are activated, resulting in systemic microvascular coagulation.[128,144] (Function of the endothelium is discussed in Chapter 22.)

Because of the release of inflammatory mediators, three major plasma enzyme cascades are activated: complement, coagulation, and kallikrein/kinin. The overall effect of the activation of these cascades is a hyperinflammatory and hypercoagulant state that maintains the edema formation, cardiovascular instability, endothelial damage, and clotting abnormalities characteristic of MODS. A massive systemic immune/inflammatory response then develops involving neutrophils, macrophages, and mast cells (Table 23-13). The pathways by which neutrophils and macrophages are acti-

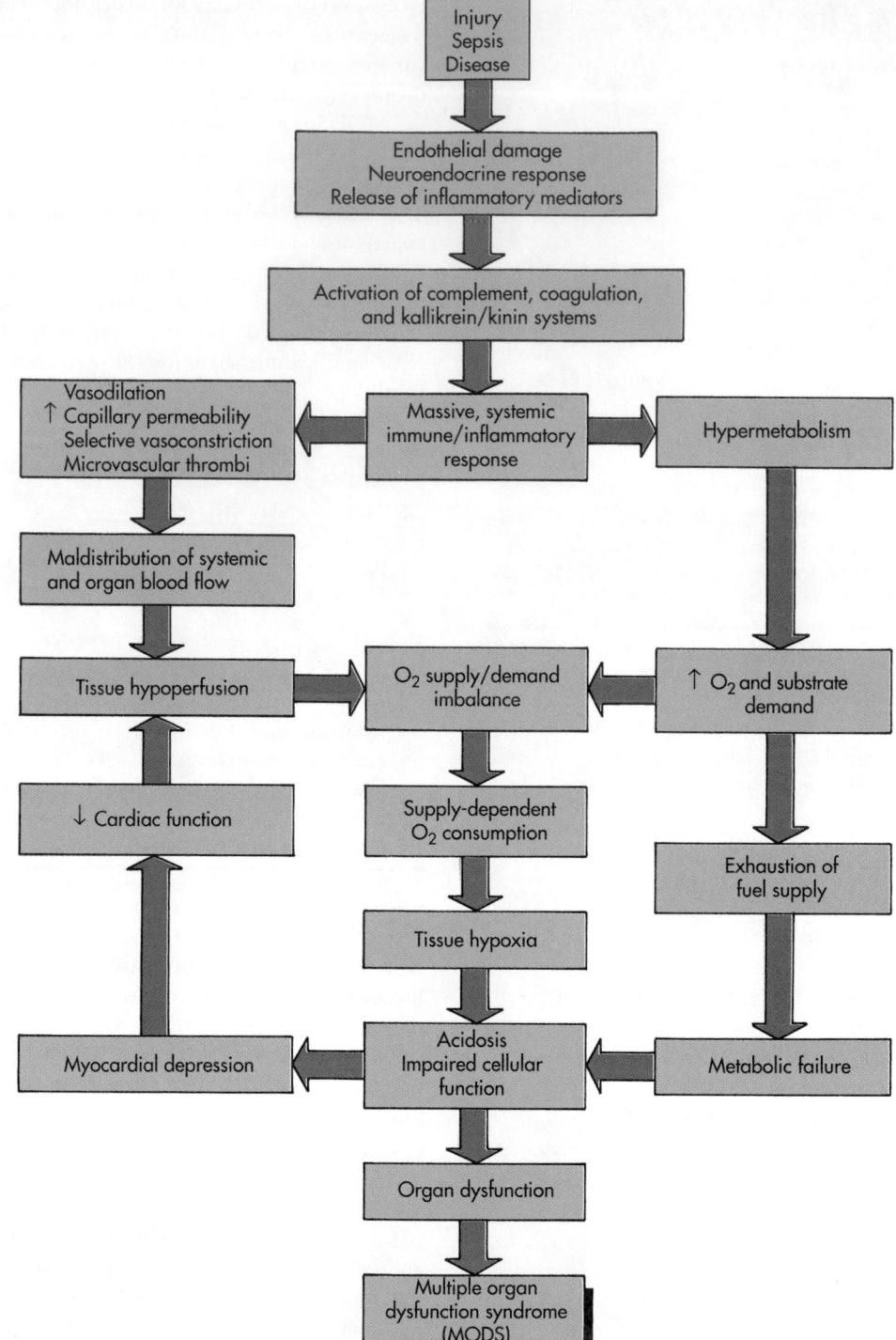

Fig. 23-48 *Pathogenesis of multiple organ dysfunction syndrome.*

vated vary and involve multiple events rather than individual triggers. The inflammatory process initiated is the same as that described in septic shock and SIRS (see p. 681) and sets the stage for MODS.[141,145,146]

The numerous inflammatory and clotting processes operating in MODS cause maldistribution of blood flow and

hypermetabolism. Oxygen delivery to the tissues decreases despite the supranormal systemic blood flow for several reasons:

1. Shunting of blood past selected regional capillary beds, which is caused when inflammatory mediators override the normal vascular tone

TABLE 23-13	Cells of Inflammation and Multiple Organ Dysfunction	
Cell	**Activators**	**Contribution to Multiple Organ Dysfunction**
Neutrophils	Complement kinins, endotoxin, clotting factors	Release of phagocytic products: toxic oxygen free radicals, superoxide ion, hydrogen peroxide, hydroxyl radicals, proteases, platelet-activating factor (PAF), arachidonic acid metabolites (prostaglandins, thromboxane, leukotrienes)
		Endothelial damage, vasodilation, vasopermeability, microvascular coagulation, selective vasoconstriction, hypotension, shock
Macrophages	Complement, endotoxin, chemotactic factors	Release of same phagocytic products as neutrophils
		Release of monokines: tumor necrosis factor (TNF), interleukin-1 (IL-1)
		TNF produces fever, anorexia, hyperglycemia, weight loss
Mast cells	Direct injury, endotoxin, complement	Release of histamine, PAF, arachidonic acid metabolites
		Vasodilation, vasopermeability, hypotension, shock

2. Interstitial edema, resulting from microvascular changes in permeability, that contributes to decreased oxygen delivery by creating a relative hypovolemia and by increasing the distance oxygen must travel to reach the cells
3. Capillary obstruction that occurs because of formation of microvascular thrombi and the aggregation of white blood cells

Hypermetabolism in MODS with accompanying alterations in carbohydrate, fat, and lipid metabolism is initially a compensatory measure to meet the body's increased demands for energy. The alterations in metabolism affect all aspects of substrate utilization. The net result of hypermetabolism is depletion of oxygen and fuel supplies.

Decreased oxygen delivery to the cells caused by maldistribution of blood flow, myocardial depression, and the hypermetabolic state combine to create an imbalance in oxygen supply and demand. This imbalance is critical in the pathogenesis of MODS because it results in a pathologic condition known as *supply-dependent oxygen consumption*.[147] Ordinarily, the amount of oxygen consumed by the cells depends only on the demands of the cells because there is an adequate reserve of oxygen that can be delivered if needed. The reserve, however, has been exhausted in MODS, and the amount of oxygen consumed becomes dependent on the amount the circulation is able to deliver; this amount is inadequate in MODS. Therefore tissue hypoxia with cellular acidosis and impaired cellular function ensue and result in the multiple organ failure.

Clinical Manifestations

There is often a predictable clinical pattern in the development of MODS,[143] although there is certainly some individual variation. After the inciting event and aggressive resuscitation for approximately 24 hours, the individual develops a low-grade fever, tachycardia, dyspnea, altered mental status, and hyperdynamic and hypermetabolic states. The lung is frequently the first organ to fail, resulting in adult respiratory distress syndrome (ARDS) (see Chapter 26). Between 7 and 10 days, the hypermetabolic and hyperdynamic states

intensify, bacteremia with enteric microorganisms is common, and signs of liver and kidney failure appear. During days 14 to 24, renal and liver failures become more severe and the gastrointestinal system shows evidence of dysfunction. Hematologic failure and myocardial failure are usually later manifestations. Encephalopathy, characterized by mental status changes ranging from confusion to deep coma, may occur at any time. Death may occur as early as 14 days or after a period of several weeks.

The clinical manifestations of individual organ failure in MODS are the result of inflammation and tissue hypoxia. Respiratory failure is characterized by tachypnea, pulmonary edema with crackles and diminished breath sounds, use of accessory muscles, and hypoxemia. Liver failure, although developing early, is not clinically detectable until later stages of MODS, at which time jaundice, abdominal distention, liver tenderness, muscle wasting, and hepatic encephalopathy appear. All facets of metabolism, substance detoxification, and immune response are impaired, albumin and clotting factor synthesis decreases, protein wastes accumulate, and liver tissue macrophages (Kupffer cells) no longer function effectively.

Progressive oliguria, azotemia, and edema mark the development of renal failure. Anuria, hyperkalemia, and metabolic acidosis may occur if renal shutdown is severe. The gastrointestinal system is very sensitive to ischemic and inflammatory injury. Clinical manifestations of bowel involvement are hemorrhage, ileus, malabsorption, diarrhea or constipation, vomiting, anorexia, and abdominal pain. Compounding the damage caused by injury to the bowel is the phenomenon of *bacterial translocation*.[148,149] When mediators and severe ischemia injure the mucosal epithelium, bacteria and toxins pass from the gut into the portal circulation. The overwhelmed liver is unable to clear these products, and they move into the systemic circulation. Thus, whether infection or some other injury was the precipitating cause of MODS, once the gut barrier is damaged, sepsis occurs.

The signs and symptoms of cardiac failure in the hypermetabolic, hyperdynamic phase of MODS are similar to those of septic shock: tachycardia, bounding pulse, increased cardiac output, decreased systemic vascular resistance, hypotension, and warm skin. In the terminal stages, hypodynamic circulation with bradycardia, profound hypotension, and ventricular dysrhythmias may develop. Ischemia and inflammation are responsible for the central nervous system manifestations, which include apprehension, confusion, disorientation, restlessness, agitation, headache, decreased cognitive ability and memory, and decreased level of consciousness. When ischemia is severe, seizures and coma can occur.

Evaluation and Treatment

Because presently there is no specific therapy for MODS, early detection is extremely important so that supportive measures can be initiated immediately. Frequent assessment of the clinical status of individuals at known risk is essential. Once organ failure develops, monitoring of laboratory values and hemodynamic parameters also can be used to assess the degree of impairment.

✓ QUICK CHECK

Why can MODS be initiated by either a septic or a non-septic insult?

Why are inflammation and clotting triggered when the vascular endothelium is injured?

Describe the mechanisms that result in decreased oxygen delivery to the tissues in MODS.

Therapeutic management of MODS consists of prevention and support. First, if the initial insult is known, it is aggressively treated and sources of infection are removed. The second priority is restoration and maintenance of tissue oxygenation and cardiovascular function. Third, nutritional support must be provided. Last, individual organs must be supported.

HEALTH ALERT

Nutritional Support to Prevent and Treat Multiple Organ Dysfunction Syndrome

Enteral nutrition (EN) has many advantages over parenteral nutrition (PN) for postoperative/posttrauma individuals. Jejunal tube feedings have advantages over gastric tube feeding: faster metabolic recovery, less vomiting, and less risk of regurgitation and aspiration. Immediate and early EN stimulates the splenic and hepatic circulations, improves mucosal blood flow, prevents intramucosal acidosis and permeability problems, and eliminates the need for stress ulcer prophylaxis. Immediate EN should be given, starting with 25 ml/hr and increasing to 100 ml/hr over 24 to 48 hours. Special attention should be given to the purity of water for the immunocompromised individual.

Data from Rolands, B.J. et al. (1998). Nutritional modulation of gut inflammation. Proceedings of the Nutrition Society, 57(3), 395-401; *Georgieff, M. et al. (1998). Positive role of immune nutrition on metabolism in sepsis and multi-organ failure.* Kidney International Supplement, 64, S80-S83.

▢ DID YOU UNDERSTAND?

Diseases of the Arteries and Veins

1. Arteriosclerosis is a thickening and hardening of the arteries, involving the intimal layer and leading to hypertension. It seems to be a part of the normal aging process, but it is a disease state when it occurs to the point of symptom development.
2. Arteriosclerosis raises the systolic pressure by decreasing arterial distensibility and lumen diameter. With arteriosclerotic changes in the artery causing narrowing and decreased elasticity, diastolic blood pressure is elevated.
3. Hypertension is the elevation of systemic arterial blood pressure resulting from increases in cardiac output or total peripheral resistance or both.
4. Hypertension can be primary, without a known cause, or secondary, caused by a primary disease.
5. The risk factors for hypertension include a positive family history, male gender, advancing age, black race, obesity, high sodium intake, diabetes mellitus, labile blood pressure, cigarette smoking, and heavy alcohol consumption.

6. The pathophysiology of hypertension includes damage and inflammation of the vessel walls that stimulate the vessels to thicken, harden, and become narrow. Narrowing causes vasoconstriction and increases the permeability of the vessel walls, leading to the influx of sodium, calcium, water, plasma proteins, and other substances. Calcium further increases smooth muscle contraction.
7. The exact cause of primary hypertension is unknown, although several hypotheses are proposed, including (a) increases in blood volume, (b) increased activity of the sympathetic nervous system, (c) increased activity of the renin-angiotensin-aldosterone system, (d) sodium and water retention by the kidneys, and (e) hormonal inhibition of sodium-potassium transport across cell walls.
8. Clinical manifestations of hypertension result from damage of organs and tissues outside the vascular system. These include heart disease, renal disease, central nervous system problems, and musculoskeletal dysfunction.

9. Hypertension is managed with both pharmacologic and nonpharmacologic methods.

10. Orthostatic hypotension is a drop in blood pressure that occurs on standing. The compensatory vasoconstriction response to standing is replaced by a marked vasodilation and blood pooling in the muscle vasculature.

11. Orthostatic hypotension may be acute or chronic. The acute form is caused by a delay in the normal regulatory mechanisms. The chronic forms are secondary to a specific disease or are idiopathic in nature.

12. The clinical manifestations of orthostatic hypotension include fainting and may involve cardiovascular symptoms, as well as impotence and bowel and bladder dysfunction.

13. An aneurysm is a localized dilation of a vessel wall, to which the aorta is particularly susceptible.

14. A thrombus is a clot that remains attached to a vascular wall. Arteriosclerosis can generate thrombus formation through roughening of the intima that activates the clotting cascade. Thrombus formation may be discrete or diffuse.

15. An embolus is a mobile aggregate of a variety of substances that occludes the vasculature. Sources of emboli include clots, air, amniotic fluid, bacteria, fat, and foreign matter. These emboli cause ischemia and necrosis when a vessel is totally blocked.

16. The most common source of arterial thrombotic emboli is the heart, as a result of mitral and aortic valvular disease and atrial fibrillation, followed by myxomas. Tissues affected include the lower extremities, the brain, and the heart.

17. Emboli to the central organs cause tissue death in lungs, kidneys, and mesentery.

18. The generation of air emboli requires a connection between the vascular compartment and a source of air.

19. Amniotic fluid may be forced into the bloodstream and generate an embolus during the labor and delivery of pregnancy.

20. Aggregates of bacteria in the vasculature may be large enough to form an embolus.

21. Fat emboli are caused mainly by trauma to the long bones, either through defective fat metabolism after trauma or through the release of fat globules from bone marrow exposed by fracture.

22. The introduction of foreign matter into the vasculature can occur with trauma and also can occur in a hospital setting in which intravenous and intraarterial lines are being used.

23. Vasospastic disorders include Raynaud disease, involving arterioles of the extremities; Prinzmetal angina, involving coronary arteries; and Buerger disease, involving arteries of the hands and feet.

24. Diabetic lesions of the arteries may be caused by a defect in glycoprotein metabolism that involves the capillary basement membranes in kidneys, retinas, and extremities.

25. Varicosities are areas of veins in which blood has pooled, usually in the saphenous veins. Varicosities may be caused by damaged valves as a result of trauma to the valve or by chronic venous distention involving gravity and venous constriction.

26. Chronic venous insufficiency is inadequate venous return over a long period of time that causes pathologic ischemic changes in the vasculature, skin, and supporting tissues.

27. Venous stasis ulcers follow the development of chronic venous insufficiency and probably develop as a result of the borderline metabolic state of the cells in the affected extremities.

28. The pathophysiology of thrombus formation in the veins is the same as for thrombus formation in the arteries.

29. Superior vena cava syndrome is a progressive occlusion of the superior vena cava that leads to venous distention in the upper extremities and head. Because this syndrome is usually caused by bronchogenic cancer, it is generally considered an oncologic emergency rather than a vascular emergency.

30. Coronary artery disease (CAD) is almost always the result of atherosclerosis that narrows or occludes the coronary arteries. Many risk factors contribute to the onset and escalation of CAD, including dyslipidemia (primarily hypercholesterolemia), smoking, hypertension, male gender, diabetes mellitus, advancing age, obesity, sedentary life-style, psychosocial factors, hyperhomocystinemia, estrogen deficiency, and heavy consumption of alcohol.

31. The three risk factors most predictive of CAD are hypercholesterolemia, cigarette smoking, and hypertension.

32. Ischemic heart disease is most commonly the result of coronary artery disease and the resultant decrease in myocardial blood supply.

33. Angina pectoris is chest pain caused by myocardial ischemia.

34. Therapeutic interventions for CAD include use of vasodilators and medications to reduce cardiac work load (e.g., β blockers), as well as surgical procedures.

35. Myocardial infarction is caused by prolonged, unrelieved ischemia that interrupts blood supply to the myocardium. After about 20 minutes of myocardial ischemia, irreversible hypoxic injury causes cellular death and tissue necrosis.

36. A transient increase in plasma enzyme levels may diagnose the occurrence of myocardial infarction and indicate its severity. Elevations of the isoenzymes creatine kinase (CK-MB), troponins, and lactic dehydrogenase (LDH-1) are most predictive of a myocardial infarction.

37. Treatment of a myocardial infarction includes bed rest, pain relief, and drug interventions to limit in-

Continued

Diseases of the Arteries and Veins—cont'd
farct size, prevent thrombus formation, and augment repair. Dysrhythmias and cardiac failure are the most common complications of acute myocardial infarction.

Disorders of the Heart Wall
1. Inflammation of the pericardium, or pericarditis, may result from several sources (infection, drug therapy, tumors). Pericarditis presents with symptoms that are physically troublesome, but in and of themselves they are not life threatening.
2. Fluid may collect within the pericardial sac (pericardial effusion). Cardiac function may be severely impaired if the accumulation of fluid occurs rapidly and involves a large volume.
3. Cardiomyopathies are a diverse group of primary myocardial disorders that are poorly understood. The cardiomyopathies are categorized as dilated (congestive), restrictive (rigid and noncompliant), and hypertrophic (asymmetric). The size of the cardiac muscle walls and chambers may increase or decrease depending on the type of cardiomyopathy, thereby altering contractile activity.
4. Hemodynamic integrity of the cardiovascular system depends to a great extent on properly functioning cardiac valves. Congenital or acquired disorders that result in stenosis or incompetence or both can structurally alter the valves.
5. Characteristic heart sounds, cardiac murmurs, and systemic complaints assist in determination of which valve is abnormal. If severely compromised function exists, a prosthetic heart valve may be surgically implanted to replace the faulty one.
6. Mitral valve prolapse (MVP) is a common finding, especially in young women. Although not grossly abnormal, the mitral valve leaflets do not position themselves properly during systole. Mitral valve prolapse may be a completely asymptomatic condition or could result in severe subjective symptoms. Afflicted valves may be at greater risk for developing infective endocarditis.
7. Rheumatic fever is an inflammatory disease that results from a delayed immune response to a streptococcal infection. The disorder usually resolves without sequelae if treated early.
8. Severe or untreated cases of rheumatic fever may progress to rheumatic heart disease, a potentially disabling cardiovascular disorder.
9. Infective endocarditis is a general term for inflammation of the endocardium, especially the cardiac valves. A wide range of conditions predispose to the development of this disorder. In the mildest cases, valvular function may be slightly impaired by vegetations that collect on the valve leaflets. If left unchecked, severe valve abnormalities, chronic bacteremia, and systemic emboli may occur as vegetations break off the valve surface and travel through the bloodstream. Antibiotic therapy can limit the extension of this disease.
10. Human immunodeficiency virus is associated with cardiac abnormalities, including myocarditis, endocarditis, pericarditis, and cardiomyopathy. Left heart failure is the most common clinical manifestation.

Manifestations of Heart Disease
1. A dysrhythmia (arrhythmia) is a disturbance of heart rhythm. Dysrhythmias range in severity from occasional missed beats or rapid beats to disturbances that impair myocardial contractility and are life threatening.
2. Dysrhythmias can occur because of an abnormal rate of impulse generation or the abnormal conduction of impulses.
3. Heart failure is an inability of the heart to supply the metabolism with adequate circulatory volume and pressure.
4. Right ventricular failure is usually the result of chronic pulmonary hypertension caused by chronic hypoxic lung disease.
5. Left heart failure (congestive heart failure) can be divided into systolic and diastolic heart failure.
6. The most common causes of left ventricular failure are myocardial infarction, fluid overload, hypertension, or valvular disease.
7. Systolic heart failure is caused by increased preload, decreased contractility, or increased afterload. These processes result in an increased left ventricular end-diastolic volume and an increase in left ventricular end-diastolic pressure that results in increased pulmonary venous pressures and pulmonary edema.
8. In addition to the hemodynamic changes of left ventricular failure, there is a neuroendocrine response that tends to exacerbate and perpetuate the condition.
9. The neuroendocrine mediators of congestive heart failure (CHF) include the sympathetic nervous system and the renin-angiotensin-aldosterone system; thus β blockers and angiotensin-converting enzyme (ACE) inhibitors are important components of the pharmacologic therapy.
10. Diastolic heart failure results from a stiff, thickened left ventricle usually caused by myocardial hypertrophy from hypertension.
11. Diastole dysfunction means that the left ventricular end-diastolic pressure is increased, even if volume and cardiac output are normal.

Shock
1. Shock is a widespread impairment of cellular metabolism involving positive feedback loops that places the individual on a downward physiologic spiral leading to multiple organ dysfunction syndrome.

◼ DID YOU UNDERSTAND? —cont'd

2. Types of shock are cardiogenic, hypovolemic, neurogenic, anaphylactic, and septic. Multiple organ dysfunction syndrome can develop from all types of shock.

3. The final common pathway in all types of shock is impaired cellular metabolism—cells switch from aerobic to anaerobic metabolism. Energy stores drop, and cellular mechanisms relative to membrane permeability, action potentials, and lysozyme release fail.

4. Anaerobic metabolism results in activation of the inflammatory response, decreased circulatory volume, and decreasing pH.

5. Impaired cellular metabolism results in cellular inability to use glucose because of impaired glucose delivery or impaired glucose intake, resulting in a shift to glycogenolysis, gluconeogenesis, and lipolysis for fuel generation.

6. Glycogenolysis is effective for about 10 hours. Gluconeogenesis results in the use of proteins necessary for structure, function, repair, and replication that leads to more impaired cellular metabolism.

7. Gluconeogenesis contributes to lactic acid, uric acid, and ammonia buildup, interstitial edema, and impairment of the immune system, as well as general muscle weakness leading to decreased respiratory function and cardiac output.

8. Cardiogenic shock is attributable to heart failure and is characterized by a decrease in cardiac output and impaired cellular metabolism.

9. Hypovolemic shock is caused by loss of blood or fluid in large amounts. The use of compensatory mechanisms may be vigorous, but tissue perfusion ultimately decreases and results in impaired cellular metabolism.

10. Neurogenic shock results from massive vasodilation, causing a relative hypovolemia, even though cardiac output may be high, and results in impaired cellular metabolism.

11. Anaphylactic shock is caused by physiologic recognition of a foreign substance. The inflammatory response is triggered, and a massive vasodilation with fluid shift into the interstitium follows. The relative hypovolemia leads to impaired cellular metabolism.

12. Septic shock begins with impaired cellular metabolism caused by uncontrolled septicemia. The infecting agent triggers the inflammatory and immune responses. Four major chemicals have been implicated in the cause of shock: (a) interleukins, (b) platelet-activating factor, (c) tumor necrosis factor, and (d) myocardial depressant factor.

13. Multiple organ dysfunction syndrome (MODS) is the progressive failure of two or more organ systems after a severe illness or injury. It can be triggered by chronic inflammation, necrotic tissue, severe trauma, burns, adult respiratory distress syndrome, acute pancreatitis, and other severe injuries.

14. The mortality of MODS is very high, ranging from 50% to 90%.

15. MODS involves the stress response; changes in the vascular endothelium resulting in microvascular coagulation; release of complement, coagulation, and kinin proteins; and numerous inflammatory processes. Consequences of all these mediators are a maldistribution of blood flow, hypermetabolism, hypoxic injury, and myocardial depression.

16. Clinical manifestations of MODS include inflammation, tissue hypoxia, and hypermetabolism. The lung is usually the first organ to fail.

KEY TERMS

Acute onset of left (congestive) heart failure, 672
Acute orthostatic hypotension, 638
Acute pericarditis, 654
Anaphylactic shock, 681
Aneurysm, 638
Angina pectoris, 645
Aortic regurgitation, 659
Aortic stenosis, 657
Arteriosclerosis, 629
Atherosclerosis, 629
Bacterial translocation, 687
Cardiogenic shock, 679
Cardiomyopathy, 656
Carditis, 661
Chronic left heart failure, 672
Chronic orthostatic hypotension, 638

Chronic venous insufficiency (CVI), 642
Complicated hypertension, 636
Complicated lesion, 630
Constrictive pericarditis (chronic pericarditis), 655
Coronary artery disease, 643
Diastolic heart failure, 674
Dissecting aneurysm, 639
Dysrhythmia (arrhythmia), 666
Embolism, 640
Embolus, 640
Endothelial injury, 629
False aneurysm, 638
Fatty streak, 629
Fibrous plaque, 630
Foam cell, 629
Heart failure, 670

Hibernating myocardium, 650
High-output failure, 675
Hypertension, 633
Hypovolemic shock, 680
Infarction, 643
Infective endocarditis, 664
Ischemia, 643
Isolated systolic hypertension, 633
Left heart failure, 671
Malignant hypertension, 636
Mitral regurgitation, 659
Mitral stenosis, 658
Mitral valve prolapse syndrome (MVPS), 660
Multiple organ dysfunction syndrome (MODS), 685
Myocardial infarction, 648

KEY TERMS

Myocardial remodeling, 650
Myocardial stunning, 650
Neurogenic shock (vasogenic shock), 680
Nonbacterial thrombotic
  endocarditis, 664
Orthostatic (postural) hypotension, 637
Percutaneous transluminal coronary
  angioplasty (PTCA), 648
Pericardial effusion, 654
Peripheral pooling, 681
Primary hypertension (essential
  hypertension, idiopathic
  hypertension), 633
Prinzmetal angina, 645
Raynaud disease, 641
Raynaud phenomenon, 641

Rheumatic fever, 660
Rheumatic heart disease, 660
Right heart failure, 675
Saccular aneurysm, 638
Secondary hypertension, 633
Septic shock, 681
Shock, 676
Silent heart attack, 648
Silent ischemia, 646
Stable angina, 645
Superior vena cava syndrome
  (SVCS), 642
Supply-dependent oxygen
  consumption, 687
Systemic inflammatory response
  syndrome (SIRS), 681

Systolic heart failure, 671
Tamponade, 655
Thromboangiitis obliterans (Buerger
  disease), 640
Thromboembolus, 639
Thrombus, 639
Tricuspid regurgitation, 660
True aneurysm, 638
Unstable angina, 645
Valvular regurgitation (valvular
  insufficiency, valvular
  incompetence), 657
Valvular stenosis, 657
Varicose vein, 641
Venous stasis ulcer, 642
Ventricular remodeling, 671

REFERENCES

1. Consigny, P.M. (1995). Pathogenesis of atherosclerosis. *American Journal of Radiology, 164,* 553-558.
2. Busse, R. & Fleming, I. (1996). Endothelial dysfunction in atherosclerosis. *Journal of Vascular Research, 33*(3), 181-194.
3. Berenson, G.S. et al. (1998). Association between multiple cardiovascular risk factors and atherosclerosis in children and young adults. The Bogalusa Heart Study. *New England Journal of Medicine, 338*(23), 1650-1656.
4. Gonzalez, E.R. (1998). Antiplatelet therapy in atherosclerotic cardiovascular disease. *Clinical Therapeutics, 20*(Suppl. B), B18-B41.
5. National Cholesterol Education Program (NCEP) Expert Panel. (1993). Summary of the second report of the National Cholesterol Expert Panel on detection, evaluation, and treatment of high blood cholesterol in adults (adult treatment panel II). *Journal of the American Medical Association, 269*(3), 3015-3023.
6. Anonymous. (1997). The sixth report of the Joint National Committee on Prevention, Detection, Evaluation, and Treatment of High Blood Pressure. *Archives of Internal Medicine, 157,* 2413-2446.
7. Winkleby, M.A. et al. (1998). Ethnic and socioeconomic differences in cardiovascular disease risk factors. *Journal of the American Medical Association, 280,* 356-362.
8. Cowley, A.W.J. (1997). Genetic and nongenetic determinants of salt sensitivity and blood pressure. *American Journal of Clinical Nutrition, 65*(2 Suppl.), 587S-593S.
9. Harrap, S.B. (1996). An appraisal of the genetic approaches to high blood pressure [review, 20 refs]. *Journal of Hypertension—Supplement, 14*(5), S111-S115.
10. Kotchen, T.A. & Kotchen, J.M. (1997). Dietary sodium and blood pressure: Interactions with other nutrients. *American Journal of Clinical Nutrition, 65*(2 Suppl.), 708S-711S.
11. Resnick, L.M. et al. (1997). Serum ionized magnesium: Relation to blood pressure and racial factors. *American Journal of Hypertension, 10,* 1420-1424.
12. Verdecchia, P. et al. (1995). Cigarette smoking, ambulatory blood pressure and cardiac hypertrophy in essential hypertension. *Journal of Hypertension, 13,* 1209-1215.
13. Vriz, O. et al. (1998). The effects of alcohol consumption on ambulatory blood pressure and target organs in subjects with borderline to mild hypertension. HARVEST Study Group. *American Journal of Hypertension, 11,* 230-234.
14. Mancia, G. et al. (1998). Early and late sympathetic activation in hypertension. *Scandinavian Cardiovascular Journal Supplement, 47,* 9-14.
15. Fyhrquist, F., Metsarinne, K., & Tikkanen, I. (1995) The role of angiotensin II in blood pressure regulation and in the pathophysiology of cardiovascular disorders. *Journal of Human Hypertension, 9*(Suppl. 5), S19-S24.
16. Malik, F.S. et al. (1997). Renin-angiotensin system: Genes to bedside. *American Heart Journal, 134,* 514-526.
17. Ghavari, A. & Klotman, P. (1998) The renin-angiotensin system as a mediator of renal injury in hypertension. *Mount Sinai Journal of Medicine, 65,* 118-124.
18. Morgan, T. & Brunner, H.R. (1996). The renin-angiotensin system and the heart: Beyond 2000. *Heart 76*(3 Suppl. 3), 98-103.

REFERENCES

19. Cowley, A.W. & Roman, R.J. (1996). The role of the kidney in hypertension. *Journal of the American Medical Association, 275,* 1581-1589.

20. Hohn, A.R. (1997). Diagnosis and management of hypertension in childhood. *Pediatric Annals, 26*(2), 105-110.

21. Wing, L.M. & Tonkin, A.L. (1997). Orthostatic blood pressure control and ageing. *Australian and New Zealand Journal of Medicine, 27,* 462-466.

22. Chen, K. et al. (1997). Acute thoracic aortic dissection: The basics. *Journal of Emergency Medicine 15,* 859-867.

23. Galla, J.D. et al. (1997). Identification of risk factors in patients undergoing thoracoabdominal aneurysm repair. *Journal of Cardiac Surgery, 12*(2 Suppl.), 292-299.

24. Englund, R. et al. (1998). Expansion rates of small abdominal aortic aneurysms. *Australian and New Zealand Journal of Surgery, 68*(1), 21-24.

25. Zarins, C.K. & Harris, E.J., Jr. (1997). Operative repair for aortic aneurysms: The gold standard. *Journal of Endovascular Surgery, 4*(3), 232-241.

26. Subramaniam, P., Bennett, R.C., & Campbell, I.A. (1998.). Infrarenal aortic aneurysm surgery in a rural surgical service: Risk factors for mortality. *Australian and New Zealand Journal of Surgery, 68*(1), 25-28.

27. Lie, J.T. (1989). The rise and fall of resurgence of thromboangiitis obliterans (Buerger's disease). *Acta Pathologica Japonica, 39*(3), 153-158.

28. Matchev, S. et al. (1997). Transcranial Doppler velocities in patients with thromboangiitis obliterans. *Angiology, 48*(6), 535-544.

29. Aerbajinai, W. et al. (1997). HLA class II DNA typing in Buerger's disease. *Internal Journal of Cardiology, 54*(Suppl.), S197-S202.

30. Lambotte, O. et al. (1997). Thromboangiitis obliterans with inaugural rheumatic manifestations. A report of three cases [see comments]. *Revue du Rhumatisme (English edition), 64*(5), 334-338.

31. Makita, S. et al. (1996). Impaired endothelium-dependent vasorelaxation in peripheral vasculature of patients with thromboangiitis obliterans (Buerger's disease). *Circulation, 94*(9 Suppl.), II211-II215.

32. VanDamme, H. et al. (1997). Thrombangiitis obliterans (Buerger's disease): Still a limb threatening disease. *Acta Chirurgica Belgica, 97*(5), 229-236.

33. Suzuki, S., Yamada, I., & Himeno, Y. (1997). Angiographic findings in Buerger disease. *International Journal of Cardiology, 54*(Suppl.), S189-S195.

34. Lau, H. & Cheng, S.W. (1997). Buerger's disease in Hong Kong: A review of 89 cases. *Australian and New Zealand Journal of Surgery, 67*(5), 264-269.

35. Valter, I. & Maricq, H. R. (1997). Prevalence of Raynaud phenomenon in Tartu and Tartumaa, southern Estonia. *Scandinavian Journal of Rheumatology, 26*(2), 117-124.

36. Ruckley, C.V. (1997). Socioeconomic impact of chronic venous insufficiency and leg ulcers. *Angiology, 48*(1), 67-69.

37. Bollinger, A. et al. (1997). Microvascular changes in venous disease: An update. *Angiology, 48*(1), 27-32.

38. Hosoi, Y. et al. (1997). A new method for the assessment of venous insufficiency in primary varicose veins using near-infrared spectroscopy. *Journal of Vascular Surgery, 26*(1), 53-60.

39. Kowallek, D.L. & De Palma, R.G. (1997). Venous ulceration: Active approaches to treatment. *Journal of Vascular Nursing, 15*(2), 50-57.

40. Mayberry, J.C. et al. (1991). Fifteen-year results of ambulatory compression therapy for chronic venous ulcers. *Surgery, 109*(5), 575-581.

41. Gloviczki, P. et al. (1997). Safety, feasibility, and early efficacy of subfascial endoscopic perforator surgery: A preliminary report from the North American Registry. *Journal of Vascular Surgery, 25*(1), 94-105.

42. Pappas, P.J. et al. (1997). Morphometric assessment of the dermal microcirculation in patients with chronic venous insufficiency. *Journal of Vascular Surgery, 26*(5), 784-795.

43. Krijnen, R.M. et al. (1997). Compression stockings and rubber floor mats: Do they benefit workers with chronic venous insufficiency and a standing profession? *Journal of Occupational and Environmental Medicine, 39*(9), 889-894.

44. Peschen, M. et al. (1997). Low-frequency ultrasound treatment of chronic venous leg ulcers in an outpatient therapy. *Acta Dermato-Venerological, 77*(4), 311-314.

45. Wakefield, T.W. et al. (1997). Pathogenesis of venous thrombosis: A new insight. *Cardiovascular Surgery, 5*(1), 6-15.

46. Ruiz, F. & Berman, D. (1998) Treatment of deep venous thrombosis with low molecular weight heparins. *Western Journal of Medicine, 168,* 186-187.

47. Chow, B.J. et al. (1997). Superior vena cava obstruction secondary to mediastinal lymphadenopathy in a patient with cystic fibrosis. *Chest, 112*(5), 1438-1441.

48. Promisloff, R.A. & Pervall-Phillips, G.P. (1997). Superior vena cava syndrome caused by a benign retrosternal multinodular goiter. *Journal of the American Osteopathic Society, 97*(7), 409-410.

49. Lai, C.L. et al. (1997). Superior vena cava syndrome caused by encapsulated pleural effusion. *European Respiratory Journal, 10*(7), 1675-1677.

50. McLaughlin, J.F., Loeser, J.D., & Roberts, T.S. (1997). Acquired hydrocephalus associated with superior vena cava syndrome in infants. *Childs Nervous System, 13*(2), 59-63.

51. Ostler, P.J. et al. (1997). Superior vena cava obstruction: A modern management strategy. *Clinical Oncology (Royal College of Radiologists) [London], 9*(2), 83-89.

REFERENCES

52. Chan, R.H. et al. (1997). Superior vena cava obstruction in small-cell lung cancer. *International Journal of Radiation, Oncology, Biology, and Physiology, 38*(3), 513-520.

53. Hoegler, D. (1997). Radiotherapy for palliation of symptoms in incurable cancer. *Current Problems in Cancer, 21*(3), 129-183.

54. Kee, S.T. et al. (1998). Superior vena cava syndrome: Treatment with catheter-directed thrombolysis and endovascular stent placement. *Radiology, 206*(1), 187-193.

55. Gross, C.M. et al. (1997). Stent implantation in patients with superior vena cava syndrome. *AJR: American Journal of Roentgenology, 169*(2), 429-432.

56. Nicholson, A.A. et al. (1997). Treatment of malignant superior vena cava obstruction: Metal stents or radiation therapy. *Journal of Vascular Intervention and Radiology, 8*(5), 781-788.

57. Hunink, M.G. et al. (1997). The recent decline in mortality from coronary heart disease, 1980-1990. *Journal of the American Medical Association, 277*, 535-542.

58. Gaziano, J.M. et al. (1997). Fasting triglycerides, high-density lipoprotein, and risk of myocardial infarction. *Circulation, 96*(8), 2520- 2525.

59. Kannel, W.B. & Wilson, P.W. (1995). An update on coronary risk factors. *Medical Clinics of North America, 79*, 951-971.

60. Stein, J.H. & McBride, P.E. (1998). Hyperhomocysteinemia and atherosclerotic vascular disease. *Archives of Internal Medicine, 158*, 1301-1306.

61. Wald, N.J. et al. (1998). Homocysteine and ischemic heart disease. *Archives of Internal Medicine, 158*, 862-867.

62. Libby, P. (1995). Molecular bases of the acute coronary syndromes. *Circulation, 91*, 2844-2850.

63. Califf, R.M. (1995). Acute ischemic syndromes. *Medical Clinics of North America, 79*, 999-1024.

64. Theroux, P. & Fuster, V. (1998). Acute coronary syndromes: Unstable angina and non-Q-wave myocardial infarction. *Circulation, 97*, 1195-1206.

65. Calnon, E.A. & Beller, G.A. (1998). Observations of silent myocardial ischemia by nuclear cardiology techniques. In S. Stern (Ed.), *Silent myocardial ischemia.* St. Louis: Mosby.

66. Langer, A. et al. (1995). Metaiodobenzylguanidine imaging in diabetes mellitus: Assessment of cardiac sympathetic denervation and its relation to autonomic and silent myocardial ischemia. *Journal of the American College of Cardiology, 25*, 610-618.

67. Shimanogata, T. et al. (1995). Scintigraphic assessment of silent myocardial ischemia after early infarction using myocardial SPECT imaging with T1 and I-MIBG. *Nuclear Medicine Communications, 16*, 893-900.

68. Gottdiener, J.S., Kop, W.J., & Krantz, D.S. (1998). Mental stress and silent myocardial ischemia: Evidence, mechanisms, and clinical implications. In S. Stern (Ed.). *Silent myocardial ischemia.* St. Louis: Mosby.

69. Deanfield, J.E. et al. (1984). Silent myocardial ischaemia due to mental stress. *Lancet, 2*, 1001-1005.

70. Rozansky, A. et al. (1988). Mental stress and the induction of silent myocardial ischemia in patients with coronary artery disease. *New England Journal of Medicine, 318*, 1005-1012.

71. Bairey, C.N., Kruntz, D.S., & Rozanski, A. (1990). Mental stress as an acute trigger of ischemic left ventricular dysfunction and blood pressure elevation in coronary artery disease. *American Journal of Cardiology, 66*, 28G-31G.

72. Blumenthal, J.A. et al. (1995). Mental-stress induced ischemia in the laboratory and ambulatory ischemia during daily life: Association and hemodynamic features. *Circulation, 92*, 2102-2108.

73. Iskander, S. & Iskandrian, A.E. (1998). Risk assessment using single-photon emission computed tomographic technetium-99m sestamibi imaging. *Journal of the American College of Cardiology, 32*, 57-62.

74. Ishikawa, K. (1998). Antiplatelet agents prevent cardiac events in patients with coronary artery disease. *Internal Medicine, 37*, 199-202.

75. Anonymous. (1998). Inhibition of the platelet glycoprotein IIb/IIIa receptor with tirofiban in unstable angina and non-Q-wave myocardial infarction. Platelet Receptor Inhibition in Ischemic Syndrome Management in Patients Limited by Unstable Signs and Symptoms (PRISM-PLUS) Study Investigators. *New England Journal of Medicine, 338*, 1488-1497.

76. Goy, J.J. & Eeckhout, E. (1998). Intracoronary stenting. *Lancet, 351*, 1943-1949.

77. Kannel, W.B. (1998). Unrecognized myocardial infarction. In S. Stern (Ed.). *Silent myocardial ischemia.* St. Louis: Mosby.

78. Kannel, W.G., Dannenberg, A.L., & Abbott, R. (1985). Unrecognized myocardial infarction: The Framingham Study. *American Heart Journal, 109*, 581-585.

79. Opie, L.H. (1996). The multifarious spectrum of ischemic left ventricular dysfunction: Relevance of new ischemic syndromes. *Journal of Molecular and Cellular Cardiology, 28*, 2403-2414.

80. Amos, D.J. & White, H.D. (1997). Remodeling after myocardial infarction: An opportunity for early intervention. *Basic Research in Cardiology, 92*, 69-71.

81. Wilson, A.T. & Channer, K.S. (1997). Hypoxaemia and supplemental oxygen therapy in the first 24 hours after myocardial infarction: The role of pulse oximetry. *Journal of the Royal College of Physicians of London, 31*(6), 657-661.

REFERENCES

82. Polanczyk, C.A. et al. (1998). Cardiac troponin I as a predictor of major cardiac events in emergency department patients with acute chest pain. *Journal of the American College of Cardiology, 32,* 8-14.

83. Coudrey, L. (1998) The troponins. *Archives of Internal Medicine, 158,* 1173-1180.

84. Laurino, J.P. et al. (1997). Thrombus precursor protein and the measurement of thrombosis in patients with acute chest pain syndrome. *Annals in Clinical Laboratory Science, 27*(5), 338-345.

85. Vinolas, X., Guindo, J., & Rodriquez, E. (1998). Sudden death and myocardial ischemia. In S. Stern (Ed.). *Silent myocardial ischemia.* St. Louis: Mosby.

86. Gershlick, A.H. & More, R.S. (1998). Treatment of myocardial infarction. *British Medical Journal, 316,* 280-284.

87. Reeder, G.S. & Gersh, B.J. (1996). Modern management of acute myocardial infarction. *Current Problems in Cardiology, 96,* 585-667.

88. Yusuf, S. et al. (1996). Treatment for acute myocardial infarction. Overview of randomized clinical trials. *European Heart Journal, 17*(Suppl. F), 16-29.

89. Lorell, B.H. (1997). Pericardial diseases. In E. Braunwald (Ed.), *Heart disease: A textbook of cardiovascular medicine* (5th ed.). Philadelphia: Saunders.

90. Marinella, M.A. (1998). Electrocardiographic manifestations and differential diagnosis of acute pericarditis. *American Family Physician, 57,* 699-704.

91. Shepherd, F.A. (1997). Malignant pericardial effusion. *Current Opinion in Oncology, 9,* 170-174.

92. Wynne, J. & Braunwald, E. (1997). The cardiomyopathies and myocarditides. In E. Braunwald (Ed.). *Heart disease: A textbook of cardiovascular medicine* (5th ed., pp. 1404-1463). Philadelphia: Saunders.

93. Carabello, B.A. & Crawford, F.A., Jr. (1997). Medical progress: Valvular heart disease. *New England Journal of Medicine, 337,* 32-41.

94. Braunwald, E. (1997) Valvular heart disease. In E. Braunwald (Ed.). *Heart disease: A textbook of cardiovascular medicine* (5th ed., pp. 1007-1076). Philadelphia: Saunders.

95. Stollerman, G.H. (1997). Rheumatic fever. *Lancet, 349,* 935-942.

96. Dajani, A.S. (1997). Rheumatic fever. In E. Braunwald (Ed.). *Heart disease: A textbook of cardiovascular medicine* (5th ed., pp. 1769-1775). Philadelphia: Saunders.

97. Markowitz, M. (1988). Evolution and critique of changes in the Jones criteria for the diagnosis of rheumatic fever. *New Zealand Medical Journal, 101,* 392-394.

98. Korzeniowski, O.M. & Kaye, D. (1997). Infective endocarditis. In E. Braunwald (Ed.). *Heart disease: A textbook of cardiovascular medicine* (5th ed.). Philadelphia: Saunders.

99. Lindner, J.R. et al. (1996). Diagnostic value of echocardiography in suspected endocarditis. An evaluation based on the pretest probability of disease. *Circulation, 93,* 730-736

100. Moon, M.R., Stinson, E.B., & Miller, D.C. (1997). Surgical treatment of endocarditis. *Progress in Cardiovascular Disease, 40*(3), 239-264.

101. Roder, B.L. et al. (1997). A study of 47 bacteremic *Staphylococcus aureus* endocarditis cases: 23 with native valves treated surgically and 24 with prosthetic valves. *Scandinavian Cardiovascular Journal, 31*(5), 305-309.

102. Dajani, A.S. et al. (1997). Prevention of bacterial endocarditis: Recommendations by the American Heart Association. *Journal of the American Medical Association, 277,* 1794-1801.

103. Michaels, A.D. et al. (1997). Cardiovascular involvement in AIDS. *Current Problems in Cardiology, 22,* 109-148.

104. Ramachandran, S. et al. (1996). The role of hypertension in the pathogenesis of heart failure. *Archives of Internal Medicine, 156,* 1789-1796.

105. Middlekauff, H.R. & Mark, A.L. (1998). The treatment of heart failure: The role of neurohumoral activation. *Internal Medicine, 37,* 112-122.

106. Colucci, W.S. & Braunwald, E. (1997). Pathophysiology of heart failure. In E. Braunwald (Ed.). *Heart disease: A textbook of cardiovascular medicine* (5th ed., pp 394-420). Philadelphia: Saunders.

107. Anonymous. (1997).The effect of digoxin on mortality and morbidity in patients with heart failure. The Digitalis Investigation Group. *New England Journal of Medicine, 336,* 525-533.

108. Anonymous. (1998). Managing the patient with advanced heart failure. Meeting proceedings of the Advanced Heart Failure Group. *American Heart Journal, 135*(6 Pt., 2 Suppl.), S201-S326.

109. Gheorghiade, M. et al. (1998). Current medical therapy for advanced heart failure. *American Heart Journal, 135*(6 Pt., 2 Suppl.), S231- S248.

110. Feuerstein, G. & Ruffolo, R.R.J. (1998). Beta-blockers in congestive heart failure: The pharmacology of carvedilol, a vasodilating beta-blocker and antioxidant, and its therapeutic utility in congestive heart failure. *Advances in Pharmacology, 42,* 611-615.

111. Constant, J. (1998). A review of why and how we may use beta-blockers in congestive heart failure. *Chest, 113,* 800-808.

112. Cash, L.A. (1996). Heart failure from diastolic dysfunction. *Dimensions of Critical Care Nursing, 15,* 170-177.

113. Dimengo, J.M. (1998). Surgical alternatives in the treatment of heart failure. *AACN Clinical Issues, 9*(2), 192-207.

REFERENCES

114. Hollenberg, S.M. & Parrillo, J.E. (1998). Shock. In A.S. Fauci et al. (Eds.). *Harrison's principles of internal medicine* (14th ed., vol. 1, pp. 214-222). St. Louis: Mosby.

115. Kilbourn, R.G., Traver, D.L., & Szabok, C. (1997). Nitric oxide and shock. *Disease-a-Month, 43*(5), 281-327.

116. Antman, E.M.K. & Braunwald, E. (1998). Acute myocardial infarction. In A.S. Fauci et al. (Eds.). *Harrison's principles of internal medicine* (14th ed., vol. 1, p. 1359). St. Louis: Mosby.

117. Berger, P.B. et al. (1997). Impact of an aggressive invasive catheterization and revascularization strategy on mortality in patients with cardiogenic shock in the global utilization of streptokinase and tissue plasminogen activator for occluded coronary arteries (GUSTO-I) trial. *Circulation, 96,* 122-127.

118. Barry, W.L. & Sarembock, I.J. (1998). Cardiogenic shock: Therapy and prevention. *Clinical Cardiology, 21,* 72-80.

119. Berger, P.B. et al. (1997). Impact of an aggressive invasive catheterization and revascularization strategy on mortality in patients with cardiogenic shock in the Global Utilization of Streptokinase and Tissue Plasminogen Activator for Occluded Coronary Arteries (GUSTO-I) trial. An observational study. *Circulation, 96,* 122-127.

120. Hollingsworth, H. (1997). Preventing insect sting anaphylaxis. *Journal of the American Medical Association, 277,* 1196-1197.

121. American College of Chest Physicians/Society of Critical Care Medicine Consensus Conference Committee. (1992). Definitions for sepsis and organ failure and guidelines for the use of innovative therapies in sepsis. *Critical Care Medicine, 20*(6), 864-874.

122. Baxter, F. (1997). Septic shock. *Canadian Anaesthetists Society Journal, 44*(1), 59-72.

123. Munford, R.S. (1998). Sepsis and septic shock. In A.S. Fauci et al. (Eds.). *Harrison's principles of internal medicine* (14th ed.). St. Louis: Mosby.

124. Abraham, E. (1997). Therapies for sepsis: Emerging therapies for sepsis and septic shock. *Western Journal of Medicine, 166,* 195-200.

125. Leibovici, L. et al. (1997). Septic shock in bacteremic patients: Risk factors, features, and prognosis. *Scandinavian Journal of Infectious Disease, 29,* 71-75.

126. Brampton, W.J. (1997). Septic shock: Current concepts. *British Journal of Hospital Medicine, 57*(40), 127-128.

127. Bone, R.C. (1997). Important new findings in sepsis. *Journal of the American Medical Association, 278*(3), 249.

128. Gando, S. et al. (1997). Participation of tissue factor and thrombin in posttraumatic systemic inflammatory syndrome. *Critical Care Medicine, 25*(11), 1820-1826.

129. Astiz, M.E. & Rackow, E.C. (1998). Septic shock. *Lancet, 351*(9114), 1501-1505.

130. Carcillo, J.A. & Cunnion, R.E. (1997). Septic shock. *Critical Care Clinics, 13*(3), 553-574.

131. Ognibene, F.P. (1997). Pathogenesis and innovative treatment of septic shock. *Advances in Internal Medicine, 42,* 313-338.

132. Baue, A.E. (1975). Multiple, progressive or sequential system failure: A syndrome for the '70s. *Archives of Surgery, 110*(7), 779.

133. Tilney, N.L., Bailey, G.L., & Morgan, A.P. (1973). Sequential system failure after rupture of abdominal aortic aneurysm: An unsolved problem in postoperative care. *Annals of Surgery, 178*(2), 117.

134. Bone, R.C. (1996). Immunologic dissonance: A continuing evolution in our understanding of the systemic inflammatory response syndrome (SIRS) and the multiple organ dysfunction syndrome (MODS). *Annals of Internal Medicine, 125*(8), 680-687.

135. Bone, R.C., Grodzin, C.J., & Balk, R.A. (1997). Sepsis: A new hypothesis for pathogenesis of the disease process. *Chest, 112*(1), 235-243.

136. Levine, J.H. et al. (1996). Multiple organ failure: Is it disappearing? *World Journal of Surgery, 20*(4), 471-473.

137. Swank, G.M. & Deitch, E.A. (1996). Role of the gut in multiple organ failure: Bacterial translocation and permeability changes. *World Journal of Surgery, 20*(4), 411-417.

138. Vincent, J.L. (1996). Prevention and therapy of multiple organ failure. *World Journal of Surgery, 20*(45), 465-470.

139. Grotz, M. et al. (1997). Rehabilitation results of patients with multiple injuries and multiple organ failure and long-term intensive care. *Journal of Trauma: Injury, Infection, and Critical Care, 42*(5), 919-926.

140. Kleinknecht, D. et al. (1996). Prognosis and mortality in patients with multiple organ system failure. *Renal Failure, 18*(3), 347-353.

141. Pastores, S.M., Katz, D.P., & Kvetan, V. (1996). Splanchnic ischemia and gut mucosal injury in sepsis and the multiple organ dysfunction syndrome. *American Journal of Gastroenterology, 91*(9), 1697-1710.

142. Bone, R.C. (1996). Toward a theory regarding the pathogenesis of the systemic inflammatory response syndrome: What we do and do not know about cytokine regulation. *Critical Care Medicine, 24*(1), 163-172.

143. Gullo, A. & Berlot, G. (1996). Ingredients of organ dysfunction or failure. *World Journal of Surgery, 20,* 40-36.

REFERENCES

144. Gawaz, M. et al. (1997). Platelet function in septic multiple organ dysfunction syndrome. *Intensive Care Medicine, 23,* 379-385.

145. Baue, A.E. (1997). Multiple organ failure, multiple organ dysfunction syndrome, and systemic inflammatory response syndrome: Why no magic bullets? *Archives of Surgery, 132*(7), 703-707.

146. Goris, R.J.A. (1996). MODS/SIRS: Result of an overwhelming inflammatory response? *World Journal of Surgery, 20,* 418-421.

147. Friedman, G. et al. (1998). Oxygen supply dependency can characterize septic shock. *Intensive Care Medicine, 24,* 118-123.

148. Aranow, J.S. & Fink, M.P. (1996). Determinants of intestinal barrier failure in critical illness. *British Journal of Anaesthesia, 77* (1), 71-81.

149. Kumar, A. (1997). Inotropes and gut mucosal perfusion: A brake on the motor of multiple organ failure? *Critical Care Medicine, 25*(8), 1266-1267.

CHAPTER

24

Alterations of Cardiovascular Function in Children

Jean Anne Connor and Kathryn L. McCance

Cardiovascular disorders in children are classified as congenital or acquired heart disease. Congenital heart disease is the most common. The diagnosis and management of congenital heart defects continue to improve with the use of fetal echocardiography and early interventional catheterization or surgical repair. Acquired heart defects in children continue to present challenges to the practitioner; although guidelines for diagnosing acquired defects are available, work is needed in developing standards of treatment and long-term follow-up.

CHAPTER OUTLINE

 Check out your CD Companion for chapter-related exercises and answers to the Quick Check questions

CONGENITAL HEART DISEASE

The incidence of *congenital heart disease (CHD)* varies from 4 to 8 per 1000 live births and is the major cause of death in the first year (other than prematurity). Several environmental and genetic risk factors are associated with the incidence of different types of CHD. Among the environmental factors are (1) maternal conditions, such as intrauterine viral infections (especially rubella), diabetes mellitus, phenylketonuria, alcoholism, hypercalcemia, drugs (e.g., thalidomide, lithium, phenytoin [Dilantin], dextroamphetamine), and complications of increased age; (2) antepartal bleeding; and (3) prematurity (Table 24-1).

Genetic factors also have been implicated in the incidence of CHD, although the mechanism of causation is often unknown (Table 24-2). The incidence of CHD is three to four times higher in siblings of affected children, and chromosomal defects account for about 6% of all cases of CHD. Down syndrome, trisomies 13 and 18, Turner syndrome, and cri du chat syndrome have been associated with a relatively high incidence of heart defects. Only a small percentage of cases of CHD are clearly linked solely to genetic or environmental factors. The cause of most defects is probably multifactorial.

Congenital heart defects can be described with respect to three principal areas:

1. *Anatomic defects* include valvular abnormalities; abnormal openings in the septa, including persistence of the foramen ovale; continued patency of the ductus arteriosus; and malformation or abnormal placement of the great vessels.

TABLE 24-1	Environmental Factors and Associated Congenital Heart Defects
Cause	**Type of Congenital Heart Defect**
Infection	
Intrauterine	Patent ductus arteriosus (PDA), pulmonary stenosis, coarctation of aorta
Systemic viral	PDA, pulmonary stenosis, coarctation of aorta
Rubella	PDA, pulmonary stenosis, coarctation of aorta
Coxsackie B5	Endocardial fibroelastosis
Radiation	Specific cardiovascular effect not known
Metabolic disorders	
Diabetes	Ventricular septal defect (VSD), cardiomegaly, transposition of the great vessels
Phenylketonuria (PKU)	Coarctation of aorta, PDA
Hypercalcemia	Supravalvular aortic stenosis, pulmonic stenosis; aortic hyperplasia
Drugs	
Thalidomide	No specific lesion
Dextroamphetamine	One case of reported transposition
Alcohol	Tetralogy of Fallot, atrial septal defect, VSD
Peripheral conditions	
Increased maternal age	VSD, tetralogy of Fallot (relationship unclear)
Antepartal bleeding	Various defects (relationship unclear)
Prematurity	PDA, VSD
High altitude	PDA, atrial septal defect (increased incidence)

TABLE 24-2	CHD in Selected Chromosomal Aberrations	
Conditions	**Incidence of CHD (%)**	**Common Defects in Decreasing Order of Frequency**
5p–(cri du chat syndrome)	25	VSD, PDA, ASD
Trisomy 13 syndrome	90	VSD, PDA, dextrocardia
Trisomy 18 syndrome	99	VSD, PDA, PS
Trisomy 21 (Down syndrome)	50	ECD, VSD
Turner syndrome (XO)	35	COA, AS, ASD
Klinefelter variant (XXXXY)	15	PDA, ASD

From Park, M.K. (1996). Pediatric cardiology for practitioners (3rd ed.). St. Louis: Mosby.
VSD, *Ventricular septal defect;* PDA, *patent ductus arteriosus;* ASD, *atrial septal defect;* PS, *pulmonary stenosis;* ECD, *endocardial cushion defect;* COA, *coarctation of the aorta;* AS, *aortic stenosis;* CHD, *congenital heart disease.*

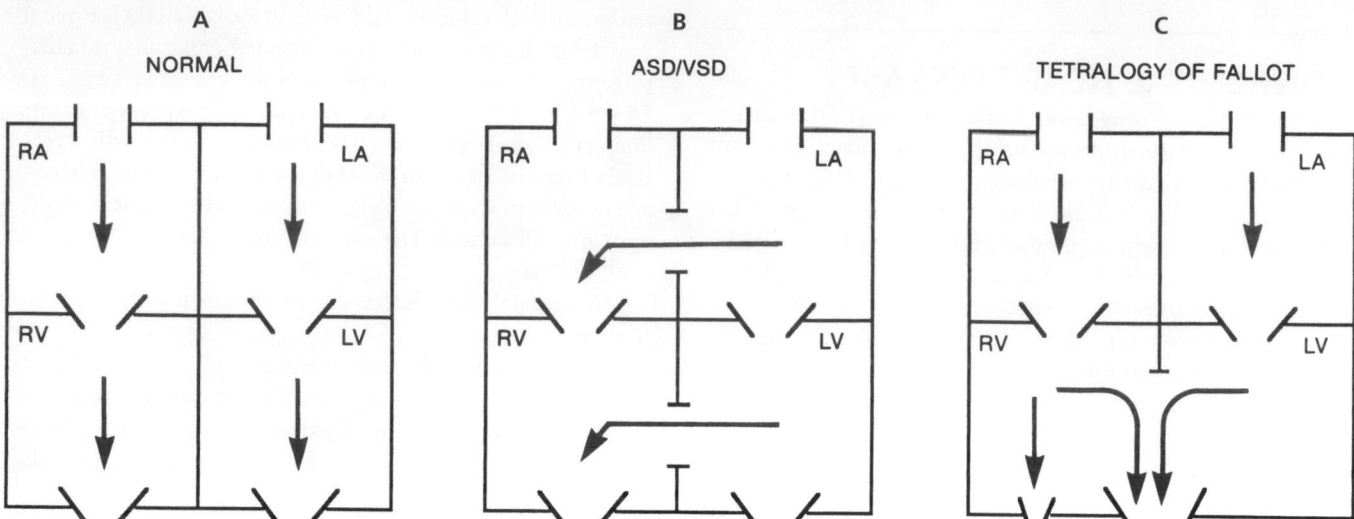

Fig. 24-1 *Shunting of blood in congenital heart disease.* **A,** Normal. **B,** Acyanotic defect. **C,** Cyanotic defect. *ASD,* Atrial septal defect; *VSD,* ventricular septal defect; *RA,* right atrium; *LA,* left atrium; *RV,* right ventricle; *LV,* left ventricle. *(From Wong, D.L. [1993].* Whaley & Wong's essentials of pediatric nursing *[4th ed.]. St. Louis: Mosby.)*

2. The *hemodynamic alterations* caused by these anatomic defects consist of (a) increases or decreases of blood flow through the pulmonary or systemic circulatory systems and (b) the mixing of pulmonary and systemic blood through an abnormal communication that permits flow between the two circulatory systems. The movement of blood between the normally separate pulmonary and systemic circulations is termed a **shunt.** Movement from the pulmonary to the systemic circulation (i.e., from the right heart to the left heart) is called a **right-to-left shunt.** Movement from the systemic to the pulmonary circulation (from the left heart to the right heart) is a **left-to-right shunt.** Shunt direction depends on relative pressures and resistances and can be obligatory or dependent. In an obligatory shunt, pressure gradients determine the direction of blood flow through an opening, whereas in a dependent shunt, vascular resistance or ventricular compliance determines the direction of flow.

3. The *status of tissue oxygenation* is gauged by the presence or absence of cyanosis. **Cyanosis** is a bluish discoloration of the skin indicating that the tissues are not receiving enough oxygen, a condition known as hypoxia. (See Chapter 26 for more discussion about cyanosis and hypoxia. Hypoxic injury to cells is described in Chapter 3.) Hypoxia may result from any disorder that prevents oxygen from reaching the body's cells. Ischemia, for example, is hypoxia from lack of blood flow. Congenital heart defects that cause hypoxia, and therefore cyanosis, involve a right-to-left shunt, which directs blood flow away from the lungs (Fig. 24-1). These defects are commonly called **cyanotic defects.** Congenital defects that do not cause cyanosis, or **acyanotic defects,** usually involve a left-to-right shunt, which directs blood toward the lungs, or no

shunt at all. Congenital heart defects can be categorized according to (a) whether they cause cyanosis, (b) whether they increase or decrease blood flow into the pulmonary circulation, and (c) shunt direction. Fig. 24-2 categorizes the congenital heart defects based on these three characteristics. A description of the most common defects follows.

Obstructive Defects
Coarctation of the aorta

Pathophysiology
Coarctation of the aorta *(COA)* is a localized narrowing near the insertion of the ductus arteriosus, resulting in increased pressure proximal to the defect (head and upper extremities) and decreased pressure distal to the obstruction (torso and lower extremities) (Fig. 24-3).

Clinical Manifestations
The location and severity of COA determine whether an infant will become symptomatic after the ductus arteriosus closes. If the COA is severe, infants will present with congestive heart failure (CHF; see p. 709), acidosis, and hypotension. Physical examination of the infant will reveal weak or absent femoral pulses with poor perfusion. A small percentage of infants with COA will remain asymptomatic after the closure of the ductus arteriosus. As they grow, older children with COA will present with unexplained hypertension. Children will usually complain of leg pain or cramping on exercise. They may also experience dizziness, headaches, fainting, or epistaxis from hypertension.[1]

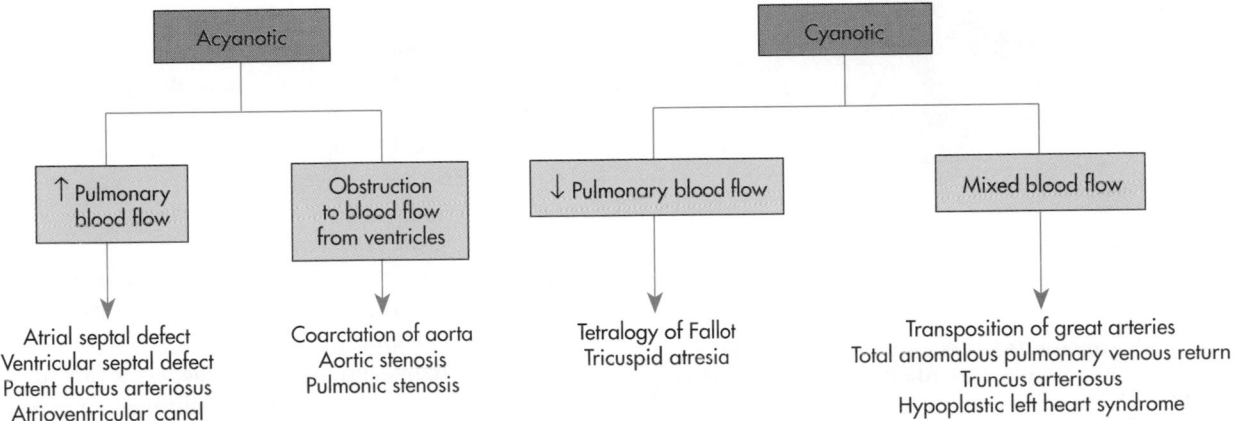

Fig. 24-2 *Comparison of acyanotic-cyanotic and hemodynamic classification systems of congenital heart disease.* *(From Wong, D.L. et al. [1999]. Whaley & Wong's nursing care of infants and children [6th ed.]. St. Louis: Mosby.)*

Fig. 24-3 *Coarctation of the aorta (COA) (postductal).* *(From Wong, D.L. et al. [1999]. Whaley & Wong's nursing care of infants and children [6th ed.]. St. Louis: Mosby.)*

Evaluation and Treatment

Physical examination and measure of upper and lower extremity blood pressure will often reveal diagnosis. Echocardiography, magnetic resonance imaging (MRI), and cardiac catheterization confirm the diagnosis. Initial treatment in the symptomatic newborn consists of continuous intravenous infusion of prostaglandin E to reopen the ductus arteriosus. Once the newborn is stabilized, surgical correction is initiated.

Surgical correction consists of either resection of the coarctated portion with an end-to-end anastomosis of the aorta or enlargement of the constricted section using a graft of prosthetic material or a portion of the left subclavian artery. Because this defect is outside the heart and pericardium, cardiopulmonary bypass is not required and a thoracotomy incision is used. Postoperative hypertension is treated with intravenous sodium nitroprusside followed by oral medications, such as captopril or hydralazine. Residual permanent hypertension after repair of COA seems to be related to age and time of repair. To prevent both hypertension at rest and exercise-provoked systemic hypertension after repair, elective surgery for COA is advised within the first 2 years of life. Multicenter studies have shown that percutaneous balloon angioplasty has been effective in reducing residual postoperative coarctation in 78% of children.[2]

Balloon angioplasty of COA as an initial intervention can and has been performed. Studies have shown that 60% to 70% of infants younger than 7 months of age have experienced recoarctation of the aorta in a short period of time. Other complications include aneurysm formation and injury to arterial access. Data exist that support balloon angioplasty as an effective therapy in infants older than 7 months of age with discrete membranous or hourglass constrictions. Data have also revealed a decreased risk of aneurysm formation in the older age-group.[2]

Aortic stenosis

Pathophysiology

Aortic stenosis (AS) is a narrowing or stricture of the aortic valve, causing resistance of blood flow from the left ventricle,

Fig. 24-4 *Aortic stenosis (AS). (From Wong, D.L. et al. [1999]. Whaley & Wong's nursing care of infants and children [6th ed.]. St. Louis: Mosby.)*

decreased cardiac output, left ventricular hypertrophy, and pulmonary vascular congestion (Fig. 24-4). The physiologic consequence of AS is the hypertrophy of the left ventricular wall, which eventually leads to increased end-diastolic pressure, resulting in pulmonary venous and pulmonary arterial hypertension. Left ventricular hypertrophy also interferes with coronary artery perfusion and may result in myocardial infarction or scarring of the papillary muscles of the left ventricle, causing mitral insufficiency. *Valvular stenosis* occurs as a result of malformed cusps resulting in a unicuspid or bicuspid valve rather than tricuspid valve or fusion of the cusps. *Subvalvular stenosis* is a stricture caused by a fibrous ring below a normal valve; supravalvular stenosis occurs infrequently. Valvular AS is a serious defect because (1) the obstruction tends to be progressive; (2) sudden episodes of myocardial ischemia, or low cardiac output, can result in sudden death; and (3) surgical repair will not result in a normal valve. This is one of the rare instances in which strenuous physical activity may be curtailed because of the cardiac condition.

Clinical Manifestations

Infants with severe defects demonstrate signs of decreased cardiac output with faint pulses, hypotension, tachycardia, and poor feeding. Children may also have complaints of exercise intolerance and chest pain. Children are at risk for bacterial endocarditis, coronary insufficiency, ventricular dysfunction, and sudden death.

Valvular aortic stenosis

Treatment

Treatment of valvular aortic stenosis varies, with nonsurgical palliation the initial treatment of choice by many interventional cardiologists. Dilation of the stenotic valve with balloon angioplasty in the cardiac catheterization laboratory

still carries a high morbidity and mortality in the critically ill neonate, but in some medical centers it compares favorably with surgical valvotomy.[3] Balloon angioplasty is, however, associated with risk of aortic regurgitation or insufficiency. Children undergoing this procedure almost always require surgical intervention at some time.

Surgical treatment for aortic valve stenosis depends on the severity of the stenosis, previous interventions, and age of the child. Aortic valve commissurotomy or closed aortic valvotomy may be used as an early intervention. Aortic valve replacement may be required if the valve is severely dysplastic. The Ross procedure, which involves moving the pulmonary valve into the aortic position and replacing it with a homograft (segments from a cadaver), has become an option. Data have shown that the pulmonary autograft has long-term durability, does not require anticoagulation, and remains uncompromised by host reactions.[2,3] Mortality for sick infants and children is between 15% and 20%. Mortality is much less for older children—approximately 1% to 2%.

Subvalvular aortic stenosis

Treatment

Surgical correction may involve incising a membrane if one exists or cutting the fibromuscular ring. If the obstruction results from narrowing of the left ventricular outflow tract and a small aortic valve annulus, a patch may be required to enlarge the entire left ventricular outflow tract and annulus and replace the aortic valve, an approach known as the *Konno procedure*. An aortic homograft (segments of cadaver aorta and pulmonary artery that are treated with antibiotics and cryopreserved) with a valve may also be used (extended aortic root replacement).

The mortality from surgical repair of subvalvular AS is less than 2%; however, about 10% of these individuals develop recurrent subaortic stenosis and require a second surgery.

Pulmonic stenosis

Pathophysiology

Pulmonic stenosis (PS) is a narrowing of the pulmonary valve at the entrance of the pulmonary artery (Fig. 24-5). Generally, a moderate to severe stenosis causes right ventricular hypertrophy. Higher pressures in the right atrium can create a right-to-left shunt across the foramen ovale. *Pulmonary atresia* is an extreme form of PS in that there is a total fusion of the commissures and blood cannot flow to the lungs. The right ventricle may be hypoplastic.

Clinical Manifestations

Most infants are asymptomatic if the stenosis is mild to moderate. Newborns with critical pulmonary stenosis will be cyanotic (from a right-to-left shunt through an ASD) and have signs and symptoms of CHF. Cardiomegaly and a decrease in pulmonary vascularity are often evident on chest x-ray.

Fig. 24-5 *A, Pulmonic stenosis (PS). B, Balloon angioplasty is used to dilate the valve.* A catheter is inserted across the stenotic pulmonic valve into the pulmonary artery, and a balloon at the end of the catheter is inflated and rapidly passed through the narrowed opening. *(From Wong, D.L. et al. [1999]. Whaley & Wong's nursing care of infants and children [6th ed.]. St. Louis: Mosby.)*

Treatment

Treatment of choice for infants with critical pulmonary stenosis is balloon angioplasty. A catheter with a special balloon device is used to dilate the area of narrowing.[2] In general, the mean systolic gradient can be reduced by 80% or more with a mortality of 0% to 6%, and surgical procedures may even be avoided in the membranous pulmonary atresia population.[3] The procedure is associated with few complications and has proved highly effective, with a 50% to 75% reduction in pressure gradient across the pulmonic valve and a low rate of complications.[4] Transventricular (closed) valvotomy (Brock) procedure is the surgical correction used in infants.

Both balloon dilation and surgical valvotomy leave the pulmonary valve incompetent because they involve opening the fused valve leaflets; however, children are usually able to tolerate pulmonary valve incompetence. Long-term problems with restenosis or valve incompetence may occur.

Defects With Increased Pulmonary Blood Flow
Patent ductus arteriosus

Pathophysiology

The pathogenesis of *patent ductus arteriosus (PDA)* is unknown. Because it is not known what causes the ductus arteriosus to close, it is difficult to pinpoint what causes it to remain open. The problem is failure of the fetal ductus arteriosus (artery connecting the aorta and pulmonary artery) to close within the first weeks of life (Fig. 24-6). The continued patency of this vessel allows blood to flow from the higher-pressure aorta to the lower-pressure pulmonary artery, causing a left-to-right shunt.

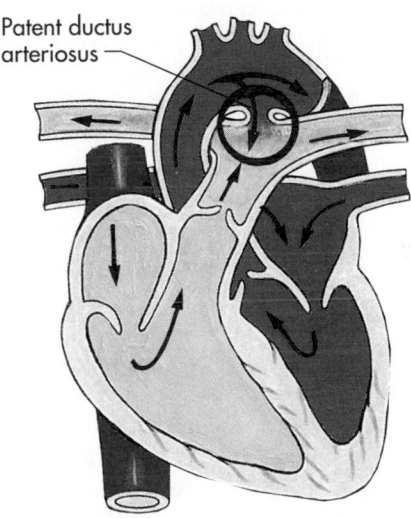

Fig. 24-6 *Patent ductus arteriosus (PDA).* *(From Wong, D.L. et al. [1999]. Whaley & Wong's nursing care of infants and children [6th ed.]. St. Louis: Mosby.)*

Clinical Manifestations

Infants may be asymptomatic or show signs of CHF. There is a characteristic machinery-like murmur. A widened pulse pressure and bounding pulses result from runoff of blood from the aorta to the pulmonary artery. Children are at risk for bacterial endocarditis and developing pulmonary hypertension in later life from chronic excessive pulmonary blood flow.

Treatment

Administration of indomethacin (a prostaglandin inhibitor) has proved successful in closing a patent ductus in premature infants and some newborns. Closure with placement of an occluder device during cardiac catheterization is done for some children. Surgical division or ligation of the patent vessel through a left thoracotomy may also be done. A new technique, visual assisted thoracoscopic surgery (VATS), uses a thoracoscope and instruments inserted through three small incisions on the left side of the chest to place a clip on the ductus. This procedure eliminates the need for a thoracotomy, thereby speeding postoperative recovery. Both surgical and nonsurgical procedures can be done at low risk, with less than 1% mortality.

Atrial septal defect

Pathophysiology

An *atrial septal defect (ASD)* is an abnormal opening in the septal wall between the two atria. This opening or communication allows blood to shunt from the higher pressure left atrium to the lower pressure right atrium. There are three types of ASDs. *Ostium primum* is an opening low in the atrial septum and may be associated with the mitral valve. *Ostium secundum* is an opening in the middle of the atrial septum and is the most common type. *Sinus venosus defect* is an opening high up in the atrial wall and may be associated with partial anomalous pulmonary venous connection.[5]

Clinical Manifestations

Children with an ASD are usually asymptomatic. Infants with a large ASD may develop CHF. Some children will experience shortness of breath with activity as they get older because extra blood shunts through the ASD into the right side of the heart and into the pulmonary circulation.

Evaluation and Treatment

Diagnosis can be confirmed by echocardiography. Repair of the defect is important. If left untreated, the child may be at risk for pulmonary hypertension, dysrhythmias, or stroke. Surgical repair involves open heart surgery with cardiopulmonary bypass. The opening is sutured closed with a Dacron patch or piece of the pericardium. Operative mortality is considered to be less than 1%. Nonsurgical intervention involves placement of a closure device performed in the cardiac catheterization laboratory.

Ventricular septal defect

Pathophysiology

A *ventricular septal defect (VSD)* is an abnormal opening of the septal wall between the ventricles. VSDs are similar to ASDs in that blood will shunt from left to right. VSDs are the most common type of congenital heart defect. VSDs are classified by the location of the opening along the septum. Premembranous VSDs, the most common type, are located high in the septal wall of the ventricle. Muscular VSDs are located low in the septal wall. VSDs can also be located in the inlet or outlet portion of the ventricle. Depending on the size and location, VSDs can spontaneously close, most often within the first 2 years of life.

Clinical Manifestations

Depending on the size, location, and degree of pulmonary vascular resistance, children may have congestive heart failure (CHF). It is important to assess for signs or symptoms of CHF or failure to thrive. If the degree of shunting is significant, the child is at risk for developing pulmonary hypertension. If shunting is left untreated, irreversible pulmonary hypertension may develop, leading to Eisenmenger syndrome, in which shunting of blood is reversed because of high pulmonary pressure.

Evaluation and Treatment

Diagnosis is confirmed by echocardiogram. Cardiac catheterization may be needed to calculate the degree of right-to-left shuting. Depending on the size of the VSD and the degree of symptoms, management may be minimal, allowing the VSD to close completely or to become small enough that surgical closure is not required. If the infant has severe CHF or failure-to-thrive that is unmanageable with medical measures, early surgical repair is performed.

Surgical repair involves open heart surgery with cardiopulmonary bypass. The opening is sutured closed with a Dacron patch. Mortality is considered low for this procedure. Nonsurgical intervention is not available at this time although devices have been developed for the muscular type of VSD occlusion.

Atrioventricular canal defect

Pathophysiology

Atrioventricular canal (AVC) defect is the incomplete fusion of endocardial cushions (Fig. 24-7). It consists of a low atrial septal defect that is continuous with a high ventricular septal defect and clefts of the mitral and tricuspid valves, cre-

Atrioventricular canal defect

Fig. 24-7 *Atrioventricular canal (AVC) defect. (From Wong, D.L. et al. [1999].* Whaley & Wong's nursing care of infants and children *[6th ed.]. St. Louis: Mosby.)*

ating a large central atrioventricular (AV) valve that allows blood to flow between all four chambers of the heart. The directions and pathways of flow are determined by pulmonary and systemic resistance, left and right ventricular pressures, and the compliance of each chamber, although flow is generally from left to right. It is the most common cardiac defect in children with Down syndrome.

Clinical Manifestations

Infants will often display moderate to severe heart failure. Some infants with pulmonary hypertension have minimal signs of CHF. There may be mild cyanosis that increases with crying. Children with AVC defects are at risk for developing irreversible pulmonary hypertension if left surgically untreated.

Treatment

Initial treatment goals include aggressive medical management of CHF. Infants are followed closely for signs or symptoms of failure-to-thrive. Complete surgical repair is performed between 6 to 12 months of age to prevent irreversible pulmonary hypertension. This procedure consists of patch closure of the septal defects and reconstruction of the AV valve tissue (either repair of the mitral valve cleft or fashioning two AV valves). If the mitral valve defect is severe, a valve replacement may be needed. Postoperative complications include heart block, CHF, mitral regurgitation, dysrhythmias, and pulmonary hypertension. Operative mortality is about 10%. A potential problem following repair is mitral regurgitation, which may later require valve replacement.

Defects With Decreased Pulmonary Blood Flow[5]
Tetralogy of Fallot

Pathophysiology

The classic form of **tetralogy of Fallot (TOF)** includes four defects: (1) ventricular septal defect, (2) pulmonic stenosis, (3) overriding aorta, and (4) right ventricular hypertrophy (Fig. 24-8). The pathophysiology varies widely, depending not only on the degree of pulmonary stenosis, but also on the size of the VSD and the pulmonary and systemic resistance to flow. If pulmonary vascular resistance is higher than systemic resistance, the shunt is from right to left. If systemic resistance is higher than pulmonary resistance, the shunt is from left to right. Stenosis decreases blood flow to the lungs and, consequently, the amount of oxygenated blood that returns to the left heart. The body attempts to compensate for hypoxia by producing more red blood cells and by increasing blood flow to the lungs through collateral bronchial vessels.

Clinical Manifestations

Some infants may be acutely cyanotic at birth; others have mild cyanosis that progresses over the first year of life as the pulmonic stenosis worsens. Acute episodes of cyanosis and hypoxia occur, called *blue spells* or *tet spells*. Anoxic spells oc-

cur when the infant's oxygen requirements exceed the blood supply, usually during crying or after feeding.

Increasing cyanosis may cause clubbing of the fingers, squatting, and poor growth in children. Children are at risk for emboli, cerebrovascular disease, brain abscess, seizures, and loss of consciousness or sudden death following an anoxic spell.

Treatment

In infants who cannot undergo primary repair, a palliative procedure to increase pulmonary blood flow and increase oxygen saturation may be performed. The preferred procedure is the *Blalock-Taussig* or *modified Blalock-Taussig shunt*, which provides blood flow to the pulmonary arteries from the left or right subclavian artery.

Elective surgical repair is usually performed in the first year of life. Indications for repair include increasing cyanosis and the development of hypercyanotic spells. Complete repair involves closure of the VSD and resection of the infundibular stenosis, with a pericardial patch to enlarge the right ventricular outflow tract. The procedure requires a median sternotomy and the use of cardiopulmonary bypass.

Operative mortality for total correction of TOF is less than 5%. With improved surgical techniques there is a lower incidence of dysrhythmias and sudden death. Surgical heart block is rare.

Tricuspid atresia

Pathophysiology

Tricuspid atresia is failure of the tricuspid valve to develop; consequently no communication occurs from right atrium to right ventricle (Fig. 24-9). Blood flows through an atrial

Fig. 24-8 *Tetralogy of Fallot (TOF). (From Wong, D.L. et al. [1999]. Whaley & Wong's nursing care of infants and children [6th ed.]. St. Louis: Mosby.)*

Fig. 24-9 *Tricuspid atresia. (From Wong, D.L. et al. [1999]. Whaley & Wong's nursing care of infants and children [6th ed.]. St. Louis: Mosby.)*

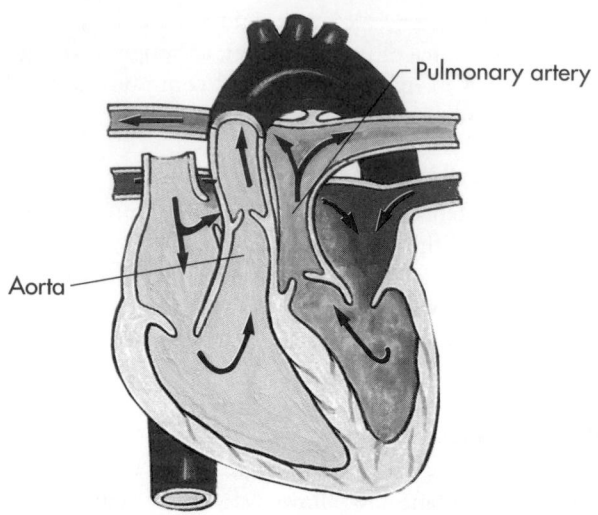

Fig. 24-10 *Transposition of the great arteries (TGA) or transposition of the great vessels (TGV). (From Wong, D.L. et al. [1999]. Whaley & Wong's nursing care of infants and children [6th ed.]. St. Louis: Mosby.)*

septal defect or a patent foramen ovale to the left side of the heart and through a ventricular septal defect to the right ventricle and out to the lungs. It is often associated with pulmonic stenosis and transposition of the great arteries. There is complete mixing of unoxygenated and oxygenated blood in the left side of the heart, resulting in systemic desaturation and varying amounts of pulmonary obstruction, causing decreased pulmonary blood flow.

Clinical Manifestations

Cyanosis is usually seen in the newborn period. Tachycardia, dyspnea, fatigue, and poor feeding may be noted. Older children have signs of chronic hypoxemia with clubbing. Children are at risk for bacterial endocarditis, brain abscess, and stroke.

Treatment

For the neonate whose pulmonary blood flow depends on the patency of the ductus arteriosus, a continuous infusion of prostaglandin E is started at 0.05 mg/kg/min until surgical intervention can be arranged. If the ASD is small, an atrial septostomy is done during cardiac catheterization. Palliative treatment is accomplished in staged procedures. Once the infant is stabilized, a shunt is placed (pulmonary-to-systemic artery anastomosis) to increase blood flow to the lungs. Some children have increased pulmonary blood flow and require pulmonary artery banding to lessen the volume of blood to the lungs.

Further palliative surgery is undertaken between 6 months and 2 years of age, depending on the child's growth and degree of cyanosis. The repair consists of the *modified Fontan procedure,* in which systemic venous return is di-

rected to the lungs without a ventricular pump through surgical connections between the right atrium and the pulmonary artery. A fenestration (opening) in the right atrial baffle is sometimes done to relieve pressure. The patient must have normal ventricular function and a low pulmonary vascular resistance for the procedure to be successful. The modified Fontan procedure separates oxygenated and unoxygenated blood inside the heart and eliminates the excess volume load on the ventricle but does not restore normal anatomy or hemodynamics.

Surgical mortality is more than 10%. Postoperative complications include dysrhythmias, systemic venous hypertension, thrombosis, pleural and pericardial effusions, elevated pulmonary vascular resistance, and ventricular dysfunction. Since the inception of the modified Fontan procedure, variations have been performed to decrease the occurrence of postoperative complications. Long-term follow-up results on survival and morbidity in children who have undergone these variations of the modified Fontan are pending.[6]

Mixed Defects[5]
Transposition of the great arteries or transposition of the great vessels

Pathophysiology

In *transposition of the great arteries (TGA)* or *transposition of the great vessels (TGV),* the pulmonary artery leaves the left ventricle and the aorta exits from the right ventricle, with no communication between the systemic and pulmonary circulations (Fig. 24-10). Associated defects, such as septal defects or patent ductus arteriosus, permit blood to enter the systemic circulation and/or the pulmonary circulation for mixing of saturated and desaturated blood. However, transposition can also produce high pulmonary blood flow under high pressure, which can result in elevated pulmonary vascular resistance.

Clinical Manifestations

Clinical manifestations depend on the type and size of the associated defects. Children with minimum communication are severely cyanotic, acidotic, and depressed at birth. Those with large septal defects or a patent ductus arteriosus may be less severely cyanotic but may have symptoms of CHF. Heart sounds vary according to the type of defect present. Cardiomegaly is usually evident a few weeks after birth.

Treatment

To provide intracardiac mixing, the administration of intravenous prostaglandin E_1 may be initiated to temporarily increase blood mixing if systemic and pulmonary mixing is inadequate to provide an oxygen saturation of 75% or to maintain cardiac output. During cardiac catheterization a balloon atrial septostomy (*Rashkind procedure*) may also be performed to increase mixing and maintain cardiac output over a longer period.

There are three types of corrective surgical repair for TGA or TGV. The most preferred type, performed in the first weeks of life, is the *arterial switch procedure*. It involves transecting the great arteries and anastomosing the main pulmonary artery to the proximal aorta (just above the aortic valve) and anastomosing the ascending aorta to the proximal pulmonary artery. The coronary arteries are switched from the proximal aorta to the proximal pulmonary artery, creating a new aorta. Reimplantation of the coronary arteries is critical to the infant's survival, and the arteries must be reattached without torsion or kinking to provide the heart with its supply of oxygen. The advantage of the arterial switch procedure is the reestablishment of normal circulation with the left ventricle acting as the systemic pump. Potential complications of the arterial switch include narrowing at the great artery anastomosis or coronary artery insufficiency.

A second type of surgical repair, performed in the first year of life, is the creation of an intraarterial baffle to divert venous blood to the mitral valve and pulmonary venous blood to the tricuspid valve using the individual's atrial septum (*Senning procedure*) or a prosthetic material (*Mustard procedure*). A disadvantage is the continuing role of the right ventricle as the systemic pump and the late development of right ventricular failure and rhythm disturbances. Other potential postoperative complications include loss of normal sinus rhythm, baffle leaks, ventricular dysfunction, and sudden death.

A third type of surgical repair, for infants with TGA, VSD, and severe pulmonic stenosis, is the *Rastelli procedure*. It involves closure of the VSD with a baffle, directing left ventricular blood through the VSD into the aorta. The pulmonic valve is then closed, and a conduit is placed from the right ventricle to the pulmonary artery, creating a physiolog-

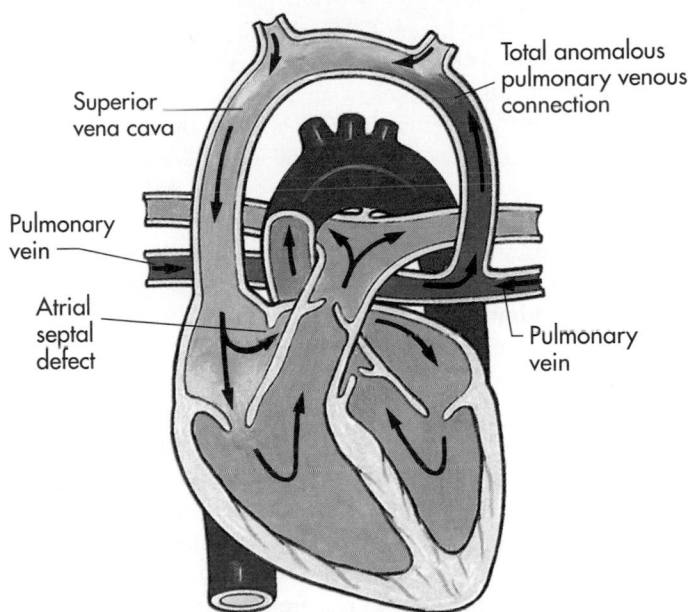

Fig. 24-11 *Total anomalous pulmonary venous connection (TAPVC).* (From Wong, D.L. et al. [1999]. Whaley & Wong's nursing care of infants and children [6th ed.]. St. Louis: Mosby.)

ically normal circulation. It is unfortunate that this procedure requires multiple conduit replacements as the child grows.

Operative mortality is about 5% to 10% with all procedures. With atrial level repairs there is later risk of dysrhythmias, ventricular dysfunction, and sudden death.

Long-term results for the arterial switch operation remain good. Two-staged arterial switch operations can also be done in children who are seen late or in whom right ventricular failure develops. Follow-up results in older children are still needed.[7]

Total anomalous pulmonary venous connection

Pathophysiology

Total anomalous pulmonary venous connection (TAPVC) is a rare defect characterized by failure of the pulmonary veins to join the left atrium. TAPVC is also called *total anomalous pulmonary venous return (TAPVR)* or *total anomalous pulmonary venous drainage (TAPVD)* (Fig. 24-11). The pulmonary veins are abnormally connected to the systemic venous circuit through the right atrium or various veins draining toward the right atrium, such as the superior vena cava. The abnormal attachment results in mixed blood being returned to the right atrium and shunted from the right to the left through an ASD. The type of TAPVC is classified according to the pulmonary venous point of attachment:
- *Supracardiac:* attachment above the diaphragm, such as to the superior vena cava (most common form)
- *Cardiac:* direct attachment to the heart, such as to the right atrium or coronary sinus

• *Infracardiac:* attachment below the diaphragm, such as to the inferior vena cava (most severe form)

The right atrium receives all the blood that normally would flow into the left atrium. As a result, the right side of the heart hypertrophies, whereas the left side, especially the left atrium, may remain small. An associated ASD or patent foramen ovale allows systemic venous blood to shunt from the higher-pressure right atrium to the left atrium and into the left side of the heart. As a result, the oxygen saturation of the blood in both sides of the heart (and ultimately, in the systemic arterial circulation) is the same. If the pulmonary blood flow is large, pulmonary venous return is also large and the amount of saturated blood is relatively high. However, if there is obstruction to pulmonary venous drainage, pulmonary venous return is impeded, pulmonary venous pressure rises, and pulmonary interstitial edema develops and eventually contributes to left heart failure. Infracardiac TAPVC often is associated with obstruction of pulmonary venous drainage and is a surgical emergency.

Fig. 24-12 *Truncus arteriosus (TA). (From Wong, D.L. et al. [1999]. Whaley & Wong's nursing care of infants and children [6th ed.]. St. Louis: Mosby.)*

Clinical Manifestations

Most infants develop cyanosis early in life. The degree of cyanosis is inversely related to the amount of pulmonary blood flow; the more pulmonary blood, the less cyanosis. Children with unobstructed TAPVC may be asymptomatic until pulmonary vascular resistance decreases during infancy, increasing pulmonary blood flow, with resulting signs of left heart failure. Cyanosis becomes worse with pulmonary vein obstruction; once obstruction occurs, the infant's condition usually deteriorates rapidly. Without intervention, cardiac failure will progress to death.

Treatment

Corrective repair is required in early infancy. The surgical approach varies with the anatomic defect. In general, however, the common pulmonary vein is anastomosed to the left atrium, the ASD is closed, and the anomalous pulmonary venous connection is ligated. The cardiac type is most easily repaired; the infracardiac type has the highest morbidity and mortality because of the higher incidence of pulmonary vein obstruction. Potential postoperative complications include reobstruction, bleeding, dysrhythmias (particularly heart block), pulmonary artery hypertension, and persistent heart failure.

The cardiac type of TAPVC has a surgical mortality of less than 5%. The incidence of morbidity is greater with the other types and increases with the presence of pulmonary vein obstruction.

Truncus arteriosus

Pathophysiology

Truncus arteriosus (TA) is failure of normal septation and division of the embryonic bulbar trunk into the pulmonary artery and the aorta, resulting in a single vessel that overrides both ventricles (Fig. 24-12). Blood from both ventricles mixes in the common great artery, causing desaturation and

hypoxemia. Blood ejected from the heart flows preferentially to the lower-pressure pulmonary arteries, causing increased pulmonary blood flow and reduced systemic blood flow. The three types are as follows:

• *Type I:* a single pulmonary trunk arises near the base of the truncus and divides into the left and right pulmonary arteries.
• *Type II:* the left and right pulmonary arteries arise separately from the posterior aspect of the truncus.
• *Type III:* the pulmonary arteries arise independently and from the lateral aspect of the truncus.

Clinical Manifestations

Most infants are asymptomatic with moderate to severe left heart failure and variable cyanosis, poor growth, and activity intolerance. Children are at risk for brain abscess and bacterial endocarditis.

Treatment

Corrective repair is a modification of the Rastelli procedure and is performed in the first few months of life. It involves closing the VSD so that the truncus arteriosus receives the outflow from the left ventricle, excising the pulmonary arteries from the aorta and attaching them to the right ventricle by means of a homograft. Currently, homografts are preferred over synthetic conduits to establish continuity between the right ventricle and pulmonary artery. Homografts are more flexible and easier to use during the procedure and appear less prone to obstruction. Postoperative complications include persistent heart failure, bleeding, pulmonary artery hypertension, dysrhythmias, and residual VSD. These children require additional procedures to replace the conduit as its size becomes inadequate in relation to growth. Mortality is more than 10%.

Fig. 24-13 *Hypoplastic left heart syndrome (HLHS). (From Wong, D.L. et al. [1999]. Whaley & Wong's nursing care of infants and children [6th ed.]. St. Louis: Mosby.)*

Hypoplastic left heart syndrome

Pathophysiology
Hypoplastic left heart syndrome (HLHS) is underdevelopment of the left side of the heart, resulting in a hypoplastic left ventricle and aortic atresia (Fig. 24-13). Most blood from the left atrium flows across the patent foramen ovale to the right atrium, to the right ventricle, and out the pulmonary artery. The descending aorta receives blood from the patent ductus arteriosus supplying systemic blood flow.

Clinical Manifestations
There is mild cyanosis and signs of left failure until the patent ductus arteriosus closes, and then there is progressive deterioration with cyanosis and decreased cardiac output, leading to cardiovascular collapse. It is usually fatal in the first months of life without intervention.

Treatment
A several-stage repair approach is used. The first stage is the *Norwood procedure,* which is anastomosis of the main pulmonary artery to the aorta to create a new aorta, shunting to provide pulmonary blood flow, and creation of a large atrial septal defect. Postoperative complications include imbalance of systemic and pulmonary blood flow, bleeding, low cardiac output, and persistent heart failure. The second stage is often a *bidirectional Glenn shunt* done at 6 to 9 months of age to relieve cyanosis and reduce the volume load on the right ventricle. The final repair is a *modified Fontan procedure.* Some believe that heart transplantation in the newborn period is the best option for these infants. Problems of neonatal transplantation include the shortage of newborn organ donors, risk of rejection, long-term problems with chronic immunosuppression, and infection.

Mortality risks are more than 25% with both surgery and transplantation. Surgical mortality for all three stages approaches 50%. Long-term (>10 year) outcome from both procedures remains uncertain.[8] Because of the high-risk nature of both surgical palliation and neonatal heart transplantation, some cardiologists continue to recommend no treatment for this defect.

Congestive Heart Failure
Congestive heart failure (CHF), classified as an acquired condition, is a common complication of many congenital heart defects. CHF occurs when the heart is unable to maintain sufficient cardiac output to meet the metabolic demands of the body. The most common causes of CHF in infancy are pressure and volume overloads secondary to congenital heart disease. (Table 24-3 lists by age the congenital heart defects that cause CHF.) Generally, 90% of children who develop CHF do so within the first 6 to 12 months of life.

In general, the pathophysiologic mechanisms of CHF in infants and children are very similar to those in adults. The same compensatory mechanisms are activated in the face of inadequate cardiac output (see Fig. 23-35).

TABLE 24-3	Causes of Congestive Heart Failure Resulting From Congenital Heart Disease
Age of Onset	**Cause**
At birth	HLHS
	Volume overload lesions
	Severe tricuspid or pulmonary insufficiency
	Large systemic AV fistula
First week	TGA
	PDA in small premature infants
	HLHS (with more favorable anatomy)
	TAPVR, particularly those with pulmonary venous obstruction
	Others
	Systemic AV fistula
	Critical AS or PS
1-4 wk	COA with associated anomalies
	Critical AS
	Large left-to-right shunt lesions (VSD, PDA) in premature infants
	All other lesions previously listed
4-6 wk	Some left-to-right shunt lesions, such as ECD
6 wk-4 mo	Large VSD
	Large PDA
	Others, such as anomalous left coronary artery from the PA

From Park, M.K. (1996). Pediatric cardiology for practitioners (3rd ed.). St. Louis: Mosby.
HLHS, *Hypoplastic left heart syndrome;* AV, *atrioventricular;* TGA, *transposition of great arteries;* PDA, *patent ductus arteriosus;* TAPVR, *total anomalous pulmonary venous return;* AS, *aortic stenosis;* PS, *pulmonic stenosis;* COA, *coarctation of the aorta;* VSD, *ventricular septal defect;* ECD, *endocardial cushion defect;* PA, *pulmonary artery.*

Clinical Manifestations of Congestive Heart Failure   BOX 24-1

IMPAIRED MYOCARDIAL FUNCTION	PULMONARY CONGESTION	SYSTEMIC VENOUS CONGESTION
Tachycardia	Tachypnea	Weight gain
Sweating (inappropriate)	Dyspnea	Hepatomegaly
Decreased urinary output	Retractions (infants)	Peripheral edema, especially peri-orbital
Fatigue	Flaring nares	Ascites
Weakness	Exercise intolerance	Neck vein distention (children)
Restlessness	Orthopnea	
Anorexia	Cough, hoarseness	
Pale, cool extremities	Cyanosis	
Weak peripheral pulses	Wheezing	
Decreased blood pressure	Grunting	
Gallop rhythm		
Cardiomegaly		

From Wong, D.L., et al. (1999). Whaley & Wong's nursing care of infants and children (6th ed.). St. Louis: Mosby.

Although CHF in children has many causes, it is often difficult to determine right or left ventricular failure. When assessing a child with CHF, a combination of symptoms generally is present. Usually, both ventricles are involved by the time signs and symptoms are apparent.[5]

Left heart failure in infants is manifested as poor feeding and sucking, often leading to failure to thrive. In left heart failure, dyspnea, tachypnea, and diaphoresis may be accompanied by retractions, grunting, nasal flaring, wheezing, coughing, and rales.[1] Common skin changes, such as pallor or mottling, are often present.

Hepatomegaly (enlargement of the liver) is typically attributable to systemic venous congestion caused by right ventricular failure. In infants, the normal liver is sharp-edged and palpable 1 to 2 cm below the costal margin. However, the absence of hepatomegaly does not rule out CHF.[1]

Puffy eyelids, periorbital edema, and weight gain without caloric increase are common manifestations of right ventricular failure in infants. Peripheral edema, which is a common finding in adults, is usually more difficult to detect in infants and young children.[1] The clinical manifestations of CHF are given in Box 24-1.

A thorough physical examination with emphasis on cardiac and pulmonary findings will often reveal the degree of CHF. Plotting the child's growth (height, weight, head circumference) is an important method of assessing failure-to-thrive. An electrocardiogram (ECG) should also be performed to determine the presence of dysrhythmias or hypertrophy. A chest x-ray is useful in assessing the presence of cardiomegaly and signs of increased pulmonary circulation.

Treatment is aimed at decreasing cardiac work load and increasing the efficiency of the heart. Medical management initially consists of diuretics, such as furosemide. Depending on the degree of CHF, other diuretics can be used in combination with furosemide to counteract potassium losses. Medications, such as digoxin (Lanoxin), an inotropic agent, are also used to increase myocardial contractility. Afterload reducers have recently been employed to further manage severe CHF.[1,9]

ACQUIRED CARDIOVASCULAR DISORDERS

Acquired heart diseases refer to disease processes or abnormalities that occur after birth. They result from various causes, such as infection, genetic disorders, autoimmune processes in response to infection, environmental factors, or autoimmune diseases. Examples of acquired heart diseases include Kawasaki disease, myocarditis, rheumatic heart disease, cardiomyopathy, and systemic hypertension. This chapter discusses Kawasaki disease and systemic hypertension. Myocarditis, rheumatic heart disease, and cardiomyopathy are discussed in Chapter 23.

Kawasaki Disease

Kawasaki disease, otherwise known as mucocutaneous lymph node syndrome, is an acute, self-limiting systemic vasculitis that may result in cardiac sequelae. It was first identified in 1967 by Dr. Tomisaku Kawasaki. Although Kawasaki disease occurs throughout the world, the greatest number of cases are seen in Japan.[10,11]

Kawasaki disease is primarily a condition of young children. Eighty percent of cases are seen in children younger than 5 years of age, with the incidence peaking in the toddler age-group. Males are affected slightly more than females. Its peak incidence is in the winter and spring.[1,12]

The etiology of Kawasaki disease remains unknown. Current etiologic theories center on an immunologic response to an infectious, toxic, or antigenic substance (including superantigen).[1,12]

 Pathophysiology

Kawasaki disease progresses pathologically and clinically in the following stages:

- *Stage I (day 0-12):* small capillaries, arterioles, and venules become inflamed, as does the heart itself.
- *Stage II (day 12-25):* inflammation spreads to larger vessels, and aneurysms of the coronary arteries develop.
- *Stage III (day 26-40):* medium-sized arteries begin the granulation process, causing coronary artery thickening; inflammation results in the microcirculation, and there is increased formation of thrombi.
- *Stage IV (day 40 and beyond):* vessels develop scarring, intimal thickening, calcification, and stenosis of coronary arteries.

Clinical Manifestations

The clinical course of the disease progresses in three stages: acute, subacute, and convalescent. In the acute phase, the child has fever, conjunctivitis, oral changes ("strawberry" tongue), rash, and lymphadenopathy and is often irritable. During this phase, myocarditis may develop. The subacute phase begins when the fever ends and continues until the clinical signs have resolved. It is at this time that the child is most at risk for coronary artery aneurysm development. Desquamation of the palms and soles occurs at this time, as well as marked thrombocytosis. The convalescent phase is marked by the continued elevation of the erythrocyte sedimentation rate and platelet count.[1,12] Arthritis still may be present. This phase continues until all laboratory values return to normal—usually about 6 to 8 weeks after onset.[1,5]

Evaluation and Treatment

The diagnosis is based on the diagnostic criteria for Kawasaki disease, which state that the child must exhibit five of six criteria, including fever (Box 24-2). These children usually have leukocytosis, increased erythrocyte sedimentation rates, marked thrombocytosis, and elevated liver enzymes. An echocardiogram is obtained at the time of diag-

---

Diagnostic Criteria for Kawasaki Disease BOX 24-2

The child must exhibit five of the following six criteria, including fever:
1. Fever for 5 or more days (often diagnosed with shorter duration of fever if other symptoms are present)
2. Bilateral conjunctival infection without exudation
3. Changes in the oral mucous membranes, such as erythema, dryness, and fissuring of the lips; oropharyngeal reddening; or "strawberry tongue"
4. Changes in the extremities, such as peripheral edema, peripheral erythema, and desquamation of palms and soles, particularly periungual peeling
5. Polymorphous rash, often accentuated in the perineal area
6. Cervical lymphadenopathy

Modified from Wong, D.L. et al. (1999). Whaley & Wong's nursing care of infants and children (6th ed.). St. Louis: Mosby.

Conditions Associated With Secondary Hypertension in Children

BOX 24-3

RENAL DISORDERS
Congenital defects
  Polycystic kidney, ectopic kidney, horseshoe kidney, etc.
  Obstructive anomalies
  Hydronephrosis
Renal tumor
  Wilms tumor
  Retrovascular
Abnormalities of renal arteries
Renal vein thrombosis
Acquired disorders
  Glomerulonephritis—acute or chronic
  Pyelonephritis
  Nephritis associated with collagen disease

CARDIOVASCULAR DISEASE
Coarctation of aorta
Arteriovenous fistulae
Patent ductus arteriosus
Aortic or mitral insufficiency

METABOLIC AND ENDOCRINE DISEASES
Adrenal tumors
  Adenoma
  Phenochromocytoma
  Neuroblastoma

Cushing syndrome
Adrenogenital syndrome
Hyperthyroidism
Aldosteronism
Hypercalcemia
Diabetes mellitus

NEUROLOGIC DISORDERS
Space-occupying lesions of cranium (increased intracranial pressure)
  Tumors, cysts, hematoma
  Cerebral edema
  Encephalitis (including Guillain-Barré and Reye syndromes)

MISCELLANEOUS CAUSES
Drugs (corticosteroids, oral contraceptives, pressor agents, amphetamines)
Burns
Genitourinary surgery
Trauma (e.g., stretching of femoral nerve with leg traction)
Insect bites (e.g., scorpion)
Intravascular overload (blood, fluid)
Hypernatremia
Toxemia of pregnancy
Heavy metal poisoning

From Wong D.L. et al. (1999). Whaley & Wong's nursing care of infants and children *(6th ed.). St. Louis: Mosby.*

nosis as a baseline to assess for coronary aneurysms or inflammation. Serial echocardiograms are obtained after treatment to assess for future development of coronary aneurysms.

The use of high-dose aspirin and intravenous immunoglobulin during the acute phase has decreased the morbidity of Kawasaki disease and has reduced the incidence of coronary abnormalities from approximately 25% to less than 65% at 6 to 8 weeks after initiation of therapy.[11,12] Most children recover completely from Kawasaki disease, including regression of aneurysms. The most common cardiovascular sequela is coronary thrombosis. Current studies are investigating long-term results of the disease.[13]

Systemic Hypertension

Hypertension (HTN) in children differs from adult hypertension in etiology and presentation. Children, when diagnosed with HTN, are often found to have some underlying disease, such as renal disease or coarctation of the aorta (Box 24-3). In recent years an increased prevalence of primary HTN in older children has been noted. Researchers are now focusing on primary HTN in older children in relation to morbidity and mortality and the presence of early atherosclerotic disease.[1,14]

Systemic hypertension in children is defined as systolic and diastolic blood pressure levels greater than the 95th percentile for age and gender on at least three occasions.[1,14] The Second Task Force on Blood Pressure Control in Children has added height as an additional criterion to the blood pressure guidelines.[15,16]

 Pathophysiology

Hypertension is classified into two categories: primary, or essential, hypertension, in which a specific cause cannot be identified; and secondary hypertension, in which a cause can be identified (see Box 24-3).[1] In infants and children a cause of HTN is almost always found. In general, the younger the child with significant hypertension, the more likely a correctable cause can be found. Therefore a thorough evaluation needs to be done.[17]

The pathophysiology of primary HTN in children is not clearly understood but may result from a complex interaction of a strong predisposing genetic component with disturbances in sympathetic vascular smooth muscle tone, humoral agents (angiotensin, catecholamines), renal sodium excretion, and cardiac output (Fig. 24-14). Ultimately these factors impair the ability of the peripheral vascular bed to adjust its own resistance to meet tissue perfusion needs.

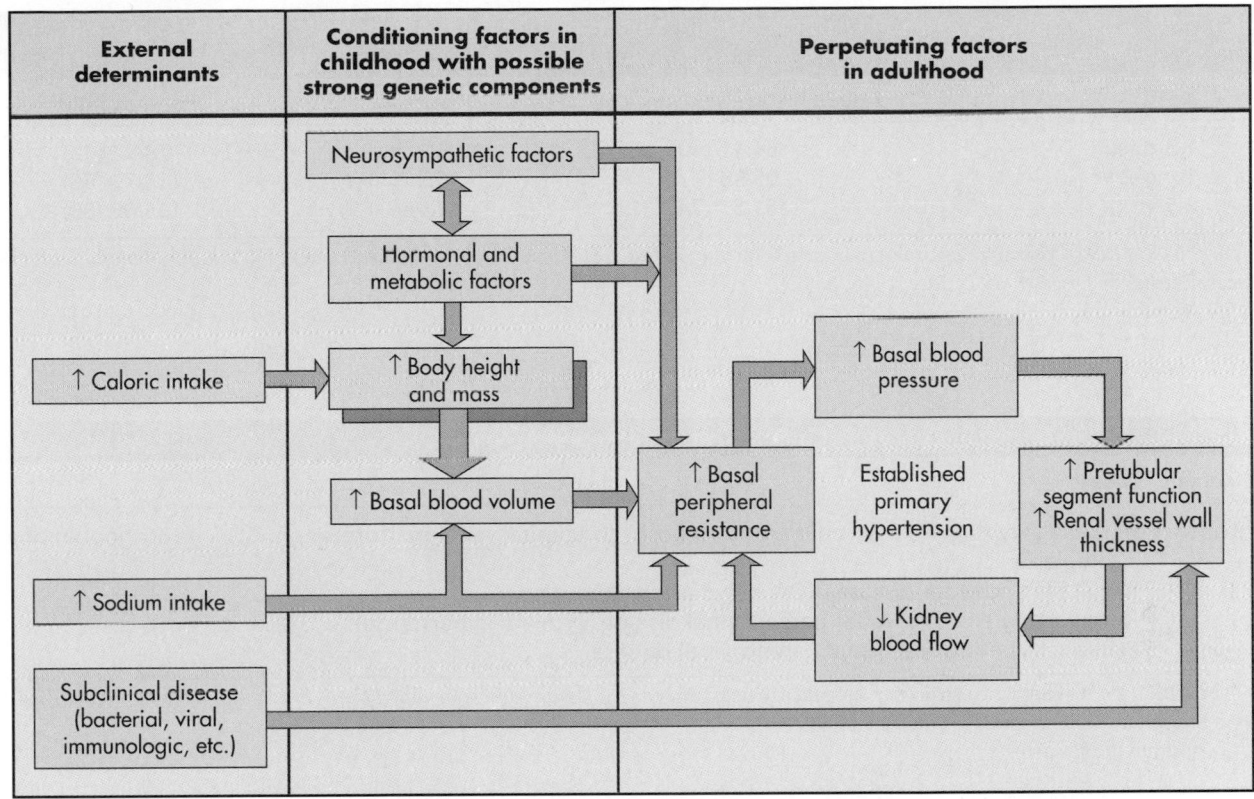

Fig. 24-14 *Mechanisms believed to influence blood pressure in children.* According to this model, a critical factor in the development of hypertension is obesity during childhood. Increased body mass, coupled with excessive sodium intake, can cause primary hypertension in children or set the stage for its development later in life. *(Modified from Voors, A.W. & Berenson, G.S. [1981]. In G. Onesti & K.E. Kin [Eds.]. Phasic pressor mechanisms: Hypertension in the young and the old. New York: Grune & Stratton.)*

TABLE 24-4	Suggested Normal BP Values (mm Hg) by Ausculatory Method (Systolic/Diastolic K5)		
Age (yrs)	Mean BP Levels	90th Percentile	95th Percentile
6-7	104/55	114/73	117/78
8-9	106/58	118/76	120/82
10-11*	108/60	120/77	124/82
12-13*	112/62	124/78	128/83
14-15			
Boys	116/66	132/80	138/86
Girls	112/68	126/80	130/83
16-18			
Boys	121/70	136/82	140/86
Girls	110/68	125/81	127/84

From Park, M.K. (1996). Pediatric cardiology for practitioners (3rd ed.). St. Louis: Mosby; modified from Goldring, D. et al. (1977). Journal of Pediatrics, 91, 884; Prineas, R.J. et al. (1980). Hypertension, 1(Suppl.), 18.

BP, *Blood pressure*; K5, *the phase V of Korotkoff sound.*

Values for ages 10-13 yr have been extrapolated from these two studies using age-related increments from other studies.

TABLE 24-5	Normative BP Levels (Systolic/Diastolic [Mean]) by Dinamap Monitor in Children 5 Yr Old and Younger		
Age	Mean BP Levels (in mm Hg)	90th Percentile	95th Percentile
1-3 days	64/41 (50)	75/49 (50)	78/52 (62)
1 mo-2 yr	95/58 (72)	106/68 (83)	110/71 (86)
2-5 yr	101/57 (74)	112/66 (82)	115/68 (85)

From Park, M.K. (1996). Pediatric cardiology for practitioners (3rd ed.). St. Louis: Mosby; modified from Park, M.K. & Menard, S.M. (1989).
American Journal of Diseases of Children, 143, 860.
BP, *Blood pressure.*

TABLE 24-6	Most Common Causes of Chronic Sustained Hypertension
Age-Group	Causes
Newborn	Renal artery thrombosis, renal artery stenosis, congenital renal malformation, COA, bronchopulmonary dysplasia
<6 yr	Renal parenchymal disease, COA, renal artery stenosis
6-10 yr	Renal artery stenosis, renal parenchymal disease, primary hypertension
>10 yr	Primary hypertension, renal parenchymal disease

From Park, M.K. (1996). Pediatric cardiology for practitioners (3rd ed.). St. Louis: Mosby; modified from (1987). Report of the Second Task Force on Blood Pressure Control in Children. Pediatrics, 79, 1-25.
COA, *Coarctation of the aorta.*

Clinical Manifestations

Most children with systemic HTN are asymptomatic. It is necessary that a thorough history and physical examination be obtained. The examination should include an accurate blood pressure measurement on three separate occasions using an appropriate-size cuff (Tables 24-4 and 24-5).[1,14,16]

Certain factors influence blood pressure in children. Children who are overweight are often hypertensive.[18] Smoking is also associated with an increased risk for HTN. The gender or race of the child has not been an associated risk factor of primary HTN.[14,16]

Evaluation and Treatment

In children, the history and physical examination should be directed at determining the etiology of HTN, such as coarctation of the aorta or renal disease (Table 24-6). If coarctation of the aorta is found, surgical or interventional correction is initiated. A complete blood count, serum chemistry levels, urinalysis, urine culture, lipid profile, and renal ultrasound are part of the routine evaluation for renal disease (Box 24-4). If HTN is found to be essential, or primary, in nature, nonpharmacologic therapy is used initially. Moderate weight loss can decrease systolic and diastolic pressures in many children. Appropriate diet, regular physical activity, and avoidance of smoking have been shown to be effective in reducing blood pressure.[1,14]

Drug therapy is controversial in children with primary hypertension; however, when nonpharmacologic therapy fails, a staged approach with the use of diuretics and/or β blockers and vasodilators is indicated.[1,19] The current emphasis on preventive cardiology, especially for children, is significant because many investigators believe signs of atherosclerosis are present from childhood.[18]

✓ QUICK CHECK

Why are the infant's height and weight important in assessment of congestive heart failure?

Why is it of critical importance to recognize and treat children during the acute phase of Kawasaki disease?

Why is the initial evaluation of significant hypertension in children important?

Routine and Special Laboratory Tests for Hypertension   BOX 24-4

Laboratory Tests	Significance of Abnormal Results
Urinalysis, urine culture, blood urea nitrogen, and creatinine levels	Renal parenchymal disease
Serum electrolyte levels (hypokalemia)	Hyperaldosteronism, primary or secondary Adrenogenital syndrome Renin-producing tumors
ECG, chest x-ray studies	Cardiac cause of hypertension, also baseline function
Intravenous pyelography (or ultrasonography, radionuclide studies, computed tomography of the kidneys)	Renal parenchymal diseases Renovascular hypertension Tumors (neuroblastoma, Wilms tumor)

Plasma renin activity, peripheral	High-renin hypertension
	   Renovascular hypertension
	   Renin-producing tumors
	   Some caused by Cushing syndrome
	   Some caused by essential hypertension
	Low-renin hypertension
	   Adrenogenital syndrome
	   Primary hyperaldosteronism

24-hr urine collection for 17-ketosteroids and 17-hydroxycorticosteroids	Cushing syndrome Adrenogenital syndrome
24-hr urine collection for catecholamine levels and vanillylmandelic acid	Pheochromocytoma Neuroblastoma
Aldosterone	Hyperaldosteronism, primary or secondary Renovascular hypertension Renin-producing tumors
Renal vein plasma renin activity	Unilateral renal parenchymal disease Renovascular hypertension
Abdominal aortogram	Renovascular hypertension Abdominal COA Unilateral renal parenchymal diseases Pheochromocytoma

From Park, M.K. (1996). Pediatric cardiology for practitioners (3rd ed.). St. Louis: Mosby.
ECG, Electrocardiogram; COA, coarctation of the aorta.

DID YOU UNDERSTAND?

Congenital Heart Disease

1. Most congenital heart defects have begun to develop by the eighth week of gestation, and most have many causes, both environmental and genetic.

2. Environmental risk factors associated with the incidence of congenital heart defects typically are maternal conditions. Maternal conditions include viral infections, diabetes, drug intake, and advanced maternal age.

3. Genetic factors associated with congenital heart defects include but are not limited to Down syndrome, trisomy 13, trisomy 18, cri du chat syndrome, and Turner syndrome.

4. Classification of congenital heart defects is based on (a) whether they cause blood flow to the lungs to increase, decrease, or remain normal and (b) whether they cause cyanosis.

5. Cyanosis, a bluish discoloration of the skin, indicates that the tissues are not receiving adequate oxygenated blood. Cyanosis can be caused by defects that (a) restrict blood flow into the pulmonary circulation; (b) overload the pulmonary circulation, causing pulmonary hypertension, pulmonary edema, and respiratory difficulty; or (c) cause large amounts of unoxygenated blood to shunt from the pulmonary to the systemic circulation.

6. Congenital defects that maintain or create direct communication between the pulmonary and systemic circulatory systems cause blood to shunt from one system to another, mixing oxygenated and unoxygenated blood and increasing blood volume and pressure on the receiving side of the shunt.

7. The direction of shunting through an abnormal communication depends on differences in pressure

Continued

▣ DID YOU UNDERSTAND? —cont'd

Congenital Heart Disease—cont'd

and resistance between the two systems. Flow is always from an area of high pressure to an area of low pressure.

8. Obstruction of ventricular outflow is commonly caused by pulmonary stenosis (right ventricle) or aortic stenosis (left ventricle).

9. Despite obstruction, ventricular outflow remains normal because of compensatory ventricular hypertrophy stimulated by increased afterload and, in postductal coarctation of the aorta, development of collateral circulation around the coarctation.

10. Left heart failure can develop as a result of right ventricular obstruction if afterload backs up into the pulmonary circulation. Left heart failure can result from left ventricular obstruction in preductal coarctation of the aorta in which left-to-right shunting through the patent ductus arteriosus greatly increases blood flow into the pulmonary circulation.

11. Acyanotic congenital defects that increase pulmonary blood flow consist of abnormal openings (atrial septal defect, ventricular septal defect, patent ductus arteriosus, endocardial cushion defect, or atrioventricular canal) that permit blood to shunt from left (systemic circulation) to right (pulmonary circulation). Cyanosis does not occur because the left-to-right shunt does not interfere with the flow of oxygenated blood through the systemic circulation.

12. If the abnormal communication between the left and right circuits is large, volume and pressure overload in the pulmonary circulation lead to left heart failure.

13. Cyanotic congenital defects in which saturated and desaturated blood mix within the heart or great arteries include truncus arteriosus, transposition of the great vessels, total anomalous pulmonary venous connection, and hypoplastic left heart syndrome.

14. In cyanotic heart defects that decrease pulmonary blood flow (tetralogy of Fallot, tricuspid atresia), myocardial hypertrophy cannot compensate for restricted right ventricular outflow. Flow to the lungs decreases, and cyanosis is caused by an insufficient volume of oxygenated blood.

15. Initial treatment for congenital heart disease, depending on the defect, is aimed at controlling the level of congestive heart failure or cyanosis. Interventional procedures in the cardiac catheterization laboratory and surgical palliation or repair are performed to restore circulation to as normal as possible.

Acquired Cardiovascular Disorders in Children

1. Examples of acquired heart disease are congestive heart failure, rheumatic heart disease, Kawasaki disease, and systemic hypertension.

2. Congestive heart failure is usually the result of congenital heart defects that increase blood volume and pressure in the pulmonary circulation. Clinical manifestations of CHF unique to children are failure-to-thrive and periorbital edema.

3. Kawasaki disease is an acute systemic vasculitis that also may result in the development of coronary artery aneurysms and thrombosis.

4. Systemic hypertension in children differs from adults in etiology and presentation. When significant hypertension is found in a child, the evaluation should rule out the presence of renal disease or coarctation.

KEY TERMS

Acyanotic defect, 700
Aortic stenosis (AS), 701
Atrial septal defect (ASD), 704
Atrioventricular canal (AVC) defect, 704
Coarctation of the aorta (COA), 700
Congenital heart disease (CHD), 699
Congestive heart failure (CHF), 709
Cyanosis, 700
Cyanotic defect, 700
Hypoplastic left heart syndrome (HLHS), 709

Kawasaki disease, 711
Left-to-right shunt, 700
Ostium primum, 704
Ostium secundum, 704
Patent ductus arteriosus (PDA), 703
Pulmonary atresia, 702
Pulmonic stenosis (PS), 702
Right-to-left shunt, 700
Shunt, 700
Sinus venosus defect, 704
Subvalvular stenosis, 702

Systemic hypertension, 712
Tetralogy of Fallot (TOF), 705
Total anomalous pulmonary venous connection (TAPVC), 707
Transposition of the great arteries (TGA; transposition of the great vessels [TGV]), 706
Tricuspid atresia, 705
Truncus arteriosus (TA), 708
Valvular stenosis, 702
Ventricular septal defect (VSD), 704

REFERENCES

1. Park, M.K. (1996). *Pediatric cardiology for practitioners* (3rd ed.). St. Louis: Mosby.
2. Reference deleted in proofs.
3. Lewis, D.A. & Tweddell, J.S. (1997). Valve repair and replacement in children. *Current Opinion in Cardiology, 12,* 63-69.
4. Radtke, W. & Lock, J.E. (1990). Balloon dilation. *Pediatric Clinics of North America, 37*(1), 193-214.
5. Wong, D. et al. (1999). *Whaley & Wong's nursing care of infants and children* (6th ed.). St. Louis: Mosby.
6. Geggel, R.L. (1997). Update on the modified Fontan procedure. *Current Opinion in Cardiology, 12,* 51-62.
7. Losay, J.A. & Hagen, T.J. (1997). Treatment of transposition of the great arteries. *Current Opinion in Cardiology, 12*(1), 84-90.
8. Cohen, D.M. & Allen, H.D. (1997). New developments in the treatment of hypoplastic left heart syndrome. *Current Opinion in Cardiology, 12,* 44-50.
9. Wong, D.L. (1995). *Whaley & Wong's nursing care of infants and children* (5th ed). St. Louis: Mosby.
10. Seymour, J.J. & Dickinson, E.G. (1998). Delayed cardiovascular sequelae from Kawasaki syndrome. *American Journal of Emergency Medicine, 16*(6), 579-581.
11. Dajani, A.S. et al. (1994). American Heart Association/Scientific statement guidelines for long-term management of patients with Kawasaki disease. *Circulation, 89*(2), 916-922.
12. Park, A.H. et al. (1997). Patterns of Kawasaki syndrome presentation. *International Journal of Pediatric Otorhinolaryngology, 40,* 41-50.
13. Nakamura, Y. et al. (1996). Mortality rates for patients with a history of Kawasaki disease in Japan. *Journal of Pediatrics, 128*(1), 75-81.
14. Emmanouilides, G.C. et al. (Eds.). (1995). *Heart disease in infants, children, and adolescents* (5th ed.). Baltimore: Williams & Wilkins.
15. Task Force on High Blood Pressure in Children and Adolescents (1987). Update on the Task Force on High Blood Pressure in Children and Adolescents: A working group from the National Blood Pressure Education Program. *Pediatrics, 98,* 649-658.
16. Sinaiko, A.R. (1996). Hypertension in children. *New England Journal of Medicine, 335*(26), 1968-1973.
17. Rudolph, A.M. et al. (1996). *Rudolph's pediatrics* (20th ed.). Stamford, Conn.: Appleton & Lange.
18. Feinstein, J.A. & Quivers, E.S. (1997). Pediatric preventive cardiology: Healthy habits now, healthy hearts later. *Current Opinion in Cardiology, 12,* 70-77.
19. Hoekelman, R.A. et al. (1997). *Primary pediatric care* (3rd ed.). St. Louis: Mosby.

CHAPTER

25

Structure and Function of the Pulmonary System

Valentina L. Brashers and Sue E. Huether

T he pulmonary system consists of the lungs, air-ways, chest wall, and pulmonary circulation. Its primary function is the exchange of gases between the environmental air and the blood. The three steps in this process are (1) ventilation, the move-ment of air into and out of the lungs; (2) diffusion, the movement of gases between air spaces in the lungs and the bloodstream; and (3) perfusion, the movement of blood into and out of the capillary beds of the lungs to body organs and tissues. The first two functions are carried out by the pulmonary system and the third by the cardiovascular system (see Chapter 22). Normally the pulmonary system functions efficiently under a variety of conditions and with little energy expenditure.

CHAPTER OUTLINE

  Check out your CD Companion for chapter-related exercises and answers to the Quick Check questions

STRUCTURES OF THE PULMONARY SYSTEM

The pulmonary system is made up of two lungs, their airways, the blood vessels that serve them (Fig. 25-1), and the chest wall, or thoracic cage. The lungs are divided into lobes: three in the right lung (upper, middle, lower) and two in the left lung (upper, lower). Each lobe is further divided into segments and lobules. The space between the lungs, which contains the heart, great vessels, and esophagus, is called the *mediastinum*. A set of tubes, or conducting airways, delivers air to each section of the lung. The lung tissue that surrounds the airways supports them, preventing their distortion or collapse as gas moves in and out during ventilation.

The lungs are protected from exogenous contaminants by a series of mechanical barriers (Table 25-1). These defense mechanisms are so effective that contamination of the lung tissue itself, particularly by infectious agents, is rare.

Conducting Airways

The conducting airways allow air into and out of the gas-exchange structures of the lung. The ***nasopharynx, oropharynx,*** and related structures are often called the *upper airway* (Fig. 25-2). These structures are lined with a ciliated mucosa that warms and humidifies inspired air and removes foreign particles from it. The mouth and oropharynx are also used for ventilation when the nose is obstructed or when increased flow is required, for example, during exercise. Filtering and humidifying are not, however, as efficient with mouth breathing.

The ***larynx*** connects the upper and lower airways and consists of the endolarynx and its surrounding triangular-shaped bony and cartilaginous structures. The endolarynx encompasses two pairs of folds—the false vocal cords (supraglottis) and the true vocal cords. The slit-shaped space between the true cords forms the glottis (see Fig. 25-2). The vestibule is the space above the false vocal cords. The laryn-

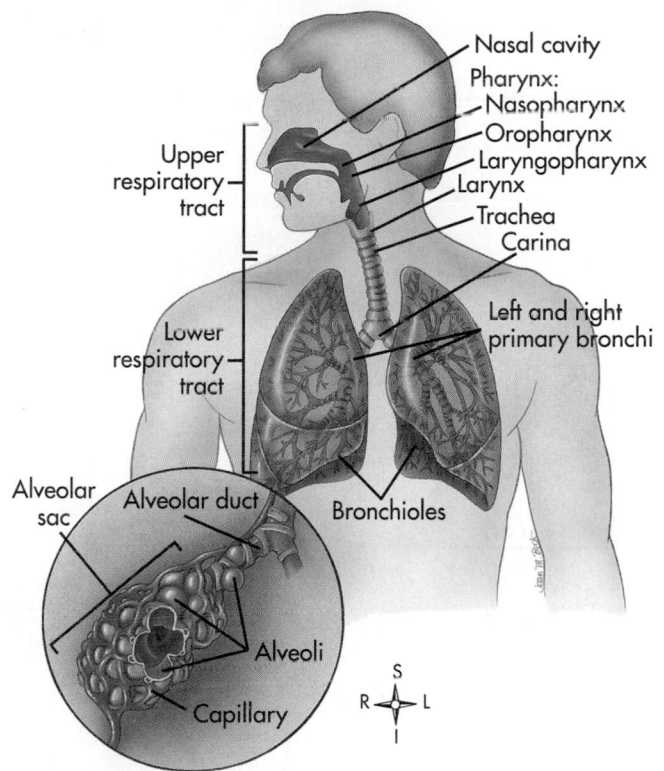

Fig. 25-1 ***Structures of the pulmonary system.*** The circle denotes the acinus, where oxygen and carbon dioxide are exchanged. *(Modified from Thibodeau, G.A. & Patton, K.T. [1999]. Anatomy & physiology [4th ed.]. St. Louis: Mosby.)*

geal box is formed of three large cartilages (epiglottis, thyroid, cricoid) and three smaller cartilages (arytenoid, corniculate, cuneiform) connected by ligaments. The supporting cartilages prevent collapse of the larynx during inspiration and swallowing. The internal laryngeal muscles control vocal cord length and tension, and the external laryngeal muscles move the larynx as a whole. Both sets of muscles are important to swallowing, ventilation, and vocalization. The

TABLE 25-1	Pulmonary Defense Mechanisms
Structure or Substance	**Mechanism of Defense**
Upper respiratory tract mucosa	Maintains constant temperature and humidification of gas entering the lungs; traps and removes foreign particles, some bacteria, and noxious gases from inspired air
Nasal hairs and turbinates	Trap and remove foreign particles, some bacteria, and noxious gases from inspired air
Mucus blanket	Protects trachea and bronchi from injury; traps most foreign particles ad bacteria that reach the lower airways
Cilia	Propel mucus blanket and entrapped particles toward the oropharynx, where they can be swallowed or expectorated
Alveolar macrophages	Ingest and remove bacteria and other foreign material from alveoli by phagocytosis (see Chapters 5 and 6)
Irritant receptors in nares (nostrils)	Stimulation by chemical or mechanical irritants triggers sneeze reflex, which results in rapid removal of irritants from nasal passages
Irritant receptors in trachea and large airways	Stimulation by chemical or mechanical irritants triggers cough reflex, which results in removal of irritants from the lower airways

NASAL WALL

PHARYNX

TRACHEA

LARYNX

Fig. 25-2 *Structures of the upper airway.* (*Modified from Thompson, J.M. et al. [1997]. Mosby's clinical nursing [4th ed.]. St. Louis: Mosby.*)

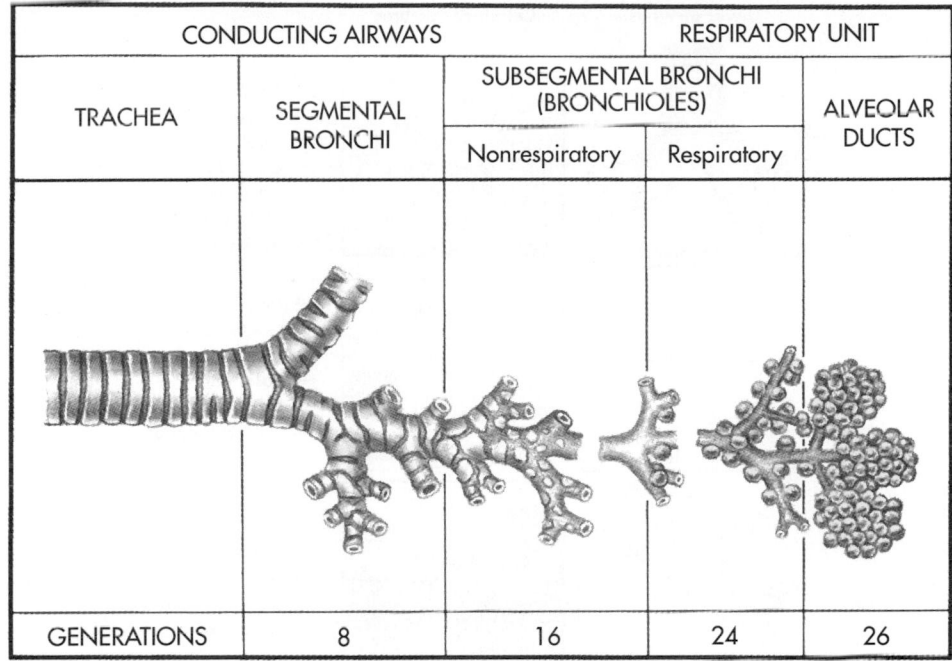

CONDUCTING AIRWAYS				RESPIRATORY UNIT
TRACHEA	SEGMENTAL BRONCHI	SUBSEGMENTAL BRONCHI (BRONCHIOLES)		ALVEOLAR DUCTS
		Nonrespiratory	Respiratory	
GENERATIONS	8	16	24	26

Fig. 25-3 *Structures of the lower airway. (From Thompson, J.M. et al. [1997]. Mosby's clinical nursing [4th ed.]. St. Louis: Mosby.)*

internal muscles contract during swallowing to prevent aspiration into the trachea and also contribute to voice pitch.

The *trachea,* which is supported by U-shaped cartilage, connects the larynx to the *bronchi,* the conducting airways of the lungs. Its two main airways, or bronchi, branch at the *carina* (see Fig. 25-1). The right and left main bronchi enter the lungs at the *hili,* or "roots" of the lungs, along with the pulmonary blood and lymphatic vessels. From the hili the main bronchi branch farther, as shown in Fig. 25-3.

The bronchial walls have three layers: an epithelial lining, a smooth muscle layer, and a connective tissue layer. The epithelial lining of the bronchi contains single-celled exocrine glands—the mucus-secreting *goblet cells*—and ciliated cells. With branching, the layers of epithelium that line the bronchi become thinner (Fig. 25-4).

Gas-Exchange Airways

The conducting airways terminate in gas-exchange airways made up of *respiratory bronchioles, alveolar ducts,* and *alveoli.* These structures together are sometimes called the *acinus* (see Figs. 25-1 and 25-3), and all of them participate in gas exchange.

The bronchioles from the sixteenth through the twenty-third divisions are called *respiratory bronchioles;* their walls are very thin. These bronchioles end in alveolar ducts, which lead to alveolar sacs made up of numerous alveoli.

The alveoli are the primary gas-exchange units of the lung, where oxygen enters the blood and carbon dioxide is removed (Fig. 25-5). Tiny passages called *pores of Kohn* permit some air to pass through the septa from alveolus to alveolus, promoting collateral ventilation and even distribution of air among the alveoli. In cross sections, alveoli appear

similar to sponges. The lungs contain approximately 25 million alveoli at birth and 300 million by adulthood.

Two major types of epithelial cells appear in the alveolus. Type I alveolar cells provide structure, and type II alveolar cells secrete *surfactant,* a lipoprotein that coats the inner surface of the alveolus and facilitates its expansion during inspiration.

Like the bronchi, alveoli contain cellular components of inflammation and immunity, particularly the mononuclear phagocytes (called *alveolar macrophages*). These cells ingest foreign material that reaches the alveolus and prepare it for removal through the lymphatics. (Phagocytosis and the mononuclear phagocyte system are described in Chapters 5 and 6.)

✓QUICK CHECK

List the major components of the pulmonary system.

What are conducting airways?

Describe an alveolus.

Pulmonary and Bronchial Circulation

The pulmonary circulation facilitates gas exchange, delivers nutrients to lung tissues, acts as a reservoir for the left ventricle, and serves as a filtering system that removes clots, air, and other debris from the circulation.

The pulmonary circulation has a lower pressure and resistance than the systemic circulation. Pulmonary arteries are exposed to about one-fifth the pressure of the systemic circulation.

Lower airways   **Cellular structures**

Fig. 25-4 *Changes in the bronchial wall with progressive branching.* (*From Wilson, S.F. & Thompson, J.M. [1990].* Respiratory disorders. *St. Louis: Mosby.*)

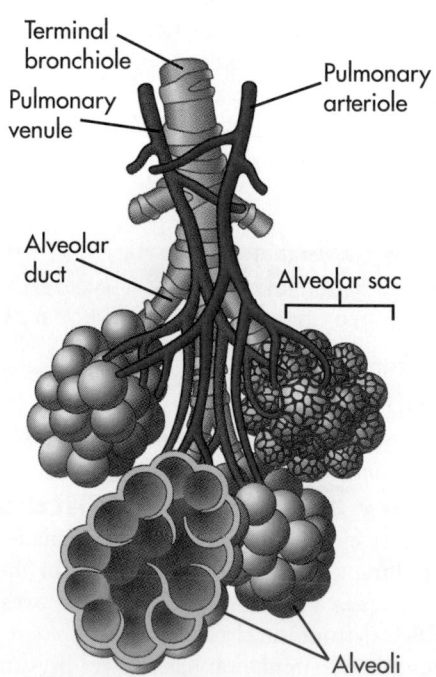

Fig. 25-5 *Alveoli.* Bronchioles subdivide to form tiny tubes called *alveolar ducts,* which end in clusters of alveoli called *alveolar sacs.* (*From Thibodeau, G.A. & Patton, K.T. [1999].* Anatomy & physiology *[4th ed.]. St. Louis: Mosby.*)

Usually about one third of the pulmonary vessels are filled with blood (perfused) at any given time. More vessels become perfused when right ventricular cardiac output increases. Therefore increased delivery of blood to the lungs does not normally increase mean pulmonary artery pressure.

The arterioles divide at the terminal bronchioles to form a network of pulmonary capillaries around the acinus. Capillary walls consist of an endothelial layer and a thin basement membrane, which often fuses with the basement membrane of the alveolar septum. Therefore very little separation exists between blood in the capillary and gas in the alveolus.

The shared alveolar and capillary walls compose the *alveolocapillary membrane* (Fig. 25-6). Gas exchange occurs across this membrane. With normal perfusion, approximately 100 ml of blood in the pulmonary capillary bed is spread very thinly over 70 to 100 m² of alveolar surface area. Any disorder that thickens the membrane impairs gas exchange.

Each pulmonary vein drains several pulmonary capillaries. Unlike the pulmonary arteries, pulmonary veins are dispersed randomly throughout the lung and then leave the lung at the hili and enter the left atrium. They have no valves.

The bronchial circulation is part of the systemic circulation, and it supplies nutrients to the conducting airways, large pulmonary vessels, and membranes (pleurae) that sur-

Fig. 25-6 *Section through the alveolar septum (gas-exchange membrane).* Inset shows a magnified view of the respiratory membrane composed of the alveolar wall (fluid coating, epithelial cells, basement membrane), interstitial fluid, and wall of a pulmonary capillary (basement membrane, endothelial cells). The gases CO_2 (carbon dioxide) and O_2 (oxygen) diffuse across the respiratory membrane.

round the lungs. Not all of its capillaries drain into its own venous system. Some empty into the pulmonary vein and contribute to the normal venous mixture of oxygenated and deoxygenated blood or right-to-left shunt (right-to-left shunts are described in Chapter 26). The bronchial circulation does not participate in gas exchange but warms and moistens inspired air and provides airway nourishment.[1]

Lung vasculature also includes deep and superficial lymphatic capillaries. Fluid and alveolar macrophages migrate from the alveoli to the terminal bronchioles, where they enter the lymphatic system. Both deep and superficial lymphatic vessels leave the lung at the hilus. The lymphatic system plays an important role in keeping the lung free of fluid. (The lymphatic system is described in Chapter 22.)

Chest Wall and Pleura

The chest wall (skin, ribs, intercostal muscles) protects the lungs from injury, and its muscles, along with the diaphragm, perform the muscular work of breathing. The ***thoracic cavity*** is contained by the chest wall and encases the lungs (Fig. 25-7). A serous membrane called the ***pleura*** adheres firmly to the lungs and then folds over itself and attaches firmly to the chest wall. The membrane covering the lungs is the visceral pleura; that lining the thoracic cavity is the parietal pleura. The area between the two pleurae is called the ***pleural space,*** or ***pleural cavity.*** Normally, only a thin layer of fluid secreted by the pleura (pleural fluid) fills

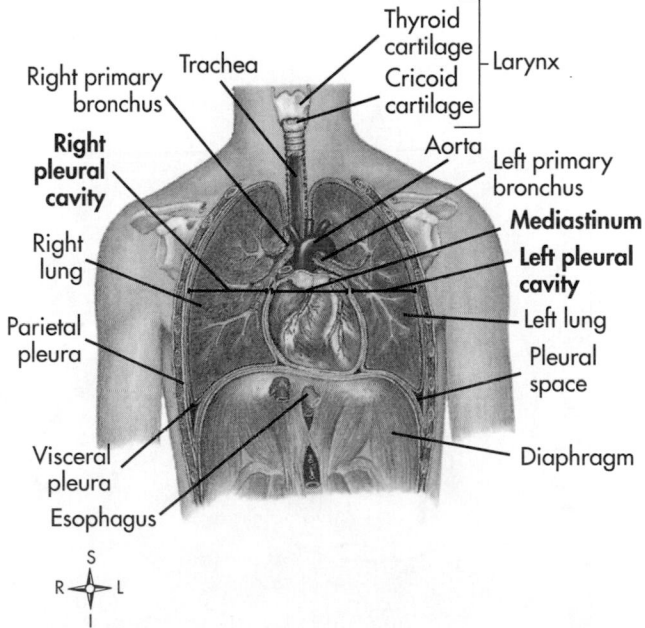

Fig. 25-7 *Thoracic (chest) cavity and related structures.* The thoracic (chest) cavity is divided into three subdivisions (left and right pleural divisions and mediastinum) by a partition formed by a serous membrane called the *pleura. (From Thibodeau, G.A. & Patton, K.T. [1999]. Anatomy & physiology [4th ed.]. St. Louis: Mosby.)*

the pleural space, lubricating the pleural surfaces and allowing the two layers to slide over each other without separating. Pressure in the pleural space is usually negative or subatmospheric (24 to 10 mm Hg).

FUNCTION OF THE PULMONARY SYSTEM

The pulmonary system functions to (1) ventilate the alveoli, (2) diffuse gases into and out of the blood, and (3) perfuse the lungs so that the organs and tissues of the body receive blood that is rich in oxygen and low in carbon dioxide. Each component of the pulmonary system contributes to one or more of these functions (Fig. 25-8).

Ventilation

Ventilation is the mechanical movement of gas or air into and out of the lungs. It is often misnamed *respiration*, which is actually the exchange of oxygen and carbon dioxide during cellular metabolism. "Respiratory rate" is actually the ventilatory rate, or the number of times gas is inspired and expired per minute.

Measurement of gas pressure

A gas is made up of millions of molecules moving randomly and colliding with each other and with the wall of the space in which they are contained. These collisions exert pressure. If the same number of gas molecules is contained in a small and a large container, the pressure is greater in the small container because more collisions occur in the smaller space (Fig. 25-9). Heat increases the speed of the molecules, which increases the number of collisions and therefore the pressure.

Fig. 25-8 *Functional components of the respiratory system.* The central nervous system responds to neurochemical stimulation of ventilation and sends signals to the chest wall musculature. The response of the respiratory system to these impulses is influenced by several factors that impact the mechanisms of breathing and, therefore, impact the adequacy of ventilation. Gas transport between the alveoli and pulmonary capillary blood depends on a variety of physical and chemical activities. Finally, the control of the pulmonary circulation plays a role in the appropriate distribution of blood flow.

Barometric pressure (P_B) (atmospheric pressure) is the pressure exerted by gas molecules in air at specific altitudes. At sea level, barometric pressure is 760 mm Hg and is the sum of the pressure exerted by each gas in the air at sea level. The portion of the total pressure exerted by any individual gas is its *partial pressure* (see Fig. 25-9). At sea level the air is made up of oxygen (20.9%), nitrogen (78.1%), and a few other trace gases. The partial pressure of oxygen is equal to

Fig. 25-9 *Relationship between number of gas molecules and pressure exerted by the gas in an enclosed space.* **A,** Theoretically, 10 molecules of the same gas exert a total pressure of 10 within the space. **B,** If the number of molecules is increased to 20, total pressure is 20. **C,** If there are different gases in the space, each gas exerts a partial pressure: here the partial pressure of nitrogen (N_2) is 20; that of oxygen (O_2) is 6; and total pressure is 26.

TABLE 25-2	Common Pulmonary Abbreviations
Symbol	**Definition**
V	Volume or amount of gas
Q	Perfusion or blood flow
P	Pressure (usually partial pressure) of a gas
S	Percentage of hemoglobin saturation with a gas (usually oxygen)
F	Fraction of gas, or gas flow (in a laboratory test)
C	Content or amount of gas
C_T	Thoracic compliance
E	Expired gas
i	Inspired gas
A	Alveolar gas
a	Arterial blood
$\bar{v}$	Mixed venous or pulmonary artery blood
D	Dead space
PaO_2	Partial pressure of oxygen in arterial blood
PAO_2	Partial pressure of oxygen in alveolar gas
$PaCO_2$	Partial pressure of carbon dioxide in arterial blood
$P\bar{v}O_2$	Partial pressure of oxygen in mixed venous or pulmonary artery blood
$P(A - a)O_2$	Difference between alveolar and arterial partial pressure of oxygen ($A - a$ gradient)
P_B	Barometric or atmospheric pressure
SaO_2	Saturation of hemoglobin (in arterial blood) with oxygen
$S\bar{v}O_2$	Saturation of hemoglobin (in mixed venous blood) with oxygen
CaO_2	Content or amount (volume) of oxygen in arterial blood
$C\bar{v}O_2$	Content of oxygen in mixed venous blood
$C(a - \bar{v})O_2$	Oxygen content difference between arterial and mixed venous blood
$\dot{V}_A$	Alveolar ventilation
$\dot{V}_D$	Dead-space ventilation
$\dot{V}_E$	Minute volume
VC	Vital capacity
V_T	Tidal volume or average breath
$\dot{Q}T$	Total perfusion or blood flow (cardiac output)
$\dot{V}/\dot{Q}$	Ratio of ventilation to perfusion
FiO_2	Fraction of inspired oxygen
FRC	Functional residual capacity
IC	Inspiratory capacity

Subscripts identify the particular gas, volume, or pressure being discussed. A dot (˙) means measurement over time, usually 1 minute.

the percentage of oxygen in the air (20.9%) times the total pressure (760 mm Hg), or 159 mm Hg (760 × 0.209 = 158.84). (Symbols used in the measurement of gas pressures and pulmonary ventilation are defined in Table 25-2.)

The amount of water vapor contained in a gas mixture is determined by the temperature of the gas and is unrelated to barometric pressure. Gas that enters the lungs becomes saturated with water vapor (humidified) as it passes through the upper airway. At body temperature (37° C), water vapor exerts a pressure of 47 mm Hg regardless of total (barometric) pressure. The partial pressure of water vapor must be subtracted from the barometric pressure before the partial pressure of other gases in the mixture can be determined. In saturated air at sea level, the partial pressure of oxygen is therefore (760 − 47) × 0.209 = 149. All pressure and volume measurements made in pulmonary function laboratories specify the temperature and humidity of a gas at the time of measurement.

Many pressure measurements are stated as variations from barometric pressure, rather than percentages of it. On such scales, barometric pressure is considered zero, and pressure varies up or down from zero. Physiologic pressure measurements that involve fluids, rather than gases, are measured as variations from barometric pressure. For example, a systolic blood pressure of 120 mm Hg indicates that systolic pressure is 120 mm Hg above barometric pressure.

✓ QUICK CHECK

List the major components of the pulmonary circulation.

What are the visceral and parietal pleurae?

What is barometric pressure? How is it related to physiologic pressure measurements?

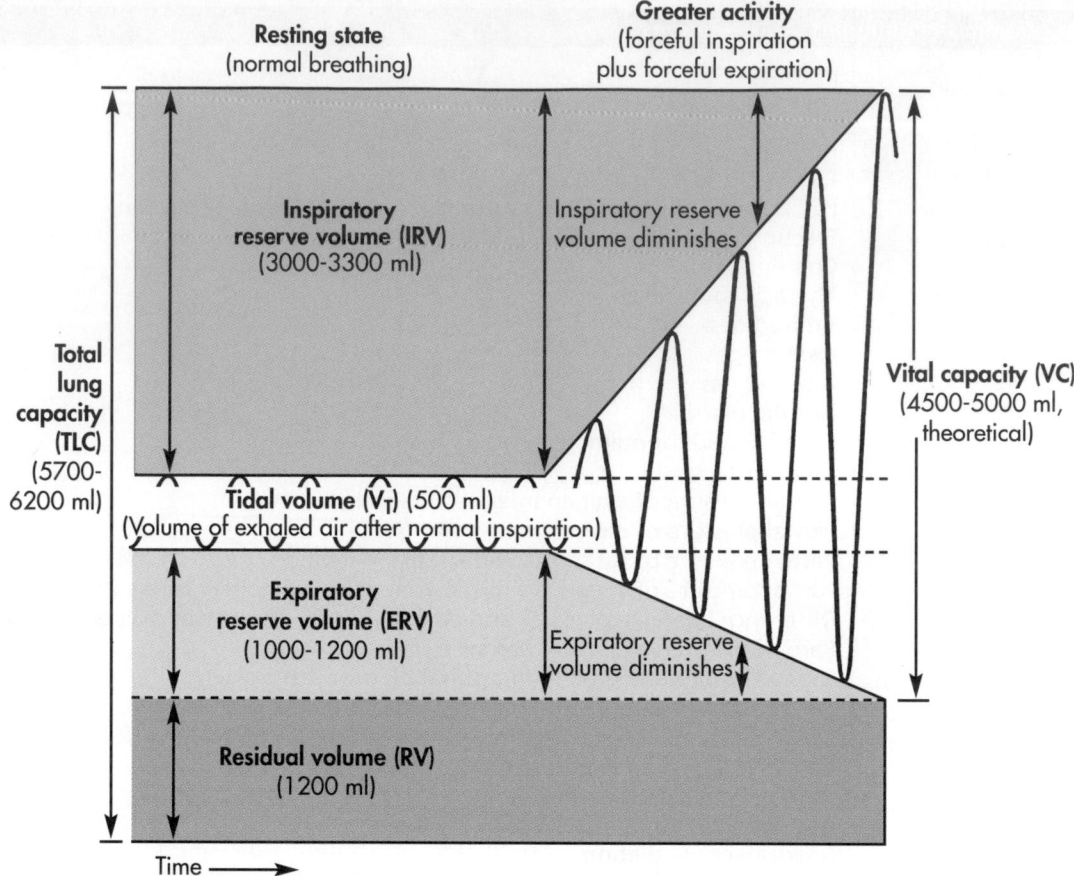

Fig. 25-10 *Spirogram.* During normal, quiet respirations the atmosphere and lungs exchange about 500 ml of air *(V_T)*. With a forcible inspiration, about 3300 ml more air can be inhaled *(IRV)*. After a normal inspiration and normal expiration, approximately 1000 ml more air can be forcibly expired *(ERV)*. Vital capacity *(VC)* is the amount of air that can be forcibly expired after a maximal inspiration and indicates, therefore, the largest amount of air that can enter and leave the lungs during respiration. Residual volume *(RV)* is the air that remains trapped in the alveoli. *(From Thibodeau, G.A. & Patton, K.T. [1999]. Anatomy & physiology [4th ed.]. St. Louis: Mosby.)*

Lung volumes and capacities

The following parameters (Fig. 25-10) should be measured:

Tidal volume (V_T): amount of gas inspired and expired during normal breathing

Inspiratory reserve volume (IRV): amount of gas that can be inspired in addition to tidal volume

Expiratory reserve volume (ERV): amount of gas that can be expired after a passive (relaxed) expiration

Residual volume (RV): volume of gas that cannot be expired and is always present in the lung

Total lung capacity (TLC): total gas volume in the lung when it is maximally inflated; sum of RV, ERV, V_T, and IRV

Vital capacity (VC): maximum amount of gas that can be displaced (expired) from the lung; sum of IRV, V_T, and ERV

Functional residual capacity (FRC): amount of gas remaining in the lung at the end of a passive expiration; sum of RV and ERV; at this point the lungs are at rest (mechanical equilibrium)

Inspiratory capacity (IC): amount of gas that can be inspired after a passive expiration (from FRC); includes V_T and IRV

Dead-space ventilation (Ḋ): volume of air that is wasted, that is, does not participate in gas exchange

Anatomic dead space: portion of tidal volume that remains in conducting airways; averages 1 ml per pound of lean body weight, or one third of each breath

Alveolar dead space: volume of gas in unperfused alveoli

Physiologic dead space: sum of normal anatomic dead space and alveolar dead space

Alveolar ventilation (Ȧ): portion of tidal volume that reaches alveoli; during expiration, part of this alveolar gas remains in the conducting airways and moves back into the alveoli with next inspiration

Lung capacities are always the sum of two or more volumes. Norms for volumes and capacities are based on age, gender, and height and are referred to as predicted values. Changes from predicted or baseline values are taken into account in diagnosing and assessing respiratory disorders.

Carbon dioxide (CO_2), the gaseous form of carbonic acid (H_2CO_3), is produced by cellular metabolism. The lung eliminates about 10,000 milliequivalents (mEq) of carbonic acid per day in the form of CO_2, which is produced at the rate of approximately 200 ml/min. Carbon dioxide is eliminated to maintain a normal arterial CO_2 ($PaCO_2$) of 40 mm Hg and normal acid-base balance.

HEALTH ALERT

Exercise and Cystic Fibrosis

Exercise is an important component in the treatment of cystic fibrosis. Although exercise tolerance may be reduced in individuals with cystic fibrosis, development of individualized programs combined with other therapies offers the opportunity to improve quality of life by greater mobility and socialization, improved self-confidence, and prolonged life expectancy.

From Balfour-Lynn, I.M. et al. (1998). A step in the right direction: Assessing exercise tolerance in cystic fibrosis [e comments]. Pediatric Pulmonology, 25(4), 278-284; Homnick, D.N. & Marks, J.H. (1998). Exercise and sports in the adolescent with chronic pulmonary disease. Adolescent Medicine, 9(3), 467-481. Moorcroft, A.J., Dodd, M.E., & Webb, A.K. (1998). Exercise limitations and training for patients with cystic fibrosis. Disability and Rehabilitation, 20(6-7), 247-253.

Neurochemical Control of Ventilation

Breathing is usually involuntary, because homeostatic changes in ventilatory rate and volume are adjusted automatically by the nervous system to maintain normal gas exchange. Voluntary breathing is necessary for talking, singing, laughing, and deliberately holding one's breath. The mechanisms that control respiration are very complex (Fig. 25-11).

The *respiratory center* in the brain stem controls respiration by transmitting impulses to the respiratory muscles, causing them to contract and relax. The respiratory center is composed of several groups of neurons: the dorsal respiratory group (DRG), the ventral respiratory group (VRG), the pneumotaxic center, and the apneustic center.[2] The basic automatic rhythm of respiration is set by the DRG, which receives afferent input from *peripheral chemoreceptors* in the carotid and aortic bodies and from several different types of receptors in the lungs. The VRG contains both inspiratory and expiratory neurons and is almost inactive during normal, quiet respiration, becoming active when increased ventilatory effort is required. The pneumotaxic center and apneustic center, situated in the pons, do not generate primary rhythm but, rather, act as modifiers of the rhythm established by the medullary centers.

Lung receptors

Three types of lung receptors send impulses from the lungs to the dorsal respiratory group:

1. *Irritant receptors* are found in the epithelium of all conducting airways. They are sensitive to noxious aerosols (vapors), gases, and particulate matter (e.g., inhaled dusts), which cause them to initiate the cough reflex. When stimulated, irritant receptors cause bronchoconstriction and increased ventilatory rate.
2. *Stretch receptors* are located in the smooth muscles of airways and are sensitive to increases in the size or volume of the lungs. They decrease ventilatory rate and volume when stimulated, an occurrence sometimes referred to as the Hering-Breuer expiratory reflex. This reflex is not thought to play a major role in the regulation of ventilation in adults, although it may be important in infants.[3]
3. *J-receptors* (juxtapulmonary capillary receptors) are located near the capillaries in the alveolar septa. They are sensitive to increased pulmonary capillary pressure, which stimulates them to initiate rapid, shallow breathing.

The lung is innervated by the autonomic nervous system (ANS). Fibers of the sympathetic division in the lung branch form the upper thoracic and cervical ganglia of the spinal cord. Fibers of the parasympathetic division of the ANS travel in the vagus nerve to the lung. (Structures and function of the ANS are covered in detail in Chapter 12.) The parasympathetic and sympathetic divisions control airway caliber (interior diameter of the airway lumen) by stimulating bronchial smooth muscle to contract or relax. The parasympathetic receptors cause smooth muscle to contract, whereas sympathetic receptors cause it to relax. Bronchial smooth muscle tone depends on equilibrium, that is, equal stimulation of contraction and relaxation. The parasympathetic division of the ANS is the main controller of airway caliber under normal conditions. Constriction occurs if the irritant receptors in the airway epithelium are stimulated by irritants in inspired air, by endogenous substances (e.g., histamine, serotonin, prostaglandins, leukotreines), by many drugs, and by humoral substances.

Chemoreceptors

Chemoreceptors monitor the pH, $PaCO_2$, and PaO_2 of arterial blood. *Central chemoreceptors* monitor arterial blood indirectly by sensing changes in the pH of cerebrospinal fluid (CSF). They are located near the respiratory center and are sensitive to hydrogen ion concentration in the CSF. (Chapter 4 describes the relationship between ions and the pH, or acid-base status, of body fluids.) The pH of the CSF reflects arterial pH because carbon dioxide in arterial blood can diffuse across the blood-brain barrier (the capillary wall separating blood from cells of the central nervous system) into the CSF until the partial pressure of carbon dioxide (PCO_2) is equal on both sides. Carbon dioxide that has entered the CSF combines with H_2O to form carbonic acid, which subsequently dissociates into hydrogen ions that are capable of stimulating the central chemoreceptors. In this way $PaCO_2$ regulates ventilation through its impact on the pH (hydrogen ion content) of the CSF.[4]

If alveolar ventilation is inadequate, $PaCO_2$ increases. Carbon dioxide diffuses across the blood-brain barrier until PCO_2 in blood and CSF reaches equilibrium. As the central

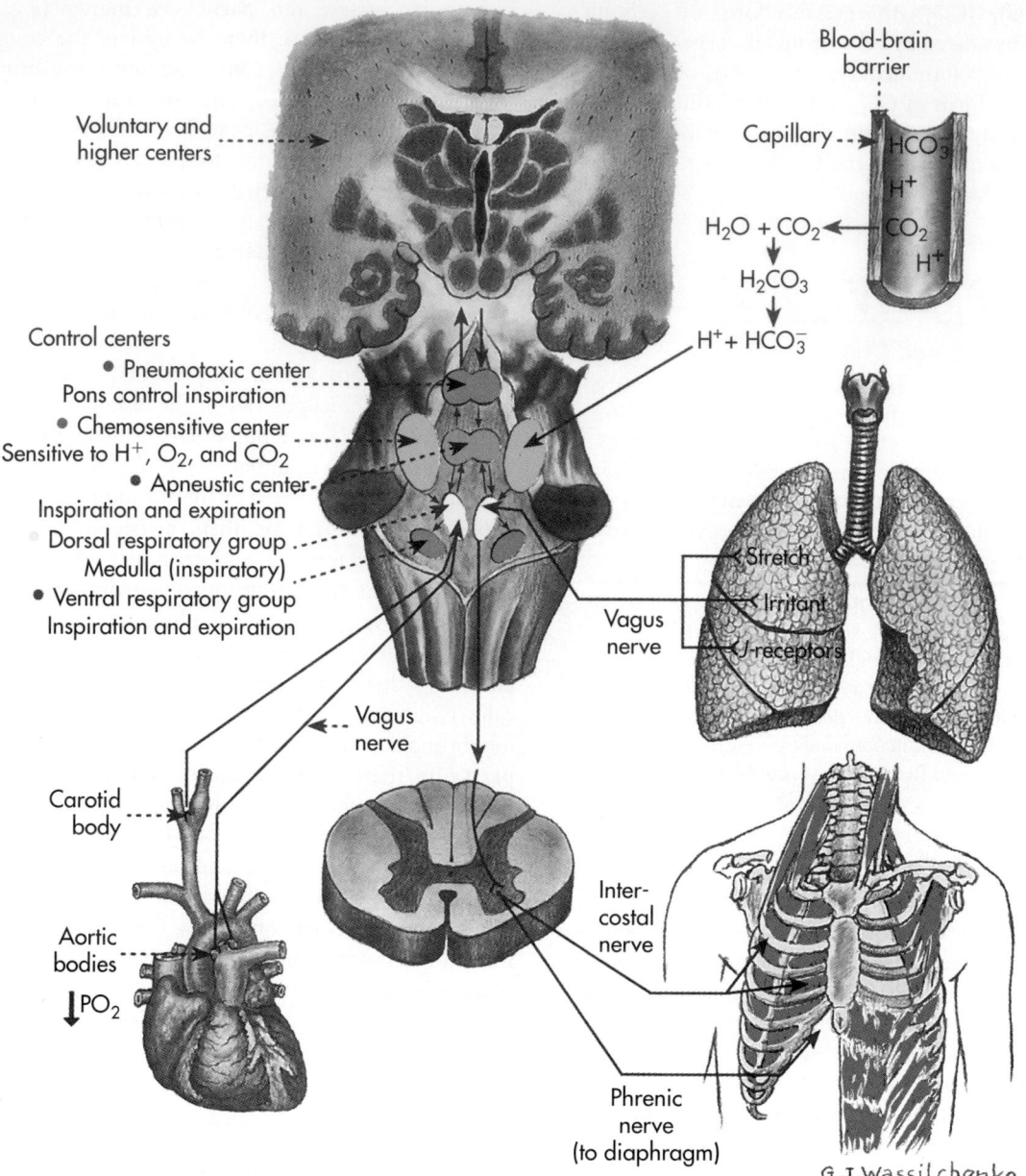

Fig. 25-11 *Neurochemical respiratory control system. (Modified from Thompson, J.M. et al. [1997]. Mosby's clinical nursing [4th ed.]. St. Louis: Mosby.)*

chemoreceptors sense the resulting decrease in pH (increase in hydrogen ion concentration), they stimulate the respiratory center to increase the depth and rate of ventilation. Increased ventilation causes the PCO_2 of arterial blood to decrease below that of the CSF, and carbon dioxide diffuses back out of the CSF, returning its pH to normal.

The central chemoreceptors are sensitive to very small changes in the pH of CSF (equivalent to a 1 to 2 mm Hg change in PCO_2) and can maintain a normal $PaCO_2$ under many different conditions, including strenuous exercise. If inadequate ventilation, or hypoventilation, is long-term (e.g., in chronic obstructive pulmonary disease), these receptors become insensitive to small changes in $PaCO_2$ and regulate ventilation poorly.

The peripheral chemoreceptors are somewhat sensitive to changes in $PaCO_2$ and pH but are sensitive primarily to oxygen levels in arterial blood (PaO_2). As PaO_2 and pH decrease, peripheral chemoreceptors, particularly in the carotid bodies, send signals to the respiratory center to increase ventilation. However, the PaO_2 must drop well below normal (to approximately 60 mm Hg) before the peripheral chemoreceptors have much influence on ventilation. If $PaCO_2$ is elevated as well, ventilation increases much more than it would in response to either abnormality alone. The peripheral chemoreceptors become the major stimulus to ventilation when the central chemoreceptors are "reset" by chronic hypoventilation.

✓ QUICK CHECK

Describe three functions of the respiratory center in the brain stem.

What are the three types of lung receptors?

How do the functions of central and peripheral chemoreceptors differ?

Mechanics of Breathing

The mechanical aspects of inspiration and expiration are known collectively as the mechanics of breathing and involve (1) major and accessory muscles of inspiration and expiration, (2) elastic properties of the lungs and chest wall, and (3) resistance to air flow through the conducting airways. Alterations in any of these properties increase the work of breathing, or the metabolic energy needed to achieve adequate ventilation and oxygenation of the blood (see p. 733).

Major and accessory muscles

The major muscles of inspiration are the diaphragm and the external intercostal muscles (muscles between the ribs) (Fig. 25-12). The diaphragm is a dome-shaped muscle that separates the abdominal and thoracic cavities. When it contracts and flattens downward, it increases the volume of the thoracic cavity, creating a negative pressure that draws gas into the lungs. Contraction of external intercostal muscles elevates the anterior portion of the ribs and increases the volume of the thoracic cavity by increasing its front-to-back (anterior-posterior [AP]) diameter. Although the external intercostals may contract during quiet breathing, inspiration at rest is usually assisted by the diaphragm only.

The accessory muscles of inspiration are the sternocleidomastoid and scalene muscles. Like the external intercostals, these muscles enlarge the thorax by increasing its AP diameter. The accessory muscles assist inspiration when minute volume (volume of air inspired and expired per minute) is very high, as during strenuous exercise, or when the work of breathing is increased because of disease. The accessory muscles do not increase the volume of the thorax as efficiently as the diaphragm does.

There are no major muscles of expiration because normal, relaxed expiration is passive and requires no muscular effort. The accessory muscles of expiration, the abdominal and internal intercostal muscles, assist expiration when minute volume is high, when expiration exceeds FRC, or when airway obstruction is present. When the abdominal muscles contract, intraabdominal pressure increases, pushing up the diaphragm and decreasing the volume of the thorax. The internal intercostal muscles pull down the anterior ribs, decreasing the AP diameter of the thorax.

Alveolar surface tension

Surface tension occurs at any gas-liquid interface and refers to the tendency for liquid molecules that are exposed to air to

Fig. 25-12 *Muscles of ventilation.* **A,** Anterior view. **B,** Posterior view. *(From Thompson, J.M. et al. [1997]. Mosby's clinical nursing [4th ed.]. St. Louis: Mosby.)*

adhere to one another. This phenomenon can be seen in the way liquids "bead" when splashed on a waterproof surface.

Within a sphere, such as an alveolus, surface tension tends to make expansion difficult. According to the law of Laplace, the pressure (P) required to inflate a sphere is equal to two times the surface tension ($2T$) divided by the radius (r) of the sphere, or $P = (2T/r)$. As the radius of the sphere (or alveolus) becomes smaller, more and more pressure is required to inflate it. If the alveoli were lined only with a waterlike fluid, taking breaths would be extremely difficult.

Alveolar ventilation, or distention, is made possible by surfactant, which lowers surface tension by coating the air-liquid interface in the alveoli. Surfactant, a lipoprotein produced by type II alveolar cells, has a detergent-like effect that separates the liquid molecules, thereby decreasing alveolar surface tension.

Surfactant lines the alveolar side of the alveolocapillary membrane and reverses the law of Laplace. As the radius of a surfactant-lined sphere (alveolus) grows smaller, the surface tension *decreases,* and as the radius grows larger, the surface tension *increases.* This occurs because the smaller radius causes surfactant molecules to crowd together and then repel one another strongly. A larger radius spreads them apart, decreasing their mutual repellence. Therefore normal alveoli are much easier to inflate at low lung volumes (i.e., after expiration) than at high volumes (i.e., after inspiration). If surfactant production is disrupted or surfactant is not produced in adequate quantities, alveolar surface tension increases and results in alveolar collapse, decreased lung expansion, increased work of breathing, and severe gas-exchange abnormalities.

The decrease in surface tension caused by surfactant is also responsible for keeping the alveoli free of fluid. In the absence of surfactant, water tends to move into the alveoli.

Elastic properties of the lung and chest wall

The lung and chest wall have elastic properties that permit expansion during inspiration and return to resting volume (FRC) during expiration. Elastin fibers in the alveolar walls and surrounding the small airways and pulmonary capillaries, as well as surface tension at the alveolar air-liquid interface, produce this effect. The *elasticity* of the chest wall is the result of the configuration of its bones and musculature.

Elastic recoil is the tendency of the lungs to return to the resting state after inspiration. Normal elastic recoil permits passive expiration, eliminating the need for major muscles of expiration. Passive elastic recoil may be insufficient during labored breathing (high minute volume), when the accessory muscles of expiration are used. The accessory muscles are also used if disease compromises elastic recoil (e.g., in emphysema) or blocks the conducting airways.

Normal elastic recoil depends on an equilibrium between opposing forces of recoil in the lungs and chest wall. Under normal conditions the chest wall tends to recoil by expanding outward. The tendency of the chest wall to recoil by expanding is balanced by the tendency of the lungs to recoil or collapse around the hili. This reaction is caused by elastic recoil and surface tension in the alveoli. The opposing forces of the chest wall and lungs create, in part, the negative intrapleural pressure.

Balance between the outward recoil of the chest wall and inward recoil of the lungs occurs at the resting level, the end of expiration, where the FRC is reached. During inspiration, the diaphragm and intercostal muscles contract, air flows into the lungs, and the chest wall expands. Muscular effort is needed to overcome the resistance of the lungs to expansion. During expiration, the muscles relax and the elastic recoil of the lungs causes the thorax to decrease in volume until, once again, balance between the chest wall and lung recoil forces is reached[5] (Fig. 25-13).

Compliance is the measure of lung and chest wall distensibility and is defined as volume change per unit of pressure change. It represents the relative ease with which these structures can be stretched and is, therefore, the opposite of elasticity. Compliance is determined by alveolar surface tension and the elastic recoil of the lung and chest wall.

Increased compliance indicates that the lungs or chest wall is abnormally easy to inflate and has lost some elastic recoil. A decrease indicates that the lungs or chest wall is abnormally stiff or difficult to inflate. Compliance is increased in normal aging and in emphysema and is decreased in adult respiratory distress syndrome, pneumonia, pulmonary edema, and fibrosis. (These disorders are described in Chapter 26.)

Airway resistance

Airway resistance, which is similar to resistance to blood flow (described in Chapter 22), is determined by the length, radius, and cross-sectional area of the airways and density, viscosity, and velocity of the gas (Poiseuille law). Resistance (R) is computed by dividing change in pressure (P) by rate of flow (F), or $R = P/F$ (Ohm law). Airway resistance is normally very low. One half to two thirds of total airway resistance occurs in the nose. The next highest resistance is in the oropharynx and larynx. There is very little resistance in the conducting airways of the lungs because of their large cross-sectional area. The most common causes of increased airway resistance are swelling (edema), obstruction (i.e., mucous plugging), and spasm of bronchial smooth muscle (bronchospasm), all of which decrease the radius of the airways. Resistance increases as the diameter of the airways (and total cross-sectional area) decreases.

Work of breathing

The work of breathing is determined by the muscular effort (and therefore oxygen and energy) required for ventilation. Normally very low, the work of breathing may increase considerably in diseases that disrupt the equilibrium between forces exerted by the lung and chest wall. More muscular effort is required when lung compliance is decreased (e.g., in pulmonary edema), chest wall compliance is decreased (e.g., in spinal deformity or obesity), or airways are obstructed by bronchospasm or mucous plugging (e.g., in asthma or bronchitis). An increase in the work of breathing can be life threatening when oxygen delivery also is impaired (e.g., in anemia).

✓ QUICK CHECK

Describe the work of the diaphragm in ventilation.

What is surfactant? What is its function?

How is elastic recoil related to compliance?

Where is airway resistance found?

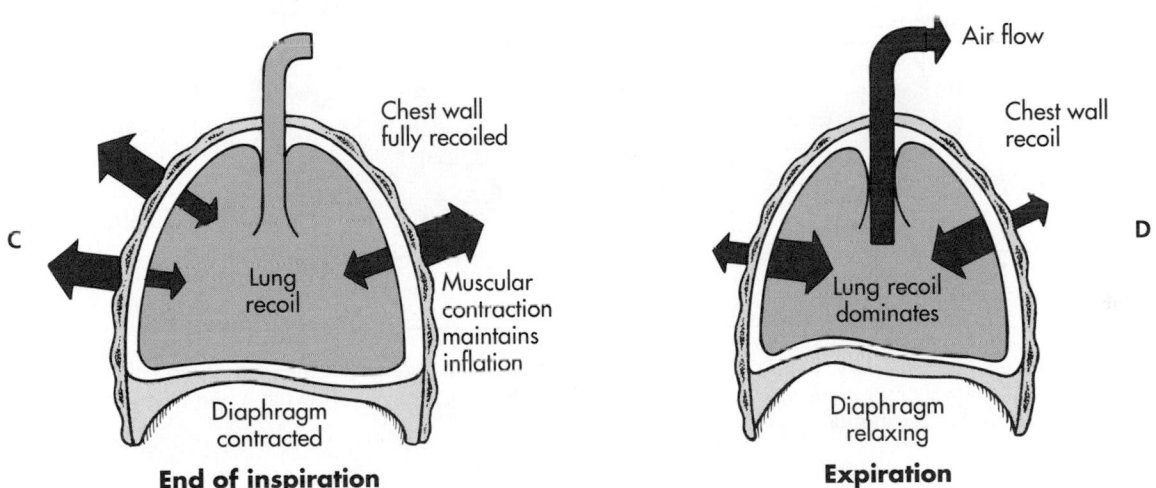

Fig. 25-13 *Interaction of forces during inspiration and expiration.* **A,** Outward recoil of the chest wall equals inward recoil of the lungs at the end of expiration. **B,** During inspiration, contraction of respiratory muscles, assisted by chest wall recoil, overcomes tendency of lungs to recoil. **C,** At the end of inspiration, respiratory muscle contraction maintains lung expansion. **D,** During expiration, respiratory muscles relax, allowing elastic recoil of the lungs to deflate the lungs.

Gas Transport

Gas transport, the delivery of oxygen to the cells of the body and the removal of carbon dioxide, has four steps: (1) ventilation of the lungs, (2) diffusion of oxygen from the alveoli into the capillary blood, (3) perfusion of systemic capillaries with oxygenated blood, and (4) diffusion of oxygen from systemic capillaries into the cells. Steps in the transport of carbon dioxide occur in reverse order: (1) diffusion of carbon dioxide from the cells into the systemic capillaries, (2) perfusion of the pulmonary capillary bed by venous blood, (3) diffusion of carbon dioxide into the alveoli, and

(4) removal of carbon dioxide from the lung by ventilation. If any step in gas transport is impaired by a respiratory or cardiovascular disorder, gas exchange at the cellular level is compromised.

Distribution of ventilation and perfusion

Effective gas exchange depends on an approximately even distribution of gas (ventilation) and blood (perfusion) in all portions of the lungs. The lungs are suspended from the hili in the thoracic cavity. When an individual is in an upright position (sitting or standing), gravity pulls the lungs down

Fig. 25-14 *Pulmonary blood flow and gravity.* The greatest volume of pulmonary blood flow normally will occur in the gravity-dependent areas of the lung. Body position has a significant effect on the distribution of pulmonary blood flow.

toward the diaphragm and compresses their lower portions or bases. The alveoli in the upper portions, or apexes, of the lungs contain a greater residual volume of gas and are larger and less numerous than those in the lower portions. Because surface tension increases as the alveoli become larger, the larger alveoli in the upper portions of the lung are more difficult to inflate (less compliant) than the smaller alveoli in the lower portions of the lung. Therefore during ventilation most of the tidal volume is distributed to the bases of the lungs, where compliance is greater.

The heart pumps against gravity to perfuse the pulmonary circulation. As blood is pumped into the lung apexes of a sitting or standing individual, some blood pressure is dissipated in overcoming gravity. As a result, blood pressure at the apexes is lower than that at the bases. Because greater pressure causes greater perfusion, the bases of the lungs are better perfused than the apexes (Fig. 25-14). Thus ventilation and perfusion are greatest in the same lung portions—the lower lobes—and depend on body position. If a standing individual assumes a supine or side-lying posi-

tion, the areas of the lungs that are then most dependent become the best ventilated and perfused.

Distribution of perfusion in the pulmonary circulation also is affected by alveolar pressure (gas pressure in the alveoli). The pulmonary capillary bed differs from the systemic capillary bed in that it is surrounded by gas-containing alveoli. If the gas pressure in the alveoli exceeds the blood pressure in the capillary, the capillary collapses and flow ceases. This is most likely to occur in portions of the lung where blood pressure is lowest and alveolar gas volume and therefore pressure are greatest, that is, at the apex of the lung.

The lungs are divided into three zones on the basis of relationships among all the factors affecting pulmonary blood flow. Alveolar pressure plus the forces of gravity, arterial blood pressure, and venous blood pressure affect the distribution of perfusion, as shown in Fig. 25-15.

In zone I alveolar pressure exceeds pulmonary arterial and venous pressures. The capillary bed collapses, and normal blood flow ceases. Normally zone I is a very small part of the lung at the apex. In zone II alveolar pressure is greater

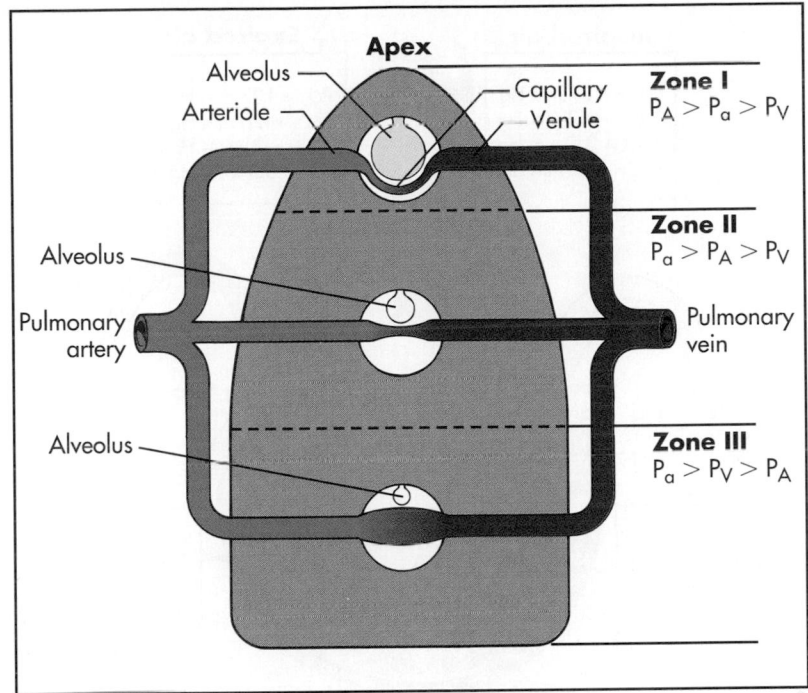

Fig. 25-15 *Gravity and alveolar pressure.* Effects of gravity and alveolar pressure on pulmonary blood flow in the three lung zones. In zone I, alveolar pressure *(P_A)* is greater than arterial and venous pressure, and no blood flow occurs. In zone II, arterial pressure *(P_a)* exceeds alveolar pressure, but alveolar pressure exceeds venous pressure *(P_V)*. Blood flow occurs in this zone, but alveolar pressure compresses the venules (venous ends of the capillaries). In zone III, both arterial and venous pressures are greater than alveolar pressure and blood flow fluctuates depending on the difference between arterial and venous pressure.

than venous pressure but not arterial pressure. Blood flows through zone II, but it is impeded to a certain extent by alveolar pressure. Zone II is normally above the level of the left atrium. In zone III both arterial and venous pressures are greater than alveolar pressure and blood flow is not affected by alveolar pressure. Zone III is in the base of the lung. Blood flow through the pulmonary capillary bed increases in regular increments from the apex to the base.

Although both blood flow and ventilation are greater at the base of the lungs than at the apexes, they are not perfectly matched in any zone. Perfusion exceeds ventilation in the bases, and ventilation exceeds perfusion in the apexes of the lung. The relationship between ventilation and perfusion is expressed as a ratio called the **ventilation-perfusion ratio** *(V̇/Q̇)*. The normal V̇/Q̇ ratio is 0.8. This is the amount by which perfusion exceeds ventilation under normal conditions.

Oxygen transport

Approximately 1000 ml (1 L) of oxygen is transported to the cells each minute. Oxygen is transported in the blood in two forms: a small amount dissolves in plasma, and the remainder binds to hemoglobin molecules. Without hemoglobin, oxygen would not reach the cells in amounts sufficient to maintain normal metabolic function. (Hemoglobin is discussed in detail in Chapter 19 and cellular metabolism in Chapter 1.)

Diffusion across the alveolocapillary membrane

The alveolocapillary membrane is ideal for oxygen diffusion because it has a large total surface area (70 to 100 m^2) and is very thin (0.5 micrometer [μm]). In addition, the partial pressure of oxygen molecules (PO_2) is much greater in alveolar gas than in capillary blood, a condition that promotes rapid diffusion down the concentration gradient from the alveolus into the capillary. The partial pressure of oxygen (oxygen tension) in mixed venous or pulmonary artery blood ($P\bar{v}O_2$) is approximately 40 mm Hg as it enters the capillary, and alveolar oxygen tension (PAO_2) is approximately 100 mm Hg at sea level. Therefore a pressure gradient of 60 mm Hg facilitates the diffusion of oxygen from the alveolus into the capillary (Fig. 25-16).

Blood remains in the pulmonary capillary for about 0.75 seconds, but only 0.25 seconds is required for oxygen concentration to equilibrate (equalize) across the alveolocapillary membrane. Therefore oxygen has ample time to diffuse into the blood, even during increased cardiac output, which speeds blood flow, shortening the time the blood remains in the capillary.

Determinants of arterial oxygenation

As oxygen diffuses across the alveolocapillary membrane, it dissolves in the plasma, where it exerts pressure (the partial

Inspired air

PO₂ = 159 mm Hg
PCO₂ = 0.3 mm Hg
PH₂O = 3.7 mm Hg
PN₂ = 597 mm Hg

Expired air

PO₂ = 127 mm Hg
PCO₂ = 28 mm Hg
PH₂O = 21 mm Hg
PN₂ = 584 mm Hg

Pulmonary artery

Pulmonary vein

From heart and systemic circulation values

PO₂ = 40 mm Hg
PCO₂ = 46 mm Hg
PH₂O = 47 mm Hg
PN₂ = 573 mm Hg

PO₂ = 104 mm Hg
PCO₂ = 40 mm Hg
PH₂O = 47 mm Hg
PN₂ = 569 mm Hg

To heart and systemic circulation values

PO₂ = 100 mm Hg
PCO₂ = 40 mm Hg
PH₂O = 47 mm Hg
PN₂ = 573 mm Hg

Tissues

PO₂ = 40 mm Hg
PCO₂ = 46 mm Hg
PH₂O = 47 mm Hg
PN₂ = 573 mm Hg

Fig. 25-16 *Partial pressure of respiratory gases in normal respiration.* The numbers shown are average values. The values of PO_2, PCO_2, and PN_2 fluctuate from breath to breath. *(Modified from Thompson, J.M. et al. [1997]. Mosby's clinical nursing [4th ed.]. St. Louis: Mosby.)*

pressure of oxygen in arterial blood, or PaO_2). As the PaO_2 increases, oxygen moves from the plasma into the red blood cells (erythrocytes) and binds with hemoglobin molecules. Oxygen continues to bind with hemoglobin until the hemoglobin binding sites are filled or *saturated.* Oxygen then continues to diffuse across the alveolocapillary membrane until the PaO_2 (oxygen dissolved in plasma) and PAO_2 equilibrate, eliminating the pressure gradient across the alveolocapillary membrane. At this point diffusion ceases (see Fig. 25-16).

Normally approximately 20 ml oxygen is transported per 100 ml blood. Because oxygen is not very soluble in plasma, most of the oxygen molecules bind with hemoglobin. Plasma carries only about 0.3 ml of oxygen per 100 ml of blood (at sea level). Although the remaining 19.7 ml is carried by hemoglobin, it is the small amount of oxygen dissolved in plasma that is responsible for oxygen's partial pressure (PaO_2) in the blood.

Although PaO_2 is important in that it provides the driving pressure that loads the hemoglobin with oxygen, it gives little information about the *amount* of oxygen carried in the blood. This amount, which is measured in milliliters per deciliter (100 ml) of blood, is the *oxygen content* of the blood. The total oxygen content of the blood depends on the amount of oxygen chemically combined with hemoglobin, as well as that dissolved in the blood. To calculate the total arterial oxygen content, one must know (1) hemoglobin concentration, or the amount of hemoglobin that is available to bind with oxygen (Hb in g/dl); (2) the *oxygen saturation* or percentage of available hemoglobin that is bound to oxygen (SaO_2); and (3) the partial pressure of oxygen (PaO_2). The maximum amount of oxygen that can be transported by hemoglobin is 1.34 ml/g. The amount of oxygen that can be physically dissolved in blood is 0.003 ml/dl per mm Hb PO_2. If these specific values are known, the oxygen content of arterial blood can be calculated[6]:

$$O_2 \text{ content} = (Hb \times SaO_2 \times 1.34) + (PaO_2 \times 0.003)$$

To calculate the oxygen content of venous blood, the partial pressure of mixed venous blood ($P\bar{v}O_2$) and venous oxygen saturation ($S\bar{v}O_2$) are substituted for the arterial values in the basic formula. Normal venous oxygen content is 15 to 16 ml/dl.

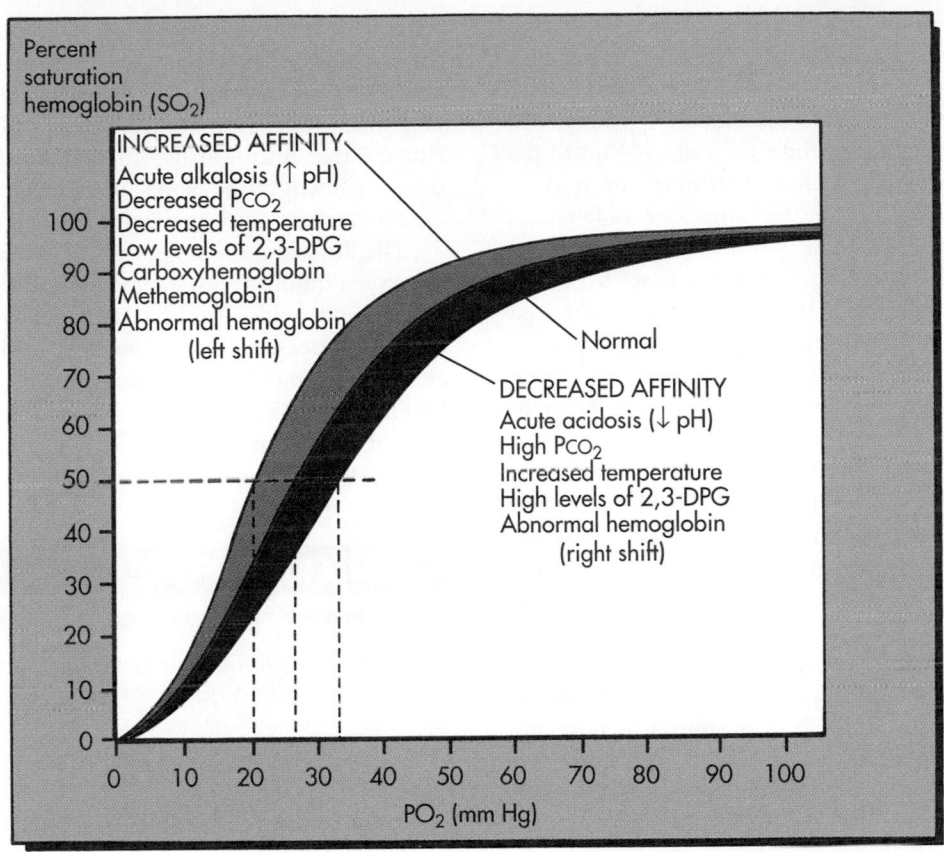

Fig. 25-17 *Oxyhemoglobin dissociation curve.* The horizontal or flat segment of the curve at the top of the graph is the arterial or association portion, or that part of the curve where oxygen is bound to hemoglobin and occurs in the lungs. This portion of the curve is flat because partial pressure changes of oxygen between 60 and 100 mm Hg do not significantly alter the percent saturation of hemoglobin with oxygen and allow adequate hemoglobin saturation at a variety of altitudes. If the relationship between SaO_2 and PaO_2 were linear (in a downward sloping straight line) instead of flat between 60 and 100 mm Hg, there would be inadequate saturation of hemoglobin with oxygen. The steep part of the oxyhemoglobin dissociation curve represents the rapid dissociation of oxygen from hemoglobin that occurs in the tissues. During this phase there is rapid diffusion of oxygen from the blood into tissue cells. The P_{50} is the PaO_2 at which hemoglobin is 50% saturated, normally 26.6 mm Hg. A lower than normal P_{50} represents increased affinity of hemoglobin for O_2; a high P_{50} is seen with decreased affinity. Note that variation from the normal is associated with decreased (low P_{50}) or increased (high P_{50}) availability of O_2 to tissues *(dotted lines)*. The shaded area shows the entire oxyhemoglobin dissociation curve under the same circumstances. *2,3-DPG,* 2,3-Diphosphoglycerate. *(From Lane, E.E. & Walker, J.F. [1987]. Clinical arterial blood gas analysis. St. Louis: Mosby.)*

Because hemoglobin transports all but a small fraction of the oxygen carried in arterial blood, changes in hemoglobin concentration affect the oxygen content of the blood. Decreases in hemoglobin concentration below the normal value of 15 ml/dl blood reduce oxygen content, and increases in hemoglobin concentration may increase oxygen content, minimizing the impact of impaired gas exchange. In fact, increased hemoglobin concentration is a major compensatory mechanism in pulmonary diseases that impair gas exchange. For this reason, measurement of hemoglobin concentration is important in assessing individuals with pulmonary disease. If cardiovascular function is normal, the body's initial response to low oxygen content is to speed up cardiac output. In individuals who also have cardiovascular disease, this compensatory mechanism does not work, making increased

hemoglobin concentration an even more important compensatory mechanism. (Hemoglobin structure and function are described in Chapter 19.)

Oxyhemoglobin association and dissociation
When hemoglobin molecules bind with oxygen, ***oxyhemoglobin (HbO_2)*** forms. Binding occurs in the lungs and is called oxyhemoglobin association or hemoglobin saturation with oxygen (SaO_2). The reverse process, where oxygen is released from hemoglobin, occurs in the body tissues at the cellular level and is called hemoglobin desaturation. When hemoglobin saturation and desaturation are plotted on a graph, the result is a distinctive S-shaped curve known as the ***oxyhemoglobin dissociation curve*** (Fig. 25-17).

Several factors can change the relationship between

PaO_2 and SaO_2, causing the oxyhemoglobin dissociation curve to shift to the right or left (see Fig. 25-17). A shift to the right depicts hemoglobin's decreased affinity for oxygen or an increase in the ease with which oxyhemoglobin dissociates and oxygen moves into the cells. A shift to the left depicts hemoglobin's increased affinity for oxygen, which promotes association in the lungs and inhibits dissociation in the tissues.

The oxyhemoglobin dissociation curve is shifted to the right by acidosis (low pH) and hypercapnia (increased $PaCO_2$). In the tissues, the increased levels of carbon dioxide and hydrogen ions produced by metabolic activity decrease the affinity of hemoglobin for oxygen. The curve is shifted to the left by alkalosis (high pH) and hypocapnia (decreased $PaCO_2$). In the lungs, as carbon dioxide diffuses from the blood into the alveoli, the blood carbon dioxide level is reduced and the affinity of hemoglobin for oxygen is increased. The shift in the oxyhemoglobin dissociation curve by changes in carbon dioxide and hydrogen ion concentrations in the blood is called the *Bohr effect*.[7]

The oxyhemoglobin curve is also shifted by changes in body temperature and increased or decreased levels of 2,3-diphosphoglycerate (2,3-DPG), a substance normally present in erythrocytes. Hyperthermia and increased 2,3-DPG levels shift the curve to the right. Hypothermia and decreased 2,3-DPG levels shift the curve to the left.

Carbon dioxide transport

Carbon dioxide is carried in the blood in three ways: (1) dissolved in plasma (PCO_2), (2) as bicarbonate, and (3) as carbamino compounds. As CO_2 diffuses out of the cells into the blood, it dissolves in the plasma. Approximately 10% of the total CO_2 in venous blood and 5% of the CO_2 in arterial blood are carried dissolved in the plasma (PCO_2). As CO_2 moves into the blood, it diffuses into the red blood cells. Within the red blood cells, CO_2, with the help of the enzyme carbonic anhydrase, combines with water to form carbonic acid and then quickly dissociates into H^+ and HCO_3^-. As carbonic acid dissociates, the H^+ binds to hemoglobin, where it is buffered, and the HCO_3^- moves out of the red blood cell into the plasma. Approximately 60% of the CO_2 in venous blood and 90% of the CO_2 in arterial blood are carried in the form of bicarbonate. The remainder combines with blood proteins, hemoglobin in particular, to form carbamino compounds. Approximately 30% of the CO_2 in venous blood and 5% of the CO_2 in arterial blood are carried as carbamino compounds (see Fig. 4-5).

CO_2 is 20 times more soluble than O_2 and diffuses very quickly from the tissue cells into the blood. The amount of CO_2 able to enter the blood is enhanced by diffusion of oxygen out of the blood and into the cells. Reduced hemoglobin (hemoglobin that is dissociated from oxygen) can carry more CO_2 than can hemoglobin that is saturated with O_2. Therefore the drop in SO_2 at the tissue level increases the ability of hemoglobin to carry CO_2 back to the lung.

The diffusion gradient for CO_2 in the lung is only approximately 6 mm Hg (venous PCO_2 = 46 mm Hg; alveolar

PCO_2 = 40 mm Hg) (see Fig. 25-16). Yet CO_2 is so soluble in the alveolocapillary membrane that the CO_2 in the blood quickly diffuses into the alveoli, where it is removed from the lung with each expiration. Diffusion of CO_2 in the lung is so efficient that diffusion defects that cause hypoxemia (low oxygen content of the blood) do not as readily cause hypercapnia (excessive carbon dioxide in the blood).

The diffusion of CO_2 out of the blood is also enhanced by oxygen binding with hemoglobin in the lung. As hemoglobin binds with O_2, the amount of CO_2 carried by the blood is decreased. Thus in the tissue capillaries, O_2 dissociation from hemoglobin facilitates the pickup of CO_2, and the binding of O_2 to hemoglobin in the lungs facilitates the release of CO_2 from the blood. This effect of oxygen on CO_2 transport is called the *Haldane effect*.[8]

Control of the Pulmonary Circulation

The caliber of pulmonary artery lumina decreases as smooth muscle in the arterial walls contracts. Contraction increases pulmonary artery pressure. Caliber increases as these muscles relax, decreasing blood pressure. Contraction (vasoconstriction) and relaxation (vasodilation) apparently occur in response to local humoral conditions, even though the pulmonary circulation is innervated by the ANS like the systemic circulation.

The most important cause of pulmonary artery constriction is a low alveolar PO_2 (PaO_2). Vasoconstriction caused by alveolar hypoxia, often termed *hypoxic vasoconstriction,* can affect only one portion of the lung (i.e., one lobe that is obstructed, decreasing its PaO_2) or the entire lung. If only one segment of the lung is involved, the arterioles to that segment constrict, shunting blood to other, well-ventilated portions of the lung. This reflex improves the lung's efficiency by better matching ventilation and perfusion. If hypoventilation affects all segments of the lung, however, pulmonary hypertension (elevated pulmonary artery pressure) can result. The pulmonary vasoconstriction caused by low alveolar PO_2 is reversible if the alveolar PO_2 is corrected. Chronic alveolar hypoxia can result in permanent pulmonary artery hypertension, which eventually leads to right heart failure (cor pulmonale).

Acidemia also causes pulmonary artery constriction. If the acidemia is corrected, the vasoconstriction is reversed. (Respiratory acidosis and metabolic acidosis are described in

Chapter 4.) An elevated $PaCO_2$ without a drop in pH does not cause pulmonary artery constriction. Other biochemical factors that affect the caliber of vessels in pulmonary circulation are histamine, prostaglandins, serotonin, and bradykinin.

✓ QUICK CHECK
What is the most important factor causing pulmonary artery constriction? What other factors are involved?

⚠ AGING & *The Pulmonary System*

ELASTICITY/CHEST WALL
Chest wall compliance decreases because ribs become ossified and joints grow stiffer.
Kyphoscoliosis may curve the vertebral column.
Elastic recoil diminishes, possibly the result of loss of elastic fibers.
Result: Increased lung compliance and reduced ventilatory capacity (VC), residual volume (RV) increases, total lung capacity (TLC) is unchanged, ventilatory reserves are reduced, ventilation-perfusion ratios fall.

GAS EXCHANGE
Decreased pulmonary capillary network.
Decreased surface area for gas exchange.
pH and PCO_2 do not change much, but Po_2 declines.
Note: Maximum PaO_2 at sea level can be estimated by multiplying person's age by 0.3 and subtracting the product from 100.

EXERCISE
Decreased Pao_2 and diminished ventilatory reserve lead to decreased exercise tolerance.
Early airway closure inhibits expiratory flow.
Changes depend on activity and fitness levels earlier in life.
Very active, physically fit individual has fewer changes in function at any age than sedentary individual.
Respiratory muscle strength and endurance decrease but can be enhanced by exercise.

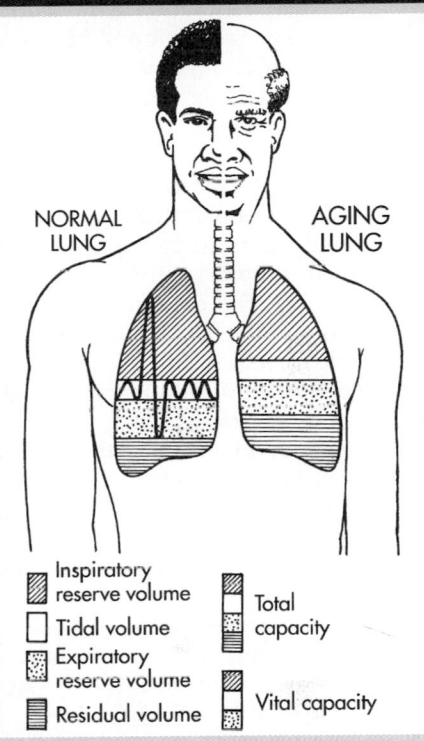

Inspiratory reserve volume
Tidal volume
Expiratory reserve volume
Residual volume
Total capacity
Vital capacity

Changes in lung volumes with aging. With aging, note particularly the decrease in vital capacity and the increase in residual volume.

From Timiras, P.S. (1994). Physiological basis of aging and geriatrics *(2nd ed.).* Boca Raton, Fla.: CRC Press.

▣ DID YOU UNDERSTAND?

Structures of the Pulmonary System
1. The pulmonary system consists of the lungs, airways, chest wall, and pulmonary and bronchial circulation.
2. Air is inspired and expired through the conducting airways, which include the nasopharynx, oropharynx, trachea, bronchi, and bronchioles to the sixteenth division.
3. Gas exchange occurs in structures beyond the sixteenth division: the respiratory bronchioles, alveolar ducts, and the alveoli. Together these structures compose the acinus.
4. The chief gas-exchange units of the lungs are the alveoli. The membrane that surrounds each alveolus and contains the pulmonary capillaries is called the *alveolocapillary membrane.*
5. The gas-exchange airways are served by the pulmonary circulation, a separate division of the circulatory system. The bronchi and other lung structures are served by a branch of the systemic circulation called the *bronchial circulation.*
6. The chest wall, which contains and protects the contents of the thoracic cavity, consists of the skin, ribs, and intercostal muscles, which lie between the ribs.
7. The chest wall is lined by a serous membrane called the *parietal pleura;* the lungs are encased in a separate membrane called the *visceral pleura.* The area where these two pleurae come into contact and slide over one another is called the *pleural space.*

Continued

DID YOU UNDERSTAND? —cont'd

Function of the Pulmonary System

1. The pulmonary system enables oxygen to diffuse into the blood and carbon dioxide to diffuse out of the blood.
2. Ventilation is the process by which air flows into and out of the gas-exchange airways.
3. Most of the time, ventilation is involuntary. It is controlled by the sympathetic and parasympathetic divisions of the autonomic nervous system, which adjust airway caliber (by causing bronchial smooth muscle to contract or relax) and control the rate and depth of ventilation.
4. Neuroreceptors in the lungs (lung receptors) monitor the mechanical aspects of ventilation. Irritant receptors sense the need to expel unwanted substances; stretch receptors sense lung volume (lung expansion); and J-receptors sense alveolar size.
5. Chemoreceptors in the circulatory system and brain stem sense the effectiveness of ventilation by monitoring the pH status of cerebrospinal fluid and the oxygen content (Po_2) of arterial blood.
6. Successful ventilation involves the mechanics of breathing: the interaction of forces and counterforces involving the muscles of inspiration and expiration, alveolar surface tension, elastic properties of the lungs and chest wall, and resistance to air flow.
7. The major muscle of inspiration is the diaphragm. When the diaphragm contracts, it moves downward in the thoracic cavity, creating a vacuum that causes air to flow into the lungs.
8. The alveoli produce surfactant, a lipoprotein that lines the alveoli. Surfactant reduces alveolar surface tension and permits the alveoli to expand as air flows in.
9. Compliance is the ease with which the lungs and chest wall expand during inspiration. Lung compliance is ensured by adequate production of surfactant, whereas chest wall expansion depends on flexibility.
10. Elastic recoil is the tendency of the lungs and chest wall to return to their resting state after inspiration. The elastic recoil forces of the lungs and chest wall are in opposition and pull on each other, creating the normally negative pressure of the pleural space.
11. Gas transport depends on ventilation of the alveoli, diffusion across the alveolocapillary membrane, perfusion of the pulmonary and systemic capillaries, and diffusion between systemic capillaries and tissue cells.
12. Efficient gas exchange depends on an even distribution of ventilation and perfusion within the lungs. Both ventilation and perfusion are greatest in the bases of the lungs because the alveoli in the bases are more compliant (their resting volume is low) and perfusion is greater in the bases as a result of gravity.
13. Almost all the oxygen that diffuses into pulmonary capillary blood is transported by hemoglobin, a protein contained within red blood cells. The remainder of the oxygen is transported dissolved in plasma.
14. Oxygen enters the body by diffusing down the concentration gradient, from high concentrations in the alveoli to lower concentrations in the capillaries. Diffusion ceases when alveolar and capillary oxygen pressures equilibrate.
15. Oxygen is loaded onto hemoglobin by the driving pressure exerted by PaO_2 in the plasma. As pressure decreases at the tissue level, oxygen dissociates from hemoglobin and enters tissue cells by diffusion, again down the concentration gradient.
16. Carbon dioxide is more soluble in plasma than oxygen is. Therefore carbon dioxide diffuses readily from tissue cells into plasma. Carbon dioxide returns to the lungs dissolved in plasma, as bicarbonate, or in carbamino compounds (e.g., bound to hemoglobin).
17. The pulmonary circulation is innervated by the autonomic nervous system (ANS), but vasodilation and vasoconstriction are controlled mainly by local and humoral factors, particularly arterial oxygenation and acid-base status.

AGING AND THE PULMONARY SYSTEM

1. Aging affects the mechanical aspects of ventilation by decreasing chest wall compliance and elastic recoil of the lungs. Changes in these elastic properties reduce ventilatory reserve.
2. Aging causes the PaO_2 to decrease but does not affect the $PaCO_2$.

KEY TERMS

Acinus, 721
Alveolar dead space, 726
Alveolar duct, 721
Alveolar ventilation ($\dot{A}$), 726
Alveolocapillary membrane, 722
Alveolus (pl., alveoli), 721
Anatomic dead space, 726
Bohr effect, 736
Bronchus (pl., bronchi), 721
Carina, 721
Central chemoreceptor, 727
Compliance, 730
Dead-space ventilation ($\dot{D}$), 726
Elastic recoil, 730
Elasticity, 730
Expiratory reserve volume (ERV), 726
Functional residual capacity (FRC), 726

Goblet cell, 721
Haldane effect, 736
Hilus (pl., hili), 721
Hypoxic vasoconstriction, 736
Inspiratory capacity (IC), 726
Inspiratory reserve volume (IRV), 726
Irritant receptor, 727
J-receptor, 727
Larynx, 719
Nasopharynx, 719
Oropharynx, 719
Oxygen content, 734
Oxygen saturation, 734
Oxyhemoglobin (HbO_2), 735
Oxyhemoglobin dissociation curve, 735
Partial pressure of a gas, 724
Peripheral chemoreceptor, 727

Physiologic dead space, 726
Pleura (pl., pleurae), 723
Pleural space (pleural cavity), 723
Residual volume (RV), 726
Respiratory bronchiole, 721
Respiratory center, 727
Stretch receptor, 727
Surface tension, 729
Surfactant, 721
Thoracic cavity, 723
Tidal volume (V_T), 726
Total lung capacity (TLC), 726
Trachea, 721
Ventilation, 724
Ventilation-perfusion ratio ($\dot{V}/\dot{Q}$), 733
Vital capacity (VC), 726

REFERENCES

1. Charan, N.B. & Carvalho, P.G. (1992). Anatomy of the normal bronchial circulatory system in humans and animals. In J. Butler (Ed.). *The bronchial circulation.* New York: Marcel Dekker.

2. Fraser, R.G. et al. (1994). *Synopsis of diseases of the chest* (2nd ed.). Philadelphia: Saunders.

3. Beachey, W. & Scanlan, C.L. (1998). Acid-base balance and the regulation of respiration. In C.L. Scanlan, C.G. Spearman, & R.L. Sheldon (Eds.). *Egan's fundamentals of respiratory care* (7th ed.). St. Louis: Mosby.

4. Seeley, R.R., Stephens, T.D., & Tate, P.P. (1995). *Anatomy and physiology* (3rd ed.). St. Louis: Mosby.

5. Scanlan, C.L. & Ruppel, G.L. (1998). Ventilation. In C.L. Scanlan, C.B. Spearman, & R.L. Sheldon (Eds.). *Egan's fundamentals of respiratory care* (7th ed.). St. Louis: Mosby.

6. Gross, G.W. & Scanlan, C.L. (1998). Gas exchange and transport. In C. Scanlan, C.B. Spearman, & R.L. Sheldon (Eds.). *Egan's fundamentals of respiratory care* (7th ed.). St. Louis: Mosby.

7. Ganong, W.F. (1997). *Review of medical physiology.* (19th ed.). Norwalk, Conn.: Appleton & Lange.

8. Guyton, A. (1996). *Textbook of medical physiology* (9th ed.). Philadelphia: Saunders.

CHAPTER

26

Alterations of Pulmonary Function

Valentina L. Brashers

Pulmonary disease is often classified as acute or chronic, obstructive or restrictive, or infectious or noninfectious and is caused by alteration in the lung or heart. Because skillful and knowledgeable clinical care plays a major role in decreasing respiratory mortality and morbidity, the clinician who has a clear understanding of the pathophysiology of common respiratory problems can greatly affect the outcome for each individual.

The lungs, with their large surface area, are constantly exposed to the external environment. Therefore lung disease is greatly influenced by conditions of the environment, occupation, and personal and social habits. Symptoms of lung disease are common and associated not only with primary lung disorders but also with diseases of other organ systems.

CHAPTER OUTLINE

 Check out your CD Companion for chapter-related exercises and answers to the Quick Check questions

CLINICAL MANIFESTATIONS OF PULMONARY ALTERATIONS
Signs and Symptoms of Pulmonary Disease

Pulmonary disease is associated with many signs and symptoms, the most common of which are cough and dyspnea. Others include chest pain, abnormal sputum, hemoptysis, altered breathing patterns, cyanosis, and fever.

Dyspnea

Dyspnea is the subjective sensation of uncomfortable breathing, the feeling of inability to get enough air. It is often described as breathlessness, air hunger, shortness of breath, labored breathing, and preoccupation with breathing.

Dyspnea is usually caused by diffuse and extensive rather than focal pulmonary disease. Disturbances of ventilation, gas exchange, or ventilation-perfusion relationships can cause dyspnea, as can increased work of breathing or diseases that severely damage lung tissue (lung parenchyma).

The signs of dyspnea include flaring of the nostrils, use of accessory muscles of respiration, and retraction (pulling back) of the intercostal spaces. In dyspnea caused by parenchymal disease (e.g., pneumonia), retractions of tissue between the ribs (subcostal and intercostal retractions) are observed more frequently than supercostal retractions (retractions of tissues above the ribs), which predominate in upper airway obstruction.

Dyspnea can occur transiently or in specific circumstances. Frequently the first episode occurs with exercise and is called *dyspnea on exertion.* Pulmonary congestion tends to cause dyspnea when the individual is lying down *(orthopnea).* The horizontal position redistributes body water, causes the abdominal contents to exert pressure on the diaphragm, or decreases the efficiency of the respiratory muscles. Orthopnea generally is relieved by sitting up in a forward-leaning posture or supporting the upper body on several pillows. Some individuals with left ventricular failure wake up at night gasping for air and have to sit up or stand to relieve the dyspnea *(paroxysmal nocturnal dyspnea [PND]).* PND results from fluid in the lungs caused by the redistribution of body water while the individual is recumbent.[1]

Abnormal breathing patterns

Normal breathing (eupnea) is rhythmic and effortless. Ventilatory rate is 8 to 16 breaths per minute, and tidal volume ranges from 400 to 800 ml. A short expiratory pause occurs with each breath, and the individual takes an occasional deeper breath, or sighs. Sigh breaths, which help to maintain normal lung function, are usually $1\frac{1}{2}$ to 2 times the normal tidal volume and occur approximately 10 to 12 times per hour.

The rate, depth, regularity, and effort of breathing undergo characteristic alterations in response to physiologic and pathophysiologic conditions. Patterns of breathing automatically adjust to minimize the work of respiratory muscles. Strenuous exercise or metabolic acidosis induces *Kussmaul respiration (hyperpnea),* which is characterized by a slightly increased ventilatory rate, very large tidal volumes, and no expiratory pause.

Labored, or obstructed, breathing occurs if the airways are obstructed, as in chronic obstructive pulmonary disease. A slow ventilatory rate, large tidal volume, increased effort, and prolonged inspiration or expiration, depending on the site of obstruction, are typical. Audible wheezing (whistling sounds) or stridor (high-pitched sounds made during inspiration) is often present.

Restricted breathing is commonly caused by disorders, such as pulmonary fibrosis, that stiffen the lungs or chest wall and decrease compliance. Small tidal volumes and rapid ventilatory rate (tachypnea) are characteristic.

Panting occurs with exercise. Shock and severe cerebral hypoxia (insufficient oxygen in the brain) contribute to gasping respirations that consist of irregular, quick inspirations with an expiratory pause. Sighing respirations consist of irregular breathing characterized by frequent, deep sighing inspirations. They are caused by anxiety.

Cheyne-Stokes respirations are characterized by alternating periods of deep and shallow breathing. Apnea lasting from 15 to 60 seconds is followed by ventilations that increase in volume until a peak is reached; then ventilation (tidal volume) decreases again to apnea. Cheyne-Stokes respirations result from any condition that slows the blood flow to the brain stem, which in turn slows impulses sending information to the respiratory centers of the brain stem. Neurologic impairment above the brain stem is also a contributing factor.

Hypoventilation/hyperventilation

Hypoventilation is inadequate alveolar ventilation in relation to metabolic demands. It is caused by alterations in pulmonary mechanics or in the neurologic control of breathing. When alveolar ventilation is normal, carbon dioxide (CO_2) is removed from the lungs at the same rate as it is produced by cellular metabolism; therefore arterial and alveolar PCO_2 values remain at normal levels (40 mm Hg). With hypoventilation, CO_2 removal does not keep up with CO_2 production and $PaCO_2$ increases, causing *hypercapnia* ($PaCO_2$ more than 44 mm Hg). (See Table 25-2 for a definition of gas partial pressures and other pulmonary abbreviations.)

Hypoventilation is often overlooked until it is severe because breathing pattern and ventilatory rate may appear to be normal. Blood gas analysis (i.e., measurement of the $PaCO_2$ of arterial blood) reveals the hypoventilation. Pronounced hypoventilation can cause somnolence or disorientation. PaO_2 may be reduced in those breathing room air.

Hyperventilation is alveolar ventilation exceeding metabolic demands. The lungs remove CO_2 faster than it is produced by cellular metabolism, resulting in decreased $PaCO_2$, or *hypocapnia* ($PaCO_2$ less than 36 mm Hg). Like hypoventilation, hyperventilation can be determined only by arterial blood gas analysis. It occurs with severe anxiety, acute head injury, and conditions that cause insufficient oxygenation of the blood.

Cough

A *cough* is a protective reflex that cleanses the lower airways by an explosive expiration. Inhaled particles, accumulated mucus, inflammation, or the presence of a foreign body initiates the cough reflex by stimulating the irritant receptors in the airway. The cough consists of inspiration, closure of the glottis and vocal cords, contraction of the expiratory muscles, and reopening of the glottis, causing a sudden, forceful expiration that removes the offending matter. The effectiveness of the cough depends on the depth of the inspiration and the degree to which the airways narrow, increasing the velocity of expiratory gas flow. Cough occurs frequently in healthy individuals.

A persistent cough indicates the presence of a disorder or disease. An acute, nonproductive cough often indicates bronchitis or viral pneumonia. Aspiration of a foreign body or irritating fumes can cause a dry cough, but persistent dry cough is commonly caused by a tumor, congestion, or hypersensitive airways. A cough that produces purulent sputum usually indicates infection, whereas one that produces nonpurulent sputum is nonspecific and merely indicates irritation. Many individuals swallow their sputum, and a lack of expectorated sputum does not mean that a cough is nonproductive.

Hemoptysis

Hemoptysis is the coughing up of blood or bloody secretions. This is sometimes confused with hematemesis, which is the vomiting of blood. Blood that is coughed up is usually bright red, has an alkaline pH, and is mixed with frothy sputum, whereas blood that is vomited is dark, has an acidic pH, and is mixed with food particles.

Hemoptysis indicates a localized abnormality, usually infection or inflammation that damages the bronchi (bronchitis, bronchiectasis) or the lung parenchyma (tuberculosis, lung abscess). Other causes include cancer and pulmonary infarction. The amount and duration of bleeding provide important clues about its source. Bronchoscopy is used to confirm the site of bleeding.

Cyanosis

Cyanosis is a bluish discoloration of the skin and mucous membranes caused by increasing amounts of desaturated or reduced hemoglobin (which is bluish) in the blood. It generally develops when 5 g of hemoglobin is desaturated, regardless of hemoglobin concentration.

Cyanosis can be caused by decreased arterial oxygenation (low PaO_2), pulmonary or cardiac right-to-left shunts, decreased cardiac output, cold environment, or anxiety. Lack of cyanosis does not necessarily indicate that oxygenation is normal. For example, severe anemia (inadequate hemoglobin concentration) and carbon monoxide poisoning (in which hemoglobin binds to carbon monoxide instead of to oxygen) can cause inadequate oxygenation of tissues without causing cyanosis. Individuals with polycythemia (an abnormal increase in numbers of red blood cells), however, may have cyanosis when oxygenation is adequate. Therefore cyanosis must be interpreted in relation to the underlying pathophysiology. If cyanosis is suggested, the PaO_2 should be measured. Central cyanosis (decreased oxygen saturation of hemoglobin in arterial blood) is best seen in buccal mucous membranes and lips. Peripheral cyanosis (slow blood circulation in fingers and toes) is best seen in nail beds.

Pain

Pain caused by pulmonary disorders originates in the pleurae, airways, or chest wall. Infection and inflammation of the parietal pleura cause pain when the pleura stretches during inspiration. The pain is usually localized to a portion of the chest wall, where a unique breath sound called a *pleural friction rub* can be heard over the painful area. Laughing or coughing makes pleural pain worse. Pleural pain is common with pulmonary infarction (tissue death) caused by pulmonary embolism and emanates from the area around the infarction.

Pulmonary pain is central chest pain that is pronounced after coughing and occurs in individuals with infection and inflammation of the trachea or bronchi (tracheitis or tracheobronchitis). It must be differentiated from cardiac pain. High blood pressure in the pulmonary circulation (pulmonary hypertension) can cause pain during exercise that is often mistaken for cardiac pain (angina pectoris).

Pain in the chest wall is muscle pain or rib pain (costochondritis). Excessive coughing, which makes the muscles sore, and rib fractures produce such pain. Chest wall pain often mimics pleural pain.

Clubbing

Clubbing is the selective bulbous enlargement of the end (distal segment) of a digit (finger or toe) (Fig. 26-1). Usually it is painless. Clubbing is commonly associated with diseases that interfere with oxygenation, such as lung cancer, bronchiectasis, cystic fibrosis, pulmonary fibrosis, lung abscess, and congenital heart disease.

Abnormal sputum

Changes in the amount and consistency of sputum provide information about progression of disease and effectiveness of therapy. The gross and microscopic appearances of sputum enable the clinician to identify cellular debris or microorganisms, which aids in diagnosis and choice of therapy.

Conditions Caused by Pulmonary Disease or Injury
Hypercapnia

Hypercapnia, or increased carbon dioxide in the arterial blood (increased $PaCO_2$), is caused by hypoventilation of the alveoli. As discussed in Chapter 25, carbon dioxide is easily diffused from the blood into the alveolar space; thus minute volume (respiratory rate times tidal volume) determines not

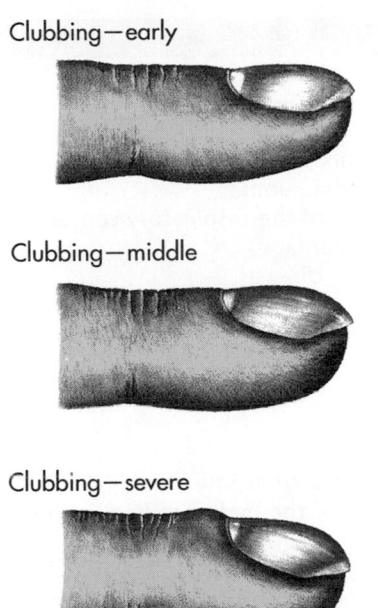

Clubbing—early

Clubbing—middle

Clubbing—severe

Fig. 26-1 *Clubbing of fingers caused by chronic hypoxemia.* *(From Seidel, H.M. et al. [1999].* Mosby's guide to physical examination *[4th ed.]. St. Louis: Mosby.)*

only alveolar ventilation but also $PaCO_2$. Hypoventilation is often overlooked because breathing pattern and ventilatory rate may appear to be normal; it is important to obtain blood gas analysis to determine the severity of hypercapnia and resultant respiratory acidosis (acid-base balance is described in Chapter 4).

There are many causes of hypercapnia. Most are a result of decreased drive to breathe or an inadequate ability to respond to ventilatory stimulation. Some of these causes include (1) depression of the respiratory center by drugs; (2) diseases of the medulla, including infections of the central nervous system or trauma; (3) abnormalities of the spinal conducting pathways, as in spinal cord disruption or poliomyelitis; (4) diseases of the neuromuscular junction or of the respiratory muscles themselves, as in myasthenia gravis or muscular dystrophy; (5) thoracic cage abnormalities, as in chest injury or congenital deformity; (6) large airway obstruction, as in tumors or sleep apnea; and (7) increased work of breathing or physiologic dead space, as in emphysema.

Hypercapnia and the associated respiratory acidosis can result in several important clinical manifestations. Of greatest concern are electrolyte abnormalities that occur in response to the low pH that may cause dysrhythmias. Individuals may also present with somnolence and even coma because of changes in intracranial pressure associated with high levels of arterial carbon dioxide, which causes cerebral vasodilation. Alveolar hypoventilation with increased alveolar CO_2 limits the amount of oxygen available for diffusion into the blood, leading to hypoxemia.

Hypoxemia

Hypoxemia, or reduced oxygenation of arterial blood (reduced PaO_2), is caused by respiratory alterations, whereas *hypoxia,* or reduced oxygenation of cells in tissues, may be caused by alterations of other systems as well. (Hypoxia can occur anywhere in the body; if it occurs in arterial blood, it is correctly called *hypoxemia.*) Although hypoxemia can lead to tissue hypoxia, tissue hypoxia can result from other abnormalities unrelated to alterations of pulmonary function, such as low cardiac output or cyanide poisoning.

There are five causes of hypoxemia: (1) decreased oxygen content (PO_2) of inspired gas, (2) hypoventilation, (3) diffusion abnormalities, (4) abnormal ventilation-perfusion ratios, and (5) pulmonary right-to-left shunt (Table 26-1). The physiologic mechanisms for each cause of hypoxemia differ, and each requires specific clinical management.

The PO_2 of arterial blood depends on the PO_2 of inspired gas (PiO_2). If PiO_2 is below normal, less oxygen is available to diffuse into the blood. The most common cause of a decreased PiO_2 is the drop in atmospheric pressure that occurs at high altitudes. The result is a decrease in PaO_2. Hypoxemia caused by high altitude is prevented by the use of supplemental oxygen.

Hypoventilation of the alveoli causes elevated $PaCO_2$ (hypercapnia). If oxygen-rich gas is not delivered to the alveoli, the oxygen content of alveolar gas (PAO_2) decreases as $PaCO_2$ increases. As PAO_2 decreases, less oxygen diffuses into the blood, causing hypoxemia. This type of hypoxemia can be completely corrected if alveolar ventilation is improved by increases in the rate and depth of breathing. Hypoventilation causes hypoxemia in unconscious persons and in individuals who have chronic obstructive pulmonary disease.

Diffusion of oxygen through the alveolocapillary membrane is impaired if the membrane is thickened or the surface area available for diffusion is decreased. Thickened membranes, as occur with edema (tissue swelling) and fibrosis (formation of fibrous lesions), increase the time required for diffusion across the alveolocapillary membrane. If diffusion is slowed enough, the PO_2 of alveolar gas and capillary blood does not have time to equilibrate during the fraction of a second that blood remains in the capillary. Destruction of alveoli, as in emphysema, decreases the surface area available for diffusion. Hypoxemia caused by impaired diffusion alone is rare, however, and hypercapnia is seldom produced by impaired diffusion because carbon dioxide diffuses so easily from capillary to alveolus that the individual with impaired diffusion would die from hypoxemia before hypercapnia could occur.

An abnormal ventilation-perfusion ratio ($\dot{V}/\dot{Q}$) is the most common cause of hypoxemia (Fig. 26-2). Normally, alveolocapillary lung units receive almost equal amounts of ventilation and perfusion. The normal $\dot{V}/\dot{Q}$ is 0.8 to 0.9 because perfusion is somewhat greater than ventilation in the lung bases and because some blood is normally shunted to the bronchial circulation. $\dot{V}/\dot{Q}$ mismatch refers to an abnormal distribution of ventilation and perfusion. Hypoxemia can be caused by inadequate ventilation of well-perfused ar-

TABLE 26-1	Causes of Hypoxemia
Mechanism	**Common Clinical Cause**
Decrease in inspired oxygen	High altitude
	Low oxygen content of gas mixture
	Enclosed breathing space (suffocation)
Hypoventilation	Lack of neurologic stimulation of the respiratory center (oversedation, drug overdose, neurologic damage)
	Chronic obstructive pulmonary disease
Alveolocapillary diffusion abnormality	Emphysema
	Fibrosis
	Edema
Ventilation-perfusion mismatch	Asthma
	Chronic bronchitis
	Pneumonia
Shunting	Acute (adult) respiratory distress syndrome
	Respiratory distress syndrome of the newborn (hyaline membrane disease)
	Atelectasis

Fig. 26-2 *Ventilation-perfusion abnormalities.*

eas of the lung (low $\dot{V}/\dot{Q}$). Mismatching of this type occurs in asthma as a result of bronchoconstriction and in pulmonary edema and pneumonia when alveoli are filled with fluid. When blood passes through portions of the pulmonary capillary bed that receive no ventilation, either because the airway leading to the alveoli is completely obstructed or because the alveoli are collapsed or filled with fluid and cellular debris, right-to-left shunt occurs, resulting in decreased systemic PaO_2 and hypoxemia. Shunting causes hypoxemia in acute (adult) respiratory distress syndrome and respiratory distress syndrome of the newborn. Hypox-

emia also can be caused by poor perfusion of well-ventilated portions of the lung (high $\dot{V}/\dot{Q}$), resulting in wasted ventilation. The most common cause of high $\dot{V}/\dot{Q}$ is a pulmonary embolus that impairs blood flow to a segment of the lung.

✓ QUICK CHECK

List the primary signs and symptoms of pulmonary disease.

What abnormal breathing patterns are seen with pulmonary disease?

What mechanisms produce hypercapnia?

What mechanisms produce hypoxemia?

Acute respiratory failure

Respiratory failure is defined as inadequate gas exchange, that is, hypoxemia, where $PaO_2 \leq 50$ mm Hg or where $PaO_2 \geq 50$ mm Hg with pH ≤ 7.25. Respiratory failure can result from direct injury to the lungs, airways, or chest wall or to another body system. It can occur in individuals who have an otherwise normal respiratory system or in those with underlying chronic pulmonary disease. Most pulmonary diseases can cause episodes of acute respiratory failure. If the respiratory failure is primarily hypercapnic, it is the result of inadequate alveolar ventilation and the individual must receive ventilatory support, such as with a bag-valve mask or mechanical ventilator. If the respiratory failure is primarily hypoxemic, it is the result of inadequate exchange of oxygen between the alveoli and the capillaries (see Hypoxemia, p. 743) and the individual must receive supplemental oxygen therapy. Many people will have a combined hypercapnic and hypoxemic respiratory failure and will require both kinds of support.

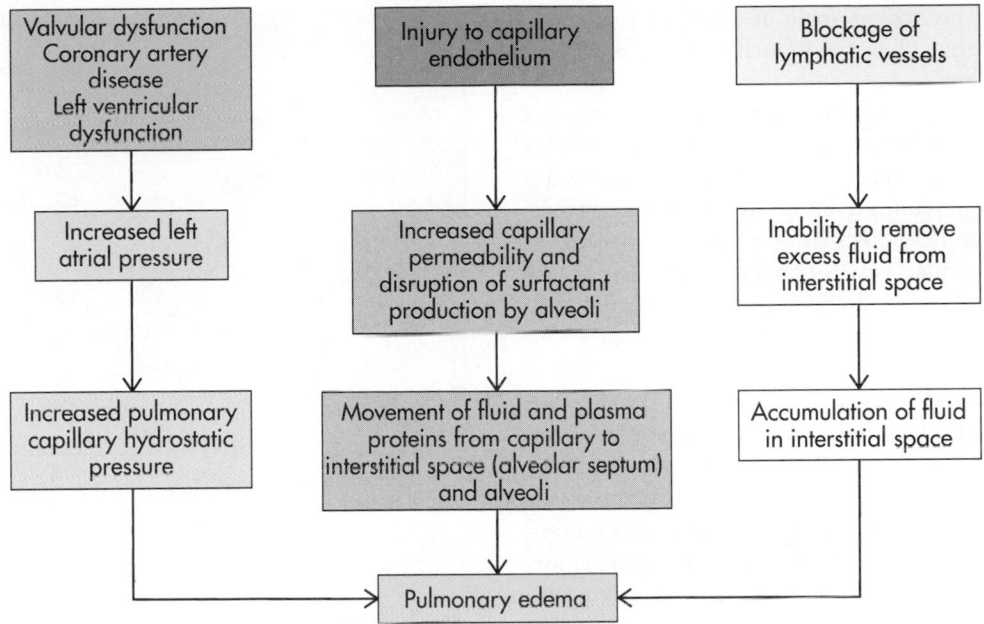

Fig. 26-3 *Pathogenesis of pulmonary edema.*

Pulmonary edema

Pulmonary edema is excess water in the lung. The normal lung is kept dry by lymphatic drainage and a balance among capillary hydrostatic pressure, capillary oncotic pressure, and capillary permeability. In addition, surfactant lining the alveoli repels water, keeping fluid from entering the alveoli. Predisposing factors for pulmonary edema include heart disease, acute (adult) respiratory distress syndrome, and inhalation of toxic gases. The pathogenesis of pulmonary edema is shown in Fig. 26-3.

The most common cause of pulmonary edema is heart disease. When the left ventricle fails, filling pressures on the left side of the heart increase and subsequently cause an increase in pulmonary capillary hydrostatic pressure. When the hydrostatic pressure push exceeds oncotic pressure, which holds fluid in the capillary, fluid moves out into the interstitium, or interstitial space (the space within the alveolar septum between alveolus and capillary). When the flow of fluid out of the capillaries exceeds the lymphatic system's ability to remove it, pulmonary edema develops.

Another cause of pulmonary edema is capillary injury that increases capillary permeability, as in cases of acute (adult) respiratory distress syndrome or inhalation of toxic gases, such as ammonia. Capillary injury causes water and plasma proteins to leak out of the capillary and move into the interstitium, increasing the interstitial oncotic pressure, which is usually very low. As the interstitial oncotic pressure begins to equal capillary oncotic pressure, water moves out of the capillary and into the lung. (This phenomenon is discussed in Chapter 4, Figs. 4-1 and 4-2.)

Pulmonary edema can also result from obstruction of the lymphatic system. Drainage can be blocked by compression of lymphatic vessels by edema, tumors, and fibrotic tissue and by increased systemic venous pressure, which elevates the hydrostatic pressure of the large pulmonary veins into which the pulmonary lymphatic system drains. This can happen in left heart failure.

Clinical manifestations of pulmonary edema include dyspnea, hypoxemia, and increased work of breathing. In severe edema, pink frothy sputum is expectorated and $PaCO_2$ increases.

The treatment of pulmonary edema depends on its cause. If the edema is caused by increased hydrostatic pressure, therapy is geared toward reducing blood pressure with diuretics, vasodilators, and drugs that improve the contraction of the heart muscle. If edema is the result of increased capillary permeability resulting from injury, the treatment is focused on removing the offending agent and supportive therapy to maintain adequate ventilation and circulation. Individuals with either type of pulmonary edema require supplemental oxygen. Positive-pressure mechanical ventilation is also used if edema significantly impairs ventilation and oxygenation.

Aspiration

Aspiration is the passage of fluid and solid particles into the lung. It tends to occur in individuals whose normal swallowing mechanism and cough reflex are impaired by a decreased level of consciousness or central nervous system abnormalities. Predisposing factors include altered level of consciousness caused by substance abuse, sedation, or anesthesia; seizure disorders; cerebrovascular accident; myasthenia gravis (a neuromuscular disorder); and Guillain-Barré syndrome (inflammation of the nerves). Aspiration is also common in children with tracheoesophageal fistula (a congenital abnormality in which the trachea and esophagus communicate; see Chapter 35). The right lung, particularly the right lower lobe, is more susceptible to aspiration than the left lung because the branching angle of the right main stem bronchus is straighter than the branching angle of the left main stem bronchus.

The aspiration of large food particles can obstruct a bronchus, resulting in bronchial inflammation and collapse of airways distal to the obstruction. If the aspirated solid is not identified and removed by bronchoscopy, a chronic, local inflammation develops that may lead to recurrent infection and bronchiectasis (permanent dilation of the bronchus). Once the pathologic process has progressed to bronchiectasis, surgical resection of the affected area is usually required.

Aspiration of acidic gastric fluid (pH <2.5) may cause severe pneumonitis (localized lung inflammation). Bronchial damage includes inflammation, loss of ciliary function, and bronchospasm. In the alveoli, acidic fluid damages the alveolocapillary membrane, allowing plasma and blood cells to move from capillaries into the alveoli, resulting in hemorrhagic pneumonitis. Movement of serous transudate into the lung causes systemic hypovolemia and hypotension. The lung becomes stiff and noncompliant as surfactant production is disrupted, leading to further edema and collapse.

Preventive measures for individuals at risk are more effective than treatment of known aspiration. Surgical patients do not receive food or fluid for several hours before surgery. Antacids are sometimes given to persons at risk to keep gastric pH above 2.5. Individuals who have difficulty swallowing are fed with extreme caution and positioned so as to minimize the likelihood of aspiration. Nasogastric tubes, which are often used to remove stomach contents, can also cause aspiration if fluid and particulate matter are regurgitated.

The rate of deaths caused by aspiration-caused pneumonitis is greater than 50%. Treatment includes supplemental oxygen and mechanical ventilation with positive end-expiratory pressure (PEEP), fluid restriction, and steroids. Bacterial pneumonia may develop as a complication of aspiration pneumonitis.

Atelectasis

Atelectasis is the collapse of lung tissue. There are two types of atelectasis:

1. **Compression atelectasis:** caused by external pressure exerted by tumor, fluid, or air in pleural space or by abdominal distention pressing on a portion of lung, causing alveoli to collapse
2. **Absorption atelectasis:** results from removal of air from obstructed or hypoventilated alveoli or from inhalation of concentrated oxygen or anesthetic agents

Clinical manifestations of atelectasis are similar to those of pulmonary infection: dyspnea, cough, fever, and leukocytosis.

Atelectasis tends to occur after surgery. Postoperative patients may have received supplemental oxygen or inhaled anesthetics, and they are usually in pain, breathe shallowly, are reluctant to change position, and produce viscous secretions that tend to pool in dependent portions of the lung. Prevention and treatment of postoperative atelectasis usually include deep breathing, frequent position changes, and early ambulation.

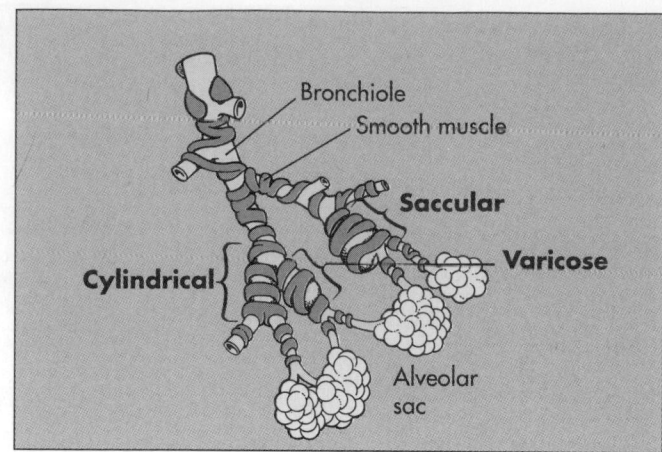

Fig. 26-4 *Types of bronchiectasis.*

Bronchiectasis

Bronchiectasis is persistent abnormal dilation of the bronchi. It usually occurs in conjunction with other respiratory conditions and can be caused by obstruction of an airway with mucus plugs, atelectasis, aspiration of a foreign body, infection, cystic fibrosis, tuberculosis, congenital weakness of the bronchial wall, or impaired defense mechanisms. Bronchiectasis is frequently associated with inflammation of the bronchi (bronchitis) and has similar symptoms (see p. 762). Bronchial dilation (Fig. 26-4) may be **cylindrical,** with symmetrically dilated airways as is commonly seen after pneumonia; **saccular,** in which the bronchi become large and balloonlike; or **varicose,** in which constrictions and dilations deform the bronchi.

The symptoms of bronchiectasis may date back to a childhood illness or infection. The disease is commonly associated with recurrent lower respiratory tract infections and expectoration of voluminous amounts of purulent sputum (measured in cupfuls). If the individual is not receiving antibiotics, the sputum has a foul odor. Hemoptysis and clubbing of the fingers are common. Pulmonary function studies show decreased vital capacity (VC) and expiratory flow rates. Bronchiectasis is often associated with bronchitis and atelectasis. Hypoxemia eventually leads to cor pulmonale (see p. 764).

Bronchiolitis

Bronchiolitis is an inflammatory obstruction of the small airways or bronchioles, occurring most commonly in children. In adults, it usually accompanies chronic bronchitis but can occur in otherwise healthy individuals in association with an infection or inhalation of toxic gases. Atelectasis or emphysematous destruction of the alveoli may develop distal to the inflammatory lesion. Bronchiolitis is usually diffuse. A decrease in the ventilation-perfusion ratio results in hypoxemia and carbon dioxide retention.

Bronchiolitis is often preceded by an upper respiratory infection and appears with rapid ventilatory rate, marked use of accessory muscles, low-grade fever, dry, nonproduc-

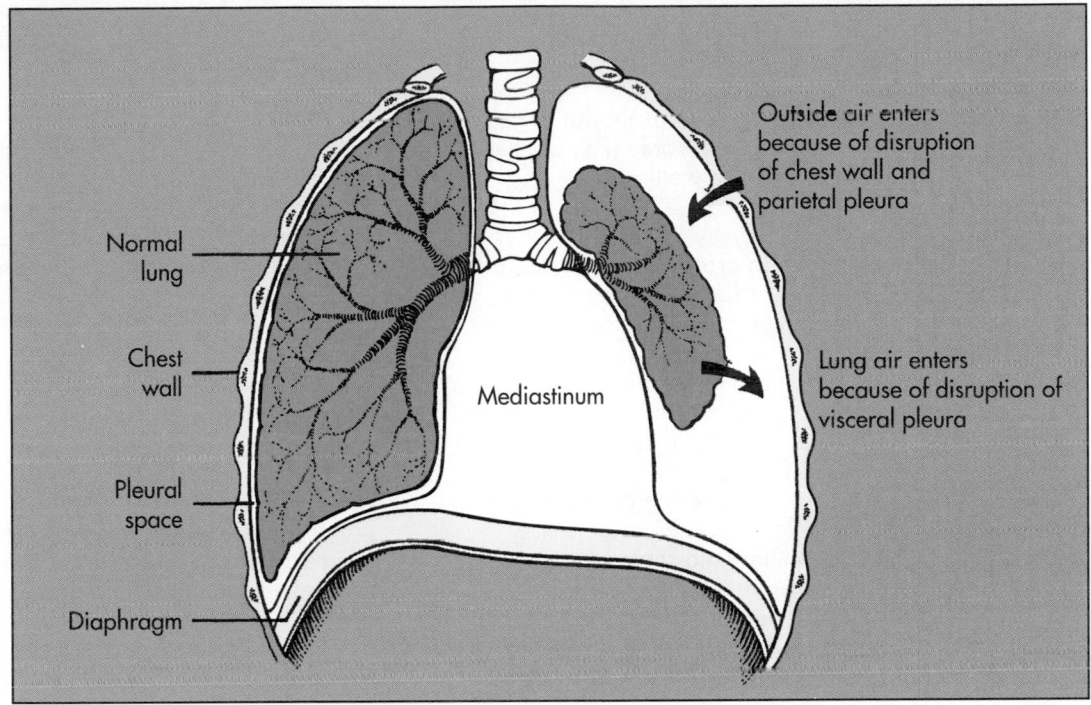

Fig. 26-5 *Pneumothorax.* Air in the pleural space causes the lung to collapse around the hilus and may push mediastinal contents (heart and great vessels) toward the other lung.

tive cough, and hyperinflated chest. If bronchiolitis is caused by an inhalation injury, pulmonary edema occurs rapidly and then quickly clears. One to two weeks later, respiratory distress develops, and infiltrates are seen on chest radiographs. Bronchiolitis is treated with appropriate antibiotics, steroids, and chest physical therapy (humidified air, coughing and deep breathing, postural drainage).

Pleural abnormalities

Pneumothorax

Pneumothorax is the presence of air or gas in the pleural space caused by a rupture in the visceral pleura (which surrounds the lungs) or the parietal pleura and chest wall.[2] As air separates the visceral and parietal pleurae, it destroys the negative pressure of the pleural space and disrupts the equilibrium between elastic recoil forces of the lung and chest wall. The lung then tends to recoil by collapsing toward the hilus (Fig. 26-5).

In *open pneumothorax (communicating pneumothorax),* air pressure in the pleural space equals barometric pressure because air that is drawn into the pleural space during inspiration (through the damaged chest wall and parietal pleura or through the lungs and damaged visceral pleura) is forced back out during expiration. In *tension pneumothorax,* however, the site of pleural rupture acts as a one-way valve, permitting air to enter on inspiration but preventing its escape by closing up during expiration. As more and more air enters the pleural space, air pressure in the pneumothorax begins to exceed barometric pressure. The pathophysiologic effects of tension pneumothorax are life threatening. Air pressure in the pleural space pushes against

the already recoiled lung, causing compression atelectasis, and against the mediastinum, compressing and displacing the heart and great vessels.

Clinical manifestations of tension pneumothorax include severe hypoxemia, dyspnea, and hypotension (low blood pressure), as well as the other signs and symptoms of pneumothorax. Deterioration occurs rapidly as venous return is decreased as a result of compression by the increasing pressure, and shock and bradycardia (reduced heart rate) may develop. Immediate treatment is required. A chest tube is placed quickly or a large-bore needle is inserted into the pleural space to decompress it until a chest tube can be placed. An outward gush of air as the needle or chest tube is inserted confirms the presence of a tension pneumothorax. The chest tube is connected to a water-seal drainage and suction until the damaged pleura is healed.

Spontaneous pneumothorax, which occurs unexpectedly in healthy individuals (usually men) between 20 and 40 years of age, is caused by the spontaneous rupture of blebs (blisterlike formations) on the visceral pleura. Bleb rupture can occur during sleep, rest, or exercise. The ruptured bleb or blebs are usually located in the apexes of the lungs. The cause of bleb formation is not known. Tension pneumothorax can develop with bleb rupture.

Clinical manifestations of spontaneous pneumothorax begin with sudden pleural pain, tachypnea, and possibly mild dyspnea. The manifestations depend on the size of the pneumothorax. Diagnosis is made with chest radiographs.

A secondary pneumothorax can be caused by chest trauma, such as a rib fracture or stab and bullet wounds that tear the pleura; rupture of a bleb or bulla (larger vesicle), as

TABLE 26-2	Mechanism of Pleural Effusion	
Type of Fluid/Effusion	**Source of Accumulation**	**Primary or Associated Disorder**
Transudate (hydrothorax)	Water fluid that diffuses out of capillaries beneath the pleurae (i.e., capillaries in lung or chest wall)	Cardiovascular disease that causes high blood pressure; liver or kidney disease that disrupts plasma protein production, causing hypoproteinemia (decreased oncotic pressure in the blood vessels)
Exudate	Fluid rich in proteins (leukocytes, plasma proteins of all kinds; see Chapter 35) that migrates out of the capillaries	Infection, inflammation, or malignancy of the pleurae that stimulates mast cells to release biochemical mediators that increase capillary permeability
Pus (empyema)	Debris of infection (microorganisms, leukocytes, cellular debris) dumped into the pleural space by blocked lymphatic vessels	Pulmonary infections, such as pneumonia; lung abscesses; infected wounds
Blood (hemothorax)	Hemorrhage into the pleural space	Traumatic injury, surgery, rupture, or malignancy that damages blood vessels
Chyle (chylothorax)	Chyle (milky fluid containing lymph and fat droplets) that is dumped by lymphatic vessels into the pleural space instead of passing from the gastrointestinal tract to the thoracic duct	Traumatic injury, infection, or disorder that disrupts lymphatic transport

The principles of diffusion are described in Chapter 1; mechanisms that increase capillary permeability and cause exudation of cells and proteins are discussed in Chapter 7.

occurs in chronic obstructive pulmonary disease; or mechanical ventilation, particularly if it includes PEEP.

The pathophysiology and clinical manifestations of secondary pneumothorax are similar to those of spontaneous pneumothorax. Occasionally air enters the mediastinum. Secondary pneumothorax (and other open pneumothoraces if large enough) is treated with a chest tube that is attached to a water-seal drainage system with suction. After the pneumothorax is evacuated and the pleural rupture is healed, the chest tube is removed.

Pleural effusion

Pleural effusion is the presence of fluid in the pleural space. The source of the fluid is usually blood vessels or lymphatic vessels lying beneath either pleura, but occasionally an abscess or other lesion is draining into the pleural space. Because the pleura is a relatively permeable membrane, fluids that accumulate in the lung can cross into the pleural space.

Like pneumothorax, pleural effusion can cause compression atelectasis and displace mediastinal contents. Unlike pneumothorax, however, pleural effusion does not cause the lung to collapse. Because there is no communication between the pleural space and environmental air, pressure in the pleural space remains negative and atelectasis is caused solely by pressure exerted by the effusion.

The most common mechanism of pleural effusion is migration of fluids and other blood components through the walls of intact capillaries bordering the pleura. Pleural effusions that enter the pleural space from the intact blood vessels

can be **transudative** (watery) or **exudative** (high concentrations of white blood cells and plasma proteins). Mechanisms of pleural effusion are summarized in Table 26-2.

Small collections of fluid normally can be drained away by the lymphatics. Dyspnea, compression atelectasis with impaired ventilation, and mediastinal shift occur with large effusions. Pleural pain is present if the pleura is inflamed, and cardiovascular manifestations occur in a large, rapidly developing hemothorax. A pleural friction rub can be heard over areas of extensive effusion.

If the effusion is causing considerable impairment of pulmonary function, thoracentesis (needle aspiration) may be performed to drain the fluid from the pleural space. A pleural effusion can contain several liters of fluid.

Empyema

Empyema (infected pleural effusion), the presence of pus in the pleural space, is a complication of respiratory infection, usually pneumonia caused by *Staphylococcus aureus*, *Escherichia coli*, anaerobic bacteria, or *Klebsiella pneumoniae*. (*Staphylococcus* is the most common cause of empyemas in children.)[3] Empyema is thought to develop when the pulmonary lymphatics become blocked, leading to an outpouring of contaminated lymphatic fluid into the pleural space.

Individuals with empyema have clinical manifestations of toxicity, including cyanosis, fever, tachycardia (rapid heart rate), cough, and pleural pain. Breath sounds are decreased directly over the empyema. Diagnosis is made by chest radiographs and thoracentesis, although positive cultures from fluids are obtained only about 50% of the time. Therefore the offending microorganism is usually identified by its preponderance in a sputum culture.

The treatment for empyema is similar to that for pneumonia (see p. 759). Antibiotics are given, and thoracentesis is performed to drain the pleural space. Chest tube placement and continuous drainage also may be required. In severe cases, instillation of thrombolytic agents into the pleural space or surgical débridement of the pleural space is performed to prevent reaccumulation.

✓ **QUICK CHECK**

Describe pulmonary edema, and list two causes.

Contrast atelectasis and bronchiectasis.

How does pneumothorax differ from pleural effusion?

What causes empyema?

Pleurisy

Pleurisy (pleuritis) is inflammation of the pleura, which become reddened and covered with an exudate of lymph, fibrin, and cellular elements. Pleural effusion may develop. The most common signs and symptoms of pleurisy are chills, fever, and pain on inspiration. Often a pleural friction rub can be heard over the affected area. Pleurisy is frequently preceded by upper respiratory infection.

Abscess formation and cavitation

An *abscess* is a circumscribed area of suppuration and destruction of lung parenchyma. Abscess formation follows *consolidation* of lung tissue, in which inflammation causes alveoli to fill with fluid, pus, and microorganisms. Necrosis (death and decay) of consolidated tissue may progress proximally until it communicates with a bronchus. If this occurs, the abscess empties into the bronchus, leaving a cavity that has a radiographic appearance similar to that of a lesion of tuberculosis. *Cavitation* is the process of abscess emptying and cavity formation. The diagnosis is made by radiography.

Pneumonia caused by aspiration, *Klebsiella,* or *Staphylococcus* is the most common cause of abscess formation. Aspiration abscess is usually associated with alcohol abuse, seizure disorders, general anesthesia, and swallowing disorders. The clinical manifestations of abscess formation are similar to those of pneumonitis: fever, cough, chills, sputum production, and pleural pain. Abscess communication with a bronchus causes a severe cough, copious amounts of often foul-smelling sputum, and occasionally hemoptysis.

Treatment includes the administration of appropriate antibiotics and chest physical therapy, including chest percussion and postural drainage. Sometimes bronchoscopy is performed to drain the abscess.

Pulmonary fibrosis

Pulmonary fibrosis is an excessive amount of fibrous or connective tissue in the lung. It can be caused by healing (for-

mation of scar tissue) after active disease (e.g., acute [adult] respiratory distress syndrome, tuberculosis) or by inhalation of harmful substances (e.g., coal dust, asbestos). When no cause for the development of fibrosis is known, it is called *idiopathic pulmonary fibrosis.*

Fibrosis causes a marked loss of lung compliance. The lung becomes stiff and difficult to ventilate, and the diffusing capacity of the alveolocapillary membrane may decrease, causing hypoxemia. Diffuse pulmonary fibrosis has a very poor prognosis.

Chest wall restriction

If the chest wall is deformed, immobilized, or made heavy by fat, the work of breathing is increased and ventilation may be compromised. The degree of ventilatory impairment depends on the severity of the chest wall abnormality. Grossly obese individuals are often dyspneic on exertion or when recumbent. Individuals with severe kyphoscoliosis (lateral bending and rotation of the spinal column, with distortion of the thoracic cage) often present with dyspnea on exertion that can progress to respiratory failure. Such individuals are also susceptible to lower respiratory tract infections. Both obesity and kyphoscoliosis are risk factors for respiratory disease in hospital patients admitted for other problems, particularly those who require surgery. Other musculoskeletal abnormalities that can impair ventilation are ankylosing spondylitis (rheumatoid arthritis of the spine; see Chapter 37) and pectus excavatum, or funnel chest (a deformity characterized by depression of the sternum).

Impairment of respiratory muscle function caused by neuromuscular disease can also restrict the chest wall and impair pulmonary function. Muscle weakness can result in hypoventilation, inability to remove secretions, and hypoxemia. The most common cause of hospital admission for individuals with neuromuscular diseases such as poliomyelitis, muscular dystrophy, myasthenia gravis, and Guillain-Barré syndrome is respiratory difficulty. (See Unit 4 for a more complete discussion of these disorders.)

Flail chest

Flail chest results from the fracture of several consecutive ribs in more than one place or the fracture of the sternum plus several consecutive ribs. These multiple fractures result in instability of a portion of the chest wall, causing paradoxic movement of the chest with breathing. During inspiration the unstable portion of the chest wall moves inward, and during expiration it moves outward, impairing movement of gas in and out of the lungs (Fig. 26-6).

The clinical manifestations of flail chest are pain, dyspnea, unequal chest expansion, hypoventilation, and hypoxemia. Treatment is internal fixation by controlled mechanical ventilation until the chest wall has stabilized.

Inhalation disorders
Exposure to toxic gases

Inhalation of gaseous irritants can cause significant respiratory dysfunction. Commonly encountered toxic gases in-

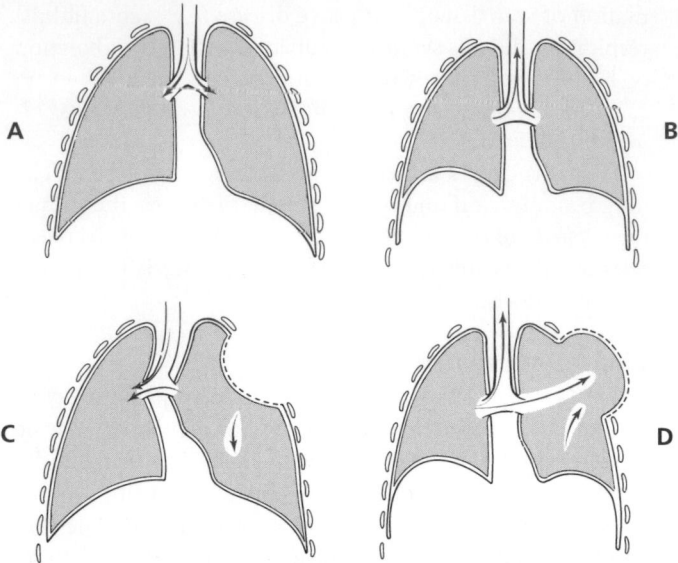

Fig. 26-6 *Flail chest.* Normal respiration: **A,** inspiration; **B,** expiration. Paradoxical motion: **C,** inspiration, area of lung underlying unstable chest wall sucks in on inspiration; **D,** expiration, unstable area balloons out. Note movement of mediastinum toward opposite lung during inspiration.

clude smoke, ammonia, hydrogen chloride, sulfur dioxide, chlorine, phosgene, and nitrogen dioxide. Inhalation of a toxic gas results in severe inflammation of the airways, alveolar and capillary damage, and pulmonary edema. Initial symptoms include burning of the eyes, nose, and throat; coughing; chest tightness; and dyspnea. Hypoxemia is common. Treatment includes supplemental oxygen, mechanical ventilation with PEEP, and support of the cardiovascular system. Steroids are sometimes used, although their effectiveness has not been well documented. Most individuals respond very quickly to therapy. Some, however, may improve initially and then deteriorate as a result of bronchiectasis or bronchiolitis (inflammation of the bronchioles).

Prolonged exposure to high concentrations of supplemental oxygen can result in a relatively rare condition known as *oxygen toxicity.* Although there is great individual variation in susceptibility to oxygen toxicity, generally the higher the concentration and longer the exposure, the more likely toxicity will occur. Oxygen concentrations of 50% to 75% for longer than 24 to 48 hours have been associated with injury to cells of the lungs. The basic underlying mechanism of injury is a severe inflammatory response mediated primarily by oxygen radicals.[4] The result is damage to alveolocapillary membranes, disruption of surfactant production, interstitial and alveolar edema, and decrease in compliance. Toxicity is often undetected because it occurs in individuals who are already in acute respiratory failure. Clinical manifestations are indistinguishable from those of adult respiratory distress syndrome (see p. 751). Treatment involves ventilatory support and reduction of inspired oxygen concentration to less than 60% as soon as tolerated by the individual.

Pneumoconiosis

Pneumoconiosis represents any change in the lung caused by inhalation of inorganic dust particles, usually in the workplace. As in all cases of environmentally acquired lung disease, the individual's history of exposure is important in determining the diagnosis. Pneumoconiosis often occurs after years of exposure to the offending dust, with progressive fibrosis of lung tissue.

The dusts of silica, asbestos, and coal are the most common causes of pneumoconiosis. Others include talc, fiberglass, clays, mica, slate, cement, cadmium, beryllium, tungsten, cobalt, aluminum, and iron. No matter what the substance, the dust deposits are permanent. Individuals may remain symptomatic for years. Clinical manifestations with advancement of disease may include cough, chronic bronchitis, dyspnea, decreased lung volumes, and hypoxemia. Treatment therefore is palliative and focuses on preventing further exposure, particularly in the workplace.[5]

Allergic alveolitis

Inhalation of organic dusts can result in an allergic inflammatory response called *extrinsic allergic alveolitis,* or *hypersensitivity pneumonitis.* Many allergens can cause this disorder, including grains, silage, bird droppings or feathers, wood dust (particularly redwood and maple), cork dust, animal pelts, coffee beans, fish meal, mushroom compost, and molds that grow on sugarcane, barley, and straw. The lung inflammation, or pneumonitis, occurs after repeated, prolonged exposure to the allergen.

Allergic alveolitis can be acute, subacute, or chronic. The acute form causes a fever, cough, and chills a few hours after exposure. In the subacute form, coughing and dyspnea are common and sometimes necessitate hospital care. Recovery is complete if the offending agent can be avoided in the future. With continued exposure, the disease becomes chronic and pulmonary fibrosis develops.

✓ QUICK CHECK

What factors inhibit chest wall compliance?

What symptoms are produced by inhalation of toxic gases?

Describe pneumoconiosis, and give two examples.

PULMONARY DISORDERS
Acute Respiratory Failure
Acute (adult) respiratory distress syndrome

Acute (adult) respiratory distress syndrome (ARDS) is a fulminant form of respiratory failure characterized by acute lung inflammation and diffuse alveolocapillary injury with noncardiogenic pulmonary edema. Identified within the past 25 years, the syndrome affects an estimated 200,000 to 250,000 people per year in the United States. New advances in

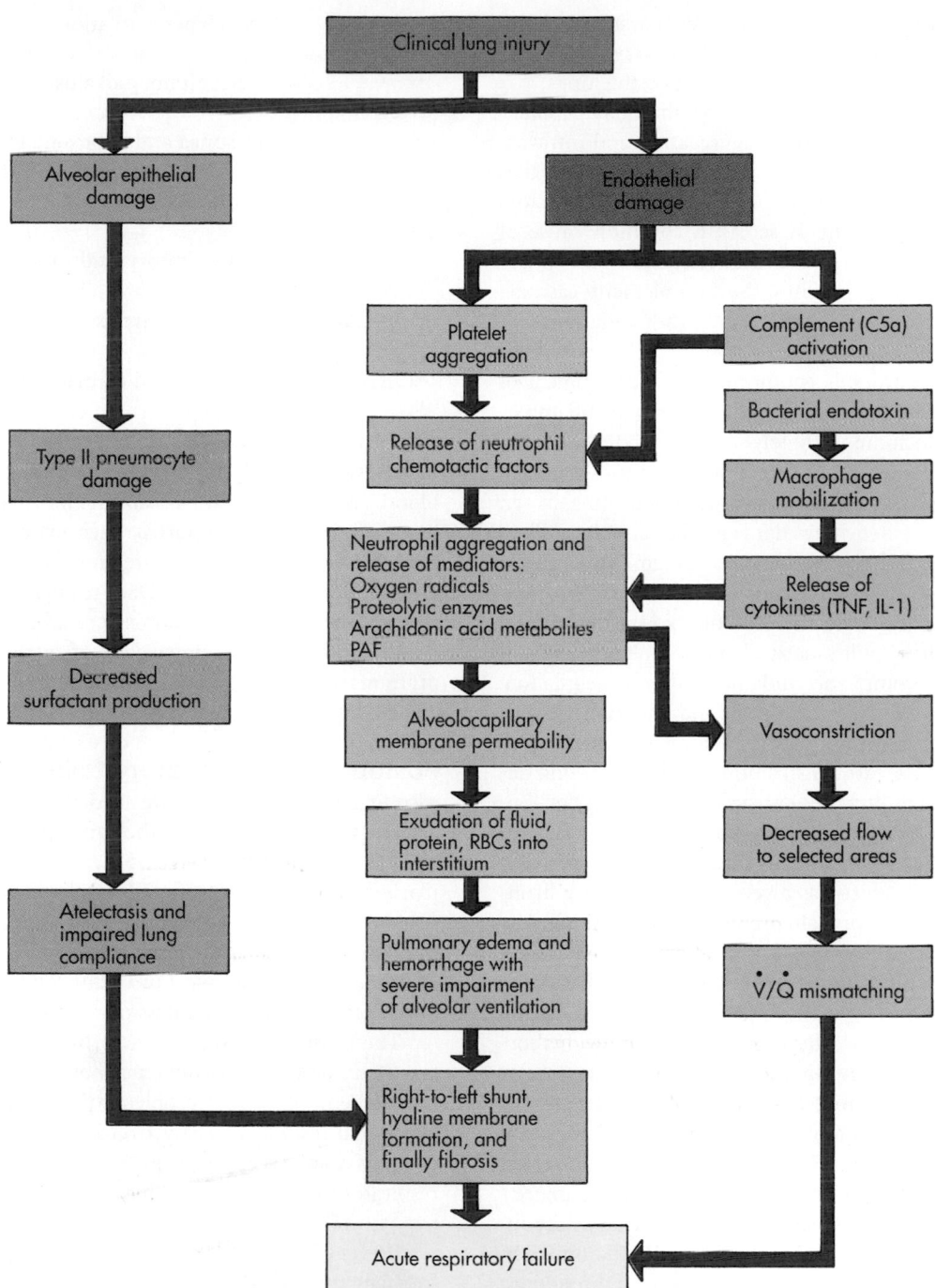

Fig. 26-7 *Pathogenesis of acute respiratory distress syndrome (ARDS).* *TNF,* Tumor necrosis factor; *IL-1,* interleukin-1; *PAF,* platelet-activating factor; *RBCs,* red blood cells.

therapy have decreased overall mortality in people younger than 60 years to approximately 40% (down from 67% in 1990), although mortality in people older than 65 years continues to be above 60%.[6] Most survivors, however, have almost normal lung function 1 year after the acute illness. ARDS is caused by injury to the lung. The most common predisposing factors are sepsis and multiple trauma (combined they cause 60% of all cases); however, there are many other causes, including pneumonia, burns, aspiration, cardiopulmonary bypass surgery, pancreatitis, massive blood transfu-

sions, drug overdose, inhalation of smoke or noxious gases, fat emboli, high concentrations of supplemental oxygen, radiation therapy, and disseminated intravascular coagulation.

Pathophysiology

All disorders causing ARDS acutely injure the alveolocapillary membrane and produce severe pulmonary edema, shunting, and hypoxemia (Fig. 26-7). The damage can occur directly, as with the aspiration of highly acidic gastric contents or the inhalation of toxic gases, or indirectly from chemical mediators released in response to systemic disorders. The common pathway for alveolocapillary membrane injury is a massive inflammatory response by the lungs.[7,8]

The initial lung injury damages the pulmonary capillary endothelium, stimulating platelet aggregation and intravascular thrombus formation. Platelets release substances that attract and activate neutrophils. Other chemotactic factors include endotoxin, present in sepsis, a common cause of ARDS; tumor necrosis factor; and interleukin-1 (IL-1). Endothelial damage also initiates the complement cascade, stimulating neutrophil activity and the inflammatory response.

The role of neutrophils is central to the development of ARDS. Activated neutrophils release a battery of inflammatory mediators, including proteolytic enzymes, toxic oxygen products, arachidonic acid metabolites (prostaglandins, thromboxanes, leukotrienes), and platelet-activating factor. These mediators extensively damage the alveolocapillary membrane and greatly increase capillary membrane permeability. This allows fluids, proteins, and blood cells to leak from the capillary bed into the pulmonary interstitium and alveoli. The resulting pulmonary edema and hemorrhage severely reduce lung compliance and impair alveolar ventilation.

Mediators released by neutrophils and macrophages also cause pulmonary vasoconstriction. Pulmonary hypertension results, and because vasoconstriction occurs to varying degrees in the vascular beds, $\dot{V}/\dot{Q}$ mismatching occurs.

The initial lung injury damages the alveolar epithelium and the vascular endothelium. Surfactant is inactivated, and its production is impaired as alveoli and respiratory bronchioles fill with fluid or collapse. The lungs become less compliant, ventilation of alveoli decreases, and pulmonary blood flow is shunted right-to-left. The work of breathing increases.

Twenty-four to forty-eight hours after the acute, hemorrhagic phase of ARDS, hyaline membranes form, and after approximately 7 days, fibrosis progressively obliterates the alveoli, respiratory bronchioles, and interstitium. Functional residual capacity declines, and more severe right-to-left shunting is seen. The end result is acute respiratory failure.[9]

The chemical mediators responsible for the alveolocapillary damage of ARDS often cause widespread inflammation, endothelial damage, and capillary permeability throughout the body resulting in the systemic inflammatory response syndrome (SIRS), which then leads to multiple organ dysfunction syndrome (MODS). In fact, death may not be caused by respiratory failure alone but by MODS associated with ARDS. (MODS is discussed in Chapter 23.)

▬ *Clinical Manifestations*

The classic signs and symptoms of ARDS are rapid, shallow breathing; respiratory alkalosis; marked dyspnea; decreased lung compliance; hypoxemia unresponsive to oxygen therapy (refractory hypoxemia); and diffuse alveolar infiltrates seen on chest radiographs, without evidence of cardiac disease. Symptoms develop progressively, as follows:

Hyperventilation
↓
Respiratory alkalosis
↓
Dyspnea and hypoxemia
↓
Metabolic acidosis
↓
Respiratory acidosis
↓
Further hypoxemia
↓
Hypotension, decreased cardiac output, death

▬ *Evaluation and Treatment*

Diagnosis is based on physical examination, analysis of blood gases, and radiologic examination. Treatment is based on early detection, supportive therapy, and prevention of complications. Many studies are underway investigating new ways to prevent or treat ARDS. Prophylactic immunotherapy, antibodies against endotoxin, inhibition of various inflammatory mediators, inhalation of nitric oxide to reduce pulmonary hypertension, antioxidants, and surfactant replacement are among the possibilities being tested.[10,11]

Postoperative respiratory failure

Although usually not as severe as ARDS, postoperative respiratory failure can result in the same pathophysiology and clinical manifestations as ARDS. Smokers are at risk, particularly if they have preexisting lung disease. Limited cardiac reserve, chronic renal failure, chronic hepatic disease, and infection also increase the tendency to develop postoperative respiratory failure. Surgical procedures involving the thorax or abdomen carry the greatest risk.

The most common postoperative pulmonary problems are atelectasis, pneumonia, pulmonary edema, and pulmonary emboli. These problems usually produce reduced functional residual capacity, decreased compliance, and decreased ventilation-perfusion ratio. Individuals in whom respiratory failure develops have generally had a period of hypotension during surgery, and many have sepsis.

Prevention of postoperative respiratory failure includes frequent turning, deep breathing, and early ambulation to prevent atelectasis and accumulation of secretions. Humidification of inspired air can help loosen secretions. Incentive spirometry gives individuals immediate feedback about tidal volumes, which encourages them to breathe deeply. Supplemental oxygen is given for hypoxemia, and antibiotics are given as appropriate to treat infection. If respiratory failure develops, the individual may require mechanical ventilation for a time. Treatment is then very similar to that for ARDS.

Obstructive Pulmonary Disease

Obstructive pulmonary disease is characterized by difficult expiration. More force (i.e., use of accessory muscles of expiration) is required to expire a given volume of air, or emp-

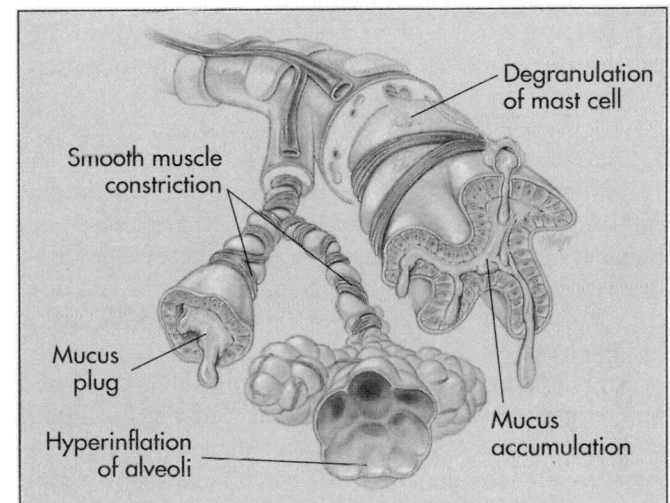

Fig. 26-8 *Airway obstruction caused by emphysema, chronic bronchitis, and asthma.* **A,** The normal lung. **B,** Emphysema: enlargement and destruction of alveolar walls with loss of elasticity and trapping of air; *(left)* panlobular emphysema showing abnormal weakening and enlargement of all air spaces distal to the terminal bronchioles (normal alveoli shown for comparison only); *(right)* centrilobular emphysema showing abnormal weakening and enlargement of the respiratory bronchioles in the proximal portion of the acinus. **C,** Chronic bronchitis: inflammation and thickening of mucous membrane with accumulation of mucus and pus leading to obstruction; characterized by cough. **D,** Bronchial asthma: thick mucus, mucosal edema, and smooth muscle spasm causing obstruction of small airways; breathing becomes labored and expiration is difficult. *(Modified from Des Jardins T. & Burton G.G. [1995]. Clinical manifestations and assessment of respiratory disease [3rd ed.]. St. Louis: Mosby.)*

tying of the lungs is slowed, or both. The most common obstructive diseases are asthma, chronic bronchitis, and emphysema. Because many individuals have both chronic bronchitis and emphysema, these diseases together are often called **chronic obstructive pulmonary disease (COPD).** Asthma is more acute and intermittent than COPD, even though it can be chronic (Fig. 26-8).

COPD is second only to heart disease as a cause of disability in adults younger than 65 years. More than one third of all patients admitted to Veterans' Administration (VA) hospitals have evidence of COPD. Its primary cause is ciga-rette smoking, with air pollution and occupational exposure to noxious dusts and gases contributing.

Asthma

Asthma is an inflammatory disease characterized by hyper-responsiveness of the airways and episodic periods of **bronchospasm** (prolonged contractions of the bronchial smooth muscle). Biochemical, autonomic, immunologic, infectious, endocrine, and psychologic factors are involved in varying degrees. Most attacks of asthmatic bronchospasm are short-lived, with freedom from symptoms between episodes, although airway inflammation is present even in asymptomatic individuals.

Asthma occurs at all ages, with approximately half of all cases developing during childhood and another one third developing before 40 years of age. It has been estimated that approximately 5% of adults and 7% to 10% of children in the United States have asthma.[12] Despite the recent increased numbers and availability of antiasthma drugs, asthma morbidity and mortality have risen in the past 20 years. Asthma is a familial disorder, and there is increasing evidence that genetics play an important and complex role in the etiology of the disease.[13] Apparently, environmental factors interact with inherited factors to increase the risk of asthma and to cause attacks of bronchospasm. For example, childhood exposure to high levels of allergens in the environment is associated with an increased likelihood of developing asthma, especially in those children with a family history of asthma. The severity of acute asthma attacks varies among individuals, over time, and with the degree of exposure to inciting factors.

Types of asthma

Asthma classification has changed in recent years. Many references still refer to *extrinsic* and *instrinsic asthma* based on whether the inflammation and airway hyperresponsiveness are mediated by immunoglobulin E (IgE). Recently, consensus groups have developed a system of asthma classification based on clinical severity (Table 26-3) (e.g., severity of symptoms, degree of activity limitation, pulmonary function tests, number of emergency room [ER] visits or hospitalizations) rather than on underlying pathophysiologic differences; this scheme correlates better with management choices and clinical outcomes.[14]

⮕ Pathophysiology

Inflammation resulting in hyperresponsiveness of the airways is the major pathologic feature of all types of asthma. Some of the most important inflammatory mediators that are released during an asthma attack are histamine, prostaglandins, and leukotrienes. In addition, chemotactic factors are produced that result in bronchial infiltration by neutrophils, eosinophils, and lymphocytes. The resulting inflammatory process produces bronchial smooth muscle spasm; vascular congestion; increased vascular permeability; edema formation; production of thick, tenacious mucus; impaired mucociliary function (see Fig. 26-8); thickening of airway walls; and increased contractile response of bronchial smooth muscle. These changes, combined with the epithelial cell damage caused by eosinophil infiltration, produce airway hyperresponsiveness and obstruction and, untreated, can lead to long-term airway damage that is irreversible.[15,16]

Airway obstruction increases resistance to air flow and decreases flow rates, primarily expiratory flow. Impaired expiration causes hyperinflation distal to obstructions and increases the work of breathing. Because of regional differences in airway resistance, the distribution of inspired air is uneven, with more air flowing to the less resistant portions.

Hyperventilation is eventually triggered by lung receptors responding to increased lung volume from air trapping and obstruction. Intrapleural and alveolar gas pressures rise and cause decreased perfusion of the alveoli. Increased alveolar gas pressure, decreased ventilation, and decreased perfusion lead to variable and uneven ventilation-perfusion relationships within different lung segments. The result is early hypoxemia without CO_2 retention (hypercapnia). Hypoxemia further increases hyperventilation by stimulating the respiratory center, so that $PaCO_2$ decreases and pH increases (respiratory alkalosis). As the obstruction becomes more severe, however, the number of alveoli being inadequately ventilated and perfused increases and CO_2 retention and respiratory acidosis develop. Respiratory acidosis signals respiratory failure.

⮕ Clinical Manifestations

During full remission, individuals are asymptomatic and pulmonary function tests are normal. During partial remission, no clinical symptoms are present but pulmonary function tests are abnormal. During attacks, individuals are dyspneic and respiratory effort is marked. Breath sounds decrease except for considerable wheezing. Because the severity of blood gas alterations is difficult to evaluate by clinical signs alone, arterial blood gas tensions should be measured.

If bronchospasm is not reversed by usual measures, the individual is considered to have severe bronchospasm or *status asthmaticus.* If status asthmaticus continues, hypoxemia worsens, expiratory flows and volumes decrease further, and the individual begins to tire. Acidosis develops as arterial PCO_2 begins to rise. Asthma becomes life threatening at this point if treatment does not reverse this process quickly. A silent chest (no audible air movement) and a PCO_2 over 70 mm Hg are ominous signs.

At the beginning of an attack, the individual experiences chest constriction, inspiratory and expiratory wheezing, dyspnea, nonproductive coughing, prolonged expiration, tachycardia, and tachypnea. Severe attacks involve the accessory muscles of respiration. As the episode resolves, coughing produces a thick, stringy, tenacious mucus. If the bronchospasm is not reversed by usual measures, a state of status asthmaticus develops with severe bronchospasm, increased work of breathing, hypoxemia, and respiratory acidosis. Asthma can be life threatening at this point.

⮕ Evaluation and Treatment

Spirometry reveals decreased expiratory flow rate, forced expiratory volume (FEV), and forced vital capacity (FVC) (see Chapter 25) with increased functional residual capacity (FRC) and total lung capacity (TLC). Blood gas analysis shows hypoxemia with early respiratory alkalosis or late respiratory acidosis. These changes are representative of obstruction to expiratory air flow with air trapping and increased lung volumes.

The most successful treatments for asthma are (1) elimination of the causative agents and (2) education. Acute

TABLE 26-3	Asthma Classification Based on Severity			
Disease Category	**Symptoms**	**Nocturnal Symptoms**	**Daily Medication for Long-term Control**	**Medication for Quick Relief**
Step 4: Severe persistent	Continual symptoms Limited physical activity Frequent exacerbations	Frequent	**Two daily medications:** Antiinflammatory agent (high-dose) inhaled glucocorticoid **and** Long acting bronchodilator (inhaled or oral β_2-agonist or theophylline) **and** Oral glucocorticoid	Short-acting, inhaled β_2-agonist Daily use or increasing use indicates need for additional long-term therapy
Step 3: Moderate persistent	Daily symptoms Daily use of inhaled, short-acting β_2-agonist Exacerbations affect activity Exacerbations at least twice weekly and may last for days	More frequent than once weekly	**One or two daily medications:** Antiinflammatory agent (medium-dose inhaled glucocorticoid) **and/or** Medium-dose inhaled glucocorticoid plus long-acting bronchodilator	Short-acting, inhaled β_2-agonist Daily use or increased use indicates need for additional long-term therapy
Step 2: Mild persistent	Symptoms more frequent than twice weekly but less than once per day Exacerbations may affect activity	More frequent than twice monthly	**One daily medication:** Antiinflammatory agent (low-dose inhaled glucocorticoid, cromolyn, or nedocromil) **or** Sustained-release theophylline *NOTE:* Leukotriene modifiers may be considered for individuals at least 12 yr old	Short-acting, inhaled β_2-agonist Daily use or increasing use indicates need for additional long-term therapy
Step 1: Mild intermittent	Symptoms no more frequent than twice weekly Asymptomatic and with normal PEFR between exacerbations Exacerbations brief (hours to days) Intensity of exacerbations varies	No more frequent than twice monthly	**No daily medication**	Short-acting, inhaled β_2-agonist Use more than twice weekly may indicate need to initiate long-term therapy

PEFR, *Peak expiratory flow rate.*

episodes are treated with drugs that are geared toward reversing bronchospasm and airway inflammation. Recommended management includes antiinflammatory therapy (inhaled corticosteroids) followed by prevention of bronchospasms (cromolyn sodium) or treatment of breakthrough symptoms with bronchodilators (β_2-agonists) as needed.[14] Education related to prevention, treatment goals, medication use, and medication side effects is essential to successful management.[17]

HEALTH ALERT

Leukotriene Inhibitors in the Treatment of Asthma

Asthma is an inflammatory disease of the airways. Left untreated, chronic airway inflammation can lead to permanent structural damage to the lungs. Inhaled corticosteroids are the primary drugs used for treating the inflammation of asthma, but they are not effective in all individuals. Some people require systemic steroids, which are associated with a large number of side effects and complications. Leukotrienes are inflammatory mediators that are especially powerful in causing bronchoconstriction and airway edema in asthma, and a new class of drugs has been approved that are receptor antagonists of these leukotrienes. The leukotriene inhibitors have been found to be very effective in treating individuals with asthma with few side effects and are especially helpful in reducing the need for systemic steroid therapy.

Data from Fabbri, L.M. et al. (1998). Physiologic consequences of long-term inflammation. American Journal of Respiratory and Critical Care Medicine, 157(5 Pt. 2), S195-S198; Horowitz, R.J., McGill, K.A., & Busse, W.W. (1998). The role of leukotriene modifiers in the treatment of asthma. American Journal of Respiratory and Critical Care Medicine, 157(5 Pt. 1), 1363-1371; O'Byrne, P.M. (1997). Leukotrienes in the pathogenesis of asthma. Chest, 111(2), 27S-34S; O'Byrne, P.M., Israel, E., & Drazen, J. (1997). Antileukotrienes in the treatment of asthma. Annals of Internal Medicine, 127, 472-480; Roche, W.R. (1998). Inflammatory and structural changes in the small airways in bronchial asthma. American Journal of Respiratory and Critical Care Medicine, 157(6 Pt. 2), S191-S194.

Chronic bronchitis

Bronchitis is inflammation of the bronchi caused by irritants (cigarette smoke, air pollutants) or infection. It can be acute or chronic and is characterized by obstruction of air flow.

Pathophysiology

Chronic bronchitis is defined as hypersecretion of mucus and chronic productive cough for at least 3 months of the year (usually the winter months) for at least 2 consecutive years. Incidence is increased in persons who smoke (up to twentyfold) and even more so in workers exposed to air pollution. It is a major health problem for elderly people. Repeated infections are common.[18]

Inspired irritants increase mucus production, as well as the size and number of mucous glands and goblet cells in the airway epithelium. Thick, tenacious mucus is produced and cannot be cleared because of impaired ciliary function. The lung's defense mechanisms are therefore compromised, increasing susceptibility to pulmonary infection and injury. The bronchial walls become inflamed and thickened from edema, accumulation of inflammatory cells, and thickened smooth muscle from chronic bronchospasm. (The pathogenesis of chronic bronchitis is shown in Fig. 26-9.)[19]

Initially this process affects only the larger bronchi, but eventually all airways are involved. Obstruction of the airways and closure result, particularly during expiration, when the airways are narrowed (Fig. 26-10). The airways collapse early in expiration, trapping gas in the distal portions of the lung. Eventually ventilation-perfusion mismatch, hypoventilation (increased $PaCO_2$), and hypoxemia occur.

Clinical Manifestations

Table 26-4 lists the common clinical manifestations of chronic bronchitis.

Evaluation and Treatment

Diagnosis is based on physical examination, chest radiograph, pulmonary function tests, and blood gas analyses; these tests reflect the progressive nature of the disease. The best "treatment" for chronic bronchitis is prevention, because pathologic changes are not reversible. By the time an individual seeks medical care for symptoms, considerable airway damage is present. If the individual stops smoking, disease progression can be halted. If smoking is stopped before symptoms occur, the risk of chronic bronchitis decreases considerably and eventually reaches that of persons who have never smoked.

Bronchodilators, expectorants, and chest physical therapy are employed as needed. Teaching of individuals includes nutritional counseling, respiratory hygiene, recognition of the early signs of infection, and techniques that relieve dyspnea, such as pursed-lip breathing. Some individuals receive prophylactic antibiotic therapy, particularly during the winter months. Steroids may be needed late in the course of the disease but should be considered a last resort.

✓ QUICK CHECK

Briefly describe the role of neutrophils in acute (adult) respiratory distress syndrome (ARDS).

What mechanisms cause obstruction in asthma?

Define chronic bronchitis.

Emphysema

Emphysema is abnormal permanent enlargement of gas-exchange airways (acini) accompanied by destruction of alveolar walls. Obstruction results from changes in lung tissues, rather than mucus production and inflammation as in

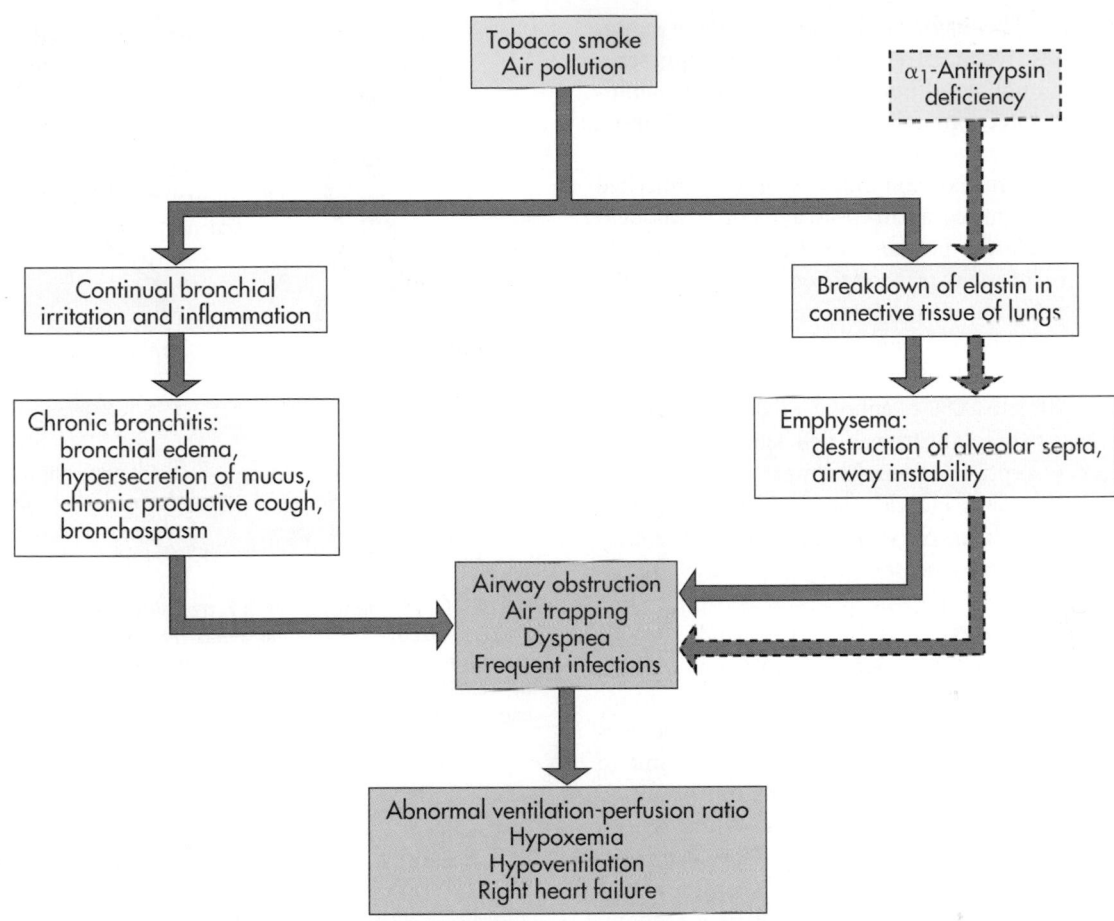

Fig. 26-9 *Pathogenesis of chronic bronchitis and emphysema (chronic obstructive pulmonary disease [COPD]).* (*Dashed arrows* indicate role of α_1-antitrypsin deficiency, if present.)

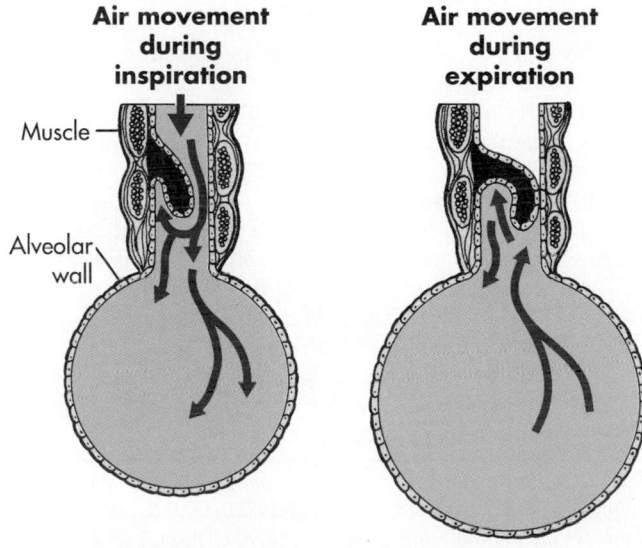

Fig. 26-10 *Mechanisms of air trapping in COPD.* Mucus plugs and narrowed airways cause air trapping and hyperinflation on expiration. During inspiration the airways enlarge, allowing gas to flow past the obstruction. During expiration the airways narrow and prevent gas flow. This mechanism of air trapping, known as "ball valving," occurs in asthma and chronic bronchitis.

TABLE 26-4	Clinical Manifestations of Chronic Obstructive Lung Disease	
Clinical Manifestations	Bronchitis	Emphysema
Productive cough	Classic sign	Late in course with infection
Dyspnea	Late in course	Common
Wheezing	Intermittent	Minimal
History of smoking	Common	Common
Barrel chest	Occasionally	Classic
Prolonged expiration	Always present	Always present
Cyanosis	Common	Uncommon
Chronic hypoventilation	Common	Late in course
Polycythemia	Common	Late in course
Cor pulmonale	Common	Late in course

chronic bronchitis. The major mechanism of air flow limitation is loss of elastic recoil.[19] The major cause of emphysema by far is cigarette smoking, although air pollution and childhood respiratory infections are known to be contributing factors.[18]

Primary emphysema is commonly linked to an inherited deficiency of the enzyme α_1-antitrypsin, a major component of α_1-globulin, a plasma protein. Normally α_1-antitrypsin inhibits the action of many proteolytic enzymes so α_1-antitrypsin deficiency (an autosomal recessive trait) produces an increased likelihood of developing emphysema because proteolysis in lung tissues is not inhibited. Homozygous individuals have a 70% to 80% likelihood of developing lung disease. Persons with α_1-antitrypsin deficiency who smoke are even more susceptible to emphysema.[20] α_1-Antitrypsin deficiency is suggested in individuals who develop emphysema before 40 years of age or in their early 40s and in nonsmokers who develop the disease.

Pathophysiology

Emphysema begins with destruction of alveolar septa, which eliminates portions of the pulmonary capillary bed and increases the volume of air in the acinus. Expiration becomes difficult because loss of elastic recoil reduces the volume of air that can be expired passively. Hyperinflation of alveoli produces large air spaces (bullae) and air spaces adjacent to pleurae (blebs). Bullae and blebs are not effective in gas exchange and result in significant ventilation-perfusion ($\dot{V}/\dot{Q}$) mismatching and hypoxemia. Septal destruction also decreases airway caliber. The combination of increased residual volume and diminished caliber causes part of each inspiration to be trapped in the acinus (Fig. 26-11). Air trapping causes hyperexpansion of the chest, which puts the muscle of respiration at a mechanical disadvantage. This results in increased work load of breathing so that late in the course of disease, many individuals will develop hypoventilation and hypercapnia.

Emphysema can be centriacinar (centrilobular) or panacinar (panlobular), depending on the site of involvement (Fig. 26-12).

1. **Centriacinar emphysema.** Septal destruction occurs in the respiratory bronchioles and alveolar ducts, causing inflammation in bronchioles. Alveolar sac intact. Tends to occur in persons who smoke and persons with chronic bronchitis.
2. **Panacinar emphysema.** Involves entire acinus, with damage more randomly distributed and involving lower lobes of lung. Tends to occur in elderly persons and persons with α_1-antitrypsin deficiency.

Clinical Manifestations

The clinical manifestations of emphysema are listed in Table 26-4.

Evaluation and Treatment

Pulmonary function testing, chest x-ray, and arterial blood gas measurement are used to diagnose emphysema. Pul-

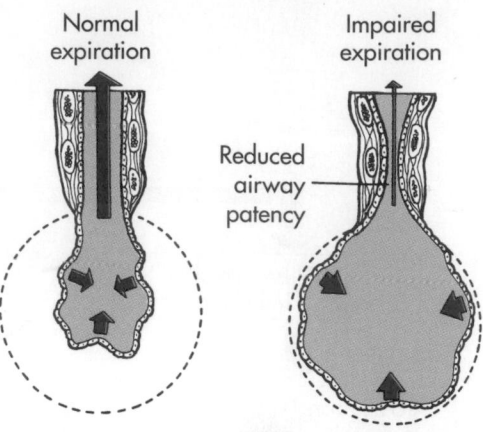

Fig. 26-11 *Mechanisms of air trapping in emphysema.* Damaged or destroyed alveolar walls no longer support and hold open the airways, and alveoli lose their property of passive elastic recoil. Both these factors contribute to collapse during expiration.

HEALTH ALERT

Guidelines for the Pharmacologic Management of COPD

In contrast to asthma, the underlying pathophysiology of emphysema does not include a large component of bronchoconstriction. Some individuals do have some element of reversible airway obstruction, however, and β_2-angonists have long been the mainstay of treatment for COPD. In recent years, the inhaled anticholinergic drug ipratropium has been found to have a longer duration of effective reversal of bronchoconstriction than β_2-angonists in COPD, has fewer side effects, and may even slow the rate of progression of the disease. For these reasons, ipratropium is now considered the first-line drug for use in individuals with COPD, with β_2-agonists used on an as-needed basis if more therapy is required. Theophylline is still indicated for some individuals, especially those with nighttime symptoms. Finally, systemic steroids are helpful in less than 20% of individuals with COPD and should be avoided unless they are of proven effectiveness in a particular individual and all other therapeutic modalities have been exhausted.

Data from Barnes, P.J. (1998). New therapies for chronic obstructive pulmonary disease. Thorax, 53(2), 137-147; Celli, B.R. (1998). Standards for the optimal management of COPD. Chest, 113(4 Suppl.), 283S-287S; Rennard, S.I. (1998). COPD: Overview of definitions, epidemiology, and factors influencing its development. Chest, 113(4 Suppl.), 235S-241S; Tsukino, M. et al. (1998). Effects of theophylline and ipratropium bromide on exercise performance in patients with stable chronic obstructive pulmonary disease. Thorax, 53(4), 269-273.

Fig. 26-12 *Types of emphysema.* **A,** Centriacinar emphysema. **B,** Panacinar emphysema. *(Micrographs from Damjanov, I. & Linder, J. [Eds.]. [1996]. Anderson's pathology [10th ed.]. St. Louis: Mosby.)*

monary function measurements are also helpful in determining a prognosis. Treatment for emphysema is similar to that for chronic bronchitis and includes smoking cessation, bronchodilating drugs, oxygen, breathing retraining, relaxation exercises, and antibiotics for acute infections. The most effective bronchodilating drug for COPD is the anticholinergic drug ipratropium, and this medication may actually slow disease progression.[18] Selected individuals with severe emphysema can benefit from lung reduction surgery or lung transplant.[21]

Respiratory Tract Infections

Respiratory tract infections are the most common cause of short-term disability in the United States. Most of these infections—the common cold, pharyngitis (sore throat), and laryngitis—involve only the upper airways. Although the lungs have direct contact with the atmosphere, they usually remain sterile. Infections of the lower respiratory tract occur most frequently in individuals whose normal defense mechanisms are impaired.

Pneumonia

Pneumonia is an acute infection of the lung caused by bacteria or viruses. More than 1 million cases of pneumonia are diagnosed each year. It occurs primarily during the winter months and is frequently associated with recent upper respiratory tract infection.

Many microorganisms carried in the oropharynx of normal individuals can cause pneumonia. The most common causal microorganisms are the following:

Gram-Positive Bacteria	Gram-Negative Bacteria	Nonbacterial Organisms
Streptococcus pneumoniae	*Escherichia coli*	*Pneumocystis carinii*
Mycoplasma pneumoniae	*Pseudomonas aeruginosa*	Fungi
Klebsiella pneumoniae	*Proteus* species	Viruses
Staphylococcus aureus	*Bacteroides* species	*Legionella* species
Streptococcus pyogenes	*Haemophilus* species	

Fungi are an uncommon cause of pneumonia, but fungal pneumonia can be caused in immunosuppressed individuals by *Candida, Mucor,* and *Aspergillus.* Fungi associated with histoplasmosis and coccidioidomycosis can infect both normal and immunosuppressed individuals.

The microorganisms that cause community-acquired pneumonia usually differ in identity, virulence, and mortality from those that cause hospital-acquired, or nosocomial, pneumonia. Community-acquired pneumonia is usually caused by *Streptococcus pneumoniae* or *Mycoplasma pneu-*

moniae. Mortality from these two organisms is very low (less than 5%). *Staphylococcus aureus, Haemophilus influenzae,* and *Klebsiella pneumoniae* cause some community-acquired disease, usually in individuals with other health problems, such as COPD or alcoholism, and can cause secondary infection in individuals with a primary viral illness. Viral pneumonia is usually caused by influenza viruses.

Most nosocomial pneumonias are caused by gram-negative bacteria, commonly *Escherichia coli, Klebsiella pneumoniae,* and *Pseudomonas aeruginosa,* although *S. aureus,* which is gram-positive, also causes pneumonia in some hospitalized individuals. The nosocomially acquired organisms result in more serious infection, with an average mortality of 50%. They are also more likely to result in lung necrosis, abscess, or empyema.

The *Legionella* species are widely distributed in water environments and are present in cooling systems and towers, condensers, shower heads, and water reservoirs. Infections may occur sporadically or in outbreaks, as was the case in the 1976 incident at the American Legion Convention in Philadelphia.

Pathophysiology

Pathogenic microorganisms can reach the lung by several routes:

- Aspiration of infected oropharyngeal secretions is the most common route of infection.
- When an infected individual coughs, sneezes, or talks, microorganisms are released into the air to be inhaled by other people.
- Microorganisms can also be inspired with aerosols (nebulized gas) from contaminated respiratory therapy equipment.
- In illness or poor dental hygiene, normal flora of the oropharynx can become pathogenic.
- *Staphylococcus* and gram-negative bacteria can be spread by the circulation from a systemic infection, by sepsis, or by contaminated needles of intravenous (IV) drug abusers.

In healthy individuals, pathogens that reach the lung are expelled or held in check by self-defense mechanisms. The cough reflex, mucociliary clearance, and phagocytosis by alveolar macrophages are backed up by the body's immune system and various components of the inflammatory response, including the release of biochemical mediators by alveolar mast cells (see Chapters 5 and 6). In susceptible individuals the invading pathogen multiplies, releasing damaging toxins and stimulating full-scale inflammatory and immune responses, both of which have damaging side effects. The antigen-antibody reaction and the endotoxins released by some microorganisms damage bronchial mucous membranes and alveolocapillary membranes. Inflammation and edema cause the acini and terminal bronchioles to fill with infectious debris and exudate, leading to ventilation-perfusion abnormalities.[20] If the pneumonia is caused by *Staphylococcus* or gram-negative bacteria, necrosis of lung parenchyma may also occur.

Pneumococcal pneumonia

In pneumococcal pneumonia, *S. pneumoniae* organisms initiate the inflammatory response, and inflammatory exudate causes alveolar edema, which leads to the other changes shown in Fig. 26-13.

Viral pneumonia

Viral pneumonia is usually mild and self-limiting but can set the stage for a secondary bacterial infection by providing an ideal environment for bacterial growth and by damaging ciliated epithelial cells, which normally prevent pathogens from reaching the lower airways. Viral pneumonia can be a primary infection or a complication of another viral illness, such as chickenpox or measles (spread from the blood). The virus not only destroys the ciliated epithelial cells but also invades the goblet cells and bronchial mucous glands. Sloughing of destroyed bronchial epithelium occurs throughout the respiratory tract, preventing mucociliary clearance. Bronchial walls become edematous and infiltrated with leukocytes. In severe cases, the alveoli are involved with decreased compliance and increased work of breathing.

Clinical Manifestations

Most cases of pneumonia are preceded by an upper respiratory infection, which is frequently viral. Individuals then develop fever, chills, productive or dry cough, malaise, pleural pain, and sometimes dyspnea and hemoptysis.

The white blood cell count is usually elevated (more than 10,000/mm³), although it may be low (less than 6000/mm³) if the individual is debilitated. Chest radiographs show infiltrates that may involve a single lobe of the lung (***lobar pneumonia***) or may be more diffuse (***bronchopneumonia***).[22]

Once the diagnosis of pneumonia has been made, the pathogen is identified by means of sputum characteristics (Gram stain, color, odor) and cultures or, if sputum is absent, blood cultures. Purulent sputum is expectorated by individuals with bacterial pneumonia, and the appearance and odor of the sputum aid in pathogen identification. Viral pneumonia and pneumonia caused by *M. pneumoniae* characteristically result in scanty sputum production. Because many pathogens exist in the normal oropharyngeal flora, the specimen may be contaminated with pathogens from oral secretions. Transtracheal aspiration is used to obtain an uncontaminated sputum specimen.

If sputum studies fail to identify the pathogen, the individual is immunocompromised, or the individual's condition worsens, further diagnostic studies may include bronchoscopy or lung biopsy. Positive identification of viruses can be difficult. Blood cultures often help to identify the virus if systemic disease is present.

Evaluation and Treatment

Diagnosis is made on the basis of physical examination, cultures of blood, and cultures of respiratory secretions. Antibiotics are used to treat bacterial pneumonia; however, resistant strains of pneumococcus are on the rise.[23] Viral pneumonia is treated with supportive therapy alone, unless

Fig. 26-13 *Pathophysiologic course of bacterial pneumonia.*

secondary bacterial infection is present. Adequate hydration and good pulmonary hygeine (e.g., deep breathing, coughing, chest physical therapy) are important aspects of treatment for all types of pneumonia.

Tuberculosis

Tuberculosis is caused by *Mycobacterium tuberculosis,* an acid-fast bacillus that usually affects the lungs but may invade other body systems. Before the advent of specific antimicrobial therapy, tuberculosis was an important cause of death and disability in North America. From 1950 to 1980 the incidence of tuberculosis decreased; from 1985 to 1992 the number of reported cases has increased alarmingly by nearly 19%; and since 1992 the incidence has decreased once again.[24] The largest increases have occurred in men 25 to 44 years old and, to a lesser extent, in children younger than 15 years and in Hispanic, black, and Asian populations. The major reason for this trend is the epidemic of acquired immunodeficiency syndrome (AIDS). Individuals with AIDS are highly susceptible to respiratory infections, including tuberculosis. A second important reason is the growing number of drug-resistant strains of tuberculosis bacillus that have developed because individuals do not consistently take their medications, allowing resistant strains to be selected and spread.[25] Emigration of infected individuals from high-prevalence areas, transmission in crowded institutional settings, homelessness, substance abuse, and lack of access to medical care have also contributed to the problem.

Pathophysiology

Like some types of pneumonia, tuberculosis is transmitted from person to person in airborne droplets. Microorganisms lodge in the lung periphery, usually in the upper lobe. Once the bacilli are inspired into the lung, they multiply and cause nonspecific pneumonitis (lung inflammation). Some bacilli migrate through the lymphatics and become lodged in the lymph nodes, where they encounter lymphocytes and initiate the immune response.

Inflammation in the lung causes neutrophils to migrate there and then alveolar macrophages. These cells are phagocytes that engulf the bacilli and begin the process by which the body's defense mechanisms isolate the bacilli, preventing their spread. The neutrophils and macrophages seal off the colonies of bacilli, forming a granulomatous lesion called a *tubercle* (see Chapter 6). Infected tissues within the tubercle die, forming cheeselike material called *caseation necrosis.* Collagenous scar tissue then grows around the tubercle, completing isolation of the bacilli. The immune response is complete after about 10 days, preventing further multiplication of the bacilli.

Once the bacilli are isolated in tubercles and immunity develops, tuberculosis may remain dormant for life. If the immune system is impaired, however, or if live bacilli escape into the bronchi, active disease occurs and may spread through the blood and lymphatics to other organs. Endogenous reactivation of dormant bacilli in the elderly population may be caused by poor nutritional status, insulin-dependent diabetes, long-term corticosteroid therapy, and other debilitating diseases.

Clinical Manifestations

In many infected individuals, tuberculosis is asymptomatic. In others, symptoms develop so gradually that they are not noticed until the disease is advanced. However, symptoms can appear in immunosuppressed individuals within weeks of exposure to the bacillus. Common clinical manifestations include fatigue, weight loss, lethargy, anorexia (loss of appetite), and a low-grade fever that usually occurs in the afternoon. A cough that produces purulent sputum develops slowly and becomes more frequent over several weeks or months. Night sweats and general anxiety are often present. Dyspnea, chest pain, and hemoptysis are uncommon findings.

Evaluation and Treatment

Tuberculosis is diagnosed by a positive tuberculin skin test, sputum culture, and chest radiographs. Tuberculosis is graded as follows to aid in evaluation and determination of appropriate therapy[26]:

0	No tuberculosis, no exposure, no infection
1	Exposure to tuberculosis, no infection
2	Tuberculosis infection, no disease
3	Tuberculosis, active disease
4	Tuberculosis, no active disease
5	Tuberculosis suspected

Treatment consists of antibiotic therapy to control active or dormant tuberculosis and prevent transmission. Today, with the increased numbers of immunosuppressed and susceptible individuals and drug-resistant bacilli, the recommended treatment includes a combination of drugs to which the organism is susceptible, including use of isoniazid, rifampin, pyrazinamide, ethambutol, and streptomycin.

✓ QUICK CHECK

What are the two major types of emphysema?

Compare pneumococcal and viral pneumonia as to severity of disease.

Describe the pathophysiologic features of tuberculosis.

In the past, individuals with active tuberculosis were isolated from the community and their families in sanitariums. Today, individuals remain at home or, rarely, in the hospital, until sputum cultures show that the active bacilli have been eliminated. This usually takes a few weeks to 2 months if antibiotics are taken conscientiously. If the individual's cooperation is in question, it is advisable for the administration of the drugs to be supervised by health care workers.[27]

Acute bronchitis

Acute bronchitis is acute infection or inflammation of the airways or bronchi that commonly follows a viral illness and is usually self-limiting. Many clinical manifestations are similar to those of pneumonia (i.e., fever, cough, chills, malaise), but chest radiographs show no infiltrates. Individuals with viral bronchitis present with a nonproductive cough that frequently occurs in paroxysms and is aggravated by cold, dry, or dusty air. Purulent sputum may be produced. Chest pain often develops from the effort of coughing. Treatment consists of rest, aspirin, humidity, and a cough suppressant, such as codeine.

Individuals with bacterial bronchitis present with a productive cough, fever, and pain behind the sternum that is aggravated by coughing. It is rare in previously healthy adults except after viral infection but is common in patients with COPD. Bacterial bronchitis is treated with rest, antipyretics, humidity, and antibiotics (usually a penicillinase-resistant penicillin). If the cough is nonproductive, a cough suppressant is given, because a dry cough can cause bronchial irritation and damage. Acute bronchitis may progress to pneumonia.

Pulmonary Vascular Disease

Blood flow through the lungs can be disrupted by disorders that occlude the vessels, increase pulmonary vascular resistance, or destroy the vascular bed. Effects of altered pulmonary blood flow may range from insignificant dysfunction to severe and life-threatening changes in ventilation-perfusion ratios. Major disorders include pulmonary embolism, pulmonary hypertension, and cor pulmonale.

Pulmonary embolism

Pulmonary embolism is occlusion of a portion of the pulmonary vascular bed by an embolus, which can be a thrombus (blood clot), tissue fragment, lipids (fats), or an air bubble. The most common emboli are thrombi dislodged from deep veins in the thigh. They can also originate in the pelvis, particularly in pregnant women.

Risk factors for *pulmonary thromboembolism,* or the obstruction of a pulmonary vessel by a thrombus, include conditions and disorders that promote blood clotting as a result of venous stasis (slowing or stagnation of blood flow through the veins), hypercoagulability (increased tendency of the blood to form clots), and injuries to the endothelial cells that line the vessels.

No matter its source, a blood clot becomes an embolus when all or part of it breaks away from the site of formation and begins to travel in the bloodstream. (Thromboembolism is described further in Chapter 20.)

Although the overall incidence of pulmonary embolism has declined in recent years, it remains an important cause of death, especially in elderly persons and hospitalized patients.[28] Emboli remain the third leading cause of death in the United States.

Pathophysiology

The impact or effect of the embolus depends on the extent of pulmonary blood flow obstruction, the size of the affected vessels, the nature of the embolus, and the secondary effects. Pulmonary emboli can occur as any of the following:

1. Massive occlusion: an embolus that occludes a major por-

Fig. 26-14 *Pathogenesis of massive pulmonary embolism caused by a thrombus (pulmonary thromboembolism).*

tion of the pulmonary circulation (i.e., main pulmonary artery embolus)

2. Embolus with infarction: an embolus that is large enough to cause infarction (death) of a portion of lung tissue
3. Embolus without infarction: an embolus that is not severe enough to cause permanent lung injury
4. Multiple pulmonary emboli: may be chronic or recurrent

The pathogenesis of pulmonary embolism caused by a thrombus is summarized in Fig. 26-14.

If the embolus does not cause infarction, the clot is dissolved by the fibrinolytic system and pulmonary function returns to normal. If pulmonary infarction occurs, shrinking and scarring develop in the affected area of the lung.

Clinical Manifestations

In most cases the clinical manifestations of pulmonary embolism are nonspecific, so evaluation of risk factors and predisposing factors is an important aspect of diagnosis.[29] More than 90% of pulmonary emboli result from clots formed in the veins of the legs and pelvis. The characteristic signs of

deep vein thrombosis are leg swelling, duskiness, and a positive Homans sign (calf pain on palpation and dorsiflexion of the foot). Sometimes the thrombus is palpable, but quite often the legs appear normal or signs are masked by superficial thrombophlebitis.

Massive occlusion causes profound shock, hypotension, tachypnea, tachycardia, severe pulmonary hypertension, and chest pain. Diagnosis can be difficult because the signs mimic those of other cardiopulmonary problems. Once these manifestations occur, death is imminent.

Manifestations of emboli that cause infarction are pleural pain, dyspnea, pleural friction rub, pleural effusion, hemoptysis, fever, and leukocytosis. On chest radiographs, the infarcted portion of the lung appears as a nonspecific infiltrate in a classic wedge shape bordering the pleura. Pulmonary infarction is most likely in individuals with underlying pulmonary disease.

Pulmonary embolism without infarction is the most common type and is the most difficult to evaluate. The individual usually presents with tachypnea, tachycardia, dyspnea, and unexplained anxiety. Occasionally syncope (fainting) or pleural pain occurs. Recurrent pulmonary emboli occur in individuals with a history of previous emboli. Recurrent emboli may not be detected until progressive incapacitation, precordial pain, anxiety, dyspnea, and right ventricular enlargement are exhibited.

Evaluation and Treatment

Routine chest radiographs and pulmonary function tests are not definitive for pulmonary embolism. Pulmonary embolism is suggested if arterial blood gas analyses demonstrate unexplained hypoxemia and hyperventilation. A perfusion scan, in which lungs are scanned after injection of a radioactive substance into the venous circulation, may indicate embolism.

The ideal treatment for pulmonary embolism is prevention through risk factor analysis and elimination of predisposing factors for individuals at risk. Venous stasis in hospital patients is minimized by leg elevation, bed exercises, position changes, early postoperative ambulation, and pneumatic calf compression. Clot formation is also prevented by prophylactic low-dose anticoagulant therapy; less anticoagulant is required to prevent a clot than to treat one.

Anticoagulant therapy is the primary treatment for pulmonary embolism. Intravenous administration of heparin is begun immediately and is followed by oral doses of coumarin. Recent studies suggest that the new low-molecular-weight heparin (enoxaparin) is as safe and effective as standard heparin but is easier to administer.[30] If massive life-threatening embolism occurs, a fibrinolytic agent, such as streptokinase, is sometimes used.

Pulmonary hypertension

Pulmonary hypertension is high blood pressure in the pulmonary arteries, specifically a rise in pulmonary artery pressure (normally pressure is 15 to 18 mm Hg) of 5 to 10 mm Hg above normal. Normally, mean pulmonary artery pressure is lower than mean systemic artery pressure.

Primary pulmonary hypertension is very rare, has no known cause, usually occurs in women between the ages of 20 and 40 years, and may be hereditary. Primary pulmonary hypertension has a very poor prognosis—most individuals die within 5 years of diagnosis.

Secondary pulmonary hypertension is more common. It can be secondary to any respiratory or cardiovascular disorder that (1) increases the volume or pressure of blood entering the pulmonary arteries or (2) narrows or obstructs the pulmonary arteries. The first cause overloads the pulmonary circulation from without; the second elevates blood pressure by increasing resistance to flow within the lungs.

Pathophysiology

In primary hypertension the small pulmonary arteries (arterioles) become narrow or obliterated as a result of hypertrophy (enlargement) of smooth muscle in the vessel walls and formation of fibrous lesions around the vessels. Pressures in the left ventricle, which receives blood from the lungs, remain normal, but high pressures generated in the lungs are transmitted to the right ventricle, which supplies the pulmonary arteries, and eventually the right ventricle fails *(cor pulmonale)*. Oxygenation is not severely affected, although mild hypoxia and cyanosis do occur. Death eventually results from cor pulmonale. (Mechanisms of heart failure are described in Chapter 23.)

There are four causes of secondary pulmonary hypertension:

1. Elevated left ventricular filling pressures, as occur in coronary artery disease and mitral valve disease
2. Increased blood flow through the pulmonary circulation (left-to-right shunts), as occurs with a ventricular septal defect or patent ductus arteriosus
3. Obliteration or obstruction of the pulmonary vascular bed by a pulmonary embolus or by chronic destruction of alveolar wall (i.e., emphysema)
4. Vasoconstriction of the vascular bed, as occurs with hypoxemia, acidosis, or their combination

Secondary pulmonary hypertension can be reversed if the primary disorder is resolved. If hypertension persists, hypertrophy occurs in the medial smooth muscle layer of the arterioles. The larger arteries stiffen, and hypertension progresses until pulmonary artery pressure equals systemic blood pressure, causing right ventricular hypertrophy and eventual cor pulmonale. The pathogenesis of heart failure caused by secondary pulmonary hypertension is shown in Fig. 26-15.

Clinical Manifestations

Pulmonary hypertension may not be detected until pulmonary artery pressure is equal to systemic blood pressure. The symptoms are often masked by primary pulmonary or cardiovascular disease. The first indication of pulmonary hypertension may be an abnormality seen on a chest radiograph (enlarged right heart border) or an electrocardiogram that shows right ventricular hypertrophy. Manifestations of fatigue, chest discomfort, tachypnea, and dyspnea, particularly with exercise, are common.

Fig. 26-15 *Pathogenesis of pulmonary hypertension and cor pulmonale.*

Evaluation and Treatment

Diagnosis of pulmonary hypertension can be made only with right heart catheterization. The diagnosis of primary pulmonary hypertension is made when all other causes of hypertension, such as mitral stenosis (see Chapter 23), COPD, and pulmonary embolus, have been ruled out.

There is no effective treatment for primary pulmonary hypertension except lung transplantation, but supplemental oxygen, digitalis, and diuretics are used as palliatives. The most effective treatment for secondary pulmonary hypertension is treatment of the primary disorder. Once pulmonary hypertension has persisted long enough for hypertrophy of the medial smooth muscle layer to develop, however, as it does with chronic hypoxemia, it is no longer reversible. Treatment often includes supplemental oxygen to reverse hypoxic vasoconstriction. Diuretics and digitalis are used judiciously to treat right ventricular failure.

Cor pulmonale

Cor pulmonale, also called *pulmonary heart disease,* consists of right ventricular enlargement (hypertrophy, dilation, or both). It is secondary to pulmonary hypertension caused by disorders of the lungs or chest wall.

Pathophysiology

Cor pulmonale develops as pulmonary hypertension creates chronic pressure overload in the right ventricle similar to that created in the left ventricle by systemic hypertension. (Systemic hypertension is discussed in Chapter 23.) Pressure overload increases the work of the right ventricle and causes hypertrophy of the normally thin-walled heart muscle.

Acute hypoxemia, as with pneumonia, can exaggerate pulmonary hypertension and dilate the ventricle as well. Right ventricular filling pressures are normal until failure occurs. The right ventricle usually fails when pulmonary artery pressure equals systemic blood pressure.

Clinical Manifestations

The clinical manifestations of cor pulmonale may be obscured by primary respiratory disease and appear only during exercise testing. The heart may appear normal at rest, but with exercise, cardiac output falls and the electrocardiogram shows right ventricular hypertrophy. Chest pain is common. The pulmonary component of the second heart sound, which represents closure of the pulmonic valve, may be accentuated, and a pulmonic valve murmur also may be present. Tricuspid valve murmur may accompany the development of right ventricular failure. Increased pressures in the systemic venous circulation may result in peripheral edema.

Evaluation and Treatment

Diagnosis is based on physical examination, radiologic examination, and electrocardiogram or echocardiography or both. The goal of treatment for cor pulmonale is to decrease the work load of the right ventricle by lowering pulmonary artery pressure. Treatment is the same as for pulmonary hypertension, and its success depends on reversal of the underlying lung disease.

> ### ✓ QUICK CHECK
>
> What factors influence the impact of an embolus?
>
> List three causes of pulmonary hypertension.
>
> What is cor pulmonale?

Lip Cancer

Cancer of the lip is more prevalent in men, with 3100 new cases per year accounting for about 1% of all cancers in men.[31] Long-term exposure to sun, wind, and cold over a period of years results in dryness, chapping, hyperkeratosis, and predisposition to malignancy. In addition, immunosuppression, such as that seen in individuals with renal transplants, increases the risk for lip cancer. The lower lip is the most common site.

Pathophysiology

The most common form of lower lip cancer is termed *exophytic*. The lesion usually develops in the outer part of the lip along the vermilion border. The lip becomes thickened and evolves to an ulcerated center with a raised border (Fig. 26-16). Verrucous-type lesions are less common. They have an irregular surface, follow cracks in the lip, and tend to extend toward the inner surface. Squamous cell carcinoma is the most common cell type. Basal cell carcinoma does not develop unless there is extension beyond the mucous membrane or vermilion border of the lip.

Fig. 26-16 *Lip cancer.* Carcinoma of lower lip with central ulceration and raised, rolled borders. *(From del Regato, J.A., Spjut, H.J., & Cox, J.D. [1985]. Ackerman and del Regato's cancer [2nd ed.]. St. Louis: Mosby.)*

Staging of Lip Cancer   BOX 26-1

STAGE 1
Primary tumor less than 2 cm; no palpable nodes

STAGE II
Primary tumor 2 to 4 cm; no palpable nodes

STAGE III
Primary tumor over 4 cm; metastatic lymph nodes

STAGE IV
Large primary tumors; nodes fixed to mandible or distant metastases

Clinical Manifestations

Malignant lesions are often preceded by the development of a blister that evolves into a superficial ulceration. There may be a history of recurrent scales that precede development of a bleeding ulceration. Metastases to the cervical lymph nodes have a low rate of occurrence (2% to 8%) and are more likely when the primary lesion is larger and exists for a longer period.

Evaluation and Treatment

Diagnosis is commonly made by clinical history and presentation of the lesion. Biopsy confirms the presence of malignant cells. The staging for lip cancer is summarized in Box 26-1. Surgical excision is effective for smaller lesions. A relatively new surgical technique, called the *Mohs micrographic surgery*, has been found to be highly effective with a low risk of local recurrence (8%).[32] Larger lesions that require extensive resection may be followed by cosmetic surgeries. The prognosis for recovery is excellent, and deaths are usually the result of inadequate treatment.

Laryngeal Cancer

Cancer of the larynx represents approximately 2% to 3% of all cancers in the United States. There are approximately 10,600 new cases per year, 8600 of them in men.[31] The risk of laryngeal cancer is increased by the amount of tobacco

Fig. 26-17 *Laryngeal cancer.* **A,** Mirror view of carcinoma of right false cord partially hiding true cord. **B,** Lateral view. *(From del Regato, J.A., Spjut, H.J., & Cox, J.D. [1985]. Ackerman and del Regato's cancer [2nd ed.]. St. Louis: Mosby.)*

smoked; risk is further heightened with the combination of smoking and alcohol consumption. The highest incidence is in men between 50 and 75 years of age.

Pathophysiology

Carcinoma of the true vocal cords (glottis) is more common than that of the supraglottic structures (epiglottis, aryepiglottic folds, arytenoids, false cords). Tumors of the subglottic area are rare. Squamous cell carcinoma is the most common cell type, although small cell carcinomas also occur (Fig. 26-17). Metastasis develops by spread to the draining lymph nodes, and distant metastasis, usually to the lung, is rare.

Clinical Manifestations

The presenting symptoms of laryngeal cancer include hoarseness, dyspnea, and cough. Progressive hoarseness is the most significant symptom and can result in voice loss. Dyspnea is rare with supraglottic tumors but can be severe in subglottic tumors. Cough occurs less commonly and may follow swallowing. Laryngeal pain or a sore throat is likely with supraglottic lesions.

Evaluation and Treatment

Evaluation of the larynx includes external inspection and palpation of the larynx and the lymph nodes of the neck. Indirect laryngoscopy provides a stereoscopic view of the structure and movement of the larynx. A biopsy can also be obtained during this procedure. Direct laryngoscopy provides specific visualization of the tumor. Plain films of the larynx and computed tomography facilitate the identification of tumor boundaries and the degree of extension to surrounding tissue.

Radiation therapy has shown good results for early carcinoma of the vocal cords and is used as an adjunct to surgery in more advanced disease. Partial laryngectomies are

the preferred treatment for small supraglottic and subglottic malignancies. Total laryngectomy is required when lesions are extensive and involve the cartilage. Efforts to preserve voice function and improve quality of life continue to be evaluated.[33]

Lung Cancer

Lung cancers (bronchogenic carcinomas) arise from the epithelium of the respiratory tract. Therefore the term *lung cancer* excludes other pulmonary tumors, including sarcomas, lymphomas, blastomas, hematomas, and mesotheliomas. Lung cancer is an epidemic in the United States, with an estimated 171,600 new cases in 1999.[31] It is the most frequent cause of cancer death, is responsible for 6% of all deaths in the United States, and, along with malignant melanoma, is the only major cancer type whose incidence is rapidly increasing. Although deaths caused by lung cancer in men have declined, the increase among women has been extraordinarily high—higher than that of any other cancer because of increased cigarette smoking by women. Deaths from lung cancer appear at ages 35 to 44 years; a sharp increase occurs between the ages of 45 and 55 years; and the incidence rate continues to increase through ages 65 to 74 years, after which it levels off and decreases among very old persons.

The most common cause of lung cancer is cigarette smoking. Approximately one in every ten smokers will develop lung cancer. Cigarette smoke contains several organ-specific carcinogens, and smoking has been causally related to carcinogenesis at several sites, including the larynx, oral cavity, esophagus, and urinary bladder. Smokers with obstructive lung disease (low FEV_1) are at even greater risk.[34] Genetic predisposition to developing lung cancer, which is evident in analysis of pedigrees, also plays a role in its pathophysiology. Risk factors for lung cancer are summarized in the Risk Factor box.

The cancer death rates for pipe and cigar users are about equal to those of cigarette smokers for cancer of the larynx, oral cavity, and esophagus. The incidence of lung cancer decreases among people who stop smoking, and it reaches a level almost as low as that of nonsmokers (those who have never smoked) 15 years after smoking has stopped. Carcinogenesis is discussed in Chapters 9 and 10.

Types of lung cancer

At least 12 different cell types of tumors are included under the broad heading of lung cancer. The four major histologic types are squamous cell carcinoma, small cell carcinoma, large cell carcinoma, and adenocarcinoma (including bronchioloalveolar cell carcinoma). For clinical and therapeutic reasons, however, lung cancers are frequently classified as small cell lung cancer (SCLC, 25% of all lung cancers) and non-SCLC (NSCLC, 75% of all lung cancers). Characteristics of these tumors, including evaluation and treatment, are listed in Table 26-5.

Non–small cell lung cancer

Squamous cell carcinoma. ***Squamous cell carcinoma*** accounts for about 30% of bronchogenic carcinomas, representing a sharp decline in incidence in the past 2 decades. These tumors are typically located near the hilus and project into bronchi (Fig. 26-18, A).

Because of the location in the central bronchi, obstructive manifestations are nonspecific and include nonproductive cough or hemoptysis. Pneumonia and atelectasis are often associated with squamous cell carcinoma (Fig. 26-18, A). Chest pain is a late symptom associated with large tumors. These tumors can remain fairly well localized and tend not to metastasize until late in the course of the disease. The preferred treatment is surgical resection, although once metastasis has taken place, total surgical resection is most difficult and survival rates dramatically decrease.

Adenocarcinoma. ***Adenocarcinoma*** (tumor arising from glands) of the lung constitutes 35% to 40% of all bron-

TABLE 26-5	**Characteristics of Common Lung Cancers**			
Tumor Type	**Growth Rate**	**Metastasis**	**Means of Diagnosis**	**Clinical Manifestations and Treatment**
Squamous cell carcinoma (30% of bronchogenic carcinomas)	Slow	Late; mostly to hilar lymph nodes	Biopsy, sputum analysis, bronchoscopy, electron microscopy, immunohistochemistry	Cough, sputum production, airway obstruction Treated surgically
Adenocarcinoma (30%-35% of bronchogenic carcinomas)	Moderate	Early	Radiography, fiberoptic bronchoscopy, electron microscopy	Pleural effusion Treated surgically
Large cell carcinoma (10%-15% of bronchogenic carcinomas)	Rapid	Early and widespread	Sputum analysis, bronchoscopy, electron microscopy (by exclusion of other cell types)	Chest wall pain, pleural effusion, cough, sputum production, hemoptysis, airway obstruction caused by pneumonia (if airways involved) Treated surgically
Small cell (oat cell) carcinoma (20%-25% of bronchogenic carcinomas)	Very rapid	Very early; to mediastinum or distally in lung	Radiography, sputum analysis, bronchoscopy, electron microscopy, immunohistochemistry, and clinical manifestations (cough, chest pain, dyspnea, hemoptysis, localized wheezing)	Airway obstruction caused by pneumonitis, signs and symptoms of excessive hormone secretion Treated by chemotherapy and ionizing radiation to thorax and central nervous system
Mesotheliomas (80% of sarcomas of pleural membrane)	Slow	Late and usually asymptomatic	Radiography, history of exposure to asbestos, thoracoscopy	Dyspnea, pleuritic pain Treated surgically

Fig. 26-18 *Lung cancer.* **A,** Squamous cell carcinoma. This hilar tumor originates from the main bronchus. **B,** Peripheral adenocarcinoma. The tumor shows prominent black pigmentation, suggestive of having evolved in an anthracotic scar. **C,** Small cell carcinoma. The tumor forms confluent nodules. On cross section, the nodules have an encephalid appearance. *(From Damjanov, I. & Linder J. [Eds.]. [1996]. Anderson's pathology [10th ed.]. St. Louis: Mosby.)*

chogenic carcinomas (Fig. 26-18, *B*). The recent increase in incidence of adenocarcinoma has been ascribed to the increasing frequency of lung cancer in women, environmental and occupational carcinogens, and changes in the histologic criteria for diagnosis. These tumors, which are usually smaller than 4 cm, more commonly arise in the peripheral regions of the pulmonary parenchyma. They may be asymptomatic and discovered by routine chest roentgenogram in the early stages, or the individual may present with pleuritic chest pain and shortness of breath from pleural involvement by the tumor.

Included in the category of adenocarcinoma is bronchioloalveolar cell carcinoma. These tumors tend to arise from the terminal bronchioles and alveoli. They are slow-growing tumors with an unpredictable pattern of metastasis. Metastasis occurs through the pulmonary arterial system and mediastinal lymph nodes. This cell type has the weakest association with smoking.

Surgical resection is possible in a high proportion of cases, but because metastasis occurs early, the 5-year survival rate is less than 10%. Newer chemotherapy agents are resulting in increased survival rates in recent studies.[35]

*Large cell carcinoma (undifferentiated). **Undifferentiated large cell carcinomas** constitute 10% and 15% of bronchogenic carcinomas. This cell type has lost all evidence of differentiation and is therefore commonly referred to as **un-***

TABLE 26-6	TNM Classification of Lung Cancer
Symbol	**Definition**
Primary tumors (T)	
T0	No evidence of primary tumor
TX	Presence of tumor proved by malignant cells in bronchopulmonary secretions but not visualized by x-ray films or bronchoscopy
Tis	Carcinoma in situ
T1	Tumor 3.0 cm or less in diameter, surrounded by lung or visceral pleura, no evidence of invasion proximal to a lobar bronchus at bronchoscopy
T2	Tumor more than 3.0 cm in diameter, or a tumor of any size that invades the visceral pleura or has associated atelectasis or obstructive pneumonitis of the hilar regions
T3	Tumor of any size with direct extension into an adjacent structure, such as chest wall, diaphragm, or mediastinum; or tumor demonstrated bronchoscopically to involve a main bronchus less than 2.0 cm to the carina; any tumor associated with atelectasis or obstructive pneumonitis of an entire lung or pleural effusion
T4	Tumor of any size with invasion of the mediastinum or involvement of heart, great vessels, trachea, esophagus, vertebral body, carina, or presence of malignant pleural effusion
Lymph node involvement (N)	
N0	No demonstrable metastasis to regional lymph nodes
N1	Metastasis to nodes in the peribronchial and/or ipsilateral hilar region
N2	Metastasis to ipsilateral lymph nodes within the mediastinum
N3	Metastasis to contralateral mediastinal or hilar lymph nodes; or contralateral ipsilateral scalene or supraclavicular nodes
Metastasis (M)	
M0	No distant metastasis
M1	Distant metastasis, such as to scalene or contralateral hilar lymph nodes, brain, bones, lung, liver

differentiated large cell anaplastic cancer. Because large cell carcinomas show none of the histologic findings of squamous cell carcinoma or adenocarcinoma, they are diagnosed by a process of exclusion. The cells are generally larger than leukocytes and contain large, darkly stained nuclei. These tumors commonly arise peripherally but are found centrally and can grow to distort the trachea and cause widening of the carina.

Once metastasis has occurred, surgical therapy is limited to palliative procedures (comfort measures) designed to relieve obstructive pneumonitis or prevent recurrence of pleural effusion. Neither radiation therapy nor chemotherapy has been successful in increasing survival.

Small cell carcinoma

Small cell carcinomas constitute 20% to 25% of bronchogenic carcinomas. It is estimated that most of these tumors are central in origin (Fig. 26-18, *C*). Cell sizes range from 6 to 8 μm. When almost no cytoplasm is present (because of density of cells) and the cells are compressed into an ovoid mass, the tumor is called *oat cell carcinoma.* This cell type has the strongest correlation with cigarette smoking. Because these tumors show a rapid rate of growth and tend to metastasize early and widely, small cell carcinomas have the worst prognosis. Survival time for untreated small cell carcinoma is usually 9 to 10 months. Fewer than 5% of individuals are alive 2 years after diagnosis.

Small cell carcinoma is most often associated with ectopic hormone production, production of hormones by tumors of nonendocrine origin, or production of an inappropriate hormone by an endocrine gland. Neuroendocrine cells (NE cells) containing neurosecretory granules exist throughout the tracheobronchial tree.[36] Ectopic hormone production is important to the clinician because resulting signs and symptoms (called *paraneoplastic syndromes*) may be the first manifestation of the underlying cancer. Small cell carcinomas commonly produce gastrin-releasing peptide, calcitonin, arginine vasopressin, and adrenocorticotropic hormone (ACTH).[37] As a result of ACTH secretion, individuals with lung cancer secrete large quantities of 17-hydroxysteroids and 17-ketosteroids, leading to the development of an atypical Cushing syndrome. Signs and symptoms related to this condition include muscular weakness, facial edema, hypokalemia, alkalosis, hyperglycemia, hypertension, and increased pigmentation. They are treated primarily with chemotherapy and radiation therapy with temporary remission.[38]

Pathophysiology

The single most important risk factor in lung cancer is tobacco smoke, which causes structural, functional, malignant,

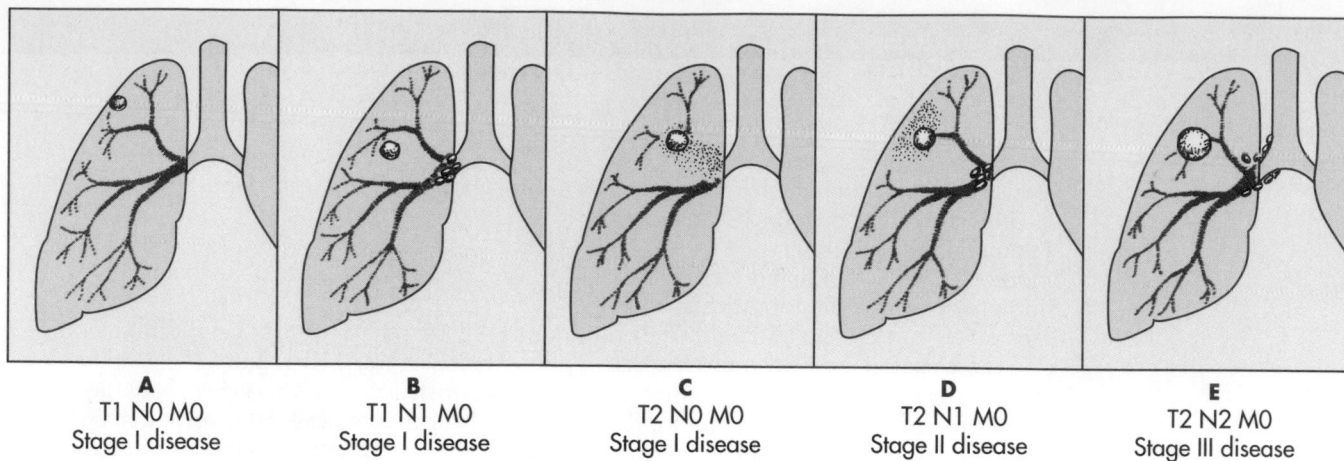

A	**B**	**C**	**D**	**E**
T1 N0 M0	T1 N1 M0	T2 N0 M0	T2 N1 M0	T2 N2 M0
Stage I disease	Stage I disease	Stage I disease	Stage II disease	Stage III disease

Fig. 26-19 *Staging of lung cancer by the TNM classification system.* **A** and **B,** Stage I disease includes tumors classified as T1, with or without metastasis to the lymph nodes in the ipsilateral hilar region. **C,** Also included in stage I are tumors classified as T2 but having no nodal or distant metastases. **D,** Stage II disease includes those tumors classified as T2, with metastasis only to the ipsilateral hilar lymph nodes. **E,** Stage III includes all tumors more extensive than T2 or any tumor with metastasis to the lymph nodes in the mediastinum or with distant metastasis.

and toxic changes. Deoxyribonucleic acid (DNA) mutating agents in cigarettes produce alterations in both oncogenes and tumor suppressor genes.[39] Individuals with lung cancer demonstrate bronchial epithelial changes progressing from squamous cell alteration or metaplasia to carcinoma in situ. Histologic changes are evident with bronchitis and emphysema. Thickening of the bronchial epithelium, mucous gland hypertrophy, and alveolar cell rupture occur more frequently in persons who smoke than in those who have never smoked. Cigarette smokers also have altered alveolar macrophage functions or phagocytosis, which may increase the risk of pulmonary infections.

Clinical Manifestations

Table 26-5 summarizes the clinical manifestations according to tumor type. By the time there are manifestations severe enough to motivate the individual to seek medical advice, the disease is usually advanced.

Evaluation and Treatment

The specific means of diagnosis and treatment for each cell type of lung cancer are summarized in Table 26-5. Of course,

the most important intervention for the population as a whole is prevention. Smoking cessation is the only proven way to reduce lung cancer risk. Trials of other measures, such as dietary modification, are underway.[40]

Staging of lung cancer

The histologic cell type and the stage of disease are the major factors that influence choice of therapy. The current accepted system for the staging of lung cancer is the *TNM classification* (Table 26-6). This system is a code in which *T* denotes the extent of the primary tumor, *N* indicates the nodal involvement, and *M* describes the extent of metastasis. Staging of lung cancer is illustrated in Fig. 26-19.

✓**QUICK CHECK**

What are the principal features of lip cancer?

Describe squamous cell carcinoma of the vocal cords.

Compare three types of lung cancer as to cause and survival.

▣ DID YOU UNDERSTAND?

Clinical Manifestations of Pulmonary Alterations

1. Dyspnea is the feeling of breathlessness and increased respiratory effort.
2. Abnormal breathing patterns are adjustments made by the body to minimize the work of respiratory muscles. They include Kussmaul, obstructed, restricted, gasping, and Cheyne-Stokes respirations, and sighing.
3. Hypoventilation is decreased alveolar ventilation caused by airway obstruction, chest wall restriction, or altered neurologic control of breathing. Hypoventilation causes increased $PaCO_2$.
4. Hyperventilation is increased alveolar ventilation produced by anxiety, head injury, or severe hypoxemia. Hyperventilation causes decreased $PaCO_2$.
5. Coughing is a protective reflex that expels secretions and irritants from the lower airways.
6. Hemoptysis is expectoration of bloody mucus, which can be caused by bronchitis, tuberculosis, abscess, neoplasms, and other conditions that cause hemorrhage from damaged vessels.
7. Cyanosis is a bluish discoloration of the skin caused by desaturation of hemoglobin, polycythemia, or peripheral vasoconstriction.
8. Chest pain can result from inflamed pleurae, trachea, bronchi, or respiratory muscles.
9. Clubbing of the fingertips is associated with diseases that interfere with oxygenation of the tissues.
10. Hypercapnia is an increased $PaCO_2$ caused by hypoventilation.
11. Hypoxemia is a reduced PaO_2 caused by (a) decreased oxygen content of inspired gas, (b) hypoventilation, (c) diffusion abnormality, (d) ventilation-perfusion mismatch, or (e) shunting.
12. Pulmonary edema is excess water in the lung caused by disturbances of capillary hydrostatic pressure, capillary oncotic pressure, or capillary permeability. A common cause is left heart failure that increases the hydrostatic pressure in the pulmonary circulation.
13. Atelectasis is the collapse of alveoli resulting from compression of lung tissue or absorption of gas from obstructed alveoli.
14. Bronchiectasis is abnormal dilation of the bronchi secondary to another pulmonary disorder, usually infection or inflammation.
15. Pneumothorax is the accumulation of air in the pleural space. It can be caused by spontaneous rupture of weakened areas of a pleura, or it can be secondary to pleural damage caused by disease, trauma, or mechanical ventilation.
16. Pleural effusion is the accumulation of fluid in the pleural space, usually resulting from disorders that promote transudation or exudation from capillaries underlying the pleura but occasionally resulting from blockage or injury that causes lymphatic vessels to drain into the pleural space.

17. Empyema is the presence of pus in the pleural space (infected pleural effusion). The source of the pus is usually lymphatic drainage from sites of bacterial pneumonia.
18. Pleurisy is inflammation of the pleura.
19. Pulmonary fibrosis is an excessive amount of connective tissue in the lung. It diminishes lung compliance and may be idiopathic or caused by disease.
20. Chest wall compliance is diminished by obesity and kyphoscoliosis, which compress the lungs, and by neuromuscular diseases that impair chest wall muscle function.
21. Flail chest results from rib or sternal fractures that disrupt the mechanics of breathing.
22. Inhalation of noxious gases or prolonged exposure to high concentrations of oxygen can damage the bronchial mucosa or alveolocapillary membrane and cause inflammation or acute respiratory failure.
23. Pneumoconiosis, which is caused by inhalation of dust particles in the workplace, can cause pulmonary fibrosis, susceptibility to lower airway infection, and tumor formation.
24. Allergic alveolitis is an allergic or hypersensitivity reaction to many allergens.
25. Bronchiolitis is the inflammatory obstruction of small airways. It is most common in children.

Pulmonary Disorders

1. Acute (adult) respiratory distress syndrome (ARDS) results from an acute, diffuse injury to the alveolocapillary membrane and decreased surfactant production, which increases membrane permeability and causes edema and atelectasis.
2. Postoperative respiratory failure is most common in surgical patients who smoke or have chronic disease.
3. Obstructive pulmonary disease is characterized by airway obstruction that causes difficult expiration. Obstructive disease can be acute or chronic in nature and includes asthma, chronic bronchitis, and emphysema.
4. In asthma, obstruction is caused by episodic attacks of bronchospasm, bronchial inflammation, mucosal edema, and increased mucus production.
5. Extrinsic asthma is caused by an immune response to allergens or other irritants.
6. Intrinsic asthma is not caused by allergens and occurs in adults older than 35 years.
7. A local imbalance between the parasympathetic and sympathetic divisions of the autonomic nervous system is thought to facilitate bronchospasm in individuals with intrinsic asthma.
8. Chronic bronchitis causes airway obstruction resulting from bronchial smooth muscle hypertrophy and production of thick, tenacious mucus.
9. In emphysema, destruction of the alveolar septa and loss of passive elastic recoil lead to airway collapse and obstruct gas flow during expiration.

Continued

▣ DID YOU UNDERSTAND?—cont'd

Pulmonary Disorders—cont'd

10. Emphysema in which septal deterioration is caused by α_1-antitrypsin deficiency or old age tends to be panacinar.

11. Emphysema in which septal deterioration results from smoking tends to be centriacinar.

12. Chronic obstructive pulmonary disease (COPD) is the coexistence of chronic bronchitis and emphysema.

13. Upper respiratory tract infections, which are the most common cause of short-term disability in the United States, include rhinitis (the common cold), pharyngitis, and laryngitis.

14. Serious lower respiratory tract infections, which occur most frequently in very old individuals and in individuals with impaired immunity or underlying disease, include pneumonia and tuberculosis.

15. Pneumococcal pneumonia is an acute lung infection resulting in an inflammatory response with four phases: (a) consolidation, (b) red hepatization, (c) gray hepatization, and (d) resolution.

16. Viral pneumonia is an acute, self-limiting lung infection usually caused by the influenza virus.

17. Tuberculosis is a lung infection caused by *Mycobacterium tuberculosis* (tubercle bacillus).

18. In tuberculosis, the inflammatory response proceeds to isolate colonies of bacilli by enclosing them in tubercles and surrounding the tubercles with scar tissue.

19. Bacilli may remain dormant within the tubercles for life or, if the immune system breaks down, cause recurrence of active disease.

20. Pulmonary vascular diseases are caused by embolism or hypertension in the pulmonary circulation.

21. Pulmonary embolism is occlusion of a portion of the pulmonary vascular bed by a thrombus (most common), tissue fragment, or air bubble. Depending on its size and location, the embolus can cause hypoxic vasoconstriction, pulmonary edema, atelectasis, pulmonary hypertension, shock, and even death.

22. Pulmonary hypertension (pulmonary artery pressure 5 to 10 mm Hg above normal) is caused by (a) elevated left ventricular pressure, (b) increased blood flow through the pulmonary circulation, (c) obliteration or obstruction of the vascular bed, or (d) active constriction of the vascular bed produced by hypoxemia or acidosis.

23. Cor pulmonale is right ventricular enlargement caused by chronic pulmonary hypertension. Cor pulmonale progresses to right ventricular failure if the pulmonary hypertension is not reversed.

24. Lip cancer is most common in men and represents about 1% of all cancers. In the most common cell type, squamous cell, metastasis is rare when lesions are diagnosed and treated early.

25. Laryngeal cancer occurs primarily in men and represents 2% to 3% of all cancers. Squamous cell carcinoma of the true vocal cords is most common and presents with a clinical symptom of progressive hoarseness.

26. Lung cancer, the most common cause of cancer death in the United States, is frequently caused by cigarette smoking.

27. Cancer cell types include squamous cell carcinoma, small cell (oat cell) carcinoma, adenocarcinoma, large cell carcinoma, bronchial adenoma, and mesothelioma. Each type arises in a characteristic site or type of tissue, causes distinctive clinical manifestations, and differs in likelihood of metastasis and prognosis.

▣ KEY TERMS

KEY TERMS

REFERENCES

1. Bradley, S.P. & Clausen, J.L. (1993). Dyspnea: Sorting through a complex differential. *Journal of Respiratory Diseases, 14*(3), 352-372.

2. Peters, J.I. & Bukowski, D. (1993). How to recognize and treat primary pneumothorax. *Journal of Respiratory Diseases, 14*(3), 459-469.

3. Sanihan, H. et al. (1998). Empyema in children. *Journal of Cardiovascular Surgery, 39*(1), 113-116.

4. Fridovich, I. (1998). Oxygen toxicity: A radical explanation. *Journal of Experimental Biology, 201*(Pt. 8), 1203-1209.

5. Tsai, W. & Morgan, W.K. (1996). The pneumoconioses. *Current Opinions in Pulmonary Medicine, 2*(2), 116-120.

6. Millberg, J.A. et al. (1995). Improved survival of patients with acute respiratory distress syndrome (ARDS): 1983-1993. *Journal of the American Medical Association, 273*(4), 306-309.

7. Kollef, M.H. & Schuster, D.P. (1995). The acute respiratory distress syndrome. *New England Journal of Medicine, 332*(1), 27-37.

8. Lechin, A.E. & Veron, J. (1994). Adult respiratory distress syndrome (ARDS): The basics. *Journal of Emergency Medicine, 12*(1), 63-68.

9. Vollman, K.M. & Aulbach, R.K. (1998). Acute respiratory distress syndrome. In *AACN clinical reference for critical care nursing* (4th ed.). St. Louis: Mosby.

10. Luce, J.M. (1998). Acute lung injury and the acute respiratory distress syndrome. *Critical Care Medicine, 26*(2), 369-376.

11. Fulkerson, W.J. et al. (1996). Pathogenesis and treatment of the adult respiratory distress syndrome. *Archives of Internal Medicine, 156*, 29-38.

12. Mannino, D.M. et al. (1998). Surveillance for asthma—United States, 1960-1995. *MMWR CDC Surveillance Summaries, 47*(1), 1-27.

13. Drazen, J.M. & Silverman, E.K. (1997). Genetics of asthma. *American Journal of Respiratory and Critical Care Medicine, 156*, 569-571.

14. Second Expert Panel on the Management of Asthma, National Heart, Lung, and Blood Institute. (1997, May). *Highlights of the expert panel report 2: Guidelines for the diagnosis and management of asthma.* Bethesda, Md.: National Institutes of Health (Pub. No. NIH97-4051A).

15. Busse, W.W. (1998). Inflammation in asthma: The cornerstone of the disease and target of therapy. *Journal of Allergy and Clinical Immunology, 102*(Pt. 2), S17-S22.

16. Roche, W.R. (1998). Inflammation and structural changes in the small airways in bronchial asthma. *American Journal of Respiratory and Critical Care Medicine, 157*, S191-S194.

17. Madge, P., McColl, J., & Patton, J. (1997). Impact of a nurse-led home management training programme in children admitted to hospital with acute asthma: A randomised controlled study. *Thorax, 52*(3), 223-228.

18. Anonymous. (1998). Strategies in preserving lung health and preventing COPD and associated diseases. The National Lung Health Education Program (NLHEP). *Chest, 113*(2 Suppl.), 123S-163S.

19. Rennard, S.I. (1998). COPD: Overview of definitions, epidemiology, and factors influencing its development. *Chest, 113*(4 Suppl.), 235S-241S.

20. Nelson, S. et al. (1995). Pathophysiology of pneumonia. *Clinics in Chest Medicine, 16*, 1-12.

21. Waddell, T.K. & Keshavjee, S. (1998). Lung transplantation for chronic obstructive pulmonary disease. *Seminars in Thoracic and Cardiovascular Surgery, 10*(3), 191-201.

22. Metlay, J.P., Kapoor, W.N., & Fine, M.J. (1997). Does this patient have community-acquired pneumonia? Diagnosing pneumonia by history and physical examination. *Journal of the American Medical Association, 278*, 1440-1445.

23. Minton, E.J. & MacFarlane, J.T. (1996). Antibiotic resistant *Streptococcus pneumoniae. Thorax, 51*(Suppl. 2), S45-S50.

24. McCray, E. et al. (1997). The epidemiology of tuberculosis in the United States. *Clinics in Chest Medicine, 18*, 99-113.

25. Mitchison, D.A. (1998). How drug resistance emerges as a result of poor compliance during short-course

REFERENCES

chemotherapy for tuberculosis. *International Journal of Tuberculosis & Lung Disease, 2,* 10-15.

26. American Thoracic Society. (1990). Diagnostic standards and classification of tuberculosis. *American Review of Respiratory Diseases, 142*(3), 725-735.

27. Chaulk, C.P. & Kazandjian, V.A. (1998) Directly observed therapy for treatment completion of pulmonary tuberculosis: Consensus statement of the Public Health Tuberculosis Guidelines Panel. *Journal of the American Medical Association, 279,* 943-984.

28. Silverstein, M.D. et al. (1998). Trends in the incidence of deep vein thrombosis and pulmonary embolism. *Archives of Internal Medicine, 158,* 585-593.

29. Oger, E. et al. (1997). The value of a risk factor analysis in clinical susceptible deep vein thrombosis. *Respiration, 64,* 326-330.

30. Litin, S.C., Heit, J.A., & Mees, K.A. (1998). Use of low-molecular-weight heparin in the treatment of venous thromboembolic disease: Answers to frequently asked questions. *Mayo Clinic Proceedings, 73,* 545-550.

31. American Cancer Society. (1999). Cancer facts and figures—1999.

32. Homkvist, K.A. & Roenigk, R.K. (1998). Squamous cell carcinoma of the lip treated with Mohs micrographic surgery: Outcome at 5 years. *Journal of the American Academy of Dermatology, 38*(6 Pt. 1), 960-966.

33. Stewart, M.G., Chen, A.Y., & Stach, C.B. (1998). Outcomes analysis of voice and quality of life in patients with laryngeal cancer. *Archives of Otolaryngology—Head & Neck Surgery, 124,* 143-148.

34. Petty, T.L. (1997). Lung cancer and chronic obstructive pulmonary disease. *Hematology/Oncology Clinics of North America, 11*(3), 531-541.

35. Bunn, P.A. & Kelly, K. (1998). New chemotherapeutic agents prolong survival and improve quality of life in non–small cell lung cancer: A review of the literature and future directions. *Clinical Cancer Research, 4*(5), 1087-1100.

36. MacKay, B., Lukeman, J.M., & Ordonez, N.G. (1991). *Tumors of the lungs.* Philadelphia: Saunders.

37. Pezza, M., Iermano, C., & Tufano, R. (1994). Nutritional support for the patient with chronic obstructive respiratory disease. *Monaldi Archives for Chest Disease, 49*(3 Suppl. 1), 33-39.

38. Sorenson, M., Lassen, U., & Hansen, H.H. (1998). Current therapy of small cell lung cancer. *Current Opinion in Oncology, 10,* 133-138.

39. Salgia, R. & Skarin, A.T. (1998). Molecular abnormalities in lung cancer. *Journal of Clinical Oncology, 16,* 1207-1217.

40. Biesalski, H.K. et al. (1998). European consensus statement on lung cancer: Risk factors and prevention. *CA: A Cancer Journal for Clinicians, 48,* 167-176.

CHAPTER

27

Alterations of Pulmonary Function in Children

Sue E. Huether

Alterations of respiratory function in children are influenced by age, development, gender, race, genetic dominance, and environmental conditions. Newborns are especially vulnerable to a variety of upper and lower airway infections caused by immunologic immaturity. Structural differences in infants and children also render them less competent to tolerate conditions causing increased work of breathing. Finally, access to medical care and timeliness of immunizations will influence the incidence and severity of pulmonary disorders.

CHAPTER OUTLINE

PULMONARY DISORDERS
Disorders of the Upper Airways
Infections (croup syndromes)

Croup syndromes are caused by infection of the upper airways. These diseases are a common cause of respiratory failure in children.

The anatomic site of infection defines the specific condition of the upper airway (Table 27-1). Because the upper airways of young children are easily occluded, croup can be life threatening. The conditions frequently referred to as croup syndrome include *viral croup, acute tracheitis, epiglottitis, laryngitis, acute laryngitis,* and *laryngotracheobronchitis (LTB)* (see Table 27-1).[1]

The actual incidence of these disorders is difficult to determine, but they comprise a significant number of respiratory illnesses in young children. In 85% of cases, croup is caused by a virus and affects children between 3 months and 5 years of age. Croup caused by bacteria (*Haemophilus influenzae, Corynebacterium diphtheriae*) occurs more rarely and in children ages 3 to 7 years. The incidence of croup is higher in males and is most common during the winter months. Approximately 15% of affected children have a strong family history of croup, with laryngitis tending to recur in the same child. Acute epiglottitis is usually caused by *H. influenzae* type B, with the peak incidence at 3.5 years of age.[2]

Pathophysiology

Airway obstruction is caused by inflammatory mucosal edema, secretions, and muscle spasm. Not only are the diameter and surface area of the immature airway relatively smaller, but also the mucous membrane is more loosely attached and more vascular in children. The glottis is small and is rapidly compromised by inflammatory edema and spasm. The negative pressure of inspiration is transmitted to the inflamed and edematous upper airway, causing it to collapse and obstruct air flow (Fig. 27-1). Turbulent air flow across inflamed vocal cords causes inspiratory stridor. The obstruction is in contrast to inflammation of the lower airways, which tend to obstruct during expiration when positive pressure inside the thorax narrows the airways, causing expiratory wheezes.

Children with viral croup (commonly parainfluenza virus types 1 and 2) may have a preceding infection of the upper respiratory passages (e.g., rhinitis or the common cold) that involves primarily the nasal mucosa. After 3 or 4 days the infection spreads to the larynx, where the true vocal cords and subglottic structures become inflamed and edematous. Spasms of smooth muscle in laryngeal walls contribute to the laryngeal obstruction.

In infections caused by *H. influenzae,* the primary site of inflammation is the **epiglottis. Epiglottitis** is a serious, life-threatening condition, because the inflammatory edema can obstruct the airway. Inflammation may spread above and below the epiglottis to involve the trachea and bronchi. If this occurs, respiratory distress is more severe and the outcome of the disease is less favorable.

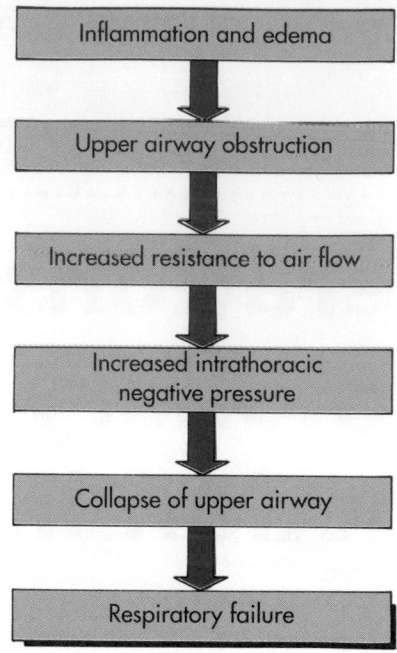

Fig. 27-1 *Upper airway obstruction with croup.*

In bacterial croup caused by *C. diphtheriae,* inflammation and infection of the upper airways, including pharyngitis and rhinitis, proceed to laryngeal inflammation. Diphtheria causes the mucosa of the larynx to become coated with a fibrous exudate, occluding the airway. Fortunately, immunization against diphtheria has made this serious disease rare in the United States.

Regardless of the causal microorganism, certain endogenous factors are believed to predispose a child to croup. Evidence for this includes (1) the tendency for croup to recur in children who have had one episode and (2) the likelihood that the same virus will cause croup in susceptible children while causing a variety of other, milder illnesses in children who are not susceptible.[3] An anatomically defective or abnormally immature larynx may be a predisposing factor for croup.

Clinical manifestations

The clinical manifestations of croup are produced by inflammatory edema and spasm (see Figs. 27-1 and 27-2). The first manifestation of inflammation *above the epiglottis* includes hoarse or muffled voice and progression to abnormal inspiratory sounds or a "quiet" respiratory effort. Use of accessory muscles with retractions (Fig. 27-3), nasal flaring, head bobbing (in infants), agitation, or fatigue may be seen with respiratory compromise. By contrast, inflammation of the glottis or below often begins with a whispery, low-volume voice and barking cough. Agitation, cyanosis or pallor, weakness, rapid pulse, low tidal volumes, and inspiratory stridor are frequently observed signs of hypoxemia. Death may occur from hypoxemia.

Most cases of croup progress only as far as stridor and slight dyspnea, and the child recovers from the acute crisis in

TABLE 27-1	**Upper Airway Infections**				
Condition	Age	Onset	Etiology	Pathophysiology	Symptoms
Acute laryngotra-cheobronchitis	6 mo-3 yr	Usually gradual	Viral	Inflammation from vocal cords to bronchial lumina	Harsh cough; low fever; may have nasal discharge, conjunctivitis
Acute tracheitis	1-12 yr	Abrupt or fol-lowing viral illness	*Staphylococcus aureus*	Inflammation of upper trachea	High fever; toxic, thick harsh cough; purulent secre-tions; may prefer head elevation
Acute epiglottitis	2-6 yr	Abrupt	*Haemophilus influenzae*	Inflammation of supraglottic structures	Severe sore throat; muffled voice; may drool; sits erect and quietly
Retropharyngeal abscess	>6 yr	Gradual, 2-5 days	*Staphylococcus aureus* Group B hemolytic streptococcus	Abscess in poste-rior pharyngeal wall	Similar to epiglottitis
Peritonsillar ab-scess	>9 yr	May be abrupt	Group B hemolytic streptococcus, *Staphylococcus aureus*	Abscess within or around tonsil	Similar to epiglottitis; may have trismus

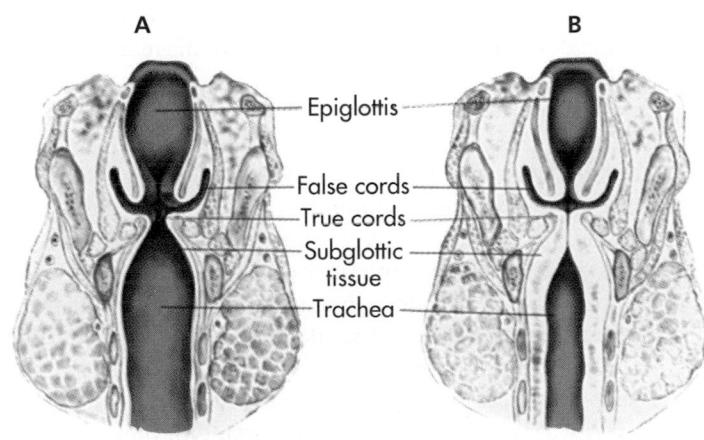

Fig. 27-2 *The larynx.* **A**, Normal larynx. **B**, Narrowing and obstruction from edema of croup. *(From Wong, D.L. et al. [1999]. Whaley & Wong's nursing care of infants and children [6th ed.]. St. Louis: Mosby.)*

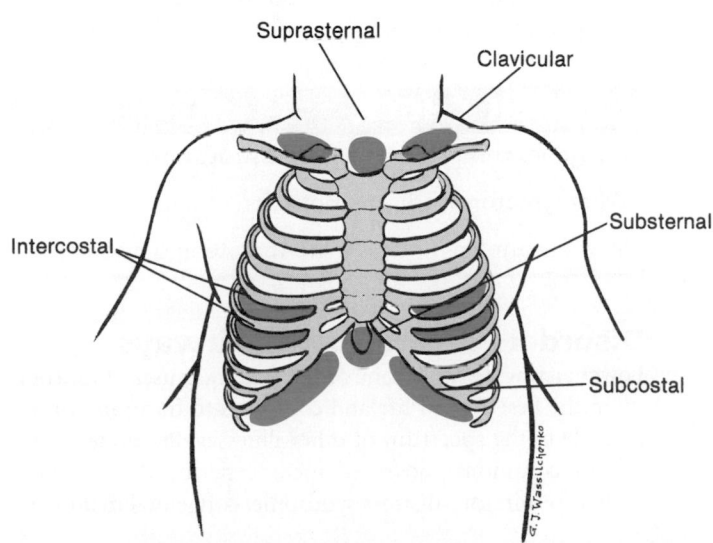

Fig. 27-3 *Areas of chest muscle retraction.* *(From Wong, D.L. et al. [1999]. Whaley & Wong's nursing care of infants and children [6th ed.]. St. Louis: Mosby.)*

a few hours. Complete recovery from croup often requires 24 to 48 hours.

Acute epiglottitis

Acute epiglottitis is a severe, life-threatening, rapidly progressive infection of the epiglottis and surrounding area. Mortality is between 8% and 12% of children admitted to hospitals. In the classic form of the disease, a child between 2 and 7 years of age suddenly develops fever, inspiratory stridor, and severe respiratory distress. The child appears anxious and has a voice that sounds muffled. Drooling and dysphagia (inability to swallow) are common. Death can occur in a few hours. Nasotracheal intubation or tracheotomy is mandatory in instances of rapidly increasing obstruction. Examination of the throat may trigger laryngospasm and cause respiratory collapse. Pneumonia, cervical lymph node inflammation, otitis, and, rarely, meningitis or septic arthritis may occur during the course of epiglottitis. The incidence of the disease is decreasing because of *H. influenzae* type B vaccination.[4]

Viral croup and acute laryngotracheobronchitis

Viral croup and acute laryngotracheobronchitis are frequently caused by the same virus. *Viral croup* usually occurs in children between the ages of 6 months and 3 years. It follows an upper respiratory infection consisting of rhinorrhea, coryza (severe infection, with discharge, of the nasal mucosa), and fever. After 2 to 3 days, the child suddenly develops symptoms of croup, with inspiratory stridor and a harsh, barking cough. Difficulty in breathing makes the child apprehensive and restless. In viral croup, the obstruction is caused by inflammatory swelling of the subglottic tissues with impingement on the airway below the level of the glottis. Spasm of the vocal cords occurs with tracheobronchitis as the inflammatory process extends.

Acute *laryngotracheobronchitis (LTB)* (acute *laryngotracheitis*) is the most common form of croup. Affected children have frequent recurrences between ages 3 and 6 years, after which airway growth decreases susceptibility. Symptoms characteristically appear worse at night. A considerable number of children with LTB require tracheotomy for the establishment of an adequate airway.

Complications occur in approximately 15% of children with viral croup or LTB. The most common complication is extension of the infection to other regions of the respiratory tract, such as the middle ear, terminal bronchioles, or lung parenchyma.

Evaluation and Treatment

Diagnosis is based on physical examination, cause of infection, and radiologic examination. Treatment for severe croup consists of (1) restricting the child's activity to avoid aggravating respiratory distress, (2) administering humidifier and oxygen (25% to 30%) to alleviate anxiety and reverse hypoxemia, (3) administering intravenous fluids to ensure adequate hydration, (4) administering aerosolized epinephrine to relieve obstruction, (5) instituting mechanical ventilation (intermittent positive-pressure breathing) with aerosol epinephrine to relieve obstruction, (6) administering antibiotics (if croup is bacterial in origin), (7) administering nebulized glucocorticoids to relieve inflammation, and (8) providing an artificial airway for obstruction.[5]

All children with epiglottitis require intubation for 1 to 3 days. Children with other airway problems are managed according to the severity of airway compromise. At no time should a child with respiratory distress be given *any* sedation unless the child's airway is protected with an endotracheal tube.

Aspiration of foreign bodies

Aspiration of foreign bodies into the airways is common among children 1 to 3 years of age. Most objects are expelled by the cough reflex, but some objects may lodge in the larynx, trachea, or bronchus. Large objects (a bite of hot dog, toy balloons, coins, bottle caps, grapes, corns, beans, nuts) may occlude the airway and are life threatening.[6] Symptoms of cough, hoarseness, and dyspnea are consistent with a foreign body in the larynx. Similar symptoms with blood-streaked sputum are associated with a foreign body in the bronchus. The obstruction can progress to atelectasis, or there can be a ball-valve effect with air accumulation distal to the obstruction. Chronic infection, bronchiectasis, asthma, or lung abscess occurs with late diagnosis. Lodged objects require endoscopic removal and treatment of the consequent problem.

Aspiration of foreign substances

Infants may aspirate amniotic fluid contaminated with meconium, bacteria, or cells from the birth canal that can cause pneumonia or respiratory distress. Aspiration of baby powder can also produce dyspnea and respiratory distress. Infants with tracheoesophageal fistulae (see Chapter 35) or gastroesophageal reflux may aspirate gastric fluids and develop chemical pneumonia. Treatment is related to the severity of the aspiration. Most important for preventing aspiration is suctioning airways when the baby's head is delivered, controlling the use of baby powder, proper positioning during feeding, and avoiding overfeeding.

✓ QUICK CHECK

How does croup cause airway obstruction?

What symptoms indicate aspiration of a foreign body?

Why is acute epiglottitis a life-threatening disorder?

Disorders of the Lower Airways

Lower airway disease is one of the leading causes of morbidity in the first year of life and continues to be an important variable in the spectrum of other illnesses. Pulmonary conditions commonly observed include perinatal conditions, such as respiratory distress syndrome; congenital malformations and conditions, such as asthma and cystic fibrosis; infections; bronchospastic disorders; aspiration syndrome; and respiratory distress syndrome.

Respiratory distress syndrome

The names *respiratory distress syndrome (RDS) of the newborn, idiopathic respiratory distress syndrome (IRDS),* and *hyaline membrane disease (HMD)* all refer to the severe lung disorder that is responsible for more neonatal deaths than any other condition. RDS of the newborn affects 5% to 10% of premature infants, or 0.05% to 0.1% of all neonates and, along with its complications, is responsible for 30% to 50% of all neonatal deaths and up to 70% of deaths in premature infants.[7] Risk factors are summarized in the Risk Factors box.

█ RISK FACTORS

RESPIRATORY DISTRESS SYNDROME OF THE NEWBORN
- Premature birth
- Male gender
- Cesarean delivery
- Diabetic mother
- Asphyxia
- Hypovolemia or hypervolemia
- Maternal antepartum hemorrhage
- Maternal shock

▰ *Pathophysiology*

During the third trimester of gestation, the final unfolding of the alveolar septum takes place, an event that significantly increases the alveolocapillary surface area of the lungs. Because alveolar septal unfolding is incomplete in premature infants, they are born with many underdeveloped and uninflatable alveoli. In addition, pulmonary blood flow is limited by fetal atelectasis and incomplete vascular development, particularly of the alveolocapillary network. Because of increased pulmonary vascular resistance, most fetal blood is shunted from the lungs through the fetal cardiac structures—the ductus arteriosus and foramen ovale.

At birth, the infant must initiate breathing and keep the previously fluid-filled lungs inflated with air. With the onset of ventilation, a marked increase in pulmonary blood flow occurs because oxygen dilates the constricted pulmonary blood vessels. Pulmonary venous return is thus increased and, consequently, so is left ventricular output. In the normal neonate, ductal closure and the decrease of pulmonary vascular resistance result in a decrease of pulmonary arterial and right ventricular pressures. At the same time, the volume of pulmonary capillary blood flow must increase approximately 10 times to provide adequate pulmonary perfusion and alter intracardiac pressure enough to close the ductus arteriosus and foramen ovale. Most full-term infants are successful in making these changes, but the premature infant with RDS is not.

The primary problem in RDS is lack of surfactant and inadequate alveolar surface area for gas exchange because of prematurity. Alveoli are small and underdeveloped. Without sufficient production of surfactant, surface tension remains high and alveoli do not adequately inflate, causing atelectasis. Infants with RDS have not developed the ability to synthesize, store, and secrete surfactant onto the alveolocapillary membrane. Without surfactant, each breath requires as much negative pressure as the initial lung expansion at birth. The infant uses more oxygen to sustain the work of breathing than is gained from ventilation. This leads to exhaustion and a decreased ability to maintain lung expansion. The pathophysiology of RDS is outlined in Fig. 27-4.

▰ *Clinical Manifestations*

Signs of RDS appear within minutes of birth. Some neonates require resuscitation at birth because of asphyxia or initial severe respiratory disease. Tachypnea (respiratory rate more than 20/min), expiratory grunting or whining, intercostal and subcostal retractions, nasal flaring, duskiness of the skin, and low body temperature are the most striking clinical manifestations of RDS. The natural course is characterized by progressive hypoxemia and dyspnea. Blood pressure and body temperature decrease. Fatigue, cyanosis, and pallor increase, and grunting decreases or disappears as the condition worsens. Apnea and irregular respirations occur as the infant tires. Edema of the extremities, ileus, and oliguria may also occur during the first 2 to 3 days of life. Signs of asphyxia as a result of apnea or partial respiratory failure indicate rapid progression of the disease. RDS can progress to death in severe cases, but in milder cases the clinical manifestations reach a peak within 3 days, after which time gradual improvement is seen. Death is rare after 3 days.

▰ *Evaluation and Treatment*

Diagnosis is based on clinical manifestations, blood gas analysis, shunting, and chest radiographs. The course of RDS can be altered dramatically by administration of exogenous surfactant, inhaled nitric oxide, and supportive treatment that maintains adequate oxygenation, circulation, acid-base balance, and nutrition.[8,9] Mechanical ventilation, often used successfully in managing RDS, can create secondary problems, such as bronchopulmonary dysplasia and chronic lung disease. Approximately 50% to 70% of infants survive with treatment.

Asthma

Asthma is an inflammatory disease characterized by hyperresponsive airways and episodes of bronchospasm.[10] It is a leading chronic illness in childhood, affecting 5% to 10% of children to some degree, and is the most frequent cause of hospital admission. Although it is unknown why childhood asthma has become more prevalent in the past 2 decades, an association exists with exposure to tobacco smoke, irritants, and respiratory infection. Inner-city black and Hispanic children have higher morbidity and mortality.[11,12] Before puberty, approximately twice as many boys as girls are affected.

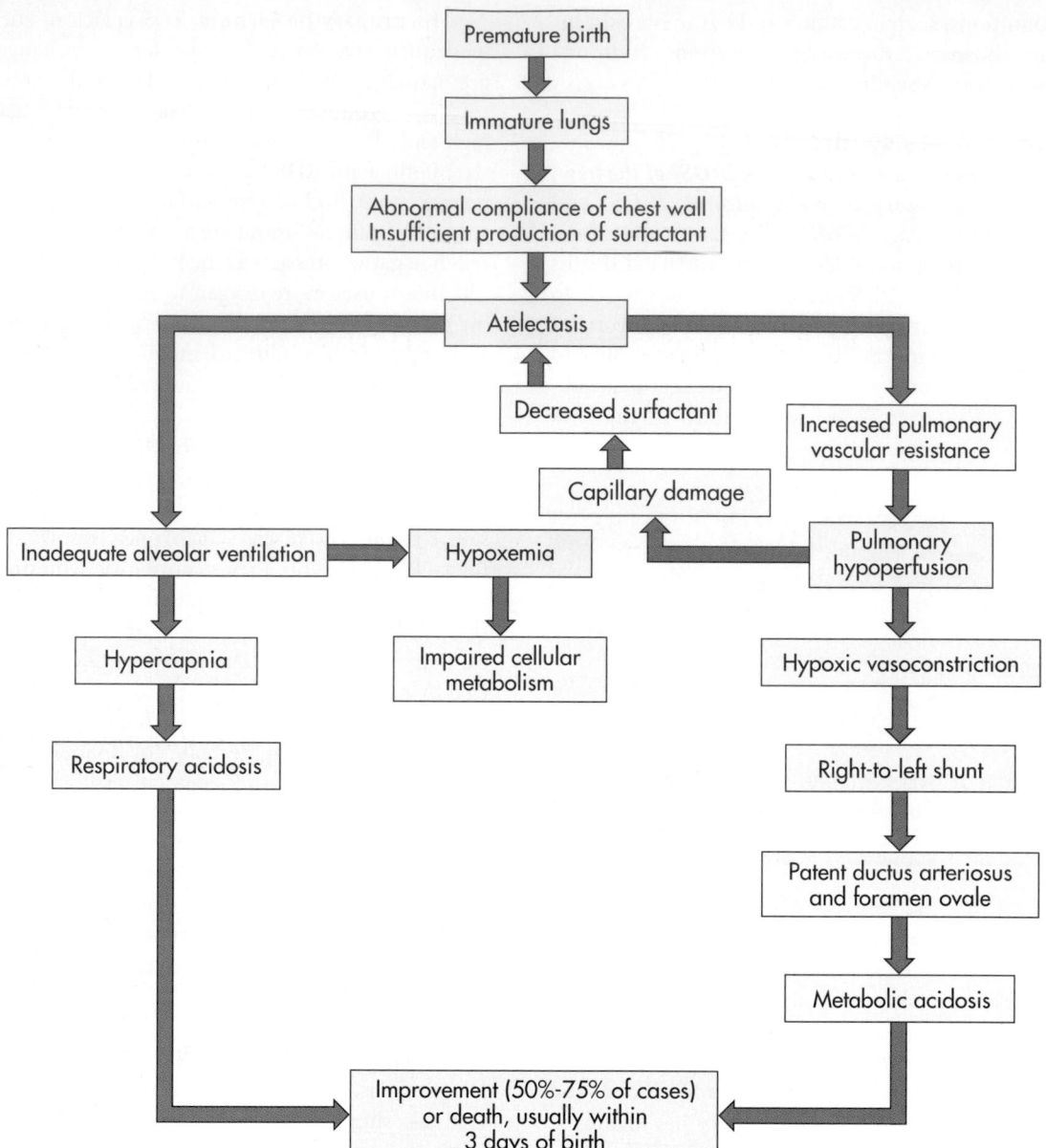

Fig. 27-4 *Pathogenesis of respiratory distress syndrome of the newborn (RDS). RDS is also known as* hyaline membrane disease.

After puberty, the incidence of asthma is evenly divided between the genders. Approximately 80% to 90% of asthmatic children have their first symptoms before 4 or 5 years of age. Children with asthma have increased wheezing during viral respiratory infections. It is estimated that asthma is inherited in 30% of cases.[13] Incidence and mortality among children and young adults with asthma increased from 1980 to 1993 (see Table 26-3 for stages of severity).[14]

Pathophysiology

Allergy, previous respiratory infection, and exercise play a major role in hyperresponsive airways and the pathogenesis and inflammatory processes of childhood asthma.[15] Allergens trigger release of immunoglobulin E (IgE), causing mast cell release of histamine and other inflammatory mediators (Fig. 27-5) (see Chapter 26). The resulting edema of the bronchial mucosa, bronchospasm, cellular infiltration, and mucus plugging vary in severity depending on the age of the child, the size and anatomy of the airways, the type of irritant that precipitates obstruction, and the duration and severity of the asthma attack. The increased work of breathing caused by use of accessory muscles and increased obstruction to air flow results in increased oxygen consumption and cardiac output.[16] This level of exertion is difficult for young children to maintain because of their small glycogen reserves and the likelihood that caloric intake is inadequate because of illness.

In most children, both larger and smaller airways are ob-

Fig. 27-5 *Pathophysiology of childhood asthma. IgE,* Immunoglobulin E; *ECF,* eosinophil chemotactic factor.

structed. The obstruction results from hypertrophy of smooth muscle, inflammatory exudate, and mucus plugs. The forced expiratory volume is diminished. Ineffective ventilation results in hypoxemia, which stimulates hyperventilation with hypocapnia and respiratory alkalosis. As obstruction becomes more severe, there is air trapping, inadequate ventilation, more severe hypoxemia, and hypercapnia with respiratory acidosis. Respiratory failure is imminent. There can be both an early and a late phase to an asthma attack (see Fig. 27-5).

In general, the younger the child, the greater the risk of morbidity and mortality. Infants in particular are at an anatomic and physiologic disadvantage because of (1) their relatively small alveolocapillary surface area; (2) the in-

creased resistance to air flow in their narrow airways; (3) the horizontal insertion angle of their diaphragm, which is mechanically disadvantageous and increases the work of breathing; (4) the relatively large number of mucous glands per square centimeter of bronchial mucosa; and (5) a deficiency in the numbers of pores of Kohn and Lambert canals that promote atelectasis distal to obstructed airways.[4] The one anatomic advantage of infants is the relatively small amount of smooth muscle in their smaller airways, making bronchospasm less severe. In infants, mechanical obstruction from edema, mucus, and inflammatory cell infiltrates, which is slow to resolve, is a more important component of airway obstruction than bronchospasm, which can be reversed with drugs.

Clinical Manifestations

In typical cases, previously well infants or young children develop what seems to be a cold with rhinorrhea, which is rapidly followed by signs and symptoms of asthma, including the high-pitched, wheezing sound heard mostly on expiration; cough, sometimes so severe as to induce gagging and vomiting; an anxious facial expression; irritability or restlessness; dyspnea; labored breathing; tachypnea; use of accessory muscles of respiration; nasal flaring; assumption of an upright posture, with raised shoulder, expanded upper chest, and arms extended behind to prop the upper torso; and, in severe attacks, cyanosis, pallor, and diaphoresis (sweating). Respiratory symptoms may be preceded by exposure to irritants, animals, molds or dusty areas, pollens, tobacco smoke, or cold air. Sometimes exercise triggers an asthma attack or the attack follows bronchitis or recurrent chest colds. Most children have only occasional attacks of mild to moderate severity and are easily treated. Chronic hyperinflation distal to an airway obstruction causes chest abnormalities, such as pectus excavatum (funnel chest) or barrel chest (an abnormal prominence of the ribs). Growth may be retarded, resulting in abnormally small stature or low weight, and puberty may be delayed.

Evaluation and Treatment

Diagnosis is determined on the basis of history, clinical manifestations, physical examination, chest x-ray, spirometry, and arterial blood gases. Treatment for mild and moderate asthma consists of avoidance of contact with allergens or irritants; hyposensitization therapy; promotion of liquefaction and expectoration of mucus through adequate hydration, administration of β-adrenergic aerosols, and oral or aerosol bronchodilators; correction of metabolic acidosis; and administration of inhaled and/or systemic corticosteroids. Between attacks, the child is encouraged to exercise, and prophylactic medication (inhaled corticosteroids, salmeterol, cromolyn sodium, or adrenergic aerosol) may be prescribed. A record of peak expiratory flow rates should be maintained to evaluate treatment effectiveness. The treatment goals are to avoid triggers, minimize symptoms, and prevent exacerbations.[17]

Respiratory infections

Children have approximately six to eight upper respiratory infections per year. The incidence of lower respiratory infections is approximately 50 infections per 1000 individuals each year for children younger than 6 years. Most of these illnesses are pneumonia.

The cause of lower airway infection depends on the infectious microorganism, the age of the child, immune function, seasonal and geographic variables, and environment. Respiratory syncytial virus (RSV) and parainfluenza 3 virus infections are most common. Ninety percent of bacterial pneumonias in children are caused by *Streptococcus pneumoniae*, with the remainder caused by *Staphylococcus* and *H. influenzae*. Vaccination is effective against *H. influenzae* and *S. pneumoniae*. Work is progressing on the development of

RSV vaccines for all age-groups.[18] Microorganisms transmitted from the maternal genital tract during childbirth, particularly gram-negative bacteria, group B streptococci, and *Chlamydia trachomatis*, can cause pulmonary infections in infants up to 3 months of age. Later in infancy and during early childhood, viral rather than bacterial infections predominate.[19]

In infants and young children, viral infections tend to be more common during the winter and early spring, with other minor peaks in the fall. During influenza epidemics, pneumonia and croup may develop in infants and children of all ages. Familial and environmental factors are associated with certain types of respiratory infection. For example, *Mycoplasma pneumoniae* infections tend to occur with overcrowding and affect multiple members of a family.

The incidence of *M. pneumoniae* infection peaks between the ages of 5 and 10 years, and as the incidence of all pneumonia decreases during adolescence, *M. pneumoniae* becomes the most common cause of bacterial pneumonia.

Pneumonia

The more common types of pneumonia in children are viral and bacterial (pneumococcal, staphylococcal, streptococcal). They are outlined in Table 27-2. All involve an inflammation of lung tissue. With appropriate antibiotic therapy instituted early in the course of illness, mortality from bacterial pneumonia is now less than 1%.[20]

Bronchitis

Bronchitis in children tends to occur in association with other conditions of the upper and lower airways, including asthma and cystic fibrosis, and is common after a respiratory illness, such as croup, pneumonia, or even a mild upper respiratory tract infection. It is aggravated by dry environmental air (e.g., in homes with forced-air heating). Viruses produce most attacks of chronic bronchitis. When the dry, hacking cough is severe enough to interfere with eating or resting, demulcents such as lollipops or cough drops are quite effective. Recurring bronchitis in childhood may be a predisposing factor for later bronchial lesions that cause chronic obstruction. Treatment of viral bronchitis is palliative, and treatment of bacterial pneumonia is related to the causative microorganism.[21]

Bronchiolitis

Bronchiolitis is a common disease of the lower respiratory tract in infants. Caused by inflammatory obstruction of the bronchioles, it tends to occur during the first 2 years of life, with a peak incidence at approximately 6 months of age, particularly during the winter and spring. Bronchiolitis is a major reason for hospital admission of infants less than 1 year of age.

RSV causes most cases of bronchiolitis, but parainfluenza 3 virus, mycoplasma, some adenoviruses, and occasionally other viruses or bacteria cause acute bronchiolitis. Infection is usually transmitted to the infant from a family member with a minor respiratory illness.

TABLE 27-2   More Common Types of Pneumonia in Children

Type	Causal Agent	Age	Onset	Signs/Symptoms	Pathophysiology
Viral pneumonia	Respiratory syncytial virus (most common)	All ages	Acute or gradual, winter and early spring	Mild to high fever, cough, rhinorrhea, malaise, fine rales, diffuse rhonchi, wheezing, diffuse areas of consolidation	Bronchiolitis with edema, increased mucus, and interstitial pneumonia
Pneumococcal pneumonia	Pneumococci (*Streptococcus pneumoniae*)	1-4 yr	Acute, follows an upper respiratory infection, winter and early spring	High fever, productive cough, pleuritic pain, increased respiration rate, decreased breath sounds in area of consolidation	Inflammation of bronchial mucosa with alveolar exudate; consolidation of all or part of a lobe. Early: red hepatization with WBCs, RBCs, and fibrin consolidation. Late: gray hepatization with fibrin and neutrophils in alveoli. Resolution: many phagocytic macrophages
Staphylococcal pneumonia	*Staphylococcus aureus* *Staphylococcus epidermidis*	1 wk-2 yr	Acute, winter months	High fever, cough, respiratory distress (retractions, nasal flaring, cyanosis, anxiety, increased respirations, grunting, shocklike state may be present)	Unilateral edema and hemorrhagic necrosis of one or more lobes, exudate on pleural surface may lead to multiple abscesses
Streptococcal pneumonia	Group A β-hemolytic streptococci	All ages	Acute, any season	High fever, chills, respiratory distress	Tracheitis, bronchitis, and interstitial pneumonia with ulcers, exudate, edema, and localized hemorrhage

WBCs, *White blood cells;* RBCs, *red blood cells.*

Pathophysiology

Viral infection causes necrosis of the bronchial epithelium and destruction of ciliated epithelial cells. As the submucosa becomes edematous, cellular debris and fibrin form plugs within the bronchioles. Edema of the bronchiolar wall, accumulation of mucus and cellular debris, and bronchospasm narrow many peripheral airways. Obstruction to air flow varies in degree and location. Atelectasis occurs in some areas of the lung and hyperinflation in others.

The mechanics of breathing are disrupted, with high tidal volume and functional residual capacity approximately twice normal. Compliance is decreased because the lungs are already highly inflated and because airway resistance within the lung is uneven and increased. These changes result in substantially increased work of breathing.

Serious alterations in gas exchange occur because of airway obstruction and patchy atelectasis. Hypoxemia and hy-percapnia develop as a result of ventilation-perfusion abnormalities, and hypercapnia is increased further because the increased work of breathing causes hypoventilation. Although pH varies, metabolic acidosis occurs more frequently than respiratory alkalosis.

Clinical Manifestations

In infants and young children, bronchiolitis is characterized by difficulty in expiration, wheezing, tachypnea, chest wall retractions, and cyanosis around the mouth. Severely affected infants appear anxious and distressed because of dyspnea. The thoracic cage is overexpanded, particularly in its anteroposterior diameter. The infant takes rapid, short breaths, and wheezing and rales are often heard on auscultation. With overexpansion of the lungs, the diaphragm is flattened, causing downward displacement of the liver and spleen. Abdominal distention results from air swallowing.

The tidal volume decreases. Some individuals have persistent airway resistance and airway hyperresponsiveness.[22]

Evaluation and Treatment

Diagnosis of bronchiolitis is based on physical examination (e.g., rhinitis, cough, wheezing, chest retractions, tachypnea) and radiologic examination. Treatment includes humidification of inspired air, hydration, and nebulized bronchodilators (albuterol).[23,24]

Some children recover from bronchiolitis within 3 to 4 days, whereas others require 1 week or more. Long-term follow-up of infants who have had bronchiolitis shows an increased incidence of asthma during childhood.[25]

Bronchiolitis obliterans

Bronchiolitis obliterans is fibrotic obstruction of the respiratory bronchioles and alveolar ducts secondary to inflammation. Most cases of bronchiolitis obliterans in children are associated with pulmonary infections (e.g., influenza, adenoviral infection, pertussis [whooping cough]) or measles. Cough, respiratory distress, and cyanosis occur initially, followed by a brief period of improvement. The progression of disease is then reflected by increasing dyspnea, cough, sputum production, and wheezing and is related to airway obstruction.[26]

There is no specific treatment for bronchiolitis obliterans. Some children deteriorate rapidly and die within weeks, whereas others follow a more chronic course.

Bronchopulmonary dysplasia

Bronchopulmonary dysplasia (BPD) is a more severe form of lung damage associated with neonatal chronic lung disease. Risk factors for BPD include premature birth and immature lungs, oxygen toxicity, positive-pressure ventilation, respiratory infection, vitamin A deficiency, α_1-antiprotease deficiency, genetic predisposition, and persistent patent ductus arteriosus.

The incidence of BPD is difficult to ascertain. The most common clinical definition of BPD includes infants who remain oxygen- and ventilator-dependent and have respiratory symptoms and radiographic abnormalities after 28 days of life.[27] The process of BPD is one of continuous injury and repair of lung tissue, causing delays in both lung and body growth (Fig. 27-6).

Episodes of atelectasis, hyperinflation, pneumothorax, and air in the interstitium are characteristic. The infant may seem to be improving but suddenly becomes apneic or develops more severe respiratory distress and cyanosis. BPD can cause death within a few weeks or can continue for months or years. Either death or recovery is possible regardless of the length of disease. The goals of treatment are to accelerate lung maturation, maintain normal oxygenation, prevent further lung damage, and promote lung repair.[28]

Cystic fibrosis

Cystic fibrosis (CF) (mucoviscidosis) is an inherited disease of the exocrine glands resulting in the production of excessive, thick mucus that obstructs the gastrointestinal system and lungs. (The gastrointestinal component of CF is discussed in Chapter 35.) Although CF is a multiorgan disease, pulmonary failure is the usual cause of death.[29] CF is the most common fatal genetic disease, and it affects about 1 of every 2500 white children; it is much less prevalent in populations of color. The disease is characterized by pancreatic enzyme deficiency, progressive obstructive infectious pulmonary disease, malabsorption, and elevated sodium chloride concentrations in the sweat. Genetic transmission follows an autosomal recessive mode of inheritance (a child must inherit a defective gene from each parent) and involves a single gene—the cystic fibrosis transmembrane conductance regulator (CFTR). Clinical manifestations are present only in homozygotes. Approximately 2% to 5% of the white population are carriers.

Pathophysiology

CF is a generalized disease with complications that affect nearly every organ system. Four alterations contribute to the presentation of the disease, and they are all related to abnormal chloride transport: thick, tenacious mucus secretions; stasis of mucus secretions; excess sodium chloride in serous secretions and sweat; and chronic respiratory tract infection.[30]

The exocrine, or mucus-producing, glands secrete an abnormally thick mucus that coagulates in the ducts of organs or the airways of the lung with obstruction and dilation that alter or destroy structure and function. Bronchiolar obstruction with thick mucus is the first stage of pulmonary involvement. The obstruction predisposes the lung to infection, primarily with *Staphylococcus aureus* and *Pseudomonas aeruginosa*. With chronic inflammation there is hyperplasia of goblet cells with enlargement and destruction of airway walls, causing bronchiectasis. The disease progresses from bronchiolitis (mucus plugging and inflammation of the small airways) to bronchitis, followed by pneumonia, peribronchial fibrosis, and bronchiectasis, the formation of large cystic dilations that involve all bronchi. Alveolar involvement ensues with infection, atelectasis, and hemorrhagic pneumonia. Recurrent pneumothorax, hemoptysis, pulmonary hypertension, and cor pulmonale are serious and life-threatening complications of severe and diffuse pulmonary disease.

Clinical Manifestations

Children with CF may have few or numerous clinical manifestations. Chronic cough and sputum production are symptomatic of lung involvement. Mucus is usually purulent. There is labored ventilation resulting in hypoxia, clubbing of the fingers, and cyanosis. The chronic pulmonary infection and malabsorption can lead to secondary manifestations of barrel chest, pectus carinatum, and kyphosis. Chronic rhinitis is common among children with CF. Although diffuse organ involvement can be characteristic of the complications of CF, the pulmonary disorders are the most common cause of morbidity and mortality.

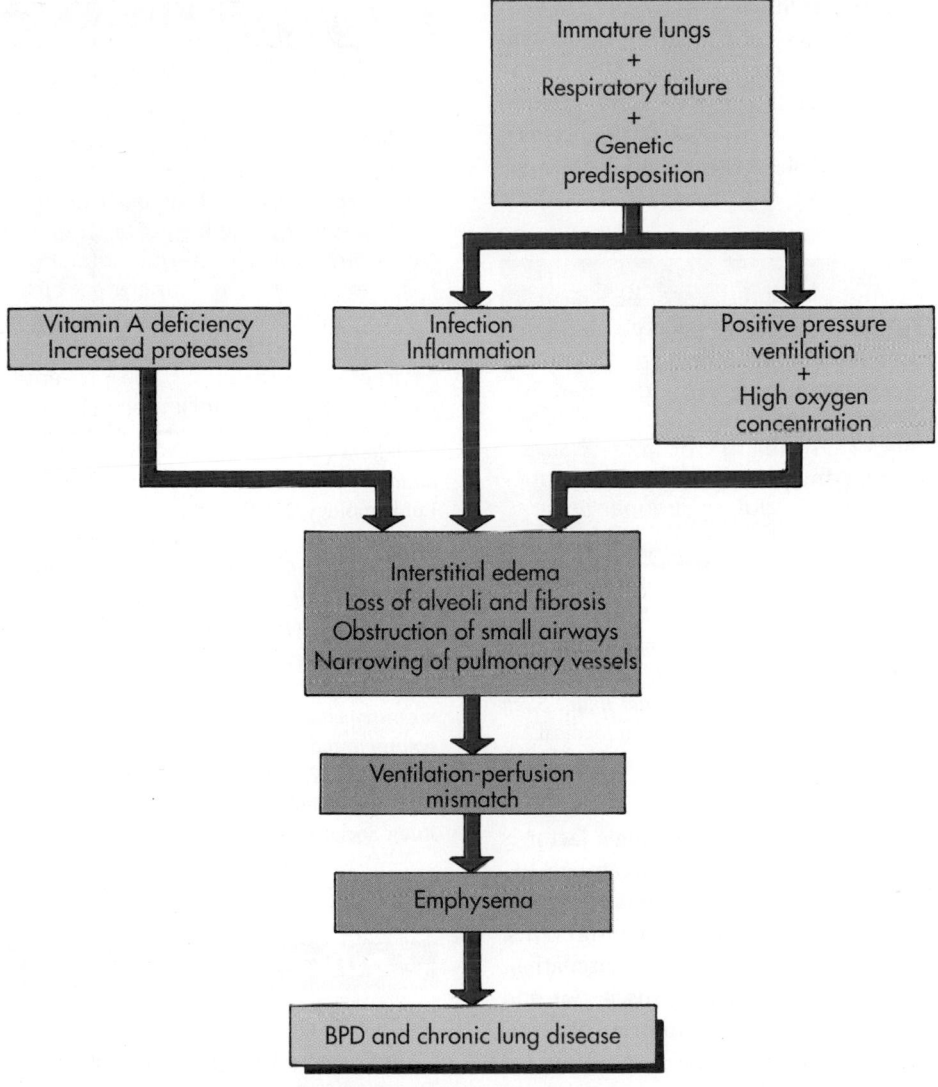

Fig. 27-6 *Pathophysiology of bronchopulmonary dysplasia (BPD).*

⬛ *Evaluation and Treatment*

Recently, new genetic markers make it possible to diagnose CF prenatally and to detect carriers in more than 70% of families with a history of CF. Cystic fibrosis is traditionally diagnosed when a sweat test discloses a sodium chloride concentration greater than 60 mEq/L. The sweat test is performed when there is a family history of CF or when there are pulmonary or gastrointestinal symptoms consistent with the disease.

Management of CF requires a multidisciplinary effort to relieve (1) symptoms from generalized organ involvement and (2) the social and financial burdens of the disease. The management plan includes judicious use of antibiotics to control pulmonary infection; aggressive pulmonary therapy with drugs to thin mucus secretions; humidified air, postural drainage, and oxygen; and lung transplantation.[30] Gene therapy is in progress.[31] Survival age is about 30 years.[32]

✓ QUICK CHECK

How is alveolar development related to RDS?

Describe the relationship between allergy and asthma.

Contrast bronchitis, bronchiolitis, and bronchiolitis obliterans.

SUDDEN INFANT DEATH SYNDROME

The greatest single cause of death among infants between 1 week and 1 year of age is *sudden infant death syndrome (SIDS),* also called *crib death* or *cot death.*[33] The syndrome refers to the sudden, unexpected death of any infant or young child in whom a postmortem examination fails to demonstrate a cause for death.

The highest incidence of SIDS is between 2 and 4 months of age; it almost always occurs during sleep, with higher frequency during the winter months. SIDS is the leading cause of postneonatal death and claims 700 to 10,000 lives each year.[34] The occurrence rate varies between 1 and 3 per 1000 live births. Risk factors for SIDS are summarized in the Risk Factors box.

RISK FACTORS

SUDDEN INFANT DEATH SYNDROME (SIDS)
Risk factors associated with SIDS include (1) prone sleeping position, (2) poor mothers younger than 20 years of age, (3) low birth weight, (4) preterm delivery, (5) multiple pregnancies, (6) sibling who dies of SIDS, (7) smoking during pregnancy, (8) significant exposure to tobacco smoke, (9) anemia during pregnancy, and (10) lack of prenatal care.

Data from Kohlendorfer, U., Kiechl, S., & Sperl, W. (1998). Sudden infant death syndrome: Risk factor profiles for distinct subgroups. American Journal of Epidemiology, 147(10), 960-968; Willinger, M. et al. (1998). Factors associated with the transition to nonprone sleep positions of infants in the United States: The National Infant Sleep Position Study [see comments]. Journal of the American Medical Association, 280(4), 329-335.

The cause of SIDS is unknown, and no single factor is predictive of the sudden death. There is no treatment because the death is sudden and unexplained. Apnea is a common finding in infants with apparent life-threatening events, and these infants have survived with successful resuscitation. Parents should be taught cardiopulmonary resuscitation and actions to take in an emergency. Home monitoring of respiratory and cardiovascular functions has been successful for infant apnea. There is also significant evidence that infants should be placed on their back, not prone or on their side, for sleeping for the first 6 months of life.[35,36]

HEALTH ALERT

Preventing Sudden Infant Death Syndrome
Sudden infant death syndrome (SIDS) is the leading cause of postnatal death in the United States. Although the specific cause of SIDS is unknown, there are strong associations with prone sleeping position, soft bedding, low infant birth weight, and low socioeconomic class. Maternal smoking during pregnancy and exposure to nicotine after birth are independent and significant risk factors for SIDS, and nicotine exposure is one of the most controllable risk factors. Parental education on the prevention of SIDS should lead to a further decline in SIDS mortality.

Data from Cooke, R.W. (1998). Smoking, intra-uterine growth retardation and sudden infant death syndrome. International Journal of Epidemiology, 27(2), 238-241; Daltveit, A.K. et al. (1998). Sociodemographic risk factors for sudden infant death syndrome associated with other risk factors. The Nordic Epidemiological SIDS Study. Acta Paediatrics, 87(3), 284-290; Henderson-Smart, D.J., Ponsonby, A.L., & Murphy, E. (1998). Reducing the risk of sudden infant death syndrome: A review of the scientific literature. Journal of Paediatric Child Health, 34(3), 213-219; Milerad, J. et al. (1998). Objective measurements of nicotine exposure in victims of sudden infant death syndrome and in other unexpected child deaths. Journal of Pediatrics, 133(2), 232-236; Wakefield, M. et al. (1998). Smoking and smoking cessation among men whose partners are pregnant: A qualitative study. Social Science Medicine, 47(5), 657-664.

✓ QUICK CHECK

Why are premature infants at risk for BPD?

Why is mucus a significant cause of obstruction in cystic fibrosis?

What are the risk factors for SIDS?

DID YOU UNDERSTAND?

Pulmonary Disorders in Children
1. Croup is a syndrome of clinical manifestations caused by acute obstruction of the larynx as a result of infection, aspiration of a foreign body, or allergy.
2. Acute epiglottitis is the most life-threatening type of croup. Acute laryngotracheobronchitis, which is less dangerous, is the most common type.
3. Aspiration of foreign bodies that lodge in the airways may cause cough, hoarseness, and dyspnea and can cause chronic infection, asthma, or lung abscess. Pneumonia and respiratory distress also can result from aspiration of contaminated fluids or gastric reflux.

4. Respiratory distress syndrome (RDS) of the newborn usually occurs in premature infants who are born before surfactant production and alveolocapillary development are complete. Atelectasis and hypoventilation cause shunting, hypoxemia, and hypercapnia.
5. The severity of asthma in children depends on the child's age (because age determines the caliber of airway lumina), the child's hypersensitivity, and the duration of the asthma attack. Children have less capacity than adults to sustain the work of breathing during asthma attacks.
6. Viral pneumonia and bacterial pneumonia cause varying degrees of illness in children; symptoms range from mild respiratory distress to rapid death.

■ DID YOU UNDERSTAND? —cont'd

7. Bronchiolitis, the inflammatory obstruction of the bronchioles, is most common in infants and is usually caused by infection by a virus that would cause only mild illness in older children or adults.

8. In bronchiolitis obliterans, the bronchioles and some small bronchi are partially or completely obliterated by nodular masses containing granulomatous or fibrous tissue.

9. Bronchopulmonary dysplasia (BPD) is an iatrogenic abnormality of pulmonary and bronchial development in premature neonates. It is caused by administration of oxygen via positive pressure, which injures tissues and delays both lung and body growth. Alterations include scarring of the alveoli and emphysema.

10. Cystic fibrosis is an autosomal recessive genetic disease characterized by excessive secretion of thick, tenacious mucus resulting in bronchiolar obstruction and infection with progression to bronchiectasis, pneumonia, pneumothorax, pulmonary hypertension, and cor pulmonale.

Sudden Infant Death Syndrome (SIDS)

1. Sudden infant death syndrome is the leading cause of postnatal death and is associated with low birth weight, prone sleeping position, and other environmental factors.

KEY TERMS

Acute laryngitis, 776
Acute tracheitis, 776
Asthma, 779
Bronchiolitis, 782
Bronchiolitis obliterans, 784
Bronchitis, 782
Bronchopulmonary dysplasia (BPD), 784

Cystic fibrosis (CF), 784
Epiglottis, 776
Epiglottitis, 776
Hyaline membrane disease (HMD), 779
Idiopathic respiratory distress syndrome (IRDS), 779
Laryngitis, 776

Laryngotracheobronchitis (LTB) (laryngotracheitis) 776, 778
Respiratory distress syndrome (RDS) of the newborn, 779
Sudden infant death syndrome (SIDS), 785
Viral croup, 776, 778

REFERENCES

1. Cressman, W.R. & Myer, C.M. (1994). Diagnosis and management of croup and epiglottitis. *Pediatric Clinics of North America, 41*(2), 265-276.

2. Behrman, R.E., Kliegman, R.M., & Arvin, A.M. (1996). *Nelson textbook of pediatrics* (15th ed.). Philadelphia: Saunders.

3. Baugh, R. & Gilmore, B.B. (1986). Infectious croup: A critical review. *Otolaryngology: Head and Neck Surgery, 95,* 40.

4. Heath, P.T. (1998). Haemophilus influenzae type b conjugate vaccines: A review of efficacy data. *Pediatric Infectious Disease Journal, 17*(9 Suppl.), S117-S122.

5. Cressman, W.R. & Myer, C.M. (1994). Diagnosis and management of croup and epiglottitis. *Pediatric Clinics of North America, 41*(2), 265-276.

6. Cataneo, A.J. et al. (1997). Foreign body in the tracheobronchial tree. *Clinical Pediatrics (Philadelphia), 36*(12), 701-706.

7. Washington Office of Technology Assessment. (1987). *Neonatal intensive care for low birthweight infants: Costs and effectiveness.* Washington, D.C.: U. S. Congress (Pub. No. OTA-HCS-38).

8. Hutchison, A.A. (1994). Respiratory disorders of the neonate. *Current Opinions in Pediatrics, 6*(2), 142-153.

9. Dekowsi, S.A. & Holtzman, R.B. (1998). An update on applications. *Pediatric Clinics of North America, 45*(3), 549-572.

10. Larsen, G.L. (1992). Asthma in children. *New England Journal of Medicine, 326*(23), 1540-1545.

11. Ertle, A.R. & London, M.R. (1998). Insights into asthma prevalence in Oregon. *Journal of Asthma, 35*(3), 281-289.

12. Huss, H., Oppenheimer, J., & Bielory, L. (1996). Asthma mortality in New Jersey residents. *New Jersey Journal of Medicine, 93*(3), 164-166.

13. Slutsky, A.S. (1998). Genetics of asthma: A primer. *Canadian Respiratory Journal, 5*(Suppl. A), 4A-8A.

14. Anonymous. (1996). Asthma mortality and hospitalization among children and young adults. *MMWR, Morbidity and Mortality Weekly Report, 45*(17), 350.

15. Sarafino, E.P., Paterson, M.E., & Murphy, E.L. (1998). Age and the impacts of triggers in childhood asthma. *Journal of Asthma, 35*(2), 213-217.

16. Murphy, S. & Kelly, W.H. (1999). *Pediatric asthma.* New York: Dekker.

17. Rabinovitch, N. & Gelfand, E.W. (1998). New approaches to the treatment of childhood asthma. *Current Opinions in Pediatrics, 10*(3), 243-249.

REFERENCES

18. Dudas, R.A. & Karron, R.A. (1998). Respiratory syncytial virus vaccines. *Clinical Microbiology Review, 11*(3), 430-439.

19. Maxson, S. & Jacobs, R.F. (1994). Guidelines for evaluating children with LRIs. *Journal of Respiratory Diseases, 15*(5), 453-463.

20. Arguedas, A.G., Stutman, H.R., & Marks, M.I. (1990). Bacterial pneumonias. In V. Chermick & E.L. Kendig (Eds.). *Disorders of the respiratory tract in children.* Philadelphia: Saunders.

21. Mäkelä, M.J., Ruuskanen, O., & Ogra, P.L. (1994). Treatment of respiratory syncytial virus infections in children. *Annals of Medicine, 26*(5), 341-343.

22. Panitch, H.B., Callahan, C.W., & Schidlow, D.V. (1993). Bronchiolitis in children. *Clinics in Chest Medicine, 14*(4), 715-731.

23. Horst, P.S. (1994). Bronchiolitis. *American Family Physician, 49*(6), 1449-1453, 1456.

24. Adcock, P.M., Sanders, C.L., & Marshall, G.S. (1998). Standardizing the care of bronchiolitis. *Archives of Pediatric and Adolescent Medicine, 152*(8), 739-744.

25. Wohl, M.G. (1990). Bronchiolitis. In V. Chermick & E.L. Kendig (Eds.). *Disorders of the respiratory tract in children.* Philadelphia: Saunders.

26. Chang, A.B., Masel, J.P., & Masters, B. (1998). Postinfectious bronchiolitis obliterans: Clinical, radiological, and pulmonary function sequelae. *Pediatric Radiology, 28*(1), 23-29.

27. Truog, W.E. (1993). Bronchopulmonary dysplasia. *Issues in Long Term Management, 14*(1), 130-147.

28. Abman, S.H. & Groothias, J.R. (1994). Pathophysiology and treatment of bronchopulmonary dysplasia: Current issues. *Pediatric Clinics of North America, 41*(2), 277-315.

29. Hillman, B.C. (1997). Genetic and immunologic aspects of cystic fibrosis. *Annals of Allergy, Asthma, and Immunology, 79*(5), 379-390.

30. Yankaskas, J.R. & Knowles, M.R. (1999). *Cystic fibrosis in adults.* Philadelphia: Lippincott-Raven.

31. Knoell, D.L. & Yiu, I.M. (1998). Human gene therapy for hereditary diseases: A review of trials. *American Journal of Health-System Pharmacy, 55*(9), 899-904.

32. Rosenstein, B.J. & Zeitlin, P.L. (1995). Prognosis in cystic fibrosis. *Current Opinions in Pulmonary Medicine, 1*(6), 444-449.

33. Anonymous. (1998). Assessment of infant sleeping position—Selected states, 1996. *MMWR, Morbidity and Mortality Weekly Report, 47*(41), 873-877.

34. Brooks, J.G. (1994). Sudden infant death syndrome. In G.M. Loughlin & H. Eigen. *Respiratory disease in children.* Baltimore: Williams & Wilkins.

35. Gibson, E. et al. (1998). Sudden infant death syndrome rates subsequent to the American Academy of Pediatrics supine sleep position. *Medical Care, 36*(6), 938-942.

36. Henderson-Smart, D.J., Ponsoby, A.L., & Murphy, E. (1998). Reducing the risk of sudden infant death syndrome: A review of the scientific literature. *Journal of Paediatrics and Child Health, 34*(3), 213-219.

CHAPTER

28

Structure and Function of the Renal and Urologic Systems

Sue E. Huether

The primary function of the kidney is to maintain a stable internal environment for optimal cell and tissue metabolism. The kidneys accomplish these life-sustaining tasks by balancing solute and water transport, excreting metabolic waste products, conserving nutrients, and regulating acids and bases. The kidney also has an endocrine function and secretes the hormones renin, erythropoietin, and 1,25-dihydroxyvitamin D_3 for regulation of blood pressure, erythrocyte production, and calcium metabolism, respectively. In times of severe fasting the kidney also can synthesize glucose from amino acids, performing the process of gluconeogenesis. The formation of urine is achieved through the process of filtration, reabsorption, and secretion by the glomeruli and tubules within the kidney. The bladder stores the urine that it receives from the kidney by way of the ureters. Urine is then removed from the body through the urethra.

CHAPTER OUTLINE

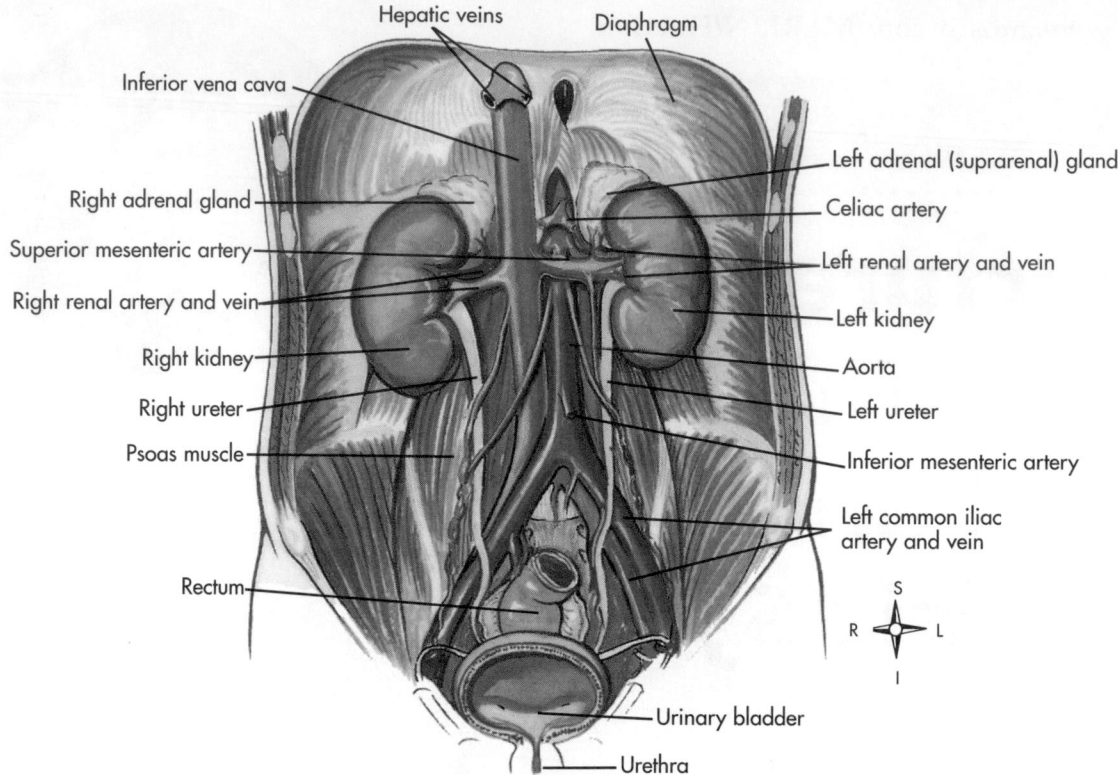

Fig. 28-1 *Organs of the urinary system.* *(From Thibodeau, G.A. & Patton, K.T. [1999]. Anatomy & physiology [4th ed.]. St. Louis: Mosby.)*

STRUCTURES OF THE RENAL SYSTEM

Structures of the Kidney

The **kidneys** are paired organs located on the posterior abdominal wall outside the peritoneal cavity. They lie on either side of the vertebral column with their upper and lower poles extending from the twelfth thoracic vertebra to the third lumbar vertebra (Fig. 28-1). Each kidney is approximately 11 cm long, 5 to 6 cm wide, and 3 to 4 cm thick. A tightly adhering capsule (the **renal capsule**) surrounds each kidney, and the kidney then is embedded in a mass of fat. The capsule and fatty layer are covered with a double layer of **renal fascia,** fibrous tissue that attaches the kidney to the posterior abdominal wall.

The cushion of fat and the position of the kidney between the abdominal organs and muscles of the back protect it from trauma. The right kidney is slightly lower than the left; it is displaced downward by the overlying liver. A medial indentation (the **hilum**) contains the entry and exit for the renal blood vessels, nerves, lymphatic vessels, and ureter.

The gross structure of the kidney can be identified in Fig. 28-2.

Nephron

The **nephron** is the functional unit of the kidney. Each kidney contains approximately 1.2 million nephrons. The

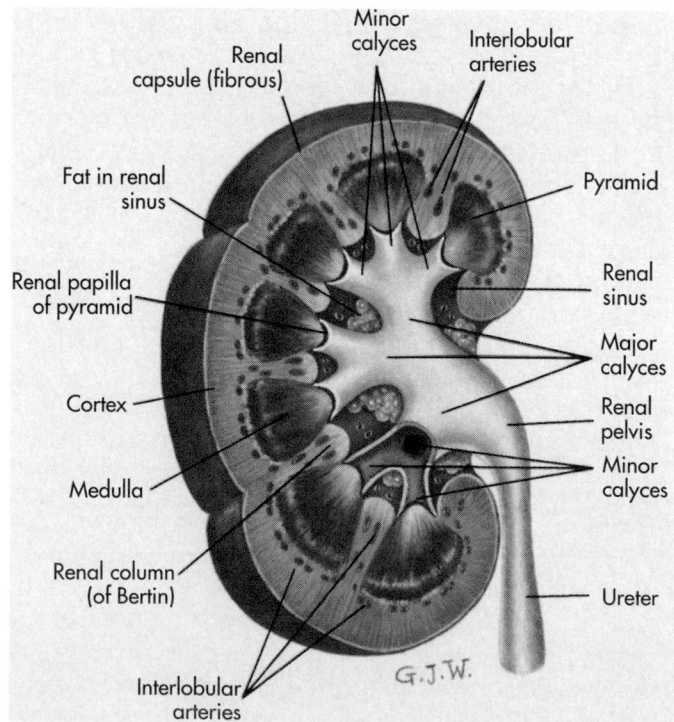

Fig. 28-2 *Kidney structure.* *(From Brundage, D.J. [1992]. Renal disorders. St. Louis: Mosby.)*

Fig. 28-3 *Components of nephron.* *(From Brundage, D.J. [1992].* Renal disorders. *St. Louis: Mosby.)*

nephron is a tubular structure with subunits that include the renal corpuscle, proximal convoluted tubule, loop of Henle, distal convoluted tubule, and collecting duct, all of which contribute to the formation of final urine (Fig. 28-3). The different structures of the epithelial cells lining various segments of the tubule facilitate the special functions of secretion and reabsorption (Fig. 28-4).

The kidney has (1) *cortical nephrons* (85% of all nephrons), which extend only partially into the medulla; and (2) *juxtamedullary nephrons,* which lie close to and extend deep into the medulla and are important for the concentration of urine (Fig. 28-5). The *glomerulus* is a tuft of capillaries that loop into *Bowman capsule,* like fingers pushed into bread dough. Together, the glomerulus and Bowman capsule are called the renal corpuscle. *Mesangial cells* (similar to monocytes) and mesangial matrix lie between and

support the capillaries. The space inside Bowman capsule is called *Bowman space.*

The *glomerular filtration membrane* filters blood components through its three layers: (1) an inner capillary endothelium, (2) a middle basement membrane, and (3) an outer layer of capillary epithelium. The capillary endothelium is composed of cells in continuous contact with the basement membrane and contains pores. The middle basement membrane is a selectively permeable network of glycoproteins and mucopolysaccharides. The epithelium has specialized cells called *podocytes* from which pedicles radiate and adhere to the basement membrane. The pedicles interlock with the pedicles of adjacent podocytes, forming an elaborate network of intercellular clefts (*filtration slits,* or slit membranes). The endothelium, basement membrane, and podocytes are covered with protein molecules bearing

Fig. 28-4 *Epithelial cells of the various segments of nephron tubules.* *(From Berne, R.M. & Levy, M.N. [Eds.]. [1993]. Physiology [3rd ed.]. St. Louis: Mosby.)*

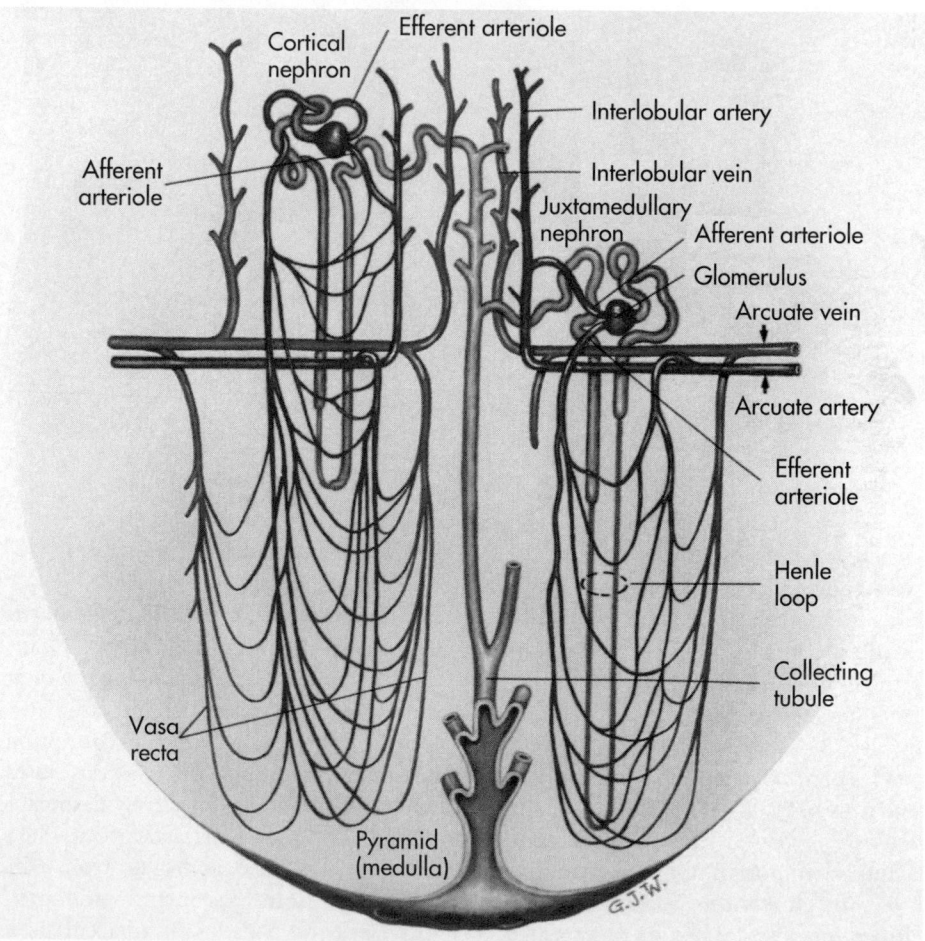

Fig. 28-5 *The nephron unit with its blood vessels.* Blood flows through nephron vessels as follows: interlobular artery, afferent arteriole, glomerulus, efferent arteriole, peritubular capillaries (around the tubules), venules, interlobular vein. *(From Brundage, D.J. [1992]. Renal disorders. St. Louis: Mosby.)*

anionic charges that retard the filtration of anionic proteins. The glomerular filtration membrane separates the blood of the glomerular capillaries from the fluid in Bowman space. The glomerular filtrate passes through the three layers of the glomerular membrane and forms the primary urine.

The glomerulus is supplied by the afferent arteriole and drained by the efferent arteriole. A group of specialized cells known as *juxtaglomerular cells* are located around the afferent arteriole where it enters the renal corpuscle (see Fig. 28-3). Between the afferent and efferent arterioles is the *macula densa* (Fig. 28-6). Together the juxtaglomerular cells and macula densa cells form the *juxtaglomerular apparatus* (see Fig. 28-3). Control of renal blood flow, glomerular filtration, and renin secretion occurs at this site.

The *proximal tubule* continues from Bowman space and has an initial convoluted segment (pars convoluta) and then a straight segment (pars recta) that descends toward the medulla (see Fig. 28-3). The proximal tubular lumen consists of one layer of cuboidal cells. This is the only surface inside the nephron where the cells are covered with microvilli (a brush border). This greatly expands the surface area of the tubule and enhances its reabsorptive function (see Fig. 28-4). The proximal tubule joins the *loop of* Henle, which extends into the medulla. The tube then loops and becomes a thickening ascending segment that extends toward the cortex. A thin segment is composed of thin squamous cells with no active transport function. The cells of the thick segment are cuboidal and actively transport several solutes.

The major structural difference between the glomeruli in the two types of nephrons is the length of the loop of Henle. In cortical nephrons, the loop is short and may not extend into the medulla. The loops of Henle for the juxtamedullary nephrons, however, may extend the whole length of the medulla (40 mm). Juxtamedullary nephrons represent about 12% of the total number of nephrons.

The *distal tubule* has straight and convoluted segments. It extends from the macula densa to the *collecting duct,* a large tubule that descends down the cortex, through the renal pyramids of the inner and outer medullae, and into the minor calyx.

Blood vessels of the kidney

The blood vessels of the kidney closely parallel nephron structure. The major vessels are as follows:

1. *Renal arteries.* Arise as the fifth branches of the abdominal aorta, divide into anterior and posterior branches at the renal hilum, then subdivide into lobar arteries supplying blood to the lower, middle, and upper thirds of the kidney.
2. *Interlobar arteries.* Further subdivisions that travel down renal columns and between pyramids; form afferent glomerular arteries.
3. *Arcuate arteries.* Branches of interlobar arteries at the cortical medullary junction; arch over the base of the pyramids and run parallel to the surface.
4. *Glomerular capillaries.* Four to eight vessels in a fistlike structure; arise from the afferent arteriole and empty into the efferent arteriole, which carries blood to the peritubular capillaries.

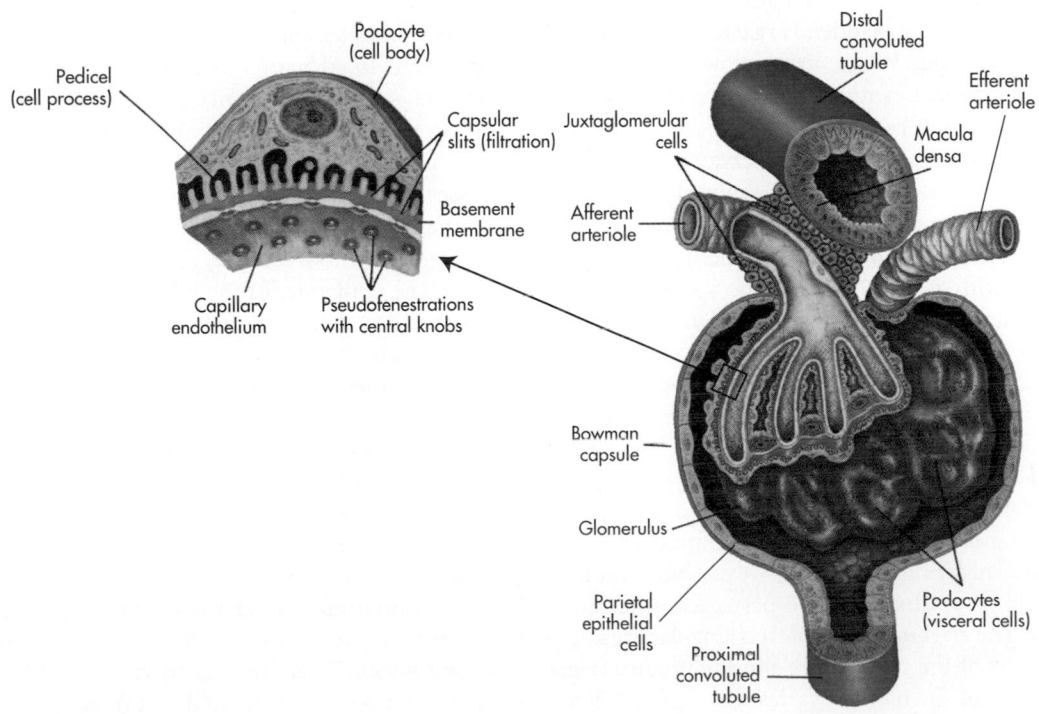

Fig. 28-6 *Anatomy of the glomerulus and juxtaglomerular apparatus. (From Brundage, D.J. [1992].* Renal disorders. *St. Louis: Mosby.)*

5. ***Peritubular capillaries.*** Surround convoluted portions of the proximal and distal tubules and the loop of Henle; adapted for cortical and juxtamedullary nephrons.
6. ***Vasa recta.*** Network of capillaries that forms loops and closely follows the loops of Henle; only blood supply to the medulla.
7. ***Renal veins.*** Follow arterial path and have same names as the arteries; eventually empty into the inferior vena cava.

Note that the lymphatic vessels tend also to follow the distribution of the blood vessels.

✓ QUICK CHECK

Describe the physical characteristics of the kidneys.

What does the nephron do?

Why are proteins not filtered at the glomerulus?

Urinary Structures

Ureters

The urine formed by the nephrons flows from the distal tubules and collecting ducts through the duct of Bellini and the ***renal papillae*** (projections of the ducts) and into the calyces and is collected in the renal pelvis (see Fig. 28-2). From the renal pelvis, urine is funneled into the ***ureters.*** Each adult ureter is approximately 30 cm long and is composed of long, intertwining muscle bundles. The lower ends pass obliquely through the posterior aspect of the bladder wall. The close approximation of muscle cells permits the direct transmission of electrical stimulation, and the resulting peristaltic activity propels urine into the bladder. Peristaltic activity is affected by urine volume. When urine flow is slow, the contraction is segmented, with downward propulsion of urine. Increasing flow rates increase peristalsis. Peristalsis is maintained even when the ureter is denervated, so ureters can be transplanted. The upper part of the ureter is innervated by the tenth thoracic nerve roots, with referred pain to the umbilicus. The innervation of lower segments arises from the sacral nerves with referred pain to the vulva or penis. Contraction of the bladder during ***micturition*** (urination) compresses the lower end of the ureter, preventing reflux. The ureters have a rich blood supply from the kidney with contributions by the lumbar and superior vesical arteries.

Bladder and urethra

The ***bladder*** is a bag of smooth muscle fibers that forms the ***detrusor muscle*** and its smooth lining of transitional epithelium. As the bladder fills with urine, it distends and the layers of transitional epithelium slide past each other and become thinner. The ***trigone*** is a smooth triangular area between the openings of the two ureters and the urethra (Fig. 28-7). The position of the bladder varies with age and gender. The bladder has a profuse blood supply, accounting for the bleeding that readily occurs with trauma, surgery, or inflammation.

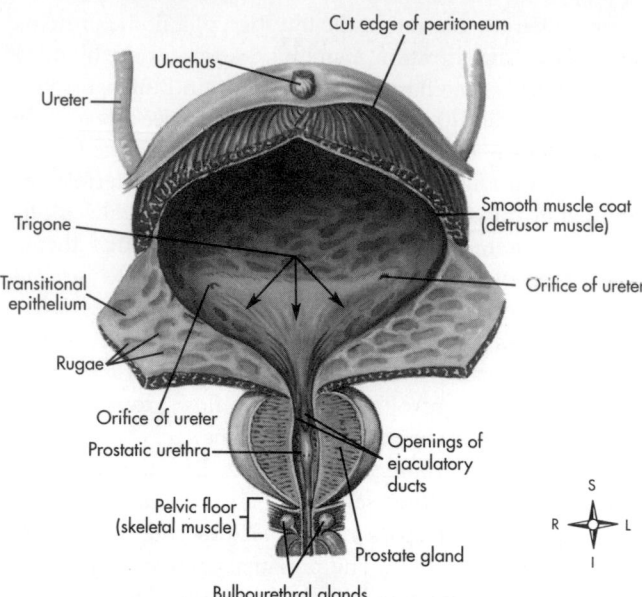

Fig. 28-7 ***Structure and location of the urinary bladder.*** Frontal view of a dissected urinary bladder (male) in a fully distended position. *(From Thibodeau, G.A. & Patton, K.T. [1999]. Anatomy & physiology [4th ed.]. St. Louis: Mosby.)*

The ***urethra*** extends from the inferior side of the bladder to the outside of the body. A ring of smooth muscle forms the ***internal urethral sphincter*** at the junction of the urethra and bladder. The ***external urethral sphincter*** is composed of striated muscles and is under voluntary control. The entire urethra is lined with mucus-secreting glands. The female urethra is short (3 to 4 cm). The male urethra is long (18 to 20 cm) and has three segments: prostatic, membranous, and cavernous. The prostatic urethra is closest to the bladder. It passes through the prostate gland and contains the openings of the ejaculatory ducts. The membranous urethra passes through the floor of the pelvis. The cavernous segment forms the remainder of the tube. It is surrounded by erectile tissue and contains the openings of the bulbourethral mucous glands.

The innervation of the bladder and internal urethral sphincter is supplied by parasympathetic fibers of the autonomic nervous system. The reflex arc required for micturition is stimulated by mechanoreceptors that respond to stretching of tissue, sensing bladder fullness and sending impulses to the sacral level of the cord. When the bladder accumulates 250 to 300 ml of urine, the bladder contracts and the internal urethral sphincter relaxes through activation of the spinal reflex arc (known as the micturition reflex). At this time a person feels the urge to void. In older children and adults, the reflex can be inhibited or facilitated by impulses coming from the brain, resulting in voluntary control of micturition by the relaxation or contraction of the external sphincter.

RENAL BLOOD FLOW

The kidneys are highly vascular organs and usually receive 1000 to 1200 ml of blood per minute, or about 20% to 25% of the cardiac output. With a normal hematocrit of 45%, about 600 to 700 ml of blood flowing through the kidney per minute is plasma. From the renal plasma flow (RPF), 20% (approximately 120 to 140 ml/min) is filtered at the glomerulus and passes into Bowman capsule. The filtration of the plasma per unit of time is known as the **_glomerular filtration rate (GFR),_** which is directly related to the perfusion pressure of the glomerular capillaries.

The remaining 80% (about 480 ml) of plasma flows through the efferent arterioles to the peritubular capillaries. The ratio of glomerular filtrate to renal plasma flow per minute (125/600 = 0.20) is called the _filtration fraction._ Normally all but 1 to 2 ml of the glomerular filtrate is reabsorbed and returned to the circulation by the peritubular capillaries.

The GFR is directly related to renal blood flow (RBF), which is regulated by intrinsic autoregulatory mechanisms, by neural regulation, and by hormonal regulation. In general, blood flow to any organ is determined by the arteriovenous pressure differences across the vascular bed. If mean arterial pressure decreases or vascular resistance increases, RBF falls.

Autoregulation

In the kidney a local mechanism tends to keep the rate of blood flow and therefore the GFR fairly constant over a range of arterial pressures between 80 and 180 mm Hg (Fig. 28-8). Changes in afferent arteriolar resistance and arteriolar pressure occur in the same direction. Therefore RBF and GFR are relatively constant, a relationship maintained by an intrinsic autoregulatory mechanism to prevent wide fluctuations in systemic arterial pressure from being transmitted to the glomerular capillaries. Solute and water excretion is thus maintained when arterial pressure changes.

As arterial pressure declines, the stretch on the afferent arteriolar wall decreases and the arteriole relaxes, with an increase in RBF; an increase in arteriolar pressure causes the arteriole to contract and decreases RBF. Another mechanism that keeps RBF and GFR constant is tubuloglomerular feedback. As the concentration of sodium chloride decreases at the macula densa of the juxtaglomerular apparatus, the afferent arterioles constrict and GFR decreases. The opposite occurs as sodium chloride at the macula densa increases.

Neural Regulation

The blood vessels of the kidney are innervated by the autonomic nervous system through sympathetic fibers that cause vasoconstriction. The innervation of the kidney comes primarily from the celiac ganglion and greater splanchnic nerve (see Fig. 12-25). The afferent and efferent arterioles are richly innervated, but nerves have not been observed in the glomerular capillaries.

When systemic arterial pressure decreases, increased renal sympathetic nerve activity is mediated reflexively

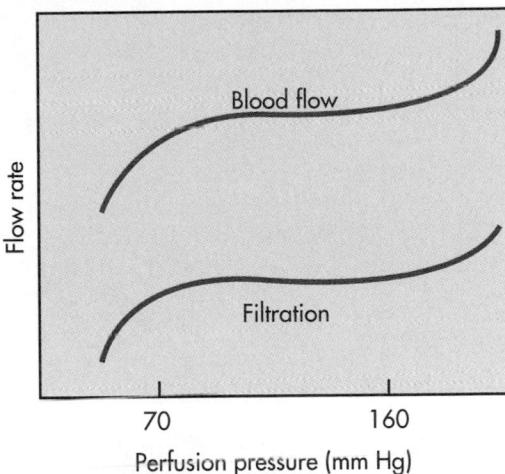

Fig. 28-8 _Renal autoregulation._ Blood flow and glomerular filtration rate are stabilized in the face of changes in perfusion pressure. _(From Berne, R.M. & Levy, M.N. [Eds.]. [1998]. Physiology [4th ed.]. St. Louis: Mosby.)_

through the carotid sinus and the baroreceptors of the aortic arch. This stimulates renal arteriolar vasoconstriction and decreases both RBF and GFR. The decreased RBF also diminishes excretion of sodium and water, promoting an increase in blood volume and thus an increase in systemic pressure.

Exercise, body position, and hypoxia also influence RBF. Exercise and change of body position activate renal sympathetic neurons and cause mild vasoconstriction. Severe hypoxia stimulates the chemoreceptors of the carotid and aortic bodies and decreases RBF by means of sympathetic stimulation. Hemorrhage induces intense sympathetic stimulation and vasoconstriction, and both GFR and blood flow are reduced.

Hormonal Regulation

A major hormonal regulator of renal blood flow is the **_renin-angiotensin system,_** which can increase systemic arterial pressure and change RBF. Renin is an enzyme formed and stored in the cells of the arterioles of the juxtaglomerular apparatus (see Fig. 28-3). Several complex physiologic mechanisms stimulate its release, including decreased blood pressure in the afferent arterioles, which reduces stretch of the juxtaglomerular cells; decreased sodium chloride concentration in the distal convoluted tubule; and sympathetic nerve stimulation of β-adrenergic receptors on the juxtaglomerular cells.[1] Numerous physiologic effects of the renin-angiotensin system serve the purpose of stabilizing systemic blood pressure and preserving the extracellular fluid volume during hypotension or hypovolemia, including sodium reabsorption, systemic vasoconstriction, sympathetic nerve stimulation, thirst stimulation, and drinking. (The effects are summarized in Fig. 28-9.)

Prostaglandins and kinins are also formed in and act on the kidneys. Other renal hormones are discussed on p. 802.

Fig. 28-9 *Cooperative roles of antidiuretic hormone (ADH) and aldosterone in regulating urine and plasma volume.* The drop in blood pressure that accompanies loss of fluid from the internal environment triggers the hypothalamus to rapidly release ADH from the posterior pituitary gland. ADH increases water reabsorption by the kidney by increasing water permeability of the distal tubules and collecting ducts. The drop in blood pressure is also detected by each nephron's juxtaglomerular apparatus, which responds by secreting renin. Renin triggers the formation of angiotensin II, which stimulates release of aldosterone from the adrenal cortex. Aldosterone then slowly boosts water reabsorption by the kidneys by increasing reabsorption of Na^+. Because angiotensin II also stimulates secretion of ADH, it serves as an additional link between the ADH and aldosterone mechanisms. *(From Thibodeau, G.A. & Patton, K.T. [1999].* Anatomy & physiology *[4th ed.]. St. Louis: Mosby.)*

✓QUICK CHECK

Where is pain from the ureters referred?

How do the bladder and urethra function in urine formation?

What is autoregulation in the kidney? What other regulatory mechanisms are at work in renal function?

KIDNEY FUNCTION
Nephron Function

The nephron can perform many functions simultaneously, as follows:

1. Filters plasma at glomerulus
2. Reabsorbs and secretes different substances along tubular structure

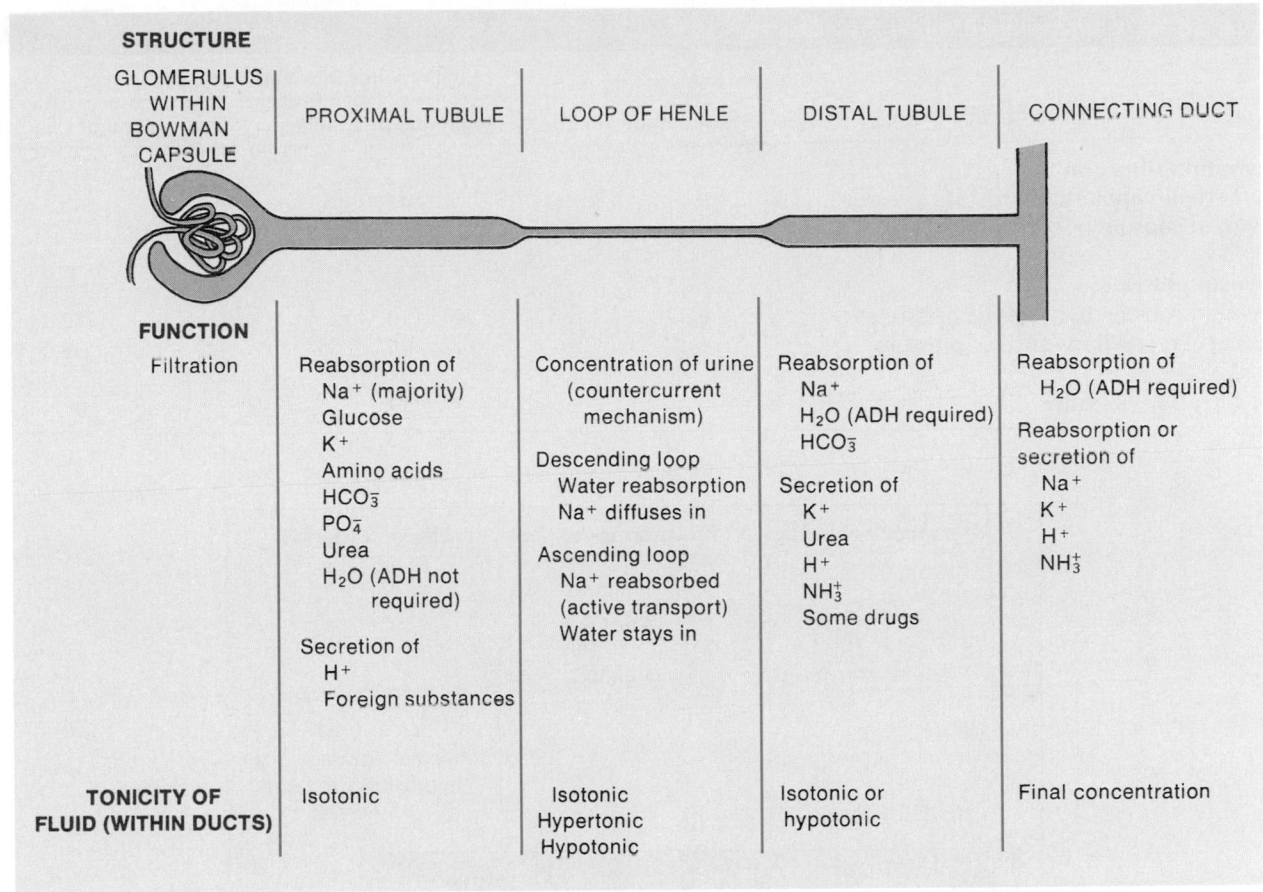

STRUCTURE

GLOMERULUS WITHIN BOWMAN CAPSULE	PROXIMAL TUBULE	LOOP OF HENLE	DISTAL TUBULE	CONNECTING DUCT

FUNCTION

| Filtration | Reabsorption of Na⁺ (majority) Glucose K⁺ Amino acids HCO₃⁻ PO₄⁻ Urea H₂O (ADH not required) Secretion of H⁺ Foreign substances | Concentration of urine (countercurrent mechanism) Descending loop Water reabsorption Na⁺ diffuses in Ascending loop Na⁺ reabsorbed (active transport) Water stays in | Reabsorption of Na⁺ H₂O (ADH required) HCO₃⁻ Secretion of K⁺ Urea H⁺ NH₃⁺ Some drugs | Reabsorption of H₂O (ADH required) Reabsorption or secretion of Na⁺ K⁺ H⁺ NH₃⁺ |

| TONICITY OF FLUID (WITHIN DUCTS) | Isotonic | Isotonic Hypertonic Hypotonic | Isotonic or hypotonic | Final concentration |

Fig. 28-10 *Major functions of nephron segments.* *ADH,* Antidiuretic hormone. *(From Wong, D.L. et al. [1999].* Whaley & Wong's nursing care of infants and children *[6th ed.]. St. Louis: Mosby.)*

3. Forms a filtrate of protein-free plasma (**ultrafiltration**)
4. Regulates the filtrate to maintain body fluid volume, electrolyte composition, and pH within narrow limits

Tubular reabsorption is the movement of fluids and solutes from the tubular lumen to the peritubular capillary plasma. Transfer of substances from the plasma of the peritubular capillary to the tubular lumen is *tubular secretion.* The transport mechanisms are both active and passive (processes defined in Chapter 4). The elimination of a substance in the final urine is known as *excretion* (Fig. 28-10).

Glomerular filtration

The fluid filtered by the glomerular capillary filtration membrane is protein free but contains electrolytes, such as sodium, chloride, and potassium, and organic molecules, such as creatinine, urea, and glucose, in the same concentrations as in plasma. Like other capillary membranes, the glomerulus is freely permeable to water and relatively impermeable to large colloids, such as plasma proteins. The molecule's size and electrical charge affect the permeability of substances crossing the glomerulus.

Capillary pressure also affects glomerular filtration. The hydrostatic pressure within the capillary is the major force

for moving water and solutes across the filtration membrane and into Bowman capsule. Two forces oppose the filtration effects of the glomerular capillary hydrostatic pressure (P_{GC}): (1) the hydrostatic pressure in Bowman space (P_{BC}) and (2) the effective oncotic pressure of the glomerular capillary blood (π_{GC}). Because the fluid in Bowman space normally contains only minute amounts of protein, it does not usually have an oncotic influence on the plasma of the glomerular capillary (Fig. 28-11).

The combined effect of forces favoring and forces opposing filtration determines the filtration pressure. The *net filtration pressure (NFP)* is the sum of forces favoring and opposing filtration. The estimated values contributing to the forces of net filtration are presented in Table 28-1.

As the protein-free fluid is filtered into Bowman capsule, the plasma oncotic pressure increases and the hydrostatic pressure decreases. The increase in glomerular capillary oncotic pressure is great enough to reduce the net filtration pressure to zero at the efferent end of the capillary and to stop the filtration process effectively. The low hydrostatic pressure and the increased oncotic pressure in the efferent arteriole then are transferred to the peritubular capillaries and facilitate reabsorption of fluid from the proximal tubules.

TABLE 28-1	Glomerular Filtration Pressures			
			Pressures (mm Hg)	
Forces		Pressures	Beginning of Capillary	End of Capillary
Promoting filtration				
Glomerular capillary hydrostatic pressure		P_{GC}	47	45
Bowman capsule oncotic pressure		π_{BC}	Negligible effect	
Opposing filtration				
Bowman capsule hydrostatic pressure		P_{BC}	10	10
Glomerular capillary oncotic pressure		π_{GC}	<u>25</u>	<u>35</u>
Net filtration pressure			12	0

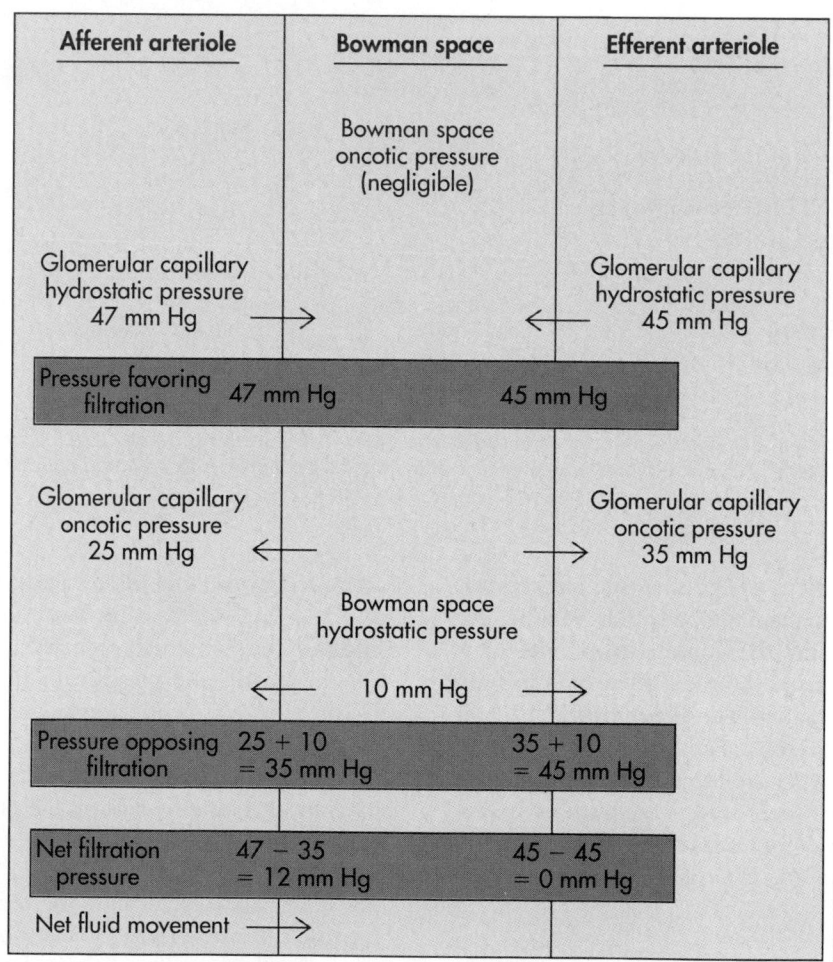

Fig. 28-11 *Glomerular filtration pressures.*

Filtration rate

The total volume of fluid filtered by the glomeruli averages 180 L/day, or approximately 120 ml/min, a phenomenal amount considering the size of the kidneys. Because only 1 to 2 L of urine is excreted per day, 99% of the filtrate is reabsorbed into the peritubular capillaries and returned to the blood. The factors determining the GFR are directly related to the pressures that favor or oppose filtration. For example, if the afferent arteriole constricts, blood flow decreases with a corresponding drop in glomerular pressure. The GFR then decreases, and body fluids are conserved. Conversely, constriction of the efferent arteriole increases the net filtration pressure and the GFR increases. When both afferent and efferent arterioles constrict, little change occurs in filtration pressure but RBF is reduced and so is the GFR.

Obstruction to the outflow of urine (caused by strictures, stones, or tumors along the urinary tract) can cause a retrograde increase in pressure at Bowman capsule and a decrease in GFR. Excessive loss of protein-free fluid from vomiting, diarrhea, use of diuretics, or excessive sweating can increase glomerular capillary oncotic pressure and decrease the GFR. Renal disease can also cause changes in pressure relationships by altering capillary permeability and the surface area available for filtration (see Chapter 29).

Tubular transport

By the end of the proximal tubule, approximately 60% to 70% of filtered sodium and water and about 50% of urea have been actively reabsorbed, along with 90% or more of potassium, glucose, bicarbonate, calcium, phosphate, amino acids, and uric acid. Chloride, water, and urea are reabsorbed passively but linked to the active transport of sodium (co-transport). Active transport in the renal tubules can be limited as the carrier molecules become saturated, a phenomenon known as **transport maximum (T_m)**. For example, when the carrier molecules for glucose become saturated, the excess will be excreted in the urine.

Proximal tubule. Active reabsorption of sodium is the primary function of the proximal tubule. Water, most electrolytes, and organic substances are co-transported with sodium. The osmotic force generated by active sodium transport promotes the passive diffusion of water out of the tubular lumen and into the peritubular capillaries. Passive transport of water is further enhanced by the elevated oncotic pressure of the blood in the peritubular capillaries. The reabsorption of water leaves an increased concentration of urea within the tubular lumen, creating a gradient for its passive diffusion to the peritubular plasma.

As the positively charged sodium ions leave the tubular lumen, negatively charged chloride ions passively follow to maintain electroneutrality. Because the inside of the tubule of the proximal tubular cell has a limited permeability to chloride, however, chloride reabsorption lags behind sodium. Hydrogen ions are actively exchanged for sodium ions. The hydrogen ions (H^+) then combine with bicarbonate (HCO_3^-). Bicarbonate is completely filtered at the glomerulus, and approximately 90% is reabsorbed in the proximal tubule. In the tubular lumen, hydrogen and bicarbonate ions form carbonic acid (H_2CO_3), which rapidly breaks down, or dissociates, to carbon dioxide (CO_2) and water (H_2O). These then diffuse into the tubular cell, where carbonic anhydrase again catalyzes the CO_2 and H_2O to form HCO_3^- and H^+. The H^+ is secreted again, and HCO_3^- combines with sodium and is transported to the peritubular capillary blood.

The bicarbonate molecule filtered at the glomerulus is not the same molecule that is reabsorbed (because it dissociates), and the hydrogen ion secreted by the proximal tubule is not excreted in the urine. Bicarbonate is thus conserved, and the hydrogen is reabsorbed as water. Therefore these ions normally do not contribute to the urinary excretion of acid or the addition of acid to the blood (Fig. 28-12).

In addition to the proximal tubular secretion of hydro-

Fig. 28-12 *Acidification of urine by tubule excretion of ammonia (NH₃).* **A,** Acidification of urine and conservation of base by distal renal tubule excretion of H^+. **B,** An amino acid (glutamine) moves into tubule cell and loses an amino group (NH₂) to form ammonia, which is secreted into the urine. In exchange, the tubule cell absorbs a basic salt (mainly $NaHCO_3$) into blood from urine. *(From Thibodeau, G.A. & Patton, K.T. [1999]. Anatomy & physiology [4th ed.]. St. Louis: Mosby.)*

gen ions, secretory transport mechanisms exist for creatinine, other organic bases, and endogenous and exogenous organic acids including para-aminohippurate (PAH) and penicillin (Box 28-1). These secretory mechanisms eliminate drugs and other exogenous chemical products from the body, frequently after conjugating them with sulfate and glucuronic acid in the liver. Many drugs and their metabolites are eliminated from the body in this way. When the renal tubules are damaged, metabolic by-products and drugs may accumulate, causing toxic levels.

Loop of Henle and distal tubule. Concentration or dilution of urine occurs principally in the loop of Henle and collecting ducts. These changes are related to the length of the loop and its depth of penetration into the medulla. The structural features of the medullary hairpin loops allow the kidney to concentrate urine and conserve water for the body. The transition of the filtrate into urine reflects the concentrating ability of the loops and final adjustments in urine composition made by the distal tubule and collecting duct.

The primary function of the loop of Henle is to establish a hyperosmotic state within the medullary interstitial fluid. It reabsorbs more solute than water into the interstitium, so the fluid leaving the ascending limb of the loop is therefore hypoosmotic, or more dilute than the fluid that entered. The distal tubule and collecting duct make final adjustments in the concentration or dilution of the excreted urine according to body needs. The vasa recta act to maintain the high osmotic gradient established by the loop of Henle.

The thin, descending segment of the loop of Henle is highly permeable to water and moderately permeable to sodium, urea, and other solutes. The thin, ascending segment is more permeable to solutes and almost impermeable to water. The thick portion of the ascending segment is highly permeable to sodium, potassium, and chloride and significantly less permeable to water and urea. The convoluted portion of the distal tubule is poorly permeable to water but readily absorbs ions and contributes to the dilution of the tubular fluid. The later, straight segment of the distal tubule and the collecting duct are permeable to water as controlled by antidiuretic hormone (ADH). Sodium is readily absorbed by the later segment of the distal tubule and collecting duct under the regulation of the hormone aldosterone (see Chapter 17). Potassium is actively secreted in these segments and is also controlled by aldosterone and other factors related to the concentration of potassium in body fluids.

Hydrogen is also secreted by the distal tubule and combines with nonbicarbonate buffers for the elimination of acids in the urine. The distal tubule thus contributes to the regulation of acid-base balance by excreting hydrogen ions into the urine and by adding new bicarbonate to the plasma. The mechanism is similar to the conservation of bicarbonate by the proximal tubule, except that the hydrogen ion is excreted in the urine. (The specific mechanisms of acid-base balance and acid excretion are described in Chapter 4.)

Glomerulotubular balance

Normally, 99% of the glomerular filtrate is reabsorbed. When the GFR decreases or increases, the renal tubules, primarily the proximal tubules, automatically adjust their rate of reabsorption of sodium and water to balance the change in GFR and regulate the quality and quantity of water delivered to the distal tubules.

Concentration and Dilution of Urine

Producing a concentrated urine involves a ***countercurrent exchange system,*** in which fluid flows in opposite directions through parallel tubes. A concentration gradient causes fluid to be exchanged across the parallel pathways. In the nephron, the fluid moves up and down the parallel sides of the hairpin loop of Henle in the medulla. The longer the loop, the greater the concentration gradient because the concentration gradient increases from the cortex to the tip of the medulla. The loops of Henle multiply the concentration gradient, and the vasa recta act as a countercurrent exchanger for maintaining the gradient.[2]

Water, sodium, and chloride

The process is initiated in the thick ascending limb of the loop of Henle with the active transport of chloride and sodium out of the tubular lumen and into the medullary interstitium (Fig. 28-13). Because the lumen of the ascending limb is impermeable to water, water cannot follow the sodium-chloride transport. This causes the ascending tubular fluid to become hypoosmotic and the medullary interstitium to become hyperosmotic. The descending limb of the loop, which receives fluid from the proximal tubule, is highly permeable to water, but it is the only place in the nephron that does not actively transport either sodium or chloride. Sodium and chloride may, however, diffuse into the descending tubule from the interstitium. The hyperosmotic interstitium causes water to move out of the descending limb, and the remaining fluid in the descending tubule becomes increasingly concentrated as it flows toward the tip of the medulla. As the tubular fluid rounds the loop and enters the ascending limb, sodium and chloride are removed and water is retained. The fluid then becomes more and more dilute as it encounters the distal tubule.

The slow rate of blood flow and the hairpin structure of the vasa recta allow blood to flow through the medullary tissue without disturbing the osmotic gradient. As blood flows into the descending limb of the vasa recta, it encounters the increasing osmotic concentration gradient of the medullary interstitium. Water moves out, and sodium and chloride diffuse into the descending vasa recta. The plasma becomes in-

Fig. 28-13 *Countercurrent mechanism for concentrating and diluting urine.* (Note: Numbers on illustration represent milliosmoles [mOsm].)

creasingly concentrated as it flows toward the tip of the medulla.

As the blood flow passes into the ascending limb and back toward the cortex, the surrounding interstitial fluid becomes comparatively more dilute. Water then moves back into the vasa recta, and sodium and chloride diffuse out. The net result is a preservation of the medullary osmotic gradient. If blood were to flow rapidly through the vasa recta, as occurs in some renal diseases, the medullary concentration gradient would be washed away and the ability to concentrate urine and conserve water would be lost. The efficiency of water conservation is related to the length of the loops: the longer the loops, the greater the ability to concentrate the urine. Many desert animals have very long loops and can reabsorb water so efficiently that they rarely need to drink.

Urea

Urea is the major constituent of urine along with water. The glomerulus freely filters urea, and tubular reabsorption depends on urine flow rate, with less reabsorption at higher flow rates. Approximately 50% of urea is excreted in the urine, and 50% is recycled within the kidney. This recycling contributes to the osmotic gradient within the medulla and is necessary for the concentration and dilution of urine. Because urea is an end-product of protein metabolism, individuals with protein deprivation cannot maximally concentrate their urine.

Urine

Urine is normally clear yellow or amber in color. Cloudiness may indicate the presence of bacteria, cells, or high solute concentration. The pH ranges from 4.6 to 8.0, but it is normally acidic, providing protection against bacteria. Specific gravity ranges from 1.001 to 1.035. Normal urine does not contain glucose or blood cells and only occasional traces of protein, usually in association with rigorous exercise.

Antidiuretic hormone

The distal tubule in the cortex receives the hypoosmotic urine from the ascending limb of the loop of Henle. The concentration of the final urine is controlled by antidiuretic hormone (ADH), which is secreted from the posterior pituitary or neurohypophysis. ADH increases water permeability and reabsorption in the last segment of the distal tubule and along the entire length of the collecting ducts, which pass through the inner and outer zones of the medulla. The water diffuses into the ascending limb of the vasa recta and returns to the systemic circulation. The excreted urine can have a high osmotic concentration, up to 1400 mOsm. The

TABLE 28-2	Action of Diuretics		
Diuretic	Site of Action	Action	Side Effects
Osmotic diuretic Mannitol Glycerol Urea	Proximal tubule	Freely filtered but not reabsorbed; osmotically attracts water and diminishes sodium reabsorption	Hypokalemia, dehydration
Carbonic anhydrase inhibitors Acetazolamide	Proximal tubule	Inhibits carbonic anhydrase; blocks hydrogen ion secretion and reabsorption of sodium and bicarbonate	Hypokalemia, systemic acidosis, alkaline urine
Inhibitors of sodium/chloride reabsorption Thiazides	Between end of ascending loop and beginning of distal tubule	Blocks sodium and chloride reabsorption; mildly suppresses carbonic anhydrase	Hypokalemia, metabolic alkalosis
Furosemide Ethacrynic acid Bumetanide	Thick ascending limb of Henle's loop	Blocks active transport of chloride, sodium, and potassium	Hypokalemia, uric acid retention
	Cortical vasodilation	Increases rate of urine formation	Hypkalemia, uric acid retention
Aldosterone antagonists Spironolactone	Distal tubule	Inhibits aldosterone, blocks sodium reabsorption, and results in potassium retention	Hyperkalemia, nausea, confusion, gynecomastia
Triamterene and amiloride	Distal tubule	Block sodium reabsorption and inhibits potassium excretion	Nausea, vomiting, headache, granulocytopenia, skin rash

volume is normally reduced to about 1% of what was filtered at the glomerulus.

ADH secretion is therefore one cause of **oliguria,** or diminished excretion of urine that is less than 400 ml/day or 30 ml/hr. Fluid imbalance may be related to the syndrome of inappropriate secretion of ADH, which is a cause of water excess (see Chapter 4). Inadequate secretion of ADH results in diabetes insipidus, the excretion of a large volume of dilute urine.

In the absence of ADH, **water diuresis,** an increase in excretion of a highly dilute urine, takes place. The distal tubules and collecting ducts become impermeable to water. Water remains in the tubular lumen and is excreted as a dilute and large volume of urine. Because ADH has no effect on sodium reabsorption, it continues to be actively transported from the distal tubule. (The mechanism for the regulation of ADH and plasma osmolality is described in Chapters 4 and 25.)

Diuretics as a factor in urine flow

A **diuretic** is any agent that enhances the flow of urine. Clinically, diuretics interfere with renal sodium reabsorption and reduce extracellular fluid volume. Diuretics are commonly used to treat hypertension and edema caused by heart failure, cirrhosis, and nephrotic syndrome.

Diuretics are divided into four general categories: (1) osmotic diuretics, (2) carbonic anhydrase inhibitors (inhibitors of urinary acidification), (3) inhibitors of loop sodium or chloride transport, and (4) aldosterone antagonists. (The physiologic mechanism related to each category is summarized in Table 28-2.)

Renal Hormones

Certain hormones are either activated or synthesized by the kidney. These hormones have significant systemic effects and include the active form of vitamin D, erythropoietin, and natriuretic hormone.

Vitamin D

Vitamin D is a hormone that can be obtained in the diet or synthesized by the action of ultraviolet radiation on cholesterol in the skin. These forms of vitamin D_3 (cholecalciferol) are inactive and require two hydroxylations to establish a metabolically active form. The first step occurs in the liver and the second in the kidneys.

Vitamin D is necessary for the absorption of calcium and phosphate by the small intestine. The renal hydroxylation step is stimulated by parathyroid hormone. A decreased plasma calcium level (less than 10 mg/dl) stimulates the secretion of parathyroid hormone. Parathyroid hormone then stimulates a sequence of events that help restore plasma calcium back toward normal:

1. Calcium mobilization from bone
2. Synthesis of 1,25-dihydroxyvitamin D_3
3. Absorption of calcium from the intestine
4. Increased renal calcium reabsorption
5. Decreased renal phosphate reabsorption

Serum phosphate fluctuations also influence the renal hydroxylation of vitamin D. Decreased levels stimulate active 1,25-dihydroxyvitamin D_3 formation, and increased levels inhibit formation. This results in compensatory changes in phosphate absorption from bone and intestine. Individuals with renal disease have a deficiency of 1,25-dihydroxyvitamin D_3 (1,25-OH_2D_3) and manifest symptoms of disturbed calcium and phosphate balance (see Chapter 4).

Erythropoietin

Erythropoietin stimulates the bone marrow to produce red blood cells in response to tissue hypoxia. (Erythrocyte production is discussed in Chapter 19.) The stimulus for erythropoietin release is decreased oxygen delivery in the kidneys.[3] The anemia of chronic renal failure, in which kidney cells have become nonfunctional, can be related to the lack of this hormone.

Atrial natriuretic factor

Atrial natriuretic factor (ANF) is secreted from cardiocytes in the right atrium when right atrial blood pressure increases. ANF directly inhibits sodium absorption in the collecting duct, increases urine formation, and decreases blood volume and blood pressure.[4]

✓ **QUICK CHECK**

Outline the process of glomerular filtration.

What types of absorption/reabsorption take place in the proximal tubule, the loops of Henle, and the distal tubule?

What is the countercurrent exchange system? What substances are involved?

What hormones are activated or synthesized by the kidney?

The Concept of Clearance

A number of specific renal functions can be measured by renal clearance. Renal clearance techniques determine how much of a substance can be cleared from the blood by the kidneys per given unit of time. The application of this principle permits an indirect measure of GFR, tubular secretion, tubular reabsorption, and RBF.

Clearance and glomerular filtration rate

The GFR provides the best estimate of functioning renal tissue. Loss or damage to nephrons leads to a corresponding decrease in GFR. The measurement of GFR requires use of a substance that has a stable plasma concentration, is freely filtered at the glomerulus, and is not secreted, reabsorbed, or metabolized by the tubules. Inulin (a fructose polysaccharide) is one substance that meets the criteria for measurement of GFR.

The accurate determination of inulin clearance requires constant infusion to maintain a stable plasma level. This is time-consuming and inconvenient. Therefore the clearance of creatinine, a natural substance produced by muscle and released into the blood at a relatively constant rate, is commonly used clinically. It is freely filtered at the glomerulus, but a small amount is secreted by the renal tubules. Therefore creatinine clearance overestimates the GFR but within tolerable limits. Creatinine clearance provides a good measure of GFR because only one blood sample is required in addition to a 24-hour volume of urine.

Substances freely filtered at the glomerulus but with a clearance less than inulin or creatinine have been reabsorbed along the tubules. For example, glucose is completely reabsorbed and has a clearance rate of nearly zero. Conversely, substances secreted by the tubules have a clearance rate greater than inulin or creatinine (i.e., greater than 1.0).

Plasma creatinine concentration

A chronic decline in the GFR over weeks or months is reflected in the *plasma creatinine (P_{cr})* concentration (normal value = 0.7 to 1.2 mg/dl). The P_{cr} concentration has a stable value when the GFR is stable, because creatinine has a constant rate of production as a product of muscle metabolism. The amount filtered is approximately equal to the amount excreted. When the GFR declines, the P_{cr} increases proportionately. Thus the GFR and P_{cr} are inversely related. If the GFR were to decrease by 50%, the filtration and excretion of creatinine would be reduced by 50% and creatinine would accumulate in plasma to twice the normal value. Therefore elevated P_{cr} values represent decreasing GFR. In the new steady state, however, the total amount of creatinine excreted in the urine would remain the same because of the proportionate decrease in GFR and increase in P_{cr}.

The application of this principle is simple and useful for monitoring progressive changes in renal function. The test is most valuable for monitoring the progress of chronic rather than acute renal disease because it takes 7 to 10 days for the plasma creatinine level to stabilize when GFR declines. Ser-

Normal Renal Function Tests

BOX 28-2

Test	Normal Value	Interpretation
Color	Amber-yellow	Drugs and foods may change color
Turbidity	Clear	Purulent matter will make cloudy
pH	4.6-8.0	Bacteria create an alkaline urine
Specific gravity		Represents concentrating ability or density of urine (i.e., higher when contains glucose or protein; lower with dilute urine)
Adult	1.010-1.025	
Infants	1.010-1.018	
Blood	Negative	Bleeding along urinary tract
MICROSCOPIC URINE		
Bacteria	None	Infection
Red blood cells	Negative	Bleeding along urinary tract
White blood cells	Negative	Urinary tract infection
Crystals	Negative	May have potential for stones
Fat	Negative	Can be associated with nephrosis
Casts	Occasional	A few are normal, may represent renal disease
URINARY CHEMISTRY		
Bilirubin	Negative	Increases may cause dark orange color
Urobilinogen	Negative	
Ketones	Negative	Represents an increase in fat metabolism
Glucose	Negative	Usually signifies hyperglycemia
Sodium	100-260 mEq/24 hr	Can increase or decrease with renal disease
Potassium	25-100 mEq/24 hr	
Protein	Negative-trace	Dysfunction of the glomerulus
NORMAL SERUM VALUES		
BUN	8-25 mg/dl	Elevated with diseased kidneys
Creatinine		Elevated with diseased kidneys
Male	0.6-1.5 mg/dl	
Female	0.6-1.1 mg/dl	
Potassium		Elevated in renal failure

ial measures can be obtained over a long time and plotted as a curve of glomerular function. The P_{cr} also becomes elevated during trauma or breakdown of muscle tissue. In such instances the value is then not useful for estimating GFR.

Blood urea nitrogen

The concentration of urea nitrogen in the blood reflects glomerular filtration and urine-concentrating capacity. Because urea is filtered at the glomerulus, blood urea nitrogen (BUN) levels increase as glomerular filtration drops. Because urea is reabsorbed by the blood through the permeable tubules, the BUN rises in states of dehydration and acute and chronic renal failure when passage of fluid through the tubules is slowed. BUN also changes as a result of altered protein intake and protein catabolism. The normal range for BUN in the adult is 10 to 20 mg/dl of blood. Normal renal function tests are listed in Box 28-2.

PEDIATRICS & Renal Function

Have higher blood flow and shorter loops to produce more dilute urine than adults.

Narrow chemical safety margin (high pH, limited ability to regulate internal environment, lowered osmotic pressure) means that any disturbance (diarrhea, infection, fasting for diagnostic tests, improper feeding) quickly produces overhydration or edema.

Greater fluid exchange rate (nearly 50% of extracellular volume) so control of hydration difficult.

⚠AGING & *Renal Function*

Number of nephrons decreases and degenerative changes occur, so are less able to concentrate urine with decreases in ability to tolerate dehydration or water loads. Response to acid-base changes and reabsorption of glucose is delayed.	Drugs eliminated by the kidney can accumulate in the plasma, causing toxic reactions. Alterations in thirst may alter water balance. Impairment in renal, hormonal regulatory systems and use of medications may alter sodium and water balance.

Data from Timiras, P. (1994). Physiological basis of aging and geriatrics (2nd ed.). Boca Raton, Fla.: CRC Press; Miller, M. (1997). Fluid and electrolyte homeostasis in the elderly: Physiological changes of aging and clinical consequences, Baillieres Clinical Endocrinology and Metabolism, *11(2), 367-387.*

▣ DID YOU UNDERSTAND?

Structures of the Renal System

1. The kidneys are paired structures lying bilaterally between the twelfth thoracic and third lumbar vertebrae.
2. The kidney is composed of an outer cortex and an inner medulla.
3. The calyces join to form the renal pelvis, which is continuous with the upper end of the ureter.
4. The nephron is the urine-forming unit of the kidney and is composed of the glomerulus, proximal tubule, hairpin loops of Henle, distal tubule, and collecting duct.
5. The glomerulus contains loops of capillaries. The capillary walls serve as a filtration membrane for the formation of the primary urine.
6. The proximal tubule is lined with microvilli to increase surface area and enhance reabsorption.
7. The hairpin loops of Henle transport solutes and water, contributing to the hypertonic state of the medulla.
8. The distal tubule adjusts acid-base balance by excreting acid into the urine and forming new bicarbonate ions.
9. The ureters extend from the renal pelvis to the posterior wall of the bladder. Urine flows through the ureters by means of peristaltic contraction of the ureteral muscles.
10. The bladder is a bag composed of the detrusor and trigone muscles and innervated by parasympathetic fibers. When accumulation of urine reaches 250 to 300 ml, mechanoreceptors, which respond to stretching of tissue, stimulate the micturition reflex.

Renal Blood Flow

1. Renal blood flows at about 1000 to 1200 ml/min, or 20% to 25% of the cardiac output.
2. Blood flow through the glomerular capillaries is maintained at a constant rate in spite of a wide range of arterial pressures.
3. The glomerular filtration rate (GFR) is the filtration of plasma per unit of time and is directly related to the perfusion pressure of renal blood flow.
4. Autoregulation of renal blood flow and neural regulation of vasoconstriction maintain a constant GFR.
5. Renin is an enzyme secreted from the juxtaglomerular apparatus and causes the generation of angiotensin, a potent vasoconstrictor. The renin-angiotensin system is thus a regulator of renal blood flow.

Kidney Function

1. The major function of the nephron is urine formation, which involves the processes of glomerular filtration, tubular reabsorption, and tubular secretion and excretion.
2. Glomerular filtration is favored by capillary hydrostatic pressure and opposed by oncotic pressure in the capillary and hydrostatic pressure in Bowman capsule. The balance of favoring and opposing filtration forces is known as net filtration pressure (NFP).
3. The GFR is approximately 120 ml/min, and 99% of the filtrate is reabsorbed.
4. The proximal tubule reabsorbs about 60% to 70% of the filtered sodium and water and 90% of other electrolytes.
5. Because most molecules are reabsorbed by active transport, the carrier mechanism can become saturated at a point known as the transport maximum (T_m). Molecules not reabsorbed are excreted with the urine.
6. The distal tubules actively reabsorb sodium and secrete potassium and hydrogen for the regulation of electrolyte and acid-base balance.
7. The concentration of the final urine is a function of the level of antidiuretic hormone (ADH) that stimulates the distal tubules and collecting ducts to reabsorb water. The countercurrent exchange system

Continued

DID YOU UNDERSTAND?—cont'd

Kidney Function—cont'd

of the long loops of Henle and their accompanying capillaries establishes a concentration gradient within the renal medulla to facilitate the reabsorption of water from the collecting duct.

8. The distal nephron regulates acid-base balance by excreting hydrogen ions and forming new bicarbonate.

9. The kidney secretes or activates a number of hormones that have systemic effects, including 1,25-dihydroxyvitamin D₃, erythropoietin, and natriuretic hormone.

10. Creatinine, a substance produced by muscle, is measured in both plasma and urine to calculate a commonly used clinical measurement of GFR.

11. Both the plasma creatinine concentration and the blood urea nitrogen (BUN) levels indicate glomerular function. Plasma creatinine is measured to monitor progressive renal dysfunction; BUN is an indicator of hydration status.

KEY TERMS

Arcuate artery, 793
Atrial natriuretic factor (ANF), 803
Bladder, 794
Bowman capsule, 791
Bowman space, 791
Collecting duct, 793
Cortical nephron, 791
Countercurrent exchange system, 800
Detrusor muscle, 794
Distal tubule, 793, 800
Diuretic, 802
Excretion, 797
External urethral sphincter, 794
Filtration slit, 791
Glomerular capillary, 793
Glomerular filtration membrane, 791
Glomerular filtration rate (GFR), 795
Glomerulus, 791

Hilum, 790
Interlobar artery, 793
Internal urethral sphincter, 794
Juxtaglomerular apparatus, 793
Juxtaglomerular cell, 793
Juxtamedullary nephron, 791
Kidney, 790
Loop of Henle, 793, 800
Macula densa, 793
Mesangial cell, 791
Micturition, 794
Nephron, 790
Net filtration pressure (NFP), 797
Oliguria, 802
Peritubular capillary, 794
Plasma creatinine (P_{cr}) concentration, 803
Podocyte, 791

Proximal tubule, 793, 799
Renal artery, 793
Renal capsule, 790
Renal fascia, 790
Renal papilla, 794
Renal vein, 794
Renin-angiotensin system, 795
Transport maximum (T_m), 799
Trigone, 794
Tubular reabsorption, 797
Tubular secretion, 797
Ultrafiltration, 797
Urea, 801
Ureter, 794
Urethra, 794
Vasa recta, 794
Water diuresis, 802

REFERENCES

1. Valtin, H. & Schafer, J.A. (1995). *Renal function* (3rd ed.). Boston: Little, Brown.

2. Koeppen, B.M. & Stanton, B.A. (1997). *Renal physiology.* St. Louis: Mosby.

3. Klausen, T. (1998). The feed-back regulation of erythropoietin production in healthy humans. *Danish Medical Bulletin, 45*(4), 345-353.

4. Vervoort, G. et al. (1998). Influence of angiotensin converting enzyme inhibition and angiotensin II type 1 receptor antagonism on renal sodium and water handling and albuminuria during infusion of atrial natriuretic factor into healthy volunteers. *Journal of Hypertension, 16*(2), 245-250.

CHAPTER 29

Alterations of Renal and Urinary Tract Function

Sue E. Huether

Renal and urinary function can be affected by a variety of disorders. The most common type of urinary dysfunction is infection of the bladder. The urinary tract also can be obstructed by stones or tumors. Renal function can be impaired by disorders of the kidney itself or by many other systemic diseases. Because the kidney filters the blood, it is directly linked to every other organ system. Renal failure, whether acute or chronic, is therefore a life-threatening condition.

URINARY TRACT OBSTRUCTION

Urinary tract obstruction, or obstructive uropathy, is an interference with the flow of urine at any site along the urinary tract (Fig. 29-1). The obstruction causes urine to accumulate behind the obstruction, leading to infection or damage to involved organs. Obstruction can be either congenital or acquired. Among the numerous causes are tumors, stones (calculi), trauma, edema, pregnancy, benign prostatic hyperplasia or carcinoma, inflammation of the gastrointestinal tract, and loss of ureteral peristaltic activity or bladder muscle function. The pathophysiology of obstructive disorders frequently can be reversed by alleviating the obstruction.

Consequences of Obstruction

The pathophysiologic consequences of urinary tract obstruction are related to (1) location within the urinary tract, (2) unilateral or bilateral involvement, (3) partial or complete obstruction, (4) acute or chronic duration, and (5) the underlying cause.

Obstruction of the ureter causes **hydroureter** (accumulation of urine in the ureter). Retrograde increases in hydrostatic pressure involving the renal pelvis and calyces produce **hydronephrosis** (accumulation of urine in the renal collecting system). Acute, complete obstructions cause an increase in pressure that is transmitted to the proximal tubule and decreases glomerular filtration. If the obstruction is complete, the glomerular filtration rate (GFR) will decline to zero, with resulting renal failure.

Chronic partial obstruction causes compression of the kidney structures from accumulation of urine, with ischemic atrophy of the papilla and medulla. Although the kidneys initially increase in size, progressive atrophy follows, with eventual loss of renal mass and smaller kidneys. The accompanying tubular damage decreases renal ability to conserve sodium and water and to excrete hydrogen ion and potassium. This may produce excessive urine volumes even though the GFR has declined. Sodium and bicarbonate are wasted with an increased risk of dehydration and metabolic acidosis.

Relief of urinary tract obstruction is usually followed by diuresis (commonly called *postobstructive diuresis*) with losses of large amounts of urine. The diuresis is related to salt and water retention during the period of obstruction and a return to a normal GFR. An uncommon result of obstruction relief is an excessive loss of sodium and water (more than 10 L/day). In some cases of chronic obstruction, diuresis may not be significant after relief of obstruction because the GFR returns to normal slowly or not at all.

Complications of urinary tract obstruction include infection and renal failure. Obstructions below the bladder cause infection because the accumulated urine enhances bacterial growth. Acute or chronic renal failure occurs with

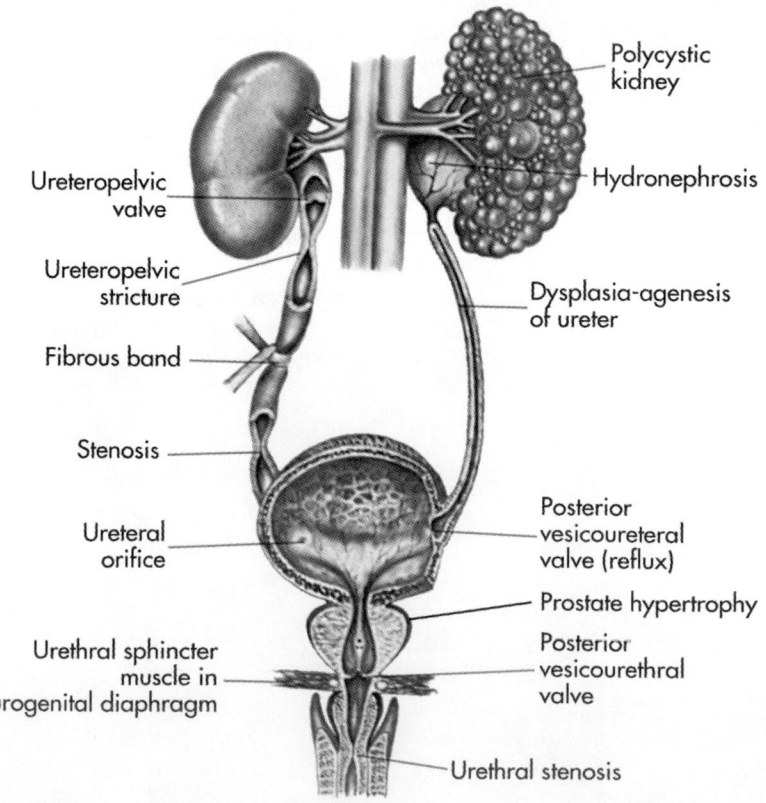

Fig. 29-1 *Major sites of urinary tract obstruction. (From Wong, D.L. et al. [1999]. Whaley & Wong's nursing care of infants and children [6th ed.]. St. Louis: Mosby.)*

prolonged bilateral obstruction (see p. 819). Acute renal failure can be prevented if the obstruction is relieved within 1 week. Chronic renal failure may be insidious.

Obstructive Disorders

Kidney stones

Calculi, or **renal stones** (nephrolithiasis), are masses of crystals and protein and are a common cause of urinary tract obstruction in adults. Renal stones occur with an incidence of approximately 10% to 20%. A significant number of patients are treated in outpatient settings. Approximately 1% of the U.S. population will have a renal stone at some time.[1]

Three major kinds of renal stones are (1) calcium oxalate or calcium phosphate (75% to 80%); (2) struvite (magnesium, ammonium, phosphate) (15%); and (3) uric acid (7%). Cystine stones are relatively rare and account for fewer than 1% of all renal stones.

Pathophysiology

The formation of stones is complicated and not entirely understood. Contributing factors include high urinary concentration of stone-forming substances, urine pH that affects solubility, facilitators and inhibitors of crystal growth, and various diseases, drugs, and diet. Inhibitors of crystal aggregation (nephrocalcin) are normally present in urine. One theory of stone formation is a reduced excretion of these inhibitors.[2]

The stone begins to form around a nucleus, or nidus. A **nidus** is a crystal that evolves in the presence of stone-forming substances such as calcium oxalate, calcium phosphate, or struvite (magnesium, ammonium, phosphate). It may become trapped within the urinary tract and accumulate other crystals, forming a stone. A high urinary saturation of stone-forming substances enhances crystal formation and stone growth (Fig. 29-2).

Some types of stone are aggregates of different substances. The pH of the urine affects the solubility of many stone-forming substances. Calcium oxalate and cystine stones form independently of the urine pH.

Stones usually grow on the papillae or in the renal tubules, calyces, renal pelvis, ureter, or bladder. Many stones are less than 5 mm in diameter and are readily passed with the urine. Large stones are sometimes called **staghorn calculi** because they grow in the pelvis and extend into the calyces to form branching stones. They are commonly associated with infection.[3] Renal failure may result unless they are surgically removed.

Calcium stones are the smallest and most common stones. They occur most commonly in middle-aged men with a familial history of stone formation. Most are formed of calcium oxalate or an aggregate of calcium oxalate and calcium phosphate. Approximately 80% are idiopathic, although they frequently are associated with hypercalciuria and hyperuricosuria (a high level of uric acid in urine). Prolonged immobilization resulting in bone demineralization can precipitate hypercalciuria and stone formation. High di-

Fig. 29-2 *Hydronephrosis.* Hydronephrosis with renal stones in renal pelvis and calyces. *(From Kissane, J.M. [Ed.]. [1990]. Anderson's pathology [9th ed.]. St. Louis: Mosby.)*

etary calcium may decrease the risk of kidney stones, and calcium supplements may increase the risk.[4] Struvite stones (magnesium, ammonium, phosphate) are precipitated by infection with urea-splitting organisms (e.g., *Pseudomonas, Proteus*) and are more common in women.

Uric acid stones are caused by gout—an increase in uric acid production and hyperuricosuria. High-purine diets (consisting of meat, fish, and poultry) also can contribute to elevated levels of uric acid. Formation of uric acid stones is enhanced by a concentrated and acidic urine.[5] Thus regional enteritis and ulcerative colitis can precipitate the formation of uric acid stones. These diseases may cause fluid loss and a metabolic acidosis that develops from loss of bicarbonate (see Chapter 4). Patients with the rare hereditary disorder cystinuria develop cystine stones. In cystinuria, an error in cystine metabolism causes decreased tubular reabsorption of cystine with an increased amount of this relatively insoluble substance in the urine.

Clinical Manifestations

Pain is the hallmark symptom of a renal stone. The location and severity vary with the site of occurrence. The pain may be in the flank or at the costovertebral angle (between the last rib and the lumbar vertebrae), or it may radiate into the groin if the stone is lower in the ureter. The pain can be exquisitely severe, requiring narcotic analgesia or ketorolac (a nonsteroidal antiinflammatory drug) for relief, and is frequently accompanied by nausea and vomiting. Colicky pain occurs as rhythmic contractions as the ureter attempts to advance the stone. Gross or microscopic hematuria (blood in the urine) may be present.

TABLE 29-1   Classification of Neurogenic Bladder

Type of Neurogenic Bladder	Cause	Neural Lesion	Clinical Manifestations	Treatment
Uninhibited (loss of cortical inhibition)	Lack of voluntary control in infancy, multiple sclerosis	Upper motor neuron	Smaller urine volume, frequency, urgency, incontinence, enuresis	Anticholinergic medication
Reflex or automatic (reflex arc maintained below lesion with spontaneous voiding)	Spinal cord transection, cord tumors, multiple sclerosis above level T_{12} of cord	Upper motor neuron	Involuntary voiding that may include incomplete emptying with retention and infection	Catheter or condom drainage; stimulation of reflex arc by stroking perineum, abdomen, or rectum
Autonomous (loss of cortical inhibition and interruption of spinal reflex arc)	Sacral cord trauma, tumors, herniated disk, abdominal surgery with transection of pelvic parasympathetic nerves	Lower motor neuron	Overflow incontinence in which bladder does not empty spontaneously with stretch fullness	Catheter, urinary diversion surgery
Motor paralysis (sensory functions intact)	Lesions at levels S_2, S_3, S_4; poliomyelitis; trauma; tumors	Lower motor neuron	Overflow incontinence caused by loss of bladder contraction	Manual compression (Credé maneuver)
Sensory paralysis (motor functions intact)	Posterior lumbar nerve roots, diabetes mellitus, tabes dorsalis	Lower motor neuron	Dribbling, overflow incontinence; loss of sensation of bladder fullness	Bladder training to empty at regular intervals (e.g., every 3 hr)

Evaluation and Treatment

The diagnosis of renal stones requires a thorough medical and family history, diet history, previous history of urinary tract disease, and use of medications. Both blood and urine tests should be performed to evaluate the presence of stone-forming substances. Urine pH and the presence of red or white blood cells should be evaluated. The GFR can be estimated by assessing the blood urea nitrogen (BUN) and plasma creatinine (see Chapter 28). A plain (flat plate) x-ray film of the abdomen and an intravenous pyelogram will identify the presence of radiopaque stones and will confirm the anatomic location.

The purpose of treatment is to prevent new stone formation, to reduce the size of stones that have already formed, and to prevent infection and obstruction. The principal components of treatment include (1) reducing the concentration of stone-forming substances by increasing the flow of urine with a high fluid intake or (2) decreasing the amount of the substance in the urine by decreasing dietary intake or endogenous production. Surgical removal is required for large stones, for obstruction, for recurrent infections, or for intractable pain. Smaller stones may pass spontaneously, or they can be extracted by instrumentation. Extracorporeal ultrasonography and laser lithotripsy are relatively noninvasive procedures that use high-frequency sound waves or laser pulses to fragment stones for excretion in the urine.[6,7]

Neurogenic bladder

Neurogenic bladder is a functional urinary tract obstruction caused by an interruption of the nerve supply to the bladder. The disruption can occur in the central nervous system or at the level of the spinal cord.

Pathophysiology

Bladder paralysis interferes with the normal flow of urine. Upper motor neuron lesions (in or below the cortex but above the sacral level of the spinal cord) cause loss of voluntary control of voiding. Lower motor neuron lesions (sacral level of the spinal cord) disrupt the sacral reflex arc and cause loss of both voluntary and involuntary control of urination.[8] The types of neurogenic bladder are reviewed in Table 29-1.

Clinical Manifestations

Infection with a neurogenic bladder may be associated with bladder distention and urine retention, placement of catheters, or the development of stones caused by bone resorption from physical immobility. Symptoms are often difficult to interpret because of disordered sensation and the presence of other neurologic disturbances. The individual may experience a burning sensation but not pain. The development of fever is frequently accompanied by chills and shivering, which aid in differentiating fever caused by other neurologic lesions.

Evaluation and Treatment

Neurogenic bladder must be properly diagnosed with uro-dynamic studies.[9] Reduction or elimination of incontinence and residual urine and maintenance of bladder pressure within normal limits are goals of treatment.

Tumors

Renal tumors

Renal adenomas (benign tumors) are uncommon but are increasing. The tumors are encapsulated and are usually located near the cortex of the kidney. Because they can become malignant, they are usually surgically removed. *Renal cell carcinoma (RCC)* is the most common renal neoplasm (85% of all renal neoplasms) and represents about 2% of cancer deaths. Renal cell carcinoma usually occurs in men (two times more frequently than in women) between 50 and 60 years of age.[10] Five-year survival is less than 50% and less than 2% with metastasis.[11]

 Pathogenesis

A moderate association has been identified between tobacco use and the incidence of renal cell carcinoma.[12] Diethyl-stilbestrol and estrogen administration is linked to renal cell carcinoma in animals.

Renal cell carcinomas are adenocarcinomas and are classified according to cell type and extent of metastasis. Clear cell tumors, the most common, present a better prognosis than granular cell or spindle tumors. Confinement within the renal capsule, together with treatment, is associated with a better survival rate. The tumors usually occur unilaterally and spread through the lymph nodes and blood vessels to the lungs, liver, lymph nodes, and bone (Fig. 29-3).[13]

 Clinical Manifestations

The classic clinical manifestations are hematuria, flank pain, palpable flank mass, and weight loss, but these symptoms occur in fewer than 10% of cases. Such signs and symptoms represent an advanced stage of disease, whereas earlier stages are often silent. The most common sites of distant metastasis are the lung, lymph nodes, liver, bone, thyroid, and central nervous system.[14,15]

Evaluation and Treatment

Diagnosis is based on the clinical symptoms, plain x-ray films of the abdomen, intravenous pyelography, renal angiography, and computed tomography. (Staging of renal cell carcinoma is presented in Table 29-2.) Treatment is usually surgical removal of the affected kidney (radical nephrectomy) with combined use of chemotherapeutic agents. Radiation therapy may also be used. Immunotherapy is promising in selected cases.[16]

Bladder tumors

Bladder tumors represent about 1% of all malignant tumors and are the fifth most common malignancy.[17,18] Approximately 54,200 people develop bladder cancer each year, and

Fig. 29-3 *Renal cell carcinoma.* Renal cell carcinomas usually are spheroidal masses composed of yellow tissue mottled with hemorrhage, necrosis, and fibrosis. *(From Damjanov, I. & Linder, J. [Eds.]. [1996]. Anderson's pathology [10th ed.]. St. Louis: Mosby.)*

TABLE 29-2	Staging of Renal Cell Carcinoma
Stage	**Metastasis**
I	Tumor confined within kidney capsule
II	Invasion through renal capsule but within surrounding fascia
III	Involvement of regional lymph nodes, renal vein, or vena cava
IV	Distant metastases

TABLE 29-3	Staging of Bladder Carcinoma
Stage	**Metastasis**
O	Limited to mucosal involvement
A	Submucosal involvement
B	Involvement of the muscularis layer
C	Invasion of the perivesical fat
D_1	Spread to regional lymph nodes
D_2	Spread to distant sites, bone, and visceral organs

12,100 die of it.[17-19] The development of bladder cancer is most common in men older than 60 years.

 Pathogenesis

The risk of primary bladder cancer is greater among people who smoke or work in the chemical, rubber, and textile industry and among women who take large amounts of phenacetin.[20] Bladder cancer results from a genetic alteration in normal bladder epithelium.[21] Metastasis is usually to lymph nodes, liver, bones, or lungs. Staging for bladder carcinoma is presented in Table 29-3. Secondary bladder cancer develops by invasion of cancer from bordering organs, such as cervical carcinoma in women or prostatic carcinoma in men.

Clinical Manifestations

Bladder tumors may be asymptomatic or accompanied by hematuria. Advanced cancers are associated with pelvic pain and frequent urination.

> **✓ QUICK CHECK**
>
> List two common complications of urinary tract obstruction, and briefly describe them.
>
> How do kidney stones form?
>
> What is neurogenic bladder?
>
> Who are at greatest risk of bladder tumors?

 Evaluation and Treatment

Diagnosis is made by cystoscopy (visual examination of the urinary tract through a cystoscope), cell studies, urograms (x-ray examinations), and transurethral biopsy. Treatment is related to the type and size of the lesion.

URINARY TRACT INFECTION
Causes of Urinary Tract Infection

Urinary tract infections (UTIs) are usually caused by bacteria. At risk are premature newborns, prepubertal children, sexually active young women, those who use diaphragm spermaticide, those with recent urologic instrumentation, those with anatomic abnormalities of the urinary tract, and elderly men and women.[22] Infections are diagnosed by culture of specific organisms with counts of 100,000 bacteria/ml of freshly voided urine. Bacterial contamination of the normally sterile urine usually occurs by retrograde movement of microorganisms or tubercular bacillus. A UTI can occur anywhere along the urinary tract, including the urethra, prostate, bladder, ureter, and kidney. Infections of the lower urinary tract may occur at least once in 50% of all women.[23]

Types of Urinary Tract Infection
Cystitis

Cystitis is an inflammation of the bladder—the most common site of UTI. The morphologic appearance of the bladder through cystoscopy describes different types of cystitis. With mild inflammation the mucosa is hyperemic (red). More advanced cases may show diffuse hemorrhage (called *hemorrhagic cystitis*) or pus formation—suppurative exudate (called *suppurative cystitis*) on the epithelial surface of the bladder. Prolonged infection may lead to sloughing of the bladder mucosa with ulcer formation (termed *ulcerative cystitis*). The most severe infections may cause necrosis of the bladder wall (termed *gangrenous cystitis*). Generally, the infections are uncomplicated and resolve spontaneously. Complicated UTIs are often antibiotic-resistant.

Pathophysiology

The most common infecting microorganism is *Escherichia coli* and less commonly *Klebsiella, Proteus, Pseudomonas,* and *Staphylococcus.* The disease may occur alone or in association with pyelonephritis or prostatitis. Cystitis is more common in women because of the shorter urethra, the closeness of the urethra to the anus, and the possibility of bacterial contamination from vaginal secretions. Introduction of bacteria and an environment that promotes bacterial growth are the common factors in cystitis. Sexually active and pregnant women, individuals with indwelling catheters, and persons with diabetes mellitus, neurogenic bladder, poor hygiene, or urinary tract obstruction are at greater risk for developing cystitis. Prostatitis and urethral obstruction from prostatic hypertrophy are predisposing factors to bacteriuria, particularly in men older than 50 years.

Clinical Manifestations

Many individuals with bacteriuria are asymptomatic. The clinical manifestations of cystitis, however, usually include frequency, urgency, dysuria (painful urination), and suprapubic and low back pain. Hematuria, cloudy urine, and flank pain are more serious symptoms. Approximately 10% of individuals with bacteriuria have no symptoms, and 30% of individuals with symptoms are abacteriuric.[24] Cystitis in the elderly population may be asymptomatic.[25]

Evaluation and Treatment

Evaluation of the urine for bacteria is the most important diagnostic procedure. Risk factors, such as urinary tract obstruction, should be identified and treated. Determining the presence of and identifying bacteria by means of urine cul-

> # *HEALTH ALERT*
> ### *Women and Urinary Tract Infections*
>
> Cystitis occurs in approximately 30% of women during their lifetime, and about one third of them will have upper urinary tract infection (UTI) (pyelonephritis). *E. coli* is the most common causative microorganism. Asymptomatic bacteriuria is common and is a particular complication of pregnancy. All pregnant women should be screened, and infection should be treated promptly to prevent maternal and infant complications. Three-day antibiotic treatment is standard for uncomplicated UTI, although a single dose with some newer drugs is proving effective. Treatment for 10 to 14 days is common for uncomplicated pyelonephritis.
>
> *Data from Faro, S. & Fenner, D. (1998). Urinary tract infections.* Clinics in Obstetrics and Gynecology, 41*(3), 744-754; Kurowski, K. (1998). The woman with dysuria.* American Family Physician, 57*(9), 2155-2164, 2169-2170; Millar, L.K. & Cox, S.M. (1997). Urinary tract infections complicating pregnancy.* Infectious Disease Clinics of North America, 11*(1), 13-26; Stein, G.E. (1998). Singledose treatment of acute cystitis with fosfomycin tromethamine.* Annals in Pharmacotherapy, 32*(92), 215-219.*

ture and sensitivity warrant treatment with an organism-specific antibiotic. Follow-up urine cultures should be obtained 1 week after initiation of treatment and again at monthly intervals for 3 months. Repeated cultures should be obtained every 3 to 4 months until 1 year after treatment for evaluation of recurrent infection.

"Nonbacterial" cystitis

A significant number of women have symptoms of cystitis but usually have a negative urine culture. This is more common in women 20 to 30 years of age and is called acute *urethral syndrome.* Its cause is obscure, but dysfunction of the external sphincter, vaginitis, urethritis, and inflammation of glands near the vagina and urethra are associated findings. Bacteria may develop in 60% of individuals up to 9 months after the initial symptoms. Symptoms frequently are relieved by a course of treatment with antibiotics, use of drugs that relax the external sphincter, or retraining of voiding habits.[26]

A persistent and chronic form of "nonbacterial" cystitis occurring primarily in women is *interstitial cystitis.* The cause is not clearly known, but autoimmune infection, neurogenic inflammation, mucosal barrier deficiency, and abnormal mast cells may cause the inflammation.[27,28] The inflammation is associated with a derangement of the bladder mucosa that makes it more susceptible to penetration by bacteria. Inflammation and fibrosis of the bladder wall are accompanied by the presence of hemorrhagic ulcers (Hunner ulcers). Characteristic symptoms include a sensation of bladder fullness, frequency, urgency, nocturia, small urine volume per voiding, and suprapelvic and urethral pain. Diagnosis can be difficult and should rule out other bladder diseases.[29] Treatment options include tricyclic antidepressants (anticholinergic and analgesic effects), antihistamines, calcium channel blockers, and bladder instillation of various drugs.

Acute pyelonephritis

Pyelonephritis is an infection of the renal pelvis and interstitium. Common causes are summarized in Table 29-4. Urinary obstruction and reflux of urine from the bladder (vesicoureteral reflux) are the most common underlying risk factors. One or both kidneys may be involved. Most cases occur in women. The responsible organism is usually *E. coli,* *Proteus,* or *Pseudomonas.* The latter two organisms are more commonly associated with infections after urethral instrumentation or urinary tract surgery. These organisms also split urea to ammonia, making an alkaline urine that increases the risk of stone formation.

Pathophysiology

The infection is probably spread by ascending organisms along the ureters, but spread also may occur by way of the bloodstream. The inflammatory process is usually focal and irregular, primarily affecting the pelvis, calyces, and medulla. The infection causes medullary infiltration of white blood cells with renal inflammation, renal edema, and purulent urine. In severe infections, localized abscesses may form in

TABLE 29-4	Common Causes of Pyelonephritis
Predisposing Factor	**Pathologic Mechanisms**
Kidney stones	Obstruction and stasis of urine contributing to bacteriuria and hydronephrosis; irritation of epithelial lining with entrapment of bacteria
Vesicoureteral reflux	Chronic reflux of urine up the ureter and into kidney during micturition, contributing to bacterial infection
Pregnancy	Dilation and relaxation of ureter with hydroureter and hydronephrosis; partly caused by obstruction from enlarged uterus and partly from ureteral relaxation caused by higher progesterone levels
Neurogenic bladder	Neurologic impairment interfering with normal bladder contraction with residual urine and ascending infection
Instrumentation	Introduction of organisms into urethra and bladder by catheters and endoscopes introduced into the urinary tract for diagnostic purposes
Female sexual trauma	Movement of organisms from the urethra into the bladder with infection and retrograde spread to kidney

the medulla and extend to the cortex. Primarily affected are the tubules; the glomeruli usually are spared. Necrosis of renal papillae can develop (Fig. 29-4). After the acute phase, healing occurs with deposition of scar tissue and atrophy of affected tubules. The number of bacteria decreases until the urine again becomes sterile. Acute pyelonephritis rarely causes renal failure.[30,31]

Clinical Manifestations

The onset of symptoms is usually acute, with fever, chills, flank or groin pain, frequency, dysuria, and costovertebral tenderness. Children and older adults may have nonspecific symptoms, such as fever and malaise.

Evaluation and Treatment

Differentiating symptoms of cystitis from those of pyelonephritis by clinical assessment alone is difficult. The specific diagnosis is established by urine culture, urinalysis, and clinical signs and symptoms.[32] White blood cell casts indicate pyelonephritis, but they are not always present in the urine.

Uncomplicated acute pyelonephritis responds well to 2 to 3 weeks of organism-specific antibiotic therapy. Follow-

Fig. 29-4 *Acute pyelonephritis.* Papillary necrosis resulting from acute pyelonephritis and obstruction. Note necrotic papillae *(arrows)*, mottled patchy cortical infiltrate of acute pyelonephritis, and congested, dilated renal pelvis. *(From Kissane, J.M. [Ed.]. [1990]. Anderson's pathology [9th ed.]. St. Louis: Mosby.)*

up urine cultures are obtained at 1 and 4 weeks after treatment if symptoms recur. Antibiotic-resistant organisms or reinfection may occur in cases of urinary tract obstruction or reflux. Intravenous pyelography and voiding cystourethrography identify surgically correctable lesions.

Chronic pyelonephritis

Chronic pyelonephritis is a persistent or recurrent autoimmune infection of the kidney with inflammation and scarring of the kidney. One or both kidneys may be involved. The specific cause of chronic pyelonephritis is difficult to determine. Recurrent infections from acute pyelonephritis may be associated with chronic pyelonephritis. Generally, chronic pyelonephritis is more likely to occur in patients who have renal infections associated with some type of obstructive pathologic condition, such as renal stones and vesicoureteral reflux.

Pathophysiology
Chronic urinary tract obstruction starts a process of progressive inflammation, altered renal pelvis and calyces, destruction of the tubules, atrophy or dilation and diffuse scarring, and finally impaired urine-concentrating ability, leading to chronic renal failure.

The lesions of chronic pyelonephritis are sometimes termed *chronic interstitial nephritis* because the inflammation and fibrosis are located in the interstitial spaces between the tubules. Causes other than chronic pyelonephritis include drug toxicity from analgesics such as phenacetin, as-

pirin, and acetaminophen; ischemia; irradiation; and immune-complex diseases.

Clinical Manifestations
The early symptoms of chronic pyelonephritis are often minimal and may include hypertension, frequency, dysuria, and flank pain. Progression leads to renal failure.

Evaluation and Treatment
Urinalysis, intravenous pyelography, and ultrasound are used diagnostically. Treatment is related to the underlying cause. Obstruction must be relieved. Antibiotics may be given, with prolonged antibiotic therapy for recurrent infection.

✓ QUICK CHECK

Why is cystitis more common in women?

What is interstitial cystitis?

How does pyelonephritis differ from cystitis?

GLOMERULAR DISORDERS
The onset of glomerular disease may be sudden or insidious. Damage to the glomerulus is the result of inflammatory processes initiated by infection, toxins, or immune responses. Damage to the glomerulus results in proteinuria, changes in GFR, and changes in capillary wall structure.[33]

Different types of glomerular disease may be associated with patterns of urinary sediment. Urine in diseases associated with a ***nephrotic sediment*** has massive amounts of protein and lipids and either only microscopic or no blood. Urine in diseases associated with ***nephritic sediment*** is characterized by the presence of blood with red cell casts, white cell casts, and varying degrees of protein, which usually is not severe. The sediment of chronic glomerular disease has waxy casts, granular casts, and less protein and blood than does nephrotic or nephritic sediment. Severe glomerular disease is usually associated with diffuse lesions and may cause oliguria, hypertension, and renal failure. Focal lesions tend to produce less severe clinical symptoms.

Reduced GFR during glomerular disease is evidenced by the plasma creatinine concentration or creatinine clearance (see Chapter 28). Glomerular damage reduces glomerular membrane surface area, glomerular capillary blood flow, and driving hydrostatic pressure. Plasma fluid tends to move to the interstitial spaces, contributing to decreased blood volume, renal blood flow, and glomerular capillary hydrostatic pressure with a decline in GFR.

Edema, caused by excessive fluid retention, may require the use of diuretics or dialysis. The volume expansion that accompanies salt and water retention leads to hypertension.

Death occurs in 2% to 5% of all persons during acute glomerular disease. During the first few weeks, the major life-threatening problems are acute renal insufficiency with fluid, electrolyte, and acid-base imbalances; acute hypertension that may cause hypertensive encephalopathy; circulatory failure; and pulmonary edema.

Glomerulonephritis

Glomerulonephritis is an inflammation of the glomerulus caused by numerous factors, including immunologic abnormalities, ischemia, free radicals, drugs, toxins, vascular disorders, and systemic diseases. Glomerular disease is the most common cause of chronic and end-stage renal failure.[34]

Types of glomerulonephritis

The classification of glomerulonephritis is arbitrary and can be described according to cause, pathologic lesions, disease progression, or clinical presentation. (Types of glomerular lesions are reviewed in Table 29-5, and features of types of glomerulonephritis are summarized in Table 29-6.) In nearly all types of glomerulonephritis, the epithelial or podocyte layer of the glomerular membrane is disturbed with loss of negative charges and changes in membrane permeability.[35]

Acute glomerulonephritis

Acute glomerulonephritis frequently is associated with a streptococcal infection (acute poststreptococcal glomerulonephritis). The disease begins abruptly and usually occurs 7 to 10 days after a streptococcal infection of the throat (5% to 10% incidence) or skin (impetigo) (25% incidence), commonly in children. Sporadic occurrences have been observed after bacterial endocarditis, which may be associated with streptococcal or staphylococcal organisms, or after viral diseases such as varicella and hepatitis B. The streptococcal antigen carries a positive charge depositing in the negatively charged glomerular basement membrane (GBM). The antigen attracts neutrophils and macrophages, initiating phagocytosis and the release of inflammatory mediators that damage epithelial and endothelial cells lying on the basement membrane.

Symptoms usually occur 10 to 21 days after infection and include hematuria, red blood cell casts, proteinuria, decreased GFR, oliguria, edema, hypertension, edema around the eyes or feet and ankles, and occasionally, ascites or pleural effusions. Immunofluorescent findings from renal biopsy indicate immune complex deposits in the glomerulus, with diffuse mesangial cell and capillary endothelial cell proliferation. The thickened glomerular membrane contributes to the decreased GFR. More severe renal disease is observed after a prolonged infection before antibiotic therapy, which prevents the spread of infection. Most individuals, especially children, recover without significant loss of renal function or recurrence of the disease.

Rapidly progressive glomerulonephritis

Rapidly progressive glomerulonephritis (RPGN) is also known as subacute, crescentic, or extracapillary glomerulonephritis. The disease affects primarily adults in their 50s and 60s and may be idiopathic or associated with a proliferative glomerular disease (with diffuse proliferation of extracapillary cells), such as poststreptococcal glomerulonephritis.

TABLE 29-5	Types of Glomerular Lesions
Lesion	Characteristics
Diffuse	Relatively uniform involvement of most (>50%) or all glomeruli; most common form of glomerulonephritis
Focal	Changes in only some glomeruli (<50%), whereas others are normal
Segmental-local	Changes in one part of the glomerulus with other parts unaffected
Mesangial	Deposits of immunoglobulins in the mesangial matrix
Membranous	Thickening of the glomerular capillary wall
Proliferative	Increase in the number of glomerular cells
Sclerotic	Glomerular scarring from previous glomerular injury
Crescentic	Accumulation of proliferating cells within Bowman space, making the appearance of a crescent

By the time RPGN is diagnosed, renal insufficiency is apparent. There is extensive proliferation of cells into Bowman space with crescent formation. Typically, the glomerular injury is accompanied by a rapid decline in glomerular function, progressing to renal failure in a few weeks or months.[36] Hematuria is common and may or may not be accompanied by proteinuria, edema, or hypertension.

Goodpasture syndrome is a type of RPGN. The disease is associated with antibody formation against both pulmonary capillary and glomerular basement membranes, with activation of complement and neutrophils that damage the GBM. Goodpasture syndrome is rare but occurs most frequently in men 20 to 30 years of age.

RPGN has a relatively poor prognosis. Pulsed methylprednisolone administration, which is given once daily for 3 to 5 days before prednisone therapy, is helpful in some cases. Anticoagulants may be of some benefit in reducing the fibrin component of crescent formation. Plasmapheresis is usually combined with prednisone and cyclophosphamide to suppress a rebound antibody production. Dialysis or transplantation is required when failure is irreversible.

Chronic glomerulonephritis

Chronic glomerulonephritis encompasses several glomerular diseases with a progressive course leading to chronic renal failure. There may be no history of renal disease before the diagnosis. Hypercholesterolemia has been associated with progressive glomerular injury. The proposed mechanism is related to glomerulosclerosis.[37] The primary cause may be difficult to establish because advanced pathologic changes may obscure specific disease characteristics (Fig.

TABLE 29-6	Features of the Common Types of Glomerulonephritis
Type and Cause	**Pathophysiology**
Poststreptococcal Group A β-hemolytic streptococcus	Deposits of immune complexes in glomerular capillary wall and infiltration of inflammatory cells with decreased capillary blood flow and GFR
Rapidly progressive or crescentic Nonspecific response to glomerular injury; can occur in any severe glomerular disease	Accumulation of inflammatory cells and debris that proliferate into Bowman space and form crescent-shaped lesions that decrease capillary blood flow and glomerular filtration Anti-glomerular membrane antibodies, which can damage the glomerulus, leading to renal failure
Membranoproliferative Usually idiopathic; associated with low complement levels	Activation of inflammatory processes that cause thickening of glomerular capillary wall, reduce glomerular blood flow and GFR
IgA nephropathy (Berger disease) Usually idiopathic; elevated IgA plasma levels	Deposits of IgA and proliferation of inflammatory cells into Bowman space with sclerosis and fibrosis of glomerulus and decreased GFR
Minimal change disease (lipoid nephrosis) Usually idiopathic	Disruption of capillary filtration membrane and loss of negative charge, which cause increased permeability, loss of protein, and nephrotic syndrome
Focal glomerulosclerosis Usually idiopathic	Similar to minimal change disease
Membranous nephropathy Usually idiopathic; can be associated with systemic diseases, i.e., hepatitis B virus, systemic lupus erythematosus, solid malignant tumors	Thickening of glomerular capillary wall from inflammatory process with increased permeability, proteinuria, and nephrotic syndrome IgG depository on epithelium of glomerular basement membrane

29-5). Diabetes mellitus and lupus erythmatosus are secondary causes of chronic glomerular injury.[38]

≋ *Pathophysiology*

Patterns of antigen-antibody complex deposition within the glomerular capillary filtration membrane have been established using light, electron, and immunofluorescent microscopy for different disease processes. The findings on light microscopy provide information about the distribution and extent of immune response injury (Table 29-7). Electron microscopy differentiates morphologic changes within the glomerular capillary wall. Staining with fluorescein identifies different antibodies (i.e., immunoglobulin G [IgG] or immunoglobulin A [IgA]) and their configurations when viewed under ultraviolet (black) light with a microscope.

Two types of immune mechanisms commonly contribute to glomerular injury: (1) deposition of circulating soluble antigen-antibody complexes and (2) formation of antibodies specific for the anti-glomerular basement membrane (anti-GBM antibodies). The severity of glomerular damage and renal insufficiency is related to the size, number, location (focal or diffuse), duration of exposure, and type of antigen-antibody complexes.

Activation of biochemical mediators of inflammation (complement, leukocytes, fibrin) begins after the antibody or antigen-antibody complexes have localized in the glomerular capillary wall. Complement is deposited with the antibodies, and its activation can serve as a chemotactic stimulus for attraction of neutrophils and monocytes. These

Fig. 29-5 *End-stage chronic glomerulonephritis.* Pebbly surface corresponds to surviving hypertrophied nephrons amid atrophy. *(From Kissane, J.M. [Ed.]. [1990]. Anderson's pathology [9th ed.]. St. Louis: Mosby.)*

further the inflammatory reaction by releasing lysosomal enzymes, which damage glomerular cell walls, and contribute to proliferation of the extracellular matrix impacting glomerular blood flow.[39]

These processes also alter membrane permeability and may cause loss of the negative electrical charge across the

TABLE 29-7	Immunologic Pathogenesis of Glomerulonephritis
Glomerular Injury	**Mechanism**
Soluble immune-complex glomerulonephritis (90%)	Formation of antibodies stimulated by the presence of endogenous or exogenous antigens results in circulating soluble antigen-antibody complexes, which are deposited in glomerular capillaries; glomerular injury occurring with complement activation and release of immunologic substances that lyse cells and increase membrane permability; immune deposits with a microscopic appearance that fluoresce in a *granular pattern* when stained with fluorescein and viewed under ultraviolet light; severity of glomerular injury related to the number of complexes formed; a type III hypersensitivity
Anti-glomerular basement membrane glomerulonephritis (5%)	Antibodies are formed and act directly against the glomerular basement membrane; immune response that causes crescent formation and a *linear pattern* of immunofluorescence; generally associated with rapidly progressive renal failure, such as Goodpasture syndrome
Alternative complement pathway	A relatively obscure mechanism associated with low levels of complement and membranoproliferative glomerulonephritis
Cell-mediated immunity	A delayed hypersensitivity response that damages the glomerulus; actual cellular mechanism not clearly understood

glomerular filtration membrane, enhancing filtration of proteins. Membrane damage can lead to platelet aggregation and degranulation, whereby platelets release substances that increase glomerular permeability, permitting the passage of protein molecules or red blood cells into the urine and causing proteinuria or hematuria. The coagulation system also may be activated and lead to fibrin deposition in Bowman space, contributing to crescent formation (deposition of substances in Bowman space). Renal blood flow is decreased, and glomerular filtration is reduced.

Clinical Manifestations

Two major changes in the urine are distinctive of glomerulonephritis: (1) hematuria with red blood cell casts and (2) proteinuria exceeding 3 to 5 g/day, with albumin as the major protein. Several disorders may produce hematuria, because bleeding can occur anywhere along the urinary tract. The characteristics of hematuria from red blood cells escaping through the glomerular membrane include a smoky brown-tinged urine, red blood cell casts, and an accompanying proteinuria. Bleeding from sites lower in the urinary tract may produce a pink- or red-colored urine. Glomerular bleeding provides prolonged contact with the acidic urine and transforms hemoglobin to methemoglobin, which has a brownish color and no blood clots. The immune-mediated inflammatory response with cellular infiltration decreases GFR, which leads to fluid retention. Salt and water are also reabsorbed, contributing to fluid volume expansion and hypertension. The history and physical examination may disclose findings that differentiate glomerular disease from another source of urinary tract bleeding. Gross proteinuria is associated with nephrotic syndrome; a decrease in urine output accompanies a decreased GFR.

After 10 to 20 years, renal insufficiency begins to develop, followed by nephrotic syndrome and an accelerated progression to end-stage renal failure. Symptom patterns vary depending on the underlying cause. Steroids usually do not change the course of the disease, and dialysis or kidney transplantation ultimately may be needed.

Evaluation and Treatment

The diagnosis of glomerular disease is confirmed by the progressive development of clinical manifestations and laboratory findings of abnormal urinalysis with proteinuria, red blood cells, white blood cells, and casts. Microscopic evaluation from renal biopsy provides a specific determination of renal injury and type of pathologic condition.

Management principles for treating glomerulonephritis are related to treating the primary disease, preventing or minimizing immune responses, and correcting accompanying problems, such as edema, hypertension, and hyperlipidemia. Specific treatment regimens are necessary for particular types of glomerulonephritis. Antibiotic therapy is essential for management of underlying infections that may be contributing to ongoing antigen-antibody responses. Corticosteroids decrease antibody synthesis and suppress inflammatory responses. Cytotoxic agents may be used cautiously because of their severe side effects. Anticoagulants may be useful for controlling fibrin crescent formation in RPGN.

Nephrotic Syndrome

Nephrotic syndrome is simply defined as the excretion of 3.5 g or more of protein in the urine per day. This large amount of urine protein is characteristic of glomerular injury. Other clinical findings associated with the proteinuria include hypoalbuminemia, edema, hyperlipidemia, and lipiduria (Table 29-8). Lipoid nephrosis (minimal change disease), membranous glomerulonephritis, and focal glomerulosclerosis are directly related to nephrotic syndrome, although

TABLE 29-8	Clinical Manifestations of Nephrotic Syndrome	
Manifestation	**Contributing Factors**	**Result**
Proteinuria	Increased glomerular permeability, decreased proximal tubule reabsorption	Edema, increased susceptibility to infection from loss of immunoglobulins
Hypoalbuminemia	Increased urinary losses of protein	Edema
Edema	Hypoalbuminemia (decreased oncotic pressure, sodium and water retention, increased aldosterone and antidiuretic hormone [ADH] secretion), unresponsiveness to atrial natriuretic peptides	Soft, pitting, generalized edema
Hyperlipidemia	Decreased serum albumin; increased hepatic synthesis of very low-density lipoproteins; increased cholesterol, phospholipids, triglycerides	Increases atherogenesis
Lipiduria	Sloughing of tubular cells containing fat (oval fat bodies); free fat from hyperlipidemia	Fat droplets that may float in urine
Decreased vitamin D	The globulin to which 1,25-vitamin D is attached for transport passes through the glomerulus and is lost in the urine	Decreased absorption of calcium from gut

these conditions can occur with other types of glomerular disease.[40] Nephrotic syndrome is more common in children than adults.

Secondary forms of nephrotic syndrome occur as a result of other organic pathologic processes. Systemic diseases include diabetes mellitus, amyloidosis, systemic lupus erythematosus, and Henoch-Schönlein purpura. Nephrotic syndrome is also seen with certain drugs, infections, malignancies, and vascular disorders. When present as a secondary complication with renal diseases, nephrotic syndrome often signifies a more serious prognosis.

Pathophysiology

Loss of plasma proteins, particularly albumin and some immunoglobulins, occurs across the injured glomerular filtration membrane. Disturbances in the glomerular basement membrane, which may be metabolic, biochemical, or physiochemical, lead to increased permeability to protein and loss of negative charge. Hypoalbuminemia results from urinary loss of albumin combined with a diminished synthesis of replacement albumin by the liver. Albumin is lost in the greatest quantity because of its high plasma concentration and low molecular weight. Loss of albumin stimulates lipoprotein synthesis by the liver and hyperlipidemia.

Even increased synthesis of plasma proteins is insufficient to compensate for losses. Decreased dietary intake of protein from anorexia or malnutrition, or accompanying liver disease may contribute to lower levels of plasma albumin. Loss of immunoglobulins may increase susceptibility to infections.

Clinical Manifestations

Proteinuria is an excessive amount of protein in the urine (up to 10 g/24 hr). Many clinical manifestations of nephrotic syndrome are related to loss of serum proteins (see Table 29-

8). They include edema, hyperlipidemia, lipiduria, and vitamin D deficiency.[41]

Evaluation and Treatment

Nephrotic syndrome is diagnosed when the protein level in a 24-hour urine collection is greater than 3.5 g. Serum albumin decreases (to less than 3 g/dl), and serum cholesterol, phospholipids, and triglycerides increase. Fat bodies may be present in the urine. The specific pathologic condition is identified by renal biopsy.

Nephrotic syndrome is commonly treated with a normal-protein, low-fat diet; salt restriction; diuretics; steroids; and occasionally, albumin replacement. Dietary protein supplements (up to 100 g) are essential, unless renal failure has occurred. Diuretics may be used. Care must be taken to observe for hypovolemia and hypokalemia or potassium toxicity in the presence of renal insufficiency. Aldactone may be combined with loop diuretics to suppress aldosterone activity and conserve potassium.

✓ QUICK CHECK

What is glomerulonephritis? List two types.

What immune mechanisms are operative in glomerulonephritis?

What causes nephrotic syndrome?

RENAL FAILURE
Classification of Renal Dysfunction

Renal insufficiency refers to a decline in renal function to about 25% of normal or a GFR of 25 to 30 ml/min. Levels of serum creatinine and urea are mildly elevated. ***Renal failure***

TABLE 29-9	Classifications of Acute Renal Failure
Area of Dysfunction	**Possible Causes**
Prerenal	Hypovolemia
	Hemorrhagic blood loss (trauma, gastrointestinal bleeding, complications of childbirth)
	Loss of plasma volume (burns, peritonitis)
	Water and electrolyte losses (severe vomiting or diarrhea, intestinal obstruction, uncontrolled diabetes mellitus, inappropriate use of diuretics)
	Hypotension or hypoperfusion
	Septic shock
	Cardiac failure or shock
	Massive pulmonary embolism
	Stenosis or clamping of renal artery
Intrarenal	Acute tubular necrosis (postischemic or nephrotoxic)
	Glomerulopathies
	Malignant hypertension
	Coagulation defects
Postrenal	Obstructive uropathies (usually bilateral)
	Ureteral destruction (edema, tumors, stones, clots)
	Bladder neck obstruction (enlarged prostate)

often refers to significant loss of renal function. When less than 10% of renal function remains, this is termed ***end-stage renal failure (ESRF)***. ***Uremia*** is a syndrome of renal failure and includes elevated blood urea and creatinine levels accompanied by fatigue, anorexia, nausea, vomiting, pruritus, and neurologic changes. ***Azotemia*** means increased serum urea levels and frequently increased creatinine levels as well. Renal insufficiency or renal failure causes azotemia. Uremia represents the numerous consequences related to renal failure, including retention of toxic wastes, deficiency states, and electrolyte disorders. Both azotemia and uremia indicate an accumulation of nitrogenous waste products in the blood.

Types of Renal Failure
Acute renal failure

Acute renal failure (ARF) is an abrupt reduction in renal function with elevation of BUN and plasma creatinine levels. It is usually associated with oliguria (urine output of less than 30 ml/hr or less than 400 ml/day), although urine output may be normal or increased. Most types of acute renal failure are reversible if diagnosed and treated early.[42] Acute renal failure can be classified as prerenal, intrarenal, or postrenal (Table 29-9).

Pathophysiology
Prerenal acute renal failure is caused by impaired renal blood flow. The GFR declines because of the decrease in filtration pressure. Poor perfusion can result from renal vasoconstriction, hypotension, hypovolemia, hemorrhage, or inadequate cardiac output. Acute prerenal failure may occur when chronic renal failure exists if a sudden stress is imposed on already marginally functioning kidneys. Failure to restore blood volume or blood pressure and oxygen delivery may cause acute tubular necrosis or acute cortical necrosis.

Intrarenal acute renal failure usually results from ***acute tubular necrosis (ATN)***. ATN caused by ischemia occurs most frequently after surgery (40% to 50% of cases) but is also associated with sepsis, obstetric complications, or severe burns. Hypotension associated with hypovolemia produces ischemia, generating toxic oxygen free radicals that cause cell swelling, injury, and necrosis.[43] Aminoglycosides (neomycin, gentamicin, tobramycin) and other antibiotics tend to accumulate in the renal cortex and may not cause renal failure until after treatment is complete. Radiocontrast media (x-ray media) also may be nephrotoxic. Dehydration, advanced age, concurrent renal insufficiency, and diabetes mellitus tend to enhance nephrotoxicity from either antibiotics or radiocontrast media. Other substances, such as excessive myoglobin (oxygen-transporting substance from muscles), carbon tetrachloride, heavy metals (mercury, arsenic), or methoxyflurane anesthesic, may promote renal failure. Necrosis caused by nephrotoxins is usually uniform and limited to the proximal tubules. Ischemic necrosis tends to be patchy and may be distributed along any part of the nephron.[44]

Three pathophysiologic explanations have been proposed to account for the oliguria of ATN. All three mechanisms probably contribute to oliguria in varying degrees throughout the course of the disease (Fig. 29-6). These theories are as follows:

1. *Tubular obstruction theory.* Necrosis of the tubules causes sloughing of cells, cast formation, or ischemic edema that results in tubular obstruction, which in turn causes a retrograde increase in pressure and reduces the GFR. Renal failure can occur within 24 hours.
2. *Back leak theory.* Glomerular filtration remains normal, but tubular reabsorption of filtrate is accelerated as a result of permeability caused by ischemia.
3. *Alterations in renal blood flow.* Afferent arteriolar constriction may be produced by intrarenal release of angiotensin II or by redistribution of blood flow from the cortex to the medulla. Changes in glomerular permeability and decreased GFR may also result from the ischemia.

Postrenal acute renal failure usually occurs with urinary tract obstruction that affects the kidneys bilaterally (e.g., bladder outlet obstruction, prostatic hypertrophy, bilateral ureteral obstruction). A pattern of several hours of anuria with flank pain followed by polyuria is a characteristic finding. This type of renal failure can occur after diagnostic catheterization of the ureters, a procedure that may cause edema of the tubular lumen.

Fig. 29-6 *Mechanisms of oliguria in acute renal failure. GFR,* Glomerular filtration rate.

Clinical Manifestations

The clinical progression of acute renal failure with recovery of renal function occurs in three phases: oliguria, diuresis, and recovery. Oliguria begins within 1 day after a hypotensive event and lasts 1 to 3 weeks, but it may regress in several hours or extend for several weeks, depending on the duration of ischemia or severity of toxic injury. From 10% to 20% of cases have nonoliguric failure. The urine output may vary in volume, but the BUN and plasma creatinine concentrations increase (plasma creatinine is inversely proportional to the GFR). Other early manifestations depend on the underlying cause of renal failure.

As renal function improves, increase in urine volume (diuresis) is progressive. During the early diuretic phase, the tubules are still damaged. Fluid and electrolyte balance must be carefully monitored and excessive urinary losses replaced.

Serial measurements of plasma creatinine provide an index of renal function during the recovery phase. Return to normal status may take from 3 to 12 months, and approximately 30% of individuals do not have full recovery of a normal GFR or tubular function.

Evaluation and Treatment

The diagnosis of ATN is related to the cause of the disease. A history of surgery, trauma, or cardiovascular disorders is common, and exposure to nephrotoxins must be considered.

The diagnostic challenge is to differentiate prerenal acute renal failure from intrarenal acute renal failure (Table 29-10).

Prevention of acute renal failure is a major treatment factor and involves maintenance of fluid volume before and after surgery or diagnostic procedures and use of mannitol.

The primary goal of therapy is to maintain the individual's life until renal function has been recovered. Management principles directly related to physiologic alterations generally include (1) correcting fluid and electrolyte disturbances, (2) treating infections, (3) maintaining nutrition, and (4) remembering that drugs or their metabolites are not excreted.

Chronic renal failure

The kidney regulates body fluid volume, solute concentration and dilution, acid-base balance, excretion of waste products, and secretion of hormones that control red blood cell production, blood pressure, and calcium metabolism. Progressive and irreversible loss of nephrons *(chronic renal failure)* decreases GFR and affects these vital processes with changes manifest throughout all organ systems. The kidneys, however, exhibit remarkable adaptive abilities, and symptomatic changes resulting from increased creatinine, urea, potassium, and alterations in salt and water balance usually do not become apparent until the renal function declines to less than 25% of normal.

TABLE 29-10	Differentation of Acute Oliguric Renal Failure					
	Urine Volume	Urine Specific Gravity	Urine Osmolality	Urine Sodium	BUN/Plasma Creatinine	FE_{Na}*
Prerenal failure	<400 ml	1.016-1.020	>500 mOsm	<10 mEq/L	>15:1	<1% (also seen in acute glomerulo-nephritis)
Acute tubular necrosis	<400 ml	1.010-1.012	<400 mOsm	>30 mEq/L	<15:1	>1% (also seen in urinary tract obstruction and renal parenchymal disease)

$$*FE_{Na} = \frac{Urine\ Na/plasma\ Na}{Urine\ creatine/plasma\ creatine} \times 100$$

TABLE 29-11	Factors Contributing to Pathophysiology of Renal Failure
Factor	Characteristics
Creatinine and urea clearance	In chronic renal failure, the GFR falls and the plasma creatinine concentration increases by a reciprocal amount; because there is no regulatory adjustment for creatinine, plasma levels continue to rise and serve as an index of changing glomerular function. As GFR declines, urea clearance increases. (NOTE: Urea is both filtered and reabsorbed and varies with the state of hydration.)
Sodium and water balance	In chronic renal failure, sodium load delivered to nephrons exceeds normal, so excretion must increase, thus less is reabsorbed. Obligatory loss occurs, leading to sodium deficits and volume depletion. As GFR is reduced, ability to concentrate and dilute urine diminishes.
Phosphate and calcium balance	Changes in acid-base balance affect phosphate and calcium balance. The major disorders associated with chronic renal failure are reduced renal phosphate excretion, decreased renal synthesis of 1,25-$(OH)_2$ vitamin D_3, and hypocalcemia. Hypocalcemia leads to secondary hyperparathyroidism, GFR falls, and progressive hyperphosphatemia, hypocalcemia, and dissolution of bone result.
Hematocrit	Because of anemia that accompanies chronic renal failure, lethargy, dizziness, and low hematocrit are common.
Potassium balance	In chronic renal failure, tubular secretion of potassium increases until oliguria develops. Use of potassium-sparing diuretics also may precipitate elevated serum potassium levels. As disease progresses, total body potassium levels can rise to life-threatening levels and dialysis is required.
Acid-base balance	In early renal insufficiency, acid excretion and bicarbonate reabsorption are increased to maintain normal pH. When GFR reaches 30% to 40%, metabolic acidosis begins. When end-stage renal failure develops, the metabolic acidosis and hyperkalemia may be severe enough to require dialysis.

GFR, *Glomerular filtration rate.*

Pathophysiology

Two theories have been proposed to account for the adaptation to loss of renal function. First, the *adaptive response* may depend on the particular location of kidney damage. For example, tubular interstitial diseases damage primarily the tubular or medullary parts of the nephron, producing problems such as renal tubular acidosis, salt wasting, and difficulty diluting or concentrating the urine. Conversely, when there is primarily vascular or glomerular damage, proteinuria, hematuria, and nephrotic syndrome are more prominent. This theory is useful for planning treatment in early stages of renal failure when symptomatic differences in renal disease may be distinct.

A second theory, the *intact nephron hypothesis*, proposes that loss of nephron mass with progressive kidney damage causes the remaining nephrons to sustain normal kidney function. These nephrons are capable of a compensatory expansion in their rates of reabsorption and secretion and can maintain a constant rate of excretion in the presence of a declining GFR. The increased work load is achieved primarily by hypertrophy and hyperfunction of the remaining nephrons.

The intact nephron hypothesis explains adaptive changes in solute and water regulation that occur with advancing renal failure. Although the urine of an individual with chronic renal failure may contain abnormal amounts of protein and red and white blood cells or casts, the major end-products of excretion are similar to those of normally functioning kidneys until advanced stages of renal failure when there is a significant reduction of functioning nephrons.

Factors involved in the pathophysiology of renal failure are outlined in Table 29-11.

■ Clinical Manifestations

The clinical manifestations of chronic renal failure are often described using the term *uremia*. Uremia refers to a number of symptoms caused by decline in renal function with the accumulation of toxins in the plasma.[45] Generally, the symptoms include hypertension, anorexia, nausea, vomiting, diarrhea, weight loss, pruritus, edema, and neurologic changes (Table 29-12).[46]

■ Evaluation and Treatment

Evaluation of chronic renal failure is based on the history and presenting signs and symptoms. Elevated serum creatinine concentrations and urea nitrogen are consistent with chronic renal failure. Ultrasound, intravenous pyelogram, or plain x-ray films will show small kidney size. Renal biopsy confirms the diagnosis.

Management involves dietary control, including protein restriction, sodium and fluid evaluation, potassium restriction, adequate caloric intake, and erythropoietin as needed.[47,48] End-stage renal failure related to diabetic nephropathy can be significantly reduced with control of hyperglycemia by intense insulin therapy, for example, four or five insulin injections per day or use of a constant infusion pump.[49] End-stage renal failure is treated with dialysis and supportive therapy.[50,51]

✓ QUICK CHECK

What mechanisms cause prerenal acute renal failure?

How does intrarenal acute renal failure differ from postrenal failure?

Briefly outline the major pathophysiologic events producing chronic renal failure.

TABLE 29-12	Systemic Effects of Uremia		
System	**Manifestations**	**Mechanisms**	**Treatment**
Skeletal	Osteitis fibrosa (bone inflammation with fibrous degeneration); bone demineralization (principally subperiosteal loss of cortical bone in the fibers, lateral ends of the clavicles, and lamina dura of the teeth); spontaneous fractures, bone pain; osteomalacia (rickets) with end-stage renal failure	Bone resorption associated with hyperparathyroidism, vitamin D deficiency, and demineralization; lowered calcium and raised phosphate levels	Control of hyperphosphatemia to reduce hyperparathyroidism; administration of calcium and aluminum hydroxide antacids, which bind phosphate in the gut, together with a phosphate-restricted diet; vitamin D replacement; avoidance of magnesium antacids because of impaired magnesium excretion
Cardiopulmonary	Hypertension, pericarditis with fever, chest pain, and pericardial friction rub, pulmonary edema, Kussmaul respirations	Extracellular volume expansion; hypersecretion of renin also associated with hypertension; fluid overload associated with pulmonary edema and acidosis leading to Kussmaul respirations	Volume reduction with diuretics that are not potassium sparing (to avoid hyperkalemia); ACE inhibitors; combination of propranolol, hydralazine, and minoxidil for those with high levels of renin; bilateral nephrectomy with dialysis or transplantation

TABLE 29-12	Systemic Effects of Uremi—cont'd		
System	**Manifestations**	**Mechanisms**	**Treatment**
Neurologic	Encephalopathy (fatigue, loss of attention, difficulty problem solving); peripheral neuropathy (pain and burning in the legs and feet, loss of vibration sense and deep tendon reflexes); loss of motor coordination, twitching, fasciculations, stupor, and coma with advanced uremia	Uremic toxins associated with end-stage renal disease	Dialysis
Hematologic	Anemia, usually normochromic normocytic; platelet disorders with prolonged bleeding times	Reduced erythropoietin secretion associated with loss of renal mass, leading to reduced red cell production in the bone marrow; uremic toxins associated with shortened red cell survival	Dialysis; recombinant human erythropoietin and iron supplementation; conjugated estrogens; DDAVP (1-desamino-8-D-arginine vasopressin); transfusion
Gastrointestinal	Anorexia, nausea, vomiting; mouth ulcers, stomatitis, urinous breath (uremic fetor), hiccups, peptic ulcers, gastrointestinal bleeding, and pancreatitis associated with end-stage renal failure	Retention of metabolic acids and other metabolic waste products	Protein-restricted diet for relief of nausea and vomiting
Integumentary	Abnormal pigmentation and pruritus	Retention of urochromes, contributing to sallow, yellow color; high plasma calcium levels and neuropathy associated with pruritus	Dialysis with control of serum calcium levels
Immunologic	Increased risk of infection that can cause death	Suppression of cell-mediated immunity; reduction in number and function of lymphocytes, diminished phagocytosis	Routine dialysis
Reproductive	Sexual dysfunction: menorrhagia, amenorrhea, infertility, and decreased libido in women; decreased testosterone levels, infertility, and decreased libido in men	Probably related to dysfunction of ovaries and testes	No specific treatment

■ DID YOU UNDERSTAND?

Urinary Tract Obstruction

1. Obstruction can occur anywhere in the urinary tract and is usually caused by renal stones or tumors. The most serious complications are hydronephrosis, hydroureter, and infection caused by accumulation of urine behind the obstruction.

2. The most common kidney stone is formed from calcium and most often causes obstruction by lodging in the urethra.

3. Obstruction can be caused by a neural lesion that interrupts innervation of the bladder. The dysfunction is called a *neurogenic bladder.*

Continued

DID YOU UNDERSTAND? —cont'd

Urinary Tract Obstruction—cont'd

4. Renal cell carcinoma is the most common renal neoplasm. The larger neoplasms tend to metastasize to the lung, liver, and bone.

5. Bladder tumors are commonly composed of transitional cells with a papillary appearance and a high rate of recurrence.

Urinary Tract Infection

1. Urinary tract infections (UTIs) are usually caused by bacteria, commonly from the retrograde movement of bacteria into the urethra and bladder.

2. Cystitis is an inflammation of the bladder commonly caused by bacteria, although types of "nonbacterial" cystitis may be caused by other conditions or by an autoimmune reaction.

3. Pyelonephritis is an acute or chronic inflammation of the renal pelvis that may cause abscess formation and scarring with an alteration in renal function. Pyelonephritis may be acute or chronic.

Glomerular Disorders

1. Glomerulonephritis is a group of related diseases of the glomerulus that can be caused by immune responses, toxins or drugs, vascular disorders, and other systemic diseases.

2. Acute glomerulonephritis commonly results from inflammatory damage to the glomerulus as a consequence of immune reactions after a streptococcal infection.

3. Rapidly progressive glomerulonephritis (RPGN) is associated with injury that results in proliferation of glomerular capillary endothelial cells and rapid loss of renal function.

4. Chronic glomerulonephritis is related to a variety of diseases that cause deterioration of the glomerulus and progressive loss of renal function.

5. Immune mechanisms in glomerulonephritis are the deposition of antigen-antibody complexes and the formation of antibodies specific for the glomerular basement membrane.

6. Nephrotic syndrome is the excretion of at least 3.5 g protein in the urine per day. Its principal signs are hypoproteinuria, hyperlipidemia, and edema. The liver cannot produce enough protein to adequately compensate for urinary loss.

7. Nephrotic syndrome is caused by a loss of plasma proteins, principally albumin and some immunoglobulins, across the injured glomerular filtration membrane.

Renal Failure

1. Acute renal failure is classified as prerenal, intrarenal, or postrenal and is usually accompanied by oliguria with an elevated plasma BUN and plasma creatinine levels.

2. Prerenal acute renal failure is caused by decreased renal perfusion with a decreased GFR, ischemia, and tubular necrosis.

3. Intrarenal acute renal failure is associated with several systemic diseases but is commonly related to acute tubular necrosis (ATN).

4. Postrenal failure is associated with diseases that obstruct the flow of urine from the kidneys.

5. Chronic renal failure represents a progressive loss of renal function. Plasma creatinine levels gradually become elevated as GFR declines; sodium is lost in the urine; potassium is retained; acidosis develops; and calcium metabolism and phosphate metabolism are altered.

KEY TERMS

Acute glomerulonephritis, 815
Acute renal failure (ARF), 819
Acute tubular necrosis (ATN), 819
Azotemia, 819
Chronic glomerulonephritis, 815
Chronic renal failure, 820
Cystitis, 812
End-stage renal failure (ESRF), 819
Glomerulonephritis, 815
Goodpasture syndrome, 815
Hydronephrosis, 808
Hydroureter, 808

Interstitial cystitis, 813
Intrarenal acute renal failure, 819
Nephritic sediment, 814
Nephrotic sediment, 814
Nephrotic syndrome, 817
Neurogenic bladder, 810
Nidus, 809
Postrenal acute renal failure, 819
Prerenal acute renal failure, 819
Pyelonephritis, 813
Rapidly progressive glomerulonephritis (RPGN), 815

Renal adenoma, 811
Renal cell carcinoma (RCC), 811
Renal failure, 818
Renal insufficiency, 818
Renal stones (calculi, nephrolithiasis), 809
Staghorn calculi, 809
Uremia, 819
Urethral syndrome, 813
Urinary tract infection (UTI), 812

REFERENCES

1. Krane, R.J., Siroky, M.B., & Fitzpatrick, J.M. (1994). *Clinical urology.* Philadelphia: Lippincott.
2. Dussol, B. & Berland, Y. (1998). Urinary kidney stone inhibitors. What is the news? *Urology International, 20*(2), 69-73.
3. Segura, J.W. (1997). Staghorn calculi, *Urologic Clinics of North America, 24*(1), 71-80.
4. Curhan, G.C. et al. (1997). Comparison of dietary calcium with supplemental calcium and other nutrients as factors affecting the risk for kidney stones in women. *Annals of Internal Medicine, 126,* 497-504.
5. Low, R.K. & Stoller, M.L. (1997). Uric acid-related nephrolithiasis. *Urologic Clinics of North America, 24*(1), 135-148.
6. Ruml, L.A., Pearle, M.S., & Pak, C.Y. (1997). Medical therapy, calcium oxalate urolithiasis. *Urologic Clinics of North America, 24*(1), 117-133.
7. Wasserstein, A.G. (1998). Nephrolithiasis: Acute management and prevention. *Disease-a-Month, 44*(5), 196-213.
8. de Groat, W.C. (1998). Anatomy of the central neural pathways controlling the lower urinary tract. *European Urology, 34*(Suppl.1), 2-5.
9. Amis, E.S., Jr. & Blaives, J.G. (1991). Neurogenic bladder simplified. *Radiologic Clinics of North America, 29*(3), 571-580.
10. Bahnson, R.R. (1994). Renal and urinary tract neoplasia. In National Kidney Foundation, *Primer on kidney diseases.* San Diego: Academic Press.
11. Erlandsson, R. (1998). Molecular genetics of renal cell carcinoma. *Cancer, Genetics, and Cytogenetics, 104*(1), 1-18.
12. Yuan, J.M. et al. (1998). Tobacco use in relation to renal cell carinoma. *Cancer Epidemiology, Biomarkers, and Prevention, 7*(5), 429-433.
13. Fidler, I.J. (1992). The biology of renal carcinoma metastasis. *Seminars in Urology, 10*(1), 3-11.
14. Vetter, J.M. (1990). Metastasis of renal-cell carcinoma: A pathologist's theoretical view. In C.G. Bollack & D. Jacqmin (Eds.). *Basic research and treatment of renal cell carcinoma metastasis.* New York: Wiley-Liss.
15. Jayson, M. & Sanders, H. (1998). Increased incidence of serendipitously discovered renal cell carcinoma. *Urology, 51*(2), 203-205.
16. Bukowski, R.M. (1997). Natural history and therapy of metastatic renal cell carcinoma: The role of interleukin-2. *Cancer, 80*(7), 1198-1220.
17. American Cancer Society (ACS). (1999). *Cancer facts and figures—1999.* Atlanta: The Author.
18. van der Meijden, A.P. (1998). Bladder cancer. *British Medical Journal, 317*(7169), 1366-1369.
19. Rozanski, T.A. & Grossman, H.B. (1994). Recent developments in the pathophysiology of bladder cancer. *AJR—American Journal of Roentgenology, 163*(4), 789-792.
20. Hall, R.R. (1994). Superficial bladder cancer. *British Medical Journal, 308*(6933), 910-913.
21. Cordon-Cardo, C. & Sheinfeld, J. (1997). Molecular and immunopathology studies of oncogenes and tumor-suppressor genes in bladder cancer. *World Journal of Urology, 15*(2), 112-119.
22. Hooton, T.M. & Stamm, W.E. (1997). Diagnosis and treatment of uncomplicated urinary tract infection. *Infectious Disease Clinics of North America, 11*(3), 551-581.
23. Barnett, B.J. & Stephens, D.S. (1997). Urinary tract infection: An overview. *American Journal of Medical Science, 314*(4), 245-249.
24. Sanford, J.P. (1975). Urinary tract symptoms and infection. *Annual Review of Medicine, 26,* 485.
25. Barnett, B.J. & Stephens, D.S. (1997). Urinary tract infection: An overview. *American Journal of Medical Science, 314*(4), 245-249.
26. Bernstein, A.M. et al. (1992). A psychophysiological evaluation of female urethral syndrome: Evidence for a muscular abnormality. *Journal of Behavioral Medicine, 15*(3), 299-312.
27. Theoharides, T.C. et al. (1995). Activation of bladder mast cells in interstitial cystitis: A light and electron microscopy study. *Journal of Urology, 153*(3, pt. 1), 629-636.
28. Ochs, R.L. (1997). Autoantibodies and interstitial cystitis. *Clinical Laboratory Medicine, 17*(3), 571-579.
29. O'Leary, M.P. et al. (1997). The interstitial cystitis symptom index and problem index. *Urology, 49*(5A, Suppl.), 58-63.
30. Ghielli, M. et al. (1998). Regeneration processes in the kidney after acute injury: Role of infiltrating cells. *Experiments in Nephrology, 6*(6), 502-507.
31. Talner, L.B. et al. (1994). Acute pyelonephritis: Can we agree on terminology? *Radiology, 192*(2), 297-305.
32. Hooten, T.M. & Stamm, W.E. (1997). Diagnosis and treatment of uncomplicated urinary tract infection. *Infectious Disease Clinics of North America, 11*(3), 551-581.
33. Gibson, I.W. & More, I.A. (1998). Glomerular pathology: Recent advances. *Journal of Pathology, 184*(2), 123-129.
34. Couser, W.G. (1998). Pathogenesis of glomerular damage in glomerulonephritis. *Nephrology, Dialysis and Transplantation, 13*(Suppl. 1), 10-15.
35. Grunfeld, J.P. et al. (1994). *Advances in nephrology* (vol. 23). St. Louis: Mosby.
36. Couser, W.G. (1988). Rapidly progressive glomerulonephritis: Classification, pathogenic mechanisms, and therapy. *American Journal of Kidney Disease, 11,* 449.
37. Neverov, N.I. et al. (1997). HDL causes mesangial cell mitogenesis through a tyrosine kinase–dependent receptor mechanism. *Journal of the American Society of Nephrology, 8*(8), 1247-1256.

REFERENCES

38. Gonick, H.C. (1997). *Current nephrology* (vol. 20). St. Louis: Mosby.

39. Nangaku, M. (1998). Complement regulatory proteins in glomerular diseases. *Kidney International, 54*(5), 1419-1428.

40. Carome, M.A. & Moore, J. (1992). Nephrotic syndrome in adults. *Postgraduate Medicine, 92*(22), 209-215, 218, 220.

41. Kaysen, G.A. (1994). Nonrenal complications of the nephrotic syndrome. *Annual Review of Medicine, 45*, 201-210.

42. Vijayan, A. & Miller, S.B. (1998). Acute renal failure: Prevention and nondialytic therapy. *Seminars in Nephrology, 18*(5), 523-532.

43. Edelstein, C.L. et al. (1997). Emerging therapies for acute renal failure. *American Journal of Kidney Disease, 30*(5, Suppl. 4), S89-S95.

44. Racusen, L.C. (1997). Pathology of acute renal failure: Structure/function correlations. *Advances in Renal Replacement Therapy, 4*(2, Suppl. 1), 3-16.

45. Robertson, K.E. & Mueller, B.A. (1996). Uremic pruritus. *American Journal of Health Systems and Pharmacology, 53*(18), 2159-2170.

46. Mailloux, L.U. & Haley, W.E. (1998). Hypertension in the ESRD patient: Pathophysiology, therapy, outcomes, and future directions. *American Journal of Kidney Disease, 32*(5), 705-719.

47. Marion, B.J. (1998). Impact of chronic renal failure on nitrogen metabolism. *Mineral and Electrolyte Metabolism, 24*(1), 34-40.

48. Winearls, C.G. (1998). Recombinant human erythropoietin: 10 years of clinical experience. *Nephrology, Dialysis and Transplantation, 13*(Suppl. 2), 3-8.

49. Molich, M.E. et al. (Diabetes Control and Complications Trial Research Group). (1993). Baseline analysis of renal function in the diabetes control and complications trial. *Kidney International, 43*, 668-674.

50. National Institutes of Health (NIH) Consensus Statement. (1994). Morbidity and mortality of renal dialysis. *Annals of Internal Medicine, 121*(1), 62-70.

51. Walker, R. (1997). General management of end stage renal disease. *British Medical Journal, 315M*(120), 1429-1432.

CHAPTER

30

Alterations of Renal and Urinary Tract Function in Children

Cyrena M. Gilman and Sue E. Huether

Some renal and urinary disorders occur in children as well as adults. In childhood, however, the kidney and genitourinary structures continue to develop, so renal dysfunction may be associated with mechanisms and manifestations that differ from those in adults. In addition, some renal and urinary disorders are congenital. Many of these involve structural anomalies of the renal system.

Kathleen Hardin Mooney, RN, PhD, contributed to this chapter in the previous edition.

CHAPTER OUTLINE

Check out your CD Companion for chapter-related exercises and answers to the Quick Check questions

STRUCTURAL ABNORMALITIES

Variations from the normal anatomic structure of the urinary tract occur in 10% to 15% of the total population. These abnormalities range from minor, nonpathologic, or easily correctable anomalies to those that are incompatible with life. For example, the kidneys may fail to ascend from the pelvis to the abdomen, causing ectopic kidneys—which usually function normally. The kidneys also may fuse as they ascend, causing a single, U-shaped **horseshoe kidney.** Approximately one third of individuals with horseshoe kidneys are asymptomatic, and the most common problems are hydronephrosis, infection, and stone formation.[1] Collectively, structural anomalies of the renal system account for approximately 45% of cases of renal failure in children.

Certain structural anomalies are commonly associated with urinary tract malformations,[2] including the following:

Low-set, malformed ears

Chromosomal disorders, especially trisomy 13 (Patau syndrome) and trisomy 18

Absent abdominal muscles (prune-belly syndrome)

Anomalies of the spinal cord and lower extremities

Imperforate anus or genital deviation

Wilms tumor

Congenital ascites

Cystic disease of the liver

Positive family history of renal disease (hereditary nephritis or cystic disease)

Fig. 30-1 *Hypospadias.* *(Courtesy M.C. Gleason, M.D., San Diego; from Novak, J.C. & Broom, B.L. [1999]. Ingalls and Salerno's maternal and child health nursing [8th ed.]. St. Louis: Mosby.)*

HEALTH ALERT

Association Between Abnormal Development Processes and Specific Diseases

Better understanding of the events involved in fetal renal and genitourinary development has led to a clear associate between abnormal development processes and specific diseases, such as renal dysplasia or cystic kidney diseases. However, other problems not associated with structural defects and manifested much later in life, such as essential hypertension, may also be the result of abnormal fetal development. In addition, many diseases have been linked to specific genes or chromosomal regions.

In utero testing, such as ultrasound or magnetic resonance imaging (MRI), permits prenatal diagnosis of many congenital renal or urologic conditions, such as hydronephrosis or cystic kidneys. Antenatal interventions, such as urinary diversions, can often preserve renal function until after birth when additional treatments are more easily done.

Data from Guillery, E.N. (1997). Fetal and neonatal nephrology. Current Opinion in Pediatrics, 9, 148-153.

Hypospadias

Hypospadias is a congenital condition in which the urethral meatus is located on the ventral side or undersurface of the penis. The meatus can be located anywhere on the glans, the penile shaft, at the base of the penis, the penoscrotal junc-

Fig. 30-2 *Hypospadias with significant chordee.* *(From Shirkey, H.C. [Ed.]. [1980]. Pediatric therapy [6th ed.]. St. Louis: Mosby.)*

tion, or the perineum (Fig. 30-1). This is the most common anomaly of the penis and occurs in about 1 in 300 infant boys. **Chordee** or penile torsion may accompany cases of hypospadias. In chordee, skin tethering and shortening of subcutaneous tissue cause the penis to bend or "bow" ventrally (Fig. 30-2).[3] Penile torsion is rotation of the penile shaft to either the right or left.[4] Partial absence of the foreskin and cryptorchidism (undescended testes, see Chapter 32) are associated with the anomaly.[5]

The goals for corrective surgery on the child with hypospadias are (1) a straight penis when erect to facilitate intercourse as an adult, (2) a uniform urethra of adequate cal-

Fig. 30-3 *Exstrophy of bladder. (Courtesy H. Gil Rushton, M.D., Children's National Medical Center, Washington DC; from Wong, D.L. [1999].* Whaley & Wong's nursing care of infants and children *[6th ed.]. St. Louis: Mosby.)*

ther to prevent spraying during urination, (3) a cosmetic appearance satisfactory to the individual, and (4) repair completed in as few procedures as possible.[6,7] Surgery is most effective, psychologically as well as physically, when performed between 6 and 12 months of age.[8]

Epispadias and Exstrophy of the Bladder

Epispadias and exstrophy of the bladder are the same congenital defect expressed to differing degrees. In male epispadias, the urethral opening is on the dorsal surface of the penis. In females, a cleft along the ventral urethra usually extends to the bladder neck. The incidence of epispadias is 1 in 40,000 to 118,000 births. Twice as many boys as girls present with this defect.[7]

In boys, the urethral opening may be small and situated behind the glans (anterior epispadias) or a fissure may extend the entire length of the penis and into the bladder neck (posterior epispadias). Children with anterior epispadias can be continent with perhaps only stress incontinence, but those with posterior epispadias will experience constant dribbling of urine.

Exstrophy of the bladder is an extensive congenital anomaly in which the lower urinary tract is exposed directly to the surface of the body (Fig. 30-3). The posterior portion of the bladder mucosa is exposed and appears bright red through a fissure in the abdominal wall. The incidence of exstrophy of the bladder is 1 in 40,000 live births. Boys are predominant by 3:1.

Exstrophy of the bladder is caused by intrauterine failure of the abdominal wall and the mesoderm of the anterior bladder to fuse. The rectus muscles below the umbilicus are separated, and the pubic rami (bony projections of the pubic bone) are not joined. This causes a waddling gait when the child first learns to walk, but most children quickly learn to compensate. Urine seeps onto the abdominal wall from the ureters, causing a constant odor of urine and excoriation

of the surrounding skin. Because the exposed bladder mucosa becomes hyperemic and edematous, it bleeds easily and is painful.

The unrepaired exstrophic bladder is cosmetically unacceptable and prone to cancerous changes as soon as 1 year after birth. Ideally, the bladder and pubic defect should be closed before the infant is 48 hours old.[8] Reconstruction of the external and internal genitalia can be done when girls reach the late teens. However, epispadias repair in boys is better done at 2 to 3 years of age, as are secondary bladder neck reconstruction, urethral reimplantation, and bladder augmentation, if it is required.[9] Objectives of management include preservation of renal function, attainment of urinary control, prevention of infection, reconstructive repair of the defect, and improvement of sexual function.

Hypoplastic/Dysplastic Kidneys

During embryologic development, the ureteric duct grows into the metanephric tissue, triggering the formation of the kidneys. If this growth does not occur, the kidney is absent—a condition called *renal aplasia.* Occasionally, a *hypoplastic kidney,* a very small normal kidney, may develop. These aberrations may be unilateral or bilateral; the occurrence may be incidental or familial. Bilateral hypoplastic kidneys are a common cause of chronic renal failure in children. Segmental hypoplasia, the Ask-Upmark kidney, is a deformity acquired secondary to intrarenal reflux.[10]

Renal dysplasia usually results from abnormal differentiation of the renal tissues; for example, primitive glomeruli and tubules, cysts, and nonrenal tissue, such as cartilage, are found in the dysplastic kidney. Dysplasia is usually also associated with obstruction of the collecting system. The obstruction may begin before birth, as in prune-belly syndrome, posterior urethral valves, or ureteroceles.

Renal Agenesis

Renal agenesis (failure of a kidney to grow or develop) may be unilateral or bilateral and randomly occurring or clearly hereditary. The kidney is usually polycystic and dysplastic. The condition may occur as an isolated entity or as a problem associated with other disorders.[11]

Unilateral renal agenesis occurs in approximately 1 of 1000 live births. Males are more often affected, and it is usually the left kidney that is absent. The single kidney is often completely normal so that the child can expect a normal, healthy life. By the time the child is several years older, the volume of this kidney may approach twice the normal size. In some instances, however, the single kidney is abnormally formed and associated with abnormalities of its collecting system. Extrarenal congenital abnormalities are relatively more common with unilateral renal agenesis.

Bilateral renal agenesis (also called *Potter syndrome*) occurs in about 1 in 3000 live births, 75% being male. The term *Potter syndrome* refers to the association with a specific group of facial anomalies (wide-set eyes, parrot-beak nose, low-set ears, and receding chin). Affected infants rarely live more than a few hours. Approximately 40% of affected infants are stillborn.

✓ QUICK CHECK

Describe hypospadias.

Why does bladder exstrophy occur?

Contrast dysplastic kidney and hypoplastic kidney.

GLOMERULAR DISORDERS
Nephrotic Syndrome

In children with nephrotic syndrome, the kidney is usually the only or the principal organ involved. This condition is termed *primary nephrotic syndrome.* If it is caused by a systemic disease or other causes (e.g., drugs, toxins), it is called *secondary nephrotic syndrome.* Primary nephrotic syndrome is found predominantly in the preschool child, with a peak incidence of onset between 2 and 3 years of age. It is rare after 8 years of age. Boys are affected more frequently than girls. No prevalent racial or geographic distributions are evident. The incidence is approximately 3 per 100,000 children per year.

Clinical Manifestations

Parents become alerted to an abnormality when they notice diminished, "frothy," or "foamy" urine output and when edema becomes pronounced with ascites, respiratory difficulty from pleural effusion, and labial or scrotal swelling. Edema of the intestinal mucosa may cause diarrhea, anorexia, and poor absorption. It often masks the malnutrition caused by malabsorption and protein loss. Because of protein deficiency, changes in the quality of hair indicate a malnourished state. Pallor, with shiny skin and prominent veins, is also common. Blood pressure is usually normal or slightly decreased. The child has an increased susceptibility to infection, especially pneumonia, peritonitis, cellulitis, and septicemia. Irritability, fatigue, and lethargy are common. Babies born with congenital nephrotic syndrome have large fontanelles and separated cranial sutures and may show gingival hyperplasia.[12]

Evaluation and Treatment

The diagnosis of nephrotic syndrome is evident from the finding of proteinuria, hyperlipidemia, and lipiduria. Several different diagnostic tests, including kidney biopsy, may be required to determine whether the cause is an intrinsic renal disease or a consequence of systemic disease. Basic management of nephrotic syndrome includes activity as tolerated; a low-sodium, well-balanced diet; glucocorticosteroids (prednisone), diuretics (furosemide, metolazone), and skin care. Immunosuppressive agents (cyclophosphamide [Cytoxan], azathioprine [Imuran]) are given to children who do not respond to steroids; paracentesis may be required for severe ascites.[13]

Glomerulonephritis

Glomerulonephritis includes a number of renal disorders in which proliferation and inflammation of the glomeruli are

Primary Glomerulonephritis in Children BOX 30-1

CAUSE
Poststreptococcal infection
Related to other bacterial or viral infection
Unknown

IMMUNOLOGIC MECHANISM
Antigen-antibody complex
Anti-GBM disease
No immunologic cause established

HISTOPATHOLOGY
No lesion
Diffuse, focal, or segmented
Membranous, proliferative, or combination of types
Lobular, exudative, necrotizing, and other types
Chronic with glomerular proliferation

CLINICAL MANIFESTATIONS OF DISEASE NEPHRITIS
Acute glomerulonephritis
Persistent (chronic) glomerulonephritis
Idiopathic nephrotic syndrome

GBM, *Glomerular basement membrane.*

secondary to an immune mechanism (Box 30-1). Chronic glomerulonephritis accounts for 53% of renal failure in children and is responsible for most school-age and teen-age children requiring dialysis and kidney transplantation.

Poststreptococcal glomerulonephritis

Acute poststreptococcal glomerulonephritis is one of the most common noninfectious renal diseases in children. The sudden onset of gross hematuria, edema, hypertension, and renal insufficiency occurs after a throat or skin infection with certain strains of group A β-hemolytic streptococci.

Pharyngeal infections are most common during cold weather; skin infections from impetigo, infected insect bites, or varicella sores usually occur during warm weather. Symptoms of varying severity develop about 1 to 3 weeks after the streptococcal infection. As many as half the children affected are asymptomatic and show only microscopic hematuria with otherwise normal renal function. The most severely affected develop acute renal failure with oliguria.

The onset of symptoms in the child is abrupt and consists of flank or midabdominal pain, irritability, general malaise, and fever. Acute hypertension may cause headache, vomiting, somnolence, and other central nervous system (CNS) manifestations, including seizures. Cardiovascular symptoms are related to circulatory overload and are compounded by hypertension. These include dyspnea, tachypnea, and an enlarged, tender liver.

The disease usually runs its course in 1 month, but urine abnormalities may be found for up to 1 year after the onset. Some children become oliguric and develop rapidly progressive glomerulonephritis, whereas others slowly progress to chronic glomerulonephritis. Prolonged proteinuria and abnormal glomerular filtration rate (GFR) indicate an unfavorable prognosis. More than 95% recover completely. Treatment is symptom-specific.

Immunoglobulin A nephropathy

Immunoglobulin A (IgA) nephropathy, the most common form of glomerulonephritis worldwide, is characterized by deposition mainly of the immunoglobulin IgA, but also some IgM, in the mesangium of the glomerular capillaries, even though no systemic immunologic disease is evident.[14] IgA neuropathy occurs almost twice as frequently in males as in females.

Children with the disease have recurrent gross hematuria, often after a respiratory infection. Most continue to have microscopic hematuria between the attacks of gross hematuria and have a mild proteinuria as well. Treatment is supportive because kidney damage is generally insignificant. Approximately 20% of affected children develop the progressive form of the disease, however, with hypertension and decreasing renal function. These children eventually require dialysis and transplantation.

Hemolytic Uremic Syndrome

Hemolytic uremic syndrome is an acute disorder characterized by hemolytic anemia originating in the microcirculation, thrombocytopenia, and acute renal failure.[15] Hemolytic uremic syndrome has been associated with bacterial and viral agents, as well as endotoxins, especially that from *Escherichia. coli* 0157:H7.[13,16] Hemolytic uremic syndrome is the most common cause of acute renal failure in children. The disease occurs most often in infants and children younger than 4 years of age but has been known to occur in adolescents and adults.[17] The prognosis has improved dramatically in recent years, with more than 90% of children surviving and most regaining normal renal function.

▰ *Pathophysiology*

In hemolytic uremic syndrome, the endothelial lining of the glomerular arterioles becomes swollen and occluded with platelets and fibrin clots. Narrowed vessels damage erythrocytes as they pass through. These damaged burr cells, helmet cells, and fragmented red blood cells are removed by the spleen, causing acute hemolytic anemia. Fibrinolysis, the process of dissolution of a clot, acts on precipitated fibrin, causing the fibrin split products to appear in serum and urine. The platelet clustering within damaged vessels, combined with the damage and removal of platelets, produces thrombocytopenia.

▰ *Clinical Manifestations*

A prodromal gastrointestinal illness (fever, vomiting, diarrhea) or, less frequently, an upper respiratory infection often precedes the onset of hemolytic uremic syndrome by 1 to 2 weeks. After a symptom-free 1- to 5-day period, the sudden onset of pallor, bruising or purpura, irritability, and oliguria heralds the onset of the disease. Slight fever, anorexia, vom-

iting, diarrhea (with the stool characteristically watery and blood stained), abdominal pain, mild jaundice, and circulatory overload are accompanying symptoms. Seizures and lethargy indicate CNS involvement. Renal failure is apparent within the first days of onset. The renal failure causes metabolic acidosis, azotemia, hyperkalemia, and often hypertension.

▰ *Evaluation and Treatment*

Clinical evaluation includes history of preexisting illness, presenting symptoms, and urine and blood analysis. Management is supportive. When renal failure occurs, early and frequent peritoneal dialysis is indicated. Blood transfusions with packed red cells are needed to maintain reasonable hemoglobin levels.

OBSTRUCTIVE DISORDERS
Urinary Tract Infections

Urinary tract infections (UTIs) are rare in newborns and are usually caused by bacteria from the bloodstream settling in the urinary tract. Urinary tract infections are most common in 7- to 11-year-old girls as a result of perineal bacteria, especially *E. coli*, ascending the urethra.[18] Individual susceptibility, bacterial virulence, and the host's anatomy (presence of reflux, obstruction, stasis, or stones) affect the severity of the disease. The abnormal urinary tract is particularly susceptible to infection.[19]

Cystitis, or infection of the bladder, results in mucosal inflammation and congestion. This causes detrusor muscle hyperactivity and a resulting decrease in bladder capacity. It may also cause distortion of the ureterovesical (UV) junction leading to transient reflux of infected urine up the ureters, causing acute or chronic pyelonephritis.[13]

Differentiating whether an infection is in the bladder or the kidneys is difficult based on symptoms alone. Infants usually develop nausea, vomiting, diarrhea, or jaundice. Children may present with fever of undetermined origin, frequency, urgency, enuresis or incontinence in a previously dry child, abdominal pain, foul-smelling urine, and sometimes hematuria. Acute pyelonephritis usually causes chills, fever, and flank or abdominal pain, along with enlarged kidney(s) caused by inflammatory edema. Chronic pyelonephritis may be asymptomatic.

Diagnosis of UTIs is by urine culture and urinalysis. Ultrasound may be necessary to rule out obstructions or abscesses.

With treatment, UTI symptoms are usually relieved in 1 to 2 days and the urine becomes sterile. Sulfonamides are the drug of choice, with the usual treatment lasting 7 to 10 days. More potent medications may be required if the child has been previously treated for UTI or has congenital abnormalities of the urinary tract, such as urethral valves. About 3 to 6 weeks after treatment is completed, all children with a first UTI should have a voiding cystourethrogram done to rule out reflux. If reflux is found, an intravenous pyelogram or DMSA (dimercaptosuccinic acid) scan may be done to check for renal damage or scarring.[18] Follow-up cultures should be

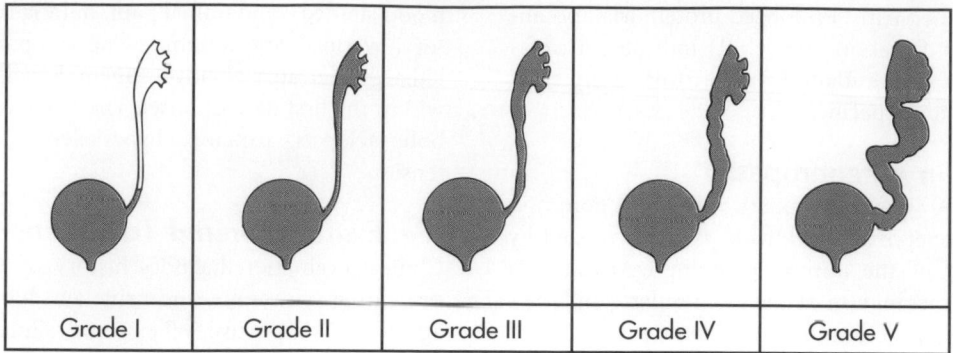

| Grade I | Grade II | Grade III | Grade IV | Grade V |

Fig. 30-4 *Grades of reflux.* *(From Retik, A. & Cukier, J. [Eds.]. [1987]. Pediatric urology. Baltimore: Williams & Wilkins.)*

done 2 to 3 weeks after the medication is completed and every 3 months for the next 1 to 2 years to monitor for recurrence, even if the child is asymptomatic.

Surgical correction of reflux or obstruction is necessary before the urinary tract can be sterilized. Children who develop frequent recurrences and who do not have surgically correctable anomalies may need prophylactic antibiotic therapy. A low dose (one-half to one-third the usual dose) of the antibiotic is given at bedtime for 1 year to keep high levels of antibiotic in bladder urine. These children also require regular cultures to rule out asymptomatic infections with resistant microorganisms.

Vesicoureteral Reflux

Vesicoureteral reflux is the retrograde flow of bladder urine into the ureters. Reflux allows infected urine from the bladder to be repeatedly swept up into the kidneys. The reflux perpetuates infection by preventing complete emptying of the bladder and allows the maximal intravesical pressure to be transmitted to the renal calyces and pyramids (Fig. 30-4). The combination of reflux and infection is an important cause of pyelonephritis, especially in children younger than 5 years.

Vesicoureteral reflux occurs more frequently in girls by a ratio of 10:1 and is uncommon in blacks. Its incidence is approximately 1 in 1000 children. Siblings of those affected have a 26% to 46% chance of having reflux, but children with parents with childhood reflux have almost a 70% chance of reflux.[20,21] Although reflux is considered abnormal at any age, the shortness of the submucosal segment of the ureter during infancy and childhood renders the antireflux mechanism relatively inefficient and delicate. Thus reflux is seen commonly in association with infections during early childhood but rarely in older children and adults.

Reflux may be unilateral or bilateral, and it can be classified or graded for comparative purposes:

Grade I: reflux into a nondilated distal ureter
Grade II: reflux into the upper collecting system without dilation
Grade III: reflux into dilated ureter or blunting of calyceal fornices

Grade IV: reflux into a grossly dilated ureter
Grade V: massive reflux with urethral dilation and tortuosity and effacement of the calyceal details

 ### *Pathophysiology*
Primary reflux results from a congenitally abnormal or ectopic insertion of the ureter into the bladder. Secondary reflux is more serious and may be transient or persistent. It develops in association with infection, malformations of the ureterovesical (UV) junction, increased intravesical pressures, and surgery on the UV junction (Fig. 30-5).

Clinical Manifestations
Children with reflux have recurrent urinary tract infection or unexplained fever, poor growth and development, irritability, and feeding problems. The family history reveals reflux or urinary tract infection, pain with voiding, and signs of urinary obstruction or neuropathy.

Evaluation and Treatment
In addition to the history of recurrent urinary tract infection and other symptoms, a voiding cystourethrogram and an intravenous pyelogram may be required for diagnosis. Most children with vesicoureteral reflux respond to nonoperative management aimed at prevention and treatment of infection. Spontaneous remission of grades I and II reflux may occur in 30% to 60% of children younger than 5 years. Children with grades III and IV reflux need careful monitoring. Recurrent infection requires surgical intervention. In cases of grade V reflux, early surgical intervention is indicated to prevent renal scarring.[22]

✓ QUICK CHECK

Describe the characteristics of poststreptococcal glomerulonephritis.

How does the cause of urinary tract infections (UTIs) in newborns differ from that in older children?

Why does vesicoureteral reflux occur?

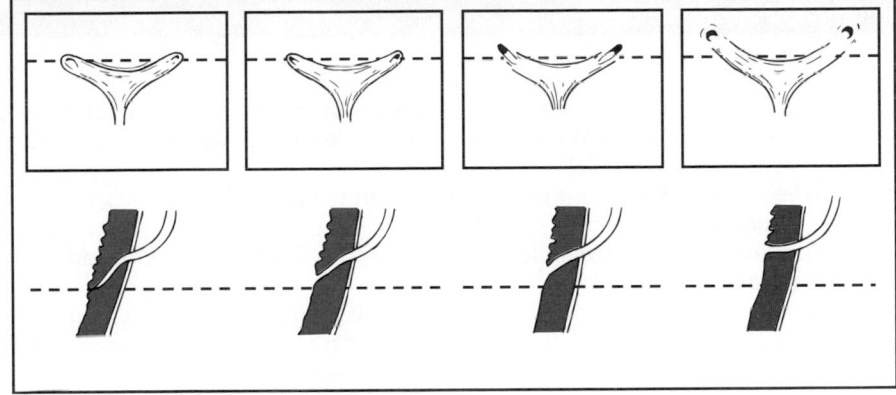

Fig. 30-5 *Normal and abnormal configuration of the ureteral orifices.* Shown from left to right, progressive lateral displacement of the ureteral orifices and shortening of the intramural tunnels. *Top,* Endoscopic appearance. *Bottom,* Sagittal view through the intramural ureter. *(From Behrman, R. et al. [Eds.]. [1992].* Nelson textbook of pediatrics. *Philadelphia: Saunders.)*

WILMS TUMOR

Wilms tumor (nephroblastoma) is an embryonal tumor of the kidney. Its incidence remains constant in the United States, with 7.8 cases per 1 million population ages 1 to 14 years. Approximately 400 children are diagnosed each year in the United States, most between 1 and 5 years of age. The peak incidence occurs between 2 and 3 years of age. Wilms tumor is the most common childhood cancer of the urinary tract. Paternal preconception toxin exposure (hydrocarbons and heavy metals) may be associated with increased risk in offspring.[23] Wilms tumor is slightly more common in black children than in white children.

Pathogenesis

Wilms tumor has both sporadic and inherited origins. The sporadic form occurs in children with no known genetic predisposition. Inherited cases, which are relatively rare, are transmitted in an autosomal dominant fashion. In both cases, Wilms tumor has been linked to the deletion or inactivation of genes on the short arm of chromosome 11, indicating the role of a tumor suppressor gene.[24]

Eighteen percent of children who have Wilms tumor also have a number of congenital anomalies. The anomalies associated with Wilms tumor are aniridia (lack of an iris in the eye), hemihypertrophy (an asymmetry of the body), and genitourinary malformations (i.e., horseshoe kidneys, hypospadias, ureteral duplication, polycystic kidneys).[25] Children with both congenital anomalies and Wilms tumor are more likely to have the inherited bilateral form of the disease.

Clinical Manifestations

Most Wilms tumors are enlarging asymptomatic abdominal masses at the time of diagnosis. Many tumors are actually discovered by the child's parent, who feels or notices an abdominal swelling, usually while dressing or bathing the child. The child appears healthy and thriving. Other presenting complaints include vague abdominal pain (37%), hematuria (21%), and fever (23%).[26] Hypertension also may be present. The reported frequency of hypertension varies from 25% to 63%.

Wilms tumor may occur in any part of the kidney and varies greatly in size at the time of diagnosis. The tumor generally appears as a solitary mass surrounded by a smooth, fibrous external capsule and also may contain cystic or hemorrhagic areas. A pseudocapsule generally separates the tumor from the renal parenchyma.

Evaluation and Treatment

On physical examination, the tumor feels firm, nontender, and smooth. The mass is generally confined to one side of the abdomen. Should the tumor be palpable past the midline of the abdomen, it may be very large or may be arising from a horseshoe or ectopic kidney. Once an abdominal mass is detected, an abdominal ultrasound may be the initial study. Abdominal computed tomography (CT) scan or MRI also may be obtained before biopsy and surgical removal of the tumor.

Diagnosis is based on surgical biopsy. Additional labora-

TABLE 30-1	Staging of Wilms Tumor
Stage	**Tumor Characteristics**
I	Tumor limited to the kidney, completely resected
II	Tumor ascending beyond the kidney but appearing to be totally resected
III	Residual nonhematogenous tumor confined to the abdomen
IV	Hematogenous metastases
V	Bilateral disease either at diagnosis or later

NOTE: Staging system of the National Wilms Tumor Study Group.

TABLE 30-2	**Classification of Incontinence**
Type	**Definition**
Total incontinence	Inability to store any urine; indicates an anatomic or functional absence of urinary sphincters (e.g., epispadias or myelomeningocele) or a bypassing of urinary sphincters (e.g., vesicovaginal fistula)
Overflow incontinence	Frequent dribbling that relieves a constantly full bladder; occurs when urinary outlet is obstructed
Urge incontinence	Sudden and uncontrollable need to void that cannot be suppressed; suggests bladder irritation
Precipitate voiding	Voiding without a preceding urge to void; suggests neurologic origin
Stress incontinence	Uncontrollable voiding that occurs when intravesical pressure momentarily exceeds intravesical resistance, as in "giggle incontinence"
Paradoxic incontinence	Incontinence in spite of normal voiding; suggests an ectopic ureteral orifice outside the urinary sphincter mechanism (e.g., a girl who is constantly wet, yet voids normally)

tory and radiologic studies are used to evaluate the presence or absence of metastasis. The most common sites of metastasis are regional lymph nodes and the lungs. Metastases also occur in the liver, brain, and bone.

Several staging systems for Wilms tumor have been developed. The most widely accepted system was developed by the National Wilms Tumor Study Group (Table 30-1). Surgical exploration and resection and chemotherapy may be used in treatment.

ENURESIS

Enuresis refers to the involuntary passage of urine by a child who is beyond the age when voluntary bladder control should have been acquired. Bladder control is accomplished by most children before the age of 4 years. Five years of age is more accurate and widely accepted, however, being largely determined by cultural beliefs and practices of parents regarding toilet training. In 80% of children, enuresis occurs at night only, in which case it is called *nocturnal enuresis.*

Types of Enuresis

In *primary enuresis,* the child has never been continent. In *secondary enuresis,* or acquired enuresis, the child has experienced a period of dryness of at least 3 to 6 months after toilet training and then becomes incontinent. Secondary enuresis may be diurnal (daytime), nocturnal, or a combination of both. (Types of incontinence are defined in Table 30-2.)

The incidence of enuresis is difficult to determine because it is not a problem that parents readily share with others and because definitions vary according to cultural norms and family practices. Some families start toilet training before 1 year of age and expect continence by the age of 1 to 1½ years, whereas other families do not expect dryness earlier than 5 years. According to research data, the incidence of enuresis in children older than 5 years ranges from 15% to 26%. Boys represent more cases of enuresis than girls by a ratio of 3:2. Teenage enuresis is usually a continuation of childhood bed-wetting.

Pathogenesis

A combination of factors is likely to be responsible for enuresis. Organic causes account for 2% to 10% of cases and include UTIs; neurologic disturbances; congenital defects of the meatus, urethra, and bladder neck; and allergies. Disorders that increase the normal output of urine, such as diabetes mellitus and diabetes insipidus, or disorders that impair the concentrating ability of the kidney, such as chronic renal failure or sickle cell disease, must be considered in the evaluation of enuresis.

Genetic factors as a cause of enuresis are speculative, but the condition does show a familial tendency. If both parents experienced enuresis as children, their children have a 70% chance of having enuresis; this decreases to a 40% chance if only one parent had enuresis.[27] Bed-wetting occurs with high frequency among siblings and other near relatives of symptomatic children. These observations are further supported by a high concordance rate in monozygotic twins with enuresis. Family studies indicate that the closer the relationship, the higher the incidence of enuresis.

A significant number of nocturnal enuretic episodes have been related to deep sleep. These children sleep more soundly than others. Many demonstrate increased frequency and magnitude of spontaneous bladder contractions during the non-rapid-eye-movement (non-REM) stage of sleep preceding bed-wetting. Nocturnal enuresis occurs as the child moves from the deeper stages of non-REM sleep into the REM stage, usually during the first two thirds of the night; children with enuresis are more difficult to rouse during this time.[28] Individuals with enuresis have also shown a lack of normal nocturnal increase in antidiuretic hormone levels and nocturnal production of large urine volumes.[29] Enuresis may also be associated with sleep apnea.[30]

In addition to physical problems associated with enuresis, such as perinatal anoxia, CNS trauma, seizures, developmental delay, UTI, radiation therapy, imperforate anus, bladder trauma or surgery, and occult spinal dysraphism, stressful psychologic situations, such as a new sibling, may cause enuresis to develop.[31,32]

Therapeutic management of enuresis includes retention control training, enuresis alarms, fluid management, diet therapy, and drugs (desmopressin, oxybutynin, imipramine). The main goals of therapy should be to have the child awaken and get up to use the toilet during the night and to preserve self-esteem in moving toward the goal.[33,34]

✓ QUICK CHECK

What is Wilms tumor, and what cellular components are involved?

What organic causes are operative in enuresis?

■ DID YOU UNDERSTAND?

Alterations in Renal Function in Children

1. Congenital renal disorders affect 10% to 15% of the population. These disorders range in severity from minor, easily correctable anomalies to those incompatible with life.
2. Hypospadias is a congenital condition in which the urethral meatus can be located anywhere on the ventral surface of the glans, the penile shaft, the midline of the scrotum, or the perineum. Epispadias is a congenital condition in which the urethral opening is located on the dorsal surface of the penis.
3. Epispadias is a mild form of exstrophy, a congenital condition that affects the urethra and bladder neck. The urethral opening in boys is on the dorsal surface of the penis.
4. Exstrophy of the bladder is a congenital malformation in which the pubic bones are separated, the lower portion of the abdominal wall and anterior wall of the bladder are missing, and the back wall of the bladder is everted through the opening.
5. A dysplastic kidney is the result of abnormal differentiation of renal tissues. The hypoplastic kidney is a very small but otherwise normal kidney.
6. Renal agenesis is the failure of a kidney to grow or develop. (The condition may be unilateral or bilateral and may occur as an isolated entity or in association with other disorders.)
7. Nephrotic syndrome is a term used to describe a symptom complex characterized by proteinuria, hypoproteinemia, hyperlipidemia, and edema. Metabolic, biochemical, or physiochemical disturbances in the glomerular basement membrane may lead to increased permeability to protein.

8. Glomerulonephritis is an inflammation of the glomeruli characterized by hematuria, edema, and hypertension. (The cause is unknown, but glomerulonephritis may follow other infections, especially those of the upper respiratory tract). Deposition of immunoglobulins in the mesangium of the glomerular capillaries leads to another type of glomerulonephritis.
9. Hemolytic uremic syndrome is an acute disorder characterized by hemolytic anemia, acute renal failure, and thrombocytopenia.
10. Urinary tract infections can result from general sepsis in the newborn but are caused by bacteria ascending the urethra in older children. The bladder alone is infected in cystitis. The infection ascends to one or both kidneys in pyelonephritis. Urinary tract anomalies must be surgically corrected to prevent frequent recurrent infections.
11. Vesicoureteral reflux, which refers to the retrograde flow of bladder urine into the ureters, provides a mechanism for pyelonephritis in children, whose ureters are shorter than those of adults.
12. Wilms tumor is an embryonal tumor of the kidney that usually presents between birth and 5 years of age. The tumor can be successfully treated by surgery, a combination of drugs, and, sometimes, radiation therapy.
13. Enuresis refers to the involuntary passage of urine.
14. Enuresis may occur during the day (diurnally) or during the night (nocturnally). The disorder tends to occur during non-REM sleep and can have a variety of organic and psychologic causes.

KEY TERMS

REFERENCES

1. McAninch, J.W. (1995). Disorders of the kidney. In E.A. Taragho & J.W. McAninch (Eds.). *Smith's general urology.* Norwalk, Conn.: Appleton & Lange.
2. Kelalis, P.P., Lowell, R.K., & Bellmam, B.A. (1992). *Clinical pediatric urology* (3rd ed.). Philadelphia: Saunders.
3. Smith, E.D. (1997). The history of hypospadias. *Pediatric Surgery International, 12,* 81-85.
4. Zaontz, M.R. & Packer, M.G. (1997). Abnormalities of the external genitalia. *Pediatric Clinics of North America, 44*(5), 1267-1297.
5. Speakman, M.J. & Azmy, A.F. (1992). Skin chordee without hypospadias—An underrecognized entity. *British Journal of Urology, 69*(4), 428-429.
6. Zaontz, M.R. & Packer, M.G. (1997). Abnormalities of the external genitalia. *Pediatric Clinics of North America, 44*(5), 1267-1297.
7. McMahon, D.R. et al. (1996). Vesical neck reconstruction in patients with the exstrophy-epispadias complex. *The Journal of Urology, 155,* 1411-1413.
8. Kass, E. et al. (1996). Timing of elective surgery on the genitalia of male children with particular reference to the risks, benefits, and psychological effects of surgery and anesthesia. *Pediatrics, 97*(4), 590-594.
9. Stein, R. et al. (1996). Social integration, sexual behaviour, and fertility in patients with bladder exstrophy—A long-term follow-up. *European Journal of Pediatrics, 155,* 678-683.
10. Holliday, M.A., Barratt, T.M., & Avner, E.D. (1994). *Pediatric nephrology* (2nd ed.). Baltimore: Williams & Wilkins.
11. Hitchcock, T. & Burge, D.M. (1994). Renal agenesis: An acquired condition? *Journal of Pediatric Surgery, 29*(3), 454-455.
12. Mattoo, T.K. (1997). Gingival hyperplasia in congenital and infantile nephrotic syndrome [letter to the editor]. *Pediatric Nephrology, 11*(3), 388.
13. Gilman, C.M. & Hoyler-Grant, C. (1998). Health challenge: Alterations in genitourinary status. In V.R. Bowden, S.B. Dickey, & C.S. Greenberg (Eds.). *Children and their families—The continuum of care* (pp. 111-1215). Philadelphia: Saunders.
14. Pan, C.G. (1997). Glomerulonephritis in childhood. *Current Opinion in Pediatrics, 9,* 154-159.
15. Moake, J.L. (1994). Haemolytic-uraemic syndrome: Basic science. *Lancet, 343*(8894), 393-397.
16. A new source of *Escherichia coli* infection. (1997). *Canadian Medical Association Journal, 156*(3), 401.
17. Siegler, R.L., Pavia, A.T., & Cook, J.B. (1997). Hemolytic-uremic syndrome in adolescents. *Archives of Pediatric and Adolescent Medicine, 151,* 165-169.
18. Miller, K.L. (1996). Urinary tract infections: Children are not little adults. *Pediatric Nursing, 22*(6), 473-480.
19. Yeung, C.K. et al. (1997). The characteristics of primary vesico-ureteric reflux in male and female infants with prenatal hydronephrosis. *British Journal of Urology, 80,* 319-327.
20. Connolly, L.P. et al. (1997). Vesicoureteral reflux in children: Incidence and severity in siblings. *The Journal of Urology, 157,* 2287-2290.
21. Belman, A.B. (1997). Vesicoureteral reflux. *Pediatric Urology, 44*(5), 1171-1190.
22. Walker, R.D. (1994). Vesicoureteral reflux update: Effect of prospective studies on current management. *Urology, 32*(3), 279-283.
23. Olsham, A.F. et al. (1993). Risk factors for Wilms tumor: Report of the national Wilms tumor study. *Cancer, 72,* 938-944.
24. Gerald, W.L. (1994). The molecular genetics of Wilms tumor: A paradigm of heterogeneity in tumor development. *Cancer Investigation, 12*(3), 350-359.
25. Breslow, N.E. & Beckwith, J.B. (1982). Epidemiological features of Wilms' tumor: Results of the national Wilms' tumor study. *Journal of the National Cancer Institute, 68,* 429-436.
26. Holliday, M.A. et al. (1993). Renal tumors in children. In *Pediatric nephrology* (3rd ed.). Baltimore: Williams & Wilkins.
27. Thomas, R. (1997). Nocturnal enuresis: A private agony. *Health Visitor, 70,* 34-35.
28. Wolfish, N.M., Pivik, R.T., & Busby, K.A. (1997). Elevated sleep arousal thresholds in enuretic boys: Clinical implications. *Acta Paediatrica, 86,* 381-384.
29. Folwell, A.J. et al. (1997). Desmopressin for nocturnal enuresis: Urinary osmolality and response. *British Journal of Urology, 80,* 480-484.
30. Wengraf, C. (1997). Management of enuresis [letter to the editor]. *Lancet, 350,* 221-222.
31. Wan, J. & Greenfield, S. (1997). Enuresis and common voiding abnormalities. *Pediatric Urology, 44*(5), 1117-1131.
32. Norgaard, J. et al. (1997). Experience and current status of research into the pathophysiology of nocturnal enuresis. *British Journal of Urology, 79,* 825-835.
33. Goin, R.P. (1998). Nocturnal enuresis in children. *Child Care and Health Development, 24*(4), 277-288.
34. Ronen, T. & Abraham, Y. (1996). Retention control training in the treatment of younger versus older enuretic children. *Nursing Research, 45*(2), 78-82.

CHAPTER

31

Structure and Function of the Reproductive Systems

Kristynia M. Robinson and Sue E. Huether

The male and female reproductive systems have several anatomic and physiologic features in common. Most obvious is their major function—reproduction—through which a 23-chromosome female gamete, the **ovum,** and a 23-chromosome male gamete, the **spermatozoon (sperm cell),** unite to form a 46-chromosome zygote that is capable of developing into a new individual. The male reproductive system produces sperm and delivers them to the female reproductive tract. The female reproductive system produces the ovum and, if the ovum is fertilized, can nurture and protect it (now called the embryo and developing fetus) and expel it at birth. These functions are determined not only by anatomic structures but also by complex hormonal, neurologic, and psychogenic factors.[1]

DEVELOPMENT OF THE REPRODUCTIVE SYSTEMS

The structure and function of both male and female reproductive systems depend on steroid hormones called *sex hormones.* Hormonal effects on the reproductive systems begin well before birth and continue for life.

Sexual Differentiation in Utero

For embryonic differentiation, the most important sex hormone is the primary male sex hormone, **testosterone.** Until the eighth week of gestation, the initial reproductive structures of male and female embryos are homologous (the same), consisting of one pair of primary sex organs, or *gonads,* and two pairs of ducts—the mesonephric ducts (wolffian ducts) and the paramesonephric ducts (müllerian

ducts) (Fig. 31-1). Both pairs of ducts empty into the urogenital sinus.

At about 8 weeks' gestation, the gonads of genetically male embryos begin to produce testosterone. Under its influence, the male gonads develop into the two testes, which produce sperm. The paramesonephric ducts degenerate, and the mesonephric ducts develop into the vas deferens—the two tubes that carry sperm from the testes to the urethra.

The presence of estrogen and the absence of testosterone cause the two female gonads to develop into ovaries, which will produce ova. In females, the mesonephric ducts deteriorate and the lower ends of the paramesonephric ducts join to become the uterus. The upper portions of the paramesonephric ducts develop into the fallopian (uterine) tubes. These two ducts carry ova from the ovaries to the uterus.

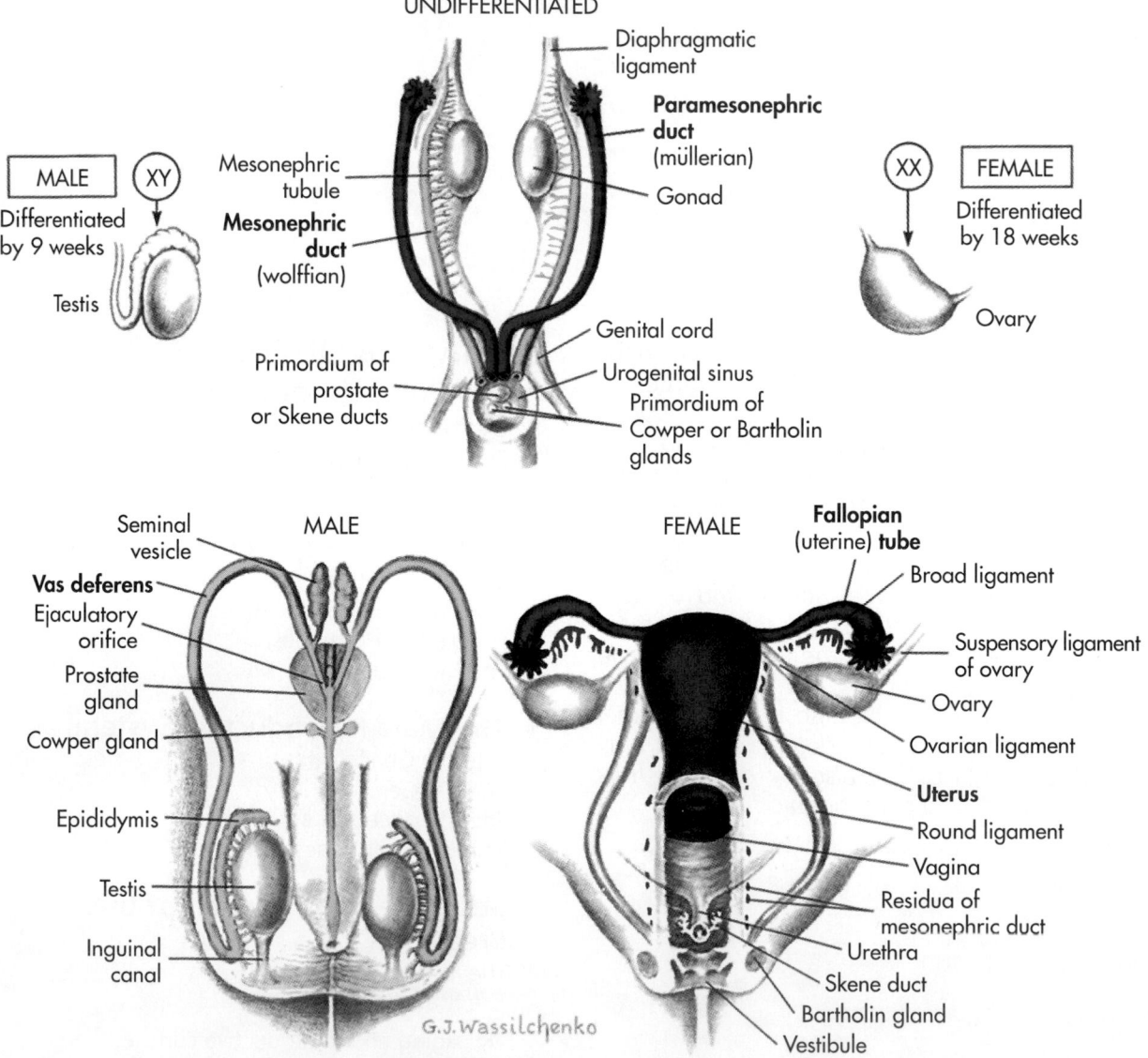

Fig. 31-1 *Internal genitalia development.* Embryonic and fetal development of the internal genitalia. *(Modified from Lowdermilk, D.L., Perry, S.E., & Bobak, I.M. [1997]. Maternity and women's health care [6th ed.]. St. Louis: Mosby.)*

Like the internal reproductive structures, the external structures develop from homologous embryonic tissues. During the first 8 weeks of gestation, both male and female embryos develop an elevated structure called the *genital tubercle* (Fig. 31-2). Testosterone is necessary for the genital tubercle to differentiate into male genitalia; otherwise, female genitalia develop. By 9 months' gestation, the internal and external genital structures are all present and the male gonads (the testes) have descended into the scrotum.[1]

Puberty

From fetal life through childhood, the testes secrete low levels of testosterone and the ovaries secrete low levels of the primary female sex hormone, *estrogen.* Between the ages of 9 and 12 years the gonads begin to produce more of the sex hormones. This triggers sexual maturation, or puberty. In girls, puberty begins at about age 10 years. In boys, it begins later—at about age 11 years. Puberty lasts 2 or 3 years and is complete when the individual is capable of reproduction.

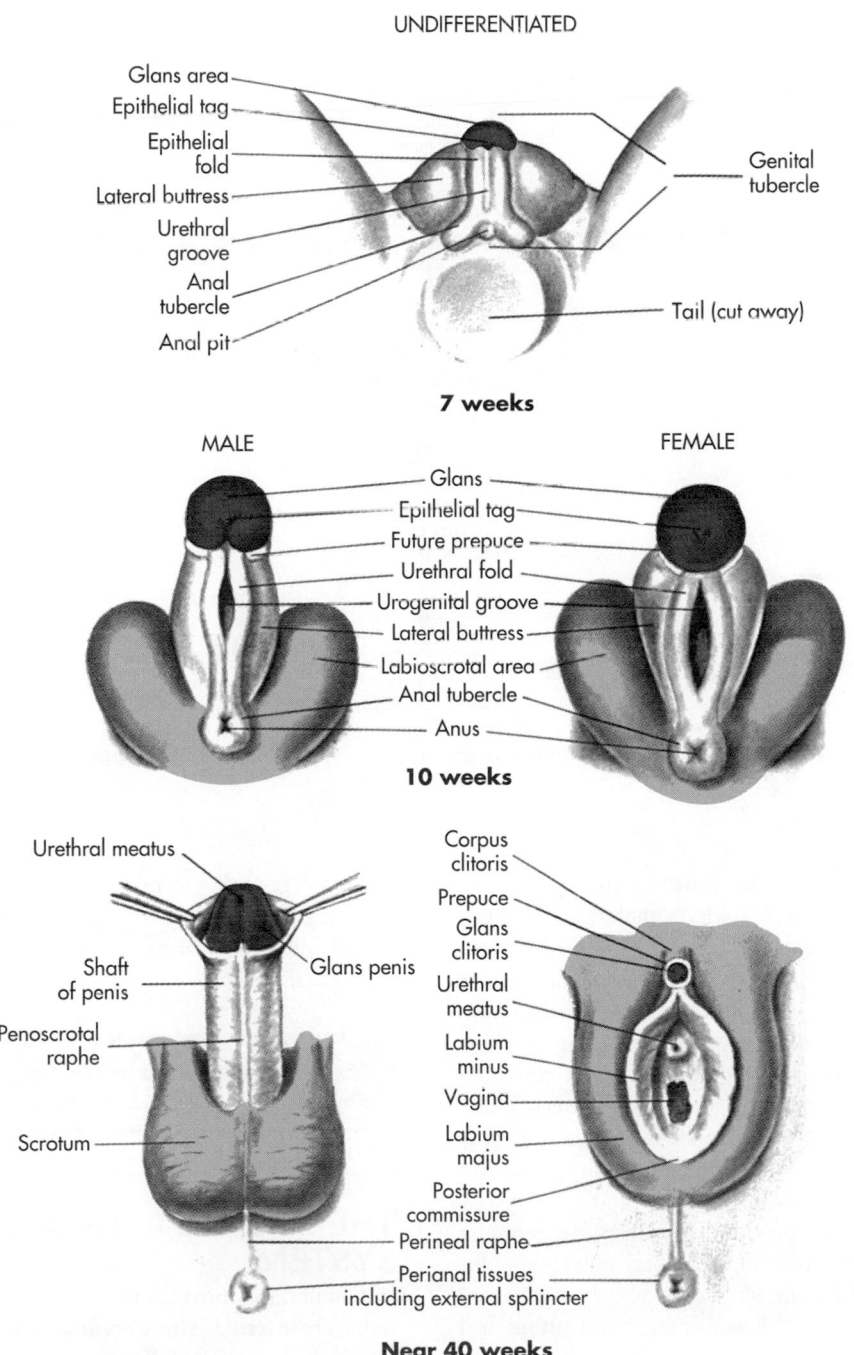

Fig. 31-2 *External genitalia development.* Embryonic and fetal development of the external genitalia. *(From Lowdermilk, D.L., Perry, S.E., & Bobak, I.M. [1997]. Maternity and women's health care [6th ed.]. St. Louis: Mosby.)*

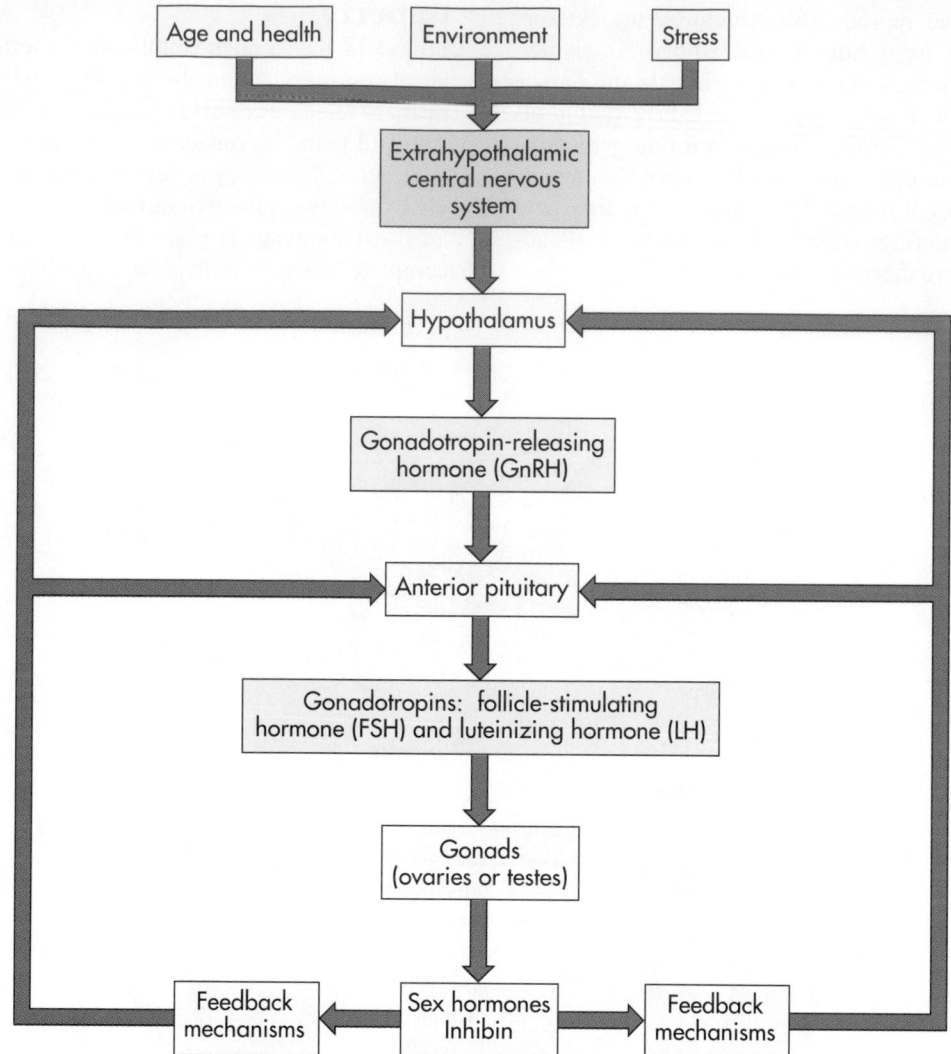

Fig. 31-3 *Hormonal stimulation of the gonads.* The hypothalamic-pituitary-gonadal axis.

Hormonal stimulation of the reproductive system involves the central nervous system (hypothalamus), the endocrine system (anterior pituitary), and the gonads themselves (ovaries and testes) (Fig. 31-3). The hypothalamus produces greater amounts of *gonadotropin-releasing hormone (GnRH),* which stimulate the anterior pituitary to increase its production of the *gonadotropins: luteinizing hormone (LH)* and *follicle-stimulating hormone (FSH).* These estrogens and testosterone then stimulate the gonads to produce more of the sex hormones (discussed in the sections on the female and male systems).

Increased sex hormone production causes the genitalia to grow into their adult proportions and stimulates the development of male and female secondary sex characteristics (beard, voice changes, breast development, and pubic and axillary hair). The most important hormonal effects occur in the gonads, however. In males, the testes begin to produce mature sperm capable of fertilizing an ovum. Male puberty is complete with the first ejaculation that contains mature sperm. In females, the ovaries begin to release mature ova. Female puberty is complete at the time of the first ovulatory menstrual period.

QUICK CHECK

Why are sex hormones crucial to reproduction?

THE FEMALE REPRODUCTIVE SYSTEM

In females, the most important reproductive organs, or genitalia, are internal. These organs are essential to reproduction and include ovaries, fallopian tubes, uterus, and vagina. The external genitalia protect body openings and play an important role in sexual functioning.[1-3]

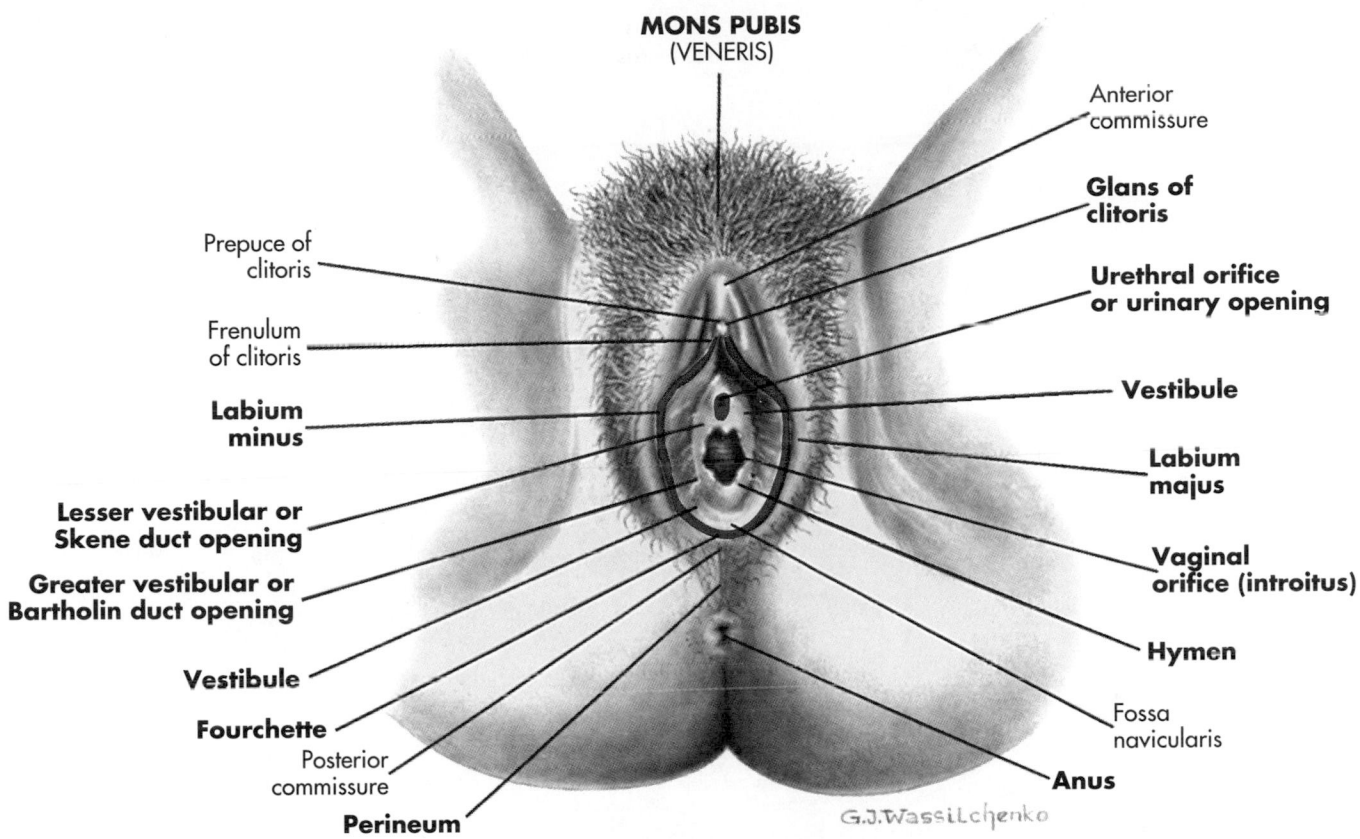

Fig. 31-4 *External female genitalia. (Modified from Lowdermilk, D.L., Perry, S.E., & Bobak, I.M. [1997]. Maternity and women's health care [6th ed.]. St. Louis: Mosby.)*

External Genitalia

Fig. 31-4 shows the external female genitalia, known collectively as the ***vulva,*** or pudendum. The major structures are as follows:

Mons pubis. Fatty layer of tissue over pubic symphysis (joint of the pubic bones); during puberty becomes covered with pubic hair and sebaceous and sweat glands become more active. Protects pubic symphysis during sexual intercourse.

Labia majora (sing., *labium majus*). Two folds of skin arising at mons pubis and extending back to fourchette, forming a cleft; during puberty amount of fatty tissue increases, pubic hair grows on lateral surfaces, and sebaceous glands on hairless medial surfaces secrete lubricants. Highly sensitive to temperature, touch, pressure, and pain; homologous to the male scrotum. Protect inner structures of vulva.

Labia minora (sing., *labium minus*). Two smaller, thinner folds of skin within labia majora that form the clitoral hood (prepuce) and frenulum, then split to enclose vestibule, and converge near anus to form fourchette. Hairless, pink, moist, well supplied with nerves, blood vessels, and sebaceous glands that secrete bactericidal fluid with distinctive odor that lubricates and waterproofs vulvar skin. Swell with blood during intercourse.

Clitoris. Richly innervated erectile organ between labia minora; has a visible glans and a shaft that lies beneath the skin, homologous to penis. Secretes smegma with unique odor that may be sexually arousing to male; fills with blood during sexual arousal. Major site of sexual stimulation and orgasm.

Vestibule. Area protected by labia minora that contains openings to vagina and urethra.

Introitus. Vaginal orifice covered by thin, perforated membrane (hymen).

Skene glands. Lesser vestibular or paraurethral glands that secrete fluids that help to lubricate the urinary meatus and vestibule and facilitate coitus.

Bartholin glands. Greater vestibular or vulvovaginal glands that secrete mucus to lubricate the inner labial surfaces and enhance the viability and motility of sperm. Also facilitate coitus.

Perineum. Area with less hair, skin, and subcutaneous tissue lying between vaginal orifice and anus; contains very little subcutaneous fat, so skin lies just above underlying muscles; stretches remarkably.

Perineal body. Fibrous structure composed of elastic fiber, connective tissue, and common attachment of bulbocavernosus, external anal sphincter, and levator ani muscles; covered by perineum.

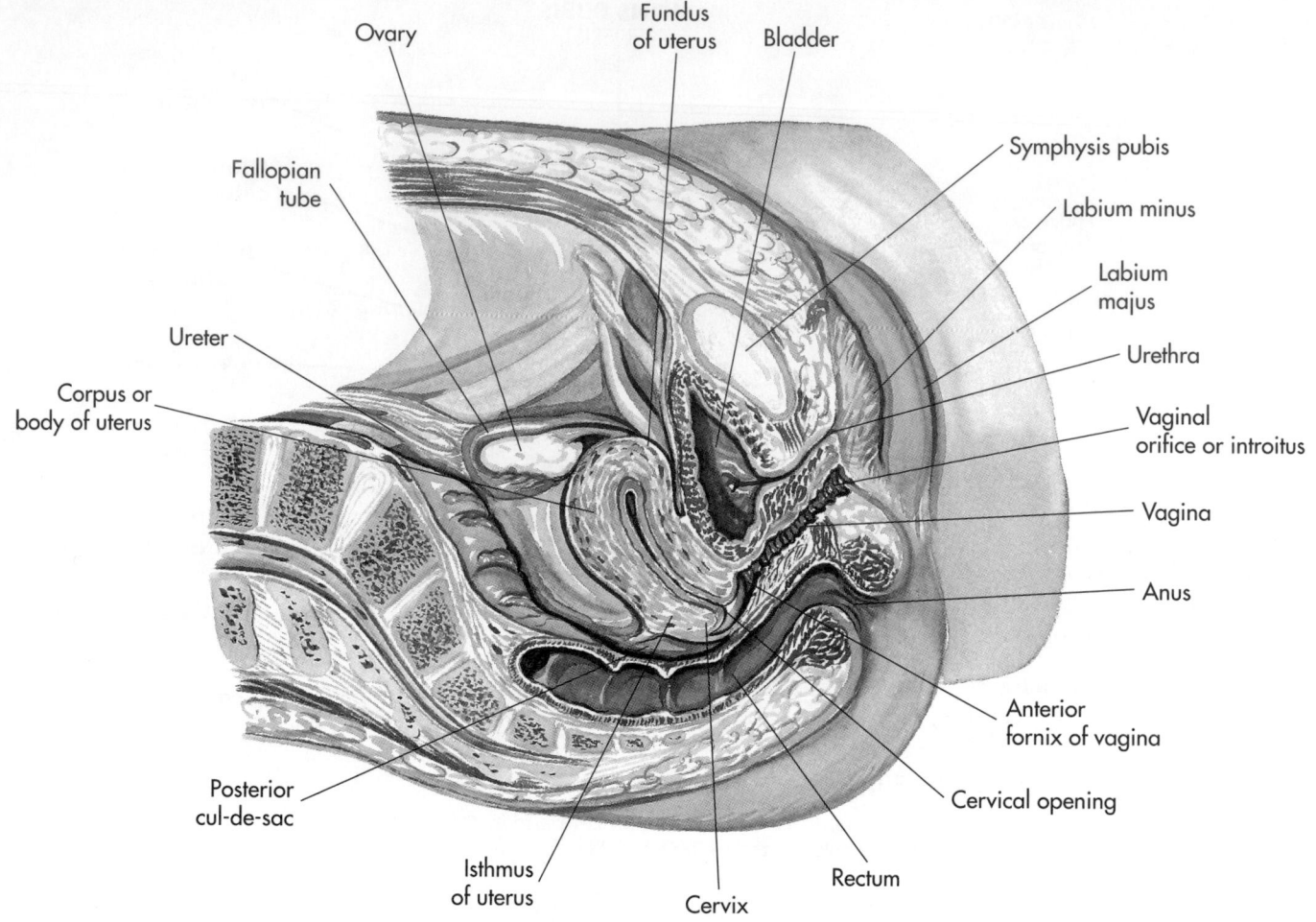

Fig. 31-5 *Internal female genitalia and other pelvic organs.* Midsagittal view, with woman lying supine. *(Modified from Lowdermilk, D.L., Perry, S.E., & Bobak, I.M. [1997].* Maternity and women's health care *[6th ed.]. St. Louis: Mosby.)*

Internal Genitalia
Vagina

The *vagina* is an elastic, fibromuscular canal that is 9 to 10 cm in length. It extends up and back from the introitus to the lower portion of the uterus. As Fig. 31-5 shows, the vagina lies between the urethra (and part of the bladder) and the rectum. Mucosal secretions from the upper genital organs, menstrual fluids, and products of conception leave the body through the vagina, which also receives the penis during coitus. During sexual excitement, the vagina lengthens and widens and the anterior third becomes congested with blood.

The vaginal wall is composed of four layers:
1. Mucous membranous lining of squamous epithelial cells that thickens and thins in response to hormones, particularly estrogen; it is continuous with the membrane that covers the lower part of the uterus. In women of reproductive age, the mucosal layer is arranged in transverse wrinkles, or folds, called *rugae* (sing., *ruga*) that permit stretching during coitus and childbirth.

2. Fibrous connective tissue containing numerous blood and lymphatic vessels.
3. Smooth muscle.
4. Connective tissue and a rich network of blood vessels.

The upper part of the vagina surrounds the cervix, the lower end of the uterus (see Fig. 31-5). The recessed space around the cervix is called the *fornix* of the vagina. The posterior fornix is "deeper" than the anterior fornix because of the angle at which the cervix meets the vaginal canal. In most women this angle is about 90 degrees. A pouch called the *cul-de-sac* separates the posterior fornix and the rectum.

Its elasticity and relatively sparse nerve supply enhance the vagina's function as the birth canal. During sexual arousal the vaginal wall becomes engorged with blood, like the labia minora and clitoris. Engorgement pushes some fluid to the surface of the mucosa, enhancing lubrication. The vaginal wall does not contain mucus-secreting glands; rather, secretions drain into the vagina from the endocervical glands or enter from the vestibule.

Two factors help to maintain the self-cleansing action of the vagina and to defend it from infection, particularly during the reproductive years. They are (1) an acid-base balance that discourages the proliferation of most pathogenic bacteria and (2) the thickness of the vaginal epithelium. Before puberty, vaginal pH is about 7.0 (neutral) and the vaginal epithelium is thin. At puberty, the pH becomes more acidic (4.0 to 5.0) and the squamous epithelial lining thickens. These changes are maintained until menopause (cessation of menstruation), when the pH rises again to more alkaline levels and the epithelium thins out. Therefore protection from infection is greatest during the years when a woman is most likely to be sexually active. Both defenses are greatest when estrogen levels are high and the vagina contains a normal population of *Lactobacillus acidophilus,* a harmless resident bacterium that helps to maintain pH at acidic levels. Any condition that causes vaginal pH to rise, such as douching or use of vaginal sprays or deodorants, low estrogen levels, or destruction of *L. acidophilus* by antibiotics, lowers vaginal defenses against infection.

Uterus

The *uterus* is a hollow, pear-shaped organ whose lower end opens into the vagina. It anchors and protects a fertilized ovum, provides an optimal environment while the ovum develops, and pushes the fetus out at birth. In addition, the uterus plays an important role in sexual response and conception. During sexual excitement, the opening of the lower uterus (the cervix) dilates slightly. At the same time, the uterus increases in size and moves upward and backward, creating a tenting effect in the midvagina that results in the cervix "sitting" in a pool of semen. During orgasm, rhythmic contractions facilitate movement of sperm through the cervical os while enhancing physical pleasure.

At puberty, the uterus attains its adult size and proportions and descends from the abdomen to the lower pelvis, between the bladder and the rectum (see Fig. 31-5). The uterus of a mature, nonpregnant female is approximately 9 cm long and 6.5 cm wide, with muscular walls 3.5 cm thick.[1] It is held loosely in position by ligaments, peritoneal tissue folds, and pressure of adjacent organs, especially the urinary bladder, sigmoid colon, and rectum. In most women the uterus is tipped forward (anteverted) so that it rests on the urinary bladder, but it may be tipped backward (retroverted). Various degrees of flexion are normal (Fig. 31-6).

The uterus has two major parts: the body, or *corpus,* and the cervix (Fig. 31-7). The top of the corpus, above the insertion of the fallopian tubes, is called the *fundus.* The diameter of the uterine cavity is widest at the fundus and narrowest at the *isthmus,* just above the *cervix* (see Fig. 31-5). The cervix, or "neck of the uterus," extends from the isthmus to the vagina. The passageway between the cervix's upper opening (the internal os) and its lower opening (the external os) is called the *endocervical canal* (see Fig. 31-7). The entire uterus, like the upper vagina, is innervated exclusively by motor and sensory fibers of the autonomic nervous system.

The uterine wall is composed of three layers (see Fig.

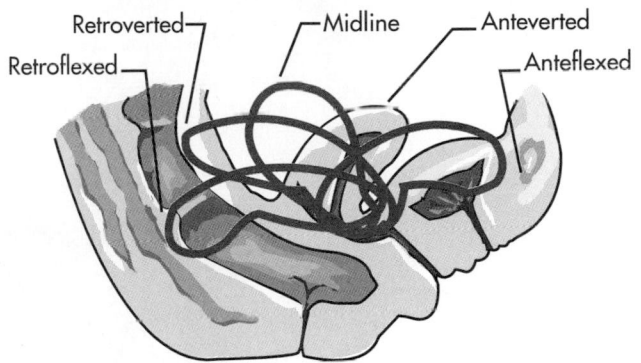

Fig. 31-6 *Variations in uterine position.*

31-7). The *perimetrium (parietal peritoneum)* is the outer serous membrane that covers the uterus. The *myometrium* is the thick, muscular middle layer. It is thickest at the fundus, apparently to facilitate birth. The *endometrium,* or uterine lining, is composed of a functional layer (superficial compact layer and spongy middle layer) and a basal layer. The functional layer of the endometrium responds to sex hormones. Between puberty and menopause, this layer proliferates and sloughs off monthly. The basal layer, which is attached to the myometrium, regenerates the functional layer after sloughing (menstruation).

The endocervical canal does not have an endometrial layer but is lined with columnar epithelial cells (see Fig. 1-29). It is continuous with the lining of the outer cervix and vagina, which are lined with squamous epithelial cells. The point where the two types of cells meet is called the *transformation zone,* or *squamous-columnar junction.* The transformation zone is the usual site of cervical dysplasia or carcinoma in situ.[1]

The cervix acts as a mechanical barrier to infectious microorganisms from the vagina. The external cervical os is a very small opening that contains thick, sticky mucus (the mucus "plug") during most of the menstrual cycle and all of pregnancy. In addition, the downward flow of cervical secretions moves microorganisms away from the cervix and uterus. In women of reproductive age, the pH of these secretions is inhospitable to most bacteria. Further, mucosal secretions contain enzymes and antibodies (mostly immunoglobulin A [IgA]) of the secretory immune system. Uterine pathophysiology includes infection, displacement of the uterus within the pelvis, benign growths of the uterine wall, and cancer.

✓ QUICK CHECK

Why are the functions of the external genitalia important?

Why does the vaginal environment change during the reproductive years?

Why does the uterine wall have three layers?

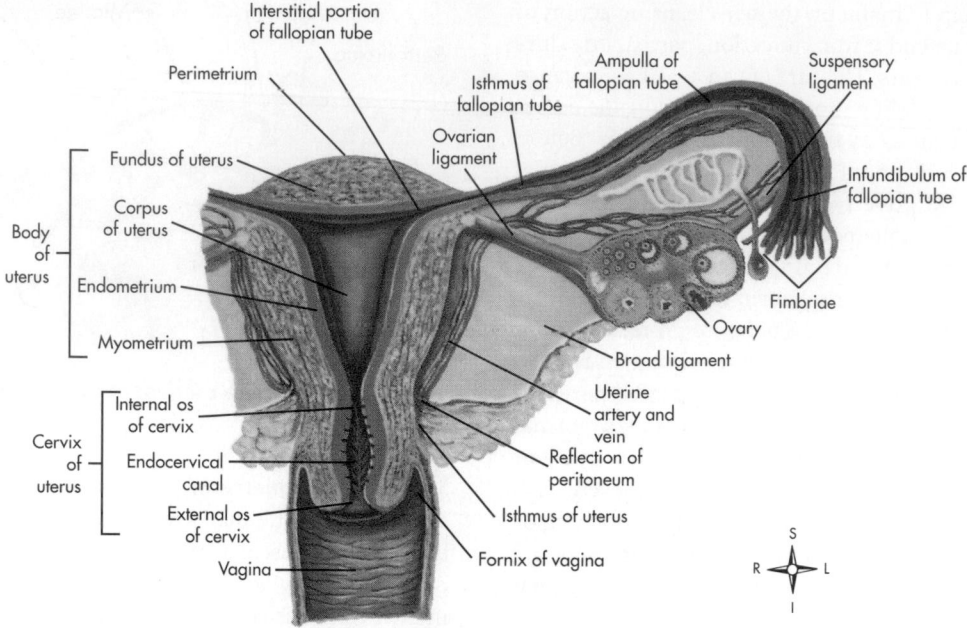

Fig. 31-7 *Cross section of uterus, fallopian tube, and ovary.* *(From Thibodeau, G.A. & Patton, K.T. [1999].* Anatomy & physiology *[4th ed.]. St. Louis: Mosby.)*

Fallopian tubes

The two *fallopian tubes* (oviducts, *uterine tubes*) enter the uterus bilaterally just beneath the fundus (see Fig. 31-7). They conduct the ova from the spaces around the ovaries to the uterus. From the uterus the fallopian tubes curve up and over the two ovaries. Each tube is 8 to 12 cm long and about 1 cm in diameter, except at its ovarian end, which flares out like the bell of a trumpet and is fringed or fimbriated *(infundibulum).* The *fimbriae* (fringes) move, creating a current that draws the ovum into the infundibulum. Once the ovum enters the fallopian tube, cilia and peristalsis (muscle contractions) keep it moving toward the uterus.

The ampulla, or distal third, of the fallopian tube is the usual site of fertilization (see Fig. 31-7). Sperm released into the vagina travel upward through the endocervical canal and uterine cavity and enter the fallopian tubes. If an ovum is present in either tube, fertilization can occur. Whether or not the ovum encounters sperm, it continues to travel through the fallopian tube to the uterus. If fertilized, the ovum (now called a *blastocyst*) implants itself in the endometrial layer of the uterine wall. If not fertilized, the ovum breaks down and leaves the uterus with menstrual fluids.

Disorders that affect the fallopian tubes (e.g., congenital malformations, infection, inflammation) block the path of both sperm and ovum and may cause infertility.

Ovaries

The *ovaries,* the female gonads, are the primary female reproductive organs. Their two main functions are secretion of female sex hormones and development and release of female gametes, or ova.

The almond-shaped ovaries are located on both sides of the uterus and are suspended and supported by the mesovarian portions of the broad ligament, ovarian ligaments, and suspensory ligaments (see Fig. 31-7). The ovaries are smaller than their male homologs, the testes. In women of reproductive age, each ovary is 3 to 5 cm long, 2.5 cm wide, and 2 cm thick and weighs 4 to 8 g. Size and weight vary somewhat from phase to phase of the menstrual cycle (see p. 847).

Fig. 31-8 shows a cross section of an ovary. At birth, the cortex of each ovary contains 200,000 to 400,000 *ova* within immature *ovarian follicles.* During puberty, some of the follicles and the ova within them begin to mature. Between puberty and menopause, the ovarian cortex always contains follicles and ova in various stages of development. Once every menstrual cycle (about every 28 days), one of the follicles reaches maturation and discharges its ovum through the ovary's outer covering, the germinal epithelium. During the reproductive years, 300 to 400 ovarian follicles mature completely and release an ovum *(ovulation).* The rest either fail to develop at all or degenerate without maturing completely.

Having ejected a mature ovum, the follicle develops into another structure, the *corpus luteum* (see Fig. 31-8). If fertilization occurs, the corpus luteum enlarges and begins to secrete hormones that maintain and support pregnancy. If fertilization does not occur, the corpus luteum secretes these hormones for approximately 14 days and then degenerates, which triggers the maturation of another follicle. The *ovarian cycle*—the process of follicular maturation, ovulation, corpus luteum development, and corpus luteum degeneration—is continuous from puberty to menopause, except during pregnancy. At menopause, this process ceases and the ovaries may

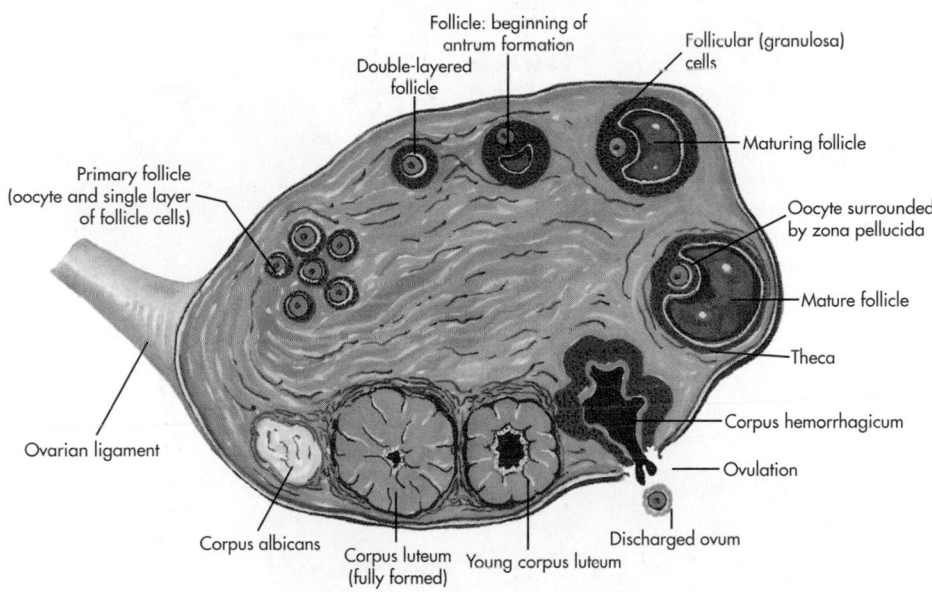

Fig. 31-8 *Cross section of ovary during reproductive years.* *(From Thibodeau, G.A. & Patton, K.T. [1999]. Anatomy & physiology [4th ed.]. St. Louis: Mosby.)*

shrink to the point that they cannot be felt during a pelvic examination.

Sex hormones are secreted by four types of cells present within the ovarian cortex: cells of the stroma, or tissue matrix; two types of cells in the ovarian follicle, *granulosa cells* and *theca cells;* and cells of the corpus luteum (Fig. 31-9). These cells all contain receptors for the gonadotropins (LH, FSH) or for the sex hormones, which are discussed in the next section.

Because ovarian function is regulated by hormones, any disorder that disrupts hormone secretion or reception by target cells can cause ovarian dysfunction and infertility. Ovarian pathologic conditions also can be caused by benign or malignant growths, cysts, infection, or inflammation.

Female Sex Hormones

The *sex hormones* are all steroid hormones; that is, they are synthesized from cholesterol (see Chapter 17). Most of them, both male and female, are present in adults of both genders all the time. The female body contains low levels of testosterone, for example, and the male body contains low levels of estrogen. The effects of the sex hormones depend on their amount and concentration in the blood.

Steroid hormones produced by the ovaries maintain female characteristics throughout life. During fetal development, infancy, and childhood, sex hormone production is low. At puberty, hormone production surges, causing sexual maturation and development of secondary sex characteristics. From puberty to menopause, the sex hormones control the ovarian-menstrual cycle, pregnancy, and lactation. The dominant female sex hormones are estrogen and proges-

terone.[1,2] These two hormones are not produced steadily. Rather, their production surges and diminishes monthly, creating the ovarian-menstrual cycle.

Estrogens

Estrogen is a generic term for any of three similar hormones: estradiol, estrone, and estriol. *Estradiol* is the most potent and plentiful of the three. The main site of estrogen production is the ovaries (ovarian follicle and corpus luteum), but limited amounts are secreted by the cortices of the adrenal glands and the placenta during pregnancy. Androgens are converted to estrogen in peripheral adipose tissue, which is the major source of estrogen in postmenopausal women and in men.

Estrogen is needed for maturation of reproductive organs, development of secondary sex characteristics, closure of long bones after the pubertal growth spurt, regulation of the ovarian-menstrual cycle, endometrial regeneration after menstruation, endometrial maintenance during pregnancy, and lactation. Estrogen also has metabolic effects on the bones, liver, blood vessels, blood, central nervous system, kidneys, and skin. During the reproductive years, estrogen helps to maintain the density of bone. The ovaries stop producing estrogen at menopause; for this reason postmenopausal women are susceptible to osteoporosis, a condition in which bone density is reduced.

Disturbances of estrogen production can be caused by abnormalities that affect (1) secretion of GnRH by the hypothalamus, (2) secretion of LH or FSH by the anterior pituitary, (3) hormonal feedback mechanisms, or (4) structural integrity of the ovaries. Estrogen's role in the menstrual cycle is described on p. 847.

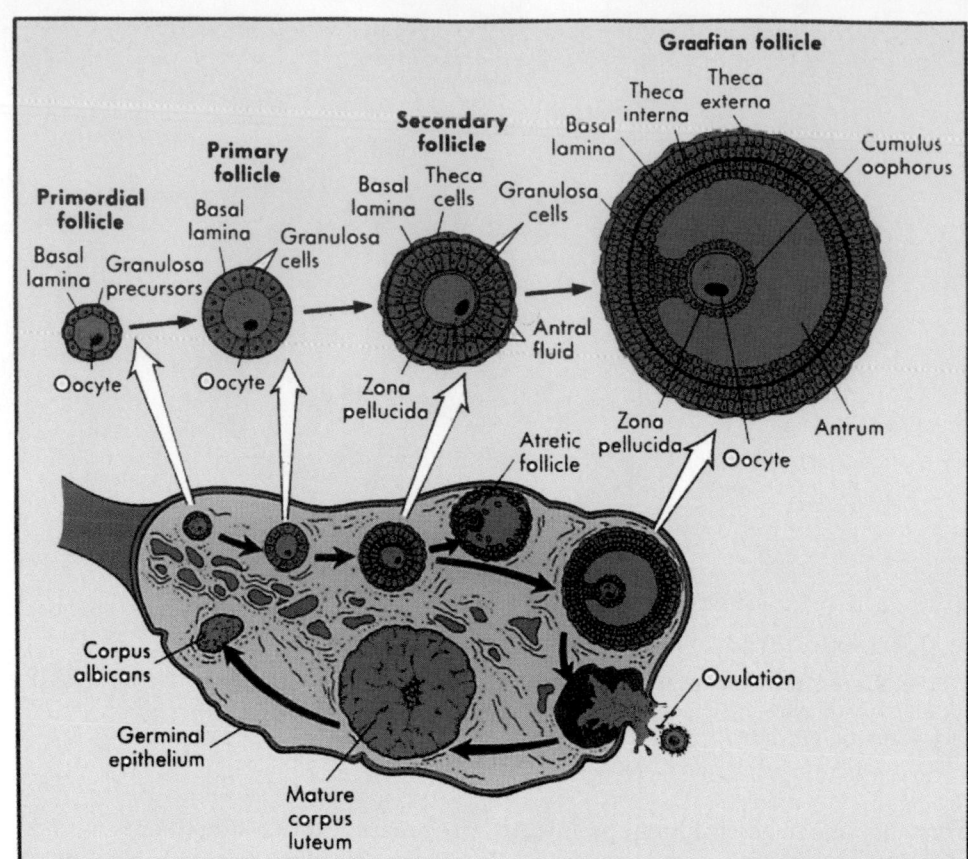

Fig. 31-9 *Development of an ovarian follicle.* Schematic representation (not to scale) of the structure of the ovary, showing the various stages in the development of the follicle and its successor structure, the corpus luteum. *(From Berne, R.M. & Levy, M.N. [Eds.]. [1998]. Physiology [4th ed.]. St. Louis: Mosby.)*

Progesterone

LH from the anterior pituitary stimulates the corpus luteum to secrete **progesterone,** the second major female sex hormone. With estrogen, progesterone controls the ovarian-menstrual cycle. Large amounts of progesterone are secreted while the corpus luteum is active, about 9 to 13 days after ovulation. Small amounts of progesterone are secreted by the adrenal cortices.

Progesterone secreted by the corpus luteum stimulates the thickened endometrium to become more complex in preparation for implantation of a blastocyte. If conception and implantation do occur, the corpus luteum persists and secretes progesterone (and estrogen) throughout pregnancy.

Progesterone is sometimes called the *hormone of pregnancy.* During pregnancy, it is produced not only by the corpus luteum but also by the placenta. Its effects in pregnancy include (1) maintenance of the thickened endometrium; (2) relaxation of smooth muscle in the myometrium, which prevents premature contractions and helps the uterus to expand; (3) thickening of the myometrium, which prepares it for the muscular work of labor; and (4) prevention of lactation until the fetus is born. Progesterone and estrogen have some opposing and complementary effects, which are summarized in Table 31-1.

Androgens

Although **androgens** are primarily male sex hormones, small amounts of them are produced in the ovaries and adrenal cortices of females. Some androgens are precursors of female sex hormones, notably estrogen and androstenedione. At puberty, androgens contribute to the skeletal growth spurt and cause growth of pubic and axillary hair. The androgens also activate sebaceous glands, accounting for some cases of acne during puberty.

✓ QUICK CHECK

Why is the ovary considered the most essential female reproductive organ?

The Menstrual Cycle

Besides pregnancy, the obvious manifestation of female reproductive functioning is menstrual bleeding (the menses), which starts with **menarche** (first menstruation) and ends with **menopause.** In the United States, the average age of first menstruation is 12.5 years, with a range from 9 to 17 years. Menarche appears to be related to body weight, especially percentage of body fat (ratio of fat to lean tissue), which may trigger a change in the metabolic rate and lead to hormonal

TABLE 31-1	Complementary and Opposing Effects of Estrogen and Progesterone	
Structure	Effect of Estrogen	Effect of Progesterone
Vaginal mucosa	Proliferation of squamous epithelium; Increase in glycogen content of cells; layering (cornification) of cells	Thinning of squamous epithelium; decornification
Cervical mucosa	Production of abundant fluid secretions that favor survival and enhance motility of sperm	Production of thick, sticky secretions that tend to "plug" the cervical os
Smooth muscle of uterus and fallopian tubes	Increased motility and ciliary action	Decreased motility and ciliary action; relaxation of myometrium
Endometrium	Stimulation of growth; increase in number of receptors for progesterone	Activation of glands and blood vessels (thus contributes to growth); accumulation of glucogen and enzymes
Breasts	Promotion of effects of prolactin (hormone that stimulates milk production); breast cell growth	Inhibition of effects of prolactin; breast cell growth

changes associated with ovulation. At first, cycles are anovulatory and may vary in length from 10 to 60 days or more. As adolescence proceeds, regular patterns of menstruation and ovulation are established at intervals ranging between 30 and 35 days. During adulthood, menstruation continues to recur in a recognizable and characteristic pattern, with the length of the menstrual cycle varying considerably among women. The commonly accepted cycle average is 28 (25 to 30) days, with rhythmic intervals of 21 to 45 days considered normal. Presumably, this strict control of menses is related to sequential ovarian secretion of estrogen and progesterone that are delivered to the endometrium during an ovulatory cycle.

Phases of the menstrual cycle

The menstrual cycle consists of three phases of one event. The event is ovulation: the release of an ovum from a mature ovarian follicle. The three phases are the follicular/proliferative phase, the luteal/secretory phase, and menstruation (Fig. 31-10).

During *menstruation (menses),* the functional layer of the endometrium disintegrates and is discharged through the vagina. Menstruation is followed by the *follicular/proliferative phase.* This phase is named for two simultaneous processes: maturation of an ovarian follicle and proliferation of the endometrium (see Fig. 31-10). During this phase, the anterior pituitary gland secretes FSH, which causes an ovarian follicle to develop. While the follicle is developing, its granulosa cells secrete estrogen and the estrogen causes cells of the endometrium to proliferate. By the time the ovarian follicle is mature, the endometrial lining is restored and ovulation occurs.

Ovulation marks the beginning of the *luteal/secretory phase* of the menstrual cycle. The ovarian follicle begins its transformation into a corpus luteum (see Fig. 31-8). LH from the anterior pituitary stimulates the corpus luteum to secrete progesterone, which in turn initiates the secretory phase of endometrial development. Glands and blood vessels in the endometrium branch and curl throughout the

functional layer, and the glands begin to secrete a thin, glycogen-containing fluid. If conception occurs, the nutrient-laden endometrium is ready for implantation. If conception and implantation do not occur, the corpus luteum degenerates and ceases its production of progesterone and estrogen. Without progesterone or estrogen to maintain it, the endometrium enters the ischemic ("blood-starved") phase and disintegrates. Then menstruation occurs, marking the beginning of another cycle.

Ovulatory cycles appear to have a minimum length of 25 to 26 days: the ovarian follicle requires 10 to 12.5 days to develop, and the luteal phase appears fixed at 14 days. Menstrual blood flow usually lasts 3 to 7 days but may last as long as 8 days or stop after 2 days and still be considered within normal limits. Bleeding is consistently scant to heavy and varies from 30 ml to 100 ml, with most blood loss occurring during the first 3 days of menses. Menstrual discharge consists of blood, mucus, and desquamated endometrial tissue and fails to clot under normal circumstances. It is usually dark and produces a characteristic musty odor on oxidation. Environmental factors (e.g., severe emotional stress, illness, malnutrition, seasonal variation) may affect the length of the menstrual cycle.

Hormonal controls

Hormonal control of the menstrual cycle depends on complex interactions among the hypothalamus, the anterior pituitary, and the ovaries (Table 31-2).[1] GnRH is secreted by the hypothalamus into the hypophyseal portal system and travels to the anterior pituitary, where it stimulates the secretion of FSH and LH. FSH and LH are released from the anterior pituitary in pulses that correspond to the secretion of GnRH.

Blood levels of estrogen and progesterone exert a feedback effect on the anterior pituitary, thereby determining how much and when FSH and LH are secreted (Table 31-2). During the early follicular phase, low levels of estrogen inhibit the FSH-secreting cells of the anterior pituitary. In addition, the developing ovarian follicle secretes *inhibin,* a

Fig. 31-10 *The menstrual cycle.* FSH, Follicle-stimulating hormone; *LH,* luteinizing hormone. *(Modified from Lowdermilk, D.L., Perry, S.E., & Bobak, I.M. [1997].* Maternity and women's health *[6th ed.]. St. Louis: Mosby.)*

protein hormone that inhibits both GnRH and FSH secretion. As the ovarian follicle grows, it produces more and more estrogen. During the late follicular phase, a rise in progesterone facilitates a positive feedback loop whereby estrogen levels begin to increase, stimulating a surge of FSH and LH secretion from the anterior pituitary. The midcycle surge of LH causes ovulation. Rising estrogen and progesterone levels during the luteal phase may inhibit the anterior pituitary and thus LH and FSH secretion. Just before menstruation, FSH and LH levels begin to increase slightly, probably because of declining estrogen and progesterone levels.

Ovarian cycle

To grow and mature, ovarian follicles require FSH, LH, and estradiol. At the end of a cycle in which pregnancy does not occur, FSH and LH levels increase slightly (see Fig. 31-10) and several ovarian follicles begin to mature. Granulosa cells

multiply, increasing the secretion of estradiol. Then one follicle becomes dominant and the others atrophy. The dominant follicle begins to secrete progressively larger amounts of estradiol, which causes the LH surge. Ovulation occurs about 16 hours after the LH surge. Progesterone, proteolytic enzymes, and prostaglandins (E and F series) trigger follicular rupture and release of the ovum.

The LH surge also transforms the granulosa cells of the ovulatory follicle into the corpus luteum. This secretes both estrogen and progesterone in amounts that depend, in part, on adequate development of the follicle before ovulation. If pregnancy does not occur, the corpus luteum persists for 14 days and then regresses and eventually disappears.

Uterine phases

Uterine phases of the menstrual cycle—the proliferative phase, the secretory phase, and menstruation—involve the

TABLE 31-2	Hormonal Feedback Mechanisms in the Menstrual Cycle		
Phase of Cycle and Ovarian Hormone Levels	**Feedback to Hypothalamus and Anterior Pituitary**	**Resultant GnRH, FSH, and LH Levels**	**Ovarian and Menstrual Events**
Early follicular phase: estrogen levels low; no progesterone secreted	Negative and inhibitory	All low	Ovarian follicle develops; endometrium proliferates
Late follicular (preovulatory) phase: estrogen levels high; minute amount of progesterone secreted	Positive and stimulatory	All surge; LH dominates	Process of ovulation begins; endometrial proliferation complete
Ovulatory phase: estrogen levels dip; progesterone levels begin to rise	Negative and inhibitory	All fall sharply	Corpus luteum begins to develop; endometrium enters secretory phase
Early luteal phase: estrogen and progesterone levels high; progesterone dominates	Negative and inhibitory	All continue to decline, but gradually	Corpus luteum fully developed; endometrium ready for implantation
Late luteal phase: estrogen and progesterone levels fall sharply	Negative and inhibitory; feedback lessens slightly	All rise slightly	Corpus luteum regresses; endometrium becomes ischemic and breaks down; menstruation begins
Menstrual phase: estrogen levels low; no progesterone secreted	Negative and inhibitory	All low	More ovarian follicles begin to develop; functional layer of endometrium is shed

GnRH, *Gonadotropin-releasing hormone;* FSH, *follicle-stimulating hormone;* LH, *luteinizing hormone.*

cyclic changes that occur in the endometrium. During the midfollicular phase, increasing levels of estrogen contribute to endometrial repair and proliferation, thus increasing endometrial thickness. Once ovulation occurs and serum progesterone levels increase, the endometrial tissue develops secretory characteristics. If implantation of a fertilized ovum does not take place, endometrial tissue begins to break down approximately 11 days after ovulation (ischemic phase of menstruation; see Fig. 31-10). Sloughing of tissue (menstrual bleeding) begins about 14 days after ovulation.

Cervical mucus also undergoes cyclic changes. During the proliferative phase, the cervical mucus is thin and watery. With the preovulatory surge of LH and estradiol, it becomes thicker and more elastic (spinnbarkeit). Increasing progesterone levels apparently contribute to the development of tiny channels in cervical mucus, providing access for sperm. Changes in the consistency of cervical mucus can be used to identify fertile intervals.

Vaginal response

The vaginal endothelium also responds to the cyclic hormonal changes of the menstrual cycle. Under the influence of estrogen, cells of the vaginal epithelium grow maximally during the follicular/proliferative phase. After ovulation, layers of keratinized cells overgrow the basal epithelium, a process known as **cornification.** Near the end of the luteal phase, leukocytes invade vaginal epithelium, removing the outer layers in a process termed **decornification.**

Body temperature

Basal body temperature (BBT) undergoes characteristic biphasic changes during menstrual cycles in which ovulation occurs. During the follicular phase, the BBT fluctuates around 98° F (37° C). During the luteal phase, the average temperature increases by 0.4° to 1.0° F (0.2° to 0.5° C). At the end of the luteal phase, 1 to 3 days before the onset of menstruation, BBT declines to follicular-phase levels. The shift in temperature is related to ovulation, corpus luteum formation, and increased serum progesterone levels. Progesterone probably acts on the thermoregulatory center of the hypothalamus to increase body temperature. Changes in BBT are used to document ovulatory cycles but are not useful to predict the exact timing of ovulation.

✓ QUICK CHECK

Why does menstruation occur?

THE MALE REPRODUCTIVE SYSTEM

In men, the external genitalia perform the major functions of reproduction. Sperm are produced in the male gonads, the testes, and delivered by the penis. The internal male genitalia have a more accessory function. They consist of conducting tubes and fluid-producing glands, all of which aid in the transport of sperm from the testes to the urethral open-

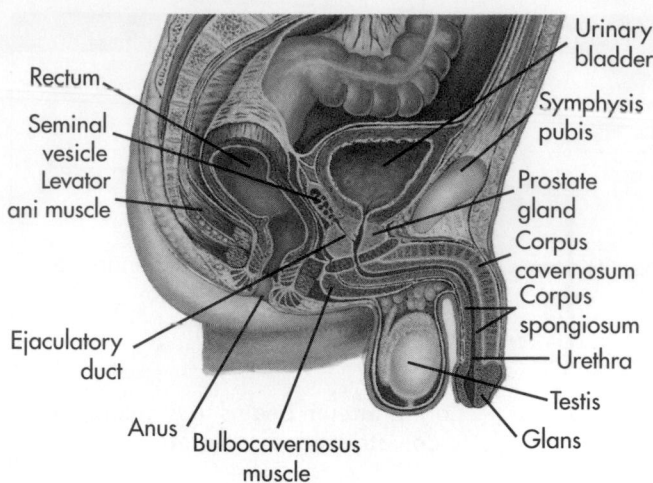

Fig. 31-11 *Structure of the male reproductive organs.* (From *Thibodeau, G.A. & Patton, K.T. [1999].* Anatomy & physiology *[4th ed.] St. Louis: Mosby.)*

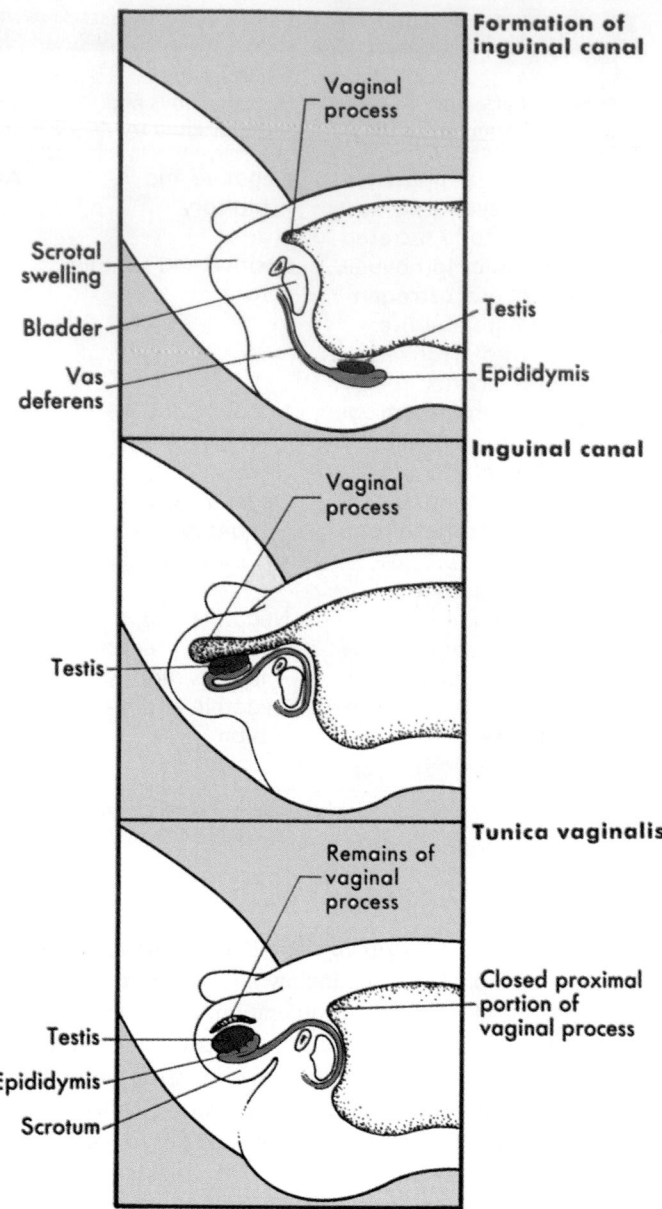

Fig. 31-12 *Descent of a testis.* The testes descend from the abdominal cavity to the scrotum during the last 3 months of fetal development.

ing of the penis. The male reproductive and urinary structures are shown in Fig. 31-11.

External Genitalia
Testes

In men, the testes are the essential organs of reproduction.[4] Like the ovaries, the testes have two functions: (1) production of gametes (i.e., sperm) and (2) production of sex hormones (i.e., androgens and testosterone). The testes are suspended outside the pelvic cavity.

During embryonic and fetal life, the testes develop within the abdomen (see Fig. 31-1). About 3 months before birth, the testes start to descend toward the developing scrotum. About 1 month before birth, they enter twin passageways called *inguinal canals.* The inguinal canals are vaginal processes created by outpouchings of the peritoneum (lining of the abdominal cavity). The descent of a *testis* is shown in Fig. 31-12. When descent is complete, the abdominal end of each vaginal process closes up and the inguinal canal disappears. Failure of the testes to descend through the inguinal canal is known as *cryptorchidism.* The scrotal end of each vaginal process becomes the outer covering of the testis, the *tunica vaginalis.*

Fig. 31-13 shows a sagittal section of a mature testis. The adult testis is ovoid and varies considerably in length (3 to 6 cm), width (2 to 3.5 cm), depth (3 to 4 cm), and weight (10 to 40 g). The testis is almost entirely surrounded by the tunica vaginalis, which separates the testis from the scrotal wall, and the *tunica albuginea.* Inward extensions of the tunica albuginea separate the testis into about 250 compartments, or lobules, each of which contains several tortuously coiled ducts called *seminiferous tubules.* Sperm are produced in these tubules. (Sperm production, termed *spermatogenesis,* is described on p. 854.) Tissue surrounding these ducts contains *Leydig cells,* which occur in clusters and produce androgens, chiefly testosterone.

The two ends of each seminiferous tubule join and leave the lobule through the *tubulus rectus.* Sperm travel from the seminiferous tubules into these straight sections, which lead to the central portion of the testis, the *rete testis.* The sperm then move through the *efferent tubules,* or vasa efferentia, to the epididymis, where they mature.

The testes are innervated by adrenergic fibers, whose sole function apparently is to regulate blood flow to the Leydig cells. The testes receive arterial blood from the internal spermatic and differential arteries. Arterial blood flows over the surface of the testes before entering the parenchyma (functional tissues). Surface flow cools the blood to temperatures that promote spermatogenesis, approximately 1° to 2° C below body core temperature.

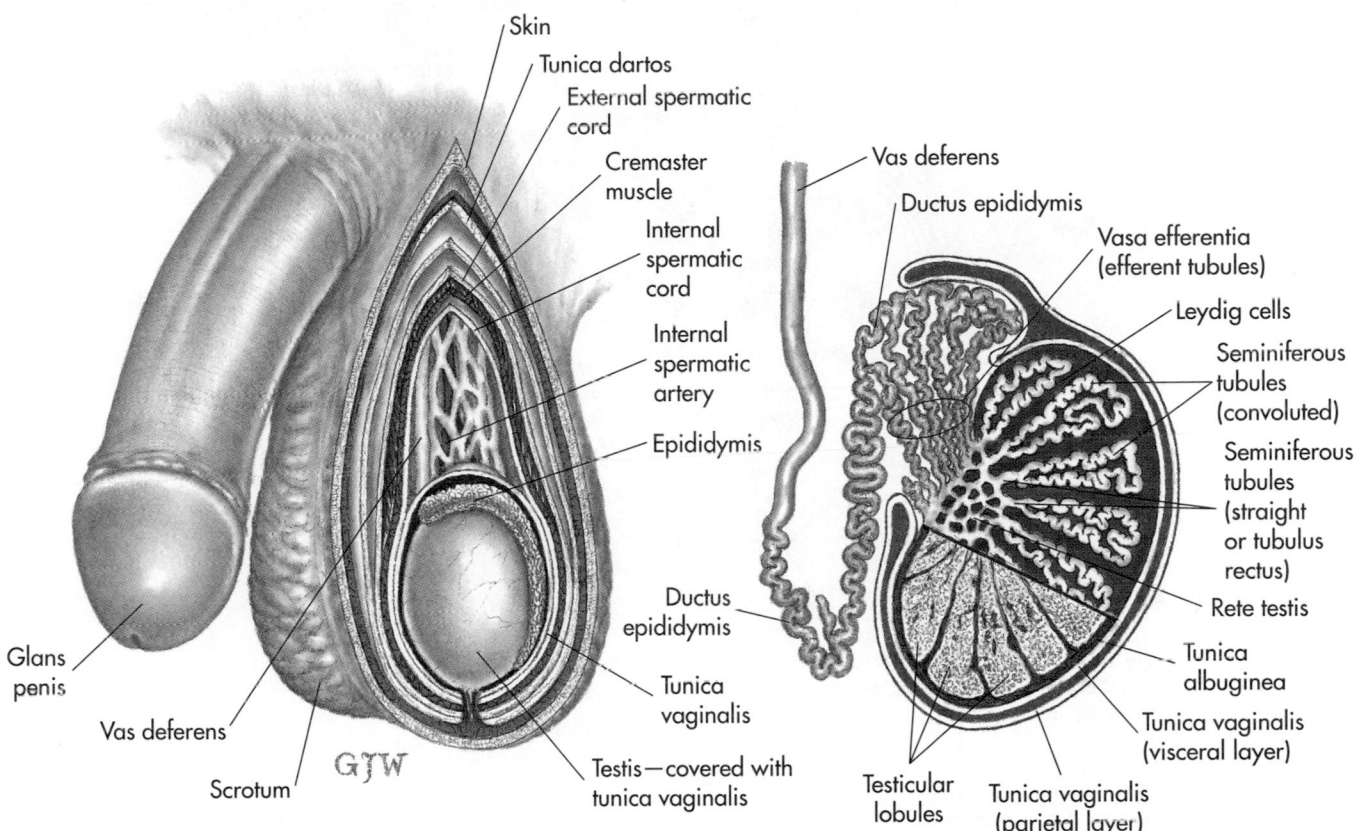

Fig. 31-13 *The testes.* External and sagittal views showing interior anatomy. *(Modified from Tanagho, E.A. & McAninch, D.W. [Eds.]. [1992]. Smith's general urology [13th ed.]. Norwalk, Conn.: Appleton & Lange.)*

Epididymis

The *epididymis* (pl., epididymides) is a comma-shaped structure that curves over the posterior portion of each testis (see Fig. 31-13). It consists of a single, 60 to 70 cm, densely packed and markedly coiled duct measuring 5 cm in length, whose structural function is to conduct sperm from the efferent tubules to the vas deferens. The epididymis has physiologic functions as well. When sperm enter the head of the epididymis, they are not fully mature or motile, nor can they fertilize an ovum. During the 12 days (or more) sperm take to travel the length of the epididymis, they receive nutrients and testosterone from the epididymal epithelium and their capacity for fertilization is enhanced.

The tail of the epididymis is continuous with the *vas deferens,* a duct with muscular layers capable of powerful peristalsis that transports sperm toward the urethra. After traveling the length of the epididymis, sperm are stored in the epididymal tail and vas deferens. The vas deferens enters the pelvic cavity through the spermatic cord (see Fig. 31-13).

Scrotum

The testes, epididymides, and spermatic cord are enclosed and protected by the *scrotum,* a skin-covered, fibromuscular sac homologous to the female labia majora (see Fig. 31-2). The skin of the scrotum is thin and has rugae (wrinkles or folds), which enable it to enlarge or relax away from the body. At puberty the scrotal skin darkens, develops active sebaceous glands, and becomes sparsely covered with hair. Just under the skin lies a layer of connective tissue (fascia) and smooth muscle, the *tunica dartos* (see Fig. 31-13). The tunica dartos also forms a septum that separates the two testes. Exposure to cold temperatures causes the tunica dartos to contract, pulling the testes close to the warm body. In warm temperatures the tunica dartos relaxes, suspending the testes away from body heat. These mechanisms promote optimal temperatures for spermatogenesis. In addition, scrotal sensitivity to touch, pressure, temperature, and pain protects the testes from potential harm. During sexual excitement, the scrotal skin and tunica thicken, the scrotum tightens and lifts, and the spermatic cords shorten, partially elevating the testes toward the body. As excitement plateaus, the engorged testes increase 50% in size, rotate anteriorly, and flatten against the body, signaling impending ejaculation.

Penis

The *penis* has two main functions: delivery of sperm and elimination of urine. (Urine formation and excretion are discussed in Chapter 28.) Embryonically, the penis is homologous to the female clitoris (see Fig. 31-2).

Fig. 31-11 shows a sagittal section of the adult penis and

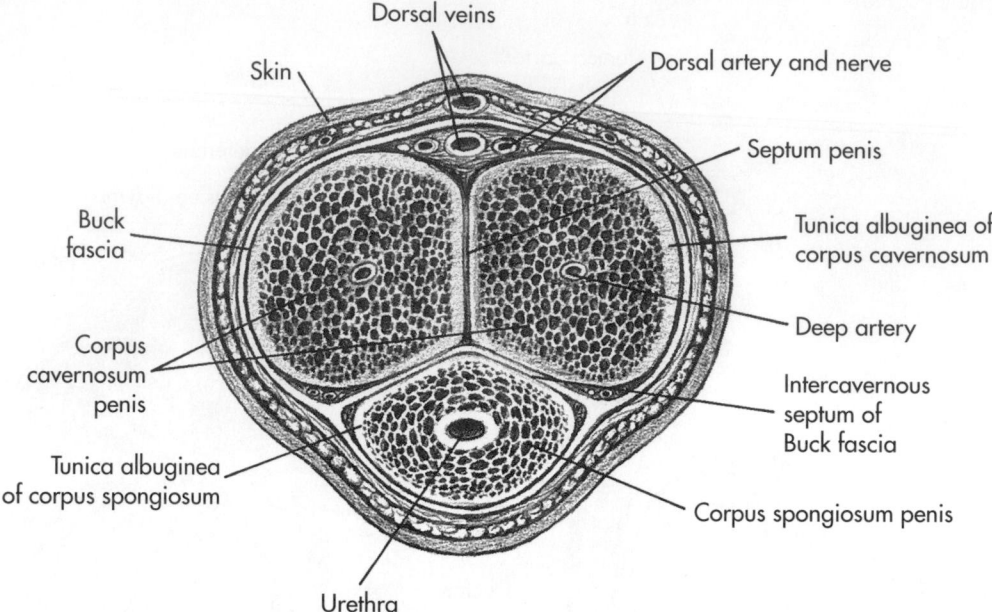

Dorsal veins

Skin

Dorsal artery and nerve

Septum penis

Buck fascia

Tunica albuginea of corpus cavernosum

Corpus cavernosum penis

Deep artery

Intercavernous septum of Buck fascia

Tunica albuginea of corpus spongiosum

Corpus spongiosum penis

Urethra

Fig. 31-14 *Cross section of the penis.* (*From Thompson, J.M. et al. [Eds.]. [1997].* Mosby's clinical nursing *[4th ed.]. St. Louis: Mosby.*)

its anatomic relation to other urogenital structures. Externally, the penis consists of a shaft with a tip, the *glans,* which contains the opening of the urethra (see Fig. 31-13). The skin of the glans folds over the tip of the penis, forming the *prepuce,* or *foreskin.* The skin of the penis is continuous with that of the groin, scrotum, and inner thighs. It is hairless, movable, and darker than surrounding skin.

Internally, the penis consists of the urethra and three compartments: two *corpora cavernosa* and the *corpus spongiosum* (Fig. 31-14) separated by Buck fascia; like the testes, the compartments are enclosed by a tunica albuginea. The *urethra* passes through the corpus spongiosum and ends at a sagittal slit in the glans. If the urethra is not completely surrounded by the corpus spongiosum, the meatus may open on the ventral surface of the penile shaft (hypospadias) or on the dorsal surface (epispadias).

Penetration of the female vagina is made possible by the *erectile reflex,* a process in which erectile tissues within the corpora cavernosa and corpus spongiosum become engorged with blood, generally 20 to 50 ml. The erectile tissues consist of vascular spaces, or chambers, supplied with blood by arterioles (small arteries). Usually, the arterioles are constricted, so that not much blood flows through the erectile tissues. Sexual stimulation, however, causes the arterioles to dilate and fill with blood, expanding the erectile tissues and causing an erection. Erection apparently is maintained by compression or constriction of veins that drain the corpora cavernosa and corpus spongiosum. When sexual stimulation ceases or orgasm and ejaculation occur, these veins open up, blood flows out of the arterioles, and the penis becomes flaccid (soft and pendulous).[5]

Erection is under the control of the autonomic nervous system but can be stimulated or inhibited by central nervous system input. Stimulation of mechanoreceptors of the penis, particularly of the glans, causes parasympathetic nerves of the autonomic nervous system to relax smooth muscle in the walls of penile arterioles. At the same time the effects of sympathetic nerves, which normally cause arteriolar smooth muscle to constrict, are inhibited.

Erections begin in utero and continue throughout life, but ejaculation does not occur until sperm production begins at puberty. Growth of the penis and scrotal contents continues well past puberty, however, and may not be complete until the late teens or early 20s. Penis size, when flaccid, varies considerably; with an erection, difference in penis size diminishes. Sexual excitement causes the corpora cavernosa to increase in length and width and become rigid; the penis becomes erect. Stimulation of the glans, which is endowed with copious sensitive nerve endings, provides maximum erotic sensation. With sexual arousal, skin color deepens, the glans doubles in size, and the urethral meatus dilates. Ejaculation occurs with frequent, strong contractions of the vas deferens, epididymis, seminal vesicles, prostate, urethra, and penis.

Internal Genitalia

Fig. 31-11 shows the anatomy of the internal genitalia and their relation to other pelvic organs. The internal genitalia consist of ducts and glands, as follows:

Ducts: consist of two vasa deferentia, ejaculatory duct, urethra; conduct sperm and glandular secretions from testes to urethral opening of the penis

Glands: consist of prostate gland, two seminal vesicles, two Cowper (bulbourethral) glands; secrete fluids that serve

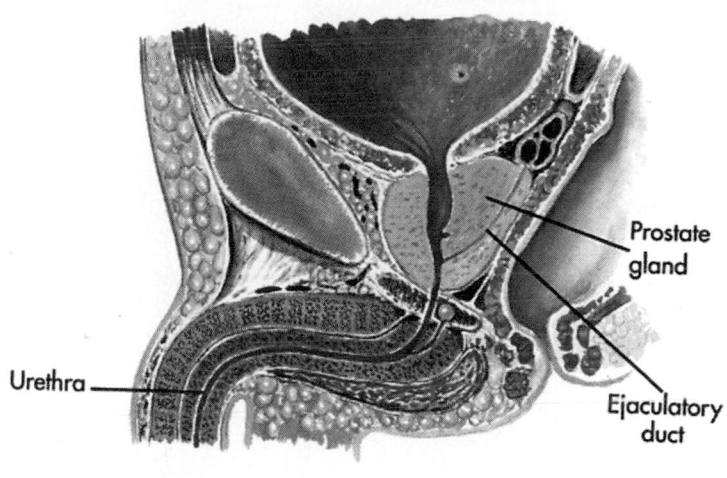

Fig. 31-15 *Anatomy of the prostate gland and seminal vesicles.* (From Seidel, H.M. et al. [1999]. Mosby's guide to physical examination [4th ed.]. St. Louis: Mosby.)

as a vehicle for sperm transport and create nutritious alkaline medium that promotes sperm motility and survival

Together the sperm and the glandular fluids compose *semen.*

Sperm leave the epididymides and travel rapidly through the internal ducts *(emission).* Emission occurs just seconds before ejaculation, at the moment when sexual arousal peaks. It always leads to ejaculation.

Emission occurs as smooth muscle in the walls of the epididymides and vasa deferentia begins to contract rhythmically, pushing sperm and epididymal secretions through the vasa deferentia. Each vas deferens is a firm, elastic, fibromuscular tube that begins at the tail of the epididymis, enters the pelvic cavity within the spermatic cord, loops up and over the bladder, and ends in the prostate gland (Figs. 31-11 and 31-15). Sperm are moved along by peristaltic contractions of smooth muscle in the walls of the vas deferens.

As sperm leave the ampulla (wide portion) of the vas deferens, the seminal vesicles secrete a nutritive, glucose-rich fluid into the ejaculate (semen). The *seminal vesicles* are glands about 4 to 6 cm long that lie behind the urinary bladder and in front of the rectum. The ducts of the seminal vesicles join the ampulla of the vas deferens to become the *ejaculatory duct,* which contracts rhythmically during emission and ejaculation. As seen in Figs. 31-11 and 31-15, the ejaculatory duct joins the urethra, where both pass through the prostate gland. During emission and ejaculation, a sphincter (muscle surrounding a duct) closes, preventing urine from entering the prostatic urethra.

The *prostate gland* is composed of alveoli and ducts embedded in fibromuscular tissue. It measures 4 cm in diameter and weighs approximately 20 g. While semen moves through the prostatic portion of the urethra, the prostate gland contracts rhythmically and secretes prostatic fluid (a thin, milky substance with an alkaline pH that helps sperm to survive in the acid environment of the female reproductive tract) into the mixture. In addition, substances in seminal and prostatic fluids help to mobilize sperm after ejaculation.

HEALTH ALERT

Prostate-Specific Antigen Testing for Prostate Cancer

Routine screening for prostate cancer is recommended in men older than 50 years. The serum prostate-specific antigen (PSA) assay is the test most commonly recommended, combined with evaluation of symptoms and digital examination. However, because PSA lacks the sensitivity and specificity to adequately distinguish between prostatic cancer and benign prostatic hyperplasia, other diagnostic markers need to be identified and randomized clinical trials need to be conducted to support routine PSA screening.

Data from Lefevre, M.L. (1998). Prostate cancer screening: More harm than good? American Family Physician, 58(2), 432-443; *Roberts, R.O. et al. (1999). Decline in prostate cancer mortality from 1980 to 1997, and an update on incidence trends in Olmsted County, Minnesota.* Journal of Urology, 161(2), 529-533.

The last pair of glands to add fluid to the ejaculate are *Cowper glands (bulbourethral glands),* whose ducts secrete mucus into the urethra near the base of the penis. Ejaculation occurs as semen reaches the base of the penis and mus-

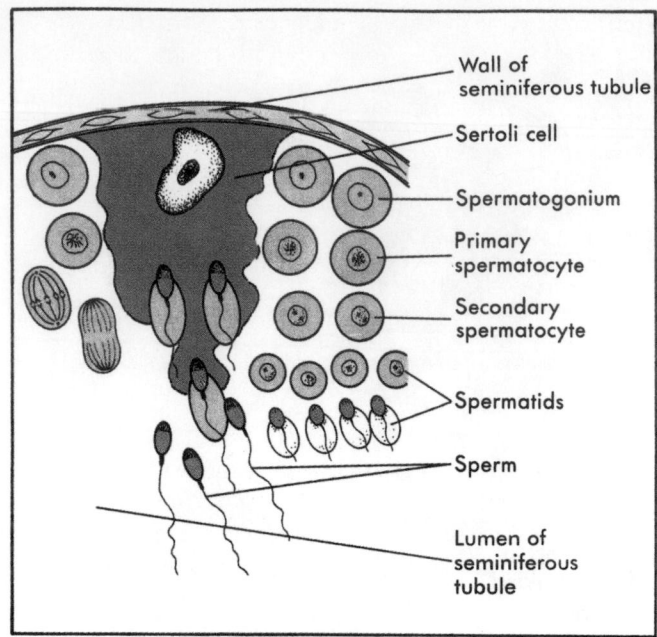

Fig. 31-16 *Spermatogenesis.* **A,** Cell division. **B,** Sperm developing within seminiferous tubule. *(From Bobak, I.M., Jensen, M.D., & Zalar, M.K. [1989].* Maternity and gynecologic care: The nurse and the family *[4th ed.]. St. Louis: Mosby.)*

cles there begin the rhythmic contractions that push semen out. Normally a man ejaculates between 2 and 6 ml of semen, containing 75 million to 400 million sperm. About 98% of the ejaculate consists of glandular fluids; 60% to 70% of volume comes from the seminal vesicles and 20% from the prostate. Therefore the ejaculate of a man who has undergone vasectomy (a surgical procedure that prevents sperm from entering the vas deferens) is reduced by only about 2%.

Spermatogenesis

Spermatogenesis begins at puberty and continues for life. In this respect, spermatogenesis differs markedly from oogenesis (production of primordial ova), which occurs during fetal life only.

Spermatogenesis takes place within the seminiferous tubules of the testes (see Fig. 31-13). The basement membrane of each seminiferous tubule is lined with diploid (46-chromosome) germ cells called *spermatogonia* (sing., spermatogonium). These cells undergo continuous mitotic division. (Mitotic division, in which a cell divides into two identical cells, is described in Chapter 1.) Some spermatogonia move away from the basement membrane and mature, becoming *primary spermatocytes* (Fig. 31-16). These undergo meiosis, a type of cell division that results in two haploid (23-chromosome) cells called *secondary spermatocytes.* (Meiosis is described and illustrated in Chapter 2.) The secondary spermatocytes then undergo meiosis, resulting in four *spermatids.* The spermatids differentiate into sperma-

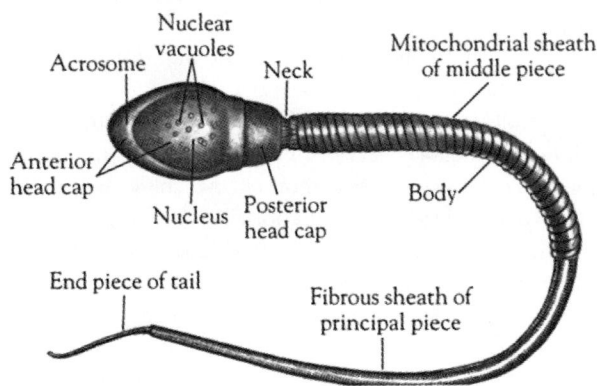

Fig. 31-17 *Mature sperm cell (spermatozoon). (From Thompson, J.M. et al. [Eds.]. [1997].* Mosby's clinical nursing *[4th ed.]. St. Louis: Mosby.)*

tozoa, or sperm, each of which contains 23 chromosomes (Fig. 31-17).

The development of spermatids into sperm depends on the presence of *Sertoli cells (nondividing support cells)* within the seminiferous tubules. The spermatids attach themselves to Sertoli cells, from which they receive the nutrients and the hormonal signals they need to develop into sperm.

The process of spermatogenesis, from mitotic division of a spermatogonium to maturation of the spermatids, takes about 70 to 80 days. Mature sperm migrate from the seminiferous tubules to the epididymides, where their capacity for fertilization continues to develop. Although they are completely mature by the time they are ejaculated, the sperm do not become motile (capable of movement) until they are activated by biochemicals in semen and in the female reproductive tract.

✓ QUICK CHECK

Why do sperm take 12 days to travel the length of the epididymis?

Male Sex Hormones

The male sex hormones are androgens. Testosterone, the primary male sex hormone, and other androgens are produced mainly by Leydig cells of the testes, but they are also produced by the adrenal glands. In men, sex hormone production is relatively constant and does not occur in a cyclic pattern, as it does in women.

The androgens' physiologic actions are related to the growth and development of male tissues and organs.[2,4,6] Androgens are responsible for the fetal differentiation and development of the male urogenital system and have some effects on the fetal brain. After birth, the Leydig cells become quiescent until activated by the gonadotropins during puberty. Then androgens cause the sex organs to grow and secondary sex characteristics to develop.

Testosterone affects nervous and skeletal tissues, bone marrow, skin and hair, and sex organs. It has an anabolic effect on skeletal muscle tissue, thereby contributing to the difference in body weight and composition between men and women. Testosterone also stimulates growth of the musculature and cartilage of the larynx, causing a permanent deepening of the voice. Testosterone directly stimulates the bone marrow and indirectly stimulates renal erythropoietin production to achieve increased hemoglobin and hematocrit levels. Because sebaceous gland activity is stimulated by testosterone, acne may develop. Hair becomes coarser in texture, and facial, axillary, and pubic hair grows in male patterns. Later in life, testosterone causes baldness in genetically susceptible individuals. Testosterone is required for spermatogenesis and for secretion of fluid by the prostate gland, seminal vesicles, and Cowper glands. Testosterone is also associated with an increase in libido (sex drive). Other, less-understood effects of testosterone include alterations in fatty acid and cholesterol metabolism.

The regulation of androgen production and spermatogenesis is achieved by a complex feedback system involving the extrahypothalamic central nervous system, the hypothalamus, the anterior pituitary, the testes, and the androgen-sensitive end organs. These relationships, which are essentially the same in women, are summarized in Fig. 31-3. Extrahypothalamic influences include such variables as physiologic and psychologic stress. These factors may inhibit or augment hypothalamic activity.

STRUCTURE AND FUNCTION OF THE BREAST

The **breasts** are modified sebaceous glands that lie on the ventral surface of the thorax, within the superficial fascia of the chest wall. They extend vertically from the second rib to the sixth or seventh intercostal space and laterally from the side of the sternum to the midaxillary line. Breast tissue also may extend into the axilla; this tissue is known as the tail of Spence.

The Female Breast

The female breast is composed of 15 to 20 pyramid-shaped lobes that are separated and supported by Cooper ligaments (Fig. 31-18). Each lobe contains 20 to 40 lobules (alveoli), which subdivide further into many functional units called *acini* (sing., acinus). Each acinus is lined with a layer of epithelial cells capable of secreting milk and a layer of subepithelial cells capable of contracting to squeeze milk from the acinus. The acini empty into a network of lobular collecting ducts, which empty into interlobular collecting and ejecting ducts. These ducts reach the skin through openings (pores) in the nipple. The lobes and lobules are surrounded and separated by muscle strands and fatty connective tissue.

An extensive capillary network surrounds the acini and is supplied by the internal and lateral thoracic arteries and the intercostal arteries. Venous return follows arterial supply, with relatively rapid emptying into the superior vena cava. The breasts receive sensory innervation from branches of the second and sixth intercostal nerves and the cervical plexus. This accounts for the fact that breast pain may be referred to the chest, back, scapula, medial arm, and neck. Lymphatic drainage of the breast occurs largely through axillary nodes, but approximately 25% occurs through transpectoral and internal mammary routes (Fig. 31-19).

The **nipple** is a pigmented, cylindrical structure usually located at the fourth or fifth intercostal space. On its surface lie multiple openings, one from each lobe. The **areola** is the pigmented, circular area around the nipple. It may be 15 to 60 mm in diameter. A number of sebaceous glands, the **glands of Montgomery,** are located within the areola and aid in lubrication of the nipple during lactation. The nipple and areola contain smooth muscles, which receive motor innervation from the sympathetic nervous system. Sexual stimulation and exposure to cold cause the nipple to become erect.

The fetal and early postnatal development of breast tissue does not depend on hormones, although fetal breast tissue does become progressively responsive to hormonal stimulation. During childhood, breast growth is latent and growth of the nipple and areola keeps pace with body surface growth. At the onset of puberty in the female, estrogen secretion stimulates mammary growth. Breast development, or **thelarche,** is usually the first sign of puberty in the female. Full differentiation and development of breast tissue are mediated by several hormones, including estrogen, proges-

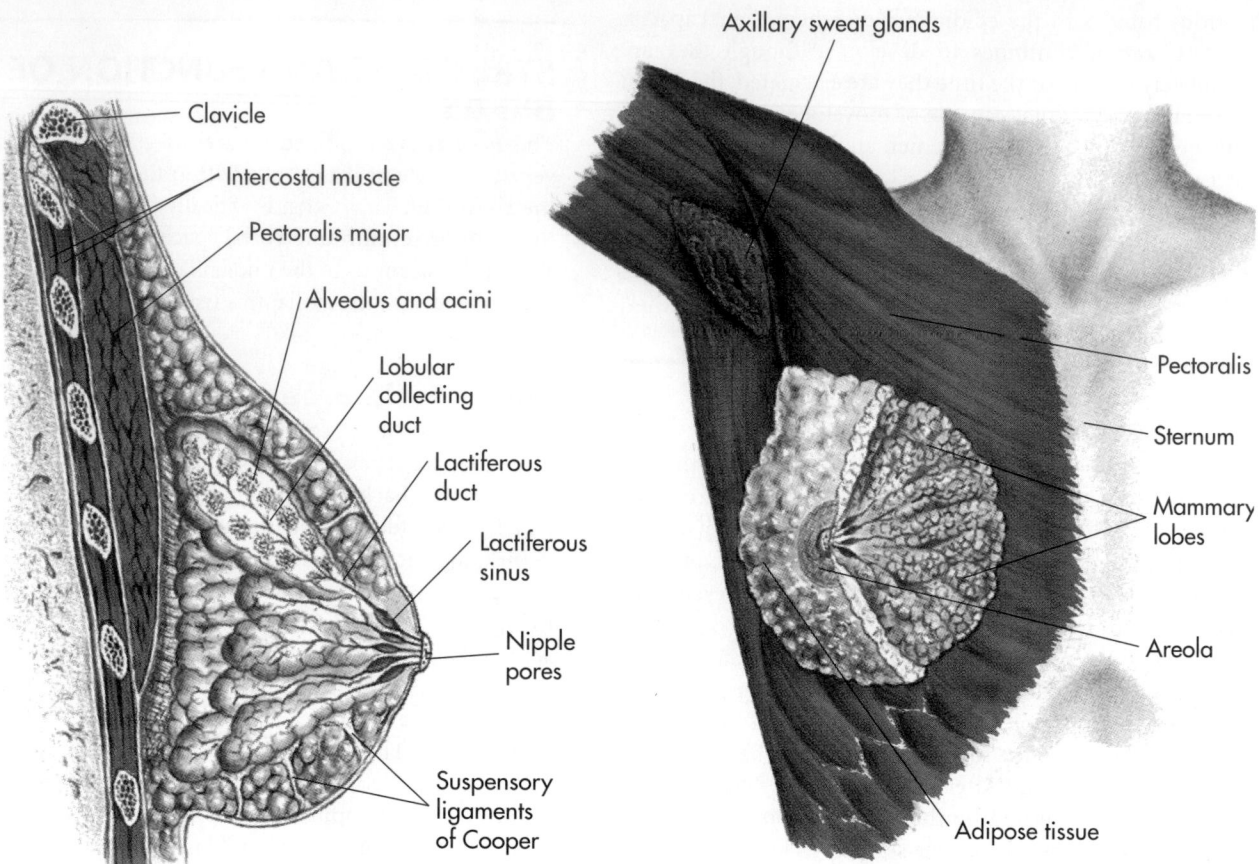

Fig. 31-18 *The female breast. (From Thompson, J.M. et al. [Eds.]. [1997].* Mosby's clinical nursing *[4th ed.]. St. Louis: Mosby.)*

terone, prolactin, growth hormone, thyroid hormone, insulin, and cortisol.

During the reproductive years, the breast undergoes cyclic changes in response to changes in the levels of estrogen and progesterone associated with the menstrual cycle. During the follicular/proliferative phase of the menstrual cycle, high estradiol levels increase the vascularity of breast tissue and stimulate proliferation of ductal and acinar tissue. This effect is sustained into the luteal/secretory phase of the cycle. During this phase, progesterone levels increase and contribute to the breast changes induced by estradiol. Specific effects of progesterone include dilation of the ducts and conversion of the acinar cells into secretory cells. Most women experience some degree of premenstrual breast fullness, tenderness, and increased breast nodularity. Breast volume may increase as much as 10 to 30 ml. Because the length of the menstrual cycle does not allow for complete regression of new cell growth, breast growth continues at a slow rate until approximately 35 years of age. Because of the cyclic changes that occur in breast tissue, breast examination should be conducted at the conclusion of or a few days after the menstrual cycle, when hormonal effects are minimal and breasts are at their smallest.

The function of the female breast is primarily to provide a source of nourishment for the newborn. Physiologically, breast milk is the most appropriate nourishment for newborns. Not only does its composition change over time to meet the changing digestive capabilities and nutritional requirements of the infant, but also breast milk contains specific immunoglobulins, especially IgA, and nonspecific antimicrobial factors, such as lysosomes and lactoferrin, which protect the infant against infection. During lactation, high prolactin levels interfere with hypothalamic-pituitary hormones that stimulate ovulation. This mechanism suppresses the menstrual cycle and prevents ovulation. In many parts of the world (underdeveloped or Third World countries), breast-feeding is the major means of contraception. Breasts are also a source of pleasurable sexual sensation and in Western cultures have become a sexual symbol.

The Male Breast

Until puberty, development of the male breast is similar to that of the female breast. In the absence of sufficiently high levels of estrogen and progesterone, the male breast does not develop any further. The normal male breast consists of a small, underdeveloped nipple; some fatty and fibrous tissue; and a few ductlike structures in the subareolar area. The male breast may appear enlarged in obese men because of accumulation of fatty tissue. During puberty, some males experience gynecomastia, a condition in which the breasts enlarge temporarily as a result of hormonal fluctuations.

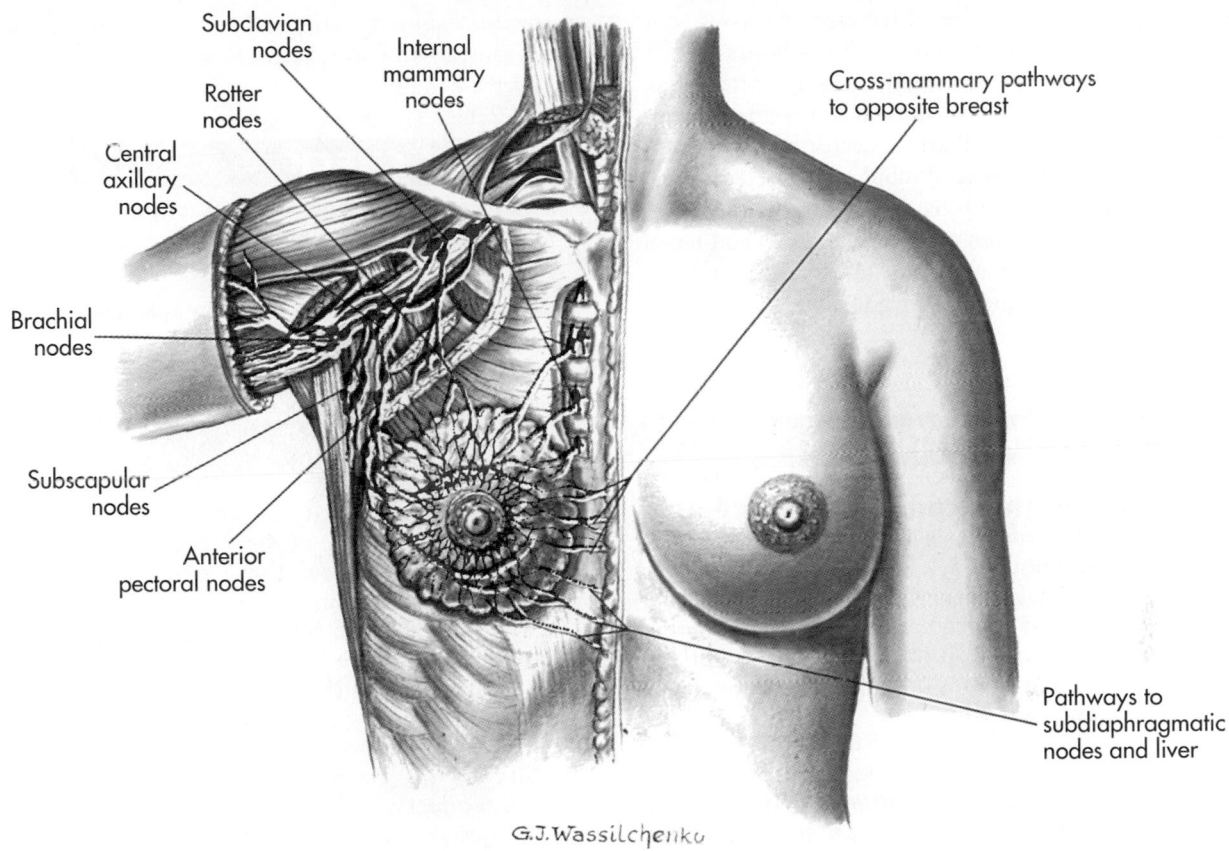

Fig. 31-19 *Lymphatic drainage of the female breast. (From Bobak, I.M., Jensen, M.D., & Zalar, M.K. [1989].* Maternity and gynecologic care: The nurse and the family *[4th ed.]. St. Louis: Mosby.)*

AGING AND REPRODUCTIVE FUNCTION

Aging and the Female Reproductive System

Menopause is a normal developmental event that is universally experienced by the average age of 50 to 51 years. It is not affected by age at menarche, childbearing, weight, socioeconomic factors, or race.

Changes are caused primarily by declining ovarian function and a resulting decrease in ovarian hormone secretion. The primary changes of menopause are as follows:

5-10 Years premenopause: extreme variability in frequency of menstruation and quality of menstrual flow; called transitional interval and occurs between 35 and 45 years of age

Ovarian changes: frequency of ovulation decreases, estrogen production is reduced, follicle and corpus luteum no longer develop

Breast tissue changes: tissue becomes involuted; fat deposits and connective tissue increase; breasts are reduced in size and firmness

Systemic changes: changes in vasomotor tone, urogenital structures, bone density, and artery walls; vasomotor flush occurs

Urogenital tract changes: ovaries shrink, uterus atrophies, vagina shortens, narrows, and loses some elasticity; lubrication of vagina diminishes; vaginal pH increases, creating higher incidence of vaginitis; cervix atrophies, cervical os shrinks; vaginal epithelium atrophies; labia major and minora become less prominent; some pubic hair is lost; urethral tone declines along with muscle tone throughout the pelvic area; urinary frequency or urgency, urinary tract infections, and incontinence may occur; regular sexual activity and orgasm may diminish some of these changes

Skeletal changes: bone mass is lost, leading to increased brittleness and porosity and possibly osteoporosis

Cardiac change: risk of coronary heart disease increases significantly

Aging and the Male Reproductive System

No known discrete event, comparable to menopause, characterizes aging of the male reproductive system. Changes do occur, however, in testicular structure and function and sexual behavior. Primary changes are summarized as follows:

Sexual drive (libido): influenced by changes in health status with aging

Erectile/ejaculatory capacity: need for longer stimulation to achieve full erection, slower and less forceful ejaculation, less pelvic muscle involvement; decreased vasocongestive response; longer refractory time, up to 24 hours

Testicular changes: decreased weight, atrophy, softening of testes; seminiferous tubules thicken in basement membrane area, have germ cell arrest, decrease in spermatogenic activity, and collapse of tubules; then sclerosis and fibrosis cause complete obstruction

Hormonal changes: hormone synthesis decreases and target tissues decline in responsiveness; testosterone levels reduce as Leydig cell numbers fall; gonadotropins increase

Associated change: functional deterioration of accessory sex organs; loss of muscle mass, strength, and endurance; decrease in libido

✓ QUICK CHECK

Why does breast development differ in adult men compared with adult women?

Why does menopause occur?

■ DID YOU UNDERSTAND?

Development of the Reproductive Systems

1. Differentiation of female and male genitalia begins in the eighth week of embryonic development, when the gonads of genetically male embryos begin to secrete male sex hormones, primarily testosterone. Until that time, the primitive reproductive organs of males and females are homologous (the same).

2. The structure and function of both male and female reproductive systems depend on interactions among the central nervous system (hypothalamus), the endocrine system (anterior pituitary), and the gonads (ovaries, testes). Accelerated production of sex hormones at puberty causes sexual maturation, making reproduction possible.

The Female Reproductive System

1. The function of the reproductive system is to produce mature ova and, when they are fertilized, to protect and nourish them through embryonic and fetal life and expel them at birth.

2. The external female genitalia are the mons pubis, labia majora, labia minora, clitoris, vestibule (urinary and vaginal openings), Bartholin glands, and Skene glands. They protect body openings and may play a role in sexual functioning.

3. The internal female genitalia are the vagina, uterus, fallopian tubes, and ovaries. Although all these organs are needed for reproduction, the ovaries are the most essential because they produce the female gametes and female sex hormones.

4. The vagina is a fibromuscular canal that receives the penis during sexual intercourse and is the exit route for menstrual fluids and products of conception. The vagina leads from the introitus (its external opening) to the cervical portion of the uterus.

5. The uterus is the hollow, muscular organ in which a fertilized ovum develops until birth. The uterine walls have three layers: the endometrium (lining), myometrium (muscular layer), and perimetrium (outer covering, which is continuous with the pelvic peritoneum). The endometrium proliferates

(thickens) and sloughs off in response to cyclic changes in levels of female sex hormones. The cervix is the narrow, lower portion of the uterus that opens into the vagina.

6. The two fallopian tubes extend from the uterus to the ovaries. Their function is to conduct ova from the spaces around the ovaries to the uterus. Fertilization normally occurs in the fallopian tubes.

7. From puberty to menopause, the ovaries are the site of (a) ovum maturation and release and (b) production of female sex hormones (estrogen, progesterone) and androgens. The female sex hormones are involved in sexual differentiation and development, the menstrual cycle, pregnancy, and lactation. Although they are primarily male sex hormones, androgens in women are precursors of female sex hormones and contribute to the prepubertal growth spurt, pubic and axillary hair growth, and activation of sebaceous glands.

8. Estrogen (primarily estradiol) is produced by cells in the developing ovarian follicle (structure that encloses the ovum). Progesterone is produced by cells of the corpus luteum, the structure that develops from the ruptured ovarian follicle after ovulation (ovum release). Androgens are produced within the ovarian follicle, adrenal glands, and adipose tissue.

9. The average menstrual cycle lasts 25 to 30 days and consists of three phases, which are named for ovarian and endometrial changes: the follicular/proliferative phase, the luteal/secretory phase, and menstruation.

10. Ovarian events of the menstrual cycle are controlled by gonadotropins and follicular secretion of inhibin. High follicle-stimulating hormone (FSH) levels stimulate follicle and ovum maturation (follicular phase); then a surge of luteinizing hormone (LH) causes ovulation, which is followed by development of the corpus luteum (luteal phase).

11. Uterine (endometrial) events of the menstrual cycle are caused by ovarian hormones. During the follicular phase of the ovarian cycle, estrogen produced by the follicle causes the endometrium to prolifer-

ate (proliferative phase). During the luteal phase, estrogen maintains the thickened endometrium while progesterone causes it to develop blood vessels and secretory glands (secretory phase). As the corpus luteum degenerates, production of both hormones drops sharply and the "starved" endometrium degenerates and sloughs off, causing menstruation.

12. Cyclic changes in hormone levels also cause thinning and thickening of the vaginal epithelium, thinning and thickening of cervical secretions, and changes in basal body temperature.

The Male Reproductive System

1. The function of the male reproductive system is to produce male gametes (sperm) and deliver them to the female reproductive tract.
2. The external male genitalia are the testes, epididymides, scrotum, and penis. The internal genitalia are the vas deferens, ejaculatory duct, prostatic and membranous sections of the urethra, seminal vesicles, prostate gland, and Cowper glands.
3. The testes (male gonads) are paired glands suspended within the scrotum. The testes have two functions: spermatogenesis (sperm production) and production of male sex hormones (androgens, chiefly testosterone).
4. The epididymis is a long, coiled tube arranged in a comma-shaped compartment that curves over the top and rear of the testis. The epididymis receives sperm from the testis and stores them while they develop further. Sperm travel the length of the epididymis and then are ejaculated into the vas deferens.
5. The scrotum is a skin-covered, fibromuscular sac that encloses the testes and epididymides, which are suspended within the scrotum by the spermatic cord. The scrotum keeps these organs at optimal temperatures for sperm survival (about 1° to 2° C lower than body temperature) by contracting in cold environments and relaxing in warm environments.
6. The penis is a cylindrical organ consisting of three longitudinal compartments (two corpora cavernosa and one corpus spongiosum) and the urethra. The urethra runs through the corpus spongiosum. The corpora cavernosa and corpus spongiosum consist of erectile tissue. Externally the penis consists of a shaft and a tip, which is called the *glans*.
7. The penis has two functions: delivery of sperm and elimination of urine.
8. Sexual intercourse is made possible by the erectile reflex, in which tactile or psychogenic stimulation of the parasympathetic nerves causes arterioles in the corpora cavernosa and corpus spongiosum to dilate and fill with blood, causing the penis to enlarge and become firm.
9. Emission, which occurs at the peak of sexual arousal, is the movement of semen from the epididymides to the penis. Ejaculation, which is a continuation of emission, is the pulsatile ejection of semen from the penis.
10. Spermatogenesis is a continuous process because spermatogonia, the primitive male gametes, undergo continuous mitosis within the seminiferous tubules of the testes. Some spermatogonia develop into primary spermatocytes, which divide meiotically into secondary spermatocytes and then spermatids. The spermatids develop into sperm with the help of nutrients and hormonal signals from Sertoli cells.
11. Production of the male sex hormones (like production of the female sex hormones) is controlled by interactions among the hypothalamus, anterior pituitary, and gonads. The male hormones are produced steadily rather than cyclically, however.

Structure and Function of the Breast

1. Until puberty the female and male breasts are similar, consisting of a small, underdeveloped nipple, some fatty and fibrous tissue, and a few ductlike structures under the areola. At puberty, however, a variety of hormones (estrogen, progesterone, prolactin, growth hormone, insulin, cortisol) cause the female breast to develop into a system of glands and ducts that is capable of producing and ejecting milk.
2. The basic functional unit of the female breast is the alveolus, or lobule, a system of ducts that branches from the nipple to milk-producing units called *acini cells*.
3. During the reproductive years, breast tissue undergoes cyclic changes in response to hormonal changes of the menstrual cycle.

KEY TERMS

Acinus (pl., acini) of breast, 855
Androgen, 846
Areola, 855
Breast, 855
Cervix, 843
Cornification, 849
Corpus cavernosum (pl., corpora cavernosa), 852
Corpus luteum, 844
Corpus spongiosum, 852
Corpus of uterus (body of uterus), 843
Cowper gland (bulbourethral gland), 853
Cul-de-sac, 842
Decornification, 849
Efferent tubule, 850
Ejaculatory duct, 853
Emission, 853
Endocervical canal, 843
Endometrium, 843
Epididymis, 851
Erectile reflex, 852
Estradiol, 845
Estrogen, 839, 845
Fallopian tube (uterine tube), 844
Fimbriae, 844
Follicle-stimulating hormone (FSH), 840
Follicular/proliferative phase, 847
Foreskin (prepuce), 852
Fornix, 842

Fundus of uterus, 843
Glands of Montgomery, 855
Glans, 852
Gonad, 838
Gonadotropin, 840
Gonadotropin-releasing hormone (GnRH), 840
Granulosa cell, 845
Infundibulum, 844
Inguinal canal, 850
Inhibin, 847
Isthmus, 843
Leydig cell, 850
Luteal/secretory phase, 847
Luteinizing hormone (LH), 840
Menarche, 846
Menopause, 846
Menstruation (menses), 847
Myometrium, 843
Nipple, 855
Ovarian cycle, 844
Ovarian follicle, 844
Ovary, 844
Ovulation, 844
Ovum (pl., ova), 837, 844
Penis, 851
Perimetrium (parietal peritoneum), 843
Prepuce, 852
Primary spermatocyte, 854
Progesterone, 846

Prostate gland, 853
Rete testis, 850
Ruga (pl., rugae; pertains to vagina and testes), 842
Scrotum, 851
Secondary spermatocyte, 854
Semen, 853
Seminal vesicle, 853
Seminiferous tubule, 850
Sertoli cell (nondividing support cell), 854
Sex hormone, 845
Spermatid, 854
Spermatogenesis, 850
Spermatogonium (pl., spermatogonia), 854
Spermatozoon (sperm cell), 837
Testis, 850
Testosterone, 838
Theca cell, 845
Thelarche, 855
Tubulus rectus, 850
Tunica albuginea, 850
Tunica dartos, 851
Tunica vaginalis, 850
Urethra, 852
Uterine tubes, 844
Uterus, 843
Vagina, 842
Vas deferens, 851
Vulva, 841

REFERENCES

1. Speroff, L., Glass, R.H., & Kase, N.G. (1994). *Clinical gynecologic endocrinology and infertility* (5th ed.). Baltimore: Williams & Wilkins.
2. Berne, R.M. & Levy, M.N. (Eds.). (1998). *Physiology* (4th ed.). St. Louis: Mosby.
3. Lowdermilk, D.L., Perry, S.E., & Bobak, I.M. (1997). *Maternity and women's health care* (6th ed.). St. Louis: Mosby.
4. Tanagho, E.A. & McAninch, D.W. (Eds.). (1992). *Smith's general urology* (13th ed.). Norwalk, Conn.: Appleton & Lange.
5. Tucker, S.M. et al. (Eds.). (1997). *Mosby's clinical nursing* (4th ed.). St. Louis: Mosby.
6. Thibodeau, G.A. & Patton, K.T. (1999). *Anatomy and physiology* (4th ed.) St. Louis: Mosby.

CHAPTER 32

Alterations of the Reproductive Systems

Including Sexually Transmitted Infections

Kristynia M. Robinson and Kathryn L. McCance

Alterations of the reproductive system span a wide range of concerns from delayed sexual development and suboptimal sexual performance to structural and functional difficulties. Many common reproductive disorders carry potentially serious physiologic or psychologic consequences. For example, sexual or reproductive dysfunction, such as impotence or infertility, can dramatically affect self-concept, relationships, and overall quality of life. In addition, prostate cancer is the most common cancer and the second leading cause of cancer deaths in men, and breast cancer is the most common cancer and the second leading cause of cancer deaths in women.[1,2] Conversely, organic and psychosocial problems, such as alcoholism, depression, situational stressors, chronic illness, and medications, can affect ovulation and menstruation, sexual performance, and fertility and may be risk factors for the development of some types of reproductive tract cancers. Diagnosis and treatment of reproductive system disorders, however, are often complicated by the stigma and symbolism associated with the reproductive organs and emotion-laden beliefs and behaviors related to reproductive health. Treatment or diagnosis for any problem may be delayed because of embarrassment, guilt, fear, or denial.

ALTERATIONS OF SEXUAL MATURATION

Various congenital and endocrine disorders can disrupt the timing of puberty, or sexual maturation. Puberty that occurs too late (delayed puberty) or too early (precocious puberty) is caused by the inappropriate onset of sex hormone production.

Delayed Puberty

The first sign of puberty in girls is thelarche, or breast development, and should begin by 13 years of age. In boys the first sign is enlargement of testes and thinning of the scrotal skin; this should happen by 14 years of age. In *delayed puberty,* these secondary sex characteristics develop later.

In 90% to 95% of cases, hormonal levels are normal, the hypothalamic-pituitary-gonadal (ovarian or testicular) axis is intact, and maturation is slow. This is much more common in boys than in girls. Treatment is seldom needed unless the delayed puberty is causing psychosocial problems.

The other 5% to 10% of cases are caused by disruption of the hypothalamic-pituitary-gonadal axis or a systemic disease. Treatment depends on the cause, and referral to a pediatric endocrinologist is necessary.[3]

Precocious Puberty

Precocious puberty is the onset of sexual maturation before the age of 8 years in girls and 9 years in boys. It is five times more common in girls than in boys, with 75% of precocity in girls being idiopathic.[4] Although boys are affected less often, the cause is more likely to be organic. See Box 32-1 for forms of precocious puberty.

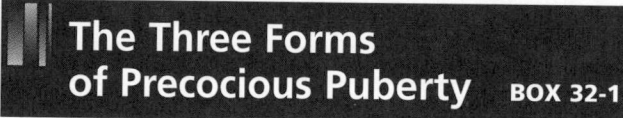

The Three Forms of Precocious Puberty   BOX 32-1

1. **Isosexual precocious puberty** is premature development of appropriate characteristics for the child's sex. The hypothalamic-pituitary-gonadal axis is working normally but prematurely. In about 10% of cases, a lethal CNS tumor may be the cause.
2. **Heterosexual precocious puberty** causes the child to develop some secondary sex characteristics of the opposite sex. Common causes are adrenal hyperplasia or androgen-secreting tumors.
3. **Incomplete precocious puberty** is the partial development of appropriate secondary sex characteristics. Premature thelarche (breast budding) is seen in girls between 6 months and 2 years of age. It does not progress to complete puberty (ovulation and menstruation). Premature adrenarche (growth of axillary and pubic hair) tends to occur between the ages of 5 and 8 years. This condition can progress to complete precocious puberty and may be caused by estrogen-secreting neoplasms or may be a varient of normal pubertal development.

All forms of precocious puberty are treated by identifying and removing the underlying cause or administering appropriate hormones. In many cases, precocious puberty can be reversed. However, *idiopathic isosexual precocity* is difficult to treat and can cause long bones to stop growing before the child has reached normal height.

DISORDERS OF THE FEMALE REPRODUCTIVE SYSTEM

Hormonal and Menstrual Alterations
Primary dysmenorrhea

Primary dysmenorrhea is painful menstruation associated with ovulation but not pelvic disease. Between 50% and 75% of women ages 15 to 25 years are affected—some (up to 15%)[4] severely enough to miss work or school. Dysmenorrhea usually begins with the onset of ovulatory cycles, around the age of 15 or 16 years. The incidence steadily rises, peaks in women in their mid-20s, and decreases slowly thereafter.

Pathophysiology

Dysmenorrhea results from excessive prostaglandin F ($PGF_{2\alpha}$) found in secretory endometrium. These lipid hormones increase myometrial contractions and constrict endometrial blood vessels, causing ischemia, endometrial bleeding, and pain. In addition, prostaglandins and prostaglandin metabolites can cause gastrointestinal complaints, headache, and syncope.

Clinical Manifestations

The chief symptom of dysmenorrhea is pelvic pain associated with the onset of menses. The severity is directly related to length and amount of menstrual flow. The pain frequently radiates into the groin and may be accompanied by backache, anorexia, vomiting, diarrhea, syncope, and headache. Usually, the discomfort begins shortly before the onset of menstruation and rarely persists beyond the second day.

Evaluation and Treatment

Primary dysmenorrhea must be differentiated from dysmenorrhea caused by disorders such as endometriosis, pelvic adhesions, inflammatory disease, or uterine fibroid. A thorough medical history and pelvic examination are completed to exclude pelvic pathologic conditions.

In women who desire contraception, primary dysmenorrhea can be relieved with oral contraceptives. Prostaglandin inhibitors work in a majority of women and should be taken at the onset of bleeding or cramping. A diet low in fat and regular exercise seem to prevent or reduce

✓ QUICK CHECK

Why does puberty occur too late or too early in some individuals?

Why do prostaglandin inhibitors decrease symptoms associated with primary dysmenorrhea?

symptoms. Other comfort measures include local application of heat, massage, relaxation techniques, and orgasm.

Primary amenorrhea

Amenorrhea means lack of menstruation. *Primary amenorrhea* is the failure of menarche and the absence of menstruation by age 14 years without the development of secondary sex characteristics or by age 16 years regardless of the presence of secondary sex characteristics. Causes include a diverse group of abnormalities, such as congenital defects of gonadotropin production; genetic disorders (Turner syndrome); congenital central nervous system (CNS) defects (e.g., hydrocephalus); congenital anatomic malformations of the reproductive system (e.g., absence of vagina or uterus); and acquired CNS lesions, including trauma, infection, and tumors.

Pathophysiology

In some congenital or acquired syndromes, the hypothalamic-pituitary-ovarian axis is dysfunctional. Because of anatomic defects of the CNS, the ovary does not receive the hormonal signals that normally initiate the development of secondary sex characteristics and menarche (beginning of menstruation). In some cases these lesions develop between the onset and conclusion of puberty. Therefore skeletal growth may occur and secondary sex characteristics may develop, but sexual maturation is interrupted before menarche.

In addition, primary amenorrhea has been associated with congenital absence or hypoplasia of the uterus and some genetic disorders, including gonadal dysgenesis (Turner syndrome), testicular feminizing syndrome (male pseudohermaphroditism), and poly-X (superfemale) syndrome. In Turner syndrome (XO), the ovaries lack gametes and ovarian failure is complete. In male pseudohermaphroditism, the individual is male genetically but female morphologically. The gonads are found either in the abdomen or in the inguinal canal and produce both androgens and estrogens. Because target tissues lack androgen receptors but have estrogen receptors, most individuals with male pseudohermaphroditism acquire female secondary sex characteristics, female external genitalia, and, except for a small vagina, absent internal female genitalia.

Clinical Manifestations

The major clinical manifestation of primary amenorrhea is the absence of menarche. The cause of the amenorrhea determines whether secondary sex characteristics and height are affected.

Evaluation and Treatment

Diagnosis of primary amenorrhea is based on history and physical examination. Laboratory studies may be required to document abnormal levels of gonadotropins and ovarian hormones. Diagnostic imaging is used to document structural abnormalities.

Treatment involves correction of any underlying disorders and hormone replacement therapy to induce the development of secondary sex characteristics. Surgical alteration of the genitalia may be undertaken to correct structural abnormalities. Hormonal manipulation or embryo transplantation may make pregnancy possible for women with primary amenorrhea.

Secondary amenorrhea

Secondary amenorrhea is the absence of menstruation for a time equivalent to 3 or more cycles or 6 months in women who have previously menstruated. Many disorders and physiologic conditions, including dramatic weight loss, are associated with secondary amenorrhea. Secondary amenorrhea is normal during early adolescence, pregnancy, lactation, and the perimenopausal period.

Pathophysiology

The pathophysiology of secondary amenorrhea is summarized in Fig. 32-1.

Clinical Manifestations

The major manifestation of secondary amenorrhea is the absence of menses. Depending on the underlying cause of the amenorrhea, infertility, vasomotor flushes, vaginal atrophy, acne, and *hirsutism* (abnormal hairiness) also may be present.

Evaluation and Treatment

Diagnosis of secondary amenorrhea involves identifying underlying hormonal or anatomic alterations. A complete history and physical examination are done, and pregnancy is ruled out before any further work-up is undertaken. Subsequent evaluation may include a progesterone challenge to induce withdrawal bleeding, or serum thyroid-stimulating hormone (TSH) or prolactin levels. Depending on the cause of the amenorrhea, treatment may involve hormone replacement therapy or a corrective procedure, such as surgical removal of pituitary tumors.

Dysfunctional uterine bleeding

Menstrual irregularity or abnormal bleeding patterns (Table 32-1) account for 33% to 69% of all gynecologic visits.[4,5] The most common cause of cycle irregularity is failure to ovulate related to age, stress, or endocrinopathy. A breakdown of common causes of abnormal bleeding based on age-group and frequency is listed in Table 32-2.

Pathophysiology

Dysfunctional uterine bleeding (DUB) is abnormal uterine bleeding resulting from a disturbance of the menstrual cycle, usually anovulation. Although it may occur at any time during the reproductive years, it is most likely to affect premenopausal women ages 40 to 50 years.

In anovulatory cycles, progesterone secretion is absent while variable amounts of estrogen continue to be secreted by the granulosa–theca cell complex. Estrogen stimulates proliferation and hyperplasia of the endometrial glands. Without the usual stromal support induced by progesterone and periodic endometrial ischemia resulting in menstruation, the endometrium attains an abnormal height with increasing hypervascularity and back-to-back glandularity.

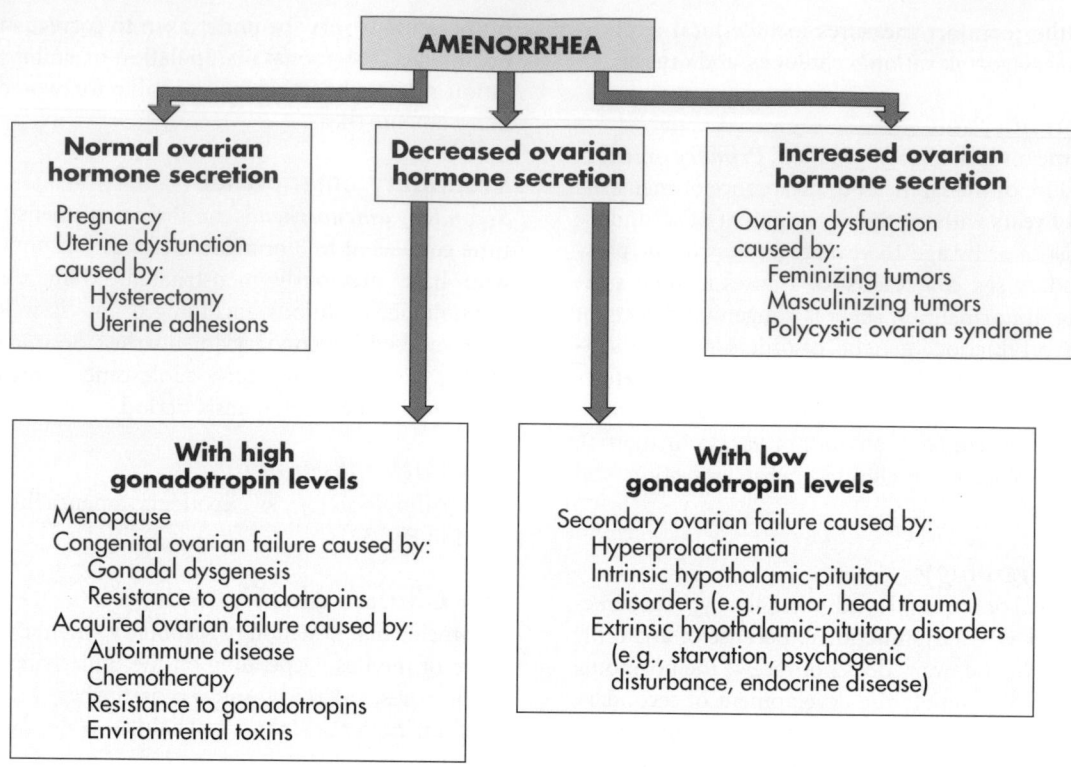

Fig. 32-1 *Causes of secondary amenorrhea.*

Random breakdown of endometrial tissue occurs, and exposure of vascular channels leads to irregular, prolonged, and excessive bleeding. In addition, unopposed estrogen induces a progression of endometrial responses that may end with atypia (atypical hyperplasia) and carcinoma.

DUB in ovulatory cycles is less common, and mechanisms underlying the bleeding are unclear. Excessive fibrinolytic activity and changes in prostaglandin production may be implicated.

Clinical Manifestations
DUB is characterized by irregular or heavy bleeding or both. Although large clots often indicate excessive blood loss, it is difficult to estimate the severity of blood loss; healthy women do not become anemic until blood loss exceeds 1.6 L over a short time.

Evaluation and Treatment
DUB is diagnosed after other organic conditions that could cause abnormal bleeding are eliminated. Goals of therapy are to control bleeding, prevent hyperplasia, prevent or treat anemia, and treat concurrent endocrine problems if present. Usual therapy is hormonal and may consist of intense progestin-estrogen therapy, short-term high-dose estrogen, cyclic low-dose contraceptives, or medroxyprogesterone acetate. Treatment for DUB with dilation and curettage (D & C) or hysterectomy is not recommended.[5]

The polycystic ovary
In women with **polycystic ovaries (PCOs),** the hypothalamic-pituitary-ovarian axis is intact and the ovary is intrinsically without defects. However, ovarian function in ovulation is inhibited by the production of excessive amounts of androgens and conversion of these androgens to estrogen in the peripheral tissues. PCO may be inherited, seemingly through transmission of an X-linked dominant disorder. Enlarged PCOs may also be associated with (1) Cushing syndrome, (2) congenital adrenal hyperplasia, (3) thyroid disease, (4) androgen-producing adrenal or ovarian tumors, and (5) syndromes with hyperprolactinemia.

Pathophysiology
The most common biochemical abnormality is inappropriate gonadotropin secretion, resulting in excessive production of both androgen and estrogen. This contributes to premature follicular atresia and persistent anovulation, leading to enlarged PCOs (Fig. 32-2). Because estrogen promotes endometrial proliferation, women with PCO are at risk for endometrial polyps and breast cancer.

Clinical Manifestations
Clinical manifestations of PCO are related to anovulation and include dysfunctional bleeding or amenorrhea, hirsutism, and infertility. Approximately 15% of women with PCO are obese.

TABLE 32-1	Abnormal Menstrual Bleeding
Term	**Definition**
Polymenorrhea	Cycles shorter than 3 wk; may indicate disturbance in endocrine control of ovulation
Oligomenorrhea	Cycles longer than 6-7 wk; may indicate disturbance in endocrine control of ovulation
Metrorrhagia	Intermenstrual bleeding or bleeding of light character occurring irregularly between cycles; may be a sign of organic disease
Hypermenorrhea	Excessive flow; may be a sign of organic disease
Menorrhea	Prolonged duration of flow
Menorrhagia	Increased amount and duration of flow
Menometrorrhagia	Prolonged flow associated with irregular and intermittent spotting between bleeding episodes

TABLE 32-2	Common Causes of Abnormal (Vaginal/Genital) Bleeding in Descending Order of Frequency	
Age-Group	**Cause**	
Prepubescence	Sexual assault	
	Trauma	
	Foreign bodies	
	Precocious puberty	
Adolescence	Anovulation (immature hypothalamic-pituitary-gonadal axis)	
	Trauma and sexual abuse	
	Pregnancy	
	Pelvic inflammatory disease	
	Coagulation disorder	
Reproductive years	Pregnancy	
	Pelvic inflammatory disease	
	Complication of contraceptives	
	Endometriosis	
	Anovulation	
Premenopause	Anovulation	
	Malignancy	
	Pregnancy	
	Endometriosis	
	Benign neoplasms (myomas, adenomyosis)	
Postmenopause	Malignancy	

**Fig. 32-2 *Polycystic ovarian disease.* *(From Symonds, E.M. & Macpherson, M.B.A. [1997].* Diagnosis in color: Obstetrics and gynecology. *London: Mosby-Wolfe.)*

An estimated 5% to 10% of menstruating women experience severe to disabling premenstrual symptoms, and 50% or more note moderately distressing symptoms. To confuse matters, it seems that (1) symptoms are experienced to some degree by all adolescent and adult women and are more likely to occur throughout all menstrual phases, (2) the presence and severity of symptoms in any one woman may be inconsistent from month to month, and (3) menstrual phase for peak symptom severity may differ depending on the population studied.[6]

Pathophysiology

The exact etiology of PMS is unknown. The cause of PMS is considered multifactorial and stress related. Currently, PMS is thought to occur when brain and nervous, immunologic, vascular, gastrointestinal, and other tissue respond abnormally to the normal hormone fluctuations of the menstrual cycle. Fluctuating estrogen and progesterone levels may trigger this biologic response but are not sufficient alone to cause PMS.

A predisposition to PMS runs in families, perhaps because of genetics or shared environment. A woman's menstrual experience tends to be similar to her mother's or her sister's experience. Further evidence supports a relationship between the severity and frequency of premenstrual symptoms and reports of low general well-being; history of major

Evaluation and Treatment

Diagnosis of PCO is based on evidence of androgen excess, chronic anovulation, and inappropriate gonadotropin secretion. Treatment includes progesterone therapy to oppose estrogen's effects and medication to stimulate ovulation. For women who do not desire pregnancy, hormonal contraception may be used to suppress androgen production.

Premenstrual syndrome

Premenstrual syndrome (PMS) is the cyclic recurrence (in the luteal phase of the menstrual cycle) of physical, psychologic, or behavioral changes distressing enough to impair interpersonal relationships or interfere with usual activities.

affective disorder and personality characteristics, such as perfectionism; increased stress; poor nutrition; lack of exercise; low self-esteem; history of sexual abuse; and family conflict. In turn, when premenstrual symptoms are perceived as distressing, the quality of interpersonal relationships and self-image are negatively affected.

Clinical Manifestations

The pattern of symptom frequency and severity is more important than specific complaints (Box 32-2). More than 200 physical, emotional, and behavioral symptoms have been attributed to PMS. Emotional symptoms, particularly depression, anger, irritability, and fatigue, have been reported as the most prominent and the most distressing, whereas physical symptoms seem to be the least prevalent and problematic. Approximately 6% of women present with classic PMS (distressing luteal symptoms), and 7% report premenstrual magnification of symptoms that are present during the entire cycle. A typical premenstrual symptom pattern may appear after the treatment of a systemic disease. Likewise, underlying physical or psychologic disease may be aggravated premenstrually.

Evaluation and Treatment

Diagnosis of PMS is based on health history and symptoms. Because the cause is complex and the occurrence and severity of PMS are mediated by life-style, social, and psychologic factors, treatment for PMS is symptomatic. Nonpharmacologic therapies, with or without medication, tend to be more effective in controlling symptoms than medication alone.

✓QUICK CHECK

Why does amenorrhea occur?

Why do anovulatory cycles lead to dysfunctional uterine bleeding?

Infection and Inflammation

Infections of the genital tract may result from exogenous or endogenous microorganisms. Exogenous pathogens are most frequently sexually transmitted. Endogenous causes of infection include microorganisms that are normally resident in the vagina, bowel, or vulva. Infection occurs if these microorganisms migrate to a new location or overproliferate or if the immune system and other defense mechanisms are impaired.

Skin disorders that can affect the vulva include reactive dermatitis, contact dermatitis, psoriasis, and impetigo. (For a discussion of skin disorders, see Chapter 39.) Most infectious disorders that affect the vulva and vagina are sexually transmitted, however. These disorders are described in Table 32-15.

Pelvic inflammatory disease

Pelvic inflammatory disease (PID) is an acute inflammatory process caused by infection (Fig. 32-3). It may involve any organ, or combination of organs, of the upper genital tract—the uterus, fallopian tubes, or ovaries—and, in its most severe form, the entire peritoneal cavity. (Infection of the fallopian tubes is termed *salpingitis* [Fig. 32-4]; infection of the ovaries is called *oophoritis.*) Most cases of PID are caused by sexually transmitted microorganisms that migrate from the vagina to the uterus, fallopian tubes, and ovaries.[7]

Pathophysiology

The development of upper genital tract infections is mediated by a number of defense mechanisms, including virulence of the organism, size of the inoculum, and defense status of the individual. PID usually is considered a polymicrobial infection, caused by mixed nongonococcal-nonchlamydial bacteria, including anaerobes (*Bacteroides* species and peptostreptococci) and facultative organisms (*Gardnerella vaginalis, Haemophilus influenzae,* and streptococci). Recovery of *Neisseria gonorrhoeae, Chlamydia trachomatis,* or both, has been reported in 50% to 60% of

---

Diagnostic and Research Criteria for PMS   BOX 32-2

1. The presence by self-report of at least one of the following somatic and affective symptoms during the 5 days before menses in each of the three prior menstrual cycles:

Affective	Somatic
Depression	Breast tenderness
Angry outbursts	Abdominal bloating
Irritability	Headache
Social withdrawal	Swollen extremities
Fatigue	

2. Relief of the above symptoms within 4 days of the onset of menses, without recurrence until at least cycle day 12.
3. The symptoms are present in the absence of any pharmacologic therapy, hormone ingestion, drug, or alcohol.
4. The symptoms occur reproducibly during two cycles of prospective recording.
5. Identifiable dysfunction in social or economic performance by one of the following criteria:
   Marital or relationship discord confirmed by partner
   Difficulties in parenting
   Poor work or school performance, attendance/tardiness
   Increased social isolation
   Legal difficulties
   Suicidal ideation
   Seeking medical attention for somatic symptom(s)

From Mortola, J.F. (1992). Issues in the diagnosis and research of premenstrual syndrome. Clinical OB/GYN, 35(30), *587-598.*

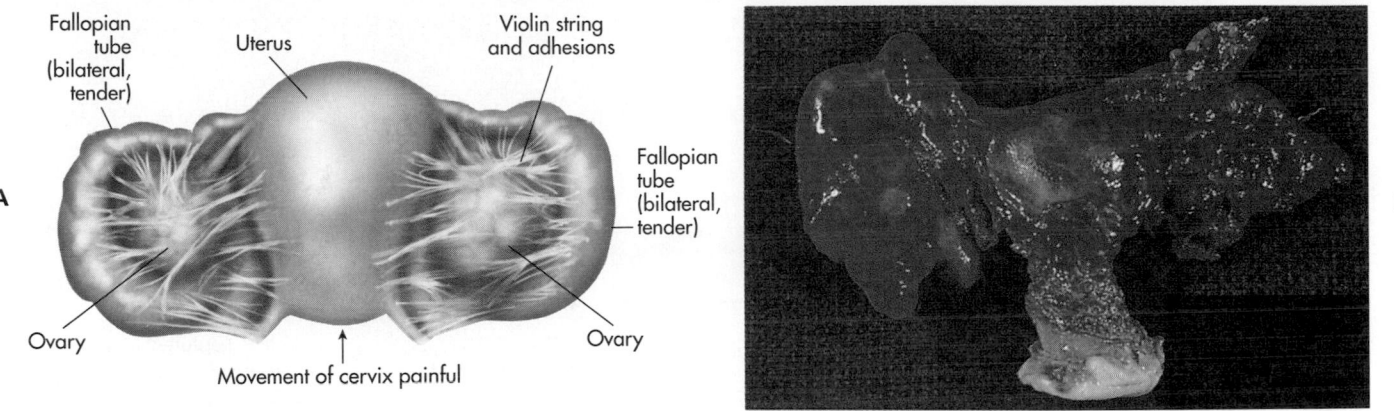

Fig. 32-3 *Pelvic inflammatory disease.* **A,** Involvement of both ovaries and fallopian tubes. **B,** Total abdominal hysterectomy and bilateral salpingo-oophorectomy specimen showing unilateral pyosalpinx. *(A from Seidel, H. et al. [1999]. Mosby's guide to physical examination [4th ed.]. St. Louis: Mosby; B from Morse, S.A., Moreland, A.A., & Holmes, K.K. [1996]. Atlas of sexually transmitted diseases and AIDS [2nd ed.]. St. Louis: Mosby-Wolfe.)*

Advanced pyosalpinx

Fig. 32-4 *Salpingitis.* **A,** Note the swollen fallopian tubes. **B,** Bilateral, retort-shaped, swollen sealed tubes and adhesions of ovaries are typical of salpingitis. *(A from Seidel, H. et al. [1999]. Mosby's guide to physical examination [4th ed.]. St. Louis: Mosby; B from Damjanov, I. & Linder, J. [Eds.]. [1996]. Anderson's pathology [10th ed.]. St. Louis: Mosby.)*

Fig. 32-5 *Algorithm or flow chart for pelvic pain.* *RUQ,* Right upper quadrant; *LUQ,* left upper quadrant; *RLQ,* right lower quadrant; *LLQ,* lower left quadrant.

women with acute PID. These organisms induce a response from the body that causes necrosis with repeated infections and predispose to PID. In addition, *Mycoplasma hominis* and *Ureaplasma urealyticum* might be etiologic agents of PID. After one episode of pelvic infection, 15% to 25% of women develop long-term sequelae, such as infertility, ectopic pregnancy, chronic pelvic pain, dyspareunia (painful intercourse), pelvic adhesions, perihepatitis, and tuboovarian (uterine tube and ovary) abscess. The incidence of complications increases markedly with repeated infections. Mortality associated with PID is 8% to 9% of cases. Most deaths resulting from PID are caused by septic shock (see Chapter 23).

Clinical Manifestations

The clinical manifestations of PID vary from sudden, severe abdominal pain with fever to no symptoms at all. An asymptomatic cervicitis may be present for some time before PID develops. Of women with salpingitis, 67% to 75% may have a subclinical infection. The first sign of the ascending infection may be the onset of low bilateral abdominal pain, often characterized as dull and steady with a gradual onset. Symptoms are more likely to develop during or immediately after menstruation. The pain of PID may worsen with walking, jumping, or intercourse. Other manifestations of PID include dysuria (difficult or painful urination) and irregular bleeding.

Evaluation and Treatment

The diagnosis of PID is based on history, abdominal tenderness, presence of uterine and cervical movement tenderness on bimanual pelvic examination, mucopurulent discharge at the cervical os, white blood cells on Gram stain or wet mount of cervical discharge, leukocytosis, and increased erythrocyte sedimentation rate. To support the diagnosis, tests for chlamydia and gonorrhea are done; sonography, laparoscopy, and culdocentesis are indicated when a woman has recurrent symptoms or symptoms unresponsive to outpatient treatment regimen, fever greater than 38° C, or an adnexal mass. Other conditions that cause pelvic pain must be excluded, including ectopic pregnancy, threatened abortion, or appendicitis (Fig. 32-5).

Treatment involves bed rest, avoidance of intercourse, and combined antibiotic therapy. From 25% to 40% of women require hospitalization for intravenous administration of antibiotics and treatment of peritonitis or a tuboovarian abscess. To prevent recurrence, sexual partners are also treated with antibiotic combinations.

Vaginitis

Vaginitis is infection of the vagina. The major causes are sexually transmitted pathogens and *Candida albicans*. The incidence of sexually transmitted vaginitis is highest in women 15 to 25 years of age.

The development of vaginitis is related to the overall health of a woman and local defense mechanisms, particularly vaginal pH. The pH of the vagina depends on cervical secretions and the presence of normal flora that help to maintain an acidic environment. Variables that alter the vaginal pH or the bactericidal nature of secretions (see Chapter 31) and predispose a woman to infection include douching; use of soaps, feminine hygiene sprays, deodorant menstrual pads or tampons; and conditions associated with increased glycogen content of vaginal secretions, such as pregnancy or diabetes.

The use of antibiotics may destroy *Lactobacillus acidophilus*, an anaerobic, gram-positive rod normally found in the vagina that helps maintain an acidic pH. In its absence, alkalinity increases and the vagina is more susceptible to trichomoniasis and bacterial vaginosis; moreover, there may be an overgrowth of *C. albicans*, causing a yeast vaginitis.

Normally, vaginal discharge is a clear, milky, or cloudy secretion with a slippery or clumpy texture. It is nonirritating, has a mild inoffensive odor, and turns yellow after drying. The amount and texture of a woman's discharge will change in response to hormonal fluctuation throughout the menstrual cycle. Vaginal secretions increase at the time of ovulation, during pregnancy, and with sexual arousal; just before menstruation, vaginal discharge becomes thick and sticky. Although the amount of vaginal discharge alone is not an indication of infection, any other change in discharge may indicate a problem. Infection is suggested with a marked change in color or if the discharge becomes malodorous or irritating.

Diagnosis is based on history, physical examination, and examination of the discharge by wet mount. Treatment involves developing and maintaining an acidic environment, relieving symptoms (usually pruritus), and administering antimicrobial or antifungal medications to eradicate the infectious organism. If the infection can be sexually transmitted, a woman's partner will also be treated.

Cervicitis

Cervicitis is an inflammation of the cervix. **Mucopurulent cervicitis (MPC)** is usually caused by one or more sexually transmitted pathogens, such as *Trichomonas*, gonorrhea, *Chlamydia*, *Mycoplasma*, or *Ureaplasma*. Infection causes the cervix to become red and edematous. A mucopurulent (mucus- and pus-containing) exudate drains from the external cervical os, and the individual may report vague pelvic pain, bleeding, or dysuria. The infectious organisms are cultured or identified by immunoassay. Definitive diagnosis is followed by oral antibiotic therapy. Sexual partners are usually treated.

Vulvitis

Inflammation of the vulva is termed *vulvitis*. Acute vulvitis is an inflammation of the skin (dermatitis) of the vulva and often of the perianal area. Vulvitis can be caused by contact with soaps, detergents, lotions, hygienic sprays, menstrual pads, or perfumed toilet paper and aggravated by nonabsorbent or tight-fitting clothes. Vulvitis is also caused by

Fig. 32-6 *Inflammation of Bartholin glands.* *(From Gardner, H.L. & Kaufman, R.H. [1969]. Benign diseases of the vulva and vagina. St. Louis: Mosby.)*

vaginal infections (e.g., candidiasis, trichomoniasis) that spread to the labia, where they cause inflammation and edema. The vulva can also be affected by other skin diseases, such as tinea cruris, psoriasis, and inflammation of the apocrine (sweat) glands (see Chapter 39).

Avoidance of irritants; wearing loose, cotton clothing; and appropriate antimicrobial/antifungal treatment for recurrent vaginitis are usually effective cures for acute vulvitis. Chronic vulvitis is usually treated with fluorinated hydrocortisone. Biopsy specimens of persistent lesions are examined for the presence of malignancy.

Bartholinitis

Bartholinitis (Bartholin cyst) is an inflammation of one or both of the ducts that lead from the introitus (vaginal opening) to Bartholin glands (Fig. 32-6). The usual causes are microorganisms that infect the lower female reproductive tract, such as streptococci, staphylococci, and sexually transmitted pathogens. Acute bartholinitis is usually preceded by an infection, such as cervicitis, vaginitis, or urethritis.

Infection or trauma causes inflammatory changes that narrow the distal portion of the duct, leading to obstruction and stasis of glandular secretions. The obstruction, or cyst, varies from 1 to 8 cm in diameter and is located in the posterolateral portion of the vulva. The affected area is usually red and painful, and pus may be visible at the opening of the duct. The individual may have fever and malaise.

Most Bartholin cysts are asymptomatic and require no treatment. Chronic bartholinitis is characterized by the presence of a small cyst that is slightly tender but otherwise is asymptomatic. Symptoms only occur if an exacerbation of infection causes an abscess to form in the gland itself.

TABLE 32-3	Cystocele, Urethrocele, and Rectocele		
Condition	**Etiology**	**Symptoms**	**Treatment**
Cystocele	Laceration, stretching, or weakening of supporting fascial tissue; usually caused by prolonged labor, multiple births, or birth of a large baby	Urinary frequency, urgency, and occasional incontinence Difficulty in complete emptying of the bladder Low backache Symptoms become problematic premenopausally or post-menopausally	Depending on age of woman and severity of the condition, includes: Isometric exercise to strengthen the pubococcygeal muscle Oral or topical estrogen to improve tone and vascularity of fascial support Pessary, a removable device that holds the bladder in position Surgical correction
Urethrocele	Pressure of fetal head on urethra and attachments beneath the symphysis pubis Familial or genetic predisposition	Asymptomatic unless it occurs in conjunction with cystocele	Isometric exercises (see cystocele)
Rectocele	Trauma to the fascia and levator muscles; usually caused by childbirth Familial or genetic predisposition	Constipation or feeling of rectal fullness Difficult defecation Pressure and sensation of fullness in the vagina	Isometric exercises Diet counseling to prevent constipation Stool softeners or laxatives Surgery

Diagnosis is based on the clinical manifestations and the identification of infectious microorganisms. Infection is treated with antibiotics, and pain is relieved with analgesics and warm sitz baths. If an abscess forms, it may be surgically drained.

Pelvic Relaxation Disorders

The bladder, urethra, and rectum are supported by the endopelvic fascia and perineal muscles. This muscular and fascial tissue loses tone and strength with aging and may fail to maintain the pelvic organs in the proper position. Uterine displacement can be caused by progressive relaxation of the pelvic support structures or trauma, such as childbirth or pelvic surgery, that damages or weakens the supporting structures. Pelvic relaxation is progressive and is related to the inherent strength or weakness of the woman's musculofascial tissue. Malpositioning of the bladder, urethra, or rectum (and hence the uterus) may occur many years after an initial injury to the supporting structure. A strong familial tendency and, perhaps, a multifactorial genetic component place some women at risk for the development of prolapse. Genital prolapse is 80 times more prevalent in whites than in blacks; and despite grand multiparity, pelvic relaxation is rare in Canadian Indians.

Fig. 32-7 shows vaginal prolapse caused by cystocele, rectocele, and enterocele. *Cystocele* is descent of the bladder and the anterior vaginal wall into the vaginal canal. In severe cases, the bladder and anterior vaginal wall bulge outside the introitus. A cystocele may cause the woman to lose urine when she laughs, sneezes, coughs, or does anything that strains the abdominal muscles. Cystocele is usually accompanied by *urethrocele,* or sagging of the urethra. Urethrocele is usually caused by the shearing effect of the fetal head on the urethra during childbirth. A *rectocele* is the bulging of the rectum and posterior vaginal wall into the vaginal canal. If this condition is severe, defecation is difficult and can be accomplished only by applying manual pressure to the posterior vaginal wall. An *enterocele* is herniation of the rectouterine pouch into the rectovaginal septum (between the rectum and posterior vaginal wall). It is usually associated with other pelvic relaxation disorders, such as uterine prolapse, cystocele, and rectocele. Table 32-3 summarizes the causes, symptoms, and treatment of cystocele, urethrocele, and rectocele.

Uterine prolapse is descent of the cervix or entire uterus into the vaginal canal (Fig. 32-8). In severe cases, the uterus falls completely through the vagina and protrudes from the introitus. First-degree uterine prolapse is not treated unless it causes discomfort. Second- and third-degree prolapses cause feelings of fullness, heaviness, and collapse through the vagina. Symptoms of other pelvic relaxation disorders also may be present. Treatment in these cases is the insertion of a *pessary,* which is a removable mechanical device that holds the uterus in position. The pelvic fascia may be strengthened through Kegel exercises—a repetitive, isometric tightening and relaxing of the pubococcygeal muscles—or by a course of estrogen therapy, particularly if the woman is past menopause. Surgical repair is the treatment of last resort. Prevention of constipation and early treatment of respiratory ailments that cause coughing may help.[8]

Fig. 32-7 *Cystocele and rectocele.* **A,** Cystocele. **B,** Large cystocele. **C,** Rectocele. **D,** Rectocele associated with ulceration of vaginal wall. *(A and C from Seidel, H. et al. [1999]. Mosby's guide to physical examination [4th ed.]. St. Louis: Mosby; B and D from Symonds, E.M. & Macpherson, M.B.A. [1994]. Color atlas of obstetrics and gynecology. London: Mosby-Wolfe.)*

Fig. 32-8 *Degrees of uterine prolapse.* **A,** Normal uterus. **B,** First-degree prolapse: descent within the vagina. **C,** Second-degree prolapse: the cervix protrudes through the introitus. **D,** Third-degree prolapse: the vagina is completely everted. *(From Seidel, H. et al. [1999]. Mosby's guide to physical examination [4th ed.]. St. Louis: Mosby.)*

Data from Consumers Union of U.S. (1997). Consumers reports on health: Guide to nutrition [Special Report]. Yonkers, N.Y.: The Author; Forrest, D.E. (1998). Common gynecologic pelvic disorders. In E.Q. Youngkin & M.S. Davis (Eds.). Women's health: A primary care clinical guide. Stamford, Conn.: Appleton & Lange.

Benign Growths and Proliferative Conditions

Benign ovarian cysts

Benign cysts of the ovary may occur at any time during the life span but are most common between puberty and menopause (Fig. 32-9). Two common causes of benign ovarian enlargement in ovulating women are follicular cysts and corpus luteum cysts. These cysts are called functional cysts because they are caused by variations of normal physiologic events. Follicular and corpus luteum cysts are unilateral. They are typically 5 to 6 cm in diameter but can grow as large as 8 to 10 cm.

A *follicular cyst* develops (1) from a dominant ovarian follicle that does not release its ovum but remains active or (2) from a degenerating follicle whose fluid is not reabsorbed. Most follicular cysts are not symptomatic, require no treatment, and either regress or rupture spontaneously within 60 days. A large follicular cyst may cause low back pain, painful intercourse (dyspareunia), chronic lower abdominal pain, and menstrual irregularities.

A *corpus luteum cyst* develops if a mature corpus luteum

persists abnormally and continues to secrete progesterone. The cyst consists of blood or fluid that accumulates in the cavity of the corpus luteum. Corpus luteum cysts are less common than follicular cysts, but luteal cysts typically cause more symptoms, particularly if they rupture. Manifestations include dull pelvic pain and amenorrhea or delayed menstruation, followed by irregular or heavier-than-normal bleeding. Rupture can cause massive bleeding with excruciating pain and require immediate surgery. Corpus luteum cysts usually regress spontaneously, however, within 2 months in nonpregnant women. Oral contraceptives may be used to prevent cysts from forming in the future.

✓ QUICK CHECK

Why is prompt treatment of pelvic inflammatory disease (PID) critical to reproductive health?

Why do benign ovarian cysts develop in women who ovulate?

Endometrial polyps

An *endometrial polyp* is a mass of endometrial tissue attached to the inner uterine lining by a pedicle (Fig. 32-10) that may be benign in younger women but tends to be malignant in postmenopausal women.[9] Polyps usually arise from the uterine fundus in response to estrogen stimulation and often coexist with endometrial hyperplasia. Polyps may be single or multiple with a narrow or broad pedicle and may vary from 0.5 to 3 cm in diameter. Although polyps most often develop in women between the ages of 40 and 49 years, they can occur at all ages.

Endometrial polyps frequently cause premenstrual spotting or intermenstrual bleeding in the premenopausal woman. These polyps consist of stromal tissue covered by either proliferative or hyperplastic mucosa. In response to

One or both sides, usually nontender

Fig. 32-9 *Ovarian cyst. (From Seidel, H. et al. [1999]. Mosby's guide to physical examination [4th ed.]. St. Louis: Mosby.)*

Fig. 32-10 *Endometrial polyp.* It is protruding through the cervical os. *(From Symonds, E.M. & Macpherson, M.B.A. [1994]. Color atlas of obstetrics and gynecology. London: Mosby-Wolfe.)*

subtle hormonal changes, irregular bleeding occurs that is nonsynchronous with the normal endometrial lining. Occasionally, significant bleeding occurs.

Diagnosis is made by hysteroscopy, hysterosalpingography, or direct examination of tissue obtained by curettage. The lesions are removed with small, curved polyp forceps. Coexistence of a separate endometrial atypical hyperplasia or adenocarcinoma is common.

Leiomyomas

Leiomyomas, commonly called *uterine fibroids,* are benign tumors that develop from smooth muscle cells in the myometrium. Leiomyomas are the most common benign tumors of the uterus, and most remain small and asymptomatic. Prevalence increases in women ages 30 to 50 years but decreases with menopause. In the United States, it is estimated that myomas develop in 30% of white and 50% of black women by the age of 50 years. The incidence of leiomyomas in black and Asian women is two to five times higher than that in white women.

The cause of uterine leiomyomas is unknown, although their size appears to be related to hormonal fluctuations. Uterine leiomyomas are not seen before menarche, and those that develop during the reproductive years generally shrink after menopause. Tumors in pregnant women enlarge rapidly but often decrease in size after termination of the pregnancy.

Pathophysiology

Most leiomyomas occur in multiples in the fundus of the uterus, although they may occur singly and throughout the uterus. Leiomyomas are classified as subserous, submucous, or intramural, according to their location within the various layers of the uterine wall (Fig. 32-11). Uterine leiomyomas are usually firm and surrounded by a pseudocapsule composed of compressed but otherwise normal uterine myometrium. Degenerative changes, such as ulceration and necrosis, may occur when the leiomyoma outgrows its blood supply and therefore are more common in larger tumors.

Clinical Manifestations

Although fibroids rarely present problems, they occasionally cause cramping, excessive bleeding, and symptoms related to pressure on nearby structures. The leiomyoma can make the uterine cavity larger, thereby increasing the endometrial surface area. This increase may account for the increased menstrual bleeding associated with leiomyomas. Pain or cramping occurs with the devascularization of larger leiomyomas and is associated with blood vessel compression that limits blood supply to adjacent structures. Because the tumor is relatively slow growing, enabling adjacent structures to adapt to pressure, symptoms of abdominal pressure develop slowly. Pressure on the bladder may contribute to urinary frequency, urgency, and dysuria. Pressure on the ureter may cause it to become distended "upstream" from the pressure point; rectosigmoid pressure may lead to constipation. A sensation of abdominal or genital heaviness may be felt with larger tumors.

Evaluation and Treatment

Uterine leiomyomas are diagnosed by physical examination. The bimanual examination discloses irregular, nontender nodularity of the uterus. Treatment depends on the symptoms, tumor size, age, reproductive status, and overall health of the individual. Most myomas can be treated conservatively. Medical treatment is aimed at shrinking the myoma with either progesterone or gonadotropin-releasing hormone (GnRH). Myomectomy may be undertaken and is the surgical treatment of choice.

Adenomyosis

Adenomyosis is the presence of endometrial glands and stroma within the uterine myometrium. It commonly develops during the late reproductive years, with the highest incidence among women in their 40s. Adenomyosis may be asymptomatic or may be associated with abnormal menstrual bleeding, dysmenorrhea, uterine enlargement, and uterine tenderness during menstruation. Treatment, when necessary, includes surgical resection of localized areas of adenomyosis or, if severe, hysterectomy.

Endometriosis

Endometriosis is the presence of functioning endometrial tissue or implants outside the uterus. Like normal endometrial tissue, the ectopic (out-of-place) endometrium responds to the hormonal fluctuations of the menstrual cycle.

Fig. 32-11 *Leiomyomas.* Uterine section showing whorl-like appearance and locations of leiomyomas, which are also called uterine fibroids. *(From Herbst, A.L. et al. [1992]. Comprehensive gynecology [2nd ed.]. St. Louis: Mosby.)*

Fig. 32-12 *Pelvic sites of endometrial implantation.* Endometrial cells may enter the pelvic cavity during retrograde menstruation. *(Modified from Herbst, A.L. et al. [1992]. Comprehensive gynecology [2nd ed.]. St. Louis: Mosby.)*

The incidence of endometriosis is difficult to determine, particularly in asymptomatic fertile women and adolescents. Between 11% and 50% of women surgically evaluated for pelvic pain, infertility, or a pelvic mass are diagnosed with endometriosis.[10] Conversely, endometriosis is found in as many as 22% of fertile asymptomatic women undergoing tubal ligation. Moreover, the frequency and severity of symptoms do not correlate with the extent or site of lesions.[11] Theories of the cause of endometriosis are contained in Box 32-3.

Pathophysiology

Endometrial implants can occur throughout the body. The most common sites of implantation are the ovaries, uterine ligaments, rectovaginal septum, and pelvic peritoneum (Fig. 32-12). Less common sites include the sigmoid colon, small intestine, rectum, appendix, bladder, uterus, vulva, vagina, cervix, lymph nodes, extremities, pleural cavity, lungs, laparotomy scars, and hernial sacs.

If the blood supply is sufficient, the ectopic endometrium proliferates, breaks down, and bleeds in conjunction with the normal menstrual cycle. The bleeding causes inflammation and pain in surrounding tissues. The inflammation may lead to fibrosis, scarring, and adhesions.

Clinical Manifestations

The clinical manifestations of endometriosis vary in frequency and severity and include infertility; abnormal vaginal bleeding; dysmenorrhea; dyschezia (pain on defecation); constipation; dyspareunia; and if implants are located within the pelvis, asymptomatic pelvic mass having irregular, movable nodules and a fixed, retroverted uterus. Most symptoms can be explained by the proliferation, breakdown, and bleeding of the ectopic endometrial tissue, with subsequent formation of adhesions. In many instances, however, the degree of endometriosis is not related to the frequency or severity of symptoms. Dysmenorrhea, for example, does not appear to be related to the degree of endometriosis. With involvement of the rectovaginal septum or the uterosacral ligaments, dyspareunia develops. Dyschezia occurs with bleeding of ectopic endometrium in the rectosigmoid musculature and subsequent fibrosis.

Approximately 25% to 35% of individuals with endometriosis are infertile, presumably because of (1) mechanical interference with ovulation or ovum transport through the fallopian tube, (2) phagocytosis of sperm by macrophages in the reproductive tract, (3) changes in prostaglandin secretion, (4) luteal phase defect, (5) unruptured luteinizing follicle syndrome, (6) hyperprolactinemia, and (7) autoimmune and genetic factors.

Evaluation and Treatment

Pelvic laparoscopy is required for definitive diagnosis of endometriosis and should be completed before beginning therapy.[8] The American Fertility Society has proposed that endometriosis be classified by the extent of the disease as stage I, mild; stage II, moderate; stage III, severe; and stage IV, extensive. All treatment is based on the stage of the disease and aimed toward prevention of disease progression, alleviation of pain, and establishment or restoration of fertility. Medical therapies include suppression of ovulation with noncyclic hormonal oral contraceptives, danazol, GnRH agonists, or gestrinone, a 19-nontestosterone derivative.[12] Conservative surgical treatment includes laparoscopic removal of endometrial implants with conventional or laser techniques and presacral neurectomy for severe dysmenorrhea. All treatments have risks or side effects, and recurrent symptoms will develop in as many as 45% of women within 5 years.[11]

Cancer

Malignant tumors of the female reproductive system are common. Endometrial carcinoma accounts for approximately 6% of all cancers in women; ovarian tumors, 4%; and cervical tumors, 2%.[13] Malignant neoplasms of the female reproductive tract account for about 1 of 8 diagnosed cancers and 1 of 12 cancer deaths in women in the United States.[14]

Cervical cancer

Invasive cancer of the cervix is the third most prevalent gynecologic cancer and accounts for approximately 2% of all cancers and 18% of gynecologic cancers. Average age for detecting and diagnosing dysplasia, or precancerous lesions, is 33 to 38 years, and 43 to 48 years for invasive cancer. Invasive carcinoma is most likely to affect women in their 50s and 60s. Whereas the overall incidence of invasive cervical cancer has decreased over the years, rates of abnormal cervical cytology have markedly increased in white women younger than 25 years, presumably because of increased infection with human papillomavirus (HPV). By age 20 years, one in eight young women will have cervical dysplasia. Incidence rates tend to be higher in women of low socioeconomic status, perhaps because of inability to access health care and poor nutrition.[13]

Because of increased prevalence of Papanicolaou (cytologic) screening, rates for invasive cancer have dropped about 5% and cervical cancer deaths by 45% since the early 1970s. Although mortality for blacks declined more rapidly than for whites, mortality risks for black women continue to be more than two times those of whites.[14]

Cervical cancer is generally considered a sexually transmitted disease. Infection of the cervix with HPV, first intercourse before age 16 years, and multiple sexual partners or a male partner with multiple partners place a woman at risk. Smoking is considered a cofactor in the development of cervical carcinoma. Poor nutrition also increases risk, perhaps by depressing the immune system. Likewise, human immunodeficiency virus (HIV)–positive women are at greater risk for developing cervical cancer.[13]

Pathophysiology

Cervical cancer is a progressive disease that is staged according to histology (Table 32-4). Premalignant lesions occur 10 to 12 years before the development of invasive carcinoma. The progressive changes of cervical cells are classified on a continuum from cervical intraepithelial neoplasia (CIN), to cervical carcinoma in situ, to invasive carcinoma. Fig. 32-13 summarizes the progressive degrees of CIN.

Clinical Manifestations

Because cervical neoplasms are asymptomatic, regular cytologic screening (Papanicolaou smear) is necessary. About 90% of cervical cancers can be detected early through the use of Pap smears. Vaginal bleeding and discharge are common symptoms. Bleeding varies and may occur after intercourse or between menstrual periods. At times, women will

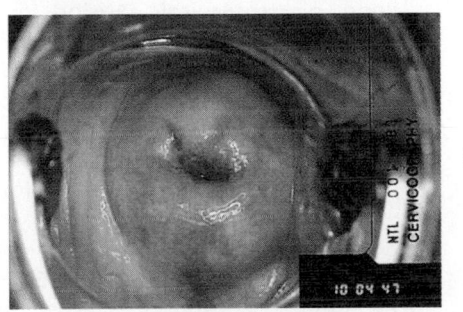

Fig. 32-13 *Cervical intraepithelial neoplasia (CIN).* **A,** Diagram of cervical endothelium showing progressive degrees of CIN. **B,** Normal multiparous cervix. *(A from Herbst, A.L. et al. [1992]. Comprehensive gynecology [2nd ed.]. St. Louis: Mosby; B from Symonds, E.M. & Macpherson, M.B.A. [1994]. Color atlas of obstetrics and gynecology. London: Mosby-Wolfe.)*

TABLE 32-4	**Clinical Staging for Cancer of the Cervix**

Stage	Characteristics
0	Cancer in situ, intraepithelial carcinoma; earliest stage of cancer; cancer confined to its original site
I	Carcinoma confined to cervix (extension to corpus disregarded)
IA	Earliest form of stage I; there is very small amount of cancer, which is visible only under a microscope
IA1	Area of invasion is < 3 mm (about 1/8 inch) deep and < 7 mm (about 1/3 inch) wide
IA2	Area of invasion is between 3 mm and 5 mm (about 1/5 inch) deep, and < 7 mm (about 1/3 inch) wide
IB	Includes cancers that can be seen without a microscope; also includes cancers seen only with a microscope that have spread deeper than 5 mm (about 1/5 inch) into connective tissue of the cervix or are wider than 7 mm
IB1	A IB cancer that is no larger than 4 cm (about 1 3/5 inches)
IB2	A IB cancer that is > 4 cm
II	Cancer has spread beyond the cervix to the upper part of the vagina; cancer does not involve the lower third of the vagina
IIA	Cancer has spread beyond the cervix to the upper part of the vagina; cancer does not involve the lower third of the vagina
IIB	Cancer has spread to the tissue next to the cervix, called the *parametrial tissue*
III	Cancer has spread to the lower part of the vagina or the pelvic wall; cancer may be blocking the ureters (tubes that carry urine from the kidneys to the bladder)
IIIA	Cancer has spread to the lower third of the vagina but not to the pelvic wall
IIIB	Cancer extends to the pelvic wall and/or blocks urine flow to the bladder
IV	Most advanced stage of cervical cancer; cancer has spread to other parts of the body
IVA	Cancer has spread to the bladder or rectum, which are organs close to the cervix
IVB	Cancer has spread to distant organs beyond the pelvic area, such as the lungs

Reprinted from the American Cancer Society's Cancer Information Database with permission.

complain of abnormal menses or postmenopausal bleeding. A less common symptom may be a serosanguineous or yellowish vaginal discharge. A new or foul odor also may be present. Severe bleeding may cause anemia. Pelvic or epigastric pain is experienced only with large lesions. Advanced disease may cause urinary or rectal symptoms.

⊟ *Evaluation and Treatment*

Cervical cytology is most accurate if cells obtained by endocervical swabbing and ectocervical scraping are examined. When dysplasia is detected, cervical biopsy and curettage are required. Colposcopy is used to identify suggestive sites for biopsy. If invasive carcinoma is found, lymphangiography, computed tomography (CT) scan, ultrasonography, or radioimmunodetection methods are used to assess lymphatic involvement.

The treatment depends on the degree of neoplastic change, the size and location of the lesion, and the extent of metastatic spread. With early detection and treatment, prognosis is excellent. Overall, the 5-year survival rate is 69% and increases to 91% with early diagnosis. A cure rate of 100% is possible for women with dysplasia or carcinoma in situ.[13,14] See Box 32-4 for recommended treatment based on staging of disease.

Vaginal cancer

Cancer of the vagina is the rarest of the female genital cancers. It can occur at any age but is found predominantly in women 60 years of age and older. More than 90% of women with vaginal cancer have squamous cell carcinoma, although melanomas, sarcomas, and adenocarcinomas are also found. (Types of tumors are described in Chapter 9.) Metastatic

cancers are more common than primary lesions in older women.

Vaginal and cervical cancers seem to have similar epidemiology. Both start as intraepithelial lesions and occur in sexually active women. HPV infection and prior carcinoma of the cervix place a woman at higher risk for developing vaginal cancer.[15] In addition, intrauterine exposure to nonsteroidal estrogens (diethylstilbestrol [DES]) has also been considered a risk factor. Between 0.14 and 1.4 cases of vaginal cancer develop per 1000 women at risk (those exposed to DES in utero). The average age at which clear cell carcinoma develops as a result of DES exposure is 19 years.

Like cervical neoplasms, vaginal cancers are classified as intraepithelial neoplasia (dysplasia), carcinoma in situ, or invasive carcinoma. The lesion usually is not invasive, and it most frequently occurs in the upper third of the vagina.

Vaginal cancer is generally asymptomatic. Therefore regular pelvic examinations, particularly for intrauterine DES exposure, are extremely important. Clinical manifestations that occur include abnormal vaginal bleeding or discharge and urinary symptoms. Pain is a symptom of advanced disease or an infected lesion.

Biopsy techniques confirm the tumor type and determine its size, location, and extent. Treatment depends on these findings and on the age of the individual. Surgery may be followed by radiation and chemotherapy.

Endometrial cancer

Carcinoma of the endometrium is the most prevalent gynecologic malignancy (Fig. 32-14). It accounts for about 6% of cancers affecting women and more than 48% of gynecologic cancers.[14,16] Estimates include 37,400 new cases in 1999, with approximately 6400 deaths.[14] Although the cause of endometrial cancer is not clear, a number of risk factors have been identified (see Risk Factor box). Ninety-five percent of endometrial cancers occur in women age 40 years or older, with an average age of 60 years at diagnosis. Whites are about 70% more likely than blacks to develop this kind of cancer, but survival rates for whites are higher than for blacks.[14]

Fig. 32-14 *Endometrial cancer.* Tumor fills the endometrial cavity. Obvious myometrial invasion is seen. *(From Damjanov, I. & Linder, J. [Eds.]. [1996]. Anderson's pathology [10th ed.]. St. Louis: Mosby.)*

RISK FACTORS

ENDOMETRIAL CANCER
- History of obesity (>30 lbs overweight)
- High-fat diet (animal fat)
- Higher socioeconomic status (may be caused by diet)
- Infertility or no pregnancies
- Early menarche (<12 years)
- Late menopause (>52 years)
- Family history of endometrial cancer
- Personal history of breast or ovarian cancer
- Prior pelvic radiotherapy
- Age ≥ 40 years
- White race
- Prolonged estrogen use or tamoxifen therapy after menopause
- Diabetes
- Hereditary nonpolyposis colon cancer
- Gallbladder disease

Data from American Cancer Society. (1999). Cancer facts and figures—1999. New York: The Author.

Delayed menarche and the use of hormonal contraception have a protective effect. After prolonged use of oral or injective contraception, protection continues for at least 10 years.

Women with postmenopausal bleeding or obese women with persistent irregular bleeding are evaluated for endometrial cancer. Screening methods for early detection of endometrial cancer are as effective as those for cervical cancer. Direct cytologic sampling of the endometrium is required for diagnosis. This may be accomplished by endometrial biopsy or fractional curettage that includes biopsies of all sectors of the uterus. Hysteroscopy and hysterography may also be used to examine the endometrium, but these methods may result in uterine perforation or enhancement of tumor cell migration if disease is advanced. Evaluation for metastasis includes routine blood work, metabolic studies, chest x-ray films, intravenous pyelography (IVP), barium enema, ultrasonography, and lymphangiography.

Treatment is based on the extent of the disease, and it includes surgical removal of the obvious tumor and radiation for control of residual microscopic disease. Chemotherapy also may be used. Five-year survival rates range from 66% to 95%.[14,16]

✓ QUICK CHECK

Why is routine screening for cervical cancer recommended by the American Cancer Society?

Ovarian cancer

Ovarian cancer ranks fifth in the number of new cases of cancer among women (Fig. 32-15).[17] The American Cancer Society (ACS) estimated 25,200 new cases and 14,500 cancer deaths in 1999.[14] In other words, ovarian cancer accounts for over 5% of all female cancer deaths and causes more deaths than any other cancer of the female reproductive system. Incidence rates increase with age and peak in the eighth decade.[17]

RISK FACTORS

OVARIAN CANCER
- Family history of ovarian, breast, uterine, pancreatic, or colon cancer
- Personal history of breast cancer
- Age: postmenopausal
- Infertility or prolonged use of fertility drugs without achieving pregnancy
- Early menarche, late menopause, or no children or first child after age 30 years
- High-fat diet
- Exposure to asbestos or talc applied to genitalia
- Genetic predisposition

Data from American Cancer Society. (1997). Ovarian cancer. New York: The Author; American Cancer Society. (1999). Cancer facts & figures—1999. New York: The Author.

Pathogenesis

The cause of ovarian cancer is unknown at present. Risk factors are presented in the Risk Factor box.

Pregnancy and childbirth decrease the risk. Hormonal contraception provides the same protection from ovarian cancer as it does from endometrial cancer. Recent studies report that women who take birth control pills for only 3 years can lower their ovarian cancer risk by 30% to 50%. Thus the protection given by birth control pills may be more than just stopping egg-related release and allowing the ovaries' outer lining to undergo less wear and tear; progestin may enhance apoptosis—allowing the body to dispose of mutated cells.[18]

Clinical Manifestations

Ovarian cancer is generally considered a silent disease, meaning that by the time the individual experiences symp-

Fig. 32-15 *Ovarian tumors.* Bilateral multicystic ovarian tumors. *(From Symonds, E.M. & Macpherson, M.B.A. [1994]. Color atlas of obstetrics and gynecology. London: Mosby-Wolfe.)*

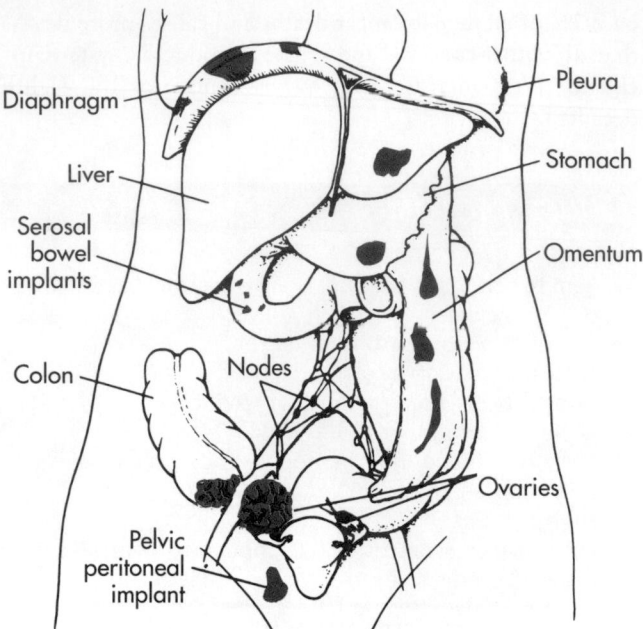

Fig. 32-16 *Metastasis of ovarian cancer.* Pattern of spread for epithelial cancer of the ovary. *(From DiSaia, P.J. & Creasman, W.T. [1993]. Clinical gynecologic oncology [4th ed.]. St. Louis: Mosby.)*

TABLE 32-5	FIGO* Staging of Carcinoma of the Ovary
Stage	**Characteristics**
I	Growth limited to the ovaries
II	Growth involving one or both ovaries with pelvic extension
III	Cancer involves one or both ovaries, and one or both of the following are present: (1) cancer has spread beyond the pelvis to the lining of the abdomen (the part of the trunk near the stomach), (2) cancer has spread to lymph nodes (glands that fight infection and produce some types of blood cells)
IV	Growth involving one or both ovaries with distant metastases; if pleural effusion is present, there must be positive cytology to allow a case to stage IV; parenchymal liver metastases indicate stage IV
Recurrent	Cancer recurred after completion of treatment

Data from American Cancer Society (ACS), (1999).
*The International Federation of Gynecologists and Obstetricians.

toms and seeks treatment, the disease has spread beyond the primary site. The most obvious symptoms are pain and abdominal swelling (ascites) that arise from the primary ovarian mass. Gastrointestinal manifestations may include dyspepsia, vomiting, and alterations in bowel habits caused by the mechanical obstruction by the tumor. Abnormal vaginal bleeding may occur if the postmenopausal endometrium is stimulated by a hormone-secreting tumor. The tumor also may cause ulcerations through the vaginal wall that result in bleeding.

Systemic manifestations of nonmetastatic malignant disease include connective tissue inflammation (dermatomyositis), abnormal pigmentation (acanthosis nigricans), and subacute cerebellar degeneration. Tumor obstruction of vascular channels can cause venous and, occasionally, arterial thrombosis. Alterations in coagulability also occur, contributing to clot formation. Metastasis frequently causes pleural effusion (Fig. 32-16).

Evaluation and Treatment

Because ovarian cancer has no early symptoms and there are no effective screening techniques to detect it, the disease is usually advanced by the time treatment is sought. Transvaginal ultrasound and a tumor marker (CA-125) may assist diagnosis but are not recommended for routine screening. Diagnosis is made after ultrasound, CT scan, magnetic resonance imaging (MRI), or other imaging techniques that enable clinicians to localize the tumor mass. The International Federation of Gynecologists and Obstetricians (FIGO) staging system is described in Table 32-5. Other preoperative studies used to determine the ex-

tent of metastasis include an upper gastrointestinal series, barium enema, intravenous pyelogram, mammography, and lymphography.

The initial approach to treatment is surgery, which is performed to determine the stage of disease and to remove as much of the tumor as possible. Radiation therapy may follow if the tumor is smaller than 2 cm in size and is confined to the abdominopelvic area without involvement of the kidneys or liver. The success of chemotherapy depends on the extent of disease, whether the tumor is a discrete mass, and whether there has been prior exposure to chemotherapeutic agents. Research into prevention and treatment of ovarian cancer is ongoing and expanding (see Health Alert box).

The mortality associated with ovarian cancer has not changed significantly over the past 20 years, mainly because the disease is already advanced at the time of diagnosis. Five-year mortality for women with regional and distant disease is 55% and 25%, respectively.[14] If ovarian cancer is diagnosed and treated early, the rate is 93%; however, less than one in four cases are detected at the localized stage.[14] The overall survival rate is 46% (Box 32-5 and Health Alert box on recovery).

Sexual Dysfunction

Increased awareness of female sexual dysfunction is relatively new, and most of what is known comes from clinical observations and anecdotal reports from women. Both organic and psychosocial disorders can be implicated in sexual dysfunction.[19] Organic problems may be the underlying cause in 10% to 20% of cases and can contribute to another 15%. Chronic illness can affect sexual functioning and re-

HEALTH ALERT

Ovarian Cancer Research

Research is constantly underway to find new ways to prevent and treat cancer. Current research into ovarian cancer includes the following:

- Studies to determine whether ovarian cancer can be identified at an earlier stage
- Investigation of new blood tests to detect tumor markers, to see if more sensitive and effective screening tests can be identified
- Further evaluation of the benefits of currently used oral contraceptives in reducing the risk of ovarian cancer
- Establishment of a national serum and tissue bank for ovarian cancer research
- Better identification of women at increased risk for ovarian cancer, including genetic research and environmental research
- Additional study of the safety and efficacy of laparoscopy for women with ovarian cancer
- Determination of the effectiveness and ideal doses of various combinations of chemotherapy drugs (including platinum, paclitaxel, topotecan, and others) in treating earlier stage disease
- A randomized study to identify the best treatments for various subsets of stage I ovarian cancer
- Reevaluation of whole abdominal radiation in certain cases
- New approaches to the treatment of advanced primary, as well as recurrent, ovarian cancer
- Measures of the quality of life in women with ovarian cancer to improve the care of patients

Data from American Cancer Society. (1997). Cervical cancer. New York: The Author.

National Organizations for Ovarian Cancer   BOX 32-5

National organizations for ovarian cancer include the following:

1. American Cancer Society
   1-800-ACS-2345
   Internet address: www.cancer.org/
2. Gynecologic Cancer Foundation
   1-800-444-4441
   Internet address: www.sgo.org/
3. National Cancer Institute
   1-800-4-CANCER
   Internet address: www.nci.nih.gov/
4. Gilda Radner Familial Ovarian Cancer Registry
   1-800-682-7426
   Internet address: rpci.med.buffalo.edu/clinic/gynonc/grwp.htm/

HEALTH ALERT

Recovery After Cancer Treatment

Recovery after cancer treatment can be enhanced through life-style changes:
- Stop tobacco use.
- Limit alcohol to < 1 drink per day.
- Improve nutrition—increase fruits, vegetables, whole grains, and high-fiber foods; limit fat, especially animal fat.
- Exercise daily.
- Rest frequently.
- Join support group and attend meetings (family members should attend support groups also).
- Communicate openly, honestly, and frequently with members of cancer care team.

Data from American Cancer Society. (1997). Ovarian cancer. New York: The Author.

sponse. Table 32-6 outlines possible effects of specified chronic diseases on female sexual functioning.

Sexual anorexia (inhibited sexual desire, decreased libido) may be a biologic manifestation of depression, alcohol or other substance abuse, prolactin-secreting pituitary tumors, or testosterone deficiency. β Adrenergic blockers used for heart disease may also inhibit sexual desire.

Vaginismus is an involuntary muscle spasm of the pubococcygeal muscle in response to attempted penetration. Common psychologic causes include prior sexual trauma and fear of sex. Organic causes are similar to those that cause dyspareunia. Even after the underlying organic problem is detected and successfully treated, vaginismus may persist.

Anorgasmia (orgasmic dysfunction) is the inability of a woman to reach or achieve orgasm. Specific disorders that may block orgasm are diabetes, alcoholism, neurologic disturbances, hormonal deficiencies, and pelvic disorders, such as infections, trauma, and surgical scarring. Other inhibitors include drugs, such as narcotics, tranquilizers, antidepressants, and antihypertensive medications.

Dyspareunia (painful intercourse) is common. Women may experience pain at any time from arousal to after intercourse. The pain may have a burning, sharp, searing, or cramping quality and may be described as external, vaginal, deep abdominal, or pelvic. A variety of psychosocial and organic causes have been identified. Inadequate lubrication may make penetration or intercourse difficult or painful. Drugs with a drying effect, such as antihistamines, certain tranquilizers, and marijuana, and disorders such as diabetes, vaginal infections, and estrogen deficiency can decrease lubrication. Other causes include skin problems around the introitus or affecting the vulva; irritation or infection of the clitoris; disorders of the vaginal opening, such as scarring from episiotomy or chronically infected hymenal remnants; intact hymen; bartholinitis; disorders of the urethra or anus; disorders of the vagina, such as infections, thinning of the walls caused by aging or decreased estrogen, or irritation

TABLE 32-6	Possible Effects of Chronic Disease on Sexual Functioning in Women
Disease	**Sexual Function**
Cerebral palsy	Intact genital sensations, decreased lubrication; difficulty with sexual activity/positioning because of muscle spasticity, rigidity, and/or weakness; pain with positioning caused by contracture of knees and hips or because of increased spasms with arousal
Cerebrovascular accident (CVA)	Difficulties in sexual positioning and sensitivity because of impaired motor strength, coordination, or paralysis; decreased sex drive with stroke on the dominant side of the brain
Diabetes	Diminished intensity of orgasm and gradual decline in ability to achieve orgasm; decreased lubrication and/or recurrent vaginal infections with resultant dyspareunia
Chronic renal failure	Decreased arousal; increasingly rare and less intense orgasms; decreased lubrication
Rheumatoid arthritis (RA)	Painful sexual activity/positions because of swollen, painful joints, muscular atrophy, and joint contracture; decreased sex drive because of pain, fatigue, and/or medication; genital sensations remain intact
Systemic lupus erythematosus (SLE)	Similar to RA; decreased lubrication and vaginal lesions result in painful penetration
Myocardial infarction (MI)	Most literature male-oriented; problems related to medications
Multiple sclerosis (MS)	Diminished genital sensitivity; decreased lubrication; declining orgasmic ability; difficulty with sexual activity because of muscle weakness, pain, or incontinence
Spinal cord injury	Reflex sexual response with injury above sacral area; disrupted response with lesion at or below sacrum; loss of sensation, decreased lubrication; spasticity, incontinence, or pain with arousal; continued orgasmic sensations or sensations diffused in general or to specific body parts, such as breast or lips

caused by spermicides or douches; and pelvic disorders, such as infection, tumors, cervical or uterine abnormalities, or torn uterine ligaments.

Sexual dysfunction may develop as a coping mechanism. Women with a history of sexual trauma—rape, incest, or molestation—frequently have problems with desire, arousal, or orgasm or experience pain with sexual activity. In extreme cases, total sexual aversion may develop. At other times, sexual dysfunction may be a symptom of marital or relationship problems. Often, unresolved anger manifests as inhibited desire or diminished arousal.

Impaired Fertility

Infertility affects approximately 15% of all couples and is defined as the inability to conceive after 1 year of unprotected intercourse. Fertility can be impaired by factors in the man or in the woman or in both partners. Male factors include diminished quality and production of sperm. Causes include infections or inflammation, endocrine or hormonal disorders, immunologic problems in which men produce antibodies to their own sperm, and environmental or lifestyle factors.[20] Female infertility factors are associated with malfunctions of the fallopian tubes, the ovaries, or the reproductive hormones. Adhesions from pelvic infection may cause blockage of one or both fallopian tubes, preventing access of the sperm to the ovum. Hormonal or local factors may disrupt ovulation or prevent a fertilized egg from implantation. Endometriosis also may contribute to infertility. A number of diagnostic procedures are required in the routine investigation of the infertile couple. Initial work-up includes semen analysis and determination of ovulation. In many instances no cause may be identified.

Treatment of infertility is aimed toward correcting problems identified during the diagnostic work-up. The best treatment for infertility is prevention of sexually transmitted infection that can result in scarring and adhesion formation in the reproductive tract of either the man or the woman.

DISORDERS OF THE MALE REPRODUCTIVE SYSTEM
Disorders of the Urethra

Urethritis and urethral strictures are common disorders of the male urethra. Urethral carcinoma, an extremely rare form of cancer, can occur in men older than 60 years.

Urethritis

Urethritis is an inflammatory process that is usually, but not always, caused by a sexually transmitted microorganism. Infectious urethritis caused by *N. gonorrhoeae* is often called gonococcal urethritis (GU); urethritis caused by other microorganisms is called nongonococcal urethritis (NGU). Nonsexual origins of urethritis include inflammation or infection as a result of urologic procedures, insertion of foreign bodies into the urethra, anatomic abnormalities, or trauma.

Noninfectious urethritis is rare and is associated with the ingestion of wood or ethyl alcohol or turpentine. It is also seen with Reiter syndrome.[21]

Symptoms of urethritis include urethral tingling or itching or a burning sensation, and frequency and urgency with urination. The individual may note a purulent or clear mucuslike discharge from the urethra. Treatment consists of appropriate antibiotic therapy for infectious urethritis and avoidance of future exposure or mechanical irritation.

Urethral strictures

A *urethral stricture* is a narrowing of the urethra caused by scarring. The scars may be congenital but are more likely to result from trauma (e.g., injury or urologic instrumentation) or untreated or severe urethral infections. Prostatitis and infection secondary to urinary stasis are common complications. Severe and prolonged obstruction can result in hydronephrosis and renal failure.

Clinical manifestations include urinary frequency and hesitancy, diminished force and caliber of the urinary stream, dribbling after voiding, and nocturia. Urethral stricture is diagnosed on the basis of history, physical examination, and cystoscopy. Treatment is usually surgical and may involve urethral dilation, urethrotomy, or a variety of open surgical techniques. The choice of surgical intervention depends on the age of the individual and the severity of the problem.

Disorders of the Penis
Phimosis and paraphimosis

Phimosis and paraphimosis are both disorders in which the foreskin (prepuce) is "too tight" to move easily over the glans penis. *Phimosis* is a condition in which the foreskin cannot be retracted back over the glans, whereas *paraphimosis* is the opposite: the foreskin is retracted and cannot be moved forward (reduced) to cover the glans (Fig. 32-17). Both conditions can cause penile pathologic conditions.

During the first 3 years of life, congenital adhesions (between the foreskin and glans) separate naturally with penile erections and are not an indication for circumcision. Phimosis can occur at any age and is most commonly caused by poor hygiene and chronic infection. It rarely occurs with normal foreskin.

Reasons for seeking treatment include edema, erythema, and tenderness of the prepuce and purulent discharge; inability to retract the foreskin is a less common complaint. Circumcision, if needed, is performed after infection has been eradicated. Complications of phimosis include inflammation of the glans (balanitis) or prepuce (posthitis) and paraphimosis. There is a higher incidence of penile carcinoma in uncircumcised males, but chronic infection and poor hygiene are usually the underlying factors in such cases.

Paraphimosis, in which the foreskin is retracted, can constrict the penis, causing edema of the glans. If the foreskin cannot be reduced manually, surgery must be performed to prevent necrosis of the glans caused by constricted blood vessels. Severe paraphimosis is a surgical emergency.

Peyronie disease

Peyronie disease ("bent nail syndrome") is a fibrotic condition that causes lateral curvature of the penis during erection (Fig. 32-18). Peyronie disease develops slowly and is characterized by tough fibrous thickening of the fascia in the erectile tissue of the corpora cavernosa. A dense, fibrous plaque is usually palpable on the dorsum of the penile shaft. The problem usually affects middle-aged men and is associated with painful erection, painful intercourse (for both partners), and poor erection distal to the involved area. In some cases, impotence or unsatisfactory penetration occurs. When the penis is flaccid, there is no pain.

A local vasculitis-like inflammatory reaction occurs, and decreased tissue oxygenation results in fibrosis and calcification. The exact cause is unknown. Peyronie disease is associated with Dupuytren contracture (a flexion deformity of the fingers or toes caused by shortening or fibrosis of the palmar or plantar fascia), diabetes, predisposition to keloids, and, in rare cases, use of β-blocker medications.[22]

There is no definitive treatment for Peyronie disease. Spontaneous remissions occur up to 50% of the time. Plication and surgical resection of the fibrous plaque followed by grafting have been successful.[21]

Priapism

Priapism is an uncommon condition of prolonged penile erection. It is usually painful and is not associated with sexual arousal (Fig. 32-19). Priapism is idiopathic in 60% of cases, whereas the remaining 40% of cases can be associated with spinal cord trauma, sickle cell disease, leukemia, pelvic tumors, or intracavernous injection therapy for impotence.

Priapism must be considered a urologic emergency. Treatment within hours is effective and prevents impotence. Conservative approaches include iced saline enemas, ketamine administration, and spinal anesthesia. Needle aspiration of blood from the corpus through the dorsal glans is often effective and is followed by catheterization and pressure dressings to maintain decompression. More aggressive surgical treatments include the creation of vascular shunts to maintain blood flow. In up to 50% of cases, erectile dysfunction results.

Balanitis

Balanitis is an inflammation of the glans penis (Fig. 32-20) and usually occurs in conjunction with posthitis, an inflammation of the prepuce. (Inflammation of the glans and the prepuce is called *balanoposthitis*.) It is associated with poor hygiene and phimosis. The accumulation under the foreskin of glandular secretions (smegma), sloughed epithelial cells, and *Mycobacterium smegmatis* can irritate the glans directly or lead to infection. Skin disorders (e.g., psoriasis, lichen planus, eczema) and candidiasis must be differentiated from inflammation resulting from poor hygienic practices. Balanitis is most commonly seen in men with poorly controlled diabetes mellitus and candidiasis. The infection is treated with antimicrobials. After the inflammation has subsided, circumcision can be considered to prevent recurrences.

Penile cancer

Carcinoma of the penis is rare in the United States, constituting less than 0.24%[14] of all malignancies in men. It can affect men 50 to 70 years of age, with 40% of diagnosed men younger than 60 years. The disease occurs almost twice as frequently in blacks as whites in the United States and tends

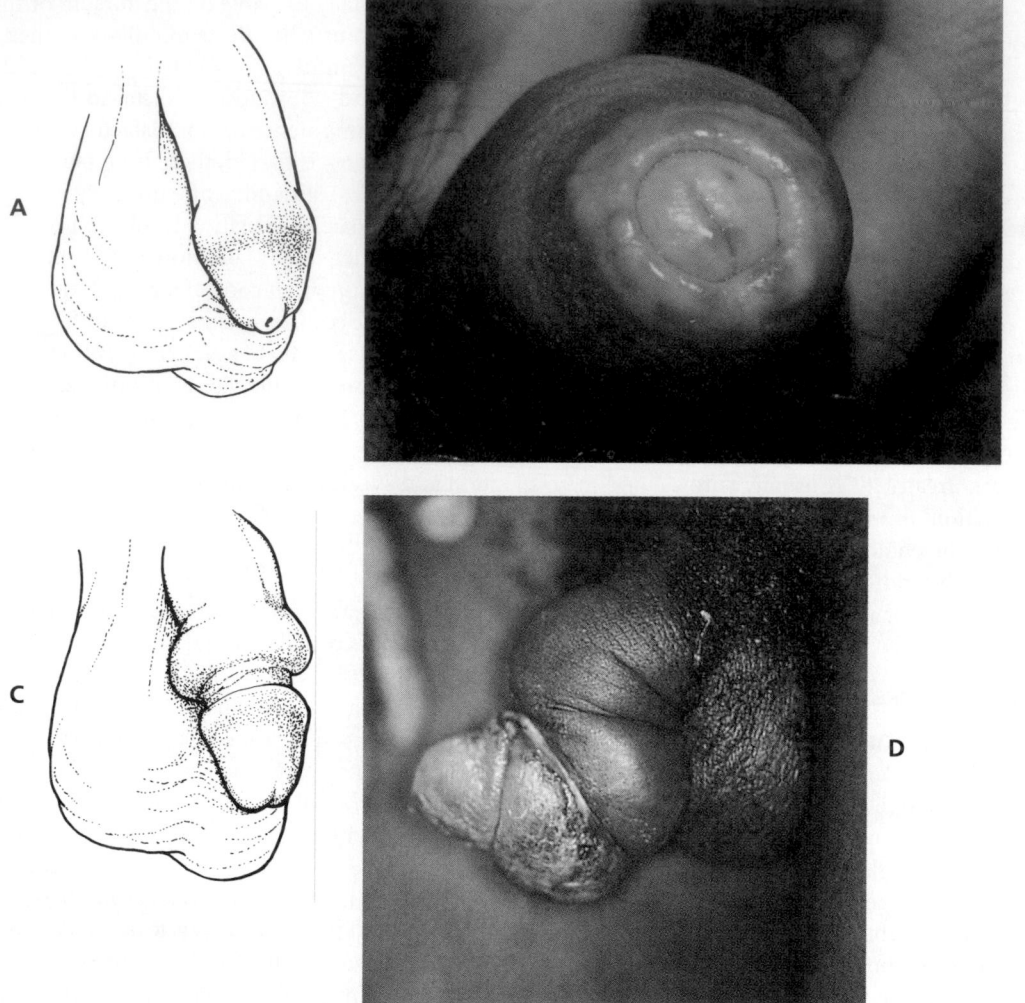

Fig. 32-17 *Phimosis and paraphimosis.* **A,** Phimosis: the foreskin has a narrow opening that is not large enough to permit retraction over the glans. **B,** Lesions on the prepuce secondary to infection cause swelling, and retraction of foreskin may be impossible. Circumcision is usually required. **C,** Paraphimosis: the foreskin is retracted over the glans but cannot be reduced to its normal position. Here it has formed a constricting band around the penis. **D,** Ulcer on the retracted prepuce with edema. *(A and C from Phipps, W.P. et al. [1995]. Medical-surgical nursing: Concepts and clinical practice [5th ed.]. London: Mosby-Wolfe; B from Taylor, P.K. [1995]. Diagnostic picture tests in sexually transmitted diseases. St. Louis: Mosby; D from Morse, S.A., Moreland, A.A., & Holmes, K.K. [1996]. Atlas of sexually transmitted diseases and AIDS [2nd ed.]. London: Mosby-Wolfe.)*

to be more common in lower socioeconomic groups. Although the exact cause is unknown, cancer of the penis is thought to develop as a result of chronic irritation caused by smegma beneath a phimotic foreskin. The incidence of penile carcinoma is highest in populations where infantile circumcision and adequate genital hygiene are not routinely practiced. In these areas, penile cancer remains a significant health problem and accounts for 10% to 20% of all malignancies in men.

Squamous cell carcinoma accounts for 95% of invasive penile cancers. Other premalignant lesions, or in situ forms of epidermal carcinoma, that occur on the penis include leukoplakia (white plaque), Paget disease (red, inflamed areas), erythroplasia of Queyrat (raised red areas), and

Buschke-Löwenstein patches (large venous areas). Condylomata (genital warts) caused by HPV may be involved in the development of precancerous lesions and squamous cell cancers.[15] At times, the penis might be the site of metastatic spread of solid tumors from the bladder, prostate, rectum, or kidney. Early squamous cell carcinoma and premalignant epidermal lesions are easily treated, but delays in seeking treatment are attributed to denial, embarrassment, failure to detect lesions under a phimotic foreskin, fear, guilt, and ignorance.

Squamous cell carcinoma usually begins as a small, fat, ulcerative or papillary lesion on the glans or foreskin that grows to involve the entire penile shaft. Extensive lesions are associated with metastases and a poor prognosis. These le-

Fig. 32-18 *Peyronie disease.* This person complained of pain and deviation of his penis to one side on erection. *(From Taylor, P.K. [1995]. Diagnostic picture tests in sexually transmitted diseases. London: Mosby-Wolfe.)*

Fig. 32-20 *Balanitis. (From Taylor, P.K. [1995]. Diagnostic picture tests in sexually transmitted diseases. London: Mosby-Wolfe.)*

Fig. 32-19 *Priapism. (From Lloyd-Davies, R.W. et al. [1994]. Color atlas of urology [2nd ed.]. London: Wolfe Medical Publications.)*

TABLE 32-7	Stages of Carcinoma of the Penis
Stage	**Definition**
I	Tumor limited to the glans or foreskin
II	Tumor extends to shaft of penis
III	Inguinal lymph nodes involved but operable
IV	Inguinal nodes inoperable, or distant metastasis has occurred

Penile carcinoma requires surgery. Palliative treatment with radiation or chemotherapy may be used when the disease is inoperable and bulky inguinal metastases have occurred. Options for individuals with carcinoma in situ include local excision, radiation, laser surgery, cryosurgery, chemosurgery, or chemotherapy with topical (5%) 5-fluorouracil. The 5-year survival rate for stage I disease is more than 80%.[23]

✓QUICK CHECK

Why are priapism and severe paraphimosis considered urologic emergencies?

What are the risk factors for cancer of the penis?

Disorders of the Scrotum, Testis, and Epididymis
Disorders of the scrotum

Varicocele, hydrocele, and spermatocele are common intrascrotal disorders.[21] A *varicocele* is an abnormal dilation of a vein within the spermatic cord and is classically described as a "bag of worms" (Fig. 32-21). Most (95%) occur on the left side and may be painful or tender. Varicocele occurs in

sions are not as painful as the amount of tissue involvement would seem to indicate. The regional femoral and iliac nodes are common metastatic sites; the urethra and bladder are rarely involved. Weight loss, fatigue, and malaise accompany chronic suppurative lesions. Untreated, progressive disease causes death within 2 years.

The specific diagnosis is made by biopsy after examination to document the location, size, and fixation of the lesion and the absence or presence of regional adenopathy. Distant metastases are uncommon. Stages of carcinoma of the penis are presented in Table 32-7.

Fig. 32-21 *Varicocele.* Dilation of veins within the spermatic cord. *(From Seidel, H. et al. [1999]. Mosby's guide to physical examination [4th ed.]. St. Louis: Mosby.)*

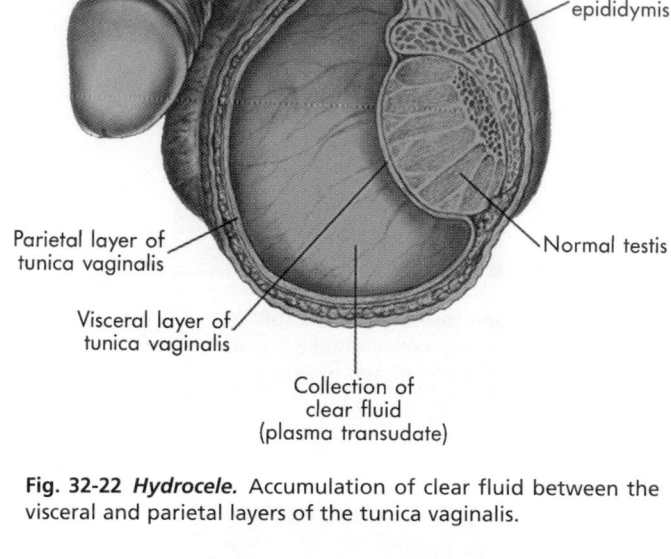

Normal epididymis

Normal testis

Parietal layer of tunica vaginalis

Visceral layer of tunica vaginalis

Collection of clear fluid (plasma transudate)

Fig. 32-22 *Hydrocele.* Accumulation of clear fluid between the visceral and parietal layers of the tunica vaginalis.

10% to 15% of males and is seen most frequently after puberty. Sudden development of a varicocele in an older man is a late sign of renal tumor. Unilateral right-sided varicoceles are rare and result from compression or obstruction of the inferior vena cava by a tumor or thrombus.

The cause of varicocele is incompetent or congenitally absent valves in the spermatic veins. Blood pools in the veins rather than flowing into the venous system. Varicocele decreases blood flow through the testis, interfering with spermatogenesis and causing infertility. If infertility is a problem, treatment consists of ligation of the spermatic vein. If varicocele is mild and fertility is not an issue, a scrotal support is usually sufficient to relieve symptoms of scrotal heaviness or "dragging."

A *hydrocele* is a collection of fluid within the tunica vaginalis (Fig. 32-22). It is the most common cause of scrotal swelling. Hydroceles in infants are congenital malformations that frequently resolve spontaneously by 1 year of age. Hydroceles in adults may be caused by an imbalance between the secreting and absorptive capacities of scrotal tissues. Hydroceles range in size from slightly larger than the testes to a grapefruit or larger and may be flaccid or tense. Compression of testicular blood supply may lead to atrophy.

The exact mechanism of idiopathic hydrocele is unknown. Secondary hydrocele may result from trauma or infection of the testis or epididymis or from a testicular tumor. Treatment for uncomplicated hydrocele is aspiration of the fluid and injection of a sclerosing drug into the scrotal sac. Recurrent hydroceles require excision of the tunica vaginalis.

A *spermatocele* is a cyst located between the head of the epididymis and the testis that is filled with milky fluid containing sperm (Fig. 32-23). Spermatoceles that cause pain or discomfort are excised. Usually, however, spermatoceles are asymptomatic or produce mild discomfort that is relieved by scrotal support. Neither hydroceles nor spermatoceles are associated with infertility.

Cryptorchidism

In *cryptorchidism* one or both testes fail to descend into the scrotum. It is the most common congenital condition involving the testes. Three percent of all full-term males and 20% of all premature males have undescended testes at birth. The testes may remain in the abdomen, or descent may be arrested in the inguinal canal or the puboscrotal junction. In approximately 75% to 90% of infants with cryptorchidism, the testes descend into the scrotum by 1 year of age, leaving a true incidence of 0.8% of the male population.

Cryptorchidism may result from a developmental delay, a defect of the testis, deficient maternal gonadotropin stimulation, or some mechanical factor that prevents descent through the inguinal canal. Mechanical possibilities include a short spermatic cord, fibrous bands or adhesions in the normal path of the testes, or a narrowed inguinal canal. Chromosomal studies do not support a genetic component.

Untreated cryptorchidism is associated with a lowered sperm count and, therefore, impaired fertility. Impaired spermatogenesis is caused by higher temperatures within the abdomen. Cryptorchidism does not prevent puberty or

Fig. 32-23 *Spermatocele*. Retention cyst of the head of the epididymis or of an aberrant tubule or tubules of the rete testis. The spermatocele lies outside the tunica vaginalis; therefore on palpation it can be readily distinguished and separated from the testis. *(From Lloyd-Davies, R.W., Parkhouse, H., Gow, J.G., & Davies, D.R. [1994]. Color atlas of urology [2nd ed.]. London: Wolfe Medical Publications.)*

Fig. 32-24 *Torsion of the testis*. The testis appear dark red and partially necrotic owing to hemorrhagic infarction. *(From Damjanov, I. & Linder, J. [Eds.]. [1996]. Anderson's pathology [10th ed.]. St. Louis: Mosby.)*

maintenance of secondary sex characteristics if the testis is otherwise normal. Undescended testes are susceptible to neoplastic processes: the risk of testicular cancer is 35 to 50 times greater for men with cryptorchidism or a history of cryptorchidism than for the general male population.

Physical examination discloses the absence of one or both testes in the scrotum. Ultrasonography or a CT scan can help clinicians locate a testis that has migrated intraabdominally. Treatment often begins with hormonal therapy. To preserve fertility, surgical correction of cryptorchidism should be attempted when the child is about 2 years of age. Orchiopexy is recommended no later than age 5 or 6 years. Placement of the cryptorchid testis into the scrotal sac does not decrease the potential for malignancy, but it does facilitate examination and tumor detection.

Torsion of the testis

In ***torsion of the testis*** the testis rotates on its vascular pedicle, interrupting its blood supply (Fig. 32-24). This event can occur at any age but is most common among neonates and adolescents, particularly at puberty. Onset may be spontaneous or follow physical exertion or trauma. Torsion twists the arteries and veins in the spermatic cord, reducing or stopping circulation to the testis. Vascular engorgement and ischemia develop, causing scrotal swelling not relieved by rest or scrotal support. Torsion of the testis is a surgical emergency. If it cannot be reduced manually, surgery must be performed within 6 hours after the onset of symptoms to preserve normal testicular function.

Orchitis

Orchitis is an acute inflammation of the testes (Fig. 32-25) and is uncommon except as a complication of systemic infection or as an extension of an associated epididymitis

Fig. 32-25 *Orchitis*. *(From Seidel, H. et al. [1999]. Mosby's guide to physical examination [4th ed.]. St. Louis: Mosby.)*

(see p. 887). Infectious organisms may reach the testes through the blood or the lymphatics or, most commonly, by ascent through the urethra, vas deferens, and epididymis. Most cases of orchitis are actually cases of epididymoorchitis. Occasionally in middle-aged men, a nonspecific, apparently noninfectious, inflammatory process (called *granulo-*

matis orchitis) can occur, apparently a granulomatous response to spermatozoa.

Mumps is the most common infectious cause of orchitis and usually affects postpubertal males. The onset is sudden, occurring 3 to 4 days after the onset of parotitis. Signs and symptoms include high fever, reaching 40° C (104° F), marked prostration, bilateral or unilateral erythema, edema and tenderness of the scrotum, and leukocytosis. An acute hydrocele may develop. Urinary signs and symptoms, which accompany epididymitis, are absent. Atrophy with irreversible damage to spermatogenesis may result in 30% of affected testes. Bilateral orchitis does not affect androgenic function but may cause permanent sterility.

Treatment is supportive and includes bed rest, scrotal support, elevation of the scrotum, hot or cold compresses, and analgesic agents for relief of pain. If an acute hydrocele develops, it is aspirated. Testicular abscess usually requires orchiectomy (removal of the testis). Appropriate antimicrobial drugs should be used for bacterial orchitis, and corticosteroids are indicated in proved cases of nonspecific granulomatous orchitis.

Cancer of the testis

Testicular cancer is among the most curable of cancers, with cure rates greater than 95%. Overall, testicular cancers are uncommon, accounting for approximately 1% of all male cancers; yet they are the most common solid tumor of young adult men. Cancer of the testis occurs most commonly in men between the ages of 15 and 35 years.[14,24] In the United States, the lifetime probability of developing testicular cancer is 0.3% for white men, an incidence that is 4.5 times higher than in blacks. Testicular tumors are slightly more common on the right side than on the left, a pattern that parallels the occurrence of cryptorchidism, and they are bilateral in 1% to 3% of cases (Fig. 32-26).

Pathophysiology

Most testicular cancers are germ cell tumors, arising from the male gametes. Germ cell tumors include seminomas, embryonal carcinomas, teratomas, and choriosarcomas. Testicular tumors also can arise from specialized cells of the gonadal stroma. These tumors, which are named for their cellular origins, are the Leydig cell, Sertoli cell, granulosa cell, and theca cell tumors.

The cause of testicular neoplasms is unknown. High levels of androgens may contribute to tumorigenesis. A genetic predisposition is suggested by the fact that the incidence is higher among brothers, identical twins, and other close male relatives. Genetic predisposition is supported further by statistics showing that the disease is relatively rare among black Africans, black Americans, Asians, and native New Zealanders. The development of testicular cancer is statistically associated with cryptorchidism. A history of trauma or infection also is associated with the development of testicular neoplasms, but it may be that coexisting testicular tumors are discovered by "accident" in men who undergo examination because of trauma or infections.

Fig. 32-26 *Testicular tumor. (From 400 Self-assessment picture tests in clinical medicine. [1984]. London: Wolfe Medical Publications.)*

Clinical Manifestations

Painless testicular enlargement commonly is the first sign of testicular cancer. Occurring gradually, it may be accompanied by a sensation of testicular heaviness or a dull ache in the lower abdomen. Occasionally acute pain occurs because of rapid growth resulting in hemorrhage and necrosis. Ten percent of affected men have epididymitis. The testicular mass is usually discovered by the individual or by his sexual partner. In about 5% of all cases of testicular cancer, gynecomastia is noted or a hydrocele is present. At the time of initial diagnosis, approximately 10% of individuals already have symptoms related to metastases. Lumbar pain also may be present and usually is caused by retroperitoneal node metastasis. Signs of metastasis to the lungs include cough, dyspnea, and bloody sputum (hemoptysis). Supraclavicular node involvement may cause difficulty swallowing (dysphagia) and neck swelling. With metastasis to the CNS, alterations in vision or mental status, papilledema, and seizures may be experienced.

Evaluation and Treatment

Evaluation begins with careful physical examination, including palpation of the scrotal contents with the individual in the erect and supine positions. Signs of testicular cancer include abnormal consistency, induration, nodularity, or irregularity of the testis. The abdomen and lymph nodes are palpated to seek evidence of metastasis, and tumor type is identified after orchiectomy. Testicular biopsy is not recommended because it may cause dissemination of the tumor and increase the risk of local recurrence. Chest x-ray films, lymphangiograms, intravenous pyelograms, abdominal ultrasound or CT scan, and measurement of serum markers (α-fetoprotein and β-subunit gonadotropin) are used in clinical staging of the disease. Besides surgery, treatment involves radiation and chemotherapy singly or in combination. Factors influencing the prognosis include histology of the tumor stage of the disease and selection of appropriate treatment. Most patients treated for cancer of the testis can expect a normal life span; some have persistent paresthesias, Raynaud phenomenon, or infertility. Almost 90% of disease-related deaths occur in the first 2 years after cessation of therapy; disease-free survival of 3 years is considered a cure. Orchiectomy does not affect sexual function.

Impairment of sperm production and quality

Spermatogenesis requires adequate secretion of follicle-stimulating hormone (FSH) and luteinizing hormone (LH) by the pituitary and sufficient secretion of testosterone by the testes. Inadequate secretion of gonadotropins may be caused by hypothyroidism, hyperadrenocortisolism, hyperprolactinemia, or hypogonadotropic hypogonadism. In the absence of adequate gonadotropin levels, the Leydig cells are not stimulated to secrete testosterone and sperm maturation is not promoted in the Sertoli cells. Spermatogenesis also depends on an appropriate response by the testes. Defects in testicular response to the gonadotropins result in decreased secretion of testosterone and high levels of circulating gonadotropins. In the absence of adequate testosterone levels, spermatogenesis is impaired. Impaired spermatogenesis also can be caused by testicular trauma, infection, atrophy of the testes, systemic illness involving high fever, ingestion of various drugs, exposure to environmental toxins, and cryptorchidism.

Fertility is adversely affected if spermatogenesis is normal but the sperm are chromosomally or morphologically abnormal or are produced in insufficient quantities. Chromosomal abnormalities are caused by genetic factors and by external variables, such as exposure to radiation or toxic substances.

Sperm motility may also affect fertility. Motility appears to be affected by characteristics of semen. Prostatic dysfunction, excessive semen viscosity, presence of drugs or toxins in the semen, and presence of antisperm antibodies are associated with impaired sperm motility. Approximately 17% of infertile males have antisperm antibodies in their semen. These antibodies may be (1) cytotoxic antibodies, which attack sperm and reduce their number in the semen, or (2) sperm-immobilizing antibodies, which impair sperm motility and reduce their ability to traverse the endocervical canal.

Treatment for impaired spermatogenesis involves correcting any underlying disorders, avoiding radiation and toxins, and using hormones to enhance spermatogenesis. In addition, semen can be modified to improve sperm motility; modifications are followed by artificial insemination.

Epididymitis

Epididymitis, or inflammation of the epididymis, generally occurs in sexually active young males (younger than 35

Fig. 32-27 *Epididymitis secondary to gonorrhea or nongonococcal urethritis.* Secondary to gonorrhea or nongonococcal urethritis, this infection spread to the testes, and rupture through the scrotal wall is threatened. *(From Taylor, P.K. [1995].* Diagnostic picture tests in sexually transmitted disease. *London: Mosby-Wolfe.)*

years) and is rare before puberty (Fig. 32-27). In young men the usual cause is a sexually transmitted microorganism, such as *N. gonorrhoeae* or *C. trachomatis*. In men older than 35 years, Enterobacteriaceae (intestinal bacteria) and *Pseudomonas aeruginosa* associated with urinary tract infections and prostatitis also may cause epididymitis. Epididymitis rarely occurs after strenuous lifting or straining or after scrotal trauma.

Pathophysiology

The pathogenic microorganism usually reaches the epididymis by ascending the vasa deferentia from an already infected urethra or bladder. The resulting inflammatory response causes symptoms of bacterial epididymitis. Epididymitis caused by heavy lifting or straining results from reflux of urine from the bladder into the vas deferens and epididymis. Urine is extremely irritating to the epididymis and initiates an inflammatory response called *chemical epididymitis.*

Clinical Manifestations

The main symptom of epididymitis is scrotal or inguinal pain caused by inflammation of the epididymis and surrounding tissues. The pain is usually acute and severe. Flank pain may occur if, as the urethra passes over the spermatic cord, edematous swelling of the cord obstructs the urethra. The individual may have pyuria, bacteriuria, and a history of

Fig. 32-28 *Benign prostatic hyperplasia.* **A,** Condition becomes a problem as prostatic tissue compresses the urethra. **B,** Gross appearance of BPH showing transition zone resulting from bulging nodules of varying size. **(A** from Seidel, H. et al. [1999]. Mosby's guide to physical examination [4th ed.]. St. Louis: Mosby; **B** from Damjanov, I. & Linder, J. [Eds.]. [1996]. Anderson's pathology [10th ed.]. St. Louis: Mosby.)

urinary symptoms, including urethral discharge. The scrotum on the involved side is red and edematous. The tail of the epididymis near the lower pole of the testis usually swells first; then swelling ascends to the head of the epididymis. The spermatic cord also may be swollen and tender.

Complications include abscess formation, infarction of the testis, recurrent infection, and infertility. Infarction is probably caused by thrombosis (obstruction by blood clots) of the prostatic vessels secondary to severe inflammation. Recurrent epididymitis may result from inadequate initial treatment or failure to identify or treat predisposing factors. Chronic epididymitis can cause scarring of the epididymal endothelium and infertility. Once scarring has occurred, treatment with antibiotics is ineffective because adequate antibiotic levels cannot be achieved within the epididymis.

Evaluation and Treatment

A history of recent urinary tract infection or urethral discharge suggests the diagnosis of epididymitis. The relief of pain when the inflamed testis and epididymis are elevated (Phren sign) is also diagnostic. Definitive diagnosis is based on culture or Gram stain of a urethral swab. Epididymal aspiration may be necessary to obtain a specimen, especially if the individual has been taking antibiotics and has sterile urine.

Treatment includes antibiotic therapy for the infection itself and various measures to provide symptomatic relief. Complete resolution of swelling and pain may take several weeks to months. The individual's sexual partner should be treated with antibiotics if the causative microorganism is a sexually transmitted pathogen.

Disorders of the Prostate Gland
Benign prostatic hyperplasia

Benign prostatic hyperplasia (BPH; benign prostatic hypertrophy) is the enlargement of the prostate gland (Fig. 32-28). This condition becomes problematic as prostatic tissue compresses the urethra, where it passes through the prostate. More than 60% of men after 60 years of age have prostatic enlargement.[25] At birth, the prostate is pea sized, and growth of the gland is gradual until puberty. At this time, there is a period of rapid development that continues until the third decade of life when the prostate reaches adult size (see Chapter 31). When the man reaches about 40 to 45 years of age, benign hyperplasia begins and continues slowly until death. Current causative theories of BPH focus on estrogen/androgen synergism or undefined prostatic growth factors with possible hormonal involvement.

BPH begins in the periurethral glands, which are the inner glands or layers of the prostate. The prostate enlarges as nodules form and grow (nodular hyperplasia) and glandular cells enlarge (hypertrophy). As nodular hyperplasia and cellular hypertrophy progress, tissues that surround the prosta-

Patient Information

Name: _____

Age: _____

Date Completed: _____

	Not at all	Less than 1 time in 5	Less than half the time	About half the time	More than half the time	Almost always
1. Over the past month, how often have you had a sensation of not emptying your bladder completely after you have finished urinating?	0	1	2	3	4	5
2. Over the past month, how often have you had to urinate again less than two hours after you finished urinating?	0	1	2	3	4	5
3. Over the past month, how often have you found you stopped and started again several times when you urinated?	0	1	2	3	4	5
4. Over the past month, how often have you found it difficult to postpone urination?	0	1	2	3	4	5
5. Over the past month, how often have you had a weak urinary stream?	0	1	2	3	4	5
6. Over the past month, how often have you had to push or strain to begin urination?	0	1	2	3	4	5
	None	1 Time	2 Times	3 Times	4 Times	5 Times
7. Over the past month, how many times did you most typically get up to urinate from the time you went to bed at night until the time you got up in the morning?	0	1	2	3	4	5

Total I-PSS Score: ____

	Delighted	Pleased	Mostly Satisfied	Mixed	Mostly Dissatisfied	Unhappy	Terrible
8. If you were to spend the rest of your life with your urinary condition just the way it is now, how would you feel about it?	0	1	2	3	4	5	6

Fig. 32-29 *International Prostate Symptom Score (I-PSS).* Questionnaires such as the I-PSS allow practitioners to quantitate an individual's BPH symptoms.

tic urethra compress it, usually but not always causing bladder outflow obstruction.

Symptoms include the urge to urinate frequently, some delay in starting urination, and decreased force of the urinary stream. As the obstruction progresses, often over several years, the bladder cannot empty all the urine and the increasing volume leads to long-term urine retention. The volume of urine retained may be great enough to produce uncontrolled "overflow incontinence" with any increase in intraabdominal pressure. At this stage, the force of the urinary stream is significantly reduced and much more time is required to initiate and complete voiding.

Progressive bladder distention causes diverticular outpouchings of the bladder wall. The ureters may be obstructed where they pass through the hypertrophied detru-

sor muscle, potentially causing hydroureter, hydronephrosis, and bladder or kidney infection.

PSA density (PSAD) is helpful in differentiating BPH from prostatic cancer. PSAD is calculated by dividing prostate-specific antigen (PSA) serum levels by the volume of prostate tissue, which is determined by transrectal ultrasound (TRUS). Treatment depends on severity of symptoms, including postvoid residual urine (PVR) and subjective symptoms score (Fig. 32-29). Thirty percent of men with mild to moderate symptoms improve with watchful waiting. Those with moderately elevated symptom scores or severe symptom scores without large PVR levels can be treated with medications, such as 5-α-reductase inhibitors (e.g., finasteride) or selective α_1-blocking agents (e.g., Prazosin). Candidates for surgical intervention include those

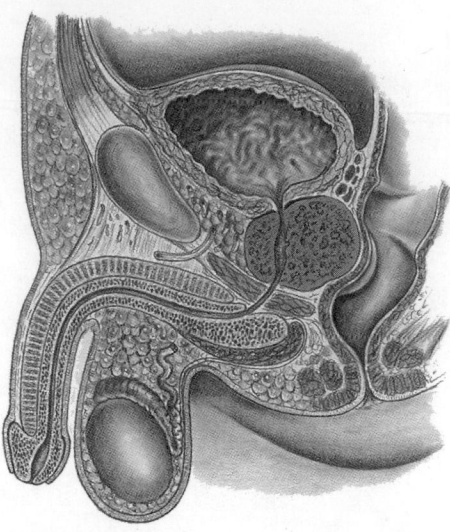

Fig. 32-30 *Prostatitis.* (*From Seidel, H. et al. [1995].* Mosby's guide to physical examination *[3rd ed.]. St. Louis: Mosby.*)

with severe symptoms, large PVR, or complications or those who fail medical therapy.[25]

Prostatitis

Prostatitis is an inflammation of the prostate. Some degree of prostatic inflammation is present in 4% to 36% of the male population, increasing to 50% in older men. Inflammation is usually limited to a few of the gland's excretory ducts (Fig. 32-30).

Prostatitis is characterized as (1) acute bacterial prostatitis, (2) chronic bacterial prostatitis, or (3) nonbacterial prostatitis. Prostatitis can be in the form of *prostatodynia* (pain in the prostate). Men with prostatodynia have the same clinical manifestations as those with nonbacterial prostatitis, but physical and laboratory examinations do not show prostatic pathologic findings. Prostatodynia may be caused by spasms in the genitourinary tract or tension in the muscles of the pelvic floor.

Defense mechanisms protecting the lower urogenital tract from infection include urethral length, micturition (urination), ejaculation, and antimicrobial substances in the prostatic fluid.

Bacterial prostatitis

Acute bacterial prostatitis is an ascending infection of the urinary tract that tends to occur in men between the ages of 30 and 50 years but is also associated with BPH in older men. Prostate infection is caused by coliform bacteria, particularly *Escherichia coli, P. aeruginosa,* and *Streptococcus faecalis,* mycoplasmas, ureaplasmas, and chlamydiae. Infection stimulates an inflammatory response in which the prostate becomes enlarged, tender, and firm. The onset of prostatitis may be acute and unrelated to previous illnesses, or it may follow catheterization or cystoscopy.

Clinical manifestations of acute bacterial prostatitis are those of urinary tract infection, including dysuria and uri-

nary frequency, which result from bacterial contamination and inflammation of the bladder, and lower abdominal and suprapubic discomfort. The individual also may have symptoms of lower urinary tract obstruction, such as slow, small urinary stream, inability to empty the bladder, and nocturia (need to urinate frequently during the night). Acute inflammatory prostatic edema can compress the urethra, causing urinary obstruction. Systemic signs of infection include sudden onset of a high fever (up to 40° C [104° F]), fatigue, arthralgia, and myalgia. Prostatic pain may occur, especially when the individual is in an upright position, because the pelvic floor muscles tighten with standing and compression of the prostate gland occurs. Some individuals experience low back pain, painful ejaculation, and rectal or perineal pain. An enlarged, extremely tender and swollen prostate that is firm, indurated, and warm may be palpated.

Because acute bacterial prostatitis is usually associated with a bladder infection caused by the same microorganism, urine cultures disclose its identity. Prostatic massage may express enough secretions from the urethra for direct bacterial examination, but massage may be painful and increases the risk that the infection will ascend to adjacent structures or enter the bloodstream and cause septicemia.

To resolve the infection and control its spread, long-term, broad-spectrum antibiotic therapy (up to 6 weeks) may be required. In severe cases the individual is hospitalized and treated with intravenous aminoglycoside and ampicillin for 7 days followed by 4 to 6 weeks of oral antibiotics. Analgesics, antipyretics, bed rest, and adequate hydration are also therapeutic. Complications include urinary retention that resolves with antibiotic therapy; prostatic abscess that may rupture into the urethra, rectum, or perineum; epididymitis; bacteremia; and septic shock. Urinary retention requiring drainage is best managed with a suprapubic catheter; Foley catheterization is contraindicated during acute infection.

Chronic bacterial prostatitis is characterized by recurrent urinary tract infections and persistence of pathogenic bacteria. This form of prostatitis is the most common recurrent urinary tract infection in men. Symptoms may be similar to those of an acute bladder infection: frequency, urgency, dysuria, perineal discomfort, low back pain, myalgia, and arthralgia. The prostate may be only slightly enlarged or boggy, but fibrosis can cause it to be firm and irregular in shape.

When the initial urine sample is bacteria free, prostatic massage is used to express secretions. Subsequently, the first 10 ml of voided urine is collected and examined microscopically. Prostatic secretions showing more than 10 white blood cells (WBCs) per high-power field (hpf) and macrophages containing fat are indicative of bacterial infection; diagnosis is confirmed by culture. A pelvic x-ray examination may show prostatic calculi.

Treatment of chronic bacterial prostatitis is difficult, mainly because damage caused by chronic inflammation blocks passage of antibiotics into prostatic tissues, making

Fig. 32-31 *Carcinoma of prostate.* **A,** Frequent sites of distant metastasis are the lymph nodes, bones, lungs, liver, and adrenals. **B,** The main tumor is present in the lateral peripheral zone as a firm, circumscribed, yellow-white mass, but multiple microscopic foci were present bilaterally in the periphery. *(A from Seidel, H. et al. [1999]. Mosby's guide to physical examination [4th ed.]. St. Louis: Mosby; B from Damjanov, I. & Linder, J. [Eds.]. [1996]. Anderson's pathology [10th ed.]. St. Louis: Mosby.)*

therapeutic levels hard to achieve. The usual treatment is a 12-week course of trimethoprim-sulfamethoxazole or a 4- to 6-week course of a fluoroquinolone agent. Men whose chronic bacterial prostatitis is not cured may require continuous, low-dose suppressive therapy or may benefit from a radical transurethral prostatectomy. Comfort measures include nonsteroidal antiinflammatory drug (NSAID) therapy and liberal use of sitz baths.

Nonbacterial prostatitis

Nonbacterial prostatitis is the most common prostatitis syndrome. It consists of prostatic inflammation without evidence of bacterial infection. The cause of nonbacterial prostatitis is not clear.[26]

Men with nonbacterial prostatitis may complain of pain or a dull ache that is continuous or spasmodic in the suprapubic, infrapubic, scrotal, penile, or inguinal area. Other symptoms are pain on ejaculation and urinary symptoms, such as frequency of urination. The prostate gland generally feels normal on palpation.

Nonbacterial prostatitis is a diagnosis by exclusion. Digital examination of the prostate, bacterial cultures of the urogenital tract, microscopic examination of expressed prostatic fluid, urethroscopy, and urodynamic studies are used to verify the diagnosis of nonbacterial prostatitis.

There is no generally accepted treatment for nonbacterial prostatitis. Symptoms can be relieved by hot sitz baths, bed rest, anticholinergics, and antiinflammatory drugs.

Cancer of the prostate

The increased incidence and slowly rising mortality of prostate cancer are becoming a major concern worldwide.[14]

Cancer of the prostate is the most common cancer in American males. It accounts for more than 14% of all cancer deaths and more than 29% of all cancers in men in the United States; only lung cancer accounts for more deaths.[2,14] Prostatic cancer rarely occurs in men younger than 50 years. Incidence increases with advancing age, with more than 75% of all prostate cancers diagnosed in men older than 65 years. About one of five American men will develop prostate cancer in their lifetime, and approximately 3% will die from it. In the United States, the incidence and mortality among blacks are two times higher than among whites.

Pathogenesis

More than 95% of prostatic neoplasms are adenocarcinomas, and most occur in the periphery of the prostate. Prostatic cancer may metastasize by local extension or through lymphatic and blood vessels. The lymph nodes, bones, lungs, liver, and adrenals are the most common sites of distant metastasis. The pelvis, lumbar spine, femur, thoracic spine, and ribs are the most common sites of bone metastasis. Local extension is usually posterior, although late in the disease the tumor may invade the rectum or encroach on the prostatic urethra and cause bladder outlet obstruction (Fig. 32-31). Prostate cancer can progress slowly, but some cases progress aggressively. New research confirms that destruction of *p27* protein (protein encoded by the *p27* gene and an inhibitor of the cell cycle) occurs commonly in the most aggressive prostate cancer.[27,28]

Clinical Manifestations

Prostatic cancer often causes no symptoms until it is far advanced. Therefore routine screening is recommended for asymptomatic men beginning at age 50 years or at age 45 years if considered high risk. The first manifestations of disease are those of bladder outlet obstruction: slow urinary stream, hesitancy, incomplete emptying, frequency, nocturia, and dysuria. Unlike the symptoms of obstruction caused by BPH, the symptoms of obstruction caused by prostatic cancer are progressive and do not remit. Local extension of prostatic cancer can obstruct the upper urinary tract ureters as well. Rectal obstruction may also occur, causing the individual to experience large bowel obstruction or difficulty in defecation. Symptoms of late disease include bone pain at sites of bone metastasis, edema of the lower extremities, enlargement of lymph nodes, liver enlargement, pathologic bone fractures, and mental confusion associated with brain metastases. Prostatic cancer and its treatment can affect sexual functioning.

Evaluation and Treatment

Screening for prostatic cancer includes digital rectal examination (DRE), prostate-specific antigen (PSA) blood tests, and transrectal ultrasound (TRUS). Cancer diagnosis is confirmed through tissue biopsy and microscopic examination of tissue. Lymphography, bone scans, and CT scans may also be used to determine metastasis to lymph, bone, or other adjacent tissue.

Treatment of prostatic cancer depends on the stage of the disease, the anticipated effects of treatment, and the age, general health, and life expectancy of the individual. Options range from hormonal or radiation therapy or chemotherapy to surgery, any combination of these, or no treatment. Palliative treatment is aimed at relieving urinary, bladder outlet, or colon obstruction, spinal cord compression, and pain.

National Organizations for Prostate Cancer   BOX 32-6

1. American Foundation for Urologic Disease
   Prostate Cancer Support Network
   300 West Pratt Street, Suite 401
   Baltimore, MD 21201-2463
   1-800-828-7866
2. National Cancer Institute
   International Cancer Information Center
   Building 82, Room 123
   Bethesda, MD 20892
   1-800-4-CANCER
   E-mail/Internet: www.nci.nih.gov
3. National Coalition for Cancer Survivorship
   1010 Wayne Avenue, 7th floor
   Silver Spring, MD 20910-5600
   1-301-650-8868
4. Patient Advocates for Advanced Cancer Treatment (PAACT)
   1143 Parmelee, N.W.
   Grand Rapids, MI 49504
   1-616-453-1477
5. US Too International, Inc.
   Prostate Cancer Survivor Support Group
   930 North York Road, Suite 50
   Hinsdale, IL 60521-2993
   1-708-323-1002 or 1-00-80-US-TOO
   (1-800-808-7866)
   Fax: 1-708-323-1993
   E-mail: usto
   Internet: http://www.ustoo.com

HEALTH ALERT

Selenium Decreases Risk of Prostate and Other Cancers

Selenium, a mineral low in many American diets, acts as an antioxidant to decrease the risk of some cancers. In a longitudinal study conducted through the Arizona Cancer Center, individuals who supplemented their diet with 200 mg of selenium experienced 63% fewer prostate cancers, 58% fewer colorectal cancers, 46% fewer lung cancers, and a 50% decrease in overall cancer deaths over a period of 4.5 years compared with individuals who received a placebo. Recommended supplementation is 100 to 200 μg/day. Good sources of selenium include fish, grains, and some yeast products.

Data from Consumers Union of U.S. (1997, November). Consumers reports on health: Guide to nutrition [Special Report]. Yonkers, N.Y.: The Author; Clark, L.C. et al. (1996). Effects of selenium supplementation for cancer prevention in patients with carcinoma of the skin. Journal of the American Medical Association, 276(24), 1957-1963; Seppa, N. (1998). Selenium averts prostate cancer. Science News, 154, 188.

Prognosis and survival rates have improved steadily over the past 50 years. Currently, the overall 5-year survival rate of all stages of prostate cancer is 87%; for cancers confined to the prostate, the 5-year survival rate is 100%[14] (Health Alert boxes and Box 32-6).

Newly diagnosed cases are staged in the following manner:

Very early: Cancer is confined to the prostate gland and cannot be felt during rectal examination.

Localized: Cancer is palpable and remains confined to the prostate gland.

Rationalized: Tumor has spread into adjacent tissues.

Advanced: Tumor has metastasized to lymph or bone.

Recurrent: Cancer has recurred in prostate or other parts of body after treatment.

Sexual Dysfunction

In males, the normal sexual response involves erection, emission, and ejaculation. *Sexual dysfunction* is the impairment of any or all of these processes and can be caused by various physiologic, psychologic, and emotional factors.

HEALTH ALERT
Prostate Cancer Research and Treatment

Research is constantly underway to find new ways to prevent and to treat all cancers. For example, current research in prostate cancer is focusing on the following areas:

Genetics:
Recent discovery of the *HPC1* gene will soon yield more information about inherited risk of prostate cancer. Further research on this gene may give scientists ideas about the chemical changes that cause prostate cancer and how to design medications to reverse those changes in inherited and sporadic (not inherited) cases. Tests to find abnormal prostate cancer genes may help identify men at high risk who would benefit from more intensive screening or from chemoprevention trials.

Diet and Chemoprevention:
Recent research has identified a high-fat diet as a risk factor for prostate cancer. Changes in hormone balance caused by dietary fat may explain this risk.

Recent research suggests that some foods contain a chemical called *lycopene* that may reduce prostate cancer risk. This chemical is an *antioxidant* (a type of chemical that prevents cell damage that can result in development of cancer). Lycopene is found in tomato sauce, raw tomatoes, grapefruit, and watermelons. Some researchers suggest eating at least two servings each week of these foods.

Monoclonal Antibodies:
These are antibodies that are engineered to carry drugs or radiation directly to the tumor and may offer a way to treat prostate cancer metastases.

Metastasis:
Metastasis is a complicated process of cells breaking away from the primary tumor, entering the blood supply, and relocating in other organs. Currently, researchers are working to define the steps that must occur before a prostate cancer tumor migrates to other locations and grows larger.

Angiogenesis:
Growth of cancers often depends on their ability to promote growth of blood vessels (angiogenesis) to nourish the cancer cells. Analysis of angiogenesis in prostate cancer specimens can help predict prognosis. New drugs are being evaluated that may be useful in stopping prostate cancer growth by preventing nourishment of the cancers by new blood vessels.

Hormone Therapy:
New drugs to block the effects of male hormones and prevent prostate cancer growth are being developed. Studies are also underway to find the most effective combination of current hormonal treatments.

Watchful Waiting (Expectant Management):
Studies are in progress to find *prognostic markers* to help predict which prostate cancers will grow very slowly and can be safely followed by watchful waiting.

Cryosurgery:
In cryosurgery, a metal probe is guided by transrectal ultrasound directly into the prostate gland and the cancer is destroyed by freezing. Because this treatment is considered experimental, researchers are still evaluating its effectiveness against prostate cancer.

Data from American Cancer Society. (1997). Prostate cancer. New York: The Author.

Until the late 1970s, most cases of male sexual dysfunction were considered psychogenic. Now there is evidence that 89% to 90% of cases involve organic factors and include (1) vascular, endocrine, and neurologic disorders; (2) chronic disease, including renal failure and diabetes mellitus; (3) penile diseases and penile trauma; and (4) iatrogenic factors, such as surgery and pharmacologic therapies. Most of these disorders cause erectile dysfunction.[29]

Pathophysiology

Sexual dysfunction can have a specific physiologic cause, can be associated with many chronic diseases and their treatment, or may be related to low energy levels, stress, or depression. For example, vascular disease may cause impotence, and endocrine disorders or conditions that cause decreased testosterone levels or testicular atrophy can diminish sexual functioning or libido. In addition, neurologic disorders and spinal cord injuries can interfere with sympathetic, parasympathetic, and CNS mechanisms required for erection, emission, and ejaculation.

Drug-induced sexual dysfunction consists of decreased desire, decreased erectile ability, or decreased ejaculatory ability. Alcohol and other CNS depressants, antihypertensives, antidepressants, antihistamines, and hormonal preparations are commonly used drugs that affect sexual functioning. Other pharmacologic agents may diminish the quality or quantity of sperm or cause priapism.

Clinical Manifestations and Treatment

Evaluation of sexual dysfunction includes a thorough history and physical examination. Particular attention is given to drug history and examination of the genitalia, prostate, and nervous system. Basic laboratory tests are used to identify the presence of endocrinopathies or other underlying disorders that can cause dysfunction. Psychologic evaluation is indicated for younger men with a sudden onset of sexual dysfunction or men of any age who can achieve but not maintain an erection. If no physiologic cause is found and the condition does not improve with psychotherapy, the man is referred for further investigation of organic causes.

Treatments for organic sexual dysfunction include both medical and surgical approaches. Nonsurgical approaches include correction of underlying disorders, particularly drug-induced dysfunction and endocrinopathy-related (e.g., reduced testosterone associated with chronic renal failure) dysfunction. Vasodilators and cessation of smoking can benefit individuals with vasculogenic erectile dysfunction. Surgical approaches include penile implants, penile revascularization, and correction of other anatomic defects contributing to sexual dysfunction.

✓ QUICK CHECK

Why is diet considered a risk factor in prostate cancer?

Why is routine screening for prostate cancer recommended?

DISORDERS OF THE BREAST
Disorders of the Female Breast
Galactorrhea

Galactorrhea (inappropriate lactation) is the persistent and sometimes excessive secretion of a milky fluid from the breasts of a woman who is not pregnant or nursing an infant. Galactorrhea, which also can occur in men, may involve one or both breasts and is not associated with breast cancer.[4]

The incidence of galactorrhea is difficult to estimate because of differences among definitions of the condition, examination techniques, and populations of women who have been studied. Prevalence has been documented as 0.1% to 32% of all women.

⬆ *Pathophysiology*

Galactorrhea is not a breast disorder but, rather, a manifestation of pathophysiologic processes elsewhere in the body. These processes are chiefly hormone imbalances caused by hypothalamic-pituitary disturbances, pituitary tumors, or neurologic damage. Exogenous causes include drugs, estrogen (e.g., in oral contraceptives), and manipulation of the nipples (Fig. 32-32).

The most common cause of galactorrhea is *nonpuerperal hyperprolactinemia,* or excessive amounts of prolactin in the blood not related to pregnancy or childbirth. Nonpuerperal hyperprolactinemia can be caused by any factor that (1) stimulates or overstimulates the prolactin-secreting units of the pituitary gland; (2) interferes with production of *prolactin-inhibiting factor (PIF),* a neurotransmitter (probably dopamine) that inhibits prolactin secretion; or (3) interferes with pituitary receptors for PIF.

Certain drugs can cause nonpuerperal hyperprolactinemia. They include the phenothiazines, reserpine, and methyldopa; exogenous estrogens, particularly in oral contraceptives; morphine; and the tricyclic antidepressants.

Hypothyroidism causes increased secretion of hypothalamic thyroid-releasing hormone (TRH), which stimulates prolactin release from the pituitary. Hypothyroidism also is associated with reduced metabolic clearance of prolactin, which prolongs its effects.

Many types of pituitary tumors cause hyperprolactinemia, particularly prolactinoma. Prolactinomas cause hyperprolactinemia by secreting prolactin, decreasing production of PIF, or putting pressure on the pituitary stalk, thus preventing delivery of PIF to the anterior pituitary. Growth hormone–secreting pituitary tumors may cause galactorrhea through the intrinsic lactogenic effect that growth hormone appears to have on mammary tissue. Prolactin-secreting lung and kidney tumors also cause hyperprolactinemia.

Galactorrhea can be induced by persistent and repeated sucking or squeezing of the nipples and has been documented in women who manipulate their breasts and nipples daily. Monthly examination of the breasts for nipple discharge usually is not associated with the development of galactorrhea.

⬆ *Clinical Manifestations*

Inappropriate lactation is manifested by the appearance of a milky breast secretion from one or both breasts of nonpregnant, nonlactating women. Most women with galactorrhea experience menstrual abnormality. If a pituitary process is involved, the woman usually experiences hirsutism and infertility; if a hypothalamic lesion is present, she may report CNS symptoms, such as intractable headache, visual field disturbances, sleep disturbances, and abnormal temperature, thirst, or appetite.[4]

⬆ *Evaluation and Treatment*

Galactorrhea in nulliparous women (women who have never been pregnant) or in parous women who have not been pregnant or have not breast-fed for 12 months must be thoroughly evaluated. Serum prolactin levels are measured, and at least two positive results are needed to diagnose hyperprolactinemia. Prolactin levels higher than 25 to 30 ng/ml (by radioimmunoassay) are considered elevated. Those in the range of 75 to 100 ng/ml are considered to be caused by a pituitary tumor until proven otherwise. Serum T_4 and TSH levels are measured to rule out hypothyroidism, and LH and FSH levels are obtained if the individual is amenorrheic. CT scans, MRI evaluations, and carotid angiography may assist in the localization of adenomas.

Treatment for galactorrhea consists of identification and treatment of the cause. Medical and surgical therapies may be involved.

Benign breast disease (fibrocystic change)

A great many terms have been used to describe benign breast lesions of epithelial origin. *Fibrocystic change (disease) (FCC; physiologic nodularity)* is perhaps most descriptive of the clinical manifestations: palpable lumps in the breast that

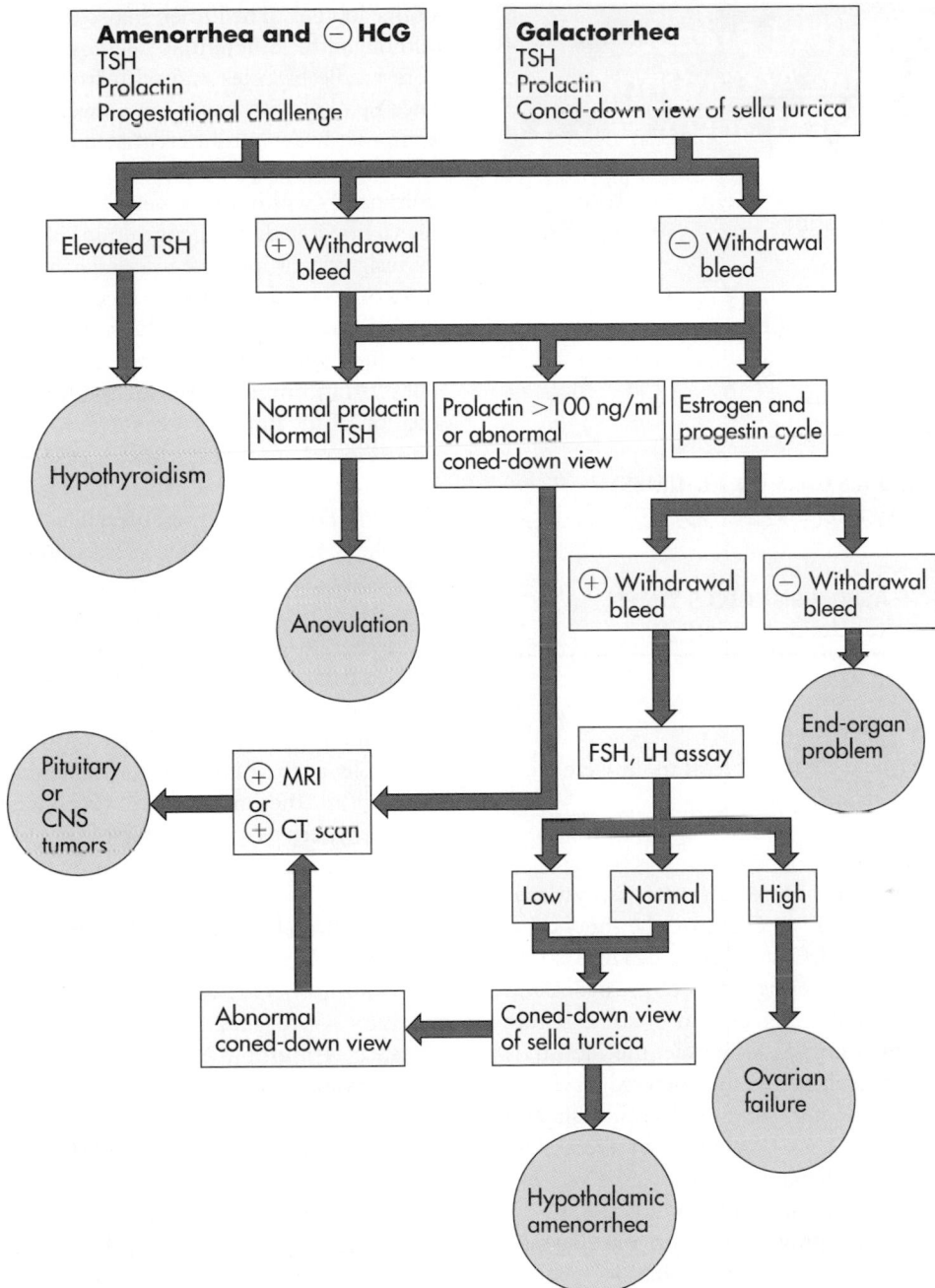

Fig. 32-32 *Flow diagram for diagnosing underlying cause of amenorrhea and galactorrhea.* *HCG,* Human chorionic gonadotropin; *TSH,* thyroid-stimulating hormone; *coned-down view,* focusing with x-ray machine; *FSH,* follicle-stimulating hormone; *LH,* luteinizing hormone; *CNS,* central nervous system; *MRI,* magnetic resonance imaging; *CT,* computed tomography.

fluctuate with the menstrual cycle and may become progressively worse until menopause. The term *fibrocystic disease* is not, however, altogether accurate. Microcysts, macrocysts, adenosis, apocrine change, fibrosis, fibroadenomas, and epithelial proliferation (hyperplasia) are all termed fibrocystic disease. The College of American Pathologists has classified biopsy tissue according to breast cancer risk. The classifications are listed in Box 32-7. Physiologic nodularity is present in approximately 50% of all menstruating women, and at least some of these pathophysiologic changes are noted in up

to 80% of all women, so it is probably a misnomer to term so widespread a process a "disease." Although FCC has been considered a risk for breast cancer, only types with epithelial proliferation (e.g., atypia hyperplasia) represent a true risk. For this reason, some authors *omit* atypical lobular hyperplasia (ALH) and atypical ductal hyperplasia (ADH) from their discussion of FCC because they may be considered precursor lesions of breast cancer. Researchers are currently working on a new test *(p53)* that would give women with FCC a better estimate of their risk of cancer. Women with an

Classification of Breast Biopsy Tissue According to Risk for Breast Cancer   BOX 32-7

NO INCREASED RISK
Adenosis (sclerosing or florid)
  Apocrine metaplasia
  Macrocysts or microcysts
  Fibroadenoma
  Fibrosis
Mild hyperplasia (3-4 cells deep)
  Mastitis or periductal mastitis
  Squamous metaplasia

SLIGHTLY INCREASED RISK (1.5 TO 2.0 TIMES)
Moderate or florid hyperplasia
  Papilloma

MODERATELY INCREASED RISK (3 TO 5 TIMES)
Atypical hyperplasia (ductal or lobular)

---

excess of a protein called *p53* in their breast tissue were more likely to develop breast cancer.[30]

Pathophysiology

Fibrocystic breast chances are of three major types: cystic, fibrous, and epithelial proliferative. Cysts are the most common feature and easily treated. Cystic change can be induced in experimental animals by altering ratios of estrogens and progesterones. It is assumed therefore that breast cysts are the result of ovarian alterations, but the exact mechanism is unknown.[31] A variety of substances are secreted into cyst fluid, including polypeptide hormones and both male and female sex steroid hormones. Cystic changes by themselves do not appear to be premalignant alterations.[31] Cysts develop more commonly in terminal ducts and lobules.

Fibrous tissue increases progressively up until menopause and regresses thereafter. The fibrosis that occurs with cysts and epithelial proliferative lesions therefore is probably a normal process.[31] In younger women, however, it is the sole abnormality in approximately 5% of benign breast biopsy specimens.[32]

Included in the category of epithelial proliferative disease are a number of structurally diverse lesions, such as sclerosing adenosis, radial scar, and the lobular and ductal hyperplasias. These changes have the most epidemiologic similarity to breast cancer of all the changes in fibrocystic change (FCC) and carry the most risk for development of a carcinoma.[31]

Sclerosing adenosis is enlargement of one or more lobular units because of an increase in the number of alveolar ducts and an increase in the density of intralobular fibrous tissue. Occasionally, a mass is produced by aggregation of adjacent lobules or uncommonly by excessive enlargement of one lobule.[31] The lumen may contain microcalcifications. Although the differential diagnosis can be difficult from core-needle biopsies and with frozen sections, the experienced pathologist, using low power microscopy, will rarely confuse it with well-differentiated carcinoma.

Ductal hyperplasia is increased numbers of cells predominantly within the lumen of the terminal ducts and lobular units. It includes a continuum of changes ranging from an insignificant increase in cellularity to features characteristics of in situ ductal carcinoma, in the latter case constituting a diagnosis of *atypical* ductal hyperplasia.

Mild hyperplasia exists when there are one or two extra but often incomplete layers of epithelial cells and little or no dilation of the lumen. Moderate and *florid hyperplasia* describes increasing degrees of epithelial proliferation with dilation and filling of the structures (Fig. 32-33).

Radial scar refers to an irregular, radial proliferation of ductlike mammary epithelial structures with dense central fibrosis. Radial scar has also been called *radial sclerosing lesions* and *sclerosing papillary proliferation*. The appearance in mammograms, as well as the gross and microscopic appearance, can cause it to be confused with infiltrating ductal carcinoma.[31]

Lobular hyperplasia refers to proliferation of small, uniform cells in the lumen of lobular units. Usually all structures within the lumen are uniformly affected. In *atypical* lobular hyperplasia the degree of proliferation and dilation approaches that of lobular carcinoma in situ.[31]

Clinical Manifestations

Pain or tenderness is the most common complaint associated with fibrocystic disease. Discomfort increases as menstruation approaches. Pain, fluctuation in lesion size, and presence of multiple lesions distinguish benign fibrocystic lesions from carcinoma.

Evaluation and Treatment

Breast biopsy is used to make a definitive diagnosis and assess an individual's risk for the development of breast cancer. Mammography may be helpful, but the very dense breast tissue frequently seen in young women can make interpretation extremely difficult. Sonography can be used to differentiate a solid mass from a cystic (fluid-filled) mass.

Treatment consists largely of relieving symptoms. The individual can minimize breast pain by wearing a brassiere that provides good support. Cystic pain is reduced by draining the cysts with the patient under local anesthesia. Many women find that the elimination or reduction of caffeine in their diet reduces both the pain and the nodularity. Women with breast pain also may benefit from a diet low in fat and high in fruits and vegetables. Danazol, a synthetic androgen, has been used to treat individuals with severe pain caused by proliferative breast disease.

Benign breast tumors include fibroadenomas, mammary duct ectasia, solitary intraductal papilloma, multiple papilloma, and fat necrosis.[33] These benign conditions are summarized in Table 32-8.

Fig. 32-33 *Hyperplasia.* **A,** Florid duct hyperplasia with massive expansion of ducts by proliferated epithelium. **B,** Radial scar with centropetal proliferation of ductlike structures and central fibrosis. *(From Damjanov, I. & Linder, J. [Eds]. [1996]. Anderson's pathology [10th ed.]. St. Louis: Mosby.)*

Breast cancer

Breast cancer, the most common cancer in American women, is the leading cause of death in women 40 to 44 years old and the second most common killer of women after lung cancer. Lifetime risk of breast cancer is 1 in 8 (Table 32-9). Between 1982 and 1987, breast cancer incidence rates for women increased about 4% per year and have since leveled off at around 110 cases per 100,000 people (Fig. 32-34). New cases among women in the United States are estimated at 175,000 in 1999. About 77% of these will occur in women older than 50 years. For all ages combined, white women are more likely to develop breast cancer than black women; yet the incidence of breast cancer is higher in blacks among women younger than 45 years. In addition, for all ages, black women are more likely to die of breast cancer (31.2/100,000) compared with white women (26/100,000).[14,34,35] Breast cancers account for about 30% of all cancer cases found in women and 16% of cancer deaths.

Risk factors and possible causes of breast cancer can be classified as reproductive, hormonal, environmental, and familial (Table 32-10). Although high-risk populations can be identified, the majority (75%) of breast cancers occur in women whose only risk factors are gender and age.[1]

Reproductive factors

A woman's age when her first child is born affects her risk for developing breast cancer. The younger she is, the lower the risk. Pregnancies that do not proceed to term apparently have no protective effect. Women who have never given birth are at greater risk than those who have. The duration of a woman's reproductive life also affects her risk of developing breast cancer. Late menarche and early menopause (i.e., a short reproductive life) reduce risk (see Pathogenesis).

Hormonal factors

The link between breast cancer and hormones is based on (1) the protective effect of an early first pregnancy; (2) the protective effect of removal of the ovaries and pituitary gland; and (3) the increased risk associated with early menarche, late menopause, and nulliparity. Estrogen replacement therapy (ERT) and combined estrogen-progestin oral contraceptives (COCs) increase breast cancer risk. Meta-analyses of hormone use and breast cancer support a causal relationship between the use of estrogens and progestins, levels of endogenous estrogens, and breast cancer incidence in postmenopausal women.[36] Long-term use (10 years or more) of ERT has been correlated with an increased risk of breast cancer. Further, a recent analysis using data from most of the large, well-designed published studies indicated that women using COCs had a slightly greater risk for developing breast cancer than women who were not users or had not used COCs for 10 years or more.[14] Hormones are discussed further in the pathogenesis section.

Environmental factors

The environmental causes of breast cancer probably affect the glandular epithelial cells of the breast during the early differential stages from undifferentiated cells to alveolar buds and lobules (see Pathogenesis). During these early phases, mitotic activity and cell division are greater than later in life.[37] High doses of ionizing radiation are associated with an increased risk of breast cancer, especially if exposure occurs during adolescence or pregnancy, when breast cells are proliferating rapidly.

A high-fat diet may increase the risk of breast cancer (see Health Alert box, p. 904). Breast cancer is rare in Japan but not in Japanese immigrants in the United States who adopt

TABLE 32-8   Benign Breast Disorders

Benign Breast Disease	Period of Greatest Risk	Pathophysiology	Clinical Manifestations of Lesion	Treatment
Fibroadenoma	Puberty, early adulthood, rare after menopause	Unknown but thought to be associated with exposure to increased estrogen levels	Painless, firm, solitary, well-circumscribed mobile mass; usually in upper outer quadrant of breast	Surgical excision of mass
Mammary duct ectasia (comedomastitis)	Menopause, postmenopause, during lactation and nursing	Subareolar ducts become dilated and fill with cellular debris, initiating inflammatory reaction; rupture of ducts may occur	Blood-stained, sticky, thick, spontaneous, multiple-duct discharge; ductal rupture creates palpable mass; burning pain, swelling of areolar area may occur	Condition usually resolves 7-10 days after onset with or without antibiotic therapy
Solitary intraductal papilloma	Age 40-50 yr	Unknown	Lesion is slow-growing and cauliflower-like and extends length of involved duct; nipple discharge from one or two ductal openings may be watery, serous, serosanguineous, or sanguineous	Surgical excision of involved duct
Multiple papillomas	Age 35-40 yr	Unknown	Similar to solitary intraductal papilloma, except that discharge is from multiple ductal openings	Depends on extent of involvement; if lesion is small, excision of that breast segment; total mastectomy if disease is widespread
Fat necrosis	Age 14-80 yr, average age 50 yr	Breast trauma, including silicone injections and breast biopsy, cause hemorrhage and induration, leading to formation of a palpable mass	Unilateral, fairly immobile breast mass, located close to the surface; mass is usually tender and painful	Mass may be reabsorbed spontaneously; biopsy, excision may be required if no reabsorption occurs

TABLE 32-9   Risk of Developing Breast Cancer

By Age (yr)	By Ratio
25	1 in 19,608
30	1 in 2525
40	1 in 217
50	1 in 50
60	1 in 26
70	1 in 14
80	1 in 15
Ever*	1 in 8

Data from American Cancer Society. (1995). Cancer response system document #407002-407038. New York: The Author.
Lifetime risk.

Western eating habits. However, studies to date are contradictory and the level of increased risk needs to be defined.[38] Alcohol use and obesity past 50 years of age have been implicated as breast cancer risks in some studies.[1,38-40]

Regular activity during both work and leisure time may reduce overall risk of breast cancer, especially in premenopausal or young postmenopausal women.[41,42] However, mechanisms for this protective effect are not known. Further research is needed.

Certain researchers link the incidence of cancer with the presence of environmental chemicals that act like hormones. Some environmental chemicals mimic estrogens and include plastics, fuels, pharmaceuticals, and chlorine-based chemicals such as DDT, polychlorinated biphenyls (PCBs), and

TABLE 32-10	Factors Associated With Increased Risk of Breast Cancer*	
Category	**Risk Factor**	**Relative Risk†**
Race	Blacks have higher incidence up to age 40 yr; whites have higher incidence over age 40 yr	1.1-1.9
Family history	Breast cancer in first-degree relative before age 60 yr	2.0-3.0
	Premenopausal or bilateral breast cancer	>4.0
	Breast cancer in two first-degree relatives	4.0-6.0
Previous medical history	Moderate or florid mammary hyperplasia	1.5-2.0
	Mammary papilloma	1.5-2.0
	Atypical mammary hyperplasia	4.0-5.0
Estrogen exposure	Early menarche (before age 12 yr)	1.1-1.9
	Late menopause (after age 55 yr)	1.1-1.9
	Postmenopausal estrogen therapy	1.4
	Oral contraceptive use	1.5
Pregnancy	Nulliparous or late first pregnancy (after age 35 yr)	1.1-1.9
Radiation exposure	Atomic bomb	3.0
	Repeated fluoroscopy	1.5-2.0
Obesity	Fat distribution Hormone levels	1.2
Alcohol abuse	See text for explanation	1.4-2.0

Normal lifetime risk in white women: 1 in 8.

†Relative risk is the incidence of the disease among individuals exposed to a risk factor divided by the incidence rate of the disease among individuals not exposed to a risk factor. A relative risk of 4.0 means the risk of dying from breast cancer increased fourfold in women with "atypia hyperplasia" compared with those without atypia.

Fig. 32-34 *Incidence and mortality of breast cancer.* Increased incidence of breast cancer but stable mortality over the past 40 years. *(Modified from Damjanov, I. & Linder, J. [Eds.]. [1996]. Anderson's pathology [10th ed.]. St. Louis: Mosby.)*

chlorofluorocarbons. They can accumulate in body fat and for years mimic the activity of estrogen in the body, including its carcinogenic effects. Some studies suggest that susceptibility to these environmental toxicants is greatest at three stages of life: before birth, during puberty, and at menopause.

Familial factors

Most women who develop a breast tumor do not have a known family history of breast cancer. A history of breast cancer, however, in first-degree relatives (mother or sister) increases a woman's risk two to three times. Risk increases even more if two first-degree relatives are involved, especially if the disease occurred before menopause and was bilateral.

A small total proportion of breast cancers (less than 7%, although the prevalence is significant) are the result of highly penetrant dominant genes (i.e., hereditary breast cancers). The most important of the dominant genes are the breast cancer susceptibility genes (*BRCA1, BRCA2*) (Box 32-8 and Fig. 32-35). *BRCA1* was cloned on chromosome 17 and *BRCA2* was mapped to chromosome 13. The *BRCA1* and *BRCA2* mutations have been estimated to account for 50% and 30%, respectively, of all inherited breast cancers.[43,44] A family history of both breast and ovarian cancer increases the risk that an individual with breast cancer carries a *BRCA1* mutation. Race is also an important distinction for genetic risk. A recent population-based study showed that whereas 3.3% of white women with breast cancer had *BRCA1* mutations, none of the 88 black women with breast cancer had a *BRCA1* mutation.[43] Carriers of the *BRCA1* gene are also at higher risk of ovarian cancer. *BRCA1* is a tumor suppressor gene; therefore any mutation in the gene may inhibit or retard its suppressor function, leading to uncontrolled cell proliferation.[45] Not much is known about *BRCA2*, except that men who develop breast cancer are more likely to have a *BRCA2* mutation than a *BRCA1* mutation.[46,47] Studies on families with multiple breast cancer cases indicate that the penetrance for breast cancer among *BRCA1* mutation carriers is about 87% by 85 years of age; the penetrance for ovarian cancer in this group is 50% by 85 years of age, 29% by 50 years, and 44% by 70 years.[48,49]

Pathogenesis

Most breast cancers arise from the ductal epithelium. Tumors of the infiltrating ductal type do not grow to a large size, but they metastasize early. This type accounts for 70% of breast cancers. Table 32-11 lists the different types of breast carcinomas and summarizes their major characteristics.

Breast cancer is a disease of the glandular epithelium and is thought to result from a mutation during the differentia-

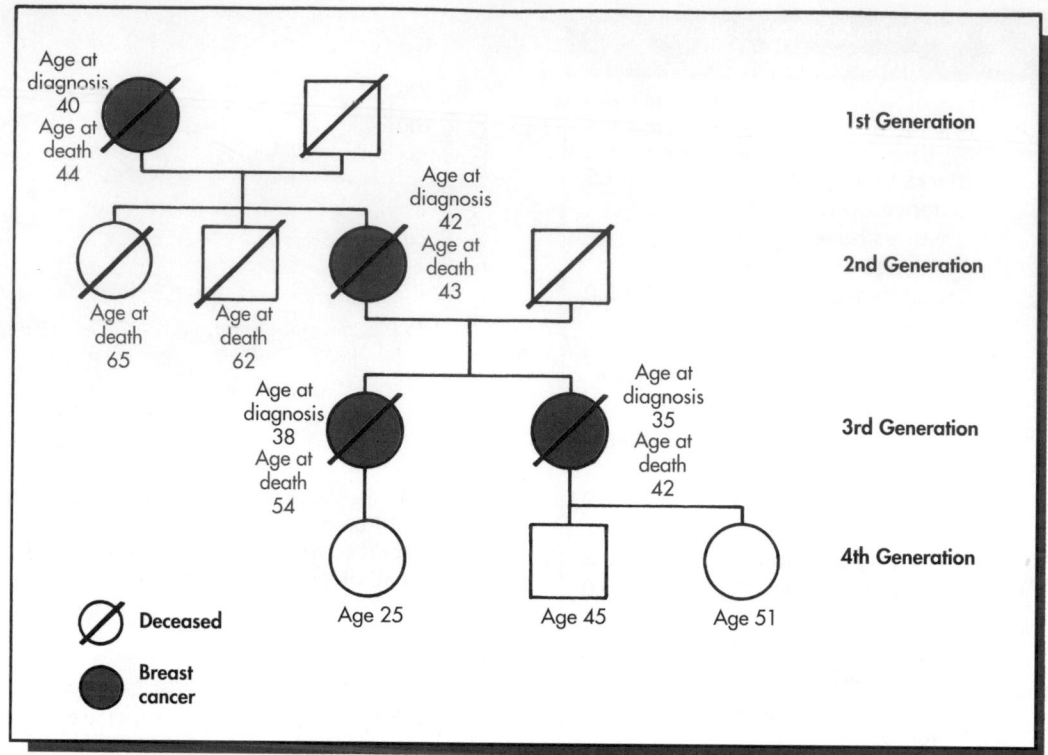

Fig. 32-35 *Example of family pedigree for breast cancer.* Family pedigree showing cases of breast cancer (●) associated with typical dominant transmission of breast cancer. *(Modified from Evans, D.G.R. et al. [1994]. Familial breast cancer.* British Medical Journal, 308, *183-187.)*

Summary: Hereditary Breast Cancer   BOX 32-8

PREVALENCE:
Approximately 12.5% of women will develop breast cancer during their lifetime. About 7% of these women have the hereditary form of breast cancer discussed here (i.e., about 1/150 to 1/200 women in the general population).

SURVIVAL
For all cases of breast cancer diagnosed in the United States from 1986 to 1992, the 5-year survival rates are 85% (whites) and 70% (blacks).

PRESENTATION
The hereditary form of breast cancer is more often bilateral and early onset (premenopausal) than nonhereditary breast cancer.

GENETICS
The mode of inheritance is autosomal dominant. Penetrance for female is 70% to 90% by age 70 years. Males also can be affected, but the penetrance is much lower. Several genes may cause hereditary breast cancer. The most important of these are the breast cancer susceptibility genes *BRCA1* and *BRCA2*. *BRCA1* has been cloned and is located on chromosome 17. Presence of this gene also increases the risk of ovarian cancer. Recently cloned, *BRCA2* has been mapped to chromosome 13.

OTHER
In general, having one first-degree female relative (i.e., mother or a sister) affected with breast cancer *doubles* a female's risk of developing a breast tumor. If two first-degree relatives develop breast tumors before age 55 years, the risk increases to 54%.

Data from American Cancer Society. (1999). Cancer facts and figures—1999. Atlanta: The Author; Lindblom, A. (1995). Breast Cancer Research and Treatment, 34(2), 171; Speroff, L., Glass, R.H., & Kase, N.G. Clinical gynecologic endocrinology and infertility (5th ed.). Baltimore: (1994). Williams & Wilkins.

TABLE 32-11	Types of Breast Carcinomas and Major Distinguishing Features
Histologic Type	**Distinguishing Features**
Carcinoma of mammary ducts	
Papillary	Well-delineated cystic masses in multiple areas; hemorrhage often present; majority appear in 40- to 60-yr age-group; often involves skin
Intraductal (comedo)	Often accompanied by evidence of infection; well-circumscribed tumors within the duct; well-differentiated tumor cells; rarely ulcerates the skin
infiltrating carcinoma	
Ductal	Fibrous, firm, glistening, gray-tan mass with chalky streaks, mixture of patterns; causes discharge from the nipple; represents about 70% of all breast cancer
Mucinous	Usually large, >3 cm in diameter, circumscribed and encapsulated, glistening appearance, varies in color; two types: pure and mixed; pure tumor is surrounded by mucin; infrequent; found in the lateral half of the breast; tends to occur in women over 70 yr
Medullary	Encapsulated and grows to be very large (7-8 cm in diameter); commonly infiltrates lymphoid tissue; occurs after age 50 yr
Tubular	Well-differentiated with orderly tubules in center (stroma) of mass; associated with noninfiltrating ductal carcinoma; occurs in women about 50 yr of age; nodal metastasis infrequent; occurrence rare
Adenoid cystic	Very rare; well-circumscribed, painless mass arising from the nipple and areola
Metaplastic	Involves cartilage or bone, mixed tumors or osteogenic sarcomas
Squamous cell	Frequent in blacks; originates in ductal epithelium
Carcinoma of mammary lobules	
Lobular carcinoma in situ	Found in individuals with fibrocystic disease; localized to upper breast quadrants; risk of 10%-35% becoming invasive; occurs frequently in mid-40s; infiltrating variety occurs in early 50s
Infiltrating lobular	Infiltrates from duct; firm mass with chalky streaks
Paget disease	Eczema of the nipple that extends to the areola; cancer usually found underneath the nipple; poorly circumscribed; large Paget cells arise from the duct and directly invade nipple; history of scaly, red rash spreading from the nipple; lesion palpable beneath the nipple, often bilateral; occurs in middle age
Inflammatory carcinoma	Not a histologic type; fairly diffuse within the breast tissue, diffuse edema of the overlying skin; extremely undifferentiated, very rare, most metastasize to axilla
sarcoma of the breast	
Cytosarcoma phyllodes	Usually large (>17 cm in diameter); mostly localized but can rupture through the skin; rarely metastasizes to lymph nodes; history of painless nodule present for years before it forms a large mass; ulceration and bleeding of skin often present; occurs in wide age range (13-77 yr)
Fibrosarcoma	Well-circumscribed, firm, and usually does not involve the skin or nipple; well-differentiated to extremely undifferentiated; arises from connective tissue; extremely rare (e.g., liposarcoma, angiosarcoma)

tion of stem cells into mature epithelial cells.[50] Pathogenesis probably involves two or three steps. First, modifications of the deoxyribonucleic acid (DNA) of the breast epithelial ductal cells are caused by genetic alterations, environmental agents, or their interactions. The initiated changes in DNA probably occur early in a woman's life—before full differentiation of the breast tissue.[37] Second, growth factors increase the rate of growth of premalignant to malignant cells—the most important of which are estrogen and progesterone. Breast cells produce other growth factors, including insulin-like growth factor (IGF), transforming growth factor-α (TGF-α), an epidermal growth factor (EGF), platelet-

derived growth factor (PGF), and TGF-β (Fig. 32-36). The production of these factors is to some degree regulated by estrogen.[37] Third is the progressive modification of specific oncogenes or the loss of specific suppressor genes leading to advanced metastatic disease.

Unlike most human organs that are differentiated at the end of fetal life, the mammary gland develops and differentiates after puberty. The mammary gland at birth is formed by primary mammary ducts that branch during childhood. At premenarche, the duct epithelium proliferates. Ductal growth (terminal duct tubular units [acini]) is stimulated by estrogen, whereas additional progesterone is required for

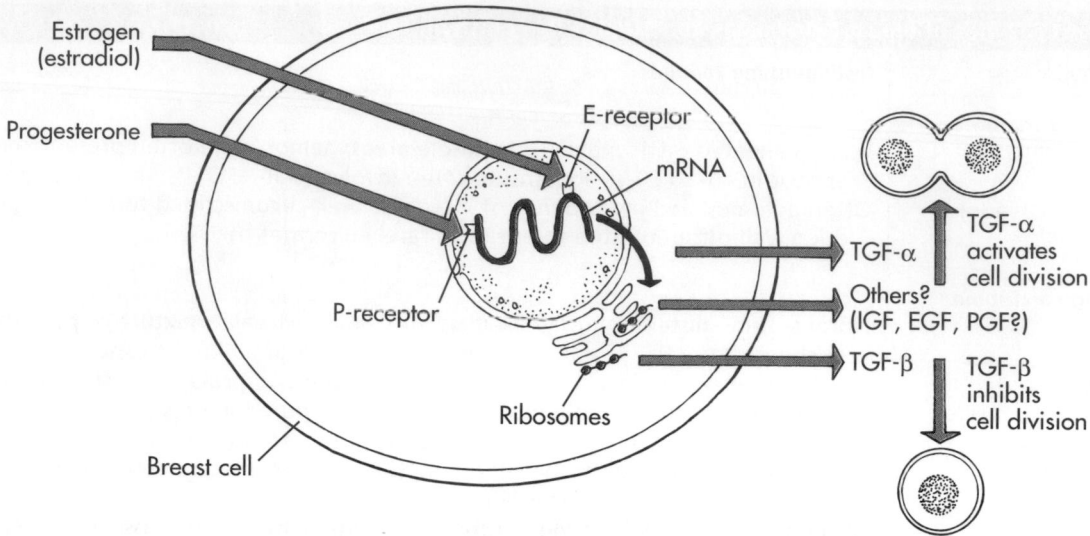

Fig. 32-36 *Control of breast cell growth.* Two levels of control of breast cell growth: (1) paracrine signaling by estrogen *(E-receptor)* and progesterone *(P-receptor)* steroids and (2) autocrine signaling by locally secreted growth factors, such as transforming growth factor (TGF-α and -β) and others, including insulin-like growth factor *(IGF)*, epidermal growth factor *(EGF)*, and platelet-derived growth factor *(PGF)*. *mRNA,* Messenger ribonucleic acid.

lobular development. Acini are the dynamic structure of the mammary gland (see Fig. 31-18). The number of these acini increases at each menstruation, with new budding structures until approximately age 35 years.[51-53]

There is an increase in the number of acini (intense lobular development) with pregnancy, resulting in full differentiation of their structure and function. When pregnancy does not happen, full differentiation of the breast may never be attained. Thus the normally "unfinished" ends of the duct system present a site of unusual sensitivity and tissue vulnerability. At menopause, acini, as well as interlobular fibrous tissues, undergo atrophy, but the large and intermediate duct system persists.[52] Involution of the glandular epithelium continues, and the breast becomes composed mainly of large ducts, increased connective tissue, and fat.

Mammary epithelial cells achieve rapid renewal by a small number of mitotic divisions of immortal stem cells. (Cell renewal is discussed in Chapters 1 and 9.) Because the number of mutations is proportional to the rate and number of stem cell divisions, factors that accelerate cell division can have a carcinogenic effect. Hormones may act as accelerators and influence the susceptibility of the breast epithelium to environmental carcinogens, because hormones control the differentiation of the mammary gland epithelium and thereby regulate the rate of stem cell division. Current knowledge of the mechanisms of differentiation of the mammary gland suggests that both estrogens and progesterone may be involved in breast carcinogenesis. This hypothesis is supported by two facts: (1) the increased incidence of breast cancer in women (i.e., 100 times more frequent in women than in men) and (2) the association of breast cancer with the events of reproductive life.

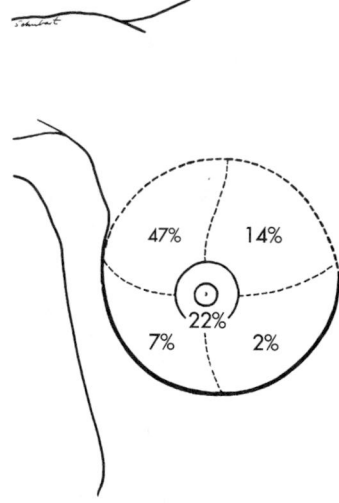

Fig. 32-37 *Distribution of carcinomas in different areas of the breast.* *(From del Regato, J.A., Spjut, H.J., & Cox, J.D. [1985]. Ackerman and del Regato's cancer: Diagnosis, treatment, and prognosis [6th ed.]. St. Louis: Mosby.)*

The majority of carcinomas of the breast occur in the upper outer quadrant, where most of the glandular tissue of the breast is located (Fig. 32-37). The lymphatic spread of cancer to the opposite breast, to lymph nodes in the base of the neck, and to the abdominal cavity is caused by obstruction of the normal lymphatic pathways or destruction of lymphatic vessels by surgery or radiotherapy (see Fig. 31-19). The less common inner quadrant tumors may spread to mediastinal nodes or Rotter nodes, which are located between the pectoral muscles (see Fig. 31-19).

TABLE 32-12	Clinical Manifestations of Breast Cancer
Clinical Manifestation	**Pathophysiology**
Local pain	Local obstruction caused by the tumor
Dimpling of the skin	Can occur with invasion of the dermal lymphatics because of retraction of Cooper ligament or involvement of the pectoralis fascia
Nipple retraction	Shortening of the mammary ducts
Skin retraction	Involvement of the suspensory ligaments
Edema	Local inflammation or lymphatic obstruction
Nipple/areolar eczema	Paget disease
Pitting of the skin (similar to the surface of an orange [peau d'orange])	Obstruction of the subcutaneous lymphatics, resulting in the accumulation of fluid
Reddened skin, local tenderness, and warmth	Inflammation
Dilated blood vessels	Obstruction of venous return by a fast-growing tumor; obstruction dilates superficial veins
Nipple discharge in a non-lactating woman	Spontaneous and intermittent discharge caused by tumor obstruction
Ulceration	Tumor necrosis
Hemorrhage	Erosion of blood vessels
Edema of the arm	Obstruction of lymphatic drainage in the axilla
Chest pain	Metastasis to the lung

Modified from Griffiths, M.J., Murray, K.H., & Russo, P.C. (1984). Oncology nursing: Pathophysiology, assessment, and intervention. New York: Macmillan.

Internal mammary chain nodes are also frequent sites of metastasis. Metastases from the vertebral veins can involve the vertebrae, pelvic bones, ribs, and skull. The lungs, kidneys, liver, adrenal glands, ovaries, and pituitary gland are also sites of metastasis.

Approximately one third of breast cancers are hormone dependent and regress in response to surgical removal of the ovaries. Estrogen and progesterone are of primary significance in maintaining some breast cancer growths. Not all breast tumors, however, are estrogen-receptor (ER) positive or progesterone-receptor (PR) positive. It is now known that estrogens, like other steroid hormones, modulate gene expression in target (e.g., breast) cells through their interaction with specific nuclear proteins (receptors). Current research, however, identifies two levels of control of cell growth: (1) paracrine signaling by estrogen and progesterone steroids and (2) autocrine signaling by locally secreted growth factors, such as transforming growth factor (TGF) (see Fig. 32-36). (Paracrine and autocrine signaling are discussed in Chapters 1 and 17. TGF is also discussed in Chapter 9.) Current evidence indicates that estrogen-dependent breast cancer growth may be regulated by positive growth stimulators, such as TGF-α and negative (inhibiting) growth stimulators, such as TGF-β.[54,55]

Clinical Manifestations

The first sign of breast cancer is usually a painless lump. Lumps caused by breast tumors do not have any classic characteristics. Other presenting signs include palpable nodes in the axilla, retraction of tissue (dimpling) (Fig. 32-38), or bone pain caused by metastasis to the vertebrae. Table 32-12

Fig. 32-38 *Retraction of nipple caused by carcinoma. (From del Regato, J.A., Spjut, H.J., & Cox, J.D. [1985]. Ackerman and del Regato's cancer: Diagnosis, treatment, and prognosis [6th ed.]. St. Louis: Mosby.)*

summarizes the clinical manifestations of breast cancers. Manifestations vary according to the type of tumor and stage of disease.

Evaluation and Treatment

Mammography, percutaneous needle aspiration, biopsy, and hormone receptor assays are generally used in evaluating breast cancer. Biopsy is the definitive diagnostic test.

Treatment is based on the extent or stage of the cancer (Box 32-9). The extent of the tumor at the primary site, the presence and extent of lymph node metastasis, and the presence of distant metastases are all evaluated to determine the stage of disease. Surgery, radiation, chemotherapy, hormone therapy, biologic therapy, and bone marrow transplantation may be used to treat breast cancer (Box 32-10).

✓ QUICK CHECK

Why is fibrocystic breast disease sometimes considered a risk factor for breast cancer?

Why have reproductive hormones been implicated as risk factors for breast cancer?

Why are reproductive factors, such as early menarche and late menopause, important for the pathogenesis of breast cancer?

HEALTH ALERT
Breast Cancer and Dietary Fats

In 1992, researchers at the Harvard School of Public Health proclaimed that dietary fat appeared to play no direct role in breast cancer risk. More recently, however, the same researchers, along with a group of Swedish colleagues, came to a different conclusion. Key was the distinction they made among fats; they found that monounsaturated fats (olive and canola oils) appear to protect against breast cancer whereas polyunsaturated fats in vegetable oils seem to increase risk. Saturated fats, a major risk factor for heart disease, had no effect. Other researchers have found another risky fat—the trans fatty acids in margarines and vegetable oils. These fats also appear to increase breast cancer risk. Persons should not add monounsaturated fats to their current diet (i.e., increasing calories), but rather they should substitute them for other fats already being eaten.

Data from Raloff, J. (1998). Unsaturated fats play yin-yang cancer role. Science News, 153, 37; Bakker, N., Van't Veer, P., & Zock, P.L. (1997). Adipose fatty acids and cancers of the breast, prostate, and colon: An ecological study. EURAMIC Study Group. International Journal of Cancer, 72(4), 587-591.

Disorders of the Male Breast
Gynecomastia

Gynecomastia is the overdevelopment of breast tissue in a male. Gynecomastia accounts for approximately 85% of all masses that develop in the male breast and affects 32% to 40% of the male population. If only one breast is involved, it is typically the left. Incidence is greatest among adolescents and men older than 50 years.

Gynecomastia results from hormonal alterations, which may be idiopathic or caused by systemic disorders, drugs, or neoplasms. Gynecomastia usually involves an imbalance of the estrogen/testosterone ratio. The normal estrogen/testosterone ratio can be altered in one of two ways. First, estrogen levels may be excessively high, although testosterone levels are normal. This is the case in drug-induced and tumor-induced hyperestrogenism. Second, testosterone levels may be extremely low, although estrogen levels are normal, as is the case in hypergonadism. Gynecomastia also can be caused by alterations in breast tissue responsiveness to hormonal stimulation. Breast tissue may have increased responsiveness to estrogen or decreased responsiveness to androgen. Alterations of responsiveness may cause many cases of idiopathic gynecomastia.

Besides puberty and aging, estrogen/testosterone imbalances are associated with hypogonadism, Klinefelter syndrome, and testicular neoplasms. Hormone-induced gynecomastia is usually bilateral. Pubertal gynecomastia is a self-limiting phenomenon that usually disappears within 4 to 6 months. Senescent gynecomastia usually regresses spontaneously within 6 to 12 months.

Systemic disorders associated with gynecomastia include cirrhosis of the liver, infectious hepatitis, chronic renal failure, chronic obstructive lung disease, hyperthyroidism, tuberculosis, and chronic malnutrition. It may be that these disorders ultimately alter the estrogen/testosterone ratio, initiating the gynecomastia.

Gynecomastia is frequently seen in males receiving estrogen therapy, either in preparation for a sex-change operation or in the treatment of prostatic carcinoma. Other drugs that can cause gynecomastia include digitalis, cimetidine, spironolactone, reserpine, thiazide, isoniazid, ergotamine, tricyclic antidepressants, amphetamines, vincristine, and busulfan. Gynecomastia is usually unilateral in these instances.

Malignancies of the testes, adrenals, or liver can cause gynecomastia if they alter the estrogen/testosterone ratio. Pituitary adenomas and lung cancer also are associated with gynecomastia.

Pathophysiology
The enlargement consists of hyperplastic stroma and ductal tissue. Hyperplasia results in a firm, palpable mass, at least 2 cm in diameter and located beneath the areola.

Evaluation and Treatment
The diagnosis of gynecomastia is based on physical examination. Identification and treatment of the cause are likely to be followed by resolution of the gynecomastia. The man should be taught to perform breast self-examination and is examined at 6- and 12-month intervals if the gynecomastia persists.

Carcinoma
Breast cancer in males accounts for 0.25% of all male cancers and less than 1% of all breast cancers. About 1300 new cases

Staging of Breast Cancer   BOX 32-9

T—Primary tumor size

TX   Primary tumor cannot be assessed

T0   No evidence of primary tumor

Tis   Carcinoma in situ: intraductal carcinoma, lobular carcinoma in situ, or Paget disease of the nipple with node

T1   Tumor 2 cm or less in greatest dimension

T2   Tumor more than 2 cm but not more than 5 cm in greatest dimension

T3   Tumor more than 5 cm in greatest dimension

T4   Tumor of any size with direct extension to chest wall or skin

NOTE: Paget disease associated with a tumor is classified according to the size of the tumor.

N—Regional lymph nodes

NX   Regional lymph nodes cannot be assessed (e.g., previously removed)

N0   No regional lymph node metastasis

N1   Metastasis to movable ipsilateral axillary lymph node(s)

N2   Metastasis to ipsilateral axillary lymph node(s) fixed to one another or to other structures

N3   Metastasis to ipsilateral internal mammary lymph node(s)

M—Distant metastasis

MX   Presence of distant metastasis cannot be assessed

M0   No distant metastasis

M1   Distant metastasis (includes metastasis to ipsilateral supraclavicular lymph node[s])

Stage grouping

Stage			
Stage	Tis	N0	M0
Stage I	T1	N0	M0
Stage IIa	T0	N0	M0
	T1	N1	M0
	T2	N0	M0
Stage IIB	T2	N1	M0
	T3	N0	M0
Stage IIIA	T0	N2	M0
	T1	N2	M0
	T2	N2	M0
	T3	N1	M0
	T3	N2	M0
Stage IIIB	T4	Any N	M0
	Any T	N3	M0
Stage IV	Any T	Any N	M1

From Beahrs, O.H., Hutter, R.V., & Kennedy, B.J. (Eds.). (1992). Breast manual for staging of cancer (45th ed.). Philadelphia: Lippincott.

Other National Organizations Addressing Breast Cancer   BOX 32-10

In addition to the American Cancer Society (1-800-ACS-2345), other sources of patient information and support include the following:

Cancer Information Service of the National Cancer Institute: 1-800-4-CANCER

National Alliance of Breast Cancer Organizations (NABCO): 1-212-719-0154

National Coalition for Cancer Survivorship: 1-301-650-8868

Susan G. Komen Foundation: 1-800-IM-AWARE

Y-ME National Organization for Breast Cancer Information and Support: 1-800-221-2141

YMCA Encore Program: 1-202-628-3636

---

of breast cancer in men are estimated in 1999.[14] It is seen most commonly after the age of 60 years, with the peak incidence between 60 and 69 years. It has, however, been reported in males as young as 6 years old and in adolescents. Possible risk factors include gynecomastia, radiation of the chest wall, and family history of breast cancer. The effects of inheritance of the breast cancer susceptibility gene (*BRCA1*) in men is unclear. Although the risk of developing breast cancer is almost nonexistent, they may have a slight increase in prostate cancer; this is still under investigation. Male carriers of the *BRCA1* gene, however, can pass the gene on to their daughters.[1,38] In terms of breast cancer susceptibility genes, men who develop breast cancer are more likely to have a *BRCA2* mutation than a *BRCA1* mutation.[47]

Male breast tumors frequently resemble carcinoma of the breast in women. Estrogen receptors have been found in up to 84% of biopsy specimens from men.[16] The malignant male breast lesion is usually a unilateral solid mass located near the nipple. Because the nipple is commonly involved, crusting and nipple discharge are typical clinical manifestations. Other findings include skin retraction, ulceration of the skin over the tumor, and axillary node involvement. Patterns of metastasis are similar to those in females.

The diagnosis of cancer is confirmed by biopsy. Because of delays in seeking treatment, male breast cancer tends to be advanced at the time of diagnosis and therefore to have a poor prognosis. Treatment protocols are similar to those for female breast cancer, but endocrine therapy is used more frequently for males because a higher percentage of male tumors are hormone-dependent. Orchiectomy is performed to treat metastatic disease.

SEXUALLY TRANSMITTED INFECTIONS

Sexually contracted infections affect more than 12 million Americans per year[56] and account for about one third of the reproductive mortality in the United States (Table 32-13).[56] Complications of sexually transmitted infections (STIs) include pelvic inflammatory disease (PID), infertility, ectopic pregnancy, chronic pelvic pain, neonatal morbidity and mortality, genital cancer, and epidemiologic synergy with HIV transmission. Long-term sequelae of untreated or undertreated STIs may be disastrous and can impact a person's physical, emotional, and financial well-being. (See color plates of STIs.)

In the past, an infection transmitted through sexual intercourse was called a *venereal disease*. Because of the limited scope, the term *venereal disease* has been replaced with *sexually transmitted disease* or *sexually transmitted infection (STI)*. Sexually transmitted diseases are infections contracted by intimate, as well as sexual, contact and include systemic infections, such as tuberculosis and hepatitis, that can spread to a sexual partner. Etiology of an STI may be bacterial, viral, protozoan, parasitic, or fungal (Table 32-14). Although the majority of STIs can be treated, viral-induced STIs are considered incurable.[56]

The current increase in severity and incidence of STIs can be attributed to demographic, life-style, and behavioral factors.[7,56] First, many infected individuals do not seek treatment because symptoms are absent, minor, or transient. Second, a rise in the number of single or never-married individuals, involvement in premarital or extramarital sexual affairs, and bisexuality contribute to an increase in number of lifetime sexual partners and increased exposure to STIs. Last, indulgence in high-risk sexual behaviors and poor health habits, such as failure to use a condom or nonmonogamous or new relationships, drug use, and douching, increases an individual's risk of exposure or the severity of infection if exposed. Perhaps partly as a result of risk-taking behavior, adolescents tend to be at highest risk for STI exposure and infection. Table 32-15 summarizes the major STIs.

TABLE 32-13	STI Statistical* Summary: United States
Each year	12 million individuals contract a sexually transmitted infection from infected partners
	Two thirds of those infected are under the age of 25 yr
	More than 4 million new cases of chlamydia are estimated to occur
	600,000 new cases of gonorrhea are estimated to occur
	16,500 new cases of syphilis were reported
Currently	Viral sexually transmitted infections affect more than 56 million people in the United States
	1 million are infected by HIV virus
	24 to 40 million are infected with the human papillomavirus (genital warts)
	31 million are infected with genital herpes
	Untreated or undertreated chlamydial infections are the primary cause of *preventable* infertility and ectopic pregnancy

*For more information, call STI hotline at 1-800-227-8922.

TABLE 32-14	Currently Recognized Sexually Transmitted Infections
Causal Microorganism	**Disease**
Bacteria	
Campylobacter	Campylobacter enteritis
Calymmatobacterium granulomatis	Granuloma inguinale
Chlamydia trachomatis	Urogenital infections; lymphogranuloma venereum
Polymicrobial	
Gardnerella vaginalis plus *Mycoplasma hominis and various anerobic bacteria*	Bacterial vaginosis
Haemophilus ducreyi	Chancroid
Mycoplasma	Mycoplasmosis
Neisseria gonorrhoeae	Gonorrhea
Shigella	Shigellosis
Treponema pallidum	Syphilis
Viruses	
Cytomegalovirus	Cytomegalic inclusion disease
Hepatitis B virus (HBV)	Hepatitis
Herpes simplex virus (HSV)	Genital herpes
Human immunodeficiency virus (HIV)	Acquired immunodeficiency syndrome (AIDS)
Human papillomavirus	Condylomata acuminata
Molluscum contagiosum virus	Molluscum contagiosum
Protozoa	
Entamoeba histolytica	Amebiasis; amebic dysentery
Giardia lamblia	Giardiasis
Trichomonas vaginalis	Trichomoniasis
Ectoparasites	
Phthirus pubis	Pediculosis pubis
Sarcoptes scabiei	Scabies
Fungus	
Candida albicans	Candidiasis

HEALTH ALERT

Treatment for Sexual Assault

Victims of sexual assault are given ceftriaxone IM, metronidazole, and azithromycin or doxycycline as prophylaxis against gonorrhea, trichomonas, bacterial vaginosis, and chlamydia. Hepatitis B vaccination is highly recommended.

TABLE 32-15	Major Sexually Transmitted Infections	
Source of Infection	**Epidemiology/Clinical Manifestations**	**Evaluation and Treatment**
Bacterial		
Bacterial vaginosis (*Haemophilus, Corynebacterium, Gardnerella vaginalis/Mycoplasma hominis*)	Occurs almost exclusively in sexually active women Risk factors include multiple or new male partners, smoking Manifestations include discharge (sometimes "fishy" odor); males generally asymptomatic; may predispose women to other STIs or preterm labor	Diagnosed from specimen of vaginal secretions (wet mount) Week-long treatment with oral or vaginal antibiotics Treatment of sex partner is controversial
Chancroid (*Haemophilus ducreyi*)	Incidence is low in United States; women are generally asymptomatic, whereas men develop inflamed, painful genital ulcer Secondary infections can occur	Definitive diagnosis is from cultured specimens Treat with antibiotics
Chlamydial infections (*Chlamydia trachomatis*)	Most common bacterial STI in United States; leading cause of infertility for both men and women and ectopic pregnancy; leading cause of blindness worldwide; often asymptomatic Acute course is fairly self-limited followed by chronic, low-grade, persistent infections over years; newborns can be infected; infections in men can cause urethritis and epididymitis; *C. trachomatis* causes acute urethral syndrome (dysuria, polyuria, pus in urine) in young women	Diagnosed by DNA or fluorescent monoclonal antibody screening of discharge; urine assay Treatment of both sexual partners with antibiotics
Gonorrhea (*Neisseria gonorrhoeae*)	Adolescents 15-19 yr at high risk; transmitted by oral, anal, or vaginal intercourse; mother to child transmission during vaginal delivery Manifestations include urethral and/or anorectal infections; vaginal discharge; bleeding or spotting and heavy menses; women may be asymptomatic	Gram-stained slides; DNA screening or culture of endocervical, pharyngeal, and anal secretions; concomitant screening for *Chlamydia* Treat both sexual partners with antibiotics
Lymphogranuloma venereum (LGV) (*C. trachomatis*)	Often confused with syphilis, herpes, or chancroid Begins as skin lesion, spreads to lymphatic tissue; appears as multivesicular ulcer on penis or scrotum in men, and vaginal wall, cervix, or labia in women; anorectal lesions, from anal intercourse, can appear in both men and women	Diagnosed through LGV complement-fixation tests, tissue culture, and monoclonal antibody tests Treated with antibiotics

NOTE: *AIDS is discussed extensively in Chapter 7.*
DNA, *Deoxyribonucleic acid;* VDRL, *Venereal Disease Research Laboratory test;* RPR, *Rapid plasma region test;* STI, *sexually transmitted infection;* IV, *intravenous.*

Continued

TABLE 32-15   Major Sexually Transmitted Infections—cont'd

Source of Infection	Epidemiology/Clinical Manifestations	Evaluation and Treatment
Bacterial—cont'd		
Syphilis (*Treponema pallidum*)	Incidence is decreasing; higher incidence in low income, minority, heterosexual couples; transmitted during first few years of infection; can occur during pregnancy to fetus "Hard chancre" develops in primary stage; systemic symptoms include low-grade fever, malaise, sore throat, hoarseness, anorexia, headache, joint pain, skin rashes; latent (tertiary) stages usually asymptomatic Neurosyphilis and life-threatening hypersensitivities can develop without treatment	Dark-field or fluorescent antibody examination of fluid from syphilitic chancre; VDRL or RPR Treatment includes penicillin injections for primary or secondary infections
Viral		
Condylomata acuminata (human papillomavirus [HPV])	Most common viral STI in United States Risk factors include multiple sexual partners, early onset of sexual activity (16-25 yr of age); increasing data link HPV with cervical and vulvar cancer in females and anorectal and squamous cell carcinoma of the penis in men; genital warts contagious; infants can be infected during delivery Warts are soft, skin-colored, whitish pink to reddish brown; may occur singly or in clusters	Diagnosis based on clinical manifestations; Pap smears aid diagnosis Treated with topical acids or cryosurgery; cervical and extensive vaginal lesions treated with 5-FU or surgical excision; treatment is cosmetic, not curative
Genital herpes (type 1 [HSV-1] or type 2 [HSV-2])	Most common cause of genital ulceration in United States; reaching epidemic status Neonatal infections can occur in utero, intrapartum, and postpartum; virus undergoes local replication in dermis and epidermis leading to vesicles; can remain in latent stage until reactivated; cause of reactivation unknown but may be related to stress, sun exposure, hormonal fluctuations	Diagnosis based on clinical manifestations Definitive diagnosis by tissue culture No curative treatment; oral acyclovir, famciclovir, or valacyclovir may be used; IV acyclovir reserved for severely immunocompromised persons
Parasitic		
Pediculosis pubis (*Phthirus pubis* [crab louse])	Commonly transmitted sexually, causes "crabs;" most common in single persons ages 15-25 yr Ranges from mild itching to severe, intolerable itching	Definitive diagnosis by examination Treated with lotion, cream, or shampoo
Scabies (*Sarcoptes scabiei*)	First human disease with *known* cause; worldwide distribution; most recent outbreak in the United States began in 1971, subsided in 1981; transmitted by close skin-to-skin contact, typically occurring within families or between sexual partners Predominant manifestation is intense itching	Diagnosed from clinical manifestations, microscopic identification Treated with topical cream or lotion
Trichomoniasis (*Trichomonas vaginalis*)	Common cause of lower genital tract infection; found in both partners; urethra most common site of infection in men, primarily involves vagina in women Manifestations range from none to severe, including pain on intercourse, dysuria, and spotting; most men remain asymptomatic	Definitive diagnosis through microscopic confirmation of trichomonads in vaginal secretions Treat with antibiotics for both sexual partners

Bacterial
Gonococcal infections

Color plate 1 *Symptomatic gonococcal urethritis.*

Color plate 2 *Endocervical gonorrhea.*

Color plate 3 *Skin lesions of disseminated gonococcal infection.*

Bacterial vaginosis

Color plate 7 *Vaginal examination with mild bacterial vaginosis.*

Syphilis

Color plate 4 *Erythematous penile plaques of secondary syphilis.*

Color plate 5 *Multiple primary syphilitic chancres of labia and perineum.*

Color plate 6 *Papular secondary syphilis.*

Lymphogranuloma

Color plate 11 *"Groove sign" in man with lymphogranuloma venereum (LV).*

Chlamydial infections

Color plate 8 *Beefy red mucosa in chlamydial infection.*

Color plate 9 *Chlamydial epididymitis.*

Color plate 10 *Chlamydial ophthalmia: erythematous conjunctiva in infant.*

Color plates from Morse, S.A., Moreland, A.A., & Holmes, K.K. (1996). Atlas of sexually transmitted diseases and AIDS (2nd ed.). London: Mosby-Wolfe.

Viral
Genital herpes

Color plate 12 *Early lesions of primary genital herpes.*

Color plate 13 *Primary vulvar herpes.*

Color plate 14 *Generalized herpes simplex in patient with atopic dermatitis.*

Human papillomavirus (HPV)

Color plate 15 *Human papillomavirus (HPV) infection of the cervix.*

Subclinical HPV infection
Cervical os
Cervical intraepithelial neoplasia
Exophytic condyloma

Color plate 16 *Exophytic (outward-growing) condyloma, subclinical human papillomavirus (HPV) infection, and high-grade cervical intraepithelial neoplasia (CIN).*

Condylomata acuminata

Color plate 17 *Condylomata acuminata: vulva and perineum.*

Color plate 18 *Condylomata acuminata: perianal.*

Color plate 19 *Condylomata acuminata: penile.*

Parasite
Trichomoniasis

Color plate 20 *"Strawberry cervix" seen with trichomoniasis.*

Scabies

Color plate 21 *Nodular lesions of scabies on male genitalia.*

Color plate 22 *Urticaria associated with scabies.*

Color plate 23 *Scabies of palm with secondary pyoderma in infant.*

Pediculosis pubis (Phthirus pubis [crablouse])

Color plate 24 *Phthirus pubis feeding on its host.*

Color plate 25 *Pubic hair with multiple nits.*

DID YOU UNDERSTAND?

Alterations of Sexual Maturation

1. Sexual maturation, or puberty, should begin in girls between the ages of 8 and 13 years and in boys between the ages of 9 and 14 years.
2. Delayed puberty is the onset of sexual maturation after these ages; precocious puberty is the onset before these ages. Treatment depends on the cause.

Disorders of the Female Reproductive System

1. The female reproductive system can be altered by hormonal imbalances, infectious microorganisms, inflammation, structural abnormalities, and benign or malignant proliferative conditions.
2. Primary dysmenorrhea is painful menstruation not associated with pelvic disease. It results from excessive synthesis of prostaglandins, which cause the myometrium to contract and constrict blood vessels, resulting in ischemic pain.
3. Primary amenorrhea is the continued absence of menarche and menstrual function by 14 years of age without the development of secondary sex characteristics or by 16 years of age if these changes have occurred.
4. Secondary amenorrhea is the absence of menstruation for a time equivalent to more than 3 cycles or 6 months in women who have previously menstruated. Secondary amenorrhea is associated with anovulation.
5. Dysfunctional uterine bleeding (DUB) is heavy or irregular bleeding caused by a disturbance of the menstrual cycle.
6. Polycystic ovary (PCO) is a condition in which excessive androgen production is triggered by inappropriate secretion of gonadotropins. This hormonal imbalance prevents ovulation and causes enlargement and cyst formation in the ovaries, excessive endometrial proliferation in the uterus, and, occasionally, hirsutism.
7. Premenstrual syndrome (PMS) is the cyclic recurrence of physical, psychologic, or behavioral changes distressing enough to disrupt normal activities or interpersonal relationships. Emotional symptoms, particularly depression, anger, irritability, and fatigue, are reported as the most distressing symptoms; physical symptoms tend to be less problematic. Treatment is symptomatic and includes self-help techniques, life-style changes, counseling, and medication.
8. Infection and inflammation of the female genitalia can result from microorganisms from the environment or overproliferation of microorganisms that normally populate the genital tract.
9. Pelvic inflammatory disease (PID) is an acute ascending infection of the upper genital tract caused by a sexually transmitted pathogen. Untreated PID can lead to infertility.
10. Vaginitis, or vaginal infection, is usually caused by sexually transmitted pathogens or *Candida albicans,* which causes candidiasis.
11. Cervicitis, which is infection of the cervix, can be acute (mucopurulent cervicitis) or chronic. Its most common cause is a sexually transmitted pathogen.
12. Vulvitis is an inflammation of the skin of the vulva. It can be caused by chemical irritants, allergens, skin disorders, irritation from tight-fitting clothing, or spread of vaginal infections, such as candidiasis.
13. Bartholinitis, also called Bartholin cyst, is an infection of the ducts that lead from the Bartholin glands to the surface of the vulva. Infection blocks the glands, preventing the outflow of glandular secretions.
14. The pelvic relaxation disorders—uterine displacement, uterine prolapse, cystocele, rectocele, and urethrocele—are caused by the relaxation of muscles and fascial supports, usually with age or after childbirth or other trauma, and are more likely to occur in women with a familial or genetic predisposition.
15. Benign ovarian cysts develop from mature ovarian follicles that do not release their ova (follicular cysts) or from a corpus luteum that persists abnormally instead of degenerating (corpus luteum cyst). Cysts usually regress spontaneously.
16. Endometrial polyps consist of overgrowths of endometrial tissue and frequently cause abnormal bleeding in the premenopausal woman.
17. Leiomyomas, also called uterine fibroids, are benign tumors arising from the muscle layer of the uterus, the myometrium. Adenomyosis is the presence of endometrial glands and stroma within the uterine myometrium.
18. Endometriosis is the presence of functional endometrial tissue (i.e., tissue that responds to hormonal stimulation) at sites outside the uterus. Endometriosis causes an inflammatory reaction at the site of implantation and is a cause of infertility.
19. Most cancers of the female genitalia involve the uterus (particularly the cervix) and the ovaries. Cancer of the vagina is rare.
20. Cervical cancer arises from the cervical epithelium and is considered a sexually transmitted infection. The progressively serious neoplastic alterations are cervical intraepithelial neoplasia (cervical dysplasia), cervical carcinoma in situ, and invasive cervical carcinoma. Smoking is a cofactor.
21. Most vaginal cancers are not invasive. Like cervical cancers, they arise from the epithelium and are identified as intraepithelial neoplasia (dysplasia), carcinoma in situ, or invasive carcinoma.
22. Risk factors for endometrial cancer include exposure to unopposed estrogen, obesity, high-fat diet, infertility or no pregnancies, late menopause, diabetes, and hypertension. Hormonal contraception protects against endometrial and ovarian cancers. Incidence of endometrial cancer is greatest among women in their 50s and early 60s.

Continued

■ DID YOU UNDERSTAND?—cont'd

Disorders of the Female Reproductive System—cont'd

23. Risk factors for ovarian cancer include family history, residence in an industrialized country, prior breast or endometrial cancer, infertility, early menopause, obesity, a high-fat diet, and exposure to asbestos or talc. Ovarian cancer causes more deaths than any other genital cancer in women.

24. Infertility, or the inability to conceive after 1 year of unprotected intercourse, affects approximately 15% of all couples. Fertility can be impaired by factors in the male, female, or both partners.

25. Chronic illness, medications, infection, sexual trauma, and a variety of psychosocial concerns have been implicated as causes of female sexual dysfunction.

Disorders of the Male Reproductive System

1. Disorders of the urethra include urethritis (infection of the urethra) and urethral strictures (narrowing or obstruction of the urethral lumen caused by scarring).

2. Most cases of urethritis result from sexually transmitted pathogens. Urologic instrumentation, foreign body insertion, trauma, or an anatomic abnormality can cause urethral inflammation with or without infection.

3. Urethritis causes urinary symptoms, including a burning sensation during urination (dysuria), frequency, urgency, urethral tingling or itching, and clear or purulent discharge.

4. The scarring that causes urethral stricture can be caused by trauma or by severe untreated urethritis.

5. Manifestations of urethral stricture include those of bladder outlet obstruction: urinary frequency and hesitancy, diminished force and caliber of the urinary stream, dribbling after voiding, and nocturia.

6. Phimosis and paraphimosis are penile disorders involving the foreskin (prepuce). In phimosis, the foreskin cannot be retracted over the glans. In paraphimosis, the foreskin is retracted and cannot be reduced (returned to its normal anatomic position over the glans). Phimosis is caused by poor hygiene and chronic infection and can lead to paraphimosis. Paraphimosis can constrict the penile blood vessels, preventing circulation to the glans.

7. Peyronie disease consists of fibrosis, affecting the corpora cavernosa, which causes penile curvature during erection. Fibrosis prevents engorgement on the affected side, causing a lateral curvature that can prevent intercourse.

8. Priapism is a prolonged, painful erection that is not stimulated by sexual arousal. The corpora cavernosa (but not the corpus spongiosum) fill with blood that does not drain out, probably because of venous obstruction. Priapism is associated with spinal cord trauma, sickle cell disease, leukemia, and pelvic tumors. It can also be idiopathic.

9. Balanitis is an inflammation of the glans penis. It is associated with phimosis, inadequate cleansing under the foreskin, skin disorders, and pathogens (e.g., *Candida albicans*).

10. Cancer of the penis is rare. Penile carcinoma in situ tends to involve the glans; invasive carcinoma of the penis involves the shaft as well.

11. A varicocele is an abnormal dilation of the veins within the spermatic cord caused by either congenital absence of valves in the internal spermatic vein or acquired valvular incompetence.

12. A hydrocele is a collection of fluid between the testicular and scrotal layers of the tunica vaginalis. Hydroceles can be idiopathic or caused by trauma or infection of the testes.

13. A spermatocele is a cyst located between the testis and epididymis that is filled with fluid and sperm.

14. Cryptorchidism is a congenital condition in which one or both testes fail to descend into the scrotum. Uncorrected cryptorchidism is associated with infertility and significantly increased risk of testicular cancer.

15. Testicular torsion is the rotation of a testis, which twists blood vessels in the spermatic cord. This interrupts the blood supply to the testis, resulting in edema and, if not corrected within 6 hours, necrosis and atrophy of testicular tissues.

16. Orchitis is an acute infection of the testes. Complications of orchitis include hydrocele and abscess formation.

17. Testicular cancer is the most common malignancy in males 15 to 35 years of age. Although its cause is unknown, high androgen levels, genetic predisposition, and history of cryptorchidism, trauma, or infection may contribute to tumorigenesis.

18. Spermatogenesis (sperm production by the testes) can be impaired by disruptions of the hypothalamic-pituitary-testicular axis that reduce testosterone secretion and by testicular trauma, infection, or atrophy from any cause. Sperm production is also impaired by neoplastic disease, cryptorchidism, or any factor that causes testicular temperature to rise (e.g., circulatory impairment, wearing tight clothing).

19. Epididymitis, an inflammation of the epididymis, is usually caused by a sexually transmitted pathogen that ascends through the vasa deferentia from an already infected urethra or bladder.

20. Benign prostatic hyperplasia (BPH), also called benign prostatic hypertrophy, is the enlargement of the prostate gland. This condition becomes symptomatic as the enlarging prostate compresses the urethra, causing symptoms of bladder outlet obstruction and urine retention.

21. Bacterial prostatitis is an infection of the prostate. Acute bacterial prostatitis causes an inflammatory response in which the prostate becomes enlarged, tender, and firm. Infection may spread to the bladder. Chronic bacterial prostatitis is recurrent prostatic infection that eventually causes fibrosis.

22. Prostate cancer is the second leading cause of cancer deaths in men (after lung cancer). Possible causes include genetic predisposition, environmental and dietary factors, and high testosterone levels. Incidence is greatest among northwestern European and North American men (particularly blacks) older than 65 years.

23. Most cancers of the prostate are adenocarcinomas that develop at the periphery of the gland. Routine screening is recommended for early detection of disease.

24. Sexual dysfunction in males can be caused by any physical or psychologic factor that impairs erection, emission, or ejaculation.

Disorders of the Breast

1. Most disorders of the breast are disorders of the mammary gland, that is, the female breast.

2. Galactorrhea, or inappropriate lactation, is the persistent secretion of a milky substance by the breasts of a woman who is not in the postpartum state or nursing an infant. Its most common cause is non-puerperal hyperprolactinemia, a rise in serum prolactin levels.

3. Fibrocystic breast disease is a catch-all term used to describe a variety of benign epithelial breast lesions, including microcysts, macrocysts, adenosis, apocrine gland change, fibroadenomas, and ductal hyperplasia. Many of these lesions are risk factors for breast cancer, and most appear to represent a response of breast tissue to estrogen stimulation.

4. The lesions of fibrocystic disease (physiologic nodularity) are nodular, are multiple, and become tender and large as menstruation approaches. They are palpable and may worsen until menopause. Symptoms tend to lessen with a diet low in fat and caffeine. Physiologic nodularity is present in about 50% of menstruating women.

5. Other benign breast lesions are fibroadenomas, mammary duct ectasia (an inflammatory condition), intraductal papillomas, and fat necrosis.

6. Breast cancer is the most common form of cancer in women and second to lung cancer as the most common cause of cancer death.

7. The major risk factors for breast cancer are environmental factors, such as obesity and alcohol consumption; reproductive factors, such as nulliparity; and familial factors, such as a family history of breast cancer.

8. Approximately one third of breast cancers are hormone dependent (progesterone-receptor positive or estrogen-receptor positive). Treatment protocols are often based on whether the tumor is receptor positive or negative.

9. Most breast cancers arise from the ductal epithelium and then may metastasize to the lymphatics, opposite breast, abdominal cavity, lungs, bones, kidneys, liver, adrenal glands, ovaries, and pituitary glands.

10. The first clinical manifestation of breast cancer is usually a small, painless lump in the breast. Other manifestations include palpable lymph nodes in the axilla, dimpling of the skin, nipple and skin retraction, nipple discharge, ulcerations, reddened skin, and bone pain associated with bony metastases.

11. Gynecomastia is the overdevelopment (hyperplasia) of breast tissue in a male. It is first seen as a firm, palpable mass at least 2 cm in diameter and is located in the subareolar area.

12. Gynecomastia affects 32% to 40% of the male population. Incidence is greatest among adolescents and men older than 50 years of age.

13. Gynecomastia is caused by hormonal or breast tissue alterations that cause estrogen to dominate. These alterations can result from systemic disorders, drugs, neoplasms, or idiopathic causes.

14. Breast cancer is relatively uncommon in males, but it has a poor prognosis because men tend to delay seeking treatment until the disease is advanced. Incidence is greatest in men in their 60s.

15. Most breast cancers in men are estrogen receptor positive.

Sexually Transmitted Infections

1. Sexually transmitted diseases are infections contracted by intimate, as well as sexual, contact and include systemic infections, such as tuberculosis and hepatitis, that can spread to a sexual partner.

2. Etiology of an STI may be bacterial, viral, protozoan, parasitic, or fungal.

3. Although the majority of STIs can be treated, viral-induced STIs are considered incurable.

KEY TERMS

Acute bacterial prostatitis, 890
Adenomyosis, 873
Amenorrhea, 863
Anorgasmia (orgasmic dysfunction), 879
Balanitis, 881
Bartholinitis (Bartholin cyst), 869
Benign prostatic hyperplasia (BPH; benign prostatic hypertrophy), 888
Cervicitis, 869
Chronic bacterial prostatitis, 890
Corpus luteum cyst, 872
Cryptorchidism, 884
Cystocele, 870
Delayed puberty, 862
Ductal hyperplasia, 896
Dysfunctional uterine bleeding (DUB), 863
Dyspareunia (painful intercourse), 879
Endometrial polyp, 872
Endometriosis, 873
Enterocele, 870
Epididymitis, 887
Fibrocystic change (disease) (FCC; physiologic nodularity), 894
Florid hyperplasia, 896

Follicular cyst, 872
Galactorrhea (inappropriate lactation), 894
Gynecomastia, 904
Heterosexual precocious puberty, 862
Hirsutism, 863
Hydrocele, 884
Idiopathic isosexual precocity, 862
Incomplete precocious puberty, 862
Infertility, 880
Isosexual precocious puberty, 862
Leiomyoma (uterine fibroid), 873
Lobular hyperplasia, 896
Mild hyperplasia, 896
Mucopurulent cervicitis (MPC), 869
Nonbacterial prostatitis, 891
Nonpuerperal hyperprolactinemia, 894
Oophoritis, 866
Orchitis, 885
Paraphimosis, 881
Pelvic inflammatory disease (PID), 866
Pessary, 870
Peyronie disease ("bent nail syndrome"), 881
Phimosis, 881
Polycystic ovary (PCO), 864

Precocious puberty, 862
Premenstrual syndrome (PMS), 865
Priapism, 881
Primary amenorrhea, 863
Primary dysmenorrhea, 862
Prolactin-inhibiting factor (PIF), 894
Prostatitis, 890
Prostatodynia, 890
Radial scar, 896
Rectocele, 870
Salpingitis, 866
Sclerosing adenosis, 896
Secondary amenorrhea, 863
Sexual anorexia (inhibited sexual desire, decreased libido), 879
Sexual dysfunction, 892
Spermatocele, 884
Torsion of the testis, 885
Urethral stricture, 881
Urethritis, 880
Urethrocele, 870
Uterine prolapse, 870
Vaginismus, 879
Vaginitis, 868
Varicocele, 883
Vulvitis, 869

REFERENCES

1. American Cancer Society. (1997). *Breast cancer.* New York: The Author.
2. American Cancer Society. (1997). *Prostate cancer.* New York: The Author.
3. Burns, C.E. et al. (1996). *Pediatric primary care: A handbook for nurse practitioners.* Philadelphia: Saunders.
4. Speroff, L., Glass, R.H., & Kase, N.G. (1994). *Clinical gynecologic endocrinology and infertility* (5th ed.). Baltimore: Williams & Wilkins.
5. Mehring, P.N. Dysfunctional uterine bleeding. (1997). *Advance for Nurse Practitioners, 5*(11), 27-32.
6. Woods, N.F. et al. (1989). *Prevalence of perimenstrual symptoms: Final report.* Seattle: University of Washington.
7. Center for Disease Control. (1998). 1998 guidelines for treatment of sexually transmitted diseases. *MMWR Morbidity and Mortality Weekly Report 47*(RR-02). URL: www.cdc.gov/epo/mmwr/mmwr_rr.html.
8. Forrest, D.E. (1998). Common gynecologic pelvic disorders. In E.Q. Youngkin & M.S. Davis (Eds.). *Women's health: A primary care clinical guide.* Stamford, Conn.: Appleton & Lange.

9. Hartenbach, E. (1998). Pelvic masses in women: Deriving a diagnosis from obscure symptoms. *Consultant, 38*(1), 161-172.
10. Berger, G.S. (1993, October). How many women are affected by endometriosis? *Contemporary OB/GYN,* 47-60.
11. Wardle, P.G. & Hull, M.G. (1993). Is endometriosis a disease? *Baillieres Clinical Obstetrics and Gynaecology, 7*(4), 673-685.
12. Shaw, R.W. (1994). A risk benefit assessment of drugs used in the treatment of endometriosis. *Drug Safety, 11*(2), 104-113.
13. American Cancer Society. (1997). *Cervical cancer.* New York: The Author.
14. American Cancer Society. (1999). *Cancer facts & figures—1998.* New York: The Author.
15. Center for Disease Prevention and Epidemiology. (1998). Anogenital papillomavirus infections. *CD Summary, 47*(2).
16. American Cancer Society. (1997). *Endometrial cancer.* New York: The Author.
17. American Cancer Society. (1997). *Ovarian cancer.* New York: The Author.

REFERENCES

18. Seppa, N. (1998). Progestin enhances an anticancer process. *Science News, 154,* 197.

19. Charlton, R.S. & Yalom, I.D. (Eds.). (1997). *Treating sexual disorders.* San Francisco: Jossey-Bass.

20. Jefferson Health System. Men's Health. (1997). Male infertility. URL: www.jeffersonhealth.org/diseases/mens_health/infertil.htm.

21. Tanagho, E.A. & McAninch, J.W. (Eds.). (1992). *Smith's general urology* (13th ed.). Norwalk, Conn.: Appleton-Lange.

22. Noble, J. (Ed.). (1996). *Textbook of primary care medicine* (2nd ed.). St. Louis: Mosby.

23. American Cancer Society. (1993). *Penile cancer.* New York: the Author.

24. American Cancer Society. (1994). *Testicular cancer.* New York: The Author.

25. Carson, C.C. (1998). Update on benign prostatic hyperplasia. *The Clinical Advisory for Nurse Practitioners, 1,* 57-65.

26. Gleich, P. (1998). Prostatis: A state-of-the-art review of diagnosis and therapy. *Consultant, 38*(2), 345-348.

27. Cordon-Cardo, C. et al. (1998). Distinct altered patterns of p27K1P1 gene expression in benign prostatic hyperplasia and prostatic carcinoma. *Journal of the National Cancer Institute, 90*(17), 1284-1291.

28. Yang, R.M., Naitoh, J., Murphy, M., et al. (1998). Low p27 expression predicts poor disease-free survival in patients with prostate cancer. *Journal of Urology, 159*(3), 941-945.

29. Jefferson Health System. Men's Health. (1997). Overview of impotence. URL: www.jeffersonhealth.org/diseases/mens_health/impotenc.htm.

30. Marmorstein, L.Y., Ouchi, T., & Aaronson, S.A. (1998). The BRCA2 gene product functionally interacts with p53 and RAD51. *Proceedings of the National Academy of Sciences of the United States of America, 95*(23), 13869-13874.

31. Sharkey, F.E., Allred, D.C., & Valente, P.T. (1996). Breast. In I. Damjanov & J. Linder (Eds.). *Anderson's pathology* (10th ed.). St. Louis: Mosby.

32. Rivera-Pomar, J.M. et al. (1980). Focal fibrous disease of breast: A common entity in younger women. *Virchow's Archiv. A, Pathological Anatomy and Histopathology, 386,* 59.

33. Branch, L.A. (1998). Breast health. In E.Q. Youngkin & M.S. Davis (Eds.). *Women's health: A primary care clinical guide.* Stamford, Conn.: Appleton-Lange.

34. Edwards, M.J. et al. (1998). Infiltrating ductal carcinoma of the breast: The survival impact of race. *Journal of Clinical Oncology, 16*(8), 2693-2699.

35. Howard, D.L., Penchansky, R., & Brown, M.B. (1998). Disaggregating the effects of race on breast cancer survival. *Family Medicine, 30*(3), 228-235.

36. Colditz, G.A. (1998). Relationship between estrogen levels, use of hormone replacement therapy, and breast cancer. *Journal of the National Cancer Institute, 90*(11), 814-823.

37. Kuller, L.H. (1995). The etiology of breast cancer—from epidemiology to prevention. *Public Health Review, 23,* 157-213.

38. American Cancer Society. (1998). Key statistics about breast cancer. URL: www.canccr.org/ben/info/brstats.htm.

39. Swanson, C.A. et al. (1997). Alcohol consumption and breast cancer risk among women under 45 years. *Epidemiology, 8,* 231-237.

40. Willett, W.C. & Stampfer, M.J. (1997). Sobering data on alcohol and breast cancer. *Epidemiology, 8,* 225-227.

41. Thune, I. et al. (1997). Physical activity and the risk of breast cancer. *New England Journal of Medicine, 336*(18), 1269-1274.

42. Gammon, M.D., John, E.M., & Britton, J.A. (1998). Recreational and occupational physical activities and risk of breast cancer. *Journal of the National Cancer Institute, 90*(2), 110-117.

43. Newman, B. et al. (1998). Frequency of breast cancer attributable to BRCA₁ in population-based series of American women. *Journal of the American Medical Association, 279*(12), 915-921.

44. Szabo, C.I. & King, M.C. (1995). Inherited breast and ovarian cancer. *Human Molecule Genetics, 4,* 1811-1817.

45. Miki, Y. et al. (1994). A strong candidate for the breast and ovarian cancer susceptibility gene, *BRCA₁. Science, 266,* 66-71.

46. McCance, K.L. & Jorde, L.B. (1998). Evaluating the genetic risk of breast cancer. *The Nurse Practitioner, 23*(8), 14-29.

47. Stratton., M.R. & Wooster, R. (1996). Hereditary predisposition to breast cancer. *Current Opinion in Genetic Development, 6,* 93-97.

48. Ford, D., Easton, D.F., & Peto, J. (1995). Estimates of the gene frequency of BRCA₁ and its contribution to breast and ovarian cancer incidence. *American Journal of Human Genetics, 57,* 1457-1462.

49. Hoskins, K.R. et al. (1995). Assessment and counseling for women with a family history of breast cancer: A guide for clinicians. *Journal of the American Medical Association, 273,* 577-585.

50. Russo, J., Tay, L.K., & Russo, I.H. (1982). Differentiation of the mammary glands and susceptibility to breast cancer. *Breast Cancer Research and Treatment, 2,* 5-73.

51. Russo, J., Tay, L.K., & Russo, I.H. (1982). Differentiation of the mammary glands and susceptibility to breast cancer. *Breast Cancer Research and Treatment, 2,* 5-73.

REFERENCES

52. Morabia, A. & Wynder, E.L. (1990). Epidemiology and natural history of breast cancer. *Surgical Clinics of North America, 70*(4), 739-752.

53. Russo, J. & Russo, I.H. (1987). Development of the human mammary gland. In M.C. Neville & C.W. Daniel (Eds.), *The mammary gland: Development, regulation, and function.* New York: Plenum.

54. Knabbe, C. et al. (1987). Evidence that transforming growth factor-B is a hormonally regulated negative growth factor in human breast cancer cells. *Cell, 48,* 417-428.

55. Waxman, J. (1991). A new understanding of the hormonal regulation of endocrine dependent cancer. *British Medical Bulletin, 47*(1), 197-208.

56. Centers for Disease Control. (1994, July). *STD surveillance.* Springfield, Va.: National Tech Informational Service.

CHAPTER

33

Structure and Function of the Digestive System

Sue E. Huether

The digestive system breaks down ingested food, prepares it for uptake by the body's cells, provides body water, and eliminates wastes. This system consists of the gastrointestinal tract and accessory organs of digestion: the liver, gallbladder, and exocrine pancreas.

Food breakdown begins in the mouth with chewing and continues in the stomach, where food is churned and mixed with acid, mucus, enzymes, and other secretions. From the stomach the fluid and partially digested food pass into the small intestine, where biochemical agents and enzymes secreted by the liver and exocrine pancreas break it down into absorbable components of proteins, carbohydrates, and fats. These nutrients pass through the walls of the small intestine into blood vessels and lymphatics that carry them to the liver for storage or further processing.

Ingested substances and secretions that are not absorbed in the small intestine pass into the large intestine, where fluid continues to be absorbed. Fluid wastes travel to the kidneys and are eliminated in the urine. Solid wastes pass into the rectum and are eliminated from the body through the anus.

Except for chewing, swallowing, and defecation of solid wastes, the movements of the digestive system (gastrointestinal motility) are all controlled by hormones and the autonomic nervous system. The autonomic innervation, both sympathetic and parasympathetic, is controlled by centers in the brain and by local stimuli that are mediated at plexuses (networks of nerve fibers) within the gastrointestinal walls.

CHAPTER OUTLINE

THE GASTROINTESTINAL TRACT

The *alimentary canal*, or *gastrointestinal tract,* consists of the mouth, esophagus, stomach, small intestine, large intestine, rectum, and anus (Fig. 33-1). It carries out the following digestive processes:

1. Ingestion of food
2. Propulsion of food and wastes from the mouth to the anus
3. Secretion of mucus, water, and enzymes
4. Mechanical digestion of food particles
5. Chemical digestion of food particles
6. Absorption of digested food
7. Elimination of waste products by defecation

Histologically, the gastrointestinal tract consists of four layers. From the inside out they are the mucosa, submucosa, muscularis, and serosa or adventitia. These concentric layers vary in thickness, and each layer has sublayers (Fig. 33-2). Intrinsic nerves are located solely within the gastrointestinal tract and are controlled by local and autonomic nervous system stimuli through the *enteric plexus* and three nerve plexuses located in different layers of the gastrointestinal walls.

Mouth and Esophagus

The *mouth* is a reservoir for the chewing and mixing of food with saliva. As food particles become smaller and move around in the mouth, the taste buds and olfactory nerves are continuously stimulated, adding to the satisfaction of eating. The tongue's surface contains thousands of chemoreceptors, or taste buds, which can distinguish salty, sour, bitter, and sweet tastes. Tastes and food odors help to initiate salivation and the secretion of gastric juice in the stomach. There are 32 permanent teeth in the adult mouth, and they are important for speech and mastication.

Salivation

The three pairs of *salivary glands,* the submandibular, sublingual, and parotid glands (Fig. 33-3), secrete about 1 L of saliva per day. *Saliva* consists mostly of water with mucus, sodium, bicarbonate, chloride, potassium, and *salivary α-amylase (ptyalin),* an enzyme that initiates carbohydrate digestion in the mouth and stomach.

Both sympathetic and parasympathetic divisions of the autonomic nervous system control salivation. Cholinergic parasympathetic fibers stimulate the salivary glands, and atropine (an anticholinergic agent) inhibits salivation and

Fig. 33-1 *Structure and function of the digestive system.* Digestion begins in the mouth with chewing, which breaks down food mechanically and mixes it with saliva. Swallowing propels chewed food through the esophagus to the stomach, where acids and stomach motility liquefy it further. Next the liquefied food enters the small intestine, where secretions of the intestinal walls, liver, gallbladder, and pancreas digest it into absorbable nutrients. Nutrients are absorbed through intestinal walls, and unabsorbed wastes enter the large intestine (colon), where fluids are removed. Solid wastes then enter the rectum and leave the body through the anus. *(From Thompson, J.M. et al. [1997]. Mosby's clinical nursing [4th ed.]. St. Louis: Mosby.)*

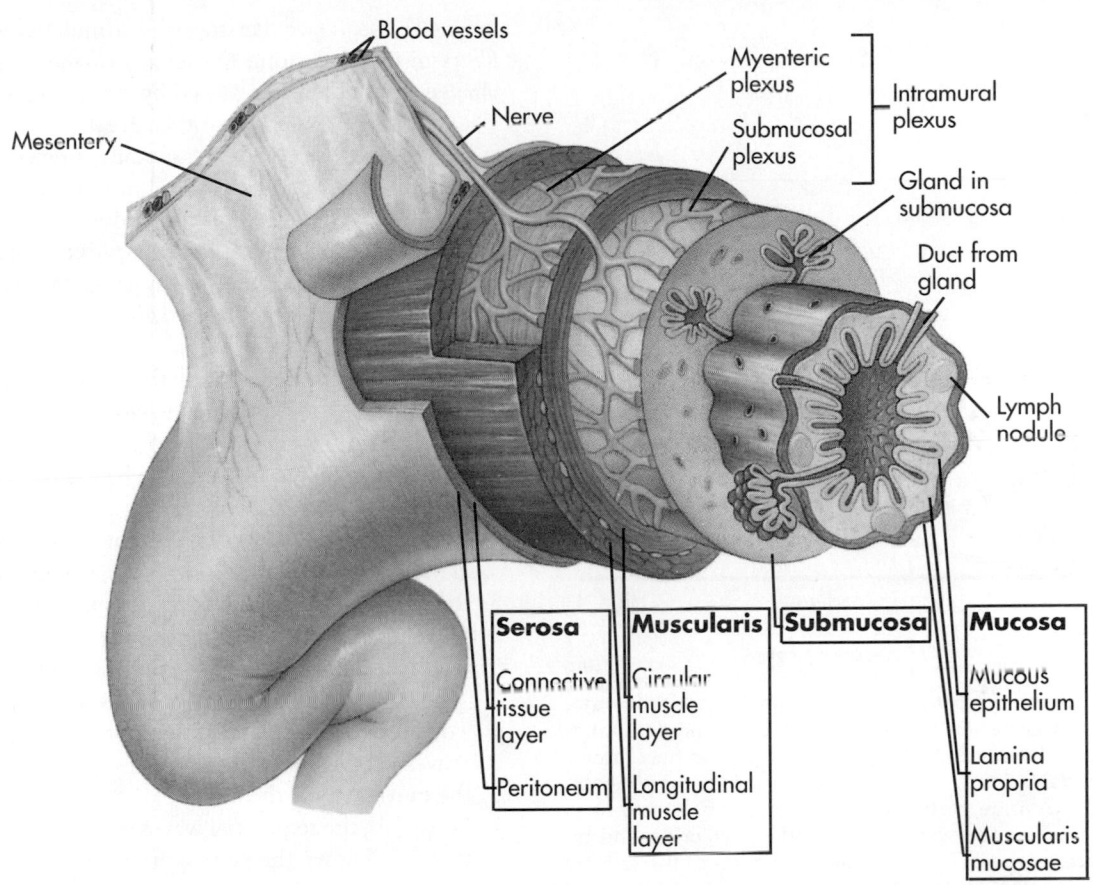

Fig. 33-2 *Wall of the gastrointestinal tract.* The wall of the gastrointestinal tract is made up of four layers with a network of nerves between the layers. Shown here is a generalized diagram of a segment of the gastrointestinal tract. Note that the serosa is continuous with a fold of serous membrane called a *mesentery*. Note also that digestive glands may empty their products into the lumen of the gastrointestinal tract by way of ducts. *(From Thibodeau, G.A. & Patton, K.T. [1999]. Anatomy & physiology [4th ed.]. St. Louis: Mosby.)*

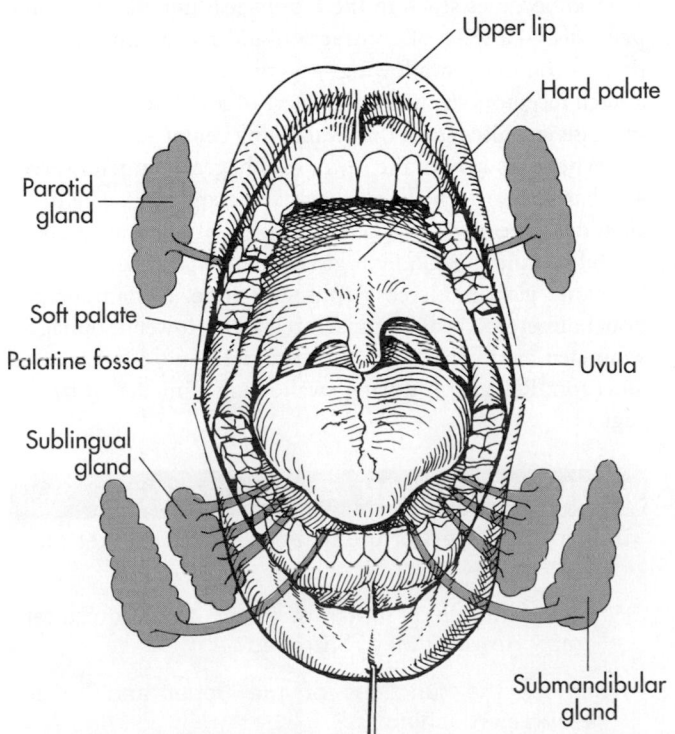

Fig. 33-3 *Structures of the mouth.* *(From Phipps, W.J. et al. [1999]. Medical-surgical nursing: Concepts and clinical practice [6th ed.]. St. Louis: Mosby.)*

Fig. 33-4 *Salivary electrolyte concentrations and flow rate.* Changes in concentration of sodium (Na^+), potassium (K^+), chloride (Cl^-), and bicarbonate (HCO_3^-) with increases in flow rate of saliva. *Black dotted line,* Sodium; *solid black line,* bicarbonate; *solid red line,* chloride; *dotted red line,* potassium. At low rates of salivary flow (i.e., between meals), sodium, chloride, and bicarbonate are reabsorbed in the collecting ducts of the salivary glands and the saliva contains fewer of these electrolytes (i.e., is more hypotonic). At higher flow rates (i.e., stimulated by food), reabsorption is decreased and saliva is hypertonic. By this mechanism, sodium, chloride, and bicarbonate are recycled until they are released to help with digestion and absorption.

makes the mouth dry. β-Adrenergic stimulation from sympathetic fibers also increases salivary secretion. The salivary glands are not regulated by hormones.

The composition of saliva depends on the rate of secretion (Fig. 33-4). Aldosterone can increase an exchange of sodium for potassium, increasing sodium conservation and potassium excretion. The bicarbonate concentration of saliva sustains a pH of about 7.4, which neutralizes bacterial acids and prevents tooth decay. Saliva also contains immunoglobulin A (IgA), which helps prevent infection. Exogenous fluoride (e.g., fluoride in drinking water) is also secreted in the saliva, providing additional protection against tooth decay.

Swallowing

The *esophagus* is a hollow, muscular tube approximately 25 cm long that conducts substances from the oropharynx to the stomach (see Fig. 33-1). Swallowed food is moved to the stomach by *peristalsis,* the sequential contraction and relaxation of outer longitudinal and inner circular layers of muscles. The upper third of the esophagus contains striated muscle (voluntary) that is directly innervated by motor neurons. The lower two thirds contains smooth muscle (involuntary) that is innervated by preganglionic cholinergic fibers from the vagus nerve. The fibers are activated in a

downward sequence. Peristalsis is stimulated when afferent fibers distributed along the length of the esophagus sense changes in wall tension caused by stretching as food passes. The greater the tension, the greater the intensity of esophageal contraction. Occasionally, intense contractions cause pain similar to "heartburn" or angina.

Each end of the esophagus is opened and closed by a sphincter. The *upper esophageal sphincter* keeps air from entering the esophagus during respiration. The *lower esophageal sphincter (cardiac sphincter)* prevents regurgitation from the stomach.

Swallowing is mediated by the swallowing center in the medulla. During the *oropharyngeal (voluntary) phase,* the following steps occur:
1. Food is segmented into a bolus by the tongue and forced posteriorly toward the pharynx.
2. The superior constrictor muscle of the pharynx contracts so the food cannot move into the nasopharynx.
3. Respiration is inhibited, and the epiglottis slides down to prevent the food from entering the larynx and trachea.
This entire sequence takes place in less than 1 second.

The *esophageal phase* proceeds as follows:
1. The bolus of food enters the esophagus.
2. Waves of relaxation travel the esophagus, preparing for the movement of the bolus.
3. Peristalsis, the sequential waves of muscular contractions that travel down the esophagus, transport the food to the lower esophageal sphincter, which is relaxed at that point.
4. The bolus enters the stomach, and the sphincter muscles return to their resting tone.
This phase takes 5 to 10 seconds, with the bolus moving 2 to 6 cm/sec.

Peristalsis that immediately follows the oropharyngeal phase of swallowing is called *primary peristalsis.* If a bolus of food becomes stuck in the esophageal lumen, *secondary peristalsis*—a wave of contraction and relaxation independent of voluntary swallowing—occurs. This is in response to stretch receptors stimulated by increased wall tension, which increase impulses from the swallowing center of the brain.

When it is closed, the lower esophageal sphincter serves as a barrier between the stomach and esophagus. The muscle tone of the lower sphincter changes with neural and hormonal stimulation. Cholinergic vagal input and the digestive hormone gastrin increase sphincter tone. Nonadrenergic, noncholinergic vagal impulses relax the lower esophageal sphincter, as do the hormones progesterone, secretin, and glucagon. Relaxation during swallowing is mediated by the vagus.[1]

✓ QUICK CHECK

Describe the layers of the walls of the gastrointestinal tract.

What are the major functions of the gastrointestinal tract? How are they controlled?

What are the functions of the upper and lower esophageal sphincters?

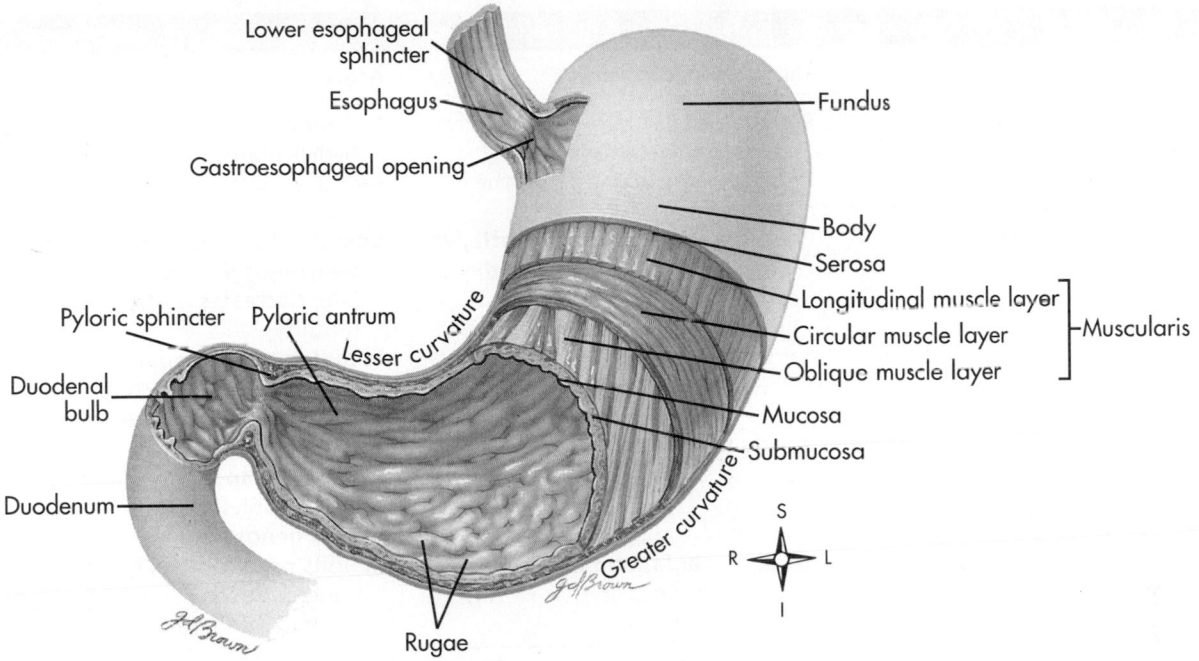

Fig 33-5 *Stomach.* A portion of the anterior wall has been cut away to reveal the muscle layers of the stomach wall. Note that the mucosa lining the stomach forms folds called *rugae. (From Thibodeau, G.A. & Patton, K.T. [1999]. Anatomy & physiology [4th ed.]. St. Louis: Mosby.)*

Stomach

The *stomach* is a hollow, muscular organ just below the diaphragm that stores food during eating, secretes digestive juices, mixes food with these juices, and propels partially digested food, called *chyme,* into the duodenum of the small intestine. The anatomy of the stomach is presented in Fig. 33-5. Its major anatomic boundaries are the lower esophageal sphincter, where food passes through the *cardiac orifice* into the stomach; the greater and lesser curvatures; and the *pyloric sphincter,* which relaxes as food is propelled through the *pylorus* into the duodenum. Functional areas are the *fundus* (upper portion), *body* (middle portion), and *antrum* (lower portion).

The tunica muscularis has a circular muscle layer and a longitudinal layer (see Fig. 33-5). The stomach wall also contains a layer of oblique muscle between the submucosa and the circular muscle layer. These layers become progressively thicker in the body and antrum. The glandular epithelium is discussed in the section about secretory functions of the stomach (see p. 922).

The stomach's blood supply is so abundant that nearly all arterial vessels must be occluded before ischemic changes occur in the stomach wall. The splenic vein drains the right side of the stomach, and the gastric vein drains the left side.

The stomach is innervated by sympathetic and parasympathetic divisions of the autonomic nervous system. Some of the autonomic fibers are extrinsic: that is, they originate outside the stomach and are controlled by nerve centers in the brain. Others are intrinsic: they originate within the stomach and also respond to local stimuli. Extrinsic sympathetic fibers reach the stomach through the celiac plexus (solar plexus), whereas extrinsic parasympathetic fibers enter through the gastric branch of the vagus nerve.

Gastric motility

In its resting state, the stomach is small and contains about 50 ml fluid. There is no wall tension, and the muscle layers in the fundus contract very little. Swallowing causes the fundus to relax (receptive relaxation) to receive a bolus of food from the esophagus. Relaxation is coordinated by efferent, nonadrenergic, noncholinergic vagal fibers and is facilitated by *gastrin* and *cholecystokinin*—two polypeptide hormones secreted by the gastrointestinal mucosa. (The actions of digestive hormones are summarized in Table 33-1.) Food is stored in vertical or oblique layers as it arrives in the fundus, whereas fluids flow relatively quickly down to the antrum.

Gastric (stomach) motility increases with the initiation of peristaltic waves, which sweep over the body of the stomach toward the antrum. The rate of peristaltic contractions is approximately three per minute and is influenced by neural and hormonal activity. Gastrin, *motilin* (an intestinal hormone), and the vagus nerve increase contraction by lowering the threshold potential of muscle fibers. (The neural and biochemical mechanisms of muscle contraction are described in Chapter 12.) Sympathetic activity and *secretin* (another intestinal hormone) are inhibitory and raise the threshold potential. The rate of peristalsis is mediated by pacemaker cells that initiate a wave of depolarization (basic electrical rhythm), which moves from the upper part of the stomach to the pylorus.

The mixing and emptying of food (chyme) from the stomach take several hours. Mixing occurs as food is pro-

TABLE 33-1	Selected Hormones and Neurotransmitters of the Digestive System		
Source	Hormone	Stimulus for Secretion	Action
Mucosa of the stomach	Gastrin	Presence of partially digested proteins in the stomach	Stimulates gastric glands to secrete hydrochloric acid and pepsinogen
Mucosa of the small intestine	Motilin	Presence of acid and fat in the duodenum	Increases gastrointestinal motility
	Secretin	Presence of chyme (acid, partially digested proteins, fats) in the duodenum	Stimulates pancreas to secrete alkaline pancreatic juice and liver to secrete bile; decreases gastrointestinal motility
	Cholecystokinin	Same as for secretin	Stimulates gallbladder to eject bile and pancreas to secrete alkaline fluid; decreases gastric motility
	Enteroglucagon	Intraluminal fats and carbohydrates	Weakly inhibits gastric and pancreatic secretion and enhances insulin release, lipolysis, ketogenesis, and glycogenolysis
	Peptide YY	Intraluminal fat and bile acids	Inhibits postpranidial gastric acid and pancreatic secretion and delays gastric and small bowel emptying

Modified from Thibodeau, G.A. & Patton K.T. (1999). Structure and function of the body (11th ed.). St. Louis: Mosby.
NOTE: *The digestive hormones are not secreted into the gastrointestinal lumen but rather into the bloodstream, in which they travel to target tissues.*

pelled toward the antrum. As food approaches the pylorus, the velocity of the peristaltic wave increases. This forces the contents back toward the body of the stomach. This **retropulsion** effectively mixes food with digestive juices, and the oscillating motion breaks down large food particles. With each peristaltic wave, a small portion of the gastric contents (chyme) passes through the pylorus and into the duodenum. The pylorus is about 1.5 cm long and is always open about 2.0 mm. It opens wider during antral contraction. Normally there is no regurgitation from the duodenum into the antrum.

The rate of **gastric emptying** (movement of gastric contents into the duodenum) depends on the volume, osmotic pressure, and chemical composition of the gastric contents. Larger volumes of food increase gastric pressure, peristalsis, and rate of emptying. Solids, fats, and nonisotonic solutions delay gastric emptying. (Osmotic pressure and tonicity are described in Chapters 1 and 4.) Products of fat digestion, which are formed in the duodenum by the action of bile from the liver and enzymes from the pancreas, stimulate the secretion of cholecystokinin. This hormone inhibits gastric motility and decreases gastric emptying so that fats are not emptied into the duodenum at a rate that exceeds the rate of bile and enzyme secretion. Osmoreceptors in the wall of the duodenum are sensitive to the osmotic pressure of duodenal contents. The arrival of hypertonic or hypotonic gastric contents activates the osmoreceptors, which delay gastric emptying to facilitate formation of an isosmotic duodenal environment. The rate at which acid enters the duodenum also influences gastric emptying. Secretions from the pancreas, liver, and duodenal mucosa neutralize gastric acid in the duodenum. The rate of emptying is adjusted to the duodenum's ability to neutralize the incoming acidity.[2]

Gastric secretion

Stimulated by eating, the stomach secretes large volumes of gastric juices or gastric secretions, including mucus, acid, enzymes, hormones, and intrinsic factor. (Intrinsic factor is necessary for the intestinal absorption of vitamin B_{12}.) The hormones are secreted into the blood and travel to target tissues in the bloodstream. The other gastric secretions are released directly into the stomach lumen.

In the fundus and body of the stomach, the **gastric glands** of the mucosa are the primary secretory units (Fig. 33-6). The composition of gastric juice depends on volume and flow rate (Fig. 33-7). Potassium remains relatively constant, but its concentration is greater in gastric juice than in plasma. The rate of secretion varies with the time of day. Generally the rate and volume of secretion are lowest in the morning and highest in the afternoon and evening. Loss of gastric juices through vomiting, drainage, or suction may decrease body stores of sodium and potassium.

Gastric secretion is inhibited by unpleasant odors and tastes and by rage, fear, or pain. A discharge of sympathetic impulses inhibits parasympathetic impulses. Increased secretions are associated with aggression or hostility and may contribute to some forms of gastric pathology.

Acid

The major functions of gastric acid are to dissolve food fibers, act as a bactericide against swallowed organisms, and convert pepsinogen to pepsin. The production of acid by the parietal cells requires the transport of hydrogen and chloride from the parietal cells to the stomach lumen. Acid is formed in the parietal cells, primarily through the hydrolysis of water (Fig. 33-8). At a high rate of gastric secretion, bicarbonate moves into the plasma, producing an "alkaline tide" in

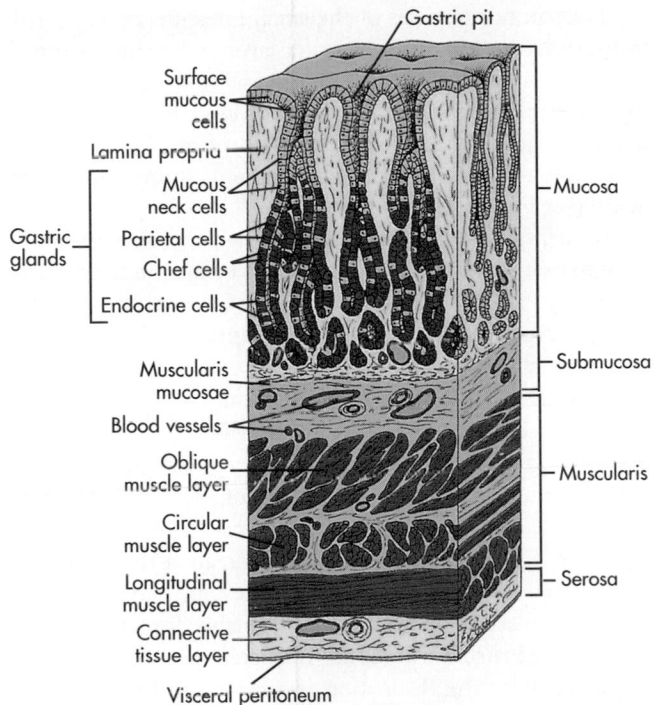

Fig. 33-6 *Gastric pits and gastric glands.* Gastric pits are depressions in the epithelial lining of the stomach. At the bottom of each pit is one or more tubular *gastric glands.* Chief cells produce the enzymes of gastric juice, such as pepsinogen, and parietal cells produce stomach acid. *(From Thibodeau, G.A. & Patton, K.T. [1999]. Anatomy & physiology [4th ed.]. St. Louis: Mosby.)*

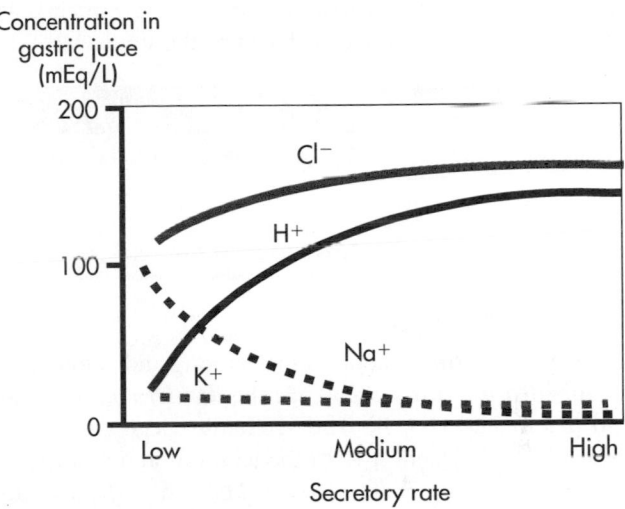

Fig. 33-7 *Relationship between secretory rate and electrolyte composition of the gastric juice.* Sodium (Na$^+$) concentration is lower in the gastric juice than in the plasma, whereas hydrogen (H$^+$), potassium (K$^+$), and chloride (Cl$^-$) concentrations are higher. *Solid red line,* Chloride; *solid black line,* hydrogen; *dotted black line,* sodium; *dotted red line,* potassium.

the venous blood, which also may result in a more alkaline urine.[3]

Acid secretion is stimulated by acetylcholine (a neurotransmitter), gastrin (a hormone), and histamine (a biochemical mediator) and is inhibited by somatostatin (a hormone). The vagus nerve releases acetylcholine and stimulates the secretion of gastrin, which stimulates release of histamine from enterochromaffin cells (mast cells; see Chapter 6) in the gastric mucosa. Prostaglandins and secretin inhibit the secretion of acid.[4]

Pepsin secretion

Acetylcholine, gastrin, and secretin stimulate the **chief cells** to release pepsinogen during eating. Pepsinogen is quickly converted to **pepsin** in the acid gastric environment (optimum pH for pepsin activation = 2.0). Pepsin is a proteolytic enzyme: that is, it breaks down protein and forms polypeptides in the stomach. Once chyme has entered the duodenum, the alkaline environment of the duodenum inactivates pepsin.

Mucus

The gastric mucosa is protected from the digestive actions of acid and pepsin by a coating of mucus called the **mucosal barrier.** The quality and quantity of mucus and the tight junctions between epithelial cells make gastric mucosa rela-

Fig. 33-8 *One mechanism for secretion of hydrochloric acid.* *(From Berne, R.M. & Levy, M.N. [Eds.]. [1996]. Principles of physiology [2nd ed.]. St. Louis: Mosby.)*

tively impermeable to acid. Prostaglandins protect the mucosal barrier by stimulating the secretion of mucus and bicarbonate and by inhibiting secretion of acid. A break in the protective barrier may occur because of exposure to *Helicobacter pylori*, aspirin, ethanol, regurgitated bile, or ischemia. Breaks cause inflammation and ulceration.

Phases of gastric secretion

The secretion of gastric juice is influenced by numerous stimuli that together facilitate the process of digestion. The phases of gastric secretion are the cephalic phase (stimulated by the thought, smell, and taste of food), the gastric phase (stimulated by distention of the stomach), and the intestinal phase (stimulated by histamine and digested protein). All phases promote the secretion of acid by the stomach.

✓ QUICK CHECK

Why are there three layers of stomach muscle?

What hormones are involved in gastric motility?

What are the phases of gastric secretion?

Small Intestine

The *small intestine* is about 5 meters long and is functionally divided into three segments: the *duodenum, jejunum,* and *ileum* (Fig. 33-9, *B*). The duodenum begins at the pylorus and ends where it joins the jejunum at a suspensory ligament called the *Treitz ligament*. The end of the jejunum and beginning of the ileum are not distinguished by an anatomic marker. These structures are not grossly different, but the jejunum has a slightly larger lumen. The *ileocecal valve,* or *sphincter,* controls the flow of digested material from the ileum into the large intestine and prevents reflux into the small intestine.[5]

The *peritoneum* is the serous membrane surrounding the organs of the abdomen and pelvic cavity. It is analogous to the pericardium and pleura, which surround the heart and lungs, respectively. The visceral peritoneum lies over the organs, and the parietal peritoneum lines the wall of the abdominal cavity. The space between these two layers is called the *peritoneal cavity* and normally contains just enough fluid to lubricate the two layers and prevent friction during organ movement.

The duodenum lies behind the peritoneum, or retroperitoneally, and is attached to the posterior abdominal wall. The ileum and jejunum are suspended in loose folds from the posterior abdominal wall by a peritoneal membrane called the *mesentery.* The mesentery facilitates intestinal motility and supports blood vessels, nerves, and lymphatics.

The arterial supply to the duodenum arises primarily from the gastroduodenal artery. The jejunum and ileum are supplied by branches of the superior mesenteric artery. The superior mesenteric vein joins the splenic vein and empties into the portal circulation to the liver. The regional lymph nodes and lymphatics drain into the thoracic duct. Both divisions of the autonomic nervous system innervate the small intestine. Secretion, motility, pain sensation, and intestinal reflexes (e.g., relaxation of the lower esophageal sphincter) are mediated by parasympathetic nerves. Sympathetic activity inhibits motility and produces vasoconstriction. Intrinsic motor innervation is mediated by the *myenteric plexus (Auerbach plexus)* and the *submucosal plexus (Meissner plexus).*

The smooth muscles of the small intestine are arranged in two layers: a longitudinal outer layer and a thicker inner circular layer (see Fig. 33-9, *A*). Mucosal folds (plica) within the small intestine slow the passage of food, thereby providing more time for digestion and absorption. The folds are most numerous and prominent in the jejunum and upper ileum (see Fig. 33-9, *B*).

Absorption occurs through *villi,* which cover the mucosal folds and are the functional units of the intestine. Each villus (see Fig. 33-9, *C*) secretes some of the enzymes necessary for digestion and absorbs nutrients. A villus is composed of absorptive columnar cells and mucus-secreting goblet cells of the mucosal epithelium. Near the surface, columnar cells closely adhere to each other at sites called *tight junctions.* Water and electrolytes are absorbed through these intercellular spaces. The surface of each columnar epithelial cell contains tiny projections called *microvilli* (see Fig. 33-9, *C*). Together the microvilli create a mucosal surface known as the *brush border.* The villi and microvilli greatly increase the surface area available for absorption. Coating the brush border is an "unstirred" layer of fluid that is important for the absorption of substances other than water and electrolytes. The *lamina propria* (a connective tissue layer of the mucous membrane) lies beneath the epithelial cells of the villi and contains lymphocytes; plasma cells, which produce immunoglobulins; and macrophages.

Central arterioles ascend within each villus and branch into a capillary array that extends around the base of the columnar cells and cascades down to the venules that lead to the portal circulation (see Fig. 33-9, *C*). A central *lacteal,* or lymphatic channel, is also contained within each villus and is important for the absorption and transport of fat molecules. Contents of the lacteals flow to regional nodes and channels that eventually drain into the thoracic duct.[6]

Between the bases of the villi are the crypts of Lieberkühn, which extend to the submucosal layer. Undifferentiated and secretory cells are located here. The undifferentiated cells arise from the base of the crypt and move toward the tip of the villus, maturing in shape and function as they progress. After becoming columnar cells and completing their migration to the tip of the villus, they function for a few days and then are sloughed into the intestinal lumen and digested. Sloughed epithelial cells are an important source of endogenous protein. The entire epithelial population is replaced about every 4 to 7 days. Many factors can influence this process of cellular proliferation. Starvation, vitamin B_{12} deficiency, and cytotoxic drugs or irradiation suppress cell division and shorten the villi. The decreased absorption that results can cause diarrhea and malnutrition. Nutrient intake and intestinal resection stimulate cell production.

Intestinal digestion and absorption

The process of digestion is initiated in the stomach by the actions of hydrochloric acid and pepsin. The chyme that passes into the duodenum is a liquid with small particles of undigested food. Digestion continues in the proximal portion of the small intestine by the action of pancreatic enzymes, in-

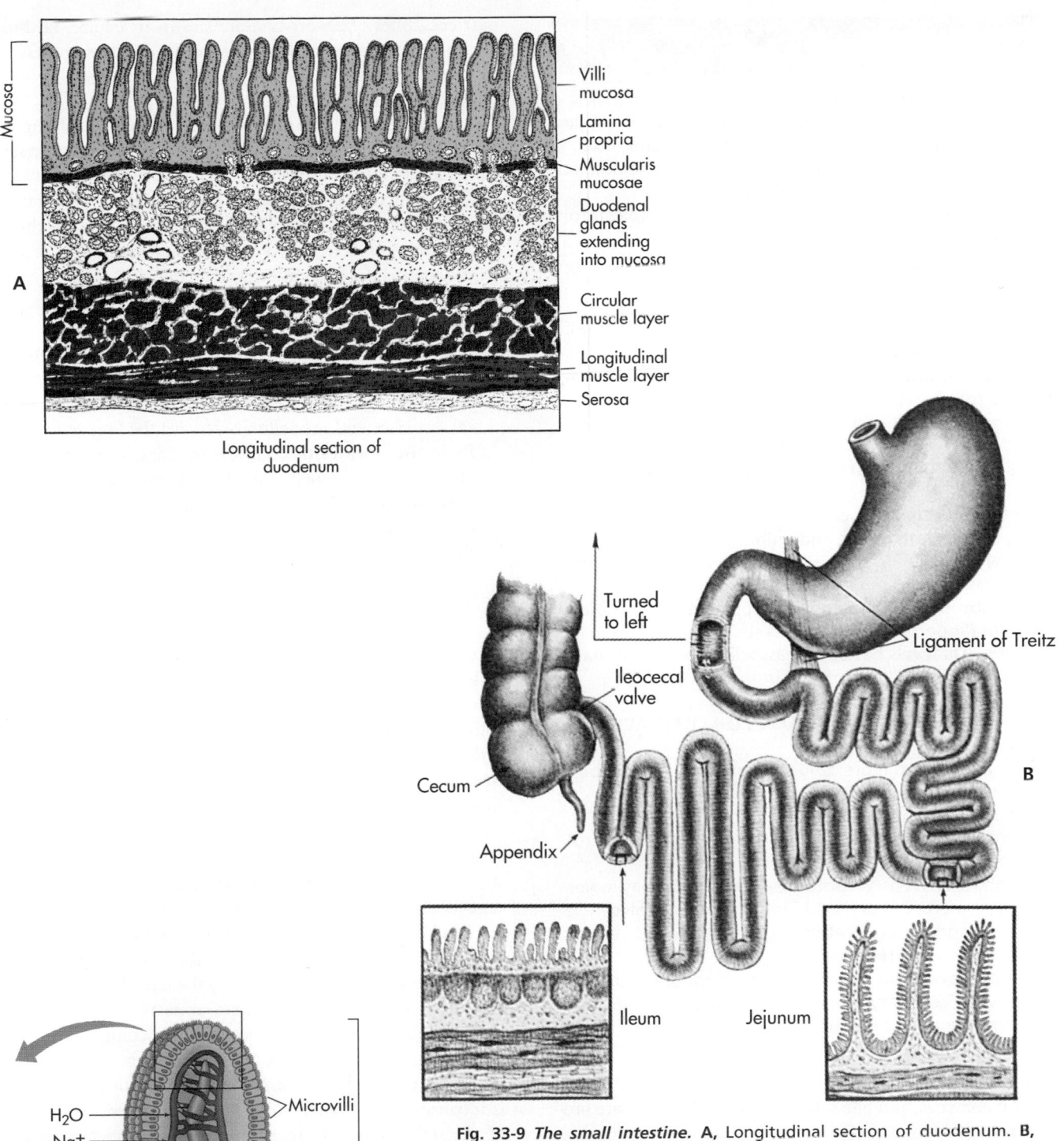

Mucosa

Villi
mucosa

Lamina
propria

Muscularis
mucosae

Duodenal
glands
extending
into mucosa

Circular
muscle layer

Longitudinal
muscle layer

Serosa

A

Longitudinal section of
duodenum

Turned
to left

Ligament of Treitz

Ileocecal
valve

Cecum

B

Appendix

Ileum   Jejunum

H_2O
Na^+
Glucose
Amino acid
Fat

Microvilli

Intestinal
villus

Epithelial
cell

Lymph
lacteal

C

Artery
Lymph duct
Vein

Muscularis mucosae

Fig. 33-9 *The small intestine.* **A**, Longitudinal section of duodenum. **B**, Duodenum, jejunum, ileum. **C**, Single villus showing lacteal, capillary, and microvilli. *(A and B from Thompson, J.M. et al. [1997]. Mosby's clinical nursing [4th ed.]. St. Louis: Mosby; C from Thibodeau, G.A. & Patton, K.T. [1999]. Anatomy & physiology [4th ed.]. St. Louis: Mosby.)*

Dietary Fat

BOX 33-1

SATURATED FATTY ACID (PALMITIC ACID [$C_{16}H_{32}O_2$])
Each carbon atom in the chain is linked by single bonds to adjacent carbon and hydrogen atoms:
1. Fats are solid at room temperature; comprise animal fat and tropical oils (coconut and palm oil).
2. Increase low-density lipoprotein (LDL) cholesterol ("bad" cholesterol) blood levels.
3. Increase the risk of coronary artery disease.

UNSATURATED FATTY ACID
Unsaturated fatty acids are soft or liquid at room temperature:
1. Omega-6 fatty acids are found in plants and vegetables (olive, canola, and peanut oils).
2. Omega-3 fatty acids are found in fish and shellfish.

MONOUNSATURATED FATTY ACIDS (OLEIC ACID [$C_{18}H_{34}O_2$])
Contain one double bond in the carbon chain:
1. Found in both plants and animals.
2. May be beneficial in reducing blood cholesterol, glucose levels, and systolic blood pressure.
3. Do not lower high-density lipoprotein (HDL) cholesterol ("good" cholesterol) level.
4. Low HDL levels have been associated with coronary heart disease.

POLYUNSATURATED FATTY ACIDS (LINOLEIC ACID [$C_{18}H_{32}O_2$])
Contain two or more double bonds in the carbon chain:
1. Found in plants and fish oils.
2. Omega-6 fatty acids lower total and LDL cholesterol blood levels.
3. High levels of polyunsaturated fatty acids may lower LDL; omega-3 fatty acids lower blood triglyceride levels and reduce platelet aggregation and reduce blood clotting tendency.
4. Are necessary for growth and development and may prevent coronary artery disease, hypertension, inflammatory and immune disorders.

---

testinal enzymes, and bile salts. Here carbohydrates are broken down to monosaccharides and disaccharides; proteins are degraded further to amino acids and peptides; and fats are emulsified and reduced to fatty acids (Box 33-1) and monoglycerides (Fig. 33-10). These nutrients, along with water, vitamins, and electrolytes, are absorbed across the intestinal mucosa by active transport, diffusion, or facilitated diffusion. Products of carbohydrate and protein breakdown move into villus capillaries and then to the liver through the portal vein. Digested fats move into the lacteals and eventually reach the liver through the systemic circulation. Intestinal motility exposes nutrients to a large mucosal surface area by mixing chyme and moving it through the lumen. Different segments of the gastrointestinal tract absorb different nutrients. Sites of absorption are shown in Fig. 33-11. Box 33-2 outlines the major nutrients involved in this process.

Intestinal motility

The movements of the small intestine facilitate both digestion and absorption. Chyme coming from the stomach stimulates intestinal movements that mix in secretions from the liver, pancreas, and intestinal glands. A churning motion brings the luminal contents into contact with the absorbing cells of the villi. Propulsive movements then advance the chyme toward the large intestine.

Intestinal motility is affected by the following two movements:

1. *Haustral segmentation*—localized rhythmic contractions of circular smooth muscles that divide and mix the chyme, bringing it into contact with the absorbent mucosal surface and propelling it toward the large intestine.
2. *Peristalsis*—waves of contraction along short segments of longitudinal smooth muscle that allow time for digestion and absorption. The intestinal villi move with contractions of the muscularis mucosae, a thin layer of muscle separating the mucosa and submucosa, with absorption promoted by the swaying of the villi in the luminal contents.

Neural reflexes along the length of the small intestine facilitate motility, digestion, and absorption. The *ileogastric reflex* inhibits gastric motility when the ileum becomes distended. This prevents the continued movement of chyme into an already distended intestine. The *intestinointestinal reflex* inhibits intestinal motility when one part of the intestine is overdistended. Both of these reflexes require extrinsic innervation. The *gastroileal reflex,* which is activated by an increase in gastric motility and secretion, stimulates an increase in ileal motility. This empties the ileum and prepares it to receive more chyme. The gastroileal reflex is probably regulated by the hormone gastrin.

During prolonged fasting or between meals, particularly overnight, slow waves sweep along the entire length of the intestinal tract from the stomach to the terminal ileum. This interdigestive myoelectric complex appears to propel residual gastric and intestinal contents into the colon.

The ileocecal valve (sphincter) marks the junction between the terminal ileum and the large intestine. This valve is intrinsically regulated and is normally closed. The arrival of peristaltic waves from the last few centimeters of the ileum causes the ileocecal valve to open, allowing a small amount of chyme to pass through. Distention of the upper large intestine causes the sphincter to constrict, preventing further distention or retrograde flow of intestinal contents.

✓ QUICK CHECK
What cells arise from the crypts of Lieberkühn?

How are fats absorbed from the small intestine?

Which reflexes inhibit intestinal motility? Which promote it?

Action	Foodstuff	Enzymes/source	Site of action

Fig. 33-10 *Digestion and absorption of foodstuffs.*

Major Nutrients Absorbed in the Intestine   BOX 33-2

WATER AND ELECTROLYTES

Approximately 85% to 90% of the water that enters the gastrointestinal tract is absorbed in the small intestine.

Sodium passes through tight junctions and is actively transported across cell membranes; it is exchanged for bicarbonate to maintain electroneutrality in the ileum; sodium absorption is enhanced by glucose transport.

Potassium moves passively across tight junctions with changes in the electrochemical gradient.

CARBOHYDRATES

Only monosaccharides are absorbed by intestinal mucosa, so complex carbohydrates must be hydrolyzed to simplest form.

Salivary and pancreatic amylases break down starches to oligosaccharides (sucrose, maltose, lactose) in stomach and duodenum; brush-border enzymes hydrolyze them in intestine so they can pass through unstirred layer by diffusion.

Fructose diffuses into the blood stream; glucose and galactose diffuse or are actively transported.

Cellulose remains undigested and stimulates large intestine motility.

PROTEINS

90% to 95% of protein is absorbed; major hydrolysis is accomplished in small intestine by pancreatic enzymes trypsin, chymotrypsin, and carboxypeptidase.

Brush-border enzymes break down into smaller peptides that can cross cell membranes, when cytosol breaks them down into amino acids, specifically, neutral amino acids, basic amino acids, and proline and hydroxyproline.

FATS

Digestion and absorption occur in four phases:

1 Emulsification and lipolysis—agents cover small fat particles and prevent them from reforming into fat droplets; then lipolysis breaks them into diglycerides, monoglycerides, free fatty acids, and glycerol.

2 Micelle formation—products are made water soluble.

3 Fat absorption—move from micelle to absorbing surface of intestinal epithelium and diffuse through resynthesis.

4 Triglycerides and phospholipids—become chylomicrons that eventually enter the systemic circulation.

MINERALS

Calcium—absorbed by passive diffusion and transported actively across cell membranes bound to a carrier protein; absorption primarily in ileum.

Magnesium—50% absorbed by active transport or passive diffusion in jejunum and ileum.

Phosphate—absorbed by passive diffusion and active transport in small intestine.

Iron—absorbed by epithelial cells of duodenum and jejunum; vitamin C facilitates.

VITAMINS

Mainly absorbed by sodium-dependent active transport, with vitamin B_{12} bound to intrinsic factor and absorbed in terminal ileum.

Large Intestine

The *large intestine* is approximately 1.5 meters long and consists of the cecum, appendix, colon (ascending, transverse, descending, and sigmoid), rectum, and anal canal (Fig. 33-12). The *cecum* is a pouch that receives chyme from the ileum. Attached to it is the *vermiform appendix,* an appendage having little or no physiologic function. From the cecum, chyme enters the *colon,* which loops upward, traverses the abdominal cavity, and descends to the anal canal. The four parts of the colon are the *ascending colon, transverse colon, descending colon,* and *sigmoid colon.* Two sphincters control the flow of intestinal contents through the cecum and colon: the ileocecal valve, which admits chyme from the ileum to the cecum, and the *O'Beirne sphincter,* which controls the movement of wastes from the sigmoid colon into the rectum. A thick (2.5 to 3 cm) portion of smooth muscle surrounds the anal canal, forming the *internal anal sphincter.* Overlapping it distally is the striated muscle of the *external anal sphincter.*

In the cecum and colon, the longitudinal muscle layer consists of three longitudinal bands called *teniae coli* (see Fig. 33-12). They are shorter than the colon and give it a "gathered" appearance. The circular muscles of the colon separate the gathers into outpouchings called *haustra.* The haustra become more or less prominent with the contractions and relaxations of the circular muscles. The mucosal surface of the colon has rugae (folds), particularly between the haustra, and *Lieberkühn crypts* but no villi. Columnar epithelial cells and mucus-secreting goblet cells form the mucosa throughout the large intestine. The columnar epithelium absorbs fluid and electrolytes, and the mucus-secreting cells lubricate the mucosa.

The myenteric plexus regulates motor and secretory activity independently of the extrinsic system. Extrinsic parasympathetic innervation occurs through the vagus and extends from the cecum up to the first part of the transverse colon. Vagal stimulation increases rhythmic contraction of the proximal colon. Extrinsic parasympathetic fibers reach the distal colon through the pelvic nerves and can increase motility throughout the colon. The internal anal sphincter is usually contracted, and its reflex response is to relax when the rectum is distended. The intrinsic nerve plexuses innervate the internal anal sphincter, which also receives sympathetic innervation to maintain contraction and parasympa-

HEALTH ALERT

Colon Cancer Risk Reduced With High-Fiber Diet

The risk for colon cancer is reduced with long-term use of a diet high in fiber. The mechanism of fiber protection is related to decreased stool transit times with decreased exposure to mutagens and a natural tumor suppressor effect of butyrate, a fermentation product of fiber.

Data from Archer, S.Y. et al. (1998). p21 (WAF1) is required for butyrate-mediated growth inhibition of human colon cancer cells. Proceedings of the National Academy of Sciences of the United States of America, 95(12), 6791-6796; Smith, J.G., Yokoyama, W.H., & German, J.B. (1998). Butyric acid from the diet: Actions at the level of gene expression. Critical Reviews in Food Science and Nutrition, 38(4), 259-297.

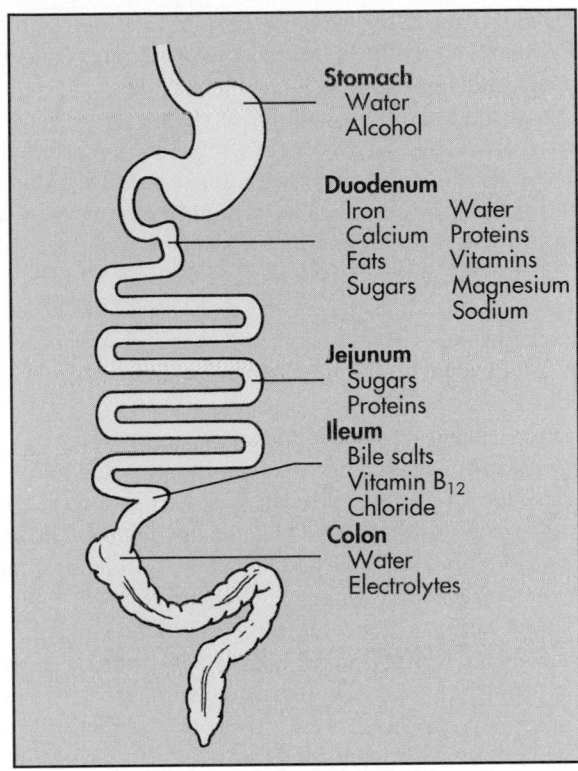

Fig. 33-11 *Sites of absorption of major nutrients.*

thetic innervation that facilitates relaxation when the rectum is full. The external anal sphincter is innervated by branches of the sacral division of the spinal cord. Sympathetic activity in the entire large intestine modulates intestinal reflexes, conveys somatic sensations of fullness and pain, participates in the defecation reflex, and constricts blood vessels. The blood supply of the large intestine and rectum is derived primarily from branches of the superior and inferior mesenteric arteries.[7]

The primary colonic movement is segmental. The circular muscles contract and relax at different sites, shuttling the intestinal contents back and forth between the haustra, most commonly during fasting. The movements massage the intestinal contents, now called **fecal mass,** and facilitate the absorption of water. Propulsive movement occurs with the proximal-to-distal contraction of several haustral units. Peristaltic movements also occur and promote the emptying of the colon. The **gastrocolic reflex** initiates propulsion in the entire colon, usually during or immediately after eating, when chyme enters from the ileum. The gastrocolic reflex

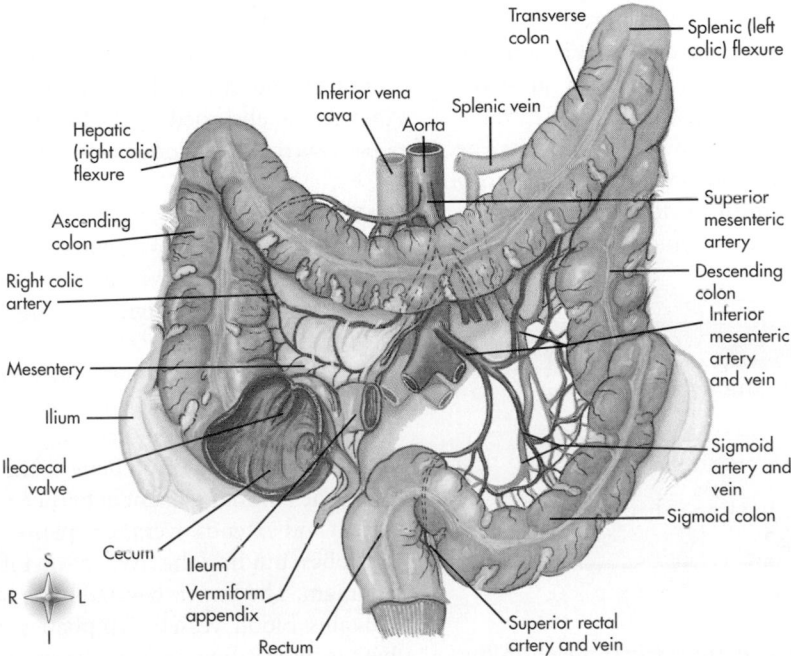

Fig. 33-12 *Division of the large intestine.* (From Thibodeau, G.A. & Patton, K.T. [1999]. Anatomy & physiology [4th ed.]. St. Louis: Mosby.)

causes the fecal mass to pass rapidly into the sigmoid colon and rectum, stimulating defecation. Gastrin may participate in stimulating this reflex.

Approximately 500 to 700 ml of chyme flows from the ileum to the cecum per day. Most of the water is absorbed in the colon by diffusion and active transport. Aldosterone increases membrane permeability to sodium, thereby increasing both the diffusion of sodium into the cell and its active transport to the interstitial fluid. (See Chapter 17 for a discussion of aldosterone secretion.) Sugars and amino acids are not absorbed by the colon, but some short-chain free fatty acids, which are produced by fermentation, are absorbed.

Absorption and epithelial transport occur in the cecum, ascending colon, transverse colon, and descending colon. By the time the fecal mass enters the sigmoid colon, the mass consists entirely of wastes and is called the *feces,* consisting of food residue, unabsorbed gastrointestinal secretions, shed epithelial cells, and bacteria.

The movement of feces into the sigmoid colon and **rectum** stimulates the **defecation reflex (rectal reflex).** The rectal wall stretches, and the tonically constricted internal anal sphincter (smooth muscle with autonomic nervous system control) relaxes, creating the urge to defecate. The defecation reflex can be overridden voluntarily by contraction of the external anal sphincter and muscles of the pelvic floor. The rectal wall gradually relaxes, reducing tension, and the urge to defecate passes. Retrograde contraction of the rectum may displace the feces out of the rectal vault until a more convenient time for evacuation. Pain or fear of pain associated with defecation (e.g., rectal fissures or hemorrhoids) can inhibit the defecation reflex.

Defecation is facilitated by squatting or sitting because these positions straighten the angle between the rectum and anal canal and increase the efficiency of straining (increasing intraabdominal pressure). Intraabdominal pressure is increased by initiating the Valsalva maneuver, that is, inhaling and forcing the diaphragm and chest muscles against the closed glottis, to increase both intrathoracic and intraabdominal pressure, which is transmitted to the rectum. (The Valsalva maneuver is lost in individuals who have undergone radical neck dissection. This group of individuals may need to alter dietary habits and rely on chemical agents to aid in defecation.)

> ### ✓ QUICK CHECK
>
> What are the two veins of the liver, and what blood flows into them?
>
> What are haustra?
>
> What two functions does the large intestine play in relation to the fecal mass?

Intestinal Bacteria

The number of bacteria increases from the stomach to the distal colon. The stomach is relatively sterile because of the secretion of acid that kills ingested pathogens or inhibits bacterial growth. Bile acid secretion, intestinal motility, and antibody production suppress bacterial growth in the duodenum, and in the duodenum and jejunum there is a low concentration of aerobes (10^{-1} to 10^{-4}/ml), primarily streptococci, lactobacilli, staphylococci, and enterobacteria. Anaerobes are found distal to the ileocecal valve but not proximal to the ileum. They constitute about 95% of the fecal flora in the colon and contribute one third of the solid bulk of feces. *Bacteroides,* clostridia, anaerobic lactobacilli, and coliforms are the most common microorganisms from the ileum to the cecum.

The intestinal tract is sterile at birth but becomes colonized with *Escherichia coli, Clostridium welchii,* and *Streptococcus* within a few hours. Within 3 to 4 weeks after birth, the normal flora is established. The intestinal bacteria do not have major digestive or absorptive functions but do play a role in metabolism of bile salts, estrogens, androgens, lipids, carbohydrates, and various nitrogenous substances and drugs.

Endogenous infections of the gastrointestinal tract occur by three major mechanisms: proliferation or overgrowth of bacteria, perforation of the intestine, and contamination of neighboring structures.

ACCESSORY ORGANS OF DIGESTION

The liver, gallbladder, and exocrine pancreas all secrete substances necessary for the digestion of chyme. These secretions are delivered to the duodenum through ducts (Fig. 33-13). The liver produces bile, which contains salts necessary for fat digestion and absorption. Between meals, bile is stored in the gallbladder. The exocrine pancreas produces (1) enzymes needed for the complete digestion of carbohydrates, proteins, and fats and (2) an alkaline fluid that neutralizes chyme, creating a duodenal pH that supports enzymatic action.

The liver also receives nutrients absorbed by the small intestine and metabolizes or synthesizes them into forms that can be absorbed by the body's cells. It then releases the nutrients into the bloodstream or stores them for later use.

Liver

The **liver** weighs 1200 to 1600 g. It is located under the right diaphragm and is divided into right and left lobes. The larger, right lobe is divided further into the caudate and quadrate lobes (Fig. 33-14). The falciform ligament separates the right and left lobes and attaches the liver to the anterior abdominal wall. The round ligament (ligamentum teres) extends along the free edge of the falciform ligament, extending from the umbilicus to the inferior surface of the liver. The coronary ligament branches from the falciform ligament and extends over the superior surface of the right and left lobes, binding the liver to the inferior surface of the diaphragm. The liver is covered by the **Glisson capsule,** which contains blood vessels, lymphatics, and nerves. When the liver is diseased or swollen, distention of the capsule causes pain and the lymphatics may ooze fluid into the peritoneal space.

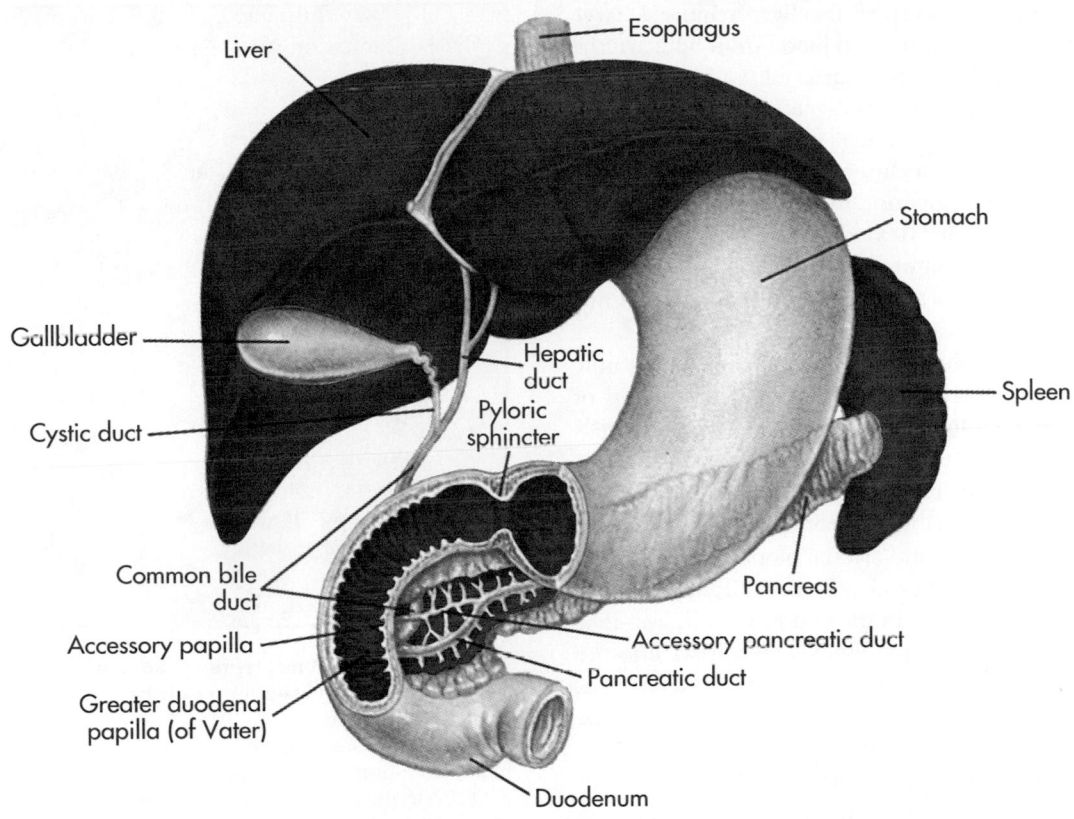

Fig. 33-13 *Location of the liver, gallbladder, and exocrine pancreas, which are the accessory organs of digestion.* *(From Thompson, J.M. et al. [1997].* Mosby's clinical nursing *[4th ed.]. St. Louis: Mosby.)*

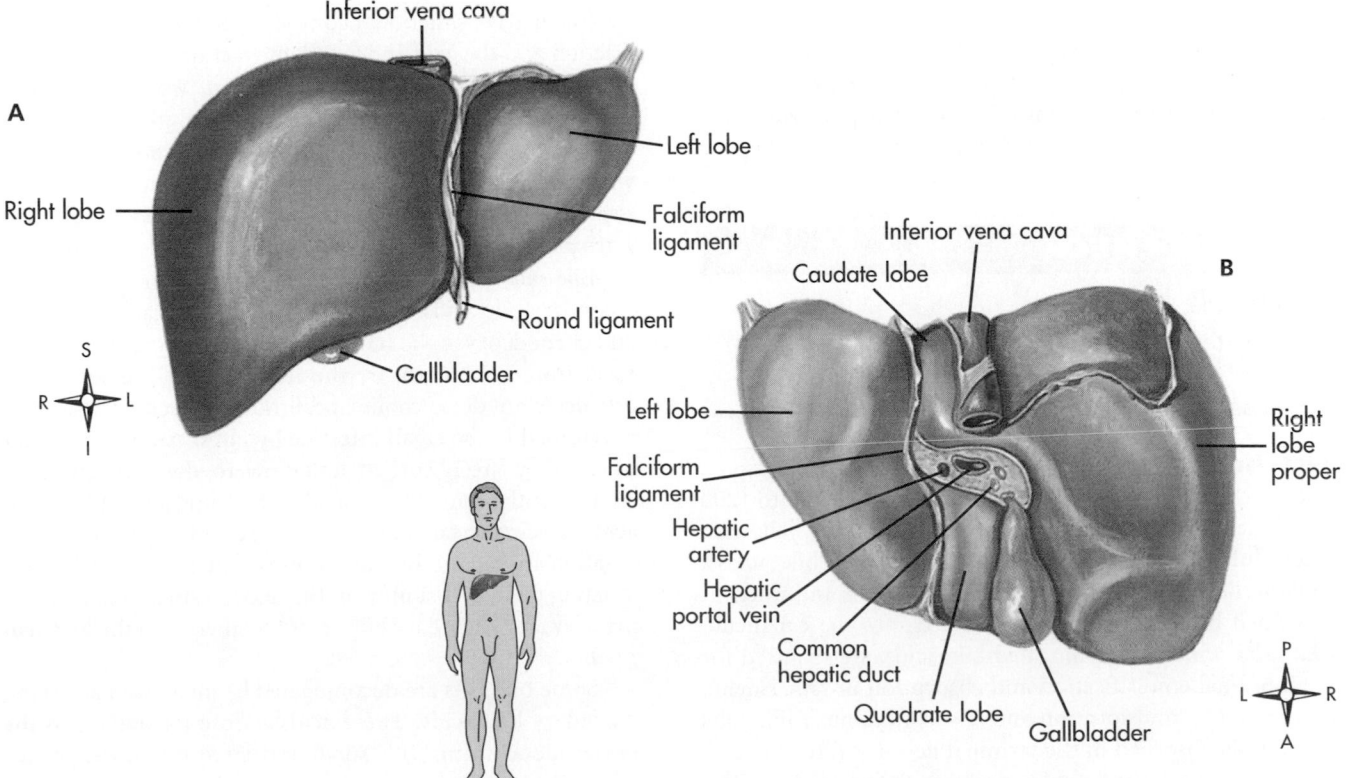

FIG. 33-14 *Gross structure of the liver.* A, Anterior view. **B,** Inferior view. *(From Thibodeau, G.A. & Patton, K.T. [1999].* Anatomy & physiology *[4th ed.]. St. Louis: Mosby.)*

The metabolic functions of the liver require a large amount of blood. The liver receives blood from both arterial and venous sources. The hepatic artery branches from the abdominal aorta and provides oxygenated blood at the rate of 400 to 500 ml/min (about 25% of the cardiac output). The hepatic portal vein, which receives deoxygenated blood from the inferior and superior mesenteric veins and the splenic vein, delivers about 1000 to 1200 ml/min to the liver. Portal venous blood constitutes 70% of the blood supply to the liver. This blood carries some oxygen and is rich in nutrients that have been absorbed from the digestive tract.

Within the liver lobes are multiple, smaller anatomic units called **liver lobules** (Fig. 33-15). They are formed of cords or plates of **hepatocytes,** which are the functional cells of the liver. These cells can regenerate; therefore damaged or resected liver tissue can regrow. Small capillaries, or **sinusoids,** are located between the plates of hepatocytes. They receive a mixture of venous and arterial blood from branches of the hepatic artery and portal vein. Blood from the sinusoids drains to a central vein in the middle of each liver lobule. Venous blood from all the lobules then flows into the hepatic vein, which empties into the inferior vena cava. Small channels (**bile canaliculi**) conduct bile, which is produced by the hepatocytes, outward to bile ducts and eventually drain into the **common bile duct** (see Fig. 33-15). This duct empties bile into the duodenum through an opening called the **major duodenal papilla** (sphincter of Oddi).

The sinusoids of the liver lobules are lined with highly permeable endothelium. This permeability enhances the transport of nutrients from the sinusoids into the hepatocytes, where they are metabolized. The sinusoids are also lined with phagocytic **Kupffer cells,** which are part of the mononuclear phagocyte system. They remove foreign substances from the blood and trap bacteria. Between the endothelial lining of the sinusoid and the hepatocyte is the **Disse space,** which drains interstitial fluid into the hepatic lymph system.

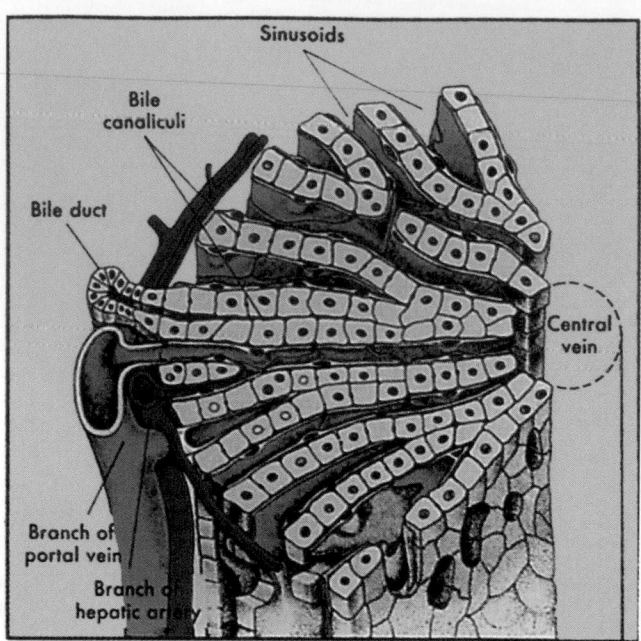

Fig. 33-15 *Diagrammatic representation of a liver lobule.* A central vein is located in the center of the lobule with plates of hepatic cells disposed radially. Branches of the portal vein and hepatic artery are located on the periphery of the lobule, and blood from both perfuses the sinusoids. Peripherally located bile ducts drain the bile canaliculi that run between the hepatocytes. *(From Berne, R.M. & Levy, M.N. [Eds.]. [1996]. Principles of physiology [3rd ed.]. St. Louis: Mosby.)*

✓ QUICK CHECK

Describe the liver.

What is the function of hepatocytes?

What are sinusoids?

Secretion of bile

The liver assists intestinal digestion by secreting 700 to 1200 ml of bile per day. **Bile** is an alkaline, bitter-tasting, yellowish green fluid that contains bile salts (conjugated bile acids), cholesterol, bilirubin (a pigment), electrolytes, and water. It is formed by hepatocytes and secreted into the canaliculi. **Bile salts,** which are conjugated bile acids, are required for the intestinal emulsification and absorption of fats. Having facilitated fat emulsification and absorption, most bile salts are actively absorbed in the terminal ileum and returned to the liver through the portal circulation for resecretion. The recycling of bile salts is termed the **enterohepatic circulation** (Fig. 33-16).

Bile has two fractional components: the acid-dependent fraction and the acid-independent fraction. Hepatocytes secrete the **bile acid–dependent fraction,** which consists of bile acids, cholesterol, lecithin (a phospholipid), and bilirubin (a bile pigment). The **bile acid–independent fraction,** which is secreted by the hepatocytes and epithelial cells of the bile canaliculi, is a bicarbonate-rich aqueous fluid that gives bile its alkaline pH.

Bile salts are conjugated in the liver from primary and secondary bile acids. The **primary bile acids** are cholic acid and chenodeoxycholic (chenic) acid. These acids are synthesized from cholesterol by the hepatocytes. The **secondary bile acids** are deoxycholic and lithocholic acid. These acids are formed in the small intestine by intestinal bacteria, after which they are absorbed and flow to the liver (see Fig. 33-16). Both forms of bile acids are conjugated with amino acids (glycine or taurine) in the liver to form bile salts. Conjugation makes the bile acids more water soluble, thus restricting their diffusion from the duodenum and ileum. The primary and secondary bile acids together form the **bile acid pool.**

Some bile salts are deconjugated by intestinal bacteria to secondary bile acids. These acids diffuse passively into the portal blood from both small and large intestines. An increase in the plasma concentration of bile acids accelerates the uptake and resecretion of bile acids and salts by the hepatocytes. The cycle of hepatic secretion, intestinal absorp-

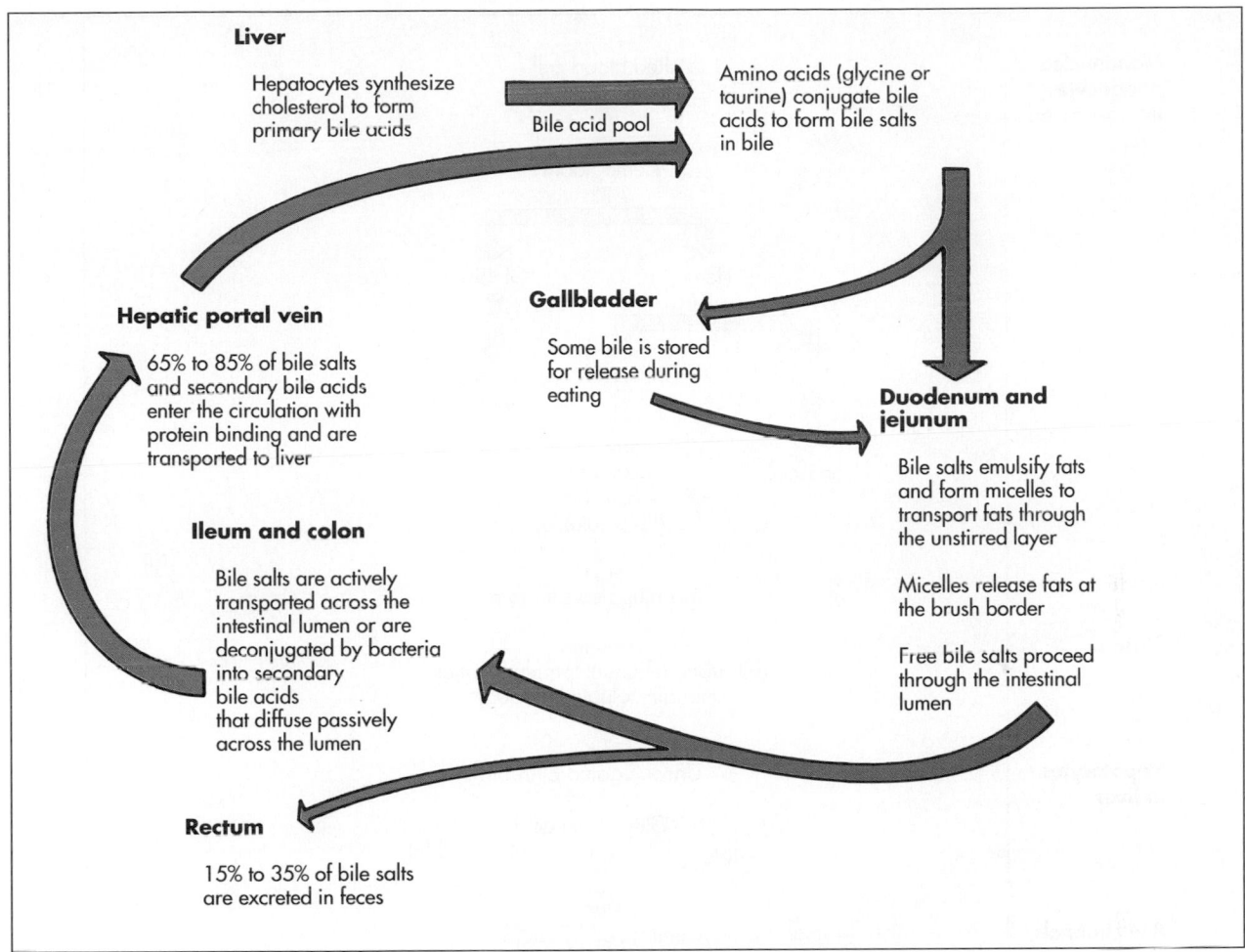

Liver

Hepatocytes synthesize cholesterol to form primary bile acids

Bile acid pool

Amino acids (glycine or taurine) conjugate bile acids to form bile salts in bile

Hepatic portal vein

65% to 85% of bile salts and secondary bile acids enter the circulation with protein binding and are transported to liver

Gallbladder

Some bile is stored for release during eating

Duodenum and jejunum

Bile salts emulsify fats and form micelles to transport fats through the unstirred layer

Micelles release fats at the brush border

Free bile salts proceed through the intestinal lumen

Ileum and colon

Bile salts are actively transported across the intestinal lumen or are deconjugated by bacteria into secondary bile acids that diffuse passively across the lumen

Rectum

15% to 35% of bile salts are excreted in feces

Fig. 33-16 *The enterohepatic circulation of bile salts.*

tion, and hepatic resecretion of bile acids completes the enterohepatic circulation.

Bile secretion is called ***choleresis.*** A ***choleretic agent*** stimulates the liver to secrete bile. One strong stimulus is a high concentration of bile salts. Other choleretics include secretin, which increases the rate of bile flow by promoting the secretion of bicarbonate from canaliculi and other intrahepatic bile ducts; cholecystokinin; and vagal stimulation.

Metabolism of bilirubin

Bilirubin is a by-product of the destruction of aged red blood cells. It gives bile a greenish black color and produces the yellow tinge of jaundice. Aged red blood cells are taken up and destroyed by macrophages of the mononuclear phagocyte system (also called the *reticuloendothelial system*), primarily in the spleen and liver. (In the liver these macrophages are Kupffer cells.) Within these cells hemoglobin is separated into its component parts, heme and globin (Fig. 33-17). The globin component is further degraded into its constituent amino acids, which are recycled to form new protein. The heme moiety is converted to biliverdin by the enzymatic cleavage of iron. The iron attaches to transferrin in the plasma and can be stored in the liver or used by the bone marrow to make new red blood cells. The biliverdin is enzy-

matically converted to bilirubin in the macrophage of the mononuclear phagocytic system and then is released into the plasma, where it binds to albumin and is known as ***unconjugated bilirubin,*** or free bilirubin, which is lipid soluble.

In the liver, unconjugated bilirubin moves from plasma in the sinusoids into the hepatocyte. Within hepatocytes it joins with glucuronic acid to form ***conjugated bilirubin.*** When conjugated bilirubin reaches the distal ileum and colon, it is deconjugated by bacteria and converted to ***urobilinogen.*** Most of the urobilinogen is then excreted in the urine, and a small amount is eliminated in feces.

Vascular and hematologic functions

Because of its extensive vascular network the liver can store a large volume of blood. The amount stored at any one time depends on pressure relationships in the arteries and veins. The liver can also release blood to maintain systemic circulatory volume in the event of hemorrhage.

Kupffer cells in the sinusoids of the liver remove bacteria and foreign particles from the portal blood. Because the liver receives all the venous blood from the gut and pancreas, the Kupffer cells play an important role in destroying intestinal bacteria and preventing infections.

The liver also has hemostatic functions. It synthesizes

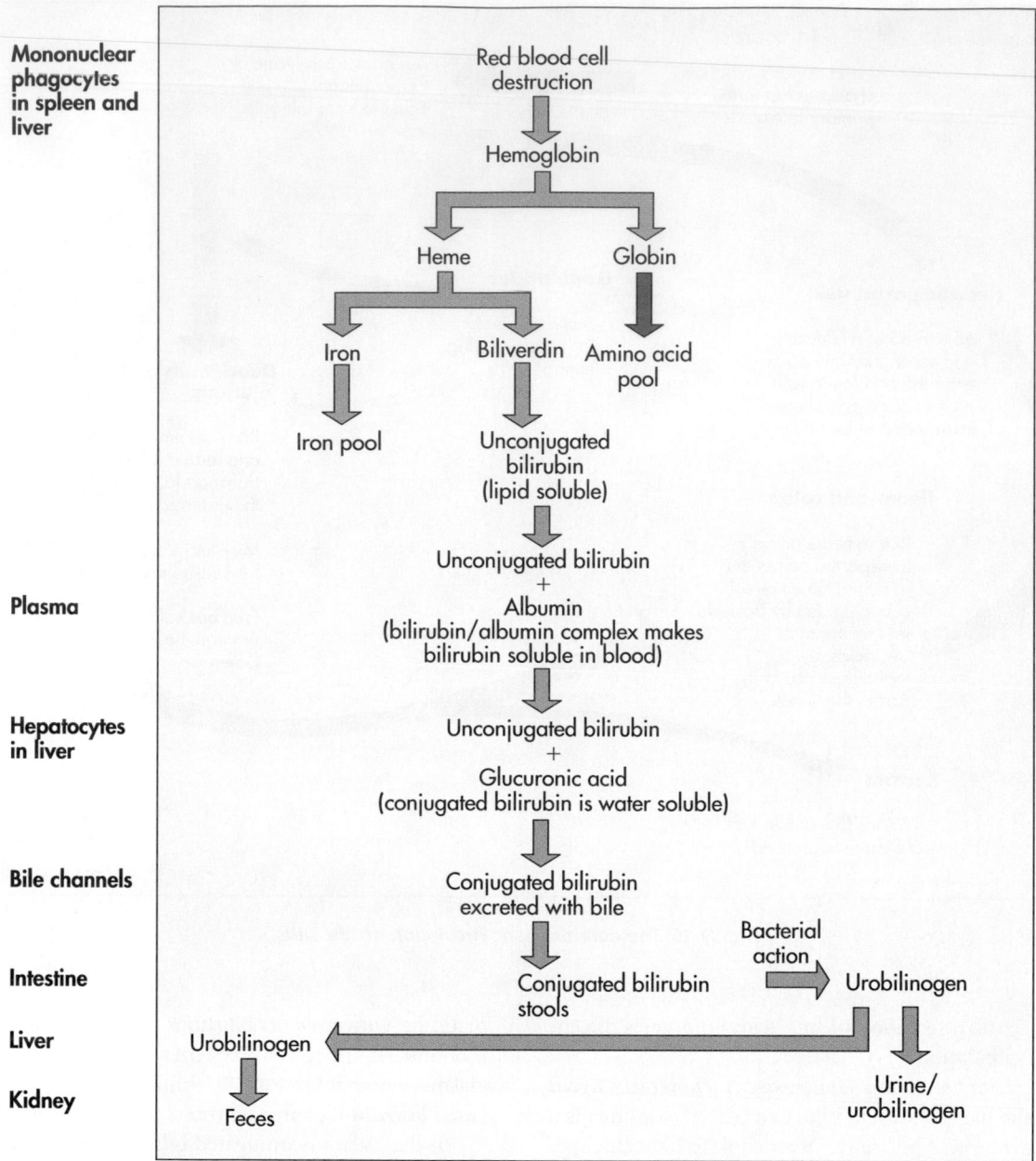

Fig. 33-17 *Bilirubin metabolism.*

prothrombin, fibrinogen, and factors I, II, VII, IX, and X, all of which are necessary for effective clotting (see Chapter 19). Vitamin K, a fat-soluble vitamin, is essential for the synthesis of other clotting factors. Because bile salts are needed for reabsorption of fats, vitamin K absorption depends on adequate bile production in the liver.

Metabolism of nutrients
Fats

Fat is synthesized from carbohydrate and protein, primarily in the liver. Fat absorbed by lacteals in the intestinal villi enters the liver through the lymphatics, primarily as triglycerides. In the liver, the triglycerides can be hydrolyzed to glycerol and free fatty acids and used to produce metabolic

energy (adenosine triphosphate [ATP]), or they can be released into the bloodstream as lipoproteins (lipids bound to proteins). The lipoproteins are carried by the blood to adipose cells for storage. The liver also synthesizes phospholipids and cholesterol, which are needed for the hepatic production of bile salts, steroid hormones, components of plasma membranes, and other special molecules.

Proteins

Protein synthesis requires the presence of all the essential amino acids (obtained only from food), as well as nonessential amino acids. Proteins perform many important roles in the body and are summarized in Table 33-2.

Within hepatocytes, amino acids are converted to carbo-

TABLE 33-2	**Proteins in the Body**
Role	**Example**
Contraction	Actin and myosin enable muscle contraction
Energy	Proteins can be metabolized for energy
Fluid balance	Albumin, a major source of plasma oncotic pressure
Protection	Antibodies and complement protect against infection and foreign substances
Regulation	Enzymes control chemical reactions; hormones regulate many physiologic processes
Structure	Collagen fibers provide structural support to many parts of the body; keratin strengthens skin, hair, and nails
Transport	Hemoglobin transports oxygen and carbon dioxide in the blood; plasma proteins serve as transport molecules; proteins in cell membranes control movement of materials into and out of cells

hydrates (ketoacids) by the removal of ammonia (NH_3), a process known as *deamination.* The ammonia is converted to urea by the liver and passes into the blood to be excreted by the kidneys. Depending on need, the ketoacids are converted to fatty acids for fat synthesis and storage or are oxidized by the Krebs tricarboxylic acid cycle (see Chapter 1) to provide energy for the liver cells.

The plasma proteins, including albumins and globulins (with the exception of γ-globulin, which is formed in lymph nodes and lymphoid tissue), are synthesized by the liver. They play an important role in maintaining blood volume and pressure by maintaining plasma oncotic pressure. The liver also synthesizes several nonessential amino acids and serum enzymes, including aspartate aminotransferase (AST; previously SGOT), alanine aminotransferase (ALT; previously SGPT), lactate dehydrogenase (LDH), and alkaline phosphatase.

Carbohydrates

The liver contributes to the stability of blood glucose levels by releasing glucose during hypoglycemia (low blood sugar) and taking up glucose during hyperglycemia (high blood sugar) and storing it as glycogen (glyconeogenesis) or converting it to fat. When all glycogen stores have been used, the liver can convert amino acids and glycerol to glucose.

Metabolic detoxification

The liver alters exogenous and endogenous chemicals (e.g., drugs), foreign molecules, and hormones to make them less toxic or less biologically active. This process, called *metabolic detoxification,* or *biotransformation,* diminishes in-

testinal or renal tubular reabsorption of potentially toxic substances and facilitates their intestinal and renal excretion. In this way alcohol, barbiturates, amphetamines, steroids, and hormones (including estrogens, aldosterone, antidiuretic hormone, and testosterone) are metabolized or detoxified, preventing excessive accumulation and adverse effects.

Although metabolic detoxification is usually protective, sometimes the end-products of metabolic detoxification become toxins. Those of alcohol metabolism, for example, are acetaldehyde and hydrogen. Excessive intake of alcohol over a prolonged period causes these end-products to damage hepatocytes. Acetaldehyde damages cellular mitochondria, and the excess hydrogen promotes fat accumulation. This is how alcohol impairs the liver's ability to function.

Storage of minerals and vitamins

The liver stores certain vitamins and minerals, including iron and copper, in times of excessive intake and releases them in times of need. The liver can store vitamins B_{12} and D for several months and vitamin A for several years. The liver also stores vitamins E and K. Iron is stored in the liver as ferritin, an iron-protein complex, and is released as needed for red blood cell production. Common tests of liver function are listed in Box 33-3.

Gallbladder

The *gallbladder* is a saclike organ on the inferior surface of the liver (Fig. 33-18). Its primary function is to store and concentrate bile between meals. Bile flows from the liver through the right or left hepatic duct into the common hepatic duct and meets resistance at the closed *sphincter of Oddi,* which controls flow into the duodenum. Bile then flows through the *cystic duct* into the gallbladder, where it is concentrated and stored. The mucosa of the gallbladder wall readily absorbs water and electrolytes, leaving a high concentration of bile salts, bile pigments, and cholesterol. The gallbladder holds about 90 ml of bile.

Within 30 minutes after eating, the gallbladder begins to contract and the sphincter of Oddi relaxes, forcing bile into the duodenum through the major duodenal papilla. During the cephalic and gastric phases of digestion, gallbladder contraction is mediated by cholinergic branches of the vagus nerve. Hormonal regulation of gallbladder contraction is derived from the release of cholecystokinin and motilin secreted by the duodenal mucosa in the presence of fat.

Exocrine Pancreas

The *pancreas* is approximately 20 cm long, with its head tucked into the curve of the duodenum and its tail touching the spleen. The body of the pancreas lies deep in the abdomen, behind the stomach (see Fig. 33-18). The pancreas is unique in that it has both endocrine and exocrine functions. The endocrine pancreas secretes hormones: insulin, glucagon, somatostatin, and pancreatic polypeptide.[8]

The *exocrine pancreas* is composed of acini and networks of ducts that secrete enzymes and alkaline fluids with important digestive functions. The acinar cells are organized

Selected Tests of Liver Function BOX 33-3

Test	Normal Value	Clinical Significance
SERUM ENZYMES		
Alkaline phosphatase	13-39 U/ml	Increases with biliary obstruction and cholestatic hepatitis
Aspartate aminotransferase (AST; previously SGOT)	5-40 U/ml	Increases with hepatocellular injury
Alanine aminotransferase (ALT; previously SGPT)	5-35 U/ml	Increases with hepatocellular injury
LDH (lactate dehydrogenase)	200-500 U/ml	Isoenzyme LD_5 is elevated with hypoxic and primary liver injury
5′-Nucleotidase	2-11 U/ml	Increases with increase in alklaine phosphatase and cholestatic disorders
BILIRUBIN METABOLISM		
Serum bilirubin		
Indirect (unconjugated)	<0.8 mg/dl	Increases with hemolysis (lysis of red blood cells)
Direct (conjugated)	0.2-0.4 mg/dl	Increases with hepatocellular injury or obstruction
Total	<1.0 mg/dl	Increases with biliary obstruction
Urine bilirubin	0	Increases with biliary obstruction
Urine urobilinogen	0-4 mg/24 hr	Increases with hemolysis or shunting of portal blood flow
SERUM PROTEINS		
Albumin	3.5-5.5 g/dl	Reduced with hepatocellular injury
Globulin	2.5-3.5 g/dl	Increases with hepatitis
Total	6-7 g/dl	
A/G ratio	1.5:1-2.5:1	Ratio reverses with chronic hepatitis or other chronic liver disease
Transferrin	250-300 μg/dl	Liver damage with decreased values, iron deficiency with increased values
α-Fetoprotein	6-20 ng/ml	Elevated values in primary hepatocellular carcinoma
BLOOD CLOTTING FUNCTIONS		
Prothrombin time	11.5-14 sec or 90%-100% of control	Increases with chronic liver disease (cirrhosis) or vitamin K deficiency
Partial thromboplastin time	25-40 sec	Increases with severe liver disease or heparin therapy
BSP (Bromsulphalein) excretion	<6% retention in 45 min	Increased retention with hepatocellular injury

into spherical lobules around small secretory ducts (see Fig. 33-18). Secretions drain into a system of ducts that leads to the *pancreatic duct (Wirsung duct),* which empties into the common bile duct at the *ampulla of Vater.* In some individuals an accessory duct (the duct of Santorini) branches off the pancreatic duct and drains directly into the duodenum at the minor duodenal papilla.

Arterial blood is supplied to the pancreas by branches of the celiac and superior mesenteric arteries. Venous blood leaves the head of the pancreas through the portal vein, with the body and tail being drained through the splenic vein. All hormonal pancreatic secretions also pass through the portal vein into the liver.

Pancreatic innervation arises from preganglionic parasympathetic fibers of the vagus nerve. These fibers activate postganglionic fibers, which stimulate enzymatic and hormonal secretion. Sympathetic postganglionic fibers from the celiac and superior mesenteric plexuses innervate the blood vessels, cause vasoconstriction, and inhibit pancreatic secretion.

The aqueous secretions of the exocrine pancreas are isotonic and contain potassium, sodium, bicarbonate, and chloride. The highly alkaline pancreatic juice neutralizes the acidic chyme that enters the duodenum from the stomach and provides the alkaline medium needed for the actions of digestive enzymes.

In the pancreas, transport of water and electrolytes through the ductal epithelium involves both active and passive mechanisms. The secretory cells of the acini actively transport hydrogen into the blood and bicarbonate into the duct lumen. Potassium and chloride are secreted by diffusion according to changes in electrochemical potential gradients. As the secretion flows down the duct, water is osmotically transported into the juice until it becomes isosmotic.

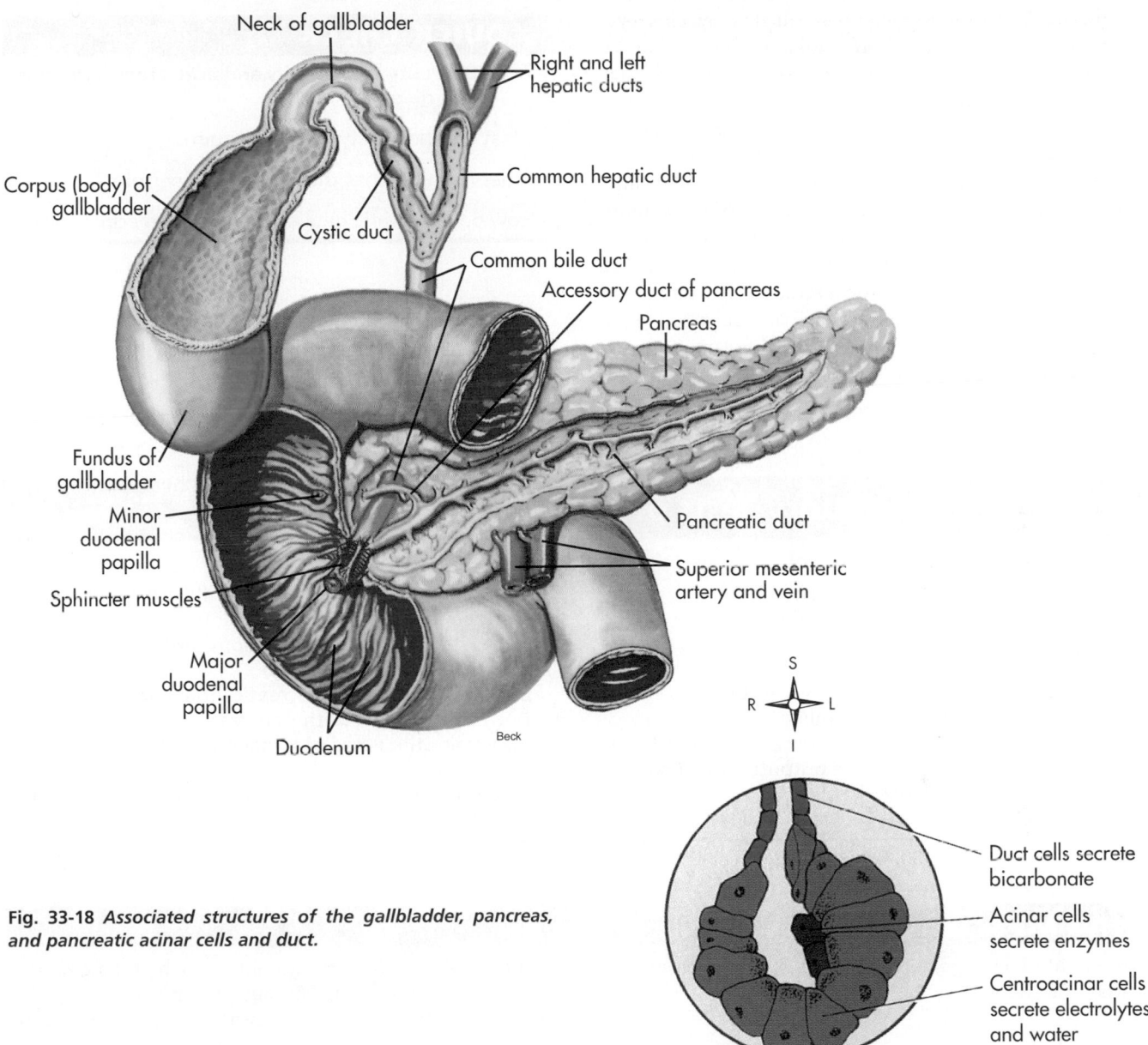

Fig. 33-18 *Associated structures of the gallbladder, pancreas, and pancreatic acinar cells and duct.*

At low flow rates, bicarbonate is exchanged passively for chloride, but at higher flow rates there is less time for this exchange and bicarbonate concentration increases. Because eating stimulates the flow of pancreatic juice, the juice is most alkaline when it needs to be: during digestion.

The pancreatic enzymes can hydrolyze proteins, carbohydrates, and fats. The proteolytic (protein-digesting) enzymes include trypsin, chymotrypsin, and carboxypeptidase. These enzymes are secreted in their inactive forms, that is, as trypsinogen, chymotrypsinogen, and procarboxypeptidase, to protect the pancreas from the digestive effects of its own enzymes. For further protection the pancreas produces **trypsin inhibitor,** which prevents the activation of proteolytic enzymes while they are in the pancreas. Once in the duodenum, the inactive forms (proenzymes) are activated by **enterokinase,** an enzyme secreted by the duodenal mucosa. Trypsinogen is the first proenzyme to be activated. Its conversion to trypsin stimulates the conversion of chymotrypsinogen to chymotrypsin and procarboxypeptidase to carboxypeptidase. Each of these enzymes cleaves specific peptide bonds to reduce polypeptides to smaller peptides.

Secretion of the aqueous and enzymatic components of pancreatic juice is controlled by hormonal and vagal stimuli. **Secretin** stimulates the acinar and duct cells to secrete the bicarbonate-rich fluid that neutralizes chyme and prepares it for enzymatic digestion. As chyme enters the duodenum, its acidity (pH of 4.5 or less) stimulates the **S cells** (secretin-producing cells) of the duodenum to release secretin, which is absorbed by the intestine and delivered to the pancreas in the bloodstream. In the pancreas, secretin causes ductal and acinar cells to release alkaline fluid. Secretin also inhibits the actions of gastrin, thereby decreasing gastric acid secretion and motility. The overall effect is to neutralize contents of the duodenum.

Enzymatic secretion follows, stimulated by cholecystokinin and acetylcholine. Cholecystokinin is released in the duodenum in response to the essential amino acids and fatty acids already present in chyme. Cholecystokinin and acetylcholine both act on the acinar cells, causing enzyme release. Once in the small intestine, activated pancreatic enzymes inhibit the release of more cholecystokinin and acetylcholine. This feedback mechanism inhibits the secretion of more pancreatic enzymes. Acetylcholine is liberated from pancreatic branches of the vagus nerve during the cephalic phase of digestion. Pancreatic polypeptide is released after eating and inhibits postprandial pancreatic exocrine secretion. (See Table 33-1 for a summary of hormonal stimulation of pancreatic secretions.) Selected tests of pancreatic function are listed in Box 33-4.

✓ QUICK CHECK

Trace the route of bile salts and acids from formation to recycling.

What are the two types of bilirubin?

What function does the gallbladder perform?

How do pancreatic beta cells differ from acinar cells?

Selected Laboratory Tests of Pancreatic Function   BOX 33-4

Test	Normal Value	Clinical Significance
Serum amylase	60-180 Somogyi units/ml	Elevated levels with pancreatic inflammation
Serum lipase	1.5 Somogyi units/ml	Elevated levels with pancreatic inflammation (may be elevated with other conditions; differentiates with amylase isoenzyme study)
Urine amylase	35-260 Somogyi units/hr	Elevated levels with pancreatic inflammation
Secretin test	Volume 1.8 ml/kg/hr Bicarbonate concentration: >80 mEq/L Bicarbonate output: >10 mEq/L/30 sec	Decreased volume with pancreatic disease because a secretin stimulates pancreatic secretion
Stool fat	2-5 g/25 hr	Measures fatty acids; decreased pancreatic lipase increases stool fat

---

⚠ AGING & *The Gastrointestinal System*

Age-related changes in gastrointestinal function include the following:

ORAL CAVITY
1 Tooth enamel and dentin wear down, so cavities are more likely.
2 Teeth are lost as a result of periodontal disease and brittle roots that break easily.
3 Taste buds decline in number.
4 Sense of smell diminishes.
5 Salivary secretion decreases.
Result: Eating in less pleasurable, appetite is reduced, and food is not chewed or lubricated enough, so swallowing is difficult.

STOMACH AND INTESTINES
1 Gastric motility and volume and acid content of gastric juice are reduced, particularly with gastric atrophy.
2 Intestinal villi become shorter and more convoluted with diminished reparative capacity.
3 Intestinal absorption, motility, and blood flow decrease, impairing nutrient absorption.
4 Nutritive substances are absorbed more slowly and in smaller amounts.
5 Rectal muscle mass is decreased, and the anal sphincter weakens.
6 Constipation is common and is related to immobility and low-fiber diet.

LIVER
1 Size and weight decrease.
2 Blood flow decreases, influencing efficiency of drug metabolism.

PANCREAS AND GALLBLADDER
1 Fibrosis, fatty acid deposits, and pancreatic atrophy occur.
2 Secretion of digestive enzymes decreases.
3 No changes in gallbladder and bile ducts occur, but there is an increased prevalence of gallstones.

From Hurwitz, A. et al. (1997). Gastric acidity in older adults, Journal of the American Medical Association, *278(8), 659-662; Timiras, P.S. (1994). Physiological basis of aging and geriatrics. Boca Raton, Fla.: CRC Press; Majumdar, A.P., Fligiel, S.E., & Jaszawski, R. (1997). Gastric mucosal injury and repair: Effect of aging,* Histology and Histopathology 12(2), 491-501.

DID YOU UNDERSTAND?

The Gastrointestinal Tract

1. The major functions of the gastrointestinal tract are the mechanical and chemical breakdown of food and the absorption of digested nutrients.

2. The gastrointestinal tract is a hollow tube that extends from the mouth to the anus.

3. The walls of the gastrointestinal tract have several layers: mucosa, muscularis mucosae, submucosa, tunica muscularis (circular muscle and longitudinal muscle), and serosa.

4. The peritoneum is a double layer of membranous tissue. The visceral layer covers the abdominal organs, and the parietal layer extends along the abdominal wall.

5. Except for swallowing and defecation, which are controlled voluntarily, the functions of the gastrointestinal tract are controlled by extrinsic and intrinsic autonomic nerves and intestinal hormones.

6. Digestion begins in the mouth, with chewing and salivation. The digestive component of saliva is α-amylase, which initiates carbohydrate digestion.

7. The esophagus is a muscular tube that transports food from the mouth to the stomach. The tunica muscularis in the upper part of the esophagus is striated muscle, and that in the lower part is smooth muscle.

8. Swallowing is controlled by the swallowing center in the reticular formation of the brain. The two phases of swallowing are the oropharyngeal phase (voluntary swallowing) and the esophageal phase (involuntary swallowing).

9. Food is propelled through the gastrointestinal tract by peristalsis: waves of sequential relaxations and contractions of the tunica muscularis.

10. The lower esophageal sphincter opens to admit swallowed food into the stomach and then closes to prevent regurgitation of food back into the esophagus.

11. The stomach is a baglike structure that secretes digestive juices, mixes and stores food, and propels partially digested food (chyme) into the duodenum.

12. The vagus nerve stimulates gastric (stomach) secretion and motility.

13. The hormones gastrin and motilin stimulate gastric emptying; the hormones secretin and cholecystokinin delay gastric emptying.

14. Mucus is secreted throughout the stomach and protects the stomach wall from acid and digestive enzymes.

15. Gastric glands in the fundus and body of the stomach secrete intrinsic factor, which is needed for vitamin B_{12} absorption, and hydrochloric acid, which dissolves food fibers, kills microorganisms, and activates the enzyme pepsin.

16. Chief cells in the stomach secrete pepsinogen, which is converted to pepsin in the acid environment created by hydrochloric acid.

17. Acid secretion is stimulated by the vagus nerve, gastrin, and histamine and inhibited by sympathetic stimulation and cholecystokinin.

18. The three phases of acid secretion by the stomach are the cephalic phase (anticipation and swallowing), the gastric phase (food in the stomach), and the intestinal phase (chyme in the intestine).

19. The small intestine is 5 meters long and has three segments: the duodenum, jejunum, and ileum.

20. The duodenum receives chyme from the stomach through the pyloric valve. The presence of chyme stimulates the liver and gallbladder to deliver bile and the pancreas to deliver digestive enzymes. Bile and enzymes flow through an opening guarded by the sphincter of Oddi.

21. Bile is produced by the liver and is necessary for fat digestion and absorption. Bile's alkalinity helps to neutralize chyme, thereby creating a pH that enables the pancreatic enzymes to digest proteins, carbohydrates, and sugars.

22. Enzymes secreted by the small intestine (maltase, sucrose, lactase), pancreatic enzymes, and bile salts act in the small intestine to digest proteins, carbohydrates, and fats.

23. Digested substances are absorbed across the intestinal wall and then transported to the liver, where they are metabolized further.

24. The ileocecal valve connects the small and large intestines and prevents reflux into the small intestine.

25. Villi are small fingerlike projections that extend from the small intestinal mucosa and increase its absorptive surface area.

26. Sugars, amino acids, and fats are absorbed primarily by the duodenum and jejunum; bile salts and vitamin B_{12} are absorbed by the ileum. Vitamin B_{12} absorption requires the presence of intrinsic factor.

27. Bile salts emulsify and hydrolyze fats and incorporate them into water-soluble micelles, which transport them through the unstirred layer to the brush border of the intestinal mucosa. The fat content of the micelles readily diffuses through the epithelium into lacteals (lymphatic ducts) in the villi. From there fats flow into lymphatics and into the systemic circulation, which delivers them to the liver.

28. Minerals and water-soluble vitamins are absorbed by both active and passive transport throughout the small intestine.

29. Peristaltic movements created by longitudinal muscles propel the chyme along the intestinal tract, and contractions of the circular muscles (haustral segmentation) mix the chyme.

30. The ileogastric reflex inhibits gastric motility when the ileum is distended.

31. The intestinointestinal reflex inhibits intestinal motility when one intestinal segment is overdistended.

32. The gastroileal reflex increases intestinal motility when gastric motility increases.

Continued

◼ DID YOU UNDERSTAND? —cont'd

The Gastrointestinal Tract—cont'd

33. The large intestine consists of the cecum, appendix, colon (ascending, transverse, descending, and sigmoid), rectum, and anal canal.

34. The teniae coli are three bands of longitudinal muscle that extend the length of the colon.

35. Haustra are pouches of colon formed with alternating contraction and relaxation of the circular muscles.

36. The mucosa of the large intestine contains mucus-secreting cells and mucosal folds, but no villi.

37. The large intestine massages the fecal mass and absorbs water and electrolytes.

38. Distention of the ileum with chyme causes the gastrocolic reflex, or the mass propulsion of feces to the rectum.

39. Defecation is stimulated when the rectum is distended with feces. The conically contracted internal anal sphincter relaxes, and, if the voluntarily regulated external sphincter relaxes, defecation occurs.

40. The largest number of intestinal bacteria are in the colon. They are anaerobes consisting of *Bacteroides,* clostridia, coliforms, and lactobacilli.

41. The intestinal tract is sterile at birth and becomes totally colonized within 3 to 4 weeks.

42. Endogenous infections of the gastrointestinal tract occur by excessive proliferation of bacteria, perforation of the intestine, or contamination from neighboring structures.

Accessory Organs of Digestion

1. The liver is the second largest organ in the body. It has digestive, metabolic, hematologic, vascular, and immunologic functions.

2. The liver is divided into the right and left lobes and is supported by the falciform, round, and coronary ligaments.

3. Liver lobules consist of plates of hepatocytes, which are the functional cells of the liver.

4. The hepatocytes synthesize 700 to 1200 ml of bile per day and secrete it into the bile canaliculi, which are small channels between the hepatocytes. The bile canaliculi drain bile into the common bile duct and then into the duodenum through an opening called the *major duodenal papilla (sphincter of Oddi).*

5. Sinusoids are capillaries located between the plates of hepatocytes. Blood from the portal vein and hepatic artery flows through the sinusoids to a central vein in each lobule and then to the hepatic vein and inferior vena cava.

6. Kupffer cells, which are part of the mononuclear phagocyte system, line the sinusoids and destroy microorganisms in sinusoidal blood.

7. The primary bile acids are synthesized from cholesterol by the hepatocytes. The primary acids are then conjugated to form bile salts. The secondary bile acids are the product of bile salt deconjugation by bacteria in the intestinal lumen.

8. Most bile salts and acids are recycled. The absorption of bile salts and acids from the terminal ileum and their return to the liver are known as the *enterohepatic circulation of bile.*

9. Bilirubin is a pigment liberated by the lysis of aged red blood cells in the liver and spleen. Unconjugated bilirubin is fat-soluble and can cross cell membranes. Unconjugated bilirubin is converted to water-soluble, conjugated bilirubin by hepatocytes and is secreted with bile.

10. The gallbladder is a saclike organ located in the inferior surface of the liver. The gallbladder stores bile between meals and ejects it when chyme enters the duodenum.

11. Stimulated by cholecystokinin, the gallbladder contracts and forces bile through the cystic duct and into the common bile duct. The sphincter of Oddi relaxes, enabling bile to flow through the major duodenal papilla into the duodenum.

12. The pancreas is a gland located behind the stomach. The endocrine pancreas produces hormones (glucagon, insulin) that facilitate the formation and cellular uptake of glucose. The exocrine pancreas secretes an alkaline solution and the enzymes (trypsin, chymotrypsin, carboxypeptidase, α-amylase, lipase) that digest proteins, carbohydrates, and fats.

13. Secretin stimulates pancreatic secretion of alkaline fluid, and cholecystokinin and acetylcholine stimulate secretion of enzymes. Pancreatic secretions originate in acini and ducts of the pancreas and empty into the duodenum through the common bile duct or an accessory duct that opens directly into the duodenum.

KEY TERMS

REFERENCES

1. Diamant, N.E. (1997). Neuromuscular mechanisms of primary peristalsis. *American Journal of Medicine, 103*(5A), 40S-43S.
2. Johnson, L.R. (1997). *Gastrointestinal physiology.* St. Louis: Mosby.
3. Helander, H.F. & Keeling, D.J. (1993). Cell biology of gastric acid secretion. *Baillieres Clinical Gastroenterology, 7*(1), 1-21.
4. Tayler, S.D. et al. (1994). Duodenal acidification and secretin, but not intraduodenal fat, inhibit human gastric acid secretion via prostaglandins. *Gastroenterology, 107*(6), 1680-1685.
5. Thomson, A.B. (1998). Small bowel review: Part 1. *Canadian Journal of Gastroenterology, 12*(7), 487-504.
6. Kvietys, P.R., Barrowman, J.A., & Granger, N.D. (1987). *Pathophysiology of the splanchnic circulation.* Boca Raton, Fla.: CRC Press.
7. Rosenblum, J.D., Boyle, C.M., & Schwartz, L.B. (1997). The mesenteric circulation: Anatomy and physiology. *Surgical Clinics of North America, 77*(2), 289-306.
8. Thibodeau, G.A. & Patton, K.T. (1999). *Anatomy and physiology* (4th ed.). St. Louis: Mosby.

CHAPTER

34

Alterations of Digestive Function

Sue E. Huether

The gastrointestinal tract is a continuous, hollow organ that extends from the mouth to the anus. It includes the esophagus, stomach, small intestine (duodenum, jejunum, ileum), large intestine (ascending, transverse, descending, and sigmoid colons), and rectum.

Disorders of the gastrointestinal tract disrupt one or more of its functions. Structural and neural abnormalities can slow, obstruct, or accelerate the movement of chyme at any level of the gastrointestinal tract. Inflammatory and ulcerative conditions of the gastrointestinal wall disrupt secretion, motility, and absorption. Many clinical manifestations of gastrointestinal tract disorders are nonspecific; that is, they can be caused by a variety of impairments. These manifestations are described in the next section.

Gale D. Danek, RN, MSN, contributed to this chapter in the previous edition.

CHAPTER OUTLINE

 Check out your CD Companion for chapter-related exercises and answers to the Quick Check questions

DISORDERS OF THE GASTROINTESTINAL TRACT
Clinical Manifestations of Gastrointestinal Dysfunction
Anorexia

Anorexia is lack of a desire to eat despite physiologic stimuli that would normally produce hunger. This nonspecific symptom is often associated with nausea, abdominal pain, and diarrhea and often accompanies disorders of other organ systems, including cancer, heart disease, and renal disease. Anorexia can also be related to psychosocial distress.

Vomiting

Vomiting is the forceful emptying of stomach and intestinal contents (chyme) through the mouth. Stimuli initiating the vomiting reflex include the presence of ipecac or copper salts in the duodenum; severe pain; distention of the stomach or duodenum; torsion or trauma affecting the ovaries, testes, uterus, bladder, or kidney; and activation of the chemoreceptor trigger zone in the medulla.

Nausea and retching usually precede vomiting. *Nausea* is a subjective experience associated with various conditions. Specific neural pathways have not been identified, but hypersalivation and tachycardia are common associated symptoms. *Retching* begins with deep inspiration. The glottis closes, intrathoracic pressure falls, and the esophagus becomes distended. Simultaneously the abdominal muscles contract, creating a pressure gradient from abdomen to thorax. The lower esophageal sphincter (LES) and body of the stomach relax, but the duodenum and antrum of the stomach go into spasm. The reverse peristalsis and pressure gradient force chyme from the stomach and duodenum up into the esophagus. Because the upper esophageal sphincter is closed, chyme does not enter the mouth. As the abdominal muscles relax, the contents of the esophagus drop back into the stomach. This process may be repeated several times before vomiting occurs. A diffuse sympathetic discharge causes the tachycardia, tachypnea, and sweating that accompany retching and vomiting. The parasympathetic system mediates copious salivation, increased gastric motility, and relaxation of the upper and lower esophageal sphincters.

Vomiting usually follows retching. The duodenum and antrum of the stomach produce retrograde peristalsis, while the body of the stomach and esophagus relax. When the stomach is full of gastric contents, the diaphragm is forced high into the thoracic cavity by strong contractions of the abdominal muscles. The higher intrathoracic pressure forces the upper esophageal sphincter to open, and chyme is expelled from the mouth. Then the stomach relaxes and the upper part of the esophagus contracts, forcing the remaining chyme back into the stomach. The lower esophageal sphincter then closes. The cycle is repeated if there is a volume of chyme remaining in the stomach.

Spontaneous vomiting not preceded by nausea or retching is called *projectile vomiting.* It is caused by direct stimulation of the vomiting center by neurologic lesions (e.g., tumors or aneurysms) involving the brain stem or can be a symptom of gastrointestinal obstruction (pyloric stenosis). The metabolic consequences of vomiting are fluid, electrolyte, and acid-base disturbances (see Chapter 4).

Constipation

Constipation is difficult or infrequent defecation. It is a common complaint caused by personal habits and various disorders and drugs. It usually means a decrease in the number of bowel movements per week, hard stools, and difficult evacuation, but the definition must be individually determined. Normal bowel habits range from two or three evacuations per day to one per week.

Pathophysiology

Constipation can be caused by neurogenic disorders of the large intestine in which neural pathways or neurotransmitters are altered.[1] A low-residue diet (the habitual consumption of highly refined foods) decreases the volume and number of stools and causes constipation. A sedentary life-style and lack of regular exercise are common causes of constipation. Hypothyroidism decreases bowel motility. Lack of access to toilet facilities and consistent suppression of the urge to empty the bowel are other causes. Excessive use of antacids containing calcium carbonate or aluminum hydroxide often results in constipation. Opiates, particularly codeine, tend to inhibit bowel motility.

Clinical Manifestations

Changes in bowel evacuation patterns, such as less frequent defecation, smaller stool volume, difficulty in evacuating the rectum, or a feeling of bowel fullness and discomfort, require investigation.

Evaluation and Treatment

The history and physical examination and stool diaries provide precise clues regarding the nature of constipation. Functional constipation, that is, constipation resulting from life-style or bowel habits, usually has a long history. Dysfunctional constipation is more likely to be sudden. Sudden-onset constipation can accompany the development of organic lesions and requires careful evaluation.

The individual's description of frequency, stool consistency, associated pain, and presence of blood is significant. In assessing frequency, it is important to discover whether evacuation was stimulated by enemas or cathartics (laxatives). Palpation discloses colonic distention, masses, and tenderness. Digital examination of the rectum is performed to assess sphincter tone and detect anal lesions. Stool transit time is evaluated. Proctosigmoidoscopy is used to visualize the lumen directly. A barium enema may be required if no lesions are directly visualized and symptoms continue after simple treatment.

The treatment for dysfunctional constipation is to manage the underlying lesion or disease. Management of functional constipation usually consists of bowel retraining, in which the individual establishes a satisfactory bowel evacuation routine without becoming preoccupied with bowel movements. The individual also may need to engage in moderate exercise, drink more fluids, and increase fiber intake. Bulk supplements (e.g., Metamucil, Konsyl), stool softeners, and laxative agents are useful for some individuals. Enemas can be used to establish bowel routine, but they should not be used habitually.

Diarrhea

Diarrhea is an increase in the frequency of defecation and the fluidity and volume of feces. Many factors determine stool volume and consistency, including water content of the colon and the presence of unabsorbed food, unabsorbable material, and intestinal secretions. Stool volume in the normal adult averages less than 200 g/day. Stool volume in children depends on age and size. An infant may pass up to 100 g/day. The adult intestine processes approximately 9 L of luminal content per day: 2 L is ingested, and the remaining 7 L consists of intestinal secretions. Of this volume, 99% of the fluid is absorbed: 90% (7 to 8 L) in the small intestine and 9% (1 to 2 L) in the colon. Normally, approximately 150 ml water is excreted daily in the stool.

Pathophysiology

Diarrhea in which the volume of feces is increased is called *large-volume diarrhea*. It generally is caused by excessive amounts of water or secretions or both in the intestines. *Small-volume diarrhea*, in which the volume of feces is not increased, usually results from excessive intestinal motility.

The three major mechanisms of diarrhea are osmotic, secretory, and motile:
1. *Osmotic diarrhea:* A nonabsorbable substance in the intestine draws excess water into the intestine and increases stool weight and volume, producing large-volume diarrhea. Causes include lactase and pancreatic enzyme deficiency and excessive ingestion of synthetic, nonabsorbable sugars.
2. *Secretory diarrhea:* Excessive mucosal secretion of fluid and electrolytes produces large-volume diarrhea. Causes include bacterial enterotoxins[2] (e.g., *Escherichia coli*), neoplasms, and excessive motility of the intestine caused by diabetic neuropathy. Small-volume diarrhea is usually caused by an inflammatory disorder of the intestine, such as ulcerative colitis or Crohn disease, but also can be the result of fecal impaction.
3. *Motility diarrhea:* Food is not mixed properly, digestion is impaired, and motility is increased. Causes include resection of the small intestine, surgical bypass of an area of the intestine, or fistula formation between loops of intestine.

Clinical Manifestations

Diarrhea can be acute or chronic, depending on its cause. Systemic effects of prolonged diarrhea are dehydration, electrolyte imbalance, and weight loss. Manifestations of acute bacterial or viral infection include fever, with or without cramping pain. Fever, cramping pain, and bloody stools accompany diarrhea caused by inflammatory bowel disease. Steatorrhea (fat in the stools) and diarrhea are common signs of malabsorption syndromes.

Evaluation and Treatment

A thorough history is taken to document the onset and frequency of diarrhea. Exposure to contaminated food or water is indicated if the individual has traveled in foreign countries or areas where drinking water might be contaminated. Iatrogenic diarrhea is suggested if the individual has undergone abdominal radiation therapy, intestinal resection, or treatment with selected drugs (e.g., antibiotics, diuretics, antihypertensives, or laxatives).[3] Physical examination helps identify underlying systemic disease. Stool culture, examination of stool specimens for blood, abdominal x-ray films, and intestinal biopsies provide more specific data.

Treatment for diarrhea includes restoration of fluid and electrolyte balance, management of distressing symptoms, and treatment of causal factors. Nutritional deficiencies need to be corrected in cases of chronic diarrhea or malabsorption.

Abdominal pain

The causal mechanisms of abdominal pain are mechanical, inflammatory, or ischemic. Generally, the abdominal organs are not sensitive to mechanical stimuli, such as cutting, tearing, or crushing. These organs are, however, sensitive to stretching and distention, which activate nerve endings in both hollow and solid structures. Pain accompanies rapid distention rather than gradual distention. Traction on the peritoneum caused by adhesions, distention of the common bile duct, or forceful peristalsis resulting from intestinal obstruction causes pain because of increased tension. Capsules that surround solid organs, such as the liver and gallbladder, contain pain fibers that are stimulated by stretching if these organs swell.

Biochemical mediators of the inflammatory response, such as histamine, bradykinin, and serotonin, stimulate organic nerve endings and produce abdominal pain. The edema and vascular congestion that accompany chemical, bacterial, or viral inflammation also cause painful stretching. Obstruction of blood flow from the distention of bowel obstruction or mesenteric vessel thrombosis produces the pain of ischemia, and increased concentrations of tissue metabolites stimulate pain receptors.

Abdominal pain can be parietal (somatic), visceral, or referred. *Parietal pain,* from the parietal peritoneum, is more localized and intense than visceral pain, which arises from the organs themselves. Parietal pain lateralizes because, at any particular point, the parietal peritoneum is innervated from only one side of the nervous system.

Visceral pain arises from a stimulus acting on an abdominal organ. It is usually poorly localized with a radiating pattern. Visceral pain is diffuse and vague because nerve endings in abdominal organs are sparse and multisegmented. Pain arising from the stomach, for example, is experienced as a sensation of fullness, cramping, or gnawing in the midepigastric area.

Referred pain is visceral pain felt at some distance from a diseased or affected organ. It is usually well localized and is felt in skin or deeper tissues that share a central afferent pathway with the affected organ. Generally, referred pain develops as the intensity of a visceral pain stimulus increases.

Gastrointestinal bleeding

Upper *gastrointestinal bleeding,* which is defined as bleeding in the esophagus, stomach, or duodenum, is characterized by frank, bright red bleeding or "coffee ground" material that has been affected by stomach acids. Upper gastrointestinal bleeding is commonly caused by bleeding varices (varicose veins) in the esophagus, peptic ulcers, or a Mallory-Weiss tear at the esophageal gastric junction from severe retching. Lower gastrointestinal bleeding, or bleeding from the jejunum, ileum, colon, or rectum, can be caused by polyps, inflammatory disease, cancer, or hemorrhoids. Acute, severe gastrointestinal bleeding is life threatening, depending on the volume and rate of blood loss, associated disease, age, and effectiveness of treatment.

The signs of gastrointestinal bleeding are defined in Table 34-1. Physiologic response to gastrointestinal bleeding depends on the amount and rate of the loss (Fig. 34-1). Changes in blood pressure and heart rate are the best indicators of massive blood loss in the gastrointestinal tract. During the early stages of blood volume depletion, the peripheral vascular compartment constricts to shunt blood to vital organs, including the brain. A sign that this is happening is postural hypotension (a drop in blood pressure that occurs with a change from the recumbent position to a sitting or upright position), lightheadedness, and loss of vision. If blood loss continues, hypovolemic shock progresses. Diminished blood flow to the kidneys causes decreased urine output and may lead to oliguria (low urine output), tubular necrosis, and renal failure. Ultimately, insufficient cerebral and coronary blood flow causes irreversible anoxia and death.

The accumulation of blood in the gastrointestinal tract is irritating and increases peristalsis, causing diarrhea. If bleeding is from the lower gastrointestinal tract, the diarrhea is frankly bloody. Bleeding from the upper gastrointestinal tract also can be rapid enough to produce **hematochezia** (bright red stools), but generally some digestion of the blood components will have occurred, producing melena—black or "tarry" stools that are sticky and have a characteristic foul odor. The digestion of blood proteins originating from massive upper gastrointestinal bleeding is reflected by an increase in blood urea nitrogen (BUN) levels (see Fig. 34-1).

The hematocrit and hemoglobin values are not the best indicators of acute gastrointestinal bleeding because plasma volume and red cell volume are lost proportionately. As the plasma volume is replaced, the hematocrit and hemoglobin values begin to reflect the extent of blood loss. The interpretation of these values is modified to account for exogenous replacement of fluids and the hydration status of the tissues.

TABLE 34-1	Presentations of Gastrointestinal Bleeding
Presentations	**Definition**
Acute bleeding	
Hematemesis	Bloody vomitus; either fresh, bright red blood or dark, grainy digested blood with "coffee grounds" appearance
Melena	Black, sticky, tarry, foul smelling stools caused by digestion of blood in the gastrointestinal tract
Hematochezia	Fresh, bright red blood passed from the rectum
Occult bleeding	Trace amounts of blood in normal-appearing stools or gastric secretions; detectable only with a guaiac test

✓ QUICK CHECK

How is visceral pain "referred"?

How does osmotic diarrhea differ from secretory diarrhea?

How do melena and hematochezia differ?

Disorders of Motility
Dysphagia

▤ *Pathophysiology*

Dysphagia is difficulty swallowing. It can result from mechanical obstruction of the esophagus or a disorder that impairs esophageal motility. Intrinsic obstructions originate in the wall of the esophageal lumen and include tumors, strictures, and diverticular herniations (outpouchings). Extrinsic mechanical obstructions originate outside the esophageal lumen and narrow the esophagus by pressing inward on the esophageal wall. The most common cause of extrinsic mechanical obstruction is tumor.

Functional dysphagia is caused by neural or muscular disorders that interfere with voluntary swallowing or peristalsis.[4] Disorders that affect the striated muscles of the upper esophagus interfere with the oropharyngeal (voluntary) phase of swallowing. Typical causes are dermatomyositis (a muscle disease) and neurologic impairments caused by cerebrovascular accidents, Parkinson disease, or achalasia.

Achalasia is a rare form of dysphagia that impairs (1) peristalsis of smooth muscle in the middle and lower portions of the esophagus and (2) lower esophageal sphincter (LES) functioning.[5] Achalasia results from neural dysfunction, probably a decrease in the number of ganglion cells in the myenteric plexus and atrophy of smooth muscle cells or lesions along the vagus nerve. Disrupted innervation results in loss of neuromuscular coordination and muscle

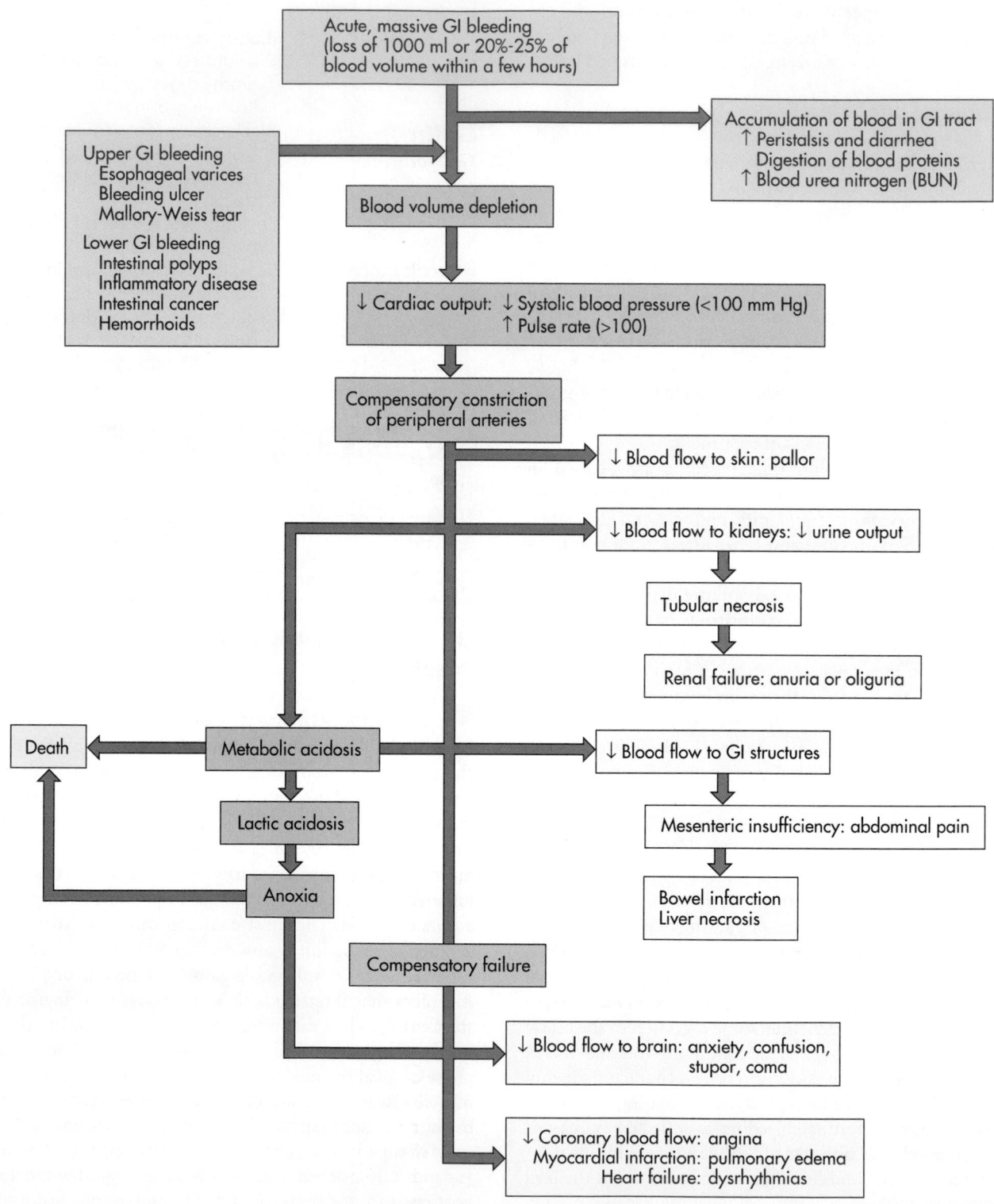

Fig. 34-1 *Pathophysiology of gastrointestinal (GI) bleeding.*

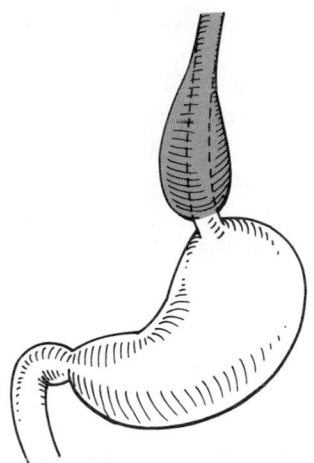

Fig. 34-2 *Achalasia.* Decreased muscle tone and peristaltic function prevent food from entering the stomach, causing esophageal distention. *(From Phipps, W.J., Sands, J.K., & Marek, J.F. [1999]. Medical-surgical nursing: Concepts and clinical practice [6th ed.]. St. Louis: Mosby.)*

tone at the lower end of the esophagus. The decreased peristalsis of the middle esophagus, loss of tone in the LES, and decreased relaxation of the LES after swallowing allow food to accumulate above the obstruction, which distends the esophagus (Fig. 34-2). As hydrostatic pressure increases, food is slowly forced past the obstruction into the stomach. Psychosocial achalasia has been documented and may be the result of life stressors.

Clinical Manifestations
Distention and spasm of the esophageal muscles during eating or drinking may cause a mild or severe stabbing pain at the level of obstruction. Discomfort occurring 2 to 4 seconds after swallowing is associated with upper esophageal obstruction. Discomfort occurring 10 to 15 seconds after swallowing is more common in obstructions of the lower esophagus. If obstruction results from a growing tumor, dysphagia begins with difficulty swallowing solids and advances to difficulty swallowing semisolids and liquids. If motor function is impaired, both solids and liquids are difficult to swallow. Regurgitation of undigested food, unpleasant taste, vomiting, and weight loss are common manifestations of all types of dysphagia.[6] Aspiration of esophageal contents can lead to pneumonia.

Evaluation and Treatment
Knowledge of the patient's history and clinical manifestations contributes significantly to a diagnosis of dysphagia. A barium swallow is used to visualize the contours of the esophagus and identify structural defects. Manometry documents the duration and amplitude of abnormal pressure changes associated with obstruction or loss of neural regulation. Esophageal endoscopy is performed to examine the esophageal mucosa and obtain biopsy specimens.

The individual is taught to manage symptoms by eating slowly, eating small meals, taking fluid with meals, and sleeping with the head elevated to prevent regurgitation and aspiration. Anticholinergic drugs (e.g., botulism toxin)[7] may alleviate achalasia. Definitive treatments include mechanical dilation of the esophageal sphincter and surgical separation of the lower esophageal muscles with a longitudinal incision (myotomy). Myotomy widens the passage into the stomach.

Gastroesophageal reflux
Gastroesophageal reflux (GER) is the reflux of chyme (acid and pepsin) from the stomach to the esophagus. The LES may relax spontaneously and transiently 1 to 2 hours after eating, permitting gastric contents to regurgitate into the esophagus. The acid is usually neutralized and cleared from the esophagus by peristaltic action within 1 to 3 minutes, and sphincter tone is restored. Gastroesophageal reflux that does not cause symptoms is known as physiologic reflux. In some individuals, however, a combination of factors causes an inflammatory response to reflux called *reflux esophagitis.*[8] GER may be a trigger for asthma.[9]

Pathophysiology
Normally the resting tone of the LES maintains a zone of high pressure that prevents GER. In individuals who develop reflux esophagitis, this pressure tends to be lower than normal. Vomiting, coughing, lifting, or bending that increases abdominal pressure can contribute to the development of reflux esophagitis. The severity of the esophagitis depends on the composition of the gastric contents and the length of time they are in contact with the esophageal mucosa. If the chyme is highly acidic or contains bile salts and pancreatic enzymes, reflux esophagitis can be severe. In individuals with weak esophageal peristalsis, refluxed chyme remains in the esophagus longer than usual. Delayed gastric emptying contributes to reflux esophagitis by (1) lengthening the period during which reflux is possible and (2) increasing the acid content of chyme. Disorders that delay emptying include gastric or duodenal ulcers, which can cause pyloric edema; strictures that narrow the pylorus; and hiatal hernia, which can weaken the LES.[10]

Reflux esophagitis causes inflammatory responses in the esophageal wall, such as hyperemia, increased capillary permeability, edema, tissue fragility, and erosion. Fibrosis and thickening may develop.

Clinical Manifestations
The clinical manifestations of reflux esophagitis are heartburn, regurgitation of acidic chyme, and upper abdominal pain within 1 hour of eating. The symptoms worsen if the individual lies down or if intraabdominal pressure increases (e.g., as a result of coughing, vomiting, or straining at stool). Edema, strictures, esophageal spasm, or decreased esophageal motility may result in dysphagia with weight loss. Alcohol or acid-containing foods, such as citrus fruits, can cause discomfort during swallowing.

Evaluation and Treatment

Diagnosis of reflux esophagitis is based on clinical manifestations, esophageal endoscopy that shows edema and erosion, and ambulatory pH monitoring. Endoscopy also allows evaluation for dysplastic changes (Barrett esophagus) and the development of esophageal carcinoma.[11] A barium swallow is used to identify associated conditions, such as hiatal hernia, gastric ulcers, and abnormal contours of the esophageal lumen.

Antacids relieve symptoms by neutralizing gastric contents. Weight reduction and cessation of smoking also help to alleviate symptoms. Proton pump inhibitors and H2 blockers are common therapies for controlling symptoms and healing esophagitis.[12,13] Sucralfate will coat ulcerated tissue; smooth muscle stimulants, such as cisapride, can increase LES gastric motility and rate of gastric emptying. If other treatments fail or if erosive esophagitis fails to heal, the LES may be narrowed with laparoscopic surgery.

Hiatal hernia

Pathophysiology

Hiatal hernia is the protrusion (herniation) of the upper part of the stomach through the diaphragm and into the thorax.[14] The two types of hiatal hernia are as follows:

1. *Sliding hiatal hernia:* The stomach slides or moves into the thoracic cavity through the esophageal hiatus; a congenitally short esophagus, trauma, or weakening of the diaphragmatic muscles at the gastroesophageal junction is contributory. Coughing, bending, tight clothing, ascites, and pregnancy accentuate the hernia. Symptoms include gastroesophageal reflux and esophagitis.
2. *Paraesophageal hiatal hernia:* The greater curvature of the stomach herniates through a secondary opening in the diaphragm and lies alongside the esophagus. Symptoms include congestion of mucosal blood flow leading to gastritis and ulcer formation. Strangulation of the hernia is a major complication.

Hiatal hernias of both types tend to occur in conjunction with several other diseases, including peptic ulcer, cholecystitis (gallbladder inflammation), cholelithiasis (gallstones), chronic pancreatitis, and diverticulosis.

Clinical Manifestations

Hiatal hernias are often asymptomatic. Generally, a wide variety of symptoms develop later in life and are associated with other gastrointestinal disorders as well. Manifestations include gastroesophageal reflux, dysphagia, heartburn, and epigastric pain. Regurgitation and substernal discomfort after eating are common.

Evaluation and Treatment

Diagnostic procedures include (1) examinations using barium as a contrast medium and (2) endoscopy. A chest x-ray film often will show the protrusion of the stomach into the thorax, indicating paraesophageal hiatal hernia.

Treatment for sliding hiatal hernia is usually conservative. The individual can diminish reflux by eating small, frequent meals and avoiding the recumbent position after eating. Abdominal supports and tight clothing are avoided, and weight control is recommended for obese individuals. Antacids alleviate reflux esophagitis. Individuals who are uncomfortable at night benefit from sleeping in a semi-Fowler position. Surgery (fundoplication) may be performed if medical management fails to control symptoms.

Pyloric obstruction

Pathophysiology

Pyloric obstruction is the narrowing or blocking of the opening between the stomach and the duodenum. This condition can be congenital (see Chapter 35) or acquired. Acquired obstruction is caused by peptic ulcer disease or carcinoma near the pylorus. Duodenal ulcers are more likely than gastric ulcers to obstruct the pylorus. Ulceration causes obstruction resulting from inflammation, edema, spasm, fibrosis, or scarring. Tumors cause obstruction by growing into the pylorus.

Clinical Manifestations

Early in the course of pyloric obstruction, the individual experiences vague epigastric fullness, which becomes more distressing after eating and later in the day. Nausea and epigastric pain may occur as the muscles of the stomach contract in attempts to force chyme past the obstruction. These symptoms disappear when the chyme finally moves into the duodenum. As obstruction progresses, anorexia develops, sometimes accompanied by weight loss. Severe obstruction causes gastric distention and atony (lack of muscle tone and gastric motility). Gastric distention stimulates gastric secretion, which increases the feeling of fullness. Rolling or jarring of the abdomen produces a sloshing sound called the *succussion splash.* At this stage vomiting is a cardinal sign of obstruction. It is usually copious and occurs several hours after eating. The vomitus contains undigested food but no bile. Prolonged vomiting leads to dehydration, which is accompanied by a hypokalemic and hypochloremic metabolic alkalosis caused by loss of potassium and gastric acid. Because food does not enter the intestine, stools are infrequent and small. Prolonged pyloric obstruction causes malnutrition, dehydration, and extreme debilitation.

Evaluation and Treatment

Diagnosis is based on clinical manifestations, a history of ulcer disease, and examination of residual gastric contents. Endoscopy is performed if gastric carcinoma is the suggested cause of pyloric obstruction. Barium studies are contraindicated.

Obstructions resulting from ulceration often resolve with conservative management. A large-bore tube is used to aspirate stomach contents and relieve distention. Then nasogastric suction is maintained for 2 to 3 days to decompress the stomach and restore normal motility. Gastric secretions that contribute to inflammation and edema can be sup-

TABLE 34-2	**Common Causes of Intestinal Obstruction**
Cause	**Pathophysiology**
Hernia	Protrusion of the Intestine through a weakness in the abdominal muscles or through the inguinal ring
Intussusception	Telescoping of one part of the intestine into another; this usually causes strangulation of the blood supply; more common in infants 10-15 mo of age than in adults
Torsion (volvulus)	Twisting of the intestine on its mesenteric pedicle, with occlusion of the blood supply; often associated with fibrous adhesions; occurs most frequently in middle-aged and elderly men
Diverticulosis	Inflamed saccular herniations (diverticuli) of the mucosa and submucosa through the tunica muscularis of the colon; diverticuli are interspersed between thick, circular, fibrous bands; most common in obese individuals older than 60 yr
Tumor	Tumor growth into the intestinal lumen; adenocarcinoma of the colon and rectum is the most common tumoral obstruction; most common in individuals older than 60 yr
Paralytic (adynamic) ileus	Loss of peristaltic motor activity in the intestine; associated with abdominal surgery, peritonitis, hypokalemia, ischemic bowel, spinal trauma, or pneumonia

TABLE 34-3	**Classification of Intestinal Obstruction**
Criteria for Classification	**Definition**
Onset	
Acute	Sudden onset; often caused by torsion, intussusception, or herniation
Chronic	Protracted onset; more commonly from tumor growth or progressive formation of strictures
Extent of obstruction	
Partial	Incomplete obstruction of intestinal lumen
Complete	Complete obstruction of intestinal lumen
Location of obstructing lesion	
Intrinsic	Obstruction develops within intestinal lumen; examples: luminal edema or hemorrhage, foreign bodies (gallstones), tumors, or intraluminal fibrosis
Extrinsic	Obstruction originates outside the intestine; examples: tumors, torsion, fibrosis, hernia, intussusception
Effects on intestinal wall	
Simple	Luminal obstruction without impairment of blood supply
Strangulated	Luminal obstruction with occlusion of blood supply
Closed loop	Obstruction at each end of a segment of the intestine
Causal factors	
Mechanical	Blockage of the intestinal lumen by intrinsic or extrinsic lesions; usually treated surgically
Functional (paralytic ileus)	Paralysis of the intestinal musculature caused by trauma, peritonitis, electrolyte imbalances, or spasmolytic agents; usually treated surgically

pressed with intravenous cimetidine. Fluids and electrolytes (saline and potassium) are given intravenously to effect rehydration and correct hypokalemia and alkalosis (see Chapter 4). Severely malnourished individuals may require parenteral hyperalimentation (intravenous nutrition). Surgery may be required to treat gastric carcinoma or persistent obstruction caused by fibrosis and scarring.

Intestinal obstruction

Intestinal obstruction can be caused by any condition that prevents the normal flow of chyme through the intestinal lumen (Table 34-2). Criteria for classifying intestinal obstruction are summarized in Table 34-3. Intestinal obstruction is classified by cause as simple or functional. Simple obstruction is mechanical blockage of the lumen by a lesion; functional obstruction is a failure of motility (paralytic ileus). Simple obstruction of the small intestine is the most common type of intestinal obstruction. Acute obstructions usually have mechanical causes, such as adhesions or hernias. Chronic or partial obstructions are more often associated with tumors or inflammatory disorders, particularly of the large intestine.

Pathophysiology

The major pathophysiologic alterations are presented in Fig. 34-3. If the obstruction is at the pylorus or high in the small intestine, metabolic alkalosis develops initially as a result of excessive loss of hydrogen ions that normally would be reabsorbed from the gastric juice. With prolonged obstruction or obstruction lower in the intestine, metabolic acidosis is more likely to occur because bicarbonate from pancreatic secretions and bile cannot be reabsorbed. Hypokalemia can be extreme, promoting acidosis and atony of the intestinal wall. Metabolic acidosis also may be accentuated by ketosis, the result of declining carbohydrate stores caused by starvation. If pressure from the distention is severe enough, it occludes the arterial circulation and causes strangulation leading to perforation. Lack of circulation permits the buildup of significant amounts of lactic acid, which worsen the metabolic acidosis. Bacteria also proliferate and may cross the mucosal barrier and cause peritonitis or sepsis.

Clinical Manifestations

Colicky pains followed by vomiting are the cardinal symptoms. Typically the pain occurs intermittently and intensifies for seconds or minutes as a peristaltic wave of muscle contraction meets the obstruction. Sweating, nausea, and hypotension occur as an autonomic response. The passing of the wave is followed by a pain-free interval. With severe distention, the pain may diminish in intensity. If strangulation occurs, the pain loses its colicky character, becoming more constant and severe as ischemia progresses to necrosis, perforation, and peritonitis.

Vomiting and distention vary, depending on the level of the obstruction. Obstruction at the pylorus causes early, profuse vomiting of clear gastric fluid. Obstruction in the proximal small intestine causes mild distention and vomiting of bile-stained fluid. Obstruction lower in the intestine causes more pronounced distention, and vomiting may not occur or may occur later and contain fecal material. Partial obstruction can cause diarrhea or constipation, but complete obstruction usually causes constipation only. Early in the course of complete obstruction, the number of bowel sounds increases, which may be tinkly and accompanied by peristaltic rushes and crampy, abdominal pain. Signs of dehydration, hypovolemia, and metabolic acidosis may be observed as early as 24 hours after the occurrence of complete obstruction. Distention may be severe enough to push against the diaphragm and decrease lung volume. This can lead to atelectasis and pneumonia, particularly in debilitated individuals.

Evaluation and Treatment

Evaluation is based on clinical manifestations. Successful management requires early identification of the site and type of obstruction. Replacement of fluid and electrolytes and decompression of the lumen with gastric or intestinal suction are essential forms of therapy. Immediate surgical intervention is required for strangulation and complete obstruction.

✓ QUICK CHECK

Why is heartburn associated with gastroesophageal reflux?

How does peritonitis develop with bowel obstruction?

Gastritis

Gastritis is an inflammatory disorder of the gastric mucosa. It can be acute or chronic and affect the fundus or antrum or both. *Acute gastritis* erodes the surface epithelium in a diffuse or localized pattern. The erosions are usually superficial.

Acute gastritis is usually the result of injury of the protective mucosal barrier caused by drugs or chemicals. Antiinflammatory drugs cause gastritis, perhaps because they inhibit prostaglandins, which normally stimulate the secretion of mucus. Alcohol, histamine, digitalis, and metabolic disorders such as uremia are contributing factors. The clinical manifestations of acute gastritis can include vague abdominal discomfort, epigastric tenderness, and bleeding. Healing usually occurs spontaneously within a few days. Discontinuing injurious drugs, using antacids, or decreasing acid secretion with cimetidine facilitates healing.

Chronic gastritis tends to occur in elderly individuals and causes thinning and degeneration of the stomach wall. Chronic gastritis is classified as type A (fundal) or type B (antral), depending on the pathogenesis and location of the lesions.

Chronic fundal gastritis, also called *atrophic gastritis*, is the most severe type. The gastric mucosa degenerates extensively in the body and fundus of the stomach, leading to gastric atrophy. Loss of chief cells and parietal cells diminishes acid secretion, so the feedback mechanism that normally inhibits gastrin secretion is impaired, causing elevated plasma levels of gastrin. Pernicious anemia develops because intrinsic factor is unavailable to facilitate vitamin B_{12} absorption.

A significant number of individuals with chronic fundal gastritis have antibodies to parietal cells, intrinsic factor, and gastric cells in their sera, suggesting that an autoimmune mechanism is involved in pathogenesis of the disease. The fact that chronic fundal gastritis occurs in association with other autoimmune diseases strengthens this association. Chronic fundal gastritis is a risk factor for gastric carcinoma, particularly in individuals who develop pernicious anemia.

Chronic antral gastritis generally involves the antrum only and occurs approximately four times more frequently than fundal gastritis. It is not associated with decreased hydrochloric acid secretion, pernicious anemia, or presence of

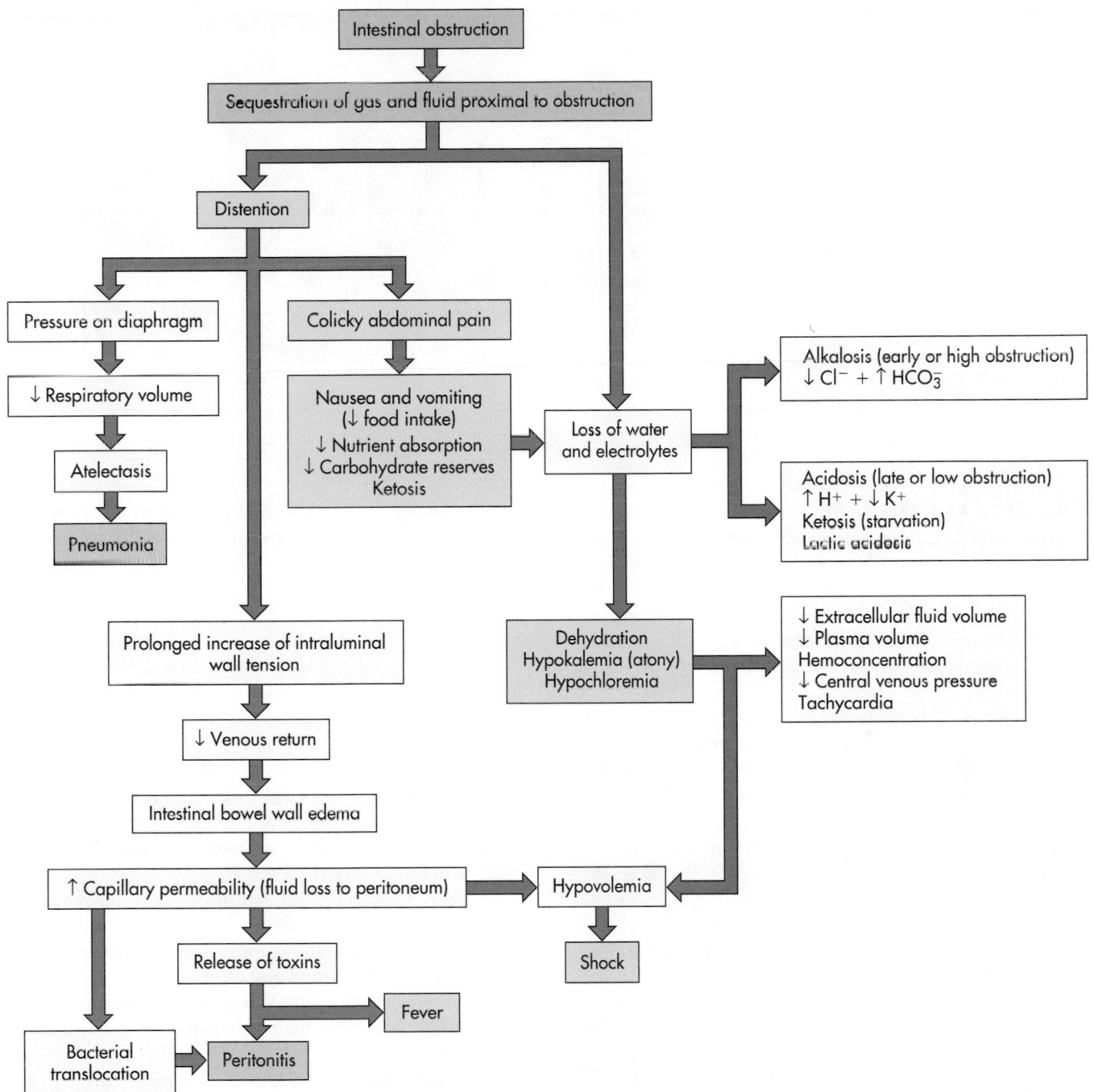

Fig. 34-3 *Pathophysiology of intestinal obstruction.*

parietal cell antibodies. *Helicobacter pylori* is a major causative factor,[15] and mucosal atrophy is rare. In approximately 10% of cases, antibodies to gastrin-secreting cells are found in the serum. Chronic reflux of bile may contribute to the gastritis by persistently disrupting the mucosal barrier (Fig. 34-4).

Signs and symptoms of chronic gastritis often do not correlate with the severity of the disease. Gastroscopic examination and biopsy may show a long-standing inflammatory process and gastric atrophy in an individual with no

history of abdominal distress. Failure to stimulate acid secretion confirms achlorhydria (diminished secretion of hydrochloric acid). The gastric secretions also can be evaluated for the presence of intrinsic factor. Individuals may report vague symptoms, including anorexia, fullness, nausea, vomiting, and epigastric pain. Gastric bleeding may be the only clinical manifestation of gastritis.

Symptoms can usually be managed with smaller meals; a soft, bland diet; and avoidance of alcohol and aspirin. Vitamin B_{12} is administered to correct pernicious anemia.

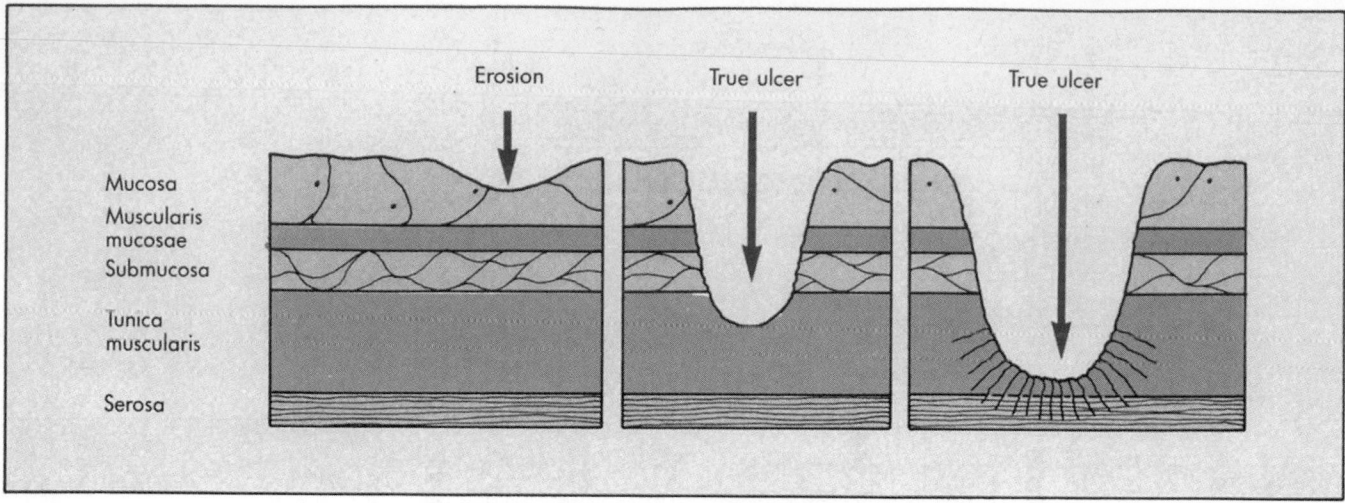

Fig. 34-4 *Lesions caused by peptic ulcer disease.*

Peptic Ulcer Disease

A *peptic ulcer* is a break, or ulceration, in the protective mucosal lining of the lower esophagus, stomach, or duodenum. Such breaks expose submucosal areas to gastric secretions and autodigestion. Peptic ulcers can be acute or chronic, superficial or deep. Superficial ulcerations are called *erosions* because they erode the mucosa but do not penetrate the muscularis mucosae (see Fig. 34-4). True ulcers extend through the muscularis mucosae and damage blood vessels, causing hemorrhage, or perforate the gastrointestinal wall.

Risk factors for peptic ulcer disease are summarized in the Risk Factors box.

> **RISK FACTORS**
>
> **PEPTIC ULCER**
> - Smoking
> - Habitual use of nonsteroidal antiinflammatory drugs (NSAIDs)
> - Alcohol
> - Chronic diseases, such as emphysema, rheumatoid arthritis, cirrhosis, and diabetes
> - Infection of the gastric and duodenal mucosa with *Helicobacter pylori*

From Henriksson, A.E. et al. (1998). Helicobacter pylori and the relation to other risk factors in patients with acute bleeding peptic ulcer. Scandinavian Journal of Gastroenterology, 33(10), 1030-1033.

Psychologic stress may be a risk factor for peptic ulcer disease, although studies of life stress and ulcer disease are inconclusive. Individuals with multiple stressors, poor coping skills, and persistent anxiety and depression in the presence of recurrent peptic ulcers may require psychiatric management.[16]

Duodenal ulcers

Duodenal ulcers occur with greater frequency than other types of peptic ulcers. The incidence of duodenal ulcers is greater among men.[17] Duodenal ulcers tend to develop in younger persons and perhaps in individuals with type O blood.[18]

Pathophysiology

Infection with *H. pylori* and nonsteroidal antiinflammatory drugs (NSAIDs) are the major cause of duodenal ulcer.[19] Hypersecretion of acid and pepsin is the primary cause of duodenal ulcers, but inadequate secretion of bicarbonate by the duodenal mucosa also may be a factor.[20] Factors that contribute to ulcer formation include the following:

1. NSAIDs inhibit prostaglandins and decrease mucus production.
2. *H. pylori* urease leads to ammonia formation, which is toxic to mucosal cells.
3. *H. pylori* phospholipases and other organism-produced enzymes damage the mucosa.
4. *H. pylori* infection stimulates gastrin production, which stimulates acid secretion and ulcer formation.[21]
5. Rapid gastric emptying occurs, which overwhelms the buffering capacity of the bicarbonate-rich pancreatic secretions.
6. There are a greater than usual number of parietal cells (acid-secreting cells) in the gastric mucosa.
7. Cigarette smoking stimulates acid production.
8. Mucosal bicarbonate secretion decreases.

All these factors, singly or in combination, cause acid and pepsin concentrations in the duodenum to penetrate the mucosal barrier and cause ulceration (Fig. 34-5).

Clinical Manifestations

The characteristic manifestation of a duodenal ulcer is chronic intermittent pain in the epigastric area. The pain begins 2 or 3 hours after eating, when the stomach is empty. It is not unusual for pain to occur in the middle of the night and disappear by morning. Pain is relieved rapidly by ingestion of food or antacids, creating a typical "pain-food-relief" pattern. Some individuals with duodenal ulcer may have no

Fig. 34-5 *Duodenal ulcer.* **A,** A deep ulceration in the duodenal wall extending as a crater through the entire mucosa and into the muscle layers. **B,** Sequence of ulcerations from normal mucosa to duodenal ulcer. **C,** Bilateral (kissing) duodenal ulcers in a person using nonsteroidal antiinflammatory drugs (NSAIDs). *(C courtesy David Bjorkman, M.D., University of Utah School of Medicine, Department of Gastroenterology.)*

TABLE 34-4	Characteristics of Gastric and Duodenal Ulcers	
Characteristics	**Gastric Ulcer**	**Duodenal Ulcer**
Incidence		
Age at onset	50-70 yr	20-50 yr
Family history	Usually negative	Positive
Gender (prevalence)	Equal in women and men	Greater in men
Stress factors	Increased	Average
Ulcerogenic drugs	Normal use	Increased use
Cancer risk	Increased	Not increased
Pathophysiology		
Abnormal mucus	May be present	May be present
Parietal cell mass	Normal or decreased	Increased
Acid production	Normal or decreased	Increased
Serum gastrin	Increased	Normal
Serum pepsinogen	Normal	Increased
Associated gastritis	More common	Usually not present
Helicobacter pylori	May be present (60%-80%)	Often present (95%-100%)
Clinical manifestations		
Pain	Located in upper abdomen	Located in upper abdomen
	Intermittent	Intermittent
	Pain-antacid-relief pattern	Pain-antacid or food-relief pattern
	Food-pain pattern	Nocturnal pain common
Clinical course	Chronic ulcer without pattern of remission and exacerbation	Pattern of remissions and exacerbations for years

symptoms; the first manifestation may be hemorrhage or perforation, particularly with history of aspirin or anticoagulant use.

Duodenal ulcers often heal spontaneously but recur within months without treatment. Exacerbations tend to develop in the spring and fall. Healing is accompanied by relief of pain. Constant, unremitting pain may be caused by complications, such as intestinal obstruction or perforation. Bleeding from duodenal ulcers causes hematemesis or melena.

Evaluation and Treatment

Several diagnostic approaches are used to differentiate duodenal ulcers from gastric ulcers or gastric carcinoma. X-ray examinations using barium may show an anatomic deformity created by the ulcer crater. If the x-ray examination is inconclusive, flexible endoscopic evaluations may be performed. Radioimmune assays of gastrin levels are evaluated to identify ulcers associated with gastric carcinomas. *H. pylori* can be detected by endoscopic evaluation or indirectly with a breath test.[22]

Management of duodenal ulcers is aimed at (1) relieving the causes and effects of hyperacidity and (2) administering antacids and drugs that suppress acid secretion (omeprazole). *H. pylori* is treated with a combination of antibiotics and proton pump inhibitors.[23] Risk of duodenal ulcer may be reduced with a high vitamin A and fiber diet.[24] Endoscopic heater probes are effective to stop bleeding.

Gastric ulcers

Gastric ulcers are ulcers of the stomach and occur about equally in males and females, usually between the ages of 55 and 65 years. They are about one fourth as common as duodenal ulcers (Table 34-4).

Pathophysiology

Use of nonsteroidal antiinflammatory drugs and *H. pylori* infection are major causes of gastric ulcer. Generally, gastric ulcers develop in the antral region, adjacent to the acid-secreting mucosa of the body. The primary defect is an abnormality that increases the mucosal barrier's permeability to hydrogen ions. Gastric secretion may be normal or less than normal.

Chronic gastritis is often associated with development of gastric ulcers and may precipitate ulcer formation by limiting the mucosa's ability to secrete a protective layer of mucus (Fig. 34-6). Other factors include the following:
1. Decreased mucosal synthesis of prostaglandin
2. Duodenal reflux of bile
3. Use of ulcerogenic drugs

An increased concentration of bile salts disrupts the gastric mucosa and may decrease the electrical potential across the gastric mucosal membrane. The break permits hydrogen ions to diffuse into the mucosa, where they disrupt permeability and cellular structure. A vicious cycle can be established as the damaged mucosa liberates histamine, which stimulates the increase of acid and pepsinogen production,

Fig. 34-6 *Pathophysiology of gastric ulcer formation.*

blood flow, and capillary permeability. The disrupted mucosa becomes edematous and loses plasma proteins. Destruction of small vessels causes bleeding.

Clinical Manifestations

The clinical manifestations of gastric ulcers are similar to those of duodenal ulcers (see Table 34-4). The pattern of "pain-food-relief" is common, but the pain of gastric ulcers also may occur immediately after eating. Gastric ulcers also tend to be chronic rather than alternating between periods of remission and exacerbation. Gastric ulcers cause more anorexia, vomiting, and weight loss than duodenal ulcers. The evaluation and treatment of gastric ulcers are similar to the evaluation and treatment of duodenal ulcers.

Stress ulcers

A ***stress ulcer*** is an acute form of peptic ulcer that tends to accompany severe illness, systemic trauma, or neural in-

jury.[25] It is not clear if emotional stress causes peptic ulcer, but some studies support this possibility.[26,27] Usually multiple sites of ulceration are distributed within the stomach or duodenum. Decreased mucosal blood flow is an important contributing event in stress ulcer formation.[28] Stress ulcers may be classified as follows:

1. ***Ischemic ulcer:*** develops within hours of events such as hemorrhage, multisystem trauma, severe burns, heart failure, or sepsis that causes ischemia of the stomach and duodenal mucosa; those that develop as a result of burn injury are frequently called *Curling ulcers*

2. ***Cushing ulcer:*** stress ulcer associated with severe head trauma or brain surgery that results from decreased mucosal blood flow and hypersecretion of acid caused by overstimulation of the vagal nuclei

   The primary clinical manifestation of stress ulcers is bleeding. Use of prophylactic antacids, sucralfate, and H2 receptor blockers and suppression of vagal stimulation with

TABLE 34-5   Surgical Management of Peptic Ulcer Disease

Procedure	Definition	Purpose
Neural surgery		
Vagotomy	Severance of the vagus nerve	Eliminate neural stimulus of acid secretion
Selective vagotomy	Severance of vagal branches supplying acid-secreting (parietal) cells	Eliminate neural stimulus of acid secretion
Gastric surgery		
Pyloroplasty	Surgical widening or removal of obstruction of the pylorus	Facilitate gastric emptying
Antrectomy (partial gastrectomy)	Removal of the antrum	Eliminate hormonal stimulus of acid secretion; that is, the gastrin-secreting cells of the antral mucosa
Subtotal gastrectomy	Removal of most of the body and all of the antrum of the stomach	Remove acid-secreting and gastrin-secreting mucosa
Anastomosis (Billroth operation)	Reattachment of stomach to duodenum (Billroth I) or jejunum (Billroth II)	Restore continuity of the gastrointestinal tract after resection

anticholinergic drugs are effective forms of therapy. Stress ulcers seldom become chronic.

Surgical treatment of ulcer

Advances in the medical treatment of peptic ulcer disease have reduced the number of cases requiring surgery to 10% to 15%. The most common indications for ulcer surgery are recurrent or uncontrolled bleeding and perforation of the stomach or duodenum. The primary objectives of surgical treatment are to reduce stimuli for acid secretion, decrease the number of acid-secreting cells in the stomach, and correct complications of ulcer disease (Table 34-5).

Acute complications of gastrectomy or anastomosis are relatively uncommon except in debilitated persons. Chronic complications, however, are likely to develop if a large portion of the stomach has been removed. These complications and their pathophysiologic mechanisms are described in the next section.

✓ QUICK CHECK

What is the most common surgical emergency of the abdomen? How does it develop?

Compare the three types of peptic ulcers.

What is Cushing ulcer?

Postgastrectomy syndromes

Postgastrectomy syndromes are a group of signs and symptoms that occur after gastric resection. They are caused by changes in motor and control functions of the stomach and upper small intestine[29] and include the following:

1. *Dumping syndrome:* rapid emptying of hypertonic chyme from surgically residual stomach (the stomach component remaining after surgical resection) into small intestine 10 to 20 minutes after eating; promoted by loss of gastric capacity, loss of emptying control when pylorus is removed, and loss of feedback control by duodenum when it is removed; responds to dietary management. Symptoms include cramping pain and diarrhea.

2. *Alkaline reflux gastritis:* stomach inflammation caused by reflux of bile and alkaline pancreatic secretions containing proteolytic enzymes that disrupt the mucosal barrier; symptoms include nausea, bilious vomiting, and sustained epigastric pain that worsens after eating and is not relieved by antacids; responds somewhat to avoidance of aspirin and alcohol, but surgical correction may be required.

3. *Afferent loop obstruction:* intermittent severe pain and epigastric fullness after eating as a result of volvulus, hernia, adhesion, or stenosis of the duodenal stump on the proximal side of the gastrojejunostomy; vomiting relieves symptoms; management includes low-fat diet, but surgery is required for complete obstruction.

4. *Diarrhea:* either frequent, persistent elimination of liquid stool or intermittent, precipitous, and unpredictable elimination of a large volume of stool; related to rapid gastric emptying, especially after large intake of high-carbohydrate liquids; small, dry meals and anticholinergic drugs are effective control measures.

5. *Weight loss:* commonly caused by inadequate food intake because individual cannot tolerate carbohydrates or a normal-size meal; stomach is also less able to mix, churn, and break down food.

6. *Anemia:* iron malabsorption may result from decreased acid secretion or lack of duodenum after Billroth II procedure; deficiencies of iron and vitamin B$_{12}$ or folate may result.

7. *Bond disorders:* related to altered calcium absorption and metabolism with increased risk for fractures and deformity.[30]

Malabsorption Syndromes

Malabsorption syndromes interfere with nutrient absorption in the small intestine. Historically they have been classified as maldigestion or malabsorption. *Maldigestion* is failure of the chemical processes of digestion that take place in the intestinal lumen or at the brush border of the intestinal mucosa. Malabsorption is failure of the intestinal mucosa to absorb (transport) the digested nutrients. Frequently these two are interrelated or occur together, making classification difficult. Generally, however, maldigestion is caused by deficiencies of the enzymes needed for digestion. Inadequate secretion of bile salts and inadequate reabsorption of bile in the ileum also contribute to maldigestion. *Malabsorption* is the result of mucosal disruption caused by gastric or intestinal resection, vascular disorders, or intestinal disease.

Pancreatic insufficiency

The pancreatic enzymes (lipase, amylase, trypsin, chymotrypsin) are required for the digestion of proteins, carbohydrates, and fats. *Pancreatic insufficiency* is the deficient production of these enzymes by the pancreas. Causes include chronic pancreatitis, pancreatic carcinoma, pancreatic resection, and cystic fibrosis. Significant damage to or loss of pancreatic tissue must occur before enzyme levels decrease sufficiently to cause maldigestion. Although pancreatic insufficiency causes poor digestion of all nutrients, fat maldigestion is the chief problem. Absence of pancreatic bicarbonate in the duodenum and jejunum causes an acidic pH that worsens maldigestion by preventing activation of the pancreatic enzymes that are present. A large amount of fat in the stool (steatorrhea) is the most common sign of pancreatic insufficiency.

Lactase deficiency

Deficiency of disaccharidase at the brush border of the small intestine is caused by a congenital defect in which a single enzyme, usually lactase, is lacking. *Lactase deficiency* inhibits the breakdown of lactose (milk sugar) into monosaccharides and therefore prevents lactose digestion and absorption across the intestinal wall. Lactase deficiency is most common in blacks and usually does not develop until adulthood. Secondary (acquired) lactase deficiency can be caused by several diseases of the intestine, including gluten-sensitive enteropathy, enteritis, and bacterial overgrowth.

The undigested lactose remains in the intestine, where bacterial fermentation causes gases to form. Undigested lactose also increases the osmotic gradient in the intestine, causing irritation and osmotic diarrhea. Clinical manifestations of lactase deficiency are bloating, crampy pain, diarrhea, and flatulence. The disorder is diagnosed by a lactose-tolerance test. Avoiding milk and adhering to a lactose-free diet relieve symptoms.

Bile salt deficiency

Conjugated bile acids (bile salts) are necessary for the digestion and absorption of fats. Bile salts are conjugated in the bile that is secreted from the liver. When bile enters the duodenum, the bile salts aggregate with fatty acids and monoglycerides to form micelles. Micelle formation solubilizes fat molecules and allows them to pass through the unstirred layer at the brush border (see Chapter 33). A minimum con-

centration of bile salts, termed the *critical micelle concentration,* is required to allow micelles to form. Therefore conditions that decrease the production or secretion of bile result in decreased micelle formation and fat malabsorption. These conditions include advanced liver disease, which decreases production of bile salts; obstruction of the common bile duct, which decreases flow of bile into the duodenum; intestinal stasis (lack of motility), which permits overgrowth of intestinal bacteria that deconjugate bile salts; and diseases of the ileum, which prevent the reabsorption and recycling of bile salts (enterohepatic circulation).

Clinical manifestations of bile salt deficiency are related to poor intestinal absorption of fat and fat-soluble vitamins (A, D, E, K). Increased fat in the stools (steatorrhea) leads to diarrhea and decreased plasma proteins. The losses of fat-soluble vitamins and their effects include the following:

1. Vitamin A deficiency results in night blindness.
2. Vitamin D deficiency results in decreased calcium absorption with bone demineralization (osteoporosis), bone pain, and fractures.
3. Vitamin K deficiency prolongs prothrombin time, leading to spontaneous development of purpura (bruising) and petechiae.
4. Vitamin E deficiency has uncertain effects but may cause testicular atrophy and neurologic defects in children.

The most effective treatment for fat-soluble vitamin deficiency is to increase medium-chain triglycerides in the diet, for example, by using coconut oil for cooking. Vitamins A, D, and K are given parenterally.

Inflammatory Bowel Disease
Ulcerative colitis

Ulcerative colitis is a chronic inflammatory disease that causes ulceration of the colonic mucosa, usually in the rectum and sigmoid colon. The lesions appear in susceptible individuals between 20 and 40 years of age. Risk factors include family history of disease and Jewish descent, and the disease is more prevalent among white populations.

Although the cause of ulcerative colitis is unknown, infectious, genetic, and immunologic factors are all suggested causes.[31] The familial tendency to develop ulcerative colitis and the occurrence of disease in identical twins support a genetic theory of causation. Perhaps most significant are humoral immunologic factors and activated macrophages associated with the disease. Anticolon antibodies have been identified in the sera of individuals with ulcerative colitis. Lymphocytes (T cells) in individuals with ulcerative colitis may have cytotoxic effects on the epithelial cells of the colon.[32] Furthermore, autoimmune disorders, such as systemic lupus erythematosus and erythema nodosum, often accompany ulcerative colitis.

Pathophysiology

The primary lesion of ulcerative colitis begins with inflammation at the base of the crypt of Lieberkühn in the large intestine. The disease is most severe in the rectum and sigmoid

TABLE 34-6 Features of Ulcerative Colitis and Crohn Disease

Feature	Ulcerative Colitis	Crohn Disease
Incidence		
Age at onset	Any age; 10-40 yr most common	Any age; 10-30 yr most common
Family history	Less common	More common
Gender (prevalence)	Equal in women and men	About equal in women and men
Cancer risk	Increased	Not increased
Pathophysiology		
Location of lesions	Large intestine, no "skip" lesions	Large or small intestine, "skip" lesions common
Inflammation and ulceration	Mucosal layer involved	Entire intestinal wall involved
Granulomas	Rare	Common
Friable mucosa	Common	Less common
Anal and perianal fistulae and abscesses	Rare	Common
Narrowed lumen and possible obstruction	Rare	Common
Clinical manifestations		
Abdominal pain	Mild to severe	Mild to severe
Diarrhea	Common	Common
Bloody stools	Common	Less common
Abdominal mass	Rare	Common
Small intestinal malabsorption	Rare	Common
Steatorrhea	Rare	Common
Clinical course	Remissions and exacerbations	Remissions and exacerbations

colon. The mucosa is hyperemic and may appear dark red and velvety. Small erosions form and coalesce into ulcers. Abscess formation, necrosis, and ragged ulceration of the mucosa ensue. Edema and thickening of the muscularis mucosae may narrow the lumen of the involved colon. Mucosal destruction causes bleeding, cramping pain, and an urge to defecate. Frequent diarrhea, with passage of small amounts of blood and purulent mucus, is common. Loss of the absorptive mucosal surface and decreased colonic transit time cause large volumes of watery diarrhea.

 ### Clinical Manifestations
The course of ulcerative colitis consists of intermittent periods of remission and exacerbation. Mild ulcerative colitis involves less mucosa, so that frequency of bowel movements, bleeding, and pain are minimal. Severe forms may involve the entire colon and are characterized by fever, elevated pulse rate, frequent diarrhea (10 to 20 stools/day), urgency, obviously bloody stools, and continuous, crampy pain. Dehydration, weight loss, anemia, and fever result from fluid loss, bleeding, and inflammation. Complications include anal fissures, hemorrhoids, and perirectal abscess. Severe hemorrhage is rare, but chronic blood loss can precipitate hypotension and shock. Edema, strictures, or fibrosis can obstruct the colon. Perforation is an unusual but possible complication. The risk of colon cancer increases significantly after 10 years of ulcerative colitis.

Evaluation and Treatment
Diagnosis of ulcerative colitis is based on the medical history and clinical manifestations. Sigmoidoscopy, barium enema, and x-ray films are used in addition to laboratory data. Infectious causes are ruled out by stool culture. The symptoms of ulcerative colitis are very similar to those of Crohn disease, making differential diagnosis difficult.

Treatment is individualized and depends on the severity of symptoms and the extent of mucosal involvement. The disease is often treated with sulfasalazine (a combination of a sulfa drug and aspirin) or mesalamine. Steroids and aminosalicylates suppress the inflammatory response and help to alleviate the cramping pain. Immunosuppression has been effective. Broad-spectrum antibiotics may be prescribed if bacterial infection is suggested. Severe, unremitting disease can require hospital admission and administration of intravenous fluids. Extreme malnutrition may require intravenous hyperalimentation. Smoking may be of some benefit.[33] Surgical resection of the colon or a colostomy may be performed if other forms of therapy are unsuccessful.[34,35]

Crohn disease
Crohn disease (granulomatous colitis, regional enteritis) is an inflammatory disorder that affects both the large and small intestines. In a small percentage of cases, Crohn disease is difficult to differentiate from ulcerative colitis (Table

34-6). The rectum is seldom involved, and the development of colon cancer is rare. Risk factors and theories of causation are the same as those for ulcerative colitis. Like ulcerative colitis, Crohn disease tends to run in families. Of affected individuals, 10% to 20% have a positive family history. Chromosome 16 may be a susceptible locus.[36] Increased suppressor T cell activity, alterations in immunoglobulin A (IgA) production, and macrophage activation are factors associated with Crohn disease.[37] Psychologic stresses have been suggested as a cause of both Crohn disease and ulcerative colitis. Although stressful events may exacerbate illness, stress is probably not a cause of disease.

Pathophysiology

The inflammation process of Crohn disease begins in the intestinal submucosa and spreads inward and outward to involve the mucosa and serosa. Activated neutrophils cause tissue injury. The ascending colon and the transverse colon are the most common sites of the disease, but both the large and small intestines may be involved. The inflammation can affect some haustral segments but not others, creating "skip lesions." One side of the intestinal wall may be affected and not the other. The ulcerations of Crohn disease produce fissures that extend inflammation into lymphoid tissue. The typical lesion is a granuloma having projections of inflamed tissue surrounded by fibrous scarring. (Granulomas are described in Chapter 6.) Fistulae may form in the perianal area between loops of intestine or extend into the bladder. Smoking increases the risk of developing severe disease.[38]

Clinical Manifestations

Individuals with Crohn disease may have no specific symptoms other than an "irritable bowel" for several years. Nonbloody diarrhea is the most common sign. Other manifestations are related to the location and extent of intestinal involvement. Weight loss and lower abdominal pain accompany Crohn disease. If the ileum is involved, the individual may be anemic as a result of malabsorption of vitamin B_{12}. There also may be deficiencies in folic acid and vitamin D absorption. In addition, proteins may be lost, leading to hypoalbuminemia. There is increased risk for colon cancer with long-standing disease.[39]

Evaluation and Treatment

The diagnosis and treatment of Crohn disease are similar to the diagnosis and treatment of ulcerative colitis. Surgery generally is performed to manage complications such as fistula, abscess, or obstruction.[40]

Diverticular disease

Diverticula are herniations or saclike outpouchings of mucosa through the muscle layers of the colon wall (Fig. 34-7). *Diverticulosis* is asymptomatic diverticular disease. *Diverticulitis* represents inflammation. Diverticular disease is most common in elderly persons, but the incidence is increasing in younger individuals, particularly in those who live in de-

Fig. 34-7 *Diverticular disease.* In diverticular disease, the outpouches *(arrows)* of mucosa seen in the sigmoid colon appear as slitlike openings from the mucosal surface of the opened bowel. *(Modified from Stevens, A. & Lowe., J. (1995). Pathology. London: Mosby.)*

veloped countries where much of the diet consists of refined foods.[41]

Pathophysiology

Although diverticula can occur anywhere in the gastrointestinal tract, the most common site is the sigmoid colon. The diverticula form at weak points in the colon wall, usually where arteries penetrate the tunica muscularis to nourish the mucosal layer. A common associated finding is thickening of the circular and longitudinal (teniae coli) muscles surrounding the diverticula.[42] Hypertrophy and contraction of these muscles increase intraluminal pressure and degree of herniation. Habitual consumption of a low-residue diet reduces fecal bulk, thus reducing the diameter of the colon. According to the law of Laplace (see Chapter 22), wall pressure increases as the diameter of a cylindrical structure decreases. Therefore pressure within the narrow lumen can increase enough to rupture the diverticula. Diverticulitis can cause abscess formation or peritonitis.[43]

Clinical Manifestations

Symptoms of diverticular disease may be vague or absent. Cramping pain of the lower abdomen can accompany constriction of the hypertrophied colonic muscles. Diarrhea, constipation, distention, or flatulence may occur. If the diverticula become inflamed or abscesses form, the individual develops fever, leukocytosis (increased white blood cell count), and tenderness of the lower left quadrant. Severe complications, such as hemorrhage, peritonitis, bowel obstruction, and fistula formation, are rare.

Evaluation and Treatment

Diverticula are often discovered during diagnostic procedures performed for other problems. Sigmoidoscopy permits direct observation of the lesions. Barium enema reveals the muscle hypertrophy, but barium may become trapped in the diverticula and form hard masses.

An increase of dietary fiber intake frequently relieves symptoms.[44] Surgical resection may be required for diverticulitis or if there are severe complications.

Appendicitis

Appendicitis is an inflammation of the vermiform appendix, which is a projection from the apex of the cecum. It is the most common surgical emergency of the abdomen and affects 7% to 12% of the population. It generally occurs between 20 and 30 years of age, although it may develop at any age.

Pathophysiology

The exact mechanism of the cause of appendicitis is controversial. Obstruction of the lumen with stool, tumors, or foreign bodies with consequent bacterial infection is the most common theory. The obstructed lumen does not allow drainage of the appendix, and as mucosal secretion continues, intraluminal pressure increases. The increased pressure decreases mucosal blood flow, and the appendix becomes hypoxic. The mucosa ulcerates, promoting bacterial or other microbial invasion with further inflammation and edema. Inflammation may involve the distal or entire appendix. Gangrene develops from thrombosis of the luminal blood vessels, followed by perforation.[45]

Clinical Manifestations

Gastric or periumbilical pain is the typical symptom of an inflamed appendix. The pain may be vague at first, increasing in intensity over 3 to 4 hours. It may subside and then recur in the right lower quadrant, indicating extension of the inflammation to the surrounding tissues. Nausea, vomiting, and anorexia follow the onset of pain, and a low-grade fever is common. Diarrhea occurs in some individuals, particularly children; others have a sensation of constipation. Perforation, peritonitis, and abscess formation are the most serious complications of appendicitis.

Evaluation and Treatment

In addition to clinical manifestations, the clinician can usually locate the painful site with one finger. Rebound tenderness is usually referred to the right lower quadrant. The white blood cell count ranges from 10,000 to 16,000 cells/mm³ with increased neutrophils. Plain films of the abdomen and computed tomography (CT) scans can assist in differentiating appendicitis from perforated ulcer or cholecystitis. Laparoscopy may be necessary in women of childbearing age.[46]

Appendectomy is the treatment for simple or perforated appendicitis. Surgery provides quick recovery for simple appendicitis. Recovery is more complicated in cases of perforation or abscess formation.[47]

Vascular Insufficiency

The stomach and intestines are supplied by three branches of the abdominal aorta: the celiac axis and the superior and inferior mesenteric arteries. Because of the rich collateral circulation, at least two of the supplying vessels must be compromised to cause ischemia.[48] Atherosclerotic lesions, thrombi, and emboli can develop in these vessels, occluding blood flow and causing ischemia or necrosis in the gastrointestinal tract.

Chronic mesenteric insufficiency can develop secondary to congestive heart failure, acute myocardial infarction, hemorrhage, stenosis, thrombus formation, or any condition that decreases arterial blood flow. Elderly individuals with arteriosclerosis are particularly susceptible. Chronic occlusion is often accompanied by formation of collateral circulation. The collateral vessels may be able to nourish the resting intestine, but after eating, when the intestine requires more blood, the arterial supply may be insufficient. Ischemia develops, causing a cramping abdominal pain (abdominal angina). Progressive vascular obstruction eventually causes continuous abdominal pain and necrosis of the intestinal tissue.

Acute occlusion of mesenteric blood flow results from dissecting aortic aneurysms or emboli. Embolic obstruction is associated with atrial fibrillation, mitral valve disease, and heart valve prostheses. The superior mesenteric artery has a more direct line of flow from the aorta; therefore emboli enter it more readily than the inferior branch, causing ischemia and necrosis of the small intestine. Ischemia and necrosis alter membrane permeability. Increased motility followed by absence of motility results. The damaged intestinal mucosa cannot produce enough mucus to protect itself from digestive enzymes.[49] Fluid moves from the blood vessels into the bowel wall and peritoneum, and its loss causes hypovolemia and further decreases intestinal blood flow. As intestinal infarction progresses, shock, fever, bloody diarrhea, leukocytosis, and abdominal distention develop. Abdominal pain may be severe.

Colicky abdominal pain after eating is a cardinal symptom of chronic mesenteric insufficiency. Some individuals suffer significant weight loss because they stop eating to control the pain. Acute mesenteric insufficiency causes severe continuous pain, rigid abdomen, and bloody diarrhea. Manifestations of unrelieved acute obstruction are distended abdomen, loss of bowel sounds, shock, peritonitis, fever, and tachycardia.

Diagnosis of mesenteric artery occlusion is based on clinical manifestations, mesenteric artery angiography, and abdominal radiography. Frequently a bruit can be heard over the occluded artery. After angiography, a vasodilating agent may be injected into the vessels to improve the circulation. Surgery is required to remove necrotic tissue or repair sclerosed vessels. Mortality is high for individuals with acute occlusion, compromised cardiac output, or coexisting systemic disease.[50]

Disorders of Nutrition
Obesity

Obesity is defined as body mass indexes that correspond to body weight of 120% or more of ideal body weight. Obesity is classified by cause as either exogenous (resulting from an excess of ingested calories) or endogenous (resulting from inherent metabolic problems).[51] Physiologically, obesity can be classified according to the structure and distribution of the adipose tissue itself. Child-onset obesity is both hyperplastic (caused by a greater-than-normal number of fat cells) and hypertrophic (caused by a greater-than-normal size of fat cells). In children, the adipose tissue is dispersed over the entire body and few metabolic abnormalities exist. Adult-onset obesity is hypertrophic; the adipose tissue is centrally located; and glucose intolerance, heart disease, and hypertension are more common. Genotype is an important predisposing factor.

Several theories have been postulated to explain the physiology of obesity:

1. Genetic theory: The obese gene product leptin is expressed in adipose tissue and may control fat stores by regulating food intake. Obese individuals have elevated leptin levels.[52,53]
2. Fat-cell theory: Individuals with hyperplastic fat (adipose) cells are overweight because they have an excessive number and size of fat cells and the number increases whenever a positive energy balance occurs.
3. Lipoprotein-lipase (LPL) theory: LPL promotes fat storage, and obese individuals have elevated levels of LPL in their fat cells, which rise even higher after weight reduction; the LPL works against the maintenance of reduced body weight and stimulates the fat cells to return to their hypertrophic size.
4. Lipostatic theory: Obese individuals have a higher "set point," which makes it difficult for them to maintain weight loss.
5. Thermogenic theory: Obese people are believed to have very few brown fat cells, which are the mitochondria-rich fat cells responsible for heat production, so they cannot burn off excess energy but, rather, store it as fat.
6. Sodium-potassium-adenosine triphosphatase (ATPase) pump theory: This enzyme pump (which transports sodium out of the cell and potassium into the cell and splits adenosine triphosphate, releasing energy) is lacking in obese individuals, leading to a lack of energy release and obesity.
7. Diabetes-associated theory: Excessive food intake stimulates hyperinsulinemia and promotes high blood levels of glucose, which is stored as glycogen in the liver or as triglycerides in the adipose cells, thereby enhancing hypertrophy and hyperplasia of fat cells in the already obese person.
8. Psychologic causation theory: Obese people are directed more by external cues, such as the sight, smell, and taste of food, than by internal cues, such as hunger and satiety; another psychologic theory postulates that eating creates the desire to eat more.

Pathophysiology

Obese individuals are at risk for a number of disorders, including coronary artery disease, diabetes, gallstones, hypertension, cardiovascular disease[54]; breast, cervical, endometrial, and liver cancer in women; and prostatic, colon, and rectal cancer in men.[55] Pulmonary function can be compromised by a large amount of adipose tissue overlying the chest cage. Gas exchange, vital capacity, and expiratory volume all decrease, causing low arterial oxygen tension and high carbon dioxide tension. Sleep apnea can occur. Exercise intolerance and pain in the fingers and weight-bearing joints, particularly the knees, are common. Joint pain may be caused by premature erosion of cartilage.

Evaluation and Treatment

Obesity is evaluated by use of height and weight tables, body mass index (ratio of weight to height), skinfold thickness, hydrostatic weighing, measurement of oxygen intake, and bioelectric impedance analysis. If excess fat interferes with physiologic or psychologic functioning, treatment may be initiated.

Obesity is a chronic condition that is managed with exercise, reduced nutrient intake, medications, surgery, and behavioral and psychologic support. Age at onset, laboratory data about metabolic function (e.g., glucose tolerance tests, serum triglyceride and cholesterol analyses), and distribution of adipose tissue determine the weight-reduction goal. Individuals with adult-onset obesity can reduce the size of their adipose cells and achieve a standard weight. Those with child-onset obesity may never achieve a standard weight.[56]

Anorexia nervosa and bulimia nervosa

Many young adults and adolescents—as many as 1% of women and adolescent girls in the United States—are affected by two complex and related eating disorders: anorexia nervosa and bulimia nervosa.[57] **Anorexia nervosa** is a psychologic and physiologic syndrome characterized by the following:

1. A fear of becoming obese despite progressive weight loss
2. A distorted body image; the perception that the body is fat when it is actually underweight
3. Body weight 15% less than normal for age and height because of refusal to eat
4. In women and girls, absence of three consecutive menstrual periods

Persons with anorexia nervosa frequently deny they have any eating problem. As the disease progresses, muscle and fat depletion give the individual a skeleton-like appearance. Postural hypotension, edema, bradycardia, hypothermia, constipation, and sleep disturbances may ensue. The loss of 25% to 30% of ideal body weight can eventually lead to death caused by starvation-induced cardiac failure. Diagnosis of anorexia nervosa involves a thorough medical history, physical and psychologic examination, and ruling out other causes of anorexia and malnutrition.

Treatment objectives for anorexia nervosa include reversing the compromised physical state, promoting insights and knowledge about the disorder, setting mutual goals, promoting interaction with family members, restoring developmental growth, modifying food habits, and restoring weight.

Correction of nutritional status can require hospitalization. When the individual demonstrates the willingness to eat food for nourishment, dietary protein, carbohydrate, and fat are introduced in tolerable amounts. Psychotherapy begins as soon as the physical symptoms are stabilized and may continue for several years.

Bulimia nervosa is characterized by binging—the consumption of normal to large amounts of food, often several thousand calories at a time—followed by self-induced vomiting or purging of the intestines with laxatives. The group at risk is the same as that for anorexia nervosa, except that bulimia nervosa tends to occur in slightly older, less affluent women. Approximately 50% of individuals with anorexia nervosa are bulimic as well.[58] Many young women stimulate vomiting inappropriately to control weight but are not classified as bulimic unless the pattern is obsessional or normal health or activity is interrupted. Diagnosis of bulimia nervosa is based on these findings:

1. Recurrent episodes of binge eating during which the individual fears not being able to stop
2. Self-induced vomiting, use of laxatives, or fasting to oppose the effect of binge eating
3. Two binge-eating episodes per week for at least 3 months

Although individuals with bulimia nervosa are afraid of gaining weight, their weight usually remains within normal range. Because of negative connotations associated with self-stimulated vomiting and purging, individuals who have bulimia nervosa binge and purge secretly. They may binge and purge as often as 20 times each day. Continual vomiting of acidic chyme can cause pitted teeth, pharyngeal and esophageal inflammation, and tracheoesophageal fistulae. Overuse of laxatives can cause rectal bleeding. Secret binging isolates the bulimic individual and leads to depression and anger that is turned inward. A vicious cycle of depression, overeating to try to feel better, vomiting and purging to maintain a normal weight, and returning depression perpetuates this eating disorder.

Because persons with bulimia are usually older than individuals with anorexia nervosa and have usually separated from a family core, individual or group counseling is the treatment focus. Individuals with bulimia nervosa rarely have physical problems requiring hospital care.

Starvation

Short-term starvation and long-term starvation have different effects.[59] Therapeutic short-term starvation is part of many weight-reduction programs because it causes an initial rapid weight loss that reinforces the individual's motivation to diet. Therapeutic long-term starvation is used in medically controlled environments to facilitate rapid weight loss in morbidly obese individuals. Pathologic long-term starvation can be caused by poverty; chronic diseases of the cardiovascular, pulmonary, hepatic, and digestive systems; malabsorption syndromes; and cancer.

Short-term starvation, or extended fasting, consists of several days of total dietary abstinence or deprivation. Once all available energy has been absorbed from the intestine,

glycogen in the liver is converted to glucose through *glycogenolysis,* the splitting of glycogen into glucose. This process peaks within 4 to 8 hours, and gluconeogenesis begins. *Gluconeogenesis* is the formation of glucose from non-carbohydrate molecules: lactate, pyruvate, amino acids, and the glycerol portion of fats. Like glycogenolysis, gluconeogenesis takes place within the liver. Both of these processes deplete stored nutrients and thus cannot meet the body's energy needs indefinitely. Proteins continue to be catabolized to a minimal degree, providing carbon for the synthesis of glucose.

Long-term starvation begins after several days of dietary abstinence and eventually causes death. The major characteristic of long-term starvation is a decreased dependence on gluconeogenesis and an increased use of ketone bodies (products of lipid and pyruvate metabolism) as a cellular energy source. Depressed insulin and glucagon levels promote lipolysis in adipose tissue. Lipolysis liberates fatty acids, which supply energy to cardiac and skeletal muscle cells, and ketone bodies, which sustain brain tissue. Fatty acid or ketone body oxidation meets most energy needs of the cells. (Some glucose is still needed as fuel for brain tissue.) Once the supply of adipose tissue is depleted, proteolysis begins. The breakdown of muscle protein is the last process to supply energy for life. Death results from severe alterations in electrolyte balance and loss of renal, pulmonary, and cardiac function.

Adequate ingestion of appropriate nutrients is the obvious treatment for starvation. In medically induced starvation, the body is maintained in a ketotic state until the desired amount of adipose tissue has been lysed. Starvation imposed by chronic disease, long-term illness, or malabsorption is treated with enteral or parenteral nutrition.

✓ QUICK CHECK

Why are Crohn disease and ulcerative colitis called inflammatory bowel diseases?

List the manifestations of anorexia nervosa.

How do child-onset obesity and adult-onset obesity differ?

DISORDERS OF THE ACCESSORY ORGANS OF DIGESTION

The accessory organs of digestion (liver, gallbladder, pancreas) secrete substances necessary for digestion and, in the case of the liver, carry out metabolic functions needed to maintain life. Causes are inflammatory disease, obstruction of ducts, and tumors. (Cancers of the digestive tract are described at the end of the chapter.)

Clinical Manifestations of Liver Disorders

Of all the accessory organ disorders, acute or chronic liver disease leads to the most systemic, life-threatening complications. These complications include portal hypertension, ascites, hepatic encephalopathy, jaundice, and hepatorenal syndrome.

Portal hypertension

Portal hypertension is abnormally high blood pressure in the portal venous system. Pressure in this system is normally 3 mm Hg; portal hypertension is an increase to at least 10 mm Hg.

Pathophysiology

Portal hypertension is caused by disorders that obstruct or impede blood flow through any component of the portal venous system or vena cava. The obstruction can occur as a result of thrombosis, inflammation, or fibrosis of the sinusoids, as occurs in cirrhosis of the liver, viral hepatitis, or schistosomiasis (a parasitic infection).[60] Portal outflow to the vena cava can be impeded by hepatic vein thrombosis or cardiac disorders that impair the pumping ability of the right heart. This causes blood to back up and increases pressure in the portal system. The most common cause of portal hypertension is obstruction caused by cirrhosis of the liver (see p. 969).

Long-term portal hypertension causes several problems that are difficult to treat and can be fatal:
1. *Varices* (distended, tortuous, collateral veins). Prolonged elevation of pressure in collateral veins causes their transformation into varices, particularly in the lower esophagus and stomach, but also in the rectum.
2. *Splenomegaly* (enlargement of the spleen) caused by increased pressure in the splenic vein, which branches from the portal vein.
3. *Ascites* (the accumulation of fluid in the peritoneal cavity) caused by increased pressure in the mesenteric tributaries of the portal vein. Hydrostatic pressure forces water out of these vessels and into the peritoneal cavity.
4. *Hepatic encephalopathy,* also called portal-systemic encephalopathy, which is characterized by central nervous system disturbances, particularly reversible alterations of consciousness.

Blood that is shunted through collateral vessels to the systemic veins bypasses the liver, where toxins, hormones, and other harmful substances normally are removed. Hepatic encephalopathy results from the presence of these substances, particularly ammonia, in blood that reaches the brain.

Clinical Manifestations

Vomiting of blood from bleeding esophageal varices is the most common clinical manifestation of portal hypertension. Slow, chronic bleeding from varices causes anemia or melena. Usually the bleeding is from varices that have developed slowly over a period of years.

Rupture of esophageal varices causes hemorrhage and voluminous vomiting of dark-colored blood. The ruptured varices are usually painless. Rupture is caused by a combination of erosion by gastric acid and elevated venous pressure. Mortality from ruptured esophageal varices ranges from 30% to 60%. Recurrent bleeding of esophageal varices indicates a poor prognosis. Most individuals die within 1 year.

Evaluation and Treatment

Portal hypertension is often diagnosed at the time of variceal bleeding and confirmed by endoscopy and evaluation of portal venous pressure. Distended collateral veins may radiate over the abdomen, giving rise to the description of caput medusae (Medusa head). The individual usually has a history of jaundice, hepatitis, or alcoholism.

Emergency management of bleeding varices includes use of vasopressors and compression of the varices with an inflatable Sengstaken-Blakemore tube, sclerotherapy, or variceal ligation. Surgical shunts may decompress the varices, but this treatment can precipitate encephalopathy or liver failure. Liver transplant is an alternative.[61]

Ascites

Ascites is the accumulation of fluid in the peritoneal cavity. Ascites traps body fluid in a "third space" from which it cannot escape. The effect is to reduce the amount of fluid available for normal physiologic functions. Cirrhosis is the most common cause of ascites, but others include heart failure, constrictive pericarditis, abdominal malignancies, nephrotic syndrome, and malnutrition.[62,63] Of individuals who develop ascites caused by cirrhosis, 25% die within 1 year. Continued heavy drinking is associated with this mortality.

Pathophysiology

Several factors contribute to the development of ascites. Impaired excretion of sodium by the kidneys promotes water retention. Portal hypertension and reduced serum albumin levels cause capillary hydrostatic pressure to exceed capillary osmotic pressure. This imbalance pushes water into the peritoneal cavity. Portal hypertension also increases the production of hepatic lymph, which "weeps" into the peritoneal cavity. Peripheral vasodilation associated with increased nitric oxide "underfills" the vascular system with hormonal stimulation that promotes renal sodium and water retention.

With cirrhosis, both portal hypertension and decreased production of albumin by hepatocytes contribute to the ascites. Besides reducing albumin synthesis, deranged liver metabolism permits the accumulation of hormones that regulate sodium and water balance. As ascites sequesters more and more body fluid, the kidneys respond by retaining sodium and water in amounts exceeding intake, particularly in response to increased aldosterone and antidiuretic hormone. This expands plasma volume, thereby accelerating portal hypertension and ascites formation.[64]

Ascites can be complicated by bacterial peritonitis, an inflammatory response that increases mesenteric capillary permeability. As plasma seeps out of the permeable mesenteric capillaries, it adds to the volume of ascitic fluid. Fig. 34-8 summarizes the mechanisms by which cirrhosis of the liver causes ascites.

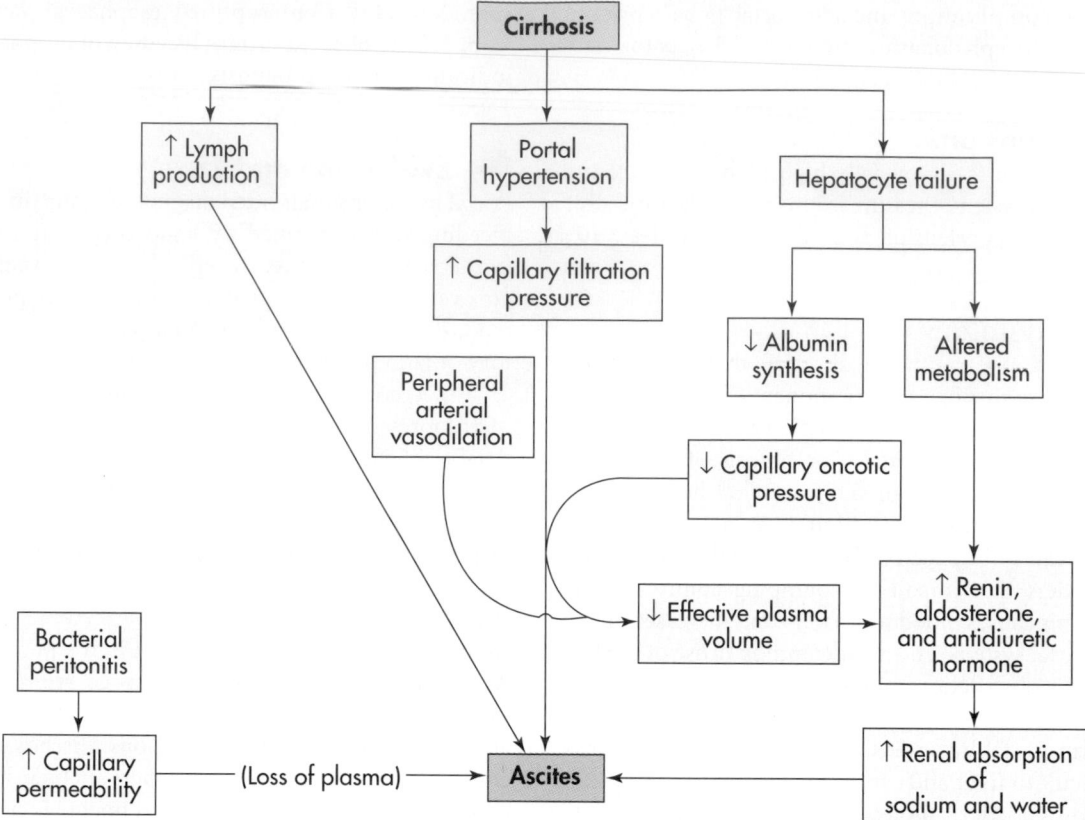

Fig. 34-8 *Mechanisms of ascites caused by cirrhosis.*

Clinical Manifestations

The accumulation of ascitic fluid causes weight gain, abdominal distention, and increased abdominal girth (Fig. 34-9). Large volumes of fluid (10 to 20 L) displace the diaphragm and cause dyspnea by decreasing lung capacity. Respiratory rate increases, and the individual assumes a semi-Fowler position to relieve the dyspnea. Approximately 10% of individuals with ascites develop bacterial peritonitis, which causes fever, chills, abdominal pain, decreased bowel sounds, and cloudy ascitic fluid.

Evaluation and Treatment

Diagnosis is usually based on clinical manifestations and identification of liver disease. Paracentesis is used to aspirate ascitic fluid for bacterial culture, biochemical analysis, and microscopic examination. The goal of treatment is to relieve discomfort. If the restoration of liver function is possible, the ascites diminishes spontaneously. In the meantime, dietary salt restriction and potassium-sparing diuretics can reduce ascites. Serum electrolytes are monitored carefully because the individual is at risk for hyponatremia and hypokalemia.

Palliative measures include paracentesis to remove 1 or 2 L of ascitic fluid and relieve respiratory distress. However, the removal of too much fluid relieves pressure on blood vessels and carries the risk of hypotension, shock, or death. Despite repeated paracentesis, ascitic fluid reaccumulates in individuals with irreversible disease. Paracentesis is also

Fig. 34-9 *Massive ascites in an individual with cirrhosis.* Distended abdomen, dilated upper abdominal veins, and inverted umbilicus are classic manifestations. *(From Prior, J.A., Silberstein, J.S., & Stang, J.M. [1981]. Physical diagnosis: The history and examination of the patient [6th ed.]. St. Louis: Mosby.)*

likely to cause peritonitis. Individuals with ascites and portal hypertension have a poor prognosis.

Hepatic encephalopathy

Hepatic encephalopathy (portal-systemic encephalopathy) is a complex neurologic syndrome characterized by impaired cerebral function, flapping tremor (asterixis), and electroencephalogram (EEG) changes. The syndrome may

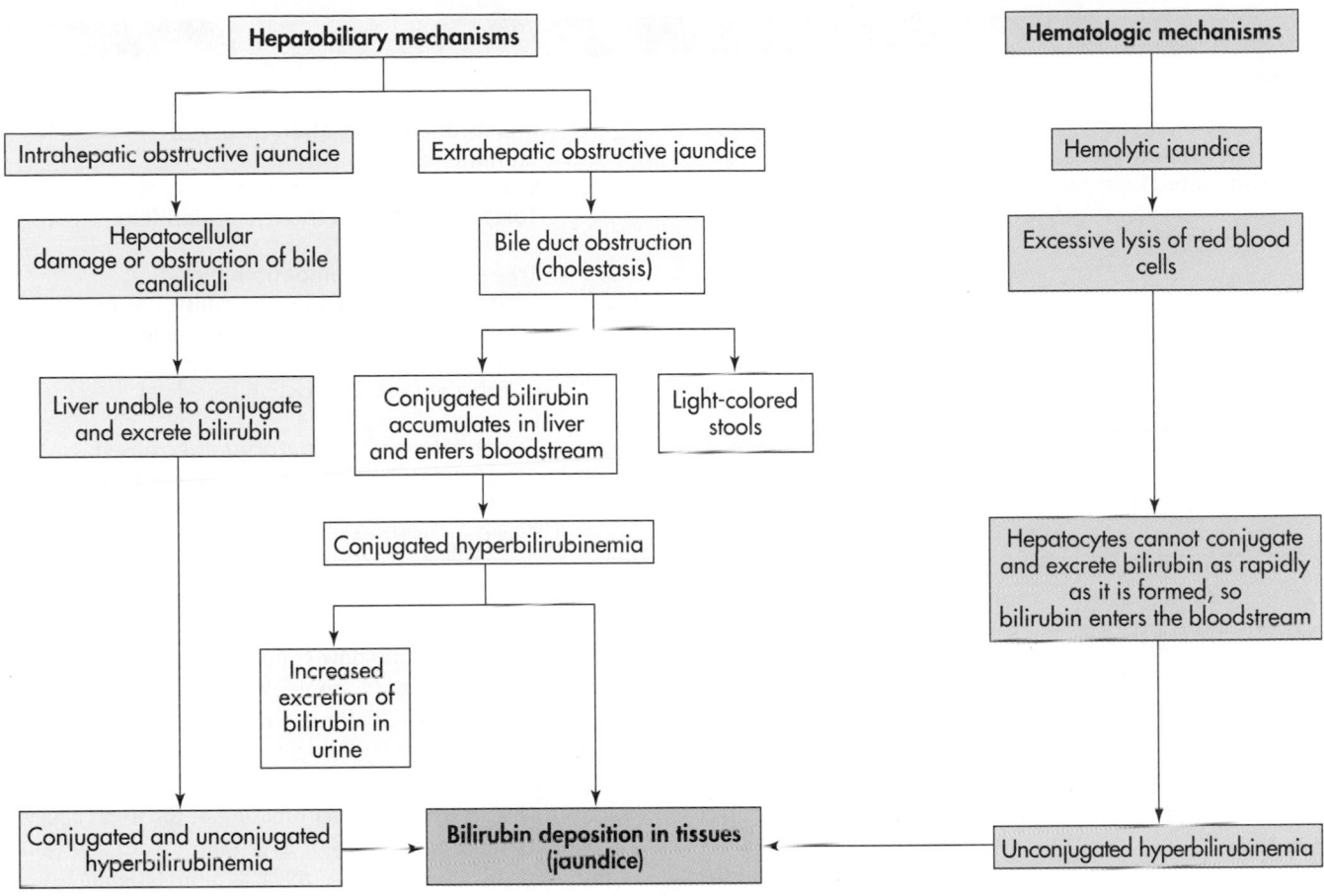

Fig. 34-10 *Mechanisms of jaundice.*

develop rapidly during acute fulminant hepatitis or slowly during the course of chronic liver disease.

Pathophysiology

Hepatic encephalopathy probably results from a combination of biochemical alterations that affect neurotransmission. Liver dysfunction and collateral vessels that shunt blood around the liver to the systemic circulation both permit toxins absorbed from the gastrointestinal tract to circulate freely to the brain. The most hazardous substances are end-products of intestinal protein digestion, particularly ammonia. Ammonia that reaches the brain may alter cerebral energy metabolism or interfere with neurotransmitters.

Blood levels of ammonia do not account for all symptoms associated with hepatic encephalopathy. The accumulation of short-chain fatty acids, serotonin, tryptophan, and false neurotransmitters probably contributes to neural derangement.[65] Infection, hemorrhage, electrolyte imbalance including zinc deficiency, sedatives, and analgesics can also precipitate stupor and coma in the presence of liver disease.[66]

Clinical Manifestations

Subtle changes in personality, memory loss, irritability, lethargy, and sleep disturbances are common initial manifestations of hepatic encephalopathy. Symptoms then can progress to confusion, flapping tremor of the hands, stupor, convulsions, and coma. Coma is usually a sign of liver failure and ultimately results in death.

Evaluation and Treatment

Diagnosis of hepatic encephalopathy is based on a history of liver disease and clinical manifestations. Electroencephalography and blood chemistry tests provide supportive data.

Correction of fluid and electrolyte imbalances and withdrawal of depressant drugs metabolized by the liver are first steps in the treatment of hepatic encephalopathy. Reduction of blood ammonia levels is accomplished by restricting dietary protein intake and eliminating intestinal bacteria. Neomycin is effective in sterilizing the bowel, but it can be nephrotoxic. Lactulose may be administered to prevent ammonia absorption in the colon.[67]

Jaundice

Jaundice, or *icterus,* is a yellow or greenish pigmentation of the skin caused by *hyperbilirubinemia* (plasma bilirubin concentrations above 1.2 mg/dl). Hyperbilirubinemia and jaundice can result from excessive hemolysis of red blood cells or disorders of the bile ducts or liver cells (Fig. 34-10). Jaundice in newborns is caused by impaired bilirubin uptake and conjugation (see Chapter 35).

TABLE 34-7	Three Common Types of Jaundice	
Type	Mechanism	Causes
Hemolytic jaundice (predominately un-conjugated bilirubin)	Destruction of erythrocytes	Membrane defect of erythrocytes Immune reaction Severe infection Toxic substances in the circulation (e.g., snake venom) Transfusion of incompatible blood
Obstructive jaundice (predominately con-jugated bilirubin)	Obstruction of passage of conjugated bilirubin from liver to intestine	Obstruction of bile duct by gallstones or tumor (extrahepatic obstructive jaundice) Obstruction of bile flow through the liver (intrahepatic obstructive jaundice) Drugs
Hepatocellular jaundice	Failure of liver cells (hepatocytes) to conjugate bilirubin and of bilirubin to pass from liver to intestine	Genetic defect of hepatocyte (decreased enzymes), such as occurs in premature infants (see Chapter 35) Severe infections

Pathophysiology

Obstructive jaundice can result from extrahepatic or intra-hepatic obstruction.[68] *Extrahepatic obstructive jaundice* develops if the common bile duct is occluded by a gallstone or tumor. Bilirubin conjugated by the hepatocytes cannot flow into the duodenum. Therefore it accumulates in the liver and enters the bloodstream, causing hyperbilirubinemia. Because conjugated bilirubin is water soluble, it appears in the urine.

Intrahepatic obstructive jaundice involves disturbances in hepatocyte function and obstruction of bile canaliculi.[69] The uptake, conjugation, and excretion of bilirubin are affected because of elevated levels of both conjugated and unconjugated bilirubin. Obstruction of bile canaliculi diminishes flow of conjugated bilirubin into the common bile duct. In mild cases, some of the bile canaliculi open. Consequently the amount of bilirubin in the intestinal tract may be only slightly decreased.

Excessive hemolysis (breakdown) of red blood cells can cause **hemolytic jaundice.** Increased unconjugated bilirubin is formed through metabolism of the heme component of destroyed red blood cells and exceeds the conjugation ability of the liver, causing blood levels of unconjugated bilirubin to rise. Unconjugated bilirubinemia is the major cause of hemolytic jaundice. Because it is not water-soluble, it is not excreted in the urine. The reserve conjugation ability of the liver usually prevents long-term unconjugated hyperbilirubinemia greater than 4 to 5 mg/dl. Severe hemolytic crisis, such as that which occurs with sickle cell disease (see Chapter 20) and hemolytic drugs, can cause jaundice. If unconjugated hyperbilirubinemia exceeds 5 mg/dl, both hemolytic and liver disorders are indicated. The causes of jaundice are summarized in Table 34-7.

Clinical Manifestations

Conjugated hyperbilirubinemia may cause the urine to darken several days before the onset of jaundice. The com-plete obstruction of bile flow from the liver to the duodenum causes light-colored stools. With partial obstruction the stools are normal in color and bilirubin is present in the urine.

Fever, chills, and pain often accompany jaundice resulting from viral or bacterial inflammation of the liver (e.g., viral hepatitis). Manifestations of liver injury from any cause commonly include anorexia, malaise, and fatigue. Yellow discoloration may first occur in the sclera of the eye and then progress to the skin. Pruritus frequently accompanies jaundice because bilirubin accumulates in the skin.

Evaluation and Treatment

Laboratory evaluation of serum establishes whether elevated plasma bilirubin is conjugated or unconjugated or both. The history and physical examination identify underlying disorders, such as alcoholism, exposure to hepatitis virus, or gall-bladder disease. The treatment for jaundice consists of correcting the cause.

Hepatorenal syndrome

Hepatorenal syndrome consists of advanced liver disease and functional renal failure with oliguria, sodium and water retention (with or without ascites and peripheral edema), hypotension, and peripheral vasodilation.[70] Renal disorders associated with liver disease can have numerous causes, but hepatorenal syndrome is usually associated with alcoholic cirrhosis and fulminant hepatitis. The renal failure is not caused by primary renal disease or other extrinsic factors, but rather by circulatory alterations.

Pathophysiology

Oliguric hepatic failure generally accompanies a sudden decrease in blood volume secondary to massive gastrointestinal bleeding or hypotension caused by failing liver function. Hypotension also can be caused by the excessive use of diuretics to treat ascites. A significant number of individuals with

TABLE 34-8	Characteristics of Viral Hepatitis				
Characteristic	**Hepatitis A**	**Hepatitis B**	**Hepatitis D**	**Hepatitis C**	**Hepatitis E**
Virus	27-nm RNA virus	42 nm DNA virus	36 nm RNA virus	30-60 nm RNA-virus	32 nm RNA virus
Antigens	HAAg	HBsAg HBcAg HBcAg	Anti-HDV	Anti-HCV	Anti-HEV
Incubation period	30 days	60-180 days	30-180 days	35-60 days	15-60 days
Route of transmission	Fecal-oral, parenteral, sexual	Parenteral, sexual	Parenteral?, fecal-oral, sexual	Parenteral, sexual	Fecal-oral
Onset	Acute with fever	Insidious	Insidious	Insidious	Acute
Carrier state	Negative	Positive	Positive	Positive	Negative
Severity	Mild	Severe; may be prolonged or chronic	Severe	Unknown	Severe in pregnant women
Chronic hepatitis	No	Yes	Yes	Yes	No
Age-group affected	Children and young adults	Any	Any	Any	Children and young adults
Prophylaxis	Hygiene, immune serum globulin	Hygiene, HBV vaccine	Hygiene, HBV vaccine	Hygiene, screening blood, interferon alpha	Hygiene, safe water

RNA, *Ribonucleic acid;* DNA, *deoxyribonucleic acid;* HAAg, *hepatitis A antigen;* HBsAG, *hepatitis B surface antigen;* HBcAg, *hepatitis B core antigen;* HDV, *hepatitis D virus;* HCV, *hepatitis C virus;* HEV, *hepatitis E virus;* HBV, *hepatitis B virus.*

advanced liver disease develop oliguria unrelated to any precipitating event. Liver failure is the apparent cause of functional renal failure in hepatorenal syndrome. Inappropriate constriction of renal arterioles is proposed as the causative mechanism for decreased glomerular filtration and oliguria. Intrarenal vasoconstriction may result from the selective effects of vasoactive substances that accumulate in the blood because of liver failure. Vasoconstriction also may be a compensatory response to portal hypotension and the pooling of blood in the splanchnic circulation. The exact reason for the vasoconstriction is unknown.

Clinical Manifestations

The onset of hepatorenal manifestations may be gradual or acute. Oliguria and complications of advanced liver disease, including jaundice, ascites, and gastrointestinal bleeding, are usually present. Systolic blood pressure is usually below 100 mm Hg. Nonspecific symptoms of hepatorenal syndrome include anorexia, weakness, and fatigue.

Evaluation and Treatment

Despite oliguria, serum potassium levels do not become dangerously elevated until the terminal stages of the hepatorenal syndrome. Blood urea increases, followed by an increase in creatinine concentration. Urine osmolality is increased, but urine sodium concentrations are below normal. Urine specific gravity is above 1.015.

The prognosis is usually poor and is related to a failing liver. Secondary problems, including fluid and electrolyte disorders, bleeding, infections, and encephalopathy, are vigorously treated.

✓ QUICK CHECK

How does portal hypertension promote ascites?

Why is unconjugated bilirubin elevated in hemolytic jaundice?

Describe hepatorenal syndrome.

Disorders of the Liver
Viral hepatitis

Viral hepatitis is a relatively common systemic disease that affects primarily the liver. Five strains of viruses cause different types of hepatitis: hepatitis A virus (HAV), hepatitis B virus (HBV), hepatitis D virus (HDV), hepatitis C virus (HCV), and hepatitis E virus (HEV). Hepatitis A formerly was known as infectious hepatitis and hepatitis B as serum hepatitis. The first five viruses can cause acute hepatitis, and types B and C also cause chronic hepatitis.[71] Hepatitis G virus (HGV) is a virus discovered in 1995 that is transmitted parenterally and sexually. It usually does not cause hepatitis or alter the cause of other liver diseases.[72] A recent report indicates it may be associated with fulminant hepatitis.[73] Characteristics of the different types of viruses that cause hepatitis are presented in Table 34-8.

Pathophysiology

All five types of viral hepatitis can cause acute, icteric illness. The pathologic lesions of hepatitis are similar to those caused by other viral infection. Hepatic cell necrosis, scarring, Kupffer cell hyperplasia, and infiltration by mononuclear phagocytes occur with varying severity. Regeneration of hepatic cells begins within 48 hours of injury. The inflammatory process can damage and obstruct bile canaliculi, leading to cholestasis and obstructive jaundice. In milder cases the liver parenchyma is not damaged. Damage tends to be most severe in cases of hepatitis B and C. Hepatitis B is also associated with acute fulminating hepatitis, a rare form of the disease that is characterized by massive hepatic necrosis. Acute fulminating hepatitis causes severe encephalopathy, which is manifested as confusion, stupor, and coma. Liver failure can occur, leading to intestinal bleeding, cardiorespiratory insufficiency, and renal failure. There is also an association between HBV and HCV and hepatocellular cancer.[74]

Clinical Manifestations

The spectrum of manifestations ranges from absence of symptoms to fulminating hepatitis, with rapid onset of liver failure and coma. Acute viral hepatitis causes abnormal liver function test results. The serum aminotransferase values, aspartate transaminase (AST) and alanine transaminase (ALT), are elevated but not consistent with the extent of cellular damage. The clinical course of hepatitis usually consists of three phases:

1. *Prodromal phase:* begins about 2 weeks after exposure and ends with the appearance of jaundice; marked by fatigue, anorexia, malaise, nausea, vomiting, headache, hyperalgia, cough, and low-grade fever; infection is highly transmissible during this phase.
2. *Icteric phase:* begins 1 to 2 weeks after prodromal phase and lasts 2 to 6 weeks; jaundice, dark urine, and clay-colored stools are common; liver is enlarged, smooth, and tender, and percussion causes pain; this is the actual phase of illness.
3. *Recovery phase:* begins with resolution of jaundice, about 6 to 8 weeks after exposure; symptoms diminish, but liver remains enlarged and tender; liver function returns to normal 2 to 12 weeks after the onset of jaundice.

Chronic active hepatitis is the persistence of clinical manifestations and liver inflammation after acute hepatitis B, hepatitis C, and hepatitis D. Liver function tests remain abnormal for longer than 6 months, and hepatitis B surface antigen (HBsAg) persists. Chronic, active hepatitis B is a predisposition to cirrhosis and primary hepatocellular carcinoma.

Evaluation and Treatment

The most specific diagnostic test for viral hepatitis is serologic analysis for HBsAg, which is the marker for HBV. Diagnosis of type A hepatitis is based on the presence of anti-HAV, as is the diagnosis of HCV. The assay for HDV is the total antibody to hepatitis D and antigen (anti-HDV). A test for HEV has not been developed. Liver function tests also can indicate other viral liver diseases, drug toxicity, or alcoholic hepatitis.

There is no specific treatment for acute viral hepatitis. For most individuals the disease is self-limiting with full recovery. Physical activity may be restricted. A low-fat, high-carbohydrate diet is beneficial if bile flow is obstructed. Alpha interferon can be useful in the treatment of chronic hepatitis B and hepatitis C, and thymosin may be a promising new treatment for HBV.[75]

To prevent transmission of hepatitis A, handwashing and use of gloves for disposing of bedpans and fecal matter are imperative. HAV may be shed in the feces for up to 3 months after onset of symptoms.[76] The administration of immune globulin before exposure or early in the incubation period can prevent hepatitis A and hepatitis B. Vaccines are available to protect against HAV and HBV infection. Prophylaxis is recommended for health care workers and others who are at risk for contact with infected body fluids, particularly children.[77]

HEALTH ALERT

Treatment for Chronic Hepatitis

Chronic hepatitis B (HBV) and C (HCV) infections affect millions of individuals in the United States and the world. Both diseases can progress to cirrhosis or hepatocellular carcinoma. Currently, alpha interferons are the only therapies approved for treatment, and approximately 50% of those with HCV and 25% with HBV do not respond and may require liver transplantation. Treatment is costly, and new antiviral agents and use of combination antivirals are being evaluated. Aggressive vaccination for prevention of hepatitis is needed.

Data from Heathcote, J. (1998). Consensus interferon: A novel interferon for the treatment of hepatitis C. Journal of Viral Hepatitis, 5(Suppl. 1), 13-18; Hoofnagle, J.H. (1998). Therapy of viral hepatitis. Digestion, 59(5), 563-578; Malaguarnera, M. et al. (1997). Interferon, cortisone, and antivirals in the treatment of chronic viral hepatitis: A review of 30 years of therapy. Pharmacology, 17(5), 998-1005; Wong, J.B. et al. (1998). Pretreatment evaluation of chronic hepatitis C: Risks, benefits, and costs. Journal of the American Medical Association, 280(24), 2088-2093.

Fulminant hepatitis

Fulminant hepatitis is a clinical syndrome resulting in severe impairment or necrosis of liver cells and potential liver failure. The disorder may occur as a complication of hepatitis C or hepatitis B, particularly HBV infection compounded by infection with the delta virus. Toxic reactions to drugs and congenital metabolic disorders also can cause fulminant hepatitis.

Edematous hepatocytes and patchy areas of necrosis and inflammatory cell infiltrates disrupt the parenchyma. The death of hepatocytes may be caused by viral or immunologic damage.

Acute liver failure usually develops within 6 to 8 weeks after the initial symptoms of viral hepatitis or a metabolic liver disorder. Anorexia, vomiting, abdominal pain, and progressive jaundice are initial signs, followed by ascites and gastrointestinal bleeding. Hepatic encephalopathy is manifested as lethargy, altered motor functions, and coma and is related to cerebral edema, ischemia, and brain stem hernia-

TABLE 34-9	Cirrhosis of the Liver	
Type and Disease Name	**Causal Mechanisms**	**Pathophysiology**
Alcoholic cirrhosis, Laennec cirrhosis, portal cirrhosis, fatty cirrhosis	Toxic effects of chronic, excessive alcohol intake; acetylaldehyde formed by alcohol metabolism damages hepatocytes	Fatty liver, inflammation (alcoholic hepatitis), and derangement of the lobular architecture by necrosis and fibrosis (cirrhosis)
Biliary cirrhosis (intrahepatic or extrahepatic obstruction of bile flow)		
Primary biliary cirrhosis	Unknown; possibly an autoimmune mechanism	Inflammation and scarring of lobular bile ducts
Secondary biliary cirrhosis	Obstruction by neoplasms, strictures, or gallstones	Inflammation and scarring of bile ducts proximal to the obstruction
Postnecrotic cirrhosis	Viral hepatitis caused by HAV or hepatitis C; drugs or more toxins; autoimmune destruction	Replacement of necrotic tissue with cirrhotic tissue, particularly fibrous, nodular scar tissue
Metabolic cirrhosis	Metabolic defects and storage disease, such as α_1-antitrypsin deficiency, glycogen storage disease, hemochromatosis, Wilson disease, galactosemia	Inflammation and scarring with specific morphologic changes related to cause

HAV, *Hepatitis A virus.*

tion. Liver function tests show elevations of both direct and indirect serum bilirubin, serum transaminases, and blood ammonia. Prothrombin time is prolonged. Renal failure and pulmonary distress can occur.[78]

Treatment of acute liver failure is supportive. The hepatic necrosis is irreversible, and 60% to 90% of affected children die. Liver transplantation may be lifesaving and should be considered early.[79] Survivors usually do not develop cirrhosis or chronic liver disease.

Cirrhosis

Cirrhosis is an irreversible inflammatory disease that disrupts liver structure and function and is a leading cause of death in the United States. Disorganization of hepatic tissues is caused by diffuse fibrosis and nodular regeneration between fibrous bands that give the liver a cobbly appearance. The liver may be larger or smaller than normal, and usually it is firm or hard when palpated. Cirrhosis is often classified by cause (Table 34-9).

Cirrhosis develops slowly over a period of years. Its severity and rate of progression depend on the cause. If toxins, such as alcohol, are involved, the rate of cell death and the severity of inflammation depend on the amount of toxin present. Removal of the toxin slows the progression of liver damage and enhances the process of regeneration.[80]

Alcoholic cirrhosis

Deaths from alcohol-related liver disease have increased over the past decade. However, high alcohol consumption among women leads to earlier and more severe cirrhosis.[81] The incidence of alcoholic cirrhosis is greatest in middle-age men. In the United States mortality resulting from cirrhosis is highest among nonwhites. Although alcoholic cirrhosis is the most prevalent of the different types of cirrhosis, the occurrence of cirrhosis among persons with alcoholism is relatively low (approximately 25%). The amount and duration of alcohol consumption are positively related to the extent of liver damage. Abuse of any type of alcoholic beverage can cause cirrhosis. Malnutrition may add to the risk of cirrhosis in alcohol abusers.[82,83]

Fatty liver is the mildest form of alcoholic liver disease. It can be caused by relatively small amounts of alcohol, may be asymptomatic, and is reversible with cessation of drinking.[84]

Alcoholic hepatitis is a precursor of cirrhosis characterized by inflammation, degeneration, and necrosis of hepatocytes and infiltration of polymorphonuclear leukocytes and lymphocytes. The injured hepatocytes contain Mallory bodies (hyaline endoplasmic reticulum), indicating the onset of fibrosis. The mechanism of hepatocyte injury is not clearly understood, but immunologic factors are suggested. Serum IgA is often elevated in individuals with alcoholic hepatitis, and liver antigens and antibodies have been identified in those with progressive alcoholic liver disease. The inflammation and necrosis caused by alcoholic hepatitis stimulate the fibrosis characteristic of the cirrhotic stage of disease.

Pathophysiology

Alcoholic cirrhosis is caused by the toxic effects of alcohol on the liver, immunologic alterations, and oxidative stress from lipid peroxidation. Alcohol is transformed to acetaldehyde, and excessive amounts significantly alter hepatocyte function. Mitochondrial function is impaired, decreasing oxidation of fatty acid. Enzyme and protein synthesis may be depressed or altered, and hormone and ammonia degradation is diminished. Acetaldehyde inhibits export of proteins from the liver, alters metabolism of vitamins and minerals, and in-

Fig. 34-11 *Clinical manifestations of cirrhosis. ADH,* Antidiuretic hormone; *AST,* aspartate transaminase; *ALT,* alanine transaminase.

duces malnutrition.[85] Cellular damage initiates an inflammatory response that, along with necrosis, results in excessive collagen formation. Fibrosis and scarring alter the structure of the liver and obstruct biliary and vascular channels.[86]

Alcoholic cirrhosis begins with fatty infiltration, fibrosis, and cirrhosis. Fat deposition (deposition of triglycerides) within the liver is caused primarily by increased lipogenesis and decreased fatty acid oxidation by hepatocytes. Lipids mobilized from adipose tissue or dietary fat intake may contribute to fat accumulation. Cessation of alcohol intake reverses the fatty accumulation, but fibrosis and liver damage are irreversible.

Clinical Manifestations

Fatty infiltration causes no specific symptoms or abnormal liver function test results. The liver is usually enlarged, however, and the individual has a history of continuous alcohol intake during the previous weeks or months. Anorexia, nausea, jaundice, and edema develop with advanced fatty infiltration or the onset of alcoholic hepatitis (Fig. 34-11).

The clinical manifestations of alcoholic hepatitis can be mild or severe. Nonspecific symptoms include fatigue, weight loss, and anorexia. Toxic effects of alcohol also can cause testicular atrophy, reduced libido, azoospermia, and decreased testosterone in men. Manifestations of acute illness include nausea, anorexia, fever, abdominal pain, and jaundice. Cirrhosis is a multiple-system disease and causes hepatomegaly, splenomegaly, ascites, gastrointestinal hemorrhage, portal hypertension, hepatic encephalopathy, and esophageal varices. Anemia results from blood loss, poor nutrition, and hypersplenism. The presence of numerous and severe manifestations increases the risk of death.

Evaluation and Treatment

The diagnosis of alcoholic hepatitis is based on the individual's history and clinical manifestations. The results of liver function tests are abnormal, and serologic studies show elevated serum enzymes and bilirubin, decreased serum albumin, and prolonged prothrombin time. Individuals with severe symptoms are treated with a regimen of corticosteroids.[87]

Liver biopsy can confirm the diagnosis of cirrhosis, but biopsy is not necessary if clinical manifestations of cirrhosis are evident. There is no specific treatment for alcoholic cirrhosis. Rest, a nutritious diet, and management of complications, such as ascites, gastrointestinal bleeding, and encephalopathy, are essential. Cessation of drinking is essential and slows the progression of liver damage, improves clinical symptoms, and prolongs life. Orthotopic liver transplantation can be successful for treatment of end-stage liver disease.[88]

Biliary cirrhosis

Biliary cirrhosis differs from alcoholic cirrhosis in that the damage and inflammation leading to cirrhosis begin in bile canaliculi and bile ducts, rather than in the hepatocytes. The two types of biliary cirrhosis are *primary* and *secondary*. Although both involve bile duct pathology, they differ with respect to cause, risk factors, and mechanisms of obstruction and inflammation as follows:

1. *Primary biliary cirrhosis:* causes inflammation and destruction of the intrahepatic bile ducts; affects women and those older than 30 years; progresses insidiously from pruritus, hyperbilirubinemia, jaundice, and light-colored stools to cirrhosis, portal hypertension, and encephalopathy; life expectancy is 5 to 10 years after onset of symptoms. Primary biliary cirrhosis can be detected by identifying the disease-specific antibody.[89] Liver transplant is highly effective.[90]

2. *Secondary biliary cirrhosis:* caused by prolonged partial or complete obstruction of common bile duct or branches by gallstones, tumors, fibrotic strictures, or chronic pancreatitis; biliary atresia and cystic fibrosis are causative in children; necrotic areas develop and lead to proliferation and inflammation of portal ducts, producing edema and fibrosis; surgery or endoscopy relieves obstruction, prolongs survival, and diminishes or resolves symptoms.

> ### ✓ QUICK CHECK
>
> What are the major pathologic differences between alcoholic and biliary cirrhosis?
>
> How does hepatits A virus (HAV) differ from hepatitis B virus (HBV)?
>
> How are varices and ascites associated with portal hypertension?

Disorders of the Gallbladder

Obstruction and inflammation are the most common disorders of the gallbladder. Obstruction is caused by *gallstones,* which are aggregates of substances in the bile. The gallstones may remain in the gallbladder or be ejected, with bile, into the cystic duct. Gallstones that become lodged in the cystic duct obstruct the flow of bile into and out of the gallbladder and cause inflammation. Gallstone formation is termed *cholelithiasis.* Inflammation of the gallbladder or cystic duct is known as *cholecystitis.*

Fig. 34-12 *Resected gallbladder containing mixed gallstones. (From Kissane, J.M. [Ed.]. [1990].* Anderson's pathology *[9th ed.]. St. Louis: Mosby.)*

Cholelithiasis

Cholelithiasis is a prevalent disorder in developed countries, where incidence is 10% to 20%, although many individuals are asymptomatic. Gallstones are of two types: cholesterol and pigmented. Cholesterol stones are the most common. Risk factors include obesity, middle age, female gender, American Indian ancestry, and gallbladder, pancreatic, or ileal disease. Pigmented stones, which are common, occur later in life and are associated with cirrhosis.[91]

Pathophysiology

Cholesterol gallstones form in bile that is supersaturated with cholesterol produced by the liver. Supersaturation sets the stage for cholesterol crystal formation, or the formation of "microstones." More crystals then aggregate on the microstones, which grow to form "macrostones." This process usually occurs in the gallbladder, which may have decreased motility. The stones may lie "silent" or become lodged in the cystic or common duct, causing pain and cholecystitis.[92] The stones can accumulate and fill the entire gallbladder (Fig. 34-12). Pigmented stones form from increased levels of unconjugated bilirubin, which binds with calcium.

Clinical Manifestations

Abdominal pain and jaundice are the cardinal manifestations of cholelithiasis. Vague symptoms include heartburn, flatulence, epigastric discomfort, and food intolerances, particularly to fats and cabbage. The pain (biliary colic) is caused by the lodging of one or more gallstones in the cystic or common duct. It can be intermittent or steady and usually occurs in the right upper quadrant, radiating to the mid-upper area of the back. Jaundice indicates that the stone is located in the common bile duct.

Evaluation and Treatment

Diagnosis is based on the history, physical examination, and radiographic evaluation. An oral cholecystogram usually outlines the stones. Intravenous cholangiography is used to differentiate cholelithiasis from other causes of extrahepatic biliary obstruction if the cholecystogram is negative. Endoscopic or percutaneous cholangiography is also a diagnostic option.

Laparoscopic cholecystectomy is the preferred treatment for gallstones that cause obstruction or inflammation. Alternative treatments are the administration of drugs that dissolve the stones and ultrasonic lithotripsy.[93]

Cholecystitis

Cholecystitis can be acute or chronic, but both forms are almost always caused by a gallstone lodged in the cystic duct.[94] The gallbladder becomes distended and inflamed, with pain similar to that caused by gallstones. Pressure against the distended wall of the gallbladder decreases blood flow and may result in ischemia, necrosis, and perforation. Fever, leukocytosis, rebound tenderness, and abdominal muscle guarding are common findings. Serum bilirubin and alkaline phosphatase levels may be elevated. The acute abdominal pain of cholecystitis must be differentiated from that caused by pancreatitis, myocardial infarction, and acute pyelonephritis of the right kidney. Cholangiography or radioactive scan can confirm the diagnosis.

Narcotics may be required to control pain, and antibiotics (e.g., gentamicin, clindamycin) often are prescribed to manage bacterial infection in severe cases. Persistent symptoms or development of chronic cholecystitis punctuated by recurrent, acute attacks usually requires gallbladder resection (cholecystectomy). If pancreatic abscesses develop, they are usually resected.[95]

Disorders of the Pancreas

Pancreatitis, or inflammation of the pancreas, is a relatively rare and potentially serious disorder that occurs equally in men and women in their 50s. Pancreatitis can be acute or chronic and is associated with conditions such as alcoholism, obstructive biliary tract disease (particularly cholelithiasis), peptic ulcers, trauma, and hyperlipidemia, as well as certain drugs.[96]

Acute pancreatitis

Pathophysiology

Acute pancreatitis (acute hemorrhagic pancreatitis) is usually a mild disease, but about 20% of those with the disease develop a severe pancreatic inflammation requiring hospital care. Although the precise pathogenic mechanism or sequence of events often is unknown, alcoholism and biliary tract obstruction are commonly associated. The most common theory is that pancreatitis develops because of obstruction to the outflow of pancreatic enzymes by bile and pancreatic duct obstruction, which permits leakage of pancreatic enzymes into pancreatic tissue. The leaked enzymes become activated, initiating autodigestion and acute pancreatitis. Gallstone obstruction of the common bile duct with bile reflux into the pancreas contributes to attacks of acute pancreatitis.[97] Toxic mediators are released into the bloodstream and cause injury to vessels and other organs, such as the lungs and kidneys. Myocardial depression and shock can develop secondary to the release of vasoactive peptides. These systemic effects are major causes of multiple organ involvement, morbidity, and mortality.[98]

Clinical Manifestations

Epigastric or midabdominal pain ranging from mild abdominal discomfort to severe, incapacitating pain is caused by (1) edema, which distends the pancreatic ducts and capsule, (2) chemical irritation and inflammation of the peritoneum, and (3) irritation or obstruction of the biliary tract. Fever and leukocytosis accompany the inflammatory response. Nausea and vomiting are caused by hypermotility or paralytic ileus secondary to the pancreatitis or peritonitis.

Abdominal distention accompanies bowel hypermotility and the accumulation of fluids in the peritoneal cavity. Hypotension and shock occur frequently because plasma volume is lost as enzymes and kinins released into the circulation increase vascular permeability and dilate vessels. Hypovolemia, hypotension, and myocardial insufficiency result. A small percentage of individuals develop tachypnea and hypoxemia secondary to pulmonary edema, atelectasis, or pleural effusions caused by circulating pancreatic enzymes. In severe cases hypovolemia decreases renal blood flow sufficiently to impair renal function. Tetany may develop as a result of calcium deposited in areas of fat necrosis or as a decreased response to parathormone. Transient hyperglycemia also can occur if glucagon is released from damaged alpha cells in the pancreatic islets. Multiple organ failure accounts for most deaths with severe acute pancreatitis.

Evaluation and Treatment

Diagnosis is based on clinical findings, identification of associated disorders, and laboratory studies. Elevated serum amylase is a characteristic but is not diagnostic of severity or specificity of disease. Serum lipase elevations are a sensitive marker of pancreatic injury, particularly of acute alcoholic pancreatitis. Newer enzyme assays are being developed.[99] Urine amylase and serum lipase are also elevated.

The goal of treatment for acute pancreatitis is to stop the process of autodigestion and prevent systemic complications. Narcotic medications may be needed to relieve pain. To decrease pancreatic secretions and "rest the gland," oral food and fluids are withheld and continuous gastric suction is instituted. Nasogastric suction may not be necessary with mild pancreatitis, but it helps to relieve pain and prevent paralytic ileus in individuals who are nauseated and vomiting. Parenteral fluids are essential to restore blood volume and prevent hypotension and shock. Parenteral hyperalimentation should be initiated to reverse the catabolic state associated with severe pancreatitis. Drugs that decrease gastric acid production (e.g., cimetidine) can decrease stimulation of the pancreas by secretin. Antibiotics may control infection. The risk of mortality increases significantly with the development of infection or pulmonary, cardiac, and renal complications.

Chronic pancreatitis

Structural or functional impairment of the pancreas leads to *chronic pancreatitis.* Chronic alcohol abuse is the most common cause.[100] Chronic pancreatitis causes continuous or intermittent abdominal pain, which usually intensifies after a meal. Occasionally manifestations of pancreatic enzyme

TABLE 34-10	Cancer of the Gut, Liver, and Pancreas			
Organ	**Deaths Out of All Cancers Combined**	**Risks**	**Cell Type**	**Common Manifestations**
Esophagus	2%	Malnutrition Alcohol Tobacco Chronic reflux	Squamous cell Adenocarcinoma	Chest pain Dysphagia
Stomach	2%	Salty food Nitrates-nitrosamines Gastric atrophy	Adenocarcinoma Squamous cell	Anorexia Malaise Weight loss Upper abdominal pain Vomiting Occult blood

Colorectal	12%	Polyps
		Ulcerative colitis
		Diverticulitis
		High-refined carbohydrates,
		    low-fiber, high-fat diet
			Adenocarcinoma (left
			    colon grows in ring;
			    right colon grows as
			    mass)
				Pain
				Mass
				Anemia
				Bloody stool
				Obstruction
				Distention

Liver	2%	HBV, HCV, HDV Cirrhosis Intestinal parasite Aflatoxin from moldy peanuts	Hepatomas Cholangiomas	Pain Anorexia Bloating Weight loss Portal hypertension Ascites ± jaundice

Pancreas	5%	Chronic pancreatitis
		Cigarette smoking
		Alcohol (?)
		Diabetic women
			Adenocarcinoma (exo-
			    crine part of gland,
			    ductal epithelium)
				Weight loss
				Weakness
				Nausea
				Vomiting
				Abdominal pain
				Depression ± jaundice
				May have insulin-secreting
				    tumors with symptoms
				    of hypoglycemia

From American Cancer Society (ACS). (1999). Cancer facts & figures—1999. Atlanta: The Society.
All the above cancers are within the top 10 causes of death from cancer.
HBV, *Hepatitis B virus;* HCV, *hepatitis C virus;* HDV, *hepatitis D virus.*

deficiency, such as steatorrhea or a malabsorption syndrome, are present. To correct enzyme deficiencies and prevent malabsorption, oral enzyme replacements are taken before and during meals. Loss of islet cell function can cause insulin-dependent diabetes. Cessation of alcohol intake is essential for the management of chronic pancreatitis.

Fibrosis, strictures, continued inflammation, and pancreatic cysts are common lesions of chronic pancreatitis. The cysts are walled-off areas or pockets of pancreatic juice, necrotic debris, or blood within or adjacent to the pancreas. Surgical drainage or partial resection of the pancreas may be required to relieve pain and to prevent cystic rupture.[101] Chronic pancreatitis is a risk factor for pancreatic cancer.

CANCER OF THE DIGESTIVE SYSTEM
Cancer of the Gastrointestinal Tract
Cancer of the esophagus

Carcinoma of the esophagus is a rare type of cancer, with an incidence of less than 1% (Table 34-10) in the United States

and Europe.[102] In the United States it occurs more in blacks than in whites and peaks at about 60 years of age.

Pathogenesis

Carcinoma of the esophagus is usually squamous cell carcinoma or, less commonly, adenocarcinoma. Adenocarcinomas are frequently secondary to infiltration by a gastric carcinoma or to the presence of Barrett epithelium (columnar rather than squamous epithelium in the lower esophagus), which is associated with chronic gastroesophageal reflux.[103] Carcinomas can occur at any level of the esophageal tract but are most common at the gastroesophageal junction.

The pathogenesis of esophageal carcinoma is facilitated by (1) alterations of esophageal structure and function that permit food and drink to remain in the esophagus for prolonged periods, (2) ulceration and metaplasia caused by esophageal reflux, and (3) chronic exposure to irritants, such as alcohol and tobacco, that cause neoplastic transformation (see Chapter 10). Chronic inadequate nutrition can impair esophageal structure and function. Nutritional deprivation, particularly deficiencies of vitamin A and zinc, produces mucosal changes and vulnerability to neoplastic changes.[104] (See Risk Factors box.)

 RISK FACTORS

ESOPHAGEAL CANCER
- Tobacco use
- Alcoholism
- Dietary factors: deficiencies of trace elements and vitamins
- Malnutrition associated with poor economic conditions or special dietary habits
- Reflux esophagitis
- Sliding hiatal hernia

 Clinical Manifestations

The two main manifestations of esophageal carcinoma are chest pain and dysphagia. The most common type of pain is heartburn (pyrosis). It is initiated by eating spicy or highly seasoned foods and by lying down. Dysphagia (pain on swallowing) is usually pressurelike and may radiate posteriorly between the scapulae. Odynophagia may be initiated by the swallowing of cold liquids. Spontaneous chest pain is more difficult to diagnose positively. Some individuals with esophageal cancer complain of a constant retrosternal pain that radiates to the back. Dysphagia usually progresses rapidly. It is mostly painless during the early stages of esophageal carcinoma.

Evaluation and Treatment

Individuals with dysphagia undergo endoscopy so that specimens can be obtained and examined for neoplastic change. Endoscopic ultrasound is also used for staging. CT studies of the thorax are also used for diagnosis. Esophageal cancer metastasizes rapidly and therefore has a poor prognosis. It is impossible to remove all lymph nodes with the tumor, but removal of the primary lesion and the local lymph nodes can benefit the individual with esophageal cancer. If the malignancy has not spread beyond these sites, cure is likely. If spread has occurred, however, an incomplete resection is of little benefit.

Cancer of the stomach

Although the incidence of gastric cancer has declined in the United States, it still represents about 1% to 2% of all new cancer cases annually.[102] In Japan, the British Isles, and Iceland, the incidence of stomach cancer has remained high consistently. Studies of Japanese immigrants to the United States show that offspring who are born and raised in the United States have an incidence rate comparable with that of other Americans. These data illustrate the importance of environmental factors, such as diet, to carcinogenesis.

The most important environmental causative factors of gastric cancer are (1) infection with *Helicobacter pylori (H. pylori)*,[105] (2) salt added to food, (3) food additives (e.g., ni-

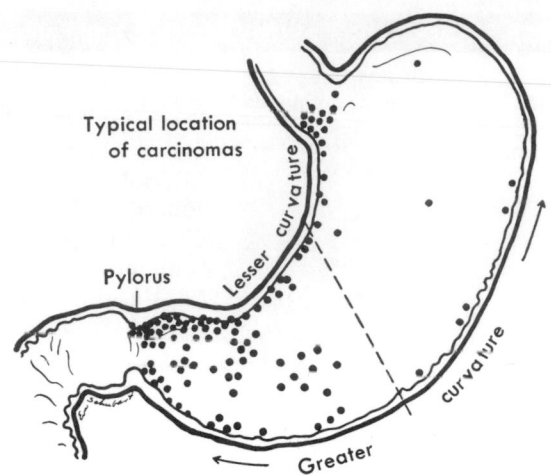

Fig. 34-13 *Typical sites of stomach cancer.* (From del Regato, J.A., Spjut, H.J., & Cox, J.D. [1985]. Cancer: Diagnosis, treatment, and prognosis [2nd ed.]. St. Louis: Mosby.)

trates) in pickled or salted foods (e.g., bacon), and (4) low intake of fruits and vegetables. Dietary salt enhances the conversion of nitrates to carcinogenic nitrosamines in the stomach. Salt is also caustic to the stomach and can cause chronic atrophic gastritis. Finally, hypertonic salt solutions delay gastric emptying. Delayed emptying increases the time during which carcinogenic nitrosamines can exert their effects on the stomach mucosa. Nitrates interact with amino acids in the stomach to form nitrosamines, enhanced at a low pH by iodides and thiocyanates. Nitrates are thought to be active only when converted to nitrites and to cause stomach cancer once atrophic gastritis has occurred. *H. pylori*–associated gastritis increases the risk for gastric cancer.[106]

The incidence of gastric cancer is greater in males than in females. Other nonenvironmental risk factors are a family history of gastric adenocarcinoma, blood type (blood group A), and pernicious anemia, which causes atrophy of the gastric mucosa in the same locations where gastric tumors arise. Loss of tumor suppressor genes may be important in gastric cancer.[107]

 Pathogenesis

Gastric cancer usually begins in the glands of the stomach mucosa. Approximately 50% develop in the prepyloric antrum (Fig. 34-13). Atrophic gastritis associated with *H. pylori* infection and intestinal metaplasia are strongly linked to the development of gastric cancer. Insufficient acid secretion by the atrophic mucosa creates a relatively alkaline environment that permits bacteria to multiply and act on nitrates. The resulting increase in nitrosoamines damages the deoxyribonucleic acid (DNA) of mucosal cells further, promoting metaplasia and neoplasia. Duodenal reflux may also contribute to intestinal metaplasia. The reflux contains caustic bile salts that destroy the mucosal barrier that normally protects the stomach.

Clinical Manifestations

The early stages of gastric cancer are generally asymptomatic or produce vague symptoms such as loss of appetite (especially for meat), malaise, and "indigestion." Later manifestations of gastric cancer include unexplained weight loss, upper abdominal pain, vomiting, change in bowel habits, and anemia caused by persistent occult bleeding. The prognosis is poor because symptoms do not occur until the tumor has penetrated the muscle layers of the stomach, spread to surrounding tissues, and entered the draining lymph nodes and veins, causing distant metastases. Generally the first manifestations of carcinoma are caused by distant metastases.

Evaluation and Treatment

Most symptoms suggest a problem in the upper gastrointestinal tract, and the lesion is shown by a barium x-ray film. Direct endoscopic visualization and biopsy usually establish the diagnosis. Another definitive technique is microscopic examination of exfoliated cells obtained by lavage during endoscopy.

Surgery is the usual treatment for gastric cancer. Staging is determined by pathologic findings after resection. Radiation therapy is generally unsuccessful, and immunotherapy is still experimental. Chemotherapy sometimes reduces the tumor. Individuals who respond well to chemotherapy generally live longer than those who do not.[108]

QUICK CHECK

How do gallstones form?

Compare acute and chronic pancreatitis.

What factors are associated with cancer of the esophagus?

Cancer of the colon and rectum

Cancer of the lower intestinal tract (colorectal cancer) is the second most common cause of cancer death in the United States, for both men and women. Colorectal cancer accounts for 10% to 15% of all cancer deaths.[102] Cancer of the colon tends to occur in individuals older than 50 years and is rare in children. Clustering in families is common; familial adenomatous polyposis has been mapped to chromosome 5, and hereditary nonpolyposis colorectal cancers are mapped to chromosomes 2 and 3. Other colorectal cancers are caused by multiple gene interactions. Worldwide, the prevalence of colorectal cancer is highest in populations with high socioeconomic standards, possibly because of dietary habits. (See Risk Factors box.) Cancer of the small intestine is rare and represents less than 1% of gastrointestinal cancers.[109]

Pathogenesis

Genetic events are associated with the development of colonic cancer. Deletion of genes is linked to the transformation of normal colon epithelial cells to benign and malignant adenomas.[110] Dietary factors, including high fat, low fiber, and low calcium, may promote somatic mutations.

RISK FACTORS

CANCER OF THE COLON AND RECTUM
- High-fat (especially egg consumption), low-fiber diet
- High consumption of alcohol
- Cigarette smoking
- Familial polyposis
- Low levels of physical activity
- Ulcerative colitis after 10 years
- Gastrectomy

From Martinez, M.E. et al. (1997). Leisure-time physical activity, body size, and colon cancer in women. Nurses' Health Study Research Group. Journal of the National Cancer Institute, 89(13), 948-955; Colditz, G.A., Cannuscio, C.C., & Frazier, A.L. (1997). Physical activity and reduced risk of colon cancer: Implications for prevention. Cancer-Causes-Control, 8(4), 649-667.

Promoting mechanisms are related to prolonged contact of the fecal mass with colon mucosa.[111]

Colorectal polyps are closely associated with development of cancer. A polyp, or papilloma, is a fingerlike projection arising from the mucosal epithelium. Most polyps are benign. Neoplastic polyps are pedunculated (stalk) adenomatous polyps or sessile (papillary or villous) adenomas (Fig. 34-14). Once the adenoma traverses the muscularis mucosae, it becomes invasive and highly malignant. Adenomas can be detected early, however, and the submucosa may not be penetrated for several years. The larger the polyp, the greater the risk of colorectal cancer. Although lesions larger than 1.5 cm occur less frequently, they are more likely to be malignant than those smaller than 1.0 cm. For other conditions commonly confused with colorectal cancer see Table 34-11.

Most colorectal cancers are moderately differentiated adenocarcinomas. These tumors have a long preinvasive phase, and when they invade, they tend to grow slowly. Colorectal carcinoma starts in the glands of the mucosal lining. Because the lymphatic channels are located under the muscularis mucosae, the lesions must traverse this layer before metastasis can occur.

Clinical Manifestations

Tumors of the right (ascending) colon and left (descending) colon evolve into two distinct tumor types.[112] On the right side the lesions are polypoid and extend along one wall of the cecum and ascending colon. Clinical manifestations include pain, palpable mass in the lower right quadrant, anemia, and dark-red or mahogany-colored blood mixed with the stool (Fig. 34-15). These large, bulky tumors become necrotic and ulcerated, contributing to persistent blood loss and anemia. Obstruction is unusual because the growth does not readily encircle the colon.

Tumors of the left, or descending, colon start as small, elevated, buttonlike masses. This type grows circumferentially and spreads along the entire bowel wall, eventually ulcerat-

Adenomatous polyp

Focal atypia
(cancer in situ)

Focal cancer
(malignant adenoma)

Focal cancer invading
stalk with some "benign"
polyp still in body

Invasive cancer con-
taining piece of polyp

Polypoid invasive cancer
without polyp remnant

Ulcerated invasive cancer
without polyp remnant

Fig. 34-14 *Development of cancer of the colon from adenomatous polyps.* The tumor becomes invasive if it penetrates the
muscularis mucosae and enters the submucosal layer. *(From del
Regato, J.A., Spjut, H.J., & Cox, J.D. [1985]. Cancer: Diagnosis,
treatment, and prognosis [2nd ed.]. St. Louis: Mosby.)*

ing in the middle as the tumor penetrates the blood supply.
Obstruction is common but occurs slowly. Manifestations
include progressive abdominal distention, pain, vomiting,
constipation, need for laxatives, cramps, and bright red
blood on the surface of the stool.

Systematic lymphatic spread occurs along the aorta to
the mesenteric and pancreatic lymph nodes. Liver metastasis
is common and follows invasion of the mesenteric veins (left
colon) or superior veins (right colon), which drain into the
portal circulation.

Rectal carcinomas are defined as tumors occurring up to
15 cm from the anal opening. Tumors of the rectum can
spread through the rectal wall to nearby structures: the
prostate in men and the vagina in women. Penetration occurs more readily in the lower third of the rectum because it
has no serosal covering. Systemic and pulmonary metastases

occur through the hemorrhoidal plexus, which drains into
the vena cava.

 Evaluation and Treatment

Screening procedures include fecal occult blood testing and
colonoscopy. Individuals with a family history of polyps
should be screened using colonoscopy with removal of
polyps when they are found.[113] A diet rich in vegetables,
grains, fruit, and calcium and low in fat can modify cancer
risk.[114] A genetic marker has been developed to identify at-
risk populations.

The staging of colorectal cancer involves endoscopic ultrasonography and operative exploration. Physical examination of the abdomen detects liver enlargement and ascites;
appropriate lymph nodes are palpated. Elevations of carcinoembryonic antigen (CEA) are often detected in the sera of
individuals with colorectal carcinoma. The amount of CEA
in the serum is a function of the stage of the disease and the
type of tumor. Operative staging consists of careful exploration during surgery and biopsy of possible metastases. The
Dukes classification for staging of colorectal cancer is as
follows:

- Stage A: cancer limited to the bowel wall
- Stage B: cancer extending through the bowel wall
- Stage C: nodal metastases regardless of extension into the
  bowel wall
- Stage D: distant metastases regardless of primary size

Treatment for cancer of the colon is always surgical. Resection and anastomosis can be performed for cancer of the
ascending, transverse, descending, or sigmoid colon and upper rectum. These surgeries are performed through abdominal incisions, and natural defecation is preserved.

Growths in the lower portion of the rectum require removal of the entire rectum. The proximal end of the descending colon is brought out through a small incision in the
abdominal wall and becomes a permanent colostomy. Resection of liver metastases can prolong survival beyond 5
years.[115] Prognosis after surgery depends on the stage and location of the tumor.

Radiation therapy is often given before surgery in the
hope that it will shrink the tumor, alter the malignant cells,
or do both, so that these cells will not survive after surgery.
Chemotherapy is used to treat metastatic disease and cases
with a high risk of recurrence. Immunotherapy can boost
the immune response.[116]

Cancer of the Accessory Organs of Digestion
Cancer of the liver

Cancer of the liver is usually caused by metastatic spread
from a primary site elsewhere in the body. Primary liver cancer is relatively rare in the United States but is common in
densely populated parts of the Far East, Southern Africa,
China, and Greece. In the United States, the incidence of primary liver cancer is higher in blacks than in whites (2 to 10
per 100,000 per year) and in males than in females. Primary

TABLE 34-11	Conditions Commonly Confused With Colorectal Cancer
Condition	**Significant Characteristics**
Diverticulitis	Left-sided pain similar to that of appendicitis; tender lower left quadrant. Associated findings: nausea, vomiting, fever, obstruction, anorexia, and leukocytosis; mucosa is intact, and perforation, peritonitis, and abscesses occur more frequently than in cancer; protosigmoidoscopy or barium enema used to distinguish from cancer
Chronic ulcerative colitis	Younger people with chronic attacks of bloody diarrhea, crampy abdominal pain, fever, malnutrition, and dehydration; usually involves the left colon and rectum; endoscopy, barium enema, and biopsy performed for definitive diagnosis
Crohn disease (granulomatous colitis)	Generally involves the right colon; chronic diarrhea with abdominal cramps, fever, weight loss, and often a palpable abdominal mass; difficult at times to distinguish Crohn disease from ulcerative colitis; endoscopic examination and barium enema used to distinguish from cancer
Appendicitis	Vague abdominal symptoms, often with a tender or nontender mass in the lower right quadrant; associated symptoms: mild fever and leukocytosis; barium enema used to distinguish cancer of the cecum from appendiceal abscess
Thrombosed hemorrhoids	Examination shows a tender, swollen, bluish painful mass in the anus; patient will have a history of hemorrhoids

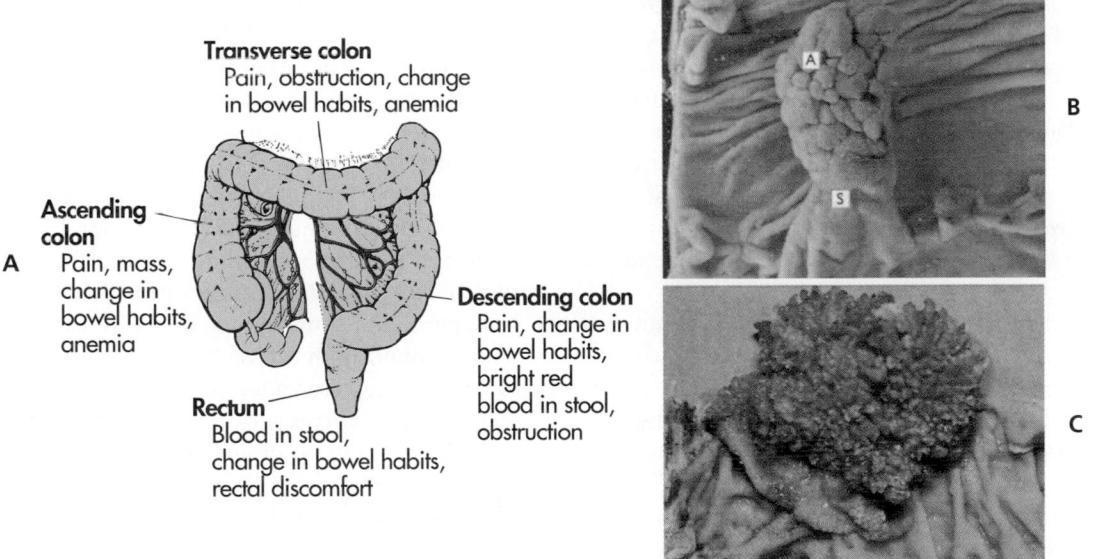

Fig. 34-15 *Signs and symptoms of colorectal cancer by location of primary lesion.* **A,** Clinical manifestations are listed in order of frequency for each region (lymphatics of colon also shown). **B,** Tubular adenomata *(A)* are rounded lesions 0.5 to 2 cm in size that are generally red and sit on a stalk *(S)* of normal mucosa that has been dragged up by traction of the polyp in the bowel lumen. **C,** Villous adenomata are frondlike lesions about 0.6 cm thick that occupy a broad area of mucosa generally 1 to 5 cm in diameter. *(B and C from Stevens, A. & Lowe, J. [1995]. Pathology. London: Mosby.)*

liver cancer is rare before the age of 40 years and is most common during the sixth decade. Together, primary and secondary liver cancers account for 1% to 2% of all cancer deaths in the United States[102] (see Risk Factors box). Chronic hepatitis (B and C) and cirrhosis are significant risk factors.[71]

RISK FACTORS

PRIMARY LIVER CANCER
- Exposure to mycotoxins. The most significant mycotoxins are the aflatoxins, particularly those produced by *Aspergillus flavus,* a mold found on spoiled corn, peanuts, and grain.
- Chronic liver disease, especially cirrhosis.
- Infection with hepatitis B virus (HBV), hepatitis C virus (HCV), and hepatitis D virus (HDV), particularly in conjunction with cirrhosis. These infections act either as carcinogens or as co-carcinogens in chronically infected hepatocytes.

 ## Pathogenesis

Primary carcinomas of the liver are hepatocellular or cholangiocellular. **Hepatocellular carcinoma (hepatocarcinoma)** develops in the hepatocytes, whereas **cholangiocellular carcinoma (cholangiocarcinoma)** develops in the bile ducts. Hepatocellular carcinoma can be nodular (consisting of multiple, discrete nodules), massive (consisting of a large tumor mass having satellite nodules), or diffuse (consisting of very small nodules distributed throughout most of the liver). It is closely associated with cirrhosis. Because carcinoma of the liver invades the hepatic and portal veins, it often spreads to the heart and lungs. Other sites of metastases are the brain, kidney, and spleen.

Cholangiocellular carcinoma occurs less frequently than hepatocellular carcinoma and is most common where liver fluke infestation is prevalent, such as Southeast China. Cholangiocellular carcinoma can occur anywhere along the bile duct and extend directly into the liver, usually as a solitary lesion. It is difficult to distinguish an invasion of cholangiocellular carcinoma from a metastatic adenocarcinoma except by neoplastic changes found in nearby ducts.

Clinical Manifestations

The clinical presentation of liver cancer in adults is characterized by vague abdominal symptoms, such as nausea and vomiting, fullness, pressure, and dull ache in the right hypochondrium. Manifestations of hepatocellular carcinoma can occur slowly or abruptly. In individuals with cirrhosis, deepening jaundice or abrupt lack of appetite is a sign of hepatocellular carcinoma. Obstruction by the tumor can cause sudden worsening of portal hypertension and development of ascites. As the tumor enlarges, it causes pain. Cholangiocellular carcinoma more commonly presents insidiously as pain, loss of appetite, weight loss, and gradual onset of jaundice. Some carcinomas of the liver rupture spontaneously, causing hemorrhage. Others are discovered accidentally during evaluation of a bone fracture or surgical exploration.

Evaluation and Treatment

There is no specific test for the diagnosis of liver cancer. The diagnosis is based on clinical manifestations, laboratory findings, radiologic examination, and exploratory laparotomy. In individuals without cirrhosis, liver scans can document filling defects. CT or ultrasonography is used to detect solid tumors, but neither can distinguish benign from malignant tumors. A liver biopsy can be diagnostic unless scattered nodules are missed by the examiner.

Surgical resection is possible only if the tumor is localized to a removable lobe of the liver. Chemotherapeutic agents are administered systemically or locally.

The overall median survival rate for those with symptomatic liver cancer is only 3 to 4 months. Surgery is hazardous and usually not undertaken if the individual has cirrhosis. Most individuals develop metastases after surgical resection, but long-term survival is possible.

Cancer of the gallbladder

Cancer of the gallbladder is more common in women than in men by a ratio of about 2 to 1. It occurs rarely before the age of 40 years and is most common between the ages of 50 and 60 years. Most gallbladder cancer is caused by metastasis. Primary carcinoma of the gallbladder is rare and usually is associated with cholelithiasis.

 ## Pathogenesis

Most primary carcinomas of the gallbladder are adenocarcinomas. A few are squamous cell carcinomas. Invasion of the liver occurs early. Spreading occurs to the cystic and periportal lymph nodes with invasion of the pancreas and retroperitoneal lymph nodes. Direct invasion of the stomach and the duodenum can cause pyloric obstruction. Infection often accompanies cancer of the gallbladder. Generalized peritonitis, gangrene, perforation, and liver abscesses are potential complications of infection.

 ## Clinical Manifestations

A typical presentation of carcinoma of the gallbladder is steady, upper right quadrant pain for about 2 months. Other manifestations include diarrhea, belching, weakness, loss of appetite, weight loss, and vomiting. Obstructive jaundice can occur if an enlarging tumor presses on the extrahepatic ducts.

 ## Evaluation and Treatment

Early diagnosis of cancer of the gallbladder is not possible. Therefore individuals with gallstones, especially older women, are evaluated carefully. Inflammatory disorders, such as cholangitis (bile duct inflammation) and peritonitis, often obscure an underlying malignancy. Diagnostic procedures include upper gastrointestinal barium study, ultrasonography, cholangiography, and CT scan.

Complete surgical resection of the gallbladder is the only

effective treatment. Because advanced malignancies cannot be resected, gallbladders containing stones are removed as a preventive measure. The prognosis of gallbladder cancer is extremely poor; most individuals die within 1 year after surgery.[117]

Cancer of the pancreas

Pancreatic cancer now ranks fifth as a cause of cancer deaths in the United States. The incidence of pancreatic cancer rises steadily with age. Males are affected slightly more often than females, and blacks more often than whites. Pancreatic cancer accounts for about 28,600 deaths annually in the United States.[99] Mortality is nearly 100%. The cause of pancreatic cancer is not known, but there are modest risks associated with cigarette smoking, certain dietary factors, diabetes mellitus, and peptic ulcer disease.[115]

Pathogenesis

Cancer of the pancreas can arise from exocrine or endocrine cells. Most pancreatic tumors arise from exocrine cells in the ducts and are called *ductal adenocarcinomas*. Tumors arising in small ducts invade nearby glandular tissue, penetrate the covering of the pancreas, and extend into surrounding tissues.[118]

Ductal adenocarcinomas can occur in the head, body, or tail of the pancreas. Tumors of the head quickly spread to obstruct the common bile duct and portal vein. These tumors can then infiltrate the superior mesenteric artery, the vena cava, and the aorta. Cancer cells that enter the blood vessels can form emboli. Tumors of the body and tail infiltrate the posterior abdominal wall. Lymphatic invasion occurs early and rapidly and involves local and regional lymph nodes. Venous invasion causes metastases to the liver. Tumor implants on the peritoneal surface can obstruct veins and promote development of ascites.

Ductal adenocarcinomas arising in the head of the pancreas cause biliary obstruction somewhat early in the disease. Individuals with such tumors survive slightly longer than those with cancer of the body and tail, presumably because they seek medical attention earlier.

Clinical Manifestations

Cancer of the body and tail of the pancreas is generally asymptomatic until there is intraductal destruction or the tumor invades adjacent tissue. Frequently vague back pain is an initial symptom. Jaundice develops in most cases, usually caused by obstruction of the bile duct.[119] Because obstruction impairs enzyme secretion and flow to the duodenum, pancreatic cancer causes fat and protein malabsorption, resulting in weight loss. Distant metastases are found in the neck nodes, the lungs, and the brain. Most individuals die of hepatic failure, malnutrition, or systemic diseases.

Evaluation and Treatment

A laparotomy is often performed, particularly if jaundice is present. Ultrasonography and CT may be needed to confirm the need for a laparotomy, especially in individuals without jaundice. Laparotomy is used to establish a definitive diagnosis, evaluate the extent of disease, and determine whether palliative bypass surgery (i.e., cholecystojejunostomy and gastrojejunostomy) is needed. Most individuals require palliative double bypass of the blocked bile ducts, as well as gastrojejunostomy to prevent duodenal obstruction.

Many surgeons recommend a total pancreatectomy because cancer of the pancreas seldom consists of a single lesion. Chemotherapy and radiation therapy are seldom beneficial, except as palliative measures. Because almost all pancreatic cancers are advanced at the time of diagnosis, staging has little relevance in determining treatment. Cancers of the gastrointestinal tract are summarized in Table 34-10.

✓ QUICK CHECK

What are the primary risk factors for gastric carcinoma?

Compare tumors of the right colon with those of the left colon.

What is the most common cause of liver cancer?

▣ DID YOU UNDERSTAND?

Disorders of the Gastrointestinal Tract

1. Anorexia (loss of appetite), vomiting, constipation, diarrhea, abdominal pain, and evidence of gastrointestinal bleeding are clinical manifestations of many disorders of the gastrointestinal tract.
2. Vomiting is the forceful emptying of the stomach effected by gastrointestinal contraction and reverse peristalsis of the esophagus. It is usually preceded by nausea and retching, with the exception of projectile vomiting, which is associated with direct stimulation of the vomiting center in the brain.
3. Constipation is frequently caused by unhealthy dietary and bowel habits combined with lack of exercise. Constipation also can result from a disorder that impairs intestinal motility or obstructs the intestinal lumen.
4. Diarrhea can be caused by excessive fluid drawn into the intestinal lumen by osmosis (osmotic diarrhea), excessive secretion of fluids by the intestinal mucosa (secretory diarrhea), or excessive gastrointestinal motility.
5. Abdominal pain is caused by stretching, inflammation, or ischemia (insufficient blood supply). Ab-

Continued

◻ DID YOU UNDERSTAND? —cont'd

Disorders of the Gastrointestinal Tract—cont'd

dominal pain originates in the organs themselves (visceral pain) or in the peritoneum (parietal pain). Visceral pain is frequently referred to the back.

6. Obvious manifestations of gastrointestinal bleeding are hematemesis (vomiting of blood), melena (dark, tarry stools), and hematochezia (frank bleeding from the rectum). Occult bleeding can be detected only by testing stools or vomitus for presence of blood.

7. Dysphagia is difficulty in swallowing. It can be caused by a mechanical or functional obstruction of the esophagus. Functional obstruction is an impairment of esophageal motility.

8. Achalasia is a form of functional dysphagia caused by loss of esophageal innervation.

9. Gastroesophageal reflux is the regurgitation of chyme from the stomach into the esophagus. An inflammatory response (reflux esophagitis) ensues if the esophageal mucosa is repeatedly exposed to acids and enzymes in the regurgitated chyme.

10. Hiatal hernia is the protrusion of the upper part of the stomach through the hiatus (esophageal opening in the diaphragm) at the gastroesophageal junction. Hiatal hernia can be sliding or paraesophageal.

11. Pyloric obstruction is the narrowing or blockage of the pylorus, which is the opening between the stomach and the duodenum. It can be caused by a congenital defect, inflammation and scarring secondary to a gastric ulcer, or tumor growth.

12. Intestinal obstruction prevents the normal movement of chyme through the intestinal tract. It is usually mechanical, that is, caused by torsion, herniation, or tumor.

13. The most severe consequences of intestinal obstruction are fluid and electrolyte losses, hypovolemia, shock, intestinal necrosis, and perforation of the intestinal wall.

14. Gastritis is an acute or chronic inflammation of the gastric mucosa.

15. Regurgitation of bile, use of antiinflammatory drugs or alcohol, and some systemic diseases are associated with gastritis.

16. Chronic gastritis of the fundus and body is the most severe form of gastritis. It can result in gastric atrophy and decreased secretion of hydrochloric acid, pepsinogen, and intrinsic factor.

17. Chronic gastritis of the antrum, the most common type, is not usually associated with impaired secretion or gastric atrophy.

18. Appendicitis is the most common surgical emergency of the abdomen. Obstruction of the lumen leads to increased pressure, ischemia, and inflammation of the appendix. Without surgical resection, inflammation may progress to gangrene, perforation, and peritonitis.

19. A peptic ulcer is a circumscribed area of mucosal inflammation and ulceration caused by excessive secretion of gastric acid, disruption of the protective mucosal barrier, or both.

20. There are three types of peptic ulcers: duodenal, gastric, and stress ulcers.

21. Duodenal ulcers, the most common peptic ulcers, are associated with increased numbers of parietal (acid-secreting) cells in the stomach, elevated gastrin levels, and rapid gastric emptying. Pain occurs when the stomach is empty, and it is relieved with food or antacids. Duodenal ulcers tend to heal spontaneously and recur frequently.

22. Gastric ulcers develop near parietal cells, generally in the antrum, and tend to become chronic. Gastric secretions may be normal or decreased, and pain may occur after eating.

23. Ischemic stress ulcers develop suddenly after severe illness, systemic trauma, or neural injury. Ulceration follows mucosal damage caused by ischemia (decreased blood flow to the gastric mucosa).

24. Cushing ulcer is a stress ulcer caused by head trauma. Ulceration follows hypersecretion of hydrochloric acid caused by overstimulation of the vagal nuclei.

25. Postgastrectomy syndromes are long-term complications that follow gastrectomy, the resection of all or part of the stomach. The postgastrectomy syndromes include dumping syndrome, alkaline reflux gastritis, afferent loop obstruction, diarrhea, weight loss, and anemia.

26. Dumping syndrome is the rapid emptying of chyme into the small intestine. It causes an osmotic shift of fluid from the vascular compartment to the intestinal lumen, which decreases plasma volume.

27. Alkaline reflux gastritis is stomach inflammation caused by the reflux of bile and pancreatic secretions from the duodenum into the stomach. These substances disrupt the mucosal barrier and cause inflammation.

28. Afferent loop obstruction is an obstruction of the duodenal stump on the proximal side of a gastrojejunostomy. Biliary and pancreatic secretions accumulate in the stump, causing distention, intermittent pain, and vomiting.

29. Malabsorption syndromes result in impaired digestion or absorption of nutrients.

30. Pancreatic insufficiency causes malabsorption associated with impaired digestion. The pancreas does not produce sufficient amounts of the enzymes that digest protein, carbohydrates, and fats into components that can be absorbed by the intestine.

31. Deficient lactase production in the brush border of the small intestine inhibits the breakdown of lactose. This prevents lactose absorption and causes osmotic diarrhea.

32. Bile salt deficiency causes fat malabsorption and steatorrhea (fatty stools). Bile salt deficiency can re-

sult from inadequate secretion of bile, excessive bacterial deconjugation of bile, or impaired reabsorption of bile salts caused by ileal disease.

33. Ulcerative colitis is an inflammatory disease that causes ulceration, abscess formation, and necrosis of the colonic and rectal mucosa. Cramping pain, bleeding, frequent diarrhea, dehydration, and weight loss accompany severe forms of the disease. A course of frequent remissions and exacerbations is common.

34. Crohn disease is similar to ulcerative colitis, but it affects both the large and small intestines and ulceration tends to involve all the layers of the lumen. "Skip lesion" fissures and granulomas are characteristic of Crohn disease. Abdominal tenderness, nonbloody diarrhea, and weight loss are the usual symptoms.

35. Diverticula are outpouchings of colonic mucosa through the muscle layers of the colon wall. Diverticulosis is the presence of these outpouchings; diverticulitis is inflammation of the diverticula.

36. Vascular insufficiency in the intestine is most often associated with occlusion or obstruction of the mesenteric vessels or insufficient arterial blood flow. The resulting ischemia and necrosis produce abdominal pain, fever, bloody diarrhea, hypovolemia, and shock.

37. Obesity can be classified as exogenous or endogenous, and adipose (fat) cells can be classified as hyperplastic or hypertrophic.

38. Susceptibility to obesity may involve an excessive number of fat cells, increased amounts of lipoprotein in fat cells, high biologic set point controlled by the hypothalamus, presence of relatively few brown (thermoregulating) fat cells, high blood glucose levels associated with type II diabetes, or decreased action of the adenosine triphosphatase (ATPase) pump.

39. Obesity increases the risk of developing coronary artery disease, cancer, and pulmonary disorders.

40. Anorexia nervosa, or self-imposed starvation, is a psychogenic disorder of adolescent and young women. It causes significant weight loss and developmental delays and can be fatal.

41. Bulimia nervosa, or binging and purging, involves eating normal or large amounts of food and then purging by inducing vomiting or abusing laxatives. Severe weight loss is rare, but frequent vomiting causes tooth decay, pharyngitis, and esophagitis.

42. Short-term starvation, or lack of dietary intake for 3 or 4 days, stimulates mobilization of stored glucose by two metabolic processes: glycogenolysis (splitting of glycogen into glucose) and gluconeogenesis (formation of glucose from noncarbohydrate molecules).

43. Long-term starvation triggers the breakdown of ketone bodies and fatty acids. Eventually proteolysis (protein breakdown) begins, and death ensues if nutrition is not restored.

Disorders of the Accessory Organs of Digestion

1. Portal hypertension, ascites, hepatic encephalopathy, jaundice, and hepatorenal syndrome are complications of many liver disorders.

2. Portal hypertension is an elevation of portal venous pressure to at least 10 mm Hg. It is caused by increased resistance to venous flow in the portal vein and its tributaries, including the sinusoids and hepatic vein.

3. Portal hypertension is the most serious complication of liver disease because it can cause potentially fatal complications, such as bleeding varices, ascites, and hepatic encephalopathy.

4. Ascites is the accumulation and sequestration of fluid in the peritoneal cavity, often as a result of portal hypertension and decreased concentrations of plasma proteins.

5. Hepatic encephalopathy (portal-systemic encephalopathy) is impaired cerebral function caused by blood-borne toxins (particularly ammonia) not metabolized by the liver. Toxin-bearing blood may bypass the liver in collateral vessels opened as a result of portal hypertension, or diseased hepatocytes may be unable to carry out their metabolic functions.

6. Manifestations of hepatic encephalopathy range from confusion and asterixis (flapping tremor of the hands) to loss of consciousness, coma, and death.

7. Jaundice (icterus) is a yellow or greenish pigmentation of the skin or sclera of the eyes caused by increases in plasma bilirubin concentration (hyperbilirubinemia).

8. Obstructive jaundice is caused by obstructed bile canaliculi (intrahepatic obstructive jaundice) or obstructed bile ducts outside the liver (extrahepatic obstructive jaundice). Bilirubin accumulates proximal to sites of obstruction, enters the bloodstream, and is carried to the skin and deposited.

9. Hemolytic jaundice is caused by destruction of red blood cells at a rate that exceeds the liver's ability to metabolize unconjugated bilirubin.

10. Hepatorenal syndrome is functional kidney failure caused by advanced liver disease, particularly cirrhosis with portal hypertension. Renal failure is caused by a sudden decrease in blood flow to the kidneys, usually caused by massive gastrointestinal hemorrhage or liver failure. Its chief clinical manifestation is oliguria.

11. Viral hepatitis is an infection of the liver caused by a strain of the hepatitis virus: hepatitis A virus (HAV), hepatitis B virus (HBV), or non-A, non B hepatitis. Although they differ with respect to modes of transmission and severity of acute illness, all cause hepatic cell necrosis, Kupffer cell hyperplasia, and infiltration of liver tissue by mononuclear phagocytes. These changes obstruct bile flow and impair hepatocyte function.

Continued

◼ DID YOU UNDERSTAND? —cont'd

Disorders of the Accessory Organs of Digestion—cont'd

12. The clinical manifestations of viral hepatitis depend on the stage of infection. Fever, malaise, anorexia, and liver enlargement and tenderness characterize the prodromal phase (stage 1). Jaundice and hyperbilirubinemia mark the icteric phase (stage 2). During the recovery phase (stage 3), symptoms resolve. Recovery takes several weeks.

13. Fulminant hepatitis is a complication of hepatitis B (with or without hepatitis D infection) or non-A, non-B hepatitis. It causes widespread hepatic necrosis and is often fatal.

14. Cirrhosis is an inflammatory disease of the liver that causes disorganization of lobular structure, fibrosis, and nodular regeneration. Cirrhosis can result from hepatitis or exposure to toxins, such as acetaldehyde (a product of alcohol metabolism). The disease causes progressive irreversible liver damage, usually over a period of years.

15. Alcoholic cirrhosis impairs the hepatocytes' ability to oxidize fatty acids, synthesize enzymes and proteins, degrade hormones, and clear portal blood of ammonia and toxins. The inflammatory response includes excessive collagen formation, fibrosis, and scarring, which obstruct bile canaliculi and sinusoids. Bile obstruction causes jaundice. Vascular obstruction causes portal hypertension, shunting, and varices.

16. Primary biliary cirrhosis is the inflammatory destruction of intrahepatic bile ducts. Its cause is unknown.

17. Secondary biliary cirrhosis develops from prolonged obstruction of bile flow with increased pressure in the hepatic bile ducts that causes pooling of bile and necrosis of tissue. Relief of obstruction relieves symptoms of jaundice and pruritus. Continued obstruction causes cirrhosis and liver failure.

18. Cholelithiasis (the formation of gallstones) is a common disorder of the gallbladder. Gallstones form in the bile as a result of the aggregation of cholesterol crystals (cholesterol stones) or precipitates of unconjugated bilirubin (pigmented stones). Gallstones that fill the gallbladder or obstruct the cystic or common bile duct cause abdominal pain and jaundice.

19. Cholecystitis is an inflammation of the gallbladder. It is usually associated with obstruction of the cystic duct by gallstones.

20. Acute pancreatitis (pancreatic inflammation) is a serious but relatively rare disorder. Some unknown factor injures the pancreatic ducts or acini. Injury permits leakage of digestive enzymes into pancreatic tissue, where they become activated and begin the process of autodigestion, inflammation, and destruction of tissues. Release of pancreatic enzymes into the bloodstream or abdominal cavity causes damage to other organs.

21. Chronic pancreatitis results from structural or functional impairment of the pancreas. It causes recurrent abdominal pain and digestive disorders.

Cancer of the Digestive System

1. Cancer of the esophagus is rare and tends to occur in people older than 60 years of age. Alcohol and tobacco use, reflux esophagitis, and nutritional deficiencies are associated with esophageal carcinoma.

2. Dysphagia and chest pain are the primary manifestations of esophageal cancer. Early treatment of tumors that have not spread into the mediastinum or lymph nodes results in a good prognosis.

3. Gastric carcinoma is associated with high salt intake, food preservatives (nitrates, nitrites), and atrophic gastritis.

4. Approximately 50% of all gastric cancers are located in the prepyloric antrum. Clinical manifestations (weight loss, upper abdominal pain, vomiting, hepatemesis, anemia) develop only after the tumor has penetrated the wall of the stomach.

5. Cancer of the colon and rectum (colorectal cancer) is the second most common cause of cancer death in the United States. Preexisting polyps are highly associated with adenocarcinoma of the colon.

6. Tumors of the right (ascending) colon are usually large and bulky; tumors of the left (descending, sigmoid) colon develop as small, buttonlike masses. Manifestations of colon tumors include pain, bloody stools, and change in bowel habits.

7. Rectal carcinoma is located up to 15 cm from the opening of the anus. The tumor spreads transmurally to the vagina in women or prostate in men.

8. Metastatic invasion of the liver is more common than primary cancer of the liver.

9. Primary liver cancers are associated with chronic liver disease (cirrhosis, hepatitis B). Hepatocellular carcinomas arise from the hepatocytes, whereas cholangiocellular carcinomas arise from the bile ducts. Primary liver cancer spreads to the heart, lungs, brain, kidney, and spleen through the circulation.

10. Cancer of the gallbladder is relatively rare and tends to occur in women older than 50 years. Adenocarcinoma is most common. Because clinical manifestations occur late in the disease, metastases to lymph channels have usually occurred by the time of diagnosis and the prognosis is poor.

11. Cancer of the pancreas now ranks fifth as a cause of cancer deaths. The one known risk factor is heavy cigarette smoking. Most tumors are adenocarcinomas that arise in the exocrine cells of ducts in the head, body, or tail of the pancreas. Symptoms may not be evident until the tumor has spread to surrounding tissues. Treatment is palliative, and mortality is nearly 100%.

KEY TERMS

REFERENCES

1. Mitolo-Chieppa, D. et al. (1998). Cholinergic stimulation and adrenergic, noncholinergic relaxation of human colonic circular muscle in idiopathic chronic constipation. *Digestive Diseases and Sciences, 43*(12), 2719-2726.

2. Sluster, L. for the *Escherichia coli* 0157.H7 Study Group. (1997). *Escherichia coli* 0157.H7 diarrhea in the United States: Clinical and epidemiologic features. *Annals of Internal Medicine, 126,* 505-513.

3. Ratnaike, R.N. & Jones, T.E. (1998). Mechanism of drug-induced diarrhoea in the elderly. *Drugs and Aging, 13*(3), 245-253.

4. Neuman, S. et al. (1995). Swallowing therapy of neurologic patients: Correlation of outcome with pretreatment variables and therapeutic methods. *Dysphagia, 10*(1), 1-5.

5. Podas, T. et al. (1998). Achalasia: A critical review of epidemiological studies. *American Journal of Gastroenterology, 93*(12), 2345-2347.

6. Cockeram, A.W. (1998). Canadian Association of Gastroenterology practice guidelines: Evaluation of dysphagia. *Canadian Journal of Enterology, 12*(6), 409-413.

7. Vaezi, M.F. & Richter, J.E. (1998). Current therapies for achalasia: Comparison and efficacy. *Journal of Clinical Gastroenterology, 27*(1), 21-35.

8. Dent, J. (1994). Rates of gastric acid and pH in the pathogenesis of gastro-esophageal reflux disease. *Scandinavian Journal of Gastroenterology—Supplement, 201,* 55-61.

9. Field, S.K. & Sutherland, L.R. (1998). Does medical antireflux therapy improve asthma in asthmatics with gastroesophageal reflux? A critical review of the literature. *Chest, 114*(1), 275-283.

10. Jones, M.P. & Shubert, M.L. (1998). Initiation and perpetuation of gastroesophageal reflux disease. *Gastroenterology, 115*(5), 1296-1298.

11. de Carle, D.J. (1998). Gastro-oesophageal reflux disease. *Medical Journal of Australia, 169*(10), 549-554.

REFERENCES

12. Song, M.W.K., Bouras, E.P., & DeVault, K.R. (1997). The esophagus. In G. Gitnick (Ed.). *Current gastroenterology* (vol. 17). St. Louis: Mosby.

13. de Carle, D.J. (1998). Gastro-esophageal reflux disease. *Medical Journal of Australia, 169*(10), 549- 554.

14. Johnson, D.A. & Ruffin, W.K. (1996). Hiatal hernia. *Gastrointestinal and Endoscopic Clinics of North America, 6*(3), 641-666.

15. Sipponen, P. et al. (1998). Review article: Pathogenesis of the transformation from gastritis to malignancy. *Alimentary Pharmacologic Therapy, 12*(Suppl. 1), 61-71.

16. Levenstein, S. et al. (1999). Stress and peptic ulcer disease. *Journal of the American Medical Association, 281*(1), 10-11.

17. Halter, F. & Brignoli, R. (1997). Epidemiology of dyspepsia: Discriminant value of smoking and *Helicobacter pylori* status as predictors of peptic lesions in primary care. *Journal of Physiology and Pharmacology, 48*(Suppl. 4), 75-83.

18. Hein, H.O., Suadicani, P., & Gyntelberg, F. (1997). Genetic markers for peptic ulcer: A study of 3387 men aged 54 to 74 years: The Copenhagen Male Study. *Scandinavian Journal of Gastroenterology, 32*(1), 16-21.

19. Barkin, J. (1998). The relation between *Helicobacter pylori* and nonsteroidal anti-inflammatory drugs. *American Journal of Medicine, 105*(5A), 22S-27S.

20. Pratha, V.S. et al. (1998). Utility of endoscopic biopsy samples to quantitate human duodenal ion transport. *Journal of Laboratory and Clinical Medicine, 132*(6), 512-518.

21. Olbe, L. et al. (1996). A mechanism by which *Helicobacter pylori* infection of the antrum contributes to the development of duodenal ulcer. *Gastroenterology, 100,* 1386-1394.

22. Ofman, J.J. et al. (1997). Management strategies for *Helicobacter pylori*–seropositive patients with dyspepsia: Clinical and economic consequences [see Comments]. *Annals of Internal Medicine, 126*(4), 280-291.

23. Ofman, J.J. et al. (1997). Management strategies for *Helicobacter pylori*–seropositive patients with dyspepsia: Clinical and economic consequences. *Annals of Internal Medicine, 126,* 288-291.

24. Aldoori, W. H. et al. (1997). Prospective study of diet and risk of duodenal ulcer in men. *American Journal of Epidemiology, 145*(1), 42-50.

25. Bobeck, M.B. & Arroliga, A.C. (1997). Stress ulcer prophylaxis: The case for a selective approach. *Cleveland Clinic Journal of Medicine, 64*(10), 533-542.

26. Aoyma, N. et al. (1998). Peptic ulcers after the Hanshin-Awaji Earthquake: Increased incidence of bleeding gastric ulcer. *American Journal of Gastroenterology, 93*(3), 311-316.

27. Feldman, M. (1998). Mental stress and peptic ulcers: An earthshaking association [editorial; comment]. *American Journal of Gastroenterology, 93*(3), 291-292.

28. Durham, R.M. & Shapiro, M.C. (1991). Stress gastritis revisited. *Surgical Clinics of North America, 71*(40), 791-810.

29. Donahue, P.E. (1994). Early postoperative and post-gastrectomy syndromes: Diagnosis, management, and prevention. *Gastroenterological Clinics of North America, 23*(2), 215-226.

30. Zittel, T.T. et al. (1997). High prevalence of bone disorders after gastrectomy. *American Journal of Surgery, 174*(4), 431-438.

31. Moses, P.L. et al. (1998). Inflammatory bowel disease. I. Origins, presentation, and course. *Postgraduate Medicine, 103*(5), 77-84.

32. Braegger, C.P. & MacDonald, T.T. (1994). Immune mechanisms in chronic inflammatory bowel disease. *Annals of Allergy, 72*(2), 135-144.

33. Thomas, G.A., Rhodes, J., & Green, J.T. (1998). Inflammatory bowel disease and smoking: A review. *American Journal of Gastroenterology, 93*(2), 144-149.

34. Hanauer, S.B. & Meyers, S. (1997). Management of Crohn's disease in adults. *American Journal of Gastroenterology, 92,* 559-566.

35. Robinson, M. (1997). Optimizing therapy for inflammatory bowel disease. *American Journal of Gastroenterology, 92*(12, suppl.), 12S-17S.

36. Brant, S.R. et al. (1998). American families with Crohn's disease have strong evidence for linkage to chromosome 16 but not chromosome 12. *Gastroenterology, 115*(5), 1056-1061.

37. MacDonald, T.T. & Murch, S.H. (1994). Aetiology and pathogenesis of chronic inflammatory bowel disease. *Baillieres Clinical Gastroenterology, 8*(1), 1-34.

38. Russel, M.G. et al. (1998). The inflammatory bowel disease: Is there any relation between smoking status and disease presentation? European Collaborative IBD Study Group. *Inflammatory Bowel Disease, 4*(3), 182-186.

39. Jain, S.K. & Peppercorn, M.A. (1997). Inflammatory bowel disease and colon cancer: A review. *Digestive Diseases, 15*(4-5), 243-252.

40. Killingback, M. (1995). Surgical treatment of Crohn's disease. In W.P. Mazier (Ed.). *Surgery of the colon, rectum, and anus.* Philadelphia: Saunders.

41. Konvolinka, C.W. (1994). Acute diverticulitis under age forty. *American Journal of Surgery, 167*(6), 562-565.

42. Wess, L. et al. (1995). Cross-linking of collagen is increased in colonic diverticulosis. *Gut, 37*(1), 91-94.

43. Jones, D.S. (1992). Diverticular disease. *British Journal of Medicine, 304,* 1435-1437.

44. Aldoori, W.H. et al. (1998). A prospective study of dietary fiber types and symptomatic diverticular disease in men. *Journal of Nutrition, 128*(4), 714-719.

45. Jones, D.S. (1992). Appendicitis. *British Journal of Medicine, 305,* 44-47.

46. Borgstein, P.J. et al. (1997). Acute appendicitis: A

REFERENCES

clear-cut case in men, a guessing game in young women. A prospective study on the role of laparoscopy. *Surgical Endoscopy, 11*(9), 923-927.

47. Styrud, J., Eriksson, S., & Granstrom, L. (1998). Treatment of perforated appendicitis: An analysis of 362 patients treated during 8 years. *Digestive Surgery, 15*(6), 683-686.

48. Patel, A., Kaleya, R.N., & Sammartano, J.R. (1992). Pathophysiology of mesenteric ischemia. *Surgical Clinics of North America, 72*(1), 31-41.

49. Kvietys, P.R., Barrowmand, A., & Granger, N.D. (1987). *Pathophysiology of the splanchnic circulation* (vol. 1). Boca Raton, Fla.: CRC Press.

50. Newman, T.S. et al. (1998). The changing face of mesenteric infarction. *American Surgeon, 64*(7), 611-616.

51. Ravussin, E. & Swinburg, G.A. (1992). Pathophysiology of obesity. *Lancet, 340,* 404-408.

52. Houseknecht, K.L. et al. (1998). The biology of leptin: A review. *Journal of Animal Science, 76*(5), 1404-1420.

53. Considine, R.V. (1997). Weight regulation, leptin and growth hormone. *Hormone Research, 48*(Suppl. 5), 116-121.

54. Schaefer, D.C. & Cheskin, L.J. (1998). Update on obesity treatment. *Gastroenterologist, 6*(2), 136-145.

55. Giovannucci, E. et al. (1995). Physical activity, obesity, and risk of colon cancer and adenoma in men. *Annals of Internal Medicine, 122*(5), 327-334.

56. Diamond, F.B., Jr. (1998). Newer aspects of the pathophysiology, evaluation, and management of obesity in childhood. *Current Opinions in Pediatrics, 10*(4), 422-427.

57. Casper, R.C. (1998). Recognizing eating disorders in women. *Psychopharmacology Bulletin, 34*(3), 267-269.

58. Garrow, J.S. & James, W.P.T. (1993). *Human nutrition and dietetics.* Edinburgh: Churchill Livingstone.

59. Yamada, T. et al. (1995). *Textbook of gastroenterology.* Philadelphia: Lippincott.

60. Bolondi, L., Gaiani, S., & Gebel, M. (1998). Protohepatic vascular pathology and liver disease: Diagnosis and monitoring. *European Journal of Ultrasound, 7*(Suppl. 3), S42-S52.

61. Neuberger, J. (1998). Transplantation for alcoholic liver disease: A perspective from Europe. *Liver Transplant Surgery, 4*(5, Suppl. 1), S52-S57.

62. McHutchison, J.G. (1997). Differential diagnosis of ascites. *Seminars in Liver Disease, 17*(3), 191-202.

63. Ginés, P., Arroyo, V., & Rodes, J. (1998). Ascites and hepatorenal syndrome: Pathogenesis and treatment strategies. In R.W. Schrier et al. (Eds.). *Advances in internal medicine* (vol. 43, pp. 99-142). St. Louis: Mosby.

64. Wong, F., Girgrah, N., & Blendis, L. (1997). Review: The controversy over the pathophysiology of ascites formation in cirrhosis. *Journal of Gastroenterology and Hepatology, 12*(6), 437-444.

65. Butterworth, R. (1994). Hepatic encephalopathy. In I.M. Arias et al. *The liver: Biology and pathobiology* (3rd ed.). New York: Raven.

66. Roberts, L.R. & Kamath, P.S. (1996). Ascites and hepatorenal syndrome: Pathophysiology and management. *Mayo Clinic Proceedings, 71*(9), 874-881.

67. Conn, H.O. (1994). Complications of portal hypertension. *Current Hepatology, 14*(8), 231-280.

68. Schiff, E., Sorrell, M.F., & Maddrey, W.C. (Eds.). (1998). *Schiff's disease of the liver* (8th ed., vol. 1). Philadelphia: Lippincott-Raven.

69. Scott-Conner, C.E. & Grogan, J.B. (1994). The pathophysiology of biliary obstruction and its effect on phagocytic and immune function. *Journal of Surgical Research, 57*(2), 316-336.

70. Wong, F. & Blendis, L. (1998). Pathophysiology and treatment of hepatorenal syndrome. *Gastroenterologist, 6*(2), 122-135.

71. Vail, B.A. (1997). Management of chronic viral hepatitis. *American Family Physician, 55*(8), 2749-2756, 2759-2761.

72. Karayiannis, P. et al. (1998). Natural history and molecular biology of hepatitis G virus/GB virus C. *Clinical Diagnosis and Virology, 10*(2-3), 103-111.

73. Sheng, L. et al. (1998). Hepatitis G virus infection in acute fulminant hepatitis: Prevalence of HGV infection and sequence analysis of a specific viral strain. *Journal of Viral Hepatitis, 5*(5), 301-306.

74. Idilman, R. et al. (1998). Pathogenesis of hepatitis B and C–induced hepatocellular carcinoma. *Journal of Viral Hepatitis, 5*(5), 285-299.

75. Hoofnagle, J.H. (1998). Therapy of viral hepatitis. *Digestion, 59*(5), 563-578.

76. Yotsuyanagi, H. et al. (1996). Prolonged fecal excretion of hepatitis A virus in adult patients with hepatitis A as determined by polymerase chain reaction. *Hepatology, 24,* 10-13.

77. Schouval, D. (1998). Vaccines for prevention of viral hepatitis. *Haemophilia, 4*(4), 587-594.

78. Lee, W.M. (1994). Acute liver failure. *American Journal of Medicine, 96*(1A), 35-95.

79. Bernstein, D. & Tripodi, J. (1998). Fulminant hepatic failure. *Critical Care Clinics, 14*(2), 181-197.

80. Hill, D.B. & Kugelmas, M. (1998). Alcoholic liver disease: Treatment strategies for the potentially reversible stages. *Postgraduate Medicine, 103*(4), 261-264, 267-268, 273-275.

81. Batey, R.B. (1992). Alcohol consumption and risk of cirrhosis. *Medical Journal of Australia, 156,* 413-416.

82. Lieber, C.S. (1991). Hepatic, metabolic, and toxic effects of ethanol: 1991 update. *Alcohol Clinical and Experimental Research, 15,* 573-592.

83. Zetterman, R.K. (1992). Modern approach to alcoholic liver disease. *Scandinavian Journal of Gastroenterology, 192*(Suppl. 27), 55-62.

84. Baraona, E. & Lieber, C.S. (1998). Alcohol and lipids. *Recent Developments in Alcoholism, 14,* 97-134.

REFERENCES

85. Ishii, H., Kurose, I., & Kato, S. (1997). Pathogenesis of alcoholic liver disease with particular emphasis on oxidative stress. *Journal of Gastroenterology and Hepatology, 12*(9-10), S272-S282.

86. Domurat, E.S. & Elias, A.N. (1992). The endocrinology and pathophysiology of alcoholic cirrhosis and renal failure. *Journal of the National Medical Association, 84*(2), 153-162.

87. McCullough, A.J. & O'Connor, J.F. (1998). Alcoholic liver disease: Proposed recommendations for the American College of Gastroenterology. *American Journal of Gastroenterology, 93*(11), 2002-2036.

88. Lucey, M.R. et al. (1992). Selection for and outcome of liver transplantation in alcoholic liver disease. *Gastroenterology, 102,* 1736-1741.

89. Metcalf, J.V. et al. (1996). Natural history of primary biliary cirrhosis. *Lancet, 348,* 1399-1402.

90. Hay, J.E. (1998). Liver transplantation for primary biliary cirrhosis and primary sclerosing cholangitis: Does medical treatment alter timing and selection? *Liver Transplant Surgery, 4*(5, Suppl. 1), S9-S17.

91. Bowen, J.C. et al. (1992). Gallstone disease: Pathophysiology, epidemiology, natural history, and treatment options. *Medical Clinics of North America, 76*(5), 1143-1157.

92. Strasberg, S.M. (1998). The pathogenesis of cholesterol gallstones, a review. *Journal of Gastrointestinal Surgery, 2*(2), 109-125.

93. Gholson, C.F., Sittig, K., & McDonald, J.C. (1994). Recent advances in the management of gallstones. *American Journal of Medical Science, 307*(4), 293-304.

94. Middelfart, H.V. et al. (1998). Pain patterns after distension of the gallbladder in patients with acute cholecystitis. *Scandinavian Journal of Gastroenterology, 33*(9), 982-987.

95. Domschke, W. (1987). Medical and/or surgical treatment of severe pancreatitis. In H.G. Berger & M. Buchler (Eds.). *Acute pancreatitis.* New York: Springer-Verlag.

96. Steer, M.L. (1992). How and where does acute pancreatitis begin? *Archives of Surgery, 127*(11), 1350-1353.

97. Lee, S.P., Nicholls, S.F., & Park, H.Z. (1992). Biliary sludge as a cause of acute pancreatitis. *New England Journal of Medicine, 326,* 589-593.

98. Norman, J. (1998). The role of cytokines in the pathogenesis of acute pancreatitis. *American Journal of Surgery, 175*(1), 76-83.

99. Kemppainen, E.A. et al. (1998). Advances in the laboratory diagnostics of acute pancreatitis. *Annals of Medicine, 30*(2), 169-175.

100. Schenker, S. & Montalvo, R. (1998). Alcohol and the pancreas. *Recent Developments in Alcoholism, 14,* 41-65.

101. Pitchumoni, C.S. (1998). Chronic pancreatitis: Pathogenesis and management of pain. *Journal of Clinical Gastroenterology, 27*(2), 101-107.

102. American Cancer Society (ACS). (1999). *Cancer facts & figures—1999.* Atlanta: The Author.

103. Cameron, A.J. (1998). Management of Barrett's esophagus. *Mayo Clinic Proceedings, 73*(5), 457-461.

104. Kjaerheim, K., Gaard, M., & Andersen, A. (1998). The role of alcohol, tobacco, and dietary factors in upper aerogastric tract cancers: A prospective study of 10,900 Norwegian men. *Cancer Causes and Control, 9*(1), 99-108.

105. McFarlane, G.A. & Munro, A. (1997). *Helicobacter pylori* and gastric cancer. *British Journal of Surgery, 84*(9), 1190-1199.

106. Kuipers, E.J. (1998). Review article: Relationship between *Helicobacter pylori,* atrophic gastritis and gastric cancer. *Alimentary Pharmacology Therapy, 12*(Suppl. 1), 25-36.

107. Wobbes, T.L. et al. (1992). Evaluation of seven tumor markers (CA 50, CA 19-9, CA 19-9 TruQuant, CA 72-4, CA 195, carcinoembryonic antigen, and tissue polypeptide antigen) in the pretreatment sera of patients with gastric carcinoma. *Cancer, 69,* 2036-2041.

108. Wils, J. (1998). Treatment of gastric cancer. *Current Opinions in Oncology, 10*(4), 357-361.

109. Gore, R.M. (1997). Small bowel cancer: Clinical and pathologic features. *Radiological Clinics of North America, 35*(2), 351-360.

110. Jorde, L.B. et al. (1999). *Medical genetics* (2nd ed.). St. Louis: Mosby.

111. Kleibeuker, J.H. et al. (1994). Calcium supplementation as a prophylaxis against colon cancer? *Digestive Diseases, 12*(2), 85-97.

112. Distler, P. & Holt, P.R. (1997). Are right- and left-sided colon neoplasms distinct tumors? *Digestive Diseases, 15*(4-5), 302-311.

113. Leiberman, D. (1998). How to screen for colon cancer. *Annual Review of Medicine, 49,* 263-272.

114. Reddy, B.S. (1993). Dietary fat, calories, and fiber in colon cancer. *Preventive Medicine, 22*(5), 738-749.

115. Yeu-Tsu, M.L. (1994). Liver metastasis of colorectal carcinoma: Diagnosis, treatment, and prognosis of resectable lesions. *Current Hepatology, 14*(7), 213-230.

116. Nordic Gastrointestinal Study Group. (1992). Expectancy or primary chemotherapy in patients with advanced asymptomatic colorectal cancer: A randomized trial. *Journal of Clinical Oncology, 10,* 904-911.

117. North, J.H., Jr. et al. (1998). Prognostic factors for adenocarcinoma of the gallbladder: An analysis of 162 cases. *American Surgeon, 64*(5), 437-440.

118. Dugan, M.C. & Sarkar, F.H. (1998). Current concepts in pancreatic cancer: Symposium summary. *Pancreas, 17*(4), 325-333.

119. Krech, R.L. & Walsh, D. (1991). Symptoms of pancreatic cancer. *Journal of Pain Symptom Management, 6*(6), 360-367.

CHAPTER
35

Alterations of Digestive Function in Children

Sue E. Huether

Disorders of the gastrointestinal tract in children include anomalies with structural and functional alterations, as well as enzyme deficiencies. Structural alterations can occur throughout the gastrointestinal tract and include cleft lip and palate, esophageal atresia, tracheoesophageal fistula, pyloric stenosis, aganglionic megacolon, and imperforate anus. Gastroesophageal reflux, hepatic and pancreatic enzyme deficiencies, and bacterial or viral invasions of the gastrointestinal tract also contribute to the diseases and gastrointestinal clinical manifestations in children.

Gale D. Danek, RN, MSN, contributed to this chapter in the previous edition.

CHAPTER OUTLINE

DISORDERS OF THE GASTROINTESTINAL TRACT
Congenital Impairment of Motility
Cleft lip and cleft palate

Cleft lip (harelip) and *cleft palate* are developmental anomalies of the first branchial arch (Fig. 35-1). These defects, which occur during embryonic development, vary in severity. In whites, the incidence of cleft lip or cleft palate ranges from 1 in 600 to 1 in 1250 births. The incidence of cleft lip, with or without cleft palate, is 1 in 1000 births, whereas the incidence of cleft palate alone is about 1 in 2500 births. Incidence is lower in black populations and higher in Japanese populations. Cleft lip, with or without cleft palate, is more common in females. Both anomalies can be unilateral or bilateral, partial or complete.

In most cases, cleft lip and cleft palate are caused by multiple factors, both genetic and nongenetic, each of which contributes only a minor developmental defect. (This phenomenon, called *multifactorial inheritance,* is discussed in Chapter 2.) Together, these factors reduce the amount of neural crest mesenchyme that migrates into the area that will develop into the face of the embryo. The cleft can be part of a syndrome determined by single mutant genes or part of a chromosomal defect, usually trisomy 13. Rarely, the cleft is caused by a teratogenic agent, such as an anticonvulsant drug.[1]

Pathophysiology

Cleft lip. Cleft lip is caused by the incomplete fusion of the nasomedial or intermaxillary process during the second month of embryonic development. The cleft causes structures of the face and mouth to develop without the normal restraints of encircling lip muscles. The facial cleft may affect not only the lip but also the external nose, nasal cartilages, nasal septum, and alveolar processes.

The cleft is usually just beneath the center of one nostril. The defect may occur bilaterally and may be symmetric or asymmetric. The more complete the cleft lip, the greater the chance that teeth in the line of the cleft will be missing or malformed.

Cleft palate. Cleft palate is often associated with cleft lip but may occur without it. The fissure may affect only the uvula and soft palate or may extend forward to the nostril and involve the hard palate and the maxillary alveolar ridge. It may be unilateral or bilateral, with the cleft occupying the midline posteriorly and as far forward as the alveolar process, where it deviates to the involved side. Clefts involving the palate only are usually but not necessarily in the midline. In some cases, the vomer and nasal septum are partly or completely undeveloped. When these facial bones are involved, the nasal cavity may freely communicate with the oral cavity.

Clinical Manifestations

Feeding the infant with cleft lip usually presents no difficulty if the cleft lip is simple and the palate intact. A baby with cleft palate usually requires large, soft nipples with cross-cut

Fig. 35-1 *Variations in clefts of the lip and palate.* **A,** Notch in vermilion border. **B,** Unilateral cleft lip and palate. **C,** Bilateral cleft lip and cleft palate. **D,** Cleft palate. *(From Wong, D.L. et al. [1999]. Whaley & Wong's nursing care of infants and children [6th ed.]. St. Louis: Mosby.)*

openings. Breast-feeding may be impossible for some infants. An orthodontic prosthesis for the roof of the mouth may facilitate sucking for some infants.

Evaluation and Treatment

Facial x-ray films confirm the extent of bone deformity. Soft tissue alterations are evaluated by history and physical examination.

The nature and extent of the cleft, the infant's condition, and the method of surgical correction proposed determine the course of treatment. Surgical correction is often planned in stages. Speech training and special attention by a prosthodontist and orthodontist are almost always required.[2]

Both before and after surgery, children with cleft palate tend to have repeated infections of the paranasal sinuses. Excessive dental decay is not unusual. Hypertrophy of tonsils and adenoids and otitis media are frequent accompaniments, and the child should be evaluated for hearing loss.[3]

Esophageal malformations

Congenital malformations of the esophagus occur in 1 of 3000 to 4500 live births. In *esophageal atresia* the esophagus ends in a blind pouch. It is usually accompanied by a fistula between the esophagus and the trachea *(tracheoesophageal fistula [TEF]).* Either defect can occur alone, however (Fig. 35-2).

Pathophysiology

Esophageal abnormalities are thought to arise from defective differentiation as the trachea separates from the esophagus during the fourth to sixth weeks of embryonic development.

Defective growth of endodermal cells leads to atresia. Incomplete fusion of the lateral walls of the foregut leads to incomplete closure of the laryngotracheal tube and fistula formation.

Clinical Manifestations

Polyhydramnios (excessive amniotic fluid) is reported to occur in 14% to 90% of mothers of affected infants because of alterations in fetal swallowing.[4] If a fistula connects the trachea with the distal esophagus, the abdomen fills with air and becomes distended, possibly interfering with breathing (see Fig. 35-2, *C* to *E*). Intermittent cyanosis may result.

Pulmonary complications are compounded by reflux of air and gastric secretions into the tracheobronchial tree through the fistula, causing severe chemical irritation. Infants with esophageal atresia but no fistula have scaphoid (boat-shaped), gasless abdomens. In fistula with atresia (see Fig. 35-2, *B*), the usual symptoms are recurrent aspiration, pneumonia, and atelectasis that remains "silent" for days or even months.

In at least 30% of infants with esophageal defects, other congenital anomalies are present as well. Cardiovascular anomalies are the most common, but other digestive tract, urinary, vertebral, and central nervous system defects can accompany esophageal atresia and tracheoesophageal fistula.

Evaluation and Treatment

Esophageal atresia is usually diagnosed at birth, when attempts to pass a catheter into the stomach fail. X-ray films will show the catheter coiled in the upper esophageal pouch.

Treatment is surgical. Esophageal continuity is restored,

Fig. 35-2 *Five types of esophageal atresias and tracheoesophageal fistulas.* **A,** Simple esophageal atresia. Proximal esophagus and distal esophagus end in blind pouches, and there is tracheal communication. Nothing enters the stomach; regurgitated food and fluid may enter the lungs. **B,** Proximal and distal esophageal segments end in blind pouches, and a fistula connects the proximal esophagus to the trachea. Nothing enters the stomach; food and fluid enter the lungs. **C,** Proximal esophagus ends in a blind pouch, and a fistula connects the trachea to the distal esophagus. Air enters the stomach; regurgitated gastric secretions enter the lungs through the fistula. **D,** Fistula connects both proximal and distal esophageal segments to the trachea. Air, food, and fluid enter the stomach and the lungs. **E,** Simple tracheoesophageal fistula between otherwise normal esophagus and trachea. Air, food, and fluid enter the stomach and the lungs. Between 85% and 90% of esophageal anomalies are type **C;** 6% to 8% are type **A;** 3% to 5% are type **E;** and fewer than 1% are type **B** or **D.** *(From Wong, D.L. et al. [1999]. Whaley & Wong's nursing care of infants and children [6th ed.]. St. Louis: Mosby.)*

and the fistula is eliminated. The child may continue to have problems with aspiration, gastroesophageal reflux, and esophagitis after surgical repair.[5] The overall survival rate for infants with esophageal defects is approximately 75%.

Pyloric stenosis

Pyloric stenosis is an obstruction of the pyloric sphincter caused by hypertrophy of the sphincter muscle and is inherited as a multifactorial trait. One of the most common disorders of early infancy, it affects infants between the ages of 1 and 2 weeks and 3 and 4 months.[6] The incidence of pyloric stenosis among males is approximately 5 in 1000, whereas that among females is only 1 in 1000. Whites are affected more frequently than blacks or Orientals, and full-term infants are affected more frequently than premature infants. Increased gastrin secretion by the mother in the last trimester of pregnancy increases the likelihood of pyloric stenosis in the infant. The overproduction of gastric secretions in the infant may be caused by stress-related factors in the mother. There is an increased incidence of pyloric stenosis in children with Down syndrome; 6.9% of children have a parent who had pyloric stenosis, and 4.9% have a close relative affected.[7]

Pathophysiology

Individual muscle fibers thicken, so the whole pyloric sphincter becomes enlarged and inelastic. The mucosal lining of the pyloric opening is folded and narrowed by the encroaching muscle. Because of the extra peristaltic effort necessary to force the gastric contents through the narrow pylorus, the muscle layers of the stomach may become hypertrophied as well.

Clinical Manifestations

Between 2 and 3 weeks after birth, an infant who has fed well and gained weight begins to vomit without apparent reason. The vomiting gradually becomes more forceful. Food is often regurgitated through the nose. The vomiting usually occurs immediately after eating, and the vomitus consists of the bulk of the feeding plus some food retained from previous feedings but is almost always free of bile.

Prolonged retention of food in the stomach is characteristic. Constipation occurs because little food reaches the intestine.

In severe, untreated cases, increased gastric peristalsis and vomiting lead to severe fluid and electrolyte imbalances, malnutrition, and weight loss that can be fatal within 4 to 6 weeks. Infants with pyloric stenosis are irritable because of hunger, and they may have esophageal discomfort caused by repeated vomiting and esophagitis. The vomitus may be blood streaked because of rupture of gastric and esophageal vessels.

Evaluation and Treatment

Diagnosis is based on the history and clinical manifestations.[8] Occasionally, gastric peristalsis is observable over the abdomen. A firm, small, movable mass, approximately the size of an olive, is felt in the right upper quadrant in 70% to 90% of infants with pyloric stenosis. Sonography clearly shows the hypertrophied pyloric muscles and narrowed pyloric channel.

The standard treatment for hypertrophic pyloric stenosis is a pyloromyotomy, in which the muscles of the pylorus are separated, or balloon dilation. Preoperative and postoperative medical management to correct fluid and electrolyte imbalance has been the key to the high success rate and low complication rates with this surgery.[9]

Some infants respond to medical and nutritional management, which is based on the theory that the pylorus will open spontaneously by 6 to 8 months of age if nutrition can be maintained. Antispasmodic drugs are given to relax the pylorospasm, and the infant is refed after vomiting.

Malrotation

In *malrotation* the colon remains in the upper right quadrant, where an abnormal membrane may press on and obstruct the duodenum. This **periduodenal band** is one of the most significant findings in malrotation. Associated abnormalities are seen in some children with duodenal and jejunal atresia.[10]

Pathophysiology

The small intestine lacks a normal posterior fixation in malrotation because it has only a rudimentary attachment near the origin of the superior mesenteric artery. Therefore the entire mass can twist when the mobile loops of intestine from the duodenojejunal junction to the middle of the transverse colon twist on themselves. The twisting is known as *volvulus*. Intestinal twisting around the rudimentary mesentery angulates and obstructs the intestinal lumen and partly or completely occludes the superior mesenteric artery, causing infarction and necrosis of the entire midgut.

Clinical Manifestations

Although most cases of malrotation-associated volvulus and infarction develop during the neonatal period (50%) or infancy (85% are younger than 1 year), some develop during childhood or even adulthood. In infants the obstruction causes intermittent or persistent bile-stained vomiting after feedings. Abdominal distention is limited initially to the epigastrium because only the stomach and duodenum are dilated. Dehydration and electrolyte imbalance may occur rapidly because large amounts of pancreatic juice, bile, and gastric secretions are lost through vomiting. Fever usually ensues. Scanty stools, diarrhea, and bloody stools are associated with progressive volvulus, vascular compression, and infarction of the intestine in infants. Intermittent or partial volvulus may be seen in older children and in adults. This condition may be asymptomatic and discovered during unrelated abdominal surgery, or it may cause minor abdominal complaints, such as nausea after meals, vomiting, or abdominal pain.

Evaluation and Treatment

Diagnosis of malrotation with volvulus and infarction is based on a review of the clinical manifestations. X-ray films of the abdomen show gas bubbles and distention proximal to the site of obstruction and barium studies.

Treatment includes laparoscopic or open surgery to reduce the volvulus.[11] Necrotic bowel may be resected and a primary anastomosis performed. When there is gangrene and question of viability of the bowel ends, an enterostomy may be performed. Second-look operations may be done to avoid resection of viable bowel. In cases of malrotation without duodenal obstruction, operative survival is 80%. Operative survival is 40% to 50% in cases of malrotation complicated by obstruction caused by periduodenal bands or other intraabdominal anomalies. Resection of large segments of the small intestine results in short bowel syndrome and its long-term sequelae.

✓ QUICK CHECK

What structures are affected in cleft palate and cleft lip?

What is esophageal atresia?

What produces pyloric stenosis?

Meconium ileus

Meconium is a substance that fills the entire intestine before birth. It consists of intestinal gland secretions and some amniotic fluid. Normally, meconium is passed from the rectum during the first 12 to 72 hours after birth.

Meconium ileus is intestinal obstruction caused by meconium formed in utero that is abnormally sticky and adheres firmly to the mucosa of the small intestine, resisting passage beyond the terminal ileum. The cause is usually a lack of digestive enzymes during fetal life. This meconium is also found to contain albumin, which is not normally found in meconium. This has been used as a screening test for cystic fibrosis. Most cases of meconium ileus are caused by cystic fibrosis.[12] In the cases *not* associated with cystic fibrosis, the cause usually is unknown. Partial aplasia of the pancreas is an associated factor, however, and one fifth of infants with meconium ileus are premature or have a history of maternal hydramnios (excessive amniotic fluid). After intestinal atresia and malrotation with volvulus, meconium ileus is the most common cause of small intestinal obstruction in newborns.

▰ *Pathophysiology*

The terminal ileum is plugged with thick, viscous meconium resulting from the formation of an insoluble, calcium-glycoprotein compound in abnormal mucus. The segment of the ileum proximal to the obstruction is distended with liquid contents, and its walls may be hypertrophied. The segment distal to the obstruction is collapsed and filled with small pellets of pale-colored stool. Meconium in the obstructed segment has the consistency of thick syrup or glue. Peristalsis fails to propel this viscous material through the ileum, and it becomes impacted. Volvulus, atresia, or perforation of the bowel sometimes accompanies meconium ileus.

▰ *Clinical Manifestations*

Abdominal distention usually develops during the first few days after birth. The infant begins to vomit within hours or days of birth. Infants with cystic fibrosis may have signs of pulmonary involvement, such as tachypnea, intercostal retractions, and grunting respirations. The distended abdomen shows patterns of dilated intestinal loops that feel doughlike when palpated. Some of the loops contain scattered, firm, movable masses. Despite hyperactive peristalsis, the rectal ampulla is empty.

▰ *Evaluation and Treatment*

Radiologic examination confirms the presence of meconium ileus. The sweat test, which is accurate in 90% of infants, is performed to detect or rule out cystic fibrosis. In approximately 50% of cases not complicated with volvulus or perforation, a hyperosmolar radiopaque enema done using fluoroscopy evacuates the meconium. If this is not possible, the meconium is removed surgically.

Survival of infants with meconium ileus is improving, with 85% to 100% survival at 1 year.[13] Mortality increases to 70% if obstruction is complicated by peritonitis. After recovery from neonatal meconium ileus, the long-term outlook depends on the severity and progression of pulmonary disease. Meconium ileus does not adversely affect the long-term nutritional outcome of cystic fibrosis.

Meconium ileus equivalent

Meconium ileus equivalent affects approximately 10% of older children with cystic fibrosis. Intestinal contents may become abnormally thick and impact the intestinal lumen, particularly after episodes of dehydration or lack of pancreatic enzymes. The child displays signs and symptoms of intestinal obstruction. In most cases, the obstruction is relieved by hypertonic enemas. Meconium ileus and meconium ileus equivalent have been shown to be risk factors for the development of cirrhosis in individuals with cystic fibrosis.[14]

Obstructions of the duodenum, jejunum, and ileum

Congenital obstruction of the duodenum can be caused by intrinsic malformations or external pressure. The duodenum can be obstructed by an annular pancreas—a defect in which the head of the pancreas surrounds part of the duodenum. Congenital obstructions of the jejunum and ileum can be attributable to atresia, stenosis, meconium ileus, megacolon (Hirschsprung disease), intussusception, Meckel diverticulum, intestinal duplication, or strangulated hernia.

In **ileal** or **jejunal atresia** the intestine ends blindly, proximal and distal to an interruption in its continuity, with or without a gap in the mesentery. Stenosis (narrowing of the lumen) causes dilation proximal to the obstruction and luminal collapse distal to it.

Congenital aganglionic megacolon

Congenital aganglionic megacolon (Hirschsprung disease) is a functional obstruction of the colon caused by inadequate motility. It is the most common cause of colon obstruction, accounting for about one third of all gastrointestinal obstructions in infants. The incidence is 1 in 5000, with a preponderance in males. There is an increased incidence in children with Down syndrome.[15]

Pathophysiology

Congenital aganglionic megacolon is caused by a malformation of the parasympathetic nervous system and is characterized by absence of the intramural ganglion cells in the enteric nerve plexuses (Meissner and Auerbach plexuses). In 80% of cases the aganglionic segment is limited to the rectal end of the sigmoid colon. In 3% of cases the entire colon lacks ganglion cells. The abnormally innervated colon obstructs fecal movements, causing the proximal colon to become distended—hence the term *megacolon* (Fig. 35-3).

Clinical Manifestations

Mild to severe constipation is the usual manifestation of congenital aganglionic megacolon. Diarrhea may be the first sign, however, because only water can travel around the impacted feces.

The most serious complication in the neonatal period is enterocolitis related to fecal impaction. Bowel dilation stretches and partly occludes the encircling blood and lymphatic vessels, causing edema, ischemia, infarction of the mucosa, and significant outflow of fluid into the bowel lumen. Copious liquid stools result. Infarction and destruction of the mucosa enable enteric microorganisms to penetrate the bowel wall. Frequently, gram-negative sepsis occurs, accompanied by fever and vomiting. Severe and rapid electrolyte changes may take place, causing collapse and death.

Evaluation and Treatment

Anorectal manometry is a reliable screening tool for the diagnosis of Hirschsprung disease. Serial manometries may be required in neonates. The definitive diagnosis is made by rectal biopsy showing an absence of ganglion cells in the submucosa of the colon. X-ray films show dilated loops of colon, and contrast films show aganglionic areas.

The involved segment is resected within the first few months of life. Alternatively, enemas are given until the lumen is clear and then stool softeners are prescribed for life. The child is not treated for diarrhea.

After surgery, enterocolitis sometimes recurs, and if it is allowed to persist, pseudopolyps may appear. Because these are essentially identical to the lesions of ulcerative colitis, they have malignant potential. Therefore a colectomy is indicated if pseudopolyps develop.

In general, the prognosis of congenital megacolon is satisfactory for children who undergo surgical treatment. Bowel training may be prolonged, but most children achieve bowel continence before puberty.

Anorectal malformations

Several congenital malformations of anorectal structures can obstruct the passage of feces. The incidence of minor abnormalities is approximately 1 in 500, and that of major anomalies is approximately 1 in 5000.

Fig. 35-3 *Congenital aganglionic megacolon (Hirschsprung disease). (From Wong, D.L. et al. [1999].* Whaley & Wong's nursing care of infants and children *[6th ed.]. St. Louis: Mosby.)*

Congenital anorectal malformations range from mild anal stenosis, which is corrected by simple dilation, to complex deformities, such as anal or rectal agenesis, atresia, and fistula (Fig. 35-4). Deformities that cause complete obstruction are known collectively as **imperforate anus.**

Approximately 40% of infants with anorectal malformations have other developmental anomalies as well. The most commonly associated major anomalies are Down syndrome, congenital heart disease, renal abnormalities, esophageal atresia, and malformations of the spine.

Imperforate anus can be detected by gentle insertion of a rectal tube. X-ray films show dilations throughout the intestinal tract. Anal stenosis can be treated by dilations, but all other anorectal malformations require surgical correction. Overall mortality is approximately 10%. Children with a low (anal) anomaly usually achieve bowel continence, but those with a high (rectal) anomaly rarely do.

Acquired Impairment of Motility
Intussusception

The most frequent cause of acquired intestinal obstruction in infants is **intussusception**—the telescoping or invagination of one portion of the intestine into another. Usually, the ileum invaginates the cecum and part of the ascending colon by collapsing through the ileocecal valve. Intussusception involving the ileum and colon (ileocolic intussusception) accounts for 80% to 90% of intestinal obstructions in infants and is two to three times more common in males than in females. Nearly 75% of intussusceptions occur before the age of 2 years; 70% occur before the age of 1 year.[16] Intussusception is rare in infants younger than 3 months of age and is uncommon after 36 months. Intussusception has occurred in children of all ages recovering from abdominal surgery

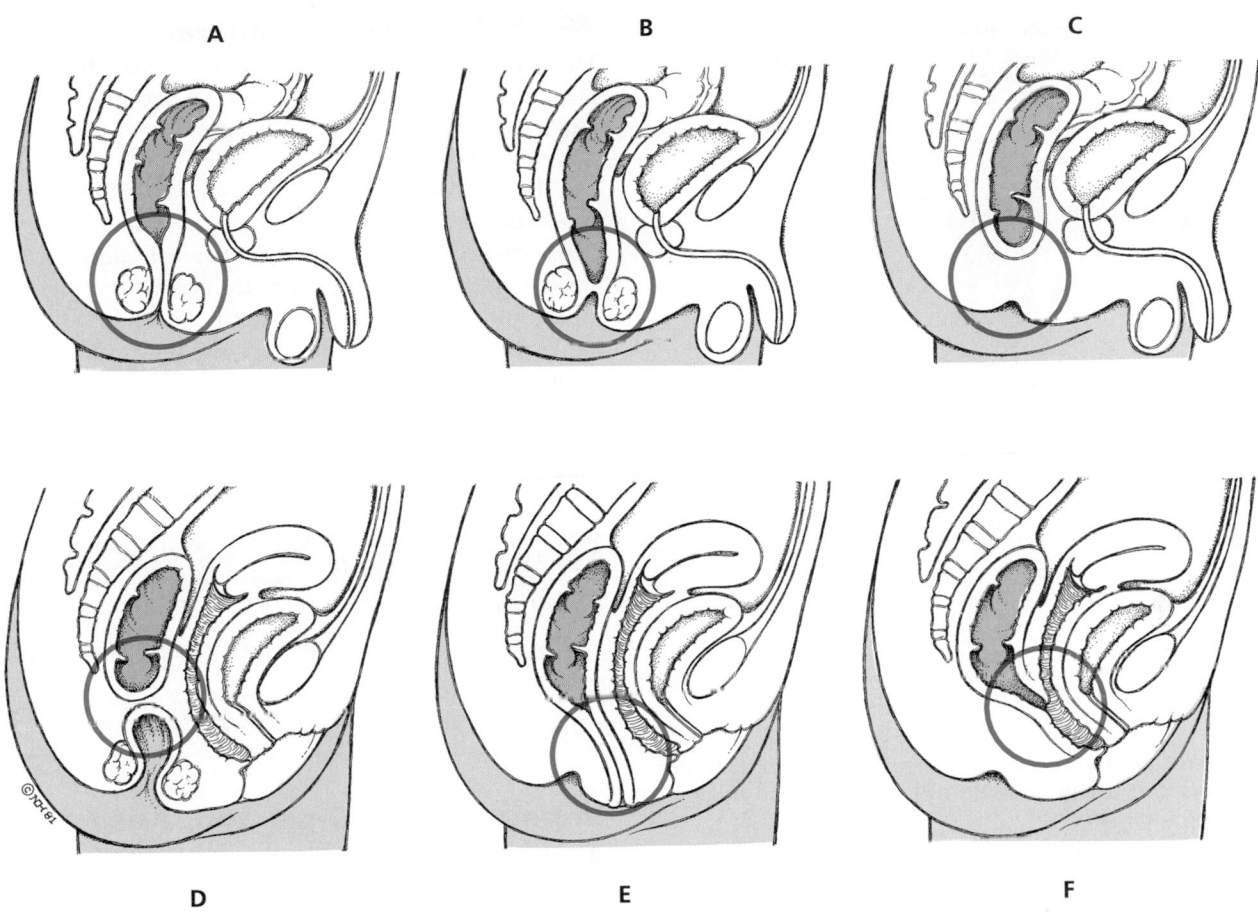

Fig. 35-4 *Anorectal stenosis and imperforate anus.* **A,** Congenital anal stenosis. **B,** Anal membrane atresia. **C,** Anal agenesis. **D,** Rectal atresia. **E,** Rectoperineal fistula. **F,** Rectovaginal fistula. *(From Wong, D.L. et al. [1999]. Whaley & Wong's nursing care of infants and children [6th ed.]. St. Louis: Mosby.)*

and has been found in children with cystic fibrosis and symptoms of bowel obstruction who were initially misdiagnosed as having meconium ileus equivalent.[17]

Pathophysiology

The proximal portion of the intestine, the intussusceptum, collapses into the distal portion, the intussuscipiens, in the direction of peristaltic flow (Fig. 35-5). The intussusceptum then drags its mesentery into the enveloping lumen. Initially, the mesentery is constricted, obstructing venous return. Compression of the mesenteric vessels between the two layers of intestinal wall and at the U-shaped angle at either end of the intussusceptum leads within hours to venous stasis, engorgement, edema, exudation, and further vascular compression. Unless the intussusception is treated, gangrene ensues. The tension of the mesentery on the intussusceptum tends to arch the bowel in a curve having its center at the mesenteric root. Edema and compression obstruct the flow of chyme through the intestine.

Clinical Manifestations

The affected infant suddenly develops abdominal pain, becomes irritable (colicky), and draws up the knees. Vomiting occurs soon afterward. A single normal stool may be passed, evacuating the colon distal to the apex of the intussusception. After that, 60% of infants pass "currant jelly" stools, which appear dark and gelatinous because of their blood and mucus content. Abdominal tenderness and distention develop as intestinal obstruction becomes more acute.

Evaluation and Treatment

Diagnosis is based on clinical manifestations, onset of symptoms, and ultrasonography. Reduction is an emergency procedure involving hydrostatic pressure exerted by an enema given under fluoroscopic guidance and is successful 60% to 70% of the time. Surgical reduction is done on children who fail or are not candidates for hydrostatic reduction. Untreated intussusception in infants is nearly always fatal. Most infants recover if the intussusception is reduced within 24 hours.[18]

Gastroesophageal reflux

Gastroesophageal reflux (GER) is the return of stomach contents into the esophagus because of relaxation or incompetence of the lower esophageal sphincter. In newborns, reflux is normal because neuromuscular control of the gastroesophageal sphincter is not fully developed. The frequency of reflux is highest in premature infants and de-

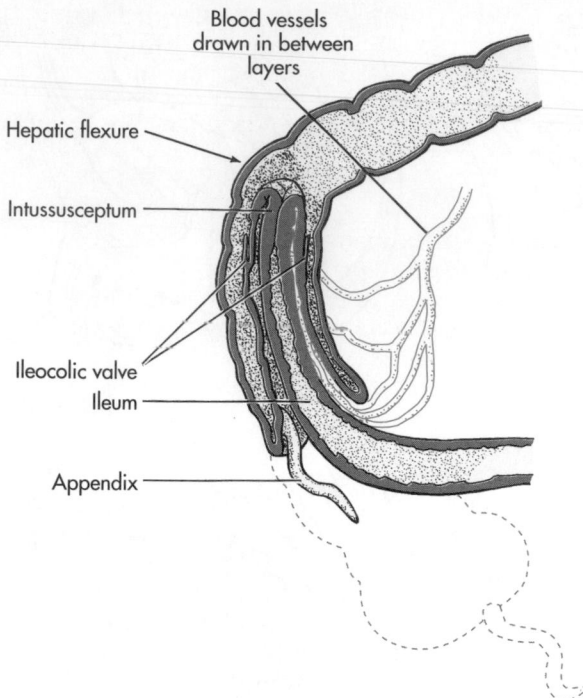

Fig. 35-5 *Ileocolic intussusception. (From Wong, D.L. et al.
[1999]. Whaley & Wong's nursing care of infants and children
[6th ed.]. St. Louis: Mosby.)*

creases during the first 6 to 12 months of life.[19] Normal infants and children have been shown to have some reflux but may be asymptomatic. Reflux is thought to be a contributing cause in infant deaths and sudden infant death syndrome.[20]

⚏ *Pathophysiology*

Delayed maturation of the lower esophageal sphincter or impaired hormonal response mechanisms are possible causes. Factors that maintain lower esophageal sphincter integrity in children include location of the gastroesophageal junction in a high-pressure zone within the abdomen, mucosal gathering within the sphincter, and the angle at which the esophagus is inserted into the stomach. Reflux persists if any of these pressure-maintaining factors is altered. Irritation of the mucosa by acidic gastric contents results in deterioration of the esophageal epithelium and stimulation of the vomiting reflex.

⚏ *Clinical Manifestations*

Of affected infants, 75% vomit excessively during the first week of life and usually have other symptoms by 6 weeks. Aspiration pneumonia develops in one third of infants with gastroesophageal reflux. In cases that persist into childhood, chronic cough, wheezing, and recurrent pneumonia are common. Inadequate retention of nutrients adversely impacts growth and weight gain. Esophagitis resulting from exposure of the esophageal mucosa to acidic gastric contents is manifested by pain, bleeding, and eventually stricture formation and abnormal motility. Approximately 25% have iron deficiency anemia caused by frank or occult blood loss.

⚏ *Evaluation and Treatment*

The clinical manifestations are often adequate to confirm a diagnosis of gastroesophageal reflux. A barium swallow and esophageal pH monitoring with a probe are useful diagnostic procedures in complex cases.

Mild gastroesophageal reflux resolves without treatment. Prone elevated positioning or upright sitting of an older child, particularly for the hour after a feeding, decreases episodes of reflux. Medications to increase motility, to increase lower esophageal sphincter pressure, or to decrease gastric acid production have been used to treat GER. If no improvement is seen with medical management or the child has life-threatening events with reflux, an antireflux surgical procedure, including gastropexy and fundoplication, is performed.[21]

✓ QUICK CHECK

Describe the pathologic defect in meconium ileus.

Why is there poor bowel motility with Hirschsprung disease?

Describe the defect in intussusception.

Impairment of Digestion, Absorption, and Nutrition

Cystic fibrosis

Cystic fibrosis (CF) of the pancreas, which is also called *mucoviscidosis* or *fibrocystic disease of the pancreas,* is a genetically transmitted disease that involves many organs and systems and usually causes death in childhood or young adulthood. It is the most frequent cause of chronic suppurative lung disease in children and is the most common life-threatening inherited disease in the white population. This section focuses on the deficiency of pancreatic enzymes. (Chapter 26 discusses the pulmonary consequences of cystic fibrosis.)

⚏ *Pathophysiology*

The pathophysiologic triad that is the hallmark of cystic fibrosis includes (1) pancreatic enzyme deficiency, which causes maldigestion; (2) overproduction of mucus in the respiratory tract and inability to clear secretions that cause progressive chronic obstructive pulmonary disease; and (3) abnormally elevated sodium and chloride concentrations in sweat. The full spectrum of involvement is evident as shown in Table 35-1.

Approximately 85% have pancreatic insufficiency.[22] Severe problems with maldigestion of proteins, carbohydrates, and fats occur because of insufficient secretion of pancreatic enzymes. Obstruction of the pancreatic ducts with thick mucus blocks the flow of pancreatic enzymes and causes degenerative and fibrotic changes in the pancreas, resulting in diabetes mellitus in some children.

⚏ *Clinical Manifestations*

Clinical manifestations are summarized in Table 35-1.

TABLE 35-1 Pathophysiology, Clinical Manifestations, and Complications of Cystic Fibrosis

Organ Involved	Secretory Dysfunction	Clinical Manifestations	Complications
Sweat glands	Elevated concentration of sodium and chloride in sweat	Hyponatremia; hypochloremia	Heat prostration; shock
Intestine			
Newborn	Viscid meconium	Meconium ileus with intestinal obstruction	Meconium peritonitis
Older child and adult	Inspissated (dried out) mucofecal masses (intestinal sludging)	Partial intestinal obstruction with severe cramping pains	Volvulus (obstruction), intussusception (prolapse)
Pancreas (enzyme deficiency)	Inspissation and precipitation of pancreatic secretions, causing obstruction of pancreatic ducts	Absence of pancreatic enzymes, causing malabsorption of food and fatty, bulky stools	Hypoproteinemia; iron deficiency anemia; malnutrition
		Decreased vitamins A, D, E, and K absorption	Vitamins A, D, E, and K deficiency and rectal prolapse
	Insulin deficiency	Glucose intolerance	Diabetes mellitus
Liver	Inspissation and precipitation of bile in biliary system	Focal biliary cirrhosis; shrunken, "hobnail" liver	Portal hypertension with esophageal varices and hematemesis
Salivary glands	Inspissation and precipitation of secretions in small ducts of submaxillary and sublingual salivary glands	Mild patchy fibrosis of salivary glands	None
Paranasal structures	Viscid mucus	Retention of mucus; clouding seen on sinus roentgenograms	Mucopyoceles (pus accumulations) with nasal deformity or orbital cavity extension
Nose	Nasal polyps	Obstruction of nasal air flow	None
Lungs	Viscid mucus in bronchioles and bronchi	Obstruction of bronchioles causing bronchiolectasis, bronchiectasis, and chronic lung infection	Hemoptysis; pneumothorax; cor pulmonale; respiratory failure
Reproductive tract			
Male	Viscid genital tract secretions during embryologic development, causing failure of formation of normal vas deferens	Sterility	None
Female	Distention of endocervical epithelial cells with cytoplasmic mucin	Decreased fertility	Polypoid cervicitis (cervical inflammation) while taking oral contraceptives

From Rudolph, A.M. & Hoffman, J.I.E. (1982). Pediatrics. Norwalk, Conn.: Appleton-Century-Crofts.

Evaluation and Treatment

Seventy-two-hour stool fat measurements are used to determine the extent of pancreatic function. Stools also may be examined for absence of pancreatic enzymes, particularly trypsin and chymotrypsin. Pancreatic replacement enzymes are administered before or with meals. High-caloric, high-protein diets with frequent snacks are used to treat the malnutrition.

Gluten-sensitive enteropathy

Gluten-sensitive enteropathy, formerly called *celiac sprue* or *celiac disease,* is the loss of mature villous epithelium caused by ingestion of gluten, the protein component of cereal grains. The gluten in wheat, rye, barley, and oats is toxic to the intestinal epithelial cells of genetically susceptible individuals.[23] The disease occurs largely in whites and has been documented in Asians from India and Pakistan but is almost

Fig. 35-6 *Pathophysiology of gluten-sensitive enteropathy.*

nonexistent in native Africans, Japanese, and Chinese. Prevalence rates in the United States have been documented as 22 per 100,000.[24]

Pathogenesis appears to be complex, involving dietary, genetic, and immunologic factors, as well as requiring exposure of susceptible individuals to environmental agents in addition to gluten.

Pathophysiology

The mucosa of the upper small intestine appears shiny, cobble-stoned, and thin in children with gluten-sensitive enteropathy. The major pathophysiologic characteristics of the disease are atrophy of villi in the upper small intestine and malabsorption of most nutrients in the presence of cereal gluten (Fig. 35-6).

Damage to the mucosa of the duodenum and jejunum exacerbates malabsorption. The secretion of intestinal hormones, such as secretin and cholecystokinin-pancreozymin, may be diminished, so secretion of pancreatic enzymes and expulsion of bile from the gallbladder decrease.

Destruction of mucosal cells causes inflammation, and water and electrolytes are secreted, leading to watery diarrhea. Potassium loss leads to muscle weakness. Magnesium and calcium malabsorption can cause seizures or tetany. Unabsorbed fatty acids combine with calcium, and secondary hyperparathyroidism increases phosphorus excretion, resulting in bone reabsorption. Calcium is no longer available to bind oxalate in the intestine and is absorbed, which causes hyperoxaluria. Gallbladder function may be abnormal, and bile salt conjugation may be decreased.

Fat malabsorption in the jejunum is the major cause of steatorrhea (fatty stools). Deficiencies of fat-soluble vitamins are common in children with gluten-sensitive enteropathy. Vitamin K malabsorption leads to hypoprothrombinemia. In one third of cases, iron and folic acid malabsorption is manifested as cheilosis, anemia, and a smooth red tongue. Vitamin B_{12} absorption is impaired in those with extensive ileal disease, and folate and iron deficiencies are common.

Clinical Manifestations

The onset of clinical manifestations of gluten-sensitive enteropathy depends on the age of the infant when gluten-containing substances are added to the diet. In 50% of affected children, onset occurs by 18 months of age, with latent intervals varying from months to years.

Diarrhea is an early sign in most infants. The stools are pale, bulky, greasy, and foul-smelling, and they may contain oil droplets. Three to five such movements occur daily. As early as 3 or 4 months of age, growth failure, anorexia, and constipation can begin. In older children, constipation is occasionally seen despite steatorrhea. Vomiting and abdominal pain are prominent in infants but unusual in older children. Anorexia is prevalent. The classic physical manifestations of organic failure to thrive, such as abdominal protuberance, wasted buttocks and limbs, and hypotonia, occur in fewer than 50% of infants with gluten-sensitive enteropathy. Growth is usually diminished.[25]

Manifestations of malabsorption, such as rickets, anemia, tetany, frank bleeding, or anemia, may be obvious.

Some children urinate more at night. The tongue is smooth and red, and the child may bruise and bleed easily. Hypomagnesemia and hypocalcemia cause irritability, tremor, convulsions, tetany, bone pain, osteomalacia, and dental abnormalities. If vitamin D deficiency is prolonged, rickets and clubbing of the terminal phalanges are likely. Eighty-six percent of older children have fingerprint changes (ridge atrophy). In older children, delayed puberty and infertility may be manifestations of otherwise subtle gluten-sensitive enteropathy.[26]

An unusual complication of gluten-sensitive enteropathy in infancy is celiac crisis. Celiac crisis is characterized by severe diarrhea, dehydration, and hypoproteinemia as a result of malabsorption and protein loss.

Evaluation and Treatment

An intestinal biopsy is mandatory to detect the classic mucosal changes caused by gluten-sensitive enteropathy. The initial biopsy is generally followed by a second intestinal biopsy to demonstrate regeneration of intestinal villi after treatment with a gluten-free diet. A wide variety of screening tests for malabsorption also may be useful. Serum immunoglobulins A and G (IgA, IgG) antigliadin (from gluten) antibodies also are measured.

Treatment consists of the immediate and permanent institution of a diet free of cereal grains (wheat, rye, barley, oats, malt). Lactose intolerance is presumed; therefore lactose (milk sugar) is also excluded from the diet. Infants are routinely given vitamin D, iron, and folic acid supplements to treat deficiencies.

Approximately 25% of children experience recurrent relapses that interfere with growth. For most children, however, the long-term prognosis is excellent. There is an increased incidence of malignant disease, particularly lymphoma, in individuals who fail to respond to gluten-free diets.

Protein energy malnutrition

Kwashiorkor and marasmus are the two most common types of malnutrition in children. These disorders are known collectively as *protein energy malnutrition (PEM)*. Both are states of long-term starvation. *Kwashiorkor* is a severe protein deficiency, and *marasmus* is a severe deficiency of all nutrients. Kwashiorkor is a widespread nutritional problem among children in developing countries and economically destitute populations. The disease usually occurs in infants or children from 1 to 4 years of age who have been weaned from breast milk to a high-starch, protein-deficient diet.

Marasmus can occur at any age, but it is common in children younger than 1 year. In marasmus, starvation is attributable to lack of protein and carbohydrates and, in neglected children, to a psychogenic basis. In developing countries and impoverished populations, early weaning of breast-fed infants to overdiluted commercial formulas is a risk factor for marasmus.

Protein energy malnutrition is also a complication of diseases, such as chronic fever, tuberculosis, malignancy, digestive and malabsorptive disorders, and psychogenic illness.

Radiation therapy and chemotherapy can also contribute to protein energy malnutrition.

Pathophysiology

In kwashiorkor, the deficit of dietary amino acids reduces protein synthesis in all tissues. Physical growth and mental growth are stunted, and maintenance of minimal life processes is in jeopardy. The lack of sufficient plasma proteins results in generalized edema with a substantial loss of potassium. The liver swells with stored fat because no hepatic proteins are synthesized to form and release lipoproteins. Pancreatic atrophy and fibrosis may be present. Kwashiorkor also causes malabsorption, reduced bone density, and impaired renal function. If the condition is not reversed, the prognosis is very poor.

Because the intake of all dietary nutrients is reduced to a minimum in marasmus, metabolic processes, including liver function, are preserved, but growth is severely retarded. Caloric intake is too low to support protein synthesis for growth or the storage of fat. Muscle wasting also occurs. Fat wasting and anemia are common and can be severe. Severe vitamin A deficiency commonly results in blindness.[27]

Clinical Manifestations

Retarded physical, mental, and psychologic development; muscle wasting; diarrhea; dermatosis; and infection characterize marasmus. The presence of subcutaneous fat, hepatomegaly, and fatty liver distinguishes kwashiorkor from marasmus.

Evaluation and Treatment

Evaluation of protein energy malnutrition is based on nutritional history and clinical manifestations. The provision of deficient nutrients will resolve clinical symptoms in 4 to 6 weeks. Physical and mental retardation may not be reversible, however. Nutritional rehabilitation with appropriate environmental stimulation for infants and young children has been shown to resolve or improve cerebral shrinkage, physical growth, and psychomotor development.[28,29]

Failure to thrive

Failure to thrive (FTT) is the inadequate physical development of an infant or child. It is manifested as a deceleration in weight gain, a low weight/height ratio, or a low weight/height/head circumference ratio. In the United States, FTT usually affects infants and young children. It is a nutritional disorder having organic or nonorganic causes. Nonorganic FTT is most common among psychosocially and economically deprived populations, whereas organic FTT occurs equally in all populations. The incidence of nonorganic FTT is more than that of organic FTT.[30]

Pathophysiology

Organic FTT has a pathophysiologic cause, for example, gastroesophageal reflux, pyloric stenosis, gastroenteritis, infection by intestinal parasites, or congenital anomalies or chronic diseases of major body systems. All these disorders reduce the availability of nutrients for maintenance and growth. A chronic disease or congenital anomaly that causes weakness or reduced stature can also create developmental problems, psychosocial problems, and emotional problems for the child.

Nonorganic FTT is a syndrome with many psychosocial causes and may be complicated by inadequate economic resources and lack of knowledge. The problem in nonorganic FTT is ineffective nurturing by primary caregivers. Infants and children are at risk for nonorganic FTT if their parents or primary caregivers are unable to provide nurturance. Various parental stressors may be involved, including the following:

- Lack of nurturance in the parents' own childhood
- Unwanted pregnancy
- Inability to bond with the infant because of health or other problems
- Postpartum depression
- Family crisis, such as the occurrence of a death or marital problems
- Stress caused by single parenthood or social isolation
- Mental, emotional, or physical illness

Clinical Manifestations

Clinical manifestations of organic FTT are retarded growth accompanied by manifestations of the underlying disease. Manifestations of nonorganic FTT are retarded growth plus reduced energy level, reduced responsiveness and interaction with the environment, social isolation, spasticity and rigidity when held or touched, inability to make eye contact or smile, refusal to eat, and rejection of foods. Weight loss and decelerated growth are accompanied by developmental retardation in many areas. Nonorganic FTT is a complex syndrome involving psychosocial, emotional, and parent-child problems that compound the pathophysiologic abnormalities.[30]

Evaluation and Treatment

FTT is suggested if a child falls below the third percentile on the growth curve or is falling off a previously established growth curve. Organic FTT is manifested in infancy by weight, height, and head circumference growth that may be parallel to but below the normal ranges. If no genetic, endocrine, or other systemic disorder is identified and if the physical and laboratory examinations show no abnormalities other than delayed growth, an environmental cause is indicated.

Hospital admission is recommended if the diagnosis is unclear or the child is in nutritional or emotional jeopardy. Eating patterns, food preferences, caloric intake, and family interactions can be assessed during the hospital stay. If the cause is environmental, the hospitalized child with FTT usually begins to gain weight.

If an organic problem has been identified, management of FTT consists of treating the cause. Management of nonorganic FTT involves the immediate total care of the child and measures to address (1) the psychosocial and emotional problems of the caregivers and (2) parent-child interactions.

Counseling, parental modeling, and long-term family support are sometimes required.[31]

Necrotizing enterocolitis

Necrotizing enterocolitis is a potentially fatal condition that, if untreated, causes bowel necrosis or perforation. Its cause is unknown. It occurs primarily in premature infants; affected infants have a mean gestational age of 31 weeks and weigh less than 1500 g.[32] The risk of necrotizing enterocolitis decreases as the gastrointestinal tract matures.

Pathophysiology

Factors contributing to the development of necrotizing enterocolitis include maternal age older than 35 years, infections, immunologic injury, perinatal stress, and the effects of medications and feeding practices. Reduced mucosal blood flow leading to hypoxic injury to intestinal mucosa is thought to be the cause. This injury allows bacterial invasion of the bowel wall.[33] Accumulation of gas in the mucosa and submucosa leads to ischemia and necrosis of intestinal segments.

Clinical Manifestations

Manifestations of necrotizing enterocolitis usually appear within 2 weeks of birth. They range from mild abdominal distention to bowel perforation, sepsis, and death. Abdominal pain, unstable temperature, bradycardia, and apnea are nonspecific signs. Affected infants have occult or grossly bloody stools (80%), gastric retention (70%), and abdominal distention (70% to 90%). Premature infants often have more severe disease and other disorders, such as hyaline membrane disease.

Evaluation and Treatment

Diagnosis is based on clinical manifestations and plain films of the abdomen that show gas accumulation in the intestine. Treatments include cessation of feeding, gastric suction to decompress the intestines, fluid and electrolyte maintenance, and administration of antibiotics to control sepsis. Surgical resection is the treatment of choice for perforation.[34] Overall mortality is 20% to 40%.[35] Low-birth-weight infants are at greatest risk of death.

Diarrhea

Diarrhea is a frequent gastrointestinal problem during infancy and early childhood. Severe diarrhea occurs one to three times during the first 3 years of life. Most episodes are self-limiting and resolve within 72 hours. The pathophysiologic mechanisms of diarrhea in children are similar to those described for adults. Prolonged diarrhea is more dangerous in children, however, because they have much smaller fluid reserves than adults. Therefore dehydration can develop rapidly if any disturbance increases fluid secretion into the gastrointestinal lumen (secretory diarrhea), draws fluid into the lumen by osmosis (osmotic diarrhea), or prevents fluid absorption in the intestine.

Infant diarrhea is of special concern because its cause may be a congenital or metabolic anomaly. Infants have low fluid reserves and relatively rapid peristalsis and metabolism. Therefore the danger of dehydration is great.

Common causes of acute diarrhea in infants include congenital aganglionic megacolon, infections, milk protein allergies, and necrotizing enterocolitis. Less common causes are adrenogenital syndrome, impaired chloride-bicarbonate exchange, congenital lactase deficiency, glucose-galactose malabsorption, and sucrase-isomaltase deficiency.

Infectious diarrhea in newborns is usually associated with nursery epidemics involving pathogens such as *Escherichia coli*, *Klebsiella*, staphylococci, *Salmonella*, and *Shigella*. Diarrhea caused by these agents has a rapid onset, and acidosis and shock can occur quickly. *Clostridium difficile*, often associated with previous antibiotic therapy, can cause acute, profuse, watery diarrhea and symptoms of colitis.[36] True milk protein allergy, which is uncommon, causes bloody, explosive stools after the introduction of bovine milk into the diet.

Acute diarrhea

Acute diarrhea in children is almost synonymous with acute viral or bacterial gastroenteritis. Viral gastroenteritis tends to be self-limiting. Bacterial gastroenteritis is treated with antibiotics if the causal pathogen can be identified. Other causes of acute diarrhea in the older child include antibiotic therapy, appendicitis, chemotherapy, inflammatory bowel disease, parasitic infestation, parenteral infections, and ingestion of toxic substances.

HEALTH ALERT

Rotavirus Vaccine

Rotavirus is the leading cause of acute gastroenteritis and diarrheal morbidity in infants and young children. The U.S. Food and Drug Administration (FDA) approved an oral rotavirus vaccine in 1998, and it is recommended for infants at 2, 4, and 6 months of age. The vaccine can be safely administered with other vaccines.

Data from American Academy of Pediatrics. (1998). Prevention of rotavirus disease: Guidelines for use of rotavirus vaccine. Pediatrics, 102(6), 1483-1491; Markwick. A.J. et al. (1998). Oral tetravalent rotavirus vaccine can be successfully coadministered with oral poliovirus vaccine and a combined diphtheria, tetanus, pertussis, and Haemophilus influenzae type b vaccine. U.S. Rhesus Rotavirus Vaccine Study Group. Pediatric Infectious Disease Journal, 38(4), 259-297.

Chronic diarrhea

Children with acute gastroenteritis frequently remain mildly symptomatic for up to 4 weeks; therefore diarrhea that persists longer than 4 weeks is considered to be chronic.

Children with chronic diarrhea can be divided into two groups: (1) otherwise well children whose growth is normal and (2) ill children whose growth is retarded. Causes of chronic diarrhea in the first group include abnormal colonic motility, lactose intolerance, encopresis, parasitic infestation, and antibiotic use. Chronic diarrhea in the second group is usually caused by a disease that impairs absorption.

Chronic nonspecific diarrhea

In **chronic nonspecific diarrhea,** uncoordinated colonic motility causes forceful expulsion of feces. In some instances, there is a family history of bowel complaints. As an infant, the child is likely to have experienced colic and diarrhea associated with teething and immunizations. In more than 90% of cases, chronic nonspecific diarrhea resolves by 40 to 50 months of age. The cure frequently accompanies toilet training. Many children with chronic nonspecific diarrhea develop irritable bowel syndrome (also called *mucous colitis*) as adults.[37] Children with chronic nonspecific diarrhea usually do well with normal food and fluid intake. Special diets and medications are used with caution.[38]

Primary lactose intolerance

Lactose intolerance, the inability to digest milk sugar, is caused by inadequate production of lactase. It is a common cause of diarrhea. The malabsorption of lactose results in osmotic diarrhea accompanied by abdominal pain, bloating, and flatulence. These symptoms begin before the age of 7 years in half of affected blacks. Hydrogen lactose breath testing provides a formal diagnosis. Treatment consists of reducing milk consumption. Some children can tolerate lactose in fermented forms, such as cheese and yogurt, or by adding soy food.[39]

DISORDERS OF THE LIVER
Disorders of Biliary Metabolism and Transport
Physiologic jaundice of the newborn

Physiologic jaundice of the newborn is usually a transient, benign icterus that occurs during the first week of life in otherwise healthy, full-term infants.[40] It is caused by mild unconjugated (indirect-reacting) hyperbilirubinemia. A high level of indirect hyperbilirubinemia (15 mg/dl) is considered pathologic. There is a risk of brain damage (kernicterus) as the bilirubin passes into brain cells and is toxic with persistent high indirect hyperbilirubinemia.

Pathophysiology

Physiologic jaundice results from the complex interaction of factors that (1) increase bilirubin production, (2) impair hepatic uptake and excretion of bilirubin, and (3) promote reabsorption of bilirubin in the small intestine. Serum bilirubin values increase to 5 to 6 mg/dl by the second to fourth day after birth in full-term infants, and to 10 to 15 mg/dl by the fifth to seventh day in premature infants.

⬛ *Clinical Manifestations*

Physiologic jaundice develops during the second or third day after birth and usually subsides in 1 to 2 weeks in full-term infants and in 2 to 4 weeks in premature infants. After this, increasing bilirubin values and persistent jaundice indicate pathologic hyperbilirubinemia. Premature infants with respiratory distress, acidosis, or sepsis are at greater risk for encephalopathy.

⬛ *Evaluation and Treatment*

Both total and direct (conjugated) bilirubin levels are measured; the direct bilirubin should not exceed 1 mg/dl.[38] Other causes of jaundice must be eliminated to confirm physiologic jaundice. Treatment depends on the degree of hyperbilirubinemia. Physiologic jaundice is usually treated by phototherapy (ultraviolet light). Pathologic jaundice requires an exchange transfusion.

Biliary atresia

Biliary atresia is a congenital malformation characterized by the absence or obstruction of intrahepatic or extrahepatic bile ducts. The cause of the intrauterine injury to the ducts is not clear but is thought to be related to chromosomal abnormality, an immune response, or viral injury. The disease expression is a continuum in which the principal process is one of bile duct destruction.

The atresia or obstruction of the bile ducts leads to plugging, inflammation, and fibrosis of the bile canaliculi. Progressive obstruction may lead to biliary cirrhosis (see Chapter 34), portal hypertension, or liver failure.[41]

Jaundice is the primary clinical manifestation of biliary atresia, along with hepatomegaly and acholic (clay-colored) stools. Fat absorption is impaired for lack of bile salts, and the infant may fail to gain weight. Cirrhosis and liver failure can lead to death.

Diagnosis of biliary atresia is based on clinical manifestations and liver biopsy. Liver function test results are abnormal. Serum transaminase and alkaline phosphatase values are elevated, and conjugated (direct) serum bilirubin levels rise progressively.

Extrahepatic atresia can be relieved by the Kasai portoenterostomy. Even with initial restoration of bile flow, however, obliteration of intrahepatic bile ducts continues and cirrhosis results. Liver transplantation is the long-term therapy for biliary atresia. Of children with biliary atresia, 80% die before the age of 3 years if not treated.[41]

Inflammatory Disorders
Hepatitis

The pathophysiology of viral and fulminant hepatitis is described in Chapter 34.

Hepatitis A

Approximately one third of the reported cases of hepatitis A occur in children,[32] particularly young children of nursery school age. Outbreaks tend to occur in day care centers with large numbers of children who are not toilet trained and staff members who practice poor handwashing techniques.[42] Hepatitis A in children is usually mild and asymptomatic, but it may involve nausea, vomiting, and diarrhea. Because jaundice is absent, infected children appear to have the flu. Almost all children recover from hepatitis A without residual liver damage.[43]

HEALTH ALERT

Hepatitis Vaccines

Hepatitis A vaccine—recommended for children 2 years and older

Hepatitis B vaccine—recommended for all unvaccinated children 0-18 years of age; for infants, the vaccines are administered at birth, 1 month, and 6 months of age

Data from American Academy of Pediatric Committee on Infectious Diseases. (1996). Prevention of hepatitis A infections: Guidelines for use of hepatitis A vaccine and immune globulin. Pediatrics, 98(6, Pt. 1), 1207-1215; Recommendations to prevent hepatitis B virus transmission—United States. (1998). MMWR—Morbidity and Mortality Weekly Report, 48(2), 33-34.

Hepatitis B

Infants of mothers who are chronic hepatitis B surface antigen (HBsAg) carriers, children with hemophilia who receive frequent blood transfusions, children who abuse parenteral drugs, and children who live in institutions for mentally retarded persons are all at risk for hepatits B virus (HBV) infection. Of newborns infected by their mothers, 90% develop chronic hepatitis and become carriers. Chronic hepatitis may develop because the infant's immune system is immature. Infected infants are at risk for cirrhosis and hepatocellular carcinoma.[44] The most serious consequence of HBV infection is fulminant hepatitis, which occurs in 1% of cases. Hepatitis D virus (HDV) infection depends on active infection with HBV. There is evidence that the risk of fulminant hepatitis is higher in individuals with combined infection of HBV and HDV than in those with HBV infection alone.[45]

Hepatitis C

Hepatitis C in children is associated primarily with blood transfusions or perinatal transmission from infected mothers. Children who received frequent transfusions before 1992 are at highest risk. The disease is usually mild in children. Between 50% and 60% of affected children develop chronic liver disease.[46]

TABLE 35-2   Galactosemia, Fructosemia, and Wilson Disease

	Galactosemia	Fructosemia	Wilson Disease
Mechanism of disease	Deficiency of galactose and phosphate uridyl transferase An autosomal recessive trait Cannot convert galactose to glucose Toxic accumulation of galactose in body tissues, liver, and brain	Deficiency of fructose-1-phosphate aldolase An autosomal recessive trait Cannot metabolize fructose, sucrose, or honey; occurs when breast milk is replaced with cow's milk Toxic accumulation of fructose in body tissues	Probably autosomal recessive Defect in copper excretion by liver Impaired transport of copper in blood caused by diminished transport protein (ceruloplasmin) Toxic accumulations of copper in liver, brain, kidney, corneas
Clinical manifestations	High levels of blood galactose Vomiting Hypoglycemia May have failure to thrive Symptoms of cirrhosis at 2-6 mo—jaundice Mental retardation if not treated Cataracts if not treated	High levels of blood fructose Vomiting Hypoglycemia May have failure to thrive Hepatomegaly Jaundice Seizures	Intention tremors Indistinct speech Dystonia Greenish yellow rings in cornea Hepatomegaly Jaundice Anorexia Renal tubular defects
Evaluation	Presence of reducing substances in urine when infant is receiving lactose	Detailed dietary history Liver or intestinal mucosa biopsy	Low plasma ceruloplasmin
Treatment	Galactose-free diet	Fructose-, sucrose-, honey-free diet Vitamin C supplementation	Chelation therapy to remove copper from body Decreased dietary intake of copper

Chronic hepatitis

Hepatitis B and hepatits C are the main causes of chronic hepatitis in children. Manifestations of chronic hepatitis include malaise, anorexia, fever, gastrointestinal bleeding, hepatomegaly, edema, and transient joint pain. Serum alanine aminotransferase and bilirubin levels are elevated. There may be evidence of impairment of synthetic functions of the liver: prolonged prothrombin time and hypoalbuminemia. Diagnosis is based on the clinical manifestations and liver biopsy. There is no effective therapy for chronic hepatitis B or chronic hepatitis C. Some success has been achieved with human alpha interferon; improvement in liver function is seen in approximately 50% of children with HBV infection treated. Young children may respond to alternate-day treatment with steroids.[38] Liver transplant may ultimately be required.

Cirrhosis

Most forms of chronic liver diseases in children can progress to cirrhosis, but they seldom do so. The complications of cirrhosis in children are the same as those in adults: portal hypertension, the opening of collateral vessels between the portal and systemic veins, and varices. In addition, children with cirrhosis experience growth failure caused by nutritional deficits, as well as developmental delay, particularly in gross motor function because of ascites and weakness. The cause of cirrhosis may influence its severity and course. Some types of cirrhosis can be stabilized if the cause is identified and treated early.[47]

Portal Hypertension

There are two basic causes of portal hypertension in children: (1) increased resistance to blood flow within the portal system and (2) increased volume of portal blood flow. The second cause is quite rare in children and is not discussed here. Increased resistance to flow can occur anywhere in the portal circulatory system. Portal hypertension can accompany cirrhosis, intraabdominal infections, portal vein thrombosis, congenital anomalies of the portal vein, and congenital hepatic fibrosis.

Types of portal hypertension
Extrahepatic portal hypertension

Extrahepatic (prehepatic) portal venous obstruction causes 50% to 70% of *extrahepatic portal* hypertension in children. In approximately two thirds of these children, no specific cause can be found.[38] Obstruction is almost always in the portal vein and is usually caused by thrombosis as a complication of abdominal trauma, pancreatitis, abdominal infections, and some systemic disorders; however, these causes are rare. The liver is usually normal in extrahepatic portal hypertension.

Intrahepatic portal hypertension

Cirrhosis is the primary cause of **intrahepatic portal hypertension.** The most common finding is fibrosis, which increases resistance to portal blood flow by constricting and reducing the compliance of the hepatic sinusoids.

Course of the disease

The important consequences of portal hypertension in children are the development of collateral circulation, with portal-systemic shunting; hypersplenism; and ascites.

Clinical Manifestations

The clinical manifestations of portal hypertension are (1) splenomegaly, (2) upper gastrointestinal bleeding, (3) ascites, and (4) hepatic encephalopathy (see Chapter 34).

Evaluation and Treatment

The objectives of the clinical investigation are to (1) locate the site of the venous block and (2) identify the disease responsible for the portal hypertension. Thorough physical examination, laboratory tests of liver function, imaging procedures, and biopsy may be included in the diagnostic evaluation. Sclerotherapy is the initial treatment of choice for severe esophageal varices in children. Surgical venous shunts are rarely performed on small children because of the high failure rate secondary to vessel occlusion, but they may be an alternative in older children.[38]

The outcome of portal hypertension depends almost entirely on its cause. Children with extrahepatic disease are expected to recover with little morbidity. For children with intrahepatic disease, the prognosis varies.

Metabolic Disorders

More than 5000 genetically determined metabolic pathways have been identified in liver tissue. The earliest possible identification of metabolic disorders is essential because (1) early treatment may prevent permanent damage to vital organs, such as the liver or brain; (2) precise genetic counseling may be possible with prenatal diagnosis; and (3) complications can be minimized, even if cure is not possible. Galactosemia, fructosemia, and Wilson disease are treatable metabolic disorders that have hepatic clinical manifestations. The mechanisms of disease, clinical manifestations, evaluation, and treatment of these disorders are contained in Table 35-2.

✓ QUICK CHECK

Why is diarrhea such a serious disorder in infants and children?

What is biliary atresia?

What are the three most common metabolic disorders that cause liver damage in children?

▣ DID YOU UNDERSTAND?

Disorders of the Gastrointestinal Tract

1. Most alterations of digestive function in children are caused by congenital obstructions of the intestinal tract; disorders of digestion, absorption, or nutrition; or liver disease.

2. Cleft lip (harelip) and cleft palate (failure of the bony palate to fuse in the midline) may occur separately or together. The fissure may affect the uvula, soft palate, hard palate, nostril, and maxillary alveolar ridge.

3. Esophageal atresia, a condition in which the esophagus ends in a blind pouch, may occur with or without tracheoesophageal fistula, or connection between the esophagus and the trachea. As the infant swallows oral secretions or ingests milk, the pouch fills, causing either drooling or aspiration into the lungs.

4. Pyloric stenosis, one of the most common disorders requiring surgery in early infancy, is an obstruction of the pyloric outlet caused by hypertrophy of circular muscles in the pyloric sphincter.

5. Malrotation of the intestine, with an obstructing band and volvulus (twisting of the bowel on itself), may partly or completely occlude the gastrointestinal tract and its blood vessels.

6. Meconium ileus is a condition in the newborn in which intestinal secretions and amniotic waste products produce a thick, tarry plug that obstructs the intestine. Of children with cystic fibrosis, 10% to 20% present with meconium ileus as a neonate.

7. Duodenal, jejunal, and ileal obstructions can be caused by meconium ileus, atresia, congenital aganglionic megacolon, and acquired obstructive disorders.

8. Congenital aganglionic megacolon (Hirschsprung disease) is caused by a malformation of the parasympathetic nervous system in a segment of the colon. It is characterized by the absence of nerves needed for peristalsis.

9. Malformations of the anus and rectum range from mild congenital stenosis of the anus to complex deformities, all of which are classified as imperforate anus.

10. The most frequent cause of acquired intestinal obstruction in infants is intussusception, a condition in which one portion of the bowel telescopes, or invaginates, into another, most commonly in the area of the ileocecal junction.

11. Gastroesophageal reflux is caused by the relaxation or incompetence of the lower esophageal sphinc-

DID YOU UNDERSTAND? —cont'd

ter. Infants are susceptible to reflux because the sphincter is not fully mature, their diet consists of liquids, and they are seldom in an upright position.

12. Cystic fibrosis is an inherited exocrine gland abnormality that causes chronic suppurative lung disease and abnormalities in other organs that contain exocrine glands.

13. The pathophysiologic triad that is the hallmark of cystic fibrosis includes pancreatic enzyme deficiency (which causes maldigestion), overproduction of mucus in the respiratory tract, and abnormally elevated sodium and chloride concentrations in sweat. Older children with cystic fibrosis also may have diabetes mellitus caused by damage to endocrine function of the pancreas and chronic liver disease. Affected individuals seldom survive beyond their 20s.

14. Gluten-sensitive enteropathy is a lifelong disease characterized by the loss of mature villous epithelium in the presence of a gluten-containing diet. It results in malabsorption and growth failure.

15. Protein energy malnutrition is a group of disorders resulting from a severe dietary deficiency of proteins, carbohydrates, or both. Starvation causes stunted mental and physical development.

16. Kwashiorkor is a severe protein deficiency that occurs in children who have stopped breast-feeding and subsist on a high-carbohydrate diet. Marasmus is a deficiency of all dietary nutrients, including carbohydrates.

17. Failure to thrive is inadequate physical growth of a child. Organic failure to thrive is caused by genetic, anatomic, or pathophysiologic factors that retard normal growth and development. Nonorganic failure to thrive is caused by nutritional deficits associated with inadequate nurturing.

18. Necrotizing enterocolitis is a disorder in neonates, particularly premature infants, thought to result from stress and anoxia of the bowel wall. Bacteria invade the mucosa and submucosa, resulting in col-

itis, necrosis, and even perforation of the intestinal wall.

19. Diarrhea in infants and children can rapidly cause dehydration and electrolyte imbalances because fluid reserves are relatively small.

20. The most common cause of acute diarrhea in children is bacterial or viral enterocolitis (infection of the gastrointestinal tract).

21. Chronic diarrhea (diarrhea persisting longer than 4 weeks) can be caused by a wide variety of underlying conditions and frequently leads to growth failure and slow development.

Disorders of the Liver

1. Physiologic jaundice of the newborn is caused by mild hyperbilirubinemia that subsides in 1 or 2 weeks. Pathologic jaundice is caused by severe hyperbilirubinemia and can cause brain damage.

2. Biliary atresia is a congenital malformation of the bile ducts that obstructs bile flow. Atresia causes jaundice, cirrhosis, and liver failure. Biliary atresia is the most common reason for liver transplantation in children.

3. Acute hepatitis has the same clinical course in children and adults, but children have milder cases of the disease. Hepatitis A is the most common form of childhood hepatitis.

4. Cirrhosis is rare in children, but it can develop from most forms of chronic liver disease.

5. Portal hypertension in children usually is caused by extrahepatic obstruction. Thrombosis of the portal vein is the most common cause of portal hypertension in children, and splenomegaly is the most frequent sign.

6. The three most common metabolic disorders that cause liver damage in children are galactosemia, fructosemia, and Wilson disease. All three are inherited as genetic traits and permit the accumulation of toxins in the liver

KEY TERMS

Biliary atresia, 1000
Chronic nonspecific diarrhea, 999
Cleft lip (harelip), 988
Cleft palate, 988
Congenital aganglionic megacolon (Hirschsprung disease), 991
Cystic fibrosis (CF), 994
Esophageal atresia, 989
Extrahepatic portal hypertension, 1001
Failure to thrive (FTT), 997
Gastroesophageal reflux (GER), 993
Gluten-sensitive enteropathy (celiac sprue), 995

Ileal atresia, 991
Imperforate anus, 992
Infant diarrhea, 999
Intrahepatic portal hypertension, 1002
Intussusception, 992
Jejunal atresia, 991
Kwashiorkor, 997
Lactose intolerance, 999
Malrotation, 990
Marasmus, 997
Meconium, 991
Meconium ileus, 991

Meconium ileus equivalent, 991
Necrotizing enterocolitis, 998
Nonorganic FTT, 998
Organic FTT, 997
Periduodenal band, 990
Physiologic jaundice of the newborn, 999
Protein energy malnutrition (PEM), 997
Pyloric stenosis, 990
Tracheoesophageal fistula (TEF), 989

REFERENCES

1. Abrishamchian, A.R., Koury, M.S., & Calle, E.E. (1994). The contribution of maternal epilepsy and its treatment to the etiology of oral clefts: A population based control study. *Genetic Epidemiology, 11*(4), 343-351.

2. Elmendorf, E.N., D'Antonio, L.L., & Hardesty, R.A. (1993). Assessment of the patient with cleft lip and palate. *Clinics in Plastic Surgery, 20*(4), 607-621.

3. Broen, P.A. et al. (1998). Acquisition of linguistic and cognitive skills by children with cleft palate. *Journal of Speech, Language, and Hearing Research, 41*(3), 676-687.

4. Kalache, K.D. et al. (1998). The upper neck pouch sign: A prenatal sonographic marker for esophageal atresia. *Ultrasound in Obstetrics and Gynecology, 119*(2), 138-140.

5. Somppi, E. et al. (1998). Outcome of patients operated on for esophageal atresia: 30 years' experience. *Journal of Pediatric Surgery, 33*(9), 1341-1346.

6. Haubrich, W.S., Schaffner, F., & Berk, J.E. (1995). *Bockus gastroenterology* (5th ed.). Philadelphia: Saunders.

7. Levy, J. (1991). The gastrointestinal tract in Down syndrome. *Progress in Clinical Biology and Research, 373,* 245-256.

8. Abbas, A.E., Weiss, S.M., & Alvear, D.T. (1999). Infantile hypertrophic pyloric stenosis: Delays in diagnosis and overutilization of imaging modalities. *American Surgeon, 65*(1), 73-76.

9. Hulka, F. et al. (1997). Complications of pyloromyotomy for infantile hypertrophic pyloric stenosis. *American Journal of Surgery, 173*(5), 450-452.

10. Bailey, P.V. et al. (1993). Congenital duodenal obstruction: A 32-year review. *Journal of Pediatric Surgery, 28*(1), 92-95.

11. Bax, N.M. & van de Zee, D.C. (1998). Laparoscopic treatment of intestinal malrotation in children. *Surgical Endoscopy, 12*(11), 1314-1316.

12. Fuchs, J.R. & Langer, J.C. (1998). Long-term outcome after neonatal meconium obstruction. *Pediatrics, 101*(4), E7.

13. Mushtaq, I. et al. (1998). Meconium ileus secondary to cystic fibrosis: The East London experience. *Pediatric Surgery International, 13*(5-6), 365-369.

14. Fitzsimmons, S.C. (1993). The changing epidemiology of cystic fibrosis. *Journal of Pediatric Surgery, 122*(1), 1-9.

15. Moore, S.W. & Johnson, A.G. (1998). Hirschsprung's disease: Genetic and functional associations of Down's and Waardenburg syndromes. *Seminars in Pediatric Surgery, 7*(3), 156-161.

16. Wang, N.L. et al. (1998). Prenatal and neonatal intussusception. *Pediatric Surgery International, 13*(4), 232-236.

17. Eggermont, E. & De-Boeck, K. (1991). Small intestinal abnormalities in cystic fibrosis patients. *European Journal of Pediatrics, 150*(12), 824-828.

18. McDermott, V.G. et al. (1994). Pneumatic reduction of intussusception: Clinical experience and factors affecting outcome. *Clinical Radiology, 49*(1), 30-34.

19. Omari, T.I. et al. (1998). Mechanisms of gastroesophageal reflux in healthy premature infants. *Journal of Pediatrics, 133*(5), 650-654.

20. Westra, S.J., Derkx, H., & Taminian, J.A. (1994) Symptomatic gastroesophageal reflux: Diagnosis with ultrasound. *Journal of Pediatric Gastroenterology and Nutrition, 19*(1), 58-64.

21. Tsou, V.M. & Bishop, P.R. (1998). Gastroesophageal reflux in children. *Otolaryngologic Clinics of North America, 31*(3), 419-434.

22. Benabdeslam, H. et al. (1998). Biochemical assessment of the nutritional status of cystic fibrosis patients related with pancreatic enzyme. *American Journal of Clinical Nutrition, 67*(5), 912-918.

23. Tracone, R., Greco, L., & Auricchio, S. (1996). Gluten-sensitive enteropathy. *Pediatric Clinics of North America, 43*(2), 355-373.

24. Talley, N.J. et al. (1994). Epidemiology of celiac sprue: A community based study. *American Journal of Gastroenterology, 89*(6), 843-846.

25. Tracone, R., Greco, L., & Auricchio, S. (1996). Gluten-sensitive enteropathy. *Pediatric Clinics of North America, 43*(2), 355-373.

26. Mariani, P. et al. (1998). The gluten-free diet: A nutritional risk factor for adolescents with celiac disease? *Journal of Pediatric Gastroenterology and Nutrition, 27*(5), 519-523.

27. Widdowson, E.M. (1991). Contemporary human diets and their relation to health and growth: Overview and conclusions. *Philosophical Transactions of the Royal Society of London, 334,* 289-295.

28. Gunston, G.D. et al. (1992). Reversible cerebral shrinkage in kwashiorkor: An MRI study. *Archives of Disease in Childhood, 67,* 1030-1032.

29. Proos, L.A. et al. (1992). A longitudinal study on anthropometric and clinical development of Indian children adopted in Sweden: Growth, morbidity, and development during two years after arrival in Sweden. *Upsala Journal of Medical Sciences, 97,* 93-106.

30. Leung, A.K., Robson, W.M., & Fagan, J.E. (1993). Assessment of the child with failure to thrive. *American Family Physician, 48*(8), 1432-1438.

31. McPhee, M., Mori, C., & Goldson, E. (1994). Change in the hospital setting: Adopting a team approach for nonorganic failure to thrive. *Journal of Pediatric Nursing, 9*(4), 218-225.

32. Avery, M.E. & First, L.R. (1994). *Pediatric medicine* (2nd ed.). Baltimore: Williams & Wilkins.

33. Sonntag, J. et al. (1998). Multisystem organ failure and capillary leak syndrome in severe necrotizing enterocolitis of very low birth weight infants. *Journal of Pediatric Surgery, 33*(93), 481-484.

34. Ladd, A.P. et al. (1998). Long-term follow-up after

REFERENCES

bowel resection for necrotizing enterocolitis: Factors affecting outcome. *Journal of Pediatric Surgery, 33*(7), 967-972.

35. Martinez-Tallo, E., Claure, N., & Bancalari, E. (1997). Necrotizing enterocolitis in full-term or near-term infants: Risk factors. *Biology of the Neonate, 71*(5), 292-298.

36. Niyogi, S.K. et al. (1991). Clostridium difficile and its cytotoxin in hospitalized children with acute diarrhea. *Indian Pediatrician, 28,* 1129-1132.

37. Levine, J.J. (1987). Chronic nonspecific diarrhea. *Pediatric Annals, 10,* 822-829.

38. Bortolotti, F. et al. (1996). Nonorgan specific autoantibodies in children with chronic hepatitis C. *Journal of Hepatology, 25*(5), 614-620.

39. Quak, S.H. & Tan, S.P. (1998). Use of soy-protein formulas and soyfood for feeding infants and children in Asia. *American Journal of Clinical Nutrition, 68*(6, Suppl.), 144S-146S.

40. Schwoebel, A. & Sakriada, S. (1997). Hyperbilirubinemia: New approaches to an old problem. *Journal of Perinatal and Neonatal Nursing, 11*(3), 78-97.

41. Bates, M.D. et al. (1998). Biliary atresia: Pathogenesis and treatment. *Seminars in Liver Disease, 18*(3), 281-293.

42. Balcarek, K.B. et al. (1995). Safety and immunogenicity of an inactivated hepatitis A vaccine in preschool children. *Journal of Infectious Diseases, 171*(Suppl. 1), S70-S72.

43. Lesnicar, C. (1988). A prospective study of viral hepatitis A and the question of chronicity. *Hepatogastroenterology, 35*(2), 69-72.

44. Balistreri, W.F. (1988). Viral hepatitis. *Pediatric Clinics of North America, 35,* 375-407.

45. Treem, W.R. (1991). Hepatic failure. In W.A. Walker et al. (Eds.). *Pediatric gastrointestinal disease.* Philadelphia: Decker.

46. Balli, F. et al. (1998). Chronic hepatitis C in children: The pathological and clinical spectrum. *Gastroenterology, 115*(6), 1525-1529.

47. Badizadegan, K. et al. (1998). Histopathology of the liver in children with chronic hepatitis C viral infection. *Hepatology, 28*(5), 1416-1423.

CHAPTER

36

Structure and Function of the Musculoskeletal System

Leona A. Mourad

The way an individual functions in daily life, moves about, or manipulates objects physically depends on the integrity of the musculoskeletal system. The musculoskeletal system is actually two systems: (1) the skeleton composed of bones and joints and (2) skeletal muscles. Each system contributes to mobility. The skeleton supports the body and provides leverage to the skeletal muscles so that movement of various parts of the body is possible. Contraction of the skeletal muscles and bending or rotation at the joints facilitate movements of the various body parts.

CHAPTER OUTLINE

Check out your CD Companion for chapter-related exercises and answers to the Quick Check questions

STRUCTURE AND FUNCTION OF BONES

Bones give form to the body, support tissues, and permit movement by providing points of attachment for muscles. Many bones meet in movable joints that determine the type and extent of movement possible. Bones also protect many of the body's vital organs. For example, the bones of the skull, thorax, and pelvis are hard exterior shields that protect the brain, heart, lungs, and reproductive and urinary organs.

The marrow cavities within certain bones serve as sites of blood cell formation. In adults, blood cells originate exclusively in the marrow cavities of the skull, vertebrae, ribs, sternum, shoulders, and pelvis. Bones also have a crucial role in mineral homeostasis, storing minerals (i.e., calcium, phosphate, carbonate, magnesium) that are essential for the proper working of many delicate cellular mechanisms.

Elements of Bone Tissue

Mature bone is a rigid connective tissue consisting of cells, fibers, a gelatinous material termed *ground substance,* and large amounts of crystallized minerals, mainly calcium, that give bone its rigidity. The structural elements of bone are summarized in Table 36-1.

Bone cells enable bone to grow, repair itself, change shape, and continuously synthesize new bone tissue and resorb (dissolve or digest) old tissue. The fibers in bone are made of collagen that give bone its tensile strength (the ability to hold itself together). Ground substance acts as a medium for the diffusion of nutrients, oxygen, metabolic wastes, biochemicals, and minerals between bone tissue and blood vessels.

Bone formation begins during fetal life with the growth of cartilage—the precursor of bone tissue. In mature bone the formation of new tissue begins with the production of an organic matrix by the bone cells. This *bone matrix* consists of ground substances, collagen, and other proteins (see Table 36-1) that take part in bone formation and maintenance.

The next step in bone formation is *calcification,* when minerals are deposited and crystallize. Minerals bind tightly to collagen fibers, producing tensile and compressional strength in bone and allowing it to withstand pressure and weight bearing.

Bone cells

Bone contains three types of cells: osteoblasts, osteocytes, and osteoclasts (Fig. 36-1). *Osteoblasts* are the bone-forming cells. Their primary function is to lay down new bone. Once this function is complete, osteoblasts become osteocytes. *Osteocytes* are osteoblasts that have become imprisoned within the mineralized bone matrix. They have an ill-defined role in maintaining the inorganic (mineral) and organic elements of bone matrix. *Osteoclasts* function primarily to resorb (remove) bone during processes of growth and repair.

Osteoblast

An *osteoblast* is a cell derived from osteogenic mesenchymal stromal cells that produces type I collagen and is the major bone-forming cell. Osteoblasts are responsive to parathyroid hormone (PTH) and produce osteocalcin when stimulated by 1,25-dihydroxyvitamin D.[1] Osteoblasts are active on the outer surfaces of bones, where they form a single layer of cells. Osteoblasts bring about new bone formation by their synthesis of osteoid (nonmineralized bone matrix). Os-

Fig. 36-1 *Bone cells.* **A,** Osteoblasts are responsible for the production of collagenous and non-collagenous proteins that compose osteoid. Active osteoblasts are lined up on the osteoid. Note the eccentrically located nuclei. **B,** Osteocyte. Scanning electron micrograph showing an osteocyte within a lacuna. The cell is surrounded by collagen fibers and mineralized bone. **C,** Osteoclasts actively resorb mineralized tissue. The scalloped surface in which the multinucleated osteoclasts rest is termed *Howship lacuna.* (*A and C from Damjanov, I. & Linder, J. [Eds.]. [1996]. Anderson's pathology [10th ed.]. St. Louis: Mosby; B from Erlandesen, S. & Magney, J. [1992]. Color atlas of histology. St. Louis: Mosby.*)

TABLE 36-1   Structural Elements of Bone

Structural Element	Function
Bone cells	
Osteoblasts	Synthesize collagen and proteoglycans; stimulate osteoclast resorptive activity
Osteocytes	Maintain bone matrix
Osteoclasts	Resorb bone; assist with mineral homeostasis
Bone matrix	
Collagen fibers	Lend support and tensile strength
Proteoglycans	Control transport of ionized materials through matrix
Bone morphogenic proteins	Induce cartilage formation
BMP-1	
BMP-2A	
BMP-3	
Glycoproteins	
Sialoprotein	Promotes calcification
Osteocalcin	Inhibits calcium-phosphate precipitation; promotes bone resorption
Laminin	Stabilizes basement membranes in bones
Osteonectin	Binds calcium in bones
Albumin	Transports essential elements to matrix; maintains osmotic pressure of bone fluid
α-Glycoprotein	Promotes calcification
Minerals (elements)	
Calcium	Crystallizes to lend rigidity and compressive strength
Phosphate	Regulates vitamin D and thereby promotes mineralization

TABLE 36-2   Effects of Selected Cytokines (Growth Factors) on Skeletal Tissues

Cytokine (Growth Factor)	Target Tissue	Formation	Resorption
Transforming growth factor-beta	Bone	+, −	+, −
	Cartilage	+, −	−
Transforming growth factor-alpha or epidermal growth factor	Bone	+, −	+
	Cartilage	+	
Insulin-like growth factor	Bone	−	0
	Cartilage	−	?
Fibroblast growth factor	Bone	+, −	0
	Cartilage		?
Platelet-derived growth factor	Bone	+	0
Colony-stimulating factors	Bone	0	+
	Cartilage	?	?
Interferon-gamma	Bone	−	−
	Cartilage	−	?
Tumor necrosis factor	Bone	−	+
	Cartilage	−	+
Interleukin-1, -3, and -6	Bone	+, −	+
	Cartilage	−	+

+, −: *Both stimulatory and inhibitory properties on the specific cell listed; 0: no effects presently known; ?: possible effects on cell listed.*

teoblasts also mineralize newly formed bone matrix.[2] Stimulation of bone formation of new bone and the orderly mineralization of bone matrix occur by concentrating some of the plasma proteins (growth factors) found in the bone matrix and by facilitating the deposit and exchange of calcium and other ions at the site. As new bone is formed, it is shaped and remodeled through the effect of transforming growth factor-beta (TGF-β), as well as other plasma proteins (growth factors) found in the bone marrow (Table 36-2).

The concept of coupling bone formation with bone resorption has been extensively studied yet is still not entirely clear. Recent studies have shown that osteoblasts release a factor the induces osteoclastic activity by stimulating osteoclastic contact (see Osteoclast). In contact with bone mineral, osteoclasts can be further stimulated by colony-stimulating factor and interleukins-1, -3, and -6 produced by macrophage cells in the presence of PTH.[3] Thus the cells of the osteoblastic lineage (osteoblasts, osteocytes) form a network of cells in bone that sense the shape and structure of bone and determine where it is appropriate that bone be formed or resorbed, according to Wolff law (bone is shaped according to its function).

Osteoblasts have an active state and a resting state. When active, osteoblasts synthesize and secrete osteoid. When in the resting state, they appear dormant. If appropriately stimulated, however, the resting osteoblasts are capable of resuming activity.

Osteoclast

Osteoclasts are large, multinucleated cells that develop from the hematopoietic monocyte-macrophage lineage. Osteoclasts are the major resorptive cells of bone. They migrate over bone surfaces to resorption areas that have been prepared and stripped of osteoid by enzymes, such as collagenases, produced by osteoblasts in the presence of PTH, which is necessary for the resorptive process.[4] Osteoclasts travel over the prepared bone surfaces, creating irregular, scalloped cavities, known as Howship lacunae or resorption bays, as they resorb bone areas.[4]

A specific area of the cell membrane forms adjacent to the bone surface and forms multiple infoldings to permit intimate contact with the resorption bay. These infoldings, known as the *ruffled border,* greatly increase the cell's surfaces under their scalloped or ruffled borders. Osteoclasts resorb bone by secretion of citric and lactic acids, which help dissolve bone minerals, and collagenases, which aid in digesting collagen, along with the action of cytokines (see Table 36-2). Osteoclasts also resorb bone through the action of lysosomes (digestive vacuoles) filled with hydrolytic enzymes in their mitochondria.

Osteoclasts bind to the bone surfaces through attachments called *integrins.* Once resorption is complete, the osteoclasts retract and loosen from the bone surface under the ruffled border through the action of calcitonin. Calcitonin binds to receptor areas of the osteoclasts' cell membranes to effectively loosen the osteoclasts from the bone surfaces.[4] Once resorption is completed, osteoclasts disappear by degeneration, either by reverting to their parent cells or through cell movements from the site where the osteoclast becomes an inactive or resting osteoclast.

Osteocyte

An *osteocyte* is a transformed osteoblast that is trapped or surrounded in osteoid as it hardens from minerals that enter during calcification (see Fig. 36-1, *B*). The osteocyte is within a space in the hardened bone matrix called a **lacuna.** Each osteocyte has a higher nucleus/cytoplasm ratio with a thin layer of nonmineralized osteoid around it, like the egg white surrounding an egg yolk.

The function of osteocytes is still somewhat unclear, but they are thought to participate in the maintenance of bone matrix by helping to concentrate nutrients in the matrix. Osteocytes obtain nutrients from capillaries in the canaliculi, which contain nutrient-rich fluids. Osteocytes also may help synthesize and replace needed elements of the matrix, thus

helping maintain mineral homeostasis with the help of PTH and osteoblast cells. Through exchanges among these cells, hormone catalysts, and minerals, optimal levels of calcium, phosphorus, and other minerals are maintained in blood plasma. The osteocyte also aids in modifying bone matrix through release of enzymes to dissolve the mineralized walls of the lacunae to prepare the bone for remodeling. Remodeling is described on p. 1012.

Bone matrix

Bone matrix is made of the *extracellular* elements of bone tissue, specifically collagen fibers, proteins, carbohydrate-protein complexes, ground substance, and minerals.

Collagen fibers

Collagen fibers make up the bulk of bone matrix. They are formed as follows:

1. Osteoblasts synthesize and secrete type I collagen.
2. Collagen molecules assemble into three thin chains (alpha chains) to form **fibrils.**
3. Fibrils organize into the staggered pattern, with each fibril overlapping its nearest neighbor by about one fourth its length. This creates gaps into which mineral crystals are deposited.
4. After mineral deposition, fibrils link together and twist to form the ropelike fibers.
5. The fibers join to form the framework that gives bone its tensile and supportive strength.

Proteoglycans

Proteoglycans are large complexes of numerous polysaccharides attached to a common protein core. They strengthen bone by forming compression-resistant networks between the collagen fibers. Proteoglycans also control the transport and distribution of electrically charged particles (ions), particularly calcium, through the bone matrix, thereby playing a role in bone calcium deposition and calcification.

Glycoproteins

Glycoproteins are carbohydrate-protein complexes that control the collagen interactions that lead to fibril formation. They may also function in calcification. Four glycoproteins are present in bone: **sialoprotein,** which binds easily with calcium; **osteocalcin,** which binds preferentially to crystallized calcium; **bone albumin,** which is identical to serum albumin and possibly transports essentials to and from bone cells and maintains the osmotic pressure of **bone fluid;** and **alpha-glycoprotein (α-glycoprotein),** which probably plays a significant role in calcification and may also facilitate bone resorption by activating osteoclasts (see Table 36-1).

Bone minerals

Mineralization (crystallization) is the final step in bone formation, after collagen synthesis and fiber formation. Mineralization has two distinct phases: (1) formation of the initial mineral deposit (initiation) and (2) proliferation or accretion of additional mineral crystals on the initial mineral de-

TABLE 36-3	Sequence of Calcium and Phosphate Compound Formation and Crystallization	
Formula	**Name**	**Abbreviation**
$Ca(HPO_4) \cdot 2 H_2O$	Dicalcium phosphate dihydrate	DCPD
$Ca_4H(PO_4)_3$	Octacalcium phosphate	OCP
$Ca_9(PO_4)_6$ (var.)	Amorphous calcium phosphate	ACP
$Ca_3(PO_4)_2$	Tricalcium phosphate	TCP
$Ca_5(PO_4)_3OH$	Hydroxyapatite	HAP

NOTE: *Compounds are listed in the order in which precipitation and crystal formation occur.*

posits (growth).[1] The majority of the mineral in the body is an analog of the naturally occurring mineral *hydroxyapatite.*

Table 36-3 lists the sequence in which calcium and phosphate form amorphous (fluid) calcium phosphate compounds that are converted, in stages, to solid hexagonal crystals of **hydroxyapatite (HAP).** As the calcium and phosphorus concentrations increase in the bone matrix, the first precipitate to form is dicalcium phosphate dihydrate (DCPD). Once DCPD precipitation begins, the remaining phases of bone crystal formation proceed until insoluble HAP is produced, with approximately 80% to 90% of the HAP incorporated into the collagen fibers. Amorphous calcium phosphate is distributed throughout the bone matrix.

Types of Bone Tissue

Bone is composed of two types of bony (osseous) tissue: **compact bone (cortical bone)** and **spongy bone (cancellous bone)** (Fig. 36-2). Both types of bone tissue contain the same structural elements, and, with a few exceptions, both compact tissue and spongy tissue are present in every bone. The major difference between the two types of tissue is the organization of the elements.

Compact bone is highly organized, solid, and extremely strong. The basic structural unit in compact bone is the **haversian system** (Fig. 36-3). Each haversian system is made up of the following:

1. A central canal called the **haversian canal**
2. Concentric layers of bone matrix called **lamellae**
3. Tiny spaces (lacunae) between the lamellae
4. Bone cells (osteocytes) within the lacunae
5. Small channels or canals called **canaliculi**

Spongy bone is less complex and lacks haversian systems. In spongy bone the lamellae are not arranged in concentric layers but in plates or bars termed **trabeculae** that branch and unite with one another to form an irregular meshwork. The pattern of the meshwork is determined by the direction of stress on the particular bone. The spaces between the trabeculae are filled with red bone marrow. The osteocyte-containing lacunae are distributed between the trabeculae and interconnected by canaliculi. Capillaries pass through the marrow to nourish the osteocytes.

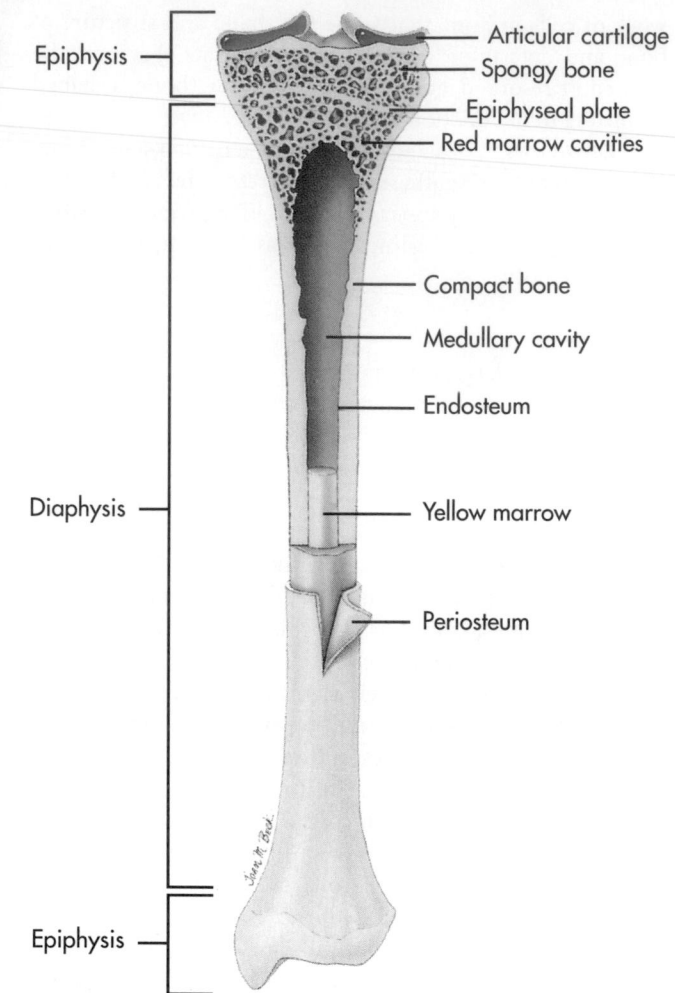

Fig. 36-2 *Cross section of bone.* Longitudinal section of long bone (tibia) showing spongy (cancellous) and compact bone. *(From Thibodeau, G.A. & Patton, K.T. [1999]. Anatomy & physiology [4th ed.]. St. Louis: Mosby.)*

All bones are covered with a double-layered connective tissue called the **periosteum.** The outer layer of the periosteum contains blood vessels and nerves, some of which penetrate to the inner structures of the bone through channels called Volkmann canals (see Fig. 36-3). The inner layer of the periosteum is anchored to the bone by collagenous fibers (Sharpey fibers) that penetrate the bone. Sharpey fibers also help hold or attach tendons and ligaments to the periosteum of bones.[5]

Characteristics of Bone

The 206 bones of the human skeleton are distributed between the axial skeleton and the appendicular skeleton. Eighty bones are in the **axial skeleton,** making up the skull, vertebral column, and thorax. The other 126 bones of the **appendicular skeleton** make up the upper and lower extremities, the shoulder girdle (pectoral girdle), and the pelvic girdle (os coxae) (Fig. 36-4). The skeleton contributes approximately 14% of an adult's body weight.

Fig. 36-3 *Structure of compact and cancellous bone.* **A,** Longitudinal section of a long bone showing both cancellous and compact bone. **B,** A magnified view of compact bone. **C,** Section of a flat bone. Outer layers of compact bone surround cancellous bone. Fine structure of compact and cancellous bone is shown to the right. *(From Thibodeau, G.A. & Patton, K.T. [1999]. Anatomy & physiology [4th ed.]. St. Louis: Mosby.)*

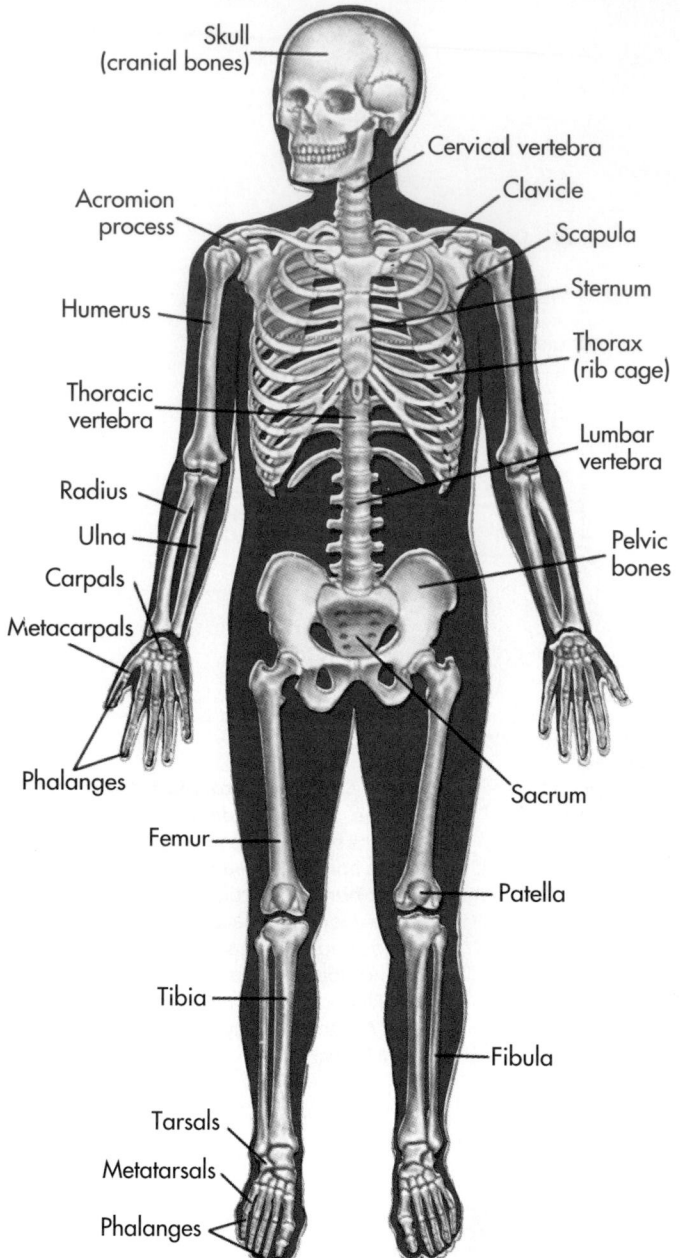

Fig. 36-4 *Axial and appendicular skeleton*. *(From Thompson, J.M. et al. [1997]. Mosby's clinical nursing [4th ed.]. St. Louis: Mosby.)*

Bones can be classified by shape as long, flat, short (cuboidal), or irregular. **Long bones** are longer than they are wide and consist of a narrow tubular midportion *(diaphysis)* that merges into a broader neck *(metaphysis)* and a broad end *(epiphysis)* (see Fig. 36-2).

The diaphysis consists of a shaft of thick, rigid compact bone that is able to tolerate bending forces. Contained within the diaphysis is the elongated marrow (medullary) cavity. The marrow cavity of the diaphysis contains primarily fatty tissue, which is referred to as *yellow marrow*. The yellow marrow assists red bone marrow in hematopoiesis only

during times of stress. The yellow marrow cavity of the diaphysis is continuous with marrow cavities in the spongy bone of the metaphysis and diaphysis. The marrow contained within the epiphysis is red because it contains primarily blood-forming tissue (see Chapter 19). A layer of connective tissue, *endosteum,* lines the outer surfaces of both types of marrow cavity.

The broadness of the epiphysis allows weight bearing to be distributed over a wide area. The epiphysis is made up of spongy bone covered by a very thin layer of compact bone. In a child, the epiphysis is separated from the metaphysis by a cartilaginous **growth plate** **(*epiphyseal plate*).** After puberty, the epiphyseal plate calcifies and the epiphysis and metaphysis merge. By adulthood, the line of demarcation between the epiphysis and metaphysis is undetectable.

In **flat bones,** such as the ribs and scapulae, two plates of compact bone are roughly parallel to each other. Between the compact bone plates is a layer of spongy bone. **Short bones (*cuboidal bones*),** such as the bones of the wrist or ankle, are often cuboidal in shape. They consist of spongy bone covered by a thin layer of compact bone.

Irregular bones, such as the vertebrae, mandibles, or other facial bones, have various shapes that include thin and thick segments. The thin part of an irregular bone consists of two plates of compact bone with spongy bone in between. The thick part consists of spongy bone surrounded by a layer of compact bone.

Maintenance of Bone Integrity
Remodeling

The internal structure of bone is maintained by *remodeling,* a three-phase process in which existing bone is resorbed and new bone is laid down to replace it. Remodeling is carried out by clusters of bone cells termed *basic multicellular units.* The basic multicellular units are made up of bone precursor cells that differentiate into osteoclasts and osteoblasts. Precursor cells are located on the free surfaces of bones and along the vascular channels (especially the marrow cavities).

In phase 1 (activation) of the remodeling cycle, a stimulus (e.g., hormone, drug, vitamin, physical stressor) activates the bone cell precursors in a localized area of bone to form osteoclasts. In phase 2 (resorption), the osteoclasts form a "cutting cone," which gradually resorbs bone, leaving behind an elongated cavity termed a *resorption cavity.* The resorption cavity in compact bone follows the longitudinal axis of the haversian system, whereas the resorption cavity in spongy bone parallels the surface of the trabeculae.

Phase 3 (formation) is the laying down of new bone, termed *secondary bone,* by osteoblasts lining the walls of the resorption cavity. Successive layers (lamellae) in compact bone are laid down, until the resorption cavity is reduced to a narrow haversian canal around a blood vessel. In this way, old haversian systems are destroyed and new haversian systems are formed. New trabeculae are formed in spongy bone. The entire process of remodeling takes about 4 months.

Fig. 36-5 *Bone remodeling.* In the remodeling sequence, bone sections are removed by bone-resorbing cells (osteoclasts) and replaced with a new section laid down by bone-forming cells (osteoblasts). The cells work in response to signals generated in that environment. The first phase of remodeling is mediated only by the multinucleated osteoclastic cells. They are activated, scoop out bone, **A**, and resorb it; then the work of the osteoblasts begins, **B**. They form new bone that replaces bone removed by the resorption process, **C**. The sequence takes 4 to 5 months. **D**, Active bone remodeling seen in the settings of primary or secondary hyperparathyroidism. Note the active osteoblasts surmounted on red-stained osteoid. Marrow fibrosis is present. *(A to C from Mundy, G.R. [1995].* Bone remodeling and its disorders. *St. Louis: Mosby; D from Damjanov, I. & Linder, J. [Eds.]. [1996].* Anderson's pathology *[10th ed.]. St. Louis: Mosby.)*

Repair

The remodeling process can repair microscopic bone injuries, but gross injuries, such as fractures and surgical wounds (osteotomies), heal by the same stages as soft tissue injuries, except that new bone, instead of scar tissue, is the final result (see Chapter 6). The stages of bone wound healing are listed here and shown in Fig. 36-5:

1. Hematoma formation
2. Procallus formation
3. Callus formation
4. Replacement, by basic multicellular units, of the callus with lamellar or trabecular bone
5. Remodeling of the periosteal and endosteal surfaces of the bone to the size and shape of the bone before injury

The speed with which bone heals depends on the severity of the bone disruption; the type and amount of bone tissue that needs to be replaced (spongy bone heals faster); blood supply and oxygen to the site; presence of growth and thyroid hormones, insulin, vitamins, and other nutrients; presence of systemic disease; effects of aging; and effective treatment, including immobilization and the prevention of complications such as infection. In general, however, hematoma formation occurs within hours of fracture or surgery; formation of procallus by osteoblasts within days; callus formation within weeks; and replacement and contour modeling within years—up to 4 years in some cases.

HEALTH ALERT

Soy Preserves Bone

Soy protein may have benefits beyond those already known—reducing a person's risk of heart disease and of breast cancer. Recent animal studies suggest that soy also helps to prevent bone loss that can lead to osteoporosis and fractures in elderly persons. Findings from a 5-week feeding study suggest that estrogen-like compounds in soy—principally the isoflavones daidzein and genistein—are responsible for its bone-sparing effects. How the compounds increase bone growth is unclear; and for soy protein to reverse bone loss, long-term consumption may be necessary.

Data from Raloff, J. (1999). Soy compounds help preserve bone. Science News, 155, 15.

STRUCTURE AND FUNCTION OF JOINTS

The site where two or more bones are attached is called a *joint,* or *articulation* (Fig. 36-6). The primary function of joints is to provide stability and mobility to the skeleton. Whether a joint provides stability or mobility depends on its location and its structure. Generally, joints that stabilize the skeleton have a simpler structure than those that enable the skeleton to move. Most joints provide both stability and mobility to some degree (Fig. 36-7).

Joints are classified based on the degree of movement they permit or on the connecting tissues that hold them together. Based on movement, a joint is classified as a *synarthrosis (immovable joint),* an *amphiarthrosis (slightly movable joint),* or a *diarthrosis (freely movable joint).* On the basis of connective structures, joints are classified broadly as fibrous, cartilaginous, or synovial. Each of these three structural classifications can be subdivided according to the shape and contour of the articulating surfaces (ends) of the bones and the type of motion the joint permits.

Fibrous Joints

A joint in which bone is united directly to bone by fibrous connective tissue is called a *fibrous joint.* Generally, fibrous joints are synarthroses (immovable), but many fibrous joints allow some movement. The degree of movement depends on the distance between the bones and the flexibility of the fibrous connective tissue.

Fibrous joints are further subdivided into three types: sutures, syndesmoses, and gomphoses. A *suture* has a thin layer of dense fibrous tissue that binds together interlocking flat bones in the skulls of young children. Sutures form an extremely tight union that permits no motion. By adulthood, the fibrous tissue has been replaced by bone. A *syndesmosis* is a joint in which the two bony surfaces are united by a ligament or membrane. The fibers of ligaments are flexible and stretch, permitting a limited amount of movement. The paired bones of the lower arm (radius and ulna) and the lower leg (tibia and fibula) and their ligaments are syndesmotic joints. A *gomphosis* is a special type of fibrous joint in which a conical projection fits into a complementary socket and is held there by a ligament. The teeth held in the maxilla or mandible are gomphosis joints.

Cartilaginous Joints

There are two types of cartilaginous joints—symphyses and synchondroses. A *symphysis* is a cartilaginous joint in which bones are united by a pad or disk of fibrocartilage. The articulating surfaces of the two bones are usually covered by a thin layer of hyaline cartilage, and the thick pad of fibrocar-

Bone

Cartilage

Muscle fiber

Tendon

Fig. 36-6 *Main tissues of a joint.* (*Micrographs from Erlandsen, S.L. & Magney, J.E. [1992].* Color atlas of histology. *St. Louis: Mosby.)*

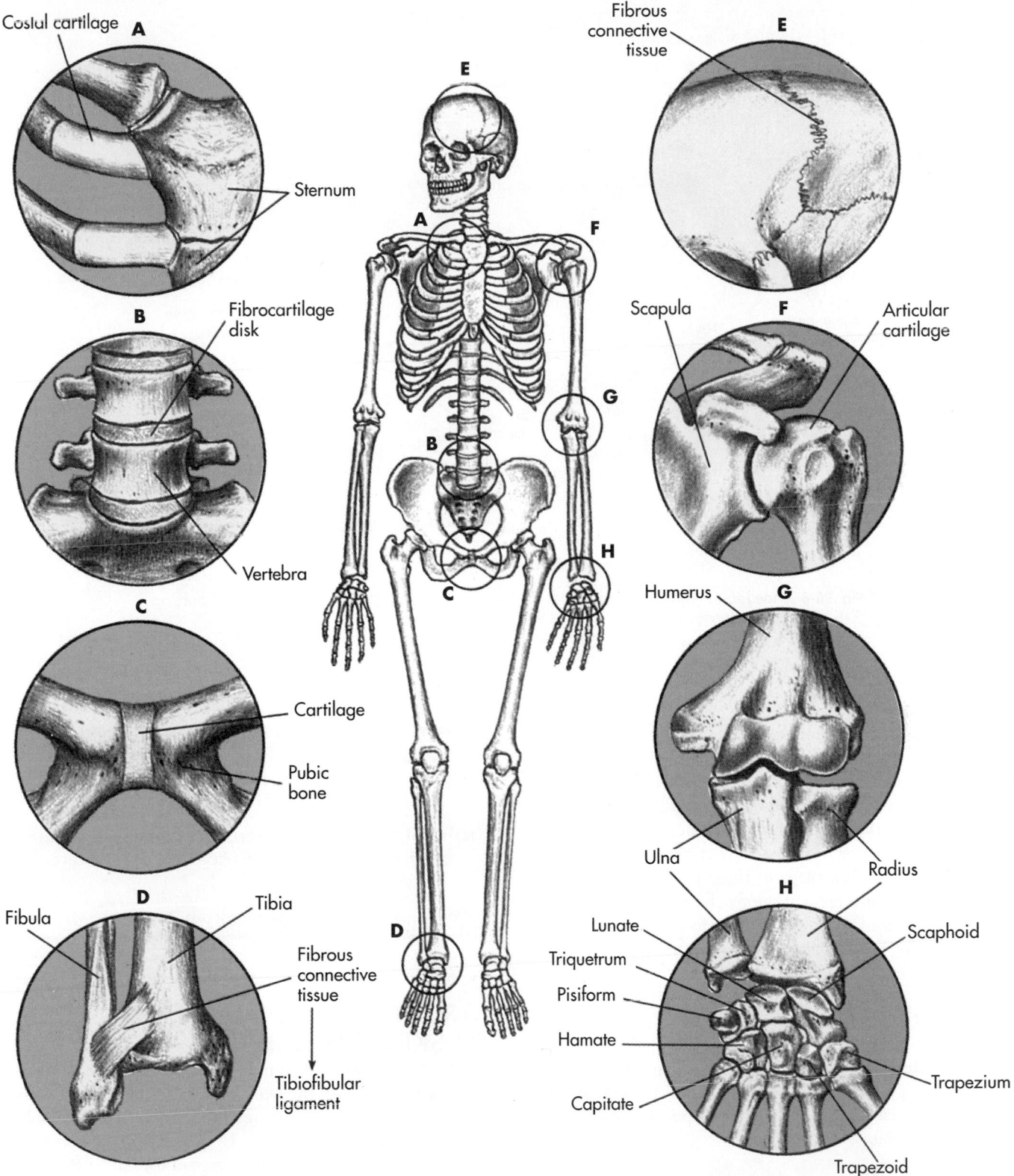

Fig. 36-7 *Types of joints.* Cartilaginous (amphiarthrodial) joints, which are slightly movable, include **(A)** a synchondrosis that attaches ribs to costal cartilage, **(B)** a symphysis that connects vertebrae, and **(C)** the symphysis that connects the two pubic bones. Fibrous (synarthrodial) joints, which are immovable, include **(D)** the syndesmosis between the tibia and fibula and **(E)** sutures that connect the skull bones and the gomphosis (not shown), which holds teeth in their sockets. The synovial joints include **(F)** the spheroid type at the shoulder, **(G)** the hinge type at the elbow, and **(H)** the gliding joints of the hand.

Fig. 36-8 *Knee joint (synovial joint).* *(From Thompson, J.M. et al. [1997]. Mosby's clinical nursing [4th ed.]. St. Louis: Mosby.)*

tilage acts as a shock absorber and stabilizer. Examples of symphyses are the symphysis pubis, which joins the two pubic bones, and the intervertebral disks, which join the bodies of the vertebrae. A *synchondrosis* is a joint in which hyaline cartilage, rather than fibrocartilage, connects the two bones. The joints between the ribs and the sternum are synchondroses. The hyaline cartilage of these joints is called *costal cartilage.* Slight movement at the synchondroses between the ribs and the sternum allows the chest to move outward and upward during breathing.

Synovial Joints
Structure of synovial joints

Synovial joints (diarthroses) are the most movable and the most complex joints in the body (Fig. 36-8). The component parts of synovial joints and their descriptions are found in Box 36-1, p. 1020.

Movement of synovial joints

Synovial joints are described as uniaxial, biaxial, or multiaxial according to the shapes of the bone ends and the type of movement occurring at the joint (Fig. 36-9). Usually, one of the bones is stable and serves as an axis for the motion of the other bone. The body movements made possible by various synovial joints are either circular or angular (Fig. 36-10).

STRUCTURE AND FUNCTION OF SKELETAL MUSCLES

The millions of individual fibers of skeletal muscle contract and relax to perform the work necessary to move the body (Fig. 36-11). Muscle constitutes 40% of adults' body weight and 50% of children's. Muscle is 75% water, 20% protein, and 5% organic and inorganic compounds. Thirty-two percent of all protein stores for energy and metabolism are contained in muscle.

Whole Muscle

There are more than 600 skeletal muscles in the body.[6] The body's muscles vary dramatically in size and shape. They range from 2 to 60 cm in length and are shaped according to

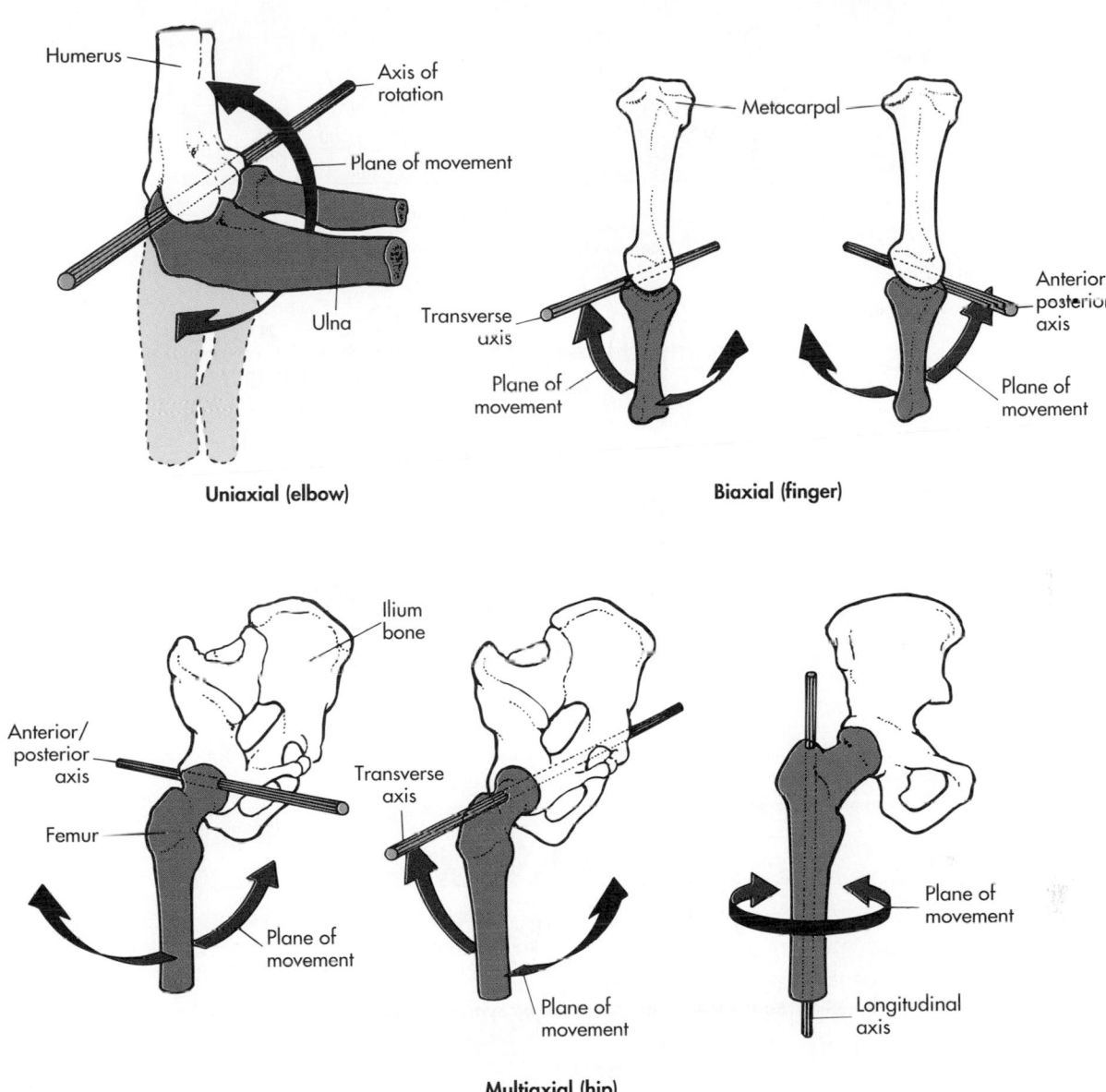

Fig. 36-9 *Movements of synovial (diarthrodial) joints.*

function. *Fusiform muscles* are elongated muscles shaped like straps and can run from one joint to another. *Pennate muscles* are broad, flat, and slightly fan shaped, with fibers running obliquely to the muscle's long axis. The multipennate deltoid muscle, which flexes and extends the arm, is a good example of a muscle shaped according to its function.

Each skeletal muscle is a separate organ, encased in a three-part connective tissue framework called *fascia.* The layers of connective tissue protect the muscle fibers, attach the muscle to bony prominences, and provide a structure for a network of nerve fibers, blood vessels, and lymphatic channels. The layers are as follows:

1. The outermost layer, the *epimysium,* is located on the surface of the muscle and tapers at each end to form the *tendon* (Fig. 36-12). Tendons allow short muscles to exert power on a distant joint where a thick muscle would interfere with the joint's mobility.

2. The *perimysium* further subdivides the muscle fibers into bundles of connective tissue, or *fascicles.*

3. The smallest unit of muscle visible without a microscope is the *endomysium,* which surrounds the muscle.

The ligaments, tendons, and fascia are made up of connective tissue that also serves to buffer the limbs from the effects of sudden strains or changes in speed. The rapid recovery necessary for strenuous exercise is supported by the elastic property of muscle and its connective tissue.

Skeletal muscle has been termed *voluntary* (controlled directly by the nervous system), *striated* (has a striped pattern when viewed under a light microscope), or *extrafusal* (to distinguish from other contractile fibers in the sensory

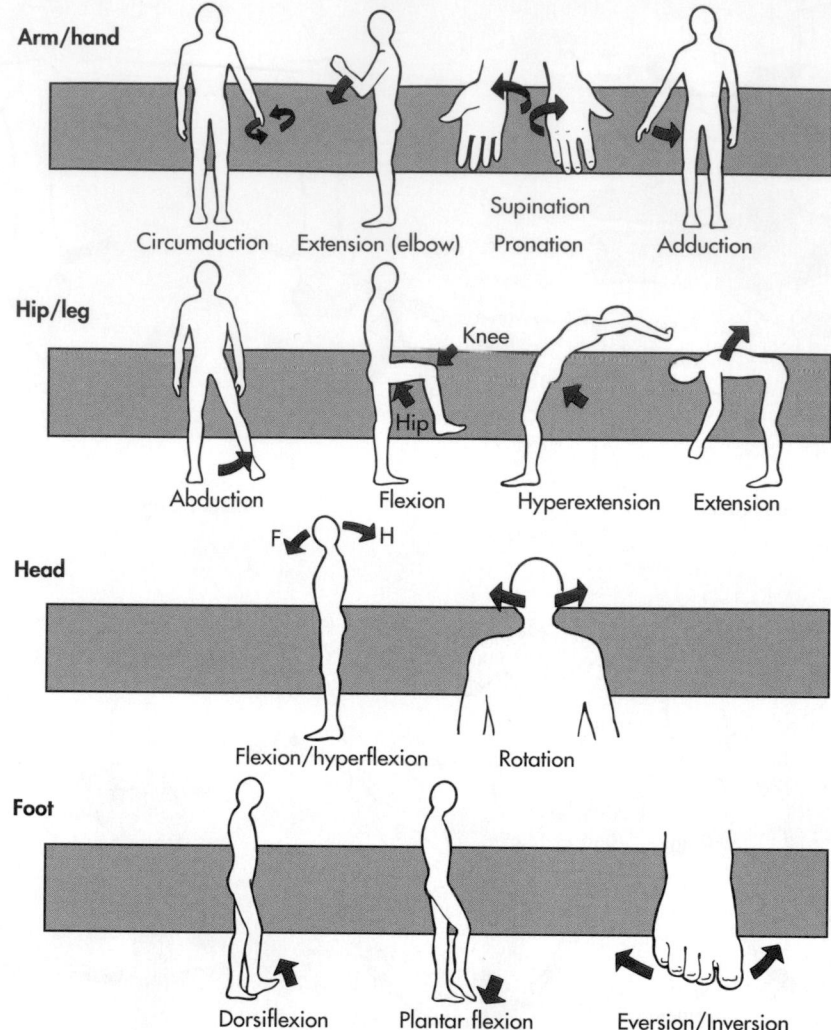

Fig. 36-10 *Body movements provided by synovial (diarthrodial) joints.*

organ of the muscle). Components that are visible on gross inspection of the whole muscle include the motor and sensory nerve fibers. These function together with the muscle, innervating portions of it and providing the electrical impulses needed for motor function.

Motor unit

From the anterior horn cell of the spinal cord, the axons of motor nerves branch out to innervate a specific group of muscle fibers. Each anterior horn cell, its axon (part of lower motor neuron; see Chapter 12), and the muscle fibers innervated by it are called a ***motor unit*** (Fig. 36-13). The motor units are composed of lower motor neurons, which extend to skeletal muscles. Often termed the functional unit of the neuromuscular system, the motor unit behaves as a single entity and contracts as a whole when it receives an electrical impulse.

The whole muscle may be controlled by several motor nerve axons. These branch to innervate many motor units

within the muscle. The whole muscle then may be made up of many motor units. The number of motor units per individual muscle varies greatly. In the calf, for example, one motor axon will innervate approximately 2000 muscle fibers, out of a total of 1,200,000 muscle fibers. This is a high innervation ratio of muscle fibers to axons, and it contrasts markedly with the low innervation ratio in the laryngeal muscles. There, two to three muscle fibers constitute each motor unit, and the innervation ratio can be of great functional significance. The greater the innervation ratio of a particular organ, the greater its endurance. Higher innervation ratios prevent fatigue, whereas lower innervation ratios allow for precision of movement.

Sensory receptors

Although muscles function as effector organs, they also contain sensory receptors and are involved in sending different signals to the central nervous system. Among these are the muscle spindles and Golgi tendon organs. ***Spindles*** are

Fig. 36-11 *Skeletal muscles of body.* **A,** Anterior view. **B,** Posterior view. *(From Thompson, J.M. et al. [1997]. Mosby's clinical nursing [4th ed.]. St. Louis: Mosby.)*

Structure, Location, and Function of Synovial Joints   BOX 36-1

JOINT (ARTICULAR) CAPSULE

Fibrous connective tissue that covers the ends of bones where they meet in a joint; Sharpey fibers firmly attach the proximal and distal capsule to the periosteum, and ligaments and tendons may also reinforce the capsule. Composed of parallel, interlacing bundles of dense, white fibrous tissue richly supplied with nerves, blood vessels, and lymphatic vessels. Nerves in and around the joint capsule are sensitive to rate and direction of motion, compression, tension, vibration, and pain.

SYNOVIAL MEMBRANE

Smooth, delicate inner lining of joint capsule; found in the nonarticular portion of synovial joint and any ligaments or tendons that traverse this cavity. Composed of two layers—vascular subintima and thin cellular intima. Vascular intima merges with the fibrous joint capsule and is composed of loose fibrous connective tissue, elastin fibers, fat cells, fibroblasts, macrophages, and mast cells; intima consists of rows of synovial cells embedded in fiber-free intercellular matrix and contains two types of cells—A and B. A cells ingest and remove (phagocytose) bacteria and particles of debris in the joint cavity; B cells secrete hyaluronate, which gives synovial fluid its viscous quality. The synovial membrane is richly supplied with blood and lymphatic vessels and is capable of rapid repair and regeneration.

JOINT (SYNOVIAL) CAVITY

Enclosed, fluid-filled space between articulating surfaces of two bones; also called joint space. Enables two bones to move "against" one another. Is surrounded by synovial membrane and filled with synovial fluid.

SYNOVIAL FLUID

Superfiltrated plasma from blood vessels that lubricates the joint surfaces, nourishes the pad of the articular cartilage, and covers the ends of the bones. Contains free-floating synovial cells and various leukocytes that phagocytose joint debris and microorganisms.

ARTICULAR CARTILAGE

A layer of hyaline cartilage that covers the end of each bone. It may be thick or thin, depending on the size of the joint, the fit of the two bone ends, and the amount of weight and shearing force the joint normally withstands. The function of articular cartilage is to reduce friction in the joint and to distribute the forces of weight bearing. Articular cartilage is composed of chondrocytes (cartilage cells) (making up about 2% of the tissue) and an intercellular matrix made up of collagen (making up about 10% to 30% of weight), protein polysaccharides (making up 5% to 10% of weight), and water. The water content ranges from 60% to almost 80% of the net weight of the cartilage, and individual molecules rapidly enter or exit the articular cartilage to contribute to the resiliency of the tissue.

At the surface of articular cartilage, the collagen fibers run parallel to the joint surface and are closely compacted into a dense, protective mat. (Loss of this dense, compacted configuration at the surface subjects the underlying fibers to splitting and thinning, in which case the cartilage is unable to tolerate weight bearing.) In the middle layer (the proliferative zone) of the cartilage, the fibers are arranged tangential to the surface, which allows them to deform and absorb some of the force of weight bearing. In the bottom layer (the hypertrophic zone) of the cartilage, the fibers are perpendicular to the joint surface, allowing them to resist shear forces, and are embedded in a calcified layer of cartilage called the tidemark. The **tidemark** anchors the collagen fibers to the underlying (subchondral) bone. Collagen fibers are important components of the cartilage matrix because they account for approximately 60% of the dry weight and because they (1) anchor the cartilage securely to underlying bone, (2) provide a taut framework for the cartilage, (3) control the loss of fluid from the cartilage, and (4) prevent the escape of protein polysaccharides (proteoglycans) from the cartilage. The proteoglycans give articular cartilage its stiff quality and regulate the movement of synovial fluid through the cartilage. The proteoglycans are macromolecules consisting of proteins, carbohydrates (glycosaminoglycans), and hyaluronic acid.

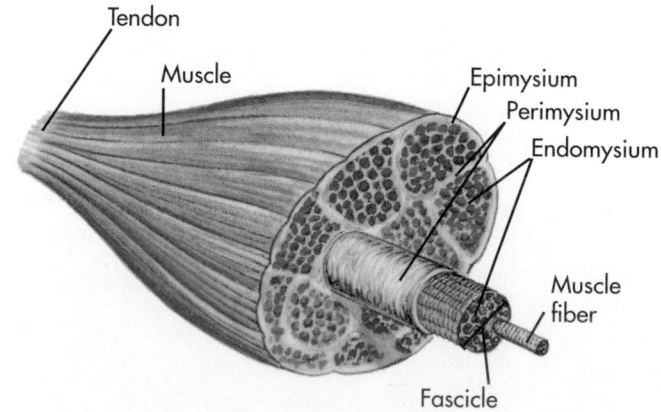

Fig. 36-12 *Cross section of skeletal muscle showing muscle fibers and their coverings.* (From Thibodeau, G.A. & Patton, K.T. [1996]. Anatomy & physiology [3rd ed.]. St. Louis: Mosby.)

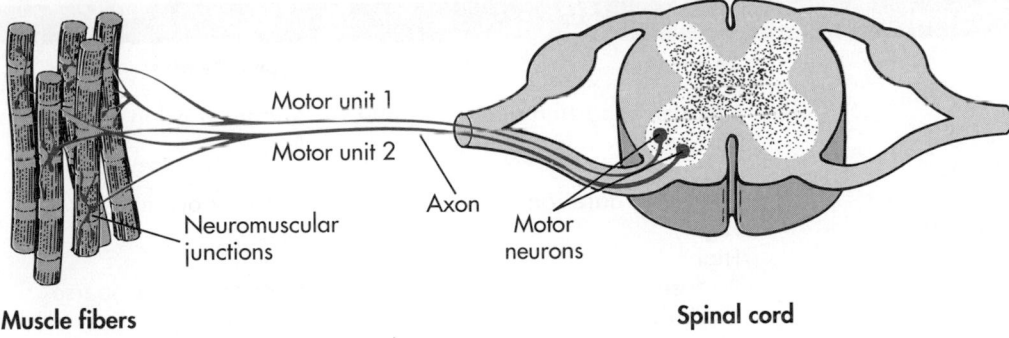

Fig. 36-13 *Motor units of a muscle.* Each motor unit consists of a motor neuron and all the muscle fibers (cells) supplied by the neuron and its axon branches.

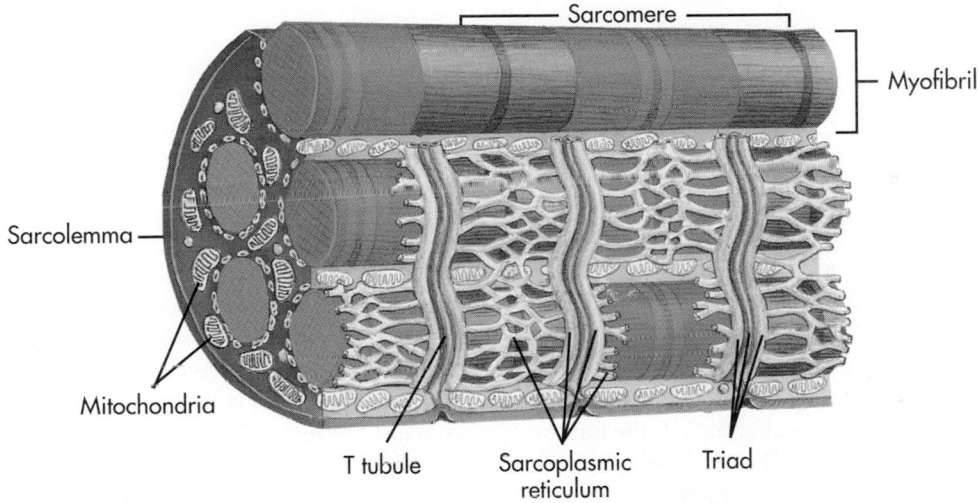

Fig. 36-14 *Myofibrils.* Myofibrils of a skeletal muscle fiber (cells) and overall organization of skeletal muscle. *(From Thibodeau, G.A. & Patton, K.T. [1999].* Anatomy & physiology *[4th ed.]. St. Louis: Mosby.)*

mechanoreceptors that lie parallel to muscle fibers and respond to muscle stretching. ***Golgi tendon organs*** are dendrites that terminate and branch to tendons near the neuromuscular junction. The muscle spindles, Golgi tendon organs, and free nerve endings provide a means of reporting changes in length, tension, velocity, and tone in the muscle. This system of afferent signals is responsible for the muscle stretch response and maintenance of normal muscle tone.

Muscle fibers

Each ***muscle fiber*** is a single ***muscle cell,*** cylindrical in structure and surrounded by a membrane capable of excitation and impulse propagation. The muscle fiber contains bundles of ***myofibrils,*** the fiber's functional subunits, in a parallel arrangement along the longitudinal axis of the muscle (Fig. 36-14). At birth, the muscle fibers have completed development from precursor cells called ***myoblasts.*** All voluntary muscles are derived from the mesodermal layer of the embryo.

The type of peripheral nerve influences the muscle fiber and motor unit considerably. Whether motor nerves are fast or slow determines the type of muscle fibers in the motor unit. White muscle (***type II fibers*** [white fast-motor fibers]) is innervated by relatively large type II alpha motor neurons with fast conduction velocities. These fibers rely on a short-term anaerobic glycolytic system for rapid energy transfer; red muscle (***type I fibers)*** depends on aerobic oxidative metabolism. Table 36-4 describes the specific characteristics of type I and type II fibers.

The overlap of muscle fibers that appears with staining gives the checkerboard appearance of muscle biopsy specimens and provides an equal distribution of fiber types throughout the muscle. This overlap also helps to compensate for muscle fiber loss and fatigue of individual motor units during activity. In spite of this, some muscles contain proportionally more of one fiber type than another. The postural muscles have more type I fibers, allowing them the high resistance to fatigue that is necessary to maintain the

TABLE 36-4	Characteristics of Muscle Fibers	
Characteristic	Type I (Red)	Type II (White)
Anatomic location	Deep axial portion of surface muscle	Surface portion of surface muscle
Contraction speed	Slow	Fast
Motor neuron type	Type I, α	Type II, A
Firing frequency	Low, long duration	Rapid, short duration
Resistance to fatigue	High	Low
Myoglobin	High	Low
Capillary supply	Profuse	Intermediate to sparse
Metabolism	Oxidative	Glycolysis
Mitochondria	Many	Few
Enzymes	Lactate dehydrogenease, types I-III	Lactate dehydrogenase, types IV and V
Creatine kinase	Cardiac type	Fast, skeletal
Example (most muscles are mixed)	Greater proportion of slow-contracting fibers in soleus	Greater proportion of fast-contracting fibers in laryngeal and ocular muscles
Glycogen content	Low	High
Intensity of contraction	Low	High
Aerobic metabolic capacity	High	Low
Fiber diameter	Small	Large
Myosin-ATPase activity	Low	High

From Spence, A.P. & Mason, E.E. (1992). Human anatomy and physiology (4th ed.). St. Paul, Minn.: West Publishing.

same position for extended periods. The ocular muscles have more type II muscle fibers, allowing them to respond rapidly to visual changes.

The number of muscle fibers varies according to location. Large muscles, such as the gastrocnemius, have more fibers (1,200,000) than smaller muscles, such as the lumbrical muscles in the hand (10,000). The diameter of muscle fibers also varies. The closely packed polygons are small (10 to 20 μm) until puberty, when they attain the normal adult diameter of 40 to 80 μm. Women usually have smaller-diameter fibers than men. Small muscles, such as the ocular muscles, are 15 μm in diameter; larger, more proximal muscles are 40 μm. Fiber size can have functional significance. Studies have shown that larger fiber diameter is associated with generation of greater forces. Fiber diameter can be increased by exercise or occupational overuse, activities that cause hypertrophied muscle.

The major components of the muscle fiber include the muscle membrane, myofibrils, sarcotubular system, sarcoplasm, and mitochondria (see Fig. 36-14). The **muscle membrane** is a two-part membrane. It includes the **sarcolemma,** which contains the plasma membrane of the muscle cell, and the cell's **basement membrane.** The sarcolemma is 7.5 μm thick and is capable of propagating electrical impulses to initiate contraction. At the motor nerve end-plate, where the nerve impulse is transmitted, the sarcolemma forms the highly convoluted synaptic cleft. The sarcolemma is made up of lipid molecules and protein systems. The protein systems perform special functions, such as transport of nutrients and protein synthesis. They also provide the sodium-potassium pump and include the cell's cholinergic receptor. The basement membrane is 50 μm thick and is composed primarily of proteins and polysaccharides. It also

serves as the cell's microskeleton and maintains the shape of the muscle cell. The basement membrane also may function in some way to restrict further diffusion of electrolytes once they have crossed the sarcolemma.

The **sarcoplasm** is the cytoplasm of the muscle cell and contains the intracellular components that are common to all cells (see Chapter 1). The sarcoplasm is an aqueous substance that provides a matrix that surrounds the myofibrils. It contains numerous enzymes and proteins that are responsible for the cell's energy production, protein synthesis, and oxygen storage. The mitochondria house enzyme systems for energy production, particularly those that regulate processes such as the citric acid cycle and adenosine triphosphate (ATP) formation. Many other structures are present in the sarcoplasm. The ribosomes are composed of primarily ribonucleic acid (RNA) and participate in the process of protein synthesis. The cell nucleus, satellite cells, glycogen granules, and lipid droplets are suspended in the sarcoplasmic matrix. Blood vessels, nerve endings, muscle spindles, and Golgi tendon organs are also directly located within this structure.

Unique to the muscle is the **sarcotubular system,** a network that includes the transverse tubules and the sarcoplasmic reticulum, which crosses the interior of the cell. The **sarcoplasmic reticulum** is made like the endoplasmic reticulum in other cells. In the muscle cells, the sarcoplasmic reticulum is involved in calcium transport, which initiates muscle contraction at the **sarcomere,** a portion of the myofibril. The sarcoplasmic reticulum is composed of tubules that run parallel to the myofibrils. The longitudinal tubules are termed **sarcotubules.** The **transverse tubules,** which are closely associated with the sarcotubules, run across the sarcoplasm and communicate with the extracellular space. Together, the

Fig. 36-15 *Muscle fibers.* **A,** Lines and bands in striated muscle. **B,** Relationships of bands, actin, myosin, and lines in relaxed and contracted muscle fibers. *(From Thompson, J.M. et al. [1993]. Mosby's clinical nursing [3rd ed.]. St. Louis: Mosby.)*

tubules of this membrane system allow for intracellular calcium uptake, regulation, release during muscle contraction, and storage of calcium during muscle relaxation.

Myofibrils

The myofibrils are the functional units of muscle contraction. Each myofibril contains sarcomeres, which appear at intervals (see Fig. 36-14). The sarcomeres are composed of two contractile proteins, *actin* and *myosin.*

The myofibrils are the most abundant subcellular muscle component, equaling 85% to 90% of the total volume. On cross section, they are irregular polygons with a mean diameter of less than 1 μm. Each myofibril is composed of serially

repeating sarcomeres, separated by Z lines, which give the muscle its striped, cross-striated appearance. Each sarcomere has a dark A band and is flanked by two light I bands (Fig. 36-15). The A band is 1.5 to 1.6 μm long and contains the thick myosin filaments. Included in the A band is a lighter zone called the H band, and in the center of the H band is the dark M band, or M line. The I band, which contains actin, is divided at the midpoint of each sarcomere by the Z line. Its length varies with the start of muscle contraction.

Myofibrils are composed of myofilaments. Each myofilament is structured in a closely packed hexagonal arrangement, with two thin filaments for every thick filament. The thick filament, along with C protein and M line protein, is

TABLE 36-5	Contractile Proteins of Skeletal Muscle Fibrils		
Name	Approximate Percentage of Myofibrillar Protein	Location	Function
Myosin	55	A band (thick filament)	Contraction; hydrolyzes ATP and develops tension
Actin	20	I band (thin filament	Contraction; activates myosin-ATPase and interacts with myosin
Troponin	7	Thin filament	Regulatory protein; in presence of Ca^{++}, promotes actin-myosin activation
Tropomyosin	5-7	Thin filament	Regulatory and structural function; links filaments, controls filament length
Alpha (α) actin	10	Z band	Regulatory and structural function; links filaments, controls filament length
Beta (β) actin	2	Z band	Regulatory and structural function; links filaments, controls filament length
M protein	2	M line (center of thick filaments)	Regulatory and structural function; provides enzyme creatine kinase
C protein	2	A band (thick filaments)	Possible structural role
Titin	Unknown	Z line (thick filament)	Links filaments to the Z line
Creatine kinase	Unknown	M line	Catalyzes the phosphorylation of ADP to form ATP
Desmin	Unknown	Z line	Structural role in Z line
Zeumatin	Unknown	Z line	Structural role in Z line

From Simon, S.R. (Ed.). (1994). Orthopaedic basic science. *Chicago: American Academy of Orthopaedic Surgeons.*
ATP, *Adenosine triphosphate;* ATPase, *adenosine triphosphatase;* ADP, *adenosine diphosphate.*

made up of myosin. Myosin has two subunits, heavy and light meromyosin, which resemble twisted golf club shafts. The thin filaments are twisted double strands made up of actin, troponin, and tropomyosin (see Chapter 22 and Fig. 22-15).

Muscle proteins

Currently, 12 proteins have been identified in the muscle fibrils.[1] (Table 36-5 outlines their distribution, location, and possible functional significance.) The contractile and regulatory functions of actin, myosin, and the troponin-tropomyosin complex (associated with actin) are the most commonly known. They also account for most of the protein found in the myofibril.

Nonprotein constituents of muscle

Substances such as nitrogen, creatine, creatinine, phosphocreatine, purines, uric acid, and amino acids all serve in the complex process of muscle metabolism. Energy is provided by glycogen and its derivatives.

Creatine metabolism and creatinine metabolism have been used to measure muscle mass. Plasma creatine is taken up by muscle and converted into the high-energy phosphate compound *phosphocreatine* by the enzyme *creatine kinase.* Creatinine is formed in muscle from creatine at a constant rate of 2%/day. (Tests for plasma creatine are discussed in Chapter 28.) Creatine excretion is increased in muscle wasting, whereas creatinine excretion is reduced. This change reflects the reduction in total body creatine stores and loss of muscle mass.

Inorganic compounds, anions (phosphate, chloride), and cations (calcium, magnesium, sodium, potassium) are important in the regulation of protein synthesis, muscle contraction, enzyme systems, and membrane stabilization. Total body potassium (TBK), measured by the K_{40} method, has been used to measure muscle mass, also called lean body mass. Total body potassium levels reflect changes in muscle mass seen during growth, malnutrition, and muscle wasting.

Components of Muscle Function

The ultimate function of muscle is to accomplish work. Although variously expressed in such measures as foot-pounds or kilogram-meters, work usually refers to the amount of energy liberated or force exerted over a distance (work = force × distance). Muscles usually contract or tense while doing work. Muscle contraction occurs on the molecular level and leads to the observable phenomenon of muscle movement.

Muscle contraction at the molecular level

The four steps of muscle contraction are (1) excitation, (2) coupling, (3) contraction, and (4) relaxation. The process involves the electrical properties of all cells and the movement of ions across the plasma membrane (see Chapter 1). The muscle fiber is an excitable tissue. At rest, an electric charge of -90 mV is continually maintained across the sarcolemma. This resting potential, generated by the separation of positive and negative charges on either side of the membrane, creates an electrochemical equilibrium caused by the selective permeability of the sarcolemma to electrolytes in the in-

TABLE 36-6	Energy Sources for Muscular Activity
Sources	**Reactions**
Short-term (anaerobic) sources	Adenosine triphosphate (ATP) $\rightarrow$ Adenosine diphosphate (ADP) + Inorganic phosphate (P_i) + Energy
	Phosphocreatine + ADP $\rightleftharpoons$ Creatine + ATP
	Glycogen/glucose + P_i + ADP $\rightarrow$ Lactate + ATP
Long-term (aerobic) sources	Glycogen/glucose + ADP + P_i + O_2 $\rightarrow$ H_2O + CO_2 + ATP
	Free fatty acids + ADP + P_i + O_2 $\rightarrow$ H_2O + CO_2 + ATP
	Creatine kinase catalyzes the reversible reaction of ATP to ADP: Creatine phosphate + ATP $\underset{}{\overset{\text{Creatine kinase}}{\rightleftharpoons}}$ Creatine + ATP

From Spence, A.P. & Mason, E.E. (1992). Human anatomy and physiology *(4th ed.). St. Paul, Minn.: West Publishing.*

tracellular and extracellular fluids, particularly potassium and sodium.

Excitation, the first step of muscle contraction, begins with the spread of an action potential from the nerve terminal to the neuromuscular junction. The rapid depolarization of the membrane initiates an electrical impulse in the muscle fiber membrane called the ***muscle fiber action potential.*** As the action potential advances along the sarcolemmal membrane, it spreads to the transverse tubules. (The velocity of conduction is much slower in muscle fibers than in myelinated nerve fibers—only 3 to 5 m/sec compared with 54 to 90 m/sec in nerve fibers.)

The second stage, ***coupling,*** follows the depolarization of the transverse tubules. This stage consists of the migration of calcium ions, which are stored in the sarcoplasmic reticulum, to the myofilaments. Calcium affects troponin and tropomyosin, muscle proteins that bind with actin when the muscle is at rest. In the presence of calcium, however, both these proteins are attracted to calcium ions, leaving the actin free to bind with myosin.

Contraction begins as the calcium ions combine with troponin, a reaction that overcomes the inhibitory function of the troponin-tropomyosin system. The thin filament, *actin,* then slides toward the thick filament, myosin. The two ends of the myofibril shorten after contraction when the myosin heads attach to the actin molecules, forming a cross-bridge that constitutes an actin-myosin complex. ATP, located on the actin-myosin complex, is released when the cross-bridges attach. This is the ***sliding filament theory*** described by A.F. Huxley in the 1950s, but it is now called the *cross-bridge theory* because of the formation of the actin-myosin cross-bridges, the process of contraction.[1] The process is so named because the actin actually slides onto the myosin, causing the sarcomere to shorten. The useful distance of contraction of a skeletal muscle is approximately 25% to 35% of the muscle's length.

The last step, ***relaxation,*** begins as the sarcoplasmic reticulum absorbs the calcium molecules, removing them from interaction with troponin. Calcium is pumped back into the sarcoplasmic reticulum by means of an active transport process. The cross-bridges detach, and the sarcomere lengthens. (The cross-bridge theory of muscle contraction is discussed in Chapter 22.)

Muscle metabolism

Skeletal muscle requires a constant supply of ATP and phosphocreatine. These substances are necessary to fuel the complex processes of muscle contraction, driving the cross-bridges of actin and myosin together and transporting calcium from the sarcoplasmic reticulum to the myofibril. Other internal processes of the muscular system that require ATP include protein synthesis, which replenishes muscle constituents and accommodates growth and repair. The rate of protein synthesis is related to hormone levels (particularly insulin), amino acid substrates, and overall nutritional status. At rest, the rate of ATP formation by oxidation of glucose or acetoacetate is sufficient to maintain internal processes, given normal nutritional status. During activity, the need for ATP increases 100-fold. The metabolic pathways for muscle activity in Table 36-6 show reactions to the immediate need for increased ATP caused by contraction. Activity lasting longer than 5 seconds expends the available stored ATP and phosphocreatine.

Stored glycogen and blood glucose are converted anaerobically to sustain brief activity without increasing the demand for oxygen. Anaerobic glycolysis is much less efficient than aerobic glycolysis, using six to eight times more glycogen to produce the same amount of ATP. With increased activity, such as intense exercise, or with ischemia, an increase in lactic acid occurs because of the breakdown of glycogen, thus causing a shift in muscle pH (see Table 36-6). This short-term mechanism "buys time" by allowing ATP formation in spite of inadequate energy stores or oxygen supply. When the anaerobic threshold is reached and more oxygen is required, physiologic changes occur, including an increase in lactic acid and increases in oxygen consumption, heart rate, respiratory rate, and muscle blood flow.

Strenuous exercise requires oxygen, which activates the

aerobic glycogen pathway for ATP formation. During maximal exercise, free fatty-acid mobilization and the aerobic glycogen pathways provide ATP over an extended time. These pathways require oxygen both to maintain maximal activity and to return the muscle to the resting state. Maximal exercise increases oxygen uptake by 15 to 20 times over the resting state. When this system becomes exhausted or inadequate to respond to the need for ATP, fatigue and weakness finally force the muscle to reduce activity with a resultant buildup of lactic acid in muscle fibers.

Sustaining maximal muscular activity accumulates an **oxygen debt,** which is the amount of oxygen needed to oxidize the residual lactic acid, convert it back to glycogen, and replenish ATP and phosphocreatine stores.[5] For example, after running at maximal speed for 10 seconds, the average person has consumed 1 L of oxygen. At rest, oxygen consumption for the same period is approximately 40 ml. As the person recovers, the measured oxygen debt is 4 L greater than the amount used during activity.

Oxygen consumption is measured to calculate the metabolic cost of activity in normal and diseased muscle. It is an indirect measure of energy expenditure, along with timed tests of activity, heart rate, and respiratory quotient (ratio of carbon dioxide to expired oxygen consumed). Energy expenditure is measured directly by heat production because heat is released whenever work is accomplished.

Another factor that changes energy requirements is muscle fiber type. Type II fibers rely on anaerobic glycolytic metabolism and fatigue readily. Type I fibers can resist fatigue for longer periods because of their capacity for oxidative metabolism.

Muscle mechanics

Muscle contraction cannot be viewed in isolation. Several factors determine how force is transmitted from the cross-bridges on individual muscle fibers to accomplish whole-muscle contraction. First, when a motor unit responds to a single nerve stimulus, it develops a phasic contraction, also called *twitch.* Because the motor unit contracts in an "all or nothing" manner, the contraction that is generated will be a maximal contraction. The central nervous system smoothly grades the force generated by "recruiting" additional motor units and varying the discharge frequency of each active motor unit. This adding of motor units within the muscle is called **repetitive discharge.**

Recruitment and repetitive discharge of motor units allow the muscle to activate the number of motor units needed to generate the desired force. The total force developed is the sum of the force generated by each motor unit. As the strength, speed, and duration of stimuli increase, the summation of contractions reaches a critical frequency called **tetanus.** When tetanus is reached, no further increase in force can be achieved.

Other variables, such as fiber type, innervation ratio, muscle temperature, and muscle shape, influence the efficiency of muscular contraction. The two muscle fiber types differ in their responses to electrical activity. Tetanus and duration of phasic contractions, which take microseconds to accomplish, are achieved more rapidly in type II than in type I muscle fibers. Low innervation ratios promote control and coordination, whereas high ratios promote strength and endurance. Muscles work best at normal body temperature, 98.6° F (37° C). Finally, muscles with a large cross-sectional area, such as the fan-shaped pennate muscles, develop greater contractile forces than smaller-diameter muscles. The initial length of a muscle and the range of shortening that occur when the muscle contracts also determine the force it can generate. The long fusiform muscles have a greater range of shortening and can contract up to 57% of their resting length. A certain amount of elongation is necessary to generate sufficient tension and muscular force. The elongation that occurs during the swing of a golf club or tennis racket is an example of how stretch improves contractile force.

Types of muscle contraction

During **isometric contraction,** the muscle maintains constant length as tension is increased (Fig 36-16). Isometric contraction occurs, for example, when the arm or leg is pushed against an immovable object. The muscle contracts, but the limb does not move. Isometric contraction is also called a **static (holding) contraction.**

During **isotonic contraction,** the muscle maintains a constant tension as it moves. Isotonic contractions can be **eccentric (lengthening)** or **concentric (shortening).** Positive work is accomplished during concentric contraction, and energy is released to exert force or lift a weight. In contrast, during an eccentric contraction the muscle lengthens and absorbs energy. Negative work is accomplished on the muscle by the load. Eccentric contraction requires less energy to accomplish and has been said to result in the development of pain and stiffness after unaccustomed exercise.

Movement of muscle groups

Muscles do not act alone but in groups, often under automatic control. When a muscle contracts and acts as a "prime mover," or **agonist,** its reciprocal muscle, or **antagonist,** relaxes. This is easily tested by holding the right arm in the horizontal position in front of the body, then bending the elbow while feeling the biceps in the front and the triceps in the back with the other hand. The biceps is firm, and the triceps is soft. As the arm is flexed, the muscles change. When the elbow is completely flexed, the biceps is soft and the triceps firm. Completing this movement causes the agonist and antagonist to change automatically; only the movement is commanded, not the alternate contraction and relaxation of the specific muscle groups.

Other associated actions may be seen during walking; as the foot leaves the ground, the paravertebral and gluteal muscles on the opposite sides of the body contract to maintain balance. One notices the loss of the associated muscle's action when paralysis offsets this process and decreases balance. If a person is paralyzed, difficulty in maintaining balance is noticeable.

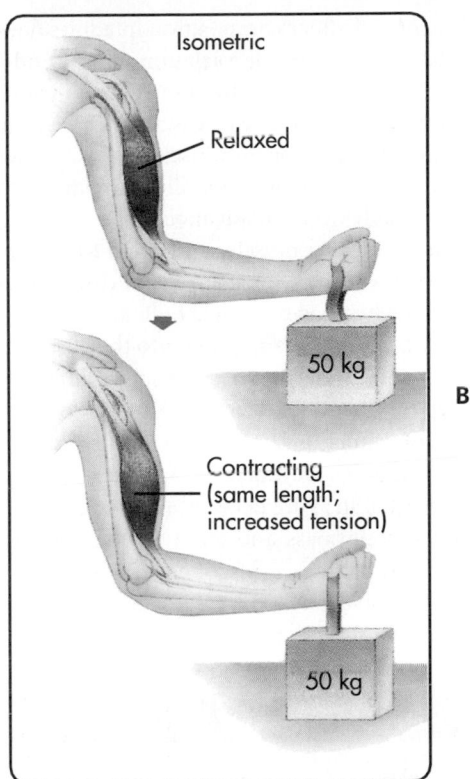

Fig. 36-16 *Isotonic and isometric contraction.* **A,** In isotonic contraction the muscle shortens, producing movement. **B,** In isometric contraction the muscle pulls forcefully against a load but does not shorten. *(From Thibodeau, G.A. & Patton, K.T. [1999].* Anatomy & physiology *[4th ed.]. St. Louis: Mosby.)*

AGING AND THE MUSCULOSKELETAL SYSTEM

Aging of Bones

Aging is accompanied by the loss of bone tissue. Bones become less stiff, less strong, and more brittle with aging. The bone remodeling cycle takes longer to complete, and the rate of mineralization also slows. With aging, women experience loss of bone density, accelerated with rapid bone loss during early menopause from increased osteoclastic bone resorption.[2] By age 70 years, susceptible women have, on the average, lost 50% of their peripheral cortical bone mass. Bone mass losses to such extent lead to deformity, pain, stiffness, and high risk for fractures. Men experience bone loss also but at later ages and much slower rates than women. Also, initial bone masses in men are approximately 30% higher than in women; therefore bone loss in men causes less risk of disability than for women. Men's peak bone mass is related to their race, heredity, hormonal factor (loss of testosterone), physical activity, and calcium intake during childhood. Bone loss in men is related to smoking, alcohol intake, and physical inactivity.[2,7] Bone mass can be gained in healthy young women up to the third decade through physical activity, intake of dietary calcium, and use of oral contraceptives.[8]

Height is also lost with aging because of increased spinal curvature.[9,10]

Stem cells in the bone marrow perform less efficiently, predisposing older persons to acute and chronic illnesses. Such illnesses cause weakness and confusion in older persons and may increase the risk of injury or falling.[11]

Aging of Joints

With aging, cartilage becomes more rigid, fragile, and susceptible to fibrillation because of more cross-linking of collagen and elastin, decreasing water content in the cartilage ground substance, and decreasing concentrations of glycosaminoglycans. Decreased range of motion of the joint is related to the changes in ligaments and muscles. Bones in joints develop evidence of osteoporosis with fewer trabeculae and thinner, less dense bones, making them prone to fractures. Intervertebral disk spaces decrease in height.[9,10] The rate of loss of height accelerates at age 70 years and beyond. Tendons shrink and harden.

Aging of Muscles

The function of skeletal muscle depends on many influences that are affected by aging, including nervous, vascular, and endocrine systems. In the young child, the development of muscle tissue depends highly on continuing neurodevelopmental maturation. Muscle fiber composition in adults does not change until late in life, but the variation among individuals increases with age. Muscle function remains trainable even into advanced age.[12] Muscle diseases have a definite association with specific age-groups. Muscular dystrophies occur in children, and muscle disabilities related to rheumatic diseases usually occur in advancing age.

Age-related loss in skeletal muscle is referred to as **sarcopenia** and is a direct cause of the age-related decrease in muscle strength. As the body ages, muscle bulk and strength decline slowly; thus strength is maintained into the 50s, with a slow decline in dynamic and isometric strength evident after age 70 years. Type II fibers also decrease. There is reduced RNA synthesis, loss of mitochondrial volume, and reduction in the size of motor units. The regenerative function of muscle tissue remains normal in aging persons. As much as 30% to 40% of skeletal muscle mass and strength may be lost from the third to ninth decades.[13] Sarcopenia is thought to be secondary to progressive neuromuscular changes and di-

minishing anabolic hormones. Recent studies demonstrated an age-related decline in synthesis of mixed proteins, myosin heavy chains, and mitochondrial protein.[14,15] Changes in these muscle proteins are related to declines in insulin-like growth factor-1 (IGF-1), testosterone, and dehydroepiandrosterone (DHEA)-sulfate.[14]

Maximal oxygen intake decreases with age. Reduced basal metabolic rate and decreased lean body mass are also seen in the aged population.

✓ QUICK CHECK

Why is one type of muscle used for lifting one's legs?

Why is adenosine triphosphate (ATP) used for muscle contraction?

Describe significant changes in the musculoskeletal system with aging.

◾ DID YOU UNDERSTAND?

Structure and Function of Bones

1. Bones provide support and protection for the body's tissues and organs and are important sources of minerals and blood cells.
2. Bone formation begins with the production of an inorganic matrix by bone cells. Bone minerals crystallize in and around collagen fibers in the matrix, giving bone its characteristic hardness and strength.
3. Bone tissue is continuously being resorbed and synthesized by basic multicellular units of osteoclasts and osteoblasts.
4. Bones in the body are made up of compact bone tissue and spongy bone tissue. Compact bone is highly organized into haversian systems that consist of concentric layers of crystallized matrix surrounding a central canal that contains blood vessels and nerves. Dispersed throughout the concentric layers of crystallized matrix are small spaces containing osteocytes. Smaller canals, called *canaliculi*, interconnect the osteocyte-containing spaces. The crystallized matrix in spongy bone is arranged in bars or plates. Spaces containing osteocytes are dispersed between the bars or plates and interconnected by canaliculi.
5. There are 206 bones in the body divided into the axial skeleton and the appendicular skeleton. Bones are classified by shape as long, short, flat, or irregular. Long bones have a broad end (epiphysis), broad neck (metaphysis), and narrow midportion (diaphysis) that contains the medullary cavity.
6. Bone injuries are repaired in stages. Hematoma formation provides the fibrin framework for formation and organization of granulation tissue. The granulation tissue provides a cartilage model for the formation and crystallization of bone matrix. Remodeling restores the original shape and size to the injured bone.

Structure and Function of Joints

1. A joint is the site where two or more bones attach. Joints provide stability and mobility to the skeleton.
2. Joints are classified as synarthroses, amphiarthroses, or diarthroses, depending on the degree of movement they allow. Joints are also classified by the type of connecting tissue holding them together. Fibrous joints are connected by dense fibrous tissue, ligaments, or membranes. Cartilaginous joints are connected by fibrocartilage or hyaline cartilage. Synovial joints are connected by a fibrous joint capsule. Within the capsule is a small fluid-filled space. The fluid in the space nourishes the articular cartilage that covers the ends of the bones meeting in the synovial joint.
3. Articular cartilage is a highly organized system of collagen fibers and proteoglycans. The fibers firmly anchor the cartilage to the bone, and the proteoglycans control the loss of fluid from the cartilage.
4. Joints help move bones and muscle.

Structure and Function of Skeletal Muscles

1. Skeletal muscle is the largest organ in the body and is made up of millions of individual fibers.
2. Whole muscles vary in size (2 cm to 60 cm) and shape (fusiform, pennate). They are encased in a three-part connective tissue framework. The fundamental concept of muscle function is the motor unit, defined as those muscle fibers innervated by a single motor nerve, its axon, and anterior horn cell.
3. Muscle fibers contain bundles of myofibrils arranged in parallel along the longitudinal axis and include the muscle membrane, myofibrils, sarcotubular system, aqueous sarcoplasm, and mitochondria. There are two types of muscle fibers, type I and type II, determined by motor nerve innervation.

DID YOU UNDERSTAND?—cont'd

4. Myofibrils and myofilaments contain the major muscle proteins, actin and myosin, which interact to form cross-bridges during muscle contraction. The nonprotein muscle constituents provide an energy source for contraction and regulate protein synthesis, enzyme systems, and membrane stabilization.

5. Muscle contraction includes excitation, coupling, contraction, and relaxation.

6. Muscle strength is graded by the "all or nothing" phenomenon and recruitment. Speed of contraction is affected by several factors: muscle fiber type, temperature, stretch, and weight of the load.

7. There are two types of muscle contraction, isometric and isotonic. Muscle shortening occurs during contraction but can be seen also during pathologic and physiologic contracture.

8. Skeletal muscle requires a constant supply of adeno-sine triphosphate (ATP) and phosphocreatine to fuel muscle contraction and for growth and repair. ATP and phosphocreatine can be generated aerobically or anaerobically.

⋀ AGING AND THE MUSCULOSKELETAL SYSTEM

1. Sarcopenia, or age-related loss in skeletal muscle, is a direct cause of decrease in muscle strength. A slow decline in dynamic and isometric strength is evident after age 70 years.

2. The regenerative function of muscle tissue remains normal in elderly persons.

3. On average, people lose about one third of a pound of muscle every year after age 40 years and gain at least as much body fat.

4. Reduced basal metabolic rate and decreased lean body mass are also noted in the elderly population.

KEY TERMS

REFERENCES

1. Simon, S.R. (Ed.). (1994). *Orthopaedic basic science.* Chicago: American Academy of Orthopaedic Surgeons.
2. Mundy, G.R. (1995). *Bone remodeling and its disorders.* London: Dunitz, Ltd.
3. Davis, L.S. et al. (1997). Immune and inflammatory responses. In W.N. Kelley et al. (Eds.). *Textbook of rheumatology* (5th ed.). Philadelphia: Saunders.
4. Rubin, C.T. & Rubin, J.E. (1997). The biology, physiology, and morphology of bone. Mankin, H.J. & Brandt, K.D. (1997). Pathogenesis of osteoarthritis. In W.N. Kelley et al. (Eds.). *Textbook of rheumatology* (5th ed.). Philadelphia: Saunders.
5. Seeley, R.R., Stephens, T.D., & Tate, P. (1997). *Anatomy and physiology* (3rd ed.). St. Louis: Mosby.
6. Dantzig. J.A. & Goldman, Y.E. (1997). Skeletal muscles. In W.N. Kelley et al. (Eds.). *Textbook of rheumatology* (5th ed.). Philadelphia: Saunders.
7. Seeman, E. (1995). The dilemma of osteoporosis in men. *American Journal of Medicine, 98*(2), 765.
8. Mourad, L.A. (1997). Musculoskeletal system. In J.M. Thompson et al. *Mosby's clinical nursing* [4th ed.]. St. Louis: Mosby.
9. Bouxsein, M.L., Myers, E.R., & Hayes, W.C. (1996). Biomechanics of age-related fractures. In R. Marcus, D. Feldman, & J. Kelsey (Eds.). *Osteoporosis.* San Diego: Academic Press.
10. Carter, D.R., vander Meulen, C.H., & Beaupré, G.S. (1996). Skeletal development: Mechanical consequences of growth, aging, and disease. In R. Marcus, D. Feldman, & J. Kelsey (Eds.). *Osteoporosis.* San Diego: Academic Press.
11. Branski, S.H. (1998). Delirium in hospitalized patients. *American Journal of Nursing, 98*(4), 16D.
12. Klippel, J.H. & Dieppe, P.A. (1998). *Rheumatology* (2nd ed.). St. Louis: Mosby.
13. Evans, W.J. (1995). Exercise, nutrition, and aging. *Clinics in Geriatric Medicine, 11*(4), 725-734.
14. Proctor, D.N., Balagopal, P., & Nair, K.S. (1998). Age-related sarcopenia in humans is associated with reduced synthetic rates of specific muscle proteins. *Journal of Nutrition, 128*(2 Suppl.), 351S-355S.
15. Roubenoff, R. (1999). The pathophysiology of wasting in the elderly. *Journal of Nutrition, 129*(15 Suppl.), 256S-259S.

CHAPTER

37

Alterations of Musculoskeletal Function

Kathryn L. McCance and Leona A. Mourad

Musculoskeletal injuries include fractures, dislocations, sprains, and strains. Fractures are the most serious. Alterations in bones, joints, and muscles may be caused by metabolic disorders, infections, inflammatory or noninflammatory diseases, or tumors.

MUSCULOSKELETAL INJURIES

Trauma is the "neglected disease."[1] It is the leading cause of death of people ages 1 to 44 years of all races and socioeconomic levels. Each year more than 100,000 persons in the United States die from accidents and 500,000 are permanently disabled.[1]

Musculoskeletal injuries have a major impact on patients, families, and society in general because of the physical and psychologic effects of limitation on daily activities, pain, and decreased quality of life; direct costs of diagnosis and treatments; and the indirect economic costs related to the loss of employment and decreased productivity.

Skeletal Trauma

Fractures

A *fracture* is a break in the continuity of a bone. A break occurs when force is applied that exceeds the tensile or compressive strength of the bone. The incidence of fractures varies for individual bones according to age and gender, with the highest incidence of fractures in young males (between the ages of 15 and 24 years) and older persons (65 years of age and older) (Box 37-1). Fractures of healthy bones, particularly the tibia, clavicle, and lower humerus, tend to occur in young persons and to be the result of trauma. Fractures of the hands and feet are usually caused by accidents in the workplace. The incidence of fractures of the upper femur, upper humerus, vertebrae, and pelvis is highest in older adults and is often associated with osteoporosis (see p. 1040). More than 250,000 fractures of the hip occur yearly in the United States alone.[2]

Classification of fractures

Fractures are classified as complete or incomplete and open or closed (Fig. 37-1). In a *complete fracture,* the bone is broken all the way through, whereas in an *incomplete fracture,* the bone is damaged but is still in one piece. Complete and incomplete fractures also can be called *open* (formerly referred to as compound) if the skin is broken and *closed* (formerly called simple) if it is not. A fracture in which a bone breaks into two or more fragments is termed a *comminuted fracture.* Fractures are also classified according to the direction of the fracture line. A *linear fracture* runs parallel to the long axis of the bone. An *oblique fracture* occurs at a 45-degree angle (oblique angle) to the shaft of the bone. A *spiral fracture* encircles the bone, and a *transverse fracture* occurs straight across the bone.

Incomplete fractures tend to occur in the more flexible, growing bones of children. The three main types of incomplete fractures are greenstick, torus, and bowing fractures. A *greenstick fracture* perforates one cortex and splinters the spongy bone. The name is derived from the damage sustained by a young tree branch (a green stick) when it is bent sharply. The outer surface is disrupted, but the inner surface remains intact. Greenstick fractures typically occur in the

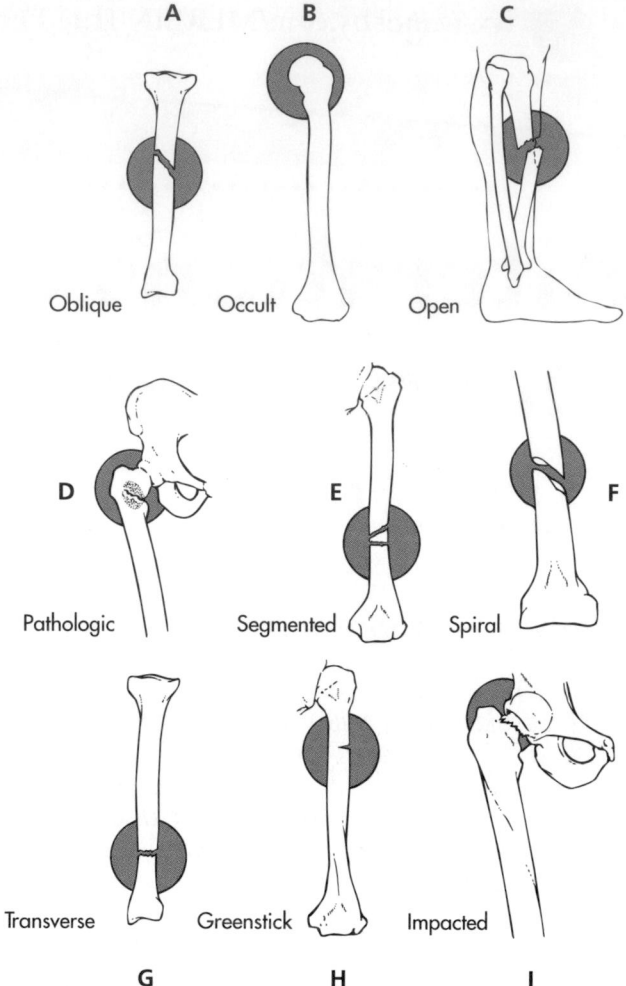

Fig. 37-1 *Examples of types of bone fractures.* **A,** Oblique: Fracture at oblique angle across both cortices. *Cause:* Direct or indirect energy, with angulation and some compression. **B,** Occult: Fracture that is hidden or not readily discernible. *Cause:* Minor force or energy. **C,** Open: Skin broken over fracture; possible soft tissue trauma. *Cause:* Moderate to severe energy that is continuous and exceeds tissue tolerances. **D,** Pathologic: Transverse, oblique, or spinal fracture of bone weakened by tumor pressure or presence. *Cause:* Minor energy or force, which may be direct or indirect. **E,** Segmented: Fracture with two or more pieces or segments. *Cause:* Direct or indirect moderate to severe force. **F,** Spiral: Fracture that curves around cortices and may become displaced by twist. *Cause:* Direct or indirect twisting energy or force with distal part held or unable to move. **G,** Transverse: Horizontal break through bone. *Cause:* Direct or indirect energy toward bone. **H,** Greenstick: Break in only one cortex of bone. *Cause:* Minor direct or indirect energy. **I,** Impacted: Fracture with one end wedged into opposite end or inside fractured fragment. *Cause:* Compressive axial energy or force directly to distal fragment. *(Redrawn from Mourad, L.A. [1997]. Musculoskeletal system. In J.M. Thompson et al. [Eds.]. Mosby's clinical nursing [4th ed.]. St. Louis: Mosby.)*

TABLE 37-1	Types of Fractures
Type	**Definition**
Typical complete fractures	
Closed fracture	Noncommunicating wound between bone and skin
Open fracture	Communicating wound between bone and skin
Comminuted fracture	Multiple bone fragments
Linear fracture	Fracture line parallel to long axis of bone
Oblique fracture	Fracture line at 45-degree angle to long axis of bone
Spiral fracture	Fracture line encircling bone (as a spiral staircase)
Transverse fracture	Fracture line perpendicular to long axis of bone
Impacted fracture	Fracture fragments pushed into each other
Pathologic fracture	Fracture at a point in the bone weakened by disease, for example, with tumors or osteoporosis
Avulsion fracture	A fragment of bone connected to a ligament or tendon breaks off from the main bone
Compression fracture	Fracture wedged or squeezed together on one side of bone
Displaced fracture	Fracture with one, both, or all fragments out of normal alignment
Extracapsular fracture	Fragment close to the joint but remains outside the joint capsule
Intracapsular fracture	Fragment within the joint capsule
Typical incomplete fractures	
Greenstick fracture	Break on one cortex of bone with splintering of inner bone surface, commonly occurs in children and elderly persons
Torus fracture	Buckling of cortex
Bowing fracture	Bending of bone
Stress fracture	Microfracture
Transchondral fracture	Separation of cartilaginous joint surface (articular cartilage) from main shaft of bone

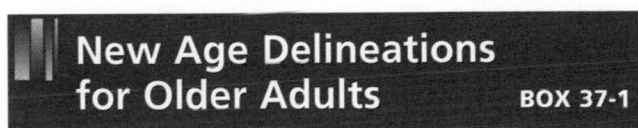

New Age Delineations for Older Adults   BOX 37-1

Ages 65-74 years: Young old
Ages 75-84 years: Old old
Ages 85 and older years: Elderly

proximal metaphysis or diaphysis of the tibia, radius, and ulna. In a *torus fracture,* the cortex buckles but does not break. Torus fractures are common in the metaphyses of persons with osteoporosis. *Bowing fractures* usually occur when longitudinal force is applied to bone. This type of fracture is common in children and usually involves the paired radius-ulna or the fibula-tibia. A complete diaphyseal fracture occurs in one of the bones of the pair, which disperses the stress sufficiently to prevent a complete fracture of the second bone, which bows. A bowing fracture resists correction (reduction) because the force necessary to reduce it must be equal to the force that bowed it. Treatment of bowing fractures is also difficult because the bowed bone interferes with reduction of the fractured bone. Types of fractures are summarized in Table 37-1.

Fractures may be further classified by cause as pathologic, stress, or transchondral fractures. A *pathologic fracture* is a break at the site of a preexisting abnormality, usually by force that would not fracture a normal bone. Any disease process that weakens a bone (especially the cortex) predisposes the bone to pathologic fracture. Pathologic fractures are commonly associated with tumors, osteoporosis, infections, and metabolic bone disorders.

Stress fractures occur in normal or abnormal bone that is subjected to repeated stress, such as occurs during athletics. The stress is less than the stress that usually causes a fracture. Two types of stress fractures are recognized: fatigue fracture and insufficiency fracture. A *fatigue fracture* is caused by abnormal stress or torque applied to a bone with normal ability to deform and recover. Fatigue fractures usually occur in individuals who engage in a new or different activity that is both strenuous and repetitive (e.g., joggers, skaters, dancers, military recruits). Because gains in muscle strength occur more rapidly than gains in bone strength, the newly developed muscles place exaggerated stress on the bones that are not ready for it. The imbalance between muscle and bone development causes microfractures to develop in the cortex. If the activity is controlled and increased gradually, new bone formation catches up to increased demands and microfractures do not occur.

Insufficiency fractures are stress fractures that occur in bones lacking normal ability to deform and recover; normal weight bearing or activity fractures the bone. Rheumatoid

Fig. 37-2 *Bone healing (schematic representation).* **A,** Bleeding at broken ends of the bone with subsequent hematoma formation. **B,** Organization of hematoma into fibrous network. **C,** Invasion of osteoblasts, lengthening of collagen strands, and deposition of calcium. **D,** Callus formation; new bone is built up as osteoclasts destroy dead bone. **E,** Remodeling is accomplished as excess callus is reabsorbed and trabecular bone is laid down. *(From Phipps, W.J. et al. [1999].* Medical-surgical nursing: Concepts and clinical practice *[6th ed.]. St. Louis: Mosby.)*

Fig. 37-3 *Exuberant callus formation following fracture. (From Rosai, J. [1996].* Ackerman's surgical pathology *[8th ed.]. St. Louis: Mosby.)*

arthritis, osteoporosis, Paget disease, osteomalacia, rickets, hyperparathyroidism, and radiation therapy cause bone to lose its normal ability to deform and recover (i.e., normal weight bearing or activity fractures the bone).

A *transchondral fracture* (also known as *osteochondritis dissecans*) consists of fragmentation and separation of a portion of the articular cartilage that covers the end of a bone at a joint. (Joint structures are defined in Chapter 36.) Single or multiple sites may be fractured, and the fragments may consist of cartilage alone or cartilage and bone. Typical sites of transchondral fracture are the head of the femur, the ankle, the knee cap, the elbow, and the wrist. Transchondral fractures are most prevalent in adolescents or in young adults participating in athletic activities.

Pathophysiology

When a bone is broken, the periosteum and blood vessels in the cortex, marrow, and surrounding soft tissues are disrupted. Bleeding occurs from the damaged ends of the bone and from the neighboring soft tissue. A clot (hematoma) forms within the medullary canal, between the fractured ends of the bone, and beneath the periosteum (Fig. 37-2). Bone tissue immediately adjacent to the fracture dies. This dead tissue (along with any debris in the fracture area) stimulates an intense inflammatory response characterized by vasodilation, exudation of plasma and leukocytes, and infiltration by inflammatory leukocytes, growth factors, and mast cells that simultaneously decalcify the fractured bone ends. Within 48 hours after the injury, vascular tissue invades the fracture area from surrounding soft tissue and the marrow cavity, and blood flow to the entire bone is increased. Bone-forming cells in the periosteum, endosteum, and marrow are activated to produce subperiosteal procallus along the outer surface of the shaft and over the broken ends of the bone (see Fig. 37-2). Osteoblasts within the procallus synthesize collagen and matrix, which becomes mineralized to form callus (woven bone). As the repair process continues, remodeling occurs, during which unnecessary callus is resorbed and trabeculae are formed along lines of stress as the repair tissues bring it in line with the tissue cells of the host (Fig. 37-3). Except for the liver, bone is unique among all body tissues in that it will form new bone, not scar tissue, when it heals after a fracture.

Clinical Manifestations

The signs and symptoms of a fracture include unnatural alignment (deformity), swelling, muscle spasm, tenderness, pain, and impaired sensation and decreased mobility. The position of the bone segments is determined by the pull of attached muscles, gravity, and the direction and magnitude of the force that caused the fracture.

Immediately after a bone is fractured, usually there is numbness in the fracture site because of trauma to the nerve or nerves at the site. The numbness may last up to 20 minutes, during which time the injured person may use the fractured bone or bones to crawl or move from the area. However, once the numbness dissipates, the subsequent pain is quite severe and incapacitating until relieved with medication and treatment of the fractured bones. The pain is related to muscle spasms at the fracture site, overriding of the fracture segments, or damage to adjacent soft tissues.

Pathologic fractures usually cause angular deformity, painless swelling, or generalized bone pain. Stress fractures are painful because of accelerated remodeling. The pain occurs during activity and is usually relieved by rest. Stress fractures also cause local tenderness and soft tissue swelling. Transchondral fractures may be entirely asymptomatic or painful during movement. Range of motion in the joint is limited, and movement may evoke audible clicking sounds (crepitus).

Evaluation and Treatment

Fracture treatment involves realigning the bone fragments (reduction) close to their normal or anatomic position and holding the fragments in place (immobilization) so that bone union can occur. Several methods are available to reduce a fracture: closed manipulation, traction, and open reduction.

Most fractures can be reduced by closed manipulation and reduction. The bone is moved or manipulated into place without opening the skin. Closed reduction is used when the contour of the bone is in fair alignment and can be maintained well with immobilization.

Traction may be used to accomplish or maintain reduction. When bone fragments are displaced (not in their anatomic position), weights are used to apply firm, steady traction (pull) and countertraction to the long axis of the bone. Traction stretches and fatigues muscles that have pulled the bone fragments out of place, allowing the distal fragment to align with the proximal fragment. Traction can be applied to the skin (skin traction) (Fig. 37-4), directly to the involved bone, or distal to the involved bone (skeletal traction). Skin traction is used when only a few pounds of pulling force are needed to realign the fragments or when the traction will be used for brief times only, such as before surgery or, for children with femoral fractures, for 3 to 7 days before applying a cast. A traction boot is applied to the skin, closed with self-adhering straps, with weights attached to the foot area of the traction boot. In skeletal traction, a pin or wire is drilled through the bone below the fracture site, and a traction bow, rope, and weights are attached to the pin or wire to apply tension and to provide the pulling force to overcome the muscle spasm and help realign the fracture fragments.

Open reduction is a surgical procedure that exposes the fracture site; the fragments are brought into alignment under direct visualization. Some form of prosthesis, screw, plate, nail, or wire usually is used to maintain the reduction (internal fixation).

Splints and plaster casts are used to immobilize and hold a reduction in place. Improper reduction or immobilization of a fractured bone may result in nonunion, delayed union, or malunion. **Nonunion** is failure of the bone ends to grow together. The gap between the broken ends of the bone fills

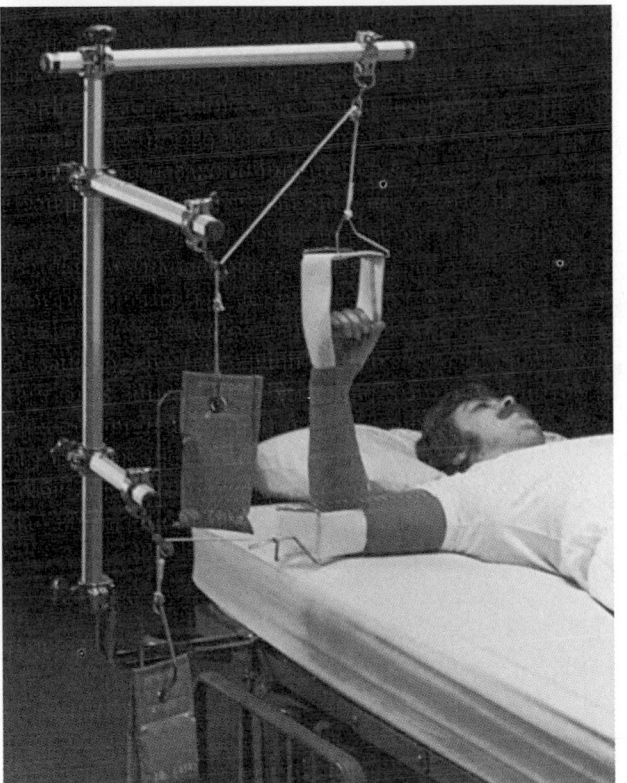

Fig. 37-4 *Two types of skin traction.* **A,** Buck extension traction. **B,** Dunlop traction. *(From Mourad, L.A. [1997]. Musculoskeletal system. In J.M. Thompson et al. [Eds.]. Mosby's clinical nursing [4th ed.]. St. Louis: Mosby.)*

with dense fibrous and fibrocartilaginous tissue instead of new bone. Occasionally, the fibrous tissue contains a fluid-filled space that resembles a joint and is termed a *false joint*, or *pseudoarthrosis*. **Delayed union** is union that does not occur until approximately 8 to 9 months after a fracture. **Malunion** is the healing of a bone in a nonanatomic position.

Dislocation and subluxation

Dislocation and subluxation are usually caused by trauma. *Dislocation* is the temporary displacement of one or more bones in a joint in which the opposing bone surfaces lose contact entirely. If the contact between the opposing bone surfaces is only partially lost, the injury is called a *subluxation.*

Dislocation and subluxation are most common in persons younger than 20 years of age and are generally associated with fractures. However, they may be the result of congenital or acquired disorders that cause (1) muscular imbalance, as occurs with congenital dislocation of the hip or neurologic disorders; (2) incongruities in the articulating surfaces of the bones, as occur with rheumatoid arthritis (see p. 1052); or (3) joint instability.

The joints most often dislocated or subluxated are the joints of the shoulder, elbow, wrist, finger, hip, and knee. The shoulder joint most frequently injured is the glenohumeral joint.

Traumatic dislocation of the elbow joint is common in the immature skeleton. In adults, an elbow dislocation is usually associated with a fracture of the ulna or head of the radius.

Traumatic dislocation of the wrist usually involves the distal ulna and carpal bones. Any one of the eight carpal bones can be dislocated after an injury.

Dislocation in the hand usually involves the metacarpophalangeal and interphalangeal joints.

Considerable trauma is needed to dislocate the hip. Anterior hip dislocation is rather rare and is caused by forced abduction, for example, when an individual lands on his or her feet from a high fall. Posterior dislocation of the hip can occur in an automobile accident in which the flexed knee strikes the dashboard, causing the head of the femur to be "pushed" posteriorly from the hip joint.

The knee is an unstable weight-bearing joint that depends heavily on the soft tissue structures around it for support. It is exposed to many different types of motion (flexion, extension, rotation) and is one of the most frequently injured joints. A knee dislocation can be anterior, posterior, lateral, medial, or rotary. It is usually the result of an injury that occurs during sports activities.

Pathophysiology

Dislocations and subluxations are often accompanied by fracture because stress is placed on areas of bone not usually subjected to stress. In addition, as the bone separates from the joint, it may bruise or tear adjacent nerves, blood vessels, ligaments, supporting structures, and soft tissue. Dislocations of the shoulder may damage the shoulder capsule and the axillary nerve. Damage to axillary nerves causes anesthesia in the sensory distribution of the nerve and paralysis of the deltoid muscle. Dislocations may also disrupt circulation, leading to ischemia and possibly permanent disability of the affected extremity tissues.

Clinical Manifestations

Signs and symptoms of dislocations or subluxations include pain, swelling, limitation of motion, and joint deformity. Pain may be caused by effusion of inflammatory exudate into the joint or associated tendon and ligament injury. Joint deformity is usually caused by muscle contractions that ex-

ert pull on the dislocated or subluxated joint. Limitation of motion results from effusion into the joint or the displacement of bones.

Evaluation and Treatment

Evaluation of dislocations and subluxations is based on clinical manifestations and roentgenograms. Treatment consists of reduction and immobilization for 2 to 6 weeks and exercises to maintain normal range of motion in the joint. Depending on the joint, healing is usually complete within months to years.

Support Structures
Sprains and strains of tendons and ligaments

Tendon and ligament injuries can accompany fractures and dislocations. A *tendon* is a fibrous connective tissue that attaches skeletal muscle to bone. A *ligament* is a band of fibrous connective tissue that connects bones where they meet in a joint. Tendons and ligaments support the bones and joints and either facilitate or limit motion. Tendons and ligaments can be torn, ruptured, or completely separated from bone at their points of attachment.

A tear in a tendon is commonly known as a *strain.* Major trauma can tear or rupture a tendon at any site in the body. Most frequently injured are the tendons of the hands and feet, the knee (patellar), the upper arm (biceps and triceps), the thigh (quadriceps), the ankle, and the heel (Achilles).

Ligament tears are commonly known as *sprains.* Ligament tears and ruptures can occur at any joint but are most common in the wrist, ankle, elbow, and knee joints. A complete separation of a tendon or ligament from its bony attachment site is known as an *avulsion* and is commonly seen in young athletes, especially sprinters, hurdlers, and runners.

Strains and sprains are classified as first degree (least severe), second degree, and third degree (most severe).

Pathophysiology

When a tendon or ligament is torn, an inflammatory exudate develops between the torn ends. Later, granulation tissue containing macrophages, fibroblasts, and capillary buds grows inward from the surrounding soft tissue and cartilage to begin the repair process. Within 4 to 5 days after the injury, collagen formation begins. At first, collagen formation is random and disorganized. As the collagen fibers interweave and connect with preexisting tendon fibers, they become organized parallel to the lines of stress. Eventually vascular fibrous tissue fuses the new and surrounding tissues into a single mass. As reorganization takes place, the healing tendon or ligament separates from the surrounding soft tissue. Usually a healing tendon or ligament lacks sufficient strength to withstand strong pull for 4 to 5 weeks after the injury. If strong muscle pull does occur during this time, the tendon or ligament ends may separate again, which causes the tendon or ligament to heal in a lengthened shape with an excessive amount of scar tissue that renders the tendon or ligament functionless.

Clinical Manifestations

Tendon and ligament injuries are painful and are usually accompanied by soft tissue swelling, changes in tendon or ligament contour, and dislocation or subluxation of bones. The pain is generally sharp and localized, and tenderness persists over the distribution of the tendon or ligament. Depending on the tendon or ligament involved, such injuries may result in decreased mobility, instability, and weakness of the affected joints, even with prompt treatment.

Evaluation and Treatment

Evaluation is based on clinical manifestations, stress radiography, arthroscopy, or arthrography. When possible, treatment consists of suturing the tendon or ligament ends in close approximation. If this is not possible because of the extent of damage, tendon or ligament grafting may be necessary. Prolonged rehabilitation exercises help ensure regaining of nearly normal functions, but recovery may be complicated by posttraumatic arthritis.

Tendinitis, epicondylitis, and bursitis

Trauma can also cause painful inflammation of tendons (tendinitis) and bursae (bursitis). Other causes of tendinitis include crystal deposits, postural misalignment, and hypermobility in a joint. Achilles tendinitis is inflammation of the Achilles tendon, one that is frequently inflamed.

Epicondylitis is inflammation of a tendon where it attaches to a bone at its origin. Epicondylar areas of the humerus, radius, or ulna, and around the knee are most frequently inflamed. *Lateral epicondylitis,* commonly called *tennis elbow,* is inflammation of the lateral epicondyle of the humerus, and *medial epicondylitis,* referred to as *golfer's elbow,* is inflammation of the medial humeral epicondyle (Fig. 37-5). Epicondylitis is also related to work activities that involve cyclic flexion and extension of the elbow, or cyclic pronation, supination, extension, and flexion of the wrist that generate loads to the elbow and forearm region.[3]

Bursae are small sacs lined with synovial membrane and filled with synovial fluid that are located between tendons, muscles, and bony prominences (Fig. 37-6). Their primary function is to separate, lubricate, and cushion these structures. Acute bursitis occurs primarily in the middle years and is caused by repeated trauma. Septic bursitis is caused by wound infection or bacterial infection of the skin overlying the bursae. The shoulder is the most common site of bursitis. Bursitis also occurs in the hip, knee, elbow, and the toe with a bunion.

Pathophysiology

Fluid from inflammation accumulates in tendinitis, causing swelling of the tendon and its enclosing sheath. Inflammatory changes cause thickening of the sheath, limiting movements and causing pain. Microtears cause bleeding, edema, and pain in the involved tendon or tendons. At times, after repeated inflammations, calcium may be deposited in the tendon origin area.

The usual bursitis is an inflammation that is reactive to overuse or excessive pressure. The inflamed bursal sac be-

Fig. 37-5 *Epicondylitis and tendinitis.* **A,** Achilles tendon, site of frequently occurring tendinitis. **B,** Medial or lateral epicondyles of humerus, site of epicondylitis. *(From Mourad, L.A. [1997]. Musculoskeletal system. In J.M. Thompson et al. [Eds.]. Mosby's clinical nursing [4th ed.]. St. Louis: Mosby.)*

Fig. 37-6 *Olecranon bursitis. (Reprinted from the Clinical Slide Collection of the Rheumatic Diseases, © 1991. Used by permission of the American College of Rheumatology.)*

comes engorged, and the inflammation can spread to adjacent tissues. The inflammation may decrease with rest, heat, and needle puncture. (Inflammation is discussed in Chapter 6.)

Clinical Manifestations

Clinical manifestations are usually localized to one side of the joint. Generally there is local or "point" tenderness (the

TABLE 37-2	Muscle Strain		
Type	**Manifestations**	**Treatment**	
First degree (example: bench press in untrained athlete)	Muscle overstretched, painful	Ice should be applied 5 or 6 times in the first 24-48 hr; gradual resumption of full weight bearing after initial rest for up to 2 wks Exercises individualized to specific injury	
Second degree (example: any muscle strain with bruising and pain)	Muscle intact with some tearing pain, mild bruising	Treatment similar to that for first-degree strains, with added mild analgesia; cryokinetics (alternating applications of heat and cold) plus progressive exercises for specific injury	
Third degree (example: traumatic injury)	Caused by tearing of fascia, muscle rupture palpable, bleeding present	Surgery to approximate ruptured edges; immobilization and non-weight bearing for 6 wk, followed by a regimen of strengthening exercises	

individual can point to the area of greatest tenderness) and more pain with active motion than with passive motion. With tendinitis, the pain is localized over the involved tendon, and movement in the affected joint is limited. The onset of pain may be gradual or sudden in bursitis, and movement in the joint is limited. Shoulder bursitis impairs arm abduction. Bursitis in the knee produces pain when climbing stairs, and crossing the legs is painful in bursitis of the hip. Lying on the side of the inflamed trochanteric bursa is also very painful. Signs of infectious bursitis may include the presence of a puncture site, prior corticosteroid injection, severe inflammation, or an adjacent source of infection, such as an infected total joint replacement.

Evaluation and Treatment

Evaluation of tendinitis, epicondylitis, and bursitis is based on clinical manifestations, physical examination, arthroscopy, arthrography, and possibly magnetic resonance imaging (MRI). Treatment includes immobilization of the joint with a sling, splint, or cast; systemic analgesics; ice or heat applications; or local injection of an anesthetic and a corticosteroid to reduce inflammation. Physical therapy to prevent loss of function begins after acute inflammation subsides.

Muscle strains

Mild injury such as *muscle strain* is usually seen after traumatic or sports injuries. Muscle strain is a general term for local muscle damage. It is often the result of sudden, forced motion causing the muscle to become stretched beyond normal capacity. Knife and gunshot wounds also cause traumatic rupture. Strains often involve the tendon as well. Muscles are ruptured more often than tendons in young people; the opposite is true in the older population. Muscle strain may be chronic when the muscle is repeatedly stretched beyond its usual capacity. There is evidence of tissue disruption with subsequent signs of muscle regeneration and connective tissue repair when a biopsy is performed. Hemorrhage into the surrounding tissue and signs of inflammation also may be present. Regardless of the cause of trauma, muscle cells are usually able to regenerate. Regeneration may take up to 6 weeks, and the affected mus-

cle should be protected during this time. (Degrees of acute muscle strain, together with their manifestations and treatment, are summarized in Table 37-2.)

A late complication of localized muscle injury is *myositis ossificans.* This condition is thought to be caused by scar tissue calcification and subsequent ossification. Examples include "rider's bone," in which the adductor muscle of the thigh of equestrians becomes calcified, and "drill bone," in which the same complication is seen in the deltoid and pectoral muscles of fencers and infantry soldiers, as well as football players after muscle injury to thigh muscles.

Myoglobinuria

Myoglobinuria, also called *rhabdomyolysis,* can be a life-threatening complication of severe muscle trauma, or secondary to malignant hyperthermia.[4] Myoglobinuria is named for the principal manifestation of the condition—an excess of myoglobin (an intracellular muscle protein) in the urine. Muscle cell damage releases the myoglobin. The most severe form is often called *crush syndrome.* Less severe and more localized forms are called *compartment syndromes,* which can lead to *Volkmann ischemic contracture* in the forearm or leg. Crush syndrome first gained notoriety in the reports of injuries seen after the London air raids in World War II. More recently it has been reported in individuals found unresponsive and immobile for long periods, usually after a drug overdose. Myoglobinuria also can be seen after viral infections, administration of certain anesthetic agents, strychnine poisoning, tetanus, heat stroke, electrolyte disturbances, and fractures. Excessive muscular activity also has been implicated in reports of myoglobinuria in athletes, such as long-distance runners, ice skaters, skiers, and military recruits. Status epilepticus, electroconvulsive therapy, and high-voltage electrical shock are also associated with severe and sometimes fatal myoglobinuria.

If the myoglobinuria is caused by fulminant malignant hyperthermia, severe muscle spasm and rhabdomyolysis can lead to renal failure. Other complications include intraoperative rigidity, tachycardia, cardiac dysrhythmias, metabolic and respiratory acidosis, and rising temperature elevations up to 43° C, which can occur at a very rapid rate. Cerebral

Fig. 37-7 *Pathogenesis of compartment syndrome and crush syndrome caused by prolonged muscle compression.* *ECF,* Extracellular fluid.

edema, cardiogenic and hypovolemic shock, pulmonary edema, and disseminated intravascular clotting can contribute to the death of an individual with *malignant hyperthermia.*

Pathophysiology

The weight of a limp extremity can generate enough pressure to produce muscle ischemia (Figs. 37-7 and 37-8). This causes edema, rising compartment pressure, and tamponade that leads to muscle infarction and neural injury, and, finally, results in cell loss. Physical interruptions in the sarcolemmal membrane, called *holes* or *delta lesions,* suggest that the sarcolemmal membrane may be the route by which muscle constituents are released. (The sarcolemmal membrane, the plasma membrane of the muscle cell, is described in Chapter 36.)

Clinical Manifestations

When myoglobin is released from the muscle cells into the circulation, it can cause a visible, dark reddish brown pigmentation of the urine. The renal threshold for myoglobin is low, approximately 0.5 mg/dl of urine, so only 200 g muscle need be damaged to cause visible changes in the urine. Along with the release of myoglobin, creatine kinase (CK) and other serum enzymes are released in massive quantities. The CK level may reach 2000 times normal (5 to 25 U/ml for women and 5 to 35 U/ml for men). The efflux of proteins and enzymes also includes loss of potassium, phosphate, nucleotides, creatinine, and creatine. Serum hypocalcemia is seen early in the course of myoglobinuria and is followed by late hypercalcemia. The risk of renal failure increases directly with the height of serum CK, potassium, and phosphorus levels.[5]

Evaluation and Treatment

Careful and thorough preoperative assessment should alert the anesthesiologist to the possibility of an individual susceptible to the possibility of malignant hyperthermia. A family history of anesthetic problems and previous untoward anesthetic experiences (muscle cramping, unexplained

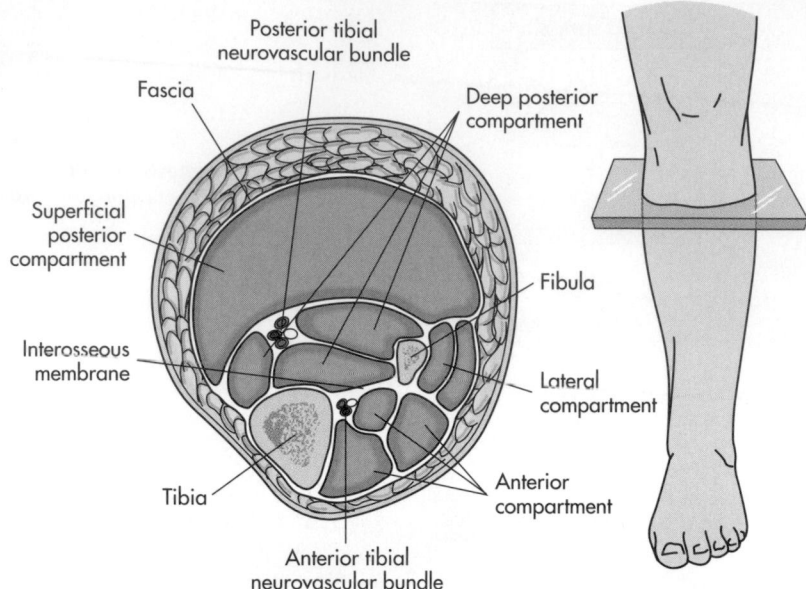

Fig. 37-8 *The muscle compartments of the lower leg.* *(From Phipps, W.J., Sands, J.K., & Marek, J.F. [1999].* Medical-surgical nursing: Concepts and clinical practice *[6th ed.]. St. Louis: Mosby.)*

fevers, dark urine) are criteria that require further clarification before administration of a volatile anesthetic, such as halothane, or of the muscle relaxant, succinylcholine.[4]

Priorities in treatment of myoglobinuria include identifying and treating the underlying disorder and preventing life-threatening renal failure. Malignant hyperthermia and myoglobinuria can be treated by infusing dantrolene sodium (Dantrium). Diluting the pigment using intravenous fluids and administration of mannitol, sodium bicarbonate, and furosemide (Lasix) to "flush" the kidney have been advocated to prevent renal failure. Secondary problems include electrolyte imbalance, volume depletion, acidosis, hyperuricemia, hyperkalemia, and calcium imbalance. These need specific treatment. Short-term dialysis also may be necessary.

Compartment syndromes may require emergency treatment when blood flow to the affected extremity is compromised because of increased venous pressure, leading to decreased arterial inflow, ischemia, and edema. When clinical evaluation is inconclusive, the rising compartment pressure can be directly measured by inserting a wick catheter, needle, or slit catheter into the muscle. Immediate fasciotomy and débridement have been advocated for pressures of more than 30 mm Hg.[6,7] Compartments frequently affected are the anterior tibial and deep posterior tibial compartments in the leg and the gluteal compartments in the buttocks.

DISORDERS OF BONES
Metabolic Bone Diseases

Metabolic bone disease is characterized by abnormal bone structure that is caused by altered or inadequate biochemical reactions, which may be attributable to genetics, diet, or hormones.

Osteoporosis

Osteoporosis is a disease in which the density or mass of bone is reduced (Fig. 37-9). The bone that remains is histologically and biochemically normal, but there is not enough of it to maintain skeletal integrity and mechanical support. The disease can be (1) generalized, involving major portions of the axial skeleton, or (2) regional, involving one segment of the appendicular skeleton. Both spongy and compact bone is lost, but spongy bone loss exceeds compact bone loss.

Healthy young women can gain bone mass up to and during the third decade of life through active physical activity, dietary calcium intake, and the use of oral contraceptives.[8] Osteoporosis is the most common metabolic disease, occurring in 50% of women in their lifetimes.[9] Because of the decreased bone mass, fractures are major risks for those persons with osteoporosis.[10] Wrist fractures in women increase during the sixth decade, and hip fractures increase exponentially from approximately age 70 years, until in the elderly population, one in three women and one in six men in the United States (up to 300,000 per year) have hip fractures.[10] Nearly 65,000 women die each year from hip fractures.[10] Vertebral fractures also occur in the latter years of

Fig. 37-9 *Osteoporotic vertebral body (right)* **shortened by compression fractures compared with a normal vertebral body.** Note that the osteoporotic vertebra has a characteristic loss of horizontal trabeculae and thickened vertical trabeculae. *(From Cotran, R.S., Kumar, V., & Collins, T. [1999]. Robbins pathologic basis of disease [6th ed.]. Philadelphia: Saunders.)*

life, mainly in the sixth and seventh decades, with possibly one in three women older than 65 years having a vertebral fracture.[11] The annual direct and indirect costs of osteoporosis are more than $13 billion.[8] Approximately half the persons with osteoporosis and fractures never walk again.[12] Osteoporosis leads to marked losses of both spongy and trabecular bone, with women losing approximately one half and men approximately one quarter of their spongy bone.

Osteoporosis is most common in whites but affects all races. Whites are more susceptible than other races to osteoporosis caused by loss of bone density with age. Blacks have only about half the fracture rate of whites, probably related to their higher peak bone mass.[13]

The cause of generalized osteoporosis remains uncertain, except in a very few cases in which the cause is known. Postmenopausal osteoporosis, which occurs in middle-aged and older women, is probably caused by decreased levels of estrogen. Before menopause, higher estrogen levels inhibit bone resorption by decreasing the sensitivity of osteoclasts to circulating parathyroid hormone (PTH). Without the inhibitory action of estrogen, PTH overstimulates osteoclasts within the basic multicellular units to initiate the remodeling cycle, which begins with resorption. (Remodeling is described in Chapter 36.) The cause of senile (age-related) osteoporosis remains unclear, but it may be that osteoblasts and osteoclasts shrink, regress to a former state, or undergo alterations that diminish their activity. Reduction in physical activity in older persons may also be a major factor in the bone loss, because preservation of bone mass depends on skeletal stress through muscle contraction and weight bearing. Active and athletic women who lose their menstrual patterns are strong candidates for bone loss.[14]

Insufficient intake or malabsorption of dietary minerals, particularly calcium, is probably a factor in the development of osteoporosis. Calcium absorption from the intestine decreases with age, and studies of individuals with osteoporosis show that their calcium intake is lower than that of age-matched controls. Deficiencies of protein and vitamins, particularly vitamins C and D, also contribute to bone loss. Excessive intakes of caffeine, alcohol, and nicotine along with low body fat have also been considered risk factors.[15,16] In addition, significant differences in the trace elements (zinc, copper, manganese) were noted in the bones and hair of unaffected individuals and those with osteoporosis.[17]

A variety of hormonal imbalances also may contribute to osteoporosis. Skeletal homeostasis depends on a very narrow range of plasma calcium and phosphate concentrations, which are maintained by the endocrine system. Therefore endocrine dysfunction ultimately can cause metabolic bone disease. The hormones most commonly associated with osteoporosis are parathyroid hormone, cortisol, thyroid hormone, and growth hormone. (Endocrine function is discussed in Unit 5.) Decreased testosterone levels contribute to male osteoporosis.[18]

Iatrogenic osteoporosis sometimes develops temporarily in individuals receiving large doses of heparin, perhaps because heparin promotes bone resorption by decreasing collagen synthesis or by increasing collagen breakdown. Osteoporosis caused by heparin therapy usually resolves when therapy ceases. Treatment with other medications may lead to development of osteoporosis, such as the use of glucocorticoid treatment for rheumatoid arthritis. Other medications inducing osteoporosis include lithium, methotrexate, anticonvulsants, cyclophosphamide, and cyclosporine.[19] Risk factors are summarized in Table 37-3.

Regional osteoporosis—osteoporosis confined to a region or segment of the appendicular skeleton—usually has a known cause. Classic regional osteoporosis is associated with disuse or immobilization of a limb because of fractures, motor paralysis, or bone or joint inflammation.[20] A negative calcium balance develops early and continues throughout the period of immobilization. After 8 weeks of immobilization, significant osteoporosis is present, although it may develop earlier in persons younger than 20 years or older than 50 years. A uniform distribution of osteoporosis has also been observed in astronauts and in individuals treated with air suspension therapy as a result of weightlessness.

Pathophysiology

Whatever the cause, osteoporosis develops when the remodeling cycle—the process of bone resorption and bone formation—is disrupted, leading to an imbalance in the coupling process. There are two mechanisms of bone loss occurring in two stages: rapid bone loss and slow bone loss. A complete remodeling cycle, consisting of basic multicellular unit activation (see Chapter 36), bone resorption, and bone formation, takes approximately 4 months in a normal, healthy adult. In an individual with osteoporosis, 2 years may be needed to complete one cycle. In normal bone, the frequency of multicellular unit activation, the rate of resorption, and the rate of new bone formation are relatively constant, so that replacement follows resorption immediately and the amount of bone replaced equals the amount of bone

TABLE 37-3 | Risk Factors for Osteoporosis

Category	Risk Factors
Genetic and constitutional	Family history of osteoporotic fracture Whites more than blacks Absence of osteoarthritis (i.e., those with osteoarthritis have decreased risk of osteoporosis) Small stature Thin (obesity appears protective), fair, pale skinned
Hormonal	Women more than men Early menopause Late menarche Nulliparity Exercise-induced amenorrhea
Life-style	Low dietary calcium Excess protein Sedentary Smoking Alcohol (has been associated with both increased and decreased bone density)
Concurrent illness and drugs	Gastrectomy, hyperparathyroidism Rheumatoid arthritis Hyperthyroidism Cushing syndrome, corticosteroid therapy Neurologic disease, cerebrovascular accident, Parkinson disease Preexisting fracture

Modified from Klippel, J.H. & Dieppe, P.A. (Eds.). (1994). Rheumatology. St. Louis: Mosby.

resorbed. In bones affected by osteoporosis, this equilibrium can be disrupted by (1) an increase in the number of basic multicellular units activated, (2) an increase in the frequency of basic multicellular unit activation, (3) an increase in the rate of resorption, (4) a delay in the rate of bone formation, or (5) a deficiency of cells in the multicellular unit. Any one of these changes causes a net decrease in total bone mass. Rapid bone loss occurs during early menopause and is osteoclast mediated, whereas slow bone loss is osteoblast mediated, occurring later after menopause.

If the number of basic multicellular units increases, resorption occurs at more sites, or loci. Loci of resorption become so numerous that new bone is destroyed along with old bone, creating a state of "runaway" resorption. If a normal number of basic multicellular units is activated with abnormal frequency, the result is a net increase in the total amount of bone lost in a given period of time.

Some hormones and drugs are thought to interfere with the relationship between osteoclast activity (bone resorption) and osteoblast activity (bone formation). Anything that causes resorption to speed up or replacement to slow down causes resorption cavities to persist, weakening the bone.

Fig. 37-10 *Kyphosis.* This elderly woman's condition was caused by a combination of spinal osteoporotic vertebral collapse and chronic degenerative changes in the vertebral column. *(From Kamal, A. & Brocklehurst, J.C. [1992]. Color atlas of geriatric medicine [2nd ed.]. St. Louis: Mosby.)*

Osteoporosis also occurs if the basic multicellular units fail to complete the three phases of the remodeling cycle. Failure occurs if the number of osteoclasts and osteoblasts in bone tissue is inadequate. Completion of the remodeling cycle requires delivery of a continuous supply of bone cell precursors from the marrow. Any interruption in the bone's vascular system will interfere with the delivery of osteoclast and osteoblast precursors to bone tissue.

Age-related bone loss occurs when bone formation decreases faster than bone resorption, particularly in the fourth decade. Men have approximately 30% more bone mass than women, which may be a factor in their later involvement with osteoporosis.[11] In addition, men have a more gradual decrease in testosterone, thereby maintaining their bone mass longer than women.

Clinical Manifestations

The specific clinical manifestations of osteoporosis depend on the bones involved. The most common manifestations, however, are pain and bone deformity. Fractures are likely to occur because the trabeculae of spongy bone become thin and sparse, and compact bone becomes porous. As the bones lose volume, they become brittle and weak and may collapse or become misshapen. Vertebral collapse causes *kyphosis* (hunchback) and diminishes height (Fig. 37-10). Fractures of the long bones (particularly the femur and humerus), distal radius, ribs, and vertebrae are most common. Fracture of the neck of the femur—the so-called broken hip—tends to occur in older or elderly women with osteoporosis. Fatal complications of fractures include fat or pulmonary embolism, pneumonia, hemorrhage, and shock. Approximately

20% of persons may die as a result of surgical complications. Male osteoporosis also is noted by hypogonadism in about 20% of persons, low plasma levels of 1,25-dihydroxyvitamin D, and malabsorption of calcium.[2]

Evaluation and Treatment

Generally, osteoporosis is detected radiographically as increased radiolucency of bone. By the time abnormalities are detected by radiologic examination, up to 25% to 30% of bone tissue may have been lost.

Types of radiologic examinations include single- or dual-photon absorptiometry and computed tomography (CT) scans. Other evaluation procedures include tests for levels of serum calcium, phosphorus, and alkaline phosphatase, and protein electrophoresis.

HEALTH ALERT

New Technique for Diagnosis of Osteoporosis

The U.S. Food and Drug Administration (FDA) has recently approved a new device that can diagnose osteoporosis in 10 seconds by scanning a person's heel using ultrasound. The new technology is remarkably faster and considerably less expensive than previous diagnostic equipment and techniques. The ultrasound procedure will cost patients about $40 per examination.

The new machine, a portable device known as the Sahara Clinical Bone Sonometer, is already in widespread use in Europe, Asia, and Latin America. It is not a screening tool but is intended for persons with high risk for bone fractures that can result from osteoporosis. Questions remain as to whether it is as precise as dual-energy x-ray or single-energy x-ray.

Data from Cimons, M. (1998). FDA OKs quick, cheap osteoporosis test. Los Angeles Times, *March 14, 1998.*

The goals of osteoporosis treatment are to slow down the rate of calcium and bone loss and to stop the disease before it progresses too far. Treatment includes increasing the dietary intake of calcium up to 1500 mg/day and vitamin D supplements to increase the intestinal absorption of calcium. Regular, moderate weight-bearing exercise can slow down the bone loss and, in some cases, reverse demineralization because the mechanical stress of exercise stimulates bone formation. Postmenopausal women may be given estrogen and progestins in addition to exercise and dietary supplements of calcium and vitamin D. It is important to reduce the risk of falls and enhance bone quality. Therefore, an exercise program to enhance rehabilitation is advised (Fig. 37-11). Etidronate disodium (Didronel) is prescribed to treat osteoporosis. New medications are currently being prescribed and evaluated to prevent or treat osteoporosis (Table 37-4). With estrogen administered cyclically with progestins, this risk is decreased and the combined estrogen-progestin therapy is given to women, particularly those in the first 10 years after menopause, to aid bone retention. However, combined estrogen-progestin therapy may be a risk factor for breast cancer (see Chapter 32).

Osteomalacia

Osteomalacia is a metabolic disease characterized by inadequate and delayed mineralization of osteoid in mature compact and spongy bone. In osteomalacia, the remodeling cycle proceeds normally through osteoid formation, but mineral calcification and deposition do not occur. Bone volume remains unchanged, but the replaced bone consists of soft osteoid instead of rigid bone. Rickets is similar to osteomalacia in pathogenesis, but it occurs in the growing bones of children, whereas osteomalacia occurs in adult bone. (Rickets is described in Chapter 38.)

Both osteomalacia and rickets are rare in the United States and western Europe but are significant health problems in Great Britain, Ethiopia, Pakistan, Iran, and India. In the United States, these diseases are prevalent in elderly persons, in premature infants of very low birth weight, and in individuals adhering to rigid macrobiotic vegetarian diets.

Many factors contribute to the development of osteomalacia, but the most important is a deficiency of vitamin D. The major risk factors in vitamin D deficiency are diets deficient in vitamin D, decreased endogenous production of vitamin D, intestinal malabsorption of vitamin D, renal tubular diseases, and anticonvulsant therapy. Classic vitamin D deficiency is rare in the United States because of the addition of synthetic vitamin D to dairy products and bread.

Disorders of the small bowel, hepatobiliary system, and pancreas are common causes of vitamin D deficiency in the United States. In malabsorptive disease of the small bowel, vitamin D and calcium absorption are decreased, so vitamin D is lost in feces. Liver disease interferes with the metabolism of vitamin D to its more active form, and diseases of the pancreas and biliary system cause a deficiency of bile salts, which are necessary for normal intestinal absorption of vitamin D.

The mechanism by which anticonvulsant drug therapy results in vitamin D deficiency is not completely understood, but researchers think that the anticonvulsants phenobarbital and phenytoin interfere with calcium absorption and increase degradation of vitamin D metabolism in the liver.[16] Renal osteodystrophy is a common cause of osteomalacia.

Pathophysiology

Crystallization of minerals in osteoid requires adequate concentrations of calcium and phosphate. When the concentrations are too low, crystallization (and hence ossification) does not proceed normally.

Vitamin D deficiency disrupts mineralization because vitamin D normally regulates and enhances the absorption of calcium ions from the intestine. A lack of vitamin D causes the plasma calcium concentrations to fall. Low plasma calcium levels stimulate increased synthesis and secretion of PTH. Although the increase in circulating PTH raises the plasma calcium concentration, it also stimulates increased renal clearance of phosphate. When the concentration of phosphate in the bone decreases below a critical level, mineralization cannot proceed normally.

Abnormalities occur in both spongy and compact bone. Trabeculae in spongy bone become thinner and fewer,

Fig. 37-11 *Osteoporosis.* A, Exercises for individuals with established osteoporosis of the spine. **B,** Additional exercises for individuals with osteoporosis. *(Modified from Klippel, J.H. & Dieppe, P.A. [1994]. Rheumatology. St. Louis: Mosby.)*

whereas haversian systems in compact bone develop large channels and become irregular. Because osteoid continues to be produced but not mineralized, abnormal quantities of osteoid build up, coating the trabeculae and the linings of the haversian canals. Excessive osteoid also can accumulate in areas beneath the periosteum. The excess of osteoid leads to gross deformities of the long bones, spine, pelvis, and skull.

Clinical Manifestations

Osteomalacia causes varying degrees of diffuse skeletal pain and tenderness. Pain is noted particularly in the hips, and the individual may be hesitant to walk. Muscular weakness is common and may contribute to a waddling gait. Bone fractures and vertebral collapse occur with minimal trauma. Low back pain may be an early complaint, but pain may also involve ribs, feet, other areas of the vertebral column, and other sites. Uremia may be present in renal osteodystrophy.

Evaluation and Treatment

Laboratory data may include elevated blood urea nitrogen (BUN) and creatinine levels, normal or low serum calcium levels, and a serum inorganic phosphate level that is usually over 5.5 mg.[16] Alkaline phosphatase and PTH levels are usually elevated. Radiographic findings show pseudofractures and radiolucent bands perpendicular to the surface of involved bones. A bone biopsy is used to evaluate the presence of renal osteodystrophy to determine bone aluminum deposits.

Treatment of osteomalacia includes the following:
1. Adjusting serum calcium and phosphorus levels to normal
2. Suppressing secondary hyperthyroidism
3. Chelating bone aluminum if needed
4. Administration of calcium carbonate to decrease hyperphosphatemia
5. Dietary supplements of vitamin D
6. Renal dialysis
7. Renal transplant for renal osteodystrophy.

Paget disease

Paget disease (osteitis deformans) is a state of increased metabolic activity in bone characterized by abnormal and excessive bone remodeling, both resorption and formation. Chronic accelerated remodeling eventually enlarges and softens the affected bones.

TABLE 37-4	New Drugs as Treatments for Osteoporosis		
Class	Dose	Benefits	Side Effects
Biphosphonates			
Alendronate	Prevention: 5 mg/day Treatment: 10 mg/day	Reduces bone loss in post-menopausal women; increases bone density at spine and hip; reduces risk of spinal or hip fractures; slows loss of height; impairs function of osteoclasts	Abdominal or musculoskeletal pain; nausea; heartburn; esophageal irritation (minimizes it if person remains upright for at least 30 min after taking)
Pamidronate*	30 mg IV every 3 mo	Increases lumbar density; decreases femoral neck fractures	Ototoxicity rare but can occur; similar effects as alendronate
Risedronate*	2.5 mg/day	Increases bone mass; aids in glucocortoid-induced osteoporosis	Unknown at present
Clodronate*	200 mg IV every month	Decrease in loss of spinal density; decrease in vertebral fracture	Unknown at present
Tiludronate*	100 mg/day	Prevents postmenopausal bone loss; decreases activity of osteoclasts in paraplegia and immobilization; preserves bone mass and a parallel increase in biomechanical bone strength	Unknown at present
Selective estrogen receptor modulator (SERM)			
Raloxifene (Evista)	60 mg/day	Decreases bone loss at spine, hip, and whole body may protect against heart disease without increasing risks of breast cancer or endometrial cancer	Hot flashes; deep vein thrombosis
Hormone			
Calcitonin	200-400 mg IV injection Nasal spray (new form of treatment)	Slows bone loss in post-menopausal women; increases spinal bone density; relieves pain associated with bone fracture; reduces risk of hip or spinal fracture	Injection may cause allergic reaction; flushing of face, hands; urinary frequency; nausea; skin rash Nasal spray may cause runny nose and itching of nasal mucosa
Other			
Sodium fluoride (sustained release)	Individualized, may be given with calcium citrate	Decreased spinal and hip fracture rates; increased femoral neck bone density; increased cancellous and trabecular bone quality	

From Licata, A.A. (1998). Biphosphonate therapy. American Journal of Medical Science, 313(1), 17.
*In clinical trials.

Paget disease can occur in any bone but most often affects the vertebrae, skull, sacrum, sternum, pelvis, and femur. The disease process may occur in one or more bones without causing significant clinical manifestations.

Paget disease can occur with equal frequency in men and women older than 40 years of age. Because it is often symptomless and can only be diagnosed by invasive procedures, few epidemiologic data are available. Autopsy data from England and Germany indicate that approximately 3% to 4% of the population older than 40 years of age have Paget disease. It is most prevalent in Australia, Great Britain, New Zealand, and the United States. Paget disease affects several members of the same family in 5% to 25% of individuals.[16]

The cause of Paget disease is unknown, but disease arises as a consequence of disorderly bone resorption and formation.[16]

Pathophysiology

Paget disease begins with excessive resorption of spongy bone. The trabeculae diminish, and bone marrow is replaced by extremely vascular fibrous tissue.

The resorption phase of Paget disease is followed by the

formation of abnormal new bone at an accelerated rate. The collagen fibers are disorganized, and glycoprotein levels in the matrix decrease. Mineralization may extend into the bone marrow. Bone formation is excessive around partially resorbed trabeculae, causing them to thicken and enlarge. Eventually, Paget disease progresses to an inactive phase, in which abnormal remodeling is minimal or absent.

Clinical Manifestations

In the skull, abnormal remodeling is first evident in the frontal or occipital regions; then it encroaches on the outer and inner surfaces of the entire skull. The skull thickens and assumes an asymmetric shape. Thickened segments of the skull may compress areas of the brain, producing altered mentality and dementia. Impingement of new bone on cranial nerves causes sensory abnormalities, impaired motor function, deafness, atrophy of the optic nerve, and obstruction of the lacrimal duct. Headache is commonly noted.

Extensive alterations of the facial bones are rare except in the jaw, where sclerosis and thickening of the maxilla and mandible displace teeth and produce malocclusion. In long bones, resorption begins in the subchondral regions of the epiphysis and extends into the metaphysis and diaphysis. Occasionally, Paget disease affects both ends of a tubular bone. In the femur, Paget disease produces an exaggerated lateral curvature. In the tibia, anterior curvature is also exaggerated. Stress fractures are common in the lower extremities.

Clinical manifestations of Paget disease in the vertebral column depend on the level of involvement and are caused by compression of adjacent structures. In the cervical spine, cord compression can lead to spastic quadriplegia. Approximately 1% of persons with Paget disease develop osteogenic sarcoma.

Evaluation and Treatment

Evaluation of Paget disease is made on the basis of radiographic findings of irregular bone trabeculae with a thickened and disorganized pattern. Early disease is detected by bone scanning that shows increased uptake of bone radionuclides. Alkaline phosphatase and urinary hydroxyproline are elevated.

Most individuals require no treatment because the disease is localized and does not cause symptoms. Treatment during active disease is for pain relief, prevention of deformity, or fracture. Etidronate disodium (Didronel), corticosteroids, calcitonin, and cytotoxic drugs are sometimes used to slow excessive resorption.

Infectious Bone Disease: Osteomyelitis

Infectious bone disease is expensive and difficult to treat and often culminates in extensive physical disability. Several factors contribute to the difficulty in treating bone infection:

1. Bone contains multiple microscopic channels that are impermeable to the cells and biochemicals of the body's natural defenses. Once bacteria gain access to these channels, they are able to proliferate unimpeded.

2. The microcirculation of bone is highly vulnerable to damage and destruction by bacterial toxins. Vessel damage causes local thrombosis (blockage) of the small vessels, which leads to ischemic necrosis (death) of bone.

3. Bone cells have a limited capacity to replace bone destroyed by infections. Initially, osteoclasts are stimulated by infection to resorb bone, which opens up isolated bone channels so that cells of the inflammatory and immune systems can gain access to the infected bone. At the same time, however, resorption weakens the structural integrity of the bone. New bone formation usually lags behind resorption, and the haversian systems in the new bone are incomplete.

Osteomyelitis is a bone infection caused by bacteria; however, fungi, parasites, and viruses also can cause bone infection (Fig. 37-12). It is further categorized according to the pathogen's mode of entry into bone tissue. *Exogenous osteomyelitis* is an infection that enters from outside the body, for example, through open fractures, penetrating wounds, or surgical procedures. In exogenous osteomyelitis, the infection spreads from soft tissues into adjacent bone. *Endoge-*

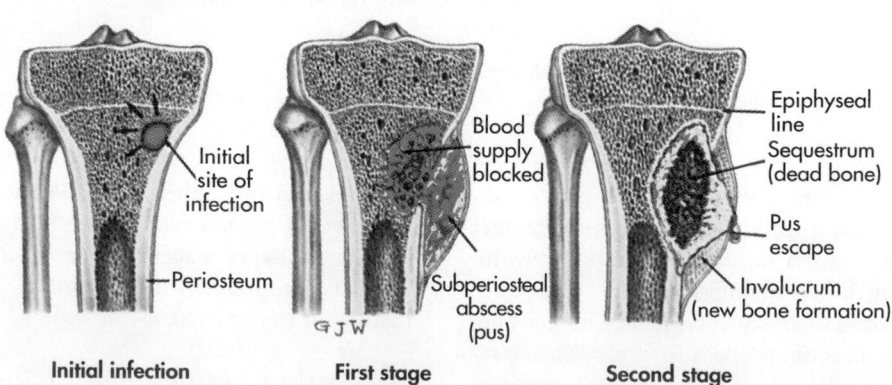

Initial infection   **First stage**   **Second stage**

Fig. 37-12 *Osteomyelitis.* Osteomyelitis of upper femur with massive bone destruction and reactive sclerosis. *(From Mourad, L.A. [1997]. Musculoskeletal system. In J.M. Thompson et al. [Eds.]. Mosby's clinical nursing [4th ed.]. St. Louis: Mosby.)*

nous (hematogenous) osteomyelitis is caused by pathogens carried in the blood from sites of infection elsewhere in the body. In hematogenous osteomyelitis, the infection spreads from bone to adjacent soft tissues. Hematogenous osteomyelitis is commonly found in infants, children, and elderly persons. (Osteomyelitis in children is discussed in Chapter 38.) In infants, incidence rates among males and females are approximately equal. In children and older adults, however, males are most commonly affected. Osteomyelitis is a common complication of sickle cell anemia and low oxygen tension.[16]

Staphylococcus aureus is the usual cause of hematogenous osteomyelitis. Other microorganisms include group B streptococcus, *Haemophilus influenzae*, *Salmonella*, and gram-negative bacteria. Group B streptococcus and *H. influenzae* tend to infect young children; *Salmonella* infection is associated with sickle cell anemia; and gram-negative infections are most common in older adults and individuals with impaired immunity.

Cutaneous, sinus, ear, and dental infections are the primary sources of bacteria in hematogenous bone infections. Soft-tissue infections, disorders of the gastrointestinal tract, infections of the genitourinary system, and respiratory infections are also sources of bacterial contamination. In addition, infections after total joint replacements are causes.

The vulnerability of specific bone depends on the anatomy of its vascular supply. In children the long bones of the extremities (tibia, humerus, femur) are particularly susceptible to hematogenous infection.

In adults, hematogenous osteomyelitis is more common in the spine, pelvis, and small bones. Microorganisms reach the vertebrae through arteries, veins, or lymphatic vessels. The spread of infection from pelvic organs to the vertebrae is well documented. Vaginal, uterine, ovarian, bladder, and intestinal infections can lead to iliac or sacral osteomyelitis.

Exogenous osteomyelitis can be caused by human bites or fist blows to the mouth. Superficial animal or human bites inoculate local soft tissue with bacteria that later spread to underlying bone. Deep bites can introduce microorganisms directly onto bone. The most common infecting organism in human bites is *S. aureus*. In animal bites, the most common infecting organism is *Pasteurella multocida*, which is part of the normal mouth flora of cats and dogs.

Direct contamination of bones with bacteria can also occur in open fractures or dislocations with an overlying skin wound. Intervertebral disk surgery and operative procedures involving implantation of large foreign objects, such as metallic plates or artificial joints, are associated with exogenous osteomyelitis. Local injections and venous punctures are significant causes of exogenous osteomyelitis. Exogenous osteomyelitis of the arm and hand bones tends to occur in persons who abuse drugs. *S. aureus* is the most common pathogen. In general, persons who are chronically ill, have diabetes or alcoholism, or are receiving large doses of steroids or immunosuppressive drugs are particularly susceptible to exogenous osteomyelitis or recurring episodes of this disease.

Pathophysiology

Regardless of the source of the pathogen, the pathologic features of bone infection are similar to those in any other body tissue (see Chapters 5 and 6). First, the invading pathogen provokes an intense inflammatory response. Inflammation in bone is characterized by vascular engorgement, edema, leukocyte activity, and abscess formation. Once inflammation is initiated, the small terminal vessels thrombose and exudate seals the bone's canaliculi. Inflammatory exudate extends into the metaphysis and the marrow cavity and through small metaphyseal openings into the cortex. In children, exudate that reaches the outer surface of the cortex forms abscesses that lift the periosteum off underlying bone. Lifting of the periosteum disrupts blood vessels that enter bone through the periosteum, which deprives underlying bone of its blood supply; this leads to necrosis and death of the area of bone infected, producing *sequestrum,* an area of devitalized bone (see Fig. 37-12). Lifting of the periosteum also stimulates an intense osteoblastic response. Osteoblasts lay down new bone that can partially or completely surround the infected bone. This layer of new bone surrounding the infected bone is called an *involucrum.* Openings in the involucrum allow the exudate to escape into surrounding soft tissue and ultimately through the skin by way of sinus tracts.

In adults, this complication is rare because the periosteum is firmly attached to the cortex and resists displacement. Instead, infection disrupts and weakens the cortex, which predisposes the bone to pathologic fracture.

Clinical Manifestations

Clinical manifestations of osteomyelitis vary with the age of the individual, the site of involvement, the initiating event, the infecting organism, and whether the infection is acute, subacute, or chronic. Acute osteomyelitis causes abrupt onset of inflammation (Fig. 37-13). If an acute infection is not completely eliminated, the disease may become subacute or chronic. In subacute osteomyelitis, signs and symptoms are usually vague. In the chronic stage, infection is indolent or silent between exacerbations. The microorganisms persist in small abscesses or fragments of necrotic bone and produce occasional flare-ups of acute osteomyelitis. The progression from acute to subacute osteomyelitis may be the result of inadequate or inappropriate therapy or the development of drug-resistant microorganisms.

In the adult, hematogenous osteomyelitis has an insidious onset. The symptoms are usually vague and include fever, malaise, anorexia, weight loss, and pain in and around the infected areas. Edema may or may not be evident. Recent infection (urinary, respiratory, skin) or instrumentation (catheterization, cystoscopy, myelography, diskography) usually precedes onset of symptoms.

Single or multiple abscesses (Brodie abscesses) characterize subacute or chronic osteomyelitis. Brodie abscesses are circumscribed lesions 1 to 4 cm in diameter, usually in the ends of long bones and surrounded by dense ossified bone matrix. The abscesses are thought to develop when the in-

Fig. 37-13 *Resected femur in a patient with draining osteomyelitis.* The drainage tract in the subperiosteal shell of viable new bone (involucrum) reveals the inner native necrotic cortex (sequestrum). *(From Cotran, R.S., Kumar, V. & Collins, T. [1999]. Robbins pathologic basis of disease [6th ed.]. Philadelphia: Saunders.)*

fectious microorganism has become less virulent or the individual's immune system is resisting the infection somewhat successfully.

In exogenous osteomyelitis, signs and symptoms of soft-tissue infection predominate. Inflammatory exudate in the soft tissues disrupts muscles and supporting structures and forms abscesses. Low-grade fever, lymphadenopathy, local pain, and swelling usually occur within days of contamination by a puncture wound.

Evaluation and Treatment

Laboratory data show an elevated white cell count. Radiographic studies include radionuclide bone scanning, tomography, and MRI. Tomography is a radiographic technique that produces an image of multiple slices through the bone. Treatment of osteomyelitis includes antibiotics and drainage of the inflammatory exudate. The use of biodegradable antibiotic-impregnated polymethylmethacrylate beads has also benefited many patients.[21] Chronic conditions may require surgical removal of the inflammatory exudate followed by continuous wound irrigation with antibiotic solutions in addition to systemic treatment with antibiotics. *Hyperbaric oxygen therapy* of 100% oxygen, given at 2 atmospheres pressure for 2 hours' duration per day for 30 treatments, is also beneficial for chronic refractory osteomyelitis.[22] Implants for total joint replacements may be removed to treat the infected joint more thoroughly.

✓ QUICK CHECK

How does osteopenia relate to osteoporosis and osteomalacia?

How does osteoporosis differ from osteomalacia? Name three differences.

DISORDERS OF JOINTS

The American Rheumatism Association recognizes 13 groups of joint disease (arthropathies). Most of these disorders can be placed into two major categories: noninflammatory joint disease and inflammatory joint disease.

Noninflammatory Joint Disease

Noninflammatory joint disease is differentiated from inflammatory joint disease by (1) the absence of synovial membrane inflammation, (2) the lack of systemic signs and symptoms, and (3) normal synovial fluid. *Degenerative joint disease (osteoarthritis)* is the most prevalent noninflammatory joint disease. Its chief pathologic feature is degeneration and loss of articular cartilage in synovial joints (Fig. 37-14). Degenerative joint disease tends to occur in men and women older than 40 years and becomes more common with increasing age. Although incidence rates are quite similar in men and women, women are more severely affected. It usually occurs in those persons who put exceptional stress on joints, as do gymnasts; long-distance runners or marathoners; basketball, soccer, or football players; and others; many develop osteoarthritis at earlier ages than usual. A previously torn anterior cruciate ligament or meniscectomy increases the risk for accelerated osteoarthritis of the knee.[23]

Types of osteoarthritis

Osteoarthritis (OA) associated with known risk factors, such as joint stress, congenital abnormalities, or joint instability caused by trauma, is referred to as *secondary* (Box 37-2). *Idiopathic,* formerly *primary,* OA is not associated with known risk factors. Both idiopathic OA and secondary OA have the same pathologic characteristics: (1) erosion of the articular cartilage; (2) sclerosis (thickening and hardening) of bone underneath the cartilage; and (3) formation of bone spurs, or *osteophytes,* which grossly alter the bony contours and enlarge the joint, possibly even leading to subluxation of the bone from the joint.

Idiopathic osteoarthritis is the most common type of noninflammatory joint disease, affecting more than 60 million persons in the United States. The joints most characteristically affected are in the hand, wrist, neck (lower cervical spine), lower back (lumbar spine, sacroiliac), hip, knees, ankles, and feet. Although the cause of osteoarthritis is unknown, aging is an important associated factor. With aging the quality and quantity of the proteoglycans in cartilage decrease in direct proportion to the severity of OA.[16] Evidence also suggests that primary osteoarthritis may be inherited as an autosomal recessive trait, suggesting that defects in one or more of the genes encoding for the structural components of articular cartilage may cause premature cartilage degeneration.[16]

Secondary OA can be caused by any condition that damages cartilage directly; subjects the joint surfaces or underlying bone to chronic, excessive, or abnormal forces; or causes instability in the joint.

Ossification and deformity of joint; erosion of cartilage

Heberden nodes

Bouchard nodes

Fig. 37-14 *Osteoarthritis (OA).* **A,** Cartilage and degeneration of the hip joint from osteoarthritis. **B,** Heberden nodes and Bouchard nodes. **C,** Severe osteoarthritis with small islands of residual articular cartilage next to exposed subchondral bone. *1,* Eburnated articular surface. *2,* Subchondral cyst. *3,* Residual articular cartilage. *(A and B from Mourad, L.A. [1997]. Musculoskeletal system. In J.M. Thompson et al. [Eds.]. Mosby's clinical nursing [4th ed.]. St. Louis: Mosby; C from Cotran, R.S., Kumar, V., & Collins, T. [1999]. Robbins pathologic basis of disease [6th ed.]. Philadelphia: Saunders.)*

Pathophysiology

The primary defect in primary and secondary OA is loss of articular cartilage. Early in the disease, the articular cartilage loses its glistening appearance, becoming yellow-gray or brownish gray. As the disease progresses, surface areas of the articular cartilage flake off and deeper layers develop longitudinal fissures (fibrillation). The cartilage becomes thin and may be absent over some areas, leaving the underlying bone (subchondral bone) unprotected. Consequently, the unprotected subchondral bone becomes sclerotic (dense and hard). Cysts sometimes develop within the subchondral bone and communicate with the longitudinal fissures in the cartilage. Pressure builds in the cysts until the cystic contents are forced into the synovial cavity, breaking through the articular cartilage on the way. As the articular cartilage erodes, cartilage-coated osteophytes may grow outward from the underlying bone and alter the bone contours and joint anatomy. These spurlike bony projections enlarge until small pieces, called *joint mice,* break off into the synovial cavity. If osteophyte fragments irritate the synovial membrane, synovitis and joint effusion result. The joint capsule also becomes thickened and at times adheres to the deformed underlying

bone, which may figure in the limitation of movement (see Fig. 37-14).

Articular cartilage is probably lost through enzymatic breakdown of the cartilage matrix—the proteoglycans, glycosaminoglycans, and collagen. First, the enzymes break down the macromolecules of proteoglycans, glycosaminoglycans, and collagen into large, diffusible fragments. Then the fragments are taken up by the cartilage cells (chondrocytes) and digested by the cell's own lysosomal enzymes. (Processes of cellular uptake and lysosomal digestion are described in Chapter 1.) The loss of proteoglycans from articular cartilage is a hallmark of the osteoarthritic process.[16]

Enzymatic destruction of articular cartilage begins in the matrix, with destruction of proteoglycans and collagen fibers. Enzymes, particularly stromelysin and acid metalloproteinase, affect proteoglycans by interfering with assembly of the proteoglycan subunit or the proteoglycan aggregate (see Chapter 36); these enzymes are markedly elevated in OA. Changes in the conformation of proteoglycans disrupt the pumping action that regulates movement of water and synovial fluid into and out of the cartilage. Without the regulatory action of the proteoglycan pump, cartilage imbibes too much fluid and becomes less able to withstand the stresses of weight bearing. With aging, the proteoglycan content is decreased, and water content in cartilage can be increased by as much as 8%, affecting the strength of the cartilage. Persons with OA, even those with fairly extensive

---

Classification of Osteoarthritis (OA) — BOX 37-2

CLASSIFICATION BY THE JOINTS INVOLVED
1. Monoarticular, oligoarticular, or polyarticular (generalized)
2. Chief joint site (index joint site) and localization within the joint
   a. Hip (superior pole, medial pole, or concentric)
   b. Knee (medial, lateral, patellofemoral compartments)
   c. Hand (interphalangeal joints and/or thumb base)
   d. Spine (apophyseal joints or intervertebral disk disease)
   e. Others

CLASSIFICATION INTO PRIMARY AND SECONDARY FORMS OF OA
Primary (idiopathic)
Secondary
1. Indicates that a likely cause can be identified
2. Metabolic causes
   a. Ochronosis
   b. Acromegaly
   c. Hemochromatosis
   d. Calcium crystal deposition
3. Anatomic causes
   a. Slipped femoral epiphysis
   b. Epiphyseal dysplasias
   c. Blount disease
   d. Perthes disease
   e. Congenital dislocation of the hip
   f. Leg length inequality
   g. Hypermobility syndromes
4. Traumatic causes
   a. Major joint trauma
   b. Fracture through a joint or osteonecrosis
   c. Joint surgery (e.g., meniscectomy)
   d. Chronic injury (occupational arthropathies)
5. Inflammatory causes
   a. Any inflammatory arthropathy
   b. Septic arthritis

CLASSIFICATION BY THE PRESENCE OF SPECIFIC FEATURES
1. Inflammatory OA
2. Erosive OA
3. Atrophic or destructive OA
4. OA with chrondrocalcinosis
5. Others

Data from Klippel, J.A. & Dieppe, P.A. (Eds.). (1994). Rheumatology. St. Louis: Mosby.

---

cartilage destruction, have elevated levels of proteoglycans/fragments in their synovial fluid, perhaps indicative of the degree of disease activity. Other studies indicate that cytokines, such as interleukin-1 (see Chapter 6 for discussion of cytokines) may play a major role in cartilage degradation as a result of release and activation of proteolytic and collagenolytic enzymes associated with an imbalance of cell responses to growth factor activity.

Enzymes that degrade collagen (i.e., collagenases) probably originate in the chondrocytes or in leukocytes. Collagen breakdown destroys the fibrils that give articular cartilage its tensile strength and exposes the chondrocytes to mechanical stress and enzyme attack. Thus a cycle of destruction begins that involves all the components of articular cartilage—proteoglycans, collagen fibers, and chondrocytes. The serum level of circulating keratin sulfate chains provides a direct measure of the rate of catabolism of the cartilage proteoglycans and is elevated in persons with generalized OA.[16]

Clinical Manifestations

Clinical manifestations of idiopathic or secondary OA typically appear during the fifth or sixth decade of life, although asymptomatic, articular surface changes are common after the age of 40 years. Pain in one or more joints, usually weight bearing or load bearing, is the first symptom of the disease. Examination usually shows general involvement of both peripheral and central joints. Peripheral joints most often involved are in the hands, wrists, knees, and feet. Central joints most often afflicted are in the lower cervical spine, lumbosacral spine, shoulders, and hips.

Joint structures are capable of generating a limited number of signs and symptoms. The primary signs and symptoms of joint disease are pain, stiffness, enlargement or swelling, tenderness, limited range of motion, muscle wasting, partial dislocation, and deformity. (See Risk Factors box.)

RISK FACTORS

OSTEOARTHRITIS
- Trauma, sprains, strains, joint dislocations, and fractures
- Long-term mechanical stress—athletics, ballet dancing, or repetitive physical tasks
- Inflammation in joint structures
- Joint instability from damage to supporting structures
- Neurologic disorders (e.g., diabetic neuropathy, Charcot neuropathic joint) in which pain and proprioceptive reflexes are diminished or lost
- Congenital or acquired skeletal deformities
- Hematologic or endocrine disorders, such as hemophilia, which causes chronic bleeding into the joints, or hyperparathyroidism, which causes bone to lose calcium
- Drugs (e.g., colchicine, indomethacin, steroids) that stimulate the collagen-digesting enzymes in the synovial membrane

Fig. 37-15 *Typical varus deformity of knee osteoarthritis. (From Doherty, M. [1994].* Color atlas and text of osteoarthritis. *London: Wolfe.)*

Pain is the predominant symptom of OA. It is usually aggravated by weight bearing or use of the joint and relieved by resting the joint. Nocturnal pain is usually not relieved by rest and may be accompanied by paresthesias (numbness, tingling, or prickling). Sometimes pain is referred to another part of the body. For example, osteoarthritis of the lumbosacral spine may mimic sciatica, causing severe pain in the back of the thigh along the course of the sciatic nerve. OA in the lower cervical spine may cause brachial neuralgia (pain in the arm) aggravated by movement of the neck. Osteoarthritic conditions in the hip cause pain that may be referred to the lower thigh and knee area. Sleep deprivation adds to the stress of the chronic pain of OA.[23]

The origin of joint stiffness is unknown. Joint stiffness is generally defined as difficulty in initiating joint movement, immobility, or a loss of range of motion. The stiffness usually occurs as joint movement begins, and it dissipates rapidly after a few minutes. Enlargement and bulging of joint contour, commonly described as swelling, may be caused by bone enlargement or the proliferation of osteophytes around the margins of the joint. Swelling also occurs if inflammatory exudate or blood enters the joint cavity, thereby increasing the volume of synovial fluid. This condition, termed *joint effusion,* is caused by (1) the presence of osteophyte fragments in the synovial cavity, (2) drainage of cysts from diseased subchondral bone, or (3) acute trauma to joint structures, resulting in hemorrhage and inflammatory exudation into the synovial cavity (see Fig. 37-14, *C).*

Range of motion is limited to some degree, depending on the extent of cartilage degeneration. Frequently, joint motion is accompanied by sounds of crepitus, creaking, or grating. Hypermobility and subluxation of joints occur in OA secondary to a neurologic disorder.

As OA of the lower extremity progresses, the person may begin to limp noticeably (Fig. 37-15). Having a limp is distressing because it affects the person's independence and ability to do usual activities of daily living. The affected joint is also more symptomatic after use, such as at the end of a period of strenuous activity.

Evaluation and Treatment

Evaluation consists of clinical assessment and radiologic studies, CT scan, arthroscopy, and MRI. Treatment is either conservative or surgical. Conservative treatment includes rest of the involved joint until inflammation, if present, subsides; range of motion to prevent joint capsule contraction; use of a cane, crutches, or walker to decrease weight bearing; weight loss if obesity is present (obese persons are five times more likely to have OA of the knees and twice as likely to have OA of the hips as normal weight persons)[24]; and analgesic and antiinflammatory drug therapy to reduce swelling and pain. Surgery is used to improve joint movement, correct deformity or malalignment, or create a new joint with artificial implants. There are more than 250,000 total hip replacements yearly in the United States, most of which are related to OA.[2]

HEALTH ALERT

Were You Aware?

Walking exerts approximately six times the body's own weight across the knee. Any increase in body weight must, therefore, be multiplied by six to determine the increased force on the knee. Obesity leads to osteoarthritis of the knee and not vice versa.

Data from Oddis, C.V. (1997). New perspectives on osteoarthritis. In W.N. Kelley et al. (Eds.). Textbook of rheumatology *(5th ed.). St. Paul, Minn.: West Publishing.*

Inflammatory Joint Disease

The second major type of joint disease is *inflammatory joint disease,* commonly termed *arthritis.* Inflammatory joint disease is characterized by inflammatory damage or destruction in the synovial membrane or articular cartilage and by systemic signs of inflammation (fever, leukocytosis, malaise, anorexia, hyperfibrinogenemia).

Inflammatory joint disease can be infectious or noninfectious. In infectious inflammatory joint disease, inflammation is caused by invasion of the joint by bacteria, mycoplasmas, viruses, fungi, or protozoa. These agents can invade the joint through a traumatic wound, surgical incision, or contaminated needle, or they can be delivered by the bloodstream from sites of infection elsewhere in the body, typically bones, heart valves, or blood vessels. In noninfectious inflammatory joint disease, which is the most common form, inflammation is caused by immune reactions or the deposition of crystals of monosodium urate in and around the joint. Rheumatoid arthritis and ankylosing spondylitis are noninfectious inflammatory diseases caused by immune reactions and possibly hypersensitivity reactions[25]; gouty arthritis is a noninfectious inflammatory disease caused by crystal deposition.

HEALTH ALERT

Hypersensitivity May Cause Some Types of Inflammatory Arthritis

In autoimmunity the immune system seems to completely "mess up," breaking through the barrier of self-tolerance and triggering inflammation when no foreign antigens appear to be present. Autoimmunity is the most prevalent mechanism to account for many diseases, such as rheumatoid arthritis. The idea that bacteria, viruses, and parasites may be the major environmental factors that initiate and sustain either autoimmunity or destructive hypersensitivity has been a central concern for research into the causes of the various types of inflammatory arthritis. Detailed studies of joint tissues of individuals have suggested that reactive arthritis may result mainly from hypersensitivity and not autoimmunity. In rheumatoid arthritis, a genetic link with major histocompatibility complex (MHC) class II genes has been established, but no evidence for associated or triggering factors has yet been found. In the absence of such clues, it is difficult to construct hypotheses that might contribute to a better understanding of pathogenesis. It may be that in some conditions currently thought to be autoimmune phenomena there is actually an immune response to a foreign invader (e.g., antigen) not easy to detect. As invaders and instigators of a hypersensitive response, bacteria and viruses need consideration. The distinction between autoimmunity and hypersensitivity has different and obvious implications for therapy because hypersensitivity would emphasize elimination of the source of antigenic stimulation. Antibiotic therapies against infectious agents could supersede the current immunosuppressive approaches used to deal with autoimmunity.

Data from Behar, S.M. & Porcelli, S.A. (1996). Science and Medicine, 3(6), 12.

Rheumatoid arthritis

Rheumatoid arthritis (RA) is a systemic autoimmune disease that causes chronic inflammation of connective tissue, primarily in the joints. (Autoimmune disease is described in Chapter 7.) The first joint tissue to be affected is the synovial membrane, which lines the joint cavity (see Chapter 36, Fig. 36-8). Eventually, inflammation may spread to the articular cartilage, fibrous joint capsule, and surrounding ligaments and tendons, causing pain, joint deformity, and loss of function (Fig. 37-16). The joints most commonly affected are in the fingers, feet, wrists, elbows, ankles, and knees, but the shoulders, hips, and cervical spine also may be involved, as well as the tissues of the lungs, heart, kidneys, and skin.

RA affects 1% to 2% of adults and, like most auto-

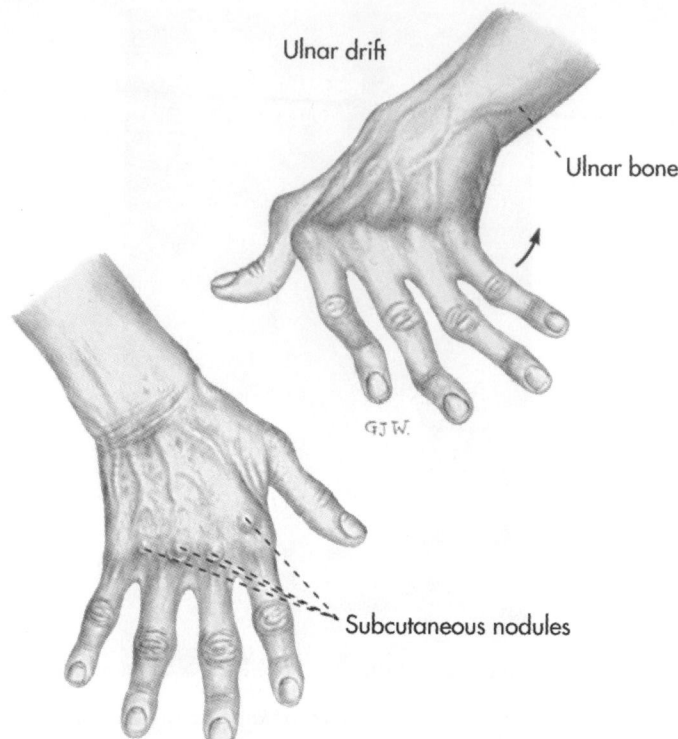

Fig. 37-16 *Rheumatoid arthritis of the hand.* Note swelling from chronic synovitis of metacarpophalangeal joints, marked ulnar drift, subcutaneous nodules, and subluxation of metacarpophalangeal joints with extension of proximal interphalangeal joints and flexion of distal joints. Note also deformed position of thumb. Hand has wasted appearance. *(From Mourad, L.A. [1997]. Musculoskeletal system. In J.M. Thompson et al. [Eds.]. Mosby's clinical nursing [4th ed.]. St. Louis: Mosby.)*

immune diseases, develops most often in women, with a female/male ratio of 3:1. The frequency of RA increases from the third decade on, affecting 5% or more of the population aged 70 years and above.[16] Besides inflammation of the joints, RA can cause fever, malaise, rash, lymph node or spleen enlargement, and Raynaud phenomenon (transient lack of circulation to the fingertips and toes).

Despite intensive research, the cause of RA remains obscure. It is probably a combination of genetic, environmental, hormonal, and reproductive factors. RA probably occurs in a genetically susceptible host because of an aberrant immune response to an unidentified antigen. A key genetic element has been localized to the HLA-DR4, HLA-DQ, and HLA-DP areas of the major histocompatibility complex.[16] Infectious microorganisms that may play a role in the cause of RA include bacteria, mycoplasmas, and viruses (especially Epstein-Barr virus). With long-term or intensive exposure to the antigen, normal antibodies (immunoglobulins [Ig]) become autoantibodies—antibodies that attack host tissues (self-antigens). Because they are usually present in individuals with RA, the transformed antibodies are termed *rheumatoid factors (RFs).* The RFs usually consist of two classes of immunoglobulin antibodies (antibodies for IgM and IgG)

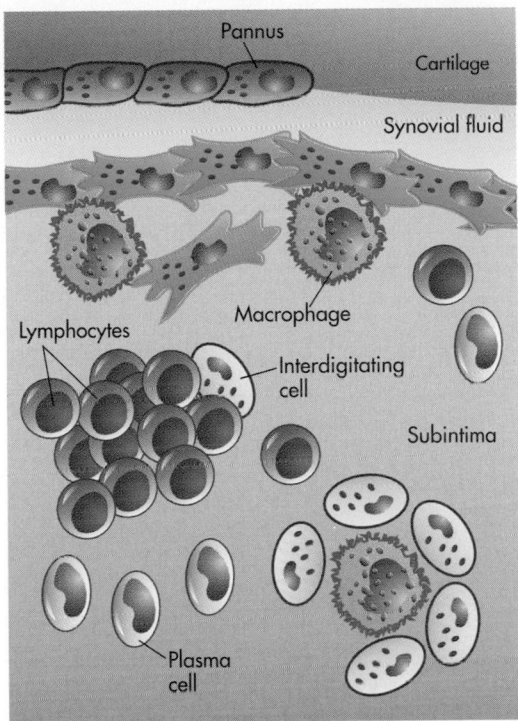

Fig. 37-17 Synovitis. Inflamed synovium showing typical arrangements of macrophages *(red)* and fibroblastic cells.

but occasionally involve antibodies for IgA. Their main antigenic targets are portions of the immunoglobulin molecules. RFs bind with their target self-antigens in blood and synovial membrane, forming immune complexes (antigen-antibody complexes). (See Chapter 5 for a discussion about antigen-antibody binding in the immune response.)

RA has a higher incidence in women, with evidence of hormonal involvement that shows that the disease symptoms lessen during pregnancy and exacerbate in the postpartal period.[14] RA also has seasonal variations, being worse in winter months.

Pathophysiology

Evidence suggests that microvascular injury and mild synovial cell proliferation are the first lesions; small blood vessels are obliterated.[16] Synovial inflammation (synovitis) occurs when immune complexes in blood and synovial tissue trigger the inflammatory response, chiefly by activating the plasma protein complement (described in Chapter 6). Complement activation stimulates kinin and prostaglandin release that increases the permeability of blood vessels in the synovial membranes and attracts leukocytes and lymphocytes to the synovial membrane.

Several types of leukocytes are attracted out of the circulation and to the synovial membrane. The phagocytes of inflammation (neutrophils, macrophages) ingest the immune complexes and, in the process of doing so, release powerful enzymes that degrade synovial tissue and articular cartilage

(Fig. 37-17). The immune system's B and T lymphocytes are also activated. The B lymphocytes are stimulated to produce more RFs, and the T lymphocytes produce enzymes that amplify and perpetuate the inflammatory response. Unlike the precipitating microorganism, which is killed off and removed from the body, the newly targeted self-antigens (immunoglobulins) are in relatively constant supply and can thus perpetuate inflammation and the formation of immune complexes indefinitely (Fig. 37-18).

Inflammatory and immune processes have several damaging effects on the synovial membrane. Along with the swelling caused by leukocyte infiltration, the synovial membrane undergoes hyperplastic thickening as its cells proliferate and enlarge abnormally. As synovial inflammation progresses to involve its blood vessels, small venules become occluded by hypertrophied endothelial cells, fibrin, platelets, and inflammatory cells, which decrease vascular flow to the synovial tissue. Compromised circulation, coupled with increased metabolic needs as a result of hypertrophy and hyperplasia, causes hypoxia and metabolic acidosis. Acidosis stimulates the release of hydrolytic enzymes from synovial cells into the surrounding tissue, initiating erosion of the articular cartilage and inflammation in the supporting ligaments and tendons.

Inflammation causes hemorrhage, coagulation, and fibrin deposition on the synovial membrane, in the intracellular matrix, and in the synovial fluid. Over denuded areas of the synovial membrane, fibrin develops into granulation tissue called *pannus.* (Granulation tissue is the earliest tissue produced in the process of healing; see Chapter 6.) Researchers disagree about whether pannus is a cause or an effect of articular cartilage involvement in RA. Some believe that, as RA progresses, pannus extends from the synovial membrane into adjacent articular cartilage and destroys the cartilage. Other researchers think that pannus forms on articular cartilage after the cartilage has been destroyed by inflammation. In any case, pannus formation does not lead to synovial or articular regeneration but rather to formation of scar tissue that immobilizes the joint.

Clinical Manifestations

The onset of RA is usually insidious, although as many as 15% of cases have an acute onset. RA begins with general systemic manifestations of inflammation, including fever, fatigue, weakness, anorexia, weight loss, and generalized aching and stiffness. Local manifestations also appear gradually over a period of weeks or months. Typically, the joints become painful, tender, and stiff. Pain early in the disease is caused by pressure from swelling. Later in the disease pain is caused by sclerosis of subchondral bone and new bone formation. Stiffness usually lasts for about 1 hour after arising in the morning and is thought to be related to synovitis. Initially the joints most commonly involved are the metacarpophalangeal (MCP) joints, proximal interphalangeal (PIP) joints, and wrists, with later involvement of larger weight-bearing joints.

Joint swelling, which is widespread and symmetric, is

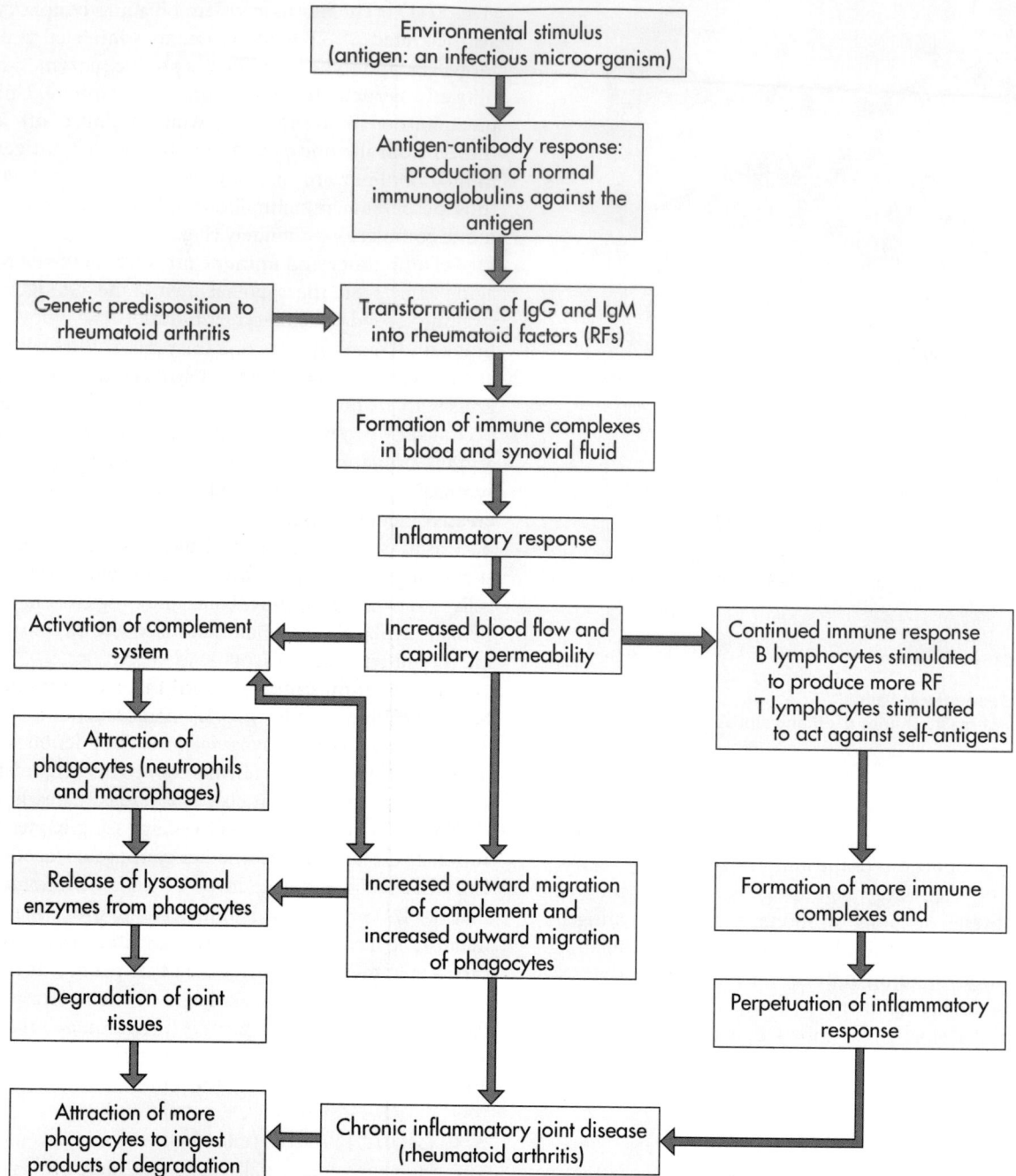

Fig. 37-18 *Probable pathogenesis of rheumatoid arthritis. IgG,* Immunoglobulin G; *IgM,* immunoglobulin M.

caused by increasing amounts of inflammatory exudate (leukocytes, plasma, plasma proteins) in the synovial membrane, hyperplasia of inflamed tissues, and formation of new bone. On palpation, the swollen joint feels warm and the synovial membrane feels "boggy." The skin over the joint may have a ruddy, cyanotic hue and may look thin and shiny.

An inflamed joint may lose some of its mobility. Even mild synovitis can lead to loss of range of motion, which becomes evident after inflammation subsides. Extension becomes limited and is eventually lost if flexion contractures

form. Loss of range of motion can progress to permanent deformities of the fingers, toes, and limbs, including ulnar deviation of the hands, boutonniere and swan-neck deformities of the finger joints, plantar subluxation of the metatarsal heads of the foot, and hallux valgus (angulation of the great toe toward the other toes). Flexion contractures of the knees and hips are also common.

Joint deformities cause the physical limitations experienced by persons with RA (Fig. 37-19). Loss of joint motion is quickly followed by secondary atrophy of the surrounding

Fig. 37-19 *Rheumatoid arthritis of the hand.* **A,** Early stage. **B,** Moderate involvement. *(From Lewis, S.M., Collier, I.C., & Heitkemper, M.M. [1996]. Medical-surgical nursing: Assessment and management of clinical problems. [4th ed.]. St. Louis: Mosby.)*

muscles. With secondary muscle atrophy the joint becomes unstable, which further aggravates joint pathology.

Two complications of chronic RA are caused by excessive amounts of inflammatory exudate in the synovial cavity. One complication is the formation of cysts in the articular cartilage or subchondral bone. Occasionally, these cysts communicate with the skin surface (usually the sole of the foot) and can drain through passages called *fistulae.* The second complication is rupture of a cyst or of the synovial joint itself, usually caused by strenuous physical activity that places excessive pressure on the joint. Rupture releases inflammatory exudate into adjacent tissues, thereby spreading inflammation.

Extrasynovial *rheumatoid nodules,* or swellings, are observed in areas of pressure or trauma in 20% of individuals with RA. Each nodule is an aggregate of inflammatory cells surrounding a central core of fibrinoid and cellular debris. T lymphocytes are the predominant leukocytes in the nodule. B lymphocytes, plasma cells, and phagocytes are found around the periphery. Nodules are most often found in subcutaneous tissue over the extensor surfaces of elbows and fingers. Less common sites are the scalp, back, feet, hands, buttocks, and knees.

Rheumatoid nodules also may invade the skin, cardiac valves, pericardium, pleura, lung parenchyma, and spleen. These nodules are identical to those encountered in some individuals with rheumatic fever and are characterized by central tissue necrosis surrounded by proliferating connective tissue. Also noted are large numbers of lymphocytes and occasional plasma cells. Acute glaucoma may result with nodules forming on the sclera. Pulmonary involvement may result in diffuse pleuritis or multiple intraparenchymal nodules. Together, the occurrence of pulmonary nodules and pneumoconiosis (chronic inflammation of the lungs from inhalation of dust) creates the syndrome called *Caplan syndrome.* Diffuse pulmonary fibrosis may occur because of immunologically mediated immune complex deposition.

Rheumatoid nodules within the heart may cause valvular deformities, particularly of the aortic valve leaflets, and pericarditis. Lymphadenopathy of the nodes close to the affected joints may develop. Rheumatoid nodules within the spleen result in splenomegaly. Involvement of blood vessels results in an acute necrotizing vasculitis, characteristic of that noted in other immunologic/inflammatory states. Thromboses of such involved vessels may give rise to myocardial infarctions, cerebrovascular occlusions, mesenteric infarction, kidney damage, and vascular insufficiency in the hands and fingers (Raynaud phenomenon). The vascular changes are primarily noted in individuals receiving steroid therapy; thus there is some concern that the therapy may play a role in initiating these lesions. Changes in skeletal muscle are often noted in the form of nonspecific atrophy secondary to joint dysfunction.

Evaluation and Treatment

Evaluation of RA is by physical examination, roentgenography of the joint, and serologic tests for rheumatoid factor and circulating immune complexes. The American Rheumatism Association lists the following diagnostic criteria for RA:

1. Morning stiffness
2. Arthritis of three or more joint areas
3. Arthritis of hand joints
4. Symmetric arthritis
5. Rheumatoid nodules
6. Serum rheumatoid factor
7. Radiographic changes

The presence of four or more criteria is diagnostic of RA. Criteria 1 through 4 with joint signs or symptoms must be present for 6 weeks.

Treatment is conservative or surgical. Conservative treatment includes rest of the inflamed joint and whole-body rest for several hours daily, use of hot and cold packs, physical therapy, antineoplastic medications, a diet high in calories and vitamins, corticosteroids, and antiinflammatory drugs taken orally or injected into the joint. Surgical synovectomy may be done early in the disease to decrease inflammatory effusion and remove pannus. Surgery is used to correct deformity or mechanical deficiency in intermediate or late stages of the disease and includes arthrodesis, arthroplasty, or total joint replacement. There is evidence that total fasting induces a substantial reduction in joint pain, swelling, morning stiffness, and other symptoms in individuals with RA.

Ankylosing spondylitis

Ankylosing spondylitis (AS) is a chronic, inflammatory joint disease characterized by stiffening and fusion (ankylosis) of the spine and sacroiliac joints. Like RA, ankylosing spondylitis is a systemic, immune inflammatory disease. Although inflammation is the primary pathologic process in both RA and ankylosing spondylitis, the two diseases differ in the primary site of inflammation and the end result. In RA the primary site of inflammation is the synovial membrane, resulting in the destruction and instability of synovial joints. In ankylosing spondylitis, the primary pathologic site is the *enthesis* (the point at which ligaments, tendons, and the joint capsule are inserted into bone) and the end result is fibrosis, ossification, and fusion of the joint, primarily the sacroiliac joints and the vertebral column.

The incidence of AS is almost equal in men and women, but the disease tends to be more severe in men. In women, AS may affect the peripheral joints of the appendicular skeleton rather than the axial skeleton, progress less rapidly, and cause less dramatic spinal changes.

The prevalence of AS in the United States is approximately 0.5% to 1% among whites, 3% to 4% among blacks, and 18% to 50% in various tribes of Native Americans. Worldwide, the disease appears to be most prevalent in whites. The prevalence of AS in males is at least 10 times more than previously considered, and the disease is more prevalent even in females. Many individuals with AS remain undiagnosed.

Primary AS usually develops in late adolescence and young adulthood, with peak incidence at about 20 years of age. Secondary AS affects older age-groups and is often associated with other inflammatory diseases (e.g., psoriatic arthropathy, inflammatory bowel disease, Reiter syndrome).

The cause of ankylosing spondylitis is unknown, but the disease is strongly associated with the presence of histocompatibility antigen HLA-B27 on the chromosome of affected individuals, suggesting a genetic predisposition to the disease. *Klebsiella* infection or other "triggers" may perpetuate the inflammatory response.[26]

Pathophysiology

Ankylosing spondylitis begins with inflammation of fibrocartilage in cartilaginous joints, primarily in the vertebrae. The fibrous tissue of the joint capsule, the cartilage that surrounds intervertebral disks, the entheses, and periosteum are infiltrated by inflammatory cells. As inflammatory cells (chiefly macrophages) and lymphocytes infiltrate and erode bone and fibrocartilage in joint structures, repair begins. Repair of cartilaginous structures begins with the proliferation of fibroblasts. Fibroblasts synthesize and secrete collagen. The collagen becomes organized into fibrous scar tissue that eventually undergoes calcification and ossification. With time, all the cartilaginous structures of the joint are replaced by ossified scar tissue, causing the joint to fuse, or lose flexibility.

Repair of eroded bone begins with osteoblast activation and proliferation. Osteoblasts lay down new bone (callus), which is remodeled and replaced by compact, lamellar bone. Bone repair changes the contour of the bone's surface because the new bone grows outward to form a new enthesis with the end of the eroded ligament. The new enthesis, which forms on top of the old one, is called *syndesmophyte.* As calcification of the spinal ligaments progresses, the vertebral bodies lose their concave anterior contour and appear square. The spine assumes the classic "bamboo spine" appearance of ankylosing spondylitis.

Clinical Manifestations

The most common signs and symptoms of early AS are low back pain and stiffness. Typically, the individual with primary disease develops low back pain during the early 20s. The pain is at first insidious but progressively becomes persistent. It is often worse after prolonged rest and is alleviated by physical activity. Early morning stiffness usually accompanies the low back pain, and the individual typically has difficulty sitting up or twisting the spine. Forward flexion, rotation, and lateral flexion of the spine are restricted and painful. Early pain and resultant loss of motion are caused by the underlying inflammation and reflex muscle spasm rather than by soft tissue or bony fusion.

As the disease progresses, the normal convex curve of the lower spine (lumbar lordosis) diminishes and concavity of the upper spine (kyphosis) increases. The individual becomes increasingly stooped. The thoracic spine becomes rounded, the head and neck are held forward on the shoulders, and the hips are flexed (Fig. 37-20).

Inflammation in the tendon insertions of the many costosternal and costovertebral muscles can cause pleuritic chest pain and restricted chest movement. The pain is usually worse on inspiration. Movement in the diaphragm is normal and full. Pressure on the anterior chest wall over the sternum, ribs, and costal cartilages may cause tenderness. Tenderness over the pelvic brim may cause discomfort at night and interfere with sleep because turning onto the iliac crests causes pain. Tenderness over the ischial tuberosities may make sitting on hard seats unbearable. Tenderness in the heels may contribute to a limp or cautious placement of the feet during walking.

Along with low back pain, many individuals have peripheral joint involvement, uveitis, fibrotic changes in the lungs, and cardiomegaly, aortic incompetence, amyloidosis, and Achilles tendinitis. Symptoms may include fatigue, weight loss, low-grade fever, hypochromic anemia, and an increased erythrocyte sedimentation rate.

Ossification of disks, joints, and ligaments of spinal column

GJW

Fig. 37-20 *Characteristic posture and sites of ankylosing spondylitis. (From Mourad, L.A. [1997]. Musculoskeletal system. In J.M. Thompson et al. [Eds.].* Mosby's clinical nursing *[4th ed.]. St. Louis: Mosby.)*

TABLE 37-5	Mean Urate Concentrations by Age and Gender
Characteristic	**Mean Urate Levels**
Prepuberty	3.5 mg/dl
Males (at puberty)	Steep rise to 5.2 mg/dl
Females (puberty to premenopause)	Slow rise to ≈ 4.0 mg/dl
Females (after menopause)	4.7 mg/dl
Hyperuricemia	
Males	7.0 mg/dl
Females	6.0 mg/dl

Gout

Gout is a syndrome caused by an inflammatory response to the formation of uric acid production or excretion resulting in high levels of uric acid in the blood (hyperuricemia) and in other body fluids, including synovial fluid. When the uric acid reaches a certain concentration in fluids, it crystallizes, forming insoluble precipitates that are deposited in connective tissues throughout the body. Crystallization in synovial fluid causes acute, painful inflammation of the joint, a condition known as **gouty arthritis.** With time, crystal deposition in subcutaneous tissues causes the formation of small, white nodules, or **tophi,** that are visible through the skin. Crystal aggregates deposited in the kidneys can form urate renal stones and lead to renal failure.

In classic gouty arthritis, monosodium urate crystals form and cause joint inflammation. Pseudogout is caused by the formation of calcium **pyrophosphate**-dihydrate crystals. The effect of either crystal is the same—the onset of an acute inflammatory response (see Chapter 6).

Gout is rare in children and premenopausal women and is uncommon in males younger than 30 years. The peak age of onset in males is between 40 and 50 years, whereas it is somewhat later in females.[27] The risk of developing gouty arthritis is similar in males and females for a particular urate concentration. Thus the lower prevalence of gout in females is likely a factor of their lower urate concentrations.[27] Therefore the plasma urate concentration is the single most important determinant of the risk of developing gout[27] (Table 37-5).

Uric acid is a weak acid that is ionized at normal body pH and thus occurs in the blood or tissues in the form of urate ion. When ionized, uric acid can form salts with various cations, but 98% of extracellular uric acid is in the form of monosodium urate (uric acid salt). At any time the proportion of uric acid or urate is pH dependent, so the ratio of these two forms varies considerably in urine.

The solubility of urate and uric acid is critical to the development of crystals. Urate is more soluble in plasma, synovial fluid, and urine than in aqueous solutions. The solubility of uric acid in urine rises dramatically as the pH increases above 4.[27] There is little change, however, in the solubility of urate within the normal pH range that exists in the plasma, synovial fluid, and other tissues. Decreasing temperatures cause both urate and uric acid solubility to fall. The pathways of production of uric acid are shown in Fig. 37-21.

Evaluation and Treatment

Diagnosis of AS is made from the history and physical examination, roentgenograms, and serum analysis for the presence of the histocompatibility antigen HLA-B27. Erythrocyte sedimentation rate is elevated throughout the disease to 10 to 15 mm/hr in males and 10 to 15 mm/hr in females (normal is 0 to 9 mm/hr in males, 0 to 2 mm/hr in females). Alkaline phosphatase levels are frequently elevated. Treatment of individuals with AS consists of physical therapy to maintain skeletal mobility and prevent the natural progression of contractures. Prevention of deformity and maintenance of mobility require a continuous program of physical therapy. Exercises are performed several times each day to maintain chest expansion, full extension of the spine, and complete range of motion in the proximal joints.

Antiinflammatory corticosteroids and analgesic medications are prescribed to suppress some of the pain and stiffness and to facilitate exercise. The medications do not prevent disease progression, but they do provide relief from symptoms. Surgical procedures, such as osteotomy, total hip replacement, and cervical spinal fusion, and radiation therapy are sometimes used to provide relief for individuals with end-stage disease or intolerable deformity. Persons should stop smoking to lessen pulmonary problems.

Synthesis   Metabolism   Elimination

Fig. 37-21 *Uric acid synthesis and elimination.* Uric acid is derived from purines ingested or synthesized from ingested foods, as well as being recycled following cell breakdown. Uric acid is then eliminated through the kidneys and gastrointestinal tract. *(Redrawn from Klippel, J.H. & Dieppe, P.A. [Eds.]. [1994].* Rheumatology. *St. Louis: Mosby.)*

Pathophysiology

The pathophysiology of gout is closely linked to purine metabolism (or cellular metabolism of purines) and kidney function. At the cellular level, purines are synthesized to purine nucleotides, which are used in the synthesis of nucleic acids, adenosine triphosphate, cyclic adenosine monophosphate (AMP), and cyclic guanosine monophosphate (GMP). Uric acid is a breakdown product of purine nucleotides (urate synthesis and elimination are illustrated in Fig. 37-22). Some individuals with gout have an accelerated rate of purine synthesis accompanied by an overproduction of uric acid. Even with restricted purine consumption, these individuals continue to overproduce uric acid. Other individuals break down purine nucleotides at an accelerated rate that also results in an overproduction of uric acid. In addition, production of uric acid can be caused by an increased turnover of nucleic acids, which is associated with an increased turnover of cells at other body sites. The increased turnover of nucleic acids leads to increased levels of uric acid with a compensatory increase in purine synthesis.

Most uric acid is eliminated from the body through the kidneys. Urate is filtered at the glomerulus and undergoes both reabsorption and excretion within the renal tubules. In primary gout, urate excretion by the kidneys is sluggish. The sluggish excretion may be the result of a decrease in glomerular filtration of urate or an acceleration in urate reabsorption. In addition, monosodium urate crystals are deposited in renal interstitial tissues, causing impaired urine flow. (Kidney function is described in Chapter 28.)

The exact process by which crystals of monosodium urate are deposited in joints and induce gouty arthritis is unknown, but several mechanisms may be involved, including the following:

1. Monosodium urate precipitates at the periphery of the body, where lower body temperatures may reduce the solubility of monosodium urate.
2. Albumin or glycosaminoglycan levels decrease, which causes decreased urate solubility.
3. Changes in ion concentration and decreases of pH enhance urate deposition.
4. Trauma promotes urate crystal precipitation.

The monosodium urate crystals may form in the synovial fluid or in the synovial membrane, cartilage, or other connective tissues in joints and elsewhere, such as in the heart, earlobes, and kidneys. Evidence suggests that an acute attack of gout is the result of the *formation* of crystals rather than the *releasing* of the crystals from connective tissues into the synovial fluid.

Monosodium urate crystals can stimulate and perpetuate the inflammatory response (see Fig. 37-22, *A* and *B*). The presence of the crystals triggers the acute inflammatory response, during which neutrophils are attracted out of the circulation and begin to phagocytose (ingest) the crystals.

Clinical Manifestations

Gout is manifested by (1) an increase in serum urate concentration (uricemia); (2) recurrent attacks of monarticular arthritis (inflammation of a single joint); (3) deposits of monosodium urate monohydrate (tophi) in and around the joints; (4) renal disease involving glomerular, tubular, and interstitial tissues and blood vessels; and (5) the formation of renal stones. These manifestations appear in three clinical stages:

1. *Asymptomatic hyperuricemia:* The serum urate level is elevated but arthritic symptoms, tophi, and renal stones are not present; may persist throughout life.
2. *Acute gouty arthritis:* Attacks develop with increased serum urate concentrations; tends to occur with sudden or sustained increases of hyperuricemia but can also be triggered by trauma, drugs, and alcohol.
3. *Tophaceous gout:* The third and chronic stage of disease; can begin as early as 3 years or as late as 40 years after the initial attack of gouty arthritis. Progressive inability to excrete uric acid expands the urate pool until urate crystal deposits (tophi) appear in cartilage, synovial membranes, tendons, and soft tissue.

Trauma is the most common aggravating factor. The great toe is subject to chronic strain in walking, and subsequently an acute gout attack may follow long walks. Trauma associated with occupations such as truck driving may also precipitate an attack.

Attacks of gouty arthritis occur abruptly, usually in a peripheral joint (see Fig. 37-22). The primary symptom is severe pain. Approximately 50% of the initial attacks occur in the metatarsophalangeal joint of the great toe. The other 50% involve the heel, ankle, instep of the foot, knee, wrist, or elbow. The pain is usually noted at night. Within a few hours the affected joint becomes hot, red, and extremely tender and may be slightly swollen. Lymphangitis and systemic signs of inflammation (leukocytosis, fever, elevated sedimentation rate) are occasionally present. Untreated, mild at-

Fig. 37-22 *Pathogenesis of acute gouty arthritis.* **A,** Depending on the urate crystal coating, a variety of cells may be stimulated to produce a wide range of inflammatory mediators. *IgG,* Immunoglobulin G; *Apo E,* apolipoprotein E; *PGE2,* prostaglandin E₂; *LTB4,* leukotreine B₄; *IL,* interleukin. **B,** Sequence of events in the production of inflammatory response to urate crystals. **C,** Gouty tophus on right foot. *(C from Dieppe, P.A. et al. [1991]. Arthritis and rheumatism in practice. London: Gower.)*

tacks usually subside in several hours but may persist for 1 or 2 days. Severe attacks may persist for several days or weeks. When the individual recovers, the symptoms resolve completely. The helix of the ear is the most common site of tophi, which are the characteristic diagnostic lesions of chronic gout.

Tophaceous deposits produce irregular swellings of the fingers, hands, knees, and feet. Tophi commonly form lumps along the ulnar surface of the forearm, the tibial surface of the leg, the Achilles tendon, and olecranon bursae. Tophi may produce marked limitation of joint movement and eventually cause grotesque deformities of the hands and feet. Although the tophi themselves are painless, they often cause progressive stiffness and persistent aching of the affected joint. Tophi in the upper extremities may cause nerve compressions, such as carpal tunnel syndrome. Tophi in the lower extremities may cause tarsal tunnel syndrome. They may also erode and drain through the skin.

Renal stones are 1000 times more prevalent in individuals with primary gout than in the general population. The stones can be the size of a grain of sand or a piece of gravel, or they can accumulate in massive deposits called *staghorn calculi.* They range in color from pale yellow to brown to reddish black, depending on their composition. Some stones consist of pure monosodium urate; others consist of calcium oxalate or calcium phosphate. Renal stones can form in the collecting tubules, pelvis, or ureters, causing obstruction, dilation, and atrophy of the more proximal tubules and leading eventually to acute renal failure. Stones deposited directly in renal interstitial tissue initiate an inflammatory reaction that leads to chronic renal disease and progressive renal failure.

Treatment

The aims of gout treatment are to terminate the acute gouty attack as promptly as possible, prevent recurring attacks, prevent or reverse complications associated with urate deposits in the joints and kidneys, and prevent formation of kidney stones. Acute gouty arthritis is treated with antiinflammatory drugs. The drugs of choice are colchicine, nonsteroidal antiinflammatory agents (NSAIDs, especially indomethacin), and allopurinol. Hydrocortisone may be injected into the joint to relieve pain. Ice also may relieve some of the inflammation of the joint. Weight bearing on the involved joint is avoided until the acute attack subsides. The individual is put on a low-purine diet, with high fluid intake to increase urinary output. Antihyperuricemic drugs are given to reduce serum urate concentrations.

✓ QUICK CHECK

How does noninflammatory joint disease differ from inflammatory joint disease? Describe two principal features of each.

How does rheumatoid arthritis affect the skin, heart, lungs, and kidneys?

How does uric acid (or urates) cause gout to develop?

DISORDERS OF SKELETAL MUSCLE

Muscle weakness and fatigue are common symptoms. In many cases, neural, traumatic, and psychogenic causes provide an adequate explanation for the failure to generate force (weakness) or sustain force (fatigue) seen in myopathies. The pathophysiologic mechanisms in some of the metabolic and inflammatory muscle diseases have been explored, but the cause of many of the myopathies remains obscure. The complex interaction between muscles and nerves affects muscular function as well. Only inherited and acquired disorders of skeletal muscles are discussed here.

Secondary Muscular Dysfunction

Muscular symptoms arise from a variety of causes unrelated to the muscle itself. Secondary muscular phenomena (contracture, stress-related muscle tension, immobility) are common disorders that influence muscular function.

Contractures

Contractures can be pathologic or physiologic. A physiologic muscle contracture occurs in the absence of a muscle action potential in the sarcolemma. Muscle shortening is explained on the basis of failure of the calcium pump in the presence of plentiful adenosine triphosphate (ATP). A physiologic contracture is seen in McArdle disease (muscle myophosphorylase deficiency) and malignant hyperthermia. The contracture is usually temporary if the underlying pathology is reversed.

A pathologic contracture is a permanent muscle shortening caused by muscle spasm or weakness. Heel cord (Achilles tendon) contractures are examples of pathologic contractures. They are associated with plentiful ATP and occur in spite of a normal action potential. The most common form of contracture is seen in conditions such as muscular dystrophy (see p. 1082) and central nervous system (CNS) injury. Contractures also may develop secondary to scar tissue contraction in the flexor tissues of a joint, for example, contracture of burned tissues in the antecubital area of the forearm leading to a flexion contracture.

Stress-induced muscle tension

Although not a uniformly recognized illness, abnormally increased muscle tension has been associated with chronic anxiety as well as a variety of stress-related muscular symptoms, including neck stiffness, back pain, and headache. Abnormalities in the CNS, reticular activating system, and autonomic nervous system (ANS) have been implicated. Although few studies have confirmed these complex interactions, the connection is intuitively plausible. For example, as an individual progressively relaxes, the amplitude of the knee jerk reflex diminishes. Conversely, individuals with absent reflexes increase tension by such maneuvers as clenching the teeth or hand grip. The underlying pathophysiology may be related to the fact that as a muscle contracts, the muscle spindle is activated. This gamma-feedback system produces a series of impulses that are transmitted to the brain by the sensitive 1A afferent fibers. Unconscious tension is thought to increase the activity of the reticular activating system as well. This influences increasing firing of the efferent loop of the gamma fibers, produces further muscle contraction, and increases muscle tension. ANS function that regulates increased blood flow to the muscle during sympathetic activity may be related to increased muscle contraction tension.

Various forms of treatment have been used to reduce the muscle tension associated with stress. Progressive relaxation training, yoga, meditation, and biofeedback are examples of stress reduction therapies. **Biofeedback** uses an integrated electromyogram (EMG) to make recordings from the skin surface. The goal is to teach the individual to control tension that has been functioning maladaptively. It is particularly useful in individuals who have a connection between skeletal muscle tension and pain. **Progressive relaxation training** emphasizes the individual's ability to perceive the difference between tension and relaxation. This technique involves sequential tensing and a relaxing environment. The individual is taught to practice this routine daily, often with the use of audiotaped instructions. By teaching the individual to recognize excessive contraction of skeletal muscle, one hopes to enhance the ability to relax specific muscle groups to relieve tension and thus reduce CNS arousal as well as ANS arousal.

Disuse atrophy

The term **disuse atrophy** describes the pathologic reduction in normal size of muscle fibers after prolonged inactivity from bed rest, trauma (casting), or local nerve damage. The effects of muscular deconditioning associated with lack of physical activity may be apparent in a matter of days. The normal individual on bed rest loses muscle strength from baseline levels at a rate of 3% per day. Bed rest also is associated with cardiovascular, skeletal, and other organ system changes. Also, as people age, their muscles atrophy and become weaker.

Measures to prevent atrophy include frequent forceful isometric muscle contractions and passive lengthening exercises. If reuse is not restored within 1 year, regeneration of muscle fibers becomes impaired.

Fibromyalgia

Fibromyalgia is a chronic musculoskeletal syndrome characterized by diffuse pain and tender points. Increased sensitivity to touch (i.e., tender points), the absence of systemic or localized inflammation, and the presence of fatigue and sleep disturbances are common. Because the symptoms are vague (see list in next column), fibromyalgia has often been misdiagnosed or completely dismissed by clinicians. A common misdiagnosis has been chronic fatigue syndrome. Eighty to ninety percent of individuals affected are women, and the peak age is 30 to 50 years. Although the incidence is unknown, the prevalence is reported to be 2% and increases with age, with a 23% prevalence in the seventh decade.[28,29] It is more common than rheumatoid arthritis, yet its cause is still unknown.[30]

The etiology of fibromyalgia has been debated for over a

TABLE 37-6	Comparison of Fibromyalgia and Myofascial Pain Syndromes	
Variable	Fibromyalgia	Myofascial Pain
Location	Generalized	Regional
Examination	Tender points	Trigger points
Response to local therapy	Not sustained	Curative
Gender	Female/male ratio: 10:1	Equal or unknown
Systemic features	Characteristic	Unknown

century. It is unlikely that it is caused by a single factor. The most common precipitating factors include the following:
- Flu-like viral illness
- Chronic fatigue syndrome
- Human immunodeficiency virus (HIV) infection
- Lyme disease
- Physical trauma
- Persistent stress
- Chronic sleep disturbance

Certain rheumatic diseases, such as RA or systemic lupus erythematosus (SLE), may coexist if not initially present with fibromyalgia (Table 37-6).[28]

Pathophysiology

It is unproven but long suspected that muscle is the end organ responsible for the pain and fatigue. Some studies have documented metabolic alterations—lower ATP, lower adenosine diphosphate (ADP), and higher concentrations of AMP—and more alterations in the number of capillaries and fiber area in individuals with fibromyalgia than in study control subjects.[28] However, these studies have not proved that these alterations are the result of muscle oxygen problems or reduced physical activity. Most studies have demonstrated that increased muscle tenderness in fibromyalgia is a result of generalized pain intolerance, possibly related to functional abnormalities within the CNS (Fig. 37-23).

It is significant that blood flow in the left and right thalami is lower in individuals with fibromyalgia than in controls.[29] The thalamus and caudate nucleus are involved in pain perception. A chronic stress response may be involved in producing lower peripheral (e.g., at the muscle site) and central levels of serotonin. Individuals with fibromyalgia may have an adrenal hyporesponsiveness.

Clinical Manifestations

The prominent symptom of fibromyalgia is diffuse, chronic pain. The locations of nine pairs of tender points for diagnostic classification of fibromyalgia are shown in Fig. 37-24. The pain often begins in one location, especially the neck and shoulders, but then becomes more generalized. People describe the pain as *burning*, or *gnawing*. Fatigue is profound. The effect on everyday life is considerable.[31] A recent study found the majority of women experienced pain and fatigue far more than 90% of their time awake.[31] Fatigue is most notable when arising from sleep and in midafternoon.

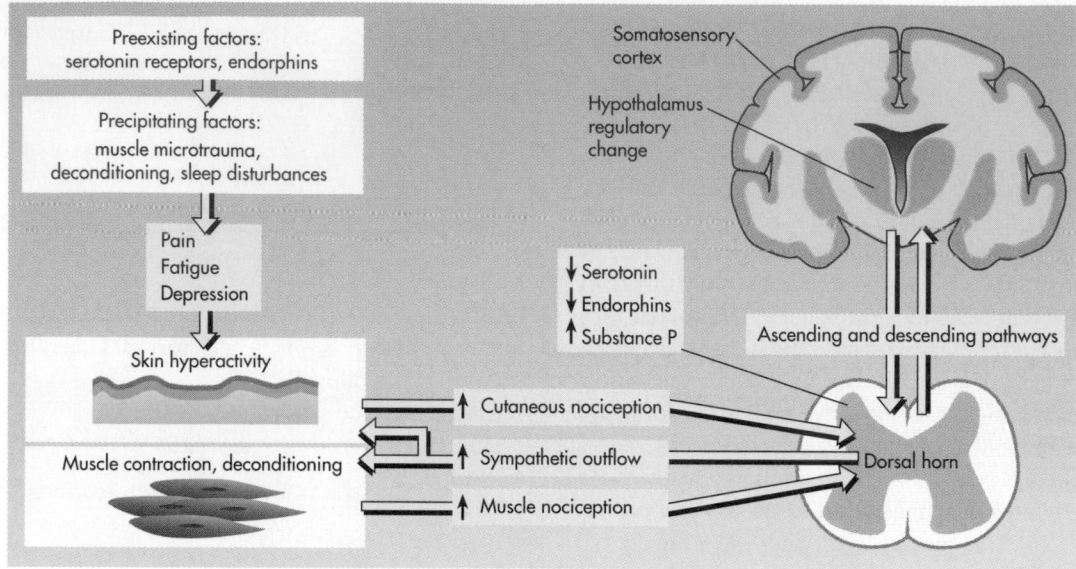

Fig. 37-23 *Theoretic pathophysiologic model of fibromyalgia.*

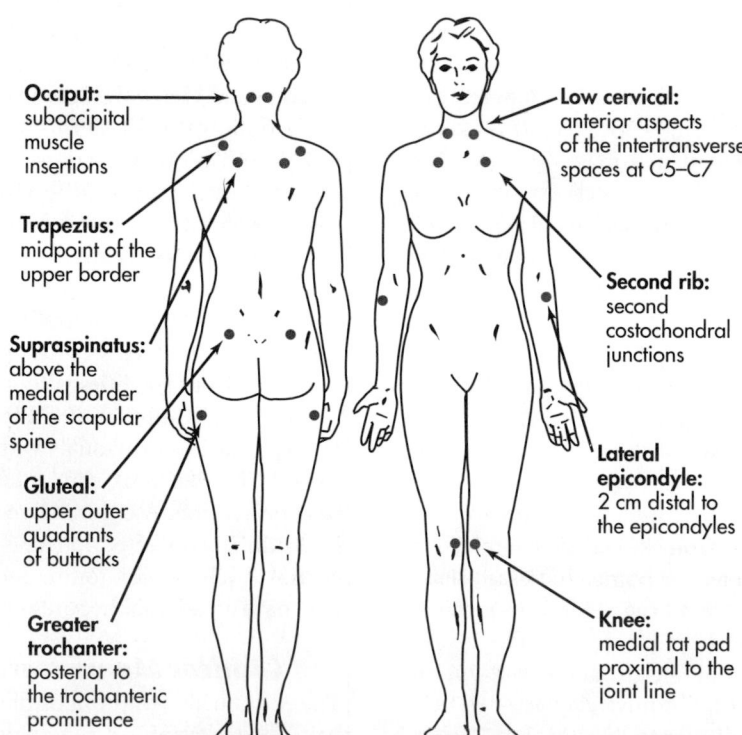

Fig. 37-24 *Location of specific tender points for diagnostic classification of fibromyalgia.* *(Redrawn from Freundlich B. & Leventhal L. [1993]. The fibromyalgia syndrome. In H.R. Schumacher, Jr, J.H. Klippel, W.J. Koopman, [Eds.]. [1993]. Primer on the rheumatic diseases [10th ed.]. Atlanta: Arthritis Foundation.)*

Headaches and memory loss are common complaints. Symptoms of irritable bowel syndrome and excess sensitivity to cold (Raynaud-like) are reported in 50% of individuals. Individuals with fibromyalgia are light sleepers and awake frequently.

Almost 25% of individuals seek psychologic support for depression. Anxiety, particularly in regard to their diagnosis and future, is almost universal.[28] Again, the only reliable finding on examination is the presence of multiple tender points.

Evaluation and Treatment

Because the manifestations of chronic, generalized pain and fatigue are present in many musculoskeletal (e.g., rheumatic) disorders, these disorders should be considered in the diagnosis of fibromyalgia.

No one regimen of medication has proved successful for fibromyalgia. Antiinflammatory medications have been used despite the fact there is no evidence of tissue inflammation. These medications have not been effective. Certain CNS-active medications, most notable the tricyclic antidepressants, amitriptyline, and cyclobenzaprine, were significantly better than placebos in controlled trials.[28] Amitriptyline significantly improved pain, morning stiffness, and sleep but not tender points. However, these successes only occurred in 25% to 45% of individuals.[28] One of the most important aspects of treatment is education and reassurance (Box 37-3).

Muscle Membrane Abnormalities

Two defects of the muscle membrane (plasma membrane of the muscle fiber) have been linked to clinical syndromes: the hyperexcitable membrane seen in the myotonic disorders and the intermittently unresponsive membrane seen in the periodic paralyses. Although these are infrequent disorders, research into the pathologic processes has led to an improved understanding of the cell membrane.

Myotonia

Myotonia is a delayed relaxation after voluntary muscle contraction, such as grip, eye closure, or muscle percussion. The distinctive "dive bomber" noise, audible on needle EMG, is caused by the prolonged depolarization of the muscle membrane. Because the depolarization is not terminated by neuromuscular blocking agents, such as curare, the abnormality has been localized at the muscle membrane, outside the neuromuscular junction and sarcotubular system. (These structures are described in Chapter 12.)

Myotonia is seen in several disorders: myotonia congenita, paramyotonia congenita, myotonic muscular dystrophy, and some forms of periodic paralysis. Most are inherited disorders and are mild in symptomatology, with the exception of myotonic muscular dystrophy (see p. 1083). Myotonia is treated by drugs that reduce muscle fiber excitability, such as procaine, procainamide, phenytoin, and quinine preparations. Recent treatments include acetazolamide, a carbonic anhydrase inhibitor, and verapamil, a calcium channel blocker.

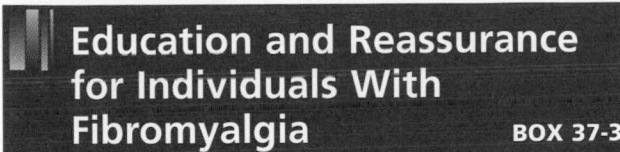

Education and Reassurance for Individuals With Fibromyalgia   BOX 37-3

Stress that the illness is real, not imagined.
Explain that fibromyalgia is probably not caused by infection.
Explain that fibromyalgia is not a deforming or deteriorating condition.
Explain that fibromyalgia is neither life-threatening nor markedly debilitating, although it is an irritating presence.
Discuss the role of sleep disturbances and the relationship of neurohormones to pain, fatigue, abnormal sleep, and mood.
Reassure that although the cause is unknown, some information is known about the physiologic changes responsible for the symptoms.
Use muscle "spasms" and, perhaps, low muscle blood flow to lay the groundwork for exercise recommendations.
Assist individual to use aerobic exercise to reduce stress and increase rapid eye movement (REM) sleep.

Periodic paralysis

Periodic paralysis is triggered by exercise and any process or medication that increases serum potassium. The disorder is often inherited in an autosomal dominant pattern, although it can be seen in hyperthyroidism. During an attack of *periodic paralysis,* the muscle membrane is unresponsive to neural stimuli and the resting membrane potential is reduced from -90 to -45 mV.

The paralysis, which leaves the individual flaccid and weak, does not affect the respiratory muscles. Many individuals have myotonia present on examination. In most cases the weakness is accompanied by a change in serum potassium, although in some individuals the change may be negligible. Cardiac dysrhythmias have been present during attacks. Although the biochemical defect remains unknown, changes in the muscle membrane and sarcoplasmic reticulum have been described.

Hypokalemic periodic paralysis is triggered by high-carbohydrate meals, prolonged bed rest, or emotional stress. (The effect of potassium on the resting membrane potential is discussed in Chapter 17.) Glucose and insulin infusions and oral potassium loading are used as provocative tests; oral and intravenous potassium can relieve acute attacks. Treatment includes thiazide diuretics and a high-salt diet. Acetazolamide and a low-salt diet are useful for long-term therapy.

Metabolic Muscle Diseases

Disorders in muscle metabolism can be caused by endocrine abnormalities or diseases of energy metabolism, such as glycogen storage disease, enzyme deficiencies, and abnormalities in lipid metabolism and mitochondrial function.

Endocrine disorders

Often the systemic effects of hormonal imbalance overshadow the individual's muscular symptoms. For example, individuals with thyrotoxicosis may have signs of proximal weakness, paresis of the extraocular muscles (exophthalmic ophthalmoplegia), and, rarely, hypokalemic periodic paralysis. Hypothyroidism is often associated with a decrease in muscle mass and strength, with weak, flabby skeletal muscles and sluggish movements.[32]

Thyroid hormone is believed to regulate muscle protein synthesis and electrolyte balance. Changes in muscle protein synthesis and electrolyte balance may therefore explain the changes in muscle mass and contractility seen in endocrine disorders. The muscular symptoms subside with appropriate treatment of the primary hormonal disorder.

Diseases of energy metabolism

Muscle relies on carbohydrates, such as glycogen and lipids (free fatty acids), for energy. When stored glycogen or lipids cannot be used because of a lack of the enzyme necessary to convert energy for contraction, the individual experiences cramps, fatigue, and exercise intolerance. Disorders of muscle metabolism can be self-limiting, such as in McArdle disease and some lipid disorders, or they can cause widespread irreparable muscle destruction, as in acid maltase deficiency.

McArdle disease

McArdle disease, or myophosphorylase deficiency, was the first myopathy in which a single enzyme defect was identified. It is now one of nine diseases identified to date that have in common an underlying defect in glycogen synthesis, glucogenolysis, or glycolysis. These diseases are often referred to as the **glycogen storage diseases (GSDs)** because each defect results in the abnormal deposition and accumulation of glycogen in skeletal muscle.[5] Individuals with McArdle disease lack muscle phosphorylase, which is responsible for the breakdown of glycogen in muscle. Normally, after the body uses the short-term ATP and phosphocreatine stores, intramuscular lactic acid accumulates as glycogen is used (see Chapter 17). The individual with McArdle disease is not able to break down glycogen or produce lactic acid.

The altered energy production manifests itself in exercise intolerance, fatigue, and painful muscle cramps. When exercise is carried to an extreme, painful muscle contracture and myoglobinuria develop. Some individuals describe a "second wind" phenomenon, in which exercise tolerance increases if they slow their pace once the initial sensation of fatigue commences. This may be caused by the use of free fatty acids as a secondary source of energy. As the disease progresses, some individuals have pronounced muscle weakness and wasting. Other organs are not involved, because the absence of phosphorylase is limited to muscle. Generally, individuals

with McArdle disease learn to adapt their daily routine to avoid muscle symptoms.

Acid maltase deficiency

Acid maltase deficiency is an uncommon glycogen storage disease associated with an accumulation of glycogen in the lysosomes of muscle cells and the cells of other tissues. The usual pathways of glycogen degradation are preserved. The absence of the enzyme acid maltase is responsible for the abnormality in glycogen metabolism, although the exact mechanism is unknown. It is an autosomal recessive disorder, with the gene located on the long arm of chromosome 17.

The infantile form is called **Pompe disease** and is recognized shortly after birth by hypotonia, dysreflexia, and an enlarged heart, tongue, and liver. Hypertrophy of these tissues is thought to be the result of glycogen deposition. Children die of cardiac or respiratory failure within 1 year of diagnosis. The adult variety becomes evident subacutely. The muscular symptoms resemble those of muscular dystrophy or polymyositis (see p. 1065). A distinguishing feature in adults may be the presence of severe respiratory muscle weakness.

Myoadenylate deaminase deficiency

An enzyme deficiency that produces changes in skeletal muscle and is associated with exercise intolerance is **myoadenylate deaminase deficiency (MDD).** Because these individuals lack myoadenylate deaminase, they have a poor capacity for sustained energy production. Myoadenylate deaminase is the catalytic enzyme that forms phosphocreatine and ATP during exercise through a metabolic pathway that binds the purine and phosphate molecules that constitute ATP. Persons with MDD differ from those with McArdle disease in that, during the ischemic exercise test, lactate production is normal when ATP and phosphocreatine are synthesized. The enzyme defect has been reported to be quite common, but in practice it may be rarely recognized as a cause of exercise intolerance.

Lipid deficiencies

Disorders of lipid metabolism are uncommon but account for severe changes in muscle metabolism. These disorders are caused by abnormalities in the transport and processing of fatty acids for energy.[5] The lipid content of muscle cells consists of the free fatty acids, which are oxidized in the mitochondria. These acids require carnitine and the enzyme carnitine palmityltransferase (CPT) to transport long-chain fatty acids to the mitochondria. CPT deficiency is an autosomal recessive disorder that invariably causes attacks of severe myalgia and myoglobinuria.[5] Carnitine deficiency causes abnormal lipid deposition in skeletal muscles.

Measuring the CPT and carnitine content in muscle aids in the diagnosis. Cells in the muscle biopsy show vacuoles and lipid deposits. Treatments with riboflavin, medium-chain triglyceride, oral carnitine, prednisone, and propranolol have been beneficial to some individuals.[5]

Inflammatory Muscle Diseases: Myositis

Viral, bacterial, and parasitic myositis

Viral, bacterial, and parasitic infections of varying severity are known to produce inflammatory changes in skeletal muscle, a group of conditions collectively described by the term *myositis*. In tuberculosis and sarcoidosis, chronic inflammatory changes and granulomas are found in muscle as well as in other affected tissues. In trichinosis, *Trichinella* larvae reside in infected pork and, after ingestion, migrate to the intestinal mucosa and from there to the lymphatics. Symptoms include severe pain, rash, and muscle stiffness. Treatment includes administration of corticosteroids, prednisone, and the antiparasitic agent thiabendazole. Toxoplasmosis, a common parasitic infection, is also associated with a generalized polymyositis that responds rapidly to therapy.

In the tropics, more prevalent disorders include bacterial infections with *Staphylococcus aureus* and parasites such as cysticercus, the larva of the tapeworm *Taenia solium*. Viral infections can be associated with an acute myositis. Muscle pain, tenderness, signs of inflammation, and creatine kinase (CK) elevation are common manifestations of viral myositis. The self-limiting symptoms of muscle aches and pains during a bout of influenza may actually be a subacute form of viral myopathy.

Polymyositis and dermatomyositis

Polymyositis (generalized muscle inflammation) and *dermatomyositis* (polymyositis accompanied by skin lesions) are the most common inflammatory muscle diseases requiring long-term care. Prevalence rates may be about 8.4 per 1,000,000 persons. The incidence appears to be increasing, although this may simply reflect more accurate diagnosis.[5]

Pathophysiology

Polymyositis and dermatomyositis are characterized by inflammation of connective tissue and muscle fibers that presumably causes the extensive necrosis and destruction of muscle fibers. The agent that causes the muscle inflammation has not been identified, but abnormalities in the immune system have been implicated. This family of diseases is now designated as autoimmune because of the presence of autoantibodies in the serum of many individuals. Studies have shown that the inflammatory cells that surround the perimysial and perivascular sites are selectively enriched in B cells and helper T cells in dermatomyositis. There is less vascular involvement in polymyositis, and most of the inflammatory cells, including B cells, T cells, and macrophages, surround the muscle fibers and fascicles. Recently, genetic markers have been located associated with polymyositis and dermatomyositis. These markers include human leukocyte antigens (HLA-B8, HLA-DR2, HLA-DRW52) in children and adults.[5]

Clinical Manifestations

The acute symptoms include many of those seen in any inflammatory process: malaise, fever, muscle swelling, pain

Fig. 37-25 *Dermatomyositis.* Heliotrope (violaceous) discoloration around the eyes and periorbital edema. *(From Habif, T.P. [1996]. Clinical dermatology [3rd ed.]. St. Louis: Mosby.)*

and tenderness, lethargy, listlessness, morning stiffness, anorexia, and weight loss. Both illnesses are usually associated with a symmetric proximal muscle weakness and can be initially confused with other myopathies. A thorough evaluation is required to exclude other disorders. Clinical features common in both polymyositis and dermatomyositis are dysphagia, reduced esophageal motility, vasculitis, Raynaud phenomenon, cardiomyopathy, and interstitial pulmonary fibrosis. Some individuals have other coexisting collagen vascular disorders, such as rheumatoid arthritis, systemic lupus erythematosus, and progressive systemic sclerosis (formerly called *scleroderma*).

The presence of skin rash, calcinosis, and eyelid edema most often suggests dermatomyositis (Fig. 37-25). The rash is often the presenting complaint and may antedate the onset of myopathic symptoms by more than 1 year.[5] The skin rash is a purple (heliotrope) color and involves the eyelids, face, chest, and extensor surfaces of the extremities. Dermatomyositis is slightly more common in children and older adults, with an onset before the age of 15 years or after the age of 50 years. The adult with dermatomyositis occasionally has underlying malignancies. Calcinosis, with calcium deposition in the subcutaneous tissue, can be a severe long-term complication of dermatomyositis.

Evaluation and Treatment

The muscle biopsy is striking in dermatomyositis, with most individuals showing inflammatory cells grouped around blood vessels and atrophy of cells in muscle fascicle. This change, perifascicular atrophy, is absent in polymyositis. CK and sedimentation rate are often extremely elevated in both disorders and are helpful indicators of disease activity. Other muscle enzymes, including aldolase, serum glutamic-oxaloacetic transaminase (SGOT), serum glutamic-pyruvic transaminase (SGPT), and lactic dehydrogenase (LDH), are also found to be elevated in most individuals.[5] Muscle biopsy is indispensable for a diagnosis of polymyositis or dermatomyositis as opposed to other myotonic disease. MRI reveals inflammation and edema of the muscles.

Treatment primarily includes immunosuppressive drugs, although they are not always successful if uniformly applied. Most clinicians choose corticosteroids initially, usually prednisone on a daily or alternating day schedule, tapering the dosage as the symptoms subside. Successful treatment with azathioprine, methotrexate, and cyclophosphamide has also been reported. Individuals with muscle weakness require careful physiotherapy to design a regular exercise program that prevents contractures and maximizes functional ability.

Toxic Myopathies

The most common cause of *toxic myopathy* is alcohol abuse. Two clinical syndromes are prevalent: (1) an acute attack of muscle weakness, pain, and swelling after a binge or (2) a more chronic, progressive proximal weakness in a drinker of long duration. The incidence of acute alcoholic myopathy has been estimated as up to 20% of individuals admitted with acute alcoholic withdrawal.

The pathologic abnormalities include necrosis of individual muscle fibers; whole segments can be found in the same stage of degeneration. The mechanism by which alcohol affects the muscle fiber is uncertain, but a direct toxic effect and nutritional deficiency have both received experimental support.

Acute alcoholic myopathy can range from benign cramps and pain resolving in a matter of hours to severe weakness and markedly increased CK associated with myoglobinuria and renal failure. Individuals are prone to repeated attacks following recovery. The only treatment is abstinence from alcohol and improved nutrition. The individual with chronic alcoholic myopathy often has coexisting peripheral neuropathy that complicates the diagnosis.

Chemical agents have also been implicated in the development of myopathy. The drug chloroquine, an antimalarial and amebicidal agent, in high doses has been associated with the development of generalized muscle weakness, particularly of the proximal muscles. Myopathy has also been caused by emetine (the major constituent of ipecac), vincristine, corticosteroids, and the toxic denatured rapeseed oil.

Rhabdomyolysis and myoglobinuria is often caused by sedatives and narcotics, particularly street heroin, clofibrate (a hypolipidemic agent), and the antifibrinolytic ϵ-aminocaproate. Drugs that induce hypokalemia, such as amphotericin B, licorice, and azathioprine, have also been reported. In addition, any drug or hormone that can raise or lower serum concentrations of sodium, potassium, calcium, phosphorus, or magnesium can induce myopathic symptoms.[5]

Repeated intramuscular injections have been associated also with changes in muscle fibers. Local necrosis of muscle fiber and elevated CK have been reported after intramuscular injections of cephalothin, lidocaine, diazepam, and digoxin; these effects were not produced with injections of saline. When drugs are injected over long periods, a chronic focal myopathy develops. Proliferation of connective tissue in both the muscle fiber and overlying skin and subcutaneous tissue has been reported. Over time, segments of the muscles, particularly the deltoid and quadriceps, are converted into fibrotic bands. Pathophysiologic mechanisms for these changes include repeated needle trauma and infection, along with the nonphysiologic acidity or alkalinity of the injected material.

✓ QUICK CHECK

How does stress affect muscle tension?

How do metabolic muscle diseases develop? What causes them?

Name one toxic myopathy, and explain why it develops.

MUSCULOSKELETAL TUMORS
Bone Tumors

Many different types of tumors involve the skeleton. *Bone tumors* may originate from bone cells, cartilage, fibrous tissue, marrow, or vascular tissue. Based on the tissue of origin, bone tumors are classified as osteogenic, chondrogenic, collagenic, or myelogenic. Each of the four types arises from one of the four stem cells that are ultimately derived from the primitive mesoderm (Fig. 37-26). In addition, bone tumors may be classified as being of histiocytic, notochordal, lipogenic, or neurogenic origin.

The mesoderm contributes the primitive fibroblast and reticulum cells. The fibroblast is the progenitor of the osteoblast and the chondroblast cell. Each cell synthesizes a specific type of intercellular ground substance, and the tumor derived from the cell is generally characterized by the type of ground substance produced by the cell. For example, osteogenic tumors usually contain cells that have the appearance of osteoblasts and produce an intercellular substance that can be recognized as osteoid. Chondrogenic tumors contain chondroblasts and produce an intercellular substance similar to chondroid (cartilage). Collagenic tumors contain fibrous tissue cells and produce an intercellular substance similar to the type of collagen found in fibrous connective tissue.

Tumors are also classified as benign or malignant. The differences between malignant and nonmalignant bone tumors are nebulous, primarily because the criteria used to differentiate them are vague (see Chapter 10). The criteria used to identify tumor cells as malignant are (1) an increased nuclear/cytoplasmic ratio, (2) an irregular nuclear border, (3) excess chromatin, (4) a prominent nucleolus, and (5) an increase in the number of cells undergoing mitosis. However, many young, rapidly growing, normal cells and cells subjected to inflammation and change in their blood supply also exhibit many of these same characteristics. (Tumor characteristics in general are described in Chapter 9.)

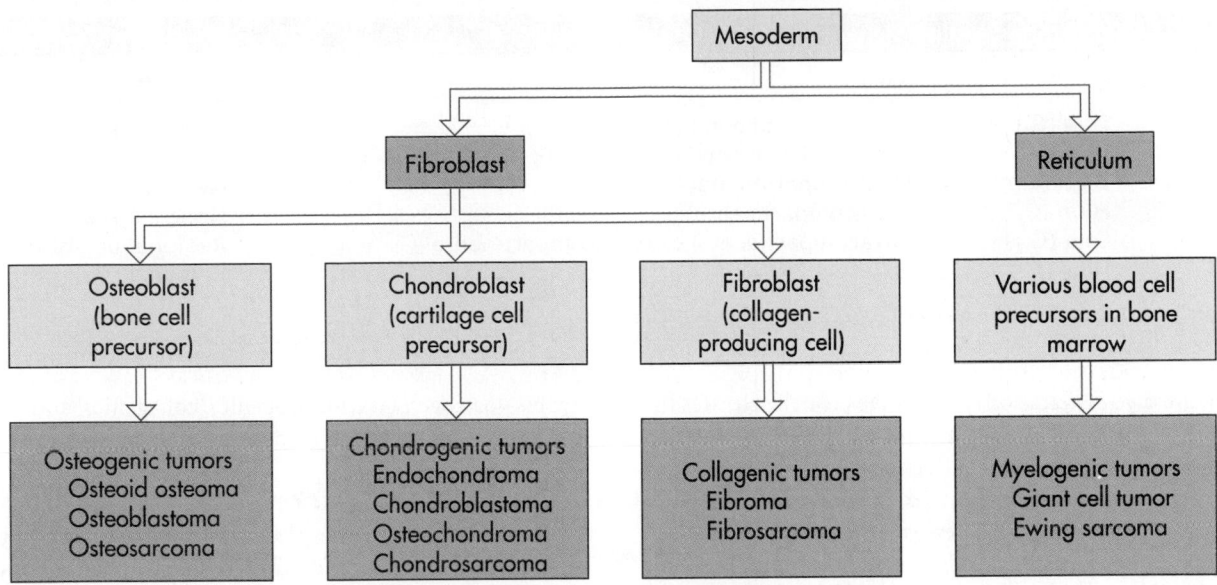

Fig. 37-26 *Derivation of bone tumors.*

TABLE 37-7	Patterns of Bone Destruction by Bone Tumors
Type	**Features**
Geographic pattern	Least aggressive type
	Generally indicative of slow-growing or benign tumor
	Well-defined margins on tumor, easily separated from surrounding normal bone
	Uniform and well-defined lytic area in bone
	Margin smooth or irregular, demarcated by short zone of transition between normal and abnormal bone tissue
Moth-eaten pattern	Characteristic of rapidly growing, malignant bone tumors
	More aggressive pattern
	Tumor margin less defined or demarcated; cannot easily be separated from normal bone
	Areas of partially destroyed bone adjacent to completely lytic areas
Permeative pattern	Caused by aggressive malignant tumor with rapid growth potential
	Margins of tumor poorly demarcated
	Abnormal bone merges imperceptibly with normal bone

Epidemiology

The incidence rate of bone tumors varies with age. In children younger than 15 years, the rate of bone tumors is relatively low, constituting approximately 3% of all malignancies. Adolescents have the highest incidence of bone tumors, and adults between the ages of 30 and 35 have the lowest incidence. After age 35 years, the incidence rate slowly increases until, at age 60 years, it equals the incidence rate in adolescents, primarily related to metastatic tumors.

Patterns of bone destruction

The general pathologic features of bone tumors include bone destruction, erosion or expansion of the cortex, and periosteal response to changes in underlying bone. The least amount of pathologic damage occurs with benign bone tumors, which push against neighboring tissue. Because they usually have a symmetric, controlled growth pattern, benign bone tumors tend to compress and displace neighboring normal bone tissue, which weakens the bone's structure until it is incapable of withstanding the stress of ordinary use, leading to pathologic fracture. Other tumors invade and destroy adjacent normal bone tissue by producing substances that promote resorption by increasing osteoclast activity or by interfering with a bone's blood supply.

Three patterns of bone destruction by bone tumors have been identified: (1) the geographic pattern, (2) the moth-eaten pattern, and (3) the permeative pattern (Table 37-7).

Tumors that erode the cortex of the bone usually stimulate a periosteal response, that is, new bone formation at the interface between the surface of the bone and the periosteum. Slow erosion of the cortex usually stimulates a uniform periosteal response. Additional layers of bone are added to the exterior surface of the bone to buttress the cortex. Eventually, the additional layers expand the bone's con-

TABLE 37-8	Surgical Staging System for Bone Tumors		
Stage	**Grade**	**Site (T)**	**Metastasis (M)**
IA	Low (G_1)	Intracompartmental (T_1)	None (M_0)
IB	Low (G_1)	Extracompartmental (T_2)	None (M_0)
IIA	High (G_2)	Intracompartmental (T_1)	None (M_0)
IIB	High (G_2)	Extracompartmental (T_2)	None (M_0)
IIIA	Low (G_1)	Intracompartmental or extracompartmental (T_1 or T_2)	Regional or distant (M_1)
IIIB	High (G_2)	Intracompartmental or extracompartmental (T_1 or T_2)	Regional or distant (M_1)

Data from Simon, S.R. (Ed.). (1994). Orthopaedic basic science. Chicago: American Academy of Orthopaedic Surgeons.

tour. Aggressive penetration of the cortex usually elevates the periosteum and stimulates erratic patterns of new bone formation. Examples of erratic patterns include concentric layers of new bone; a sunburst pattern, in which delicate rays of new bone radiate toward the periosteum from a single focus on the underlying surface; and rays of new bone that grow perpendicularly, creating a brush or bristle pattern.

Evaluation

A malignant bone tumor must be identified early to allow the survival of the individual and the preservation of the affected limb. However, individuals frequently have only vague symptoms that may be attributed to minor trauma, degenerative changes, or inflammatory conditions. In addition, other conditions may obscure the diagnosis.

Thorough diagnostic studies are needed to determine the exact type and extent of bone tumor present, which also helps determine the optimal treatment regimen. Serum alkaline phosphatase levels are elevated in bone lytic tumors and significantly elevated in osteosarcoma. Radiologic studies include plain radiologic films, a CT scan, and an MRI, which has become the examination of choice for the local staging of bone tumors, especially the staging of peripheral osteosarcomas (see Table 37-7). MRI is also used to monitor the response of osteosarcomas to radiation or chemotherapy and to detect recurrent disease. A CT scan can evaluate involvement of osteosarcoma in flat bones when the tumor is not well defined on a plain film, can assist in differentiating the tumor, and can locate pulmonary metastases. Radionucleotide bone scans show an increased uptake at the tumor site.

Additional diagnostic studies done for specific bone tumors include a complete blood count and erythrocyte sedimentation rate (to rule out infection or myeloma) and serum levels of calcium and phosphorus to detect hypercalcemia. Serum glucose levels may be elevated in chondrosarcoma. Acid phosphatase may show moderate elevations in bone metastases, multiple myeloma, and advanced Paget disease. Serum protein electrophoresis and immunoelectrophoresis are done to rule out other diseases. Fine needle biopsy is done, usually at the time of surgery, to determine the exact tumor type.

Types

A very large number of lesions are classified as bone tumors. The bone tumors most representative of the four derivative types—osteogenic, chondrogenic, collagenic, and myelogenic tumors—are described here (Table 37-8).

Osteogenic tumors: osteosarcoma

Osteogenic (bone-forming) tumors are characterized by the formation of bone or osteoid tissue with a sarcomatous tissue. The tissue can have the appearance of callus or compact or spongy bone. The most common malignant bone-forming tumor is the osteosarcoma.

Osteosarcomas account for 38% of bone tumors. The male/female ratio is 3:2, and osteosarcoma occurs predominantly in adolescents and young adults. Sixty percent of osteosarcomas occur in persons younger than 20 years. A secondary peak incidence for osteosarcoma occurs in the 50- to 60-year age-group, primarily in individuals with a history of radiation therapy several years previously for pelvic or other malignancies (Fig. 37-27).

Osteosarcoma is a malignant bone-forming tumor. It is large, destructive, and most often found in bone marrow; it has a moth-eaten pattern of bone destruction. The borders of the tumor are indistinct and merge into adjacent normal bone. Osteosarcomas always contain osteoid and callus, produced by anaplastic stromal cells, which are atypical, abnormal cells not seen in normal developing bone; they are neither normal nor embryonal. The osteosarcoma may also contain chondroid (cartilage) and fibrinoid tissue that may form the bulk of the tumor. The osteoid is deposited as thick masses or "streamers" between the trabeculae of callus, which infiltrate the normal compact bone, destroy it, and replace it with dense callus and masses of osteoid. Demonstrating the presence of osteoid aids in the diagnosis of osteosarcoma. Bone tissue produced by osteosarcomas never matures to compact bone.

Ninety percent of osteosarcomas are located in the metaphyses of long bones, especially the distal femoral metaphysis, with 50% around the knee area. The tumor typically breaks through the cortex, lifts the periosteum, and forms a soft tissue mass that is *not* covered by a smooth shell of new bone. Lifting of the periosteum stimulates bizarre patterns of new bone formation called a *periosteal reaction*. Distinct osteosarcomas occur on the surface of long bones, called parosteal, periosteal, and high-grade surface osteosarcomas; dedifferentiated parosteal and central osteosarcomas also occur.

The most common initial symptoms are pain and

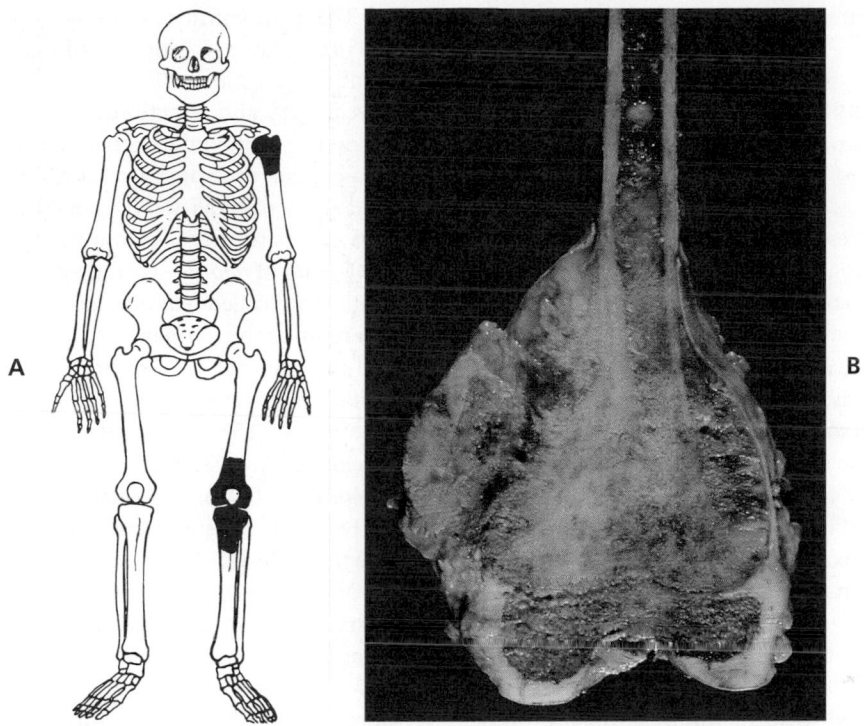

Fig. 37-27 *Osteosarcoma.* **A,** Common locations of osteosarcoma. **B,** Femur has a large mass involving the metaphysis of the bone; the tumor has destroyed the cortex, forming a soft tissue component. *(From Damjanov, I. & Linder, J. [Eds.]. [1996]. Anderson's pathology [10th ed.]. St. Louis: Mosby.)*

swelling. Initially, the pain is slight and intermittent, but within a short time the pain increases in severity and duration. Pain is usually worse at night and gradually requires medication. Systemic symptoms are uncommon. Usually, a coincidental history of trauma is noted. Occasionally, the individual may present with a pathologic fracture.

Surgery is a major treatment of choice, with the location of the tumor, its size, malignancy grade, and evidence of metastasis dictating the type and extent of surgery (see Table 37-8). Preoperative chemotherapy has greatly increased the number of individuals qualifying for limb salvage surgery. Limb-salvaging procedures have been made possible by advances in reconstructive techniques and endoprosthetics. Limb salvage ultimately may be successful in as many as 80% of persons. Individuals must have achieved most of their bone growth to be a candidate for limb salvage procedures.

If an amputation is done, individuals are monitored closely with chest roentgenograms and CT. Pulmonary metastases are surgically resected, and chemotherapy is now a common therapy given both before and after operation, using combinations of chemotherapeutic agents.

Chondrogenic tumors: chondrosarcoma

Chondrogenic (cartilage-forming) tumors produce cartilage or *chondroid,* a primitive cartilage or cartilage-like substance. The most common chondrogenic tumor is chondrosarcoma.

Chondrosarcoma is a tumor of middle-age and older adults. Most cases of primary chondrosarcoma are found in persons between 50 and 70 years of age. Secondary chondrosarcoma (a chondrosarcoma derived from an **endochondroma**) occurs most frequently in young adults between 20 and 30 years of age. The tumor is found more frequently in men than in women.

A chondrosarcoma is a large, ill-defined malignant tumor that infiltrates trabeculae in spongy bone. It occurs most often in the metaphysis or diaphysis of long bones, especially the femur, and in the bones of the pelvis. If located near the end of the bone, the tumor will infiltrate into the joint space. The tumor expands and enlarges the contour of the bone, causes extensive erosion of the cortex, and expands into the soft tissues.

Symptoms associated with the chondrosarcoma have an insidious onset. Local swelling and pain are the usual presenting symptoms. At first the pain is dull and intermittent; then it gradually intensifies and becomes constant. It may waken the person at night.

Diagnostic studies include radiographs, which must be reviewed carefully for an accurate diagnosis. Biopsy is done at the time of surgery. (If biopsy is done before scheduled surgical incision, seeding of tumor cells could occur.) Sufficient tumor material must be obtained to facilitate an accurate diagnosis.

Surgical excision is generally regarded as the treatment of choice. Many surgically treated individuals demonstrate recurrences, however, so amputation is becoming one treatment of choice. Therefore individuals with tumors located in the limbs have a better prognosis than those with pelvic lesions.

Collagenic tumors: fibrosarcoma

Collagenic (collagen-forming) tumors produce fibrous connective tissue. The most typical collagenic tumor is the fibrosarcoma.

Fibrosarcomas represent 4% of the primary malignant bone tumors, with a broad age distribution. They may occur at any age but are most common in adults between 30 and 50 years of age. The incidence is slightly greater in females. Fibrosarcoma may also be a secondary complication of radiation therapy, Paget disease, and long-standing osteomyelitis.

Fibrosarcoma is a solitary tumor that most frequently affects the metaphyseal region of the femur or tibia. The tumor is composed of a firm fibrous mass of tissue that contains collagen, malignant fibroblasts, and occasional osteoclast-like giant cells.

The tumor begins in the marrow cavity of the bone and infiltrates the trabeculae. It demonstrates a permeative growth pattern, destroys the cortex, and extends into the soft tissue. Metastasis to the lung is common.

Symptoms associated with the tumor have an insidious onset, which delays diagnosis. Pain and swelling are the usual presenting symptoms and usually indicate that the tumor has broken through the cortex. Local tenderness, a palpable mass, and limitation of motion also may be present. A pathologic fracture in the affected bone is frequently the reason for seeking medical help. Diagnostic studies include radiographs and MRI.

Radical surgery and amputation are the treatments of choice for fibrosarcoma. Radiation therapy is generally considered ineffective treatment for this tumor.

Myelogenic tumors

Myelogenic tumors originate from various bone marrow cells. Two types of myelogenic tumors are giant cell tumor and myeloma.

Giant cell tumor. **Giant cell tumor** is the sixth most common of the primary bone tumors, accounting for 4% to 5% of bone tumors. Giant cell tumors have a wide age distribution; however, they are rare in persons younger than 10 years or older than 70 years. Most giant cell tumors are found in persons between 20 and 40 years of age. Unlike most other bone tumors, giant cell tumors affect females more frequently than males.

The giant cell tumor is a solitary, circumscribed tumor that causes extensive bone resorption because of its osteoclastic origin. The giant cell tumor is located in the center of the epiphysis in the femur, tibia, radius, or humerus. The tumor has a slow, relentless growth rate and is usually contained within the original contour of the affected bone. It may, however, extend into the articular cartilage. When the tumor extends, it is usually covered by periosteum or periosteal bone growth. The tumor also may extend into local soft tissue, but it has a low rate of metastasis to other organs or tissues, although it has a high recurrence rate.

The most common symptoms associated with the giant cell tumor are pain, local swelling, and limitation of movement. Diagnostic studies include radiographs, CT, and MRI. Cryosurgery and resection of the tumor with the use of adjuvant polymethylmethacrylate (PMMA) for bone grafts decrease recurrence and are more successful treatments than curettage and radiation. Depending on the extent of the tumor and its recurrence, amputation may be necessary.

Myeloma. **Myeloma** is a neoplastic proliferation of immunocytes called *plasma cells*. The myeloma is the most common of the primary malignant tumors of the skeleton and accounts for 27% of bone tumors. The tumor may be solitary or multifocal (known as a *multiple myeloma*). Approximately 15% of the detected myelomas are multiple myelomas (see Chapter 10). The myeloma is common in persons older than 40 years of age. Males are affected twice as frequently as females, and blacks have a higher incidence rate than whites.

Myelomas characteristically cause cortical and medullary bone lysis and infiltrate the bone marrow. The most common initiating symptom of myeloma is pain, which may be felt in a single bone or the entire skeleton. The usual sites of pain are the lower back, upper spine, pelvis, ribs, and sternum. The pain is initially aching, intermittent, and aggravated by weight bearing. As the disease progresses, the pain becomes severe and prolonged. It is common for the individual with myeloma to be treated for a slipped disk or arthritis before the correct diagnosis of myeloma is established. In addition to pain, the individual may also experience weakness, fatigue, weight loss, and anorexia.

Persons with myeloma have a poor prognosis, and the treatment is generally palliative. Pain is relieved with narcotics, and special beds are used to lessen pain and prevent pathologic fractures. Cord decompression may be necessary in persons with spinal myeloma. Radiotherapy and chemotherapy have very limited success.

Muscle Tumors

Rhabdomyoma

Rhabdomyoma is an extremely rare benign tumor of muscle that generally occurs in the tongue, neck muscles, larynx, uvula, nasal cavity, axilla, vulva, and heart. These tumors are usually treated by surgical excision and do not recur.

Rhabdomyosarcoma

The malignant tumor of striated muscle is called **rhabdomyosarcoma.** This tumor is highly malignant with rapid metastasis. Rhabdomyosarcomas are located in the muscle tissue of the head, neck, and genitourinary tract in 75% of cases. The remainder are in the trunk and extremities.

Three types of rhabdomyosarcoma are differentiated on pathologic section: pleomorphic, embryonal, and alveolar. The pleomorphic, or spindle cell, type is considered to be one of the most highly malignant tumors of the extremities seen in adulthood. Once believed to be a common sarcoma, it is now believed to be very rare.[33] Embryonal tumors are most frequently seen in childhood and appear to be shaped like a tadpole or tennis racquet. Alveolar-type tumors appear latticelike and look like lung tissue alveoli.

The diagnosis of rhabdomyosarcoma is made by incisional biopsy and examination of the specimen by a pathologist. CT scan also helps define the tissue borders. Staging is based on pathologic grade of the tumor and is helpful in determining prognosis and treatment.

Treatment consists of a combination of surgical excision, radiation therapy, and systemic chemotherapy. Cure with distant metastasis is unlikely.

Other tumors

Metastatic deposits of tumors in muscles are rare in spite of the extensive vascular supply of skeletal muscles. It is sug-

gested that local pH or metabolic changes prevent metastatic involvement from other tumors. When adjacent carcinomas do cause muscle damage, it is usually related to the compression of tissue and resultant muscle atrophy.

✓ QUICK CHECK

From what cells do bone tumors originate?

Compare five major characteristics of benign bone tumors with those of malignant bone tumors.

How does the presence of metastatic tumors affect treatment options and prognosis of persons with osteosarcoma?

■ DID YOU UNDERSTAND?

Musculoskeletal Injuries

1. One of ten persons in the United States experiences an acute musculoskeletal injury each year.
2. The most serious musculoskeletal injury is a fracture. A bone can be completely or incompletely fractured. A closed fracture leaves the skin intact. An open fracture has an overlying skin wound. The direction of the fracture line can be linear, oblique, spiral, or transverse. Greenstick, torus, and bowing fractures are examples of incomplete fractures that occur in children. Stress fractures occur in normal or abnormal bone that is subjected to repeated stress. Fatigue fractures occur in normal bone subjected to abnormal stress. Normal weight bearing can cause an insufficiency fracture in abnormal bone.
3. Dislocation is complete loss of contact between the surfaces of two bones. Subluxation is partial loss of contact between two bones. As a bone separates from a joint, it may damage adjacent nerves, blood vessels, ligaments, tendons, and muscle.
4. Tendon tears are called *strains,* and ligament tears are called *sprains.* A complete separation of a tendon or ligament from its attachment is called an *avulsion.*

Disorders of Bones

1. Metabolic bone diseases are characterized by abnormal bone structure. In osteoporosis the density or mass of bone is reduced because the bone-remodeling cycle is disrupted. Osteomalacia is a metabolic bone disease characterized by inadequate bone mineralization. Excessive and abnormal bone remodeling occurs in Paget disease.
2. Osteomyelitis is a bone infection caused *most frequently* by bacteria. Bacteria can enter bone from outside the body (exogenous osteomyelitis) or from infection sites within the body (hematogenous osteomyelitis).

Disorders of Joints

1. Noninflammatory joint disease is differentiated from inflammatory joint disease by the absence of synovial membrane inflammation, the absence of systemic signs and symptoms, and the presence of normal synovial fluid.
2. Osteoarthritis is a noninflammatory joint disease characterized by the degeneration and loss of articular cartilage, sclerosis of underlying bone, and formation of bone spurs (osteophytes).
3. Rheumatoid arthritis is an inflammatory joint disease characterized by inflammatory destruction of the synovial membrane, articular cartilage, joint capsule, and surrounding ligaments and tendons. Rheumatoid nodules may also invade the skin, lung, and spleen and involve small and large arteries. Rheumatoid arthritis is a systemic disease that affects the heart, lungs, kidneys, and skin, as well as the joints.
4. Ankylosing spondylitis is a chronic, inflammatory joint disease characterized by stiffening and fusion of the spine and sacroiliac joints.
5. Gout is a metabolic disorder associated with high levels of uric acid in the blood and body fluids. Uric acid crystallizes in the connective tissue of a joint where it initiates inflammatory destruction of the joint.

Disorders of Skeletal Muscle

1. A pathologic contracture is permanent muscle shortening caused by muscle spasticity, as seen in central nervous system (CNS) injury or severe muscle weakness.
2. Stress-induced muscle tension is presumably caused by increased activity in the reticular activating system and gamma loop in the muscle fiber. The use of progressive relaxation training and biofeedback has been advocated to reduce muscle tension.

Continued

▣ DID YOU UNDERSTAND? —cont'd

Disorders of Skeletal Muscle—cont'd

3. Fibromyalgia is a chronic musculoskeletal syndrome characterized by diffuse pain and tender points. Unknown but suspected is that muscle is the end-organ responsible for the pain and fatigue. Most cases are women, and the peak age is 30 to 50 years of age.

4. Atrophy of muscle fibers and overall diminished size of the muscle are seen after prolonged inactivity. Isometric contractions and passive lengthening exercises decrease atrophy to some degree in immobilized patients.

5. Hyperexcitable membranes cause the physical and electrical phenomenon of myotonia. The disorder is treated with drugs that reduce muscle fiber excitability. Periodic paralysis is caused by an unresponsive muscle membrane and is accompanied by changes in serum potassium. The biochemical defect is possibly related to changes in the muscle membrane and sarcoplasmic reticulum.

6. Metabolic muscle diseases are caused by endocrine disorders, glycogen storage diseases, enzyme deficiencies, and abnormal lipid function. The muscle depends on a complex system of carbohydrates and fats converted by enzymes to produce energy for the muscle cell. Abnormalities in these pathways can inhibit function or cause damage to the muscle fiber. These illnesses are rare, yet account for significant functional abnormalities.

7. Viral, bacterial, and parasitic infections of muscles produce the characteristic clinical and pathologic changes associated with inflammation. These are usually treatable and self-limiting disorders.

8. Polymyositis (generalized muscle inflammation) and dermatomyositis (polymyositis accompanied by skin rash) are characterized by inflammation of connective tissue and muscle fibers and muscle fiber necrosis. Cell-mediated and humoral immune factors have been implicated. Treatment with immunosuppressive agents is effective in many cases.

9. The most common toxic myopathy is caused by alcohol abuse. Direct toxic effects of alcohol-producing necrosis of muscle fibers and nutritional deficiency have been suggested. The only treatment is abstinence and improved nutrition. The toxic effects of many drugs on muscle fibers cause local trauma to the muscle fibers caused by direct effects of the needle, secondary infection, and changes caused by nonphysiologic acidity and alkalinity in the fibers.

Musculoskeletal Tumors

1. Sarcomas of muscle tissue are rare. Rhabdomyosarcoma has a uniformly poor prognosis because of an aggressive invasion and early, widespread dissemination. The usual treatment includes surgical excision, radiation therapy, and systemic chemotherapy.

2. Bone tumors originate from bone cells, cartilage cells, fibrous tissue cells, or vascular marrow cells. Each cell produces a specific type of ground substance that is used to classify the tumor as osteogenic (bone cell), chondrogenic (cartilage cell), collagenic (fibrous tissue cell), or myelogenic (vascular marrow cell). Malignant bone tumors are usually large, aggressively destroy surrounding bone, invade surrounding tissue, and initiate independent growth outside the site of origin. Benign bone tumors are less destructive, limit their growth to the anatomic confines of the bone, and have a well-demarcated border.

KEY TERMS

Acid maltase deficiency, 1064
Acute gouty arthritis, 1058
Ankylosing spondylitis (AS), 1056
Asymptomatic hyperuricemia, 1058
Avulsion, 1036
Biofeedback, 1061
Bone tumor, 1066
Bowing fracture, 1033
Bursae, 1037
Caplan syndrome, 1055
Chondrogenic (cartilage-forming)
　tumor, 1069
Chondroid, 1069
Chondrosarcoma, 1069
Closed (simple) fracture, 1032
Collagenic (collagen-forming)
　tumor, 1070
Comminuted fracture, 1032

Compartment syndrome, 1038
Complete fracture, 1032
Contracture, 1060
Degenerative joint disease
　(osteoarthritis), 1048
Delayed union, 1035
Dermatomyositis, 1065
Dislocation, 1035
Disuse atrophy, 1061
Endochondroma, 1069
Endogenous (hematogenous)
　osteomyelitis, 1046
Enthesis, 1056
Epicondylitis, 1037
Exogenous osteomyelitis, 1046
Fatigue fracture, 1033
Fibromyalgia, 1061
Fibrosarcoma, 1070

Fracture, 1032
Giant cell tumor, 1070
Glycogen storage disease (GSD), 1064
Gout, 1057
Gouty arthritis, 1057
Greenstick fracture, 1032
Hyperbaric oxygen therapy, 1048
Idiopathic (primary)
　osteoarthritis, 1048
Incomplete fracture, 1032
Inflammatory joint disease
　(arthritis), 1051
Insufficiency fracture, 1033
Involucrum, 1047
Joint effusion, 1051
Kyphosis, 1042
Lateral epicondylitis (tennis
　elbow), 1037

KEY TERMS

REFERENCES

1. Skinner, H.B. et al. (1997). Musculoskeletal trauma surgery. In W.N. Kelley et al. (Eds.). *Textbook of rheumatology* (5th ed.). St. Paul, Minn.: West Publishing.

2. Willhite, L. (1998). Osteoporosis in women: Prevention and treatment. *Journal of the American Pharmacology Association, 38*(5), 614-623 [Quiz 623-624].

3. Bernard, B.P. (Ed.). (1997). *Musculoskeletal disorders and workplace factors.* Washington, D.C.: U.S. Department of Health & Human Services.

4. Vermette, E. (1998). Malignant hyperthermia. In W.N. Kelley et al. (Eds.). *Textbook of rheumatology* (5th ed.). St. Paul, Minn.: West Publishing.

5. Wortmann, R.L. (1997). Inflammatory disease of muscle and other myopathies. In W.N. Kelley et al. (Eds.). *Textbook of rheumatology* (5th ed.). St. Paul, Minn.: West Publishing.

6. Yamaguchi, S. & Viegas, S.F. (1998). Causes of upper extremity compartment syndrome. *Hand Clinics, 14*(3), 365-370.

7. Trice, M. & Colwell, C.W. (1998). A historical review of compartment syndrome and Volkmann's ischemic contracture. *Hand Clinics, 14*(3), 335-341.

8. Notelovitz, M. (1997). Estrogen therapy and osteoporosis: Principles and practice. *American Journal of Medical Science, 313*(1), 2.

9. Atkins, M. (1996). Preventing osteoporosis. *Ohio Nurses Review, 17*(1), 11-14.

10. Avioli, L.V. (Ed.). (1993). *The osteoporotic syndrome: Detection, prevention, and treatment* (3rd ed.). New York: Wiley-Liss.

11. Center, J. & Eisman, J. (1997). The epidemiology and pathogenesis of osteoporosis. *Baillieres Clinical Endocrinology and Metabolism, 11*(1), 23-62.

12. Mann, M. (1996). *Petition letter.* Washington D.C.: National Osteoporosis Foundation.

13. Physicians Committee for Responsible Medicine. (1997). Are dietary guidelines racially biased? *Good Medicine, 6*(4), 12.

14. De-Cree, C. (1998). Sex steroid metabolism and menstrual irregularities in the exercising female: A review. *Sports Medicine, 25*(6), 369-406.

15. Clark, K. & Sowers, M.R. (1996). Alcohol dependence, smoking status, reproductive characteristics, and bone mineral density in premenopausal women. *Research in Nursing and Health, 19*(5), 399-408.

16. Simon, S.R. (Ed.). (1994). *Orthopaedic basic science.* Chicago: American Academy of Orthopaedic Surgeons.

17. Cashman, K. & Flynn, A. (1998). Trace elements and bone metabolism. *Bibliotheca Nutritio et Dieta, 54,* 150-164.

18. Lauritzen, J.B. (1997). Hip fracture: Epidemiology, risk factors, falls, energy absorption, hip protectors, and prevention. *Danish Medical Bulletin, 44*(2), 155-168.

19. LeBoff, N.S. (1997). Metabolic bone disease. In W.N. Kelley et al. (Eds.). *Textbook of rheumatology* (5th ed.). St. Paul, Minn.: West Publishing.

20. Cattermole, H.C. et al. (1997). Bone mineral changes during tibial fracture healing. *Clinical Orthopaedics and Related Research, 339,* 190.

21. Calhoun, J.M. & Mader, J.T. (1997). Treatment of osteomyelitis with a biodegradable antibiotic implant. *Clinical Orthopaedics and Related Research, 341,* 206.

22. Mourad, L.A. (1997). Musculoskeletal system. In J.M. Thompson et al. (Eds.). *Mosby's clinical nursing* (4th ed.). St. Louis: Mosby.

REFERENCES

23. Roos, E.M. et al. (1998). Knee injury and osteoarthritis outcome score (KOOS)—Development of a self-administered outcome measure. *Journal of Orthopedics and Sports Physical Therapy, 28*(2), 88-96.

24. Fumento, M. (1997). Weight after 50. *Modern Maturity, 41R*(3), 34.

25. Kiely, P.D. (1998). The Th1-Th2 model—What relevance to inflammatory arthritis. *Annals of Rheumatology and Disease, 57*(6), 328-330.

26. van der Linden, S. (1997). Ankylosing spondylitis. In W.N. Kelley et al. (Eds.). *Textbook of rheumatology* (5th ed.). St. Paul, Minn.: West Publishing.

27. Cohen, M.G. & Emmerson, B.T. (1998). Gout. In J.H. Klippel & P.A. Dieppe (Eds.). *Rheumatology* (2nd ed.). St. Louis: Mosby.

28. Goldenberg, D.L. (1998). Fibromyalgia and related syndromes. In J.H. Klippel & P.A. Dieppe (Eds.). *Rheumatology* (2nd ed.). St. Louis: Mosby.

29. Olsen, N.J. & Park, J.H. (1998). Skeletal muscle abnormalities in patients with fibromyalgia. *American Journal of Medical Science, 315*(6), 351-358.

30. Gordon, S. & Morrison, C. (1998). Fibromyalgia and its primary care implications. *Medical-Surgical Nursing, 7*(4), 207-213, 216.

31. Henricksson, C. & Burckhardt, C. (1996). Impact of fibromyalgia on everyday life: A study of women in the USA and Sweden. *Disability and Rehabilitation, 18*(5), 241-248.

32. Seeley, R.R., Stephens, T.D., & Tate, P. (1995). *Anatomy and physiology* (3rd ed.). St. Louis: Mosby.

33. Miettinen, M. & Weiss, S.W. (1996). Soft tissue tumors. In I. Damjanov & J. Linder (Eds.). *Anderson's pathology* (10th ed.). St. Louis: Mosby.

CHAPTER 38

Alterations of Musculoskeletal Function in Children

Kathryn L. McCance

Musculoskeletal alterations in children are very common. They may be congenital, such as clubfoot; hereditary, such as muscular dystrophy; or acquired, such as Legg-Calvé-Perthes disease. Some of these disorders are acute and the child will recover completely, and others are chronic or, in some cases, terminal.

Frances Lynn McCullough, RNP, MNSc, contributed to this chapter in the previous edition.

CHAPTER OUTLINE

CONGENITAL DEFECTS

Developmental Dysplasia of the Hip

Developmental dysplasia of the hip (DDH), formerly called *congenital dislocation of the hip,* is an abnormality in the development of the proximal femur, acetabulum, or both. Although most often present at birth, it may occur at any time in the newborn or infant period. Risk factors include family history, first pregnancies with accompanying oligohydramnios (deficient volume of amniotic fluid), and any other conditions that limit movement, placing the hips in a position of flexion and adduction, such as breech positions in utero. The presence of other anomalies, such as foot deformities and torticollis, also increases the risk. Treatment depends on the age of the child, severity of dysplasia, and duration of dysplasia. Nonoperative treatment involves bracing, traction, casts, or a combination of these; surgery is required for dislocations discovered in walking-age children.[1,2]

Deformities of the Foot

Foot deformities are common in children and may result from intrauterine positioning or true embryonic malformations. Metatarsus adductus is the most common foot deformity; talipes equinovarus (clubfoot) is another common deformity. In both, arrested or abnormal embryonic development has been implicated. In *metatarsus adductus,* the forefoot is adducted and in varus, giving the foot a kidney bean shape. *Talipes equinovarus (clubfoot)* involves both the bony structures and the soft tissues of the foot. The forefoot is adducted (turned inward), and the hindfoot is in varus and inverted. The entire foot is in equinus (pointing downward). True clubfoot is rigid and cannot be corrected passively. Metatarsus adductus may resolve without treatment, although in most cases stretching exercises are combined with bracing to bring the foot into a neutral position. Treatment of talipes equinovarus begins in the newborn nursery with manipulation, weekly casting, and surgery if needed.[1-4]

ABNORMAL DENSITY OF MODELING OF THE SKELETON

Osteogenesis Imperfecta

Osteogenesis imperfecta (brittle bone disease) is an inherited disorder of connective tissues that affects primarily bone. The major errors in osteogenesis imperfecta lie in the synthesis and structures of collagen, with recent findings indicating the encoding for collagen to be "remarkable feeble." The majority of individuals have mutations of one of two genetic loci that encode type I collagen.[5] The mutant collagen molecules severely impair the formation of the extracellular matrix, causing an abnormal architecture of dermis and bone.[6] The classic clinical manifestations of osteogenesis imperfecta are bone fractures; osteoporosis; abnormally short, bowed, and deformed limbs; short stature; curvature of the spine; and bluish discoloration of the sclera (white of the eye) (Fig. 38-1). Four syndromes of varying severity in clinical manifestations have been identified: types II and III are the most severe; types I and IV are slightly more common and less severe, inherited as autosomal dominant traits. Treatments range from orthopedic measures such as splinting to supplements of calcium or fluoride, vitamin C, or magnesium oxide.[2,7]

Scoliosis

Scoliosis is a structural or nonstructural lateral curvature of the spine (Fig. 38-2). *Nonstructural scoliosis* results from a cause other than the spine itself, such as posture, leg length discrepancy, or pain. *Structural scoliosis* is curvature associated with vertebral rotation. Nonstructural scoliosis can become structural if the underlying cause is not found and treated.

Structural scoliosis can result from congenital skeletal abnormalities; neuromuscular diseases; trauma; extraspinal contractures; bone infections that involve the vertebrae; metabolic bone disorders such as rickets, osteoporosis, or osteogenesis imperfecta; joint disease; or tumors. Structural scoliosis with no known cause, termed *idiopathic scoliosis,* accounts for at least 65% of cases and may be genetically linked.

Individuals with adolescent scoliosis may have an abnormality of the central nervous system involving the balance mechanism in the midbrain. Postural and equilibrium dysfunctions, along with vestibular dysfunction, also have been implicated.

The earliest pathologic changes, which are actually secondary changes, occur in the soft tissues. The muscles, ligaments, and other soft tissues become shortened on the concave side of the curve long before bone deformities occur. Progressive deformities of the vertebral column and ribs develop. In growing children, lateral deviation of the spinal column ceases and one-sided compression of the vertebral bodies on the concave side of the curve begins. Vertebral deformity occurs as asymmetric forces are applied to the epiphyseal center of the ossification by shortened and tight soft tissues on the concave side.

Clinically, this appears as mild spinal curvature with prominence of one hip or rounded shoulders. The curve disappears with forward flexion of the spine, lying down, or traction of the head. Spinal curvature is usually visible or palpable, and the muscles on one side of the lower back (the convex side) may be prominent or bulging. Most cases of idiopathic scoliosis are noted during school screening programs. Diagnosis is made by x-ray examination. Treatment involves bracing or surgery, depending on the size of the spinal curvature.[1,8,9]

BONE INFECTION: OSTEOMYELITIS

Osteomyelitis is an inflammation of the bone and the bone marrow. Occurring twice as often in males as females, acute osteomyelitis may affect infants and children of any age but occurs most frequently between 3 and 12 years of age.[10]

Fig. 38-1 *Osteogenesis imperfecta treated with osteotomies and telescoping medullary rods.*
A, Severe deformity of both femurs. **B,** Same individual after multiple osteotomies with telescoping medullary rod fixation. **C,** Same individual 4 years later demonstrating growth of femurs,
no recurrence of deformity, and elongation of rods. (Plaster casts are in place for immobilization
of tibial osteotomies.) *(From Crenshaw, A.H. [Ed.]. [1992]. Campbell's operative orthopaedics [8th
ed., vol. 3]. St. Louis: Mosby.)*

Fig. 38-2 *Scoliosis in children.* Normal spinal alignment and abnormal spinal curvatures associated with scoliosis. **A,** Normal. **B,** Mild. **C,** Severe. **D,** Rotation and curvature of scoliosis.

In children, the long bones of the extremities (tibia, humerus, femur) are particularly susceptible to hematogenous infection. The bacteria pass through the bone's branching blood vessels until they reach the terminal capillaries on the metaphyseal side of the growth plate. In this area, the circulation is sluggish, creating an ideal site for bacterial growth and multiplication. The bacteria lodge in the small vascular channels, where they can initiate inflammation. The rich phagocytic mechanism frequently prevents most of the bacteria from establishing an infectious state. In some cases, however, the bacteria lodge at the end of the arterial loops beneath the epiphyseal plate and infection develops because there are no phagocytic cells to remove the bacteria (Fig. 38-3).[2,11]

Although bacterial blood infections are common in children, not all infections result in osteomyelitis. Possible mechanisms responsible for osteomyelitis may also be related to trauma, an associated factor in some children. Osteomyelitis can be induced with a subclinical bacterial infection by making a small crack in the epiphyseal plate. The same bacteria without the injury produce a rare, subclinical form of osteomyelitis that appears to heal spontaneously. Thus trauma may be a precursor or causative factor that allows the bacteria to settle in the bone or joint.

The organism responsible for osteomyelitis varies and is related to the age of the child. Factors that predispose to the development of osteomyelitis include impetigo, furunculosis, infected lesions of varicella (chickenpox), infected burns, cerebral abscesses, immunization with bacillus Calmette-Guérin (BCG) vaccine, prolonged intravenous or central parenteral alimentation, drug addiction, and direct trauma to the area adjacent to the site of the osteomyelitis.

Osteomyelitis usually begins as a bloody abscess in the metaphysis of the bone. The abscess ruptures under the periosteum and spreads along the bone shaft or into the bone marrow cavity if untreated. Infection usually first gains entrance to the subperiosteal space in the metaphysis, the path of least resistance because the cortex of the bone in this area is porous or mazelike, and the inflammatory response blocks spread within the bone. Debris accumulates, causing the periosteum to separate and form a shell of new bone around the infected portion of the shaft. Because the periosteum is separated from an adequate blood supply, sections of the bone die, becoming *sequestrum.* The periosteum that maintains a blood supply generates new bone and is responsible for the appearance of the periosteal new bone, or *involucrum.* The presence of the sequestra and involucrum indicates that the disease has progressed to subperiosteal abscess formation.

When the infection in the metaphysis occurs near a joint, the accumulating pus (bacteria, white blood cells, fluid) creates increasing pressure that may cause a rupture into the joint cavity. If this occurs, the pus causes inflammation and *secondary suppurative arthritis.* Osteomyelitis in infants is frequently associated with septic arthritis because the infant's bone has blood vessels that perforate the growth plate (Fig. 38-4). Normal anatomic variations in infants allow infection to spread directly to the epiphysis, which causes both joint disease and permanent epiphyseal disease.

Why are children susceptible to joint involvement? First, capillaries penetrate the epiphyseal plate and provide direct communication between the metaphysis of the bone and the joint cavity during the first month of life. Second, the capsules of the hip joints attach directly to the femur. Because of these two structural differences during infancy, infections originating in the metaphysis of the bone can spread rapidly to the joint cavity. The reverse may also occur—infections of

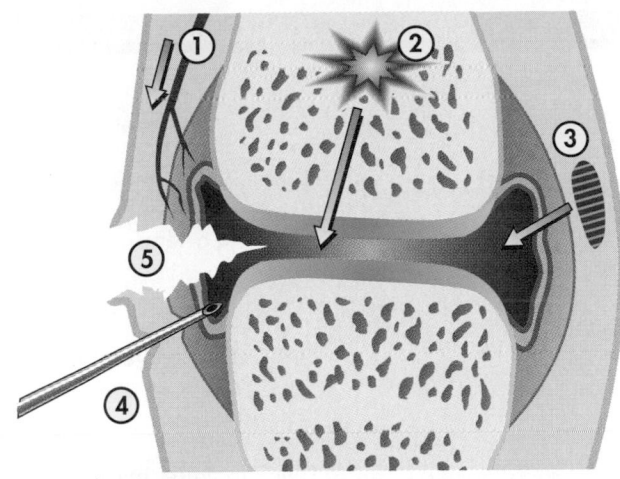

Fig. 38-4 *The routes of infection to the joint. 1,* The hematogenous route. *2,* Dissemination from osteomyelitis. *3,* Spread from an adjacent soft tissue infection. *4,* Diagnostic or therapeutic measures. *5,* Penetrating damage by puncture or cutting.

Fig. 38-3 *Pathogenesis of acute osteomyelitis differs with age.* **A,** In infants younger than 1 year the epiphysis is nourished by penetrating arteries through the physis, allowing development of the condition within the epiphysis. **B,** In children up to 15 years of age the infection is restricted to below the physis because of interruption of the vessels.

the joint cavity can spread to the bone's metaphysis. In extreme cases, bone growth may be completely arrested. Infantile osteomyelitis is characterized by permanent arrest in bone growth and involvement of multiple sites within the same bone or in multiple bones.

In children, osteomyelitis is usually an abrupt illness characterized by fever and systemic signs of toxicity. Sometimes the illness is subacute, with the child complaining of swelling, redness, tenderness, and slow movement of the affected bone or bones. Most frequently the long bones are affected, but osteomyelitis may also be found in the pelvis and small bones of the hands and feet. Clinical manifestations include elevated white blood cell counts and elevated erythrocyte sedimentation rates.

Treatment involves administration of the appropriate antibiotic, drainage of infected bone, and symptomatic relief of pain and discomfort. Death is rare, but serious complications can result, including dislocations of joint and arrest of bone joint growth.

HEALTH ALERT

New Treatment and Evaluation Trends for Osteomyelitis

Recent data about osteomyelitis highlight new treatment and evaluation trends. In many children, acute staphylococcal osteomyelitis may be better treated and at reduced cost by minimizing surgical methods, by shortening the duration of antibiotic courses and hospital stays, by switching quickly to an oral route for antibiotics, and by not using serum bactericidal levels. In addition, C-reactive protein (CRP), an acute-phase protein (so-called because of its ability to bind to the C-protein of pneumococci), promotes uptake by phagocytes; thus CRP is an opsonin that promotes phagocytosis. C-reactive protein also appears to be a better laboratory study than sedimentation rate in the diagnosis of bone or joint infection and in monitoring a person's clinical response to antibiotics.

Data from Wall, E.J. (1998). Childhood osteomyelitis and septic arthritis. Current Opinions in Pediatrics, 10(1), 73-76.

JUVENILE RHEUMATOID ARTHRITIS

The rheumatic diseases are a group of diverse conditions having in common the inflammation of connective tissues (see Chapter 37). They include rheumatoid arthritis, systemic lupus erythematosus, dermatomyositis, progressive systemic sclerosis, and polyarthritis.

Juvenile rheumatoid arthritis (JRA) is the childhood form of rheumatoid arthritis and is often accompanied by systemic manifestations. It affects about 250,000 children in the United States.

Although the basic pathophysiology of JRA is the same

TABLE 38-1   Characteristics of Juvenile Rheumatoid Arthritis (JRA) Related to Mode of Onset

	Systemic Onset	Pauciarticular (Two or Three Subtypes)	Polyarticular (Two Subtypes)
Percentage of patients	30%	45%	25%
Age at onset	Bimodal distribution 1-3 yr of age 8-10 yr of age	Type I: less than 10 yr Type II: over 10 yr	Throughout childhood and adolescence
Sex ratio (female/male)	1.5:1	Type I: Almost all female Type II: 1:9	Mostly female
Joints involved	Any Only 20% have joint involvement at time of diagnosis	Usually confined to lower extremities—knee, ankle, and eventually sacroiliac; sometimes elbow	Any joints: usually symmetric involvement of small joints Hip involvement in 50% Spine involvement in 50%
Extraarticular manifestations	Fever, malaise, myalgia, rash, pleuritis or pericarditis, adenomegaly, splenomegaly, hepatomegaly	Type I: chronic iridocyclitis; mucocutaneous lesions Type II: acute iridocyclitis; sacroiliitis common; eventual ankylosing spondylitis in many Type III: arthritis only	Systemic signs minimal Possible low-grade fever, malaise, weight loss, rheumatoid nodules, and/or vasculitis
Laboratory tests	Elevated ESR, RF negative; ANA rarely positive; anemia; leukocytosis	Elevated ESR; ANA positive Type I: HLA-DRW5 positive Type II: HLA-B27 positive Type III: HLA-TMo positive	Elevated ESR Type I: RF positive Type II; RF negative
Long-term prognosis	Mortality—1%-2% of all JRA patients Joint destruction in 40%	Continuous disease; eventual remission in 60% Type I: ocular damage; functional blindness in 10% Type II: ankylosing spondylitis Type III: best outlook for recovery	Longer duration; more crippling; remission in 25% Type I: high incidence of disabling arthritis Type II: outlook good

From Wong, D.L. et al. (1999). Whaley & Wong's nursing care of infants and children (6th ed.). St. Louis: Mosby.
ESR, *Erythrocyte sedimentation rate;* RF, *rheumatoid factor;* ANA, *antinuclear antibody;* HLA, *human leukocyte antigen.*

as that of adult rheumatoid arthritis, JRA differs in the following points:

1. Mode of onset has three distinct forms:
   a. Arthritis in fewer than five joints (pauciarticular)
   b. Arthritis in more than five joints (polyarthritis)
   c. Systemic disease (most common)
2. The large joints are predominantly affected.
3. Subluxation and ankylosis of the cervical spine are common.
4. Joint pain is not as severe as the adult type.
5. Chronic uveitis is common.
6. Serologic tests often detect antinuclear antibody.
7. Serologic tests seldom detect rheumatoid factor.

Rheumatoid nodules are not limited to subcutaneous tissue but are found in the heart, lungs, eyes, and other organs.

Treatment for children with JRA is supportive but not curative—its aims are to control inflammation and other clinical manifestations of the disease and to minimize deformity.[12-14] Future directions for treatment will include anticy-

tokine therapies.[15] Table 38-1 summarizes the characteristics of JRA related to mode of onset.

✓ QUICK CHECK

Why does a mutation of type I collagen cause osteogenesis imperfecta?

Why is the metaphyseal site of the growth plate susceptible to osteomyelitis?

How does juvenile rheumatoid arthritis differ from the adult form?

AVASCULAR DISEASES OF THE BONE: OSTEOCHONDROSES

The avascular diseases of the bone, the *osteochondroses,* are caused by insufficient blood supply to growing bones. Currently, vascular impairment and trauma, coupled with un-

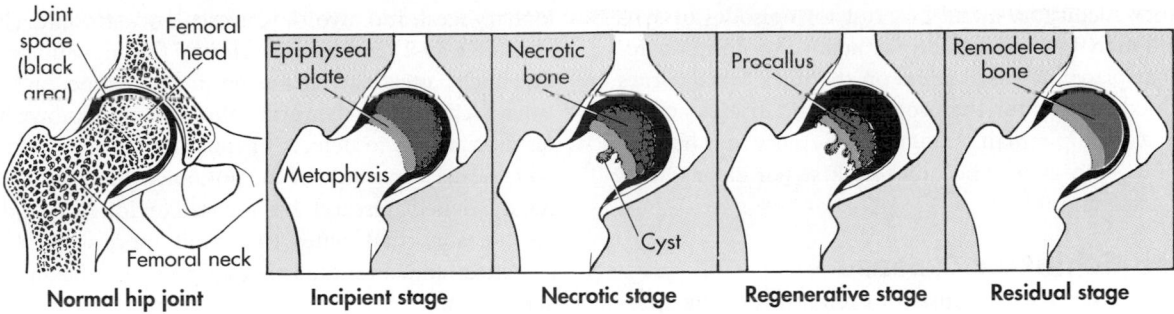

Fig. 38-5 *Stages of Legg-Calvé-Perthes disease, a form of osteochondrosis.*

derlying development or genetic predisposition, have been identified as probable causes of osteochondroses. The most common osteochondroses involve the head of the femur, the capital femoral epiphysis (Legg-Calvé-Perthes disease); the epiphyses of the vertebral bodies (Scheuermann disease); the proximal bones of the feet (tarsal navicular bones; Köhler bone disease); the proximal tibial epiphysis (Blount disease); the tibial tuberosity (Osgood-Schlatter disease); and the calcaneus.

The classic clinical course of the osteochondroses consists of three overlapping stages: (1) avascular necrosis, or death of newly formed bone or cartilage associated with diminished blood supply; (2) an acute inflammatory response in tissues adjacent to areas of necrosis; and (3) healing and repair.

Synovitis is often the cause of the first clinical manifestations—pain and muscle spasm. Deformities become evident during the second or intermediate stage of osteochondrosis. Necrosis and articular damage are followed by processes of healing: ingrowth of new blood vessels and the appearance of primitive mesenchymal tissues that later differentiate into osteoblasts and contribute to the proliferation of reparative cells and new bone. Cysts in the articular cartilage and endochondral bone affect articular contour and congruity and future function and growth. Cysts disappear, and bone and articular remodeling are completed.

Legg-Calvé-Perthes Disease

Legg-Calvé-Perthes disease (coxa plana) is a common osteochondrosis usually occurring in children between the ages of 3 and 12 years, with a peak incidence at 6 years. The disorder is bilateral in 10% to 20% of children, and boys are affected three to five times more often than girls. This self-limited disease of the hip, which runs its natural course in 2 to 5 years, is presumably produced by recurrent interruption of the blood supply to the femoral head. The ossification center first becomes necrotic (osteonecrosis) and then is gradually replaced by live bone.

Several causative theories have been proposed, including a generalized disorder of epiphyseal cartilage growth, thyroid deficiency, trauma, and infection. A plausible theory is that acute synovitis (infection of the synovial membrane)

and increased hydrostatic pressure in the hip joint compress blood vessels that supply the femoral head.

Among the important constitutional factors are birth weight (much lower than in unaffected children), skeletal maturation (delayed), and height (affected children are between 2.5 and 7 cm shorter than unaffected children). Familial occurrence is common. The disease is rare in blacks and frequent in children of Japanese and Central European ancestry.

In the first stage, the soft tissues of the hip (synovial membrane and joint capsule) are swollen, edematous, and hyperemic, often with fluid present in the joint (Fig. 38-5). In the second, or active vascular necrotic, stage, the entire or anterior half of the epiphysis of the femoral head is dead and the metaphyseal bone at the junction of the femoral neck and capital epiphyseal plate is softened because of increased blood supply and decalcification. Soon granulation tissue (procallus) and blood vessels invade the dead bone. The third, or regenerative healing, stage ordinarily lasts 2 to 4 years. The dead femoral head is replaced by procallus, and new bone is laid down. Collapse and flattening of the femoral head occur, and the femoral neck becomes short and wide (see Fig. 38-5). In the fourth, or residual, stage, remodeling takes place and the newly formed bone is organized into a live spongy bone.

Injury or trauma precedes the onset of the clinical manifestations in approximately one third of children with Legg-Calvé-Perthes disease. For several months the child complains of a limp and pain that is referred to the knee, inner thigh, and the groin, following the path of the obturator nerve. The pain is usually aggravated by activity and relieved by rest.

The typical physical findings include spasm on rotation of the hip in extension, limitation of internal rotation and abduction, and hip flexion-abduction deformity. If the child is walking, an abnormal gait termed an **antalgic abductor lurch** is apparent. If the hip pain or limp has been present for a prolonged period, muscles of the hip and thigh atrophy.

The goals of treatment are to preserve normal congruity of the femoral head and acetabulum (hip socket) and maintain spasm-free and pain-free range of motion in the hip joint. Currently, most children can be managed with antiinflammatory medications and bed rest for episodes of synovitis, and activity modification (avoidance of jumping activities that place increased stress on the hip). Serial x-rays are obtained to monitor the progress of the disease and to ensure that the hip remains congruent. Surgery may be necessary if the femoral head becomes subluxed or incongruent with the acetabulum.[1,2,16]

Osgood-Schlatter Disease

Osgood-Schlatter disease consists of tendinitis of the anterior patellar tendon, within which the patella (kneecap) is embedded, and associated osteochondrosis of the tubercle of the tibia. Osgood-Schlatter disease occurs most frequently in preadolescents and adolescents who participate in sports and is more prevalent in boys than in girls.

The severity of the lesion varies from mild tendinitis to a complete separation of the anterior extension of the tibial epiphysis, which is the part of the epiphysis that contributes to growth of the tibial tubercle. The mildest form of Osgood-Schlatter disease causes ischemic (avascular) necrosis in the region of the bony tibial tubercle, with hypertrophic cartilage formation during the stages of repair. In more severe cases the abnormality involves a true epiphyseal separation of the tibial tubercle with avascular necrosis.

The child complains of pain and swelling in the region around the patellar tendon and tibial tubercle, which becomes prominent and is tender to direct pressure. The pain is most severe after physical activity that involves vigorous quadriceps contraction or direct local trauma to the tibial tubercle area. Sudden onset of pain is caused by a pathologic fracture through an area of ischemic necrosis.

The goal of treatment for Osgood-Schlatter disease is to decrease the stress at the tubercle. Often a period of 4 to 8 weeks of restriction from strenuous physical activity, especially activities requiring deep knee bending, is sufficient. If relief from pain is not achieved, a cast is required to immobilize the knee, a situation that is particularly difficult if the condition is bilateral.

Gradual resumption of activity is permitted after 8 weeks, but return to unrestricted athletic participation requires an additional 8 weeks to allow for revascularization, healing, and ossification of the tibial tubercle.[1,17]

MUSCULAR DYSTROPHY

The *muscular dystrophies* are a group of familial disorders that cause degeneration of skeletal muscle fibers. The most prevalent of the muscle diseases in childhood, the muscular dystrophies are characterized by progressive, symmetric weakness and wasting of skeletal muscle groups, with increasing disability and deformity.

The muscular dystrophies are classified according to age of onset, rate of progression, distribution of muscular involvement, and inheritance patterns. The major types that are clinically and genetically distinct are the pseudohypertrophic (Duchenne), facioscapulohumeral, limb girdle, ocu-

lopharyngeal, and myotonic muscular dystrophies (Fig. 38-6 and Table 38-2). Because the clinical findings and genetic inheritance patterns are consistent for each type, each may involve a separate biochemical defect, as yet unknown. Current research points to defects in muscle fiber membrane as either a cause or result of an unknown biochemical abnormality. Genetic research has focused on identifying the locus for the abnormal genes to permit more accurate carrier detection and, eventually, description of the biochemical aberration.[2,3]

The physiology of all types of muscular dystrophy is more or less the same. The genetic abnormality may cause an abnormality in the intracellular metabolism of the muscle fibers, perhaps in an enzyme system within the muscle cell or in muscle metabolism, so that the ability to absorb or metabolize a substance vital to muscular function is impaired. Creatine metabolism is defective, and levels of intramuscular enzymes in the glycolytic system are decreased.

Muscle cells show necrosis and phagocytosis, and fibers are eventually replaced with fat (causing fatty infiltration) and connective tissues (causing fibrosis). The involved muscle fibers are randomly distributed—there is no distinct pattern.

Duchenne Muscular Dystrophy

In 1868 the French neurologist G.B.A. Duchenne described a pseudohypertrophic muscular paralysis associated with large amounts of fat and connective tissue. Today, *Duchenne muscular dystrophy (DMD)*, the most severe type, is the most common muscular dystrophy, occurring in approximately 1 in 3500 male births. This prevalence figure is similar among all ethnic groups studies so far.[16] It is a myopathy caused by mutations in the dystrophin gene located on the short arm of the X chromosome. A protein called *dystrophin* is present in normal muscle cells; it is abnormal in structure, reduced, or absent in Duchenne muscular dystrophy (Fig. 38-7). Dystrophin is thought to be involved in maintaining the structural integrity of the cell's cytoskeleton. Dystrophin also occurs in the brain, and about one third of people with DMD show metal retardation. As an X-linked inherited disorder, it affects only boys.

Duchenne muscular dystrophy causes muscle bulk to diminish, and in later stages a predominant pink or yellowish pink replaces the dark red staining of normal muscle. Interstitial fibrous connective tissue and fat eventually replace muscle fibers. Although fibers regenerate in the younger child, they are abnormal in many ways and become nonfunctional with time.

Duchenne muscular dystrophy is usually identified at about 3 years of age, with parents noting slow motor development with progressive weakness and muscle wasting. Sitting, standing, and walking are delayed, and the child is clumsy, falls frequently, and has difficulty climbing stairs.

Muscular weakness always begins in the pelvic girdle, causing a "waddling" gait. Hypertrophy of the calf muscles is apparent in 80% of cases. The method of rising from the

TABLE 38-2   Major Muscular Dystrophy Syndromes

Disease	Mode of Inheritance	Age at Clinical Onset	Usual Distribution	Rate of Progression	Mental Retardation	Distinguishing Findings
Duchenne muscular dystrophy (DMD)	X-linked recessive, sporadic	1-3 yr	Hips and shoulders, quadriceps femoris, gastrocnemius (pseudohypertrophy)	Rapid	Frequent	Elevated serum enzymes (CK, LDH, AST [formerly SGOT], aldolase)
Facioscapulohumeral (FSH) dystrophy	Autosomal dominant	Early adolescence; over 8 yr	Shoulder girdle, neck, face, pelvic girdle (late)	Moderate	Occasional	Several distinct muscle pathologic conditions
Limb girdle (LG) dystrophy	Poorly defined or recessive	Late childhood or during adolescence; over 8 yr	Pelvic and shoulder girdles	Variable	Variable	Collection of several diseases
Myotonic dystrophy (MyD)	Autosomal dominant	Variable—birth to fifth decade	Distal extensor muscle, eyelids, face, neck, hands, pharynx	Slow, related to age at clinical onset, faster with younger patients	Frequent	Percussion myotonia, cataracts, diabetic GTT despite increased insulin, testicular atrophy, decreased IgG

CK, Creatine kinase; LDH, lactic dehydrogenase; AST, aspartate transaminase; SGOT, serum glutamic oxaloacetic transaminase; GTT, glucose tolerance test, IgC, immunoglobulin C.

Fig. 38-6 *Initial muscle groups involved in three types of muscular dystrophy.* **A,** Pseudohypertrophic. **B,** Facioscapulohumeral. **C,** Limb girdle. *(From Wong, D.L. et al. [1999].* Whaley & Wong's nursing care of infants and children *[6th ed.]. St. Louis: Mosby.)*

Fig. 38-7 *Duchenne muscular dystrophy.* **A,** Patient with late-stage Duchenne muscular dystrophy showing severe muscle loss. **B,** Transverse section of gastrocnemius muscle from a normal boy. **C,** Transverse section of gastrocnemius muscle from a boy with Duchenne muscular dystrophy. Normal muscle fiber is replaced with fat and connective tissue. *(From Jorde, L.B. et al. [1999]. Medical genetics [2nd ed.]. St. Louis: Mosby.)*

floor by "climbing up the legs" (Gowers sign) is characteristic and is caused by weakness of the lumbar and gluteal muscles. The foot assumes a talipes equinovarus position, and the child tends to walk on the toes because of weakness of the anterior tibial and peroneal muscles. Within 3 to 5 years, muscles of the shoulder girdle become involved. The deep tendon reflexes are usually depressed or absent. Contractures and wasting of the muscles contribute to muscular atrophy and deformity of the skeleton. Because the disease is progressive, incapacitation often occurs by adolescence.

Duchenne muscular dystrophy has the following serious complications:

Pulmonary function: greatly compromised because of marked kyphoscoliosis ("humped" upper spine combined with scoliosis), which usually develops after the child is confined to a wheelchair

Cardiac involvement: occurs in as many as 95% of affected children, with chronic heart failure in as many as 50%

Mental retardation: affects about one third of individuals, with mean IQ approximately 80

Smooth muscle dysfunction: causes megacolon, volvulus, cramping pain, and malabsorption in the gastrointestinal tract

Diagnosis is confirmed by measurement of serum enzymes, electromyography (EMG), muscle biopsy, and radiologic studies. The serum enzymes, especially creatine kinase (CK), are increased to more than 20 times normal, even during infancy and before the onset of weakness. As muscle cells die, CK leaks into the bloodstream. Histologic changes in muscle include degeneration of muscle fibers, with varied fiber size and central nuclei.

Two methods are available for prenatal diagnosis: transabdominal amniocentesis and chorionic villus biopsy sampling. Because prenatal diagnosis with chorionic villus sampling is possible much earlier than with amniocentesis, if pregnancy termination has to be carried out, it is therefore likely to be much less upsetting for the parents.[17] Elevated CK levels at birth are diagnostic indicators of Duchenne muscular dystrophy. Identification of female carriers of the disease cannot be achieved with certainty, but serum CK is elevated in 60% to 80% of carriers.

Although there is no effective treatment for Duchenne muscular dystrophy, maintaining function in unaffected muscle groups for as long as possible is the primary goal. Activity fosters maintenance of muscle function, but strenuous exercise may hasten the breakdown of muscle fibers. Range-of-motion exercises, bracing, and surgical release of contracture deformities are used to maintain normal function for as long as possible. Genetic counseling is recommended. With X-linked inheritance, male siblings of an affected child have a 50% chance of being affected and female siblings have a 50% chance of being carriers.

Progressive weakness leads to wheelchair confinement between the ages of 8 and 15 years, after which obesity or excessive thinness, kyphoscoliosis, and other complications of immobility develop. Death, usually resulting from respiratory or cardiac muscle weakness, occurs before 20 years of age. Only 25% of children with Duchenne muscular dystrophy reach the age of 21 years.[18]

✓ QUICK CHECK

What is the most common osteochrondrosis?

Why are only boys affected with Duchenne muscular dystrophy?

Why is a deficiency of dystrophin significant to the development of Duchenne muscular dystrophy?

MUSCULOSKELETAL TUMORS
Bone Tumors

Bone tumors are uncommon tumors in childhood, accounting for fewer than 5% of childhood malignancies and occurring mostly during adolescence. The two main tumors are osteosarcoma and Ewing sarcoma. Children very rarely develop fibrosarcoma, chondrosarcoma, or non-Hodgkin lymphoma of the bone.[19]

Osteosarcoma

Osteosarcoma, accounting for 60% of childhood bone tumors, is the most common bone tumor during childhood and originates in bone-producing mesenchymal cells. Tumors can be broadly classified as those arising within the bone and those arising on the surface of bone. Three fourths occur between the ages of 10 and 25 years, with most diagnosed between 15 and 19 years of age. Therefore osteosarcoma is predominantly a tumor that develops during the adolescent growth spurt. Incidence before age 15 years is the same for males and females.

Osteosarcoma may develop as a result of rapid local growth, which increases the likelihood of mutation. It can be induced by ionizing radiation, even with relatively low doses, and can be a tragic consequence of therapeutic radiation for other forms of cancer. The latent period after radiation exposure is 5 to 40 years. There has also been a link to individuals with retinoblastoma (a hereditary eye tumor). In fact, osteosarcoma is more likely to occur if the individual has bilateral retinoblastoma, confirming a genetic transmission of the eye tumor rather than a spontaneous mutation in the genes. The link between retinoblastoma and subsequent osteosarcoma occurs whether or not radiation has been part of the treatment for retinoblastoma. Osteosarcoma has been associated with a few other medical syndromes. The most well-established association involves older individuals with Paget disease of the bone and is not seen during childhood.

Osteosarcoma has not been linked to chemical carcinogens or viruses. No deoxyribonucleic acid (DNA) or ribonucleic acid (RNA) virus has been isolated.

Molecular analysis has demonstrated deletion of genetic material on the long arm of chromosome 13, which led to the identification of a tumor suppressor gene as part of the mechanism for tumor development. The oncogene *src* has also been associated with osteosarcoma.

≋ *Pathophysiology*

Osteosarcoma occurs mainly in the metaphyses of long bones, sites of active epiphyseal growth. Most tumors arise in bones involved with the knee joint at the distal end of the femur or proximal end of the tibia. As a tumor of mesenchymal cells, osteosarcoma demonstrates production of osteoid cells.

Osteosarcoma is a bulky tumor that extends beyond the bone into a soft tissue mass. It may encircle the bone and destroy the trabeculae of the diseased area. Osteosarcoma disseminates through the bloodstream, usually to the lung. As many as 25% of children diagnosed with osteosarcoma exhibit lung metastases at diagnosis. Other sites of metastatic spread include other bones and visceral organs.

≋ *Clinical Manifestations*

The most common presenting complaint is pain. The pain can be intermittent at first, but it continues and increases in severity. There may be swelling, warmth, and redness caused by the vascularity of the tumor. Symptoms may also include cough, dyspnea, and chest pain if lung metastasis is present. If a lower extremity is involved, a child may limp or suffer a pathologic fracture. Although osteosarcoma is not the result of trauma, trauma may call attention to a preexisting tumor.

≋ *Evaluation and Treatment*

The five histologic types of osteosarcoma are determined by the predominant cell type. The tumor is graded according to degree of malignancy; the higher the number, the worse the prognosis.

Surgery and chemotherapy are the primary treatments for osteosarcoma. The tumor is resistant to radiation. Traditionally, surgery includes amputation at the joint above the involved bone; however, more recent limb salvage procedures have gained acceptance, and amputation may be avoided in most children.

Chemotherapy is an important component of treatment because as many as 80% of children treated with surgery alone eventually develop metastatic disease. Currently, methotrexate, citrovorum factor rescue, adriamycin, and combinations of bleomycin, actinomycin, cyclophosphamide, ifosfamide, and cisplatin are used. These will change,

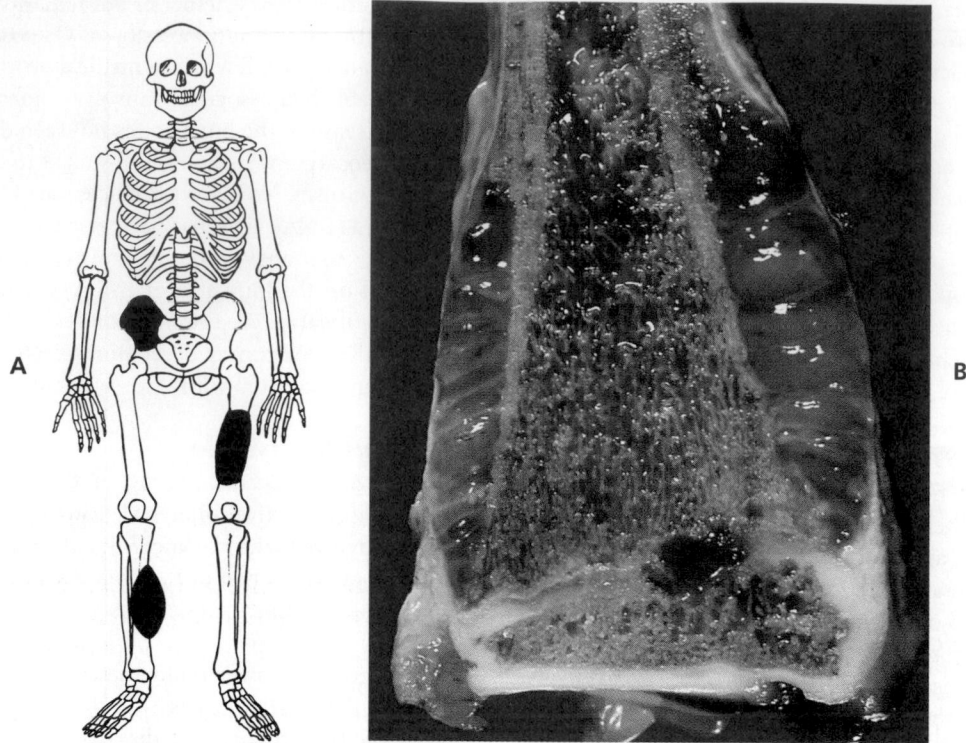

Fig. 38-8 *Ewing sarcoma.* **A,** Most common anatomic sites. **B,** Close-up view of Ewing sarcoma of the distal end of the tibia. Tumor extends into the soft tissue. *(From Damjanov, I. & Linder, J. [Eds.]. [1996]. Anderson's pathology [10th ed.]. St. Louis: Mosby.)*

however, as newer drugs are developed and found to be more effective. The role of preoperative chemotherapy is being evaluated. The use of chemotherapy with surgery has increased the 5-year survival rate to 50% or more.

A number of approaches have been used to treat pulmonary metastases. Because pulmonary metastases are generally solitary, focal lesions, thoracotomy with wedge resection has proven to be the most effective treatment.

Ewing sarcoma

Ewing sarcoma is the second most common and most lethal malignant bone tumor during childhood. This tumor is named after James Ewing, who first identified it as a separate clinical diagnosis in 1921. Ewing sarcoma probably originates from cells within the bone marrow space and does not involve bone-forming cells. The most common period of diagnosis is between 5 and 15 years of age; it is rare after age 30 years. Like osteosarcoma, Ewing sarcoma is slightly more common in males than females, and the cause is also unknown. Also like osteosarcoma, there is a link with periods of rapid bone growth. Evidence for hereditary links has not been firmly established; however, Ewing sarcoma is very rare in blacks, in both the United States and Africa, perhaps indicating some genetic resistance.

Pathophysiology

Ewing sarcoma is most commonly located in the midshaft of long bones or in flat bones. The most common sites include the femur (most common), pelvis (second most common), and humerus (Fig. 38-8). It can occur in any bone.

Arising from bone marrow, Ewing sarcoma can break through the cortex of the bone to form a soft tissue mass. Although the tumor does not form osteoid, it often contains areas of blood vessels and hemorrhage. Ewing sarcoma metastasizes to nearly every organ. Metastasis occurs early and is usually apparent at diagnosis or within 1 year. The most common sites are the lung, other bones, lymph nodes, bone marrow, liver, spleen, and central nervous system.

Clinical Manifestations

Like osteosarcoma, the most common complaint is pain that increases in severity. A soft tissue mass is often present. Additional symptoms may include fever, malaise, and anorexia.

Evaluation and Treatment

No specific laboratory test is diagnostic; however, the sedimentation rate will be elevated and lactic dehydrogenase (LDH) often is elevated, which is a poor prognostic sign. Biopsy is used to conclusively establish the diagnosis.

Previously, radiation of approximately 1500 rads was the primary treatment modality. The use of multidrug chemotherapy has improved survival rates. Recent treatment protocols call for preoperative chemotherapy followed by radiation or surgical resection, or both, with continuation of chemotherapy for 12 to 18 months afterward.

Ewing sarcoma has had a dismal prognosis with 5-year

survival rates no better than 5% to 10%. Combinations of aggressive radiation, chemotherapy, and surgical resection have, however, improved the survival rate for localized disease to more than 60%. The major predictor of prognosis appears to be the location of the primary tumor and whether metastases are present at diagnosis. The most favorable sites of involvement are the extremities; the worst prognosis involves tumors of the trunk and particularly tumors in the pelvis.

Nonossifying fibroma

The *nonossifying fibroma,* which may be a defect in ossification rather than a true tumor, makes up approximately 50% of benign bone tumors. It may begin as a fibrous, cyst-like lesion, called a *fibrous cortical defect,* in children younger than 2 years. Most fibrous cortical defects resolve spontaneously or are obliterated by reparative ossification or remodeling. In some cases, however, the fibrous cortical defect persists and proliferates, becoming a fibroma. Ninety percent of these tumors occur in persons younger than 20 years.

Nonossifying fibroma is a sharply demarcated tumor surrounded by a dense border of hardened bone. The tumor itself consists of fibrocytes arranged in whorled bundles, fibroblastic tissue, and osteoclast-like giant cells. As the tumor evolves, the fibrocytes imbibe lipids and assume a foamy appearance; thus they are known as foam cells. The tumor also contains extensive deposits of hemosiderin pigment. The tumor is characteristically located in the metaphyseal region of the bone and may cause a slight bulging of the cortex. The long axis of the tumor parallels the long axis of the bone.

The nonossifying fibroma is usually asymptomatic and is found coincidentally. If the tumor is large enough, it may cause slight swelling or localized pain. An active adolescent may first be seen with a pathologic fracture.

The fibroma is generally not treated until it occupies more than 50% of the diameter of the bone or extends more than 3 to 4 cm into the cortex. Then it is removed by curettage and the area is packed with bone chips.

Muscle Tumors

Most soft tissue tumors in children are benign. Only two malignant soft tissue tumors occur with any frequency—rhabdomyosarcoma in the younger child and synovial cell sarcoma in the teenager. Both of these occur rarely. Soft tissue tumors originate from the primitive mesenchymal cells that normally give rise to muscle, tendons, blood vessels, lymphatic structures, fibrous and connective tissue, and bursa and fascia. Table 38-3 identifies the classification of soft tissue tumors depending on origin. All malignant soft tissue tumors are highly aggressive, invade surrounding structures, and metastasize early.[19]

Rhabdomyosarcoma (RMS) is the most common soft tissue sarcoma of childhood and accounts for more than 50% of soft tissue tumors but less than 3% of all childhood cancers. RMS arises from embryonal rhabdomyoblasts that normally differentiate into mature striated muscle. The five subclassifications of RMS are (1) embryonal (most com-

TABLE 38-3	Classification of Tumors by Origin
Tissue	**Tumor**
Muscle	
Striated	Rhabdomyosarcoma
Smooth	Leiomyosarcoma
Adipose	Liposarcoma
Fibrous	Fibrosarcoma
Synovial mesothelium	Synovial sarcoma
Lymphatic structures	Lymphangiosarcoma
Blood vessels	Hemangiopericytoma
Nerve sheath	Neurogenic sarcoma

mon), (2) botryoid, (3) alveolar, (4) pleomorphic, and (5) undifferentiated cell types I or II (rare). The pleomorphic variety of RMS occurs in adults but is uncommon in children.

RMS can develop anywhere striated muscle is located. The primary locations and percentage ranges of incidence are (1) the head and neck (including the orbit), 61% to 36%; (2) the trunk, 33% to 8%; (3) the extremities, 24% to 14%; and (4) the genitourinary tract, 17% to 10%. Two age ranges (2 to 6 years of age and 15 to 19 years of age) are associated with RMS. More than two thirds of children with RMS are diagnosed by 10 years of age, and RMS is slightly more common in males than females.

Although RMS can be induced in laboratory animals with viruses, chemical carcinogens, and heavy metal compounds, similar links have not been established in humans. On rare occasions, familial cases have been reported, sometimes associated with congenital malformations. RMS also has been reported to be a complication of neurofibromatosis and has been associated with breast cancer. Embryonal tumors of rhabdomyosarcoma are characterized by abnormalities (e.g., gene deletions) on chromosome 11, whereas alveolar tumors are characterized by a translocation between chromosomes 2 and 13. Studies to date indicate association between *p53* (a tumor suppressor gene) mutations and sporadic childhood RMS.[20]

Pathophysiology

Rhabdomyosarcoma generally appears as a firm, fleshy, grayish white mass. It sometimes exhibits variations, particularly with the botryoid subclassification, which appears as a cystic polypoid mass. Depending on the phase of differentiation of the rhabdomyoblast, this tumor may have round or spindle-shaped, tadpole-shaped, or multinucleated giant cells.

The *embryonal subclass of RMS* is the most common, and the cells are generally round or spindle shaped because of their primitive stage. These tumors do not show striations and are consistent with the appearance of developing muscle in the 7- to 10-week-old fetus. Embryonal RMS is more common in younger children and is usually found in the head and neck region.

The *botryoid subclass of RMS* is very similar to the embryonal subclass. The gross appearance is often a bizarre polypoid, glistening, edematous "cluster of grapes" that is a mass of stroma and dilated blood vessels. Botryoid RMS is most common in young children and favors hollow viscera, including the bladder, vagina, common bile duct, ear, nasopharynx, and uterus.

The *alveolar subclass of RMS* is the most common type of RMS in adolescents. It generally involves an extremity or the perineal and perirectal areas and appears firmer than the embryonal and botryoid types. The tumor is composed of clusters of small, round rhabdomyoblasts and may have multinucleated giant cells. The alveolar subclass represents a higher degree of cellular differentiation than the embryonal or botryoid subtypes. The cell pattern is consistent with the hollow tube stage of normal muscle development seen in the 10- to 12-week-old fetus.

The *pleomorphic subclass of RMS* accounts for only 2% of pediatric RMS and is sometimes seen in adults during the third to fifth decade. It is composed of multinucleated giant cells and racket-shaped cells. The tumor cells appear as mature striated muscle that has become dedifferentiated.

The *undifferentiated cell types of RMS* are a relatively new subclass. Similar in appearance to Ewing sarcoma (a bone tumor), they are most commonly found in the extremities.

RMS spreads by rapid local infiltration, as well as through the bloodstream and lymphatic system. At least 20% of children with RMS have metastatic disease at diagnosis. The preferred sites of metastases include the lungs, lymph nodes, bone marrow, liver, brain, and bone.

Clinical Manifestations

The signs and symptoms of RMS depend on the anatomic location of the primary tumor and presence of symptomatic metastases. The tumors are usually painless, and early detection of RMS is facilitated by the presence of a palpable or visible mass. Deep-seated tumors cause functional impairment. The clinical manifestations of RMS are outlined in Table 38-4.

Evaluation and Treatment

Staging of RMS is based on the classification system of the Intergroup Rhabdomyosarcoma Study, a national cooperative study group. Four stages are proposed based on the resectability of the tumor. Approximately 15% of children have stage I disease (localized disease, completely resected); approximately 28% of children have stage II disease (grossly resected tumor with microscopic residual or regional disease that is totally resected); approximately 36% of children have stage III disease (gross residual disease); and approximately 20% of children have stage IV disease (metastatic disease present). Rhabdomyosarcoma is treated by a combination of surgery, radiation, and chemotherapy. Complete surgical resection provides the greatest assurance that cure can be achieved; however, cure occurs in only 16% of children. If surgical resection leads to serious disfigurement or functional disability (e.g., enucleation for orbital tumors or cys-

TABLE 38-4	Clinical Manifestations of Rhabdomyosarcoma
Location	**Manifestation**
Head and neck	
Orbit	Ptosis
	Exophthalmos
	Proptosis
Paranasal sinuses	Nasal obstruction
	Epistaxis
	Swelling
	Chronic sinusitis
Nasopharynx	Hypernasal speech
	Nasal discharge
	Visible polypoid mass
Oropharyngeal	Dysphagia
	Painful mastication
Middle ear	Chronic serous otitis media
	Discharge from affected ear
	Facial nerve palsy
	Conduction hearing loss
	Visible polypoid mass
Extremities	
All locations	Deep-seated, fixed palpable mass
Retroperitoneal	
All locations	Usually asymptomatic
	May have vague abdominal pain
	Bowel or genitourinary obstruction (late)
	Possible palpable mass
Genitourinary	
Vaginal	Abnormal vaginal bleeding
	Protruding polypoid mass
Prostate	Urinary tract obstruction
Bladder	Urinary retention
	Straining to void
	Hematuria
Paratesticular	Mass in scrotum that may be painful

tectomy for bladder tumors), chemotherapy and radiation serve as the primary treatment and surgery is avoided. If there is a high likelihood of local recurrence, however, as is the case for testicular and prostate tumors, radical orchiectomies and hemiscrotectomy will be used. For all tumors except stage I disease, local radiation therapy is given. A variety of combination chemotherapies are used with RMS. Agents shown to be effective include vincristine, actinomycin D, cisplatin, VP-16, carboplatin, etoposide, and cyclophosphamide. Chemotherapy for stage I or II disease is given for 1 year if there is no disease recurrence. For stage III or IV, treatment continues an additional year combined with radiation therapy. Intrathecal chemotherapy is given to children whose tumor locations favor central nervous system spread.

The primary prognostic factor in RMS is the degree of residual disease that remains after surgical resection. Children with localized disease (stages I and II) have long-term survival rates reported at 70% to 80%. If widespread disease is present, long-term survival rates drop to 20%. Orbital tumors have an overall favorable prognosis, probably because of the lack of lymphatics in the area and early physical signs of disease.

✓ QUICK CHECK

Why is rapid growth associated with osteosarcoma?

What are the two main bone tumors in children?

Why would mutation of *p53* be related to the development of rhabdomyosarcoma?

▣ DID YOU UNDERSTAND?

Musculoskeletal Alterations in Children

1. Developmental dysplasia of the hip is an abnormality in the development of the proximal femur, acetabulum, or both. It is a serious and disabling condition in children if not diagnosed and treated.
2. Foot deformities are common in children and may result from intrauterine positioning or embryonic malformations. Two common deformities include metatarsus adductus and talipes equinovarus.
3. Osteogenesis imperfecta (brittle bone disease) is an inherited disorder of collagen that affects primarily bones and results in serious fractures of many bones.
4. Scoliosis is a lateral curvature of the spinal column that can be caused by congenital malformations of the spine, poliomyelitis, skeletal dysplasias, spastic paralysis, and unequal leg length, but it is most often idiopathic.
5. Osteomyelitis is a local or generalized bacterial infection of bone and bone marrow. Bacteria are usually introduced by direct extension from a nearby infection, through the bloodstream, or by trauma.
6. Juvenile rheumatoid arthritis is an inflammatory joint disorder characterized by pain and swelling.
7. Avascular diseases of the bone are collectively referred to as osteochondroses and are caused by an insufficient blood supply to growing bones.
8. Legg-Calvé-Perthes disease is one of the most common osteochondroses. This disorder is characterized by epiphyseal necrosis or degeneration of the head of the femur followed by regeneration or recalcification.
9. Osgood-Schlatter disease is characterized by inflammation or partial separation of the tibial tubercle caused by chronic irritation, usually as a result of overuse of the quadriceps muscles. The condition is seen primarily in muscular, athletic adolescent males.
10. The muscular dystrophies are a group of genetically transmitted diseases characterized by progressive atrophy of symmetric groups of skeletal muscles without evidence of involvement or degeneration of neural tissue. There is an insidious loss of strength in all forms of the disorder with increasing disability and deformity.
11. The two main types of malignant childhood bone tumors are osteosarcoma and Ewing sarcoma.
12. Osteosarcoma, the most common malignant childhood bone tumor, originates in bone-producing mesenchymal cells and is most often located in the distal end of the femur or proximal end of the tibia.
13. Most childhood osteosarcoma cases are diagnosed between 15 and 19 years of age and occur equally in males and females.
14. Ewing sarcoma originates from cells within the bone marrow space and is most often located in the midshaft of long bones or in flat bones.
15. Ewing sarcoma is more common in males and is most frequently diagnosed between the ages of 5 and 15 years.
16. Pain is the usual presenting symptom for either osteosarcoma or Ewing sarcoma.
17. The primary treatments for osteosarcoma are surgery and chemotherapy. The primary treatment for Ewing sarcoma is a combination of chemotherapy, radiation, and surgery.
18. The most common type of childhood soft tissue tumor is rhabdomyosarcoma.
19. Rhabdomyosarcoma originates from embryonal rhabdomyoblasts that normally differentiate into mature striated muscle. There are five subtypes.
20. Clinical manifestations of rhabdomyosarcoma depend on the anatomic location; superficial tumors exhibit a painless palpable mass, whereas deep-seated tumors cause functional impairment.
21. Rhabdomyosarcoma is treated with a combination of surgery, radiation, and chemotherapy.

KEY TERMS

Alveolar subclass of RMS, 1088
Antalgic abductor lurch, 1081
Botryoid subclass of RMS, 1087
Developmental dysplasia of the hip (DDH), 1076
Duchenne muscular dystrophy (DMD), 1082
Dystrophin, 1082
Embryonal subclass of RMS, 1087
Ewing sarcoma, 1086
Idiopathic scoliosis, 1076

Involucrum, 1078
Juvenile rheumatoid arthritis (JRA), 1079
Legg-Calvé-Perthes disease, 1081
Metatarsus adductus, 1076
Muscular dystrophy, 1082
Nonossifying fibroma, 1087
Nonstructural scoliosis, 1076
Osgood-Schlatter disease, 1082
Osteochondrosis, 1080
Osteogenesis imperfecta (brittle bone disease), 1076

Osteomyelitis, 1076
Osteosarcoma, 1085
Pleomorphic subclass of RMS, 1088
Rhabdomyosarcoma (RMS), 1087
Secondary suppurative arthritis, 1078
Sequestrum (pl., sequestra), 1078
Structural scoliosis, 1076
Talipes equinovarus (clubfoot), 1076
Undifferentiated cell types of RMS, 1088

REFERENCES

1. McCullough, L. & Lyman, K.S. (1998). Musculoskeletal considerations across the life span. In S.J. Gates & P.A. Mooar (Eds.). *Musculoskeletal primary care* (pp. 1-47). Philadelphia: Lippincott.
2. Morrissy, R. & Weinstein, S. (Eds.). (1996). *Lovell and Winter's pediatric orthopaedics* (4th ed.). Philadelphia: Lippincott-Raven.
3. Cummings, R.J. & Lovell, W.W. (1988). Operative treatment of congenital idiopathic club foot. *Journal of Bone and Joint Surgery, 70A*(7), 1108-1112.
4. Kyzer, S.P. & Stark, S.L. (1995). Congenital idiopathic clubfoot deformities. *AORN Journal, 61*(3), 492-506.
5. Minch, C.M. & Kruse, R.W. (1998). Osteogenesis imperfecta: A review of basic science and diagnosis. *Orthopedics, 21*(5), 558-568; quiz, 568-569.
6. Cole. W.G. (1997). The Nicholas Andry Award–1996. The molecular pathology of osteogenesis imperfecta. *Clinical Orthopedics, 343*, 243-248.
7. Kocher, M.S. & Shapiro, F. (1998). Osteogenesis imperfecta. *Journal of the American Academy of Orthopaedic Surgeons, 6*(4), 225-236.
8. Cordover, A.M. et al. (1997). Natural history of adolescent thoracolumbar and lumbar idiopathic scoliosis into adulthood. *Journal of Spinal Disorders, 10*(3), 193-196.
9. Sawark, J.F. & Kramer, A. (1998). Pediatric spinal deformity. *Current Opinions in Pediatrics, 10*(1), 82-86.
10. Spencer, C.H. (1998). Bone and joint infections in children. *Current Opinions in Rheumatology, 10*(5), 494-497.
11. Shetty, A.K. & Gedalia, A. (1998). Septic arthritis in children. *Rheumatic Disease Clinics of North America, 24*(2), 287-304.
12. Sathananthan, R. & David, J. (1997). The adolescent with rheumatic disease. *Archives of Disease in Childhood, 77*(4), 355-358.
13. Schaller, J.G. (1997). Juvenile rheumatoid arthritis. *Pediatrics in Review, 18*(10), 337-349.
14. Jarvis, J.N. (1998). Pathogenesis and mechanisms of inflammation in the childhood rheumatic diseases. *Current Opinions in Rheumatology, 10*(5), 459-467.
15. Mangge, H. & Schauenstein, K. (1998). Cytokines in juvenile rheumatoid arthritis (JRA). *Cytokine, 10*(6), 471-480.
16. Jorde, L.B. et al. (1999). *Medical genetics* (2nd ed.). St. Louis: Mosby.
17. Kaeding, C.C. & Whitehead, R. (1998). Musculoskeletal injuries in adolescents. *Primary Care, 25*(1), 211-223.
18. Jones, K.J. & North, K.N. (1997). Recent advances in diagnosis of the childhood muscular dystrophies. *Journal of Paediatrics and Child Health, 33*(93), 195-201.
19. Heinrich, S.D. & Scarborough, M.T. (Eds.). (1996). Evaluation of the child with a bone or soft-tissue neoplasm. *Orthopedic Clinics of North America, 27*(3), 431-451.
20. Dehner, L.P. (1998). The evolution of the diagnosis and understanding of primitive and embryonic neoplasms in children: Living through an epoch. *Modern Pathology, 11*(7), 669-685.

CHAPTER

39

Structure, Function, and Disorders of the Integument

Sue E. Huether

The skin is the largest organ of the body. Combined with the accessory structures of hair, nails, and glands, it forms the integumentary system. The skin covers the entire body and accounts for approximately 20% of the body's weight. The primary function of the skin is to protect the body from the environment by serving as a barrier against microorganisms, ultraviolet radiation, loss of body fluids, and the stress of mechanical forces. The skin also regulates body temperature within a very narrow range and is involved in the production of vitamin D. Touch and pressure receptors provide important protective functions and pleasurable sensations.

CHAPTER OUTLINE

STRUCTURE AND FUNCTION OF THE SKIN

Layers of the Skin

The skin is formed of two major layers: (1) a superficial or outer layer of *epidermis* and (2) a deeper layer of *dermis* (the true skin) (Fig. 39-1). The *hypodermis* is an underlying layer of connective tissue that contains macrophages, fibroblasts, and fat cells. Each skin layer contains cells that represent progressive stages of skin cell differentiation as the skin grows. These are summarized in Table 39-1.

HEALTH ALERT

Tissue Adhesives for Closure of Skin Lacerations

Tissue adhesives or glue (octylcyanoacrylate) is a pliable, waterproof adhesive film that can be applied to a laceration and left in place until it disintegrates in 7 to 14 days. It is appropriate for use in simple lacerations in areas where there is not excessive mobility or tension. The adhesives are particularly useful in children because they are painless and easy to apply and have good cosmetic results when compared with monofilament sutures.

Data from Burns, T.B. et al. (1998). A new tissue adhesive for laceration repair in children. Journal of Pediatrics, *132(6), 1067-1070; Penoff, J. (1999). Skin closures using cyanoacrylate tissue adhesives.* Plastic Surgery Educational Foundation DATA Committee. Device and technique assessment. *Plastic and Reconstructive Surgery, 103(2), 730-731.*

Dermal appendages

The *dermal appendages* include the nails, hair, *sebaceous glands,* and the eccrine and apocrine *sweat glands.* The nails are protective keratinized plates that appear at the ends of fingers and toes. They have four structural units: (1) the proximal nail fold, (2) the matrix from which the nail grows, (3) the hyponychium (the nail bed), and (4) the nail plate (Fig. 39-2). Nail growth continues throughout life at 1 mm or less per day.

Hair color, density, grain, and pattern of distribution vary considerably and depend on age, gender, and race. Hair follicles arise from the matrix (or bulb) located deep in the dermis. They extend from the dermis at an angle and have an erector pili muscle attached near the middermis that straightens the follicle when contracted, causing the hair to stand up. Hair growth begins in the bulb, with cellular differentiation occurring as the hair progresses up the follicle. Hair is fully hardened, or cornified, by the time it emerges at the skin surface. Hair growth is cyclic, with periods of growth and rest that vary over different body surfaces.

The *sebaceous glands* open onto the surface of the skin through a canal. They are found in greatest numbers on the face, chest, and back, with modified glands on the eyelids, lips, nipples, glans penis, and prepuce. Sebaceous glands se-

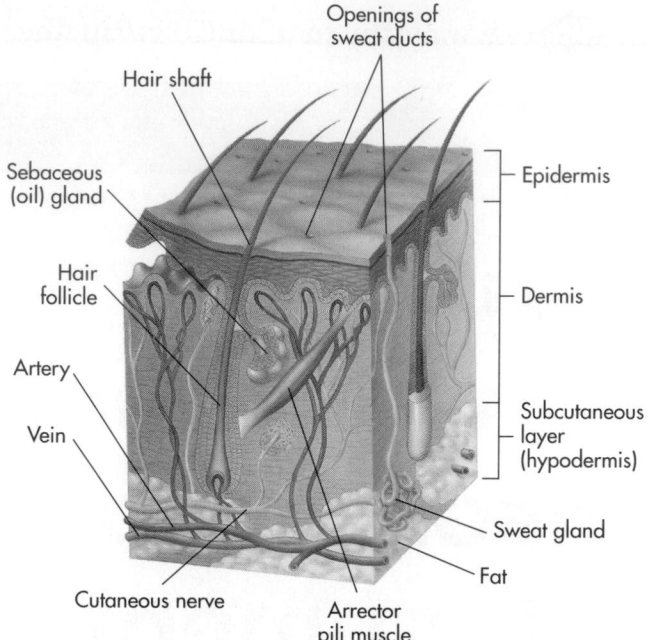

Fig. 39-1 *Structure of the skin. (From Thibodeau, G.A. & Patton, K.T. [1999].* Anatomy & physiology *[4th ed.]. St. Louis: Mosby.)*

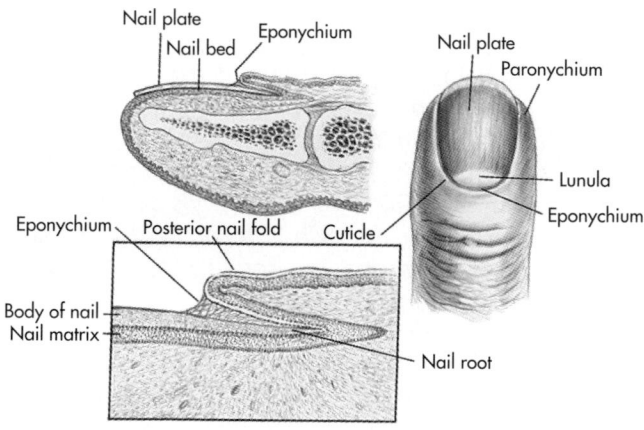

Fig. 39-2 *Structures of the nail. (From Thompson, J.M. et al. [1997].* Mosby's clinical nursing *[4th ed.]. St. Louis: Mosby.)*

crete sebum, composed primarily of lipids, which oils the skin and hair and prevents drying. Growth of sebaceous glands is stimulated by testosterone, and their enlargement is an early sign of puberty.

The *eccrine sweat glands* are distributed over the body, with the greatest numbers in the palms of the hands, soles of the feet, and forehead. They are important in thermoregulation and cooling of the body through evaporation. The *apocrine sweat glands* are fewer in number and are located in the axillae, scalp, face, abdomen, and genital area.

Blood supply and innervation

The blood supply to the skin is limited to the *papillary capillaries,* or plexus, of the dermis. These capillary loops are

TABLE 39-1   Layers of the Skin

Structure	Cell Types	Characteristics
Epidermis	Keratinocytes and melanocytes	Most important layer of skin; normally very thin (0.12 mm) but can thicken and form corns or calluses with constant pressure or friction
	Langerhans cells	Cells with dendrite process and immune functions
Stratum corneum	Keratinocytes and melanocytes	Tough superficial layer covering the body
Stratum lucidum	Keratinocytes and melanocytes	Clear layer of cells containing eleidin, which becomes keratin as cells move up to corneum layer
Stratum granulosum	Keratinocytes and melanocytes	Keratohyalin gives a granular appearance to this layer
Stratum spinosum	New keratinocytes	Polygonal-shaped with spinous processes projecting between adjacent keratinocytes
Stratum germinativum	Keratinocytes	Basal layer where keratinocytes divide and move upward to replace cells shed from the surface
Dermis Papillary layer Reticular layer	Collagen, elastin, reticulin, ground substance	Irregular connective tissue layer with rich blood, lymphatic, and nerve supply; contains sensory receptors and special glands
Hypodermis		Subcutaneous tissue or superficial fascia of varying thickness that connects the overlying dermis to underlying muscle

supplied by a deeper arterial plexus. Branches from the deep plexus also supply hair follicles and sweat glands. A subpapillary network of veins drains the capillary loops. Arteriovenous anastomoses in the dermis facilitate the regulation of body temperature. Heat loss can be regulated by varying blood flow through the skin by opening and closing the arteriovenous anastomoses in conjunction with evaporative heat loss of sweat. The sympathetic nervous system regulates both vasoconstriction and vasodilation. Only α-adrenergic receptors are in the skin. The lymphatic vessels of the skin arise in the papillary dermis and drain into larger subcutaneous trunks, removing cells, proteins, and immunologic mediators.

✓ QUICK CHECK

Describe the two layers of the skin.

How do the skin blood vessels regulate body temperature?

What cells of the skin regulate immune function?

Clinical Manifestations of Skin Dysfunction
Lesions

Identification of the morphologic structure and appearance of the skin in combination with a health history is necessary to identify underlying pathophysiology. Table 39-2 describes and illustrates the basic lesions of the skin. Special skin lesions are described in Table 39-3.

Pressure ulcers

Pressure ulcers, or pressure sores, are ischemic ulcers resulting from pressure and shearing forces. The term *decubitus*

Ⓐ AGING & *Changes in Skin Integrity*

Skin becomes thinner, dryer, and wrinkled

Epidermal cells contain less moisture and change shape

Dermoepidermal border flattens, shortening and decreasing number of capillary loops

Fewer melanocytes, giving decreased protection from ultraviolet radiation and leading to graying of hair

Irregular pigmentation

Loss of the rete pegs, giving smooth, shiny appearance

Loss of elastin, producing wrinkling

Dermis thins, producing translucent, paper-thin quality

Loss of flexibility of collagen fibers, so skin cannot stretch and regain shape as readily

Barrier function of strateum corneum reduced

Dermis more permeable and less able to clear substances, so they accumulate and cause irritation

Atrophy of eccrine, apocrine, and sebaceous glands, causing dry skin

Significantly decreased Langerhans cells, reducing the skin's immune response

Pressure and touch receptors and free nerve endings decrease, causing reduced sensory perception

Decreased wound healing as a result of decreased blood flow and slower rate of basal cell turnover

With compromised temperature regulation, loss of cutaneous vasomotion and decreased eccrine sweat production, there is increased risk of heat stroke and hypothermia

Thinning of nail plate and more brittle nails

Data from Timiras, P.S. (1994). Physiological basis of aging and geriatrics. Boca Raton, Fla.: CRC Press; Gilchrest, B.A. (1996). A review of skin aging and its medical therapy. British Journal of Dermatology, 135(6), 867-875.

Text continued on p. 1099

TABLE 39-2	Primary and Secondary Skin Lesions	
Primary Skin Lesions	**Examples**	

Macule
A flat, circumscribed area that is a change in the color of the skin; less than 1 cm in diameter

Freckles, flat moles (nevi), petechiae, measles, scarlet fever

Macules[c]

Papule
An elevated, firm, circumscribed area less than 1 cm in diameter

Wart (verruca), elevated moles, lichen planus

Flat warts[c]
(Courtesy Dr. E. Sahn.)

Patch
A flat, nonpalpable, irregular-shaped macule more than 1 cm in diameter

Vitiligo, port-wine stains, mongolian spots, café au lait spot

Vitiligo[h]

Plaque
Elevated, firm, and rough lesion with flat top surface more than 1 cm in diameter

Psoriasis, seborrheic and actinic keratoses

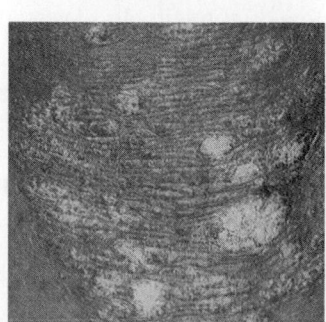

Plaque[e]

TABLE 39-2	Primary and Secondary Skin Lesions—cont'd		
Primary Skin Lesions	**Examples**		
Wheal Elevated, irregular-shaped area of cutaneous edema; solid, transient; variable diameter	Insect bites, urticaria, allergic reaction		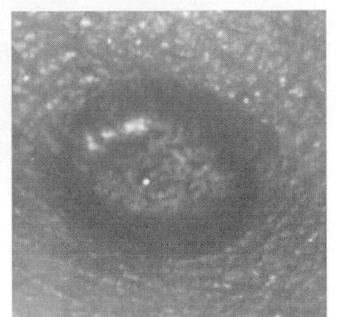 **Wheal**[c]
Nodule Elevated, firm, circumscribed lesion; deeper in dermis than a papule; 1-2 cm in diameter	Erythema nodosum, lipomas		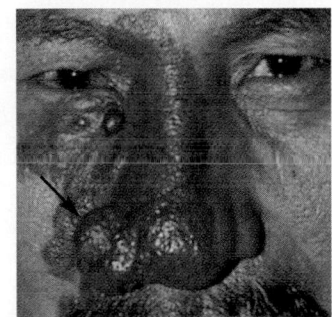 **Hypertrophic nodule**[d]
Tumor Elevated, solid lesion; may be clearly demarcated; deeper in dermis; more than 2 cm in diameter	Neoplasms, benign tumor, lipoma, hemangioma		 **Hemangioma**[h]
Vesicle Elevated, circumscribed, superficial, not into dermis; filled with serous fluid; less than 1 cm in diameter	Varicella (chickenpox), herpes zoster (shingles)		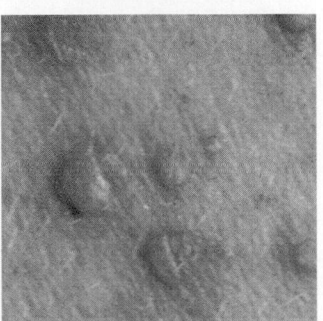 **Vesicles**[c]

Continued

TABLE 39-2 Primary and Secondary Skin Lesions—cont'd

Primary Skin Lesions	Examples		
Bulla Vesicle more than 1 cm in diameter	Blister, pemphigus vulgaris		 **Bulla**[c] **(Courtesy Dr. K.A. Riley.)**
Pustule Elevated, superficial lesion; similar to a vesicle but filled with purulent fluid	Impetigo, acne		 **Acne**[h]
Cyst Elevated, circumscribed, encapsulated lesion; in dermis or subcutaneous layer; filled with liquid or semisolid material	Sebaceous cyst, cystic acne		 **Sebaceous cyst**[h]
Telangiectasia Fine, irregular red lines produced by capillary dilation	Telangiectasia in rosacea		 **Telangiectasia**[d]

TABLE 39-2	Primary and Secondary Skin Lesions—cont'd		
Secondary Skin Lesions	**Examples**		
Scale Heaped-up, keratinized cells; flaky skin; irregular; thick or thin; dry or oily; variation in size	Flaking of skin with seborrheic dermatitis following scarlet fever, or flaking of skin following a drug reaction; dry skin		**Fine scaling**[a]
Lichenification Rough, thickened epidermis secondary to persistent rubbing, itching, or skin irritation; often involves flexor surface of extremity	Chronic dermatitis		**Stasis dermatitis in early stage**[f]
Keloid Irregular-shaped, elevated, progressively enlarging scar; grows beyond the boundaries of the wound; caused by excessive collagen formation during healing	Keloid formation following surgery		**Keloid**[h]
Scar Thin to thick fibrous tissue that replaces normal skin following injury or laceration to the dermis	Healed wound or surgical incision		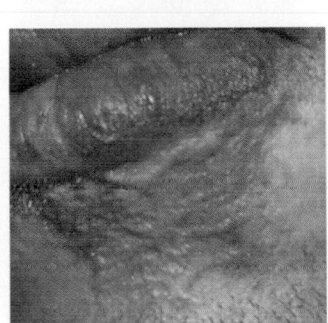 **Hypertrophic scar**[d]

Continued

TABLE 39-2	Primary and Secondary Skin Lesions—cont'd		
Secondary Skin Lesions	**Examples**		
Excoriation Loss of the epidermis; linear, hollowed-out, crusted area	Abrasion or scratch, scabies		 **Scabies**[h]
Fissure Linear crack or break from the epidermis to the dermis; may be moist or dry	Athlete's foot, cracks at the corner of the mouth		 **Fissures**[d]
Erosion Loss of part of the epidermis; depressed, moist, glistening; follows rupture of a vesicle or bulla	Varicella, variola after rupture		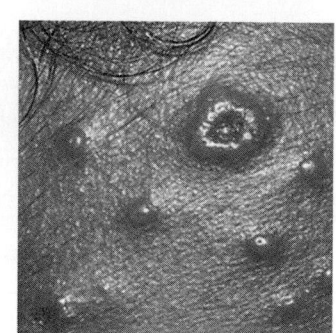 **Erosion**[b]
Ulcer Loss of epidermis and dermis; concave; varies in size	Decubiti, stasis ulcers		 **Stasis ulcer**[e]

TABLE 39-2	**Primary and Secondary Skin Lesions—cont'd**	
Secondary Skin Lesions	**Examples**	
Atrophy		
Thinning of the skin surface and loss of skin markings; skin appears translucent and paper-like	Aged skin, striae	

Aged skin[g]

From Thompson, J.M. & Wilson S.F. (1996). Health assessment for nursing practice. *St. Louis: Mosby.*

[a]Baran, R., Dawber, R.R., & Levene, G.M. (1991). Color atlas of the hair, scalp, and nails. *St. Louis: Mosby.*

[b]Cohen, B.A. (1993). Pediatric dermatology. *London: Wolfe.*

[c]Farrar, W.E. et al. (1992). Infectious diseases (2nd ed.). *London: Gower.*

[d]Goldman, M.P. & Fitzpatrick, R.E. (1998). Cutaneous laser surgery: The art and science of selective photo thermolysis (2nd ed.). *St. Louis: Mosby.*

[e]Habif, T.P. (1996). Clinical dermatology (3rd ed.). *St. Louis: Mosby.*

[f]Marks, J.G. Jr. & DeLeo, V.A. (1991). Contact and occupational dermatitis. *St. Louis: Mosby.*

[g]Seidel, H.M. et al. (1999). Mosby's guide to physical examination (4th ed.). *St. Louis: Mosby.*

[h]Weston, W.L., Lane, A.T., & Morelli, J.G. (1996). Color textbook of pediatric dermatology (2nd ed.). *St. Louis: Mosby.*

TABLE 39-3	**Special Skin Lesions**
Type	**Clinical Manifestations**
Comedone	A plug of sebaceous and keratin material lodged in the opening of a hair follicle; an open comedone has a dilated orifice (blackhead), and a closed comedone has a narrow opening (whitehead)
Burrow	A narrow, raised, irregular channel caused by a parasite
Petechiae	A circumscribed area of blood less than 0.5 cm in diameter
Purpura	A circumscribed area of blood greater than 0.5 cm in diameter
Telangiectasia	Dilated, superficial blood vessels

RISK FACTORS

PRESSURE ULCER
- Elderly persons in hospitals and nursing homes
- Neurologic disorders (spinal cord injuries, dementia, or cerebrovascular disease)
- Immobilization
- Incontinence
- Fractured femur
- Debilitation
- Lying in bed without changing position or relieving pressure over an extended period
- Lying for hours on hard x-ray and operating tables
- Chronic diseases accompanied by anemia, edema, renal failure, malnutrition, sepsis, and urinary or fecal incontinence
- Coarse bed sheets used for turning by dragging, which produces a shearing force

ulcer refers to ulcers or pressure sores that develop when an individual lies in the recumbent position for a long time. The risks for pressure ulcers are summarized in the Risk Factors box.[1]

Pressure sores usually develop over bony prominences, such as the sacrum, heels, ischia, and greater trochanters. Continuous pressure on tissue between the bony prominence and a resistant outside surface distorts capillaries and occludes the blood supply. If the pressure is relieved within a few hours, a brief period of reactive hyperemia (redness) occurs with no lasting tissue damage. If the pressure continues unrelieved, the endothelial cells lining the capillaries become disrupted with platelet aggregation, forming microthrombi

that block blood flow and cause anoxic necrosis of surrounding tissues. Pressure ulcers can be classified by stages[2]:

I. Nonblanchable erythema of intact skin

II. Partial-thickness skin loss involving epidermis or dermis

III. Full-thickness skin loss involving damage or necrosis of subcutaneous tissue that may extend to, but not through, underlying fascia

IV. Full-thickness skin loss with extensive destruction, tissue necrosis, or damage to muscle, bone, or supporting structures

A layer of dead tissue forms that appears as a blister when there is superficial damage or as a reddish blue discoloration when there is deeper tissue damage. Superficial sores are more common on the sacrum as a result of shearing or friction forces (forces parallel to the skin). Deep sores develop closer to the bone as a result of tissue distortion and vascular occlusion from pressure perpendicular to the tissue (over the heels, trochanter, and ischia).

The necrotic tissue initiates an inflammatory response, with pain, fever, and leukocytosis. Although bacteria colonize the dead tissue, the infection is usually localized and self-limiting. Proteolytic enzymes from bacteria and macrophages dissolve necrotic tissues and cause a foul-smelling discharge that resembles, but is not, pus.

Pressure sores are painful and cause an inflammatory response with hyperemia, fever, and increased white blood cell count. If the ulceration is large, toxicity and pain lead to loss of appetite, debility, and renal insufficiency. Individuals who are immunosuppressed or have diabetes mellitus may develop infection and inflammation of adjacent tissues (cellulitis) or septicemia.

The primary goal for those at risk for pressure ulcers is prevention. Turning every 2 hours and use of flotation devices and alternating pressure mattresses are effective preventive techniques. Nutrition, oxygenation, and fluid balance must be maintained.

Superficial ulcers should be covered with flat, nonbulky dressings that cannot wrinkle and cause increased pressure or friction. Spontaneous healing occurs more quickly in a moist environment.[3] Successful healing requires continued adequate relief of pressure. Large, deep pressure ulcers may require surgical débridement of necrotic tissue and opening of deep pockets for drainage.

Keloids

Keloids are sharply elevated, irregularly shaped, progressively enlarging scars caused by excessive amounts of collagen in the corneum during connective tissue repair. Seemingly inconsequential trauma may result in a keloidal reaction, particularly in blacks and Orientals. Burns incite this reaction more commonly than other types of injury.

Excessive or poorly aligned tension on a wound, introduction of foreign material into the skin, and certain types of trauma (e.g., burns) are all provocative factors. Those parts of the body at risk include shoulders, back, chin, ears, and lower legs. Most keloids appear within 1 year of trauma. Individuals 10 to 30 years of age develop lesions much more commonly than do children before puberty or older adults. A familial tendency for keloid formation has been found, with both autosomal recessive and autosomal dominant inheritance patterns being reported.

Keloids start as pink or red, firm, well-defined, rubbery plaques that persist for several months after trauma. Later, uncontrolled overgrowth causes extension beyond the site of the original wound and the tumor becomes smoother, irregularly shaped, hyperpigmented, harder, and more sympto-

Fig. 39-3 *Keloid formation. (Courtesy Department of Dermatology, School of Medicine, University of Utah.)*

matic. The fibrous tissue that accumulates in keloids is associated with increased cellularity and metabolic activity of fibroblasts. The tendency to send out *clawlike prolongations* is typical (Fig. 39-3).

Preventive measures, such as avoiding unnecessary, elective surgeries, are of paramount importance. When surgery is necessary for cosmetic reasons, having it done in early childhood is best. Scalpel surgery with strict aseptic technique and avoidance of wound tension is required. Electrosurgery or chemosurgery should be avoided. Injection of corticosteroids into the lesion often brings excellent results and is the treatment of choice.

Pruritus

Pruritus, or itching, is a symptom associated with many primary skin disorders, such as eczema or lice infestations, or it can be a manifestation of systemic disease (e.g., chronic renal failure, cholestatic liver disease, thyroid disorders, iron deficiency), or the use of opiate drugs. It may be localized or generalized and may move from one location to another.[4]

Multiple stimuli can produce itching, including substance P, histamine, heat, and electrical stimulation with a fine probe. Substance P, a neurotransmitter present throughout the nervous system, induces histamine release and wheal formation with itching when injected into the skin. Antihistamines and local anesthetics block substance P–induced itching. Lymphocytes are also present in many itching skin diseases, and lymphokines may be involved in the pathogenesis of itching. Major nerve pathways for itching are not well defined, but they may involve C fibers.[5,6]

Management of localized itching depends on the cause, and the primary condition must be treated. Symptomatic relief may be obtained from antihistamines, which also have a sedative effect. Minor tranquilizers, such as promethazine, may be effective for some causes of pruritus. Itching related to dry, rough skin (xerosis) can be managed with applications of emollients and increased environmental humidity. Topical steroids are immediately effective with some occurrences of pruritus; however, some pruritus is resistant to any type of therapy.

DISORDERS OF THE SKIN

Disruptions in skin integrity may be precipitated by trauma, abnormal cellular function, infection and inflammation, and systemic diseases.

Inflammatory Disorders

The most common inflammatory disorder of the skin is *eczema* (eczematous inflammation), an inflammatory response of the skin caused by endogenous and exogenous agents; it is often considered synonymous with dermatitis. Endogenous eczemas include atopic dermatitis and seborrheic dermatitis. Exogenous eczemas include irritant dermatitis and allergic contact dermatitis. Eczematous dermatitis is characterized by erythema, vesicles, scales, and itching. Edema, serous discharge, and crusting occur with continued irritation and scratching. In chronic eczema, the skin becomes thickened, leathery, and hyperpigmented from recurrent irritation and scratching. The location of eczema is related to the underlying cause. Eczematous inflammations need to be differentiated from other rashes and dermatoses, particularly psoriasis.

Allergic contact dermatitis

Allergic contact dermatitis is a common form of cell-mediated or delayed hypersensitivity. (See Chapter 7 for different types of allergic responses.) The response is an interaction of skin barrier function, reaction to irritants, and neuronal responses, such as itching.[7] Various allergens (e.g., microorganisms, chemicals, foreign proteins, latex, drugs, metals) can form the sensitizing antigen. Contact with poison ivy is a common example (Fig. 39-4). As the allergen comes in contact with the skin, the allergen is bound to a carrier protein, forming a sensitizing antigen. The Langerhans cells process the antigen and carry it to T cells, which then become sensitized to the antigen. Keratinocytes also may activate lymphocytes and endothelial cells in allergic contact dermatitis.[8] In latex allergy there is an increase in immunoglobulin E (IgE) antibodies.[9]

Delayed hypersensitivity is characterized by the passing of several hours before an immunologic response is apparent. The T cells play an important role because they differentiate and secrete lymphokines that affect macrophage movement and aggregation, coagulation, and other inflammatory responses (see Chapter 6). Sensitization usually develops with first exposure to the antigen, and symptoms of dermatitis occur with reexposure.

The manifestations of allergic contact dermatitis include

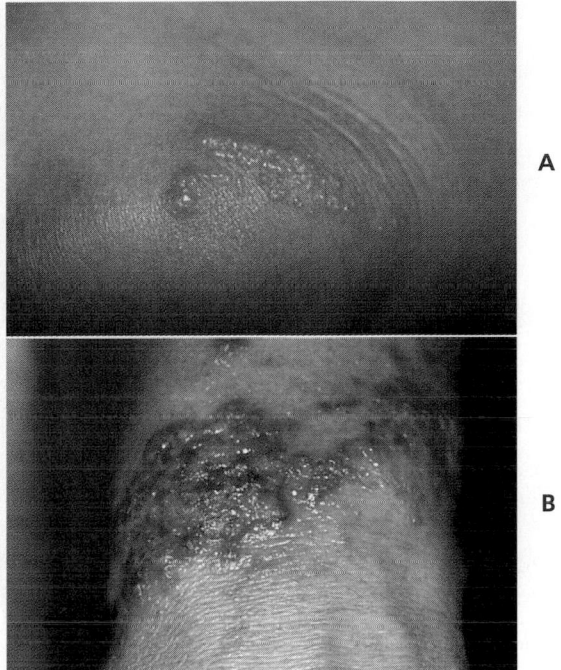

Fig. 39-4 *Poison ivy.* A, Poison ivy on knee. **B,** Poison ivy dermatitis. *(Courtesy Department of Dermatology, School of Medicine, University of Utah.)*

erythema and swelling with pruritic (itching) vesicular lesions in the areas of allergen contact. The pattern of distribution provides clues to the source of the antigen (i.e., hands exposed to chemical solutions or boundaries from rings and bracelets). Removal of the irritant is necessary for the inflammatory response to resolve and tissue repair to begin. Topical or systemic steroids may be required for treatment.

Irritant contact dermatitis

Irritant contact dermatitis is a nonimmunologically mediated inflammation of the skin. Chemical irritation from acids and prolonged exposure to soaps, detergents, and various agents used in industry can cause inflammatory lesions. The skin lesions resemble allergic contact dermatitis. Removing the source of irritation and using topical agents provide effective treatment.

Atopic dermatitis

Atopic dermatitis affects 9% to 12% of the population and has increased in incidence in the last 30 years.[10] It is more common in infancy and childhood; however, some individuals are affected throughout life. A family history of asthma, allergic rhinitis, dry skin, and eczema accompanies this disorder. The dermatitis results from the complex activation of mast cells, T lymphocytes, Langerhans cells, monocytes, IgE production by B cells, and other inflammatory cells that release histamine, lymphokines, and other inflammatory mediators (Fig. 39-5).[10,11]

During adolescence and adulthood, the lesions are usu-

Fig. 39-5 *Atopic dermatitis. (Courtesy Department of Dermatology, School of Medicine, University of Utah.)*

Fig. 39-6 *Stasis ulcer. (Courtesy Department of Dermatology, School of Medicine, University of Utah.)*

ally localized to the hands and feet or flexor surfaces (i.e., antecubital fossa, popliteal space) of the arms and legs. The erythema, scaling, and lichenification (thickened and leatherlike skin) are exacerbated by scratching, because the lesions are manifest by itching. The scratching increases susceptibility to infection from *Staphylococcus aureus* and predisposition to cutaneous dissemination of viruses, particularly herpes simplex and vaccinia. Affected individuals also have a higher incidence of cataracts.

Management of atopic dermatitis includes (1) avoidance of known irritants, (2) good lubrication, (3) preservation of skin moisture, (4) control of inflammation with steroids, (5) treatment of infection, and (6) control of itching. New treatments are directed toward normalizing immune responsiveness (i.e., topical tacrolimus).

Stasis dermatitis

Stasis dermatitis usually occurs on the legs as a result of venous stasis and edema and is associated with varicosities, phlebitis, and vascular trauma. First, erythema and pruritus develop and then scaling, petechiae, and hyperpigmentation. Progressive lesions become ulcerated, particularly around the ankles and tibia (Fig. 39-6).

Treatment includes elevating the legs as often as possible, not wearing tight clothes around the legs, and not standing for long periods. Acute inflammations are treated with antibiotics. Chronic lesions with ulceration are treated with wet dressings of Burow solution or silver nitrate. Edema is controlled with external compression.

Seborrheic dermatitis

Seborrheic dermatitis is a common chronic inflammation of the skin involving the scalp, eyebrows, eyelids, ear canals,

nasolabial folds, axillae, chest, and back (Fig. 39-7). In infants it is known as *cradle cap*. The cause is unknown, and the lesions appear from infancy to old age with periods of remission and exacerbation. The lesions appear as scaly, white or yellowish inflammatory plaques with mild pruritus. Mild cases are treated with shampoos containing sulfur, salicylic acid, or tar. Corticosteroid applications are useful for suppression of severe symptoms but should not be used for maintenance therapy.

Papulosquamous Disorders

Psoriasis, pityriasis rosea, and lichen planus are characterized by papules, scales, plaques, and erythema. Collectively they are described as *papulosquamous disorders.*

Psoriasis

Psoriasis is a chronic, relapsing, proliferative skin disorder that occurs at any age and affects 1% to 2% of the population. The onset is generally established by 20 years of age. Genetic, immunologic, and biochemical alterations and triggering agents have been investigated. T cells are thought to play a pathogenic role through cytokine production.[12] A family history of psoriasis is often established, and an HLA-associated inheritance is likely.[13]

Both the dermis and epidermis are thickened with cellular proliferation and inflammation. The turnover time for shedding the epidermis is decreased to 3 to 4 days, with many more germinative cells and increased transit time through the dermis. Cell maturation and keratinization are bypassed, and the epidermis thickens and plaques form. The loosely cohesive keratin gives the lesion a silvery appearance. Capillary dilation and increased vascularization accommodate the increased cell metabolism but also cause erythema.

Fig. 39-7 *Seborrheic dermatitis. (Courtesy Department of Dermatology, School of Medicine, University of Utah.)*

Fig. 39-8 *Psoriasis.* Typical oval plaque with well-defined borders and silvery scale. *(Courtesy Department of Dermatology, School of Medicine, University of Utah.)*

The disease can be mild, moderate, or severe, depending on the size, distribution, and inflammation of the lesions. Psoriasis is marked by remissions and exacerbations. Arthritis develops in approximately 5% of individuals with psoriasis.

The typical psoriatic lesion is a well-demarcated, thick, silvery, scaly, erythematous plaque surrounded by normal skin (Fig. 39-8). Small erythematous papules enlarge and coalesce into larger inflammatory lesions on the face, scalp, elbows, and knees and at sites of trauma. Lesions that develop in skin folds are smooth and have a deep red color. The scales are usually loosely adherent and may cause small bleeding points when removed.

In guttate psoriasis, small papules appear suddenly on the trunk and extremities (Fig. 39-9) a few weeks after a streptococcal respiratory infection. Guttate psoriasis may resolve spontaneously in weeks or months.

Treatment is related to reducing epidermal cell turnover. Mild lesions are usually treated with emollients, keratolytic agents, and corticosteroids. Moderate to severe lesions may respond to ultraviolet light, methotrexate, acitretin, and cyclosporin.[14] Severe disease may require hospitalization. Lesions of the scalp, nails, and genitalia are treated with different lotions and shampoos.

Pityriasis rosea

Pityriasis rosea is a self-limiting inflammatory disorder that occurs more frequently in young adults, usually during the winter months. The cause is thought to be a virus.[15] Pityriasis rosea begins as a single lesion *(herald patch)* that is circular, demarcated, and salmon-pink, approximately 3 to 4 cm in diameter, and usually located on the trunk. Early lesions are macular and papular. Secondary lesions develop within 14 to 21 days and extend over the trunk and upper part of the extremities (Fig. 39-10), although rarely on the face. The small erythematous papules expand into characteristic oval lesions. The pattern of distribution follows the skin lines around the trunk and resembles a drooping pine tree. As scales flake off from the margin of the lesions, a col-

Fig. 39-9 *Guttate psoriasis following streptococcal infection.* Numerous uniformly small lesions may abruptly occur following streptococcal pharyngitis. *(Courtesy Department of Dermatology, School of Medicine, University of Utah.)*

larette pattern is formed. Itching is the most common symptom. Occasionally headache, fatigue, or sore throat precedes the development of the lesions.[16]

The diagnosis of pityriasis rosea is made by the clinical appearance of the lesion. It can be confused with secondary syphilis, psoriasis, or seborrheic dermatitis. The disorder is usually self-limiting and resolves in a few months with symptomatic treatment for pruritus. Ultraviolet light or systemic corticosteroids may be used to control itching. Sun exposure facilitates resolution of the lesions.

Lichen planus

Lichen planus is a benign inflammatory disorder of the skin and mucous membranes. Some individuals develop lichenoid lesions after exposure to drugs or film processing chemicals. The age of onset is usually between 30 and 70 years. The disorder begins with nonscaling, violet-colored pruritic papules, 2 to 10 mm in size, usually located on the wrists, ankles, lower legs, and genitalia (Fig. 39-11). The

Fig. 39-10 *Pityriasis rosea herald patch.* A collarette pattern has formed around the margins. *(Courtesy Department of Dermatology, School of Medicine, University of Utah.)*

Fig. 39-11 *Hypertrophic lichen planus on arms. (Courtesy Department of Dermatology, School of Medicine, University of Utah.)*

papules are flat topped and have a polygonal shape, often with a small central depression. New lesions are pale pink and evolve into a dark violet color. Persistent lesions may be thickened and red, forming hypertrophic lichen planus. The lesions often involve the oral mucous membranes, appearing as lacy white rings that must be differentiated from leukoplakia or oral candidiasis. Mucous membrane lesions also can develop on the penis and vulvovaginal area. Usually, oral lesions do not ulcerate, but localized or extensive painful ulcerations can occur. Chronic ulcerated lesions become malignant in 1% of individuals with the disease. Thinning and splitting of nails are common, and part or all of the nail may be shed.[17]

Pruritus is the most distressing symptom. The lesions are self-limiting and may last for months or years, with an average duration of 12 to 18 months. Hyperpigmentation resulting from the inflammation is a common consequence of the lesion. Approximately 20% of individuals have a recurrence. Diagnosis is made by the clinical appearance of the lesion. Antihistamines may be given for itching, and topical or systemic corticosteroids may be used to control inflammation. Acitretin is a first-line therapy with cutaneous lesions.[18]

✓ QUICK CHECK

Why is there inflammation with contact dermatitis?

What factors are associated with atopic dermatitis?

What lesions are associated with papulosquamous disorders?

Give three examples of papulosquamous disorders.

Acne vulgaris

Acne vulgaris is an inflammatory disorder of the pilosebaceous follicle (the sebaceous gland contiguous with a hair follicle) that usually occurs during adolescence. It is discussed with pediatric skin disorders in Chapter 40.

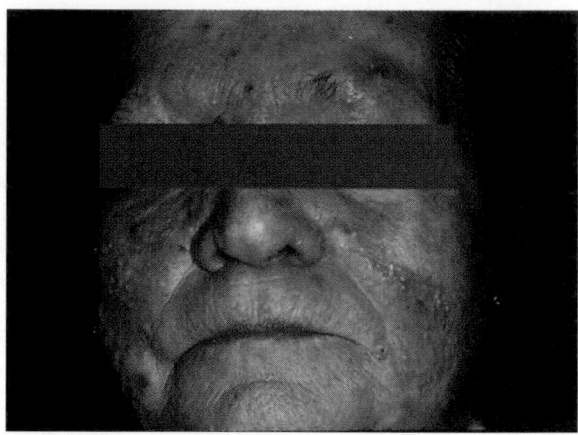

Fig. 39-12 *Granulomatous rosacea.* Pustules and erythema occur on the forehead, cheeks, and nose. *(Courtesy Department of Dermatology, School of Medicine, University of Utah.)*

Acne rosacea

Acne rosacea is a chronic inflammation of the skin that develops in middle-age adults.[19] The cause is unknown. The most common lesions are erythema, papules, pustules, and telangiectasia. They occur in the middle third of the face, including the forehead, nose, cheeks, and chin (Fig. 39-12). The lesions are associated with chronic flushing and sensitivity to the sun. Hypertrophy of the sebaceous glands may be severe enough to produce an irreversible bulbous appearance of the nose (rhinophyma). Disorders of the eye frequently accompany rosacea, particularly conjunctivitis and keratitis. Facial application of fluorinated topical steroids may precipitate rosacea-like lesions that are difficult to treat.

Hot drinks or alcohol should be taken cautiously because the heat and vasodilation accentuate erythema. Tetracycline is the drug of choice for treatment, and a low maintenance dose may be required after the most severe lesions are controlled. Surgical excision of excessive tissue may be required for rhinophyma.[20]

Lupus erythematosus

Lupus erythematosus is an inflammatory disease that expresses cutaneous manifestations. Discoid, or cutaneous, lupus erythematosus (DLE) is limited to the skin and can lead to systemic lupus erythematosus. (Systemic lupus erythematosus [SLE], a diffuse, multisystem disease, is discussed in Chapter 7.)

Discoid lupus erythematosus

Discoid lupus erythematosus (DLE) usually occurs in adults, particularly women in their late 30s or early 40s, but any age can be affected. The lesions may be single or multiple and of various sizes. Often the lesions are located on light-exposed areas of the skin, and photosensitivity is common. The face is the most common site, with a characteristic butterfly distribution over the cheeks and bridge of the nose.

The cause is thought to be an altered immune response. DLE may be described as a subset of SLE, with cutaneous manifestations as the only symptom[21] (Fig. 39-13). On skin biopsy with immunofluorescent observation, there are lumpy deposits of immunoglobulins, especially IgM.

The early lesion is asymmetric, with a 1- to 2-cm raised red plaque with a brownish scale. The scale penetrates the hair follicle and leaves a carpet-tack appearance when removed. The lesions persist for months and then resolve spontaneously or atrophy. Healing progresses from the center of the lesion, with a residual telangiectasia and hypopigmented scarring. Atrophy of the dermis and epidermis can cause a depressed scar. Scalp lesions may lead to hair loss. Other symptoms of cutaneous lupus erythematosus include alopecia (hair loss), telangiectasias, urticaria, and Raynaud phenomenon. Raynaud phenomenon is characterized by an initial stage of vasospasm that leads to white, numb, and cold digits followed by cyanosis and then a reactive hyperemia as the vasospasm relaxes.

Diagnosis of DLE is made from the presenting symptoms, biopsy of skin lesions, and Wood tests. Individuals with DLE should use sunscreen or limit direct exposure to the sun. Initial treatment with topical steroids relieves symptoms. Systemic therapy with antimalarial drugs (i.e., chloroquine sulfate, sulfasalazine) usually leads to clinical improvement within 1 to 3 months.[22] Thalidomide is effective in severe refractory cases[23] but must not be used in women who may become pregnant.

Vesiculobullous Disorders

Vesiculobullous skin disorders share a common characteristic of vesicle, or blister, formation. Two such diseases are pemphigus and erythema multiforme.

Pemphigus

Pemphigus is a chronic blister-forming disease of the skin and oral mucous membranes. The disease is relatively rare and can occur in all age-groups but is more prevalent between 40 and 50 years of age (Fig. 39-14).

Fig. 39-13 *Subacute cutaneous lupus (discoid lupus erythematosus). (Courtesy Department of Dermatology, School of Medicine, University of Utah.)*

Fig. 39-14 *Bullous pemphigoid.* Generalized eruption with blisters arising from an edematous, erythematous annular base. *(Courtesy Department of Dermatology, School of Medicine, University of Utah.)*

Pemphigus is an autoimmune disease caused by circulating IgG autoantibodies. Serum autoantibodies react with the intracellular cement or substance that holds the epidermal cells together. The antibody reaction is thought to cause the intraepidermal blister formation and acantholysis (loss of cohesion between epidermal cells) characteristic of pemphigus.[24]

The types of pemphigus are as follows:

1. *Pemphigus vulgaris:* most common form; epidermis separated above basal layer with blister formation; usually

begins with sore in mouth or on scalp, developing in 6 months to 1 year into flaccid bullous lesions that rupture easily, leaving crusty denuded skin; lesions spread to face, back, chest, umbilicus, and groin; pressure on a blister causes it to spread (Nikolsky sign); complicated by secondary infection

2. *Pemphigus foliaceus* and *pemphigus erythematosus:* less severe forms of disease; oral lesions usually absent; erythema with crusting, scaling, and bullae develops more locally; blisters in horizontal plane of stratum corneum and rupture easily, forming crusts; can spread to become more generalized

3. *Paraneoplastic pemphigus:* a recently recognized mucocutaneous form of pemphigus with intractable cutaneous lesions, distinct autoantibodies, and associated hematologic malignancies[25]

The diagnosis of pemphigus is made from the clinical manifestations and histologic examination of the skin. Immunofluorescence demonstrates the presence of antibodies at the site of blister formation. The clinical course of the disease may range from rapidly fatal to relatively benign. The primary treatment for pemphigus is systemic corticosteroids, usually in high doses during acute episodes or when there is widespread involvement. Azathioprine or mycophenolate also may be used and decreases the steroid dosage requirement. Newer methods of treatment and a clearer understanding of the pathogenesis have improved the prognosis.[26,27]

Erythema multiforme

Erythema multiforme is an acute, recurrent, inflammatory disorder of the skin and mucous membranes, often associated with immunologic or toxic reactions to herpesvirus.[28] It can occur at any age but occurs more frequently between 20 and 40 years of age. Immune complex formation and deposition of C3, IgM, and fibrinogen around the superficial dermal blood vessels, basement membrane, and keratinocytes are found in most individuals with erythema multiforme. Edema develops in the superficial dermis, so vesicles and bullae form. The lesions vary in clinical presentation and may involve the skin or mucous membranes or both. The characteristic "bull's-eye," or "target," lesions occur on the skin surface with a central erythematous region surrounded by concentric rings or alternating edema and inflammation. The lesions usually occur suddenly in groups over a period of 2 to 3 weeks. Urticarial plaques, 1 to 2 cm in diameter, can develop without the target lesion. A vesiculobullous form is characterized by mucous membrane lesions and erythematous plaques on the extensor surfaces of the extremities. Single or multiple vesicles or bullae may arise on a part of the plaque accompanied by pruritus and burning. The lesions heal within 3 to 4 weeks.

The most common form in children and young adults is *Stevens-Johnson syndrome* (severe bullous form), in which numerous erythematous bullous lesions occur on the skin and mucous membranes. An immune mechanism is probably related to drug reactions.[29] Prodromal symptoms of fever, headache, malaise, sore throat, and cough develop in approximately one third of the cases. The bullous lesions form erosions and crusts when they rupture. The mouth, air passages, esophagus, urethra, and conjunctiva may be involved. Blindness can result from corneal ulcerations. Difficulty eating, breathing, and urinating may develop with severe manifestations. The disease can involve the kidneys and extend from the upper respiratory passages into the lungs. Severe forms of the disease can be fatal.

Diagnosis is made by (1) recognition of the target lesion or by skin biopsy if the target lesion is absent and (2) medication history. Mild acute forms of the disease last 10 to 14 days and require no treatment. Ongoing drug therapy should be reevaluated and underlying infections treated. Fluid and electrolyte balance should be monitored in severe forms of the disease, and mucous membranes should be carefully managed with a bland diet, warm saline eyewashes, topical anesthetics, or corticosteroids to maintain comfort and prevent infection. Cutaneous blisters can be treated with wet compresses of Burow solution. Ophthalmic, kidney, and lung involvement require special care. Resolution occurs in 8 to 10 days, usually without scarring. Mucosal lesions may take 6 weeks to heal.

✓ QUICK CHECK

Describe the inflammatory lesion associated with lupus erythematosus.

Compare the three forms of pemphigus.

What is Stevens-Johnson syndrome?

Infections

Cutaneous infections are common forms of skin disease. They generally remain localized, although serious complications can develop with systemic involvement. The types of skin infection include bacterial, viral, and fungal. Most infections occur superficially; however, systemic signs and symptoms occasionally develop and can be life threatening. The normal flora of the skin consists of aerobes, yeast, and anaerobes. These flora often provide protection against pathogens that cause skin infections, including *Staphylococcus* and *Streptococcus.*

Bacterial infections

Most bacterial infections of the skin are caused by local invasion of pathogens. Coagulase-positive *S. aureus* and, less frequently, β-hemolytic streptococci are the common causative microorganisms.

Folliculitis

Folliculitis is a bacterial infection of the hair follicle. *S. aureus* commonly causes the infection, which develops from proliferation of the microorganism around the opening of the follicle with spread into the follicle. Inflammation is caused by the release of chemotactic factors and enzymes from the bacteria. The lesions appear as pustules with a surrounding area of erythema. They are most prominent on the scalp and extremities and rarely cause systemic symptoms. Prolonged skin moisture, skin trauma, and poor hygiene are associated contributing factors. Cleaning with soap and water and topical application of antibiotics are effective treatments.

Furuncles and carbuncles

Furuncles, or "boils," are inflammations of hair follicles (Fig. 39-15). They may develop after folliculitis that spreads through the follicular wall into the surrounding dermis. The invading microorganism is usually *S. aureus.* The infecting strain may spread to the skin from the anterior nares. Any skin area with hair can be infected, and one or several lesions may be present. The initial lesion is a deep, firm, red, painful nodule 1 to 5 cm in diameter. Within a few days, the erythematous nodules change to a large fluctuant and tender cystic nodule accompanied by cellulitis. No systemic symptoms are present, and the lesion may drain large amounts of pus and necrotic tissue.

Carbuncles are a collection of infected hair follicles and usually occur on the back of the neck, the upper back, and the lateral thighs. The lesion begins in the subcutaneous tissue and lower dermis as a firm mass that evolves into an erythematous, painful, swollen mass that drains through many openings. Abscesses may develop. Chills, fever, and malaise can occur during the early stages of lesion development.

Furuncles and carbuncles are treated with warm compresses to provide comfort and promote localization and spontaneous drainage. Abscess formation requires incision and drainage, and recurrent infections are treated with systemic antibiotics.

Cellulitis

Cellulitis is an infection of the dermis and subcutaneous tissue usually caused by *Staphylococcus.* Cellulitis can occur as an extension of a skin wound, as an ulcer, or from furuncles or carbuncles. The infected area is erythematous, swollen, and painful. The infection responds to systemic antibiotics, as well as Burow soaks to relieve pain.

Erysipelas

Erysipelas is an acute superficial infection of the skin most often caused by group A streptococci. The face, ears, and lower legs are involved. Chills, fever, and malaise precede the onset of lesions by 4 hours to 20 days. The initial lesions appear as firm, red spots that enlarge and coalesce to form a clearly circumscribed, advancing, bright red, hot lesion with a raised border. Vesicles may appear over the lesion and at the border. Itching, burning, and tenderness are present. Cold compresses provide symptomatic relief, and systemic antibiotics are required to arrest the infection.

Impetigo

Impetigo is a superficial lesion of the skin that is caused by coagulase-positive *Staphylococcus* or β-hemolytic strepto-

Fig. 39-15 *Furuncle of the forearm. (Courtesy Department of Dermatology, School of Medicine, University of Utah.)*

cocci. The disease occurs in adults but is more common in children (see Chapter 40).

Viral infections

Herpes simplex virus

There are six types of **herpes simplex virus (HSV):** HSV-1 (type 1), HSV-2 (type 2), cytomegalovirus (CMV), varicella-zoster virus, Epstein-Barr virus, and human herpes virus 6 (HHV-6).[30] A cold sore or fever blister is the most common manifestation of the herpes simplex virus.[31] HSV-1 usually occurs in nongenital sites and causes infection of the cornea (herpes keratitis), mouth (gingivostomatitis), and labia (labialis). Individuals receiving cytotoxic therapy for cancer are at risk. Genital infections are more commonly caused by HSV-2 (see Chapter 32). After penetrating the skin, HSV is established in the sensory nerve ganglion innervating the primary site. The primary infection is asymptomatic and can be determined only by a rising antibody titer.[32]

The incubation period ranges from 2 to 14 days, and clinical symptoms last 1 to 3 weeks. An individual then continues to shed the virus for 2 to 6 weeks. The virus remains dormant within sensory or autonomic nerve ganglia and can lead to recurrence of the disease with sun exposure, fever, or stress. Lesions are usually located at or near the primary site. Because anti-HSV antibodies develop in response to infection, recurrence is also related to the amount of antibodies present.

The lesions of HSV-1 appear as a rash or clusters of inflamed and painful vesicles within the mouth, over the tongue, or on the lips and around the nose (Fig. 39-16). Increased sensitivity, paresthesias, and mild burning may occur before onset of the lesion. The vesicles rupture, forming a crust. Lesions may last 2 to 6 weeks. Occasionally, there is an associated upper respiratory infection. Treatment is symptomatic, and the lesions usually resolve within 2 weeks.

Herpes zoster and varicella

Herpes zoster (shingles) and *varicella (chickenpox)* are caused by the same herpesvirus, varicella-zoster virus (VZV). Varicella occurs as a primary infection followed

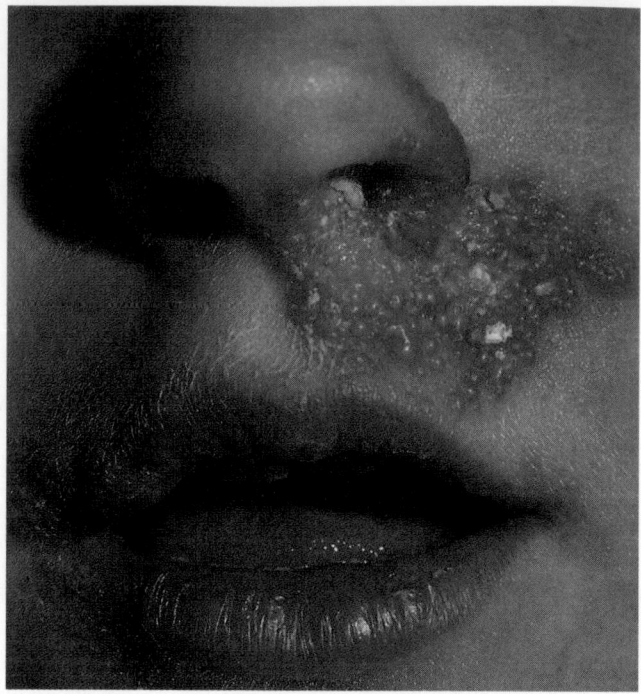

Fig. 39-16 *Herpes simplex labialis.* Typical presentation with tense vesicles appearing on the lips and extending onto the skin. *(From Habif, T.B. [1996]. Clinical dermatology: A color guide to diagnosis and therapy [3rd ed.]. St. Louis: Mosby.)*

Fig. 39-17 *Herpes zoster.* Diffuse involvement of a dermatome. *(Courtesy Department of Dermatology, School of Medicine, University of Utah.)*

Fig. 39-18 *Verruca vulgaris.* *(Courtesy Department of Dermatology, School of Medicine, University of Utah.)*

years later by herpes zoster virus. Chickenpox usually occurs in children (see Chapter 40).

Herpes zoster has initial symptoms of pain and paresthesia localized to the affected dermatome (the cutaneous area innervated by a single spinal nerve; see Chapter 12), followed by vesicular eruptions that follow along a facial, cervical, or thoracic lumbar dermatome (Fig. 39-17). Local symptoms are alleviated with compresses, calamine lotion, or baking soda. Antiviral drugs (vidarabine, acyclovir) are useful.[33] Approximately 20% of individuals experience postherpetic neuralgia (i.e., pain) treated with tricyclic antidepressants.[34]

Warts

Warts (verrucae) are benign lesions of the skin caused by the human papillomavirus(HPV). The lesions are round and elevated with a rough, grayish surface, and they can occur anywhere on the skin. Warts are transmitted by touch. Common warts (verruca vulgaris) occur most frequently in children and are usually on the fingers, although they may be located on any skin surface or mucous membrane. Warts vary in shape, size (flat, round, or fusiform), and location. Plantar warts are usually located at pressure points on the bottom of the feet (Fig. 39-18).

Condylomata acuminata (venereal warts) are cauliflower-like lesions that occur in moist areas, along the glans of the penis, vulva, and anus (see Chapter 32). Epidermodysplasia verruciformis is a rare condition and is associated with warts all over the body.

Diagnosis of warts is by visualization. Treatment considers the age of the individual and the size and location of the lesion. Warts can be removed by freezing with liquid nitrogen, electrocautery, vaporization with lasers, application of keratolytics, or application of irritants and corrosives, such as salicylic acid, formaldehyde, interferons, or saturated solution of potassium iodide.[35] Recurrence is not unusual, and many warts resolve spontaneously.

Fungal infections

The fungi causing superficial skin infections are called *dermatophytes,* and they thrive on keratin (stratum corneum, hair, nails). Fungal disorders are known as *mycoses;* when caused by dermatophytes, the mycoses are termed *tinea* (dermatophytosis or ringworm). *Tinea pedis* is a chronic, superficial fungal infection of the skin of the foot common in adults (Fig. 39-19). In prepubertal children most scaling disorders of the toes and feet are eczema. *Tinea corporis (ringworm)* and *tinea capitis* (a fungal infection of the scalp) are much more common in children than adults (see Chapter 40).

TABLE 39-4   **Common Sites of Tinea Infections**

Site	Clinical Manifestations
Tinea capitis (scalp)	Scaly, pruritic scalp with bald areas; hair breaks easily
Tinea corporis (skin areas, excluding scalp, face, hands, feet, groin)	Circular, clearly circumscribed, mildly erythematous scaly patches with a slightly elevated ringlike border; some forms are dry and macular, and other forms are moist and vesicular
Tinea cruris (groin, also known as "jock itch")	Small erythematous and scaling vesicular patches with a well-defined border that spreads over the inner and upper surfaces of the thighs; occurs with heat and high humidity
Tinea pedis (foot, also known as "athlete's foot")	Occurs between the toes and may spread to the soles of feet, nails, and skin or toes; slight scaling; macerated, painful skin, occasionally with fissures and vesiculation
Tinea manus (hand)	Dry, scaly, erythematous lesions, or moist, vesicular lesions that begin with clusters of intensely itching, clear vesicles; often associated with fungal infection of the feet
Tinea unguium or onychomycosis (nails)	A superficial or deep inflammation of the nail that develops yellow-brown accumulations of brittle keratin over all or portions of the nail

Fig. 39-19 *Tinea pedis.* Inflammation has extended from the web area onto the dorsum of the foot. *(Courtesy Department of Dermatology, School of Medicine, University of Utah.)*

Tinea infections

Tinea infections are classified according to their location on the body. The most common sites are summarized in Table 39-4. These infestations are common in children.[36] Tinea is diagnosed by culture, microscopic examination of skin scrapings prepared with potassium hydroxide wet mount, or observation of the skin with an ultraviolet light (Wood lamp). Cultures establish the particular type of fungus and are necessary for hair and nail infections. Fungi have characteristic spores and filaments known as **hyphae** that are more prominent when prepared in potassium hydroxide. The spores fluoresce blue-green when exposed to ultraviolet light. Treatment is related to the type of fungi and includes both topical and systemic antifungal medication.

Candidiasis

Candidiasis is caused by the yeastlike fungus *Candida albicans* and normally can be found on mucous membranes, on the skin, in the gastrointestinal tract, and in the vagina. *C. albicans* can, under certain circumstances, change from a commensal microorganism to a pathogen, particularly when the immune system is depressed. Among those factors that predispose to infection are (1) local environment of moisture, warmth, maceration, or occlusion; (2) the systemic administration of antibiotics; (3) pregnancy; (4) diabetes mellitus; (5) Cushing disease; (6) debilitated states; (7) infants younger than 6 months of age, as a result of decreased immune reactivity; (8) immunosuppressed persons; and (9) certain neoplastic diseases of the blood and monocyte/macrophage system. The resident bacteria on the skin, mainly cocci, inhibit proliferation of *C. albicans*. *C. albicans* can activate the complement system by the alternative pathway and produce small abscesses. Candidiasis affects only the outer layers of mucous membranes and skin and occurs in the mouth, vagina, uncircumcised penis, and large skin folds. Table 39-5 lists the differentiation of different sites of candidiasis.

The initial lesion is a thin-walled pustule that extends under the stratum corneum with an inflammatory base that may burn or itch. The accumulation of inflammatory cells and scale produces a whitish yellow curdlike substance over the infected area. The lesion ceases to spread when it reaches dry skin.[37]

Vascular Disorders

Vascular abnormalities are commonly associated with skin diseases, may be congenital, or may involve vascular responses to local or systemic vasoactive substances. Blood vessels may increase in number, dilate, constrict, or become obliterated by disease processes.

TABLE 39-5	Sites of Candidiasis		
	Risk Factors	**Clinical Manifestations**	**Treatment**
Vagina (vulvovaginitis)	Heat, moisture, occlusive clothing Pregnancy Systemic antibiotic therapy Diabetes mellitus Sexual intercourse with infected male	Vaginal itching; white, watery, or creamy discharge Red and swollen vaginal and labial membranes with erosions Lesions may spread to anus and groin	Miconazole cream Clotrimazole tablets or cream Nystatin tablets Ketoconazole cream Loose cotton clothing
Penis (balanitis)	Uncircumcised Sexual intercourse with infected female	Pinpoint red, tender papules and pustules on glans and shaft of penis	Any of creams listed above Topical steroids for severe inflammation
Mouth	Diabetes mellitus Immunosuppressive therapy Inhaled steroids	Red, swollen, painful tongue and oral mucous membranes Localized erosions and plaques appear with chronic infection	Nystatin oral suspension Clotrimazole troches Ketoconazole

Cutaneous vasculitis

Vasculitis (angiitis) is an inflammation of the blood vessels. The initiating site may be the blood, the vessel wall, or the adjacent tissue. Small vessels are usually affected. Immune complexes, which initiate an uncontrolled inflammatory response, often cause damage, and the lesions are frequently polymorphic.

Cutaneous vasculitis develops from the deposit of immune complexes in small blood vessels as a toxic response to drugs (phenothiazines, barbiturates, sulfonamides) or allergens or as a response to streptococcal or viral infection. The deposit activates complement, which is chemotactic for polymorphonuclear leukocytes. The cutaneous form usually resolves in a few weeks and is treated with steroids.

The disorder is also known as *allergic vasculitis* in adults. A systemic form (cutaneous systemic vasculitis) can involve other organs, including the kidneys, lungs, and gastrointestinal tract. The lower legs and feet have palpable purpura (from the leakage of blood from damaged vessels) that progress to hemorrhagic bullae with necrosis and ulceration from occlusion of the vessel. Lesions appear in clusters and remain from 1 to 4 weeks. Recurrences are common. Biopsy may disclose the presence of complement or immunoglobulins in the vessel walls.

Identifying and removing the antigen (chemical, drug, or source of infection) are the first steps of treatment. Prednisone may be used when symptoms are severe.

Urticaria

Urticarial lesions are most commonly associated with type 1 hypersensitivity reactions to drugs (penicillin, aspirin), certain foods (strawberries, shellfish), systemic diseases (intestinal parasites, lupus erythematosus), or physical agents (heat or cold)[38] (see Chapter 7). The lesions are mediated by histamine release, which causes the endothelial cells of skin blood vessels to contract. The leak of fluid from the vessel appears as wheals, welts, or hives, and there may be few or many and distributed over the entire body. Most lesions resolve spontaneously within 24 hours, but new lesions may appear. All possible causes should be removed. Antihistamines usually reduce hives and provide relief of itching. Corticosteroids and β-adrenergic agonists may be required for severe attacks. Chronic urticaria is probably an autoimmune disease.[39,40]

Scleroderma

Scleroderma means sclerosis of the skin. The disease is more prominent in women. It may affect the visceral organs or remain localized to the skin. Systemic scleroderma involves the connective tissues of many organs, including the kidneys, gastrointestinal tract, and lungs. The cutaneous lesions are most often on the face and hands, the neck, and the upper chest, although the entire skin can be involved.

There are massive deposits of collagen with fibrosis, accompanied by inflammatory reactions, vascular changes in the capillary network with a decrease in the number of capillary loops, and dilation of the remaining capillaries.[41] Autoimmunity and an immune reaction to a toxic substance are both possible initiating mechanisms of the disease, and autoantibodies are often recovered from the skin and serum of individuals with scleroderma.[42]

The skin is hard, hypopigmented, taut, shiny, and tightly connected to the underlying tissue. The tightness of the facial skin projects an immobile masklike appearance, and the mouth may not open completely. The nose may assume a beaklike appearance. The hands are shiny and sometimes red and edematous. The fingers become tapered and flexed, often with depressed scars and loss of fingertips from atrophy. Raynaud phenomenon with episodic arteriolar vasoconstriction of the fingers contributes to ulcer formation. The nails may be shed (Fig. 39-20). Calcium deposits develop in the subcutaneous tissue and erupt through the skin. Pro-

Fig. 39-20 *Scleroderma (acrosclerosis).* Note inflammation and shiny skin. *(Courtesy Department of Dermatology, School of Medicine, University of Utah.)*

gression to body organs may occur, and death is caused by subsequent respiratory failure, renal failure, cardiac dysrhythmias, or esophageal or intestinal obstruction or perforation.[43] There is no specific treatment, and 50% of individuals die within 5 years from onset.

Suitable clothing and a warm environment are essential for protecting the hands. Trauma and smoking should be avoided. Vasodilator drugs or sympathectomy rarely has lasting effects. Symptomatic treatment is required for involved organs (i.e., intestinal resection for obstruction, antibiotics for pneumonitis, and regulation of hypertension).[44]

✓ **QUICK CHECK**

Name two bacterial skin infections, and describe the typical lesions.

Compare herpes zoster and varicella.

What features distinguish urticarial lesions?

Insect Bites
Ticks
Ticks are significant vectors of transmitted diseases, including Rocky Mountain spotted fever and other rickettsial diseases, tularemia, and Lyme disease. Ticks vary in size from 1 cm to about the size of a comma on this printed page. They embed their heads in the skin to obtain blood. As they gorge themselves, they enlarge to many times their normal size and may release toxins or transmit microorganisms during feeding. In most instances, tick bite causes only a papular urticaria. If mouth parts remain in the skin when the tick is removed, the persistent nodule may require excision; the tick should be removed intact. Irritant substances, such as camphor, gasoline, soft wax, or heat from a match, may stimulate the tick to withdraw its head. Applying tick repellant, such as

diethyltoluamide (DEET), butopyronoxyl (Indalone), or benzyl benzoate, helps to prevent tick bites.

Lyme disease is a multisystem inflammatory disease caused by the spirochete *Borrelia burgdorferi* transmitted by tick bites. The highest incidence is among children, and 50% of infected individuals are symptom free. The incidence is increasing.[45] The disease occurs in stages, and the mechanisms of injury are not well understood:
1. Soon after bite, localized infection (rash—erythema migrans with or without flu-like illness)
2. Nine months later, disseminated infection (secondary erythema migrans, arthralgias, meningitis, neuritis, carditis)
3. Late persistent infection continuing for years (arthritis, encephalopathy, polyneuropathy)

The microorganism is difficult to culture.

The diagnosis of Lyme disease is based on the clinical presentation and history of tick bite, if known. Serologic tests may confirm the diagnosis. Antibiotics are used for treatment with good success, although the response may be slow. A safe vaccine for prevention of Lyme disease has been developed.[46]

Mosquitoes and flies
There are thousands of species of *mosquitoes* throughout the world. Species from the Culicidae family are responsible for malaria, yellow fever, dengue fever, filariasis, and St. Louis encephalitis. Mosquitoes can bite through thin, loose clothing and are attracted by warmth and sweat. The edema, pruritus, and papular lesions of the mosquito bite are caused by the disruption of the skin from the insertion of a blood tube by a female mosquito. Irritating salivary secretions also contain anticoagulants. Reactions vary depending on the sensitivity of the victim.

Several species of flies are blood suckers. The black fly (Simuliidae family) is usually found in swarms, near moving bodies of water in the late spring and early summer, and is a vicious biter. The initial bite is painless because the fly injects an anesthetic with it. Subsequent lesions are painful and accompanied by significant swelling of surrounding tissues. Systemic reactions, such as fever, headache, and nausea, are common.

Very small flies of the Ceratopogonidae family, also known as *no-see-ums, midges, punkies,* or *sand fleas,* are also blood suckers. The bite of the female is particularly miserable and produces immediate pain, erythema, and vesicles. Itching and vesicular reactions may persist for weeks.

The fiercest blood-sucking flies are the Tabanidae, or horseflies, deerflies, gadflies, greenheads, and clegs. These flies vary in size from 1 to 5 cm and produce painful, bleeding bites because of their large mouth parts. The bites produce urticaria that may be accompanied by weakness, dizziness, and wheezing.

Wounds produced by biting insects should be cleansed with soap and water and a local antiseptic applied. Local applications of steroid creams or antihistamine will reduce symptoms. Systemic reactions require more specific care.

Benign Tumors

Most benign tumors of the skin are associated with aging. Benign tumors include seborrheic keratosis, keratoacanthoma, actinic keratosis, and moles.

Seborrheic keratosis

Seborrheic keratosis is a benign proliferation of basal cells that produces elevated lesions that may be smooth or warty in appearance. They are usually seen in older people and occur as multiple lesions on the chest, back, and face. The color varies from tan to waxy yellow, flesh-colored, or dark brown-black. Lesion size varies from a few millimeters to several centimeters, and they are often oval and greasy appearing with a hyperkeratotic scale (Fig. 39-21). Cryotherapy with liquid nitrogen is effective treatment, and the lesions usually slough 2 to 3 weeks after treatment.

Keratoacanthoma

A keratoacanthoma is a benign, self-limiting tumor that arises from hair follicles. It usually occurs on sun-exposed surfaces and develops between 60 and 65 years of age. The most commonly affected sites are the face, back of the hands, forearms, neck, and legs. The lesion develops in stages with a histologic pattern resembling squamous cell carcinoma[47]:

1. *Proliferative stage:* rapid-growing, dome-shaped nodule with central crust
2. *Mature stage:* lesion fills with whitish-colored keratin and requires differentiation from squamous cell carcinoma
3. *Involution stage:* occurs over a 3- to 4-month period with regression of lesion

Although the lesions will resolve spontaneously, they can be removed by curettage or excision to improve cosmetic appearance.

Actinic keratosis

Actinic keratosis is a premalignant lesion found on skin surfaces exposed to the ultraviolet radiation of the sun. The prevalence is highest in individuals with unprotected, light-colored skin and rare in those with black skin. The lesions appear as pigmented patches of rough, adherent scale. Surrounding areas may have telangiectasias. Freezing with liquid nitrogen provides quick, effective treatment. Excisions also may be performed, providing tissue for cellular analysis. The lesions should continue to be evaluated for progression to squamous cell carcinoma. Protection from the sun with clothing or a sun-blocking agent to prevent lesions from developing elsewhere is advised.

Nevi (moles)

Nevi are pigmented or nonpigmented lesions that form from melanocytes beginning at ages 3 to 5 years. During the early stages of development, the cells accumulate at the junction of the dermis and epidermis and are macular lesions. Over time the cells move down into the dermis and the nevi become nodular and palpable. Nevi may appear on any part of the skin and vary in size. They occur singly or in groups and are not disfiguring. Nevi may undergo transition to ma-

Fig. 39-21 *Seborrheic keratosis.* Typical lesion that is broad, flat, and comparatively smooth surfaced. *(Courtesy Department of Dermatology, School of Medicine, University of Utah.)*

lignant melanoma (see p. 1114). Nevi irritated by clothing should be excised.

(see p. 1114)

> ## ✓ QUICK CHECK
>
> List two diseases caused by insect bites.
>
> Compare keratoacanthoma and actinic keratosis.

Cancer

Because many cancerous skin lesions are treated and not reported, statistics on the incidence of skin cancer are difficult to obtain. It is estimated that skin cancers are the most prevalent form of cancer and nearly all persons living beyond age 65 years will have had at least one skin cancer. The most common types are basal cell carcinoma and squamous cell carcinoma. These carcinomas are 50% more common in men than in women, and incidence increases steadily with age. Malignant melanoma is the most serious skin cancer with 44,200 new cases per year and increasing at a rate of 3.4% per year.[48] An estimated 9200 people die of skin cancer each year, 7300 from malignant melanoma.[48] Important trends related to skin cancer are described in Box 39-1.

Solar radiation causes most skin cancers.[49] Protection from the sun during the first 10 to 20 years of life significantly reduces the risk of skin cancer.[50] Areas widely exposed to the sun's rays—the face, neck, and hands—are highly vulnerable for such lesions. Outdoor workers (farmers, sailors, fishermen) are high-risk skin cancer populations. Risk factors for skin cancer are contained in the Risk Factors box.

> ## ∎ *RISK FACTORS*
>
> **SKIN CANCER**
> - Excessive exposure to ultraviolet radiation from the sun or tanning salons
> - Fair complexion
> - Occupational exposure to coal tar, pitch, creosote, arsenic compounds, and radium
> - Cancer is negligible in blacks because of heavy skin pigmentation

INCIDENCE

Approximately 1 million cases per year with the majority being the highly curable **basal** or **squamous cell** cancers; not as common is the most serious **malignant melanoma** with an estimated 44,200 cases per year

MORTALITY

Total estimated deaths in 1999 were 9200; 7300 from malignant melanoma, 1900 from other skin cancers

WARNING SIGNALS

Any unusual skin condition, especially a change in the size or color of a mole or other darkly pigmented growth or spot

PREVENTION AND EARLY DETECTION

Avoidance of sun when ultraviolet light is strongest (e.g., 10:00 AM and 3:00 PM); use sunscreen preparations, especially those containing ingredients such as PABA (para-aminobenzoic acid); basal and squamous cell skin cancers often form a pale, waxlike, pearly nodule or a red, scaly, sharply outlined patch; melanomas are usually dark brown or black pigmentation; they start as small molelike growths that increase in size, change color, become ulcerated, and bleed easily from a slight injury

TREATMENT

There are four methods of treatment; surgery, electrodesiccation (tissue destruction by heat), radiation therapy, or cryosurgery (tissue destruction by freezing); for malignant melanomas, wide and often deep excisions and removal of nearby lymph nodes are required

SURVIVAL

For basal cell and squamous cell cancers, cure is virtually ensured with early detection and treatment; malignant melanoma, however, metastasizes quickly; this accounts for a lower 5-year survival rate for white patients with this disease

Fig. 39-22 *Basal cell carcinoma.* Center has ulcerated. (*Courtesy Department of Dermatology, School of Medicine, University of Utah.*)

posed, the face and neck. In dark-skinned persons, basal cells contain the pigment *melanin*, a protective factor against sun exposure. Although ultraviolet radiation seems to be the primary causative agent, arsenic and genetic factors are also implicated.

The growth rate for these tumors is quite slow. The lesion starts as a nodule (more than 5 mm across) that is pearly or ivory in appearance and slightly elevated above the skin surface with small blood vessels on the surface. As the lesion grows, it often ulcerates, develops crusting, and is firm to the touch. If left untreated, basal cell lesions invade surrounding tissues and, over months or years, can destroy a nose, eyelid, or ear (for treatment, see Box 39-1).

Squamous cell carcinoma

Squamous cell carcinoma is a tumor of the epidermis characterized by two types: in situ and invasive. Because of the invasive nature of some tumors, squamous cell carcinoma is significantly more malignant if left untreated.[51]

Sunlight causes squamous cell carcinoma. Areas affected are the head and neck (75%) and the hands (15%), with 10% of cases elsewhere on the body.[52] In countries where arsenic is higher in drinking water, these tumors are more predominant. X-rays and gamma rays are also associated with squamous cell carcinoma. In addition, individuals who are immunosuppressed experience a greater occurrence.

The exact mechanism for producing squamous cell carcinoma is unknown. It is unclear whether ultraviolet light produces its harmful effects because of problems in deoxyribonucleic acid (DNA) synthesis, repair, or replication.

Invasive squamous cell carcinoma can arise from premalignant lesions of the skin and rarely develops from normal-appearing skin. The premalignant lesions include sun-damaged skin or dysplasias (actinic dermatitis); leukoplakia, or whitish discolored areas; scars; radiation-induced keratosis; tar and oil keratosis; and chronic ulcers and sinuses. The invasive type grows more rapidly than basal cell carcinomas and can spread to regional lymph nodes. These tumors are firm and increase in both elevation and diameter. The surface may be granular and bleed easily (Fig. 39-23).

Basal cell carcinoma

Basal cell carcinoma is a surface epithelial tumor of the skin and is the most common skin cancer. The tumors grow upward and laterally or downward to the dermal/epidermal junction (Fig. 39-22). They usually have depressed centers and rolled borders. Early tumors are so small they are not clinically apparent. Generally, these tumors do not invade blood or lymph vessels; thus they do not metastasize beyond the skin but grow by direct extension to adjacent structures.

The risk for basal cell carcinoma is sunlight exposure in fair-skinned individuals. Lesions are seen most frequently in regions with intense sunlight and on those areas most ex-

Fig. 39-23 *Squamous cell carcinoma.* The sun-exposed ear is a common site for squamous cell carcinoma. *(Courtesy Department of Dermatology, School of Medicine, University of Utah.)*

Fig. 39-24 *Lentigo malignant melanoma. (Courtesy Department of Dermatology, School of Medicine, University of Utah.)*

In situ squamous cell carcinoma is usually confined to the epidermis (intraepidermal) but may extend into the dermis. Common premalignant skin lesions are actinic (solar) keratosis and Bowen disease. Bowen disease is a dysplasia of the basal layer of the dermis or carcinoma in situ often found on unexposed areas of the body and demonstrated by flat, reddish, scaly patches. These lesions may enlarge to more than 1 cm in diameter, rarely invading surrounding tissue and almost never metastasizing. Other cellular components in the skin (e.g., sweat glands, hair follicles) can give rise to skin cancer, but these are relatively uncommon.

Malignant melanoma

Melanoma is a malignant tumor of the skin originating from melanocytes, or cells that synthesize the pigment melanin. The long-continuing increase in melanoma-related deaths appears to be slowing, particularly in women.[53] Early recognition of cutaneous melanomas can have a major impact on surgical cure of this disease. The ABCD rule is used as a guide (*A*symmetry, *B*order irregularity, *C*olor variation, *D*iameter larger than 6 mm).[54]

Causative factors implicated in melanoma induction include genetic predisposition, solar radiation, and steroid hormone activity. Sunlight is an important promotional factor. Melanomas arise as a result of malignant degeneration of melanocytes located either along the basal layer of the epidermis or in a benign melanocytic nevus. The relationship between nevi and melanoma makes it important for the clinician to understand the various neval forms (Table 39-6). Most nevi never become suspicious; however, suspicious pigmented nevi need removal.[55] Indications for biopsy include color change, size change, irregular notched margin, itching, bleeding or oozing, nodularity, scab formation, and ulceration. The clinical varieties of cutaneous melanoma include lentigo malignant melanoma (LMM) (Fig. 39-24), superficial spreading melanoma (SSM), and primary nodular melanoma (PNM).

Treatment of melanoma with no evidence of metastatic disease involves surgical excision to the primary lesion site and regional lymph nodes, radiation therapy, chemotherapy, and biologic response modifiers. Lesions of the extremities have the best surgical prognosis, next best are head and neck lesions, and trunk lesions have the poorest prognosis. Only 20% to 40% of patients with regional lymph node involvement are alive and cured at 5 years.

Kaposi sarcoma

Kaposi sarcoma (KS) is a vascular malignancy associated with immunodeficiency states and occurs among kidney transplant recipients taking immunosuppressive drugs. A rapidly progressive form of KS appears with acquired immunodeficiency syndrome (AIDS) (see Chapter 32). KS is also common among middle-age black males in equatorial Africa and persons of Mediterranean or Jewish descent. Two forms of the disease have been described—classic and epidemic.[56] Proliferation of the tumor depends on the presence of platelet-derived growth factors.[57]

The human immunodeficiency virus and cytomegalovirus have been proposed as cofactors in the development of KS.[58] Human herpesvirus 8 has also been found in almost all cases of KS.[59] The endothelial cell is thought to be the progenitor of KS. The lesions emerge as purplish brown macules and develop into plaques and nodules with angioproliferation. They tend to be multifocal rather than spreading by metastasis. The lesions initially appear over the lower extremities in the classic form (Fig. 39-25). The rapidly progressive form associated with AIDS tends to spread symmetrically over the upper body, particularly the face and oral mucosa. The lesions are often pruritic and painful. About 75% of individuals with epidemic KS have involvement of lymph nodes, particularly in the gastrointestinal tract and lungs. Organ involvement is much less common in the classic form. The rapidly progressive form has a poor prognosis and shorter survival rates than the classic form. (See Chapter 32 for a further discussion of AIDS.)

Diagnosis is by skin biopsy, with a high index of suspicion for those with immunodeficiency. Local lesions can be excised. Multiple disseminated lesions may be treated with a

TABLE 39-6	Classification of Nevi
Type	Common Characteristics
Junctional nevus	Flat, well-circumscribed, vary in size up to 2 cm, dark color, hairs may be present; originate in basal layer of epidermis and can eventually reach the cutaneous surface; most likely to develop into a melanoma
Compound nevus	Most common in adolescents and are the majority of pigmented lesions in children; rarely does this lesion develop to melanoma; usually 1 cm in size; hairs may be present; surface is elevated and smooth
Intradermal nevus	Small, less than 1 cm, with regular edges and bristlelike hairs; color ranges from skin tone to light brown; has a slight likelihood of developing into a melanoma

Fig. 39-25 *Kaposi sarcoma.* The purple lesion commonly seen on the skin. *(Courtesy Department of Dermatology, School of Medicine, University of Utah.)*

combination of α-interferon, radiotherapy, and cytotoxic drugs. General response to treatment is poor, but a 2-year survival rate is better in individuals with KS alone than in those with KS and an opportunistic infection.

✓ QUICK CHECK

What is the most common skin cancer?

What malignancy can arise from melanocytes?

How is Kaposi sarcoma related to AIDS?

Burns

About 1.25 million people are burned in the United States each year,[60] with 60,000 people hospitalized and 10,000 burn-related deaths.[61] Most significant burns occur in the home, and the highest percentage of deaths (70%) are from home fires.[62]

The total burn incidence in the United States has dropped 37.5%, from 2 million burn injuries in 1971 to 1.25 million in 1991. Deaths from fire and burn injuries have decreased 50% to an estimated 5500 burn deaths in 1991, compared with 9000 burn-associated deaths in 1971.[63]

Burns may be caused by thermal or nonthermal sources including chemical, electrical, or radioactive. Thermal injuries result from exposure to direct flames, hot liquids, or radiation. Direct contact, inhalation, and ingestion of acids, alkalis, or blistering agents cause chemical burns. Electrical burns occur with the passage of electrical current through the body to the ground. Associated electrical flames or flashes also can burn the skin.

Burn wound depth

The depth of injury identifies the level of tissue destruction, the extent of injury determines mortality. Depth of the burn is divided into four categories (Table 39-7).

First-degree burns are a *partial-thickness injury* involving only the epidermis, without injury to the underlying dermal or subcutaneous tissue. The skin maintains water vapor and bacterial barrier functions. Many instances of sunburn are first-degree injuries caused by the exposure of skin to the ultraviolet radiation from the sun. Initially, there is local pain and erythema, but no blisters appear for about 24 hours. An extensive first-degree burn may cause systemic responses, such as chills, headache, localized edema, and nausea or vomiting. No treatment of extensive first-degree burns is required unless the person is elderly or an infant, in which case severe nausea and vomiting may lead to inadequate fluid intake and dehydration. Therapy consists of intravenous hydration until the nausea and vomiting subside at 24 to 72 hours after burn injury. Comfort measures for previously healthy children or adults with extensive first-degree burns consist of aspirin for adults or acetaminophen for children every 4 hours in age-appropriate dosages and frequent application of a water-soluble lotion. First-degree burns heal in 3 to 5 days without scarring.

Second-degree burns describe two categories of burn depth with markedly different characteristics. These are partial-thickness injuries, but they evoke vastly different responses. The hallmark of *superficial partial-thickness injury* is the appearance of thin-walled, fluid-filled blisters that develop within just a few minutes after injury. Another dominant characteristic of superficial injury is pain. As blisters break or are removed, nerve endings are exposed to air (Fig. 39-26). Tactile and pain sensors remain intact throughout the healing process, with each wound care procedure causing extreme pain. Wounds heal in 3 to 4 weeks, provided the individual is adequately nourished and no complications develop (Fig. 39-27). Scar formation is unusual with this injury.

TABLE 39-7	Depth of Burn Injury			
		Second Degree		**Third Degree**
Characteristic	**First Degree**	**Superficial Partial-Thickness**	**Deep Partial-Thickness**	**Full-Thickness**
Morphology	Destruction of epidermis only	Destruction of epidermis and some dermis	Destruction of epidermis and dermis, leaving only skin appendages	Destruction of epidermis, dermis, and underlying subcutaneous tissue
Skin function	Intact	Absent	Absent	Absent
Tactile and pain sensors	Intact	Intact	Intact but diminished	Absent
Blisters	Present only after first 24 hr	Present within minutes, thin-walled and fluid-filled	May or may not appear as fluid-filled blisters; often is layer of flat, dehydrated "tissue paper" that lifts off in sheets	Blisters rare; usually is a layer of flat, dehydrated "tissue paper" that lifts off easily
Appearance of wound after initial débridement	Skin peels at 24-48 hr, normal or slightly red underneath	Red to pale ivory, moist surface	Mottled with areas of waxy, white, dry surface	White, cherry red, or black, may contain visible thrombosed veins; dry, hard, leathery surface
Healing time	3-5 days	21-28 days	30 days to many months	Will not heal; may close from edges as secondary healing if wound is small
Scarring	None	May be present, low incidence influenced by genetic predisposition	Highest incidence because of slow healing rate promoting scar tissue development, also influenced by genetic predisposition	Skin graft; scarring minimized by early excision and grafting, influenced by genetic predisposition

Fig. 39-26 *Superficial partial-thickness injury.* Scald injury following débridement of overlying blister and nonadherent epithelium. *(Courtesy Intermountain Burn Center, University of Utah.)*

Fig. 39-27 *Axillary burn scar contracture.* Note the blanching of the anterior axillary fold and small ulceration, both indicating the diminished range of motion. *(Courtesy Intermountain Burn Center, University of Utah.)*

Fig. 39-28 *Deep partial-thickness wound.* Note pale appearance and minimal exudate. *(Courtesy Intermountain Burn Center, University of Utah.)*

Fig. 39-29 *Full-thickness thermal injury.* The wound is dry and insensate. *(Courtesy Intermountain Burn Center, University of Utah.)*

Deep partial-thickness burns involve the entire dermis, sparing skin appendages such as hair follicles and sweat glands (see Table 39-7 and Fig. 39-28). These wounds take weeks to heal, and current therapy consists of surgical removal of the burn wound (excision) followed by application of the person's own unburned skin from another body area (autograft). The ultimate healing of deep partial-thickness burns commonly results in hypertrophic scarring with poor functional and cosmetic results.

Third-degree burns, or *full-thickness burns,* involve destruction of the entire epidermis, dermis, and often underlying subcutaneous tissue (see Table 39-7). On occasion, all underlying subcutaneous tissue is destroyed and muscle or bone may be destroyed. Elasticity of the dermis is destroyed, giving the wound a dry, leathery appearance (Fig. 39-29). As marked edema forms, distal circulation may be compromised in areas of circumferential burns. *Escharotomies* (cutting through the burned skin) are performed to release pressure. Full-thickness burns are painless because all nerve endings have been destroyed by the injury.

The extent of the *total body surface area (TBSA)* burn is estimated using either the "rule of nines" (Fig. 39-30) or the Lund and Browder chart[64] (Fig. 39-31). Severity of burn injury is a combination of many factors, including age, medical history, extent and depth of injury, and body area involved. The American Burn Association has defined criteria to assist health care professionals to identify who should be cared for at a specialized burn center (Box 39-2).

Pathophysiology and Clinical Manifestations

Burn injury results in dramatic changes in most physiologic functions of the body within the first few minutes after the event. The effect of burn depends on two parameters: first, the extent of body surface affected and, second, the depth of cutaneous injury. Burns exceeding 20% TBSA in most adults are considered to be major burn injuries and are associated with massive evaporative water losses and flux of large

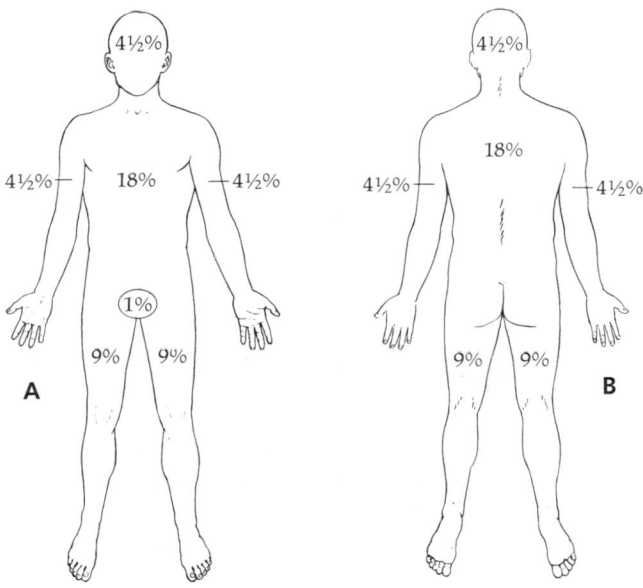

Fig. 39-30 *Estimation of burn injury: Rule of nines.* A commonly used assessment tool with estimates of the percentages (in multiples of 9) of the total body surface area burned. **A,** Adults *(anterior view).* **B,** Adults *(posterior view). (From Thompson, J.M. et al. [1997]. Mosby's clinical nursing [4th ed.]. St. Louis: Mosby.)*

amounts of fluid and electrolytes in the body tissues, manifested as generalized edema and circulatory hypovolemia.

With a major burn injury, a systemic pathophysiology ensues that requires therapeutic intervention to sustain life. The immediate (acute) physiologic consequences of major burn injury center around the profound, life-threatening hypovolemic shock that occurs in conjunction with cellular and immunologic disruption within a few minutes of injury (Fig. 39-32). *Burn shock* is a phenomenon consisting of both a hypovolemic cardiovascular component and a cellular component.

Hypovolemia associated with burn shock is the result of massive fluid losses from the circulating blood volume. The

Relative percentages of areas affected by growth (age in years)

	0	1	5	10	15	Adult
A: half of head	9½	8½	6½	5½	4½	3½
B: half of thigh	2¾	3¼	4	4¼	4½	4¾
C: half of leg	2½	2½	2¾	3	3¼	3½

Second degree _____ and

Third degree _____ =

Total percent burned__

Fig. 39-31 *Estimation of burn injury: Lund and Browder chart.* Areas designated by letters (*A, B,* and *C*) represent percentages of body surface area that vary according to age. Accompanying table indicates relative percentages of these areas at various stages in life. *(From Sabiston, D.C., Jr. [Ed.]. [1977]. Textbook of surgery: The biological basis of modern surgical practice [11th ed.]. Philadelphia: Saunders.)*

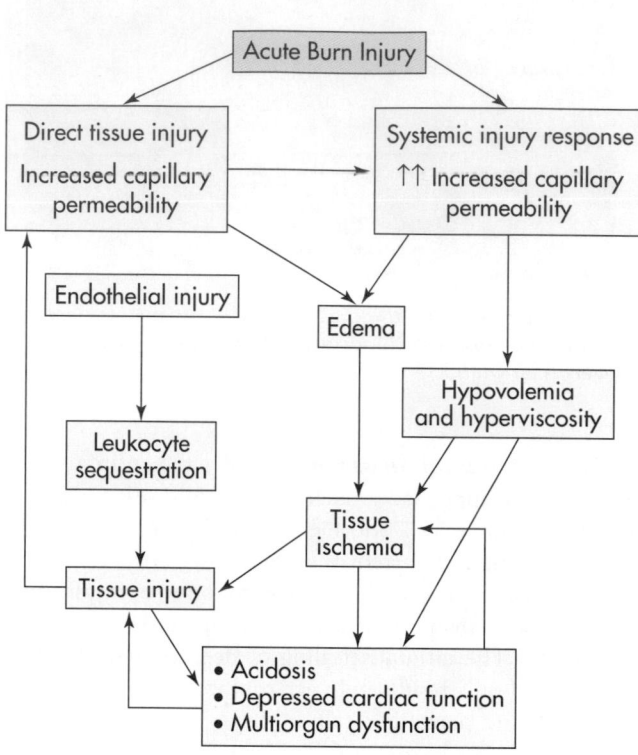

Fig. 39-32 *Immediate cellular and immunologic alterations of burn shock.*

losses are caused by an increase in capillary permeability that persists for approximately 24 hours after burn injury. *Fluid resuscitation* (Box 39-3) is the administration of intravenous fluids, often lactated Ringer solution, in an effort to restore the circulating blood volume during the period of increasing capillary permeability. In addition to hypovolemia, most other organ systems are affected. Cardiac contractility is diminished during the initial 24-hour resuscitation period with shunting of blood away from the liver, kidney, and gut, and other viscera with attendant decreased function of these organs.

There is also evidence that cellular metabolism is disrupted with onset of the burn wound, resulting in altered cell membrane permeability and loss of normal electrolyte homeostasis. Many mediators of inflammation (prostaglandins, thromboxanes, histamine, serotonin) and myocardial depressant factor play a role in the vascular response to burns.

Cardiovascular response to burn injury

The severity of hypovolemic shock is directly related to the extent of the burn. The fluid and protein movement out of the vascular compartment results in an elevated hematocrit and white blood cell count and hypoproteinemia. If not treated immediately, profound hypovolemic shock leads to irreversible shock and death within a few hours. Restoration of capillary integrity and a functional lymphatic system are required for resolution of the edema. Usually this occurs within 24 hours, but in extensive burns, it may take days or weeks. After the individual has reached the end point of burn shock, the term used to describe the person's condition is *capillary seal.*

Cellular response to burn injury

In addition to capillary endothelial permeability changes resulting in vascular fluid losses, there are transmembrane potential changes in cells not directly damaged by heat. Such membrane potential changes may be caused by a circulating shock factor.[65] Other changes can be categorized as (1) metabolic responses or (2) immunologic responses to the burn injury. Evaporative water loss must also be managed.

American Burn Association Burn Center Referral Criteria   BOX 39-2

SECOND- AND THIRD-DEGREE BURNS
>10% BSA burned for age <10 years or >50 years
>20% BSA burned for ages 10 to 50 years
Face, hands, feet, genitalia, perineum, and major
  joints

THIRD-DEGREE BURNS
>5% BSA involved in any age-group

OTHER BURNS
Electrical
Chemical
With smoke inhalation injury

OTHER CONDITIONS
Coexisting trauma
Preexisting disease
Circumferential burns of an extremity or chest

From American Burn Association. (1990). *Journal of Burn Care and Rehabilitation, 11*(2), 98.
BSA, *Body surface area.*

Maintenance Fluid Replacements Following Major Burn Injury*   BOX 39-3

1. *Basal fluid* replacements per day
   1500 ml/day/m² body surface area = 24-hour requirements
2. *Evaporative water loss* from burn wound
   a. Adults: (25 + % total body surface area burn)
      (m² body surface area) = ml/hr
   b. Children: (35 + % total body surface area burn)
      (m² body surface area) = ml/hr
3. *Total hourly maintenance fluids*
   Basal fluid requirements per day ÷ 24 hours +
   evaporative water loss per hour = ml/hr maintenance fluids

Example: A 70-kg adult with a 50% total body sur-
  face area burn and a body surface area of 2 m re-
  quires the following:
  Basal = (1500 ml/day)(2 m² body surface area) =
    3000 ml/24 hr, or **125 ml/hr**
  Evaporative = (25 + 50% total body surface burn)
    (2 m² total body surface area) = (75) (2) = **150
    ml/hr**
  Total maintenance fluids = **125 ml + 150 ml = 275
    ml/hr**

*From end of burn shock until wound closure is achieved.

The cellular dysfunction of burn injury extends beyond the transmembrane potential disruption and the sodium-potassium pump impairment to include a loss of intracellular magnesium and phosphate[66] and elevated serum lactic dehydrogenase (LDH) levels.[67] Thus impairments of basic cellular function may be the underlying cause of the diminished membrane potentials.

Metabolic reactions to the stress of a major burn injury involve the response of the sympathetic nervous system and other homeostatic regulators. Catecholamines are found in elevated amounts in both the serum and urine of burned individuals. Cortisol, glucagon, and insulin levels are elevated with a corresponding increase in gluconeogenesis, lipolysis, and proteolysis. Changes in lipid metabolism are reflected as an elevation in plasma free fatty acids (FFAs) and a decrease in plasma cholesterol and phospholipids.[68] Glucose and lactate kinetics are altered after burn injury. Although tissue hypoxia produces lactic acidosis, its persistence in the presence of adequate tissue perfusion suggests an increased rate of glycogenolysis.[69]

Burn injury induces an almost immediate hypermetabolic state that persists until wound closure. The metabolic rate increased with burn size in a curvilinear relationship with oxygen consumption rarely exceeding two times basal levels. Evaporative water loss and surface cooling are not the primary stimulus for the hypermetabolic state; rather, the hypermetabolism is related to an increase and resetting of the thermal regulatory set point. A core body temperature of 38.5° C is typical.

The inflammatory response at the wound level is magnified into a generalized systemic inflammatory response that is often deleterious.[70-72] Vasodilation, increased capillary permeability, and edema occur to facilitate healing of the local area.

Immunologic response

The immunologic/inflammatory response to burn injury is immediate, prolonged, and severe. The end result in individuals surviving burn shock is a dysregulation of immune mediators and cells with increased susceptibility to potentially fatal systemic burn wound sepsis. White blood cells are altered at a time when their need to inhibit sepsis is vital.[73] Phagocytosis is impaired, and cellular and humoral immunity is abnormal. Macrophages and neutrophils also release large amounts of inflammatory cytokines and, when combined with bacterial products, produce distant organ dysfunction and multiple organ failure.[74] Normally, opsonin renders bacteria susceptible to phagocytosis, but the burn injury triggers a consumptive decrease in opsonins with a greater risk for infection. Individuals with altered immuno-

Fig. 39-33 *Hypertrophic scarring.* Deep partial-thickness thermal injury can result in extensive hypertrophic scarring. *(Courtesy Intermountain Burn Center, University of Utah.)*

Fig. 39-34 *Application of cultured epithelial autografts.* The thin sheets of keratinocytes are attached to gauze backing to allow application onto the clean, excised thigh. *(Courtesy Intermountain Burn Center, University of Utah.)*

competence or chronic disease before burn injury are at additional risk for complications.[75]

Evaporative water loss

One of the major purposes of intact skin is to serve as a barrier to evaporative water loss (EWL) from the body. With major burn injury, this ability of the skin to regulate evaporative water loss is totally disrupted. Calculation of the amount of fluid lost by evaporative water loss includes losses from all sources. Normally, the skin is the major source of insensible loss (75%) and the lungs are minor sources (25%), with a total loss of only approximately 600 to 800 ml/day. This changes dramatically with burns because not only does skin loss increase but also lung loss increases because of hypermetabolism and hyperventilation, especially in an intubated individual. Total evaporative losses exceed many liters per day in an adult with large burn wounds. Replacement of the loss is mandatory to prevent volume deficit.

 Evaluation and Treatment

Burn recovery is long and stormy, with complications the rule rather than the exception. The goal of burn management is wound closure in a manner that promotes survival. Scar formation with contractures is often a consequence of healing in deep partial-thickness and third-degree burns (Fig. 39-33).

The three essential elements of survival of major burn injury are (1) meticulous wound management, (2) adequate fluids and nutrition, and (3) early surgical excision and grafting (Fig. 39-34).[76] Burn pain is almost always acute, and treatment strategies usually differ from strategies for chronic pain. In addition to opioid-based agents, new strategies for treatment may include antianxiety agents, hypnosis, and relaxation techniques.[77]

Frostbite

Frostbite is injury to the skin caused by exposure to extreme cold. The most common areas affected are fingers, toes, ears, nose, and cheeks. The mechanism of injury appears to be related to direct cold injury to cells, indirect injury from ice crystal formation, and impaired circulation with anoxia to the exposed area.[78] Frozen skin becomes white or yellowish and is waxy. There is numbness and no sensation of pain.

Redness and discomfort are seen with mild frostbite during rewarming followed by a return to normal in a few hours. Cyanosis and mottling develop followed by redness, swelling, and burning pain on rewarming in more severe cases. Within 24 to 48 hours, vesicles and bullae appear that resolve into crusts that eventually slough off, leaving thin, newly formed skin. The most severe cases result in gangrene with loss of the affected part. Frostbite may be classified by depth of injury: superficial includes partial skin freezing (first degree) and full-thickness skin freezing (second degree); deep includes full-thickness skin and subcutaneous freezing (third degree) and deep tissue freezing (fourth degree).[79]

Immediate treatment of frostbite is to cover affected areas with other body surfaces and warm clothing. The area should not be rubbed or massaged. Immersion in a warm water bath (40° C to 44° C) until frozen tissue is thawed is the best treatment. Pain is severe and should be treated with potent analgesics. Gentle cleansing and no pressure on the skin should be maintained during healing. Amputation of necrotic tissue is delayed until a clear line of demarcation is established.[61]

DISORDERS OF THE HAIR
Alopecia
Male-pattern alopecia (androcentric alopecia)

Alopecia means loss of hair. Localized hair loss in men is not a disease but a genetically predisposed response to androgens. Within the distribution of hair over the scalp, androgen-sensitive hair follicles are on top and androgen-insensitive follicles are on the sides and back. In genetically predisposed men, the androgen-sensitive follicles are transformed into vellus follicles. The normal hair is shed and replaced by fine, light, short hair. Male-pattern baldness begins with frontotemporal recession and progresses to loss of hair over the top of the scalp. Minoxidil is used to stimulate hair growth.[80] Affected men may choose to wear wigs, have hair transplants, or undergo plastic surgery.

Female-pattern alopecia

Some women in their 20s and 30s experience progressive thinning and loss of hair over the central part of the scalp. Contrary to male-pattern baldness, there is no loss of hair along the frontal hairline. Many of these women have elevated levels of serum adrenal androgen dehydroepiandrosterone sulfate (DHEAS).[81]

Alopecia areata

Alopecia areata is rapid onset of hair loss in multiple areas of the scalp, usually in round patches. The eyebrows, eyelashes, beard, and other areas of body hair are rarely involved. Stressful events, cell-mediated immune factors, genetic susceptibility, and metabolic disorders, such as Addison disease, thyroid disease, and lupus erythematosus, are associated with alopecia areata.[82,83]

The affected areas of skin are smooth or may have short shafts of hair. The hair shaft is poorly developed and breaks at the surface. Regrowth occurs within 1 to 3 months, but there may be recurrent hair loss at the same site. There is usually permanent regrowth of hair. Some young people experience total loss of hair (alopecia totalis), and the long-term prognosis for regrowth is poor.

Diagnosis is made by observation of the pattern of hair loss. Biopsy may show a lymphocytic infiltrate around the follicle. Intralesional steroids may be used to stimulate hair growth when there are a few small areas of hair loss. Systemic steroids are used for larger areas of alopecia. Topical applications of anthralin are also used to stimulate hair growth. Minoxidil has been tested for use in resistant cases and has been found effective in approximately 18% of cases with severe alopecia areata.[84]

Hirsutism

Hirsutism occurs in women and is the growth and distribution of hair on the face, body, and pubic area in a male pattern. There is also frontotemporal hair recession. These areas of hair growth are androgen sensitive. Variations of hair growth in women are great, and a male pattern may be normal. Women who develop hirsutism may be secreting hormones associated with ovarian or adrenal disease, and such women should be evaluated for polycystic ovaries, adrenal hyperplasia, or adrenal tumors. If no hormonal pathologic conditions exist, treatment may include cosmetic removal of hair, oral contraceptives, glucocorticoids, or cimetidine.

DISORDERS OF THE NAIL
Paronychia

Paronychia is an acute or chronic infection of the cuticle. Acute paronychia is manifest by the rapid onset of painful inflammation of the cuticle, usually after minor trauma. An abscess may develop requiring incision and drainage for relief of pain. The most common causative microorganisms are staphylococci and streptococci. Occasionally *Candida* is present.

Chronic paronychia develops slowly, with tenderness and swelling around the proximal or lateral nail folds. One or more fingers or toes may be involved. Individuals whose hands are frequently exposed to moisture are at greatest risk. Manipulation of the cuticle opens the space between the proximal nail fold and nail plate, leaving a moist, warm medium for the incubation of pathogenic microorganisms. The skin around the nail becomes more edematous and painful with progressive infection. Pus may be expressed from the proximal nail fold. The nail plate is usually not affected, although it can become discolored with ridges.

Treatment includes keeping the hands dry. Oral antibiotics are not very effective because they do not penetrate the affected tissues. Topical application of thymol is usually effective.

Onychomycosis

Onychomycosis is a fungal or dermatophyte infection of the nail plate. The most common pattern is a nail plate that turns yellow or white and becomes elevated with the accumulation of hyperkeratotic debris within the plate. Fungal infections of the nail are differentiated from psoriasis by culture and microscopy and the absence of pitting on the nail surface, which is characteristic of psoriasis. Treatment is difficult because topical or systemic antifungal agents do not penetrate the nail plate readily. New antifungal drugs are more effective.[85] Surgical excision of the nail may be required.

✓ QUICK CHECK

Describe the three degrees of burn injury.

What dangers accompany frostbite?

What is alopecia? Compare the different types.

What disorders of the nail are seen?

DID YOU UNDERSTAND?

Structure and Function of the Skin

1. Skin is the largest organ of the body and equals 20% of body weight.
2. The skin has two layers—the dermis and epidermis.
3. The underlying epidermis contains a basal and spinous layer with melanocytes, Langerhans cells, and Merkel cells.
4. The dermis is composed of connective tissue elements, hair follicles, sweat glands, sebaceous glands, blood vessels, nerves, and lymphatic vessels.
5. The papillary capillaries provide the major blood supply to the skin, arising from deeper arterial plexuses.
6. Heat loss and heat conservation are regulated by arteriovenous anastomoses that lead to the papillary capillaries.
7. Pressure ulcers develop from pressure and shearing forces that occlude capillary blood flow with resulting ischemia and necrosis. Areas at greatest risk are pressure points over bony prominences, such as the greater trochanters, sacrum, ischia, and heels. Immobilized individuals with fractures and neurologic deficits are most prone to develop pressure ulcers.
8. Pruritus is itching and is associated with many skin disorders. The exact neurologic mechanism is unknown, but pain receptors with low-intensity stimulation are one theory of irritation.

Disorders of the Skin

1. Contact dermatitis is a form of delayed hypersensitivity that develops with sensitization to allergies, such as metal, chemicals, or poison ivy.
2. Irritant contact dermatitis develops from prolonged exposure to chemicals, such as acids or soaps.
3. Atopic or allergic dermatitis is associated with a family history of allergies, hay fever, elevated IgE levels, and increased histamine sensitivity. Pruritus and scratching predispose the skin to infection, scaling, and thickening.
4. Stasis dermatitis occurs on the legs and results from venous stasis and edema.
5. Seborrheic dermatitis involves scaly, yellowish, inflammatory plaques of the scalp, eyebrows, eyelids, ear canals, chest, axillae, and back. The cause is unknown.
6. Papulosquamous disorders are characterized by papules, scales, plaques, and erythema.
7. Psoriasis is a chronic skin disease with thickening of both the epidermis and dermis, characterized by scaly, erythematous, pruritic plaques.
8. Pityriasis rosea is a self-limiting disease characterized by oval lesions with scales around the edges located along skin lines of the trunk.
9. Lichen planus is a papular, violet-colored inflammatory lesion of unknown origin manifest by severe pruritus.
10. Acne vulgaris is an inflammation of the pilosebaceous follicle.
11. Acne rosacea develops on the middle third of the face with hypertrophy and inflammation of the sebaceous glands.
12. Lupus erythematosus can affect only the skin (discoid) or have a systemic presentation. The inflammatory lesions usually occur in sun-exposed areas with a butterfly distribution over the nose and cheeks.
13. Pemphigus is a chronic, autoimmune, blistering disease that begins in the mouth or on the scalp and spreads to other parts of the body, often with a fatal outcome. There are two forms—pemphigus vulgaris and bullous pemphigus.
14. Erythema multiforme is an acute inflammation of the skin and mucous membranes with lesions that appear targetlike with alternating rings of edema and inflammation, often associated with allergic reactions to drugs. Stevens-Johnson syndrome is a severe form that also involves the mucous membranes.
15. Folliculitis is a bacterial infection of the hair follicle.
16. A furuncle is an infection of the hair follicle that extends to the surrounding tissue.
17. A carbuncle is a collection of infected hair follicles that forms a draining abscess.
18. Cellulitis is a diffuse infection of the dermis and subcutaneous tissue.
19. Erysipelas is a superficial streptococcal infection of the skin commonly affecting the face, ears, and lower legs.
20. Impetigo may have a bullous or an ulcerative form and is caused by *Staphylococcus* or *Streptococcus.*
21. Herpes simplex virus type 1 (HSV-1) causes cold sores but can infect the cornea, mouth, and labia. HSV-2 causes genital lesions and is usually spread by sexual contact.
22. Herpes zoster and varicella are both caused by the same herpesvirus.
23. Warts are benign, rough, elevated lesions caused by papillomavirus. Condylomata acuminata, or venereal warts, are spread by sexual contact.
24. Tinea infections (fungal infections) can occur anywhere on the body and are classified by location (i.e., tinea pedis, tinea corporis, tinea capitis).
25. Candidiasis is a yeastlike fungal infection occurring on skin, mucous membranes, and the gastrointestinal tract.
26. Cutaneous vasculitis is an inflammation of skin blood vessels with purpura, ischemia, and necrosis resulting from vessel necrosis.
27. Urticarial lesions are associated with hypersensitivity responses and appear as wheals, welts, or hives.
28. Scleroderma is a sclerosis of the skin that may also affect systemic organs and cause renal failure, bowel obstruction, or cardiac dysrhythmias.

DID YOU UNDERSTAND? —cont'd

29. Ticks cause a local reaction and can cause systemic disease when mouth parts pierce the skin and remain embedded in the tissue.

30. Lyme disease is a multisystem inflammatory disease caused by *Borrelia burgdorferi* transmitted by tick bites.

31. Mosquitoes can transmit infectious diseases, and the saliva from their bite produces the characteristic itching and wheal formation.

32. Blood-sucking flies are represented by many species, including Ceratopogonidae ("no-see-ums"), Tabanidae (horseflies), and Simuliidae (blackflies). Their bites are usually painful and produce bleeding, and the itching and local reactions may last for days with systemic symptoms of fever and malaise.

33. Seborrheic keratosis is a proliferation of basal cells that produce elevated, smooth, or warty lesions of varying size. They are most common among the elderly population.

34. Keratoacanthoma arises from hair follicles on sun-exposed areas. Three stages of development characterize the lesion, which results in a dome-shaped, crusty lesion filled with keratin that resolves in 3 to 4 months.

35. Actinic keratosis is a pigmented scaly lesion that develops in sun-exposed individuals with fair skin. The lesion may become malignant in the form of a squamous cell carcinoma.

36. Nevi arise from melanocytes and may be pigmented or fleshy pink. They occur singly or in groups and may undergo transition to malignant melanoma.

37. Basal cell carcinoma is the most common skin cancer and occurs most frequently on sun-exposed areas.

38. Squamous cell carcinoma is a tumor of the epidermis and can be localized (in situ) or invasive.

39. Malignant melanoma arises from melanocytes, and if not excised early, metastasis occurs through the lymph nodes.

40. Kaposi sarcoma is a vascular malignancy associated with immunodeficiency states.

41. Burns are classified according to depth and extent of injury.

42. First-degree burns involve the superficial skin without loss of protective function.

43. Second-degree burns are superficial (blister formation) or superficial partial-thickness with a waxy white appearance and no involvement of dermal appendages.

44. Third-degree burns involve full skin thickness and often underlying tissues. They are painless and can be life threatening as a result of hypovolemic shock and metabolic and immunologic responses.

45. Severe burns cause profound edema and burn shock related to an inflammatory response throughout the cardiovascular system; consequently, distant organ function is affected, and immune protection is altered with increased risks for sepsis.

46. Keloids are sharply elevated scars that extend beyond the border of traumatized skin.

47. Frostbite usually occurs on cheeks and digits, with direct injury to cells and impaired circulation.

Disorders of the Hair

1. Male-pattern alopecia is an inherited form of irreversible baldness with hair loss in the central scalp and recession of the temporofrontal hairline.

2. Female-pattern alopecia is a thinning of the central hair of the scalp beginning in women at 20 to 30 years of age.

3. Alopecia areata is patchy loss of hair usually associated with stress or metabolic diseases; it is usually reversible.

4. Hirsutism is a male pattern of hair growth in women that may be normal or the result of excessive secretion of androgenic hormones.

Disorders of the Nail

1. Paronychia is an inflammation of the cuticle that can be acute or chronic and is usually caused by staphylococci or streptococci.

2. Onychomycosis is a fungal infection of the nail plate.

KEY TERMS

Acne rosacea, 1104
Acne vulgaris, 1104
Allergic contact dermatitis, 1101
Alopecia, 1120
Alopecia areata, 1121
Apocrine sweat gland, 1092
Atopic dermatitis, 1101
Basal cell carcinoma, 1113
Burn shock, 1117

Candidiasis, 1109
Capillary seal, 1118
Carbuncle, 1107
Cellulitis, 1107
Clawlike prolongation, 1100
Condylomata acuminata, 1108
Cutaneous vasculitis, 1110
Deep partial-thickness burn, 1117
Dermal appendage, 1092

Dermis, 1092
Discoid lupus erythematosus (DLE), 1105
Eccrine sweat gland, 1092
Eczema, 1101
Epidermis, 1092
Erysipelas, 1107
Erythema multiforme, 1106
Escharotomy, 1117

KEY TERMS

First-degree burn, 1115
Fluid resuscitation, 1118
Folliculitis, 1106
Frostbite, 1120
Furuncle, 1107
Herald patch, 1103
Herpes simplex virus (HSV), 1107
Herpes zoster, 1107
Hirsutism, 1121
Hyphae, 1109
Hypodermis, 1092
Impetigo, 1107
Irritant contact dermatitis, 1101
Kaposi sarcoma (KS), 1114
Keloid, 1100
Lichen planus, 1103
Lupus erythematosus, 1105

Lyme disease, 1111
Melanoma, 1114
Mosquito, 1111
Onychomycosis, 1121
Papillary capillary, 1092
Papulosquamous disorder, 1102
Paraneoplastic pemphigus, 1106
Paronychia, 1121
Partial-thickness injury, 1115
Pemphigus, 1105
Pemphigus erythematosus, 1106
Pemphigus foliaceus, 1106
Pemphigus vulgaris, 1105
Pityriasis rosea, 1103
Psoriasis, 1102
Scleroderma, 1110
Sebaceous gland, 1092

Seborrheic dermatitis, 1102
Second-degree burn, 1115
Squamous cell carcinoma, 1113
Stasis dermatitis, 1102
Stevens-Johnson syndrome, 1106
Superficial partial-thickness injury, 1115
Sweat gland, 1092
Third-degree burn (full-thickness burn), 1117
Tinea capitis, 1108
Tinea corporis (ringworm), 1108
Tinea infection, 1109
Tinea pedis, 1108
Total body surface area (TBSA), 1117
Urticarial lesion, 1110
Varicella, 1107
Wart, 1108

REFERENCES

1. Berlowitz, D.R., Brandeis, G.H., & Anderson, J. (1997). Predictors of pressure ulcer healing among long-term care residents. *Journal of the American Geriatric Society, 45*, 30-34.

2. Cox, K.R., Laird, M., & Brown, J.M. (1998). Predicting and preventing pressure ulcers in adults. *Nursing Management, 29*(7), 41-45.

3. Yarkony, G.M. (1994). Pressure ulcers: A review. *Archives of Physical Medicine and Rehabilitation, 75*(8), 908-917.

4. Klecz, R.J. & Schwartz, R.A. (1992). Pruritus. *American Family Physician, 45*(6), 2681-2686.

5. Greaves, M.W. and Wall, P.D. (1996). Pathophysiology of itching. *Lancet, 348*(9032), 938-940.

6. Schmeltz, M. et al. (1997). Specific C-receptors for itch in human skin. *Journal of Neuroscience, 17*(20), 8003-8008.

7. Muizzuddin, N., Marenus, K.D., & Maes, D.H. (1998). Factors defining sensitive skin and its treatment. *American Journal of Contact Dermatitis, 9*(3), 170-175.

8. Barker, J.N. (1992). Role of keratinocytes in allergic contact dermatitis. *Contact Dermatitis, 26*(3), 145-148.

9. Mahmoudi, M., Dineen, A.M., & Hunt, L.W. (1998). Simultaneous IgE-mediated urticaria and contact dermatitis from latex. *Allergy, 53*(10), 1009-1010.

10. Kim, H.J. & Honig, P.J. (1998). Atopic dermatitis. *Current Opinions in Pediatrics, 10*(4), 387-392.

11. Graham-Brown, R.A.C. (1997). Therapeutics in atopic dermatitis. In W.D. James et al. *Advances in dermatology* (vol. 13, pp. 3-31). St. Louis: Mosby.

12. Szabo, S.K. et al. (1998). Identification and quantitation of interferon-gamma producing T cells in psoriatic lesions: Localization to both CD4+ and CD8+ subsets. *Journal of Investigative Dermatology, 111*(6), 1072-1078.

13. Bhalerao, J. & Bowcock, A.M. (1998). The genetics of psoriasis: A complex disorder of the skin and immune system. *Human Molecular Genetics, 7*(10), 1537-1545.

14. Spuls, P.I. et al. (1998). The development of practice guidelines for the treatment of severe plaque from psoriasis. *Archives of Dermatology, 134*(12), 1591-1596.

15. Drago, F. et al. (1997). Human herpesvirus 7 in patients with pityriasis rosea: Electron microscopy investigations and polymerase chain reaction in mononuclear cells, plasma, and skin. *Dermatology, 195*(4), 374-378.

16. Allen, R.A., Janniger, C.K., & Schwartz, R.A. (1995). Pityriasis rosea. *Cutis, 56*(4), 198-202.

17. Tosti, A. et al. (1998). Lichen planus of the nails and fingertips. *European Journal of Dermatology, 8*(6), 447-448.

18. Cribier, B., Frances, C., & Chosidow, O. (1998). Treatment of lichen planus. An evidence-based medicine analysis of efficiency. *Archives of Dermatology, 134*(12), 1521-1530.

19. Wilkin, J.K. (1994). Rosacea: Pathophysiology and treatment. *Archives of Dermatology, 130*(3), 359-362.

20. Webster, G.F. (1998). Acne and rosacea. *Medical Clinics of North America, 82*(5), 1145-1154, vi.

21. Yell, J.A., Mbuagbaw, J., & Burge, S.M. (1996). Cutaneous manifestations of systemic lupus erythematosus. *British Journal of Dermatology, 135*, 355-362.

22. Bulman, P.M. & Hunder, G. (1998). New approaches for treatment of systemic lupus erythematosus [news]. *Annals of Internal Medicine, 129*(12), 1095-1096.

23. Stevens, R.J. et al. (1997). Thalidomide in the treatment of cutaneous manifestations of lupus erythematosus:

REFERENCES

Experience in sixteen consecutive patients. *British Journal of Rheumatology, 36*(3), 353-359.

24. Eyre, R.W. & Stanley, J.R. (1989). Biochemical differentiation of types of pemphigus. *Immunology & Serology, 46*, 317-331.

25. Schoen, H. et al. (1998). Immunoapheresis in paraneoplastic pemphigus. *Archives of Dermatology, 134*(6), 706-710.

26. Fleischli, M.E., Valek, R.H., & Pandya, A.G. (1999). Pulse intravenous cyclophosphamide therapy in pemphigus. *Archives of Dermatology, 135*(1), 57-61.

27. Enk, A.H. & Knop, J. (1999). Mycophenolate is effective in the treatment of pemphigus vulgaris. *Archives of Dermatology, 135*(1), 54-56.

28. Aurelian, L., Kokuba, H., & Burnett, J.W. (1998). Understanding the pathogenesis of HSV-associated erythema multiforme. *Dermatology, 197*(3), 219-222.

29. Roujeau, J.C. (1997). Stevens-Johnson syndrome and toxic epidermal necrolysis are severity variants of the same disease which differs from erythema multiforme. *Journal of Dermatology, 24*(11), 726-729.

30. Wahren, B. & Linde, A. (1991). Virological and clinical characteristics of human herpes virus 6. *Scandinavian Journal of Infectious Disease, 80*(Suppl.), 105-109.

31. Crumpacker, C.S. (1987). Herpes simplex. In T.B. Fitzpatrick et al. (Eds.). *Dermatology in general medicine* (3rd ed.). New York: McGraw-Hill.

32. Mindel, A. (1991). Cutaneous herpes simplex infection. *Scandinavian Journal of Infectious Disease, 80*(Suppl.), 47-52.

33. Morgan, R. & King, D. (1998). Shingles: A review of diagnosis and management. *Hospital Medicine, 59*(10), 770-776.

34. Volmink, J. et al. (1996). Treatments for postherpes neuralgia—A systemic review of randomized controlled trials. *Family Practitioner, 13*(1), 84-91.

35. Jablonska, S. (1998). Traditional therapies for the treatment of condylomata acuminata (genital warts). *Australasian Journal of Dermatology, 39*(Suppl. 1), S2-S4.

36. Stein, D.H. (1998). Tineas—Superficial dermatophyte infections. *Pediatric Review, 19*(11), 368-372.

37. Levitz, S.M. (1992). Overview of host defenses in fungal infections. *Clinics in Infectious Disease, 14*(Suppl. 1), 537-542.

38. Zuberbier, T. et al. (1996). Clinical aspects and therapeutic responsiveness. *Acta Dermato-Venereologica, 76*, 295-297.

39. Henz, B.M. & Zuberbier, T. (1998). Most chronic urticaria is food-dependent, and not idiopathic. *Experimental Dermatology, 7*(40), 139-142.

40. Leznoff, A. (1998). Chronic urticaria. *Canadian Family Physician, 44*, 2170-2176.

41. Steen, V.D. (1998). Clinical manifestations of systemic sclerosis. *Seminars in Cutaneous Medicine and Surgery, 17*(1), 48-54.

42. Haustein, U.F. & Anderegg, U. (1998). Pathophysiology of scleroderma: An update. *Journal of the European Academy of Dermatology and Venereology, 11*(1), 1-8.

43. Lee, P. (1993). Clinical aspects of systemic and localized sclerosis. *Current Opinions in Rheumatology, 5*(6), 785-791.

44. White, B. (1998). Clinical approach to scleroderma. *Seminars in Cutaneous Medicine and Surgery, 17*(3), 213-218.

45. Evans, J. (1998). Lyme disease. *Current Opinions in Rheumatology, 10*(4), 339-346.

46. Van Hoecke, C. et al. (1998). Clinical and immunological assessment of a candidate Lyme disease vaccine in health adults: Antibody persistence and effect of a booster dose at month 12. *Vaccine, 16*(17), 1688-1692.

47. Binder, M. et al. (1998). Estimation of volume-weighted mean nuclear volume discriminates keratoacanthoma from squamous cell carcinoma. *American Journal of Dermatopathology, 20*(5), 453-458.

48. American Cancer Society (ACS). (1999). *Cancer facts and figures—1999.* Atlanta: The Author.

49. English, D.R. et al. (1997). Sunlight and cancer. *Cancer Causes and Control, 8*(3), 271-283.

50. Truhan, A.P. (1991). Sun protection in childhood. *Clinical Pediatrics, 30*(12), 676-681.

51. Goldman, G.D. (1998). Squamous cell cancer: A practical approach. *Seminars in Cutaneous Medicine and Surgery, 17*(20), 80-95.

52. Franceschi, S. et al. (1996). Site distribution of different types of skin cancer: New aetiologic clues. *International Journal of Cancer, 67*, 24-28.

53. Berwick, M. & Halpern, A. (1997). Melanoma epidemiology. *Current Opinions in Oncology, 9*(2), 178-182.

54. Koh, H.K. et al. (1996). Prevention and early detection strategies for melanoma and skin cancer: Current status. *Archives of Dermatology, 132*, 436-443.

55. Williams, M.L. & Sagebiel, R.W. (1994). Melanoma risk factors and atypical moles. *Western Journal of Medicine, 160*(4), 343-350.

56. Safai, B. (1987). Pathophysiology and epidemiology of epidemic Kaposi's sarcoma. *Seminars in Oncology, 14*(2, Suppl. 3), 7.

57. Sturzl, M. et al. (1992). Expression of platelet-derived growth factor and its receptor in AIDS-related Kaposi sarcoma in vivo suggests paracrine and autocrine mechanisms of tumor maintenance. *Proceedings of the National Academy of Science of the United States of America, 89*(15), 7046-7050.

58. Goopman, J. (1987). Neoplasms in the acquired immune deficiency syndrome: The multidisciplinary approach. *Seminars in Oncology, 14*(2, Suppl. 3), 1-6.

59. Li, N., Anderson, W.K., & Bahwan, J. (1998). Further confirmation of the association of human herpesvirus 8 with Kaposi's sarcoma. *Journal of Cutaneous Pathology, 25*(8), 413-419.

REFERENCES

60. Brigham, P.A. & McLoughlin, E. (1996). Burn incidence and medical care use in the United States: Estimates, trends, and data sources. *Journal of Burn Care and Rehabilitation, 17*(2), 95-107.

61. Greenfield, L.J. et al. (1997). *Surgery: Scientific principles and practice* (2nd ed.). Philadelphia: Lippincott-Raven.

62. Pruitt, B.A., Goodwin, C.W., & Cioffi, W.G. (1995). Thermal injuries. In J.H. Davis & G.F. Sheldon. *Surgery: A problem-solving approach* (2nd ed.). St. Louis: Mosby.

63. Brigham, P.A. & McLoughlin, E. (1996). Burn incidence and medical care use in the United States: Estimates, trends, and data sources. *Journal of Burn Care and Rehabilitation, 17*(2), 95.

64. Miller, S.F. et al. (1991). Burn size estimate reliability: A study. *Journal of Burn Care and Rehabilitation, 12*(6), 546-559.

65. Evans, J.A., Darlington, D.N., & Gann, D.S. (1991). A circulating factor(s) mediates cell depolarization in hemorrhagic shock. *Annals of Surgery, 312*(6), 549-557.

66. Klein, G.L. & Herndon, D.N. (1998). Magnesium deficit in major burns: Role in hypoparathyroidism and end-organ parathyroid hormone resistance. *Magnesium Research, 11*(2), 103-109.

67. Deets. D.D. & Glaviano, V.V. (1973). Plasma and cardiac lactic dehydrogenase activity in burn shock. *Proceedings of the Society of Experimental Biology and Medicine, 142*, 412-416.

68. Okamoto, R., Glaviano, V.V., & Pindok, M. (1971). Myocardial lipases and catecholamines in burn shock. *Proceedings of the Society of Experimental and Biological Medicine, 137*, 347-353.

69. Wilmore, D.W., Aulick, H.L., & Goodwin, C.W. (1979). Glucose metabolism following severe injury. *Acta Chirurgica Scandinavica, 498*, 3-47.

70. Gump, F.E., Price, J.B., Jr., & Kinney, J.M. (1970). Blood flow and oxygen consumption in patients with severe burns. *Surgery, Gynecology, and Obstetrics, 130*, 23-28.

71. Wilmore, D.W. et al. (1977). Influence of the burn wound on local and systemic responses to injury. *Annals of Surgery, 186*, 444-458.

72. Wilmore, D.W. et al. (1980). Effect of injury and infection on visceral metabolism and circulation. *Annals of Surgery, 192*, 491-500.

73. Griswold, J.A. (1993). White blood cell response to burn injury. *Seminars in Nephrology, 13*(4), 409-415.

74. Garner, W.L. et al. (1994). Acute skin injury releases neutrophil chemoattractants. *Surgery, 116*(1), 42-48.

75. Kelly, D. & Lynch, J.B. (1992). Burns in alcohol and drug users result in longer treatment times with more complications. *Journal of Burn Care and Rehabilitation, 13*, 218-220.

76. Nguyen, T.T. et al. (1996). Current treatment of severely burned patients. *Annals of Surgery, 223*(1), 14-25.

77. Patterson, D.R. (1995). Nonopioid-based approaches to burn pain. *Journal of Burn Care and Rehabilitation, 16*(2, pt. 2), 372-376.

78. Grandberg, P.O. (1991). Freezing cold injury. *Arctic Medical Research, 50*(Suppl. 6), 76-79.

79. Fisher, R.P., Souba, W.W., & Ford, E.G. (1988). Temperature associated injuries and syndromes. In K.L. Mattox, E.E. Moore, & D.V. Feliciano (Eds.). *Trauma.* Norwalk, Conn.: Appleton & Lange.

80. Savin, R.C. & Atton, A.V. (1993). Minoxidil: Update on its clinical role. *Dermatologic Clinics, 11*(1), 55-64.

81. Rushton, D.H. (1993). Management of hair loss in women. *Dermatologic Clinics, 11*(1), 47-53.

82. Ghersetich, I., Campanile, G., & Lotti, T. (1996). Alopecia areata: Immunohistochemistry and ultrastructure of infiltrate and identification of adhesion molecule receptors. *International Journal of Dermatology, 35*, 28-33.

83. Gupta, M.A., Gupta, A.K., & Watteel, G.N. (1997). Stress and alopecia areata. *Acta Dermato-Venereologica, 77*, 297-298.

84. Feidler-Weiss, V.C., et al. (1987). Evaluation of oral minoxidil in the treatment of alopecia areata. *Archives of Dermatology, 123*, 1488-1490.

85. Elewski, B.E. (1998). Onychomycosis: Pathogenesis, diagnosis, and management. *Clinical Microbiology Review, 11*(93), 415-429.

www.mosby.com/MERLIN/Huether

CHAPTER

40

Alterations of the Integument in Children

Sue E. Huether

Children frequently develop alterations in the skin. The lesions may be minor or severe and localized or generalized. There are often no prodromal symptoms. Skin diseases in children may have different mechanisms than in adults, although the causative mechanisms may be similar. Many diseases resolve spontaneously and require no treatment. Diagnosis is commonly made from the history, appearance, and distribution of the lesion or lesions. Common skin diseases of childhood are presented here.

Noreen Heer Nicol, RN, MS, FNP, contributed to this chapter in the previous edition.

CHAPTER OUTLINE

* **Acne Vulgaris,** 1128

* **Dermatitis,** 1128
  Atopic Dermatitis, 1128
  Diaper Dermatitis, 1129

* **Infections of the Skin,** 1129
  Bacterial Infections, 1129
  Fungal Infections, 1130
  Viral Infections, 1131

* **Insect Bites and Parasites,** 1134
  Scabies, 1134
  Pediculosis (Lice Infestation), 1135
  Fleas, 1135
  Bedbugs, 1136

* **Vascular Disorders,** 1136
  Strawberry Hemangioma, 1136
  Cavernous Hemangiomas, 1136
  Salmon Patches, 1137
  Port-Wine Stain, 1137

* **Other Skin Disorders,** 1137
  Miliaria, 1137
  Erythema Toxicum Neonatorum, 1137

Check out your CD Companion for chapter-related exercises and answers to the Quick Check questions

1127

ACNE VULGARIS

Acne vulgaris is the most common skin disease and affects 85% of the population between the ages of 12 and 25 years. Genetic influences may determine an individual's susceptibility and severity of the disease. The incidence of acne is the same in both genders, although severe disease affects males more frequently.

Acne develops at distinctive pilosebaceous units known as *sebaceous follicles.* Located primarily on the face and upper parts of the chest and back, these follicles have many large sebaceous glands, a small vellus hair, and a dilated follicular canal that is visible as a "pore" on the skin surface. Acne lesions may be inflammatory or noninflammatory (Fig. 40-1). In **noninflammatory acne,** the comedones are open (blackheads) and closed (whiteheads), with the accumulated material causing distention of the follicle and thinning of follicular canal walls. **Inflammatory acne** develops in closed comedones when the follicular wall ruptures, expelling sebum into the surrounding dermis and initiating inflammation. Pustules form when the inflammation is close to the surface; papules and cystic nodules can develop when the inflammation is deeper, causing mild to severe scarring. Both types of lesions may exist in the same individual.

The principal causative factors are abnormal keratinization of the follicular epithelium, excessive sebum production, and proliferation of *Propionibacterium acnes.* Androgenic hormones are involved. Dihydrotestosterone increases the size and productivity of the sebaceous glands.[1] Sebum accumulation obstructs the pilosebaceous unit until the accumulated material and bacteria within the follicle (see Fig. 40-1) produce inflammation when it is exposed to the dermis with rupture of a follicle.

Acne conglobata is a highly inflammatory form of acne with communicating cysts and abscesses beneath the skin.

Remissions tend to occur during the summer, perhaps from more exposure to sunlight.

Topical treatment, including benzoyl peroxide, salicylic acid, and tretinoin, should be the first line of therapy because it is the least invasive. Use of systemic therapies, including oral antibiotics, sex hormones, corticosteroids, and isotretinoin, may be limited by side effects. Acne surgery, including comedo extraction, intralesional steroids, and cryosurgery, is useful in selected patients. Severe scarring may be treated with dermabrasion.[2]

DERMATITIS
Atopic Dermatitis

Atopic dermatitis (AD) is the most common cause of eczema in children, with a prevalence of up to 12%.[3] From 75% to 80% of individuals with atopic dermatitis have a personal or family history of asthma or allergic rhinitis (hay fever). Onset is usually from 2 to 6 months of age, and 85% of cases occur within the first 5 years of life. There are no specific laboratory features of AD that can be used for diagnostic purposes. An increased serum immunoglobulin E (IgE) level and positive skin tests to a variety of common food and inhalant allergens are seen in approximately 80% of individuals.[4] Similarly, blood eosinophilia is a common finding in AD.

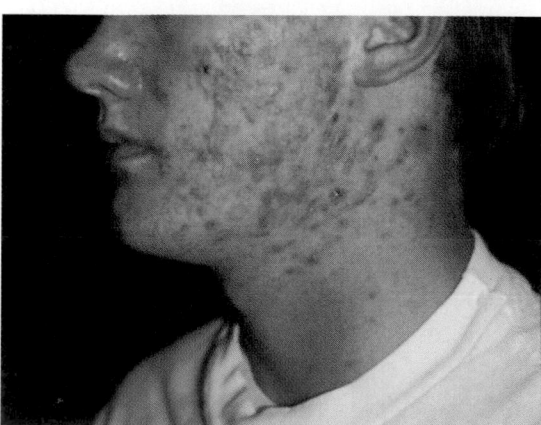

Fig. 40-1 *Cystic acne.* Multiple pustules (erythematous papules and pustules) are present, and several have become confluent. Note areas of scarring. *(Courtesy Department of Dermatology, School of Medicine, University of Utah.)*

Fig. 40-2 *Atopic dermatitis.* Characteristic lesions with crusting from irritation and scratching over knees and around ankles. *(Courtesy Department of Dermatology, School of Medicine, University of Utah.)*

AD has a constellation of clinical features that include severe pruritus, chronic course with frequent exacerbations, and characteristic eczematoid appearance and age-dependent distribution of skin lesions. The skin becomes increasingly dry, sensitive, itchy, and easily irritated because the barrier function is impaired. Microscopic epidermal cracks that let water out and irritants and allergens in lead to further drying and cracking, which results in rubbing and scratching. Rubbing and scratching to relieve the itch are actually responsible for many of the clinical changes seen. In young children, the rash appears primarily on the face, scalp, trunk, and extensor surfaces of the arms and legs (Fig. 40-2). In older children and adults, the rash tends to be found on the neck, antecubital and popliteal fossae, and hands and feet. Individuals with AD also tend to develop viral, bacterial, and fungal skin infections in the eczematous areas.

Management of patients with AD includes accurate diagnosis, identification and elimination of exacerbating factors, such as irritants and allergens, and reduction of emotional stresses. Hydration of the skin is the key to good therapy. Antiinflammatory agents, such as topical corticosteroids or tar preparations, are necessary during active flares of eczema. Systemic therapy includes the use of sedating antihistamines and antibiotics.

Diaper Dermatitis

Diaper dermatitis is probably the most common skin disorder of infancy and early childhood. This collection of inflammatory disorders affects the lower aspect of the abdomen, genitalia, buttock, and upper portion of the thigh. It is a form of contact dermatitis initiated by a combination of factors including prolonged exposure to and irritation by urine and feces, maceration by wet diapers, and airtight plastic diaper covers. Frequently, diaper dermatitis is secondarily infected with *Candida albicans.*

The lesions vary from mild erythema to erythematous papular lesions. Candidal (monilial) diaper dermatitis is usually very erythematous, with sharp margination and pustulovesicular satellite lesions (Fig. 40-3).

Fig. 40-3 *Diaper dermatitis.* **A,** Diaper dermatitis with erosions. **B,** Diaper dermatitis with *Candida albicans* secondary infection. *(Courtesy Department of Dermatology, School of Medicine, University of Utah.)*

✓ QUICK CHECK

What causes the inflammation of acne vulgaris?

What lesions are typical of atopic dermatitis in children?

What causes diaper dermatitis?

Treatment is frequently changing diapers to keep the area clean and dry or frequently exposing the perineal area to air. Topical antifungal medication is used to treat *C. albicans.* Short-term use of low-potency topical steroids alternately with antifungals at each diaper change helps to reduce the inflammation. Use of various topical medications to provide a barrier from the irritating agents promotes healing.

INFECTIONS OF THE SKIN

Infectious diseases caused by bacteria, viruses, and fungi constitute the major forms of skin disease. Most infections tend to occur superficially; however, systemic signs and symptoms develop occasionally and can be life threatening.

Bacterial Infections

Impetigo contagiosum

Impetigo is a common bacterial skin infection in infants and children, usually caused by staphylococcus and streptococcus.[5] The disease is more common in midsummer to late summer, with a higher incidence in hot, humid climates. Impetigo is particularly infectious among people living in crowded conditions with poor sanitary facilities. It affects children in good health, but conditions such as anemia and malnutrition are predisposing factors. There are two types of impetigo: bullous and vesicular (Box 40-1). Both start as vesicles with a very thin vesicular roof composed of stratum corneum (Fig. 40-4).

The treatment of choice for both types of impetigo is systemic antibiotics. Prompt treatment avoids complications, such as glomerulonephritis. Removal of crusts and scrubbing the lesions with antibacterial soaps have not been effective.[6] Good handwashing techniques and isolation of the infected child's washcloth, towels, drinking glass, and linen are important.

Fig. 40-4 *Impetigo and herpes simplex virus (HSV) of upper lip.* Note weeping and crusting lesions. *(Courtesy Department of Dermatology, School of Medicine, University of Utah.)*

Staphylococcal scalded-skin syndrome

Staphylococcal scalded-skin syndrome (SSSS) is the most serious staphylococcal infection that affects the skin. It is caused by infection with group II staphylococci, which produce a toxin—an epidermolysin that causes a separation of the skin just below the granular layer of the epidermis. The syndrome is more common in children younger than 10 years than in adults. Adults have circulating antistaphylococcal antibodies and are better able to metabolize and excrete the toxin. Neonates are at the highest risk because of their lack of immunity, not having prior exposure to the toxin.

The clinical symptoms begin with fever, malaise, rhinorrhea, and irritability followed by generalized erythema with exquisite tenderness of the skin. There may be an associated impetigo, but the infection often begins in the throat or chest. The erythema spreads from the face and trunk to cover the entire body except the palms, soles, and mucous membranes. Within 48 hours, blisters and bullae may form and the pain is severe (Fig. 40-5). Fluid loss from ruptured blisters and water evaporation from denuded areas may cause dehydration. Perioral and nasolabial crusting and fissures develop. In severe cases, the skin of the entire body may slough. When secondary infection can be prevented, healing of the involved skin occurs in 10 to 14 days, usually without scarring. Before medical intervention is initiated, culture, histology, or exfoliative cytology must be done to differentiate SSSS from toxic epidermal necrolysis (TEN). When the infection is confirmed, treatment with oral or intravenous antibiotics is begun. The skin should be treated the same as a severe burn, with meticulous aseptic technique. Special care is required when there is involvement of the lips and eyelids.

Fungal Infections
Tinea capitis

Tinea capitis, a fungal infection of the scalp, is the most common fungal infection of childhood. It rarely affects infants and is seen in children between 2 and 10 years of age. Primary organisms responsible for this disease are *Microspo-*

Impetigo
BOX 40-1

BULLOUS IMPETIGO
Caused by *Staphylococcus aureus*
Bacterial toxin produced (exfoliative toxin [ET]) causes disruption in cellular adhesion
Occurs in neonates
Is highly contagious
Source is family member with pustule or asymptomatic carrier with pathogen in anterior nares, perineal region, or fingernails
Transmitted by contact with individual or contaminated equipment
Presents with vesicles that enlarge or coalesce to form superficial bullae, few localized lesions or many scattered over the skin surface; as bullae rupture, thin, flat, honey-colored crust appears (hallmark of impetigo)
Lesions found on face around the nose and mouth; hands and other exposed areas also susceptible

VESICULAR IMPETIGO
Contagious, acute, superficial, vesiculopustular form
Caused by group A *Streptococcus pyogenes* (alone or with *S. aureus*)
Spread by direct physical contact with other infected individuals or through insect bites
Presents as small vesicles with a honey-colored serum; yellow to white-brown crusts form as vesicles rupture and extend radially
Untreated lesions last for weeks and cover large area
Regional lymphadenitis common
Most significant complication is acute glomerulonephritis
Treatment is aggressive in light of this complication

---

rum canis and *Trichophyton tonsurans. M. canis* is found on cats, dogs, and certain rodents. Humans appear to be a terminal host for *M. canis,* and children who handle such animals are possible hosts. Human-to-human transmission does not occur. *T. tonsurans* conversely is transmitted human-to-human, with areas of crowding the most prevalent environments. Frequently, the lesions are circular and manifest by broken hairs 1 to 3 mm above the scalp, leaving a partial alopecia from 1 to 5 cm in diameter (Fig. 40-6). A slight erythema and scaling with raised borders can be observed.

Diagnosis is best confirmed by performing Wood light examination, potassium hydroxide (KOH) examination, and fungal culture, in that order. Oral griseofulvin is the treatment of choice, and new agents are being tested for resistant strains.[7]

Tinea corporis

Tinea corporis is a common superficial dermatophyte infection in children. The organisms most commonly responsible for this disease are *M. canis* and *Trichophyton mentagro-*

Fig. 40-5 *Staphylococcal scalded-skin syndrome (SSSS).* The skin lesions, showing desquamation and wrinkling of the skin margins, appeared 1 day after drainage of a staphylococcal abscess. *(From Levine, G. & Norden, C. [1972]. New England Journal of Medicine, 287, 1339.)*

Fig. 40-6 *Tinea capitis. (Courtesy Department of Dermatology, School of Medicine, University of Utah.)*

phytes. As in tinea capitis, contact with young kittens and puppies is a common source of the disorder. Tinea corporis preferentially affects the nonhairy parts of the face, trunk, and limbs. Lesions are often erythematous, round or oval scaling patches that spread peripherally with clearing in the center, creating the "ring" appearance, which is why this disease is commonly referred to as *ringworm.* The lesions are distributed asymmetrically, and multiple lesions, when present, overlap. Potassium hydroxide examination of the scale from the border of the lesions confirms the diagnosis. Most lesions respond well to applications of appropriate topical antifungal medications.[8]

Thrush

Thrush is the term used to describe the presence of *Candida* in the mucous membranes of the mouth of infants and, less commonly, adults. Thrush is characterized by the formation of white plaques or spots in the mouth that lead to shallow ulcers caused by keratolytic proteases from the microorganism. The tongue may have a dense, white covering. The underlying mucous membrane is red and tender and may bleed when the plaques are removed. The disease is often accompanied by fever and gastrointestinal irritation. The infection commonly spreads to the groin, buttocks, and other parts of the body. Treatment may be difficult and may include oral antifungal washes, such as nystatin oral suspension. Simultaneous treatment of a *Candida* nipple infection or vaginitis in the mother is helpful in reducing the *C. albicans* surface colonization of the infant. Feeding bottles and nipples should be sterilized to prevent reinfection. The diaper area should be kept clean and dry.

Viral Infections

Viral infections of the skin in children are caused by poxvirus, papovavirus, and herpesvirus.

Molluscum contagiosum

Molluscum contagiosum is a common, highly contagious viral infection of the skin and, occasionally, conjunctiva that affects primarily children. A poxvirus that induces epidermal cell proliferation causes this disease. The epidermis grows down into the dermis to form saccules containing clusters of virus. The characteristic molluscum body is composed of mature, immature, and incomplete viruses and cellular debris.[9]

The lesions of molluscum are discrete, slightly umbilicated, dome-shaped papules 1 to 5 mm in diameter that appear anywhere on the skin or conjunctiva. The lesions are mainly on the trunk, face, and extremities in children (Fig. 40-7). There is usually no inflammation surrounding mol-

Fig. 40-7 *Molluscum contagiosum.* Waxy pink globules with umbilicated centers. *(From Habif, T.P. [1996]. Clinical dermatology: A color guide to diagnosis and therapy [3rd ed.]. St. Louis: Mosby.)*

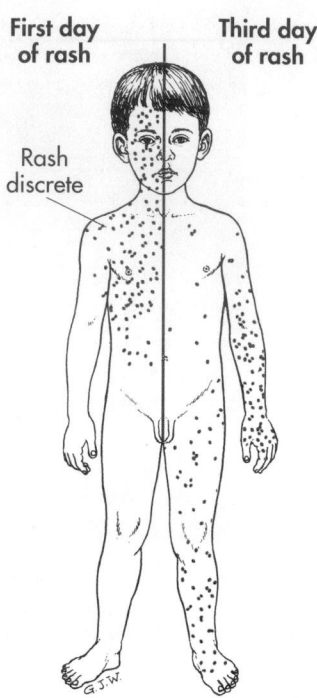

Fig. 40-8 *Measles.* Full-blown maculopapular rash with tendency to coalesce. *(From Wehrle, P.F. & Top, F.H., Sr. [1981]. Communicable and infectious diseases [9th ed.]. St. Louis: Mosby.)*

luscum lesions unless they are traumatized or secondary infection occurs. Scarring occurs with healing.

The best three diagnostic procedures are (1) staining smears of the expressed molluscum body, (2) examining a biopsy specimen, or (3) inoculating a molluscum suspension into cell cultures to demonstrate the cytotoxic reactions. Most lesions are self-limiting and clear in 6 to 9 months if not manipulated. The papules can be removed by curette or destroyed with liquid nitrogen.[10] If multiple lesions are present, however, these procedures are painful to small children and are not justified. Topical cantharidin can be used to treat these lesions. Measures to prevent spread of infection must be taken. Recurrences are common.

Rubella (German or 3-day measles)

Rubella is a common communicable disease of children and young adults caused by a ribonucleic acid (RNA) virus that enters the bloodstream through the respiratory route. This disease is mild in most children. The incubation period ranges from 14 to 21 days. Prodromal symptoms include enlarged cervical and postauricular lymph nodes, low-grade fever, headache, sore throat, runny nose, and cough. A faint-pink to red coalescing maculopapular rash develops on the face with spread to the trunk and extremities 1 to 4 days after the onset of initial symptoms (Fig. 40-8). The rash is thought to be the result of virus dissemination to the skin. The rash subsides after 2 to 3 days, usually without complication. Children are usually not contagious after development of the rash (Table 40-1).

Vaccination for rubella is usually combined with vaccines for mumps and measles (rubeola) (MMR). Recommendations now state that MMR vaccine should be given at 12 to 15 months of age, so there will not be interference from maternal measles antibody, and again at either 4 to 6 years or 11 to 12 years.[11] Measles is known to occur in previously immunized children.[12]

Women of childbearing age are immunized if their rubella hemagglutination-inhibition titer is low. Pregnancy should be avoided for 3 months after vaccination because the attenuated virus in the vaccine may remain for this period. Pregnant women who have rubella early in the first trimester may have a fetus that develops congenital defects. There is no specific treatment. Recovery is spontaneous, although lymph nodes may remain enlarged for weeks. Supportive therapy includes rest, fluids, and use of a vaporizer. In rare cases, a mild encephalitis or peripheral neuritis may follow rubella.

Rubeola (red measles)

Rubeola is a highly contagious, acute viral disease of children. Transmitted by direct contact with droplets from in-

TABLE 40-1	Differential Presentation of Viral Diseases Producing Rashes			
Viral Disease	**Incubation**	**Prodromal Symptoms**	**Duration/Characteristics**	**Clinical Symptoms**
Rubella (German measles)	14-21 days	1-2 days Mild fever Malaise Respiratory symptoms	1-3 days Pink-red maculopapular Face and trunk	Enlarged and tender occipital and periauricular nodes
Rubeola (measles)	7-12 days	2-5 days Fever Cough Respiratory symptoms	3-5 days Purple-red to brown maculopapular Face, trunk, extremities	Koplik spots 1-3 days before rash
Roseola (exanthema subitum)	5-15 days	2-5 days High fever	1-3 days Red macular Neck and trunk	Rash develops when fever subsides
Varicella (chickenpox)	11-20 days	1-2 days Low-grade fever Cough May be asymptomatic	7-14 days Red papules, vesicles, pustules in clusters	Eruption of new lesions for 4-5 days Occasional ulcerative lesion in the mouth

fected persons, rubeola is caused by an RNA-containing paramyxovirus with an incubation period of 7 to 12 days, during which there are no symptoms. Prodromal symptoms include high fever (up to 40.5° C), malaise, enlarged lymph nodes, runny nose, conjunctivitis, and "barking" cough. Within 3 to 4 days, an erythematous maculopapular rash develops over the head and spreads distally over the trunk, extremities, hands, and feet. Early lesions blanch with pressure, followed by a brownish hue that does not blanch as the rash fades. Characteristic pinpoint white spots surrounded by an erythematous ring develop over the buccal mucosa and are known as *Koplik spots.* These spots precede the rash by 1 to 2 days. The rash then subsides within 3 to 5 days.

Complications associated with measles may be caused by the primary infection or by a secondary bacterial infection. Measles encephalitis occurs in about 1 of 800 cases, and most children recover completely. Only a small minority develop permanent brain damage or die. Bacterial complications include otitis media and pneumonia, usually caused by group A hemolytic streptococcus, *Haemophilus influenzae,* or *S. aureus* infection.

Measles is prevented by a single vaccination of live attenuated measles virus. There is no specific treatment for measles, and supportive therapy is the same as for rubella. Antibiotic therapy is initiated if secondary bacterial infections develop.

Roseola (exanthema subitum)

Roseola is a presumed viral infection of infants between 6 months and 2 years of age and can be seen in children up to 4 years of age. The incubation period is 5 to 15 days, followed by the sudden onset of fever (38.9° to 40.5° C) that lasts for 3 to 5 days. After the fever, an erythematous macular rash that lasts about 24 hours develops primarily over the trunk and neck. Children usually feel well, eat normally, and have few other symptoms. There is usually no treatment.

Chickenpox, herpes zoster, and smallpox
Chickenpox

Chickenpox is a disease of early childhood, with 90% of children contracting the disease during the first decade of life. Being a highly contagious virus, chickenpox is spread by close person-to-person contact and by airborne droplets. Introduction of an infected person into a household results in 90% possibility of susceptible persons developing the disease within the incubation period, usually 14 days. Children are contagious for at least 1 day before development of the rash. Transmission of the virus may occur until approximately 5 to 6 days after the onset of the first skin lesions in normal children. In immunocompromised children, the virus is recoverable for a longer period, but they must be considered contagious for at least 7 to 10 days. Chickenpox occurs most commonly in the late winter and early spring. Transmission occurs more readily in temperate climates than in tropical climates.

Normally, children who develop chickenpox have no prodromal symptoms. The first sign of illness may be itching or the appearance of vesicles, usually on the trunk, scalp, or face. The rash later spreads to the extremities. Characteristically, lesions can be seen in various stages of maturation with macules, papules, and vesicles present in a particular area at the same time (Fig. 40-9). The vesicular lesions are superficial and can be easily ruptured. New lesions will erupt for 4 to 5 days, until there are approximately 100 to 300 in different stages of development. The vesicles become crusted, with only the crust remaining, although there may be an occasional vesicle on the palm later in the disease. Although uncommon, ulcerative lesions are sometimes seen in the mouth and, less commonly, on the conjunctiva and pharynx. Fever usually lasts 2 to 3 days and ranges from 38.5° to 40° C.

Complications are rare in children but more common in adults. They can include transient hematuria (from rupture of vesicles in the bladder), epistaxis, laryngeal edema, and

Rash relatively profuse on trunk

Rash sparse distally

Fig. 40-9 *Chickenpox.* Generalized, polymorphous eruption. *(From Wehrle, P.F. & Top, F.H., Sr. [1981]. Communicable and infectious diseases [9th ed.]. St. Louis: Mosby.)*

varicella pneumonia. One case of chickenpox produces almost complete immunity against a second attack. The fetus may be malformed if chickenpox develops in the first trimester of pregnancy.[13] Infants whose mothers have chickenpox at any stage of pregnancy have a higher risk of developing herpes zoster during the first few years of life.

Uncomplicated chickenpox requires no specific therapy. Baths, wet dressings, and oral antihistamines are occasionally helpful to relieve itching and to prevent secondary infection from developing as a result of scratching. Oral antistaphylococcal drugs should be given if secondary bacterial infection is present. Zoster immune globulin may be administered to immunodeficient individuals if given within 72 hours after exposure to chickenpox. Oral acyclovir may be valuable in immunosuppressed or other select groups of children. The use and role of the varicella vaccine in the United States remain unclear.

Herpes zoster

Although **herpes zoster (shingles)** occurs mainly in adults, approximately 5% of cases are in children younger than 15 years. The course of the disease in children with an immune defect is more complicated and requires intravenous treatment with acyclovir.[14] The chickenpox virus persists for life in sensory nerve ganglia and reactivates to cause herpes zoster. The eruption of zoster consists of groups of vesicles situated on an inflammatory base and following the course of a sensory nerve. Common dermatomal distribution in childhood is thoracic. The base of the lesions frequently appears hemorrhagic, and some of the lesions may become

necrotic and ulcerative. Therapy is similar to that for chickenpox unless it is ophthalmic or disseminated zoster, for which acyclovir is indicated.

Smallpox

Smallpox (variola) was a highly contagious and deadly but preventable disease. It was caused by poxvirus variolae. Because of worldwide mass immunizations, the world is now virtually free of smallpox.[15]

> ✓**QUICK CHECK**
>
> Compare impetigo and staphylococcal scalded-skin syndrome as to cause and presentation.
>
> Describe rubella and rubeola.
>
> How are chickenpox and herpes zoster related?

INSECT BITES AND PARASITES

Insect bites and infestations are common causes of skin disorders in children and adults. Skin damage occurs by various mechanisms, including trauma of bites and stings, allergic reactions, transmission of disease, injection of substances that cause local or systemic reactions, and inflammatory reactions from retained mouth parts.

Scabies

Scabies is a contagious disease caused by the itch mite, *Sarcoptes scabiei* (Fig. 40-10, *A*). It is transmitted by close personal contact and by infected clothing and bedding. Scabies is frequently epidemic in areas of overcrowded housing and poor sanitation. Infestation is initiated by a female mite that tunnels into the stratum corneum, depositing eggs and creating a burrow several millimeters to 1 centimeter long. Over a 3-week period, the eggs mature into adult mites, which sometimes can be recognized as tiny dots at the ends of intact burrows.

Symptoms appear 3 to 5 weeks after infestation. The primary lesions are burrows, papules, and vesicular lesions, with severe itching that worsens at night. Itching is thought to be related to sensitization to the larval stages of the parasite. In older children and adults, the lesions occur in the webs of fingers; axillae; creases of the arms and wrists; along the belt line; and around the nipples, genitalia, and lower buttocks. Infants and young children have a different pattern of distribution, with involvement of the palms, soles, head, neck, and face (Fig. 40-10, *B*). Secondary infections and crusting develop from scratching and eczematous changes.

Diagnosis of scabies is made by observation of the tunnels and burrows and scraping of the skin with microscopic examination of the mite or its eggs or feces. Treatment is the application of a scabicide and is curative. All clothing and linens should be washed and dried in hot cycles or dry cleaned.

Fig. 40-10 *Scabies.* **A,** Scabies mite, as seen clinically when removed from its burrow. **B,** Characteristic scabies bites. *(Courtesy Department of Dermatology, School of Medicine, University of Utah.)*

Pediculosis (Lice Infestation)

The three known types of human lice are (1) the head louse *(Pediculus capitis)*, (2) the body louse *(Pediculus corporis)*, and (3) the crab or pubic louse *(Phthirus pubis)*. They are parasites and survive by sucking blood. The female louse reproduces every 2 weeks, producing hundreds of nits as newly hatched lice mate with old. The mouth parts are shaped for piercing and sucking and attach to the skin while feeding. When piercing the skin, the louse secretes a toxic saliva, and the mechanical trauma and toxin produce a pruritic dermatitis. Head and body lice are acquired by personal contact, combs, or brushes. Crab lice are spread by body contact, such as contact with an infected adult (see Chapter 32). Sharing clothing is also a common source of transmission.

Itching is the major symptom of lice. With head lice, the ova attach to hairs above the ears and in the occipital region. The primary lesion of the body louse is a pinpoint red macule, papule, or wheal with a hemorrhagic puncture site. The primary lesion is often not seen, because it is masked by excoriations, wheals, and crusts. The crab louse is found on pubic hairs but may also involve other body hair, such as eyelashes, mustache, beard, and axillae. Young children particularly may become infected with crab lice on their eyebrows or eyelashes.

The live louse, 2 to 3 mm long, is rarely observed, although the ova, or nits, can be observed as oval, yellowish, pinpoint specks fastened to a hair shaft. The ova will fluoresce under an ultraviolet light (Wood lamp) and can be best observed with a microscope. Use of lindane shampoo (Kwell), applied for 5 minutes and rinsed out, is effective for treating head lice. Lindane lotion is used for body and crab lice and is left on for 12 hours with retreatment in 1 week if ova are still visible. All clothes, towels, bedding, combs, and brushes should be washed and dried in hot air or boiled, or clothes should be ironed. Individuals who have close personal contact also should be treated.

Fig. 40-11 *Flea bites.* Flea bite producing an urticarial wheal with central puncture.

Fleas

Young children are very susceptible to *flea bites,* and the most common are the bites of cat, dog, and human fleas.[16] Bites occur in clusters along the arms and legs or where there are tight-fitting clothes. The bite produces an urticarial wheal with a central hemorrhagic puncture (Fig. 40-11). Treatment includes spraying carpets, crevices, and furniture with malathion or lindane powder. Infected animals should be treated, and clothes and bedding should be washed in hot water.

Bedbugs

Bedbugs live in the crevices and cracks of floors, walls, and furniture and in bedding or furniture stuffing. They are 3 to 5 mm long and reddish brown. Bedbugs emerge to feed in darkness and attach to the skin to suck blood. Feeding occurs for 5 to 15 minutes, and the bedbug then leaves. It will move long distances to search for food and can travel from house to house.

Two or three bites, commonly referred to as "breakfast, lunch, and dinner," usually appear in a line on exposed areas of the skin. If the host has not been previously sensitized, the only symptom is a red macule that develops into a nodule, lasting up to 14 days. In sensitized children and adults, pruritic wheals, papules, and vesicles may form. Secondary infections require treatment. Bedbugs are eliminated by spraying with chlordane or lindane and by cleaning or disposing of bedding, mattresses, and furniture.

VASCULAR DISORDERS

Congenital vascular malformations occur in 10% of all infants.[17] The lesions are developmental in origin, with islands of angioblastic tissue failing to communicate with normal adjacent blood vessels. The most common disorders are strawberry hemangioma, cavernous hemangioma, nevus flammeus, and salmon patches. They are known collectively as *vascular nevi*.

Strawberry Hemangioma

The *strawberry hemangioma* is a distinct, raised vascular lesion that may be present at birth but usually emerges 3 to 5 weeks later. It proliferates and becomes bright red and elevated with minute capillary projections that give it a strawberry appearance. There is usually only one lesion, and it is located on the head and neck area or trunk (Fig. 40-12). After the initial growth, the lesion grows at the same rate as the child and then starts to involute at 12 to 16 months of age. Approximately 90% of strawberry hemangiomas involute by 5 to 6 years of age, usually without scarring.[18]

Cavernous Hemangiomas

Cavernous hemangiomas are present at birth and have larger and more mature vessels within the lesion than strawberry hemangiomas. Some lesions, however, are composed of a mixture of strawberry and cavernous hemangiomas. They appear primarily on the head and neck area and have a bluish red color with less distinct borders (Fig. 40-13). Cavernous hemangiomas grow rapidly up to 6 months of age and mature by 1 year of age. A period of involution begins and proceeds for 6 to 12 months, with complete involution by 2 to 3 years in 30% of children and by 9 years of age in 90% of children.

Hemangiomas that require treatment are near structures such as the eye, nares, auditory canal, or pharynx or grow rapidly and are susceptible to trauma or secondary infection. No form of treatment is entirely satisfactory. Surgery, liquid nitrogen, or laser ablation can control bleeding or reduce the size of the lesion, however. The best cosmetic results are obtained when there is spontaneous involution. Ulceration, bleeding, and infection are relatively rare, but cleansing and use of topical antibiotics are effective when they do occur. Open lesions do better when left open to the air, and Telfa dressings are recommended if bandages are required.

Fig. 40-12 *Strawberry hemangioma. (From Stewart, W.D., Danto, J.L., & Maddin, S. [1978]. Dermatology: Diagnosis and treatment of cutaneous disorders [4th ed.]. St. Louis: Mosby.)*

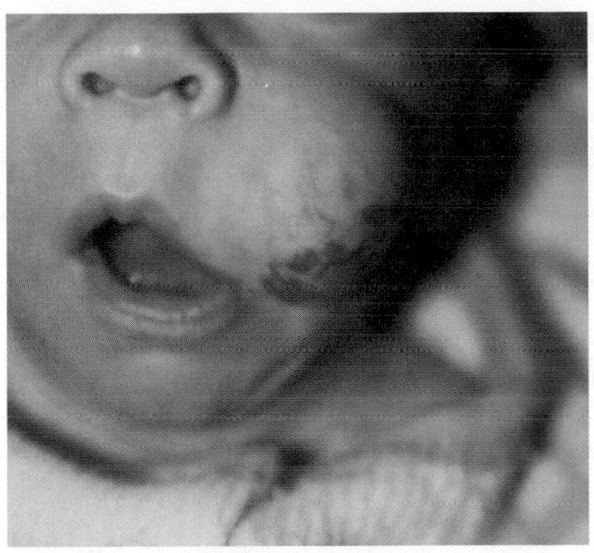

Fig. 40-13 *Cavernous hemangioma*. *(Courtesy Department of Dermatology, School of Medicine, University of Utah.)*

Fig. 40-14 *Port-wine hemangioma*. Port-wine hemangioma in a child. *(Courtesy Department of Dermatology, School of Medicine, University of Utah.)*

Salmon Patches

Salmon patches are macular, pink lesions present at birth and located on the nape of the neck (stork bites), forehead, upper eyelids, or nasolabial fold region. The pink color results from distended dermal capillaries, and 95% fade by 1 year of age. They generally do not present a cosmetic problem.

Fig. 40-15 *Miliaria rubra*. Note discrete erythematous papules or papulovesicles. *(Courtesy Department of Dermatology, School of Medicine, University of Utah.)*

Port-Wine Stain

Port-wine stain (nevus flammeus) is a congenital malformation of the dermal capillaries. The lesions are flat, and their color ranges from pink to dark reddish purple. They are present at birth or within a few days after birth and do not fade with age. Involvement of the face and other body surfaces is common, and the lesions may be large (Fig. 40-14). During adolescence and later adult years, the port-wine stain may become papular and cavernous. Treatments using cryosurgery or tattooing are not very satisfactory. The pulsed dye laser has been used most recently to successfully lighten the color and flatten the more nodular and cavernous lesions.[19] Waterproof cosmetics may be used to cover the lesions.

OTHER SKIN DISORDERS
Miliaria

Miliaria is a dermatosis commonly seen in infants that is characterized by a vesicular eruption after prolonged exposure to perspiration with subsequent obstruction of the eccrine ducts. There are two forms of miliaria: *miliaria crystallina* and *miliaria rubra*. In miliaria crystallina, ductal rupture occurs within the stratum corneum and appears as 1- to 2-mm clear vesicles without erythema. They rupture within 24 to 48 hours and leave a white scale. In miliaria rubra, the ductal rupture occurs in the lower epidermis with inflammatory cells attracted to the site of the rupture. Miliaria rubra (prickly heat) is characterized by 2- to 4-mm discrete erythematous papules or papulovesicles (Fig. 40-15). Both forms may become secondarily infected, requiring systemic antibiotics. The key to management is avoidance of excessive heat and humidity, which cause sweating. Light clothing, cool baths, and air conditioning assist in keeping the skin surface dry and cool.

Erythema Toxicum Neonatorum

Erythema toxicum neonatorum (toxic erythema of the newborn) is a benign, erythematous accumulation of macules, papules, or pustules that appear at birth or 3 to 4 days after birth. The lesions first appear as a blotchy, macular erythematous rash. The macules vary from 1 mm to 1 cm. When papules or pustules develop, they are light yellow or white and 1 to 3 mm in diameter. There may be few or several hundred lesions, and any body surface can be affected, with the exception of the palms and soles, where there are no pilosebaceous follicles. The cause of the lesion is unknown, and it is self-limiting. No treatment is required.

✓QUICK CHECK

Give two examples of insect bites or parasites that affect children. What features are seen in each?

Compare a strawberry hemangioma and a cavernous hemangioma.

▣ DID YOU UNDERSTAND?

Acne Vulgaris

1. Acne is a common disorder that affects susceptible pilosebaceous follicles, primarily of the face, neck, and upper trunk. It is characterized by both noninflammatory and inflammatory lesions.

Dermatitis

1. Atopic dermatitis is associated with elevated IgE levels and a family history of asthma and hay fever. Red, scaly lesions commonly occur on the face, cheeks, and flexor surfaces of the extremities in infants and young children.
2. Diaper dermatitis is a type of contact dermatitis that develops from prolonged exposure to urine and feces and frequently becomes secondarily infected with *Candida albicans.*

Infections of the Skin

1. Impetigo is a contagious bacterial disease occurring in two forms—bullous and vesicular. The toxins from the bacteria produce a weeping lesion with a honey-colored crust.
2. Staphylococcal scalded-skin syndrome (SSSS) is a staphylococcal skin infection that occurs more commonly in young children with low titers of antistaphylococcal antibody. Painful blisters and bullae form over large areas of the skin, requiring systemic antibiotics for treatment.
3. Thrush is a fungal infection of the mouth caused by *Candida albicans.*
4. Tinea capitis and tinea corporis are fungal infections of the scalp and body caused by dermatophytes.
5. Molluscum contagiosum is a poxvirus of the skin that produces pale papular lesions filled with viral and cellular debris.
6. Rubella (3-day measles) is a communicable disease characterized by fever, sore throat, enlarged cervical and postauricular nodes, and a generalized maculopapular rash that lasts 1 to 4 days.
7. Rubeola is a contagious disease with symptoms of high fever, enlarged lymph nodes, conjunctivitis, and a red rash that begins on the head, spreads to the trunk and extremities, and lasts 3 to 5 days. Both bacterial and viral complications may accompany rubeola.
8. Roseola is a benign disease of infants with a sudden onset of fever that lasts 3 to 5 days, followed by a rash that lasts 24 hours.
9. Chickenpox (varicella) is a highly contagious disease caused by the varicella-zoster virus. Vesicular lesions occur on the skin and mucous membranes. Individuals are contagious from 1 day before the development of the rash until about 5 to 6 days after the rash develops.
10. Herpes zoster (shingles) is a viral eruption of vesicles on the skin along the distribution of a sensory nerve. Children with immune suppression develop more serious complications.
11. Smallpox (variola) was a highly contagious, deadly disease that has been eradicated worldwide by vaccination.

Insect Bites and Parasites

1. Scabies is an itching lesion caused by the itch mite, which burrows into the skin forming papules and vesicles. The mite is very contagious and is transmitted by direct contact.
2. Pediculosis (lice infestation) is caused by bloodsucking parasites that secrete a toxic saliva and damage the skin to produce a pruritic dermatitis. Lice are spread by direct contact and are recognized by the ova or nits that attach to the shafts of body hairs.
3. Flea bites produce a pruritic wheal with a central puncture site and occur as clusters in areas of tight-fitting clothing.
4. Bedbugs are blood-sucking parasites that live in cracks of floors, furniture, or bedding and feed at night. They produce pruritic wheals and nodules.

Vascular Disorders

1. A strawberry hemangioma is a vascular lesion present at birth that proliferates in size and then grows at the same rate as the child. Most lesions resolve spontaneously by 5 years of age.
2. A cavernous hemangioma is present at birth, with larger vessels than a strawberry hemangioma, and is bluish red. Cavernous hemangiomas usually involute by 9 years of age and may require surgical removal if located near the eyes, nares, or genitalia.

DID YOU UNDERSTAND? —cont'd

3. Salmon patches are macular pink lesions with dilated capillaries that usually resolve by 1 year of age.

4. Port-wine stains are congenital malformations of dermal capillaries that do not fade with age.

5. Miliaria is small pruritic papules or vesicles that result from closure of the sweat duct opening in infants.

6. Erythema toxicum neonatorum is a benign accumulation of macules, papules, and pustules that spontaneously resolves within a few weeks after birth.

KEY TERMS

REFERENCES

1. Lucky, A.W. (1998). A review of infantile and pediatric acne. *Dermatology, 196*(1), 95-97.
2. Nyguyen, Q.H., Kim, Y.A., & Schwartz, R.A. (1994). Management of acne vulgaris. *American Family Physician, 50*(1), 89-95, 99-100.
3. Jones, S.M. & Sampson, H.A. (1993). The role of allergens in atopic dermatitis. *Clinical Reviews in Allergy, 11*(4), 471-490.
4. Kim, H.J. & Honig, P.J. (1998). Atopic dermatitis. *Current Opinions in Pediatrics, 10*(4) 387-392.
5. Brook, I., Frazier, E.H., & Yeager, J.K. (1997). Microbiology of nonbullous impetigo. *Pediatric Dermatology, 14*(3), 192-195.
6. Hacker, S.M. (1994). Common infections of the skin: Characteristics, causes, and cures. *Postgraduate Medicine, 96*(2), 43-46, 49-52.
7. Friedlander, S.F. & Suarez, S. (1998). Pediatric antifungal therapy. *Dermatology Clinics, 16*(3), 527-537.
8. Noble, S.L., Forbes, T.C., & Stamm, P.L. (1998). Diagnosis and management of common tinea infections. *American Family Physician, 58*(1), 163-174, 177-178.
9. Prasad, S.M. (1996). Molluscum contagiosum. *Pediatric Review, 17*(4), 118.
10. Ronnerfalt, L., Fransson, J., & Wahlgren, C.F. (1998). EMLA cream provides rapid relief for the curettage of molluscum contagiosum in children with atopic dermatitis without causing serious application-site reactions. *Pediatric Dermatology, 15*(4), 309-312.
11. Watson, J.C. et al. (1998). Measles, mumps, and rubella—Vaccine use and strategies for elimination of measles, rubella, and congenital rubella syndrome and control of mumps: Recommendations of the Advisory Committee on Immunization Practices (ACIP). *MMWR—Morbidity and Mortality Weekly Report, 47*(RR-8), 1-57.
12. Poland, G.A. & Jacobson, R.M. (1994). Failure to reach the goal of measles elimination: Apparent paradox of measles infection in immunized persons. *Archives of Internal Medicine, 154*(16), 1815.
13. Wheller, T.H. (1983). Varicella and herpes zoster: Changing concepts of the natural history, control, and importance of a not-so-benign virus. *New England Journal of Medicine, 309,* 1434.
14. Kakourou, T. et al. (1998). Herpes zoster in children. *Journal of the American Academy of Dermatologists, 39*(Pt. 1), 207-210.
15. Ellner, P.D. (1998). Smallpox: Gone but not forgotten. *Infection, 26*(5), 263-269.
16. Howard, R. & Frieden, I.J. (1996). Papular urticaria in children. *Pediatric Dermatology, 13*(3), 246-249.
17. Jacobs, A.H. & Watson, R.G. (1976). The incidence of birthmarks in the neonate. *Pediatrics, 58,* 218.
18. Low, D.W. (1994). Hemangiomas and vascular malformations. *Seminars in Pediatric Surgery, 3*(2), 40-61.
19. Troilius, A., Wrangsjo, B., & Ljunggeren, B. (1998). Potential psychological benefits from early treatment of port-wine stains in children. *British Journal of Dermatology, 139*(1), 59-65.

Appendix

Conversion Factors to International System of Units (SI Units)

Component	Normal Range in Units as Customarily Reported	Conversion Factor	Normal Range in SI Units, Molecular Units, International Units, or Decimal Fractions
Biochemical components of blood*			
Acetoacetic acid (S)	0.2-1.0 mg/dl	98	19.6-98.0 μmol/L
Acetone (S)	0.3-2.0 mg/dl	172	51.6-344.0 μmol/L
Albumin (S)	3.2-4.5 g/dl	10	32-45 g/L
Ammonia (P)	20-120 μg/dl	0.588	11.7-70.5 μmol/L
Amylase (S)	60-160 Somogyi units/dl	1.85	111-296 U/L
Base, total (S)	145-160 mEq/L	1	145-160 mmol/L
Bicarbonate (P)	21-28 mEq/L	1	21-28 mmol/L
Bile acids (S)	0.3-3.0 mg/dl	10	3-30 mg.L
		2.547	0.8-7.6 μmol/L
Bilirubin, direct (S)	Up to 0.3 mg/dl	17.1	Up to 5.1 μmol/L
Bilirubin, indirect (S)	0.1-1.0 mg/dl	17.1	1.7-17.1 μmol/L
Blood gases (B)			
P_{CO_2} arterial	35-40 mm Hg	0.133	4.66-5.32 kPa
P_{O_2} arterial	95-100 mm Hg	0.133	12.64-13.30 kPa
Calcium (S)	8.5-10.5 mg/dl	0.25	2.1-2.6 mmol/L
Chloride (S)	95-103 mEq/L	1	95-103 mmol/L
Creatine (S)	0.1-0.4 mg/dl	76.3	7.6-30.5 μmol/L
Creatinine (S)	0.6-1.2 mg/dl	88.4	53-106 μmol/L
Creatinine clearance (P)	107-139 ml/min	0.0167	1.78-2.32 ml/s
Fatty acids (total) (S)	8-20 mg/dl	0.01	0.08-2.00 mg/L
Fibrinogen (P)	200-400 mg/dl	0.01	2.00-4.00 g/L
Gamma globulin (S)	0.5-1.6 g/dl	10	5-16 g/L
Globulins (total) (S)	2.3-3.5 g/dl	10	23-35 g/L
Glucose (fasting) (S)	70-110 mg/dl	0.055	3.85-6.05 mmol/L
Insulin (radioimmunoassay) (P)	4.24 μlU/ml	0.0417	0.17-1.00 μg/L
	0.20-0.84 μg/L	172.2	35-145 pmol/L
Iodine, BEI (S)	3.5-6.5 μg/dl	0.079	0.28-0.51 μmol/L
Iodine, PBI (S)	4.0-8.0 μg/dl	0.079	0.32-0.63 μmol/L
Iron, total (S)	60-150 μg/dl	0.179	11-27 μmol/L
Iron-binding capacity (S)	300-360 μg/dl	0.179	54-64 μmol/L
17-Ketosteroids (P)	25-125 μg/dl	0.01	0.25-1.25 mg/L
Lactic dehydrogenase (S)	80-120 units at 30° C	0.48	38-62 U/L at 30° C
	Lactate $\rightarrow$ pyruvate		
	100-190 U/L at 37° C	1	100-190 U/L at 37° C
Lipase (S)	0-1.5 U/ml (Cherry-Crandall)	278	0-417 U/L

From Thibodeau, G.A., Patton, K.T. (1999). Anthony's textbook of anatomy & physiology (16th ed.). St. Louis: Mosby.

*This is a selected (not a complete) list of biochemical components. The ranges listed may differ from those accepted in some laboratories and are shown to illustrate the conversion factor and the method of expression in SI molecular units.

S, Serum; P, plasma

Component	Normal Range in Units as Customarily Reported	Conversion Factor	Normal Range in SI Units, Molecular Units, International Units, or Decimal Fractions
Lipids (total) (S)	400-800 mg/dl	0.01	4.00-8.00 g/L
Cholesterol	150-250 mg/dl	0.026	3.9-6.5 mmol/L
Triglycerides	75-165 mg/dl	0.0114	0.85-1.89 mmol/L
Phospholipids	150-380 mg/dl	0.01	1.50-3.80 g/L
Free fatty acids	9.0-15.0 mM/L	1	9.0-15.0 mmol/L
Nonprotein nitrogen (S)	20-35 mg/dl	0.714	14.3-25.0 mmol/L
Phosphatase (P)			
Acid (units/dl)	Cherry-Crandall	2.77	0-5.5 U/L
	King-Armstrong	1.77	0-5.5 U/L
	Bodansky	5.37	0-5.5 U/L
Alkaline (units/dl)	King-Armstrong	1.77	30-120 U/L
	Bodansky	5.37	30-120 U/L
	Bessey-Lowry-Brock	16.67	30-120 U/L
Phosphorus, inorganic (S)	3.0-4.5 mg/dl	0.323	0.97-1.45 mmol/L
Potassium (P)	3.8-5.0 mEq/L	1	3.8-5.0 mmol/L
Proteins, total (S)	6.0-7.8 g/dl	10	60-78 g/L
Albumin	3.2-4.5 g/dl	10	32-45 g/L
Globulin	2.3-3.5 g/dl	10	23-35 g/L
Sodium (P)	136-142 mEq/L	1	136-142 mmol/L
Testosterone: Male (S)	300-1200 ng/dl	0.035	10.5-42.0 nmol/L
Female	30-95 ng/dl	0.035	1.0-3.3 nmol/L
Thyroid tests (S)			
Thyroxine (T_4)	4-11 μg/dl	12.87	51-142 nmol/L
T_4 expressed as iodine	3.2-7.2 μg/dl	79.0	253-569 nmol/L
T_3 resin uptake	25%-38% relative uptake	0.01	0.25%-0.38% relative uptake
TSH (S)	10 μU/mL	1	$<10^{-3}$ IU/L
Urea nitrogen (S)	8-23 mg/dl	0.357	2.9-8.2 mmol/L
Uric acid (S)	2-6 mg/dl	59.5	0.120-0.360 mmol/L
Vitamin B_{12} (S)	160-950 pg/ml	0.74	118-703 pmol/L
Hematology values*			
Red cell volume (male)	25-35 mL/kg body weight	0.001	0.025-0.035 L/kg body weight
Hematocrit	40%-50%	0.01	0.40-0.50
Hemoglobin	13.5-18.0 g/dl	10	135-180 g/L
Hemoglobin	13.5-18.0 g/dl	0.155	2.09-2.79 mmol/L
RBC count	4.2-6 $\times$ 10^6/μL	1	4.6-6 $\times$ 10^{12}/L
WBC count	5.0-10 $\times$ 10^3/μL	1	4.5-10 $\times$ 10^9/L
Mean corpuscular volume	80-96 μm^3	1	80-96 fL

The International Committee for Standardization in Hematology recommends that the numbers remain the same but that the units change, so that hemoglobin is expressed as grams per deciliter (g/dl) even though other measurements are expressed as units per liter (U/L).

INDEX

*Syndromes and disorders appear in **boldface** type.*

Prefixes and Suffixes Commonly Used in Medical Terminology

Prefix	Meaning	Suffix	Meaning
a-	Without, not	-al, -ac	Pertaining to
af-	Toward	-algia	Pain
an-	Without, not	-aps, -apt	Fit, fasten
ante-	Before	-arche	Beginning, origin
anti-	Against, resisting	-ase	Signifies an enzyme
auto-	Self	-blast	Sprout, make
bi-	Two, double	-centesis	A piercing
circum-	Around	-cide	To kill
co-, con-	With, together	-clast	Break, destroy
contra-	Against	-crine	Release, secrete
de-	Down from, undoing	-ectomy	A cutting out
dia-	Across, through	-emesis	Vomiting
dipl-	Twofold, double	-emia	Refers to blood condition
dys-	Bad, disordered, difficult	-flux	Flow
ectop-	Displaced	-gen	Creates, forms
ef-	Away from	-genesis	Creation, production
em-, en-	In, into	-gram	Something written
endo-	Within	-graph(y)	To write, draw
epi-	Upon	-hydrate	Containing H_2O (water)
eu-	Good	-ia, -sia	Condition, process
ex-, exo-	Out of, out from	-iasis	Abnormal condition
extra-	Outside of	-ic, -ac	Pertaining to
hapl-	Single	-in	Signifies a protein
hem-, hemat-	Blood	-ism	Signifies "condition of"
hemi-	Half	-itis	Signifies "inflammation of"
hom(e)o-	Same, equal	-lemma	Rind, peel
hyper-	Over, above	-lepsy	Seizure
hypo-	Under, below	-lith	Stone, rock
infra-	Below, beneath	-logy	Study of
inter-	Between	-lunar	Moon, moonlike
intra-	Within	-malacia	Softening
iso-	Same, equal	-megaly	Enlargement
macro-	Large	-metric, -metry	Measurement, length
mega-	Large, millionth	-oid	Like, in the shape of
mes-	Middle	-oma	Tumor
meta-	Beyond, after	-opia	Vision, vision condition
micro-	Small, millionth	-oscopy	Viewing
milli-	Thousandth	-ose	Signifies a carbohydrate (especially sugar)
mono-	One (single)		
neo-	New	-osis	Condition, process
non-	Not	-ostomy	Formation of an opening
oligo-	Few, scanty	-otomy	Cut
ortho-	Straight, correct, normal	-penia	Lack
para-	By the side of, near	-philic	Loving
per-	Through	-phobic	Fearing
peri-	Around, surrounding	-phragm	Partition
poly-	Many	-plasia	Growth, formation
post-	After	-plasm	Substance, matter
pre-	Before	-plasty	Shape, make
pro-	First, promoting	-plegia	Paralysis
quadr-	Four	-pnea	Breath, breathing
re-	Back again	-(r)rhage, -(r)rhagia	Breaking out, discharge
retro-	Behind	-(r)rhaphy	Sew, suture
semi-	Half	-(r)rhea	Flow
sub-	Under	-some	Body
super-, supra-	Over, above, excessive	-tensin, -tension	Pressure
trans-	Across, through	-tonic	Pressure, tension
tri-	Three, triple	-tripsy	Crushing
		-ule	Small, little
		-uria	Refers to urine condition

From Thibodeau, G.A., Patton, K.T. (1999). Anthony's text-book of anatomy & physiology *(16th ed.). St. Louis: Mosby.*